Neuromuscular Disorders

Notice

Neuromuscular Disorders

SECOND EDITION

Anthony A. Amato, MD
Vice-Chairman
Department of Neurology
Chief
Neuromuscular Division
Brigham and Women's Hospital
Boston, Massachusetts
Professor of Neurology
Harvard Medical School
Boston, Massachusetts

James A. Russell, DO, FAAN
Vice Chairman
Department of Neurology
Lahey Hospital & Medical Center
Director
ALS Clinic
Lahey Hospital & Medical Center
Chairman, Ethics Section
Lahey Hospital & Medical Center
Clinical Professor of Neurology
Tufts University School of Medicine
Boston, Massachusetts

Mc Graw Hill Education

New York Chicago San Francisco Athens London Madrid
Mexico City Milan New Delhi Singapore Sydney Toronto

Neuromuscular Disorders, Second Edition

1 2 3 4 5 6 7 8 9 0 CTP/CTP 19 18 17 16 15

ISBN 978-0-07-175250-3
MHID 0-07-175250-1

This book was set in Minion Pro by Aptara, Inc.
The editors were Alyssa K. Fried and Robert Pancotti.
The production supervisor was Catherine H. Saggese.
The illustration manager was Armen Ovsepyan.
Illustrations were created by Renee L. Cannon, MA, CMI.
Project management was provided by Indu Jawwad, Aptara, Inc.
The cover designer was Thomas De Pierro.
China Translation & Printing Services, Ltd. was the printer and binder.

Library of Congress Cataloging-in-Publication Data

Amato, Anthony A., 1960- , author.
Neuromuscular disorders / Anthony A. Amato, James A. Russell. – Second edition.
p. ; cm.
Preceded by: Neuromuscular disorders / [edited by] Anthony A. Amato, James A. Russell. c2008.
Includes bibliographical references and index.
ISBN 978-0-07-175250-3 (hardcover) – ISBN 0-07-175250-1 (hardcover)
I. Russell, James A. (James Adams), 1951- , author. II. Neuromuscular disorders (Amato) Preceded by (work): III. Title.
[DNLM: 1. Neuromuscular Diseases–diagnosis. 2. Diagnosis, Differential. 3. Diagnostic Techniques, Neurological. 4. Medical History Taking. WE 550]
RC925
616.7′44–dc23

2015008911

I want to express my gratitude to my mentors and colleagues who have taught me the art of neuromuscular medicine and continue to do so. I would be remiss if I did not thank all the patients whom I have had the honor to learn from all these years. Most of all I would like to thank and dedicate this book to my wife, Mary, and my children, Joseph, Erin, Michael, and Katie, for their unconditional love and support over the years.

— Anthony A. Amato, MD —

To the newest addition to our lives, Isabel Reagle Russell, in the hope that someday you will see this undertaking as a source of both pride and motivation.

— James A. Russell, DO, FAAN —

CONTENTS

CONTRIBUTORS

Erik Ensrud, MD
Director, Neuromuscular Center and EMG Laboratory
Boston Veterans Affairs Health Care System
Director, Neuromuscular Rehabilitation Clinic
Brigham and Women's Hospital
Boston, Massachusetts

Sabrina Paganoni, MD, PhD
Instructor in Physical Medicine and Rehabilitation
Harvard Medical School
Neurological Clinical Research Institute (NCRI)
Massachusetts General Hospital
Spaulding Rehabilitation Hospital
Boston Veterans Affairs Health Care System
Boston, Massachusetts

FOREWORD

Textbooks that have a lasting influence are rare. In neurology, such examples are *Merritt's Neurology* and *Adams and Victor's Principles of Neurology,* both now in print for decades and continually updated. I believe the second edition of Amato and Russell's *Neuromuscular Disorders* is such a textbook. Immediately on the publication of the first edition, it became the primary textbook source of information for study of neuromuscular disease. *Neuromuscular Disorders* filled a large gap in the field. Until that time, there was no single text that covered the principles of motor neuron disease, nerve disease, neuromuscular junction disorders, and muscle disorders. *Neuromuscular Disorders* covers all these areas superbly. It is written primarily through the voice of two authors, Tony Amato and Jim Russell, and this provides a wonderfully consistent message and makes the book easy to read. In the second edition, there are guest authors for some specialty areas involving rehabilitative medicine, Erik Ensrud and Sabrina Paganoni, and their chapters are outstanding and the fluent voice is maintained.

The book has gained many fans because it addresses neuromuscular disorders from the clinician's perspective rather than from that of bench scientists. In addition, the book brings together muscle and nerve pathology and electrodiagnostic medicine as extensions of the clinician's approach to the patient. Readers can go to one text to find the principles of the various neuromuscular disorders and find information on pathology and neurophysiology that will enable clinicians to help their patients. *Neuromuscular Disorders* not only can aid the clinician in diagnosing patients but also includes up-to-date information on therapeutic approaches. For all these reasons, Amato and Russell's *Neuromuscular Disorders* has been adopted as the primary source book in the field for residents, fellows, and practicing physicians in academia and in the private setting. I am certain that the second edition will continue to gain many fans among neurologists, physical medicine and rehabilitation specialists, and other health care providers.

I feel confident that this impressive book may well follow in the footsteps of classics like Merritt's and Adams and Victor's and will be a source of essential practical information in our field for years to come. This book can be counted on to provide what is needed to help our patients who have serious neuromuscular health issues. We are all indebted to the authors for providing us with an updated edition of this wonderful book.

Richard J. Barohn, MD
Chairman, Department of Neurology
Gertrude and Dewey Ziegler Professor of Neurology
University Distinguished Professor
Vice Chancellor for Research
President, Research Institute
University of Kansas Medical Center
Kansas City, Kansas

PREFACE

It has been seven years since the publication of the first edition of this book. Much has changed, particularly in our knowledge of the imaging, genetic, and immunologic tools at our disposal that aid in our ability to understand and diagnose many neuromuscular disorders. We have attempted to read and consider as much of this information as possible and translate it into a text that attempts to bridge the gap between translational science and practical application at the bedside. Once again, we attempt to blend our understanding of evidence-based medicine with our personal experiences as "seasoned" clinicians to provide a resource that is of pragmatic value to others.

All chapters in the book have been rewritten, in many cases extensively with the assimilation of contemporary citations. We have chosen to divide a singular chapter on neuromuscular transmission disorders into two chapters, one devoted solely to autoimmune myasthenia and a second devoted to other disorders of the neuromuscular junction. In addition, we have expanded the book by the addition of three new chapters. Because immunomodulating treatments compose a large part of the therapeutic armamentarium of the neuromuscular clinician, Chapter 4 was created to describe the general principles of immunosuppressants and modulating treatments and the commonly used modalities. Although all successful neuromuscular clinicians require a fundamental understanding of physiatry, we have called on colleagues more knowledgeable than we, Drs. Sabrina Paganoni and Erik Ensrud, to enhance this book by writing chapters on the rehabilitation of neuromuscular diseases and on other disorders that may confound the clinician as neuromuscular mimics.

What remains unchanged, however, is the fundamental principle that optimal patient care depends on accurate diagnosis. Judicious use of tests, prescription of effective treatment(s) and avoidance of potentially harmful ones, recognition of potential comorbidities, and accurate patient counseling are all dependent on this principle. For the foreseeable future, the focal point of accurate diagnosis will be at the bedside and will depend on the skills of the master clinician who recognizes and formulates information. This book is written in respect of and support for this time-honored and effective clinical approach.

SECTION I

EVALUATION AND MANAGEMENT OF PATIENTS WITH NEUROMUSCULAR DISEASE

CHAPTER 1

Approach to Patients with Neuromuscular Disease

▶ GENERAL PRINCIPLES

The evaluation of patients with suspected neurologic disease remains first and foremost a bedside exercise. Accurate diagnosis requires consideration of individual patient and disease differences. Despite the benefits of evidence-based medicine, conclusions are more relevant to populations than to individuals. Confounding variables that are part of the human experience may be overlooked or overemphasized by testing algorithms. This textbook will repeatedly emphasize the strongly held philosophy of its authors, that is, patient management flows from an accurate diagnosis. An accurate diagnosis is most likely to be obtained based on a differential diagnosis driven by clinical assessment and hypotheses. These hypotheses should be formulated on the basis of the principles of neurologic localization, the correlation of the chronologic course of symptom development with the behaviors of differing disease conditions, and the application of risk factor analysis. Ideally, the tests described in the subsequent two chapters and throughout the text would be utilized with the primary intent of resolving a clinically established differential diagnosis ideally to prove a working diagnosis. As all tests are potentially fallible, the credibility of their results diminishes when they are used as screening procedures. A laboratory abnormality, occurring without the context of clinical correlation, fails to establish the desired confidence in a cause and effect relationship with the patient's complaint(s). Metaphorically, laboratory tests are analogous to a carpenter's tools. They are of great value when placed in the hands of a skillful artisan, but are potentially damaging if used injudiciously.

In this book, a neuromuscular disorder will refer to any condition that affects the structure and/or function of any component of the neuromuscular system, beginning and working centrifugally from the cell bodies of the anterior horn and dorsal root ganglion. This will include disorders of nerve root, plexus, nerve, neuromuscular junction and muscle. In essence, with the exception of disorders affecting small, poorly, or unmyelinated nerve fibers such as the small fiber or pure autonomic neuropathies, a neuromuscular disorder may alternatively be defined as one that can be potentially detected by electromyography and nerve conduction studies. Disorders affecting the peripheral autonomic system or cranial nerves will be discussed only as necessary to better understand diseases affecting their somatic and spinal counterparts.

Many neuromuscular disorders are the result of or are influenced by single gene or complex genetic mutations. Many of these patients will not recognize the hereditary nature of their disease. This may be due to a recessive inheritance pattern, spontaneous mutation, false paternity, or incomplete or delayed penetrance. Frequently, it is due to a lack of familiarity with the medical issues of other family members. In suspected hereditary disease, acquisition of family history, particularly if done in a cursory fashion, may be insufficient. Examination of other family members, even if only briefly, is strongly recommended when heritable diseases are considered.

The differential diagnosis of disorders of the neuromuscular system is in part age-dependent. The differential diagnosis of neuromuscular conditions in infants, children, and adolescents is both overlapping and unique in comparison to their adult counterparts (Tables 1-1 to 1-3).[1,2] The applied diagnostic principles are similar although both the examination and review of symptoms may be hampered in infants. In the pediatric population, parents must be questioned with great care and sensitivity. The heightened concern of the parents may cause them to unconsciously omit important details of the patient's status or assume a benign attribution as the cause of the symptom. Parents may also bring a considerable amount of guilt to the examination, which may limit their willingness to share information. The parents' fears and associated guilt should be addressed. If necessary, professional counseling should be offered in addition to treating the patient. Often, when a child is ill, the entire family is affected, which can in turn have profound repercussions on the entire family from both a physical and a psychological standpoint.

The nature of neurologic practice is such that many patients evaluated by a neurologist will have complaints that are attributable neither to a specific neuromuscular disorder nor to the nervous system in general. Confidence in the ability to exclude neuromuscular disorders from consideration is enhanced by a thorough knowledge of how these conditions behave. The strategies outlined in this chapter are based on the general principle that diagnostic accuracy is enhanced by correlation of the patient's signs and symptoms, with knowledge of the natural history and behavior of the ever-expanding menu of neuromuscular diseases. In our opinion, adherence to these principles will improve diagnostic accuracy. This chapter will attempt to focus on information that is important to elicit, and also on an organizational framework to allow accurate interpretation.

▶ TABLE 1-1. DIFFERENTIAL DIAGNOSIS OF THE FLOPPY INFANT

Central nervous system disorders (most common etiology)

Anterior horn cell
- Spinal muscular atrophy types I and II

Peripheral neuropathy
- CMT III (Dejerine–Sottas, congenital hypomyelinating/amyelinating neuropathy)
- CMT I and CMT II—rare
- Giant axonal neuropathy

Neuromuscular junction
- Infantile botulism
- Transient neonatal myasthenia gravis
- Congenital myasthenic syndromes

Myopathy
- Congenital myopathies (all of them can present in infancy)
- Muscular dystrophies
  - Congenital muscular dystrophies
  - Dystrophinopathy/sarcoglycanopathy (rare)
  - Congenital myotonic dystrophy
- Metabolic myopathies
  - Glycogen storage defects
    - Acid maltase deficiency
    - Debrancher deficiency
    - Branching enzyme deficiency
    - Myophosphorylase deficiency (rare)
  - Disorders of lipid metabolism
    - Carnitine deficiency
    - Other fatty acid/acyl-CoA dehydrogenase deficiencies
- Mitochondrial myopathies
  - Benign and fatal infantile myopathy
  - Leigh's syndrome
- Endocrine myopathies (e.g., hypothyroidism)

Modified with permission from Dumitru D, Amato AA. Introduction to myopathies and muscle tissue's reaction to injury. In: Dumitru D, Amato AA, Swartz MJ, eds. *Electrodiagnostic Medicine*. 2nd ed. Philadelphia, PA: Hanley & Belfus; 2002.

▶ TABLE 1-2. NEUROMUSCULAR CAUSES OF WEAKNESS PRESENTING IN CHILDHOOD OR EARLY ADULTHOOD

Anterior horn cell
- Spinal muscular atrophy type III
- Poliomyelitis
- Amyotrophic lateral sclerosis

Peripheral neuropathy
- Acute or chronic inflammatory demyelinating polyneuropathy
- Hereditary neuropathies

Neuromuscular junction
- Botulism
- Myasthenia gravis
- Congenital myasthenic syndromes
- Lambert–Eaton syndrome

Myopathy
- Congenital myopathies
  - Central core
  - Multicore
  - Centronuclear
  - Nemaline
- Muscular dystrophies
  - Dystrophinopathy (Duchenne or Becker)
  - Limb-girdle muscular dystrophies
  - Myofibrillar myopathy
  - Myotonic dystrophy
  - Other dystrophies (e.g., FSHD and EDMD)
- Metabolic myopathies
  - Glycogen storage defects
    - Acid maltase deficiency
    - Debrancher and branching enzyme deficiency
  - Disorders of lipid metabolism
    - Carnitine deficiency
    - Other fatty acid/acyl-CoA dehydrogenase deficiencies
- Mitochondrial myopathies
- Periodic paralysis
- Electrolyte imbalance
  - Hyperkalemia
  - Hypokalemia
  - Hypophosphatemia
  - Hypercalcemia
- Endocrine myopathies
- Toxic myopathies
- Inflammatory myopathies
  - Dermatomyositis
  - Polymyositis (after the age of 20 years)
  - Infectious myositis

FSHD, facioscapulohumeral muscular dystrophy; EDMD, Emery–Dreifuss muscular dystrophy.
Modified with permission from Dumitru D, Amato AA. Introduction to myopathies and muscle tissue's reaction to injury. In Dumitru D, Amato AA, Swartz MJ. eds. *Electrodiagnostic Medicine*. 2nd ed. Philadelphia, PA: Hanley & Belfus; 2002.

▶ DOES THE PATIENT HAVE A NEUROMUSCULAR PROBLEM?

HISTORY TAKING

Neuromuscular diseases manifest themselves through some symptoms or combination of symptoms attributable directly or indirectly to the dysfunction of peripheral motor, sensory and autonomic nerves, neuromuscular junction or muscle. Motor symptoms are typically expressed in a "negative" fashion (weakness or atrophy). Occasionally, "positive" symptoms referable to overactivity [e.g., muscle cramps and fasciculations with LMN involvement and stiffness or flexor spasms in upper motor neuron (UMN) involvement] may dominate the clinical presentation. Sensory symptoms may also manifest with either a positive (e.g., paresthesia) or a negative (e.g., numbness or sensory ataxia) manner. Although pain may be considered a positive sensory symptom, it will be considered as an independent symptom in this text as it is neither a common or dominant feature in many neuromuscular conditions.

Neuromuscular disorders which manifest themselves solely within the domain of the motor system typically originate from anterior horn cells, the neuromuscular junction,

TABLE 1-3. NEUROMUSCULAR CAUSES OF WEAKNESS PRESENTING IN MIDDLE TO LATE ADULTHOOD

Anterior horn cell
- Spinal muscular atrophy type III
- Kennedy disease
- Poliomyelitis
- Amyotrophic lateral sclerosis

Peripheral neuropathy
- Hereditary neuropathies
- Acute or chronic inflammatory demyelinating polyneuropathy
- Drug-induced or toxic neuropathies
- Diabetic neuropathy
- Amyloid
- Vasculitis

Neuromuscular junction
- Botulism
- Myasthenia gravis
- Lambert–Eaton syndrome

Myopathy
- Muscular dystrophies
  - Dystrophinopathy (Becker)
  - Limb-girdle muscular dystrophies
  - Myofibrillar myopathy
  - Oculopharyngeal dystrophy
  - Bent spine/dropped head syndrome
- Metabolic myopathies
  - Glycogen storage defects
    - Acid maltase deficiency
    - Debrancher deficiency
  - Disorders of lipid metabolism (rare)
- Congenital myopathies
  - Sporadic late onset nemaline myopathy
- Mitochondrial myopathies
- Periodic paralysis
  - Familial hypo-KPP manifest within the first three decades
  - Familial hyper-KPP usually manifests in the first decade
- Electrolyte imbalance
  - Hyperkalemia
  - Hypokalemia
  - Hypophosphatemia
  - Hypercalcemia
- Endocrine myopathies
- Toxic myopathies
- Myopathy associated with systemic disease (e.g., cancer), poor nutrition, and disuse
- Amyloid myopathy
- Inflammatory myopathies
  - Inclusion body myositis (most common inflammatory myopathy after the age of 50 years)
  - Dermatomyositis
  - Polymyositis (after the age of 20 years)
  - Infectious myositis

hypo-KPP, hypokalemic periodic paralysis; hyper-KPP, hyperkalemic periodic paralysis.
Modified with permission from Dumitru D, Amato AA. Introduction to myopathies and muscle tissue's reaction to injury. In: Dumitru D, Amato AA, Swartz MJ, eds. *Electrodiagnostic Medicine.* 2nd ed. Philadelphia, PA: Hanley & Belfus; 2002.

muscle or rarely motor nerve fibers. Sensory symptoms typically imply a disorder of nerve root, dorsal root ganglion, plexus, or one or more peripheral nerve trunks. During history acquisition, there is considerable value in identifying both the location and the nature of the initial symptom(s), including the context in which that symptom developed. The subsequent evolution of symptoms should then be developed in a chronologic fashion with particular attention to the topographical distribution. The value of this approach may be illustrated with the example of multifocal neuropathy. At the time of their initial neurologic assessment, the patient's deficits may have become confluent and indistinguishable from a length-dependent neuropathy and its far more extensive differential diagnosis. Identifying that the initial symptom occurred in a focal nerve distribution limits the differential diagnosis and improves diagnostic accuracy. The benefit of defining the chronologic course is that the differential diagnosis of acute neuromuscular disorders is notably disparate from that of its chronic counterparts (Tables 1-4 to 1-6).

TABLE 1-4. NEUROMUSCULAR DISORDERS PRESENTING WITH ACUTE OR SUBACUTE PROXIMAL OR GENERALIZED WEAKNESS

Anterior horn cell
- Poliomyelitis

Peripheral neuropathy
- Guillain–Barré syndrome
- Porphyria
- Diphtheria
- Tick paralysis
- Toxic neuropathies
- Diabetic amyotrophy
- Vasculitis
- Carcinomatous infiltration (e.g., leukemia and lymphoma)
- Paraneoplastic neuropathy

Neuromuscular junction
- Botulism
- Lambert–Eaton syndrome
- Myasthenia gravis

Myopathy
- Periodic paralysis
- Electrolyte imbalance
- Endocrinopathies
- Inflammatory myopathies
  - Dermatomyositis
  - Polymyositis
  - Infectious myositis
  - Immune mediated necrotizing myopathy
- Toxic myopathies
- Metabolic myopathies
  - Glycogen and lipid disorders

Neuromyopathy
- Critical illness neuromyopathy

Reroduced with permission from Dumitru D, Amato AA. Introduction to myopathies and muscle tissue's reaction to injury. In: Dumitru D, Amato AA, Swartz MJ, eds. *Electrodiagnostic Medicine.* 2nd ed. Philadelphia, PA: Hanley & Belfus; 2002.

TABLE 1-5. DIFFERENTIAL DIAGNOSIS OF CHRONIC PROGRESSIVE PROXIMAL WEAKNESS

Anterior horn cell
- Amyotrophic lateral sclerosis
- Spinal muscular atrophy type III
- Kennedy disease

Peripheral neuropathy
- Chronic inflammatory demyelinating polyneuropathy
- Multifocal motor neuropathy
- Toxic neuropathies
- Neuropathy associated with systemic disorders
  - Connective tissue disease (e.g., vasculitis)
  - Diabetes mellitus
  - Amyloidosis
- Paraneoplastic
- Carcinomatous infiltration (e.g., leukemia and lymphoma)

Neuromuscular junction
- Lambert–Eaton syndrome
- Myasthenia gravis

Myopathy
- Muscular dystrophy
- Periodic paralysis
- Electrolyte imbalance
- Endocrinopathies
- Inflammatory myopathies
  - Dermatomyositis
  - Polymyositis
  - Infectious myositis
- Toxic myopathies
- Metabolic myopathies
  - Glycogen and lipid disorders

Miscellaneous: Tick paralysis, hypophosphatemia; hypokalemia

Reproduced with permission from Dumitru D, Amato AA. Introduction to myopathies and muscle tissue's reaction to injury. In: Dumitru D, Amato AA, Swartz MJ, eds. *Electrodiagnostic Medicine*. 2nd ed. Philadelphia, PA: Hanley & Belfus; 2002.

TABLE 1-6. NEUROMUSCULAR CAUSES OF CHRONIC DISTAL WEAKNESS CAUSING BILATERAL FOOT AND/OR HEEL DROP

Anterior horn cell
- ALS[a]

Distal spinal muscular atrophy
- Polio and other enterovirus[a]
- Conus medullaris syndrome—e.g., myelodysplasia, ependymoma, syringomyelia
- Scapuloperoneal form of SMA

Nerve
- Charcot–Marie–Tooth disease
- Multifocal neuropathies[a]—infiltrative (neoplastic, amyloid, sarcoid, neurofibromatosis), vasculitic, immune mediated (MADSAM, MMN)

NMJ
- Autoimmune myasthenia gravis (rare)
- Congenital myasthenia

Muscle
- Distal myopathies—Nonaka, Miyoshi, Udd, Welander, Laing
- Muscular dystrophies—scapuloperoneal, fascioscapuloperoneal, Emery–Dreifuss, oculopharyngeal distal myopathy, calveolinopathy
- Congenital myopathies—nemaline, central core, nemaline
- Glycogen storage diseases—brancher, debrancher/polyglucosan body disease, Pompe, phosphorylase B kinase deficiency
- Lipid storage disorders—neutral lipid storage myopathy, multiple acyl-coA dehydrogenase deficiency
- Myofibrillar myopathy
- Inflammatory—inclusion body myositis[a]

[a]Usual notable asymmetries.

In the history acquisition, it is imperative not to accept words at face value and to explore what that word means to a patient. For example, it is not uncommon for patients to say numb when they mean weak, and weak when they mean numb. The mechanism of impaired function should be explored. For example, questions should be formulated to determine whether a fall is due to proximal weakness resulting in failure of antigravity muscles, tripping due to a foot drop, or loss of balance due to impaired proprioception, vestibular function, or disordered postural reflexes originating at the central nervous system level. Detailed questioning may be required to determine whether the inability to get out of the chair is due to proximal weakness or impaired central nervous initiation.

It is important to identify symptoms not only referable to the peripheral neuromuscular system but to symptoms relating to impairment of higher cortical or cranial nerve function. In addition, a major discriminator in the development of a differential diagnosis is the presence or absence of symptoms referable to involvement of other organ systems. A careful system review is important in an attempt not only to achieve a diagnosis but also to fully anticipate the scope of its potential morbidity. For example, the recognition of orthostasis either by history or examination can provide insight that an evolving, otherwise nonspecific neuropathy pattern may be attributable to amyloidosis. Symptoms referable to cardiomyopathy or cardiac conduction defects, impaired GI motility, cutaneous change, and contractures may clarify the differential diagnosis in the heritable myopathies.

As muscle weakness is usually the most objective manifestation of neuromuscular disease, emphasis is placed not only on its existence but on its characteristics (e.g., upper or lower motor neuron) and on the pattern of involvement (Tables 1-4 to 1-7). The existence of weakness may be apparent either through history taking or, more commonly, by examination. Even though muscle weakness is the hallmark of neuromuscular disease, patients frequently identify weakness by its functional consequences. Patients with proximal upper extremity weakness commonly complain of activities of daily living (ADLs) that involve use of the arms at or above shoulder level. Shaving or drying hair, obtaining objects off

▶ TABLE 1-7. **PATTERNS OF MUSCLE WEAKNESS AND CORRELATIONS WITH NEUROMUSCULAR LOCALIZATION**

Patterns of Weakness	Localization
• Weakness of extensor muscles in the upper extremities, flexors in the lower extremities	UMN
• Hemiparesis	UMN
• Multifocal, asymmetric weakness without sensory involvement	MND Multifocal motor neuropathy MG (uncommon)
• Multifocal, asymmetric weakness with sensory involvement	Polyradiculopathy; multifocal CIDP (Lewis–Sumner syndrome or MADSAM) Multifocal neuropathy
• Multifocal sensory loss	Dorsal root ganglionopathy
• Symmetric weakness, proximal or generalized without sensory involvement	Myopathy MND DNMT
• Generalized motor > sensory	Polyradiculoneuropathy
• Asymmetric cranial nerve ± limbs	MG
• Distal symmetric—motor only	Distal myopathies Distal spinal muscular atrophy
• Distal symmetric—sensory > motor	LDPN
• Multiple nerve—asymmetric	Multifocal neuropathy
• Multiple root—asymmetric	Polyradiculopathy
• Multiple nerves and roots, single extremity	Plexopathy
• Single root	Monoradiculopathy
• Single nerve	Mononeuropathy

UMN, upper motor neuron; MND, motor neuron disease; MG, myasthenia gravis; LDPN, length-dependent polyneuropathy; PN, polyneuropathy; DNMT, disorders of neuromuscular transmission.

shelves, or getting arms in coat sleeves are notable examples. Distal upper extremity weakness interferes with a wide variety of activities such as diminished grip strength, difficulty with opening flip tops on beverage cans, buttoning or using nail clippers. Patients with hip flexor weakness have trouble going up stairs or getting their legs into vehicles. Patients with hip or knee extensor weakness have troubles with stairs in either direction, getting up from a squat or a deep chair. Patients with foot dorsiflexion weakness may trip whereas patients with plantar flexion weakness cannot run or walk as fast and cannot reach for objects as effectively.

Conversely, the complaint of weakness is more commonly used by patients as a synonym for asthenia—a more pervasive, generalized complaint due to a number of different conditions. History taking pertaining to muscle weakness should focus on the identification of specific functions or activities that the patient finds difficult. If a patient who claims to be weak cannot describe a specific activity that is problematic for them, the existence of true muscle weakness remains suspect unless subsequently corroborated by the physical examination. Conversely, it is not rare for a disorder such as Lambert–Eaton myasthenic syndrome where credible functional impairments due to muscle weakness appear disproportionate to actual weakness found on bedside examination.

At times, weakness may present with pain rather than with symptoms directly attributable to weakness. For example, patients with trapezius weakness commonly present with shoulder pain, presumably due to traction on pain-sensitive structures resulting from their "shoulder drop." Pain originating from strain on joints or soft tissues, as a secondary consequence of neuromuscular disease and the weakness it produces, is not uncommon.

UMN involvement needs to be considered in patients with potential neuromuscular disease, either as an alternative explanation for symptoms, or as a component of their neuromuscular condition. UMN pathology interferes with the synergistic functions of multiple muscle groups. As a result, functional activities highly dependent on coordinated muscle actions are commonly impaired early in the disease course. Impaired running and hand dexterity are notable examples. In addition, positive motor symptoms that occur commonly in UMN disease such as limb stiffness or spasms are readily recognized. They may complain of a tendency to drag one or both lower extremities. If the corticobulbar tracts are affected, swallowing and articulation are affected early and prominently, as these functions are dependent on the coordinated interplay of multiple muscle groups. The speech pattern that results is often halting, effortful, and "strangled" in its characteristics. Patients may lose their ability to effectively sniff or blow their nose. Patients with corticobulbar tract involvement may also develop lability of affect known as pseudobulbar palsy or forced yawning.

In contrast, as the final common pathway, lower motor neuron disorders express themselves in a limited number of ways, typically as a direct effect of functional loss due to weakness. Depending on a patient's handedness, vocation or hobbies, this may not be noticed until the weakness is substantial. Less commonly, the patient's initial complaints pertaining to lower motor neuron loss may reflect awareness of atrophy, fasciculations, or cramps.

Patients with weakness of hip flexion will have difficulty getting in and out of a car without manually lifting their thighs. Unless there is concomitant knee extensor weakness, patients will have more difficulty going upstairs than down as the former requires active hip flexion against gravity. Patients with weakness of hip abductors will waddle as a compensatory maneuver to maintain their center of gravity and balance. Patients with chronic weakness of hip extension will have difficulty rising from a chair and a tendency to have exaggerated lumbar lordosis as well, the latter resulting from posterior displacement of the shoulders for the same compensatory reasons. Knee extension weakness will result in difficulty getting up from a squat or out of deep chairs and commonly results in falls due to buckling of one or both knees. These patients may hyperextend their knees in order to prevent this while standing or walking (i.e., genu recurvatum). Ankle dorsiflexion weakness often results in tripping. Ankle plantar flexion weakness affects the efficiency of walking and deprives individuals from the ability to stand on their toes and run effectively.

In the upper extremity, people with weakness of the shoulder girdle will have difficulty with antigravity movements such as washing their hair, lifting heavy pans, inserting arms into coat sleeves, or retrieving objects from shelves. Weakness of elbow flexion and extension often goes unnoticed until fairly severe but may be recognized while attempting to open doors that require pull and push, respectively. Wrist and digit weaknesses interfere with grip and dexterity, which may impair multiple ADLs, including opening of bottles and cans, grasping zipper tabs, turning ignition keys, or buttoning buttons.

Neuromuscular disorders often affect the motor and to a lesser extent sensory functions of cranial nerves. Extraocular muscle involvement is a key discriminating factor in working through the differential diagnosis of neuromuscular disorders. For example, the extraocular muscles are rarely affected in motor neuron disease (MND), the majority of polyneuropathies or acquired inflammatory myopathies. Conversely, they may represent prominent manifestations of the inflammatory demyelinating polyneuropathies, disorders of neuromuscular transmission, and a finite list of muscle diseases, typically heritable in nature.

Patients typically become aware of ptosis by personal or family observation (Table 1-8). Occasionally, they first become aware when their vision is impaired by the drooping eyelid. Extraocular muscle involvement is typically expressed as diplopia, although patients with slowly progressive, symmetric involvement of the extraocular muscles such as in chronic progressive external ophthalmoplegia may have limited awareness of their deficit.

Patients with acute onset of unilateral facial weakness are usually very aware of the existence and nature of their problem. In many neuromuscular disorders, facial weakness is often chronic and symmetric, and as a result, the patient may not be aware of their deficit (Table 1-9). It is not rare for chronic bifacial weakness to be recognized for the first time on a routine neurologic examination. Questions pertaining to a tendency to sleep with eyes incompletely closed, the ability to blow up balloons or whistle may help to estimate the duration of a problem in situations such as these.

Symptomatic jaw weakness is an infrequent neuromuscular complaint. When present, it is often overshadowed by symptoms referable to muscles concomitantly affecting speech, swallowing, and breathing. Difficulty with chewing should nonetheless be inquired about, as it may sometimes be the initial or key symptom in a limited number of disorders such as myasthenia or Kennedy disease.

Symptoms referable to tongue weakness are common in many neuromuscular disorders. Patients typically become aware of tongue weakness as a result of dysarthria. Other issues may include the inability to manipulate food properly within their mouth. This kind of detail is uncommonly

TABLE 1-8. NEUROMUSCULAR CAUSES OF PTOSIS OR OPHTHALMOPLEGIA

Peripheral neuropathy
Guillain–Barré syndrome
Miller–Fisher syndrome
CANOMAD
Mitochondrial (SANDO)
Neuromuscular junction
Botulism
Lambert–Eaton syndrome (ptosis only)
Myasthenia gravis (pupil sparing)
Congenital myasthenia
Myopathy
Mitochondrial myopathies
Kearn–Sayres syndrome
Progressive external ophthalmoplegia
Oculopharyngeal and oculopharyngodistal muscular dystrophy
Myotonic dystrophy (ptosis only)
Congenital myopathy
Myotubular
Nemaline (ptosis only)
Congenital fiber type disproportion
Multiminicore disease
Hyperthyroidism/Graves disease (ophthalmoplegia without ptosis)
Hereditary inclusion body myopathy type III
Notable exceptions: anterior horn cell diseases; acquired inflammatory myopathies

CANOMAD, chronic ataxic neuropathy ophthalmology IgM paraprotein cold agglutinins disialosyl antibodies; SANDO, sensory ataxic neuropathy, dysarthria, ophthalmoplegia.
Modified with permission from Dumitru D, Amato AA. Introduction to myopathies and muscle tissue's reaction to injury. In: Dumitru D, Amato AA, Swartz MJ, eds. *Electrodiagnostic Medicine*. 2nd edn. Philadelphia, PA: Hanley & Belfus; 2002.

TABLE 1-9. NEUROMUSCULAR DISORDERS ASSOCIATED WITH FACIAL WEAKNESS[29]

Anterior horn cell
Amyotrophic lateral sclerosis
Spinal muscular atrophy
Kennedy disease
Polycranialradiculoneuropathy
Lyme
Sarcoidosis
Neoplastic meningitis
Chronic meningitis
GBS
CIDP
Neuromuscular junction
Autoimmune myasthenia gravis
Congenital myasthenia gravis
Lambert–Eaton myasthenia gravis
Botulism
Muscle
Facioscapulohumeral muscular dystrophy
Congenital myopathies
Myotonic muscular dystrophy
Inclusion body myositis
Oculopharyngeal distal myopathy

volunteered by the patient and is more frequently elucidated by detailed questioning.

Weakness of the neck muscles may be noticed by patients or their families when the neck extensors can no longer support the weight of the head and head drop develops by the development of head drop (Table 1-10). This is often accompanied by nuchal discomfort, presumably due to the constant and unaccustomed traction on posterior cervical ligamentous structures. Neck discomfort from head drop may be distinguished from other, more common causes of neck pain, by the relief allowed by neck support. Head drop may contribute to dysphagia as well. Trapezius weakness is most commonly symptomatic when acute and unilateral and is usually a result of a mononeuropathy of the accessory nerve. As discussed above, trapezius weakness is usually presents with shoulder pain as the index symptoms. Shoulder drop can be easily missed unless the patient is viewed from the rear, with the back exposed.

Weakness of the scapula can result from weakness of either the trapezius or serratus anterior muscles (Table 1-11). Scapular winging interferes with both shoulder-girdle strength and mobility. Patients may note either difficulty in raising an arm above the head or an inability to push with the accustomed force, for example, while doing pushups.

The symptoms of ventilatory muscle weakness represent an ominous, occasionally initial manifestation of a selective group of neuromuscular disorders (Table 1-12).[3] In this text, ventilation will refer to the mechanical act of air exchange from atmosphere to alveoli as opposed to respiration, the act of gas exchange between alveoli and the circulation. Dyspnea on exertion is the typical symptom of hypoventilation but may not become evident in this population due to the limited ability of patients to exert themselves. Diaphragmatic weakness is more symptomatic in the supine position leading to orthopnea. Symptomatic hypoventilation

TABLE 1-10. NEUROMUSCULAR DISORDERS ASSOCIATED WITH HEAD DROP[7–24]

Anterior horn cell
Amyotrophic lateral sclerosis
Radiation myelopathy
Syringomyelia
Neuromuscular junction
Autoimmune myasthenia gravis
Neuropathy
Guillain-Barré syndrome
CIDP
Muscle
Polymyositis
Inclusion body myositis
Focal myositis
Sporadic late onset nemaline myopathy (SLONM)
Hereditary inclusion body myopathy
Laminopathy
Selenoproteinopathy
Isolated neck extensor myopathy
Proximal myotonic myopathy
Carnitine deficiency
Facioscapulohumeral muscular dystrophy
Mitochondrial myopathy
Hyperparathyroidism
Hypokalemia
Myofibrillar myopathy (desmin)

TABLE 1-11. NEUROMUSCULAR DISORDERS ASSOCIATED WITH SCAPULAR WINGING[25]

Anterior horn cell
Scapuloperoneal spinal muscular atrophy
Nerve
Accessory nerve palsy
Long thoracic nerve palsy
Davidenkow's syndrome
Muscle
Facioscapulohumeral muscular dystrophy
Scapuloperoneal muscular dystrophy
Limb-girdle muscular dystrophy (e.g., calpainopathy)
Acid maltase deficiency
Neuromuscular diseases where scapular winging occurs uncommonly
Myotonic muscular dystrophy
Emery–Dreifuss muscular dystrophy
Myotubular myopathy
Nemaline rod myopathy
Central core myopathy
Phosphofructokinase deficiency

TABLE 1-12. NEUROMUSCULAR DISORDERS ASSOCIATED WITH VENTILATORY MUSCLE WEAKNESS[26–28,32]

Anterior horn cell
Motor neuron disease/amyotrophic lateral sclerosis
Poliomyelitis
West Nile virus
Nerve
Bilateral phrenic neuropathies (brachial plexus neuritis)
Critical illness neuropathy
Guillain–Barré syndrome
CIDP (consider POEMS)
CMT2 C
Multifocal motor neuropathy with phrenic neuropathy (rare)
Amyloidosis
Porphyria
Toxins (thallium, lead, arsenic, organophosphates, vincristine)
Neuromuscular junction
Autoimmune myasthenia gravis
Congenital myasthenia
Botulism
Lambert–Eaton myasthenic syndrome
Envenomations (reptile, insect, marine)
Tick paralysis
Muscle
Myotonic muscular dystrophy
Dystrophinopathies
Limb-girdle muscular dystrophy (2C–F, 2I)
Emery–Dreifuss muscular dystrophy
Acid maltase deficiency
Phosphofructokinase deficiency (rare)
Carnitine deficiency
Poly/dermatomyositis (rare)
Myotubular myopathy
Multiminicore disease with rigid spine (SEPN-1)
Carnitine palmitoyl transferase deficiency and rhabdomyolysis
Nemaline rod myopathy
Congenital fiber type disproportion
Critical illness myopathy
Mitochondrial myopathy (rare)
Myofibrillar myopathy (desmin)
Necrotizing myopathy
Myopathy associated with signal recognizing protein (SRP) antibodies
Metabolic (hypokalemia, hypophosphatemia)

in the neuromuscular disorders often presents in a protean fashion with nonspecific, frequently nocturnal and unrecognized symptoms.[4] The nocturnal predilection may be multifactorial. In addition to orthopnea from diaphragmatic weakness, the supine position also places more of the surface area of the chest wall against surfaces that add further resistance to chest wall expansion. Weakness of pharyngeal musculature may diminish the support of the upper airway further compromising the upper airway integrity during inspiration. Patients who are dependent on accessory muscles, paralyzed during REM sleep, will experience further compromise of ventilation during this stage of sleep. Resulting nocturnal hypercarbia may interrupt normal sleep cycling and promote nocturnal restlessness and diurnal fatigue. Early morning headache and confusion due to carbon dioxide retention are usually late symptoms that clearly warrant the provision of positive pressure airway support.

With the sensory history, there is great value in allowing the patient to identify the topographic area of involvement which is frequently more accurately identified by the patient than by the examining physician. For example, paresthesia confined to one or two contiguous digits would, in the vast majority of cases, indicate a disorder of the neuromuscular system that may be difficult to corroborate even by a detailed sensory examination conducted by an experienced physician. With the sensory history, it is also important to identify any associated morbidity, for example, loss of balance or ability to identify a coin in a pocket due to proprioceptive loss.

Disorders that affect sensory neurons may lead to a variety of perceived sensations that may in part be related to the size of the sensory axons affected and the duration of the illness. Paresthesias (a positive or abnormal spontaneous sensation) may be described as tingling, prickly, burning, shooting or electrical sensations, often with an unpleasant or painful characteristic. The latter three sensations are thought to indicate preferential involvement of small unmyelinated sensory nerve endings. Other abnormal although probably less specific perceptions include coldness as well as itching. If large myelinated sensory fibers are affected, the patient may describe a band-like, wrapped, swollen, "pad-like," or wooden sensation. They may feel as though they have cotton stuffed between their toes or that their body parts are encased in plastic, dried glue, or that their skin is foreign to them. Pain associated with large diameter nerve fibers is often deep, dull, and aching in characteristic.

Numbness can be conceptualized as a loss of sensation, that is, a negative sensory symptom. In actuality, it is really a sign in that it may not be recognized by the patient until the affected body region is touched. It is largely held that unrecognized numbness unaccompanied by paresthesia is indicative of a very chronic, slowly progressive process. As an example, unrecognized sensory loss without paresthesia is one of the characteristic features of Charcot–Marie–Tooth disease.

As with the motor history, it is important to explore the functional consequences of sensory loss although these may be less specific. In the authors' experience, the complaint of "dropping things" from the hands has poor discriminating value in the separation of definable from nondefinable neurologic disease. Conversely, impaired balance from large fiber sensory loss, that is, sensory ataxia, is an important symptom associated with significant morbidity. Inquiries should be made regarding nocturnal balance, the use of a night-light, and balance in the shower while hair washing.

Impaired autonomic system function occurs in certain causes of peripheral neuropathy as well as in presynaptic disorders of neuromuscular transmission. Identification of dysautonomia may aid greatly in focusing the differential diagnosis. Common symptoms include orthostatic intolerance with faintness and nuchal discomfort, constipation, diarrhea, or early satiety, urinary retention, incontinence, erectile dysfunction, sweating abnormalities including dry cracked feet, blurred vision, dry eyes, or dry mouth.

Perception of pain is dependent on nerve function but results from injury to other tissues. Pain caused by nerve injury or dysfunction, is referred to as neuropathic pain. Neuropathic pain is recognized by its characteristics or by its association with objective evidence of relevant nerve injury. It is often linear in its orientation and often, but not always has burning, lancinating, deep boring or electrical characteristics. Allodynia, or cutaneous pain triggered by a normally innocuous stimulus, for example, the touch of bed clothes may occur in patterns not typically recognized as typical nerve or nerve root distributions. The truncal neuropathy of diabetes is a notable example of this. Muscle pain is also a common complaint brought to the attention of the neuromuscular clinician. Along similar lines, myalgia without a definable trigger, associated weakness, or some other objective finding is unlikely to be of neuromuscular causation. As mentioned previously, pain commonly occurs as a consequence of neuromuscular disease, frequently mechanical in nature and related to imbalanced forces on joints and other connective tissues promoted by muscle weakness or impaired sensation.

THE EXAMINATION

Time constraints are a medical reality. Examining clothed patients represents an understandable but unfortunate response to this inconvenience. In neuromuscular medicine, this short cut is not a viable option. As emphasized later in this section, there are numerous observations that can be made only by direct observation of exposed body parts that provide clues integral to accurate diagnosis.

The strategy of the neuromuscular examination is to identify patterns of weakness and sensory loss and correlate them with typical patterns of specific disorders. In certain cases, such as a multifocal neuropathy, the patterns are more readily identifiable early in the disease, whereas in others, for example, ALS, some degree of disease evolution may be required for the diagnosis to become apparent. Either by history or examination but ideally by both, involvement of motor, sensory and/or autonomic systems should be sought. Recognized patterns such as distal symmetric, that is length-dependent, proximal symmetric, UMN, single or multiple peripheral nerve patterns, and single or multiple nerve root patterns should be sought for and ideally recognized. In an analogous manner, sensory loss should be characterized as small fiber, large fiber or both. If possible, the recognition of length-dependent, multifocal, single nerve and single nerve root distribution of sensory signs, and symptoms will provide an invaluable diagnostic clue.

The motor examination of cranial nerves begins with observation. In childhood spinal muscular atrophies the upper lip may have a tented configuration. A number of myopathies will produce "myopathic facies" with a transverse smile with little or no elevation of the corners of the mouth. With severe weakness of muscles of mastication, the jaw may be slack and hang open. Patients with facial weakness affecting the obicularis oculi may have ptosis of the lower lid resulting in visible sclera between the lower limbus of the cornea and the margin of the lower eye lid. These same patients may be observed not to oppose their eyelids completely while blinking. More subtle facial weakness may be noticeable when the eyelids are not completely "buried" when the patient is asked to squeeze their eyes shut as hard as they can.

Atrophy in muscles innervated by cranial nerves may be evident in the temporalis, sternocleidomastoid, and particularly in the tongue. The former two are common features of myotonic muscular dystrophy. Tongue atrophy can be seen in a number of neuromuscular disorders most notably the MNDs. Fasciculations of the face and tongue are key diagnostic features, particularly in the evaluation of bulbar syndromes, and should be actively sought for in suspected amyotrophic lateral sclerosis (ALS) and the spinal muscular atrophies. As with any other muscle, it is important to examine the muscle in a relaxed rather than partially contracted state as muscle movement in the latter situation may be readily misinterpreted as fasciculations. It is also important to distinguish a generalized tremulousness of the tongue, which occurs frequently in normal patients from the random twitching of individual motor units that represent fasciculations.

Manual muscle testing in cranial innervated muscle is an integral part of the neuromuscular examination. Facial weakness can be assessed by attempting to pry the tightly closed eyes and/or lips apart. We grade facial weakness on a mild, moderate, and severe scale. Mild weakness means that the eyelids oppose and generate some but inadequate strength with an attempt to open them. Moderate weakness means that the eyelids oppose but offer minimal resistant whereas severe weakness means that the eyelids cannot completely oppose. With the lips, mild weakness is determined by the ability to blow up the cheeks with air but the inability to prevent air leakage when the cheeks are compressed. Moderate weakness is the ability to oppose the lips but not puff out the cheeks whereas severe weakness is the inability to oppose the lips.

Jaw strength can be tested by looking for lateral chin deviation upon opening or by trying to pry open the fully closed jaw by placing the fingers on the back of the neck and applying downward pressure with the thumbs. Attempting to assess jaw opening strength should be done with caution as inadvertent trauma to the teeth may occur if the jaw snaps shut inadvertently.

Tongue strength is best tested by having the patient "pocket" each cheek with manual pressure being placed on the cheek and indirectly on the tongue attempting to force it back to the midline. Again we use a mild, moderate, and severe scale. Mild weakness is a retained ability to pocket but an inability to resist pressure. Moderate weakness is the ability to pocket the cheek in a limited fashion with little or no resistance to pressure. Severe weakness refers to little or no tongue movement. Neck flexion and extension strength is tested in the customary isometric manner by having the patient resist full neck flexion and extension, respectively, with or without the use of a dynamometer.

Myotonia and paramyotonia of eyelid opening and closing, as well as in limb muscles, may be sought for in the appropriate context, particularly in suspected paramyotonia myotonia and myotonia congenita. In assessing for eyelid myotonia or paramyotonia, the patient is asked to repetitively close their eyes tightly and open them quickly. With myotonia, the delay in opening is most apparent with the first attempt whereas in paramyotonia, it gets worse with subsequent efforts. The examiner can also ask the patient to look up for several seconds and then rapidly look back down to the primary position. If the eyelid does not return to the primary position as fast as the globe, myotonia of the eyelid elevators may be considered along with other causes of lid lag. Myotonia can also be sought for by percussing the tongue with the assistance of gauze and two tongue blades but this is cumbersome procedure that and probably adds little to the assessment of myotonia through grip or percussion of limb muscles. An additional eyelid sign of potential use in neuromuscular disease is the Cogan eyelid twitch. The patient is asked to look down, and then rapidly saccade to mid-position. A positive result is identified by an overshoot of the upper lid followed by a few oscillatory movements of the upper lid until it settles back to its normal relationship with the globe.

Relevant to this is our belief that ptosis, proptosis, and to a certain extent facial weakness are best recognized by understanding the normal anatomic relationship between the eyelids and the globe. Typically, the lower margin of the upper lid covers the upper 2 to 3 mm of the limbus whereas the upper margin of the lower lid typically intersects the lower limbus. The observation of sclera between the upper lid and the limbus indicates eyelid retraction or proptosis. The observation of sclera between the lower lid and the limbus represents obicularis oculi weakness or proptosis. A narrowed palpebral fissure represents squinting, blepharospasm, atrophy, or retraction of the globe.

Observation of the eyebrow position is also helpful in the interpretation of abnormal eyelid positioning. If the lower margin of the upper lid is lower than it should be due to ptosis, the eyebrow is typically elevated in a compensatory attempt of the frontalis muscle to elevate it unless the frontalis is weak as well, for example, myasthenia. Conversely, if the upper lid position is lowered by squinting from blepharospasm, the eyebrow is usually lower than the opposite side if uninvolved.

The pupils should be examined, preferably, at least initially, in a dimly lit room to assess for the possibility of Horner's syndrome. The lack of pupillary reactivity may represent an autonomic component of the patient's disorder. Perhaps, the greatest value of the pupil examination in neuromuscular disease is to distinguish neuromuscular disorders causing ophthalmoparesis that spare the pupil from those that do not. Myasthenia, most diabetic third nerve palsies, and myopathic causes of ophthalmoparesis fit into the former category. Ophthalmoparesis with pupillary involvement may occur as a consequence of Guillain–Barré syndrome and its variants and also due to presynaptic disorders of neuromuscular transmission such as botulism.

Examination of limb and trunk muscles also begins with observation. Again, it is our strongly held belief that although the patient should be gowned with appropriate undergarments, that every part of the body should be available to direct observation. There are many potential clues that can be obtained in this manner. Muscle atrophy, focal or generalized, and muscle hypertrophy should be sought for. Viewing the shoulder girdles from the back may identify shoulder drop from trapezius weakness or overt scapular winging. Viewing the chest in males may disclose gynecomastia. Viewing the shoulder girdles from the front may disclose a crease in the pectoralis, an elevated scapula producing a pseudohypertrophic appearance of the trapezius or a horizontally oriented clavicle all resulting from weakness of periscapular muscles. In a similar vein, abnormal scapular positioning may affect the positioning of the arms which may be internally rotated so that back of the hand rather than the thumb is anteriorly oriented producing a simian posture. Arm movement during conversation, that is, gesticulation may identify diminished spontaneous movements of one or both upper extremities due to proximal weakness, limitation of joint movement, or central nervous system disease. Conversely, the physician may notice completely normal spontaneous movement under these conditions which is subsequently found to be incongruous with the patient's inability (or unwillingness) to use the limb properly during the examination, implicating decreased effort from pain, apraxia, or psychogenic etiology.

Muscles should be closely observed for adventitious movements such as tremor, fasciculations, myokymia, or rippling. In our experience, benign fasciculations tend to be felt by the patient more frequently than they are seen, are most commonly seen in the calves and feet, and occur briefly and repetitively in a single spot before disappearing. Postural tremor is not rare in neuromuscular disease and may be a notable feature of Charcot–Marie–Tooth disease, CIDP, or spinal muscular atrophy. Fasciculations that occur in multiple locations in multiple muscles simultaneously are more ominous and suggest excessive cholinesterase inhibitor effect, a nerve hyperexcitability disorder, or most commonly, a motor system disease.

Muscle contractures (nonphysiologic) or other dysmorphic features may be noted either by observation or during passive movement of limbs. Contractures may be

▶ **TABLE 1-13. NEUROMUSCULAR DISORDERS ASSOCIATED WITH EARLY JOINT CONTRACTURES**

Anterior horn cell
Arthrogryposis multiplex congenita
SMA
Nerve
CMT3
Neuromuscular junction
Congenital myasthenia gravis—rapsyn
Muscle
Central core disease
Nemaline myopathy
Congenital fiber type disproportion
Bethlem myopathy
Ullrich congenital muscular dystrophy
Dystrophinopathy
Emery–Dreifuss muscular dystrophy types I–III
Dominant myopathy with ankle contractures and high CK
Juvenile dermatomyositis

seen in a number of neuromuscular conditions as listed in Table 1-13 and may provide key diagnostic clues. Dysmorphic features such as long thin facies, high-arched palates, kyphoscoliosis, exaggerated lumbar lordosis, cavus foot deformities, and hammer toes are also key diagnostic clues. Cavus foot deformities are usually indicative of long-standing disorders dating to childhood and are frequent accompaniments of Charcot–Marie–Tooth disease, distal forms of spinal muscular atrophy, hereditary spastic paraparesis, and Friedreich ataxia. There are many neuromuscular conditions with accompanying dermal or epidermal changes. These include the ecchymoses of Cushing disease, the angiokeratomas of Fabry disease, the skin changes of POEMS syndrome, the skin and nail bed changes of dermatomyositis, Mee's lines in finger and toe nails representing growth arrest in response to arsenic or lead intoxication among others.

The identification of scapular winging may require provocative posturing as well as observation. It is an important and easily overlooked diagnostic clue in the assessment of neuromuscular disease. Affected patients will be unable to raise their hand over their head effectively. Scapular winging may be evident by simply looking at the patient from the rear. It may be accentuated by a number of maneuvers depending on which muscles are weak. Scapular winging due to weakness of the serratus anterior results in the inferior-medial angle of the scapula being elevated more off the ribcage and migrating further away from the midline than its superior-medial counterpart. It can be accentuated by having the patient push against a wall or by putting downward pressure on the humerus when the arm is flexed at the shoulder. With scapular winging resulting from trapezius weakness, the entire medial border is elevated. Winging is accentuated by attempted external rotation, or abduction of the arm at the shoulder against resistance. The dynamics of scapular winging resulting from the more diffuse myopathic and motor neuron disorders are more complex.

Provocative muscle testing should also be performed when relevant. Percussion myotonia is most commonly tested in the extensor digitorum communis (EDC) and thenar eminence. In the former, the forearm is supported by the examiner in a pronated position, allowing the wrist and fingers to hang limply. The EDC is percussed just distal to the head of the radius. A normal response is no movement or a minimal brief flicker of digit extension. The presence of myotonia is suggested when one or more of the digits extends at the metacarpal phalangeal joints and sustains this posture for a second or so. Percussion of the thenar eminence is performed in a similar manner with the wrist and forearm supported while the forearm is fully supinated. The thumb should be maintained limply in the same plane as the palm. Myotonia is identified when the thumb abducts notably in response to a brief percussive strike to the abductor pollicis brevis muscle. Grip myotonia is sought for by having the patient tightly grip an object, for example the examiners index and middle finger for a few seconds, then rapidly release the grip. A slow and deliberate extension of the fingers indicates myotonia. Typical myotonia improves with repeated trials. Paradoxical myotonia worsens with repeated trials. Myoedema refers to a mounding of muscle in response to percussion of a muscle belly that represents an uncommon finding in some muscle diseases.

The foundation of the neuromuscular examination is the assessment for the presence and pattern of muscle weakness. Two strategies are typically employed: isometric manual muscle resistance and functional testing. Ideally, suspected weakness identified by the first method, for example, reduced resistance of foot dorsiflexors, would be confirmed by the latter, that is, the inability to walk on the heels. There is an art to manual muscle testing, which is undoubtedly improved upon by experience, particularly in the distinction of true weakness as opposed to that due to impaired effort. Muscles are typically tested in an isometric fashion that is a contracted position with the patient asked to resist the force applied by the examiner. For example, elbow flexors are tested with the patient's fist resting against his or her shoulder. The patient is held by the examiner in such a way that the muscle(s) tested are isolated to the extent possible. Again, in the case of the elbow flexors, the examiner would place the hand that delivers the force just proximal to the wrist to produce the greatest mechanical advantage, while at the same time removing wrist movement from consideration. The other hand, which serves to stabilize, is placed on the biceps just proximal to the elbow.

In order to obtain full patient effort, the patient has to have confidence that the examiner will not harm them. The examiner should sustain full effort long enough to detect either true weakness with its smooth characteristics or "give way" weakness with its ratchety and inconsistent character. It is important however, to relinquish effort before the full range of motion is exhausted so as to avoid injury. Along similar lines, great caution should be exercised to avoid pathologic fracture in any patient with cancer potentially metastatic to bone.

Mild degrees of weakness may easily go unrecognized by both patient and examiner alike. This is particularly true in strong muscles like the quadriceps and the gastrocnemius, or when the strength or effort of examiner is limited. It is imperative that the examiner place themselves at the greatest mechanical advantage and gives an appropriate effort so as to avoid a false-negative result. For example, ideal examination of neck flexion, elbow flexion, knee extension, and trunk flexion, the patient should be tested in the supine position, where the patient has to move against gravity and resistance. Testing a patient on their side is ideal for testing hip abduction and the prone position optimal for elbow, hip and neck extension, and knee flexion.

It is in these same strong muscles where functional testing is particularly useful. For example, hip and knee extension strength can be assessed by the patient's ability to get up from a deep chair or their ability to perform a partial squat or hop on one leg. Foot plantar flexion strength can be assessed by having the patient elevate their heel while standing on one leg.

Once weakness is recognized, two characteristics are of paramount importance: its pattern and its severity. The primary importance of the pattern of weakness is in the formulation of the initial diagnosis. Pattern recognition as a diagnostic tool is addressed in Tables 1-4 to 1-7 and will be elaborated on repeatedly in this and subsequent chapters. The importance of the degree of weakness may also contribute to the diagnosis, for example, demonstrating progression both within and between different muscle groups is a key in the diagnosis of ALS. In addition, and perhaps more importantly, establishing the degree of weakness is also key in establishing treatment responsiveness.

To this end, accurate quantitative measurements of strength are paramount. Historically, the Medical Research Council (MRC) scale has been used by most institutions for this purpose. This is a 0–5 scale, with 5 representing normal strength and 0 representing no discernible muscle movement. By definition, the MRC scale requires muscles be examined against gravity. An MRC grade of 3 preserves ability to move the joint through a full range of motion against gravity but with negligible resistance to the examiner. An MRC grade of 2 represents movement through a complete range of motion with gravity eliminated. An MRC grade of 1 represents observed muscle contraction with little or no limb or digit movement. With the MRC scale, the majority of weak muscles will fall into the four (modest weakness) range. For this reason, the MRC scale has been modified to include a 4− and 4+ category to expand this largest group of weak muscles.

The MRC scale is problematic, as it may be insensitive, qualitative, and subjective.[5] The potential exists for considerable inter-examiner variability. It has been documented that patients may lose 80% or more of their motor units in a given muscle before they receive a 3 or less MRC rating.[5] In the opinion of the authors', it is a poor tool to measure motor deficits in UMN disease where functional impairment may be more on the basis of altered coordination and tone rather than loss of strength. Increasingly in clinical trials, and to some extent in clinical practice, tools such as hand-held dynamometry are used in an attempt to measure strength in a more objective, linear, and reproducible manner. As an example, in the experience of the authors' most men can generate 40 or more kilograms of force in the majority of upper extremity muscles. An MRC grade of 3 approximates a force of 10 kg, implying that a modified MRC grade between 4− and 4+ represents approximately 75% of the weakness spectrum in these muscle groups.

Ventilation can be assessed at the bedside by a number of techniques. There is value in asking the patient to generate a forceful sniff or cough. Use of accessory muscles should be noted as well as a tendency for the patient to interrupt sentences to catch their breath. Shallow breathing can be detected by auscultation. The vital capacity can be roughly estimated in the cooperative patients by having them inspire fully and then count out loud at the rate of 1 per second until that single breath is exhausted. That number multiplied by a hundred will estimate their vital capacity measured in cubic centimeters. There may be value as well in examining the patient in the supine position to assess for paradoxical abdominal movements (outward abdominal movement in response to inspiration) as an indicator of diaphragmatic weakness.

UMN signs in the cranial nerve distribution are limited in number and in specificity. An enhanced jaw jerk or gag reflex, the presence of a snout reflex, forced yawning and a pseudobulbar affect are all accepted UMN signs. Reduction in the speed in which a patient is able to repetitively blink or wiggle their tongue back and forth, in the absence of weakness or mechanical restriction of the respective muscles probably represents central nervous system dysfunction but is unlikely to specify corticobulbar tract pathology. The same is likely true for synkinesis of two muscles innervated by different cranial nerves, for example the inability to keep the jaw from moving side to side when the requested task is wiggling the tongue back and forth in the horizontal plane.

Impaired motor function of corticospinal tract origin may include weakness, particularly if acute in onset, but tends to be dominated by impaired coordination and function. Clumsiness disproportionate to the degree of weakness is a sensitive, albeit nonspecific indicator of UMN disease. UMN weakness may also be suspected on the basis of topographic pattern of involvement. A hemiparetic pattern, even in ALS (also known as the Mill's variant) is rarely LMN in nature. A paraparetic or quadriparetic pattern often occurs as a result of corticospinal involvement of the spinal cord but may just as easily occur in a neuromuscular disorder as well. UMN weakness when limited in distribution is often more distal than proximal, particularly in the upper extremity. Often, UMN weakness can be implicated when flexors are stronger than extensors in the upper limbs and the opposite in the lower extremities. For example, weakness of hip flexion, knee flexion, and foot dorsiflexion in combination strongly suggests UMN disease. Impaired motor function of central nervous system origin can often be deduced by observation, that is, the reduced spontaneous use of a body part such as diminished gesturing of an arm during talking.

UMN disease is also implicated when deep tendon reflexes are exaggerated, or with the existence of pathologic reflexes or spastic tone. The detection of hyperactive deep tendon reflexes can be somewhat subjective. Sustained clonus is undoubtedly pathologic in all cases. Deep tendon reflexes that persist in a limb that is weak and atrophic, unsustained clonus, and reflex spread are all suggestive of UMN pathology but are probably not pathognomonic. Babinski signs are universally accepted as a marker of UMN pathology but bilateral Hoffman's signs and absent abdominal reflexes need to be interpreted with some caution.

Like its motor counterpart, the results of the sensory examination are most credible when they are concordant with both the history and available functional tests of sensation. There are many sensory examination strategies. In the authors' experience, the application of sensory stimuli in a random fashion with subsequent attempts to identify the boundaries of the sensory loss is often difficult to interpret and may produce false-positive results. An alternative technique is a hypothesis-driven approach in which the examiner attempts to prove or disprove a specified pattern of sensory loss, for example, a length-dependent pattern in a patient with numb feet. As examiners can apply stimuli with different intensities inadvertently and as patients have different thresholds for what they consider reduced (or increased), it is important to perform sensory testing in a reproducible and as unbiased manner as is possible. For this reason, there is a benefit from testing with the patient's eyes closed and with the addition of random null stimuli. This is particularly true with vibration where patients commonly confuse the touch of the tuning fork with vibration as the sensation in question. Using the tip of the examiner's finger as a random substitute for the tuning fork is a means to ensure that the patient is responding positively to vibration and not simply to pressure.

There are a few important points to recognize in performing the sensory examination. As already emphasized, it is not uncommon to be unable to convincingly demonstrate sensory loss in a symptomatic region in a person with credible sensory complaints. Conversely and somewhat paradoxically, it is not uncommon to find patients in the setting of a partial nerve injury who claim to react to a stimulus in a hypersensitive manner in an area that they claim to be numb. Finally, it is important to realize that the topographical area where sensory symptoms are perceived and sensory loss is found is often far smaller than published anatomical charts would suggest for any nerve or dermatomal distribution. Presumably, this is the result of the considerable overlap between contiguous nerve territories.

There are a limited number of functional sensory tests to corroborate the findings on the direct sensory examination. The best known of these is the Romberg test, which assesses proprioceptive (or less likely bilateral vestibular) dysfunction in the lower extremities arising from either the peripheral or the central nervous system. The finger–nose test, also done with the eyes closed, is an analogous test for proprioceptive loss in the upper extremities. Stereognosis testing can be helpful at times. Even with severe nerve injuries, absolute anesthesia is rare. Patients who claim to feel absolutely nothing in the hands yet can readily manipulate an object in that hand with their eyes closed are unlikely to have the degree of sensory loss that is claimed.

Common bedside screening tests of autonomic function include observation of pupillary responses as described above. The feet should be observed for the presence of dry, cracked skin suggesting the possibility of anhydrosis. Pulse variation in response to deep breathing is a test of parasympathetic function. Arguably, the most commonly performed and valuable bedside autonomic test is orthostatic blood pressure and pulse measurements. They should be done after a few minutes in the supine position. Both blood pressure and pulse should be measured immediately on standing (or sitting) and at 1-minute intervals for at least 3 minutes, depending on the index of suspicion and the result.

Examination of young children, particularly infants, can be a challenge. Infants can be placed in a prone position to observe if they are capable of extending their head. An inability to do so suggests weakness of the neck extensor muscles. Most infants have considerable subcutaneous fat that makes muscle palpation quite difficult. Palpating neck extensor muscles is a good place to attempt this evaluation as little subcutaneous fat overlies this muscle group. Neck flexion strength can be assessed as the child is pulled by the arms from a supine to a sitting position. Crying during the examination allows the opportunity to assess the child's vocalization (e.g., presence of a weak cry) and fatigability to the physical examination. Muscle weakness in infants is usually characterized by an overall decrease in muscle tone and many children with profound weakness are characterized as "floppy." This terminology does not necessarily imply a neuromuscular disorder. In fact, most floppy infants result from a central nervous system problem. In view of prominent subcutaneous tissue, fasciculations may be visible only in the tongue. Observation of tremor is important as it may be a feature of spinal muscular atrophy and some hereditary neuropathies. It is important to examine the parents of floppy infants for the possibility of a neuromuscular disorder. This is particularly important in children suspected of having myotonic dystrophy. In addition, weakness can transiently develop in infants born to mothers with myasthenia gravis.

▶ WHAT IS NEUROMUSCULAR PROBLEM?

The following section will attempt to summarize the patterns of motor and sensory involvement that typify the diseases described in this text, in an attempt to facilitate the localization process (Table 1-6). Further formulation of the differential diagnosis will require knowledge of the behaviors and natural histories of the disorders that are addressed in Tables 1-1 to 1-3 and described in detail in subsequent chapters of this book.

MOTOR NEURON DISEASES

The hallmark of the MND, also known as anterior horn cell diseases or motor neuronopathies, is painless weakness and atrophy frequently accompanied by the positive symptoms of cramps and fasciculations. Although cramps and fasciculations may occur in apparent absence of disease, and can be seen with any peripheral nerve disorder, they are far more prevalent in disorders of the anterior horn. As mentioned above, benign fasciculations are commonly evanescent and confined to a singular area at any given time. Conversely, fasciculations seen in numerous locations on a continuous or near continuous basis is almost always the result of a motor neuron disorder. The absence of fasciculations does not preclude a motor neuron localization, particularly where there is considerable subcutaneous tissue that may obscure their observation, infants and those with an elevated body mass index being the most notable examples. Sensory symptoms and sensory loss do not typically occur in MND except in Kennedy disease. Nonetheless, it may occasionally occur in ALS due to other unrelated problems or potentially as a consequence of the occasional multisystem variants of this disorder.[6]

Most motor neuron disorders are hereditary/degenerative in nature and as a result have an insidiously progressive course. The rate of progression varies both with and between different MND, ALS, and spinal muscular atrophy type I having the most virulent courses. The pattern of weakness varies with the disorder. With ALS, onset is typically focal and asymmetric, for example, foot drop. Even early in the course however, weakness can be recognized as being multisegmental and outside of a single nerve or nerve root distribution. Poliomyelitis and other neurotropic viruses may present focally as well with marked asymmetry or with a more generalized presentation. The spinal muscular atrophies tend to have a symmetric presentation that is generalized or proximally predominant in both the X-linked bulbospinal (Kennedy disease) and infantile forms. The more uncommon distal spinal muscular atrophies have a distal, symmetric pattern of weakness that may mimic neuropathies or distal myopathies. Juvenile segmental spinal muscular atrophy (Hirayama disease) presents focally in the distal aspect of first one and at times the other upper extremity.

The recognition of MND is also aided by the identification of functions that are spared. Most notably, patients with MND virtually never experience ptosis or ophthalmoparesis except in the rare cases of ALS that behave more like a multisystem disorder. Impaired bulbar function (i.e., speech and swallowing) is common in many MND. Facial and jaw weakness may occur but are typically less prominent than the weakness of the tongue and throat muscles. Deep tendon reflexes tend to be lost unless there is concomitant UMN disease such as in ALS.

DORSAL ROOT GANGLIONOPATHIES

These disorders, also known as sensory neuronopathies, are characterized by non–length-dependent, multi-focal sensory signs and symptoms. Like many nerve diseases, distal aspects of limbs tend to be more afflicted than proximal, thus potentially mimicking the far more common length-dependent polyneuropathy pattern. Careful history taking may be required to identify the non–length-dependent or asymmetric features. Both the resulting chronologic course and the presence or absence of pain is variable and in large part dependent on etiology. Electrodiagnosis is useful to demonstrate that sensory fibers alone are affected. In polyneuropathies, there is almost always some indication of motor involvement, even when not apparent clinically, particularly if fibrillation potentials within intrinsic foot muscles are sought for. Sensory ataxia is a common manifestation of these disorders. Dorsal root ganglionopathies may be autoimmune, toxic, infectious, or at times degenerative in etiology.

MONORADICULOPATHIES

Monoradiculopathies are among the most common neurologic problems, commonly due to some mechanism associated with degenerative spine and disc disease. Their phenotype is in turn dependent on the mechanism and acuity of nerve root compression. The prototypical symptom of an acute monoradiculopathy, usually related to disc herniation is pain, limited to one extremity, and following the course of the involved dermatome. The pain may not affect the entire dermatome simultaneously, for example, buttock and anterolateral leg pain sparing the thigh in an L5 radiculopathy. Contrary to common belief, the pain usually begins in the scapular and the buttock area rather than the neck or back. Sensory and motor deficits are not universal, but when present, should be confined to a single segment. Weakness should be confined to a single myotome but involve more than one peripheral nerve distribution. For example, in a C7 monoradiculopathy, both elbow extension (C7/radial) and wrist flexion (C7/median) are often involved. Conversely, weakness may not be detectable in all muscles innervated by that particular myotome. For example, demonstrating weakness only in the extensor hallicus longus is not uncommon in an L5 monoradiculopathy. A helpful caveat is the recognition that a given muscle is virtually never completely paralyzed from a single nerve root lesion as virtually all muscles have multiple segmental innervation.

In a similar fashion, sensory symptoms and deficits virtually always involve a smaller region than is predicted from dermatomal maps due to overlap of territories from contiguous dermatomes. For example, patients with C6 radiculopathies describe their numbness or paresthesias as affecting only the tip of their thumb.

A deep tendon reflex(s) may be diminished if appropriate to the involved root. The pain of a monoradiculopathy in the lower extremity may be reproduced by the straight-leg or reverse straight-leg raising signs or by lateral bending toward the affected extremity. In the cervical region, it may be reproduced by extending and laterally bending the head and neck toward the symptomatic side in an attempt to promote foraminal compression.

In chronic radiculopathies, pain may be intermittent and position/activity dependent such as in lumbar spinal stenosis, or may be minimal or nonexistent. Chronic radiculopathies typically occur from some component of spondylotic spine disease resulting from bone spurs or hypertrophied ligaments. Multiple rather than single nerve roots are more commonly affected by this process and motor and sensory deficits may be less dramatic in their manifestations.

POLYRADICULOPATHY

The typical phenotype of polyradiculopathy is the sequential development of motor and sensory signs and symptoms involving more than one spinal segment in one or more extremities. These disorders are typically painful, and with certain etiologies, involve cranial nerves as well.

The etiologies are heterogeneous and in many cases involve diseases with a predilection for cerebrospinal fluid, the meninges, or neural foramen nerve roots and cranial nerves pass through on their journey from spinal cord to limbs, head, and trunk. The most common cause of polyradiculopathy is lumbosacral spinal stenosis typically presenting with back and lower extremity pain provoked by standing and walking. Diabetic radiculoplexopathy can be another common cause of what may be considered a polyradiculopathy. This typically presents as an acute painful disorder affecting the L2–L4 innervated muscles in one leg. Some patients will have their other leg affected on a delayed basis. Other causes of polyradiculopathy are relatively uncommon and are typically related to inflammatory, infectious, or neoplastic disorders that produce a chronic meningitis. Cranial nerves, both motor and sensory, are commonly affected in these disorders.

PLEXOPATHY

A plexopathy is suspected when sensory and motor deficits are restricted to a single limb, the deficits being more widespread than can be explained on the basis of a single nerve or nerve root dysfunction. Pain is the rule rather than the exception, as the causes of plexopathy are most commonly traumatic, inflammatory, or neoplastic which either compress, infiltrate or inflame nerve. Occasionally, most notably with acute brachial plexus neuritis, or diabetic radiculoplexopathy, sensory signs and symptoms may be modest or nonexistent. The reasons for this may be multifactorial. Acute brachial plexus neuritis has a predilection affecting purely motor nerves, for example, the long thoracic or anterior interosseous nerves. In fact, it is this multifocal nerve pattern confined to one upper extremity or adjacent cranial or upper cervical nerves that often serves as a diagnostic clue. The motor predominant nature of acute brachial plexopathy may be related to a demyelinating pathophysiology that may preferentially affect motor function in a manner similar to the Guillain–Barré syndrome.

MONONEUROPATHY

Mononeuropathy syndromes are usually readily recognizable due to their frequency and relative homogeneity of presentation for a particular compression or entrapment syndrome. They most commonly result from the anatomic vulnerability to compression (external forces—e.g., Saturday night palsy) or entrapment (internal forces—e.g., carpal tunnel syndrome) of particular nerves at specific locations. The mode of presentation between different mononeuropathies is variable, in part due to the constituency of the nerve, for example, pure sensory nerves such as the lateral femoral cutaneous nerve. More commonly, the mode of presentation varies due to pathophysiology which may be primarily axonal or due to differing mechanisms of demyelination. In the case of carpal tunnel syndrome and ulnar neuropathies at the elbow, sensory symptoms tend to initially predominate. Common peroneal or radial neuropathies at the spiral groove tend to have more of a motor predominance. Pain may or may not be an issue. Pain without motor, sensory, or reflex signs or symptoms is uncommonly due to a definable mononeuropathy despite descriptions of alleged mononeuropathy syndromes such as the piriformis and pronator syndromes.

In any event, signs and symptoms should be restricted to the distribution of a single peripheral nerve, distal to the site of nerve injury. The converse is not always true. For example, it may be very difficult to demonstrate weakness of ulnar forearm muscles, which are at risk from ulnar neuropathies at the elbow. This phenomenon has been attributed to selective fascicular involvement. As nerve fibers destined for the same muscle tend to sequester themselves in the same fascicle even in proximal locations, these fascicles may be relatively spared from a compression or entrapment process that may affect certain fascicles more than others. Alternatively, weakness of ulnar wrist flexion may be obscured by the preservation of median wrist flexion.

LENGTH-DEPENDENT POLYNEUROPATHY

Length-dependent polyneuropathy is one of the most common neuromuscular problems encountered both by neurologists and other physicians. Long, narrow axons are presumably vulnerable to the axonal transport mechanisms on which they are dependent, and the 200 or more etiologies that can adversely affect them. Despite a phenotype that usually begins with symmetric motor and/or sensory involvement of the toes and feet, there is considerable heterogeneity in clinical expression. Conceptually, the majority of these disorders result from toxic, metabolic, or hereditary disturbances of cell body metabolism or myelin growth resulting in impaired axon transport or nerve impulse transmission. This provides a cogent explanation for preferential involvement of most distal aspects of the longest nerves in the body affected in a symmetric, "length-dependent" fashion. Usually, sensory, motor, and reflex functions are all impaired in this length-dependent pattern although sensory signs and symptoms typically predominate. The best explanation for this phenomenon is that sensory nerve endings of the feet have no backup system. Denervation of intrinsic foot muscles that flex and extend the toes however, is clinically masked by leg muscles providing the same function. The inability to spread the toes provides a nonspecific but sensitive means of clinically suspecting motor involvement in length-dependent neuropathies. Identifying fibrillation potentials or low amplitude compound muscle action potentials in intrinsic foot muscles may be the only reliable way to detect early motor involvement in many length-dependent polyneuropathies. Again, it is important to plot the evolution of sensory symptoms to ensure that they are not asymmetric or non–length-dependent in pattern suggesting a different anatomic localization such as multifocal neuropathy, polyradiculopathy, or sensory neuronopathy.

POLYRADICULONEUROPATHY

Polyradiculoneuropathy refers to a disorder that affects multiple nerves both at the nerve and nerve root level. The most commonly encountered polyradiculoneuropathies are acquired, inflammatory, and demyelinating in nature, for example, the Guillain–Barré syndrome and chronic inflammatory demyelinating polyneuropathy (CIDP). Uncommonly, this pattern may occur as an axon loss process secondary to a disorder like acute intermittent porphyria or Lyme disease.

Polyradiculoneuropathies are usually readily distinguished from length-dependent polyneuropathy. They tend to be motor rather than sensory predominant. The pattern of involvement is typically symmetric but is usually more generalized and non–length-dependent. There may be cranial nerve involvement, which would be an extremely rare occurrence in most causes of length-dependent polyneuropathy. Reflex loss is typically generalized rather than length dependent. This is a consequence of the demyelinating pathophysiology with differential slowing in different fibers within the same nerve that desynchronizes impulse transmission rendering functions dependent on synchronous impulse transmission such as deep tendon reflexes and vibration perception impaired.

▶ MULTIFOCAL NEUROPATHY

Multifocal neuropathy has been historically referred to as mononeuritis multiplex or multiple mononeuropathies. It is not a universally accepted term but will be the preferred term in this chapter for the following reasons. Multiple mononeuropathy is an equally accurate descriptor but may imply to some a more benign multifocal compressive syndrome in contrast to many causes of multifocal neuropathy which tend to be systemic in nature. Mononeuritis multiplex is a frequently used designation but is unsatisfactory to us in that it implies an inflammatory pathology that may not exist or may go unproven. For this reason, we have chosen to avoid it.

The deficits of multifocal neuropathy are often abrupt and painful, occurring haphazardly (although usually distally) and asymmetrically, with weakness and sensory loss being mapped to individual peripheral nerve distributions in more than one extremity. As described above, clinical recognition may depend on examination of the patient early in the disease, or obtaining an accurate history of early disease evolution, prior to the inevitable confluence of deficits.

Multifocal neuropathy is often the result of disorders that infiltrate (sarcoidosis, lymphoma, amyloidosis) or infarct (vasculitis, diabetes) nerve, or provide susceptibility to compressive and/or demyelinating nerve injury (multifocal motor neuropathy, multifocal acquired demyelinating sensory and motor neuropathy, hereditary liability to pressure palsy).

▶ NEUROMUSCULAR TRANSMISSION DISORDERS

These disorders are difficult to lump together from a clinical perspective, as there is phenotypic variability. Like MND and myopathy, the signs and symptoms are attributable exclusively to the motor domain. As the neuromuscular junction is a more physiologically dynamic structure than nerve or muscle, fluctuations in strength and stamina are hallmarks of these disorders. In acquired disorders of neuromuscular transmission, muscle atrophy is notable for its absence.

In postsynaptic disorders of neuromuscular transmission like myasthenia, for reasons not clearly understood, there is a predilection for cranial innervated musculature. Ptosis, diplopia, dysarthria, dysphagia, and chewing difficulties are common complaints. The deficits can be quite asymmetric and at times remarkably focal. Rarely, myasthenia may present with limb weakness with little, if any, oculobulbar involvement. This can also be either symmetric in nature mimicking a myopathy or focal such as a finger or foot drop, thus potentially mimicking an MND. Postsynaptic disorders of neuromuscular transmission do not affect the cholinergic receptors of the autonomic nervous system. Pupils should be spared even with complete ophthalmoparesis. Deep tendon reflexes are commonly spared in myasthenia gravis unless involved muscles are significantly weak.

Signs and symptoms of cholinergic dysautonomia are commonplace in presynaptic disorders of neuromuscular transmission such as botulism and the Lambert–Eaton myasthenic syndrome. Weakness in these two disorders tends to be symmetric and is often proximally predominant and generalized. Cranial nerve involvement is very common in botulism. It does occur in the Lambert–Eaton myasthenic syndrome, although not as prominently as in botulism or myasthenia gravis. Deep tendon reflexes are commonly lost in a generalized pattern in any presynaptic disorder of neuromuscular transmission.

▶ MYOPATHIES

Myopathy is suspected in three different clinical settings, fixed, typically painless and symmetric weakness, periodic weakness due to disorders of ion channels, and exercise-induced muscle pain, fatigue, and stiffness due to disorders of muscle energy metabolism. With fixed weakness, symmetry is a relative term. Minor asymmetries are common in disorders such as facioscapulohumeral muscular dystrophy and inclusion body myositis (IBM). The distribution of weakness is often proximal, but there are many notable exceptions. Myopathies presenting with symmetric, distally predominant weakness are not rare. These usually begin in the lower extremities but may begin in the hands as well. Myopathies, particularly those of a hereditary nature (e.g., facioscapulohumeral or oculopharyngeal dystrophy) and IBM, may also be recognized by regional patterns of weakness. Weakness in neck flexors and extensors should be sought in all neuromuscular disease but are particularly common in myopathy in addition to disorders of neuromuscular transmission and anterior horn cells. Cranial muscle involvement is variable. Dysphagia, ptosis, ophthalmoparesis, facial, jaw, and tongue weakness may occur and aid in the differential diagnosis of myopathic disorders. Reflexes may be lost or preserved, depending on the pattern and severity of muscle involvement.

Attention to other elements of the examination may aid in the identification of the existence, type, and potential complications of muscle disease. Percussion, grip, or electrical myotonia will serve to identify a select group of myopathies (Table 2-1, Chapter 2). A number of myopathies may associate with joint contractures or skeletal abnormalities. Muscle hypertrophy is a constant feature of the dystrophinopathies and may occur with certain limb-girdle dystrophy phenotypes as well as infiltrative disorders of muscle such as amyloid myopathy. Involvement of ventilatory and cardiac muscle as well as other organ systems may aid in diagnosis and allow anticipation of future morbidity (Table 1-12).

RHABDOMYOLYSIS/MYOGLOBINURIA

The clinical phenotypes related to ion channel disorders and metabolic muscle diseases that may differ from the fixed weakness that typify most muscle disease will be discussed in the relevant chapters that follow. As rhabdomyolysis and myoglobinuria may result from numerous causes, it will be more convenient to discuss the topic here. Rhabdomyolysis and myoglobinuria, although conceptually different, are terms that are often used interchangeably. In this book, they will be discussed as a singular clinical and laboratory entity (RHB/MGU).[33] Although discussed later in this book in the context of individual diseases, it is addressed here in order to provide an overview and strategic approach to the problem. Rhabdomyolysis refers to an acute, large scale breakdown of striated muscle fibers whereas myoglobinuria implicates the urinary excretion of the pigment myoglobin released into the bloodstream as a consequence. Attempts have been made to define these terms quantitatively. Myoglobin is visible in the urine when its concentration exceeds 100 μg/dL or when plasma levels exceed 1.5 mg/dL but is an insensitive means to detect small or chronic CK elevations and usually becomes undetectable within hours, long before serum CK normalizes. Rhabdomyolysis has been defined by serum CK levels exceeding five times the upper limits of normal. As there are many patients who may carry CK levels in excess of this chronically and even asymptomatically, this quantitative definition fails to conceptually capture the acute and potentially catastrophic nature of the RHB/MGU syndrome. The RHB/MGU syndrome is most commonly associated with serum CK levels in tens of thousands.

There are numerous potential causes of RHB/MGU that are typically monophasic and result from toxic, traumatic, or infectious insults (Table 1-14). In addition, a number of heritable metabolic myopathies pose a risk for recurrent episodes. There is some evidence that there may be genetic susceptibility underlying some individuals who experience RHB/MGU in apparent response to an environmental provocation.[34] Unfortunately, many cases remained undiagnosed despite intensive evaluation.

The symptoms of RHB/MGU are often nonspecific. There is often a nonspecific fever and malaise, usually accompanied by the more specific myalgias, muscle swelling, tenderness, and a generalized sense of weakness (asthenia). In the author's experience, it can be difficult to discern the cause of diminished patient movement. Both muscle pain and actual weakness may play a role, the former seemingly being the primary mechanism in most cases. The release of myofiber contents into the blood stream can lead to nausea and vomiting, cardiac arrhythmia (hyperkalemia), and even CNS side effects such as confusion and coma. Rhabdomyolysis, if severe enough, can lead to enough movement of fluid into muscle to cause intravascular volume depletion and hypotension. Rhabdomyolysis can trigger the coagulation cascade and lead to disseminated intravascular coagulation. The most notorious complication is the development of acute tubular necrosis secondary accumulation of myoglobin and case formation within renal tubules. Ventilatory failure due to involvement of diaphragm and chest wall muscles is a rare complication of rhabdomyolysis secondary to carnitine palmitoyl transferase deficiency.[32]

The pathophysiology of RHB/MGU is not fully understood. The intracellular migration of sodium and water may lead to a secondary exchange of intracellular sodium with

▶ **TABLE 1-14. CAUSES OF RHABDOMYOLYSIS/ MYOGLOBINURIA[30,31,38]**

Toxic
Envenomation—specific species of snake, bees, spiders
Ingestion—(1) animals who have ingested toxins—e.g., Haff disease (fish), quail that have eaten hemlock, (2) certain mushroom species
Recreational drugs—cocaine, heroin, alcohol, amphetamines, LSD, loxapine, hemlock, mercuric chloride, phencyclidine, strychnine, terbutaline
Environmental exposure—monensin, chlorophenoxy herbicides, toluene, pentaborane
Medications—amiodarone, emetine, cholesterol lowering agents, epsilon amino caproic acid, isoniazid, lamotrigine, pentamidine, propofol, proton pump inhibitors, valproate, zidovudine, neuroleptic malignant syndrome
Metabolic
Hypokalemia
Hyperthermia
Hyperosmolality (hyperglycemia)
Hypophosphatemia
Infectious (more common in children)
Bacteria (tetanus, salmonella, Legionella, group A beta hemolytic strep)
Virus (influenza, EBV, CMV, HIV)
Parasites (malaria)
Rickettsial
Ischemic—acute peripheral arterial occlusion
Traumatic
Crush injury
Compartment syndrome
Miscellaneous
Status epilepticus
Delirium tremens
High voltage electrical shock
Excessive exercise in the deconditioned
Heritable
Mitochondrial—cytochrome c oxidase deficiency, complex I deficiency, primary coenzyme Q10 deficiency, cytochrome b deficiency, lipoamide dehydrogenase, succinate dehydrogenase and aconitase
Glycogen storage disease—myophosphorylase, phosphofructokinase, phosphoglycerate mutase and kinase, LDH deficiency, phosphorylase B kinase deficiency
Lipid storage disease—carnitine palmitoyl transferase deficiency, carnitine translocase, acyl-CoA dehydrogenase deficiency
Channelopathies—malignant hyperthermia types I–VI, hypokalemic periodic paralysis
Congenital myopathies—King–Denborough syndrome, central core disease
Muscular dystrophy—DM1 (rare), dystrophinopathy (rare) LGMI 2I
Inflammatory—dermatomyositis (rare)

extracellular calcium in muscle fibers that remain viable. This in turn may lead to persistent activation of the myofiber contractile apparatus that may perpetuate muscle injury. The need to pump sodium out of cells may deplete ATP as an additional adverse effect of this cascade. Furthermore, injury may occur as a consequence of the ischemia created by increased compartmental pressure, even in the absence of crush injury, by the fluid migration described above. The biochemical milieu created by muscle breakdown may in itself be toxic either through the release of the normally sequestered contents of the muscle fibers, from calcium-dependent proteases and phospholipases, or from the cytokines release by the customary inflammatory response to injury.

Recognition of RHB/MGU may or may not be obvious. A high index of suspicion should be maintained with predisposing conditions such as crush injury, prolonged immobilization, or introduction of potentially myotoxic drugs. Myoglobinuria and acute, diffuse myalgias are obvious clues but are not always readily evident, particularly when detailed history is not readily available. Patients typically have a leukocytosis. The measurement of serum CK is the most efficient and direct diagnostic tool. A positive urine dipstick for (which detects both myoglobin and hemoglobin) in the absence of red blood cells on microscopic examination of the urine strongly suggests myoglobinuria.

Diagnosis of the underlying cause may also be obvious or remain enigmatic despite extensive evaluation. In most series, drugs and metabolic disturbances are the most common identified cause of RHB/MGU.[35] It is estimated that approximately a third to a half of patients who do not have an obvious cause of their RHB/MGU, will be found to have an identifiable enzymatic deficiency or underlying muscle disease as a cause of their syndrome.[36] The yield will be predictably higher in patients who have had recurrent episodes.[37]

In RHB/MGU, CK levels typically peak in 12–24 hours and remain at peak levels for a few days. In response to minor muscle injury such as EMG examinations, CK levels typically normalize in a week. In more protracted causes of muscle injury such as infection or with very high CK elevations, it would be prudent to wait a few weeks to determine if CK has normalized. Once the CK peaks, it can be anticipated that it will drop by 50% every 48 hours. This is a potentially valuable diagnostic tool as normalization of CK should suggest a monophasic cause of RHB/MGU or carnitine palmitoyl transferase deficiency. Persistent elevations, although not universally found, would be more in keeping with glycogen storage disease or other pre-existing and persistent myopathic disorders.

The forearm exercise test is a valuable screening tool for those glycogen storage disorders characterized by exercise-induced symptomatology and the potential for RHB/MGU. Its yield will be greatest in those individuals whose RHB/MGU is provoked by brief periods of intense exercise. Its yield will be less in individuals whose RHB/MGU appears to occur sporadically, on a delayed basis after more protracted exertion, or following fasting. In these circumstances, CPT deficiency will be the most common hereditary etiology. Forearm exercise testing will be described in detail in the section on glycogen storage disease. In summary, baseline determinations of venous lactate and ammonia obtained. Forearm muscles are then repetitively and forcefully exercised, typically with a grip dynamometer. Using a blood pressure cuff to render the forearm ischemic is no longer done by the majority of neuromuscular specialists as the risk of patient injury is felt to exceed any additional diagnostic yield. Serial measurements of venous lactate and ammonia are obtained from the ipsilateral basilic or cephalic veins in the antecubital fossa. In patients with glycogen storage disease, these measurements are often superfluous as the affected patient will develop a sustained painful "contracture" of the forearm muscles often leading to a dystonic posture with forearm pronation, wrist flexion with ulnar deviation, and finger flexion. A three-fold elevation or more above baseline of either lactate or ammonia signifies adequate effort. With glycogen storage disease, ammonia will elevate but lactate will not. The converse will occur with myoadenylate deaminase deficiency, the clinical significance of which remains controversial. In young adults experiencing RHB/MGU during or after protracted exercise, particularly if recurrent or with normalization of CK following the acute episode, we commonly obtain genetic testing for CPT deficiency.

It is difficult to provide dogmatic advice regarding the role of muscle biopsy in the evaluation of RHB/MGU. Muscle biopsy in the acute setting is to be avoided. Random myofiber necrosis in similar stages of degeneration, affecting both type I and type II fibers, without any specific diagnostic features is the anticipated outcome. Whether muscle biopsy should be performed subsequent to the RHB/MGU episode is a more difficult question to answer. The yield in identifying the exact cause of RHB/MGU is extremely low, and the cost of providing a comprehensive analysis of the muscle biopsy can be substantial. In our opinion, muscle biopsy in RHB/MGU should be reserved for those individuals with recurrent episodes of RHB/MGU of indeterminate cause with negative exercise forearm testing and genetic analysis for CPT deficiency.

Hydration is the most important therapeutic intervention. Six to twelve liters of intravenous fluids in the first 24 hours are recommended in the absence of comorbidities. Urine output should ideally be in the 200–300 mL/h range. The fluid should not be hypotonic. Mannitol and sodium bicarbonate are frequently added although there is limited evidence to support their efficacy. Vigorous diuresis with furosemide represents a mainstay of treatment as well. A high index of suspicion for compartment syndrome should be maintained and fasciotomy considered when clinically appropriate. Hypokalemia, hypocalcemia, and hypophosphatemia should be screened for and treated if necessary. Awareness of adult respiratory distress syndrome, ischemic bowel, and the possibility of hemorrhage secondary to DIC should be maintained. Alkalinization should be utilized where appropriate.

▶ SUMMARY

Diagnostic accuracy is in large part dependent on a clinician's ability to elicit and formulate pertinent information from three domains of the patient's history and examination, these being anatomic localization, definition of the disease course, and relevant risk factors. The astute clinician will learn to discard information that is not germane to the patient's current problem, and formulate a differential diagnosis by accurately matching the information from the three domains mentioned above to the known behaviors of different diseases. An accurate diagnosis may be evident solely from this clinical process, or may require further testing to confirm or refute the differential diagnosis generated by this process. This chapter has addressed the strategies that serve as the foundation for this problem-solving approach. Subsequent chapters will discuss the features of the neuromuscular diseases in an attempt to complete this diagnostic and hopefully therapeutic endeavor.

REFERENCES

1. David WS, Jones HR Jr. Electromyography and biopsy correlation with suggested protocol for evaluation of the floppy infant. *Muscle Nerve.* 1994;17(4):424–430.
2. Dumitru D, Amato AA. Introduction to myopathies and muscle tissue's reaction to injury. In Dumitru D, Amato AA, Swartz MJ, eds. *Electrodiagnostic Medicine.* 2nd ed. Philadelphia, PA: Hanley & Belfus; 2002:1229–1264.
3. Shoesmith CL, Findlater K, Rowe A, Strong MJ. Prognosis of amyotrophic lateral sclerosis with respiratory onset. *J Neurol Neurosurg Psychiatry.* 2007;78:629–631.
4. Chokroverty S. Sleep-disordered breathing in neuromuscular disorders: A condition in search of recognition. *Muscle Nerve.* 2001;24(4):451–455.
5. Cudkowicz ME, Qureshi M, Shefner J. Measure and markers in amyotrophic lateral sclerosis. *NeuroRx.* 2004;1:273–283.
6. Isaacs JD, Dean AF, Shaw CE, Al-Chalabi A, Mills KR, Leigh PN. Amyotrophic lateral sclerosis with sensory neuropathy: Part of a multisystem disorder? *J Neurol Neurosurg Psychiatry.* 2007;78:750–753.
7. Wolfe GI, Bank WJ. Pseudokyphosis in motor neuron disease corrected by the pocket sign [abstract]. *Muscle Nerve.* 1994; 17:1091.
8. Van Gerpen JA. Camptocormia secondary to early amyotrophic lateral sclerosis. *Mov Disord.* 2001;16:358–360.
9. Hoffman D, Gutmann L. The dropped head syndrome with chronic inflammatory demyelinating polyneuropathy. *Muscle Nerve.* 1994;17:808–810.
10. Keating JM, Yapundich RA, Claussen GC, Oh SJ. Head drop syndrome as a presenting feature of polymyositis [abstract]. *Muscle Nerve.* 1996;9:1190.
11. Hund E, Heckl R, Goebel HH, Meinck UM. Inclusion body myositis presenting with isolated erector spinae paresis. *Neurology.* 1995;45:993–994.
12. Biran I, Cohen O, Diment J, Peyser A, Bahnof R, Steiner I. Focal, steroid responsive myositis causing dropped head syndrome. *Muscle Nerve.* 1999;22:769–771.
13. Lomen-Hoerth C, Simmons ML, Dearmond SJ, Layzer RB. Adult-onset nemaline myopathy: another cause of dropped head. *Muscle Nerve.* 1999;22:1146–1150.
14. Chanin N, Selcen D, Engel AG. Sporadic late onset nemaline myopathy. *Neurology.* 2005;65:1158–1164.
15. Katirji B, Hachwi R, Al-Shekhlee A, Cohen ML, Bohlmann HH. Isolated head drop due to adult- onset nemaline myopathy treated by posterior fusion. *Neurology.* 2005;65:1504–1505.

16. Luque FA, Rosenkilde C, Valsamis M, Danon MJ. Inclusion body myositis (IBM) presenting as the "dropped head syndrome" (DHS) [abstract]. *Brain Pathol.* 1994;4:568.
17. Evidente VG, Cook A. Floppy head syndrome resulting from proximal myotonic dystrophy [abstract]. *Ann Neurol.* 1997;42:417.
18. Serratrice J, Weiller PJ, Pouget J, Serratrice G. [An unrecognized cause of camptocormia: proximal myotonic myopathy]. *Presse Med.* 2000;29(20):1121–1123. French.
19. Karpati G, Carpenter S, Engel AG, et al. The syndrome of systemic carnitine deficiency: clinical, morphologic, biochemical, and pathophysiologic features. *Neurology.* 1975;25:16–24.
20. Umapathi T, Chaudhry V, Cornblath D, Drachman D, Griffin J, Kuncl R. Head drop and camptocormia. *J Neurol Neurosurg Psychiatry.* 2002;73:1–7.
21. Baquis GD, Moral L, Sorrell M. Neck extensor myopathy: a mitochondrial disease [abstract]. *Neurology.* 1997;48(suppl 2):A443.
22. Berenbaum F, Rajzbaum G, Bonnichon P, Amor B. Une hyperparathyroidie revelee par une chute de la tete. *Rev Rheum Ed Fr.* 1993;60:467–469.
23. Beekman R, Tijssen CC, Visser LH, Schellens RL. Dropped head as the presenting symptom of primary hyperparathyroidism. *J Neurol.* 2002;249(12):1738–1739.
24. Yoshida S, Takayama Y. Licorice-induced hypokalemia as a treatable cause of dropped head syndrome. *Clin Neurol Neurosurg.* 2003;105(4):286–287.
25. Barohn RL, McVey AL, DiMauro S. Adult acid maltase deficiency. *Muscle Nerve.* 1993;16:672–676.
26. Serrano MC, Rabinstein AA. Cause and outcomes of acute neuromuscular respiratory failure. *Arch Neurol.* 2010;67(9):1089–1094.
27. Hughes RA, Bihari D. Acute neuromuscular respiratory paralysis. *J Neurol Neurosurg Psych.* 1993;56(4):334–343.
28. Nicolle MW, Stewart DJ, Remtulla H, Chen R, Bolton CF. Lambert-Eaton myasthenic syndrome presenting with severe respiratory failure. *Muscle Nerve.* 1996;19:1328–1333.
29. Durmus H, Laval SH, Deymeer F, et al. Oculopharyngodistal myopathy is a distinct entity: clinical and genetic features of 47 patients. *Neurology.* 2011;76:227–235.
30. Huerta-Alardín AL, Varon J, Marik PE. Bench-to-bedside review: rhabdomyolysis- an overview for clinicians. *Crit Care.* 2005;9(2):158–169.
31. Mathews KD, Stephan CM, Laubenthal K, et al. Myoglobinuria and muscle pain are common in patients with limb-girdle muscular dystrophy 2I. *Neurology.* 2011;76:194–195.
32. Berardo A, DiMauro S, Hirano M. A diagnostic algorithm for metabolic myopathies. *Curr Neurol Neuroscience Rep.* 2010; 10:118–126.
33. Warren JD, Blumbergs PC, Thompson PD. Rhabdomyolysis: a review. *Muscle Nerve.* 2002;25:332–347.
34. Vladutiu GD, Simmons Z, Isackson PJ, et al. Genetic risk factors associated with lipid-lowering drug-induced myopathies. *Muscle Nerve.* 2006;34(2):153–162.
35. Melli G, Chaudhry V, Cornblath DR. Rhabdomyolysis: an evaluation of 475 hospitalized patients. *Medicine (Baltimore).* 2005 84:377–385.
36. Gabow PA, Kaehny WD, Kelleher SP. The spectrum of rhabdomyolysis. *Medicine.* 1982;61:141–152.
37. Lofberg M, Jankala H, Paetau A, Harkonen M, Sormer H. Metabolic causes of recurrent rhabdomyolysis. *Acta Neurol Scand.* 1998;98:268–275.
38. Rose MR, Kissel JT, Bickley LS, Griggs RC. Sustained myoglobinuria: the presenting manifestation of dermatomyositis. *Neurology.* 1996;47:119–123.

CHAPTER 2

Testing in Neuromuscular Disease

The role of laboratory testing in the diagnosis of neuromuscular disease is described in the first chapter. Tests are ideally used to support a clinically established working diagnosis, not in a random search process. False-positive test results occur with some frequency, and can easily lead to unnecessary testing and interventions as well as potential harm if not measured against pensive clinical analysis.

This chapter will focus on nonhistologic tests that are readily available to most clinicians and potentially useful to the neuromuscular physicians in their assessment of patients. In keeping with the philosophy of this text, emphasis will be placed on tests that have pragmatic application. The science behind the testing will be provided only to the extent necessary to understand the utility, performance, interpretation, and limitations of a test within a given clinical context. The following topics will be addressed:

- Electromyography (EMG) and nerve conduction studies (NCS), collectively known as electrodiagnosis (EDX)
- Quantitative sensory testing (QST)
- Autonomic nervous system testing (ANST)
- Routine laboratory (blood) testing
- DNA mutational analysis
- Biochemical testing for inborn errors of metabolism
- Serologic testing
- Cerebrospinal fluid (CSF) analysis
- Nerve and muscle imaging

► EMG AND NCS (EDX)

BASIC PRINCIPLES

Physician Skill and Knowledge

Like all tests, EDX has limitations, as do the people who order, perform, and interpret them. The most satisfactory results occur when the requesting physician understands the tests' value and limitations, and posits specific questions to the electromyographer that the test is capable of answering. A satisfactory result is also dependent on an electromyographer who examines the patient, understands the differential diagnosis of the clinical problem, and tailors the electrodiagnostic examination to adequately explore those possibilities. In keeping with this philosophy, it is readily understandable that the nerves tested during NCS and the muscles selected for EMG, although often guided by algorithm, are frequently modified both on a case-by-case basis both prior to and during its performance.

Temperature Considerations

Attention to detail is important in EDX. One notable example is attention to limb temperature. As a general rule, hand temperatures of >33°C and foot temperatures of >31°C are desirable. Although warm water baths and heating lamps may be used, in our experience, reusable microwaveable heating pads applied to the limbs are the most effective technique for obtaining and maintaining this thermal environment.

With cold limbs, amplitudes of both compound motor action potentials (CMAP) and sensory nerve action potentials (SNAP) are increased. Abnormally low CMAP and SNAP amplitudes could be potentially normalized. Conversely, conduction speeds are reduced, including slowing of conduction velocities and prolongation of distal, F wave, and H reflex latencies (Fig. 2-1). Repetitive stimulation techniques are also affected by limb temperature. Limb cooling diminishes the degree of the decremental response in patients with disorders of neuromuscular transmission (DNMT). Failure to maintain adequate limb or facial temperature could readily lead to a false-negative result. Although it would be unusual for fibrillation potentials to disappear with limb cooling, their prevalence and therefore their detection may be hampered by cool body temperatures as well. In summary, with the exception of cold-induced myotonic discharges in paramyotonia congenita (PMC) and repetitive stimulation techniques in certain muscle channelopathies described below, the accuracy of EDX is improved upon by establishing and maintaining adequate limb warmth of at least 32°C.

Safety Considerations

Patients and their physicians are concerned about the potential EDX risks in patients who have pacemakers, defibrillators, central lines and altered hemostasis. In general, although testing under these circumstances is not risk free, available published data would suggest that the risk is limited if appropriate precautions are taken. Like most medical decisions, the potential benefits of EDX testing in a patient with any of these situations should be balanced against the risks.

The risk of performing NCS in patients with external wires leading to the heart is unknown but is considered a relative if not absolute contraindication.[1] There is a paucity of

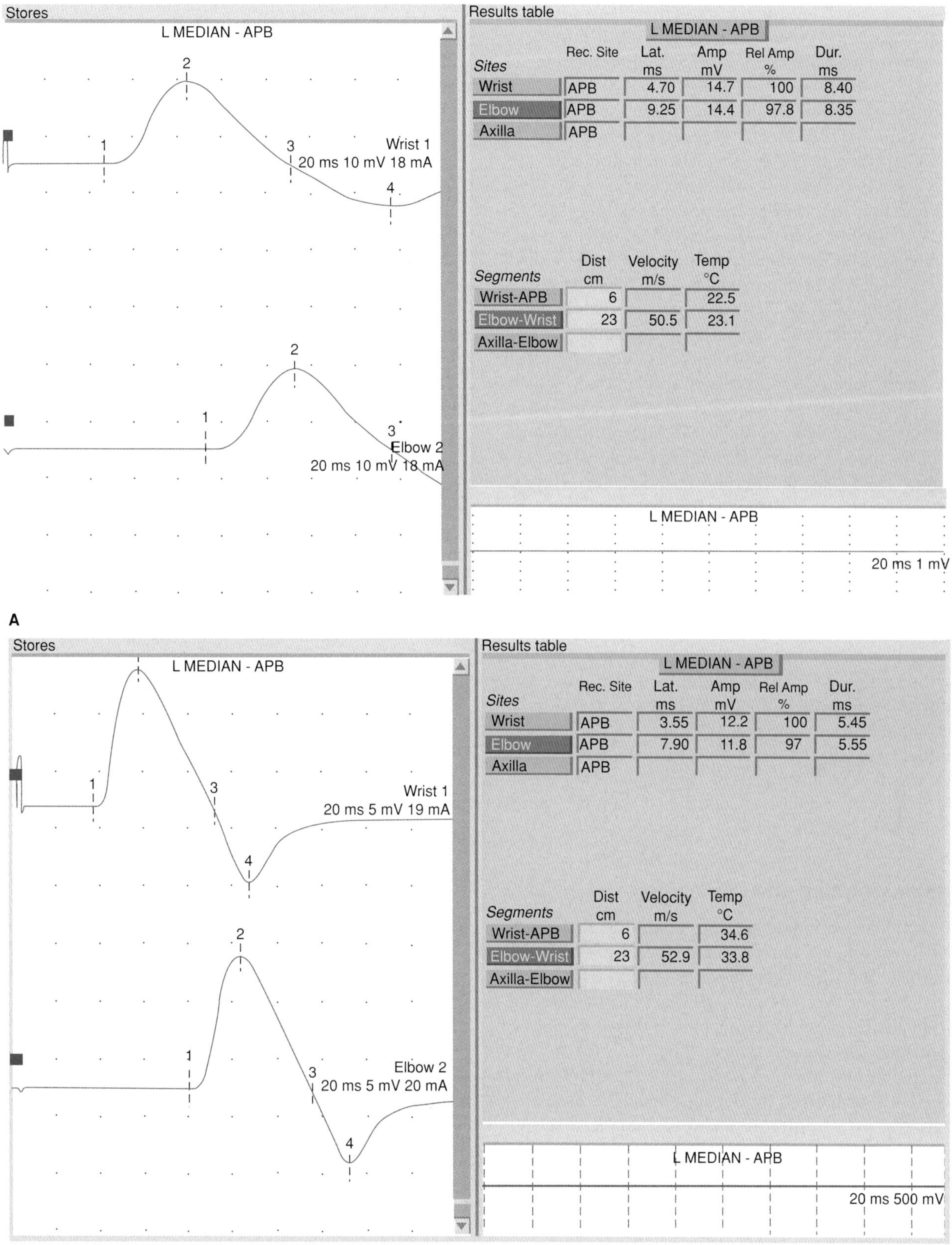

B

Figure 2-1. Effect of cool limb temperature on motor nerve conduction studies—median CMAPs (compound muscle action potentials) demonstrating factitiously significant increase in distal latency, slightly decreased conduction velocity, prolonged CMAP duration and increased amplitude (note different gain settings) following cooling **(A)** and corrected by limb warming **(B)**.

information as well regarding the risk to patients with central lines, pacemakers, and defibrillators. Both experience and theory suggest the risk is small and nerve conductions appear safe if the stimulus is not delivered in topographical proximity (within 6 cm) to the tubing or wire and a stimulation of 0.2 ms or less is used.[2–4] Even less is known about the safety of repetitive nerve stimulation techniques in this setting. A study to address this issue is underway.

Regarding the needle examination and hemostasis, the risk of bleeding or hematoma formation in patients taking anticoagulants or antiplatelet drugs also appears small and is estimated to be approximately 1.5%.[5] When present, the risk of clinically significant bleeding also appears to be small. On the other hand, compartment syndrome has been reported in patients with normal hemostasis although its risk is generally considered minimal.[6] Available, albeit limited, evidence would support the performance of needle examination in patients who are therapeutically anticoagulated. Caution should be exercised when the international normalized ratio (INR) is supratherapeutic (i.e., >3), platelet count is less than 20,000, or in deep muscles where hematoma formation may not be readily evident or easily compressible. If needle examination is to be done, the smallest diameter that is feasible should be utilized. Needle EMG also poses the risk of pneumothorax, particularly when studying the serratus anterior and diaphragm.[4] These muscles, in particular, should be studied by those well versed in anatomy, who are well experienced in the technique, and then only when clinical circumstances warrant. EMG poses a risk to electromyographers as well, largely in the form of the potential transmission of infectious agents through inadvertent needle sticks. The most common preventable reason for these accidents appears to be a hurried and harried examiner who is not adequately attentive.[7]

Test Construction and Reporting

Opinions differ regarding the role of clinical assessment in the construction and reporting of the EDX evaluation. Purists believe that EDX conclusions should be based solely on the results of the study and should not be influenced by clinical bias. The argument in support of this philosophy is the potential risk that meaningful EDX observations will be ignored if they do not conform to a preexisting clinical belief. This potential bias is valid and should be considered and avoided by introspective electromyographers. Having said that, it is the strongly held belief of the authors that clinical perspective in the EDX evaluation is integral to the efficient construction and accurate interpretation of the study. There are a number of lines of reasoning to support this perspective.

For example, there are disorders that share identical electrodiagnostic signatures but have differing etiologies, natural histories, and treatment potentials. Early amyotrophic lateral sclerosis (ALS) affecting the lower extremities, polyradiculopathy of severe lumbosacral spinal stenosis or a dural arteriovenous malformation may be electrodiagnostically indistinguishable.[8–10] The EDX conclusions in this case should be appropriately weighted by clinical insight. In addition, patients may have more than one disorder affecting the same components of the neuromuscular system. If this is the case, accurate EDX conclusions will be confounded without the clinical insights necessary to distinguish which abnormal EDX parameters are and which are not germane to the problem at hand. A third argument in support of coupling EDX impressions with clinical insight is the realization that in some cases, pathology may be subclinical. It is not uncommon to find mild median nerve conduction slowing across the wrist in individual with a vocation that involves repetitive hand use whose complaints bear no resemblance to the clinical phenotype of carpal tunnel syndrome (CTS). Reporting based solely on EDX result risks unnecessary surgery in patients whose morbidity rests primarily on tendon or joint injury.

Normative Data

With the improvements and uniformity provided by contemporary electrodiagnostic equipment, it can be argued that it is no longer necessary for each laboratory to establish their own normative data. Assuming that attention is paid to accurate measurement, adequate temperature maintenance, and standardized distances for distal latency measurements, normative data provided by a number of reliable published sources are likely to be adequate. It is important however, to recognize the potential pitfalls of population-based "normal" values. Normative data are influenced by age. EDX in infants has to be interpreted by a completely different set of norms than are used in adults. By the same token, conduction studies have to be more cautiously interpreted in the elderly, particularly lower extremity sensory conductions. Although sural and superficial peroneal SNAPs are elicitable in many older patients, they can be absent in otherwise normal patients 60 years of age and older. This may confound the distinction between two common problems in this age group, peripheral neuropathy and lumbosacral polyradiculopathy due to spinal stenosis, the distinction of which relies heavily on evaluation of SNAPs.

Another age-related misinterpretive risk stems from the recognition that larger motor unit potentials (MUPs) may be seen in seemingly normal elderly individuals, particularly in intrinsic hand and foot muscles. This has been attributed to reinnervation resulting from (1) the wear and tear of the process in intrinsic hand or foot muscles, (2) motor unit loss resulting as a normal component of aging, or (3) in response to remotely symptomatic or asymptomatic spondylosis of the lumbar or cervical spine.

There is considerable heterogeneity in normative values for NCS within healthy populations. Any parameter measured may be normal within population based norms but may be differ from the patient's frequently unknown baseline values. For this reason, focal or unilateral problems are best studied by comparing results with the analogous nerve of the opposite extremity rather than utilizing population norms. In most laboratories, a side-to-side amplitude difference of more than 50% is considered abnormal. Even this represents a potentially insensitive means to detect subtle nerve pathology.

Timing

Timing considerations in EDX are critical. In general, it is estimated that complete Wallerian degeneration requires 3–5 days to produce a noticeable decline in CMAP amplitudes, with the nadir occurring between days 7 and 9. Wallerian degeneration in sensory nerves lags slightly behind with amplitude loss becoming apparent between the fifth and seventh days. The SNAP amplitude reaches its lowest point in a monophasic nerve injury by the 10th or 11th day.[11] For this reason, an interval of 10 days to 2 weeks between injury and the performance of NCS is ideal in most instances. There is a risk of false interpretation if NCS are preformed prematurely.

This is particularly true with conduction block. In most circumstances, a significant CMAP amplitude above but not below a focal nerve lesion suggests a demyelinating conduction block. This conclusion would implicate a limited number of peripheral nerve disorders with the potential for full and relatively rapid recovery in many cases. If motor conductions are performed hyperacutely within the aforementioned 9-day window before Wallerian degeneration is complete, an axon loss lesion may be falsely interpreted as demyelinating conduction block resulting in erroneous differential diagnostic and prognostic considerations.

The interpretation of the needle portion of the EDX examination is also subject to timing considerations. Fibrillation potentials and positive waves occurring in a muscle at rest, the most sensitive indicator of ongoing denervation on EMG, may develop within days in muscles that are in close anatomic proximity to the site of nerve injury. Three weeks may be required however, for these to develop within all muscles at risk. As many patients may be reluctant to undergo multiple examinations, the EDX should be ideally postponed for 3 weeks after disease onset in most circumstances.

There are at least two circumstances in which it may be preferable to perform EDX earlier than the normal 3-week recommendation. One of these occurs when there is the suspicion or knowledge of a preexisting nerve injury. It may be important for either legal or medical reasons to identify preexisting abnormalities before new ones develop. Performing two examinations, one as early as possible and then a second examination a month or more later, would be best suited to address this issue. A second scenario would be a suspected Guillain–Barré syndrome (GBS) where rapid EDX support for the diagnosis is desired. As in other neuromuscular disorders, it may require days or weeks for the complete EDX signature of GBS to fully develop. Nonetheless, the rapid evolution of NCS abnormalities, even if not diagnostic, in the absence of findings characteristic of other potential causes of acute generalized weakness, can be reassuring to the clinician and guide management decisions in the critical first week of the illness.

Additional Considerations

EMG is often performed in the evaluation of patients who may eventually undergo muscle biopsy. In order to avoid the potentially confounding variable of needle artifact, it is our practice to restrict the needle examination to one side of the body if muscle biopsy is a consideration. The most appropriate muscle on the opposite side is then recommended to the referring physician. Needle EMG can also elevate serum CK values and potentially introduce another confounding variable in the evaluation of the patient with neuromuscular disease. For this reason, blood should be ideally drawn prior to, immediately after, or greater than 72 hours after EMG performance.[12]

PERFORMANCE OF THE ELECTRODIAGNOSTIC EXAMINATION

The routine EMG/NCS examination traditionally consists of motor NCS, sensory NCS, and the needle electromyographic examination. F waves and H reflexes are also commonly tested although in most cases provide complementary rather than novel information. As previously mentioned, nerves and muscles should be selected on a case-by-case basis. Initial selection is based on the diagnostic question posed, the clinical information available, and may be modified as the test unfolds. It is appropriate to emphasize that techniques used to detect DNMT such as repetitive motor nerve stimulation (RNS) testing and single fiber EMG (SFEMG) are not part of the routine evaluation in most laboratories. Once again, the importance of clinical surveillance in test construction is emphasized.

NERVE CONDUCTION STUDIES

Motor Nerve Conductions

Motor nerve conductions are performed by applying an active surface recording electrode to the midportion of a muscle belly and stimulating the nerve innervating it at one or more locations. The active electrode position is chosen to overly the motor point, that is, the confluence of neuromuscular junctions. This allows for a biphasic waveform known as the compound muscle action potential (CMAP) with a well-defined take off point for accurate measure of latency, waveform amplitude, and area. In addition, a reference electrode is used, placed off the muscle belly and usually on the muscle tendon. The CMAP is obtained by stimulating the nerve in question at anatomically accessible points. To elicit the desired response, the intensity of the electrical stimuli applied to the nerve is increased until all involved axons and muscle fibers are activated and the maximal response is obtained. This is referred to as the supramaximal stimulus and is the desired effect in all routine motor and sensory conduction studies. Each nerve tested may be stimulated at one or more locations, limited only by anatomical accessibility and patient tolerance.

Readily testable motor nerves are the median, ulnar, radial, accessory, facial, tibial, and common peroneal. The phrenic, femoral, axillary, and musculocutaneous nerves can be tested, although in each case technical issues may make reliable and reproducible information more difficult to obtain. The CMAP amplitude of the H response stimulating tibial nerve and recording from soleus represents another motor conduction parameter. The CMAP waveform that is obtained represents the sum of all the individual single muscle fiber action potentials (SFMAPs) within that muscle activated by the nerve stimulus. Because different fibers within a nerve have different conduction velocities, the waveform is dome like rather than spiked in its configuration. The proximal or left-hand side of the waveform represents the action potentials of the fibers innervated by the fastest conducting axons. The trailing aspect of the dome represents the action potentials of the muscle fibers innervated by the slowest conducting motor axons (Fig. 2-1). As stimuli are delivered at increasing distances from the target muscle, that is, more proximal locations, the distance between the initial and terminal aspects of the CMAP waveform widens. This results in an increasing duration of the CMAP waveform without a reduction in the area under the curve, the number of activated nerve and muscle fibers being identical. This is the basis of the normal physiologic waveform dispersion described below.

Typically, three parameters are measured with an additional parameter assessed more subjectively. The baseline to peak amplitude and the area under the curve of the CMAP waveform are proportionate to the number of viable muscle fibers that are activated within the recording radius of the active recording electrode. These parameters represent an indirect measure of the number of viable and excitable axons that innervate them. Reduction in CMAP amplitude results from axon loss anywhere between anterior horn cell and neuromuscular junction, impaired neuromuscular transmission (particularly presynaptic), or of loss of muscle. In some instances, the CMAP amplitude may be adversely affected by diseases that preferentially affect the integrity of the myelin sheath producing conduction block or temporal dispersion. This will be described subsequently.

The other two parameters routinely measured are distal latency (time between stimulus delivery and lead edge of CMAP and conduction velocity. These parameters are measures of conduction speed and therefore primarily reflect myelin integrity. Conduction velocity and distal latency are reported separately in motor conduction studies for a number of reasons. The distal latency reflects conduction along different segments of nerve (wrist to hand or ankle to foot) than the conduction velocity (elbow to wrist or knee to ankle). In certain pathologic conditions, one parameter may be abnormal whereas the other remains unaffected. Distal latency and conduction velocity are also reported differently for purposes of technical accuracy. Distal latency measures not only nerve conduction but neuromuscular transmission time as well. In addition, terminal nerve twigs attenuate in diameter and have a conduction velocity that does not accurately reflect conduction speed in the more proximal nerve.

The last parameter to be assessed on a more subjective basis is CMAP appearance. Although morphologic changes can be measured by comparing ratios of CMAP duration to amplitude, these are usually made on a qualitative rather than quantitative basis. Subtle changes may occur in normal individuals when CMAPs are obtained from stimulation at different points along the course of a nerve. As previously described, this is referred to as physiologic dispersion. With physiologic dispersion, it is estimated and modeled that the CMAP amplitude with proximal stimulation should never drop below 80% of that obtained from the most distal stimulus site. Nerve root stimulation sites provide the notable exception to this rule.[13] More dramatic reductions of CMAP amplitude, particularly over short segments of nerve, suggest demyelinating pathology due to conduction block or temporal dispersion, anatomic variants such as a median to ulnar crossover, or alternatively technical error (Figs. 2-2A,B and 2-3).

CMAP afterdischarges represent one other potential alteration of CMAP morphology. When present, these repetitive CMAPs follow single or repetitive supramaximal nerve stimuli. They appear as one or more additional negative peaks in the immediate aftermath of initial CMAP detectable either with routine motor conductions, with repetitive stimulation or with F wave assessment. The afterdischarges may actually interfere with F wave identification. Afterdischarges are not uniform with consecutive stimuli and have much smaller amplitudes than the initial supramaximal response (Figs. 2-4 and 2-5). They are uncommon, typically identified in disorders of nerve hyperexcitability in which nerve or muscle depolarization persists or repolarization is delayed **(Chapter 10).** They are commonly associated with continuous motor unit activity at rest with needle EMG. There is a spectrum of these spontaneous discharges ranging from single random MUP discharges (i.e., fasciculation potentials), to doublets or other multiplets which when discharging rhythmically or semirhythmically appear as myokymic discharges. At the extreme of these spontaneous discharges are high-frequency decrescendo waveforms known as neuromyotonic discharges. The generators of these discharges are believed to reside within motor nerve, probably within terminal twigs.

The clinical value of afterdischarge identification is derived from their specificity. They are associated with a limited number of disorders that may affect nerve, neuromuscular transmission, or muscle. Neuromyotonia, also known as Isaac syndrome or the syndrome of continuous muscle fiber activity is the most notable form of nerve

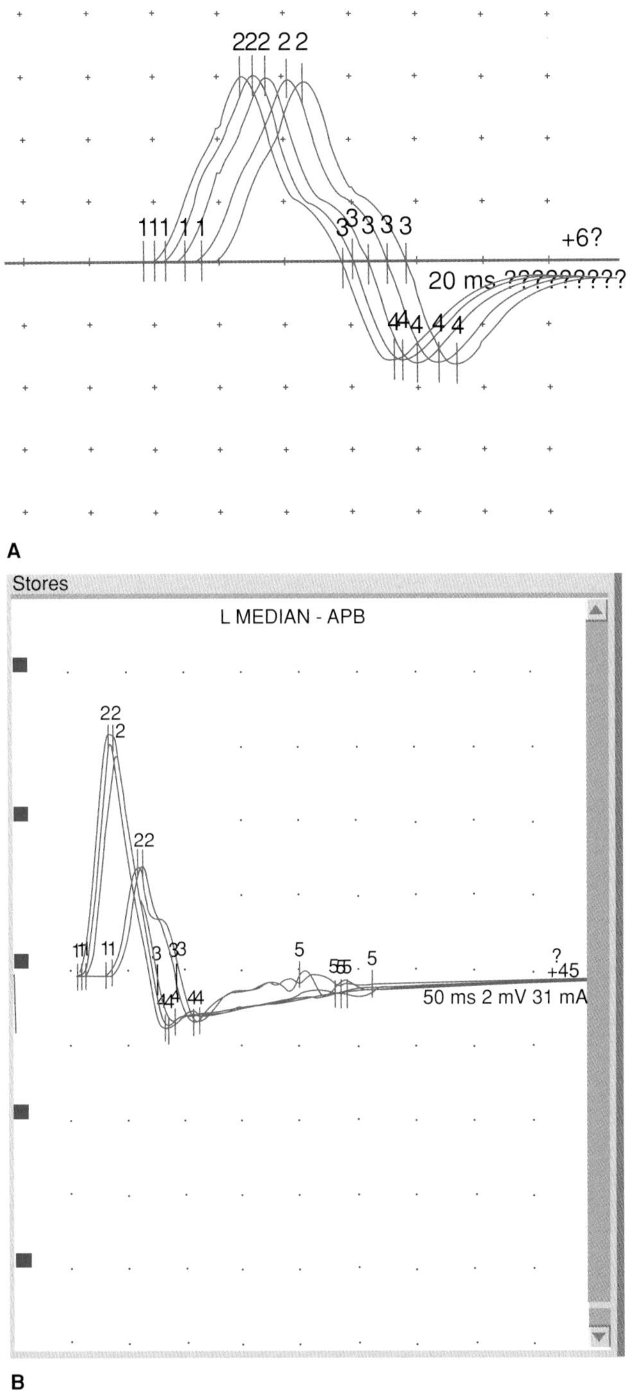

Figure 2-2. **(A)** Short segmental incremental stimulation in normal individual demonstrating identical CMAP (compound muscle action potential) waveforms with equivalent spacing between consecutive waveforms and **(B)** ulnar neuropathy at the elbow with focal demyelination with conduction block (amplitude reduction between responses 3 and 4), focal slowing (widening baseline interval between responses 3 and 4), and mild temporal dispersion (increased CMAP duration between responses 3 and 4).

hyperexcitability.[14–17] Our current understanding implicates malfunction of nerve potassium channels by antibodies directed against contactin-associated protein-like 2 (Caspr2). Presumptively, the afterdischarges result from prolonged nerve depolarization due to impaired potassium channel function resulting in the inability of nerves to rapidly repolarize.

In addition, afterdischarges may occur in disorders in which there is prolonged cholinergic activity at neuromuscular junctions such as toxic exposures to organophosphates, anticholinesterases or congenital acetylcholinesterase deficiency, and slow channel syndrome.[18] These afterdischarges appear similar to those that occur in disorders of nerve hyperexcitability in that they occur following a single supramaximal stimulus delivered to a motor or mixed nerve. The physiologic basis for these afterdischarges appears to be prolongation of the end-plate potential at the neuromuscular junction, unrelated to the delayed neurotoxic effects that frequently occur with toxic organophosphate exposure.

A different type of afterdischarge of muscular rather than nerve origin referred to as post-exercise myotonic potentials (PEMPs) may occur with myopathy associated with impaired sodium channel, particularly PMC, and to a lesser extent chloride channel function, that is, myotonia congenita (MC).[19,20] PEMPs are not seen in sodium or calcium ion channel disorders that produce periodic paralysis phenotypes.[19] These afterdischarges can be differentiated from those of neural origin as they do not occur after a single supramaximal motor stimulation but only in the context of the short exercise testing that is described below. They persist if repetitive stimulation is delivered immediately post-exercise but dissipate as the interval between exercise and stimuli evolves, whether or not the stimuli are repetitive or individual.

Sensory Nerve Conductions

Sensory conduction studies are also performed with surface electrodes in most instances. Unlike motor conductions, the recording electrodes are placed over nerve not muscle. Nerve rather than muscle action potentials are measured, with maximal amplitudes measured in micro- rather than millivolts: making them more technically difficult to obtain. The resulting wave form is referred to as an SNAP. The same disc recording electrodes, or in the case of the median and ulnar nerves, ring electrodes on digits are utilized. The tested nerve is then stimulated at either a more proximal or a distal location than the recording site. The former technique is described as antidromic, as the impulse travels in the direction opposite to that of normal centripetal physiologic conduction in sensory nerve fibers. With stimuli delivered distal to the recording site in sensory or mixed nerves, conduction is considered orthodromic. Nerves routinely studied include the median, ulnar, dorsal cutaneous ulnar, radial, medial antebrachial cutaneous, lateral antebrachial cutaneous, sural, and superficial peroneal. The lateral femoral cutaneous, saphenous, posterior cutaneous nerve of the forearm, medial

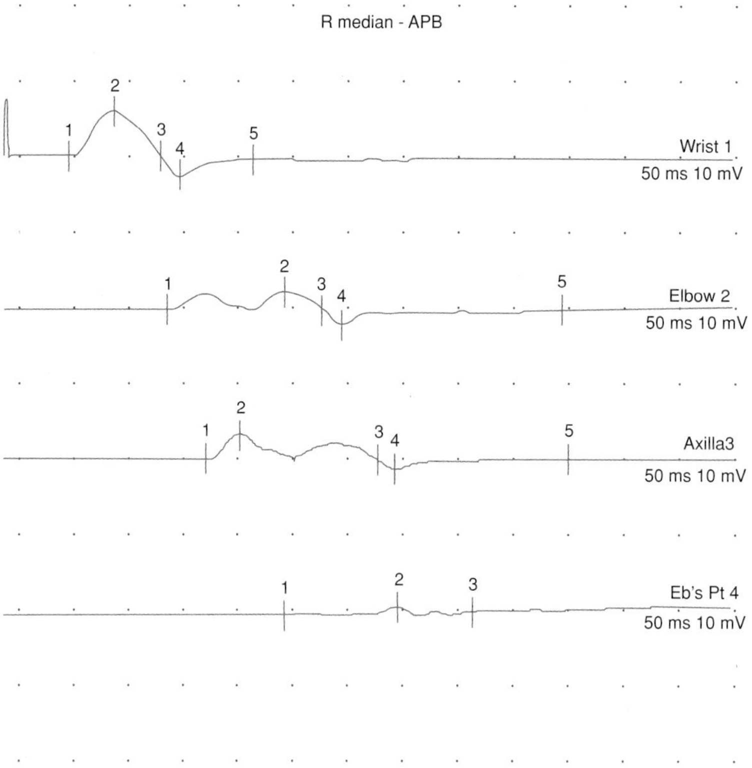

Figure 2-3. Median motor nerve conduction at four different points of stimulation demonstrating differential slowing (temporal dispersion) in patient with multifocal motor neuropathy.

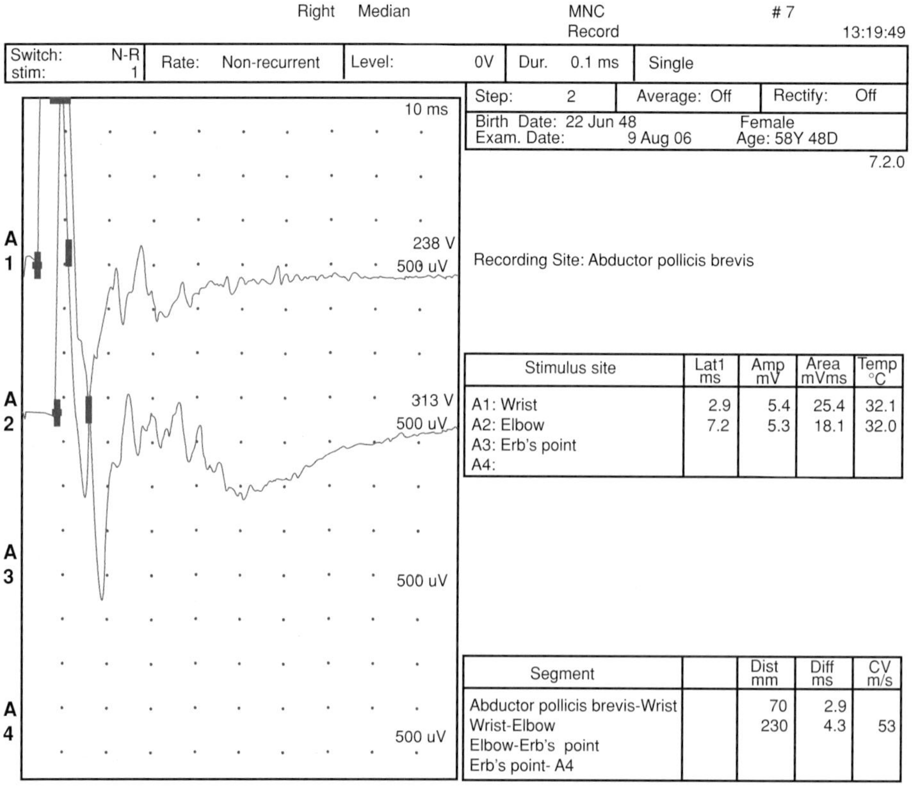

Figure 2-4. After discharges in neuromyotonia with routine motor conduction studies. (Used with permission of Drs. Alpa Shah and Steven Vernino, University of Texas Southwestern.)

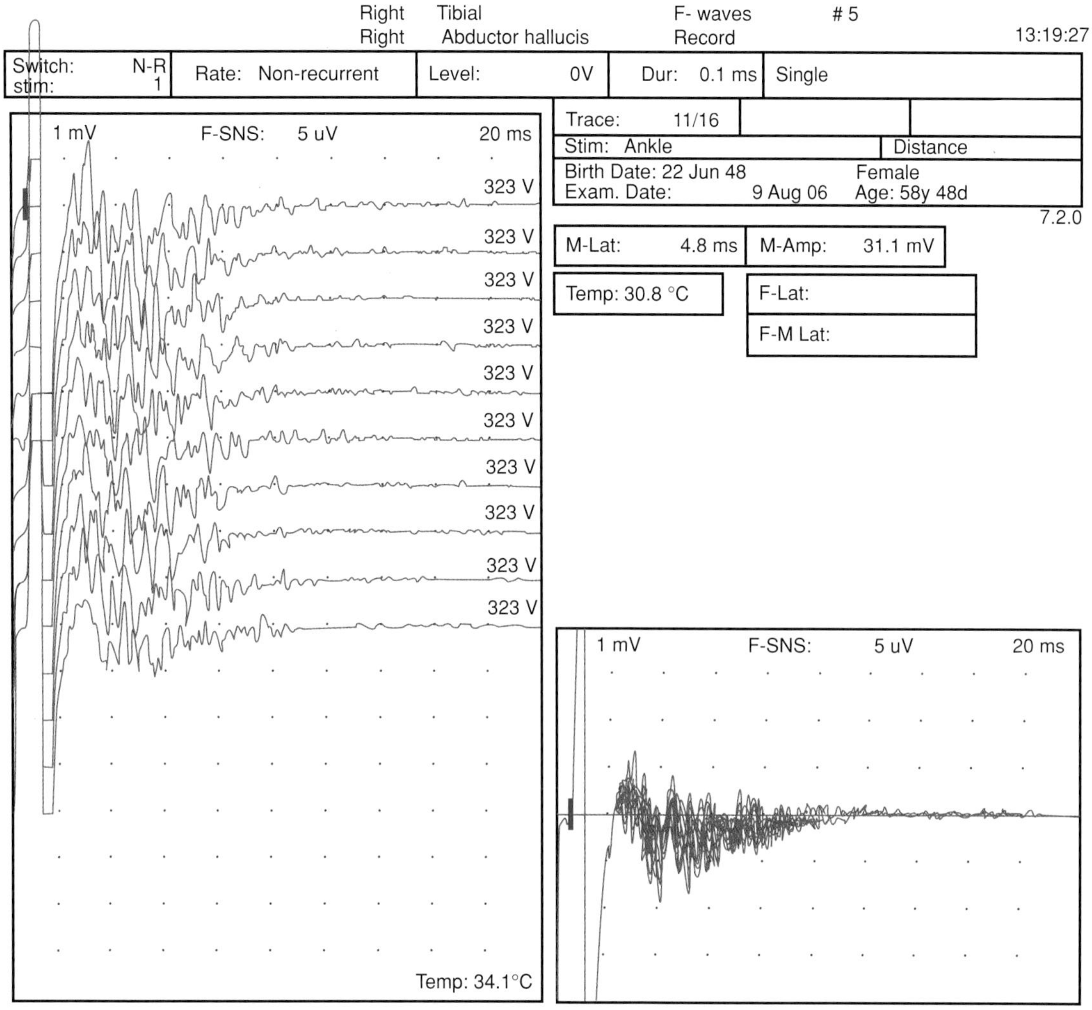

Figure 2-5. After discharges in neuromyotonia with F wave determinations. (Used with permission of Drs. Alpa Shah and Steven Vernino, University of Texas Southwestern.)

and lateral plantar nerves, and median and ulnar studies with less commonly used digits are less frequently tested. Many of these latter studies are fairly easy to obtain in the young, healthy, slender, and nonedematous but can be technically difficult in those with the opposite characteristics.

In many laboratories, only two parameters are measured; SNAP amplitude and either distal latency or conduction velocity (Fig. 2-6). As there are no neuromuscular junctions to contend with in sensory nerves, both the distal latency and the conduction velocity are measures of nerve conduction speed, differing only in the segment of nerve tested and the units with which it is reported. With motor conductions, there are some disorders in which distal latencies are prolonged disproportionate to forearm or leg conduction velocities. As there are few, if any, recognized conditions in which conduction speed is consistently more affected in one segment of sensory nerves than another, it can be argued that the reporting of distal latency as the sole measurement of sensory conduction speed is adequate. With motor distal latencies, the onset of the waveform is used for measurement, thereby identifying the fastest conducting axons. With SNAPs, the distal latency is typically measured from the waveform peak rather than the onset. This is done for technical reasons, as the onset of the SNAP waveform may be difficult to reproducibly identify. Sensory conduction velocities are however measured utilizing the SNAP takeoff from baseline rather than peak.

The second, and in the majority of situations, more important SNAP parameter is amplitude. As SNAPS are nerve rather than muscle action potentials, amplitude reduction does not occur on the basis of impaired neuromuscular transmission or myofiber atrophy/loss. With the exception of certain types of demyelinating pathology described below, reduced SNAP amplitude indicates either advanced age, excessive subcutaneous tissue or fluid, poor technique, or, most commonly, loss of peripheral sensory axons; the pathology occurring anywhere at or distal to the dorsal root ganglia.

Detecting morphologic change of SNAP waveforms is of limited value. Waveforms obtained with proximal stimuli

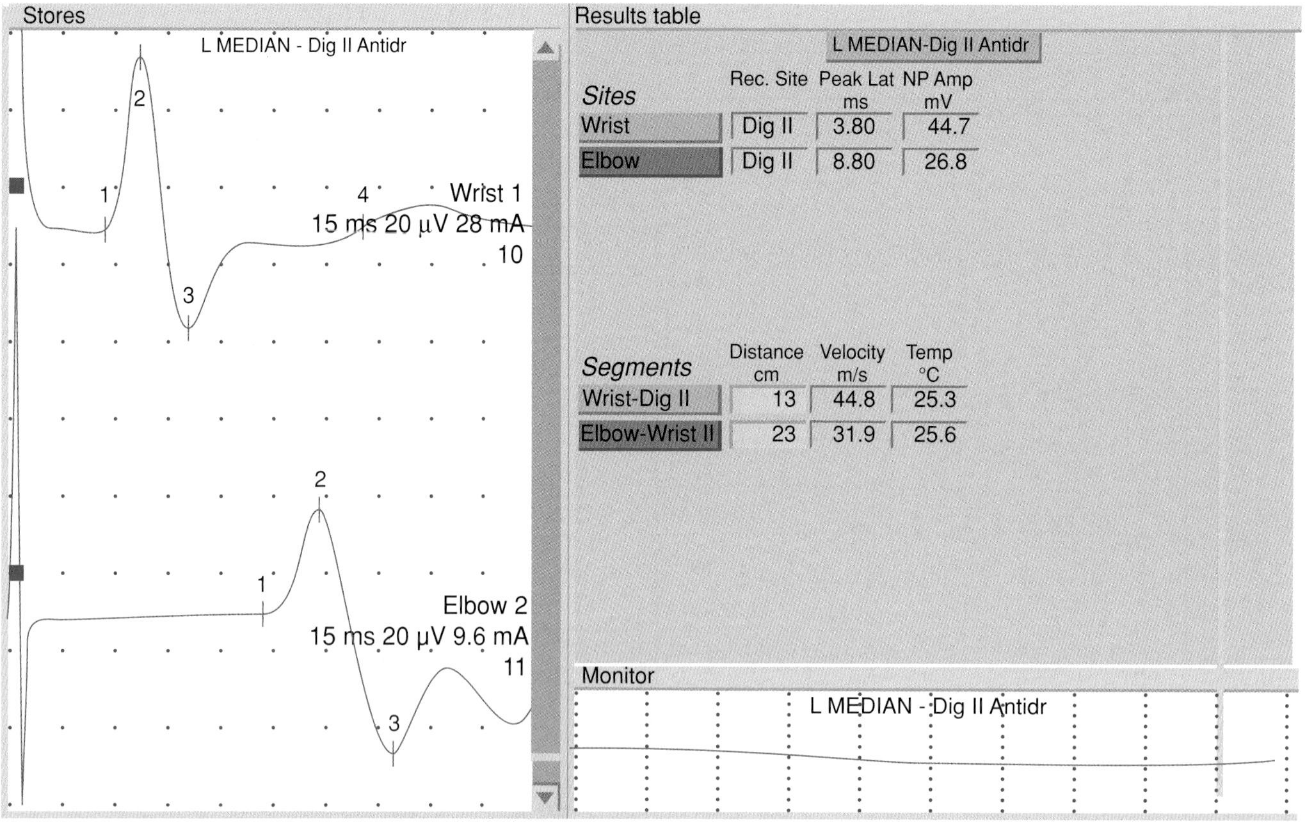

Figure 2-6. Sensory nerve action potentials in a normal individual demonstrating normal physiologic dispersion over distance with decreased amplitude and prolonged duration of median SNAP (sensory nerve action potential) waveform stimulating at elbow (bottom) as compared to stimulating at the wrist (top).

are typically significantly reduced in amplitude and prolonged in duration in comparison to their distally obtained counterparts (Fig. 2-6). This is due to the same principle of physiologic dispersion described above. This phenomenon is more pronounced than its motor counterpart due to the far wider range of conduction velocities in sensory nerves. As a result, attempts to identify demyelinating conduction block or significant morphologic differences in SNAP waveforms are not routinely attempted, particularly with stimuli delivered at wide interval distances.

F Waves and H Reflexes

Motor and sensory conduction studies are typically performed in the below elbow and knee segments where nerves are more anatomically accessible. F waves and H reflexes have potential value as a result of their ability to assess conduction in more proximally located nerve segments. F waves can be obtained by delivering supramaximal stimulation to any motor or mixed nerve in a normal individual, in most instances. F waves can be difficult to obtain in certain nerves, for example, common peroneal, even in the apparent absence of pathology. For that reason, it can be perilous to suggest the existence of nerve injury based solely on the absence of an F response from a single nerve. In normal adults, H reflexes can be elicited from the soleus muscle while stimulating the tibial nerve and, on occasion, from the flexor carpi radialis. Identification of H reflexes in other nerve/muscle pairs implies the existence of upper motor neuron disease due to decreased central nervous system inhibition on the reflex arc, analogous to a hyperactive deep tendon reflex.

The relevant anatomy and physiology of an F response can be described in the following manner. When a supramaximal stimulus is delivered to a nerve, the primary orthodromic response is the CMAP (M wave) as previously described. In addition, the initial nerve depolarization also produces an antidromic action potential traveling centripetally toward the spinal cord. At the level of the corresponding anterior cell(s), this antidromic action potential establishes a persistent or second action potential at the level of either the perikaryon or its axon hillock. This supplemental action potential is carried in a centrifugal or orthodromic direction along the entire length of one or more of the same motor axon(s) back to the original target muscle. As a result, the muscle is depolarized twice in response to a single stimulus, the second muscle action potential (F wave) having understandably a much longer latency and smaller amplitude. Unlike the initial CMAP, which represents the action potentials all of the responsive muscle fibers, each (F) response represents the action potentials of muscle fibers belonging to a single motor

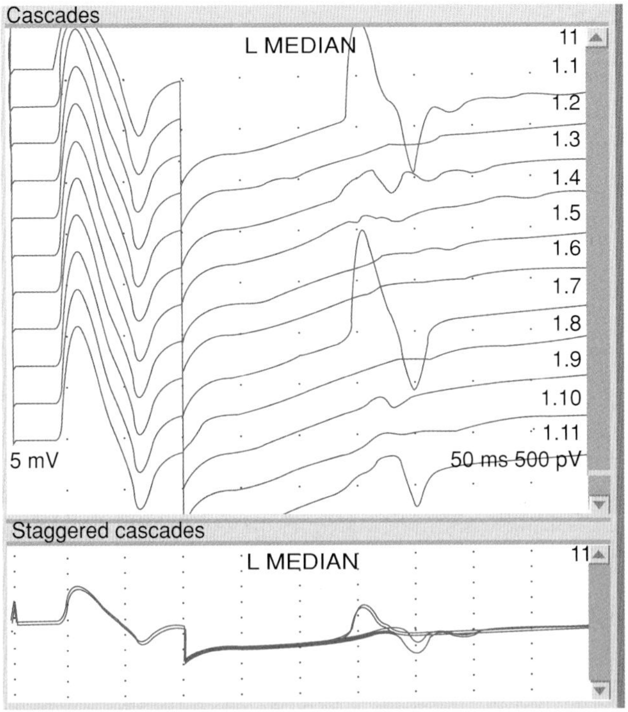

Figure 2-7. F waves—11 consecutive supramaximal stimuli delivered to the median nerve at the wrist in a normal individual while recording from the abductor pollicis brevis muscle demonstrating uniform CMAPs (compound muscle action potentials) but typical F wave behavior, that is, waveforms that are variable in occurrence, latency, and morphology.

unit. With each sequential stimulus, different motor units are typically activated. As a result, sequential F wave responses have varying latencies and morphologies in comparison to those occurring with the previous or subsequent stimuli.

F waves have significant limitations. Even in a normal nerve/muscle pair, F waves do not result from each stimulus. Amplitude measurements are of no particular value, as these represent the action potentials of only a small and varying proportion of single muscle fibers. There is heterogeneity of F wave latencies as sequential responses rarely arise from motor axons with identical conduction velocities (Fig. 2-7). A number of latency measurements can be made, the response with the shortest latency typically being the parameter reported. The potential value of F waves is their ability to detect conduction slowing over the segments of nerve not tested by routine conduction velocity measurements, that is, the proximal to elbow and knee segments. This value is most apparent early in the course of acquired demyelinating neuropathies, where prolonged F wave latencies may occur because of disease predilection for nerve roots, prior to slowing of conduction velocity or prolongation of distal latency in more distal nerve segments. In most cases however, F waves are either absent, or prolonged in the setting of slowed conduction velocities. Simultaneous slowing of conduction velocities and F waves has no localizing value, as the slowing of the F latency in this circumstance may represent slowing in the same distal aspect of the nerve where the conduction velocity is measured.

The H reflex represents the electrophysiologic analog of the Achilles deep tendon reflex. As in the F response, the stimulus applied to the tibial nerve in the popliteal fossa will travel in two directions. Unlike F waves, the H reflex is obtained with submaximal stimulus intensity. With delivery of stimuli of low intensity and long duration (1 ms), the lower-threshold 1 A sensory fibers within the tibial nerve are preferentially activated. As a result, the initial action potentials are propagated solely within thickly myelinated sensory nerve fibers. These impulses travel both centrifugally, where they have no known clinical or diagnostic consequence, and centripetally (orthodromically) along tibial and sciatic sensory fibers. Impulse transmission through the dorsal root of the S1 segment allows completion of a monosynaptic reflex to S1 anterior horn cells. Activation of these produces the H reflex representing a long latency CMAP originating from the soleus muscle. Typically, the H reflex has a latency in the high 20 to mid-30 μs range, depending on patient height.

As the intensity of the stimulus delivered to the tibial nerve increases, characteristic H reflex behavior is demonstrable. Action potentials will develop within the higher-threshold tibial motor fibers in addition to the 1 A sensory fibers already activated. These motor nerve action potentials also travel bidirectionally. The orthodromic impulses will activate the soleus muscle producing a typical CMAP. This has a far shorter latency than the H reflex and does not typically make its appearance until the H reflex is well established. The antidromic action potentials created in tibial motor fibers have a different effect. These will collide in a proximal location with the action potentials responsible for the H reflex. As the stimulus intensity increases, more tibial motor axons are depolarized resulting in increasing soleus CMAP amplitude but declining H reflex amplitude. Eventually, the H reflex will disappear while the CMAP will become supramaximal.

In summary, in response to sequential stimuli of 0.5–1-ms duration delivered to the tibial nerve in the popliteal fossa with increasing intensities, the H reflex appears first. Subsequently, the CMAP or M wave appears and enlarges to its supramaximal amplitude while the H reflex declines in amplitude and disappears. The tibial motor fibers distal to the stimulus site are depolarized twice, whereas both the tibial sensory fibers and the tibial motor fibers proximal to the stimulation site are depolarized once in response to a single stimulus (Fig. 2-8).

Both the maximal amplitude and the latency of the H reflex can be measured. The former estimates the number of viable motor units and muscle fibers within the S1 segment/soleus muscle complex and is typically greater than 1 mV in size. The latter provides at least an estimate of conduction speed within the motor and sensory fibers of the S1 segment. As in the case of F waves, H reflexes have greatest utility and localization value when these are abnormal in the setting of

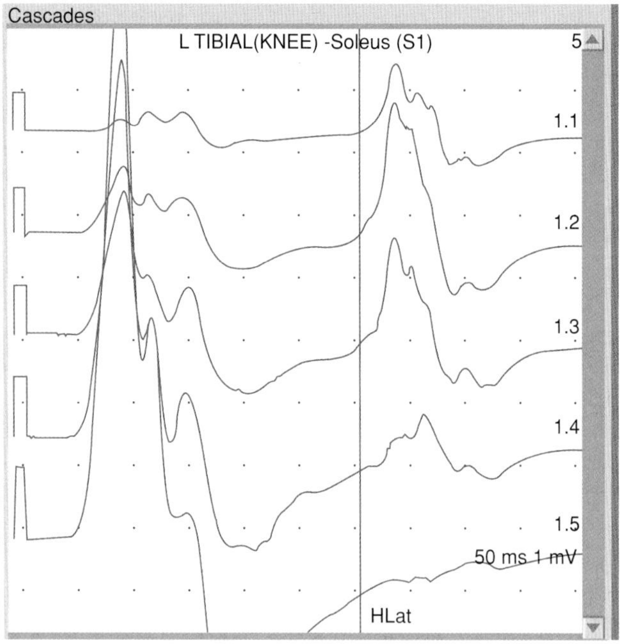

Figure 2-8. H reflex—five consecutive and increasing stimuli to the tibial nerve in the popliteal fossa in a normal individual, recording from the soleus demonstrating a typical H reflex pattern, that is, H reflex amplitude initially > M response amplitude, subsequent peaking than decline, and eventual absence of H reflex, associated with gradual increase to supramaximal M response. Note uniform H reflex latency.

normal routine conduction parameters. This applies most frequently early in the course of acquired demyelinating polyneuropathies. In addition, H reflex amplitudes have value in the assessment of S1 radiculopathies. If an H reflex is absent more than a week after symptom onset in the setting of normal routine conduction parameters and reduced recruitment in S1 innervated muscles, proximal conduction block in the tibial nerve, sciatic nerve, sacral plexus, or S1 nerve root can be inferred. Focal slowing of nerve conduction in a proximal location is theoretically detectable by H reflex assessment. In reality, this slowing is usually obscured by normal conduction speed in the other normal and more extensive parts of the S1 reflex arc. Attempts to provide an anatomic diagnosis of a focal neuropathy or radiculopathy on the basis of by F and H responses alone should be discouraged.

Repetitive Nerve Stimulation

Performance and interpretation of RNS techniques evolves from an understanding of the normal physiology of neuromuscular transmission. Muscle end-plate potentials (EPPs) are the precursors of muscle fiber action potentials. Unlike nerve or muscle action potentials that are all or none events that precede and follow EPPs respectively, EPPs are graded. Their amplitudes are proportionate to the number of successful interactions between acetylcholine (Ach) molecules and muscle end-plate receptor sites. Quantal release of ACh decreases with successive stimuli delivered in intervals of greater than 200 μs (e.g., <5 Hz). Under normal circumstances, this quantal and resultant EPP decline is of no practical importance, as there is a considerable physiologic reserve. With disease states that alter either the presynaptic release of ACh or postsynaptic receptor responsiveness, this reserve becomes inadequate. The EPP at individual neuromuscular junctions may fall below the threshold for myofiber action potential generation, and both CMAP amplitude and muscle strength may decline. As a result, slow (2–5 Hz) repetitive stimulation may produce a successive decline or decrement in CMAP amplitude in both pre- and postsynaptic (Fig. 2-9) DNMT. To avoid false-positive results based on technical factors, a decrement of at least 10% is required to be considered abnormal although a smaller decrement in a technically pristine study is suspicious. This decremental response has both clinical and single fiber analogues, that is, fatigable weakness and blocking of single fiber action potentials, respectively.

The recording and stimulating electrode placement in RNS is identical to routine motor conductions. Only the manner of stimulus delivery is altered. As mentioned above, the diagnostic yield of RNS will improve by ensuring that the tested muscle is warm and by removing drugs that augment neuromuscular transmission such as pyridostigmine prior to testing. RNS often produces unwanted movement artifact, which may require limb immobilization in order to secure a technically reliable study. Unfortunately the muscles with the highest diagnostic yield are also those most prone to movement and technical artifact.

False-positive decremental responses due to technical error are commonplace. In order for a decremental response to be considered pathologic, it must be reproducible and conform to the typical pattern. This pattern is best understood by understanding its physiologic basis. Pathologic decrements are not linear. Typically, the CMAP decline between two consecutive responses is greatest between the first and second stimuli and reaches its nadir by the fourth response. The reason for this latter phenomenon is the mobilization of ACh stores in the presynaptic neuron that allows delayed restoration of the immediate release pool. This allows for partial augmentation of the EPP after the fourth or fifth consecutive stimulus. With subsequent stimuli, the CMAP amplitude then begins to increase slightly although it never reaches the size of the initial response. If a train of 8–10 stimuli are delivered, the resulting configuration will have an asymmetric saucer-like appearance, with the left edge being higher. This configuration is of particular importance in distinguishing variation in CMAP amplitude due to disease from that due to technical considerations which are commonplace and easily misinterpreted by the unwary.

The electrophysiologic basis of the incremental response is closely related to calcium's role in the presynaptic release of ACh. When presynaptic ACh release is impaired by disease, it can be enhanced by augmenting the concentration of calcium in the presynaptic terminal. In a seemingly paradoxical manner, this can be accomplished by the delivery of

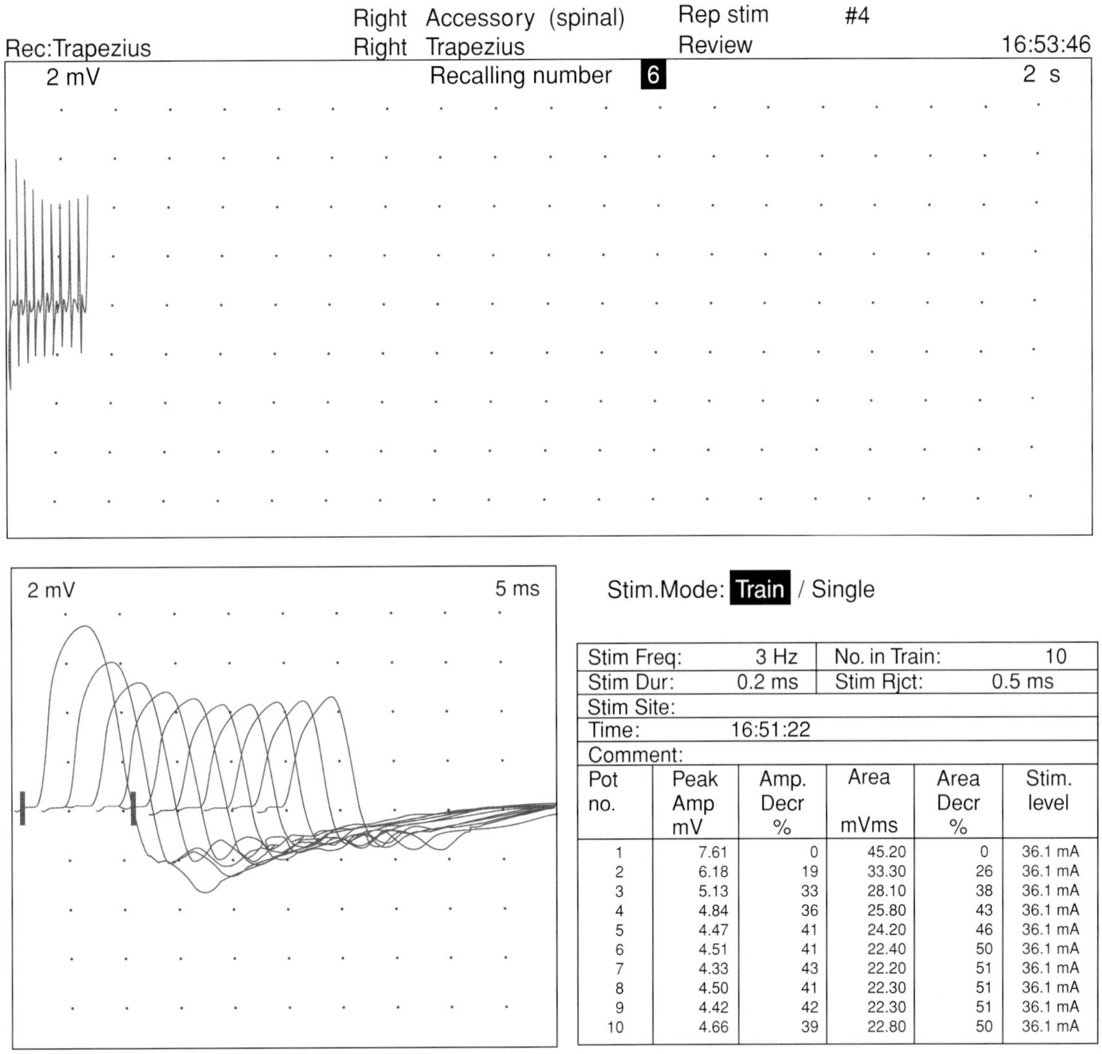

Stim Freq:	3 Hz	No. in Train:	10
Stim Dur:	0.2 ms	Stim Rjct:	0.5 ms
Stim Site:			
Time:	16:51:22		
Comment:			

Pot no.	Peak Amp mV	Amp. Decr %	Area mVms	Area Decr %	Stim. level
1	7.61	0	45.20	0	36.1 mA
2	6.18	19	33.30	26	36.1 mA
3	5.13	33	28.10	38	36.1 mA
4	4.84	36	25.80	43	36.1 mA
5	4.47	41	24.20	46	36.1 mA
6	4.51	41	22.40	50	36.1 mA
7	4.33	43	22.20	51	36.1 mA
8	4.50	41	22.30	51	36.1 mA
9	4.42	42	22.30	51	36.1 mA
10	4.66	39	22.80	50	36.1 mA

Figure 2-9. Decremental response to slow (3 Hz) repetitive stimulation with typical pattern in myasthenia gravis (note normal initial CMAP amplitude of 7.61 mV).

repetitive stimuli at a frequency of greater than 5 Hz. Stated in a different way, this is accomplished with stimuli delivered at intervals shorter than 200 μs. In presynaptic DNMTs, the baseline CMAP is typically reduced, at times dramatically. This is the most notable difference between pre- and postsynaptic disorders and sets the stage for the ability to demonstrate an incremental response. The initial low amplitude CMAP can be increased by a factor of 100% or more by either "fast" repetitive stimulation (5–50 Hz) or more humanely by brief exercise of the muscle being studied (Fig. 2-10A and B). With the brief exercise technique, a supramaximal stimulus is followed by 10 seconds of isometric exercise to the muscle being studied, and then immediately by a second post-exercise supramaximal stimulus. Trains of fast repetitive stimulation are typically reserved for those who cannot perform or cooperate with the post-exercise technique.

An incremental response is defined by a >100% increase in CMAP amplitude comparing the post-exercise response to the baseline. The degree of increment cannot exceed the difference between the baseline and premorbid CMAP amplitude for that muscle. A physiologic increment (i.e., higher amplitude, shorter duration, identical area under the curve) may occur in normal patients but typically does not exceed 40% of the baseline. It implies a more synchronous discharge of the component SFMAPs that constitute that CMAP waveform.

The electrodiagnostic approach to a patient with a suspected DNMT is dependent on the clinical context and on the initial, supramaximal CMAP amplitude. To overly simplify the concept, if it is small, try to make it bigger, and if it is big, try to make it smaller. In other words, in the case of either a reduced initial CMAP amplitude or a decrement in response to slow repetitive stimulation, an attempt to increase the CMAP amplitude is made. This can be accomplished by brief exercise, fast repetitive stimulation (10–50 Hz) or by administration of an anticholinesterase medication. Conversely,

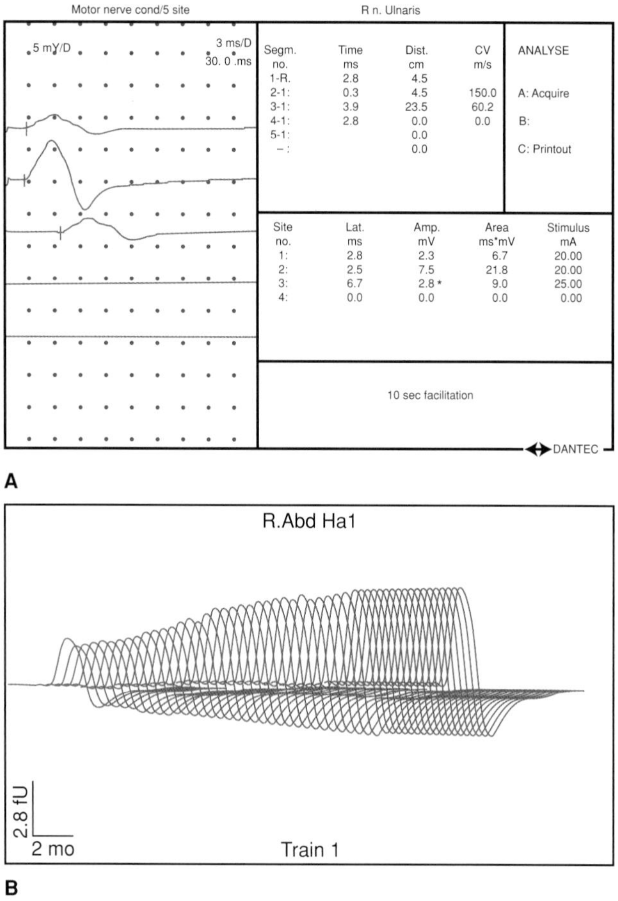

Figure 2-10. Incremental response to brief (10 seconds) exercise in patient with LEMS **(A)** (trace 1 ulnar CMAP at baseline stimulating at wrist, trace 2 ulnar CMAP immediately after 10 seconds of isometrically resisted finger abduction stimulating at wrist, trace 3 ulnar CMAP 1 minute later stimulating at elbow). Incremental response to 20 Hz fast repetitive stimulation **(B)**. CMAP, compound muscle action potential; LEMS, Lambert–Eaton myasthenic syndrome.

when faced with a normal initial CMAP amplitude and a suspected DNMT, the electrodiagnostician should seek to produce a decrement by slow repetitive stimulation without, or if necessary, with 1 minute of isometric exercise.

To elaborate, presynaptic DNMT have electrophysiologic properties that are both shared and distinctive in comparison to their postsynaptic counterparts. In suspected myasthenia gravis (MG), the initial CMAP amplitude is typically normal. The first step is to try and demonstrate a decremental response to slow repetitive stimulation. Ideally, for the sake of efficiency, RNS would be performed on a clinically weak muscle that has been warmed. The absence of decremental response to slow repetitive stimulation in a weak muscle would effectively preclude the diagnosis of autoimmune MG as the cause of that weakness. If a decrement is demonstrated, the train of stimulation can be repeated following 10 seconds of exercise to look for post-exercise facilitation or decrement repair. If a decrement is not demonstrable at baseline, repeating the train once a minute for 5 minutes following 1 minute of exercise applied to that muscle may improve diagnostic yield. This phenomenon is referred to as post-exercise exhaustion.

Presynaptic DNMT also decrement with low rates of repetitive stimulation. Early in the course, this may be the only abnormality found with nerve conductions. Presynaptic DNMT are usually distinguished from MG electrodiagnostically on the basis of low baseline CMAP amplitudes. In this case, the initial response from the electrodiagnostician should be to attempt to elicit an incremental response. This is easily done in a cooperative patient by exercising the appropriate muscle for 10 seconds and then immediately delivering a second supramaximal stimulus as described above. If the patient is not cooperative, a train of fast repetitive stimuli (10–50 Hz) may be used as a surrogate. If an increment is demonstrated, a subsequent train of stimuli delivered at 2–3 Hz will produce a characteristic decrement and further solidify the diagnosis of a neuromuscular transmission defect.

Short- and Long-Exercise Tests

The nondystrophic muscle channelopathies constitute a complex, overlapping group of disorders related to gene mutations of chloride, calcium, sodium, and potassium (Andersen–Tawil syndrome) channels in muscle. They will be described in detail in Chapter 30. As a result of their pathophysiologies, the phenotypes are typically dominated at least initially by episodic symptoms, either stiffness related to myotonia, weakness related to periodic paralysis, or a combination of both. Stiffness is felt to result from persistent muscle fiber depolarization and contraction whereas periodic weakness is felt to represent a more severe degree of depolarization rendering the muscle inexcitable. In chronic stages, particularly in the periodic paralyses, persistent weakness may develop.

Electrophysiologic testing of the nondystrophic myotonias involves detection of afterdischarges known as PEMPs as previously described in both routine motor conductions and F wave determinations, the presence or absence of myotonic discharges on needle EMG, response to repetitive nerve stimulation, and in particular, responses to short- and long-exercise testing which will be the focus of this section. Short- and long-exercise tests offer diagnostic support for both the existence and type of muscle channelopathy.[19,21] The tests are variations of standard motor NCS which utilize the ulnar or common peroneal nerves recording from the abductor digiti minimi or extensor digitorum brevis muscles, respectively. Both forms of exercise testing require careful attention to uniform patient positioning, limb temperature, muscle relaxation, and stimulus intensity.

Both short- and long-exercise tests are performed by maintaining limb temperature at 32–34°C and establishing a stable baseline, supramaximal CMAP amplitude. With the

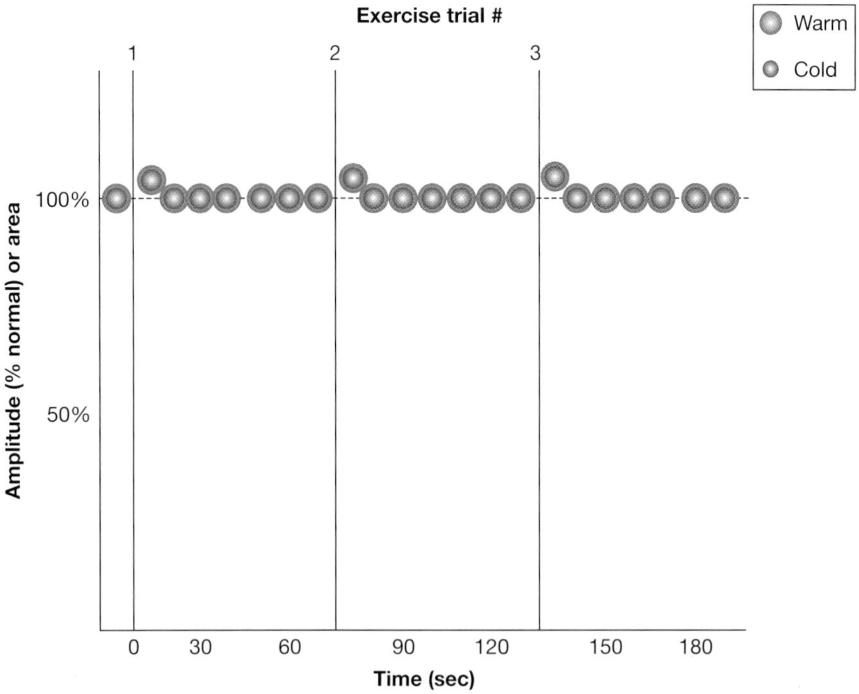

Figure 2-11. Short-exercise test—normal.

short-exercise test, a single supramaximal stimulus is delivered, the tested muscle is isometrically exercised for 10 seconds, followed by an immediate post-exercise supramaximal stimulus and six additional single stimuli every 8 seconds are delivered over the course of the next 50 seconds. After a 10-second rest period between trials, two subsequent, identical trials are performed, each preceded by 10 seconds of isometric exercise. Five patterns of abnormality have been described, the first three of which utilize the short-exercise test alone. The other two patterns are defined by a combination of the long- and short-exercise tests.

In normal individuals, there is a slight CMAP amplitude and/or area increment immediately following exercise that rapidly returns to baseline during the first trial and does not differ with the second and third trials.[19] The CMAP amplitude rapidly returns to baseline by the second or third stimulus of the first trial (Fig. 2-11).[19,21] The mean increment in immediate post-exercise CMAP amplitude is 4% (range −28 to +27) and the mean increment of CMAP area is +3% (range −58 to +84).[21] An increment of <10% or decrement <20% in CMAP amplitude and/or area compared to baseline is considered normal.[21] The short-exercise test has been further refined by using the same algorithm following limb cooling and rewarming, utilizing a combination of both amplitude and area to improve both the sensitivity and specificity of increment or decrement measurements.[21] Cooling is typically delivered for 7 minutes with a target cutaneous temperature of 15°C. In normal individuals, cooling with or without rewarming the limb does not alter the normal pattern.[20,21]

The long-exercise test is performed with identical electrode application.[21] The muscle to be studied is isometrically exercised for 5 minutes. During the period of exercise, single supramaximal stimuli are delivered at 1-minute intervals. Subsequent to the exercise, single supramaximal stimuli are then delivered immediately, every minute for 5–6 minutes, and then every 2–5 minutes for 40–50 minutes. The long-exercise test is of the greatest utility in the identification of the periodic paralyses. Normal patients may demonstrate a minimal initial decrement in CMAP amplitude and/or area with a rapid return to baseline (Fig. 2-12). In African-Caribbean controls the mean decrement may be slightly greater. Authorities recommend that an abnormal decrement on long-exercise testing for amplitude and area exceeds 40%.[21]

The response patterns with repetitive stimulation seen in the dystrophic or nondystrophic myotonic disorders differ from those seen in pre- and post-synaptic DNMT. In general, because of discomfort, repetitive stimulation is performed in suspected nondystrophic myotonia cases only when the remainder of the electrodiagnostic assessment is inconclusive. The major value of repetitive stimulation in this setting is increased sensitivity, particularly in recessively inherited MC.[22] In the nondystrophic myotonias, there is typically no decremental response prior to exercise. Depending on the specific disorder, and the frequency of repetitive stimulation, there may be either a decrescendo pattern in which the CMAP amplitude continuously declines (10-Hz stimulation in a warm limb in MC, or 10-Hz stimulation following limb cooling in PMC) or a pattern in which there is an initial dramatic reduction

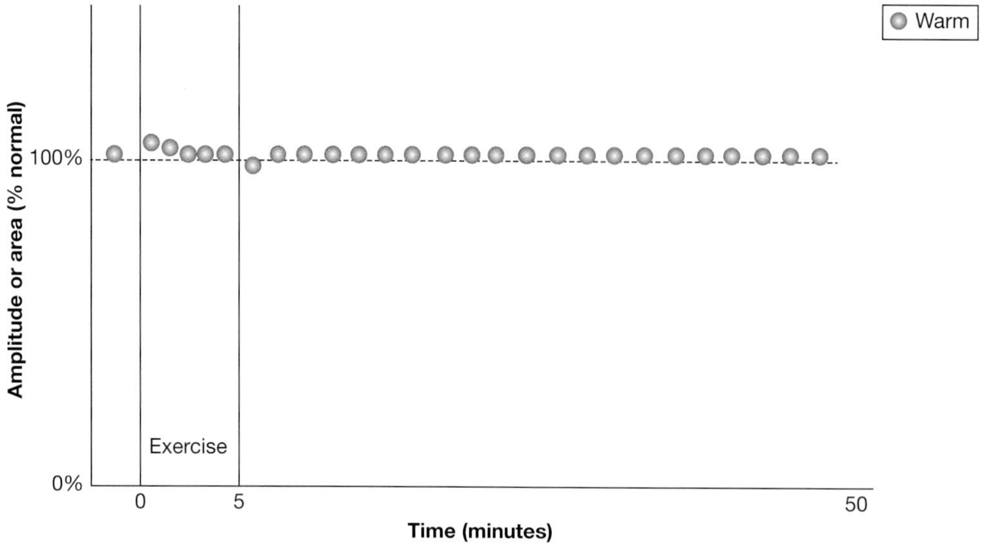

Figure 2-12. Long-exercise test—normal.

in CMAP amplitude following exercise which then declines further and then gradually increases with 3-Hz stimulation in PMC) (Fig. 2-13).[19,22,23]

The following is a summary of the typically patterns of abnormalities seen in MC phenotype associated with chloride channel mutations, PMC, potassium-aggravated myotonia (PAM), sodium channel myotonia (SCM), and hyperkalemic periodic paralysis (hyperKPP) associated with sodium channel mutations, and hypokalemic periodic paralysis associated with both calcium (hypoKPP1) and sodium channel (hypoKPP2) mutations. The reader is referred to Table 2-1 and Chapter 30 for summary and complete description of these disorders.

In MC with short-exercise testing, CMAP amplitude and area decrement is the greatest in the initial response following exercise (Figs. 2-14 and 2-15). If it exceeds 40% of baseline, it is considered pathognomonic of a chloride channel disorder.[21] With the next six stimuli delivered over the ensuing 50 seconds, the decrement lessens and the CMAP amplitudes and areas gradually approach baseline thus rendering a curve with an ascending positive slope. With the subsequent two trials, the magnitude of the decrement lessens but the trajectory of the curves remains the same. With cooling, the magnitude the decrement increases slightly, particularly in dominantly inherited disease. Although this *type 2* pattern is seen with both recessively and dominantly

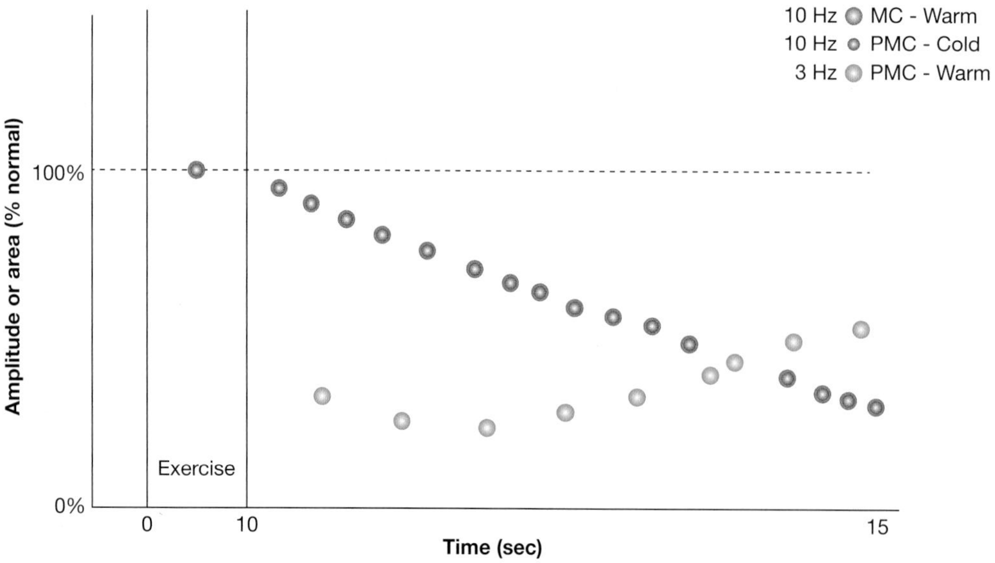

Figure 2-13. Repetitive stimulation in nondystrophic myotonia.

▶ TABLE 2-1. SHORT- AND LONG-EXERCISE TESTS IN THE NONDYSTROPHIC MYOTONIAS AND PERIODIC PARALYSES

Phenotype	Channel	Short-Exercise Effect on CMAP Amplitude	Post-Exercise Myotonic Potentials	Response to Repeat Short Exercise	Response to Cooling and Repeat Short Exercise	Long Exercise Effect on CMAP Amplitude	Myotonic Discharges on EMG	Other Disorders in Which This Pattern Can Be Identified
MC (type 2 pattern)	Cl^-	Immediate ↓ with subsequent repair	Yes	Less prominent CMAP ↓	1. AR – no change 2. AD- exaggerated ↓ CMAP amplitude	No change	Yes	1. PAM 2. MD 1 & 2
PMC (type 1 pattern)	Na^+	Immediate ↓ but less than type 2 but with longer effect[a]	Yes	More prominent ↓ CMAP amplitude	Even further ↓ CMAP amplitude	Prolonged and significant ↓ amplitude	Yes	None to date
Other sodium channel myotonias (type 3 pattern)	Na^+	No change	No	No change	Variable	No change	Yes	None to date
HyperKPP (type 4 pattern)	Na^+	Immediate ↑ that persists	No	Further ↑ CMAP amplitude	Unknown	↑ amplitude immediately that ↓ over time	Yes (not universal)	HypoKK-2
HypoPP-1 (type 5 pattern)	Ca^{++}	No change	No	No change	Unknown	↓ amplitude immediately that ↓ further over time	No	HypoKK-2
HypoPP-2 (type 4 or 5 patterns)	Na^+	Type 4 or 5	No	Type 4 or 5	Unknown	Type 4 or 5	No	HyperKPP HypoPP-1

[a]Exceptions with Q270 K^+ mutation.
MC, myotonia congenital; PMC, paramyotonia congenita; HypoPP, hypokalemic periodic paralysis; HyperKPP, hyperkalemic periodic paralysis; DM, myotonic dystrophy; EMG, electromyography; CMAP, compound muscle action potential.

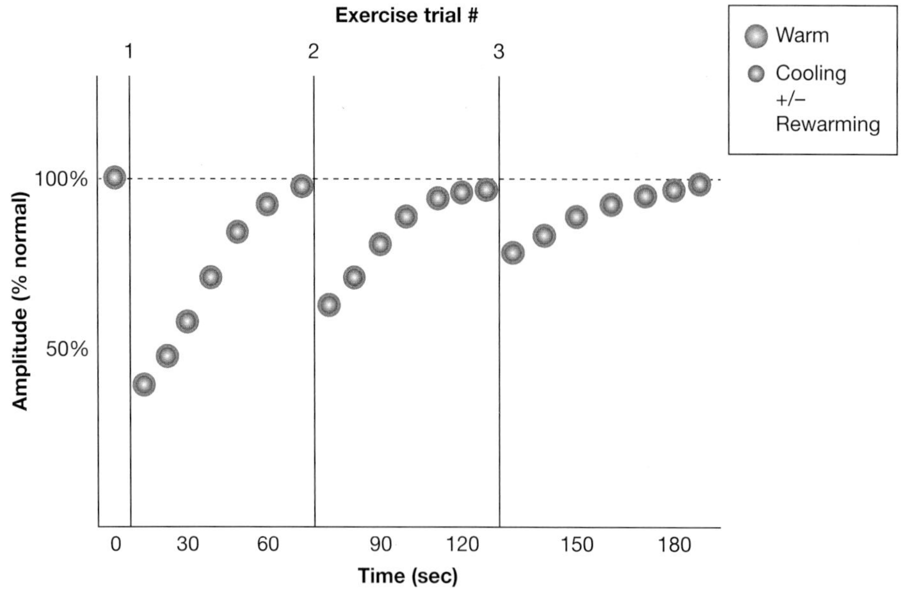

Figure 2-14. Short-exercise test—type 2 pattern—recessive inheritance.

inherited forms of MC, the decrement is far more dramatic in the former (Fig. 2-14).[20] This pattern is seen in approximately 83% of patients with confirmed chloride channel mutations with traditional amplitude comparisons but improves to 100% if amplitude and area comparisons are done concordantly [19,21] PEMPs in the short-exercise test in response to single or repetitive stimuli are found in approximately one-third of individuals with MC. Myotonic discharges with EMG are found in essentially all patients with MC.

A *type 2* pattern is seen predominantly in patients with MC but has been identified in sodium channel mutations associated with PAM, hyperKPP with myotonia, and both myotonic muscular dystrophy types 1 and 2.[19,20] In myotonic muscular dystrophy, the short-exercise testing with and without cooling produces a similar pattern of lesser magnitude than recessively inherited MC. Long-exercise testing in MC patients produces a pattern indistinguishable from controls.

Short-exercise testing in PMC produces a different configuration. There is little or no decrement in CMAP amplitude and area immediately following exercise. With the subsequent six stimuli however, the amplitude increasingly

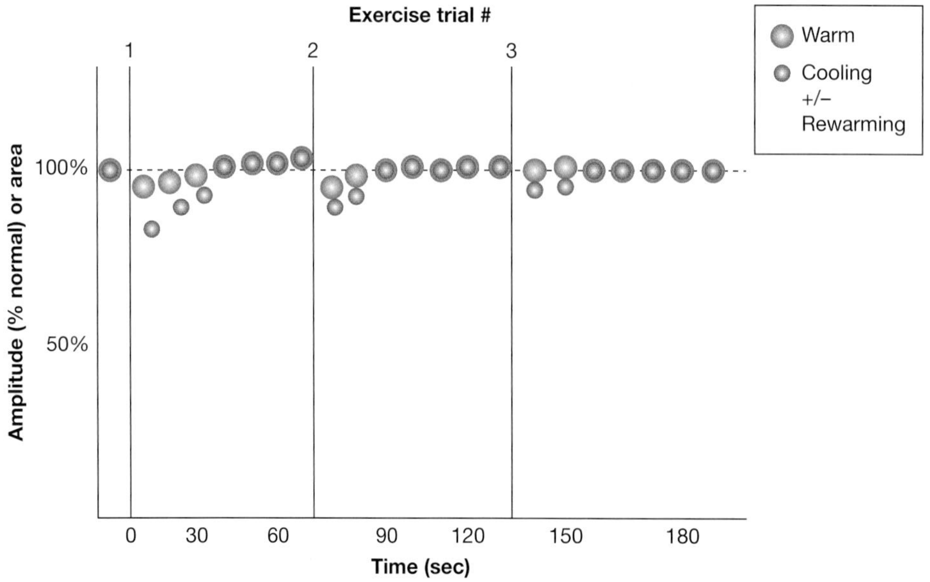

Figure 2-15. Short-exercise test—type 2 pattern—dominant inheritance.

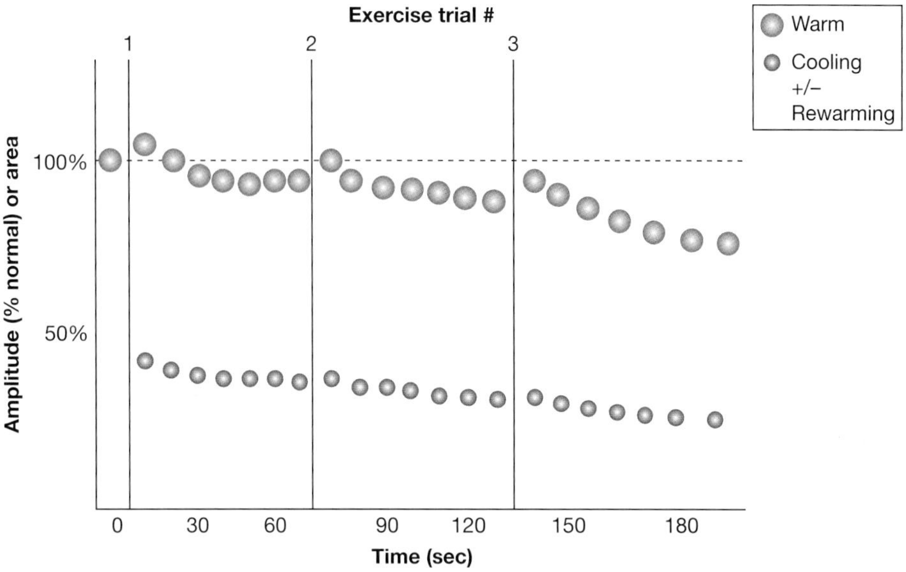

Figure 2-16. Short-exercise test—type 1 pattern.

declines, providing a curve with a negative rather than positive slope. The magnitude of this response becomes more dramatic in the second and third trials. In this *type 1* pattern, the most dramatic effect occurs following limb cooling, or rewarming following cooling.[19,21] Although the configuration of the curves remains the same, the magnitude of CMAP amplitude and/or area decrement is even more dramatic. A CMAP amplitude and area decrement of >20% in response to cooling with or without rewarming is thought to be pathognomonic of PMC[21] (Fig. 2-16).

Post-exercise myotonic potentials in response to single or repetitive stimuli following brief exercise are found in essentially all PMC patients. They dissipate both within an individual trial and between subsequent short-exercise trials. Pattern 1 has been exclusively associated with the PMC phenotypes/genotypes to date. The result of long-exercise testing in PMC also differs considerably from MC. A significant and persistent CMAP amplitude and area decrement occurs averaging a 66% reduction in comparison to baseline. The clinical weakness associated with the long-exercise test may preclude its completion. Myotonic discharges with EMG are anticipated in patients with PMC.

One specific sodium channel gene mutation resulting in the PMC phenotype (Q270 K) has an apparent unique short-exercise test signature.[20] Short-exercise testing without cooling demonstrates a *type 2* pattern essentially identical to that seen in MC, that is, an initial CMAP amplitude and/or area decrement immediately post-exercise that improves within the first trial and then between subsequent trials. After limb cooling, the pattern reverts to approximate the type1 pattern typically seen in PMC, that is CMAP amplitudes and/or areas decrement with a downward slope within the first trial that worsens with each of the subsequent two trials.

In most PAM and other myotonia/periodic paralysis syndromes associated with other sodium channel mutations, short-exercise testing is essentially normal although cold-induced reduction in CMAP amplitudes have been described in at least two genotypes.[20] PEMPs are rarely described in PAM and the SCMs, disorders that clinically overlap PMC and MC.[19,21] There is no significant CMAP amplitude and area decrement with short exercise, either prior to or subsequent to limb cooling.[19] This has been referred to as the *type 3* pattern (Fig. 2-17). No significant change in CMAP amplitude or area is seen in response to long-exercise testing in PAM. Myotonic discharges with EMG are anticipated in these disorders.

In hyperKPP, different authors describe different short-exercise test results. Fournier et al. describe an immediate CMAP amplitude and area increment that exceeds that seen in controls both in amplitude and in duration of effect (Fig. 2-18).[19] It persists throughout the entire minute of the study. With repetitive trials of short exercise, the CMAP amplitude and area increments in comparison to baseline by an average of 64%.[19] According to Tan et al. however, short-exercise testing does not differ from normals in either hyperKPP or hypoKPP-1 patients.[21]

Distinguishing between hyperKPP and hypoKPP electrophysiologically may be either relatively easy or hard depending on the response to short-exercise testing and the presence or absence of myotonic discharges. According to Fournier and colleagues, the *type 4* pattern is characteristic of hyperKPP or some hypoKPP-2 patients (Fig. 2-17). It is defined by occasional myotonic discharges in some hyperKPP patients, an absence of PEMPs, an incremental CMAP amplitude pattern in short-exercise testing as described in the previous paragraph, and the long slow decrement in response to long-exercise testing.[19] A decrement of at least

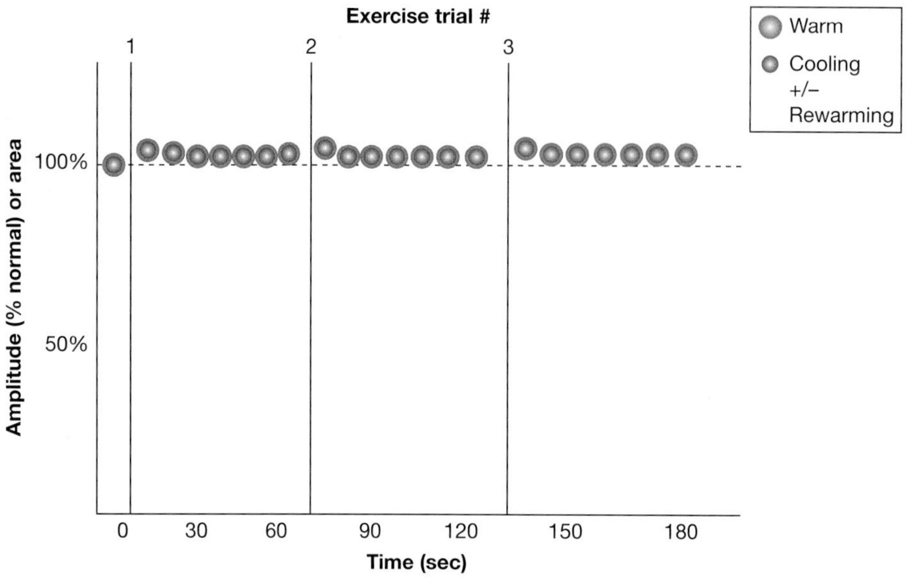

Figure 2-17. Short-exercise test—type 3 pattern.

40% of CMAP amplitude and area with long-exercise testing is found in a majority of periodic paralysis patients and may be seen in Andersen–Tawil syndrome patients as well.[21] The mean time to reach an abnormal decrement in periodic paralysis is approximately 25 minutes but may take the full 50 minutes of the test to appear, or perhaps even longer in hypoKPP-2.[21] The *type 5* pattern is the typical signature of hypoKPP-1 or occasional hypoKPP-2 patients (Fig. 2-19).[19] Neither myotonic discharges nor PEMPs are seen. The short-exercise test is normal and the long-exercise test demonstrates the same slowly developing decremental pattern that is seen in the type 4 pattern.[19]

Motor Unit Number Estimates

Considerable loss of motor units may occur without clinically evident weakness. This is particularly true in slowly progressive disorders where collateral sprouting and reinnervation are at least partially compensatory. In patients with ALS, it has been shown that the CMAP amplitude may not

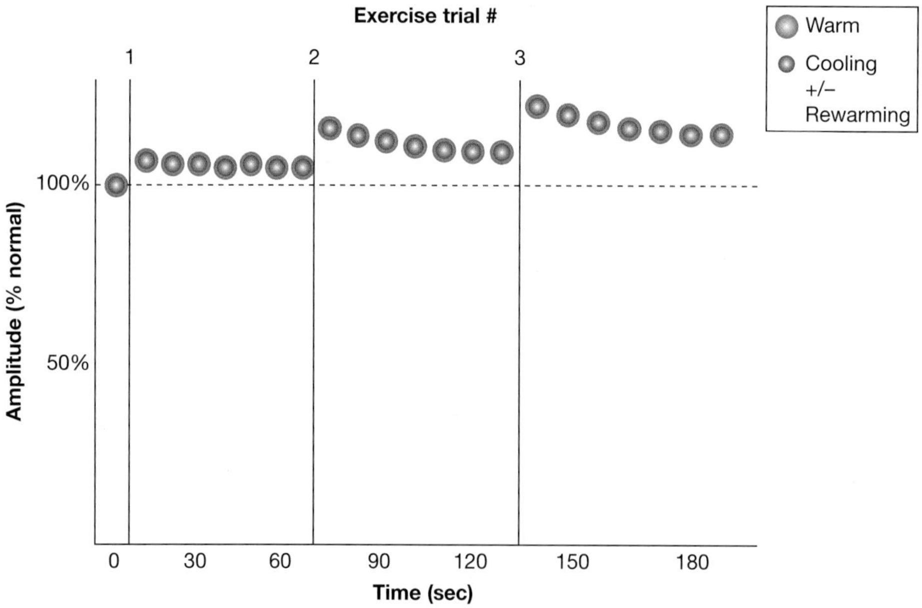

Figure 2-18. Short-exercise testing—type 4 pattern.

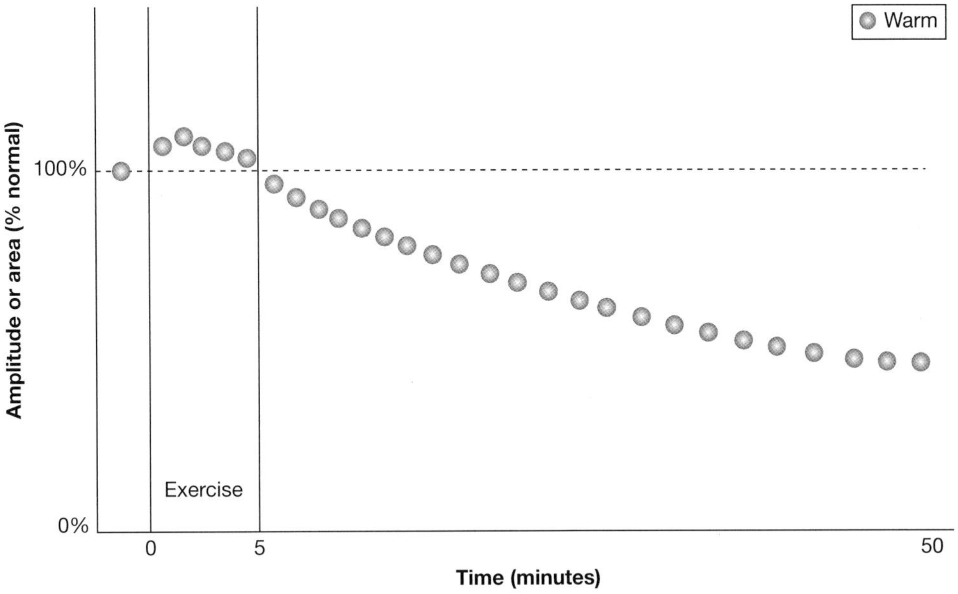

Figure 2-19. Long-exercise testing—type 4 or 5 pattern.

reliably decline until the estimated number of motor units drops below 10% of normal.[24] Numerous motor unit number estimation (MUNE) techniques have been developed in an attempt to count the number of viable motor units in a given muscle.[25] This has been done with the belief that MUNE would represent a more accurate means to monitor disease course or to detect a response to treatment than measurements of strength. All techniques attempt to estimate motor unit number by estimating the average size of the amplitude generated by a single motor unit, and then dividing this number into the maximal CMAP amplitude for the entire muscle.

MUNE is, in large part, a research technique, with limited application in the daily practice of neuromuscular disease. It can be time consuming and, with some techniques, technically challenging due to unstable neuromuscular transmission that may occur with reinnervation. Unlike standard EDX techniques, which can offer a panoramic perspective on multiple nerves and multiple muscles, MUNE is typically done on one or at most a limited number of nerves in a single setting. In addition, individual techniques have their limitations including the nerve/muscle pairs that are accessible to them.[25] MUNE has probably been most frequently used in the ALS population and has been successfully utilized in at least two clinical trials.[26–28] Multiple authors have demonstrated that MUNE decline and the size of individual MUPs increase sequentially in patients with ALS, consistent with our understanding of the denervating/reinnervating process.[24,27–32]

NEEDLE EMG

Needle EMG is performed by inserting a recording electrode into muscle and assessing the electrical waveforms both at rest and with voluntary muscle activation. EMG is interpreted by determining the type of abnormality within a specific muscle, identifying the pattern of muscles in which those abnormalities occur, and then correlating these results with those of NCS as well as the clinical context. Muscles are typically evaluated under three conditions: at rest assessing insertional and spontaneous activity, with minimal voluntary activation assessing motor unit action potential (MUAP) morphology and stability, and with a gradual increase in muscle activation assessing MUAP recruitment.

Insertional and Spontaneous Activity

Spontaneous activity and insertional activity are similar but not synonymous concepts. Insertional activity refers to the immediate response to needle movement. A brief burst of insertional activity occurring with each needle movement within viable muscle is the means by which the examiner is certain that they are in muscle. Increased insertion can refer to a protracted and nonspecific response to needle movement seen immediately after axon loss as a harbinger of the abnormal spontaneous activity in the form of positive waves and fibrillation potentials in muscles tested early after nerve injury. A number of the forms of abnormal spontaneous activity such as complex repetitive and myotonic discharges are often triggered by needle insertion. In disease, and in numerous other situations, increased insertional and abnormal spontaneous activities occur together.

Spontaneous activity refers to activity that occurs independently of needle movement. It may occur with or without a provoking needle movement but is sustained long after any provoking stimulus ceases. To further emphasize the subtle, but meaningful differences in the terminology, it is possible to have a situation in which there is increased spontaneous activity in the setting of decreased insertional activity, a concept

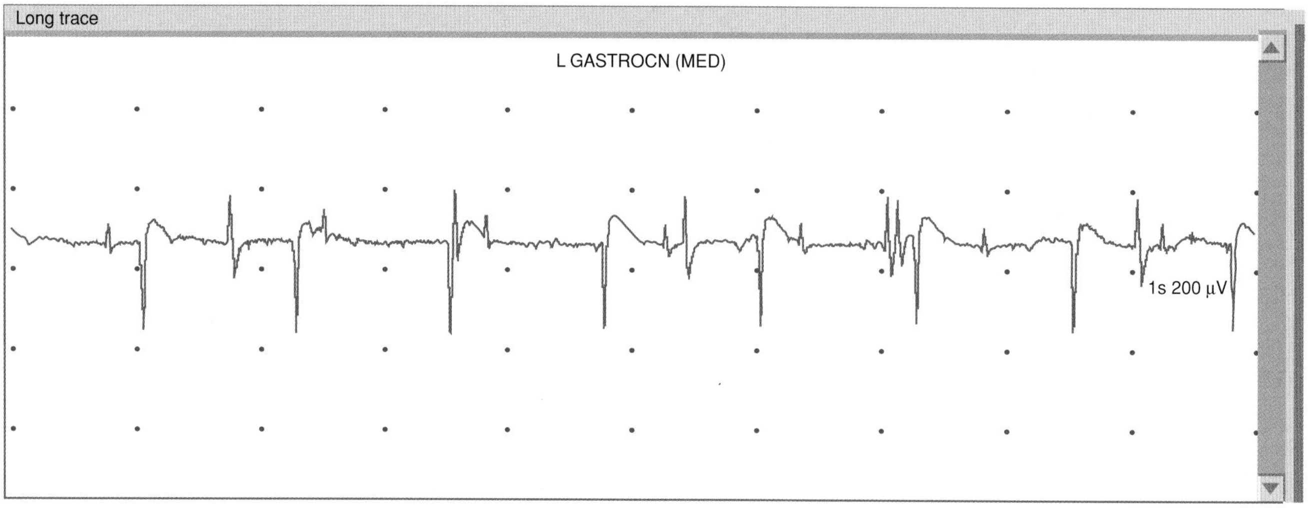

Figure 2-20. Fibrillation potentials and positive waves—single action potentials that usually fire with metronomic frequency; fibrillation potentials have short duration, positive waves with characteristic configuration and longer duration. The sound produced by fibrillations can be described as a "ticking." Positive waves have a more nonspecific, duller sound than fibrillation potentials, with recognition based more on their firing pattern and characteristic shape. These waveforms may occur in isolation or concurrently as in this figure.

that at first glance may seem counterintuitive. For example, it is not uncommon to experience this scenario while studying intrinsic foot muscles in patients with chronic polyneuropathies. There is often reduced insertional activity, presumably due to replacement of viable muscle by connective tissue. By the same token, there are isolated areas in that muscle where fibrillation potentials can be found, presumably representing isolated, viable, and nonreinnervated muscle fibers.

Spontaneous activity can be normal. End-plate spikes and end-plate noise represent miniature EPPs and are seen in normal muscles at rest when the needle is in proximity to the motor endplate. In contrast, there are a number of abnormal waveforms that may occur in an abnormal muscle at rest. These include fibrillation potentials and positive sharp waves, cramp potentials, myokymic discharges, myotonic discharges, complex repetitive discharges, and neuromyotonic discharges (Figs. 2-20 to 2-24). Of these, fibrillation potentials and positive sharp waves are the most prevalent (Fig. 2-20). They are recognized by their metronomic and regular firing pattern. When present, these suggest that

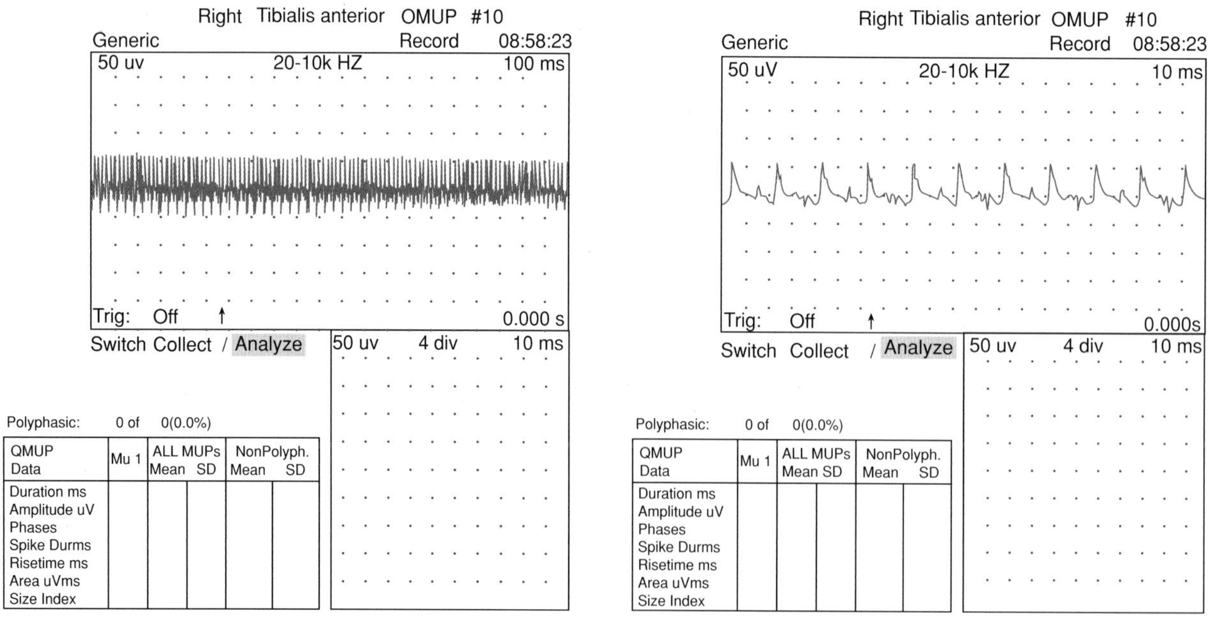

Figure 2-21. Complex repetitive discharges—a discharge with abrupt onset and cessation, the sound produced frequently described as "machinery like."

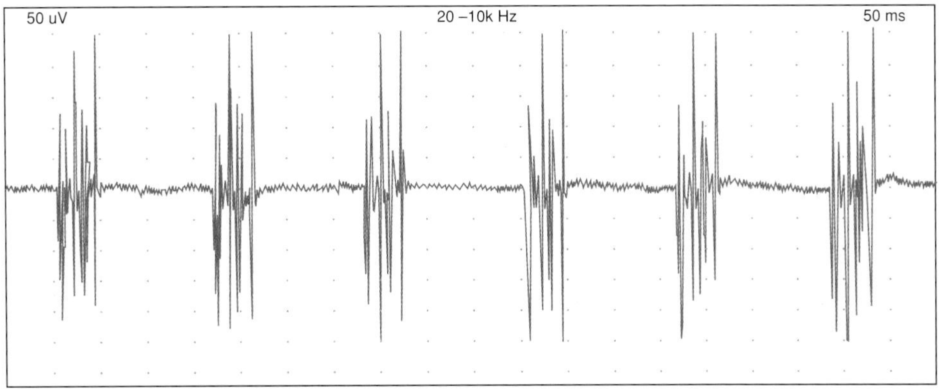

Figure 2-22. Myokymic discharges—semirhythmic grouped discharges, the sound produced frequently likened to the troops marching. (Used with permission of Dr. Devon Rubin, Mayo Clinic, Jacksonville.)

anatomic continuity has been lost between a muscle fiber and its innervating axon. Less commonly, they may result from myopathies associated with muscle membrane instability. Fibrillation potentials and positive waves occur most commonly from denervation in association with axon loss at any location from anterior horn cell to terminal twig (Table 2-2).[33] They do not occur in demyelinating neuropathies in the absence of axon loss.

Fibrillation potentials and positive waves are not however, specific for axon loss Table 2-2. They may be observed in both DNMT and certain muscle diseases. In the former, the axon may be effectively separated from its target muscle by ablation of the neuromuscular junction. In myopathy, particularly those associated with the pathologic features of segmental necrosis of muscle or fiber splitting, viable segments of muscle may be separated from segment of muscle containing the neuromuscular junction. By doing so, the myopathic process has effectively denervated segments of viable muscle. There are a number of myopathies, notably the channelopathies, and some of the congenital and mitochondrial myopathies, where these forms of abnormal spontaneous activity occur without clear explanation of the denervating mechanism. Presumably, muscle membrane instability provides an alternative explanation for this form of waveform generation.

Other forms of abnormal spontaneous activity are less common. As some of these discharges have clinical concomitants that go by the same name, this text will follow the convention used by others. The clinical observation will be referred to by the name alone, for example, fasciculation whereas the waveform will be referred to as a potential or discharge, for example, fasciculation potential. Complex repetitive discharges are nonspecific and occur in both chronic nerve and muscle disorders (Fig. 2-22). Although usually considered an indication of nerve or muscle pathology, current thinking suggests that they may be occasionally identified as a normal finding in both the biceps and more commonly, the iliopsoas muscles. Complex repetitive discharges have a machinery-like sound that typically starts and stops abruptly. Whether related to nerve or muscle disease, they are thought to originate from a reverberating circuit that develops within contiguous myofibers. Complex repetitive discharges are typically unassociated with any observable clinical concomitant.

Myotonic discharges also appear to originate from muscle and are primarily associated with heritable muscle

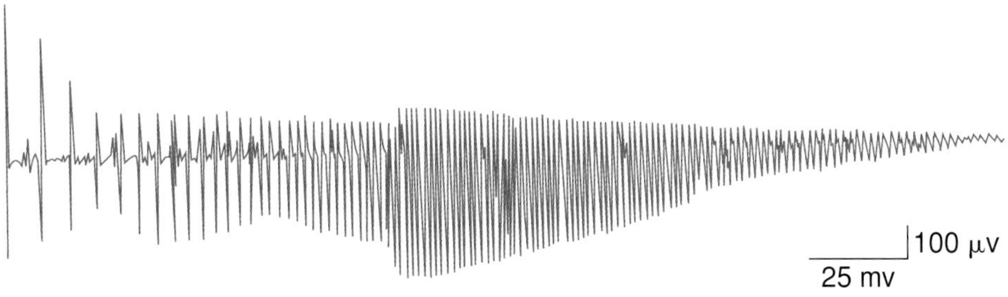

Figure 2-23. Myotonic discharges—with variable waveform amplitude and frequency, producing a waxing and waning discharge likened to an accelerating and decelerating chain saw or motorbike motor.

▶ TABLE 2-2. DISORDERS ASSOCIATED WITH POSITIVE WAVES AND FIBRILLATION POTENTIALS[33]

Site	Type	Examples
Anterior horn	Axon loss	ALS, SMA, poliomyelitis, syringomyelia, spinal cord infarction
Ventral root	Axon loss	Spinal stenosis, neoplastic meningitis
Plexus	Axon loss	Trauma, tumor, brachial plexus neuritis, diabetic radiculoplexopathy
Peripheral Nerve	Axon loss	Toxic, metabolic, hereditary, entrapment, and compression
NMJ	Pre-synaptic	Botulism, LEMS[a]
	Post-synaptic	Autoimmune myasthenia gravis
Muscle	Inflammatory	Dermatomyositis, polymyositis, inclusion body myositis
	Infiltrative	Amyloidosis, sarcoidosis
	Dystrophic	Dystrophinopathy, limb girdle, myotonic dystrophy
	Toxic	Cholesterol lowering agents, chloroquine
	Necrotizing	Anti-signal recognizing protein
	Inherited metabolic	α glucosidase deficiency
	Congenital myopathies (certain)	Myotubular myopathy, late onset Nemaline
	Infectious	HIV, other viral, trichinosis

[a]Uncommon.

disease (Fig. 2-23). These produce a waxing and waning sound historically likened to a dive bomber. From a more contemporary perspective, a revving chain saw or motor bike may represent a more apt simile. Myotonic discharges do not sustain themselves and typically dissipate until such time that they are provoked by the next needle movement or muscle contraction. Their presence often obscures the ability to adequately study MUAPs or assess other forms of abnormal spontaneous activity. Myotonic discharges are the major EDX signature of myotonic muscular dystrophies, (particularly DM1) the nondystrophic myotonias associated with chloride and certain sodium channel disorders, and in some patients with hyperKPP.[33,34] These are also seen in certain glycogen storage disorders, most notably acid maltase deficiency, branching and debranching enzyme deficiencies, myofibrillar myopathy, and occasionally in toxic and inflammatory myopathies (Table 2-3). Myotonic discharges are not clinically observable but are commonly associated with muscle stiffness.

Other forms of abnormal spontaneous activity appear to be generated by nerve such as fasciculations potentials, myokymic and neuromyotonic discharges. All of them can be conceptualized as part of nerve hyperexcitability spectrum disorders.[15] Fasciculation potentials are singular, spontaneous discharges of single MUPs that represent the electrophysiologic correlate of the fasciculations that can often be seen while observing the muscle with the naked eye. They can be seemingly benign (or at least associated with subclinical pathology) or associated with any one of a number of nerve diseases. They are most closely linked and probably most commonly seen in anterior horn cell diseases. Numerous authors have attempted to identify the morphologic or behavioral characteristics of fasciculation potentials that would distinguish benign from more ominous forms. There have been recent publications that promote the concept that complex and unstable fasciculation potentials correlate with pathology and can be used as a surrogate marker for fibrillation potentials and positive waves in the electrodiagnostic evaluation of ALS patients.[35–37] Ironically, a contributing author to one of these papers has studied fasciculation potentials and has concluded that there are no characteristics that confidently allow the distinction of benign from pathologic fasciculations.[38] The ability to observe clinical fasciculations, in association with fasciculation potentials, is undoubtedly

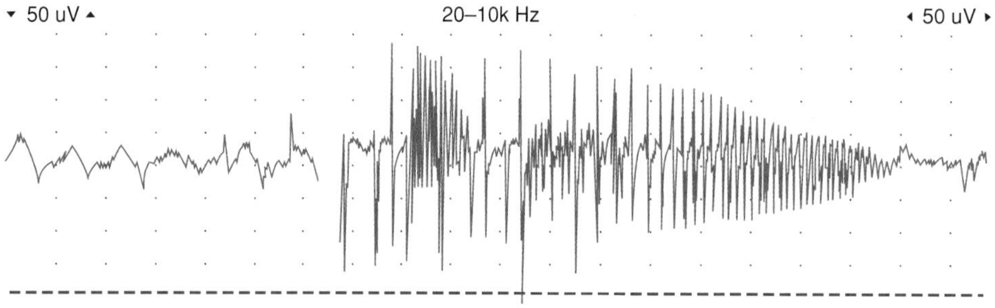

Figure 2-24. Neuromyotonic discharges—very high-pitched discharges with sound likened to "screaming formula one race car" engine. (Used with permission of Dr. Devon Rubin, Mayo Clinic, Jacksonville.)

TABLE 2-3. DISORDERS ASSOCIATED WITH MYOTONIC DISCHARGES

Myotonic muscular dystrophy types 1 and 2
Myotonia congenita
Paramyotonia congenita
Other nondystrophic myotonias, e.g., potassium-aggravated myotonia
Hyperkalemic periodic paralysis
Azacholesterol
Monocarboxylic acids
Colchicine myopathy
Cholesterol lowering agent myopathy
Hypothyroidism
Inflammatory myopathies (rare)
Acid maltase deficiency
Branching enzyme deficiency myopathy
Debranching enzyme deficiency myopathy
Hereditary vacuolar myopathies (Danon disease and X-linked myopathy with excessive autophagy)
Myofibrillar myopathy and other distal myopathies with rimmed vacuoles
Welander myopathy

related to the thickness of subcutaneous tissue, the depth of the muscle, and whether the fasciculations arise from superficially placed motor units within that muscle.

Cramp potentials are groups of spontaneously firing, otherwise normal MUPs that discharge in a sputtering pattern, typically with abrupt onset and cessation. Like fasciculations, they are typically neurogenic in origin and may have either a benign or pathologic significance. They are commonly found in chronic neuropathic conditions such as motor neuron diseases, radiculopathy, or polyneuropathy but can occur in any of the nerve hyperexcitability syndromes discussed subsequently in the following paragraphs on myokymic and neuromyotonic discharges or in a number of metabolic disturbances including pregnancy, uremia, and hypothyroidism.[33] Cramp potentials are typically associated with clinical cramping.

Myokymic discharges are grouped discharges of two or more MUPs that fire repeatedly in a semirhythmic manner with interval gaps of electrical silence. The intraburst frequency is between 40 and 150 Hz. The sound produced has been likened to troops marching. These probably result from ephaptic transmission between injured, contiguous axons. Myokymic discharges can be seen in a number of different etiologies of nerve disease (Fig. 2-21 and Table 2-4). These may be associated with disorders as mundane as CTS or as unusual as rattlesnake envenomation. In the cranial musculature, these are most commonly associated with multiple sclerosis, GBS, and brainstem neoplasms. These are common in disorders of neural overactivity such as the cramp fasciculation syndrome and Isaac's syndrome. Myokymic discharges are most commonly associated with radiation-induced nerve injury. Myokymic discharges may or may not be associated with the recognition of clinical myokymia.

TABLE 2-4. DISORDERS ASSOCIATED WITH MYOKYMIC DISCHARGES[33]

Location	Disorder
Facial muscles	Multiple sclerosis
	Brainstem glioma
	Guillain–Barré syndrome
	Bells palsy
	Head and neck radiation
Limb muscles	Radiation
	Chronic nerve compression, e.g., CTS
	Isaac's syndrome and its differential diagnosis (see Table 2-5)

Neuromyotonic discharges are infrequently seen (Fig. 2-24). They are commonly associated with other waveforms such as myokymic discharges, cramp discharges, and fasciculation potentials that occur in disorders of neural hyperexcitability. Their duration is brief as their high frequency (150–300 Hz) precludes them from sustaining themselves for protracted periods. Their sound has been likened to the scream of a formula-one race car engine. These are most closely linked to the disorder known by the names neuromyotonia, Isaac's syndrome, or the syndrome of continuous muscle fiber activity. Neuromyotonic discharges are nonspecific and may be associated with a number of neurogenic disorders, some of which are paraneoplastic (Table 2-5).[21,33,39] Although initially some of these cases were attributed to antibodies directed against voltage-gated potassium channels(VGKCs), subsequent studies have revealed that these antibodies actually are directed against Caspr2.[17] An analogous discharge, the neurotonic discharge, may be recorded from muscles

TABLE 2-5. DISORDERS ASSOCIATED WITH NEUROMYOTONIC DISCHARGES[15,21,33,39,40]

Acquired	Isaac's or Morvan syndrome
	Cramp fasciculation syndrome
	Paraneoplastic (thymoma, thyroid carcinoma)
	Multifocal motor neuropathy
	IgM kappa paraproteinemic neuropathy
	Diabetic neuropathy
	Copper deficiency
	Creutzfeld–Jakob disease
	Intraoperative nerve irritation
	Anticholinesterase poisoning
	Timber rattlesnake envenomation
	Radiation
Hereditary	Charcot–Marie–Tooth disease
	ALS
	Distal spinal muscular atrophy
	Kennedy disease
	Paramyotonia congenita

during intraoperative monitoring, particularly with acoustic nerve surgery, as a means of detecting potential injury to the facial nerve.

Motor Unit Action Potential Analysis

The purpose of examining the muscle with minimal levels of voluntary activation is to assess the morphology and stability of individual MUAPs. The motor unit consists of an anterior horn cell, its axon, and all of the muscle fibers it innervates. The MUAP refers to the collection of all single fiber action potentials, arising from the muscle fibers of that MUP, that are within the recording radius of the needle. MUAPs become smaller when there is a loss or physiologic nonparticipation of muscle fibers within the motor unit. This typically occurs in disorders of muscle and neuromuscular transmission. In the former, the number of fibers within the motor unit decreases as a result of myofiber degeneration. Alternatively, the size of the action potential that each fiber generates decreases as a result of myofiber atrophy. In DNMT, the amplitude and/or duration of the MUAP may decrease from blockade of neuromuscular transmission, physiologically reducing the number of single fiber muscle action potentials (SFMAPs) contributing to that MUAP.

Conversely, MUAPs typically become larger following chronic denervation and reinnervation typically occurring between 3 and 6 months after disease onset.[33] An orphaned muscle fiber deprived of its axon supply may be reinnervated by a collateral nerve twig belonging to a neighboring viable motor unit. As a result, surviving motor units in the aftermath of axon loss will typically grow both in amplitude and in duration. Normal values for both amplitude and duration are available but vary depending on patient age and the muscle studied. In general, most MUAPs in most limb muscles are between 8 and 15 μs in duration and less than 2 mV in amplitude. MUAP morphology does not change in a substantive manner in a purely demyelinating nerve disorder, although both increased duration and polyphasia may result from variable conduction slowing in terminal nerve twigs.

MUAPs typically have triphasic configurations, although occasional MUAPs with a few extra turns or phases are common. Polyphasic or serrated MUAP morphology implies that the individual SFMAP components of that MUP have become desynchronized. Satellite potentials, that is, waveforms that are separate from but time-locked to the primary MUAP waveform, are considered as a subtype of polyphasia. An abundance of polyphasic MUAPs implies that the process, if monophasic is subacute, that is, of weeks' to months' duration.[33] Polyphasic MUAPs have no etiologic specificity and can be seen in myopathies, axon loss, and demyelinating nerve disease. Polyphasic motor units will eventually reconfigure themselves into a triphasic configuration, even in those MUPs that have been exceptionally enlarged in remote denervating and reinnervating disease such as polio.

The concepts outlined in the preceding three paragraphs are generally accurate but have exceptions. Large motor units reminiscent of reinnervation following denervation occur in chronic myopathies, particularly inclusion body myositis.[33,41,42] Long-duration MUAPs in myopathy have been hypothetically attributed to three different mechanisms all of which are related to regenerating fibers. The nerve fibers that innervate regenerating muscle fibers may have slow conduction velocities relating to their immaturity. Regenerating muscle fibers may have neuromuscular junctions scattered along their length rather than condensed near a single motor point. Either of these may lead to delayed arrival of the muscle fiber action potential between the site of its origin and the site of the recording electrode, thus dispersing the SFMAP components within the MUP. Lastly, the conduction velocity of the regenerating muscle fiber itself may have this same dispersal effect.[42]

Conversely, in certain axon loss disorders, small motor units referred to as nascent units may be seen. These occur because of a concomitant reduction in MUP size and MUP number. A severe monophasic nerve injury with reinnervation that allows for only a limited number of myofibers to be initially incorporated into the motor unit is probably the most common situation in which nascent units occur. These may also be seen in rapidly evolving denervating disorders in which effective reinnervation does not occur, and in which degeneration of terminal twigs occurs early in the disease course. The familial form of ALS associated with the A4 V mutation of the SOD1 gene is perhaps the most notable example of this latter mechanism. In either case, small motor units from nerve and muscle diseases are most readily distinguished from one another by their characteristic decreased and increased recruitment patterns respectively as described below.

MUP variability or instability refers to the alteration of MUP morphology on consecutive discharges (Fig. 2-25). Under normal circumstances, every single fiber action

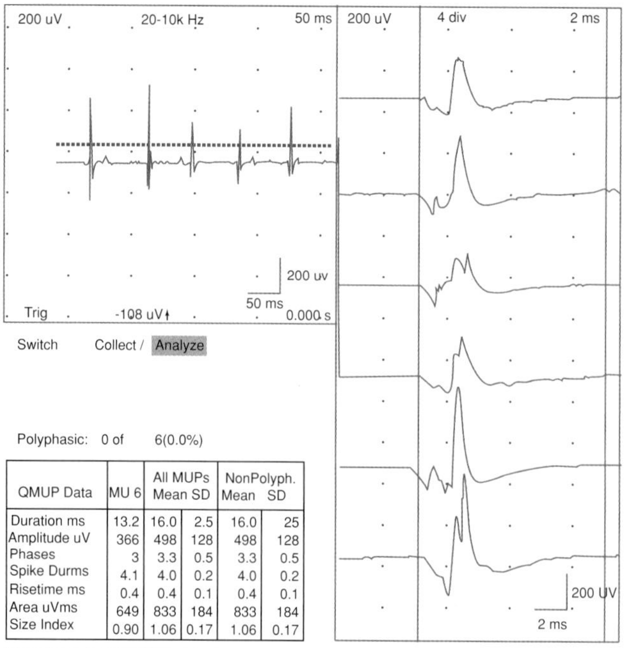

QMUP Data	MU 6	All MUPs Mean	SD	NonPolyph. Mean	SD
Duration ms	13.2	16.0	2.5	16.0	25
Amplitude uV	366	498	128	498	128
Phases	3	3.3	0.5	3.3	0.5
Spike Durms	4.1	4.0	0.2	4.0	0.2
Risetime ms	0.4	0.4	0.1	0.4	0.1
Area uVms	649	833	184	833	184
Size Index	0.90	1.06	0.17	1.06	0.17

Figure 2-25. Motor unit potential (MUP) variability.

potential within a given motor unit discharge in a near concordant fashion. As a result, as long as the needle position is stable, the MUAP will have an identical configuration each time it discharges. With disordered neuromuscular transmission of any cause, transmission at one or more individual neuromuscular junctions may be delayed or actually fail. As this is a physiologic rather than a direct structural effect, this provides a dynamic process affecting different neuromuscular junctions variably with consecutive discharges. As a result, the configuration of the MUP may change quite dramatically with consecutive discharges. Variability of amplitude is best demonstrated by having the patient minimally activate the muscle being tested, in order to isolate an individual MUP while using slow sweep speeds (50–100 ms/division) and high settings on low-frequency filters, similar to what is deployed in SFEMG. This allows the examiner to visualize the same MUP multiple times on the same screen. MUP variability is most closely associated with DNMT. It can often be seen however, in early reinnervation where neuromuscular junctions are immature. Traumatic nerve injury and ALS are notable examples.

Motor Unit Action Potential Recruitment

As the last component of the needle examination, the examiner attempts to estimate the number of MUAPs that the patient is capable (or willing) to activate. This is done by having the patient gradually increase the amount of isometric resistance in the muscle being tested. Under normal circumstances, an increasing number of MUPs will be recruited, that is, seen and heard on the EMG machine display. Each has its own distinctive sound and configuration as the makeup and topographical relationship of each MUAP to the recording electrode differs with any needle location.

In axon loss, and in demyelinating neuropathies with conduction block, there are a reduced number MUAPs that can be recruited. As a result, the remaining activatable MUAPs that fire do so with a greater frequency than normal in an attempt to compensate for MUAP loss. This is referred to as reduced recruitment. Reduced recruitment is one cause of a reduced interference pattern. Again, these are two terms that are related, but not synonymous. A reduced interference pattern may also occur as a result of a patient's inability or unwillingness to fully activate all MUAPs at their disposal due to disorders of the central nervous system, pain, or malingering. In this case, there will be no rapidly firing MUAPs identified despite a reduced number of MUAPs on the screen as there is no stimulus to do so.

Many strategies are utilized in an attempt to quantitate MUAP loss. More often than not, reduced recruitment is estimated by training one's ear to detect MUAPs firing at rates that are excessive. The ear is quite sensitive in its ability to detect rapidly firing MUAPs in response to motor unit loss. Many electromyographers can accurately estimate the firing frequency of an MUAP to within 2 Hz, certainly within 5 Hz. With full recruitment resulting in a full interference pattern, there will be an amorphous blending of the sound created by all activated motor units. With reduced recruitment, rapidly firing individual MUAPs can be detected by hearing the distinctive sound that each MUAP firing at an accelerated pace produces. This effect has been likened to the sound produced by a baseball card placed in the spokes of a child's moving bicycle wheel. This can be done at very low levels of recruitment by estimating the firing frequency of the first MUAP when the second MUAP is recruited, and the firing frequency of the second MUAP when the third MUAP is recruited and so on. Typically, firing frequency of an MUAP at onset is 6–8 Hz. The second MUAP is typically recruited by the time this MUAP is firing at 10 or 12 Hz. If a single MUP is firing at a rate greater than 12 Hz (in limb muscles) and no other MUAP is recruited, this is an objective measure of decreased recruitment. Hearing MUAP firing faster than this is an accurate indicator of axon loss or demyelinating conduction block. This is the method espoused by Daube and Rubin and represents the preferred method by the authors because of its combined accuracy and efficiency.[33]

There are more objective methods that can be utilized by someone who has not yet developed a trained ear. The recruitment ratio is an alternative method This involves identifying the rate of the fastest firing MUP and dividing it by the number of MUAPs that have been activated. This number should never exceed 5 in normal circumstances. For example, if the most rapidly firing of two recruited MUAPS were discharging at a rate of 15 Hz, and only two MUPs were activated, this ratio of 7–1/2 would represent reduced recruitment.

In myopathies or DNMT, the problem is not a reduced number of motor units but reduced MUAP size. As the amount of force generated by individual MUAPs is often reduced, more motor units need to be recruited earlier than normal to generate the same amount of force. The firing rates of these MUAPs remain normal. This effect has been termed as early or increased recruitment. In general, increased recruitment, proportionate to effort rendered, is a subjective and fairly insensitive EDX measure and is usually not recognized until other EDX features of muscle disease or DNMT are evident.

SFEMG and Other Specialized Techniques of Motor Unit Analysis

SFEMG has a number of potential applications. Its primary clinical application is to enhance the sensitivity of DNMT testing. Unfortunately, what is gained in sensitivity is often lost in specificity. For this reason, its greatest utility lies in its ability to discriminate between subtle presentations of DNMT from nonneuromuscular diseases. It is limited in its ability to distinguish one neuromuscular disorder from another. In general however, large jitter values associated with frequent neuromuscular blocking is more likely to represent a DNMT than in diseases of the anterior horn cell, nerve, or muscle.

The basic goal of SFEMG is to capture and analyze two or more SFMAPs belonging to the same MUAP. In order to do so, it is necessary to limit MUAP recruitment to be able to see, hear, and cleanly record these SFMAPs. In cooperative patients, this can be accomplished on a voluntary basis. In patients who are unable to activate a limited number of MUAPs and maintain a stable level of recruitment for any reason, stimulated SFEMG, as described below, may well represent a better option. Historically, there are two significant technical differences between SFEMG and standard EMG recordings. Both involve limiting the recording radius of the needle so as to facilitate SFMAP acquisition and analysis. Limiting the recording radius involves increasing the low-frequency (high-pass) filter setting to 500 Hz. The second means to limit the recording radius is to use a special SFEMG needle whose recording radius is smaller than its concentric or monopolar counterparts. In part due to the cost and inconvenience involved in the use of SFEMG needles, that require both repeated sterilization and sharpening, electromyographers are now utilizing standard, disposable concentric EMG needles. Normative jitter data for concentric needles are approximately 5 μs less at any given age for any given muscle, in comparison to published norms using SFEMG needles.[221]

The primary parameter measured by SFEMG is jitter which represents the variation in the interval between two SFMAPs belonging to the same MUAP. Jitter is a property of normal neuromuscular transmission. Its physiologic basis is derived from the variable nature of the EPP as was described in the section on repetitive nerve stimulation. The key to understanding the origin of jitter is the knowledge that the slope of the rise in membrane potential that occurs between the resting membrane potential and action potential threshold is proportionate to the amplitude of the EPP. In other words, the higher the EPP, the steeper the slope and the shorter the interval between the inciting nerve and the resulting muscle fiber action potential. As a result, the interval between consecutive discharges of two SFMAPs belonging to the same motor unit will fluctuate with the normal variation in quantal ACH release and resultant EPP amplitude and slope.

In practice, two (or more) SFMAPS are captured by using a triggered delay line. To do so, the electrodiagnostician will carefully manipulate the EMG needle until it is within an acceptable recording distance from at least one SFMAP. The optimal needle position is determined by listening for generation of the sharp, crisp sound that is generated by this proximity and then confirming the proximity by assuring that the rise time of the waveform is less than 300 μs with an amplitude that is greater than 200 μV. Typically, this is done with a sweep speed of 1 ms/division and a gain of 100–200 μV/division.

Once this SFMAP is isolated, subtle movements of the electrode are made in an attempt to find a second SFMAP belonging to the same motor unit, identified by its "time-locked" characteristics. The interval between the two (or more) spikes should be far enough apart to be measurable but not farther than 4 ms, for purposes of measurement accuracy. Ideally, a steady, low level of contraction will allow the recording of a 100 consecutive discharges of this fiber pair. At least 50 of these 100 discharges must be captured to allow for accurate statistical analysis. Under normal circumstances, the waveforms representing the second of the two SFMAP waveforms will be nearly overlapping with each other but will not be perfectly superimposed. This variation between the first and fluctuating second single muscle fiber action potentials is the basis of normal jitter. (Fig. 2-26). This variation in interpotential interval is usually expressed as the mean consecutive difference (MCD), a calculation readily computed by most contemporary EMG machines. The mean sorted difference (MSD) is also calculated and is a more accurate measure of jitter if the MCD/MSD ratio exceeds 1.25.

Assuming constant positioning of the needle in relation to the muscle fiber pair, there are five normal physiologic and anatomical factors that contribute to the interpotential interval: (1) the length of the terminal twigs, (2) the conduction velocity of the terminal twigs, (3) neuromuscular transmission time, (4) the distance between muscle fiber and recording needle, and (5) the velocity of muscle fiber action potential propagation. Of these, only three are physiologic and therefore potentially capable of varying from discharge to discharge. As long as firing rate is kept relatively constant, and the interpotential interval does not exceed 4 ms, jitter occurs almost exclusively on the basis of variable neuromuscular transmission time.

Normal values for jitter vary with patient age and the muscle selected but are typically in the 15–45-μs range. Twenty fiber pairs are usually acquired and analyzed to provide adequate statistical significance. The need to acquire this amount of data stems from the observation that MG can be as patchy electrophysiologically as it is clinically. Abnormally high jitter values can also be declared if 10% or 2 of the 20 fiber pairs have jitter values that exceed a second higher set of normative values that are also age and muscle specific. The benefit of this second set of norms is that it allows this sometimes labor-intensive test to be terminated early when strikingly abnormal.

Abnormally low jitter values are also potentially pathologic. For example, reduced jitter has been in disorders associated with myofiber splitting. Reduced jitter is uncommonly recognized as disorders with reduced jitter values are uncommonly tested with this methodology.

The second parameter that is typically sought after is neuromuscular blocking. Blocking does not typically occur until jitter values are high, typically with MCD values in excess of 100 μs. Blocking is recognized when a triggering potential, identical in morphology to previous and successive triggering potentials, is unaccompanied by a second, time-locked SFMAP (Fig. 2-26). It is of course possible that the triggering potential itself is blocked, but it is likely that this occurrence would go unrecognized. Blocking rarely occurs in seemingly normal, older individuals.

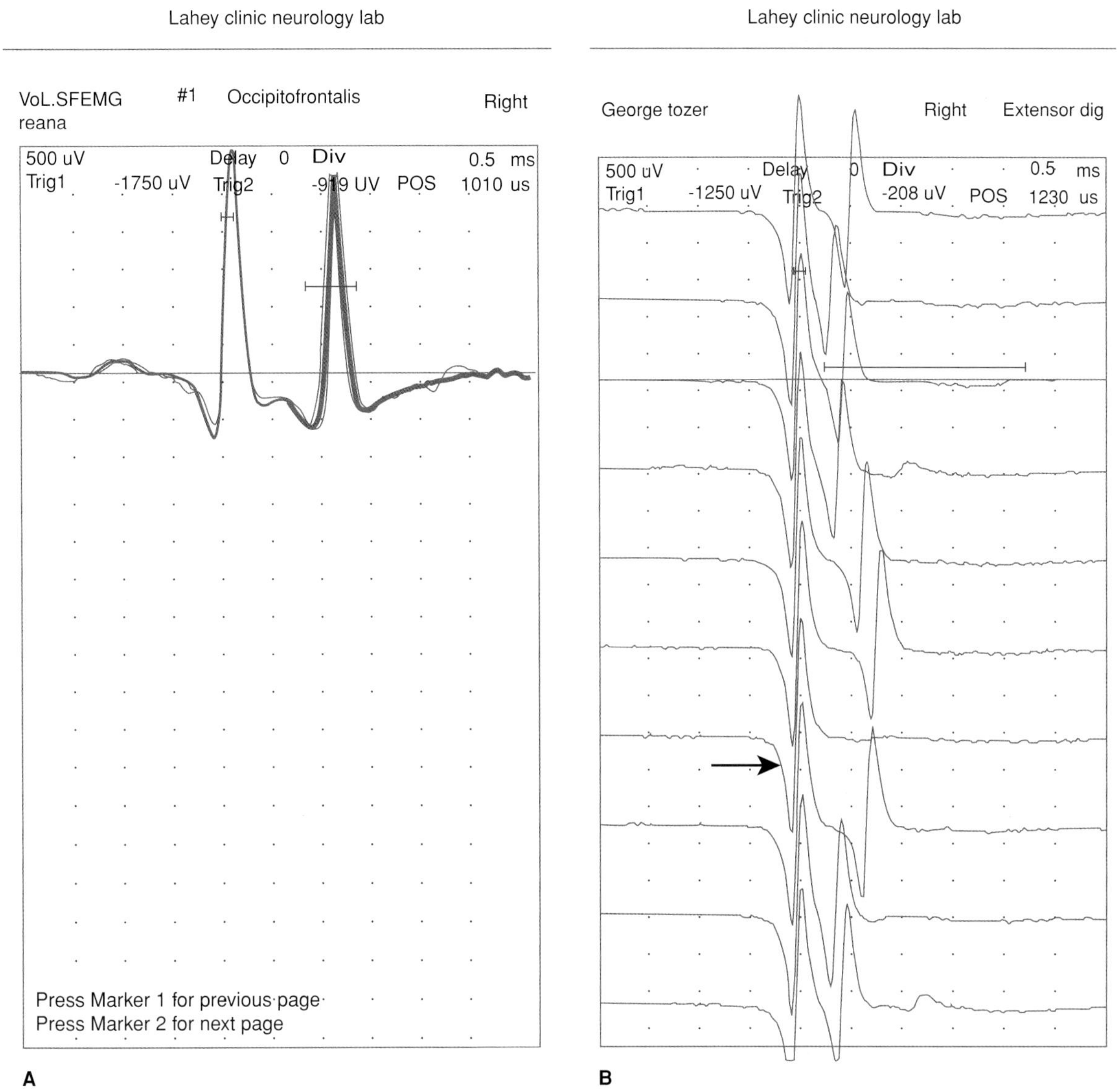

Figure 2-26. Single fiber electromyography demonstrating a normal recording (A) and increased jitter and blocking (seventh pair from top—*arrow*) (B).

Another parameter that can be measured by the SFEMG needle is fiber density, the electrophysiologic analog of reinnervation and type grouping seen on muscle biopsy. Fiber density is not as commonly used as a clinical tool as are assessments of jitter and blocking. Under normal circumstances, a random placement of the SFEMG needle will reveal only a single fiber action potential from a given motor unit 60% of the time. A couplet, that is, two SFMAPs belonging to the same motor unit will be identified in 35% of insertions and a triplet only 5% of the time. The technique for fiber density determination differs slightly from jitter measurements. The SFEMG needle is manipulated so as to obtain maximal amplitude from the first single fiber action potential that is obtained. Once that is accomplished, the number of single fiber potentials, regardless of size, that are time linked to the index potential are counted. This is done for at least an additional 19 potentials. The total number of fiber potentials is then divided by the number of test sites. For example, if 30 potentials are identified at 20 sites, the fiber density will be 1.5. Fiber density is considered an index of successful reinnervation and differs from jitter, which in denervating diseases is considered an index of immature reinnervation. Contrasting jitter values with fiber density values is one way to estimate how complete the reinnervation process is. High fiber density values with normal jitter are an indication that the reinnervation process has matured. Normative values for fiber density again vary with patient age and muscle selected and are based on measurements made with SFEMG needles.

There is another form of SFEMG referred to as stimulated SFEMG. In this technique small electrical stimuli are delivered, by a needle electrode, to a nerve fiber within the tested muscle. Jitter is then recorded from a single muscle fiber innervated by the same nerve. There are both advantages and disadvantages of this technique. As it does not depend on voluntary muscle activation, it is more readily performed on those who cannot (or will not) cooperate. As the stimulus rate does not vary as opposed to voluntary activation, a spurious MCD value secondary to varying firing rates will not occur. The time-consuming effort of finding a fiber pair is removed from consideration. Drawbacks include the recognition that normal values for jitter are less than voluntary SFEMG. The optimal frequency of stimulation has to be adjusted to ensure accurate jitter measurements; too low a rate of stimulation will produce falsely high MCD values. There is also the possibility of falsely reduced jitter values if the muscle fiber is stimulated directly, eliminating neuromuscular transmission from the equation.

The primary value of SFEMG is its enhanced sensitivity and its ability to detect delays rather than overt failure of neuromuscular transmission through the identification of increased jitter values, prior to the development of actual muscle weakness. Once a DNMT is severe enough to be produce weakness, a decremental response to repetitive nerve stimulation will be found in that muscle. As SFEMG is typically more labor intensive than RNS, SFEMG becomes superfluous unless the muscle is not readily accessible by RNS techniques. SFEMG, in a weak muscle, will demonstrate not only increased jitter (delayed neuromuscular transmission) but actual blocking or failure of neuromuscular transmission at multiple neuromuscular junctions within that muscle. Blocking is typically seen only when jitter values exceed 100 μs. As implied above, the other advantage of SFEMG other than its increased sensitivity in identifying abnormalities in muscles that are not weak is that it is a needle rather than nerve conduction technique. Accordingly, the anatomic limitations imposed by RNS are not as relevant to SFEMG where numerous muscles are readily available for study.

There are other EMG techniques that are uncommonly used in clinical settings. Macro EMG involves the use of a specialized needle with multiple recording ports. This allows waveform acquisition over a far wider recording radius than with conventional concentric or monopolar EMG needles. Macro EMG is used primarily in research settings to assess the size and distribution of SFMAP components of MUAPs.

MUAPs of increased duration and amplitude are often so strikingly different from normal MUAPs that these may be readily identified by subjective means. The distinction between normal MUAPs that are small and pathologic MUAPs that are reduced in amplitude and duration is more difficult to assess subjectively. MUAP analysis or quantitation is a technique that has been used to objectively measure the average amplitude and duration of a population of MUAPs. An abnormal result is determined by comparison of the average size of an MUAP in a studied muscle to normative data. These norms account for MUAP size variability based on patient age and muscle selected. MUAP quantitation may be used as both a clinical and, more commonly, a research tool in laboratories that offer it.

THE PATHOPHYSIOLOGY OF NERVE INJURY—ELECTRODIAGNOSTIC AND CLINICAL CORRELATES

The pathophysiology of peripheral nerve lesions can be inferred from EDX data, as can the clinical symptoms that the pathophysiologic process produces. Four different pathophysiologies can be considered from an EDX perspective, axon loss, and three forms of demyelination. The latter have been referred to as focal or uniform slowing, differential slowing also known as temporal dispersion, and conduction block. More than one of these mechanisms may coexist with any given disease or injury. There is a fifth pathophysiology of nerve to consider from at least a theoretical if not a practical basis, that being disordered function of ion channels. Neuropathies due to certain marine toxins, drugs and autoantibodies are hypothesized to produce symptoms by impaired ion channel function.

Loss of CMAP and SNAP amplitudes are the primary nerve conduction manifestations of axon loss. With axon loss, conduction slowing may occur if the largest, fastest conducting axons degenerate. Conduction slowing tends to be modest with axon loss alone unless severe. In pure axon loss, focal conduction abnormalities do not typically occur unless conduction studies are done hyperacutely before axonal degeneration takes place. The needle examination in axon loss is characterized by abnormal spontaneous activity within 1–3 weeks of disease onset, reduced motor unit recruitment immediately and enlarged, reinnervated MUPs within a matter of months. Axon loss leads to muscle atrophy and weakness, loss of all sensory modalities, and loss of deep tendon reflexes within the territories of nerves that are affected.

Demyelination may cause uniform slowing of nerve conduction. Conceptually, in uniform slowing, conduction is slowed equally in all fibers within the affected segment(s) of nerve. As all impulses traverse the affected portion of nerve synchronously, the only clinical consequence of such a lesion is paresthesia, with or without pain. Uniform slowing may occur in a focal segment of nerve as a consequence of mechanical injury. It is a common EDX signature of CTS and some ulnar neuropathies at the elbow. It may occur along the entire course of multiple nerves in the hereditary demyelinating and dysmyelinating disorders. It may occur as a consequence of disordered ion channel function as well. Historically phenytoin, a sodium channel blocker, was identified as the cause of peripheral neuropathy. This association seems to be based predominantly, if not solely, on the basis of slowed nerve conduction velocities. Clinical neuropathy associated with phenytoin use seems to be a rare event.

Differential slowing and demyelinating conduction block are almost always associated with acquired nerve disease and may occur in either a focal or a multifocal distribution. Conceptually, differential slowing results from different degrees of slowing within different nerve fibers within the same segment of nerve. Conceptually, all impulses traverse the damaged segment of the nerve successfully but at different speeds. As a result, the CMAP waveform broadens and becomes dispersed, with a resulting loss of amplitude and increased CMAP duration. Typically, the waveform takes on a serrated rather than smooth contour (Fig. 2-3). Theoretically, as all axons are conducting and all muscle fibers activated, the area under the curve remains the same. Differential slowing may occur either from mechanical nerve injury in a mononeuropathy or in a multifocal fashion in the acquired demyelinating polyradiculoneuropathies such as GBS and chronic inflammatory demyelinating polyradiculoneuropathy (CIDP). Clinically, differential slowing primarily affects clinical modalities that require synchronous impulse transmission, notably deep tendon reflexes and vibratory perception.

Conduction block usually implies demyelination affecting consecutive myelin internodes precluding effective action potential transmission in affected fibers. It is most accurately recognized when stimuli can be delivered sequentially over short segments of nerve. When a nerve is stimulated distal to the affected area, the CMAP amplitude is normal as demyelinating lesions have no upstream or downstream effect on axon viability and nerve conduction. Stimulation above the block results in a drop in CMAP amplitude and area proportionate to the number of fibers affected (Fig. 2-2B). This same phenomenon may also occur without overt demyelination, presumably on the basis of immune-mediated ion channel dysfunction.

Clinically, conduction block produces neither significant muscle atrophy, loss of the so-called small fiber modalities including autonomic functions, nor perception of pain and temperature. Significant atrophy does not occur as the trophic influence of preserved axons remains. The latter functions are preserved as small poorly myelinated or unmyelinated fibers remain relatively unscathed, as demyelinating lesions have little or no influence on these fiber types. Conduction block is the only type of demyelinating pathology that results in muscle weakness.

THE VALUE AND LIMITATIONS OF EDX

EDX studies are very helpful in certain circumstances and of limited utility in others. In essence, these can, with varying degrees of confidence, determine the following:

- The existence of a problem within the neuromuscular system.
- Where within an individual nerve the problem lies.
- The topographic pattern of that problem, for example, single nerve, single root, length-dependent, etc.
- The pathophysiology of the problem and the expected clinical consequences.
- Insight into the severity and, to a lesser extent, the prognosis of the problem.

Although disease etiology may be implied by the electrodiagnostic findings, it is rarely, if ever, defined as a direct result of EDX interpreted in isolation. Although the EDX examination is fairly sensitive and can provide support for the existence of most neuromuscular disorders, there are notable exceptions. One of these is the increasingly accepted concept of small fiber peripheral neuropathy, typically presenting with burning, hypersensitive feet. Conventional EDX techniques exclusively test large myelinated fibers. They do not adequately assess disorders that exclusively affect small myelinated or unmyelinated fibers producing distortions in perception of pain and thermal sense with or without impaired autonomic function. Other tests, described later in this chapter, in the subsequent chapter on histologic testing, and in the chapter on distal symmetric polyneuropathy (DSPN) have been used in attempts to assess small fiber integrity.

Another arena in which EDX is insensitive is in muscle disorders where both the existence and classification of myopathy may be challenging. Myopathies in which the pathology consists solely of myofiber atrophy or nondestructive internal changes of myofiber architecture can be particularly difficult. Certain endocrine, congenital, and mitochondrial myopathies are examples of this. In the myopathy of excessive corticosteroid use characterized by type II myofiber atrophy, the abnormal type II MUAPs are not detectable, as these are obscured by their initially recruited type I counterparts.

As previously mentioned, an additional drawback of EDX is the time required for the full complement of EDX abnormalities to develop following nerve injury. In addition with traumatic injuries, EDX cannot adequately distinguish between complete severance of axons with preservation of the connective tissue sheath and complete nerve transaction. This is of pragmatic importance as the current standard of care would be to attempt primary nerve reanastomosis acutely if complete nerve transaction had occurred. Another potential problem related to timing and prognosis is falsely identifying a lesion as demyelinating conduction block when it is actually axon loss in nature, a phenomenon known as pseudo-conduction block. This may occur if motor nerve conductions are performed within 5 days of injury, prior to Wallerian degeneration. In this situation, the amplitude below the lesion may be initially preserved but reduced above the lesion, thus mimicking conduction block and suggesting an inappropriately optimistic prognosis.

ELECTRODIAGNOSTIC LOCALIZATION WITHIN THE NEUROMUSCULAR SYSTEM

EDX is capable, in many cases, of clarifying or reinforcing the localization of the pathologic process within the neuromuscular system (Table 2-6). The strategy is similar to the same pattern recognition methods used clinically at the bedside. Differential diagnosis is greatly facilitated in nerve disease by anatomic categorization, that is, identifying the problem as a mononeuropathy, a monoradiculopathy, a polyradiculopathy, a polyradiculoneuropathy, a plexopathy, a multifocal

▶ **TABLE 2-6. ELECTRODIAGNOSTIC LOCALIZATION (TYPICAL PRESENTATIONS)**

Diagnosis	CMAP Amp	Cond Slow	Disp/ CB	SNAP Amp	Fibs/ PW	Other Abnl Spon Act	Prsp dnrv	MUP Size	MUP No.	Pattern
Mononeuropathy	↓	+/−	+/−	↓	Yes	+/−	No	↑	↓	Single nerve
Multifocal neuropathy	↓	No	+/−	+/−	Yes	+/−	No	+/−	↓	Multiple nerves
LD polyneuropathy	+/−	+/−	No	↓↓	Yes	No	No	↑	↓	LD symmetric LE > UE
Polyradiculoneuropathy (demyelinating)	↓	No	Yes	↓	+/−	No	+/−	+/−	↓	Diffuse non-LD
Monoradiculopathy	+/−	No	No	NL	Yes	+/−	Yes	↑	↓	Monosegmental
Polyradiculopathy	↓	No	No	NL	Yes	+/−	Yes	↑↑	↓	Polysegmental
Plexopathy	↓	No	No	↓↓	Yes	Occ Myk	No	↑↑	↓	Multiple nerves and roots in single extremity
Sensory neuronopathy	NL	No	No	↓↓	No	No	No	NL	NL	Diffuse non-LD
Motor neuron disease	↓↓	+/−	No	NL	No	+/−	Yes	↑↑	↓↓	Diffuse non-LD
Presynaptic DNMT	↓↓	No	No	NL	+/−	No	+/−		NL	Diffuse
Postsynaptic DNMT	NL	No	No	NL	+/−	No	+/−	↓	NL	Diffuse
Myopathy without abnormal spont act	+/−	No	No	NL	No	No	No	↓	NL	Diffuse or proximally predominant
Myopathy with fibs and positive waves	+/−	No	No	NL	Yes	No	Yes	↓	NL	Diffuse or proximally predominant
Myopathy with myotonia	+/−	No	No	NL	+/−	Myt	+/−	↓	NL	Diffuse, may affect facial and distal muscles

Amp, amplitude; Slow, slowing; Disp, dispersion; CB, conduction block; Abnl spon act, abnormal spontaneous activity; Prsp dnrv, paraspinal denervation; LD, length dependent; LE, lower extremity; Myt, myotonic potentials; Myk, myokymic potentials; Occ, occasional; UE, upper extremity; +/−, may or may not occur depending on severity or pathophysiology (e.g., axonal or demyelinating) of disorder.

neuropathy, a DSPN (length-dependent polyneuropathy-LDPN), or a motor or sensory neuronopathy. Neuronopathy refers to a disorder affecting the cell bodies, i.e. the anterior horn cells or dorsal root ganglia, respectively. Myopathies and DNMT have distinctive EDX signatures in most cases that allow localization to these structures as well.

Regarding localization within a nerve, there are a number of considerations. There are essentially three means to predict pathologic localization in focal nerve disease. The first involves identification of CMAP and SNAP amplitude abnormalities and understanding their localization significance. Sensory nerve conductions are abnormal in axon loss lesions affecting the dorsal root ganglion, the plexus, or the peripheral nerve. They are normal in disorders of the anterior horn, the neuromuscular junction, and muscle. They are usually normal as well in disorders affecting nerve roots, despite clinical sensory symptoms. The reason for this is not intuitive. An axon separated from its nucleus will degenerate. In disorders of the dorsal root, Wallerian degeneration takes place in a centripetal fashion, that is, toward and within the posterior column of the spinal cord. As a result, the peripheral sensory axon remains viable and capable of conducting externally applied impulses in a normal fashion, even within symptomatic regions. A normal SNAP in a clinically affected territory implies that the patient's sensory symptoms are attributable to small fiber involvement, which cannot be detected by standard NCS techniques, that the patient is feigning symptoms, or that the pathology is proximal to the dorsal root ganglia. Abnormal SNAP amplitudes in both upper and lower extremities with normal CMAP amplitudes imply disorders of the dorsal root ganglia.

Conversely, abnormal CMAP amplitudes with spared SNAPs imply a localization to anterior horn, ventral root, neuromuscular junction, muscle, or those uncommon disorders that exclusively affect motor nerve fibers within the peripheral nerve trunk. The latter possibility is most readily defined by the identification of demyelinating features confined to motor nerves. Reduced CMAP and SNAP amplitudes together imply disorders of peripheral nerve or plexus, which are in turn distinguished by the pattern of involvement within and between limbs.

The second and most precise means of localization occurs when a focal demyelinating lesion exists and is detectable. Detection requires the ability to stimulate both above and below the site of the nerve lesion. Specifically, an abrupt change in waveform latency, amplitude, or configuration occurring over a short segment of nerve implies demyelinating pathology as long as it is identified more than 7 days following symptom onset. The ability to identify these changes is however limited by anatomy and nerve accessibility. Deeply situated nerves in proximal locations are in large part inaccessible, or if accessible, cannot be stimulated comfortably or in isolation. If the lesion is purely axonal, or if the lesion is in an area that is difficult to access with NCS, nerve conductions will be able to localize the problem to the nerve but not within the nerve.

There are situations where demyelinating pathology can be implied but not proven. If a muscle is clinically weak but has a normal CMAP from all accessible points of stimulation of the nerve that innervates it, an absent F wave from that nerve and muscle suggests proximal conduction block. In a similar context, if the conduction velocity and distal latencies of a motor conduction study are normal but the F latency is prolonged, a demyelinating lesion with focal slowing at a proximal location is suggested. The third scenario arises when needle EMG is performed in a weak muscle that has a normal CMAP amplitude. Reduced recruitment occurring in the absence of abnormal spontaneous activity or morphologic changes in MUAPs implies a demyelinating conduction block pathophysiology as well. To implicate predominantly demyelinating pathophysiology in all of these situations, testing would have to occur at an interval after potential Wallerian degeneration and the development of fibrillation potentials would have had a chance to occur.

The third localization opportunity occurs in axon loss lesions in which localization can be inferred by the pattern of denervation. Here the electromyographer is hampered by at least three aspects of anatomy. Localization is limited by the anatomical location and distribution of branch points to individual muscles and their location along the course of a given nerve. In the ulnar nerve, for example, branches occur only in the hand and at the elbow, with none in the arm and forearm segments. Localization in this manner is also hindered by the tendency for fibers designated for certain muscles to be sequestered in selected fascicles. For example, it is common for ulnar forearm muscles to be spared with ulnar neuropathies occurring at the elbow. The presumption is that the fascicles containing the fibers supplying forearm muscles are rendered less vulnerable to nerve entrapment or compression by their position within the nerve, a concept referred to as selective fascicular involvement. Finally, most muscles are innervated by multiple roots. This benefits the patient but potentially confounds the electromyographer. This overlap may make it difficult to provide single root localization. As an example, most muscles innervated by the C5 myotome are also innervated by the C6 myotome and vice versa, making discrimination between these two monoradiculopathies potentially challenging.

A mononeuropathy is defined by NCS and/or EMG abnormalities confined to a single nerve distribution. Mononeuropathies are most frequently caused by external nerve compression or by entrapment within a normally existing anatomical structure rendered abnormal from mechanical or other factors. Mononeuropathies may be associated with all of the pathophysiologic processes defined above, with the possible exception of ion channel dysfunction, often in combination. Prognosis is determined by etiology as well as by the type and relative degree of pathophysiology.

A monoradiculopathy is defined when sensory conductions are normal and denervation exists in a myotomal or segmental pattern. In other words, all affected muscles should share the same root innervation but include innervations from more than one peripheral nerve. For example, in a C7 radiculopathy, denervation would be expected in both the triceps and the flexor carpi radialis muscles. Both have singular root but different nerve innervation. CMAP amplitudes are usually spared in monoradiculopathies for the following reasons. Many of the commonly affected nerve roots, particularly in the upper extremities, do not correspond to the same segments as the routinely performed conduction studies. In addition, most muscles have multiple root innervations. Even if there is significant axon loss within a given segment, potential loss of CMAP amplitude is buffered by the contribution(s) of other unaffected segments. Lastly, if root pathophysiology is predominantly demyelinating, it will not alter routine motor nerve conduction parameters.

Conceptually, all mono- or polyradiculopathies, that have some degree of axon loss and affect ventral roots, should manifest paraspinal denervation. In reality, this may not always be demonstrable. It is not uncommon to identify a segmental (myotomal) pattern of denervation with normal SNAPs in the same segment in the apparent absence of paraspinal denervation. In this situation, the electrodiagnostician should not be dissuaded from rendering an anatomic diagnosis of radiculopathy, particularly in the appropriate clinical context. In this context, it is important to realize that intraspinal pathology of any cause, for example ALS, can have an identical electrodiagnostic signature, which can be falsely localized to root disease if clinical context is not considered and a more extensive needle examination not performed.

For the most part, monoradiculopathies are most readily recognized when there is axon loss. For the reasons described above, demyelinating radiculopathies can only be inferred, may only have subtle electrodiagnostic findings, and therefore may go unrecognized.

Polyradiculopathy is defined by denervation in the distribution of multiple segments and their corresponding paraspinal musculature. Again, sensory potentials should be spared. CMAP amplitudes are more likely to be affected than monoradiculopathies, as the buffering provided by multiple root innervations is not as pronounced. As already mentioned, polyradiculopathies may be electrodiagnostically indistinguishable from early motor neuron disease, as in both cases the pattern of denervation is polysegmental with paraspinal involvement, occurring with sparing of sensory conduction parameters.

Rarely, a purely sensory polyradiculopathy affecting dorsal roots exists that can present with multifocal sensory symptoms, including sensory ataxia.[44] In these cases, localization is postulated based on imaging, somatosensory-evoked potential abnormalities, and/or dorsal rootlet biopsy result. SNAPS are normal in the symptomatic regions. H reflexes are typically absent if the S1 segments are affected. In reported cases, motor conduction studies and needle examination were normal in the majority of patients in keeping with the proposed dorsal root localization.[44]

Polyradiculoneuropathy differs conceptually from polyradiculopathy, involving nerve trunk as well as nerve root. This distinction is usually made electrodiagnostically although maybe confirmed by gadolinium-enhanced magnetic resonance (MR) imaging. The electrodiagnostic signature of polyradiculopathy is the concomitant involvement of SNAPs and paraspinal denervation. Although there are a number of potential etiologies, the most readily recognized causes of polyradiculoneuropathies are the acquired inflammatory demyelinating polyradiculoneuropathies, that is, GBS and CIDP. In these disorders, motor conduction studies are commonly replete with demyelinating features, including uniform and differential slowing (temporal dispersion) and conduction block. Some degree of axon loss is common in most cases although pure axon loss variants of GBS and CIDP do exist, making EDX more complicated. In addition, there are axonal forms of polyradiculoneuropathy, for example porphyria. In the inflammatory, demyelinating polyradiculoneuropathies, sensory conductions are affected although "sural sparing" may occur. Sural sparing refers to a non–length-dependent pattern of SNAP abnormalities where upper extremity SNAP abnormalities occur with preservation, or relative preservation of the sural, and/or superficial peroneal sensory responses. Denervation, when present in polyradiculoneuropathies, occurs on a generalized basis without length dependency and by definition affects the paraspinal muscles.

Plexopathies are typically defined when both sensory and motor abnormalities affect more than one nerve and nerve root distribution confined to a single limb, both clinically and electrodiagnostically. There are exceptions. Specific etiologies of plexopathy such as acute brachial plexus neuritis may affect more than one limb, in either a clinically evident or an occult basis. Plexopathies affect both SNAP and CMAP amplitudes. In most cases, SNAPS are affected to a greater degree than CMAPS although brachial plexus neuritis with a predilection toward pure motor nerves such as the long thoracic or anterior interosseous provides a notable exception to this generalization. In this disorder, the pattern may actually conform more to multifocal neuropathy confined to the upper limb, rather than to an anatomically defined plexopathy. In acute brachial plexus neuritis, the pathology may extend beyond the boundaries of the brachial plexus to involve other nerves such as the recurrent laryngeal and phrenic. When the CMAP amplitudes are affected disproportionately to the SNAPS, concomitant involvement of the ventral roots should be considered. The pattern of denervation in plexopathy varies with etiology. A plexopathy is best defined electrodiagnostically when the pattern of abnormalities identifies and is only explained by pathology in a distinct plexus element, for example, the upper trunk of the brachial plexus. In traumatic and inflammatory plexopathies, localization to a single plexus component is the exception rather than the rule. In a true anatomic plexopathy, sparing of paraspinal musculature is expected.

Polyneuropathies will be discussed here in four categorical domains: multifocal neuropathy, DSPN, sensory neuronopathy, and motor neuronopathy, a.k.a. motor neuron disease. Although it is unusual to discuss motor neuron diseases in the context of polyneuropathies, it is done so here as it is conceptually difficult to discuss disorders affecting dorsal root ganglia (which can phenotypically resemble polyneuropathy) without discussing disorders of their anterior horn cell counterparts.

Multifocal neuropathy is a pattern of neuropathy that has been referred to as mononeuritis multiplex or multiple mononeuropathies by others. As described in Chapter 1, we have purposely avoided the use of mononeuritis multiplex as it has the pathologic implication of inflammation that may not exist. We have avoided the term multiple mononeuropathies as it may imply to some a benign disorder of multiple nerve compression or entrapments. The value of the multifocal neuropathy construct is that it implies a readily recognizable pattern of neuropathy affecting multiple nerves in multiple locations. Multifocal neuropathy typically results from a limited number of disorders that are capable of either infarcting or infiltrating peripheral nerve, often occurring in the context of an associated systemic disease. It is diagnosed when EDX abnormalities occur in multiple nerve distributions, typically in an asymmetric fashion. Typically, there is both sensory and motor involvement, although both pure motor and perhaps pure sensory variants exist. When multifocal neuropathies are either pure motor or sensory, distinction from the neuronopathies may be difficult. The pathophysiology is usually axonal. If the pattern is demyelinating, hereditary liability to pressure palsy (HNPP), multifocal-acquired demyelinating sensory and motor neuropathy (MADSAM or the Lewis–Sumner syndrome), or if purely motor, multifocal motor neuropathy (MMN) should be considered. Electrodiagnostic definition of multifocal neuropathy often requires a careful historical review as well as an extensive electrodiagnostic examination with fastidious attention to detail.

DSPN is the most common polyneuropathy phenotype. Signs and symptoms first occur in the most distal aspects of the longest nerves in a symmetric or near-symmetric fashion. DSPN is defined electrodiagnostically when both sensory and motor abnormalities are identified in a symmetric, length-dependent fashion. For example, muscles innervated by the L5 and S1 myotomes in the foot should be affected to a greater extent than their analogs in the leg which in turn should be affected more than L5–S1 innervated muscles in the thigh or hip region. As the etiologies of DSPN are usually toxic, metabolic, or hereditary, an axonal pathophysiology usually predominates. A predominantly demyelinating DSPN pattern is most commonly seen in hereditary neuropathies and in a few acquired neuropathies such as those associated with IgM monoclonal proteins. Other acquired demyelinating neuropathies such as AIDP and CIDP are more correctly categorized as polyradiculoneuropathies and can be commonly distinguished from length-dependent DSPN through features such as sural sparing.

Many DSPNs appear to be predominantly sensory in nature, both from a clinical and nerve conduction study basis. There are at least three potential reasons for this. SNAPs are typically affected earlier and to a greater extent than their

CMAP counterparts. The second potential explanation is anatomical. At onset, involvement of sensory nerve endings in the toes commonly produce symptoms that are typically positive (pain and paresthesias) and are therefore easily recognized. Conversely, clinical detection of motor abnormalities in the intrinsic foot muscles is rendered difficult by the duplicate function of leg muscles which also contribute to toe flexion and extension. Only toe abduction/adduction, a function difficult to clinically assess, is controlled solely by intrinsic foot muscles. Lastly, the detection of motor involvement in DSPN may be obscured by an electromyographic bias. In the author's experience, many patients with normal CMAP amplitudes in intrinsic foot muscles and no detectable weakness will be found to have fibrillation potentials and/or positive wave in intrinsic foot muscles. As the intrinsic foot muscles are frequently avoided by many electromyographers, the opportunity to identify subclinical motor involvement may be overlooked.

Sensory neuronopathies or dorsal root ganglionopathies, as these are sometimes called, are typically caused by toxic, inflammatory, or infectious mechanisms. Although there is a tendency toward length dependency, asymmetric and often subtle non–length-dependent areas of abnormality are key to their detection, either by clinical or by EDX means. Multifocal reductions in SNAP amplitudes are the hallmark of these disorders. The most readily definable pattern of sensory neuronopathy is when upper extremity SNAPs are reduced to the same extent or more than their lower extremity counterparts, without involvement of lower extremity CMAPs. This pattern of sensory nerve conduction abnormalities is analogous to the pattern of sural sparing described above. In sensory neuronopathies however, unlike the inflammatory myelinating polyradiculoneuropathies, both motor conduction and needle EMG abnormalities are by definition absent.

Motor neuronopathies or motor neuron diseases are commonly degenerative, hereditary, or infectious. The pattern of weakness varies with cause. Sensory conductions are normal except in Kennedy disease or when there is a second, potentially confounding disorder. The pathophysiology appears to be that of axon loss, occurring in a polysegmental pattern early in the disease or diffusely when the disease is more established. Denervation occurring in a nerve or length-dependent distribution pattern should suggest an uncommon motor neuropathy. Once again, with the exception of the potential of prolonged H reflex, latencies polyradiculopathy, the NCS and EMG pattern of motor neuronopathies and polyradiculopathy may be electrodiagnostically indistinguishable.

Presynaptic DNMTs are usually multifocal if not diffuse in their topographic distribution, both clinically and electrodiagnostically. They are more likely to be symmetric in manifestation than their postsynaptic counterparts Their hallmark is CMAP amplitude reduction with SNAP sparing. As described above, the hallmark of presynaptic DNMTs are CMAP amplitudes that increment after brief exercise or in response to repetitive stimulation at rates of 5 Hz or more. A decremental response to slow repetitive stimulation may be demonstrated if sought for. Fibrillation potentials occur in botulism but are infrequent in the Lambert–Eaton myasthenic syndrome (LEMS). MUAPs may be normal or reduced in size, that is, small in amplitude, short in duration, and polyphasic in configuration. Like all DNMT, motor unit variability will be demonstrable in a clinically affected muscle if sought for. Recruitment may be concomitantly increased.

Postsynaptic DNMTs have an electrodiagnostic signature that overlaps with its presynaptic counterpart. As a general rule abnormalities may be more focal and therefore more difficult to identify in postsynaptic disorders. The major discriminator is that CMAP amplitudes are typically normal at rest in post-synaptic disorders except in the most severe cases. The typical EDX strategy in post-synaptic disorders is to perform routine conductions and needle examination first to potentially identify other pure motor disorders. In postsynaptic DNMT, routine conductions are typically normal. Decremental responses are then sought for at rest, and if necessary with 1 minute of intervening exercise. The latter will increase the probability of demonstrating a pathologic decrement if not evident at rest. If demonstrated, a decrement can be repaired by brief exercise (10 seconds), fast repetitive stimulation (10–50 Hz), or by the administration of edrophonium. The latter requires proper monitoring precautions.

A clinically weak muscle in MG should demonstrate a decremental response to 2–5-Hz repetitive stimulation in all cases, as the decrement is the EDX analog of clinical weakness. This may be easy to accomplish in generalized MG but elusive in patients whose signs and symptoms are restricted to the oculomotor system. As in the case of presynaptic DNMT, MG spares sensory potentials and may be associated with small MUPs. Fibrillation potentials are uncommon but may occur when receptor sites are damaged sufficiently to essentially denervate muscle fibers.

EDX AS A PROGNOSTIC TOOL

The extent to which EDX is used as a prognostic tool undoubtedly varies from laboratory to laboratory. EDX assessment of prognosis can be ascertained in many different ways.[45] In general, demyelinating lesions are likely to resolve quickly (weeks to months) and completely if their cause is eliminated. There are certain disorders such as radiation injury and MMN in which conduction block may persist. The prognosis for axon loss lesions is more uncertain and depends on the degree and location of the injury, as well as the age and comorbidities of the patient. The severity of the lesion is best judged by the amplitudes of the SNAP and CMAP responses. Severely reduced CMAP amplitudes, in the absence of demyelinating conduction block, imply that a limited number of residual axons are available for collateral sprouting, and a large number of orphaned muscle fibers are in need of reinnervation. Prognosis for significant recovery in these situations is guarded. Prognosis is also determined in axon loss lesions by the distance between the injury and the target. For example, in brachial plexus injuries, improvement in biceps and deltoid function occur far more frequently than return of hand function. Although fibrillation potentials in neurogenic disease indicate axon loss, grading systems for fibrillation potentials are not adequately linear or quantitative enough to utilize in disease prognostication.

In ALS, rapid disease progression correlates with at least three recognized electrodiagnostic patterns. These are an abundance of fibrillation potentials associated with modest changes of chronic denervation and reinnervation, prominent MUP variability, and rapid MUNE decline.[29,46]

Prognosis in the GBS had been linked to a composite of CMAP amplitudes. Although reduced CMAP amplitudes could represent demyelinating conduction block in terminal nerve twigs, they are more likely to represent axon loss with the more pessimistic prognosis for rapid recovery that it portends.[47] The identification of conduction block at the elbow in combination with a normal CMAP when stimulating distally suggests an 86% likelihood of full subjective recovery from an ulnar neuropathy at the elbow.[48]

QUANTITATIVE SENSORY TESTING

QST is used in both clinical and research settings, in an attempt to provide measurements of small myelinated and unmyelinated nerve functions.[48–52] Peripheral neuropathies, in most cases, are thought to be pathologically indiscriminate and affect peripheral nerve fibers of all sizes. The concept of small fiber neuropathy (SFN) recognizes the existence of a select group of neuropathy patients in whom the signs and symptoms suggest preferential injury to small, poorly myelinated (A-delta) or unmyelinated (C) peripheral nerve fibers less than 7 μm in diameter.[53–55] As mentioned above, conventional EDX does not assess small fiber viability and function and is therefore of limited utility in SFN unless larger myelinated fibers are concomitantly affected. Quantitative sensory techniques represent an attempt to fill this diagnostic gap as well as to provide a potential tool for epidemiologic studies and therapeutic trials. It also provides a potential means to screen for subclinical neuropathy in industries where the potential for neurotoxic exposure exists.[49,50,56] Two other techniques that may also be used in SFN assessment, autonomic testing and the assessment of intraepidermal nerve fiber density (INFD) via skin biopsy, will be discussed in the next section and next chapter, respectively. The latter technique is reported to have a sensitivity of 88% and a specificity of 91% in the diagnosis of SFN.[57] This sensitivity may exceed that of QST and ANST although the test results may not be concordant, implying the potential benefit of using multiple testing modalities in SFN suspects.[57–60]

Clinically, SFN, as discussed in detail in Chapter 21, is considered to be DSPN subtype. SFN is estimated to represent 5% of the DSPN population.[54,58,61] The natural history of SFN may include evolution into a more typical DSPN phenotype with both small and large fiber involvement.[57] Other patterns of SFN involvement are suspected, although there is no current diagnostic gold standard to define the limits of phenotypic expression. Typically, patients complain of painful, often burning paresthesias with associated cutaneous hypersensitivity. In its purest form, the only abnormalities on clinical examination in SFN, if any, are diminished perception of thermal sensation and either diminished or enhanced response to painful stimuli. Vibratory perception is either normal for age or diminished mildly at the toes. Motor, reflex, and EDX examinations are commonly normal unless large fiber involvement is also present.[53,58,61]

QST is a psychophysical test whose accuracy is dependent on optimal control of multiple environmental variables including patient understanding and cooperation.[50] Understandably there are certain patient populations in whom testing is unlikely to succeed. Although the stimuli delivered are quantified, the patient responses are largely subjective. There are numerous testing algorithms, used by different commercial vendors, that have been developed in an attempt to make QST as accurate, reproducible, and efficient as possible.[62] It is unclear which existing algorithm achieves these goals with the most success. Results are very much dependent on the patient population studied, the environment in which they are studied, as well as the equipment and testing algorithm used.[50,63] QST should not be used as the sole means to detect nerve pathology nor should it be relied upon for dispute resolution in a medical–legal venue.[64]

It is beyond the scope of this chapter to provide a detailed discussion of QST algorithms. There are a number of different paradigms used in terms of both stimulus threshold and reproducibility of result. Threshold algorithms attempt to identify the smallest stimulus intensity perceived, the smallest difference in stimulus intensity perceived, or the lowest stimulus intensity that provides a given magnitude of response, for example, pain. Reproducibility algorithms are dynamic paradigms, which involves ramping stimulus intensity up or down until identical thresholds are identified. Results are considered abnormal when these exceed 95% of age-matched norms. In contrast to threshold testing algorithms, static stimuli are delivered as individual stimuli of set duration and intensity. Either flanking or forced choice algorithms can be used. The 4–2–1 paradigm is the most frequently used flanking algorithm. If a stimulus is perceived, the stimulus is reduced by four orders of magnitudes at a time until no longer perceived, then increased by two levels of magnitude until recognized, and then reduced by one order of magnitude. In a sense, the process "zeros in" on the threshold. The forced choice paradigm provides paired stimuli, one of which is null. The true stimulus varies in intensity, and the null stimulus varies randomly in its order of delivery.[33]

The most commonly used QST testing algorithms assess thresholds for cooling and vibration, particularly in a diabetic population.[65] In SFN, the expectation is that thermal thresholds would be affected disproportionately to those for vibration. Although QST is used predominantly for suspected peripheral neuropathy, one of its limitations is that it tests the entirety of the somatosensory system. Accordingly, abnormal test results have no localizing value. One potentially beneficial, although unvalidated, application of QST is its use in topographical areas not readily accessible to conventional EDX.[66] For example, provides a theoretical means to evaluate sensory complaints of the trunk or genitalia.

QST has been studied in a number of clinical applications. Thermal testing may be abnormal in diabetic patients before the onset of symptoms or abnormal EDX.[56,67–69] In uremic patients, altered vibratory thresholds seem to be more prevalent than their thermal counterparts in presumed neuropathy.[70] Conversely, impaired thermal threshold may be the first abnormality to occur, and the paradoxical heat perception resulting from a cold stimulus may also occur in the uremic population.[71,72] QST is frequently applied in the evaluation of the frequently painful distal sensory neuropathy in the HIV population.[64,73]

In studies conducted to date, QST sensitivity for the detection of SFN has ranged from 60% to 85%. In general, this sensitivity in the detection of small fiber pathology is similar to both quantitative sudomotor axon reflex testing (QSART) discussed below and epidermal nerve fiber density discussed in the following chapter.[53]At least one study has suggested that INFD provides a more sensitive means to confirm small fiber involvement.[58] In general however, the information derived from different testing modalities utilized in an attempt to identify SFN are universally more complementary than overlapping. Accordingly, multiple modalities may be required both to identify small fiber dysfunction, and to convince the physician that an abnormal result is valid.[74] As QST abnormalities may reflect either peripheral or central nervous system pathology, and in consideration of their apparently similar thresholds for detection of abnormalities within the peripheral nervous system, abnormal QST coupled with normal epidermal nerve fiber density should provoke consideration of central nervous system pathology.[54]

AUTONOMIC NERVOUS SYSTEM TESTING

Symptoms that implicate dysautonomia can be classified as either cholinergic, adrenergic, or as sudomotor in nature. Orthostatic intolerance manifested as lightheadedness or fainting, fading of visual or auditory perception, and fatigue or nuchal discomfort are all symptoms that may result from impaired sympathetic vasomotor tone. In an older population, orthostatic intolerance may manifest as cognitive change without the perception of lightheadedness.[75] Other symptoms of impaired sympathetic function include ptosis and impaired ejaculation. Symptoms of cholinergic dysautonomia include blurred vision and photophobia from impaired pupillary constriction, impotence, resting tachycardia, the sicca complex of dry eyes and dry mouth, urinary retention, gastroparesis, and intestinal pseudo-obstruction. Symptoms of sudomotor dysfunction relate to disordered sweating. The latter may manifest as dry feet or somewhat paradoxically by hyperhidrosis in unaffected areas in an attempt to compensate for hypohidrosis in other topographic distributions.

Detecting pathologic involvement of the autonomic nervous system provides at least three potential applications in the evaluation of patients with neuromuscular disease. In patients with suspected neuropathic pain without signs of large fiber neuropathy, for example, burning feet and suspected SFN, ANST provides a means to document small myelinated (A-delta) or unmyelinated (C) nerve fiber involvement. In patients with large fiber, sensory motor neuropathies, ANST may allow documentation of autonomic involvement. By doing so, it may limit differential diagnostic considerations and focus evaluation.[44,76,77] As there are a limited number of diseases that have combined somatic and autonomic neuropathy, ANST can facilitate this strategic approach (Table 2-7).[78–82] Finally, the coexistence of dysautonomia with somatic peripheral neuropathy provides potential prognostic insight. In diabetic neuropathy in particular, dysautonomia significantly contributes to morbidity and adversely affects life expectancy.[83]

The pharmacology of the autonomic nervous system is complex but integral to the understanding of ANST. In way of brief and simplified review, all preganglionic neurons of both the parasympathetic and the sympathetic nervous

▶ TABLE 2-7. PERIPHERAL NEUROPATHY ASSOCIATED WITH DYSAUTONOMIA

Idiopathic

Immune mediated
- Paraneoplasia
- Guillain–Barré syndrome

Infiltrative
- Primary systemic amyloidosis

Metabolic
- Porphyria
- Diabetes mellitus

Toxic
- *cis*-Platinum
- Vinca alkaloids
- Perhexilene
- Hexacarbons
- Thallium
- Arsenic
- Acrylamide
- Taxol
- Lead
- Pesticides
- Pyridoxine toxicity

Hereditary
- Familial amyloidosis
- Hereditary sensory and autonomic neuropathy types I–IV
- Fabry's disease
- Tangier's disease
- Mitochondrial disorders

systems are thinly myelinated and use ACh as their primary neurotransmitter. The postganglionic receptors which these affect are populated by nicotinic receptors whose activation is blocked by hexamethonium. These ganglionic receptors are thought to represent the targets for circulating autoantibodies found in the serum of approximately half of autoimmune autonomic neuropathy patients.[75] Although nonautonomic cholinergic receptors on skeletal muscle are also nicotinic, they differ pharmacologically. These receptors are blocked by curare and are the target of different antibodies, particularly the ACh receptor antibodies of MG.

The postganglionic parasympathetic fibers synapse with muscarinic cholinergic receptors on the end organs that they innervate. There are at least three types of muscarinic receptors in the body. M1 receptors are found in the cerebral cortex and 5% of sympathetic ganglia, M2 receptors are found primarily in the heart, and M3 receptors populate secretory glands.[84] Atropine is the primary antagonist at these receptors.

The majority of postganglionic sympathetic neurons release norepinephrine as their primary neurotransmitter. The notable exceptions to this rule are sweat glands, smooth muscle fibers within the walls of blood vessels populating skeletal muscle that promote vasodilatation, and some of the chromaffin cells of the adrenal medulla. All of these are cholinergic in nature. There are four currently recognized types of adrenergic receptors, two alpha and two beta. Alpha-1 receptors mediate vasoconstriction, intestinal relaxation, and pupillary dilation, components of the primordial flight response. Alpha-2 receptors are presynaptic in location and inhibit norepinephrine release. Activation of beta-1 receptors, which may be induced by both epinephrine and norepinephrine, increase both heart rate and contractility. Beta-2 receptors are primarily receptive to the effects of epinephrine and are most prevalent in the smooth muscle of blood vessels within muscle. Stimulation of beta-2 receptors results in vasodilatation.

ANST provides a means by which to detect cardiovagal, adrenergic, and postganglionic sudomotor dysfunction.[85] ANST encompasses an extensive list of testing modalities that are capable of assessing autonomic nervous system function, most of which are beyond the scope of this chapter.[63,86] The most commonly utilized tests assess cardiovagal function through heart rate responses to deep breathing, the Valsalva maneuver, and tilt table testing, adrenergic function through blood pressure responses to the Valsalva maneuver and tilt table testing, and sudomotor function through QSART. Illustrations of normal and abnormal responses to these tests are provided in Figures 2-27 to 2-29.

In normal individuals, the heart rate will accelerate in response to inspiration and the associated increased venous return to the right heart and will decelerate in response to expiration (sinus arrhythmia). This response will diminish as a normal consequence of aging. The afferent receptors for this reflex include pulmonary stretch receptors, cardiac mechanoreceptors, and possibly baroreceptors.[86] Sinus arrhythmia is a consequence of normal, parasympathetic, cardiovagal tone. There are numerous protocols that address both the performance and the measurement of heart rate variability. Commonly the patient is positioned with the head up 30 degrees from supine. The patient is asked to breath slowly and steadily at a rate of 6/min (5-second inspirations and 5-second expirations), usually for a period of 1 minute. Heart rate response to deep breathing can be measured either by the greatest difference between the fastest and slowest rate that occur during this interval or by the calculation of an *E* (expiration) to *I* (inspiration) ratio. In our laboratory, and in our illustrations, the average of the greatest difference between the fastest and slowest rate for the six trials is utilized. The E:I ratio is calculated by measuring the shortest (*I*) and longest (*E*) intervals between QRS complexes (R–R interval) as a singular, summed, or averaged value. As the heart rate is the slowest during expiration, the R–R interval increases accordingly resulting in an *E:I* ratio of >1. There are published, age-matched normative data for both of these parameters. The mean heart rate variation in heart rate in a teenager is 30 beats per minute (bpm) with the 5th to 95th percentile range being 14 to 41 bpm. Between 60 and 69 years of age, the mean heart rate variation is closer to 18 with the 90% of normals being in the 7–27 bpm range.[77,78]

The physiology of the Valsalva maneuver is more complex. The patient is asked to sustain a constant expiratory pressure of 40 mm Hg for approximately 15 seconds by exhaling into a mouth piece attached to a manometer. A slow leak in the system is provided. Both heart rate and blood pressure responses are monitored during and in the immediate aftermath of this maneuver. Four distinct phases are discernible, the first and third and the first part of the second phase (IIA) are mechanical in nature and phase IIB and IV result from autonomic nervous system response to these mechanical events. During the first phase, there is a transient increase in blood pressure resulting from direct mechanical compression of the aorta to increased intrathoracic pressure. Phase IIA also results from increased intrathoracic pressure and is defined by a drop in blood pressure occurring from reduced venous return to the heart. Phase III is initiated with glottic release and a resultant decline in intrathoracic pressures. Blood pressure transiently declines as relatively collapsed intrathoracic venous structures can now readily refill and temporarily limit venous return.

Phase IIB is normally identified by rising blood pressure that approaches baseline. This is promoted by increased vasomotor tone mediated by the increased alpha adrenergic output of the sympathetic nervous system. During the entirety of phase II, heart rate increases as a consequence of cardiovagal withdrawal. During phase IV, blood pressure rises and pulse declines under normal circumstances, with over- and undershoots of their respective baseline values. Increasing blood pressure is due to increased venous return and cardiac output coupled with the persistent effects of increased, sympathetically mediated vasomotor tone. The cardiovagal effects that are measured during the Valsalva maneuver can be quantitated by calculating the Valsalva ratio, the fastest heart rate

Test Results

Analysis type : HRDB **Analysis ID** : 423
Analysis date : 08/25/2006 **Analyst** : HRDB
Analysis comments:

Max rate	Min rate	Rate difference
75.0	58.0	17.0
78.0	57.0	21.0
76.0	58.0	18.0
76.0	65.0	11.0
76.0	62.0	14.0
77.0	63.0	14.0
	Avarage HR difference:	15.8

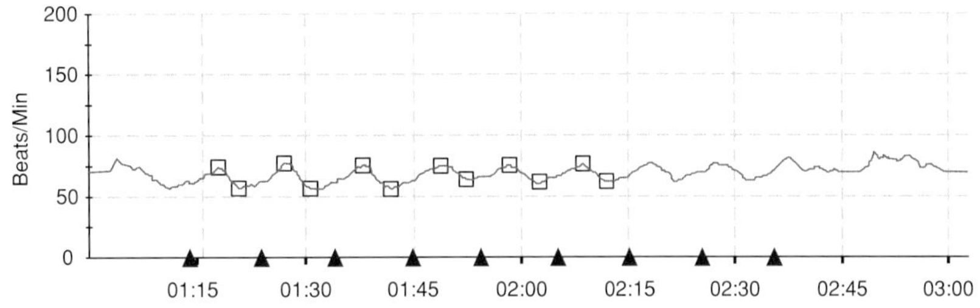

A

Test Results

Analysis type : HRDB **Analysis ID** : 63
Analysis date : 01/31/2007 **Analyst** : HRDB
Analysis comments :

Max rate	Min rate	Rate difference
61.0	52.0	9.0
62.0	54.0	8.0
59.0	55.0	4.0
60.0	56.0	4.0
60.0	57.0	3.0
59.0	57.0	2.0
	Average HR difference:	5.0

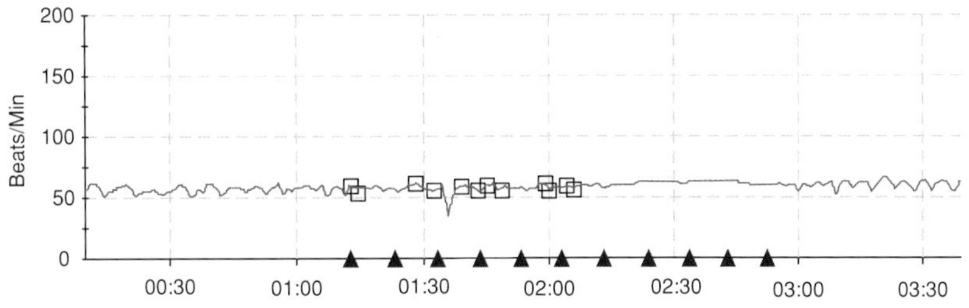

B

Figure 2-27. Normal (average heart rate difference 15.8) **(A)** and abnormal (average heart rate difference 5.0) **(B)** heart rate responses to deep breathing.

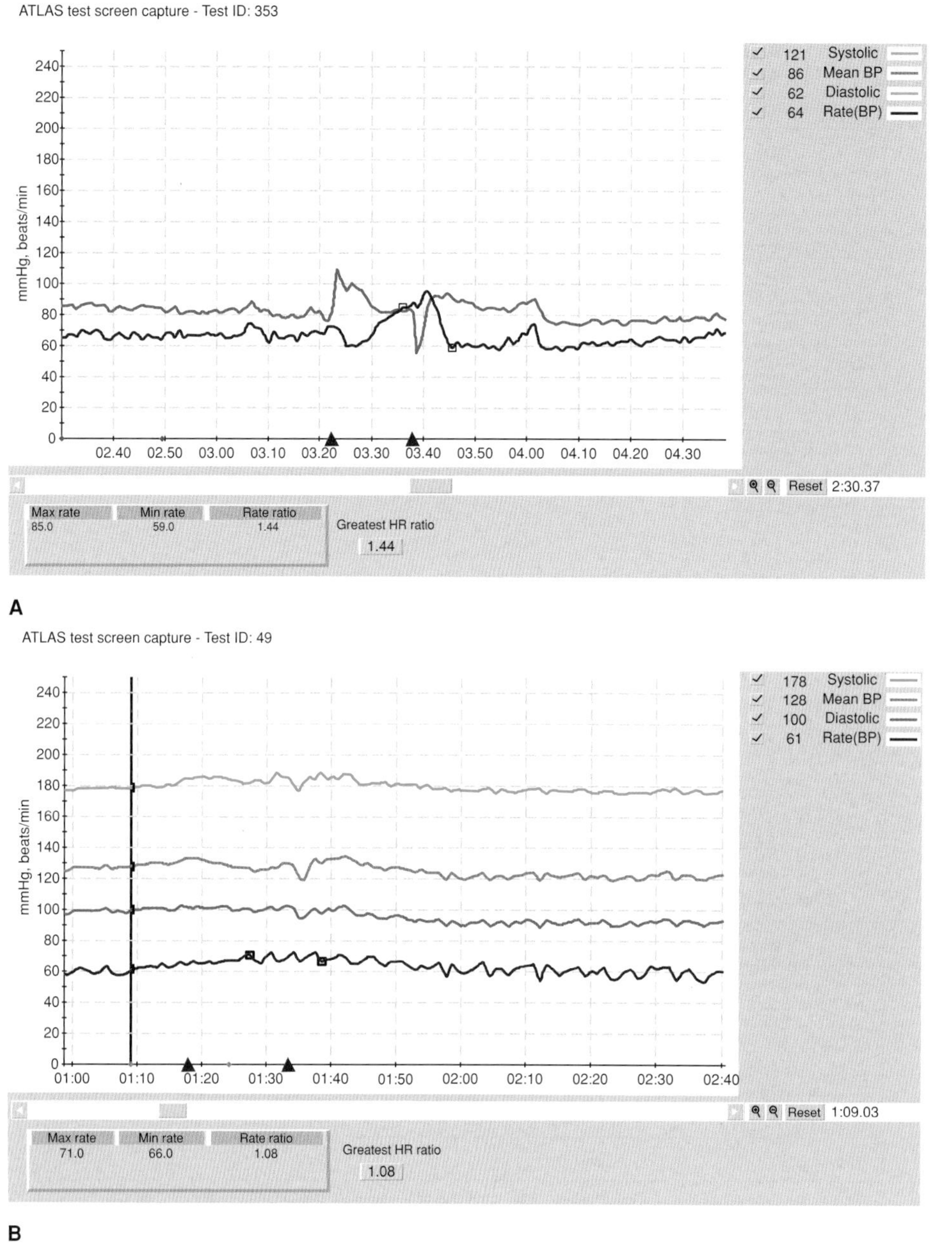

Figure 2-28. Normal **(A)** and abnormal **(B)** responses to the Valsalva maneuver. *Red line,* heart rate; *green line,* mean arterial blood pressure. First *pink triangle,* glottic closure; second *pink arrow,* glottic release.

during phase II divided by the slowest rate recorded during phase IV. Normative data for the Valsalva ratio are readily available.[77] The ratio does not change as dramatically with age and gender as do other autonomic parameters. A normal ratio averages 1.6 for males and 1.5 for females during their teenage years. Abnormal sympathetic responses are best identified by a failure of both blood pressure rise during phase IIB and blood pressure overshoot during phase IV to occur.[86]

Tilt table testing is used to assess heart rate and blood pressure in response to standing in a controlled but somewhat artificial environment. The primary utility is to explore potential mechanisms of syncope or near syncope. Normally, despite a 25–30% shift in venous blood from central to peripheral compartments with assumption of the upright position, rapid compensatory responses from the autonomic nervous system preclude major changes in either pulse or blood pressure.[86] Orthostatic hypotension is frequently defined as a drop in either systolic blood pressure of $\geq$20 or diastolic blood pressure of $\geq$10 mm Hg. Typically, symptoms do not develop until systolic blood pressure drops of 30 or diastolic pressures of 15 mm Hg occur. Orthostatic hypotension usually occurs either immediately or within a few minutes of standing. A drop in blood pressure with an associated tachycardia suggests hypovolemia of whatever cause.

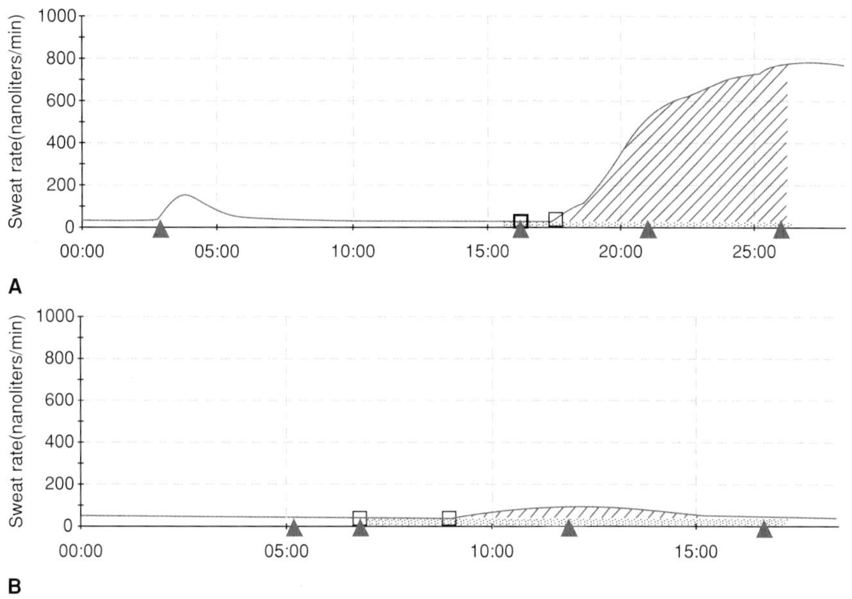

Figure 2-29. Normal **(A)** and abnormal **(B)** responses to quantitative sudomotor axon reflex testing. First *green triangle*, ACh injection; second *green triangle*, 2 mA stimulus begins; third *green arrow*, stimulus ceases; fourth *green arrow*, 5 minutes post stimulus cessation.

A drop in blood pressure without compensatory tachycardia implicates dysautonomia due to disease or drug effect. Symptomatic tachycardia with a heart rate ≥30 bpm above baseline without a significant drop in blood pressure is the signature of the postural orthostatic tachycardia syndrome. Finally, prolonged tilt table monitoring may be utilized in an attempt to reproduce symptoms in patients believed to suffer from neurocardiogenic syncope (vasovagal syncope). In these patients, symptoms of impaired CNS blood flow are accompanied by hypotension and paradoxical bradycardia.

QSART is a means to assess cholinergic, postganglionic sympathetic sudomotor function.[87,88] It is particularly attractive as a test for SFN and other DSPNs with dysautonomic components. It can be applied in numerous topographical locations and is therefore potentially capable of identifying a length-dependent pattern of hypohydrosis. Typically, QSART is performed by placing sweat capsules in four standardized locations: the dorsum of the foot, shin, thigh, and forearm. These capsules measure the humidity produced by sweat production emanating from the tested skin surface in response to an injected intradermal cholinergic stimulus. The sensitivity of QSART in the detection of SFN has been quoted as being 60–80%, similar to QST.[53,58,89–92] In diabetic patients, there are similar rates of both sensitivity and concordance regarding results of the heart rate response to deep breathing, the Valsalva maneuver, and QSART.[93] Normative data for QSART also varies by gender, age and area tested.[77] Mean values range between 1 and 3 μL/cm squared.

ANST, perhaps more than any other testing modality, requires adequate control of environmental variables that may readily confound the accuracy of test results. Normative data vary considerably with patient age. Ideally, testing would be performed in some who is adequately hydrated, has not eaten for 8 hours, nor smoked tobacco, drank ethanol or caffeine, and has not been recently physically or emotionally stressed. Drugs that potentially react with adrenergic or cholinergic receptors are to be avoided if possible, including those with indirect autonomic effects such as insulin. Extremes of temperature or pressure stockings can adversely affect the outcome of testing procedure.[77]

Currently, ANST is recommended as a consideration in patients with suspected SFN or autonomic neuropathy phenotypes.[85] Neither the American Academy of Neurology, nor the authors recommend ANST as part of the routine evaluation of patients with DSPN without clinical suggestion of autonomic nervous system involvement. Heart rate variability to deep breathing is felt to have a greater than 90% sensitivity and greater than 97% specificity for the identification of dysautonomia in a diabetic neuropathy cohort, in the absence of confounding cardiac disease.[85] QSART is reported to have a sensitivity exceeding 75% in detecting sudomotor abnormalities in a population with a SFN phenotype.[85] Like QST, it is felt that both the sensitivity and specificity of ANST is improved upon either performance of a battery of tests rather than a single test.[85]

BLOOD TESTING

There is limited evidence that to identify a sensitive, specific, and cost-effective laboratory evaluation strategy for most neuromuscular syndromes. As evaluations for specific neuromuscular syndromes will be addressed in detail in subsequent chapters of this book, they will be mentioned here only in summary terms. An ideal blood test would be cost effective, and accurate in identifying or excluding a specific disorder in a tested population. There are few tests that conform to this description, ACh receptor (AChR) binding antibodies being arguably the best example.

ROUTINE BLOOD TESTING FOR PERIPHERAL NEUROPATHY

Peripheral neuropathy is a common neuromuscular problem, often associated with a nonspecific phenotype, and associated with an extensive list of potential causes. Numerous publications and clinical experience indicate that a significant number of these individuals will go undiagnosed despite extensive evaluation.[94,96] Understandably, there is an incentive to test extensively in an attempt to fill in this gap. There are many published algorithms that attempt to provide neurologists with an ideal battery of screening tests for peripheral neuropathy.[31,65,95,97,98] One of these is a recent practice parameter constructed by the American Academy of Neurology.[85,99] Their recommendations are that fasting blood sugar, vitamin B12 levels and serum protein electrophoresis are the only blood tests currently recommended in the patient with a typical, sensory predominant, axonal DSPN. A more extensive evaluation is justified when there are atypical phenotypic features.[95] Specifically, a neuropathy with acute–subacute onset, a multifocal or non–length-dependent pattern, associated with significant sensory ataxia or with associated systemic symptoms is worthy of a more aggressive diagnostic approach that could include more extensive blood work, CSF analysis, imaging or histological analysis of nerve or other relevant tissues.[75] As the selection of additional tests is dependent on both the neuropathy phenotype, as well as in the context in which the neuropathy occurs, recommendations concerning selection of other tests will be provided in the following paragraphs, rather than in a algorithmic format.

Deficiency of vitamin B1, B6, B12, E, and folic acid are potentially causally related to peripheral neuropathy. In addition, a sensory neuropathy/neuronopathy may occur with vitamin B6 toxicity in daily doses that are estimated to exceed 200 mg.[100] Other than for B12, testing for vitamin deficiency is generally not recommended on a routine basis and is generally reserved for those patients perceived to be at higher risk.[98] This group would include patients with a sensory predominant neuropathy who are at risk of nutritional deficiency due to alcoholism, dietary anomalies, isoniazid exposure, and malabsorption from bariatric surgery or enteral disease such as celiac sprue. Symptom onset in the hands may indicate a myeloneuropathy, a common presentation of vitamin B12 deficiency. Measurements of serum levels of methylmalonic acid may improve detection of this latter disorder when B12 levels are in the borderline 200–300 ng/L range. As copper deficiency produces a phenotype in many ways identical to B12 deficiency, determination of serum copper and ceruloplasmin levels are recommended with any evaluation for myeloneuropathy.

Serum monoclonal proteins (MCPs) have been recognized to occur with an increased prevalence in patients with polyneuropathy for decades. Most MCPs associated with peripheral neuropathy will initially be designated as being of unknown significance (MGUS). The neuropathy associated with MGUS may vary depending on MCP type but is typically a nonspecific, sensory > motor, and length-dependent phenotype. Both the clinical and EDX features implicate a primarily axonal, DSPN phenotype in neuropathies associated with IgG and IgA MCPs.[101,102] In these cases, the association between the neuropathy and MGUS is statistical; a causal relationship remains unproven.

The best evidence for a causal relationship for MGUS exists in patients with an IgM kappa MCP. IgM kappa-related neuropathy has a very distinctive demyelinating sensory-predominant phenotype, frequently with sensory ataxia. This is in turn often associated with antibodies directed toward myelin-associated glycoprotein in a significant percentage of cases. These antibodies will be discussed further in the following section.

A small percentage of patients with an MCP at the time of initial evaluation and a larger percentage subsequently will have a secondary cause. Multiple myeloma, amyloidosis, lymphoma, cryoglobulinemia, or POEMS syndrome are noteworthy examples. A lambda, rather than a kappa, light chain increases the probability of a secondary cause of an MCP. Secondary causes of MCP-related neuropathy often have more distinctive phenotypes. For example, polyneuropathy, organomegaly, endocrinopathy, monoclonal protein and skin changes (POEMS) syndrome is often associated with a motor-predominant, demyelinating, non–length-dependent CIDP phenotype. Serum measurements of vascular endothelial growth factor (VEGF) may represent a serum marker for this disease and may aid discriminating POEMS from other disorders associated with neuropathy, an MCP and multi-organ involvement.[103,104] Amyloidosis may manifest with a number of phenotypes such as a small fiber phenotype with prominent dysautonomia or as a severe multifocal, axonal, sensorimotor neuropathy[105] MCPs or light chains can be detected in these disorders in serum and/or urine by immunoelectrophoresis or preferably by immunofixation. The latter is more sensitive but is also more labor intensive. For these reasons, it is not used as a default screening procedure by many laboratories.

Diabetic neuropathy is common and is associated with multiple phenotypes. It is estimated to be the cause of neuropathy in 15–30% of North American patients.[97,98,106] The diagnosis of diabetic neuropathy is dependent on the fulfillment of criteria outlined by the American Diabetes Association and by the association with one or more of the characteristic clinical and EDX diabetic neuropathy phenotypes.[107] Although thickening of the basal membranes of the vasa nervorum demonstrable by nerve biopsy is characteristic of diabetes, the role of basement membrane thickening in the pathogenesis of diabetic nerve injury remains uncertain. A direct causal relationship between diabetes and neuropathy is only suggested pathologically. Alternative causes of peripheral neuropathy should always be considered in diabetic patients, particularly if the phenotype is atypical. The American Diabetes Association indicate that an elevated (fasting blood sugar) ($\geq$124 mg/dL) an abnormal 2-hour glucose tolerance test ($\geq$200 mg/dL), or an elevated hemoglobin AIC ($\geq$6.5%) are diagnostic of diabetes mellitus.[94] Traditionally, neuropathy was not readily attributed to diabetes unless the diagnosis of diabetes was well established. More recently, a statistical association has been demonstrated between impaired glucose tolerance (FBS 110–125 mg/dL, GTT 140–199 mg/dL, hemoglobin A1 C between 5.7 and 6.4%) and a SFN phenotype.[108–111]

In patients with a multifocal neuropathy pattern, particularly those of acute to subacute onset, screening blood tests relevant to this pattern of neuropathy are recommended. The odds of identifying an underlying cause, particularly a systemic disease, is much higher in this phenotype than in DSPN. Notable considerations include serum and urine immunofixation, sedimentation rate and/or c-reactive protein, eosinophil count and tests for anti-cytoplasmic neutrophilic antibodies, rheumatoid factor, SS-A and SS-B antibodies, angiotensin converting enzyme, and Lyme and HIV serology.[112] In these patients, relevant imaging, CSF evaluation for potential neoplastic meningitis which may mimic a multifocal neuropathy, and potential nerve biopsy should be additional considerations.

Blood testing for heavy metals known to cause peripheral neuropathy (arsenic, lead, mercury and thallium) has a limited role in the evaluation of patients with peripheral neuropathy. The reasons are, both the rarity of the conditions and the short circulating half-life of the toxic substances. Neuropathies resulting from heavy metal exposure are frequently motor predominant and commonly coexist with central nervous system and systemic symptoms such as abdominal pain, hair, skin, and nail changes. Blood testing is most likely to be helpful in the setting of an acute monophasic exposure. Urine, nail, and hair assessments are more likely to be positive with chronic low-level exposures. One particular pitfall is the possibility of false-positive urine arsenic testing resulting from seafood ingestion. Many seafood species contain significant amounts of the relatively innocuous pentavalent forms of arsenate as opposed to the more toxic trivalent arsenate species.

ROUTINE BLOOD TESTING FOR MYOPATHY

Measurement of serum creatine kinase (CK) is a valuable adjunct in the evaluation of patients with neuromuscular disease.[113] Although considered to be primarily a marker of muscle disease, increased serum CK levels commonly occur in ALS and other neurogenic disorders. Conversely, elevated CK levels do not occur in all myopathies. In normal individuals, levels may reach 5× the upper limits of normal following EDX or other invasive medical procedures and perhaps as high as 50× the upper limits of normal in extreme, protracted exercise. Levels increased by any of these provocations should return to normal by 1 week after the event but have been reported to remain elevated for 3 weeks following eccentric exercise involving protracted muscle contraction.[114,115] The level of CK does not appear to correlate with the degree of muscle destruction or weakness.

Elevations of serum CK may occur in asymptomatic individuals. Normal CK levels vary with gender, race, age, muscle mass, and physical activity. A recent population study demonstrated that 13% of whites, 23% of South Asians, and 49% blacks had CK measurements at rest that exceeded manufacturer's upper limits of normal.[116] At the extreme, the upper limits of normal (97.5th percentile) for serum CK in their black male population was 801 IU.[116] What may appear to be an abnormality may not be so in an individual when normative data for gender and race are considered. As neuromuscular specialists commonly evaluate patients with elevated CK levels, both with and without statin exposure, knowledge of this variability in normal populations becomes quite important.

Recognizing that a certain percentage of patients with hyperCKemia are likely to be normal, there are undoubtedly inherited neuromuscular conditions in which elevated serum CK levels may be pre-penetrant, that is exist in individuals with disease causing mutations who have yet to develop recognizable signs or symptoms. It is equally plausible that many of these patients with "idiopathic hyperCKemia" harbor sequence alterations in various muscle proteins that are not "disease causing" but capable of causing CK "leak."

There are other blood tests that may be helpful in the identification of specific muscle diseases. Measurement of serum lactate, although neither sensitive nor specific, provides a screening test for certain mitochondrial myopathies. Serum carnitine levels may be extremely low in primary carnitine deficiency. A plasma acylcarnitine profile may be helpful in suspected disorders of lipid metabolism, particularly multiple acyl-dehydrogenase deficiency. A peripheral blood smear may be helpful in identifying lipid-containing vacuoles within leukocytes known as Jordan bodies which may be found in neutral lipid storage disorders.

DNA MUTATIONAL ANALYSIS

Genetic testing is an evolving and complex diagnostic tool for neuromuscular disease. There are many nuances associated with genetic testing that the neuromuscular clinician should be familiar with before ordering DNA testing, This is particularly true with an asymptomatic patient at perceived risk. This is also true when attempting to counsel a patient regarding the implications of their genetic test result, whether it be positive or negative. Many of the heritable disorders discussed in this book are Mendelian in nature, that is, a single gene mutation is sufficient to cause disease. Increasingly, the cryptic world of complex genetics is coming slowly into focus. There are probably far more mutations that confer increased risk for disease development in concert with some other genetic or environmental influence, than cause disease independently in a Mendelian fashion. A specific example of genetic complexity, even within the domain of Mendelian genetics, is the recognition that specific mutations may behave differently in those with different ethnic origins. For example the G90A mutation of the SOD1 gene causes an ALS phenotype in Scandinavians only in the homozygotes. In non-Scandinavians, it behaves as a dominantly inherited disease.

Another complexity is the recognition that not all sequence alterations within known disease-related genes are mutations that will cause disease. Such sequence alterations may represent benign polymorphisms and some occur so infrequently that we are not yet aware whether they are pathogenic or not. In addition, incomplete penetrance must be considered. That is, not all patients carrying a known disease producing mutation will become symptomatic during their lifetime.

Genotype–phenotype correlations are also complex. As mentioned above, differing phenotypes may evolve from mutations of a single gene. For example, mutations of the lamin A/C gene may cause distinctive phenotypes including Charcot–Marie–Tooth disease (CMT), Emery–Dreifuss muscular dystrophy, congenital muscular dystrophy, and an adult onset limb-girdle muscular dystrophy phenotype. Conversely, many similar, if not identical, phenotypes arise from mutations arising from different genes on multiple chromosomes. For example, there are now over 35 recognized genotypes of CMT. Both the identification and exclusion of pathologic mutations may be rendered difficult for a number of reasons. We do not know all of the pathologic mutations for most diseases. Even with known genotypes, there are multiple mutation mechanisms, not all of which may be identified by the technology used by the laboratory called upon to detect it.

DNA mutational analysis is most commonly employed to diagnose symptomatic individuals. These tests may also be applied to individuals who are understandably concerned about future risk. When used in these latter situations, it is incumbent upon the ordering physician to be fully cognizant of all potential ramifications of the testing result and to provide fully informed consent. This would include the implications of both positive and negative results. It must also consider the potential impact on other family members whose genotype may be inadvertently illuminated. Both patient and physician should be aware that these costly tests are often not reimbursed by third party payers in presymptomatic individuals.

In the neuromuscular realm, mutational analysis is available for selected genotypes of an increasing number of motor neuron, peripheral nerve, neuromuscular junction and muscle diseases. Disorders for which testing is readily available are listed in Table 2-8. The web site www.genetests.org represents an updated, valuable resource to identify laboratories capable of performing genetic testing in specific diseases. Other mutational analyses may be available in research laboratories. Specific genetic disorders and testing are discussed in detail in subsequent chapters of this book.

Increasingly, physicians, institutions, payers, and patients are struggling to identify the appropriate paradigm for genetic testing, one that balances the considerable cost with the value to patient, physician, and society as a whole. Ideally, precise phenotyping would allow for genetic confirmation or exclusion by utilizing a single test or rational algorithm, making cost considerations more manageable. Attempts have been undertaken, for example in Charcot–Marie–Tooth (CMT) disease, to provide logical, while at the same time, cost-effective strategies with which to approach this problem.[99,117,118] There are clear benefits provided by confirming a disorder to have a genetic etiology. These include diagnostic closure, thus eliminating the need for further diagnostic and for the most part therapeutic intervention. In addition, the opportunity for more accurate genetic counseling is provided. Nonetheless, current realities are that genotype identification rarely alters either patient management or the natural history of the patient's disease. The ethical dilemma of distributional justice, that is, whether the cost of genetic testing is justified by these limited benefits to both patient and society is a rhetoric question that will remain unanswered by the authors.

Most hereditary neuropathies fall within the boundaries of CMT and produce morbidity largely limited to the peripheral nervous system, There are also inherited neuropathic syndromes, largely confined to the peripheral nervous system that do not conform to the CMT phenotype. These include seven recognized mutations producing five different phenotypes of hereditary sensory and autonomic neuropathy, the hereditary motor neuropathies (distal spinal muscular atrophy), and familial brachial plexus neuropathies.[119]

BIOCHEMICAL TESTING FOR INBORN ERRORS OF METABOLISM

There are numerous but uncommon inherited metabolic diseases, many of which may have neuromuscular manifestations. Axons of peripheral nerves axons and their surrounding myelin sheaths appear to be particularly vulnerable to heritable, metabolic disturbances. This is presumably due to their configuration and the complex metabolic requirements necessary to maintain the health of a structure that may exceed 1 m in length.[119] Although DNA mutational analysis may be utilized in some cases, diagnostic confirmation is usually achieved by biochemical or at times by pathologic means. In many cases, reduced levels of the gene product are sought, for example, reduced alpha-galactosidase levels in Fabry disease. In other cases, elevated levels of a substance resulting from the "synthetic or degradation road block"

▶ TABLE 2-8. **COMMERCIALLY AVAILABLE DNA ANALYSES FOR NEUROMUSCULAR DISEASE (BLOOD)**

Disease Category	Type	Gene Location	Gene Product
Motor neuron disease	fALS 1 (20%)	AD 21q	Superoxide dismutase 1
	fALS 4	AD 9q34	Senataxin
	fALS 6 (4%)	AD/AR 16p11.2	Fusion in sarcoma (FUS)
	fALS 8	AD 20q13.3	Vesicle associated binding protein (VABP)
	fALS 9	AD 14q11.2	Angiogenin (ANG)
	fALS 10 (4%)	AD 1p36.2	TDP43
	fALS 11	AD 6q21	FIG-4
	fALS/FTD (25%)	AD9p21.2	C9ORF72
	SMA I-IV	AR 5q	Survival motor neuron gene 1
	X-linked spinobulbar muscular atrophy	X 11q	Androgen receptor gene
Muscular dystrophy	Duchenne/Beckers	X 21p	Dystrophin
	Limb girdle 2 A	AR 15q	Calpain 3
	Limb girdle 2B	AR 2p	Dysferlin
	Limb girdle 2 C	AR 13q	Gamma sarcoglycan
	Limb girdle 2D	AR 17q	Alpha sarcoglycan
	Limb girdle 2E	AR 4q	Beta sarcoglycan
	Limb girdle 2 F	AR 5q	Delta sarcoglycan
	Limb girdle 2I	AR 19q13.3	Fukutin-related protein
	Limb girdle 1B	AD 1q21.2	Lamin-A/C
	Limb girdle 1 C	AD 3p	Caveolin 3
	Myotonic DM1	AD 19	Dystrophica myotonia protein kinase
	Myotonic DM2	AD 3	Zinc finger protein 9
	FSH	AD 4q35	D4Z4 locus
	Oculopharyngeal	AD 14q	Polyadenylate-binding protein nuclear 2
	Emery–Dreifuss	X 28q	Emerin
		AD 1q	Lamin-A/C
		Xq27.2	FHLM1
Congenital muscular dystrophy	Bethlem myopathy	AD 2q37, 21q22.3	Collagen type VI
	Ullrich congenital muscular dystrophy	AR 2q37, 21q22.3	Collagen type VI
	LMNA related	AR 1q21.2	Lamin A/C (LMNA)
	Rigid spine syndrome	AR 1p36–p35	Selenoprotein
	CMD with integrin α7 mutations	AR 12q13	Integrin α7
	Walker–Warburg syndrome CMD type 1 C	AR 19q13.3	Fukutin-related protein
	Fukuyama CMD	AR 9q31	Fukutin
	Merosin deficiency CMD	AR 6q22–23	Laminin α2
Channelopathies	Myotonia congenita	AD 7q	Chloride channel protein—CLCN1
	Potassium-aggravated myotonia	AD 17q23.1–q25.3	Sodium channel protein type 4 subunit alpha
	Paramyotonia congenita	AD 17q23.1–q25.3	Sodium channel protein type 4 subunit alpha
	Schwartz–Jampel syndrome 1 (chondrodystrophic myotonia)	AR 1p36.1	Basement membrane-specific heparan sulfate proteoglycan core protein
	Hyperkalemic periodic paralysis	AD 17q23.1–q25.3	Sodium channel protein type 4 subunit alpha
	Hypokalemic periodic paralysis 1	AR 1q32	Voltage-dependent L-type calcium channel subunit alpha-1 S
	Hypokalemic periodic paralysis 2	AD	Sodium channel protein type 4 subunit alpha
Glycogen storage disease	*Type II:* Pompe disease	AR 17q	Acid alpha 1–4 glucosidase
	Type IIB: Danon disease (x-linked vacuolar cardiomyopathy and myopathy	Xq24	Lysosome-associated membrane glycoprotein 2
	Type IV: Forbes–Cori disease	AR 1p21	Glycogen debranching enzyme
	Type IV: GBE1-related disorders *(polyglucosan disease, congenital hypotonia, isolated adult myopathy)*	AR 3p12	1,4-alpha-glucan-branching enzyme
	Type V: McArdle disease	AR 11q	Myophosphorylase
	*Type VII:*Tarui disease	AR 12q13.3	Phosphofructokinase

(continued)

▶ TABLE 2-8. **(CONTINUED)**

Disease Category	Type	Gene Location	Gene Product
	Type IX: Phosphorylase b kinase deficiency	Xq13 Xp22.2–22.1 AR 16q12–13 AR 16p12.1–11.2	Phosphorylase b kinase
	Type X: Phosphoglycerate mutase deficiency	AR 7p13-p12.3	Phosphoglycerate mutase 2
	Type XI: Lactate dehydrogenase A deficiency	11p15	Lactate dehydrogenase A
	Type XIII: Enolase 3 deficiency	17pter-p12	Beta enolase
Lipid storage myopathy	Carnitine deficiency	AR 5q31.1	Solute carrier family 22 member 5
	Carnitine palmitoyltransferase deficiency IA	AR 11q	Carnitine palmitoyltransferase I
	Carnitine palmitoyltransferase deficiency II	AR 1p	Carnitine palmitoyltransferase 2
	Neutral lipid storage disease with myopathy	AR 11p15.5	Patatin-like phospholipase domain-containing protein 2
	3-hydroxyacyl-CoA dehydrogenase deficiency	AR 4q22–26	Hydroxyacyl-CoA dehydrogenase
	Acyl–CoA dehydrogenase deficiency, shot/branched chain	AR 10q25–26	Short/branched chain specific acyl-CoA dehydrogenase
	Long-chain 3-hydroxyacyl-CoA dehydrogenase deficiency	AR 2p23	Trifunctional enzyme subunit alpha
	Multiple acyl-0CoA dehydrogenase deficiency (glutaric aciduria II)	AR 15q23–25 AR 19q13.3 AR 4q23-qter	Electron transfer flavoprotein
	Short-chain acyl-CoA dehydrogenase deficiency	AR 12q22-qter	Short-chain specific acyl-CoA dehydrogenase deficiency
	Long-chain 3-hydroxyacyl-CoA dehydrogenase deficiency	AR 17p13	Long-chain specific hydroxyacyl-CoA dehydrogenase
Mitochondrial myopathies	Kearns–Sayre syndrome	Maternal mtDNA	
	PEO with mitochondrial DNA deletions PEOA1	AD 15q25	DNA polymerase gamma 1
	MELAS	Maternal mtDNA	NADH-ubiquinone oxidoreductase chain 1 or mitochondrial tRNA leucine 1
	MNGIE	AR 15q25	DNA polymerase gamma 1
	NARP	MT-ATP6 Nucleotide 8993	ATPase synthase subunit a
	SANDO MIRAS	AR 15q25	DNA polymerase gamma 1
Neuropathy CMT	Type 1 A	AD 17p11.2	Peripheral myelin protein 22 (duplication)
	Type 1B	AD 1q	Myelin protein 0
	Type 1 C	AD 16p	Lipopolysaccharide-tumor necrosis factor-alpha factor
	Type 1D	AD 10q	Early growth response protein 2
	Type 1E	AD 17p	Peripheral myelin protein 22
	Type 1 F	AD 8p	Neurofilament triplet L protein
	Type 2A1	AD 1p36.2	Kinesin-like protein
	Type 2A2	AD 1p36.2	Mitofusin
	Type 2B1 (EDMD2) (LGMD1B) (CMD)	AD 1q21.2	Lamin A/C
	Type 2 B2	AD 19q13.3	Mediator of RNA polymerase II transcription subunit 25
	Type 2 C	AD 12q24.1	Transient receptor potential cation subfamily V member 4

▶ TABLE 2-8. **(CONTINUED)**

Disease Category	Type	Gene Location	Gene Product
	Type 2D (dSMA V)	AD 7p15	Glycyl-t RNA synthetase
	Type 2E/1 F	AD 8p21	Neurofilament light polypeptide
	Type 2 F	AD 7q11.2	Heat shock protein beta-1
	Type 2 H/2 K	AD 8q13–21.1	Ganglioside-induced differentiation-associated protein 1
	Type 2I	AD 1q22	Myelin protein 0
	Type 2 J	AD 1q	Myelin protein 0
	Type 2 L	AD 12q24	Heat shock protein beta-8
	Type 2 N	AD 16q22	Alanyl-tRNA synthetase
	Type 4 A	AR 8q13–21.1	Ganglioside-induced differentiation-associated protein 1
	Type 4B1	AR 11q22	Myotubularin-related protein 2
	Type 4 B2	AR 11p15	Myotubularin-related protein 13
	Type 4 C	AR 5q32	SH3 domain and tetratricopeptide repeats-containing protein 2
	Type 4D	AR 8q24.3	Protein NDRG1
	Type 4E	AR 10q21.1–22.1	Early growth response protein 2
	Type 4 F	AR 19q31.1–13.2	Periaxin
	Type 4 H	AR 12p11.2–13.1	FYVE, RhoGEF, and PH domain-containing protein 4
	Type 4 J	AR 6q21	Polyphosphoinositide phosphatase mitofusin 2
	Type 6 (with optic atrophy)	AR 1p36.2	
	X-linked type 1	Xq13.1	Gap junction beta-1 protein
	X-linked type 5	Xq22–24	Ribose-phosphate pyrophosphokinase 1
	DNM2-related	AD 19p13.2	Dynamin-2
	HNPP	AD17p11.2	Peripheral myelin protein 22 (deletion)
Familial amyloid polyneuropathy		AD18q11.2–12.1	Transthyretin
Congenital myasthenic syndromes	AGRN-related CMS (familial limb girdle myasthenia)	AR 1pter-p32	Agrin
	CHAT-related CMS	AR 10q11.2	Choline O-acetyltransferase
	CHRNA1-related CMS (slow and fast channel syndromes)	AR or AD 2q24–32	Acetylcholine receptor subunit alpha
	CHRNB1-related CMS (slow channel syndrome)	AR or AD 17p12–11	Acetylcholine receptor subunit beta
	CHRND-related CMS (slow and fast channel syndromes)	AR or AD 2q33–34	Acetylcholine receptor subunit delta
	CHRNE-related CMS (slow channel syndrome)	AR or AD 17p13–p12	Acetylcholine receptor subunit epsilon
	COLQ-related CMS	AR 3p25	Acetylcholinesterase collagenic tail peptide
	DOK7-related CMS (familial limb girdle myasthenia)	AR 4p16.2	Protein DOK7
	MuSK-related CMS	AR 9q31.3–32	Muscle skeletal receptor tyrosine protein kinase (rapsyn)
	RAPSN-related CMS	AR 11p11.2–11.1	43-kDa receptor-associated protein of the synapse
	SCN4 A-related CMS	AR 17q23.1–25.3	Sodium channel protein type 4 subunit alpha
Congenital myopathies	ACTA1-related CFTD	AD 1q42.1	Actin
	SEPN1-related CFTD	AR 1p36–35	Selenoprotein N
	TPM-related CFTD	AR or AD 1q22–23	Tropomyosin alpha-3 chain
	ACTA1-related nemaline myopathy	1q42.1	Actin
	CFL2-related nemaline myopathy	14q12	Coflilin-2
	NEB-related nemaline myopathy	AR 2q22	Nebulin
	TNNT1-related nemaline myopathy	AR 19q13.4	Troponin T
	TPM2-related nemaline myopathy	AD 9p13.2–13.1	Tropomyosin beta chain

(continued)

▶ TABLE 2-8. (CONTINUED)

Disease Category	Type	Gene Location	Gene Product
	TPM3-related nemaline myopathy	AD or AR1q22–23	Tropomyosin alpha-3 chain
	Myotubular	AD 19p13.2	Dynamin-2
	Myotubular	AR 2q14	Myc box-dependent-interacting protein 1
	Myotubular	Xq28	Myotubularin
	Central core disease	AD 19q13.1	Ryanodine receptor 1
	RYR-1-related multiminicore disease	AR 19q13.1	Ryanodine receptor 1
	SEPN-1 multiminicore disease (rigid spine)	AR 1p36–35	Selenoprotein N
Myofibrillar myopathy	Alpha-B crystallinopathy	AD 11q22.3–23.1	Alpha crystalline B chain
	BAG3-related myofibrillar myopathy	AD 10q25.2–26.2	BAG family molecular chaperone regulator 3
	Desminopathy	AD or AR 2q35	Desmin
	Filaminopathy	AD 7q32	Filamin-C
	Myotilinopathy	AD 5q31	Myotilin
	Zaspopathy	AD 10q22.2–23.3	LIM domain-binding protein 3

fALS, familial amyotrophic lateral sclerosis; SMA, spinal muscular atrophy; FSH, facioscapulohumeral; MELAS, mitochondrial encephalomyopathy, lactic acidosis and stroke-like episodes; CMT, Charcot–Marie–Tooth; HNPP, hereditary liability to pressure palsy; SPG, spastic paraplegia gene; MNGIE, mitochondrial neurogastrointestinal encephalomyopathy; CPEO, chronic progressive external ophthalmoplegia; NARP, neuropathy, ataxia, retinitis pigmentosa; SANDO, sensory ataxia neuropathy, dysarthria and ophthalmoplegia; MIRAS, mitochondrial recessive ataxia syndrome; dSMA, distal SMA; LGMD, limb girdle muscular dystrophy; EDMD, Emery–Dreifuss muscular dystrophy; CMD, congenital muscular dystrophy; CMS, congenital myasthenic syndrome; CFTD, congenital fiber type disproportion.

created by the deficient gene product may be the means by which the diagnosis is achieved. Phytanic acid buildup due to phytanic acid oxidase deficiency in Refsum disease is an example of the latter. The major inherited disorders that may associate with peripheral neuropathy and the most common means to achieve diagnostic confirmation are summarized in Table 2-9. DNA mutational analysis for many of these disorders is available only through research laboratories. Again, www.genetests.org is a valuable resource in this regard.

Biochemical testing to confirm the diagnosis of an inherited neuromuscular disorder is not confined to the realm of peripheral neuropathy. Western blot for dysferlin may be performed on peripheral monocytes for evaluation of LGMD2B or Miyoshi myopathy. Dried blood spot analysis for alpha-glucosidase activity is an outstanding screening test for Pompe disease (acid maltase deficiency). Some advocate that this test should be done routinely on all newborns, as there is now enzyme replacement therapy available for this lethal disease. The test should be considered for all children and adults with myopathy and prominent ventilatory failure or limb-girdle pattern of weakness.[120]

SEROLOGIC TESTING

There is a wide spectrum in the value of serologic tests available in the evaluation of neuromuscular disease.[121] At one end of the spectrum are ACh receptor binding antibodies that are sensitive, specific and undoubtedly of pathophysiologic relevance. On the other hand, there are commercially available antibodies that have at best a tenuous relationship to disease causation and any phenotype. Like all testing, the specificity of antibody testing is increased when a hypothesis-driven approach is used. Ideally, a specific test is ordered to support or confirm a clinically suspected diagnosis. When large panels are ordered indiscriminately, an opportunity facilitated by industry marketing practices, the probability of a false-positive result increases.[61,67,119]

This section will address those antibody tests that are commercially available, that appear to represent legitimate markers of specific neuromuscular phenotypes, and have adequate sensitivity to warrant their use when clinically indicated. Tests with limited sensitivity and/or specificity are purposefully omitted. In the patients with peripheral neuropathy, the yield of antibody tests will increase in patients with subacute courses, demyelinating pathophysiology, multifocal distributions, and phenotypes restricted to either a motor, sensory, or autonomic domain.[75] Chronic neuropathies that are length dependent, predominantly axonal, and sensorimotor in their characteristics are less likely to associate with abnormal serologic tests of diagnostic significance.

Current evidence would support this clinically driven approach. In one study of 79 patients with cryptogenic polyneuropathy, 6% were found to have significant titers of one of the four commonly tested antibodies (anti-Hu, anti-GM1, anti-MAG, and antisulfatide).[122] Two of these five individuals had nonspecific phenotypes not typically correlated with the detected antibody considered to represent false-positive results. With neurologic paraneoplastic antibodies, significant antibody titers were found in less than 1% of cases considered to be at high risk of paraneoplastic syndromes.

Paraneoplastic Antibodies

It is estimated that approximately 5% of patients with peripheral neuropathy will be found to have cancer with aggressive

▶ TABLE 2-9. **INHERITED METABOLIC DISEASES ASSOCIATED WITH PERIPHERAL NEUROPATHY**[119]

Category	Disorder	Locus	Gene Product	Test[a]
Familial amyloid polyneuropathy		AD18q11	Transthyretin	DNA sequencing Tissue diagnosis
		AD11q23	Apolipoprotein A-1	Tissue diagnosis
		AD9q34	Gelsolin	Tissue diagnosis
Leukodystrophy	Metachromatic	AR22q13	Arylsulfatase	Arylsulfatase A deficiency in leukocytes Sulfatide excretion in urine Tissue deposition of metachromatic lipid deposits DNA sequencing or targeted mutation analysis
	Krabbe	14q31	Galactocerebrosidase	Galactocerebroside deficiency in leukocytes DNA sequencing or targeted mutation analysis
	Adrenal	XR	ATP-binding cassette subfamily D member 1	C26–C22 long chain fatty acid ratio DNA sequencing or duplication/deletion analysis
Peroxisomal	Refsum	AR10pter-p11.2 AR6q22-q24	Phytanoyl-coA hydroxylase (90%) PEX7 (10%)	Phytanic acid Phytanoyl-coA hydroxylase enzyme activity (fibroblasts) DNA sequencing
	Fabry	XRq22	Alpha galactosidase A	Alpha galactosidase A DNA sequencing
Lipoprotein deficiency	Tangiers	XR9q22	ATPase-binding cassette 1	↓ HDL ↑ triglycerides
	Cerebrotendinous xanthomatosis	AR2q33	CYP27A1	↑ cholestanol ↓ cholesterol ↑ bile alcohols DNA sequencing
	Abetalipoproteinemia			↓ beta-lipoproteins, LDL, and VLDL
Porphyria	Acute intermittent	AD11q	Porphobilinogen deaminase	↑ urinary delta amino levulinic acid/porphobilinogen Erythrocyte hydroxymethylbilane synthase/porphobilinogen deaminase activity DNA sequencing and mutation scanning
Defective DNA maintenance	Xeroderma pigmentosa	AR3p25	XPC	DNA sequencing
	Ataxia telangiectasia	AR11q22	ATM	↑ alpha-fetoprotein ATM protein immunoblotting DNA sequencing and mutation scanning
Mitochondrial	MNGIE	AR ECGF1	Thymidine phosphorylase	↑ thymidine ↓ thymidine phosphorylase (leukocytes) DNA sequencing
Miscellaneous	Giant axonal neuropathy	AR16q24	Gigaxonin	Nerve biopsy DNA sequencing
	Neurofibromatosis type 1	AD17q11	Neurofibromin	Protein truncation testing DNA sequencing Nerve biopsy
	Neurofibromatosis type 2	22q12	Merlin	DNA sequencing DNA mutation scanning Nerve biopsy

[a]All tests use blood unless otherwise designated.
MNGIE, mitochondrial neurogastrointestinal encephalomyopathy; HDL, high density lipoprotein; LDL, low-density lipoprotein; VLDL, very low density lipoprotein.

investigation.[123] In most cases, the neuropathy will conform to a nonspecific DSPN phenotype. Accordingly, there is uncertainty as to whether the relationship is causal or coincidental. A subacute course, recognition of a suspicious phenotype such as sensory neuronopathy, and in particular, identification of a "paraneoplastic antibody" increases the likelihood that the cancer and neuropathy are related. Paraneoplastic antibodies associated with peripheral neuropathy include those directed against the antineuronal nuclear type 1 (ANNA-1 or anti-Hu), the anti-neuronal nuclear types 2 and 3, the collapsing response-mediator protein 5 (CRMP-5), amphiphysin, and N-type calcium channel antigens.[75] In general, "paraneoplastic" antibodies are a marker of the existence and type of cancer, and do not specifically correlate with a singular phenotype.[122]

Of these antibodies, anti-Hu (ANNA-1) has the most clearly defined phenotype and is the paraneoplastic antibody most commonly found in disorders of the peripheral nervous system.[124] Hu refers to an antigen found within the nuclei of dorsal root ganglia, the central nervous system, the myenteric plexus, and in certain cancers, most notably small cell carcinoma of the lung (SCCL).[76,125,126] Although many of the phenotypes associated with Hu antibody correlate with the locations of Hu antigen, the weight of existing evidence does not provide a direct pathogenetic role for these antibodies.[127] Detecting anti-Hu antibodies in the serum will lead to the detection of an underlying malignancy in greater than 90% of cases. Some of these may not be initially detectable by conventional imaging methods.

Anti-Hu antibodies are most closely correlated with a sensory neuronopathy phenotype, that is, a non–length-dependent, multifocal syndrome of sensory loss that frequently includes pain and sensory ataxia. In a cohort of patients with anti-Hu antibodies in the serum, neuropathy represents 70–80% of all neurologic complications.[75] Having said that, only 1% of patients with SCCL will develop a sensory neuronopathy.[75] Conversely, it is estimated that 20% of patients presenting with a sensory neuronopathy will be found to have an underlying malignancy. Not all neuropathies associated with anti-Hu antibodies however, will conform to a sensory neuronopathy phenotype. Some will be found to have a DSPN, a motor predominant phenotype, or an acute autonomic neuropathy.[128] The latter may approximate the clinical features of the nonparaneoplastic immune-mediated autonomic neuropathy associated with antibodies directed against the ganglionic ACh receptor as described below. Impaired enteric motility is the most common manifestation of the paraneoplastic form of acute autonomic neuropathy, frequently presenting as constipation, vomiting, early satiety, or abdominal pain.[75] Cerebellar degeneration, and limbic and brainstem encephalitis are other notable Hu-related syndromes.[129] Testing for anti-Hu antibodies is recommended in the appropriate clinical context, that is, a subacute sensory syndrome occurring in a smoker, with or without other symptoms suggesting neoplasia or other concomitant paraneoplastic syndromes.

Antibodies directed against the collapsing response-mediator protein 5 or anti-CV2 have an even more diverse association with neurologic and nonneurologic syndromes.[105] An axonal, sensory predominant neuropathy is found in approximately a half of patients with these antibodies. Unlike the anti-Hu syndrome, sensory axons rather than sensory nuclei within the dorsal root ganglia appear to be the target of the suspected immune-mediated injury.[75,130] Other manifestations include cerebellar degeneration, MG, uveitis, optic neuropathy, chorea, and dysgeusia/dysosmia. Again, the presence of these antibodies correlates best with small cell lung cancer. An association with thymoma has been reported as well.[131] Antibodies directed against N-type voltage-gated channel antibodies, distinct from the P/Q type associated with the LEMS, may also represent a marker for paraneoplastic neuropathy.[75]

Nicotinic ganglionic ACh receptor autoantibodies (α3-AChR) target the receptors that mediate synaptic transmission in autonomic ganglion. As mentioned above, their presence in the serum often correlates with a syndrome of subacute dysautonomia. The phenotype may include orthostatic hypotension, erectile dysfunction in males, sicca symptoms, heat intolerance secondary to anhidrosis, abnormal pupillary responses, impaired gastrointestinal motility with gastroparesis and constipation, and urinary retention secondary to neurogenic bladder.[75,78,129,132] Other neurologic manifestations associated with these antibodies may include peripheral neuropathy in approximately 36% of individuals and encephalopathy in 13%.[237] Like LEMS, these autoantibodies may be either paraneoplastic or nonparaneoplastic.[237] They are identified in approximately 50% of patients with an acute or subacute autonomic neuropathy. When paraneoplastic, they are often associated with adenocarcinoma of the breast, prostate, lung or GI tract.[133]

Antibodies Directed Toward Glycolipid and Glycoprotein Components of Peripheral Nerves

At least a dozen glycoproteins and glycoproteins are constituents of peripheral nerve. Although they represent a minor quantitative component of peripheral nerve, they provide potential pathophysiologic relevance. As they are exclusively found in peripheral nerve, and are frequently superficially positioned, they provide an exposed and potentially specific antigenic target for an autoimmune attack.[75] In addition, some of these antigens share epitopes with bacterial species that may be relevant to the pathogenesis of neuropathies such as GBS.

Antibodies directed against myelin-associated glycoprotein, first described in 1980, have a very well defined phenotype and are the most likely of all currently available peripheral neuropathy antibody tests to have a direct pathogenic role.[134,135] Typically, MAG associated neuropathy, referred to by the DADS acronym (distal acquired demyelinating sensory neuropathy), is a slowly progressive disorder that affects males more than females. Middle-aged and older individuals are at risk. It is characterized by large fiber sensory loss and sensory ataxia, global areflexia, demyelinating neurophysiology and often by tremor. Distal weakness, when present, develops later in the course.

In nerve biopsies from patients with this disorder, immunofluorescent staining has detected radiolabeled antibody bound to peripheral nerve myelin. This is associated with the distinctive pathologic feature of myelin membrane separation. MAG antibodies are found in 50–70% of patients with the characteristic phenotype associated with an IgM kappa MCP.[136–138] Conversely, approximately 85% of patients with this phenotype and anti-MAG antibodies will have a detectable IgM MCP.[139] In the author's experience, serum immunoelectrophoresis should be repeated in patients with the typical clinical and electrophysiologic manifestations of DADS if no MCP is initially identified. The presence or absence of anti-MAG activity in patients with the DADS phenotype and an IgM MCP does not appear to change either natural history or treatment responsiveness.[82] In light of this, it can be argued that testing for anti-MAG antibodies is superfluous in patients who have the characteristic clinical syndrome, EDX pattern, and presence of an IgM kappa MCP. If anti-MAG activity is sought, it is important to be aware of the potential for false-positive test results for the enzyme-linked immunosorbent assay (ELISA) screening technique. Conversely, the specificity for the Western Blot confirmatory test has been reported to be as high as 80–90%.[139,140]

IgM antibodies directed against the GM1 ganglioside, first described in 1984, correlate with the syndrome of MMN, with or without detectable demyelinating conduction block.[141–149] Although the GM1 glycolipid exists in motor nerves, there is no convincing evidence to date that these antibodies are pathogenic. In high titer, these appear to be fairly specific for MMN.[73,150,152] Their specificity declines in low titer, being detectable in motor neuron disease, inflammatory demyelinating neuropathy, and normal individuals. The utility of anti-GM1 antibody testing is greatest in the clinical setting of a lower motor neuron syndrome in which demyelinating conduction block cannot be demonstrated. Identification of high titers of IgM anti-GM1 antibodies in this population support the diagnosis of a treatable motor neuropathy and distinguish it from a treatment-resistant, degenerative, or hereditary motor neuron disease. Although the sensitivity of this test has been quoted to be as high as 85%, their absence does not preclude treatment responsiveness as their sensitivity is generally quoted to be in a more modest 40–60% range.[75,144,153] Testing for anti-GM1 antibodies in lower motor neuron syndromes accompanied by definite upper motor neuron and/or bulbar features has a low yield and is not generally recommended.[148]

IgG anti-GM1 antibodies have been linked to the classic demyelinating form of GBS may also have serologic evidence of *Campylobacter jejuni* infection, thus providing a potential antigenic link between these two entities. IgG GD1 autoantibodies have been specifically linked to the acute motor axonal neuropathy (AMAN) variant of GBS in the Chinese but not to *C. jejuni* infection.[75] In general, testing for either of these antibodies adds little to the traditional clinical, EDX and CSF diagnostic evaluation for GBS.

Testing for antibodies directed against the GQ1b ganglioside is helpful in the appropriate clinical setting as a marker for GBS and its Miller Fisher variant in patients presenting with acute ophthalmoparesis, providing high levels of sensitivity and specificity.[75,154,155] They are found in the serum of 80–100% of patients with the Miller Fisher syndrome.[156,157] The apparent relevance of anti-GQ1b antibodies is made even more attractive by the demonstration that this antigen is abundantly expressed in the paranodes of the cranial nerves affecting oculomotor function.[155] The GQ1b antigen can be found in certain strains of *C. jejuni*.

IgM antibodies directed against the sulfatide moiety of peripheral nerve correlates with a chronic, axonal, sensory predominant phenotype that may be painful. These antibodies however, are found in less than 1% of patients with typical DPSN.[75,158] Approximately half of patients with antisulfatide activity will be found to have an associated monoclonal protein. As these antibodies occur infrequently, are of uncertain pathophysiologic significance, and do not define an apparent treatable condition, they have limited clinical utility in the author's estimation.

Antibody Testing for DNMT

The basis for antibody testing in MG has evolved from the initial pathogenetic observations of Patrick and Lindstrom in 1973.[159] Testing for the presence of antibodies directed at various components of the nicotinic, postsynaptic anti-ACH receptor remains the most accurate of neuromuscular antibody tests. Most of these antibodies have an unequivocal pathogenetic role in MG. There are five different antibodies that are commercially available, have potential diagnostic relevance for autoimmune MG, and are related directly or indirectly to disease pathogenesis. These include ACh receptor binding, blocking and modulating antibodies, antibodies directed against muscle-specific kinase (MuSK), and striated muscle auto antibodies. The role of each of these antibodies will be briefly discussed.

Identification of AChR binding antibodies in the serum is the primary means by which the diagnosis of autoimmune MG is serologically confirmed. Detection of these antibodies is a highly specific and reasonably sensitive test. The incidence of false-negative testing varies depending on how limited or generalized the disease is. The incidence of AChR antibodies in generalized myasthenia is estimated at approximately 80–90%, whereas the incidence in ocular myasthenia is quoted to be in the 50–70% range.[55,160] This is unfortunate as the incidence of false-negative tests is therefore greatest in the myasthenic population most difficult to diagnose by other means. The accuracy of AChR antibodies detection is also dependent on the type of assay and source of receptor antigen used. Radioimmunoprecipitation of human AChR harvested from amputated limbs is the preferred methodology.[161,162]

False-positive AChR antibodies tests are uncommon but have been reported to occur. These may be found in LEMS, graft versus host disease, autoimmune hepatitis, healthy relatives of patients with myasthenia, patients with thymoma, and rare patients with lung cancer and motor neuron disease.[160] There is no correlation between antibody titer and the severity of MG nor is there a difference in phenotype or treatment responsiveness between seronegative and seropositive individuals. AChR antibodies have no utility in monitoring treatment response, as titers do not reliably decline coincident with successful treatment and as antibodies may remain in patients who enjoy clinical remission. Occasionally, patients with MG will seroconvert so that repeating the test in someone who is initially seronegative may be of potential value.

ACh receptor blocking and modulating antibodies have limited clinical utility. It is generally estimated that modulating antibodies may be detected in a significant titer in approximately 5% of patients who lack AChR binding antibodies.[160] In view of low yield and cost considerations, it is reasonable to postpone this test until after the AChR binding and MuSK antibody testing, and EDX evaluation fail to provide diagnostic confirmation. This test is reported on a percentage basis and should be considered significant only when present at a high percentile. Minimally positive test results in normal patients occur. AChR blocking antibodies are highly specific. False positives have rarely been reported in the LEMS and in patients exposed to curare-like drugs. Blocking antibodies however, are essentially never present in otherwise seronegative patients. Accordingly, they have no role in screening, their primary role being to aid in the identification of a potential false-positive result.[160]

Antistriated muscle antibodies or striational antibodies have virtually no utility in the diagnosis of MG. Their presence however, suggests at least a predisposition toward autoimmunity in patients with symptoms suggestive of MG who are otherwise seronegative. Nonetheless, in the authors' experience, striational antibodies in high titre are not uncommonly found in individuals without clinical evidence of myasthenia or imaging evidence of thymic abnormality. Striational antibodies are present in approximately 80% of myasthenics with thymoma and have their greatest utility in the detection of this tumor.[163] Striational autoantibodies cross-react with a number of different striated muscle components including actin, actinin, myosin, the ryanodine receptor, and titin (connectin).[164] The specificity of these antibodies is somewhat limited. These antibodies may occur in patients with MG without thymoma, thymoma without MG, LEMS, autoimmune liver disease, or in patients treated with penicillamine.[165,166] Striational autoantibodies are of probable limited utility in patients with imaging evidence of thymoma. Their sensitivity in detecting thymoma has been reported to be similar to that of computed tomography (CT) imaging of the chest.[167] Following titers of antistriated muscle antibodies in an effort to detect recurrent tumor in patients who have had thymectomy is a rational but unproven strategy.[168] Titin antibodies are also found in the sera of 80% of patients with thymoma and 11% of patients with MG without thymoma. In the latter group, disease onset is essentially always after the age of 60 years.[66] Titin antibody testing is not commercially available.

Although delayed onset of a congenital myasthenia syndrome is always a consideration, the majority of evidence suggests that most seronegative MG have an autoimmune etiology well. This conclusion is based on similar alterations of ACh receptor morphology, passive transfer experiments, and equivalent responses to immunomodulating treatments. Other antibodies have been sought to fill this diagnostic gap.[55,169,170] In 2001, antibodies directed against muscle-specific tyrosine kinase (MuSK) were identified in between 40 and 70% of seronegative myasthenic patie nts.[109,171–176] Unlike AChR antibody positive MG, the severity of anti-MuSK MG appears to correlate with antibody concentration.[177] Initially, these antibodies were thought to exist only in the sera ACh binding autoantibody seronegative patients,[178] but an overlap is now known to exist, at least in some ethnic groups.[179] MuSK appears to have a role in the clustering of nicotinic ACh receptors during embryogenesis.[161] Although MuSK antibodies appear to be a specific marker for the MG phenotype,[171] it has yet to be demonstrated that these alter either the anatomy or the physiology of the neuromuscular junction or are causally related to weakness produced by this or other mechanisms.[161,180]

Rippling muscle syndrome is a rare disorder often found in patients with inherited myopathies, particularly the limb-girdle dystrophy phenotype associated with caveolin deficiency. It may also occur as an acquired disorder in association with MG, thymoma, and AChR antibodies.[181,182]

The LEMS is an immune-mediated, presynaptic disorder neuromuscular transmission. It may occur as an isolated disorder in young women but most frequently occurs as a paraneoplastic condition in older individuals. The associated neoplasm is SCCL in the majority of the affected individuals. Detection of an underlying malignancy has been reported to occur at a frequency between 43% and 69% of individuals with the LEMS phenotype.[183] Autoantibodies directed against the P/Q type of voltage-gated calcium channels are pathogenetic and represent a highly sensitive and specific marker for this disease. These antibodies do not block calcium channels but rather bind to them, resulting in downregulation through endocytosis. This in turn reduces the number of active zones in the presynaptic region and result in diminished quantal release. These antibodies were originally estimated to occur in high titer in virtually 100% of paraneoplastic LEMS and in greater than 90% of LEMS occurring independent of any underlying malignancy.[184,185] As in seronegative MG, seronegative LEMS appears to be an antibody-mediated autoimmune disorder. The phenotype can be induced by passive transfer experiments in animals.[183] False-positive test results are rare and usually occur in low titer. They are reported to occur in MG, motor neuron disease, other neurologic paraneoplastic syndromes, and small cell lung cancer without an associated neurologic syndrome.[160,184] Anti-glial nuclear antibodies

(SOX-1) directed against the Bergmann glia of the cerebellum have been identified as a marker of neoplasia in LEMS. In one study, SOX-1 autoantibodies have been found in 64% of LEMS patients with small cell lung cancer, but in none of the patients with apparent idiopathic LEMS.[186] To the best of our knowledge, this antibody test is not commercially available.

Serologic Testing for Muscle Disease

There is no consensus regarding the role of myositis-specific (MSA) and myositis-associated (MAA) antibodies in the evaluation of patients with suspected immune-mediated myopathies (IMM). These tests are utilized more frequently by rheumatologists than neuromuscular medicine specialists.[160,187,188] In our opinion, only a few of these antibodies have added diagnostic value to a careful clinical and pathologic assessment of patients with IMM. Although autoantibodies have been reported to occur in 60–80% of these patients, those that are myositis specific appear to occur far less frequently.[160,187] MAA typically occur in individuals with other connective tissue diseases, with or without an associated myositis. These patients are usually associated with good treatment responsiveness.[187]

There are a few potential benefits that derive from the acquisition of MSA.[189–192] There are cases in which inflammation is not apparent in IIM, presumably due to sampling error or to a necrotizing as opposed to an inflammatory mechanism of disease. Conversely, there are cases in which inflammation is present in myopathies not felt to be immune mediated, for example, certain muscular dystrophies. In either case, the presence of one or more of these antibodies may help to determine whether immune modulating treatment is a rational option. In addition, the presence of specific types of antibodies may predict patterns of organ involvement in addition to skeletal muscle, as well as the potential for treatment responsiveness.

Only three antibodies that arguably have the most significant clinical value will be described here. A more comprehensive list can be found in other resources.[188] The anti-histidyl-tRNA synthetase or Jo-1 antibody, is found in 20–30% of patients with polymyositis or dermatomyositis. Its presence correlates with the presence of interstitial lung disease or mechanics hands in approximately 75% of inflammatory myopathy patients. Antibodies directed against signal recognition protein (SRP) occur in around 3% of IIM patients. Although initially these SRP antibodies were associated with polymyositis, most biopsies reveal features of a necrotizing myopathy without significant inflammatory cell infiltrate. SRP antibody positive necrotizing myopathy is more common in blacks with acute onset, prominent cardiac involvement and poor responsiveness to immunomodulating treatment.[190] Mi-2 autoantibodies are seen predominantly if not exclusively in approximately 8% of pediatric and adult dermatomyositis cases and typically predict treatment responsiveness.[188,191] Of importance, none of these autoantibodies has been associated with inclusion body myositis, or the granulomatous, HIV-associated, or graft versus host disease forms of IIM.[188]

Two other, as of yet commercially unavailable autoantibodies, deserve mention. The 200/100 autoantibody that targets the 3-hydroxy-3-methylglutaryl-coenzyme A reductase (HMG-CoA) receptor is a potential biomarker of the necrotizing myopathy associated with statin drugs.[193,194] The 155/140 autoantibody is seen in dermatomyositis and appears to be a marker for underlying malignancy.[195]

Serologic Testing for Infectious Causes of Neuromuscular Disease

Lyme disease is a cause of a number of neuromuscular syndromes, including cranial neuropathy and polyradiculopathy.[192] Serology is the primary testing method for confirmation as a result of the difficulties inherent in the culture of the *Borrelia burgdorferi* spirochete. There are a number of controversies. In most laboratories, initial screening is performed on serum by ELISA methodology, a test with high sensitivity but limited specificity.[196–199] ELISA is estimated to have a 5% false-positive rate. False negatives are typically due to early testing, delayed seroconversion that requires 2–8 weeks to occur, or to early antimicrobial exposure. By the time neurologic manifestations occur in the early disseminated phase of the disease, false-negative results are unexpected. If the ELISA screen is positive, confirmation is achieved by Western blot detection of IgM and IgG antibodies directed at specific Lyme antigens.[200] There is no recognized role for Western blotting in the setting of a negative ELISA screen. Despite its specificity, the use of Western blotting alone without ELISA screening provides some risk of a false-negative result. Polymerase chain reaction, C6 ELISA antigen detection in urine, detection of immune complex disruption, and B lymphocyte chemoattractant have either not been adequately tested or not achieved adequate levels of sensitivity and/or specificity to be routinely applied to either serum or CSF.[201] In the CSF, demonstrating IgG and IgM Lyme antibodies in concentrations greater than those found in serum is currently the recommended means to confirm central nervous system involvement. The detection of Lyme antibodies in the spinal fluid may lack sensitivity, and CSF pleocytosis and/or elevation of protein levels in the appropriate clinical context is considered sufficient by some to identify CNS Lyme disease.[202–204] Rare cases of seronegative (blood) CNS Lyme detectable only with CSF examination have been reported.[192]

HIV is a neurotropic virus with a number of potential neuromuscular manifestations.[205–208] Serologic testing is based on the detection of IgG antibodies directed against the p24 nucleocapsid and gp41 and 120 envelope proteins. These antibodies appear within 6 weeks in the majority of infected individuals and within 6 months in 95%. They persist for life.[209,210] A positive test requires detection of two of these three antigens and has a detected sensitivity and specificity of over 99%.[211] As in Lyme disease, serologic testing for HIV typically consists of an ELISA screen followed by Western blot confirmation. HIV antigens can be detected in the CSF in patients with CNS involvement.[212]

Other Serologic Tests in Neuromuscular Disease

Neuropathy is estimated to occur in approximately 10% of patients with Sjögren and/or the sicca syndrome. There are a number of reported neuropathy phenotypes that occur with this condition.[75,213,214] A sensory neuronopathy syndrome with or without an associated trigeminal neuropathy, is the most distinctive of these. As trigeminal neuropathy is infrequent in paraneoplastic sensory neuropathy, its identification serves as a potentially helpful clue in distinguishing between these two disorders.[75] A SFN phenotype may be the most common neuromuscular condition associated with Sjögren syndrome. Multifocal neuropathy or multiple cranial neuropathies may occur as well.[215,216] Anti-Ro (SS-A) and Anti-LA (SS-B) antibodies represent a reasonable screening test in patients with a neuropathy with sicca symptomatology or a typical Sjögren phenotype. These are detectable in approximately 60% of patients.[75] Detection of antinuclear antibodies or the rheumatoid factor provides less specific support for a Sjögren diagnosis. The diagnosis of seronegative Sjögren or sicca-related neuropathy is dependent on tissue analysis, usually provided by lip biopsy that will reveal an inflammatory response directed against minor salivary glands.

The potential association between celiac sprue and polyneuropathy is controversial.[217,218] Celiac disease is estimated to occur in 2–1/2% of individuals with an apparent idiopathic polyneuropathy, seemingly exceeding the prevalence of the disease in age-matched controls without neuropathy.[217] The neuropathy pattern is typically DSPN, that is sensory predominant, axonal, and length dependent.[219,220] The neuropathy is reported to occur at times in the absence of gastrointestinal symptoms. Gliadin, transglutaminase, and endomysial antibody tests are all potential screening tests for this disorder, the former having the least specificity. IgA, rather than IgG gliadin antibodies are felt to be more specific for celiac disease. When these are detected in neuropathy patients, it is usually in individuals with sprue, thus limiting the utility as a screening tool in idiopathic neuropathy patients.[217] At best, these antibodies represent screening tools and the diagnosis is ultimately dependent upon the demonstration of malabsorption and typical small bowel pathology. Neuropathy response to dietary and immunomodulating treatment has been disappointing to date, suggesting that the neuropathy is due to alternative mechanism, or that nerves are irreparably damaged.

Vasculitic neuropathy may occur in either a multifocal or DSPN pattern. The latter may represent the confluence of a multifocal neuropathy syndrome. Neuropathy occurs in approximately half of the patients with systemic necrotizing vasculitis with the greatest prevalence in polyarteritis nodosa, eosinophilic granulomatosis with polyangiitis (EGPA), and granulomatosis with polyangiitis (GPA). It is often the initial organ-specific manifestation of these disorders. Antineutrophilic cytoplasmic antibodies (ANCA) are markers for these disorders. P-ANCA directed against myeloperoxidase represents a marker for the former two disorders. C-ANCA directed against antiproteinase 3 is highly specific for GPA.[75] In one series, 8% of 166 neuropathy patients had positive blood tests for ANCA.[221] Approximately half of these patients were found to have systemic vasculitis. As this series was derived from a major peripheral neuropathy referral center, it is not clear whether its application to a more general neuropathy population would result in a similar yield. Vasculitis and neuropathy also occurs as a consequence of vasculitis in association with rheumatoid arthritis. Titers of rheumatoid factor tend to be high in this setting, which occurs infrequently. Typically, patients have long-standing rheumatoid arthritis, usually with associated signs and symptoms of systemic disease including palpable purpura. Predictably, the yield and accuracy of ANCA and rheumatoid factor testing will be greatest in patients with acute to subacute painful multifocal neuropathy patterns who have signs and symptoms of an underlying systemic disease.

Some patients with disorders of peripheral nerve hyperexcitability (e.g., Isaacs syndrome, neuromyotonia, cramp-fasciculation syndrome) have antibodies both in serum and CSF that were initially attributed to VGKC antibodies.[15,39,222] Recent studies, suggest that the true antigen is Casp2 which has a role in concentrating VGKCs in the juxtaparanodal regions of central and peripheral nervous systems.[17] These antibodies are more commonly associated with limbic encephalitis than with a disorder of the peripheral neuromuscular system.[222] The classic peripheral phenotype associated with these disorders is known as Isaac syndrome that can be conceptualized as part of the spectrum of a peripheral nerve hyperexcitability syndrome.[39] As in LEMS, Isaac's syndrome is an autoimmune disorder that can occur in isolation, in association with other autoimmune diseases or as a paraneoplastic syndrome.[15,39,185,223,224] When Isaac's syndrome is associated with concomitant CNS pathology, usually a behavioral syndrome, it has been historically referred to as Morvan syndrome.

In summary, in keeping with the theme of this book, blood testing in neuromuscular disease should be applied judiciously in the evaluation of neuromuscular disease. The majority of the tests that have been discussed are ideally acquired when relevant to the clinical context of an individual patient, not as routine screening tools. In typical length-dependent, sensory predominant neuropathies, we routinely adhere to AAN guidelines and test only for the presence of a monoclonal protein, abnormal glucose metabolism, and B12 deficiency. In patients with a sensory neuronopathy or sensory ataxia phenotype, we recommend the additional testing for anti-Hu, anti-nuclear, SSA and SSB antibodies, and rheumatoid factor as well as vitamin B6 levels. In patients with a multifocal neuropathy phenotype, we would obtain an additional nonspecific marker of systemic inflammation such as sedimentation rate or CRP, ANCA, and potentially a genetic test for the PMP-22 deletion if clinically relevant. In any patient with a purely motor disorder, we would routinely obtain a measurement of serum CK, antibody testing for the Ach binding receptor and would have a low threshold for obtaining antibodies directed against the GM-1 ganglioside and voltage-gated calcium channel. Genetic testing for familial ALS, Kennedy disease and/or SMN spinal muscular atrophy would be considered in the appropriate clinical context.

CSF ANALYSIS

CSF analysis is a helpful evaluation in select groups of patients with neuromuscular disease. From an anatomic perspective, an abnormal CSF result implies the existence of pathology in the central nervous system or within the nerve roots. As such, these are diagnostically helpful from a number of different perspectives. An elevated CSF protein level without a cellular response is paradoxically is the hallmark of the acute and chronic inflammatory demyelinating polyneuropathies (AIDP) and CIDP. This profile can also be seen in structural disorders of nerve root such as disc herniations and spinal stenosis, mitochondrial disorders, paraneoplastic disorders, spinal cord infarction, and a third to half of ALS cases.[124] In suspected mitochondrial disorders, CSF lactate measurements may be helpful as well. A CSF pleocytosis is expected in infectious disorders affecting nerve roots and/or spinal cord such as Lyme, syphilis, poliomyelitis, West Nile virus, enterovirus, CMV, and HIV infections. Serologic tests for these organisms can provide a specific diagnosis. A CSF pleocytosis is also seen in most cases of neoplastic meningitis, which can be confirmed through cytologic or flow cytometric evaluations. Paraneoplastic disorders affecting both the peripheral and/or central nervous system are frequently associated with some combination of pleocytosis, elevated CSF protein, or oligoclonal banding.[124] It is hoped that the emerging field of proteomics will allow for identification of a specific biomarker(s) within spinal fluid that will allow for early diagnosis in disorders such as ALS where there is currently no confirmatory test. Detection of a reliable biomarker also holds promise of identifying an effective response to treatment.

NERVE AND MUSCLE IMAGING

Imaging of nerve and muscle is being used with increased frequency in the evaluation of patients with neuromuscular disorders.[225–227] Arguably, this role will continue to evolve as resolution of the images and neurologist's familiarity with the benefits of a number of different applications expand. The advantages provided by MR over computerized tomography include increased resolution, the ability to easily image in multiple planes, and the availability of a noniodinated contrast agent. In addition, MR has the potential advantage over CT in terms of timing of injury. For example, chronic nerve and muscle diseases are both associated with fatty replacement of muscle manifesting as increased signal in T1-weighted images. Acutely denervated muscle will demonstrate little if any signal change with T1 sequencing.[228] T2-weighted images however, accentuate the signal produced by water. Increased T2 signal occurs within acutely denervated muscle. It is generally felt to correlate with the pathologic features of edema, inflammation, and myofiber necrosis.[150,167,174,229–233]

For these reasons MRI has supplanted CT as the imaging modality of choice in most cases of suspected nerve or muscle pathology except in those who cannot receive or tolerate MR due to financial considerations, their size, MR availability, claustrophobic tendencies, or contraindications such as pacemakers. Nonetheless, CT is not without value in neuromuscular disease. It can differentiate nerve from muscle disease, not only based on the pattern of muscular involvement but based on the basis of x-ray attenuation changes within individual muscles as well.[151] CT has been demonstrated to be 85% sensitive in detecting neuromuscular pathology in general, using muscle histology as the comparative gold standard.[234] Traditional roles of imaging, for example detection of a herniated disc, a Pancoast tumor, or a retroperitoneal hematoma will not be addressed in this chapter. Ideally, future imaging techniques will provide a means to track axonal regrowth following injury or intervention, as well as development of specific imaging markers that would allow detection of substances such as amyloid within nerve or muscle.

Imaging of muscle has numerous potential applications.[235,236] For example, in the dropped head or bent spine syndromes, fatty replacement of paraspinal muscles readily detectable on MRI can define a neuromuscular as opposed to an extrapyramidal or orthopedic cause of the patient's abnormal posture (Fig. 2-30). Uncommonly, MRI of the spine may demonstrate unexpected abnormalities within paraspinal muscles identifying a neuromuscular rather than etiology as the cause of the patient's back or neck pain. MRI has been reported to be 89–97% sensitive and 89% specific in detecting abnormalities in the inflammatory myopathies.[167,229] Signal changes have also been documented to occur coincident with treatment responsiveness in these disorders.[229,237] As in EDX, it has been used to detect asymptomatic muscle involvement in patients with a characteristic rash and to aid in the distinction of muscle weakness due to steroids as opposed to the underlying disease.[150,229] The pattern of muscle involvement may also be helpful in the identification of certain muscle diseases such as the muscular dystrophies and inclusion body myositis where specific patterns of muscle involvement are known to occur.[167] Although the authors do not routinely use MR imaging in the selection of an appropriate muscle to biopsy, it can be a very helpful tool in the appropriate clinical context. For example, certain patients with neuromuscular disease may have muscles that are at the extremes of the spectrum, that is, either end-stage or normal. In this context, MRI may allow detection of a modestly affected muscle suitable for biopsy. Although of limited pragmatic benefit, rhabdomyolysis is associated with a diffuse pattern of increased signal on T2 or short tau inversion recovery (STIR) sequences.[174,238] Gadolinium has

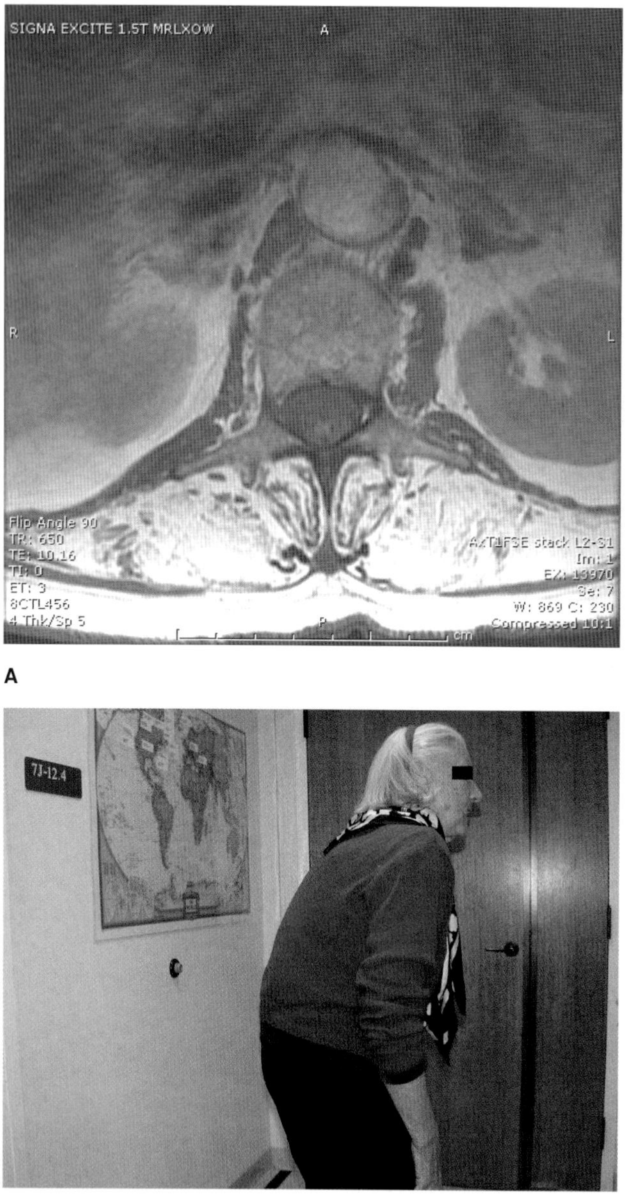

A

B

Figure 2-30. **(A)** MRI (T1 sequence) demonstrating fatty replacement and atrophy of the lumbar paraspinal musculature in **(B)** an older woman with bent spine syndrome.

a limited role in MRI of muscle and is used predominantly for the assessment of suspected primary or metastatic muscle tumors.[235] MRI can be helpful as well in the detection of the relatively rare conditions of muscle infarction, muscle hemorrhage, or rhabdomyosarcomas.

MRI has a number of beneficial applications in nerve disease as well. MRI imaging may identify a pattern of muscle involvement that defines a specific nerve lesion while at the same time implicating the site of lesion within the nerve. Normal nerve is isointense to muscle on both T1- and T2-weighted sequences. An axonal injury will have increased signal characteristics within nerve on cross-sectional images using STIR and T2 fast spin echo sequences both at and distal to the injury site, that will also enhance with gadolinium.[228] STIR enjoys the benefit of more intense signal characteristics and fat signal suppression but does not provide the image resolution of its T2 fast spin echo counterpart. Acutely denervated muscle will also have increased signal characteristics on STIR and T2 fast spin echo sequences that may precede the development of acute denervation on the EDX examination. Chronic denervation produces fatty infiltration of denervated muscle.[225] Signal changes do not take place in muscles associated with purely demyelinating nerve injuries.[225] Ideally, MRI could accurately identify nerve transaction or avulsion in traumatic injury to expedite surgical intervention in these cases. Unfortunately, current imaging resolution and evolution of signal changes within nerve and muscle do not provide this capability.

MRI imaging has been used to detect focal nerve entrapment or compression syndromes. One potential benefit of MRI imaging in this context is its potential ability to identify a secondary pathology as a contributor to the syndrome, for example, a ganglion cyst within Guyon's canal (Fig. 2-31). In the case of CTS, MRI has not usurped the traditional role of EDX in most institutions as CTS has a demyelinating pathophysiology in most if not all cases and is therefore readily detectable.[239] There is the potential for a greater role for MRI in the evaluation of ulnar neuropathy at the elbow. It has been estimated that up to one-half of ulnar neuropathies have a predominantly axonal pathophysiology, which usually precludes precise EDX localization. MRI has been

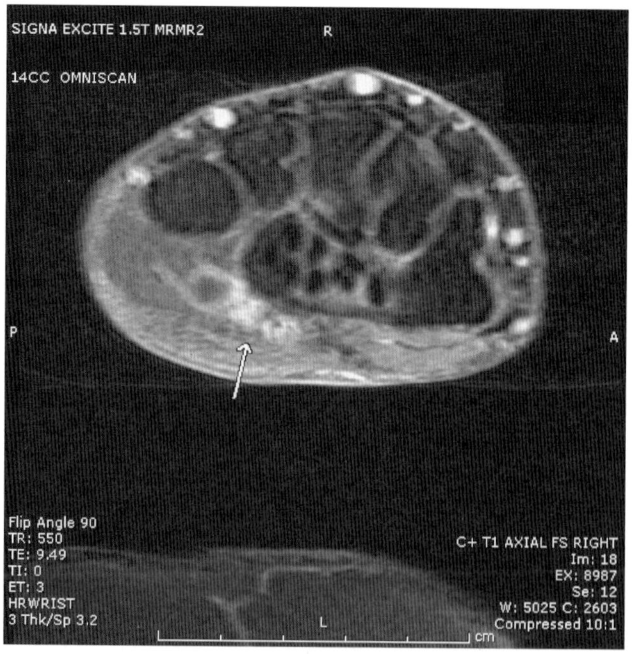

Figure 2-31. MRI (T1 sequence with gadolinium) demonstrating enhancing mass (*arrow*) in Guyon's canal (ganglion cyst) in a young female presenting with painless weakness and atrophy restricted to intrinsic right-hand muscles innervated exclusively by the ulnar nerve.

shown to identify increased signal in areas consistent with ulnar nerve injury at least in some cases and may do so when EDX is normal.[240] MRI has been reported to be occasionally beneficial in other less frequent and at times controversial mononeuropathies including thoracic outlet, piriformis syndromes, and tarsal tunnel syndromes, as well as posterior interosseous and peroneal neuropathies.[225] It would be prudent to interpret subtle imaging abnormalities cautiously in these aforementioned contexts and to accept their validity only when congruent with clinical and EDX data.

MRI is the current diagnostic modality of choice to identify peripheral nerve tumors (Fig. 2-32). Virtually all of these, regardless of histology, demonstrate gadolinium enhancement. Benign histology cannot reliably be distinguished from its malignant counterpart by MRI, although positron emission tomography may be helpful in this regard. A potentially vexing clinical problem, the separation of recurrent tumor versus radiation-induced plexus injury, may be solved in some cases by different MR characteristics. Recurrent tumor tends to be focal, irregular, and enhancing. Radiation-induced nerve injury tends to produce either uniform enlargement or focal atrophy.[225]

MRI is capable of identifying areas of presumed inflammation, edema, and demyelination in the acquired inflammatory demyelinating neuropathies, including MMN, GBS, and CIDP,[241–245] and in brachial plexus neuritis.[246,247] In some cases, nerve roots are preferentially involved in keeping with known pathologic data.[241] T2 signal abnormalities in brachial plexus elements may be seen in both CIDP and MMN.[245] Other than for symmetry, these changes are identical. These may be of considerable utility, however, allowing for the discrimination of MMN and other, presumed degenerative and untreatable lower motor neuron syndromes. This latter application may be particularly helpful as it can detect abnormalities of peripheral nerve in locations proximal to where NCS are easily applied. Although insightful in the appropriate clinical context, neither the location, signal characteristics, nor the morphology of imaging abnormality predict pathology in these disorders. Similar changes, particularly in nerve roots, may be seen in infectious, neoplastic, or other inflammatory diseases (e.g., sarcoidosis) with affinity for peripheral nerve.[226] MRI may be capable of identifying hypertrophic nerves seen in conditions such as CMT disease,[248] particularly within the spinal canal where these may lead to the clinical syndrome of neurogenic claudication.

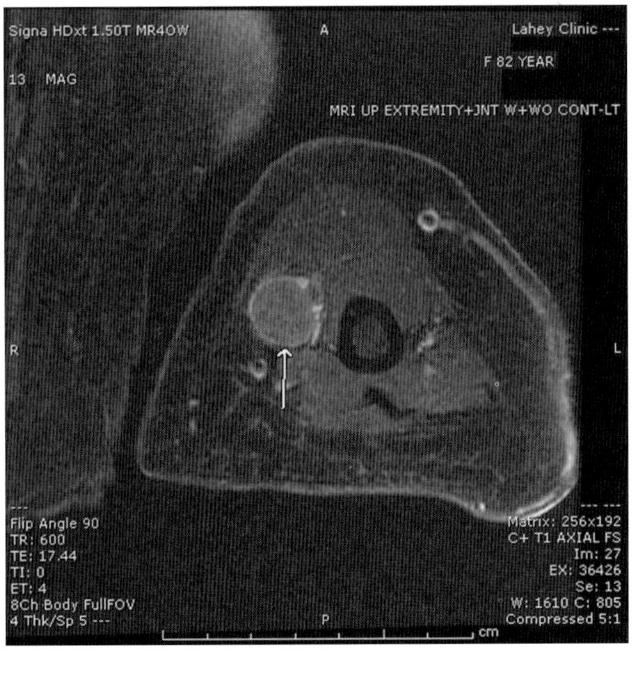

Figure 2-32. MRI (T1 sequence with fat saturation and gadolinium) axial image of the humerus demonstrating an enlarged and enhancing median nerve due to biopsy proven metastatic lymphoma.

MRI can provide valuable insight into the cause of intramedullary disorders of the spinal cord whose phenotypes may overlap with neuromuscular syndromes (Figs. 2-33A,B and 2-34). Syringomyelia, spinal cord infarction, intramedullary neoplasms, vitamin B12 and copper deficiency are notable examples.[249–251]

Ultrasonography is an emerging neuromuscular diagnostic tool that it is readily available, relatively inexpensive, quick, and painless.[252,253] It is limited by specificity and its ability to visualize deep structures particularly in individuals with a large body habitus. Measured parameters include the cross-sectional area of nerve in comparison to normative values and in comparison to unaffected nerve segments. In general, the cross-sectional area of the nerve will normally increase at proximal sites, in taller individuals, and at sites of nerve entrapment. Ultrasound has been used to identify nerve transaction and has demonstrated an 89% sensitivity and 95% specificity under experimental conditions.[254] Nerve ultrasound has been utilized in the evaluation of patients with known or suspected entrapment/compression mononeuropathies including CTS, ulnar neuropathy at the elbow and peroneal neuropathy at the fibular head.[255–260] Ultrasound can be used to demonstrate an increase in nerve cross-sectional area as a common feature in either inherited or acquired demyelinating neuropathy whereas this same parameter is commonly reduced in axonal neuropathies.[261] Ultrasound has been utilized to detect nerve root hypertrophy in CIDP.[262,263]

Muscle ultrasound has been used in an attempt to identify fibrillation potentials in muscle. Sensitivity has been reported to be 45% and specificity 60% in this application.[264] It has been applied as a potential diagnostic tool in both muscular dystrophy and inflammatory myopathy.[265–267] It is capable of detecting altered echogenicity within muscle indicative of pathology as well as defining the existence and pattern of muscle atrophy or hypertrophy. Like MRI, it can be applied to identify an ideal muscle to biopsy.[226] This may be particularly relevant with young children where the identification of a moderately involved muscle may be problematic either through clinical or electrodiagnostic assessment.[268]

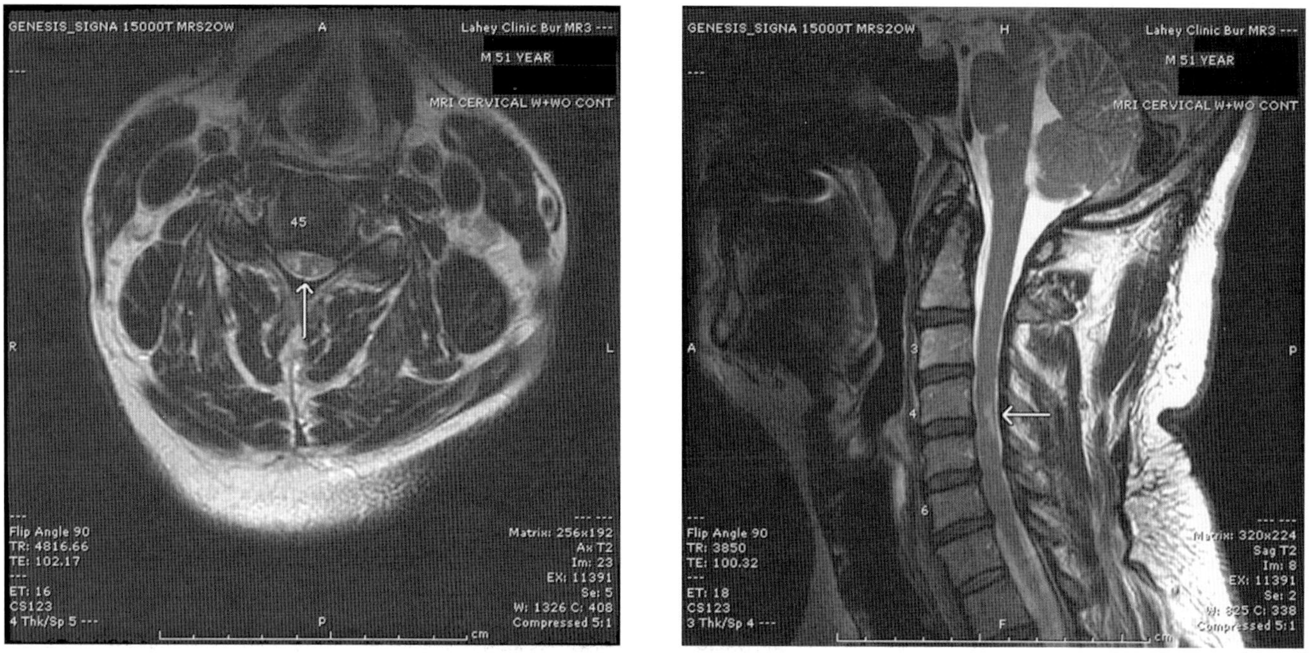

A B

Figure 2-33. T2 sequence axial plane **(A)** and T2 image sagittal plane **(B)** demonstrating increased signal of the gray matter at the C4–C5 interspace in a man with painless weakness and atrophy of the shoulder girdle.

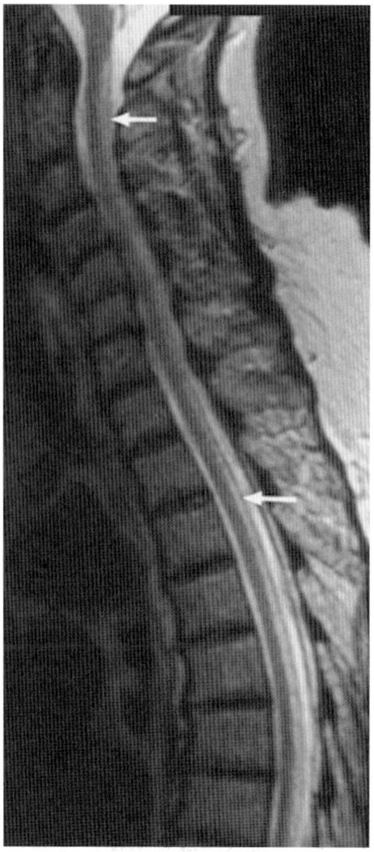

A

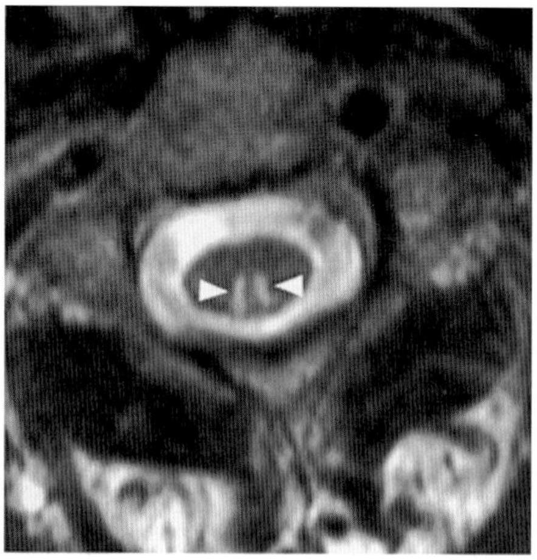

B

Figure 2-34. T2 sequence axial **(A)** and sagittal planes **(B)** demonstrating increased signal within the posterior columns in an individual with cyanocobalamin deficiency.

▶ SUMMARY

This chapter has attempted to provide an even and practical description of many of the ancillary tests available to the neuromuscular clinician. It has attempted to fairly emphasize both the strengths and the weaknesses of each modality. Again, these tests represent a proverbial double-edged sword that may achieve either a desired or an undesired effect dependent on the skill, knowledge, and particularly judgment of the individual that utilizes them.

REFERENCES

1. LaBan MM, Petty D, Hauser AM, Taylor RS. Peripheral nerve conduction stimulation: Its effect on cardiac pacemakers. *Arch Phys Med Rehabil.* 1988;69(5):358–362.
2. Mellion ML, Buxton AE, Iyer V, Almahameed S, Lorvidhaya P, Gilchrist JM. Safety of nerve conduction studies in patients with peripheral intravenous lines. *Muscle & Nerve.* 2010;42(2):189–191.
3. Schoeck AP, Mellion ML, Gilchrist JM, Christian FV. Safety of nerve conduction studies in patients with implanted cardiac devices. *Muscle & Nerve.* 2007;35(4):521–524.
4. Al-Shekhlee L, Shekhlee A, Shapiro BE, Preston DC. Iatrogenic complications and risks of nerve conduction studies and needle electromyography. *Muscle Nerve.* 2003;27(5):517–526.
5. Caress JB, Little AA, Zaebarah V, Albers JW. Survey of electrodiagnostic laboratories regarding hemorrhagic complications from needle electromyography. *Muscle Nerve.* 2006;34:356–358.
6. Lynch SL, Boon AJ, Smith J, Harper CH Jr., Tanaka EM. Complications of needle electromyography: hematoma risk and correlation with anticoagulant and antiplatelet therapy. *Muscle Nerve.* 2008;38:1225–1230.
7. Mateen FJ, Grant IA, Sorenson EJ. Needlestick injuries among electromyographers. *Muscle Nerve.* 2008;38:1541–1545.
8. Daube JR, Armon C. Electrophysiological signs of arteriovenous malformations of the spinal cord. *J Neurol Neurosurg Psychiatry.* 1989;52:1176–1181.
9. Linden D, Berlit P. Spinal arteriovenous malformations: Clinical and neurophysiologic findings. *J Neurol.* 1996; 243:9–12.
10. Schrader V, Koenig E, Thron A, Dichgans J. Neurophysiologic characteristics of spinal arteriovenous malformations. *Electro Clin Neurophys.* 1989;29:169–177.
11. Chaudhry V, Cornblath DR. Wallerian degeneration in human nerves: Serial electrophysiological studies. *Muscle Nerve.* 1992; 15:687–693.
12. Levin R, Pascuzzi RM, Bruns DE, Boyd JC, Toly TM, Phillips LH II. The time course of creatine kinase elevation following concentric needle EMG. *Muscle Nerve.* 1987;10:242–245.
13. Raynor EM, Shefner JM, Ross MH, Logigian EL, Hinchey JA. Root stimulation studies in the evaluation of patients with motor neuron disease. *Neurology.* 1998;50:1907–1909.
14. Auger RG, Daube JR, Gomez MR, Lambert EH. Hereditary form of sustained muscle activity of peripheral nerve origin causing generalized myokymia and muscle stiffness. *Ann Neurol.* 1985;15:13–21.
15. Merchut MP. Management of voltage-gated potassium channel antibody disorders. *Neurol Clin.* 2010;28(4):941–959.
16. Dhand UK. Isaacs' syndrome: clinical and electrophysiological response to gabapentin. *Muscle Nerve.* 2006;34:646–650.
17. Lancaster E, Huijbers MG, Bar V, et al. Investigations of Caspr2, an autoantigen of encephalitis and neuromyotonia. *Ann Neurol.* 2011;69:303–311.
18. Maselli RA, Soliven BC. Analysis of the organophosphate-induced electromyographic response to repetitive nerve stimulation: paradoxical response to edrophonium and D-tubocurarine. *Muscle Nerve.* 1991;14:1182–1188.
19. Fournier E, Arzel M, Sternberg D, et al. Electromyography guides toward subgroups of mutations in muscle channelopathies. *Ann Neurol.* 2004;56(5):650–661.
20. Fournier E, Viala K, Gervais H, et al. Cold extends electromyography distinction between ion channel mutations causing myotonia. *Ann Neurol.* 2006;60:356–365.
21. Tan SV, Matthews E, Barber M, et al. Refined exercise testing and a DNA-based diagnosis in muscle channelopathies. *Ann Neurol.* 2011;69(2):328–340.
22. Michel P, Sternberg D, Jeannet PY, et al. Comparative efficacy of repetitive nerve stimulation, exercise, and cold in differentiating myotonic disorders. *Muscle Nerve.* 2007;36: 643–650.
23. Streib EW. AAEM minimonongraph #27: Differential diagnosis of myotonic syndromes. *Muscle Nerve.* 1987;10:603–615.
24. Cudkowicz M, Qureshi M, Shefner J. Measures and markers in amyotrophic lateral sclerosis. *NeuroRx.* 2004;1(2):273–283.
25. Gooch CL, Shefner JM. ALS surrogate markers. *MUNE . Amyotroph Lateral Scler Other Motor Neuron Disord.* 2004;5 (Suppl 1):104–107.
26. Cudkowicz ME, Shefner JM, Schoenfeld DA, et al; The Northeast ALS Consortium. Trial of celecoxib in amyotrophic lateral sclerosis. *Ann Neurol.* 2006;60(1):22–31.
27. Shefner JM, Cudkowicz ME, Schoenfeld D, et al; NEALS Consortium. A clinical trial of creatine in ALS. *Neurology.* 2004;63(9):1656–1661.
28. Shefner JM, Cudkowicz ME, Zhang H, Schoenfeld D, Jillapalli D, Russell JA; Northeast ALS Consortium. The use of statistical MUNE in a multicenter clinical trial. *Muscle Nerve.* 2004;30:463–469.
29. Armon C, Brandstater ME. Motor unit number estimate-based rates of progression of ALS predict patient survival. *Muscle Nerve.* 1999;22(11):1571–1575.
30. Bromberg MB, Larson WL. Relationships between motor-unit number estimates and isometric strength in distal muscles in ALS/MND. *J Neurol Sci.* 1996;139(Suppl):38–42.
31. Felice KJ. A longitudinal study comparing thenar motor unit number estimates to other quantitative tests in patients with amyotrophic lateral sclerosis. *Muscle Nerve.* 1997;20(2):179–185.
32. Yuen EC, Olney RK. Longitudinal study of fiber density and motor unit number estimate in patients with amyotrophic lateral sclerosis. *Neurology.* 1997;49:573–578.
33. Daube JR, Rubin DI. Needle electromyography. *Muscle Nerve.* 2009;39:244–270.
34. Young NP, Daube JR, Sorenson E, Milone M. Absent, minimal and unrecognized myotonic discharges in myotonic muscular dystrophy type 2. *Muscle Nerve.* 2010;41:758–762.
35. de Carvalho M, Dengler R, Eisen A, et al. Electrodiagnostic criteria for ALS. *Clin Neurophysiol.* 2008;119:497–503.
36. de Carvalho M, Swash M. Awaji diagnostic algorithm increases sensitivity of El Escorial criteria for ALS diagnosis. *Amyotroph Lateral Scler.* 2009;10:53–57.

37. Douglass CP, Kandler RH, Shaw PJ, McDermott CJ. An evaluation of neurophysiological criteria used in the diagnosis of motor neuron disease. *J Neurol Neurosurg Psychiatry.* 2010;81:646–649.
38. Mills KR. Characteristics of fasciculations in amyotrophic lateral sclerosis and the benign fasciculation syndrome. *Brain.* 2010;133:3458–3469.
39. Rubio-Agusti I, Perez-Miralles F, Sevilla T, et al. Peripheral nerve hyperexcitability: A clinical and immunologic study of 38 patients. *Neurology.* 2011;76:172–178.
40. Weiss N, Behin A, Psimaras D, Delattre JY. Postirradiation neuromyotonia of spinal accessory nerves. *Neurology.* 2011;75:1188–1189.
41. Dabby R, Lange DJ, Trojaborg W, et al. Inclusion body myositis mimicking motor neuron disease. *Arch Neurol.* 2001;58: 1253–1256.
42. Uncini A, Lange DJ, Lovelace RE, Solomon M, Hays A. Long-duration polyphasic motor unit potentials in myopathies: A quantitative study with pathological correlation. *Muscle Nerve.* 1990;13:263–267.
43. Stålberg EV, Sanders DB. Jitter recordings with concentric needle electrodes. *Muscle Nerve.* 2009;4:331–339.
44. Sinnreich M, Klein CJ, Daube JR, Engelstad J, Spinner RJ, Dyck PJ. Chronic immune sensory polyradiculopathy. *Neurology.* 2004;63:1662–1669.
45. Gilchrist JM, Sachs GM. Electrodiagnostic studies in the management and prognosis of neuromuscular disorders. *Muscle Nerve.* 2004;29:165–190.
46. Daube JR. Electrophysiologic studies in diagnosis and prognosis of motor neuron diseases. *Neurol Clin.* 1985;3:473–493.
47. Cornblath DR, Mellits ED, Griffin JW, et al. Motor conduction studies in Guillain-Barré syndrome: Description and prognostic value. *Ann Neurol.* 1988;23:354–359.
48. Friedrich JM, Robinson LR. Prognostic indicators from electrodiagnostic studies for ulnar neuropathy at the elbow. *Muscle Nerve.* 2011;43:596–600.
49. Dyck PJ, Zimmerman IR, O'Brien PC, et al. Introduction of automated systems to evaluate touch-pressure, vibration, and thermal cutaneous sensation in man. *Ann Neurol.* 1978;4:502–510.
50. Dyck PJ, O'Brien PC. Quantitative sensation testing in epidemiological studies of peripheral neuropathy. *Muscle Nerve.* 1999;22:659–662.
51. Shy ME, Frohman EM, So YT, et al. Quantitative sensory testing. *Neurology.* 2003;60:898–904.
52. Peripheral Neuropathy Association. Quantitative sensory testing: A consensus report. *Neurology.* 1993;43:1050–1052.
53. Lacomis D. Small-fiber neuropathy. *Muscle Nerve.* 2002;26: 173–188.
54. Løseth S, Lindal S, Stålberg E, Mellgren SI. Intraepidermal nerve fibre density, quantitative sensory testing and nerve conduction studies in a patient material with symptoms and signs of sensory polyneuropathy. *Eur J Neurol.* 2006;13:105–111.
55. Soliven BC, Lange DJ, Penn AS, et al. Seronegative myasthenia gravis. *Neurology.* 1988;38:514–517.
56. Bird SJ, Brown MJ, Spino C, Watling S, Foyt HL. Value of repeated measures of nerve conduction and quantitative sensory testing in a diabetic neuropathy trial. *Muscle Nerve.* 2006;34:214–224.
57. Walk D, Zaretskaya M, Parry GJ. Symptom duration and clinical features in painful sensory neuropathy with and without nerve conduction abnormalities. *J Neurol Sci.* 2003;214:3–6.
58. Periquet MI, Novak V, Collins MP, et al. Painful sensory neuropathy: Prospective evaluation using skin biopsy. *Neurology.* 1999;53:1641–1647.
59. Singer W, Spies JM, McArthur J, et al. Prospective evaluation of somatic and autonomic small fibers in selected neuropathies. *Neurology.* 2004;62:612–618.
60. Walk D, Wendelschafer-Crabb G, Davey C, Kennedy WR. Concordance between epidermal nerve fiber density and sensory examination in patients with symptoms of idiopathic small fiber neuropathy. *J Neurol Sci.* 2007;255(1–2):23–26.
61. Wolfe GI, Baker NS, Amato AA, et al. Chronic cryptogenic sensory polyneuropathy: Clinical and laboratory characteristics. *Arch Neurol.* 1999;56(5):540–547.
62. Yarnitsky D. Quantitative sensory testing. *Muscle Nerve.* 1997; 20:198–204.
63. Gibbons C, Freeman R. The evaluation of small fiber function—autonomic and quantitative sensory testing. *Neurol Clin.* 2004;22:683–702.
64. Simpson DM, Kitch D, Evans SR, et al; The ACTG A5117 Study Group. HIV neuropathy natural history cohort study: Assessment measures and risk factors. *Neurology.* 2006;66(11): 1679–1687.
65. Dyck PJ, Kratz KM, Lehman KA, et al. The Rochester diabetic neuropathy study: Design, criteria for types of neuropathy, selection bias, and reproducibility of neuropathic tests. *Neurology.* 1991;41:799–807.
66. Yamamoto AN, Gajdos P, Eymard B, et al. Anti-titin antibodies in myasthenia gravis: Tight association with thymoma and heterogeneity of nonthymoma patients. *Arch Neurol.* 2001;58:885–890.
67. Jensen TS, Bach FW, Kastrup J, Dejgaard A, Brennum J. Vibratory and thermal thresholds in diabetes with and without clinical neuropathy. *Acta Neurol Scand.* 1991;84:326–333.
68. Ziegler D, Mayer P, Gries FA. Evaluation of thermal, pain, and vibration sensation thresholds in newly diagnosed type 1 diabetic patients. *J Neurol Neurosurg Psychiatry.* 1998;51:1420–1424.
69. Bravenboer B, Van Dam PS, Hop J, Steenhoven J, Erkelens DW. Thermal threshold testing for the assessment of small fibre dysfunction: Normal values and reproducibility. *Diabetic Med.* 1992;9:546–549.
70. Lindblom U, Tegner R. Thermal sensitivity in uremic neuropathy. *Acta Neurol Scand.* 1985;71:290–294.
71. Angus-Lepman H, Burke D. The function of large and small nerve fibers in renal failure. *Muscle Nerve.* 1992;15:288–294.
72. Yosipovitch G, Yarnitsky D, Reiss J, et al. Paradoxical heat sensation in uremic polyneuropathy. *Muscle Nerve.* 1995;16: 768–771.
73. Winer JB, Bang B, Clarke JR, et al. A study of neuropathy in HIV infection. *Q J Med.* 1992;302:473–488.
74. Gibbons CH, Freeman R, Veves A. Diabetic neuropathy: A cross-sectional study of the relationships among tests of neurophysiology. *Diabetes Care.* 2010;33:2629–2634.
75. Vernino S, Wolfe GI. Antibody testing in peripheral neuropathies. *Neurol Clin.* 2007;25:29–46.
76. Kissel JT. Autoantibody testing in the evaluation of peripheral neuropathy. *Semin Neurol.* 1998;18:83–94.
77. Low PA, Denq JC, Opfer-Gehrking TL, Dyck PJ, O'Brien PC, Slezak JM. Effect of age and gender on sudomotor and cardiovagal function and blood pressure response to tilt in normal subjects. *Muscle Nerve.* 1997;20:1561–1568.
78. Klein CJ, Vernino S, Lennon VA, et al. The spectrum of autoimmune autonomic neuropathies. *Ann Neurol.* 2003;53:752–758.

79. Low PA, Vernino S, Suarez G. Autonomic dysfunction in peripheral nerve disease. *Muscle Nerve*. 2003;27:646–661.
80. McLeod JG. Invited review: Autonomic dysfunction in peripheral nerve disease. *Muscle Nerve*. 1992;15:3–13.
81. McLeod JG. Autonomic dysfunction in peripheral nerve disease. *J Clin Neurophysiol*. 1993;10(1):51–60.
82. Sandroni P, Vernino S, Klein CM, et al. Idiopathic autonomic neuropathy; comparison of cases seropositive and seronegative for ganglionic acetylcholine receptor antibodies. *Arch Neurol*. 2004;61:44–48.
83. Ewing DJ, Campbell IW, Clarke BI. Mortality in diabetic autonomic neuropathy. *Lancet*. 1976;1:601–603.
84. Goyal RK. Muscarinic receptor subtypes: Physiology and clinical implications. *N Engl J Med*. 1989;321:1022–1029.
85. England JD, Gronseth GS, Franklin G, et al. Practice parameter: evaluation of distal symmetric polyneuropathy: role of autonomic testing, nerve biopsy, and skin biopsy (an evidence-based review). *Neurology*. 2009;72:177–184.
86. Novak V, Freimer ML, Kissel JT, et al. Autonomic impairment in painful neuropathy. *Neurology*. 2001;56:861–868.
87. Kennedy WR, Sakuta M, Sutherland D, Goetz FC. Quantitation of the sweating deficiency in diabetes mellitus. *Ann Neurol*. 1984;15:482–488.
88. Low PA, Caskey PE, Tuck RR, Fealey RD, Dyck PJ. Quantitative sudomotor axon reflex test in normal and neuropathic subjects. *Ann Neurol*. 1983;14:573–580.
89. Harati Y, Low PA. Autonomic peripheral neuropathies: Diagnosis and clinical presentation. In: Appel S ed. *Current Neurology*. Chapter 3. Boston, MA: Houghton Mifflin; 1990.
90. Ravits JM. AAEM Minimonograph #48 autonomic nervous system testing. *Muscle Nerve*. 1997;20:919–937.
91. Giuliani MJ, Steward JD, Low PA. Distal small-fiber neuropathy. In: Low PA ed. *Clinical Autonomic Disorders*. 2nd ed. Philadelphia, PA: Lippincott-Raven; 1997:699–714.
92. Stewart KD, Low PA, Fealey RD. Distal small-fiber neuropathy: Results of tests of sweating and autonomic cardiovascular reflexes. *Muscle Nerve*. 1992;15:661–665.
93. Tobin K, Giuliani MJ, Lacomis D. Comparison of different modalities for detection of small-fiber neuropathy. *Clin Neurophys*. 1999;110:1909–1912.
94. Dyck PJ, Oviatt RF, Lambert EH. Intensive evaluation of referred unclassified neuropathy yields improved diagnosis. *Ann Neurol*. 1981;10:222–226.
95. Burns TM, Bauermann ML. The evaluation of polyneuropathies. *Neurology*. 2011;76:S6–S13.
96. Fagius J. Chronic cryptogenic polyneuropathy; the search for a cause. *Acta Neurol Scand*. 1983;67:173–180.
97. Low PA, Zimmerman BR, Dyck PJ. Comparison of distal sympathetic with vagal function in diabetic neuropathy. *Muscle Nerve*. 1986;9:592–596.
98. Lubec D, Mulbacher W, Finsterer J, Mamoli B. Diagnostic work-up in peripheral neuropathy: An analysis of 171 cases. *Postgrad Med J*. 1999;75:723–727.
99. England JD, Gronseth GS, Franklin G, et al. Practice parameter: evaluation of distal symmetric polyneuropathy: role of laboratory and genetic testing (an evidence-based review). *Neurology*. 2009;72:185–192.
100. Saperstein DS. Selecting diagnostic tests in peripheral neuropathy patients. In Course #7FC 002. Peripheral Neuropathy Annual Meeting of the American Academy of Neurology. San Diego, CA; 2006.
101. Schaumburg H, Kaplan J, Windebank A, et al. Sensory neuropathy from pyridoxine abuse. A new megavitamin syndrome. *N Engl J Med*. 1983;309(8):445–448.
102. Kelly JJ, Kyle RA, O'Brien PC, Dyck PJ. Prevalence of monoclonal protein in peripheral neuropathy. *Neurology*. 1981;31:1480–1483.
103. Nobile-Orazio E., Terenghi F, Giannotta C, Ballia F, Nozza A. Serum VEGF levels in POEMS syndrome and in immune-mediated neuropathies. *Neurology*. 2009;72(11):1024–1026.
104. Briani C, Fabrizi GM, Ruggero S, et al. Vascular endothelial growth factor helps differentiate neuropathies in rare plasma cell dyscrasias. *Muscle Nerve*. 2011;43:164–167.
105. Vrethem M, Cruz M, Wen-Xin H, Malm C, Holmgren H, Ernerudh J. Clinical, neurophysiological and immunopathological evidence of polyneuropathy in patients with monoclonal gammopathies. *J Neurol Sci*. 1993;34:130–135.
106. Saperstein DS, Katz JS, Amato AA, Barohn RJ. Clinical spectrum of chronic acquired demyelinating polyneuropathies. *Muscle Nerve*. 2001;24:311–324.
107. Proceedings of a consensus development conference on standardized measures in diabetic neuropathy. *Diabetes Care*. 1992;15:1080–1108.
108. Pourmand R. Evaluating patients with suspected peripheral neuropathy: Do the right thing, not everything. *Muscle Nerve*. 2002;26:288–290.
109. Novella SP, Inzucchi SE, Goldstein JM. The frequency of undiagnosed diabetes and impaired glucose tolerance in patients with idiopathic sensory neuropathy. *Muscle Nerve*. 2001;24:1229–1231.
110. Russell JW, Feldman EL. Impaired glucose tolerance—does it cause neuropathy? *Muscle Nerve*. 2001;24(9):1109–1112.
111. Singleton JR, Smith AG, Bromberg MB. Painful sensory polyneuropathy associated with impaired glucose tolerance. *Muscle Nerve*. 2001;24:1225–1228.
112. Hansen K, Legech A-M. The clinical and epidemiological profile of Lyme neuroborreliosis in Denmark 1985–1990. *Brain*. 1992;115:399–423.
113. Katirji B, Al-Jaberi MM. Creatine kinase revisited. *J Clin Neuromusc Dis*. 2001;2:158–163.
114. Sumner CJ, Sheth S, Griffin JW, Cornblath DR, Polydefkis M. The spectrum of neuropathy in diabetes and impaired glucose tolerance. *Neurology*. 2003;60:108–111.
115. Nicholson GA, McLeod JG, Morgan G, et al. Variable distributions of serum creatine kinase reference values. Relationship to exercise activity. *J Neurol Sci*. 1985;71:233–245.
116. Brewster LM, Mairuhu G, Sturk A, van Montfrans GA. Distribution of creatine kinase in the general population: Implications for statin therapy. *Am Heart J*. 2007;154:655–661.
117. Saporta AS, Sottilel SL, Miller LJ, Feely MS, Siskind SE, Shy ME. Charcot-Marie-Tooth disease uptight and genetic testing strategies. *Ann Neurol*. 2011;69:22–33.
118. Amato AA, Reilly ME. The death panel for Charcot-Marie-Tooth panels. *Ann Neurol*. 2011;69:22–33.
119. Klein CJ. The inherited neuropathies. *Neurol Clin*. 2007;25:173–207.
120. Amato AA, Hunderfund ANL, Selcen D, Keegan M. A 49-year-old woman with progressive shortness of breath. *Neurology*. 2011;76:830–836.
121. Wolfe GI, Kaminski HJ. Antibody testing in neuromuscular disorders, part 1: Peripheral neuropathies. *J Clin Neuromusc Dis*. 2000;2:84–95.

122. Pittock SJ, Kryzer TJ, Lennon VA. Paraneoplastic antibodies coexist and predict cancer, not neurologic syndrome. *Ann Neurol.* 2004;56:715–719.
123. Antoine JC, Mosnier JF, Absi L, Convers P, Honnorat J, Michel D. Carcinoma associated paraneoplastic peripheral neuropathies in patients with and without anti-onconeural antibodies. *J. Neurol Neurosurg Psychiatry.* 1999;67:7–14.
124. Psimaras D, Carpentier AF, Rossi C; PNS Euronetwork. Cerebrospinal fluid study and paraneoplastic syndromes. *J Neurol Neurosurg Psychiatry.* 2010;81:42–45.
125. Dalmau J, Furneaux HM, Rosenblum MK, Graus F, Posner JB. Detection of anti-Hu antibody in specific regions of the nervous system and tumor from patients with paraneoplastic encephalomyelitis/sensory neuropathy. *Neurology.* 1991;41: 1757–1764.
126. Camdessanche JP, Antoine JC, Honnorat J, et al. Paraneoplastic peripheral neuropathy associated with anti-Hu antibodies. A clinical and electrophysiological study of 20 patients. *Brain.* 2002;125:166–175.
127. Wolfe GI, El-Feky WH, Katz JS, Bryan WW, Wians FH Jr., Barohn RJ. Antibody panels in idiopathic polyneuropathy and motor neuron disease. *Muscle Nerve.* 1997;20:1275–1283.
128. Dalmau J, Graus F, Rosenblum MK, Posner JB. Anti-Hu-associated paraneoplastic encephalomyelitis/sensory neuronopathy. A clinical study of 71 patients. *Medicine.* 1992;71:59–72.
129. Oh SJ, Gurtekin Y, Dropcho EJ, King P, Claussen GC. Anti-Hu antibody neuropathy: A clinical, electrophysiological, and pathological study. *Clin Neurophysiol.* 2005;116:28–34.
130. Yu Z, Kryzer TJ, Griesmann GE, Kim K, Benarroch EE, Lennon VA. CRMP-5 neuronal autoantibody: Marker of lung cancer and thymoma-related autoimmunity. *Ann Neurol.* 2001;49: 146–154.
131. Luchinetti CF, Kimmel DW, Lennon VA. Paraneoplastic and oncologic profiles of patients seropositive for type 1 antineuronal nuclear autoantibodies. *Neurology.* 1998;50:652–657.
132. Grant IA, Hunder GG, Homburger HA, Dyck PJ. Peripheral neuropathy associated with sicca complex. *Neurology.* 1997;48:855–862.
133. McKeon A., Lennon VA, Lachance DH, Fealey RD, Pittock SJ. Ganglionic acetylcholine receptor autoantibody: Oncologic, neurological, and serological accompaniments. *Arch Neurol.* 2009;66(6):735–741.
134. Yuki N, Sato S, Tsuji S, Ohsawa T, Miyatake T. Frequent presence of anti-GQ1b antibody in Fisher's syndrome. *Neurology.* 1993;43:414–417.
135. Nobile-Orazio E, Francomano E, Daverio R, et al. Anti-myelin-associated glycoprotein IgM antibody titers in neuropathy associated with macroglobulinemia. *Ann Neurol.* 1989;26:543–550.
136. Latov N, Sherman WH, Nemni R, et al. Plasma-cell dyscrasia and peripheral neuropathy with a monoclonal antibody to peripheral-nerve myelin. *N Engl J Med.* 1980;303:618–621.
137. Gosselin S, Kyle RA, Dyck PJ. Neuropathy associated with monoclonal gammopathy of undetermined significance. *Ann Neurol.* 1991;30:54–61.
138. Katz JS, Saperstein DS, Gronseth G, Amato AA, Barohn RJ. Distal acquired demyelinating symmetric neuropathy. *Neurology.* 2000;54:615–620.
139. Nobile-Orazio E, Manfredini E, Carpo M, et al. Frequency and clinical correlates of anti-neural IgM antibodies in neuropathy associated with IgM monoclonal gammopathy. *Ann Neurol.* 1994;36:416–424.
140. Nobile-Orazio E, Latov N, Takatsu M, et al. Neuropathy and anti-MAG antibodies without detectable serum M-protein. *Neurology.* 1984;34:218–221.
141. Antoine JC, Honnorat J, Camdessanche JP, et al. Paraneoplastic anti-CV2 antibodies react with peripheral nerve and are associated with a mixed axonal and demyelinating peripheral neuropathy. *Ann Neurol.* 2001;49:214–221.
142. Carpo M, Allaria S, Scarlato G, Nobile-Orazio E. Marginally improved detection of GM1 antibodies by Covalink ELISA in multifocal motor neuropathy. *Neurology.* 1999;53:2206–2207.
143. Freddo L, Yu RK, Latov N, et al. Gangliosides GM1 and GD1b are antigens for IgM M-protein in a patient with motor neuron disease. *Neurology.* 1986;36:454–458.
144. Kinsella LJ, Lange DJ, Trojaborg W, Sadiq SA, Younger DS, Latov N. Clinical and electrophysiologic correlates of elevated anti-GM-1 antibody titers. *Neurology.* 1994;44:1278–1282.
145. Nobile-Orazio E, Cappellari A, Priori A. Multifocal motor neuropathy: Current concepts and controversies. *Muscle Nerve.* 2005;31:663–680.
146. Pestronk A, Chaudhry V, Feldman EL, et al. Lower motor neuron syndromes defined by patterns of weakness, nerve conduction abnormalities, and high titres of antiglycolipid antibodies. *Ann Neurol.* 1990;27:316–326.
147. Taylor BV, Gross I, Windebank AJ. The sensitivity and specificity of anti-GM1 antibody testing. *Neurology.* 1996;47:951–955.
148. Gooch CL, Amato AA. Are anti-ganglioside antibodies of clinical value in multifocal motor neuropathy? *Neurology.* 2010;75:1950–1951.
149. Cats EA, Jacobs BC, Yuki N, et al. Multifocal motor neuropathy: association of anti-GM1 IgM antibodies with clinical features. *Neurology.* 2010;75:1961–1967.
150. von Schaik IN, Bossuyt PM, Brand A, Vermeulen M. Diagnostic value of GM1 antibodies in motor neuron disorders and neuropathies: A meta-analysis. *Neurology.* 1995;45:1570–1577.
151. Park JH, Olsen NJ, King L Jr., et al. Use of magnetic resonance imaging and P-31 magnetic resonance spectroscopy to detect and quantify muscle dysfunction in the amyopathic and myopathic variants of dermatomyositis. *Arthritis Rheum.* 1995;38:68–77.
152. Parry GJ. Antiganglioside antibodies do not necessarily play a role in multifocal motor neuropathy. *Muscle Nerve.* 1994;17: 97–99.
153. Swash M, Brown MM, Thakkar C. CT muscle imaging and the clinical assessment of neuromuscular disease. *Muscle Nerve.* 1995;18:708–714.
154. Pestronk A, Choksi R. Multifocal motor neuropathy. Serum IgM anti-GM1 ganglioside antibodies in most patients detected using covalent linkage of GM1 to ELISA plates. *Neurology.* 1997;49:1289–1292.
155. Carpo M, Pedotti R, Allaria S, et al. Clinical presentation and outcome of Guillain–Barré and related syndromes in relation to anti-ganglioside antibodies. *J Neurol Sci.* 1999;168:78–84.
156. Chiba A, Kusunoki S, Obata H, Machinami R, Kanazawa I. Serum anti-GQ1b IgG antibody is associated with ophthalmoplegia in Miller Fisher syndrome and Guillain Barre syndrome: Clinical and immunohistochemical studies. *Neurology.* 1993;43:414–417.
157. Willison HJ, Veitch J, Paterson G, Kennedy PG. Miller Fisher syndrome is associated with serum antibodies to GQ1b ganglioside. *J Neurol Neurosurg Psychiatry.* 1993;56:204–206.
158. Lopate G, Parks BJ, Goldstein JM, Yee WC, Friesenhahn GM, Pestronk A. Polyneuropathies associated with high titre antisulfatide antibodies: characteristics of patients with and

without serum monoclonal proteins. *J Neurol Neurosurg Psychiatry*. 1997;62:581–585.
159. Pestronk A, Li F, Bieser K, et al. Anti-MAG antibodies: Major effects of antigen purity and antibody cross-reactivity on ELISA results and clinical correlation. *Neurology*. 1994;44:1131–1137.
160. Patrick J, Lindstrom J. Autoimmune response to acetylcholine receptor. *Science*. 1973;180:871–872.
161. Kaminski HJ, Sanantilan C, Wolfe GI. Antibody testing in neuromuscular disorders, part 2: Neuromuscular junction, hyperexcitability and muscle disorders. *J Clin Neuromusc Dis*. 2000;2:96–105.
162. Lindstrom JM, Seybold ME, Lennon VA, Whittingham S, Duane DD. Antibody to acetylcholine receptor in myasthenia gravis. Prevalence, clinical correlates, and diagnostic value. *Neurology*. 1976;26:1054–1059.
163. Vincent A, Newsom-Davis J. Acetylcholine receptor antibody as a diagnostic test for myasthenia gravis: Results in 153 validated cases and 2967 diagnostic assays. *J Neurol Neurosurg Psychiatry*. 1985;48:1246–1252.
164. Lanska DJ. Diagnosis of thymoma in myasthenics using anti-striated muscle antibodies: Predictive value and gain in diagnostic certainty. *Neurology*. 1991;41:520–524.
165. Aarli JA. Titin, thymoma, and myasthenia gravis. *Arch Neurol*. 2001;58:869–870.
166. Romi F, Skeie GO, Aarli JA, Gilhus NE. Muscle autoantibodies in subgroups of myasthenia gravis patients. *J Neurol*. 2000;247:369–375.
167. Lennon VA. Serological diagnosis of myasthenia gravis and the Lambert–Eaton myasthenic syndrome. In: Dekker M ed. *Handbook of Myasthenia Gravis and Myasthenic Syndromes*. New York, NY: Marcel Dekker; 1994:149–164.
168. Reimers CD, Schedel H, Fleckenstein JL, et al. Magnetic resonance imaging of skeletal muscles in idiopathic inflammatory myopathies of adults. *J Neurol*. 1994;241:306–314.
169. Cikes N, Momoi M, Williams CL, et al. Striational autoantibodies: Quantitative detection by enzyme immunoassay in myasthenia gravis, thymoma and recipients of d-penicillamine and allogeneic bone marrow. *Mayo Clin Proc*. 1988;63:474–481.
170. Burges J, Vincent A, Molennar PC, Newsom-Davis J, Peers C, Wray D. Passive transfer of seronegative myasthenia gravis to mice. *Muscle Nerve*. 1994;17:1393–1400.
171. Evoli A, Batocchi AP, Lo Monaco M, et al. Clinical heterogeneity of seronegative myasthenia gravis. *Neuromuscul Disord*. 1996;6:155–161.
172. Hoch W, McConville J, Helms S, Newsom-Davis J, Melms A, Vincent A. Autoantibodies to the receptor tyrosine kinase MuSK in patients with myasthenia gravis without acetylcholine receptor antibodies. *Nat Med*. 2001;7:365–368.
173. Deymeer F, Gungor-Tuncer O, Yilmaz V, et al. Clinical comparison of anti-MuSK- vs anti-AchR-positive and seronegative myasthenia gravis. *Neurology*. 2007;68:609–611.
174. Evoli A, Padua L, Monaco ML, et al. Clinical correlates with anti-MuSK antibodies in generalized seronegative myasthenia gravis. *Brain*. 2003;126:2304–2311.
175. Zhou L, McConville J, Chaudhry V, et al. Clinical comparison of muscle-specific tyrosine kinase (MuSK) antibody-positive and -negative myasthenic patients. *Muscle Nerve*. 2004;30: 55–60.
176. Sanders DB, El-Salem K, Massey JM, McConville J, Vincent A. Clinical aspects of MuSK antibody positive seronegative MG. *Neurology*. 2003;60:1978–1980.
177. Zagoria RJ, Karstardt N, Konbes TD. MR imaging of rhabdomyolysis. *J Comput Assist Tomogr*. 1986;10:268–277.
178. Bartoccioni E, Scuderi F, Minicuci GM, Marion M, Ciaraffa F, Evoli A. Anti-MuSK antibodies: Correlation with myasthenia gravis severity. *Neurology*. 2006;67:505–507.
179. Abicht A, Lochmuller H. What's in the serum of seronegative MG and LEMS: MuSK et al. *Neurology*. 2002;59:1672–1673.
180. Ohta K, Shigemoto K, Kubo S, et al. MuSK antibodies in AchR AB-seropositive MG vs. Ach R Ab-seronegative MG. *Neurology*. 2004;62:2132–2133.
181. Selcen D, Fukuda T, Shen XM, Engel AG. Are MuSk antibodies the primary cause of myasthenic symptoms? *Neurology*. 2004;62:1945–1950.
182. Ansevin C, Agamanolis D. Thymoma and myasthenia gravis with rippling muscles. *Arch Neurol*. 1996;53:197–199.
183. Mueller-Felber W, Ansevin C, Ricker K, et al. Immunosuppressive treatment of rippling muscles in patients with myasthenia gravis. *Neuromuscul Disord*. 1999;9:604–607.
184. Nakao YK, Motomura M, Fukudome T, et al. Seronegative Lambert–Eaton myasthenic syndrome: Study of 110 Japanese patients. *Neurology*. 2002;59:1773–1775.
185. Lennon VA, Kryzer TJ, Griesmann GE, et al. Calcium-channel antibodies in the Lambert–Eaton syndrome and other paraneoplastic syndromes. *N Engl J Med*. 1995;332:1467–1474.
186. Sabater L., Titulaer M., Saiz A., Verschururen J., Güre AO, Graus F. SOX1 antibodies are markers of paraneoplastic Lambert-Eaton myasthenic syndrome. *Neurology*. 2008;70:924–928.
187. Newsom-Davis J, Mills KR. Immunological associations of acquired neuromyotonia (Isaacs' syndrome). *Brain*. 1993;116: 453–469.
188. Oskarsson B. Myopathy: Five new things. *Neurology*. 2011; 76(suppl 2):S14–S19.
189. Lacomis D, Oddis CV. Myositis-specific and – associated autoantibodies: A review from the clinical perspective. *J Clin Neuromusc Dis*. 2000;2:34–40.
190. Amato AA, Barohn RJ. Inflammatory myopathies: Dermatomyositis, polymyositis, inclusion body myositis, and related diseases. In: Schapira AHV, Griggs RC eds. *Muscle Diseases*. Boston, MA: Butterworth Heinemann; 1999:299–338.
191. Love L, Leff R, Fraser D, et al. A new approach to the classification of idiopathic inflammatory myopathy: Myositis-specific autoantibodies define useful homogeneous patient groups. *Medicine*. 1991;70:360–374.
192. Mimori T. Autoantibodies in connective tissue disease: Clinical significance and analysis of target autoantigens. *Intern Med*. 1999;38:523–532.
193. Mammen AL, Chung T, Christopher-Stine L, et al. Autoantibodies against 3-hydroxy-3-methylglutaryl-coenzyme A reductase in patients with statin-associated autoimmune myopathy. *Arthritis Rheum*. 2011;63:713–721.
194. Christopher-Seine L, Casciola-Rosen LA, Hong G, Chung T, Corse AM, Mammen AL. A novel autoantibody recognizing 200-KD and 100-kd proteins is associated with an immune mediated necrotizing myopathy. *Arthritis Rheum*. 2010;62:2757–2766.
195. Targoff IN, Mamyrova G, Trieu EP, et al. A novel auto-antibody to 155-kd protein is associated with dermatomyositis. *Arthritis Rheum*. 2006; 54:3682–3689.
196. Halperin JJ. Lyme disease and the peripheral nervous system. *Muscle Nerve*. 2003;28(2):133–143.

197. American College of Physicians. Guidelines for laboratory evaluation in the diagnosis of Lyme disease. *Ann Intern Med.* 1998;128:1106.
198. Halperin JJ, Logigian EL, Finkel MF, Pearl RA. Practice parameters for the diagnosis of patients with nervous system Lyme borreliosis (Lyme disease). *Neurology.* 1996;46:619–627.
199. Tugwell P, Dennis DT, Weinstein A, et al. Laboratory evaluation in the diagnosis of Lyme disease. *Ann Intern Med.* 1997;1127:1106.
200. Wormser GP, Dattwyler RJ, Shapiro ED, et al. The clinical assessment, treatment and prevention of Lyme disease, human granulocytic anaplasmosis, and babesiosis: Clinical practice guidelines by the Infectious Diseases Society of America. *Clin Infect Dis.* 2006;43:1089.
201. Dressler F, Whalen JA, Reinhardt BN, Steere AC. Western blotting in the serodiagnosis of Lyme disease. *J Infect Dis.* 1993;167(2):392–400.
202. Nocton JJ, Bloom BJ, Rutledge BJ, et al. Detection of Borrelia burgdorferi DNA by polymerase chain reaction in cerebrospinal fluid in Lyme neuroborreliosis. *J Infect Dis.* 1996;174:623–627.
203. Coyle PK, Schutzer SE, Deng Z, et al. Detection of Borrelia burgdorferi-specific antigen in antibody-negative cerebrospinal fluid in neurologic Lyme disease. *Neurology.* 1995;45(11):2010–2015.
204. Halperin JJ, Luft BJ, Anand AK, et al. Lyme neuroborreliosis: Central nervous system manifestations. *Neurology.* 1989;39(6):753–759.
205. Logigian EL, Kaplan RF, Steere AC. Chronic neurologic manifestations of Lyme disease. *N Engl J Med.* 1990;323(21):1438–1444.
206. Brew BJ. The peripheral nerve complications of human immunodeficiency virus (HIV) infection. *Muscle Nerve.* 2003;28:542–552.
207. Dalakas MC, Pezeshkpour GH. Neuromuscular diseases associated with human immunodeficiency virus infection. *Ann Neurol.* 1988;23(suppl):S38–S48.
208. Robinson-Papp J, Simpson DM. Neuromuscular diseases associated with HIV-infection. *Muscle Nerve.* 2009;40:1043–1053.
209. Lange DJ, Britton CB, Younger DS, Hays AP. The neuromuscular manifestations of human immunodeficiency virus infections. *Arch Neurol.* 1988;45:1084–1048.
210. Allain JP, Laurian Y, Paul DA, Senn D. Serological markers in early stages of human immunodeficiency virus infection in haemophiliacs. *Lancet.* 1986;2:1233.
211. Horsburgh CR, Ou CY, Jason J, et al. Duration of human immunodeficiency virus infection before detection of antibody. *Lancet.* 1989;2:637.
212. Centers for Disease Control (CDC). Update: Serologic testing for HIV-1 antibody – United States, 1988 and 1989. *MMWR Morb Mortal Wkly Rep.* 1990;39:380.
213. Hollander H, Levy JA. Neurologic abnormalities and recovery of human immunodeficiency virus from cerebrospinal fluid. *Ann Intern Med.* 1987;106:692–695.
214. Sène D, Jallouli M, Lefaucheur JP, et al. Peripheral neuropathies associated with primary Sjögren syndrome immunologic profiles of nonataxic sensory neuropathy and sensorimotor neuropathy. *Medicine.* 2011;90:133–138.
215. Font J, Ramos-Casals M, de la Red G, et al. Pure sensory neuropathy in primary Sjögren's syndrome. Long term prospective follow up and review of the literature. *J Rheumatol.* 2003;30:1552–1557.
216. Chai J, Hermman D, Stanton M, Barbano RL, Logigian EL. Painful small-fiber neuropathy in Sjögren syndrome. *Neurology.* 2005;65:925–927.
217. Sandroni P, Low PA. Autonomic peripheral neuropathies: Clinical presentation, diagnosis, and treatment. *J Clin Neuromusc Dis.* 2001;2:147–157.
218. Chin RL, Sander HW, Brannagan TH, et al. Celiac neuropathy. *Neurology.* 2003;60:1581–1585.
219. Cross AH, Golumbek PT. Neurologic manifestations of celiac disease: Proven, or just a gut feeling. *Neurology.* 2003;60:1566–1568.
220. Hadjivassiliou M, Grunewald RA, Davies-Jones GA. Gluten sensitivity as a neurological illness. *J Neurol Neurosurg Psychiatry.* 2002;72:560–563.
221. Wills A, Hovell CJ. Neurological complications of enteric disease. *Gut.* 1996;39:501–504.
222. Tan KM, Lennon VA, Klein CJ, Boeve EF, Pittock SJ. Clinical spectrum of voltage-gated potassium channel autoimmunity. *Neurology.* 2008; 70:1883–1890.
223. Chalk CH, Homburger HA, Dyck PJ. Anti-neutrophil cytoplasmic antibodies in vasculitic peripheral neuropathy. *Neurology.* 1993;43:1826–1827.
224. Hart IK. Acquired neuromyotonia: A new autoantibody-mediated neuronal potassium channelopathy. *Am J Med Sci.* 2000;319:209–216.
225. Shilito P, Molenaar PC, Vincent A, et al. Acquired neuromyotonia: Evidence for autoantibodies directed against K+ channels of peripheral nerves. *Ann Neurol.* 1995;38:714–722.
226. Grant GA, Britz GW, Goodkin R, Jarvik JG, Maravilla K, Kliot M. The utility of magnetic resonance imaging in evaluating peripheral nerve lesions. *Muscle Nerve.* 2002;25:314–331.
227. Filler AG, Maravilla KR, Tsuruda JS. MR neurography and muscle MR imaging for image diagnosis of disorders affecting the peripheral nerves and musculature. *Neurol Clin.* 2004;22:643–682.
228. vd Vliet AM, Thijsssen HO, Joosten E, Merx JL. CAT in neuromuscular disorders as comparison of CT and histology. *Neuroradiology.* 1988;30:421–425.
229. Koltzenburg M, Bendszus M. Imaging of peripheral nerve lesions. *Curr Opin Neurol.* 2004;17:621–626.
230. Fraser DD, Frank JA, Dalakas M, Miller FW, Hicks JE, Plotz P. Magnetic resonance imaging in the idiopathic inflammatory myopathies. *J Rheumatol.* 1991;18:1693–1700.
231. Hernandez RJ, Sullivan DB, Chenevert TL, Keim DR. MR imaging in children with dermatomyositis: Musculoskeletal findings and correlation with clinical and laboratory findings. *Am J Roentgenol.* 1993;161:359–366.
232. Keim DR, Hernandez RJ, Sullivan DB. Serial magnetic resonance imaging in juvenile dermatomyositis. *Arthritis Rheum.* 1991;34:1580–1584.
233. Murphy WA, Totty WG, Carrole JC. MRI of normal and pathological skeletal muscle. *Am J Radiol.* 1986;146:565–574.
234. Cartwright MS, Chloros GD, Walker FO, Wiesler ER, Campbell WW. Diagnostic ultrasound for nerve transaction. *Muscle Nerve.* 2007;35:796–799.
235. Stonecipher MR, Jorizzo JL, Monu J, Walker F, Sutej PG. Dermatomyositis with normal muscle enzyme concentrations. A single-blind study of the diagnostic value of magnetic resonance imaging and ultrasound. *Arch Dermatol.* 1994;130:1294–1299.

236. Olsen NJ, Qi J, Park JH. Imaging and skeletal muscle disease. *Curr Rheumatol Rep*. 2005;7:106–114.
237. Scott DL, Kingsley GH. Use of imaging to assess patients with muscle disease. *Curr Opin Rheumatol*. 2004;16:678–683.
238. Chapman S, Sopiuthwood TR, Fowler J, Ryder CA. Rapid changes in magnetic resonance imaging of muscle during the treatment of juvenile dermatomyositis. *Br J Rheumatol*. 1994;33:184–186.
239. Fleckenstein JL, Archer BT, Barker BA, Vaughan JT, Parkey RW, Peshock RM. Fast short-tau inversion-recovery MR imaging. *Radiology*. 1991;179:499–504.
240. Britz GW, Haynor DR, Kuntz C, et al. Ulnar nerve entrapment at the elbow: Correlation of magnetic resonance imaging, clinical, electrodiagnostic, and intraoperative findings. *Neurosurgery*. 1996;38:458–465.
241. Bertorini T, Halford G, Lawrence J, Vo D, Wassef M. Contrast-enhanced magnetic resonance imaging of the lumbosacral roots in the dysimmune inflammatory polyneuropathies. *J Neuroimaging*. 1995;5:9–15.
242. Kuwabara SK, Nakajima M, Matsuda S, Hattori T. Magnetic resonance imaging at the demyelinative foci in chronic inflammatory demyelinating polyneuropathy. *Neurology*. 1997;48:874–877.
243. Midroni G, de Tilly LN, Gray B, Vajsar J. MRI of the cauda equina in CIDP: Clinical correlations. *J Neurol Sci*. 1999;170:36–44.
244. Parry GJ. AAEM case report #30: Multifocal motor neuropathy. *Muscle Nerve*. 1996;19:269–276.
245. Cosgrove JC. Magnetic resonance imaging in the evaluation of carpal tunnel syndrome: A literature review. *J Clin Neuromusc Dis*. 2000;1:175–183.
246. Vernino S, Low PA, Fealey RD, Stewart JD, Farrugia G, Lennon VA. Autoantibodies to ganglionic acetylcholine receptors in autoimmune autonomic neuropathy. *N Engl J Med*. 2000;343:847–845.
247. Zhou L, Yousem DM, Chaudhry V. Role of magnetic resonance neurography in brachial plexus lesions. *Muscle Nerve*. 2004;30:305–309.
248. Ellegala DB, Lankerovich L, Haynor D, Bird T, Goodkin R, Kliot M. Characterization of genetically defined types of Charcot–Marie–Tooth neuropathies using magnetic resonance neurography. *Neurosurgery*. 1998;43:655–721.
249. Jaiser SR, Winston GP. Copper deficiency myelopathy (review). *J Neurol*. 2010;257(6):869–881.
250. Kumar N, Ahlskog JE, Klein CJ, Port JD. Imaging features of copper deficiency myelopathy: a study of 25 cases. *Neuroradiology*. 2006;48(2):78–83.
251. Locatelli ER, Laureno R, Ballard P, Mark AS. MRI in vitamin B12 deficiency myelopathy. *Can J Neurol Sci*. 1999;26(1):60–63.
252. Halford H, Graves A, Bertorinie T. Muscle and nerve imaging techniques in neuromuscular diseases. *J Clin Neuromusc Dis*. 2000;2:41–51.
253. Walker FO, Alter KE, Boon AJ, et al. Qualifications for practitioners of neuromuscular ultrasound: Position statement of the American Association of Neuromuscular and Electrodiagnostic Medicine. *Muscle & Nerve*. 2010;42(3):442–444.
254. Walker FO, Cartwright MS, Wiesler ER, Caress J. Ultrasound of nerve and muscle. *Clin Neurophysiol*. 2004;115:495–507.
255. Hobson-Webb LD, Massey JM, Juel VC, Sanders DB. The ultrasonographic wrist-to- forearm median nerve area ratio in carpal tunnel syndrome. *Clin Neurophysiol*. 2008;119: 1353–1357.
256. Claes F, Meulstee J, Claessen-Oude Luttikhuis TT, Huygen PL, Verhagen WI. Usefulness of additional measurements of the median nerve with ultrasonography. *Neurol Sci*. 2010;31(6):721–725.
257. Yoon JS, Walker FO, Cartwright MS. Ultrasonographic swelling ratio in the diagnosis of ulnar neuropathy at the elbow. *Muscle Nerve*. 2008;38:1231–1235.
258. Visser LH. High-resolution sonography of the common peroneal nerve: Detection of intraneural ganglia. *Neurology*. 2006; 167:1473–1475.
259. Beekman R, Visser LH. Sonography in the diagnosis of carpal tunnel syndrome: A critical review of the literature. *Muscle Nerve*. 2003; 27:26–33.
260. Beekman R, Wokke JH, Schoemaker MC, Lee ML, Visser LH. Ulnar neuropathy at the elbow: Followup in prognostic factors determining outcome. *Neurology*. 2004;63:1675–1680.
261. Zaidman CM, Al-Lozi M, Pestronk A. Peripheral nerve size in normals and patients with polyneuropathy: an ultrasound study. *Muscle Nerve*. 2009;40(6):960–966.
262. Matsuoka N, Kohriyama T, Ochi K, et al. Detection of cervical nerve root hypertrophy by ultrasonography and chronic inflammatory demyelinating polyradiculoneuropathy. *J Neurol Sci*. 2004;219:15–21.
263. Taniguchi N, Itoh K, Wang Y, et al. Sonographic detection of diffuse peripheral nerve hypertrophy and chronic inflammatory demyelinating polyradiculoneuropathy. *J Clin Ultrasound*. 2000;28(9)488–491.
264. Van Alfen N, Nienhuis M, Zwarts MJ, Pillen S. Detection of fibrillations using muscle ultrasound: diagnostic accuracy and identification of pitfalls. *Muscle Nerve*. 2011;43:178–182.
265. Heckmatt JZ, Dubowitz V, Leeman S. Detection of pathological change in dystrophic muscle with B-scan ultrasound imaging. *Lancet*. 1980;1:1389–1390.
266. Reimers CD, Fleckenstein JL, Wiltt TN, Muller-Felber W, Pongratz DE. Muscular ultrasound in idiopathic inflammatory myopathies of adults. *J Neurol Sci*. 1993;116:82–92.
267. Reimers CD, Schlotter B, Eicke BM, Witt TN. Enlargement in neuromuscular diseases: A quantitative ultrasound study in 350 patients and review of the literature. *J Neurol Sci*. 1996;143:46–56.
268. Wu JS, Darras BT, Rutkove SB. Assessing spinal muscular atrophy with quantitative ultrasound. *Neurology*. 2010;75: 526–531.

CHAPTER 3

Muscle and Nerve Histopathology

Muscle and nerve biopsies can be extremely useful in the evaluation of patients with myopathies and neuropathies. That said, not everyone suspected of having a muscle or nerve disorder needs a biopsy. In this chapter, we discuss the indications and limitations for muscle and nerve biopsies, how specific muscle or nerves are selected for biopsy, and various aspects of specimen handling. Further, we review the routine stains that are performed on muscle and nerve tissue, other stains or studies that can be performed on the tissue, and when to order them. We also mention the role of skin biopsy to assess epidermal nerve fibers in the evaluation of patients with peripheral neuropathy. This chapter is not designed to make the reader a neuropathologist. However, clinicians who take care of patients with neuromuscular disease and order biopsies should have at least a working knowledge of muscle and nerve histopathology.

▶ MUSCLE BIOPSIES

Muscle biopsies are studied through a combination of various histochemistry stains on frozen sections and paraffin-embedded tissue, electron microscopy (EM), and molecular studies (e.g., enzyme assay, protein analysis by Western blot, mitochondrial DNA mutations).[1–5] It is important to correlate the histopathologic findings with clinical history, neuromuscular examination, and electrodiagnostic findings.

▶ INDICATIONS FOR MUSCLE BIOPSY

A muscle biopsy may be helpful when the patient has objective muscle weakness, abnormal muscle enzymes (e.g., elevated serum creatine kinase [CK] levels), abnormal skeletal muscle magnetic resonance imaging, or myopathic electromyography (EMG) findings. These findings may point to a myopathy but not the exact etiology, and therefore a muscle biopsy may be indicated. That said, if the diagnosis is suspected on the basis of the phenotype and can be made by less invasive means, we generally opt for this first. For example, in a young boy with proximal weakness and large calves, we would first do genetic testing for a dystrophinopathy. Muscle biopsies are less helpful in evaluating patients with only myalgias, subjective weakness, or just slight elevations of CK in the absence of objective abnormalities.[6]

▶ TECHNIQUES

Muscle tissue can be obtained through an open (minor surgical procedure) or needle biopsy. A larger sample of tissue can be biopsied by the open surgery technique, and we prefer this method in patients who may have patchy pathology (e.g., inflammatory myopathies) or myopathies that require metabolic analysis (e.g., mitochondrial disorders or glycogen storage diseases), molecular studies (e.g., Western blotting and direct genetic analysis), or EM. Needle biopsy can also be technically difficult in patients with substantial subcutaneous tissue or whose muscles are atrophic and/or fibrotic. However, the yield of a needle biopsy can be quite high in laboratories that are experienced in handling the small amount of tissue obtained by this technique.[7–10] The advantage of a needle biopsy is that it allows for the examination of multiple sites within the muscle and it is a less invasive procedure than an open muscle biopsy.

We select the specific muscle to biopsy based on the clinical examination, or occasionally based on skeletal muscle magnetic resonance imaging or EMG guidance. If the requesting physician is not the person who performs the surgery (the usual situation), communication between the two is essential to ensure that the proper site is chosen. Preferably, one should biopsy a mildly weak muscle in the Medical Research Council (MRC) grade 4/5 range to increase the yield. If the muscle is too weak (i.e., MRC grade 3 or less), the tissue typically has end-stage damage. It is often impossible to discern a myopathic process from severe neurogenic atrophy under these conditions. In patients with little, if any, weakness on examination, or those who might only have weakness in muscles that are not easily accessible to biopsy (e.g., iliopsoas muscle in a patient with only hip flexor weakness), needle EMG or skeletal muscle magnetic resonance imaging are used to select the muscle to biopsy. However, it is important to biopsy the contralateral muscle to the needle examination in order to avoid artifact from needle EMG.

We find that the easiest muscle to biopsy with open surgery is the biceps brachii and is our first choice if clinically affected. Other muscles that are commonly biopsied are the deltoid, triceps, and quadriceps. We occasionally biopsy the

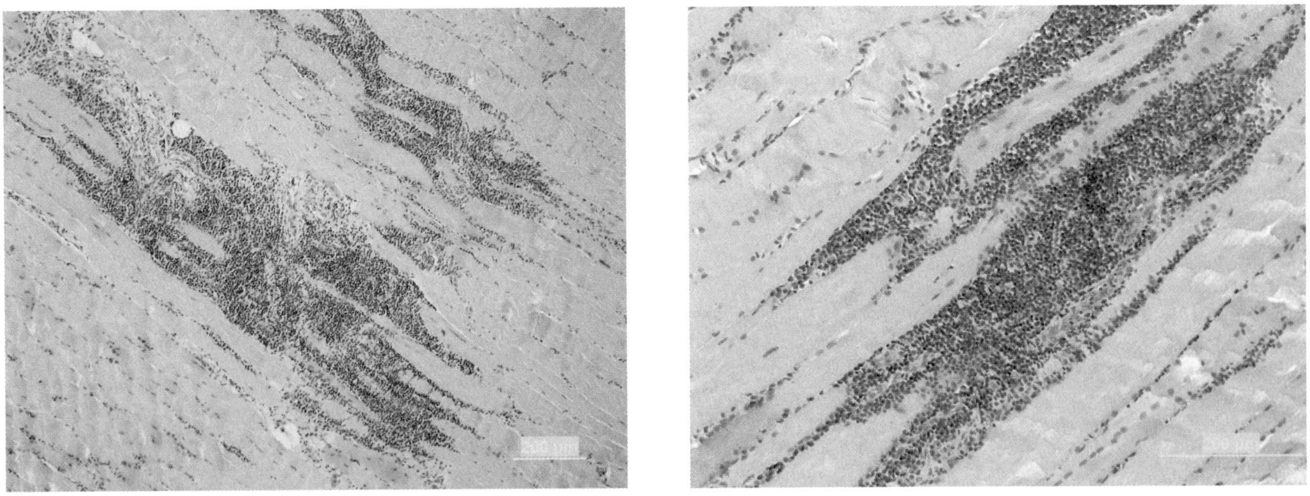

A B

Figure 3-1. Paraffin sections are useful because large, longitudinal segments of muscle fibers can be cut and stained compared to frozen sections. Marked endomysial inflammatory cell infiltrate in this biopsy of a patient with polymyositis **(A)**. On higher power, inflammatory cell infiltrates can be seen to invade the necrotic segments **(B)**. Paraffin sections, hematoxylin and eosin (H&E).

cervical paraspinals in patients with isolated neck extensor weakness or bent spine syndrome. The peroneus brevis muscle is useful to biopsy along with the overlying superficial peroneal nerve in patients suspected of having vasculitis. In patients with suspected distal myopathies, we have found the tibialis anterior, gastrocnemius, and forearm extensor muscles easy to biopsy. Otherwise, we tend to avoid the gastrocnemius or tibialis anterior muscle, because asymptomatic radiculopathies or unrelated axonal polyneuropathies may give a false impression that the primary abnormality is a neurogenic process and therefore overshadow an underlying myopathy.

In adults, muscle biopsies are performed under local anesthesia, but young children require sedation or general anesthesia. The biopsies are taken from the belly of the muscle, and it is important to avoid the region of the tendon. Each specimen should be about 1–2 cm in length and 0.5 cm in width. The specimens should be wrapped in slightly moist gauze and placed in separate labeled sterile containers until they reach the laboratory. It is important not to place the specimens in a container of saline else this will lead to artifact. Nor should the entire specimen be placed in fixative else the important histochemistry stains, protein/enzyme analysis, and mutation analysis cannot be performed. Again, this information needs to be communicated with the surgeon and the pathology laboratory. Because muscle disorders can be multifocal (e.g., inflammatory myopathies), we obtain at least two separate specimens, which are immediately frozen in isopentane cooled in liquid nitrogen. The frozen tissue is then sectioned and stained for routine histochemistry. In patients with prominent myalgias and tenderness, we may biopsy a piece of the overlying fascia to assess for fasciitis. Separate specimens may also be taken and again frozen immediately for biochemical analysis (e.g., for glycogen or lipid storage disorders and mitochondrial myopathies), mitochondrial DNA analysis, or for Western blot (e.g., in various forms of muscular dystrophy).

In addition, a separate piece of muscle tissue is fixed in formalin or Bouin's fluid for paraffin sections. Paraffin sections can be particularly useful in inflammatory myopathies and vasculitis, as it allows for the examination of a somewhat larger piece of tissue than that used for histochemistry in cross section and longitudinal section and assesses inflammatory cells and vasculature more effectively (Fig. 3-1). However, due to shrinkage of the muscle tissue associated with the processing, the muscle fibers in paraffin sections are often appear cracked and are not ideal for the evaluation of histochemical abnormalities. Finally, an additional piece of muscle is usually taken for possible ultrastructural examination by EM. This small piece of muscle tissue is secured on a clamp or stretched out by suturing the muscle over a tongue blade, in order to prevent hypercontraction artifact. This tissue is fixed in glutaraldehyde for plastic (resin) embedding for EM.

A standard battery of histochemical stains is used for light-microscopic evaluation of frozen sections (Table 3-1).[1–5] Hematoxylin and eosin (H&E) and modified Gomori-trichrome stains assess the size, shape, and cytoarchitecture of the muscle fibers, presence of internalized nuclei, destruction of fibers (e.g., necrosis) and regeneration, as well as the supporting connective tissue (e.g., increased endomysial connective tissue as seen in dystrophies) and vasculature (vasculitis) (Figs. 3-2 and 3-3). Inflammatory cell infiltration is easily appreciated with these stains. In addition, some specific abnormalities are well demonstrated with modified Gomori-trichrome stain: ragged red fibers associated with mitochondrial myopathies (Fig. 3-4A), nemaline rods (Fig. 3-4B), tubular

▶ TABLE 3-1. **MUSCLE FIBER-TYPE CHARACTERISTICS**

	Type 1	Type 2A	Type 2B
Gross appearance			
Color	Dark	Dark	Pale
Capillary density	High	High	Low
Muscle fiber diameter	Smallest	Large	Largest
Comparative histochemical activity			
ATPase 4.3	Strong	Weak	Weak
ATPase 4.6	Strong	Weak	Strong
ATPase 9.4	Weak	Strong	Strong
Adult myosin heavy chain—fast	Weak	Strong	Strong
Adult myosin heavy chain—slow	Strong	Weak	Weak
NADH-TR	Strong	Strong	Weak
SDH	Strong	Weak	Weak
Cytochrome oxidase	Strong	Weak	Weak
Glycogen content	Low	High	High
Glycogen phosphorylase	Weak	Strong	Strong
Myoglobin content	High	High	Low
Lipid content	High	High	Low
Modified Gomori trichrome	Strong	Weak	Weak
Electron microscopy			
Mitochondria	Numerous	Numerous	Few
Z-disc	Intermediate	Wide	Narrow
Physiologic characteristics			
Twitch speed	Slow	Fast	Fast
Fatigability	Resistant	Resistant	Susceptible
Axons			
Diameter	Smallest		Largest
Conduction velocity	Slowest		Fastest
Other classifications			
	Intermediate (Red)	Red	White
	S	FR	FF
	SO	FOG	FG
	B	C	A

FR, fast, resistant; FF, fast, fatigable; S, slow; FOG, fast, oxidative glycolytic; FG, fast, glycolytic; SO, slow oxidative; NADH-TR, nicotinamide adenine dinucleotide tetrazolium reductase.
Modified with permission from Carpenter S, Karpati G. *Pathology of Skeletal Muscle*. 2nd ed. New York, NY: Oxford; 2001.

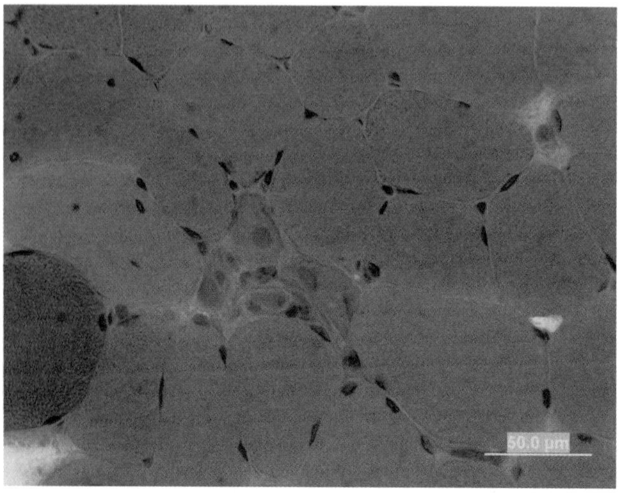

Figure 3-2. A cluster of regenerating muscle fibers are apparent on this H&E stain.

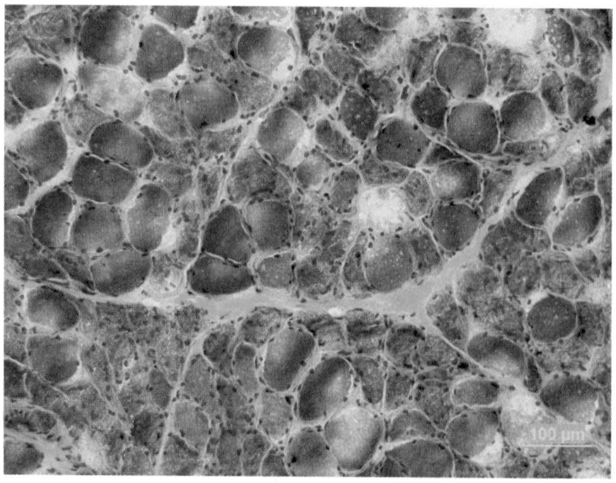

Figure 3-3. Muscle biopsy in a patient with acute quadriplegic myopathy reveals marked atrophy and degeneration of muscle fibers on this modified Gomori-trichrome stain.

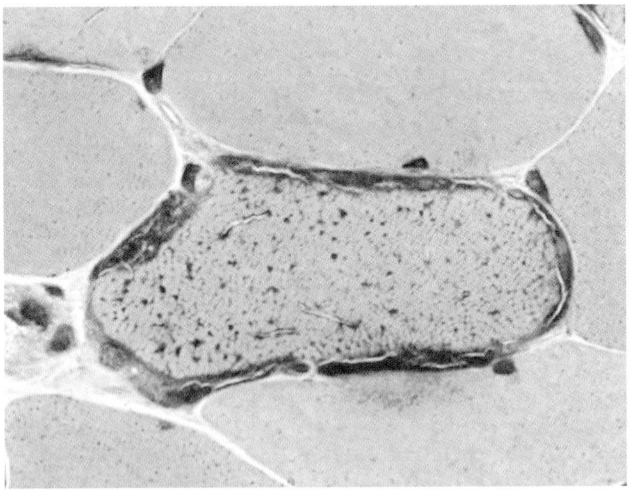

A

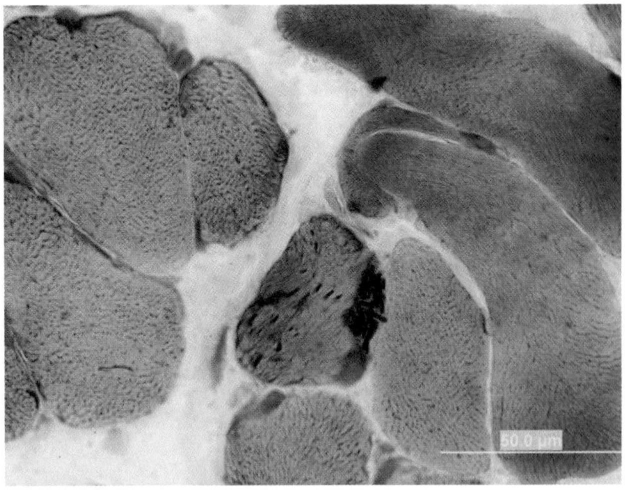

B

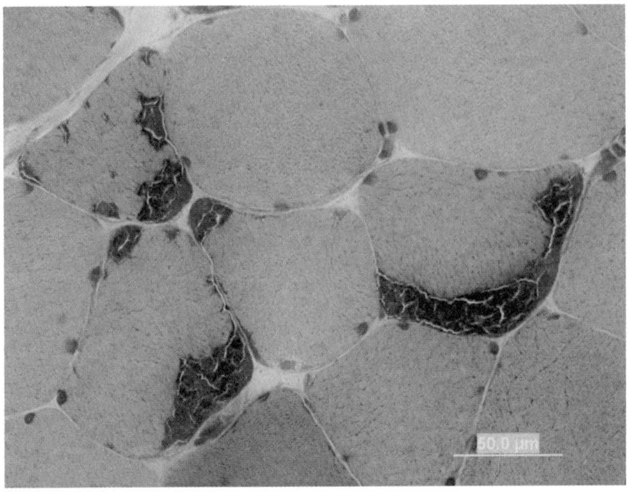

C

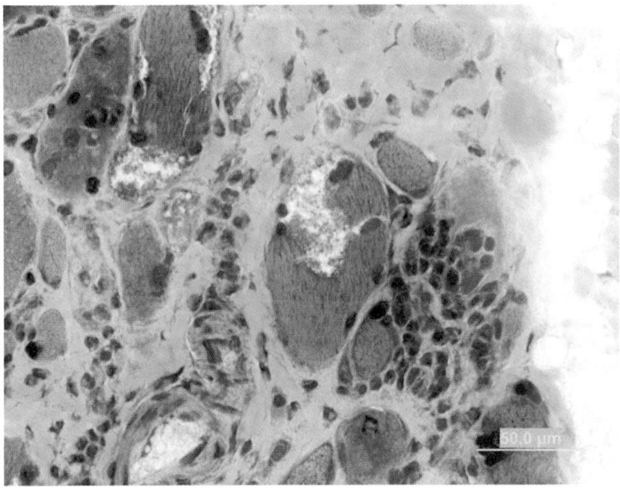

D

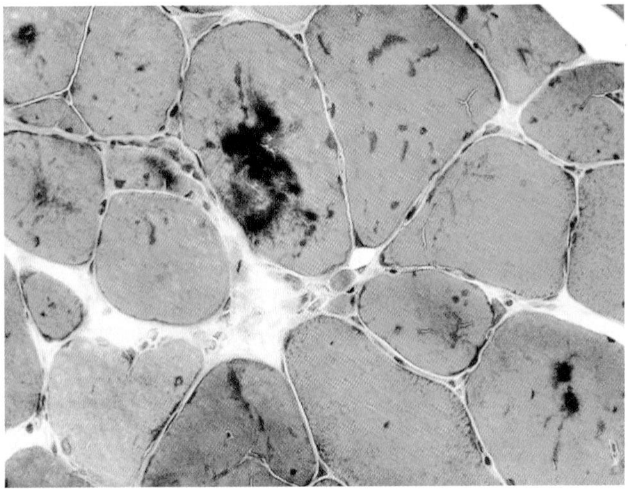

E

Figure 3-4. Modified Gomori-trichrome stain reveals a ragged red fiber in a patient with a mitochondrial myopathy **(A)**, nemaline rods in a patient with congenital myopathy **(B)**, tubular aggregates in a patient with myalgias **(C)**, and rimmed vacuoles filled with debri in a patient with IBM **(D)**. Myofibrillar myopathy is best recognized on the modified Gomori-trichrome stain as amorphous accumulation of dark green or bluish-purple debri and more distinct, denser cytoplasmic inclusions **(E)**.

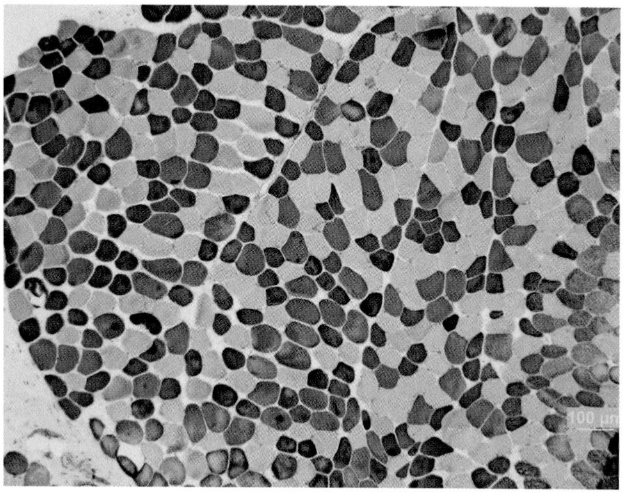

A

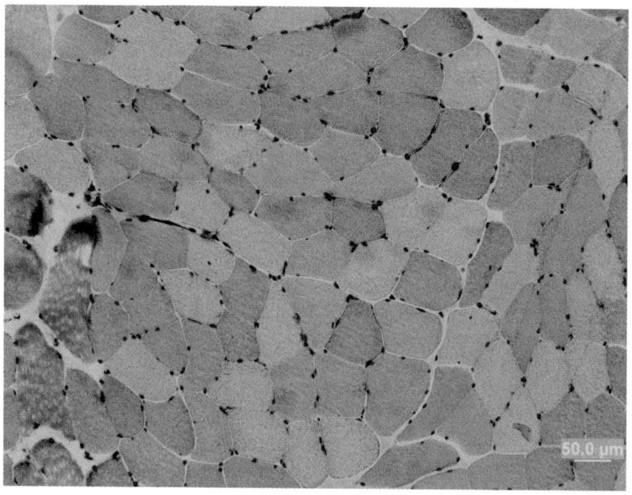

B

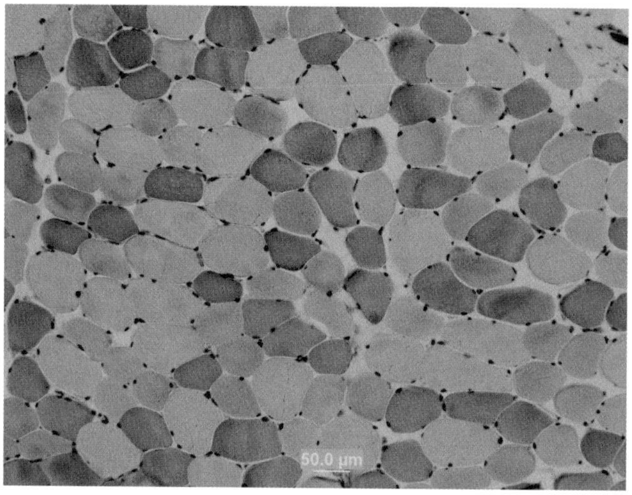

C

Figure 3-5. The myofibrillar adenosine triphosphatase (ATPase) is typically performed at three pHs: 4.3, 4.6, and 9.4. Type 1 fibers are lightly stained, whereas type 2 fibers are dark on ATPase 9.4 stain **(A)**. Type 1 fibers are dark, whereas type 2 fibers are light on ATPase 4.3 stain **(B)**. The ATPase 4.6 stains type 1 fibers dark, type 2 A fibers light, and type 2B fibers in between **(C)**.

aggregates (Fig. 3-4C), rimmed vacuoles (Fig. 3-4D), and features of myofibrillar myopathy (Fig. 3-4E).

The myofibrillar adenosine triphosphatase (ATPase) is typically performed at three pHs, 4.3, 4.6, and 9.4, in order to assess the size and distribution of different muscle fiber types (Table 3-1 and Fig. 3-5). Individual muscle fibers can be classified into four different fiber types on the basis of their staining characteristics and physiologic properties: types 1 (slow twitch, fatigue resistant, and oxidative metabolism), 2A (fast twitch, intermediate fatigue resistance, and oxidative and glycolytic metabolism), 2B (fast twitch, poor fatigue resistance, and glycolytic metabolism), and 2C (undifferentiated and embryonic). In adults, only about 1–2% of muscle fibers are the undifferentiated type 2C fibers.[11] The specific muscle fiber type is determined by the innervating motor neuron. The different muscle fiber types are normally distributed randomly, forming a so-called checkerboard pattern. Alterations in the random distribution of fiber such as seen with fiber-type grouping are a sign of denervation with subsequent reinnervation. Some myopathies are associated with a predominance or atrophy of a specific fiber type. For example, some congenital myopathies are associated with a predominance of type 1 fibers, which are also smaller in diameter than normal. Disuse and steroid myopathy are associated with preferential atrophy of type 2B fibers.

Periodic acid–Schiff (PAS) stain is used to assess glycogen content, which may be increased in the glycogen storage disorders (Fig. 3-6). If there is abnormal PAS staining then a PAS with diastase should be performed, as glycogen is removed with diastase but more complex carbohydrates (such as polyglucosan bodies) are resistant to digestion with diastase. Loss of some enzyme activities associated with some metabolic myopathies can be detected by specific staining protocols (e.g., myophosphorylase and phosphofructokinase). Sometimes in polyglucosan body neuropathy, PAS-positive inclusions are evident in small intramuscular nerves on muscle biopsies (Fig. 3-7). Acid phosphatase stains can highlight

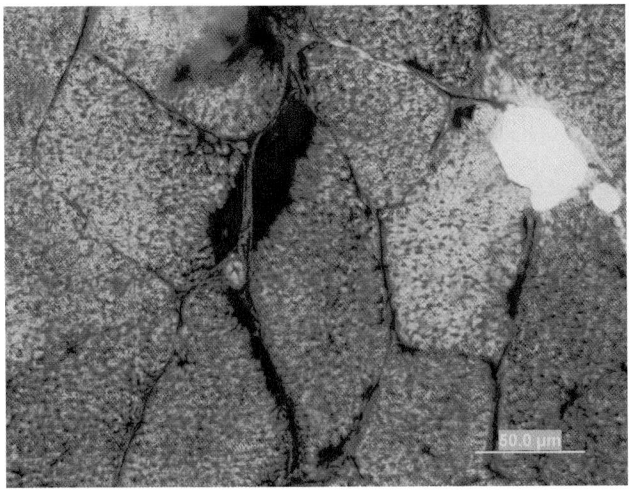

A

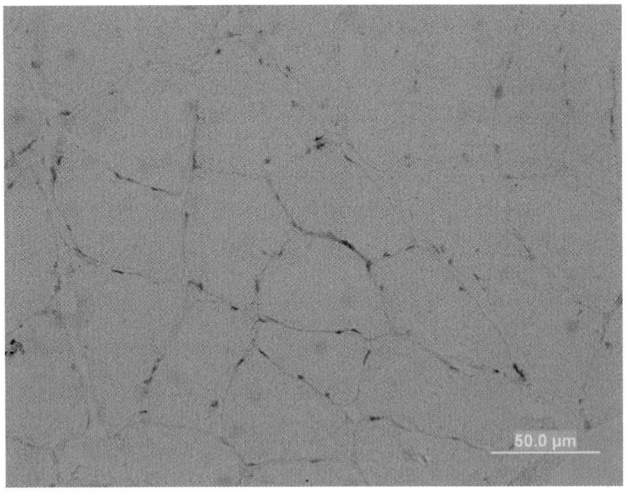

B

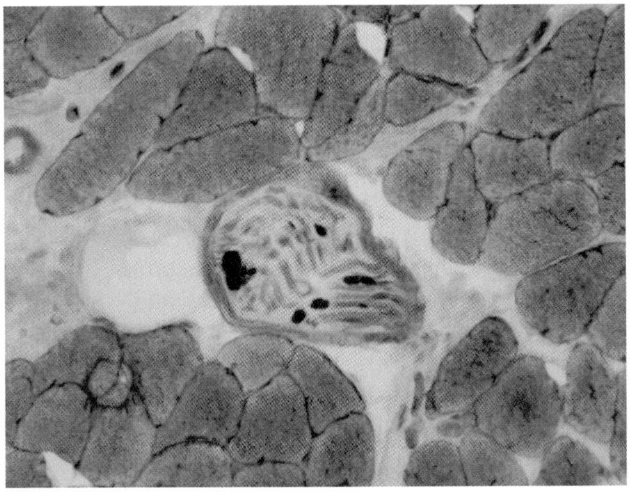

C

Figure 3-6. Scattered muscle fibers have small foci of increased glycogen deposition in subsarcolemmal regions in a patient with McArdle disease **(A)**, periodic acid–Schiff (PAS) stain. When diastase is added to the PAS stain the abnormal accumulations are no longer evident, suggesting that the deposits were glycogen **(B)**. PAS stain may also detect polyglucosan bodies in intramuscular nerve twigs in muscle biopsy in patients with polyglucosan body neuropathy **(C)**.

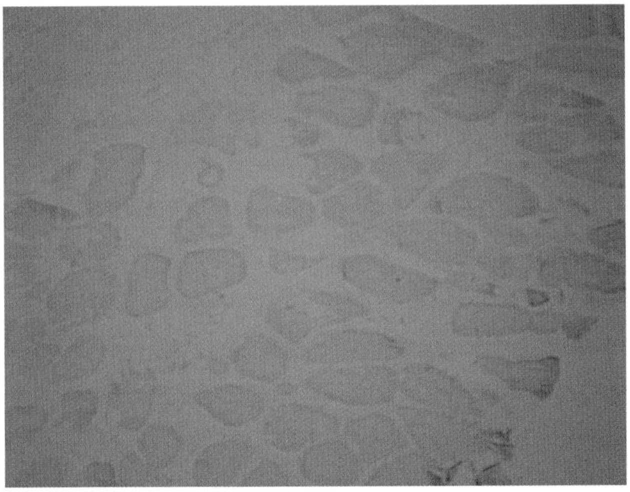

A

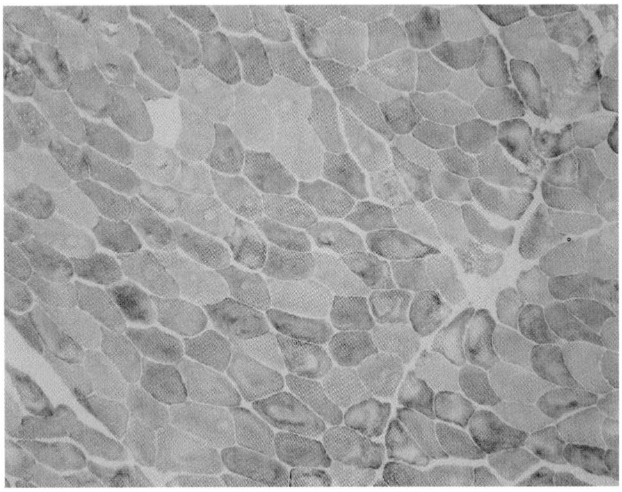

B

Figure 3-7. Myophosphorylase stain demonstrates absent myophosphorylase activity in a patient with McArdle disease **(A)**. Myophosphorylase activity in a healthy control biopsy **(B)**. Type 2 fibers that contain more myophosphorylase stain are darker than type 1 fibers.

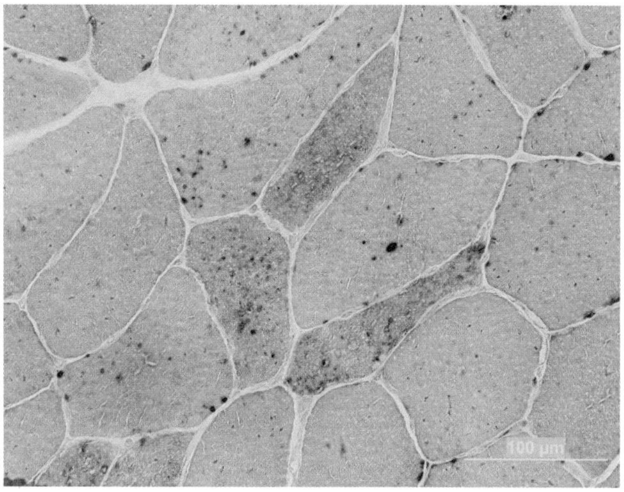

Figure 3-8. Acid phosphatase stains macrophages and muscle fibers lysosomes. In patients with Pompe disease, a lysosomal glycogen storage disorder, increased lysosomes are evident and brought out by acid phosphatase stain even when vacuoles may be difficult to appreciate on other routine stains such as H&E and modified Gomori trichrome.

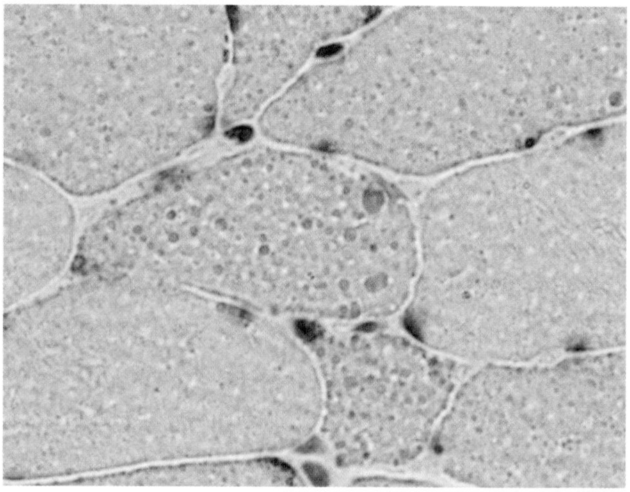

Figure 3-9. Increased lipid droplets in muscle fibers are evident on this oil red O stain in a case of a lipid storage myopathy.

lysosomes that are increased in certain disorders (e.g., Pompe disease) as well as macrophages that may be present in muscle tissue (Fig. 3-8). In addition, oil red O or Sudan black can evaluate lipid content, which may be increased in patients with lipid storage myopathies (Fig. 3-9). Oxidative enzyme stains (nicotinamide adenine dinucleotide tetrazolium reductase or NADH-TR, succinate dehydrogenase or SDH, cytochrome-C oxidase or COX) are useful for identifying mitochondrial and intermyofibrillar network abnormalities (Figs. 3-10 A and B). The SDH and COX stains can be combined to highly SDH-positive, COX-negative fibers characteristic of disorders associated with mitochondrial DNA mutations (Fig. 3-10C). Target fibers and central cores are also particularly well seen with the NADH-TR stain (discussed later). In addition, a so-called trabeculated or lobulated staining pattern is seen on NADH-TR in some dystrophies, although this is not a disease-specific abnormality (Fig. 3-10D). Various stains (Congo red, crystal violet, cresyl violet, and Alcian blue) can be performed to assess for amyloid deposition (Fig. 3-11).

Immunohistochemistry is important in evaluating specific types of muscular dystrophies (e.g., dystrophin staining for Duchenne and Becker muscular dystrophy; merosin and

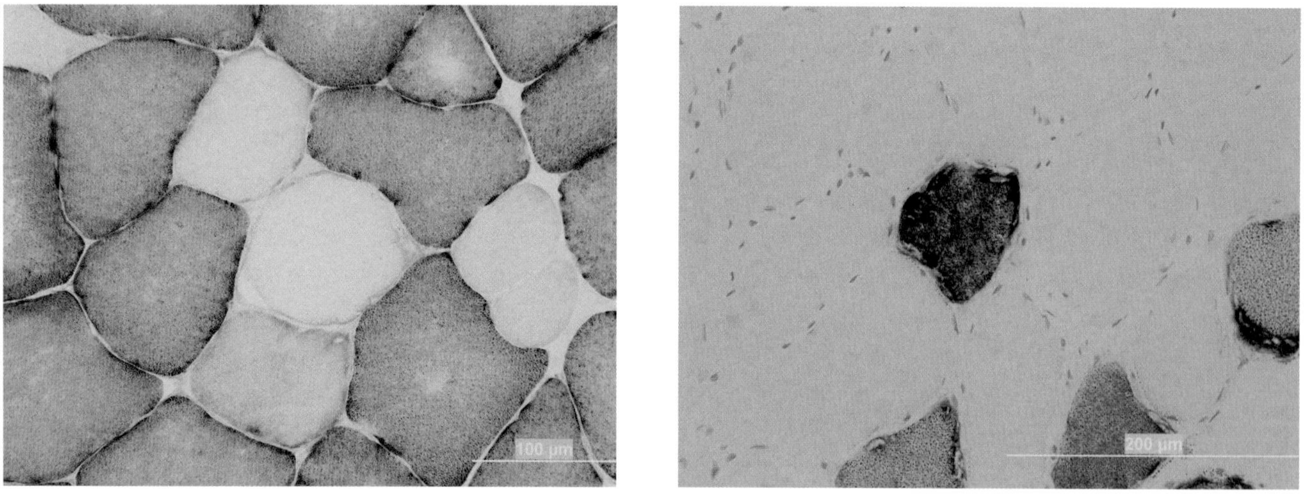

A B

Figure 3-10. In addition to ragged red fibers seen on modified Gomori-trichrome stain (Fig. 3-4 A), mitochondrial myopathies may demonstrate muscle fibers with absent or reduced cytochrome oxidase staining (COX) **(A)** or increased succinic dehydrogenase staining (SDH) **(B)**. *(continued)*

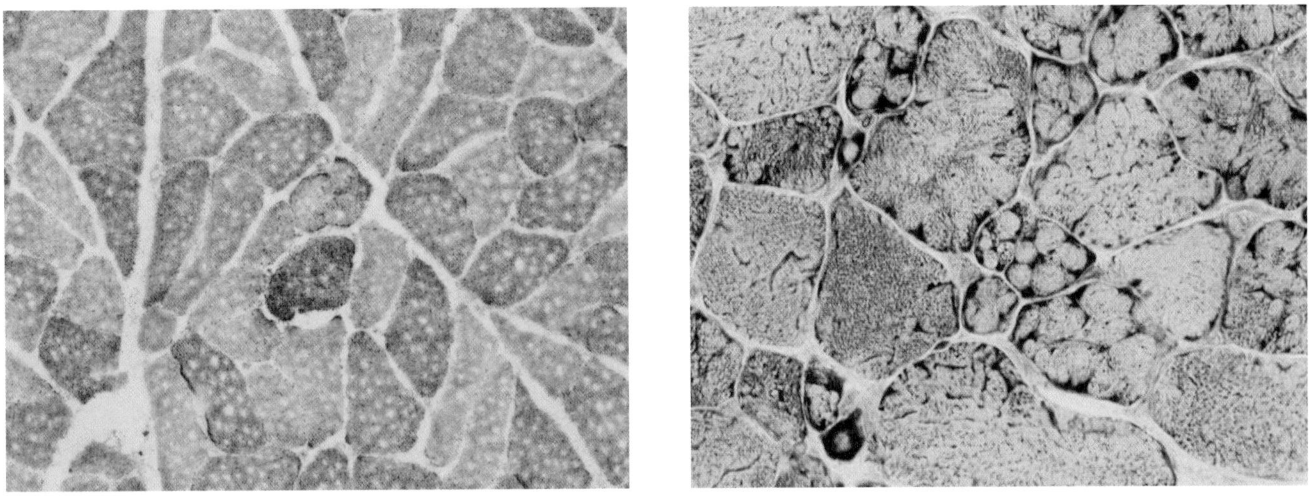

C D

Figure 3-10. (*Continued*) The COX and SDH stains can be combined such that COX-negative fibers that are SDH-positive show up intensely blue **(C)**. These stains are useful because ragged red fibers that are COX negative but SDH positive are usually associated with mitochondrial DNA mutations—though the primary mutation may still involve nuclear encoded genes that govern mitochondrial DNA. NADH-TR stain also highlights trabeculated or lobulated fibers as seen in this biopsy in a patient with muscular dystrophy **(D)**.

alpha-dystroglycan staining for congenital muscular dystrophy; sarcoglycans, caveolin, and dysferlin for limb girdle muscular dystrophies; and emerin for X-linked Emery-Dreifuss muscular dystrophy) (Fig. 3-12). Immunohistochemistry can also be valuable in inflammatory myopathies and vasculitis (e.g., stains for major histocompatibility antigens, complement, membrane attack complex, immunoglobulins, and appropriate inflammatory cell markers) (Fig. 3-13).

EM is used to assess the ultrastructural components of muscle fibers (e.g., the sarcolemma, sarcomeres, nuclei, and mitochondria) and vasculature (e.g., tubulofilaments in capillaries in dermatomyositis).[12] Various myopathies have specific ultrastructural abnormalities that are more readily characterized by EM (e.g., nemaline rods, central cores, proliferation of abnormal appearing mitochondria, myofibrillar degeneration, vacuoles, and filamentous inclusions in nuclei and sarcoplasm) (Fig. 3-14).

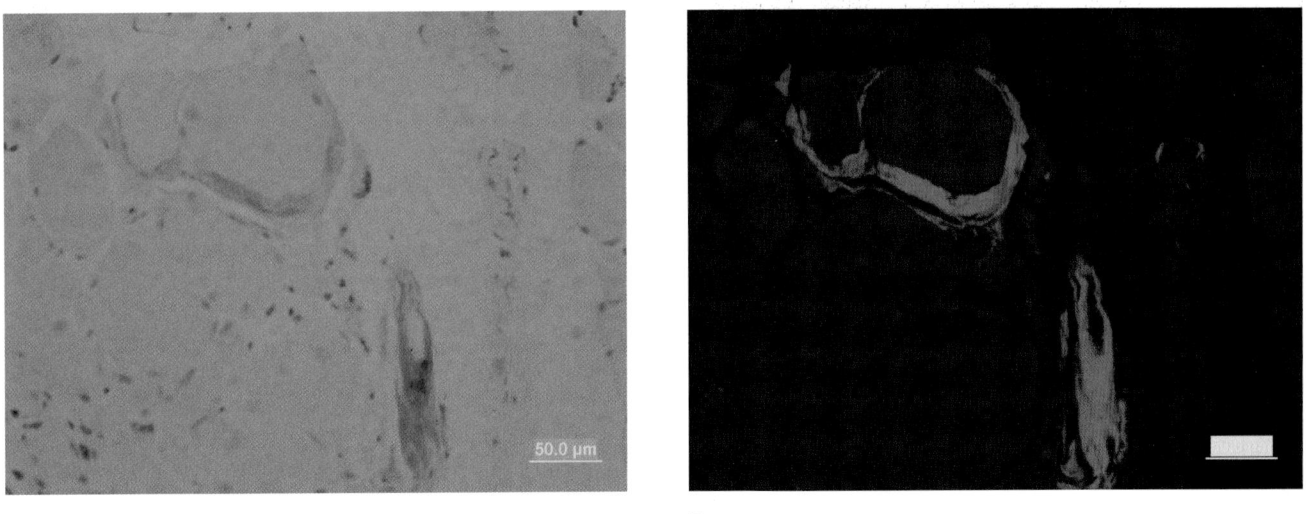

A B

Figure 3-11. Congo red stain demonstrates amyloid deposition surrounding muscle fibers and blood vessels. Under routine light microscopy, the amyloid deposition is pinkish red staining **(A)**, apple green under polarized light, but is most easily appreciated as bright red using rhodamine optics **(B)**.

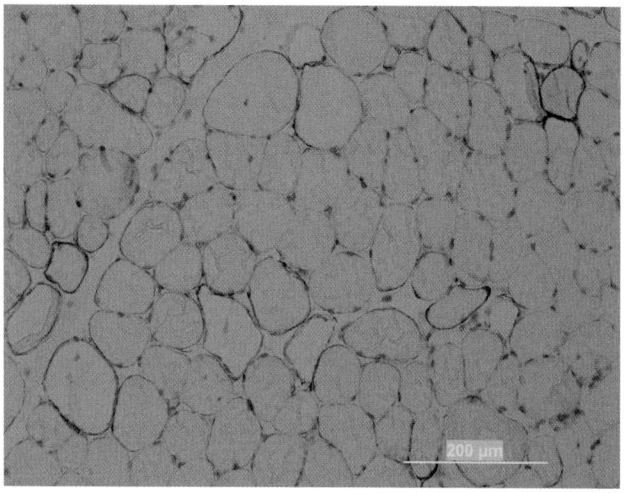

A

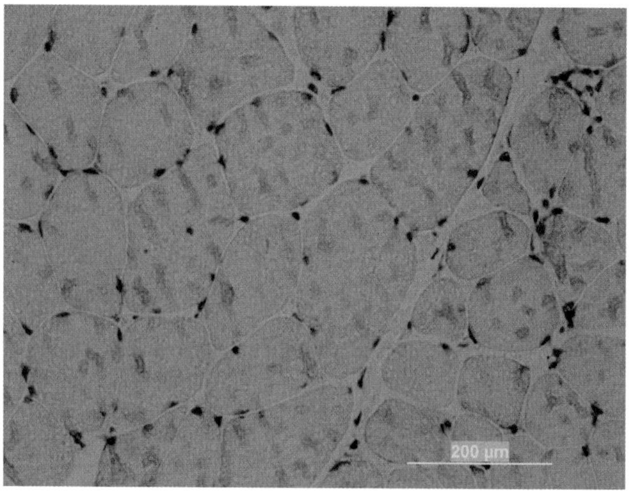

B

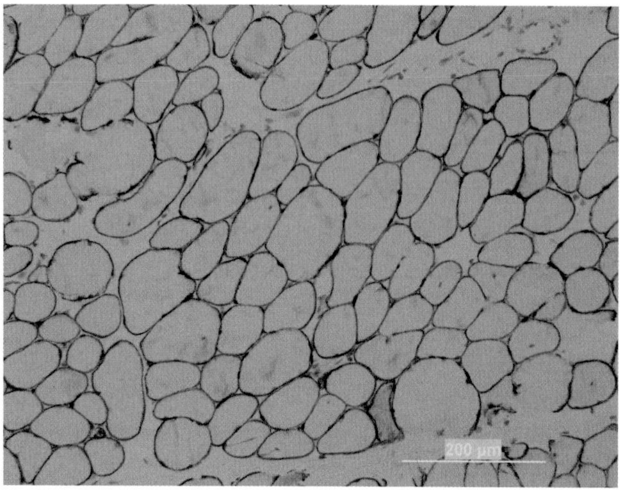

C

Figure 3-12. LGMD 2I. Muscle biopsies demonstrate reduced or patchy merosin staining **(A)**, absent alpha-dystroglycan staining **(B)**, but normal dystrophin staining **(C)** around the sarcolemma. Immunoperoxidase stains.

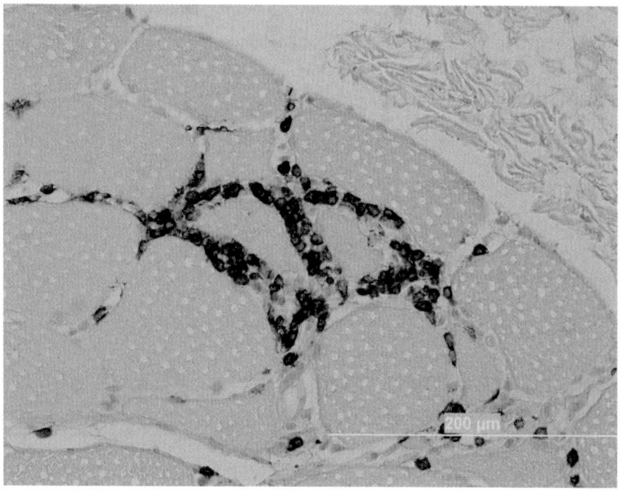

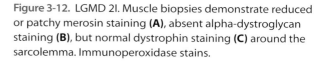

Figure 3-13. Specific types of inflammatory cells, in this case CD8+ T lymphocytes can be seen in the endomysium surrounding muscle fibers in polymyositis. Immunoperoxidase stain.

▶ STRUCTURE OF NORMAL SKELETAL MUSCLE

Skeletal muscle is a syncytial tissue composed of sheets of individual muscle fibers with multiple nuclei. The connective tissue within muscles include the endomysium that surrounds individual muscle fibers, the perimysium that groups muscle fibers into primary and secondary bundles (fasciculi), and the epimysium that envelops single muscles or large groups of fibers. Normally, myonuclei are located adjacent to the muscle membrane (sarcolemma) and are oriented parallel to the length of the fiber. These are oval in shape and contain evenly distributed chromatin and inconspicuous nucleoli. In approximately 3% of normal adult fibers, the myonuclei lie more internal within the cytoplasm (sarcoplasm). Increased internalized nuclei are a nonspecific abnormality, as these are seen in different types of myopathies as well as in neurogenic disorders.

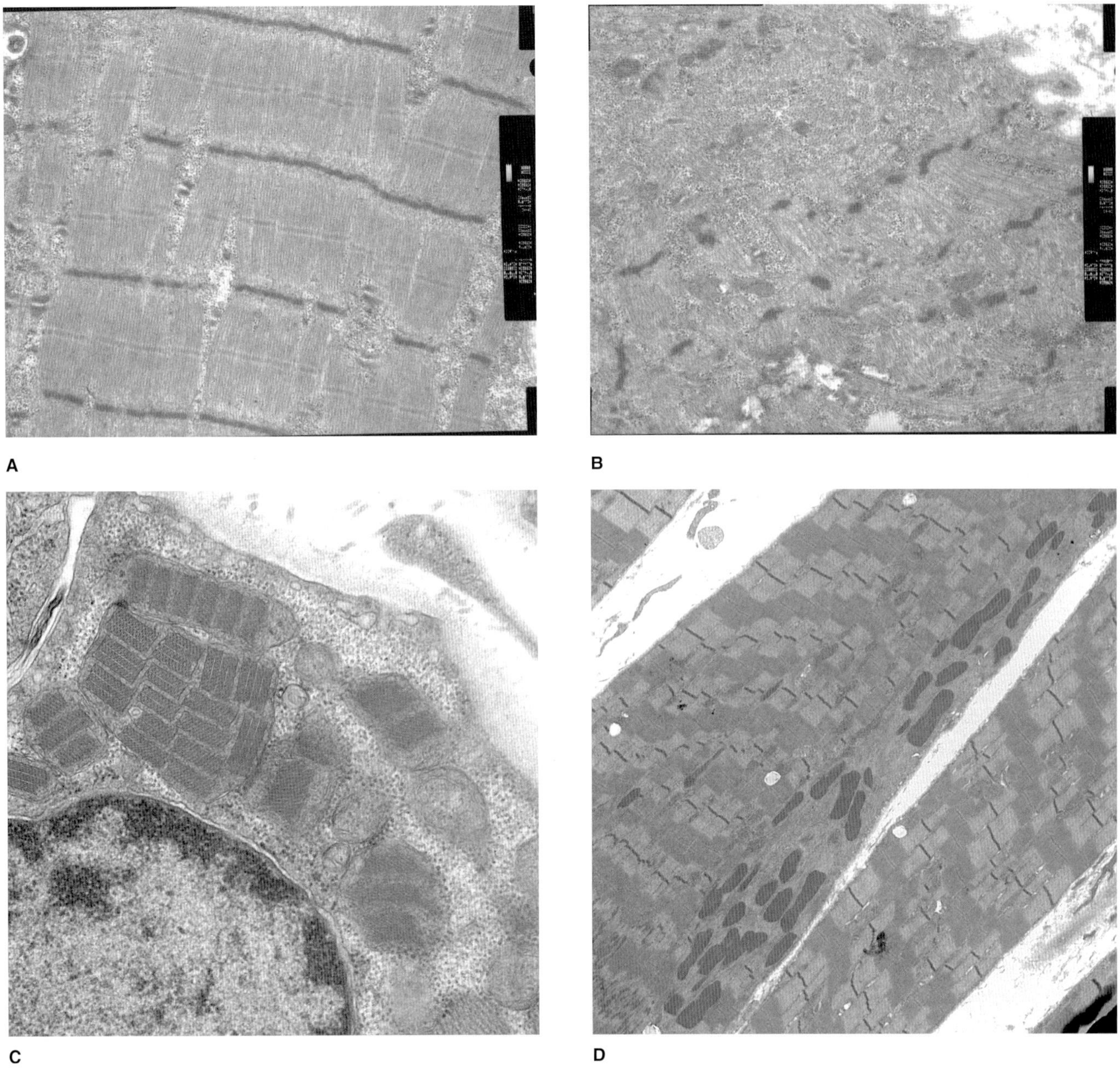

Figure 3-14. Electron microscopy is useful in assessing ultrastructural abnormalities. Normal sarcomere can be appreciated with Z-disc, thick and thin filaments, glycogen granules and mitochondria **(A)**. In critical illness myopathy, severe disruption of the sarcomere is evident with loss of the myosin thick filaments **(B)**. Abnormal proliferation of mitochondrial with paracrystalline inclusions in this muscle biopsy of a patient with mitochondrial myopathy **(C)** and rods as evident in a biopsy of a patient with nemaline myopathy **(D)**.

Satellite cells are present next to the sarcolemma and are enveloped by basement membrane that surrounds the muscle fibers. Most of the sarcoplasm of the muscle fiber contains myofilaments, which form the contractile apparatus and supporting structures. Individual muscle fibers contain repeating units (sarcomeres) of interlaced, longitudinally directed thin filaments and thick filaments and perpendicularly oriented Z bands to which the thin filaments are connected (Fig. 3-14A). The sarcomere is connected to the sarcolemma via filamentous actin. The sarcolemma is composed of various protein complexes and is connected to the extracellular matrix. Greater detail of the sarcolemmal proteins and extracellular matrix is discussed in Chapter 27.

The T tubules are composed of invaginations of the sarcolemmal membrane into the interior of the muscle fibers. Their course is parallel to the Z bands and they are surrounded on each site by the sarcoplasmic reticulum. The T tubules allow for rapid depolarization of muscle membrane deep within muscle fiber cells and the accelerated release of calcium from the sarcoplasmic reticulum during excitation.

Adult muscle fibers are polygonal in appearance but are more rounded in shape in infancy and early childhood. The cross-sectional diameter of individual fibers varies depending on the specific muscle, fiber type, and age of the individual. The motor unit comprises the motor neuron and the muscle fibers it innervates . The individual muscle fibers of a motor unit are normally randomly distributed as previously mentioned, within a sector approximating 30% of the muscle's cross-sectional diameter.

The percentages of type 1, 2A, and 2B fibers differ in various muscle groups, and it is important to be aware of the normal percentages of these fibers in the biopsied muscle for accurate assessment.[13] The most commonly biopsied muscles (i.e., biceps brachii, triceps, and quadriceps) have approximately equal amounts of the three major fiber types, although the deltoid muscle has more type 1 fibers than type 2A and 2B. Because muscle fibers from a single motor unit are randomly distributed among muscle fibers of different motor units and fiber types, a checkerboard or mosaic pattern is appreciated on ATPase stains (Fig. 3-5).

Although ATPase stain is primarily used to assess fiber type, we can often ascertain the fiber types from other standard stains (Table 3-1). For example, type 1 fibers stain more intensely with modified Gomori-trichrome, lipid, and oxidative enzyme stains than type 2 fibers because of the increased number of mitochondria and oxidative metabolism associated with type 1 fibers. In contrast, type 2 fibers, which are involved with glycolytic metabolism, stain more intensely with PAS, as these contain more glycogen but are lighter staining on modified Gomori-trichrome, lipid, and oxidative enzyme stains.

The diameters of individual muscle fibers are assessed in order to characterize their size. Quantitative analysis is performed by measuring the mean and range of the diameters for each different fiber type.[14–17] Importantly, the diameters of muscle fibers increase to a point during childhood until the early teens. At 1 year of age the mean muscle fiber diameter is approximately 16 μm. The size increases by about 2 μm/yr until the age of 5 years and subsequently by 3 μm/yr until 9 years of age. By 10 years of age, mean muscle diameters range from 38 to 42 μm. Normal adult size is reached between the ages of 12 and 15 years.[17] There is usually less than 12% difference in the largest mean fiber diameters between the major fiber types. Both types 1 and 2 adult muscle fibers are larger in men than in women. Type 2 fibers are usually larger than type 1 fibers in men; type 1 fibers are larger than type 2 fibers in women. The diameter of muscle fibers is also dependent on the specific muscle biopsied. For example, in adults, the diameters of muscle fibers in the biceps brachii are as follows: type 1 fibers 64.3 +/− 3.7 μm and type 2 fibers 72.7 +/− 5.3 μm in men and type 1 fibers 56.8 +/− 4.8 μm and type 2 fibers 54.6 +/− 7.0 μm in women. In the vastus lateralis, the diameters of muscle fibers are slightly different: type 1 fibers 59.5 +/− 6.4 μm and type 2 fibers 64.8 +/− 8.1 μm in men and type 1 fibers 58.8 +/− 6.1 μm and type 2 fibers 49.9 +/− 6.2 μm in women.[14]

▶ REACTIONS TO INJURY

Muscle abnormalities may be classified on histopathologic and etiologic grounds into three major categories: (1) neurogenic atrophy: a pattern of muscle pathology consequent to denervation, and if present, reinnervation; (2) myopathies: inherited and acquired diseases characterized by abnormalities in the muscle fiber itself; these include dystrophies, congenital, inflammatory, metabolic, and toxic myopathies; and (3) disorders of the neuromuscular junction. Patients with neuromuscular junction defects usually have only slight and nonspecific alterations apparent on routine light microscopy and are rarely biopsied except at very specialized centers.[1–5]

Upon review of muscle biopsy slides, specific features on various stains are important to note. It is essential to assess the size and variability of muscle fibers, the distribution of fiber types, the size and location of the myonuclei, the presence of necrotic and regenerating muscle fibers, other alterations in the cytoarchitecture and organelles (e.g., the presence of target fibers, cores, vacuoles, tubular aggregates, and ragged red fibers), and any abnormal accumulation of glycogen or lipid. Besides the muscle fibers, we evaluate the surrounding vasculature (is there evidence of vasculitis and thickened basement membranes?) and the supportive tissue (is there increased endomysial connective tissue, edema, or amyloidosis?). One should characterize any inflammatory cell infiltrate making note of the type (lymphocytes, plasma cells, eosinophils, and macrophages), the location (endomysial, perimysial, and perivascular), and if there is cellular invasion of nonnecrotic or just necrotic appearing fibers. We discuss some of the common abnormalities seen on muscle biopsy in the following section, but in more detail in the subsequent chapters where specific disorders and their characteristic histologic features are described.

In the setting of axonal degeneration, the muscle fibers within that motor unit lose their neural input and undergo denervation atrophy. This leads to decreased synthesis of myofilaments, degeneration of myofibrils, and a reduction in the size of the muscle fiber.[18] The atrophic fibers lose their polygonal appearance and look angulated in shape (Fig. 3-15). Neurogenic disorders affect motor nerves that innervate both type 1 and 2 fibers. Therefore, in early denervation, muscle biopsies reveal scattered, atrophic angulated muscle fibers of both fiber types. As more motor nerves degenerate, rather than seeing isolated atrophic angulated fibers, there are groups of adjacent muscle fibers that are

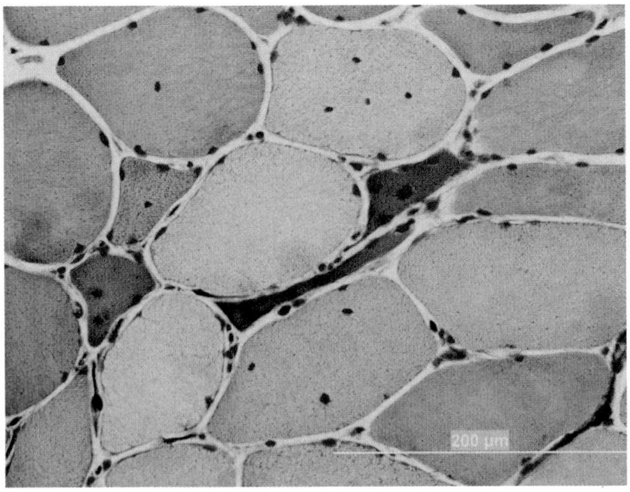

A

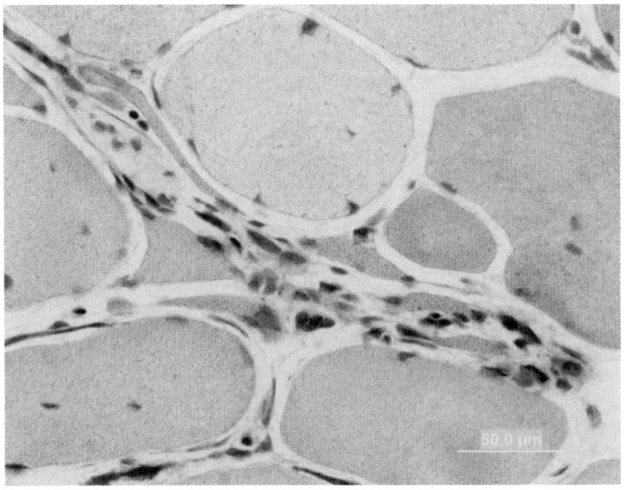

B

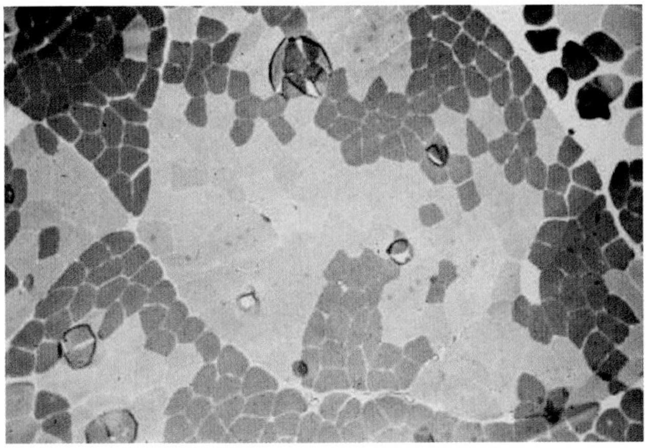

C

Figure 3-15. Neurogenic atrophy. Denervation results in muscle fibers becoming atrophic and angulated in appearance **(A)**. Several atrophic and angulated fibers clustered together are referred to as group atrophy **(B)**. If surrounding nerve fibers sprout and reinnervate nearby denervated muscle fibers, the newly reinnervated fibers assume the fiber type of the motor nerve that now innervates them. This leads to the loss of the mosaic pattern on ATPase stains and the appearance of fiber-type grouping **(C)**. ATPase 4.3.

atrophic (grouped atrophy). A feature of denervation is the presence of the so-called target fibers. Reorganization of the cytoarchitecture within muscle cells results in a rounded central zone of disorganized filaments that contain fewer mitochondrial and glycogen. Target fibers have three zones that are circumferentially oriented, which are best seen on NADH-TR staining (Figs. 3-16A and B). The innermost zone is devoid of mitochondrial, glycogen, phosphorylase, and ATPase enzymatic activity; the second zone has increased enzymatic activity, whereas the third zone exhibits intermediate enzymatic activity. Target fibers occur in neurogenic disorders in the course of reinnervation and need to be distinguished from central cores in which there are just two zones of staining (Fig. 3-16C). Central cores are specific for the congenital myopathy central core disease. The so-called moth-eaten or targetoid fibers resemble targets and cores on the NADH-TR stain but have less circumscribed patches of reduced oxidative enzyme staining again without a distinct intermediate zone of enzyme activity. Moth-eaten targetoid fibers (Fig. 3-16D) are nonspecific and can be seen in myopathic and neurogenic disorders. Both central cores and target fibers preferentially affect type 1 fibers. In contrast to central core myopathy in which the cores are present in the majority of type 1 fibers, the percentages of fibers with target and targetoid abnormalities are less abundant. Target fibers and central cores can also be appreciated on other stains such as the ATPase, PAS, and modified Gomori-trichrome stains (Fig. 3-16E).

Denervated muscle fibers send out trophic signals that lead nearby unaffected axons to sprout collateral branches, in an attempt to reinnervate the newly denervated muscle fibers. Once successful reinnervation is accomplished, the newly reinnervated muscle fiber assumes the physiologic properties of the reinnervating neuron. This may lead a type 1 fiber to become a type 2A fiber or a type 2B fiber to become a type 1 fiber. As a consequence, the normal checkerboard appearance of muscle tissue is replaced by large groups of single muscle fibers, all with the same fiber type (e.g., fiber-type grouping) (Fig. 3-15C). If these larger motor nerves subsequently degenerate, large areas of atrophic fibers of the same fiber type are seen—a different type of grouped atrophy.

In contrast to neurogenic atrophy, myopathic disorders are associated with a wider spectrum of histopathologic alterations

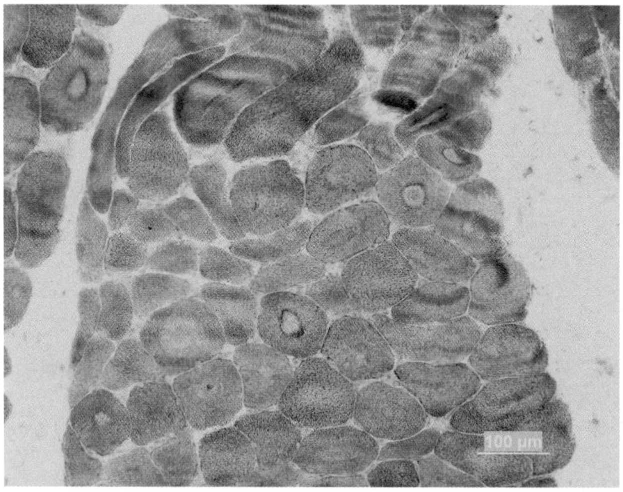

A

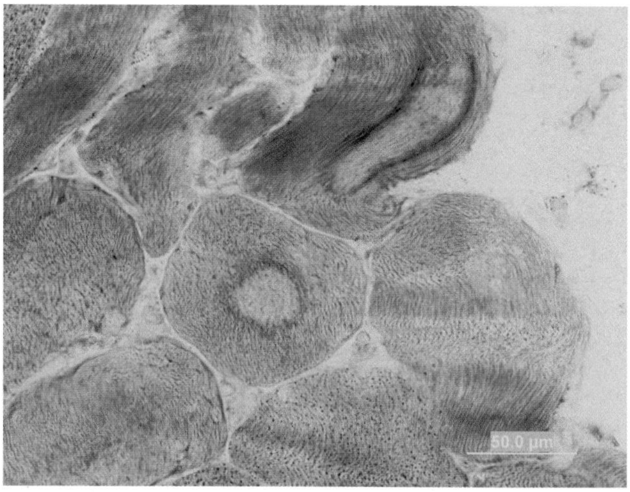

B

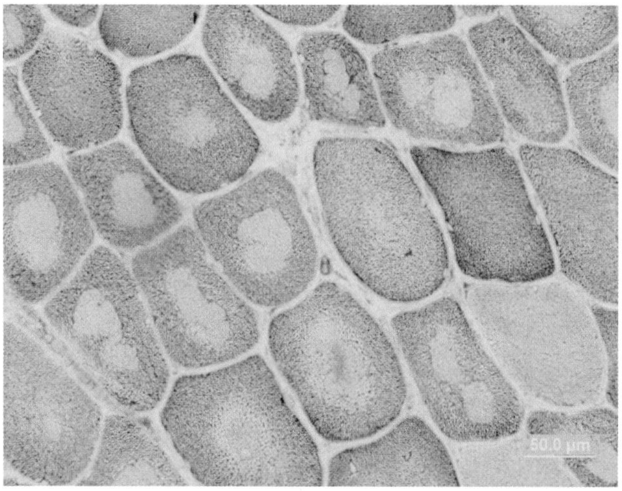

C

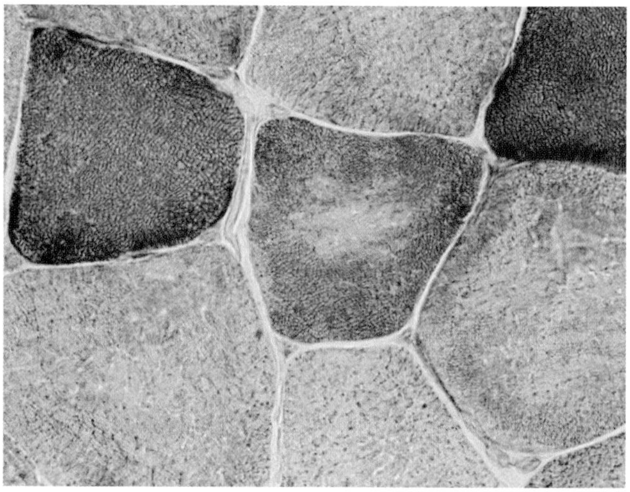

D

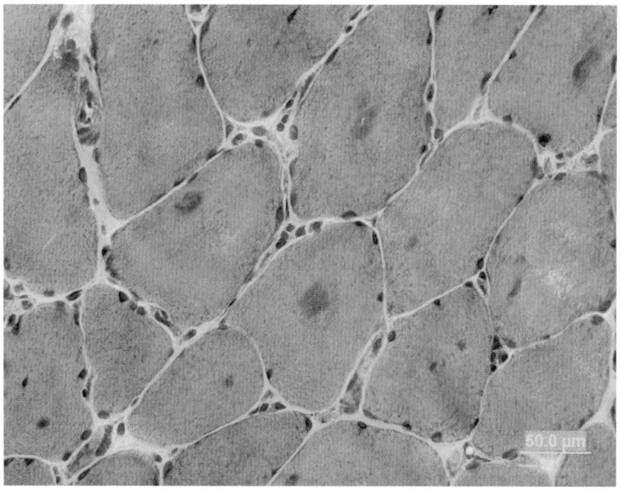

E

Figure 3-16. In the course of reinnervation, target fibers may develop. True target fibers have three zones in the center of the muscle fibers that are best seen on NADH-TR staining, at low power **(A)**, and at higher power **(B)**. The innermost zone is pale; the second zone has increased enzymatic activity, whereas the third zone exhibits intermediate enzymatic activity. Central cores resemble targets, but there is not a second zone with increased enzyme activity **(C)**. In targetoid or the so-called moth-eaten fibers the zones of reduced activity are even less distinct **(D)**. Target fibers and cores can also be appreciated on other stains such as the modified Gomori-trichrome stain **(E)**. On the Gomori-trichrome stain, the center of the target fibers stain dark and are surround by pale staining zone.

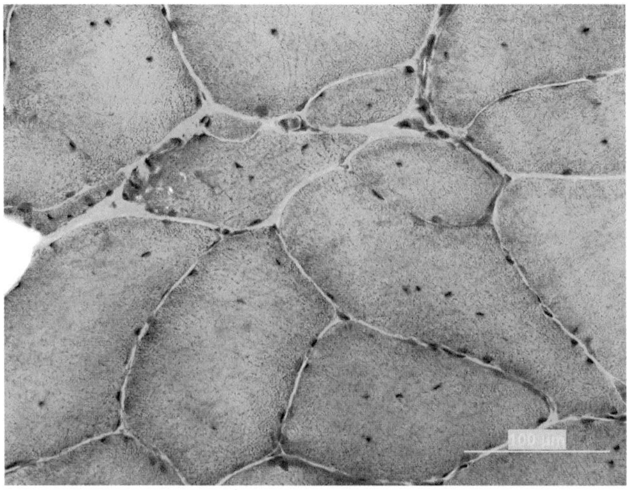

Figure 3-17. Variability in muscle fiber size, increased internalized nuclei, muscle fiber splitting, and small intracytoplasmic vacuoles are nonspecific myopathy features appreciated on this modified Gomori-trichrome stain.

(Fig. 3-17). Remember that muscle is a syncytium formed from the fusion of thousands of myoblasts. Because of its syncytial nature, histopathologic abnormalities may be focal rather than occurring along the entire length of a muscle fiber (e.g., segmental necrosis). Genetic disorders can manifest discrete abnormalities, with other regions of the single fiber appearing relatively normal. An example of this can be seen in mitochondrial myopathies in which the histopathologic alterations are dependent on the degree of abnormal mitochondria, which in turn is a reflection of the percentage of mutated mitochondrial DNA in the region. Thus, when cut longitudinally, one may appreciate segments of the muscle fiber with a ragged red appearance, which do not stain with cytochrome oxidase, whereas other nearby segments of the same fiber may be normal. In dystrophies, one often sees scattered necrotic muscle fibers on the cross section. However, if the tissue is cut longitudinally, one sees that necrosis is segmental in nature. Likewise, inflammatory myopathies are multifocal, resulting in infiltrates surrounding and invading segments of muscle fibers along their length.

Myopathies are usually associated with a random loss of muscle fibers belonging to different motor units. Atrophy of muscle fibers is a common histopathologic feature in myopathies, but rather than fibers becoming angular as in neurogenic atrophy, these usually become more rounded in appearance in myopathic disorders. Small groups of atrophic fibers of similar type may be observed in myopathies due to muscle fiber splitting, degeneration, and regeneration; however, large areas of group atrophy or fiber-type grouping are more typical of neurogenic atrophy. Preferential atrophy or hypotrophy of type 1 fibers is seen in certain myopathic disorders (e.g., myotonic dystrophy and various congenital myopathies). On the other hand, preferential type 2 fiber atrophy can be seen in certain endocrine disorders (e.g., steroid myopathy), as well as a complication of disuse.

Besides atrophy of muscle fibers, hypertrophy can develop in response to increased load, either in the setting of exercise or in pathologic conditions where other muscle fibers are injured. Large fibers may divide along a segment (muscle fiber splitting) so that, in cross section, a single large fiber contains a cell membrane traversing its diameter. Because both chronic myopathic and neurogenic disorders can be associated with a mixture of atrophic and hypertrophic fibers, increased variability of muscle fiber size is a nonspecific abnormality.

Necrosis is a feature more common in myopathies, but it can also occur in denervated muscle fibers (Fig. 3-18).

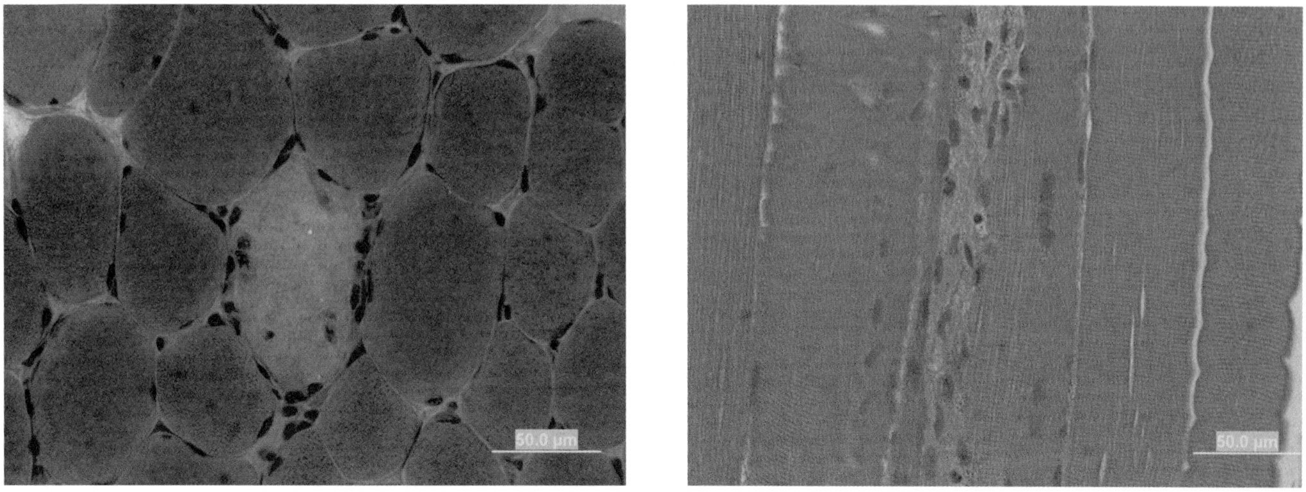

A B

Figure 3-18. A necrotic muscle fiber is pale staining in comparison to surrounding muscle fibers in cross section, H&E stain. **(A)** Segmental necrosis is often well appreciated on paraffin sections in which large, longitudinal segments can be visualized. The striations of the sarcomeres can be appreciated in normal fibers, whereas the necrotic segment of an adjacent fiber loses the striations. The necrotic segment is invaded by macrophages **(B)**. Paraffin section, H&E stain.

A single muscle fiber can undergo either total necrosis or segmental necrosis, but again, given the syncytial nature of muscle, atrophy along the entire fiber length is rare. The more common form of muscle tissue loss is referred to as segmental necrosis in which a relatively small segment of the single muscle fiber is affected. The site of necrosis may be focal at first, but it extends longitudinally along the muscle fiber with disease progression. Segmental necrosis is best appreciated on paraffin or semithin sections of muscle fibers cut longitudinally. With segmental necrosis, the affected portion of the single muscle fiber becomes more rounded and the sarcoplasm begins to have a featureless ground-glass appearance. Semithin and EM sections reveal degeneration of the Z disc and myofibrillar network as well as abnormal mitochondria. Macrophages are recruited into the area and infiltrate the necrotic segments in order to digest the disintegrating muscle tissue and damaged tissue. In certain diseases (polymyositis and inclusion body myositis [IBM]), macrophages and lymphocytes may invade nonnecrotic tissue such that a muscle fiber can be "severed" into distinct segments.

Repair of necrotic segments can occur and begins with the proliferation of adjacent satellite cells in the region of the destroyed portion of the fiber.[19] The satellite cells align next to each other to form myotubes. Several myotubes form per segment and adhere to the surrounding basal lamina. The expansion of myotubes occurs laterally and longitudinally, eventually reaching and fusing with the healthy muscle tissue stumps. The regenerating muscle fibers can be appreciated by their large internalized nuclei with prominent nucleoli, and their basophilic cytoplasm that is laden with ribonucleic acid (RNA) (Fig. 3-19). Old damage can be ascertained by the increase in the number of internalized nuclei (Fig. 3-17). Myonuclei, which usually lie along the subsarcolemmal membrane, are more internalized in regenerated segments.

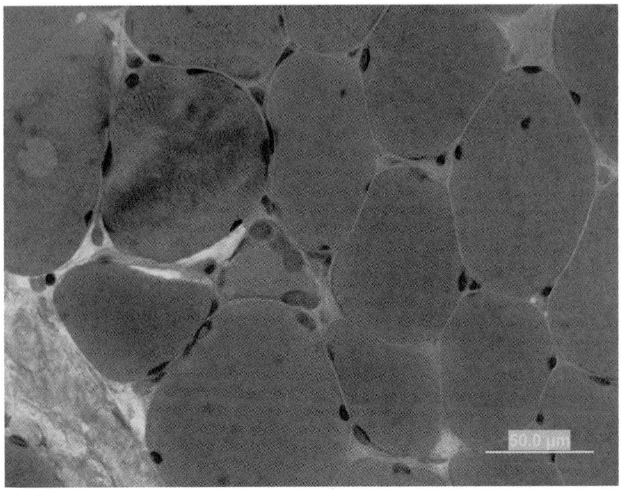

Figure 3-19. Regenerating muscle fibers are smaller and more basophilic than normal fibers and contain enlarged nuclei sometimes with nucleoli, as these are very active in trying to replenish necessary muscle proteins. H&E stain.

Other characteristics of myopathic injury include alterations in structural proteins or organelles, formation of vacuoles, and accumulation of intracytoplasmic deposits. Increased endomysial connective tissue is a common feature of muscular dystrophies but is also seen in chronic inflammatory myopathies and severe end-stage neurogenic atrophy. One of the most common reasons for a muscle biopsy in adults is to assist in diagnosis of a primary inflammatory myopathy. The characteristic histopathologic features on muscle biopsies in dermatomyositis are perifascicular atrophy and perivascular, perimysial inflammatory cell infiltrate with many plasmacytoid dendritic cells (Fig. 3-20A). On the other hand, polymyositis is associated with endomysial T cells that surround and often appear to invade nonnecrotic muscle fibers (Fig. 3-20B). IBM shares these features with polymyositis, but in addition there is often rimmed vacuoles and various inclusions apparent on light microscopy and EM (Fig. 3-20C). It is important to note that rimmed vacuoles and inclusions are not seen in at least 20% of any given IBM biopsy so the diagnosis of IBM cannot be excluded in the absence of these findings. Furthermore, one will not see rimmed vacuoles on paraffin sections, only on frozen sections—so it is imperative to do histochemistry staining of frozen section and not just paraffin sections. Immune-mediated necrotizing myopathy is associated with scattered necrotic and regenerating muscle fibers in the absence of significant inflammatory cell infiltrate (Fig. 3-18). Less common forms of inflammatory myopathy include granulomatous or giant cell myositis (Fig. 3-20D) and eosinophilic myositis (Fig. 3-20E). A precautionary note is that inflammatory cell infiltrates are seen in dystrophies and other types of myopathy and thus are not specific for an immune-mediated process.

► NERVE BIOPSIES

As is true for muscle biopsies, the interpretation of a nerve biopsy requires correlation of histologic changes, with clinical information including the results of electrophysiologic investigations. Nerve biopsies are generally less useful than muscle biopsies because the pathologic abnormalities are often nonspecific and frequently do not help distinguish one form of peripheral neuropathy from the other.[20–23] In addition, there is increased morbidity associated with the removal of a segment of sensory nerve, which leads to permanent numbness in the corresponding cutaneous distribution. Also, nerve biopsies can be complicated by significant neuropathic pain in the distribution of the nerve for several months and the potential for growth of painful neuromas. Therefore, we do not recommend nerve biopsies just because the patient has a generalized neuropathy of undetermined etiology despite an extensive laboratory evaluation. This situation is quite common, as discussed in Chapter 22.

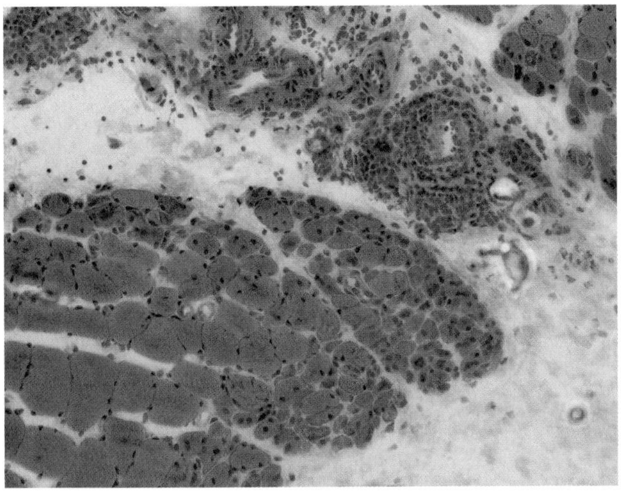
A

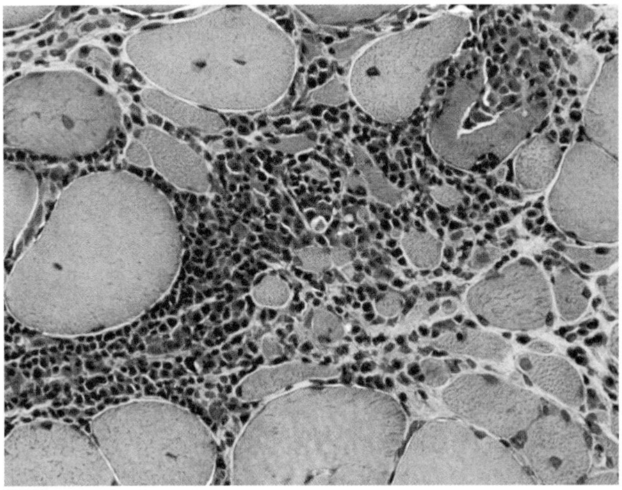
B

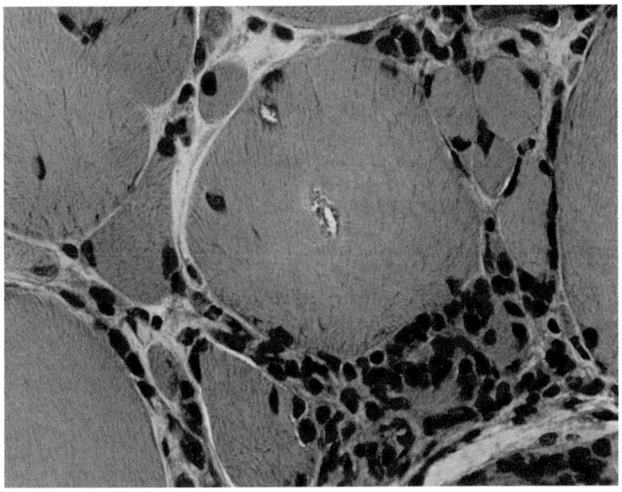
C

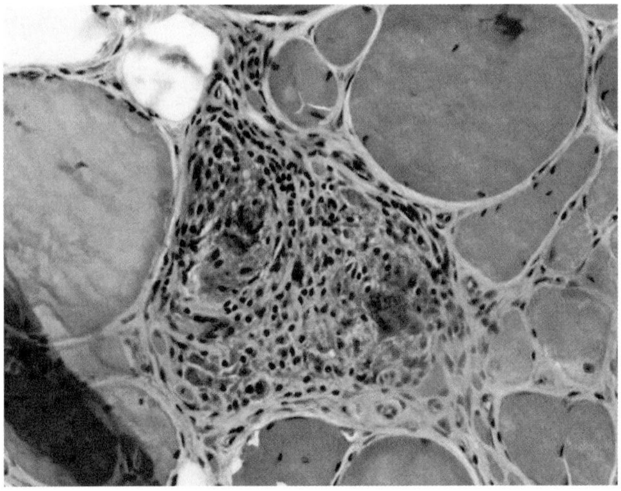
D

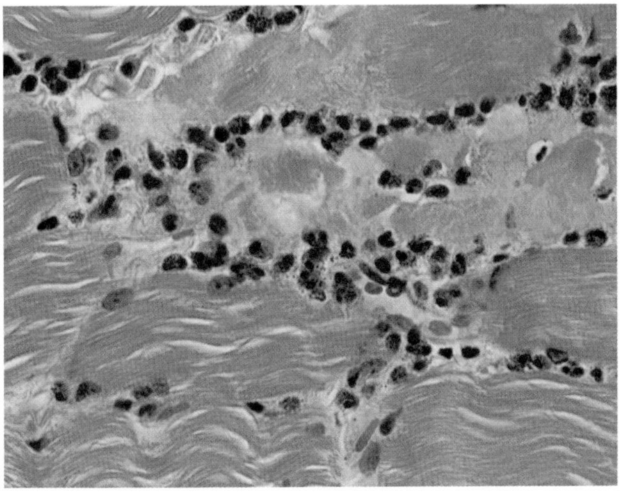
E

Figure 3-20. The characteristic feature of dermatomyositis is perifascicular atrophy and perivascular, perimysial inflammation **(A)**, H&E stain. Polymyositis is associated with endomysial inflammatory cell infiltrates surrounding and often appearing to invade nonnecrotic muscle fibers **(B)**, H&E stain. Inclusion body myositis likewise has features of polymyositis but rimmed vacuoles are often apparent **(C)**, H&E stain. In sarcoidosis and granuolomatous myositis the biopsies reveal granulomas **(D)**, H&E stain. Eosinophils are prominent among the inflammatory cells in eosinophilic myositis, but these cells may rarely also seen in inflammatory dystrophies **(E)**, H&E stain.

▶ INDICATIONS FOR NERVE BIOPSY

Suspected amyloidosis and vasculitis are the major indications for nerve biopsy. Amyloidosis should be considered in patients with a monoclonal gammopathy, autonomic neuropathy, systemic signs of amyloidosis (e.g., renal insufficiency or cardiomyopathy), or a family history of amyloidosis. Vasculitic neuropathy is in the differential diagnosis in people presenting with a history of multiple mononeuropathies, particularly when of acute onset and painful, and when there is an underlying connective tissue disease (e.g., systemic lupus erythematosus and rheumatoid arthritis), eosinophilia or late-onset asthma (Churg–Strauss syndrome), renal failure or chronic sinusitis, hepatitis B or C, an elevated erythrocyte sedimentation rate, or antinuclear cytoplasmic antibody. Additional indications for nerve biopsy include other autoimmune inflammatory conditions (e.g., sarcoidosis), possible infectious processes (e.g., leprosy), and tumor infiltration (e.g., lymphoma and leukemia). Also, a nerve biopsy may be required for the diagnosis of a tumor of the peripheral nerve (e.g., perineurioma). Less commonly, nerve biopsy may be warranted to diagnose uncommon forms of hereditary neuropathy when DNA testing is not available or is negative (e.g., giant axonal neuropathy and polyglucosan body neuropathy).

▶ TECHNIQUES

We usually biopsy a superficial sensory nerve that is clinically affected and also abnormal on sensory nerve conduction studies. The most common nerve biopsied is the sural nerve. We prefer to biopsy the sural nerve in the mid-shin approximately one-third to one-fourth of the distance from ankle to knee, as opposed to the lateral ankle itself where the nerve may be more prone to trauma and healing may not be as good (Fig. 3-21). Patients should be warned that following

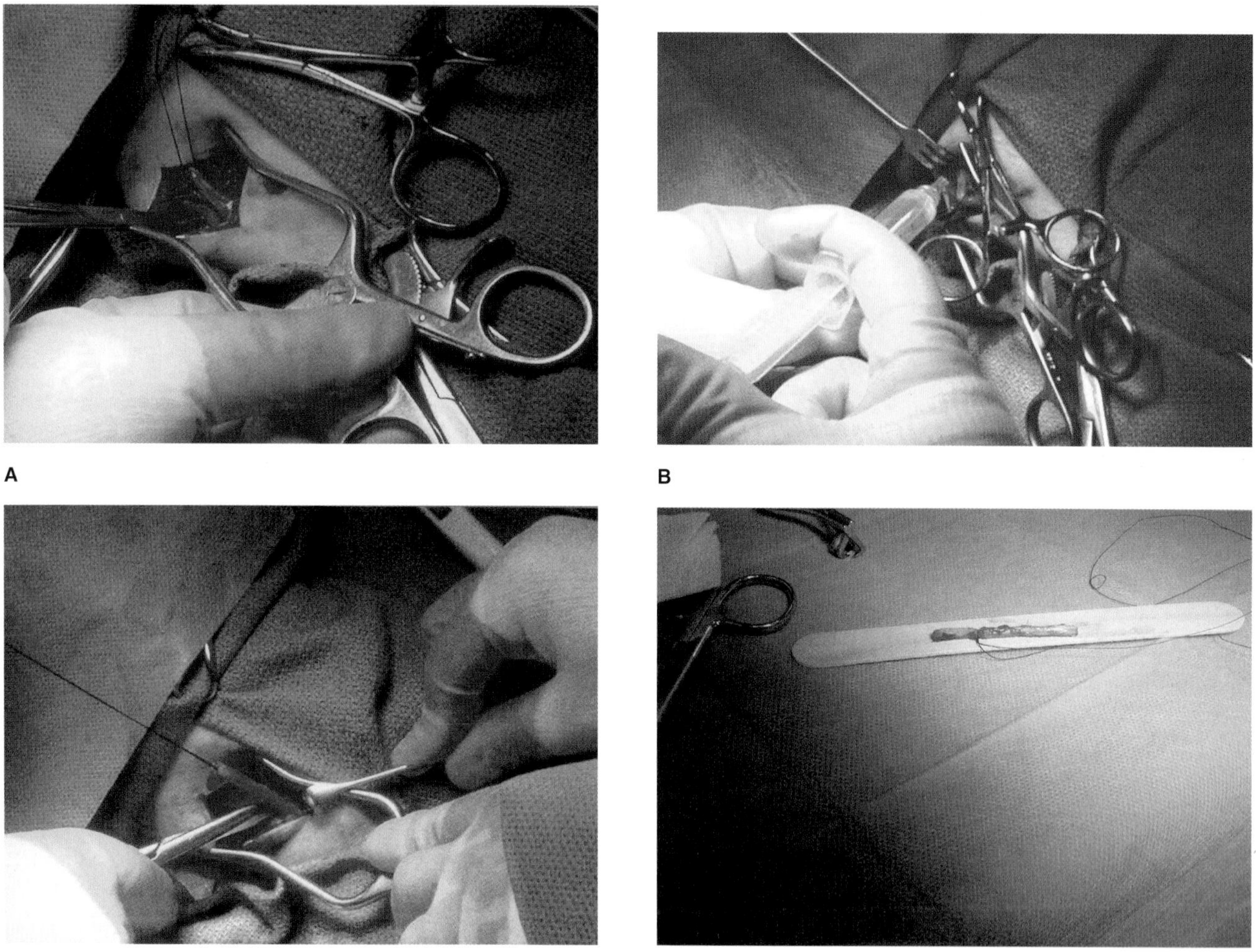

A B C D

Figure 3-21. The sural nerve is usually biopsied approximately one-third up from the ankle just lateral to the midline in the grove made by the Achilles' tendon. It is important for the surgeon to isolate and distinguish the saphenous vein from the sural nerve as they lie next to each other. The saphenous vein can look nearly identical to the sural nerve, often leading to an erroneous "nerve biopsy" with a lumen if care is not taken. A silk suture is gently lifting the sural nerve away from the saphenous vein **(A)**. The nerve is injected proximally with lidocaine **(B)**, and then is dissected away from the surrounding tissue **(C)**. A 4-cm segment is biopsied and divided into separate specimens for frozen section, paraffin embedding, semithin, EM, and teased fiber preparations **(D)**.

the sural nerve biopsy, there is often pain for several months as well permanent loss of sensation on the lateral aspect of the ankle and foot.[20] A superficial peroneal nerve biopsy is particularly useful when vasculitic neuropathy is suspected and there is foot drop, because the underlying peroneus brevis muscle can also be biopsied through the same incision site, thereby increasing the diagnostic yield (Fig. 3-22). Biopsy of the superficial peroneal nerve will lead to numbness of the dorsum of the foot and again often neuropathic pain for several months.[20] If only the upper extremities are involved, the superficial radial nerve can be biopsied; however, this leads to numbness of the dorsum of the hand, which is problematic for most patients. Importantly, because of sampling error, the single small segment of distal sensory nerve may not be representative of focal disease processes elsewhere in the peripheral nervous system, especially in processes with predominant motor involvement. On rare occasions when a patient has a multifocal process and the lesion appears proximal (e.g., amyloidomas, inflammatory process, and tumors), a fascicular nerve biopsy of a lesion in the root, plexus, or proximal nerve may be required. This procedure should only be performed, however, by neurosurgeons experienced in the technique and where the tissue can be processed appropriately in the neuropathology laboratory.

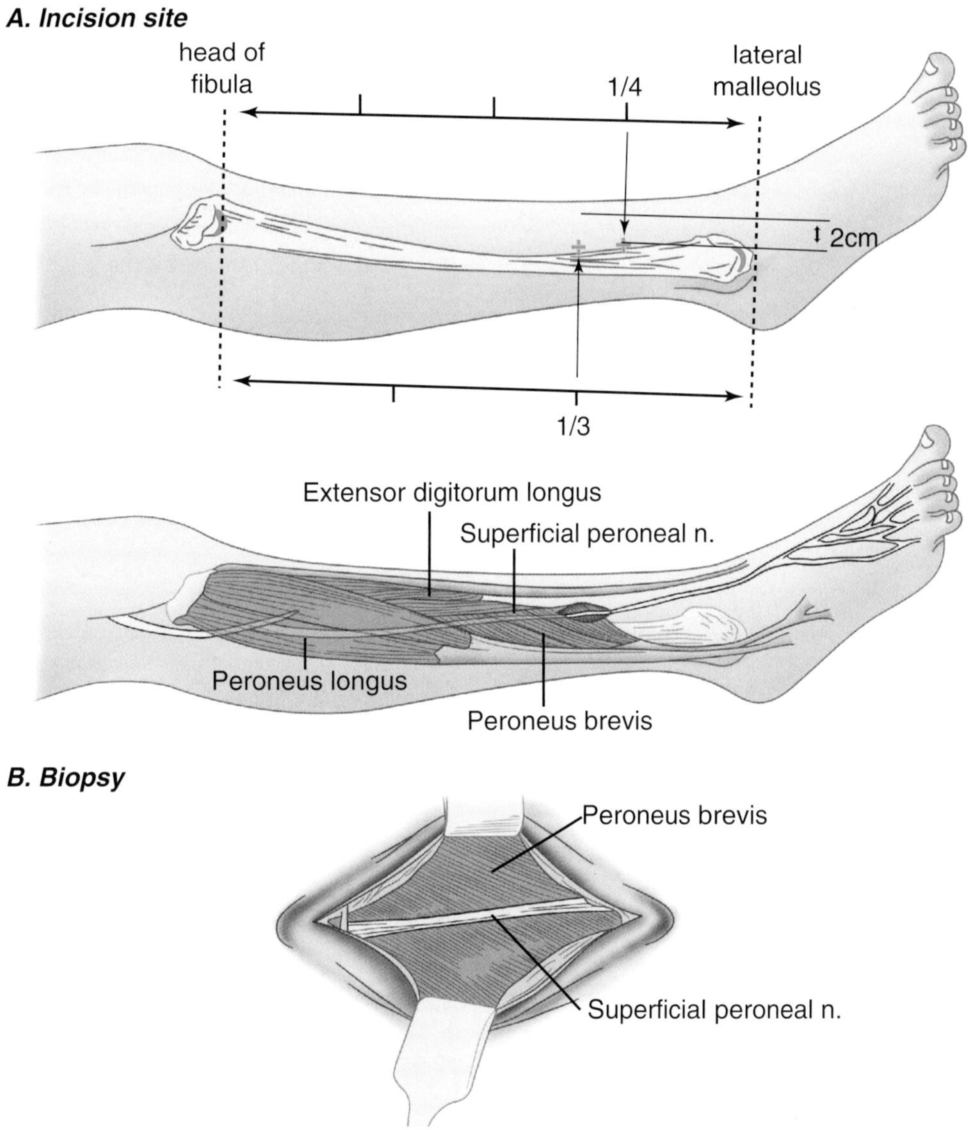

Figure 3-22. A combined superficial peroneal nerve and muscle biopsy is useful when looking for vasculitis. The nerve is typically found between one-third and one-fourth up from the lateral malleolus and approximately 1–1.5 cm anterior to the fibula. The nerve in this position can lie above or beneath the fascia overlying the peroneus brevis muscle, so both can be taken from a single incision. (Modified with permission from Mendell JR, Erdem S, Agamonolis DR. Peripheral nerve and skin biopsies. In: Mendell JR, Kissel JT, Cornblath DR, eds. *Diagnosis and Management of Peripheral Nerve Disorders*. New York, NY: Oxford University Press; 2001.)

Nerve biopsies are performed under local anesthesia in adults; general anesthesia is often required to obtain an adequate specimen from children or when a proximal nerve segment needs to be biopsied (e.g., root, plexus, or proximal nerve). The pathology laboratory should be contacted in advance of the surgery so that the tissue can be picked up directly from the operating room and processed immediately. Local anesthetic should be injected into the nerve just proximal to the site of transection in awake patients in order to reduce pain associated with sectioning the nerve (Fig. 3-21B). A 4–5-cm long section of nerve should be excised. The specimen can be wrapped in a saline-moistened gauze (not drenching wet).

The nerve biopsy is divided into several portions so that different types of studies can be performed (Fig. 3-21E). We generally take a small piece at the most proximal end for the frozen section. This piece is rapidly frozen in mounting medium for immunofluorescence studies. These studies can reveal the deposition of immunoglobulins or other inflammatory markers, such as complement or fibrinogen. Routine paraffin embedding (following fixation in formalin) is performed on a portion of tissue taken from the proximal and distal segments of the nerve biopsy (approximately 1 cm in length at both ends). The paraffin sections can be stained with H&E, trichrome, Luxol fast blue (stains myelin blue), Bodian stain or neurofilament stains for axons Fig. 3-23).[3,21,24–27] Congo red, Alcian blue, or cresyl violet should be done to look for amyloid (Fig. 3-24). A PAS stain is useful when polyglucosan body neuropathy is a consideration (Fig. 3-25, and a Fite stain can be done to look for the acid-fast bacilli, if lepromatous neuropathy is possible

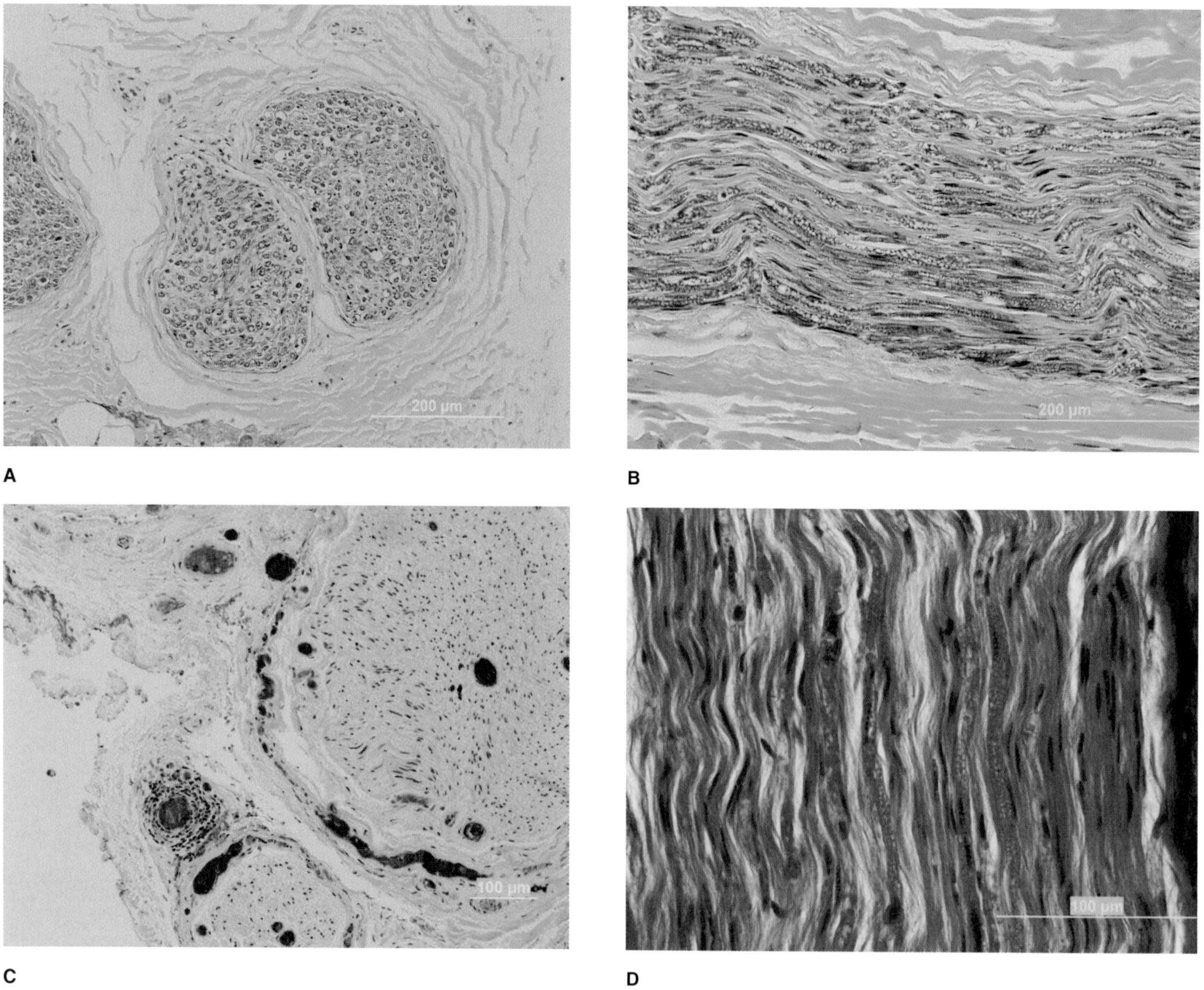

Figure 3-23. Paraffin sections of nerve biopsy. Myelin stains pink on modified Gomori trichrome in this normal nerve seen in cross section **(A)** and longitudinally **(B)**. A reduction in myelinated fibers is apparent by the loss of pink stain on this modified Gomori-trichrome stain **(C)** and as blue staining myelinated nerve fibers on a Luxal fast blue stain **(D)**; however, it is not possible to tell if this is due to primary demyelinating neuropathy or secondary demyelination from a primary axonopathy. (*continued*)

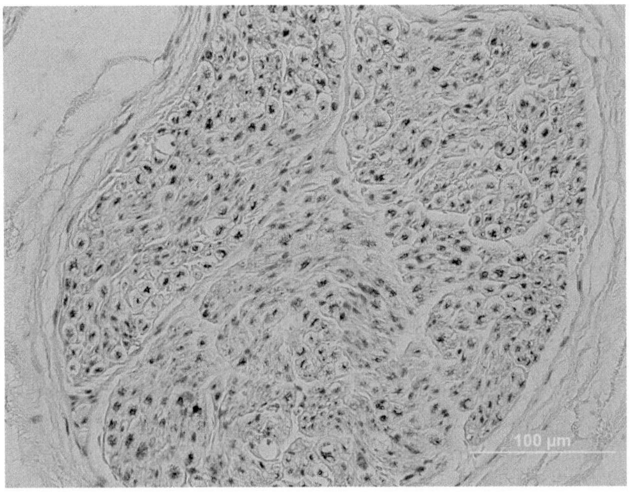

E

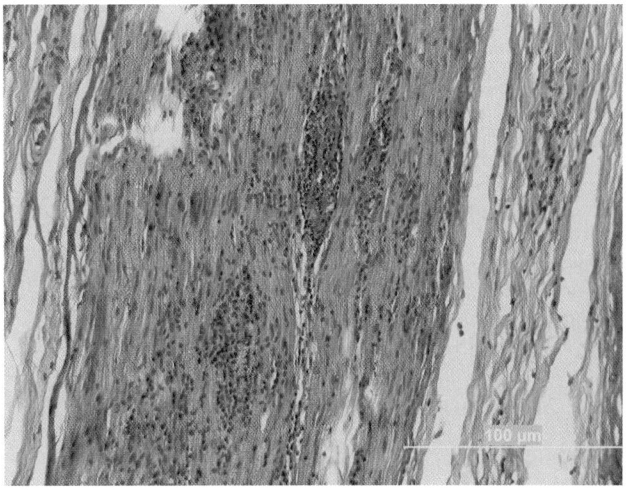

F

Figure 3-23. (*Continued*) SMI-31 stains phosphorylated neurofilaments that are abundant in normal axons, as seen in this normal nerve **(E)**. H&E stain does not distinguish myelinated axons very well, but is useful to look for vasculitis and other inflammatory cell infiltrates, as seen in this biopsy of a patient with lymphoma **(F)**.

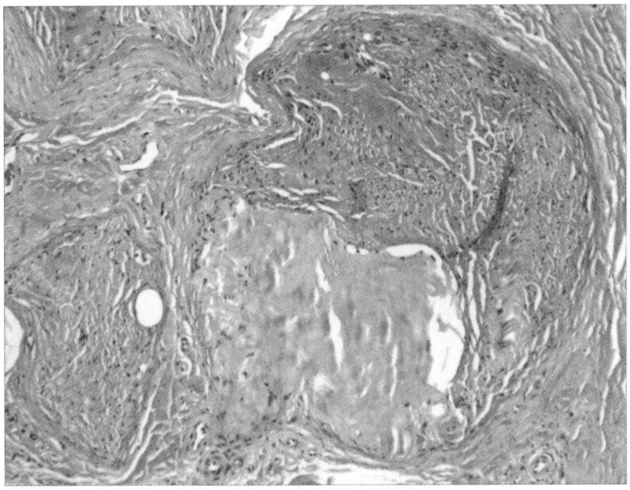

A

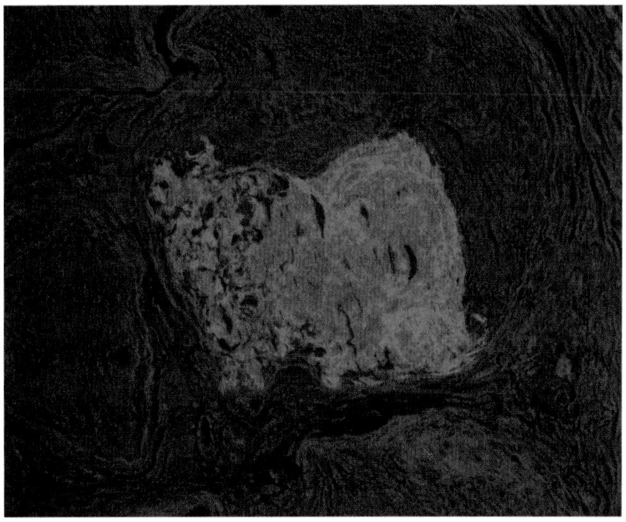

B

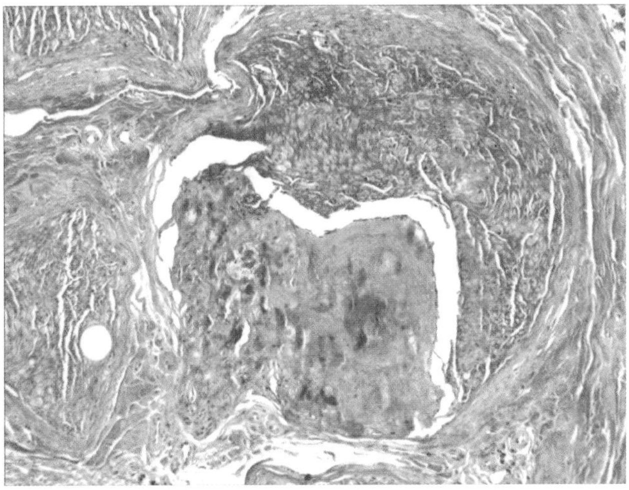

C

Figure 3-24. Familial amyloid polyneuropathy. Nerve biopsy demonstrates abnormal accumulation of amyloidogenic material in the endoneurium in the biopsy of a patient with a transthyretin mutation. The material stains faintly pink on H&E **(A)**. With Congo red under routine light microscopy, amyloid stains intensely red when viewed under rhodamine optics **(B)**. Amyloid stains blue with Alcian blue stain **(C)**.

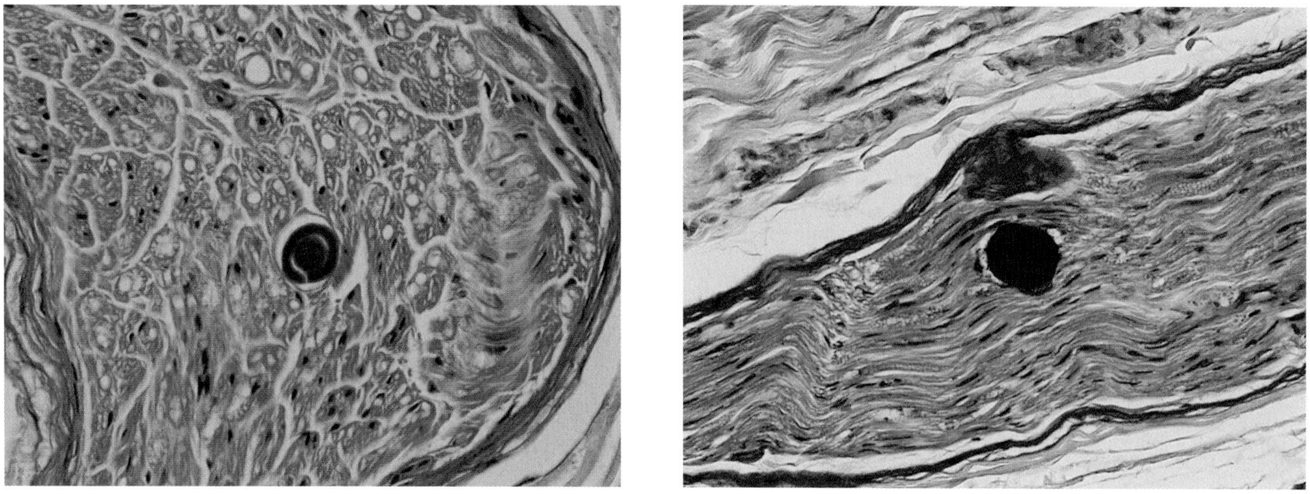

A B

Figure 3-25. PAS stain demonstrates polyglucosan bodies within the axons in polyglucosan body neuropathy, as seen in cross section **(A)** and longitudinal section **(B)**.

(Fig. 3-26). Immunohistochemistry studies can be done to better assess inflammatory cell infiltrates (Fig. 3-27), and other specific stains can be done to better evaluate Schwann cells and perineurial cells when indicated. For example, immunoreactivity against the Schwann cell marker S-100 is useful for schwannomas and neurofibromas (Fig. 3-28), whereas immunoreactivity to epithelial membrane antigen (EMA), which is present on perineurial cells, is helpful in diagnosing perineuriomas. The paraffin-embedded tissue is most useful for evaluating signs of vasculitis, other inflammatory cell infiltrates including granulomas and lymphoma, infection (e.g., leprosy), and amyloidosis. Because the pathology can be multifocal, we like to take sections for paraffin embedding at the proximal and distal ends of the biopsy segment (Fig. 3-21E). In addition, loss of myelinated nerve fibers can be appreciated with various stains of paraffin-embedded tissue.

The remainder of the tissue is stretched delicately on a tongue blade or kept isometric with sutures and fixed in glutaraldehyde or other fixatives (e.g., Karnovsky's fixative). Some of this tissue will then be embedded in plastic and processed for toluidine blue-stained semithin sections (10 μm) and thin sections (1 μm) for EM.[3,21,24–28] The semithin and EM analyses are most important in assess-

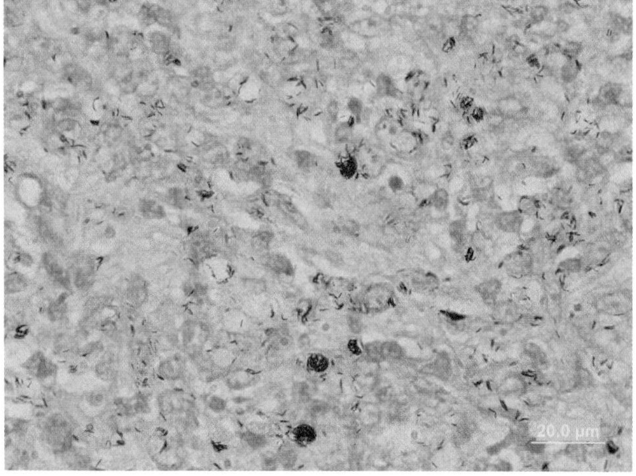

Figure 3-26. Borderline leprosy. Nerve biopsy in a patient with leprosy reveals red staining bacilli using the Fite stain on paraffin sections.

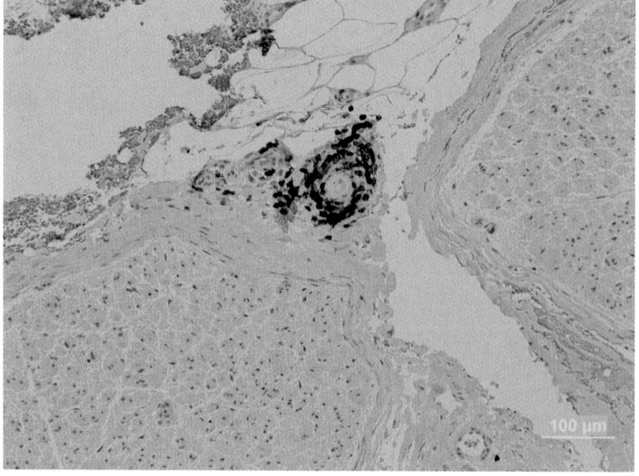

Figure 3-27. Immunoperoxidase stain reveals perivascular CD3+ T lymphocytes in a nerve biopsy in a patient with chronic inflammatory demyelinating polyneuropathy (CIDP).

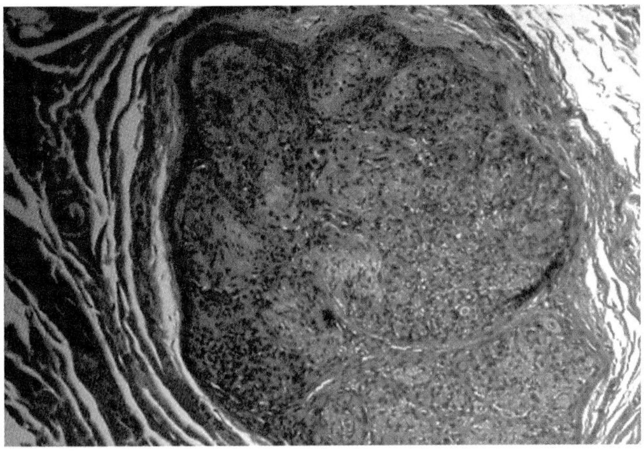

A

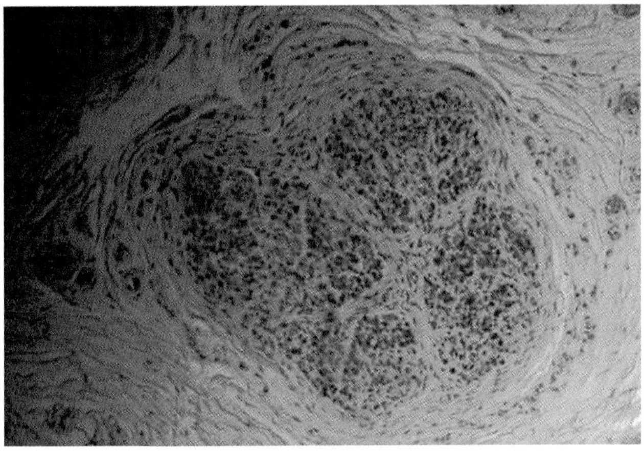

B

Figure 3-28. Neurofibroma. The nerve fascicle has a lobulated appearance, H&E stain **(A)**. The cells have wavy, elongated nuclei, and the background material is loosely arranged and myxoid. Bands of thick collagen are apparent in the center of the tumor. Some of the proliferating tumor cells are immunoreactive for S-100, suggesting Schwann cell origin **(B)**.

ing the axons, Schwann cells, and myelin sheath of myelinated nerve fibers as well as in looking at abnormalities in small unmyelinated nerve fibers (Fig. 3-29). Quantitative morphometric methods can be employed to assess numbers of individual large or small myelinated and unmyelinated fibers in the biopsy, as certain neuropathies have a predilection for certain nerve fiber types. However, this is not routinely done as it is time consuming and often of limited value. Other portions of this fixed material may be used for teased nerve fiber analysis (Fig. 3-30). With this method, individual myelinated fibers are separated from the nerve fascicles and lightly stained, allowing examination of the integrity and thickness of the myelin sheath as well as revealing alterations in internode length. Thus, one can better quantify the degree of demyelinated or thinly myelinated axon, axons with increased or redundant myelin, and axons undergoing active Wallerian degeneration.

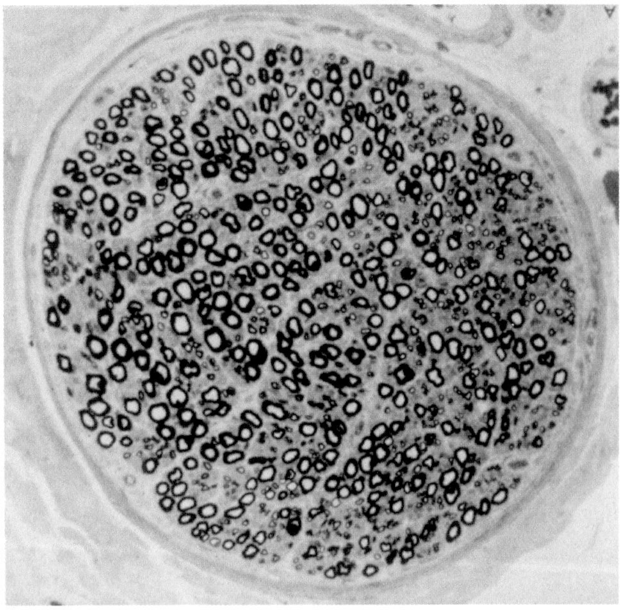

Figure 3-29. Semithin section reveals a normal nerve fascicle.

Teased fiber preparation, however, is very labor intensive and often does not add much to what can be assessed from the semithin and EM sections; thus, it is reserved for more difficult cases (e.g., question of CIDP in biopsy with mild or nonspecific abnormalities on semithin or EM).

► STRUCTURE OF NORMAL NERVE

Peripheral nerves are composed of axons, Schwann cells, myelin sheaths, and supporting tissue. Individual nerve fibers are surrounded by endoneurial connective tissue and grouped into fascicles encased by perineurial sheaths. All the fascicles within a nerve in turn are surrounded by epineurial connective tissue. A blood–nerve barrier is created between the perineurial cells and endoneurial capillaries derived from the vasa nervorum, both of which form tight junctions. The blood–nerve barrier appears to be relatively less competent within nerve roots, dorsal root ganglia, autonomic ganglia, and terminal twigs. The nerve–CSF barrier is formed by the tight junctions between the cells that form the outer layer of the arachnoid membrane. These cells fuse with the perineurium of the roots and cranial nerves as these leave the subarachnoid space.

Myelinated and unmyelinated nerve fibers intermingle within each fascicle. Further, along the course of the entire nerve, individual nerve fibers course in and out of different fascicles. In the sural nerve, which is most commonly biopsied, myelinated fibers range between 2 and 15 μm in diameter and have a bimodal distribution. There are approximately twice as many small myelinated axons as there are large myelinated fibers. Segments of myelinated

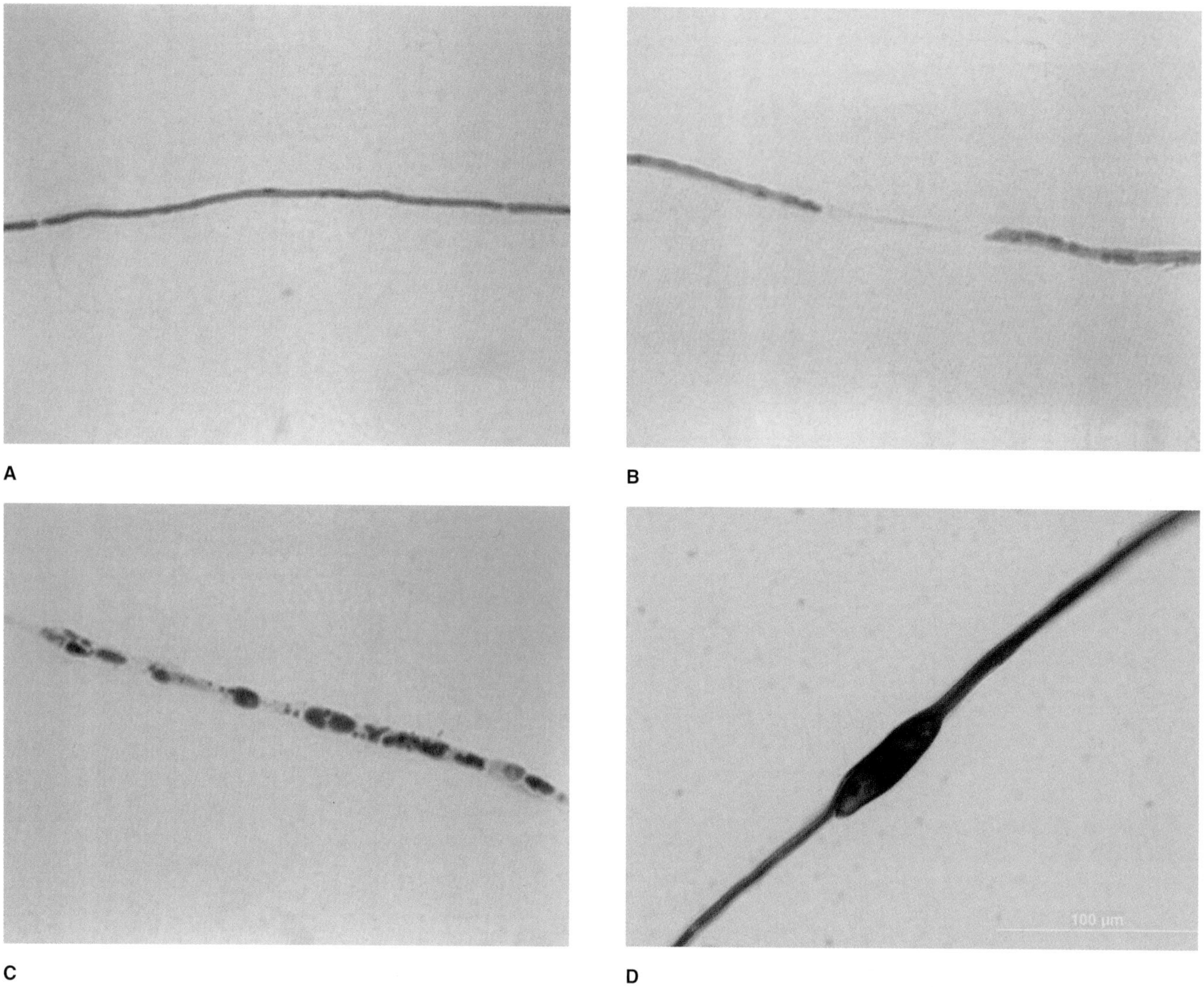

Figure 3-30. Teased nerve fibers. A normal teased fiber internode is seen **(A)** as well as a short, demyelinated internode **(B)**. A teased nerve fiber segment undergoing Wallerian degeneration with myelin ovoids is appreciated in **(C)**. Redundant folds of myelin lead to formation of tomacula (Latin for sausage) that are best appreciated on teased fiber preparations **(D)** and are commonly seen in hereditary neuropathy with liability to pressure palsies and occasionally in other forms of Charcot–Marie–Tooth disease.

fibers (internodes) are separated by nodes of Ranvier. A single Schwann cell supplies the myelin sheath for each internode. The thickness of the myelin sheath is directly proportional to the diameter of the axon, and the larger the axon diameter, the longer the internodal distance. The ratio of the diameter of the axon to the diameter of the entire nerve fiber (axon plus its surrounding myelin) or G-ratio is approximately 0.6. A higher-than-normal diameter ratio implies that the axons are thinly myelinated. In contrast, lower G ratios are seen in axonopathies with axonal atrophy or rare conductions with redundant myelin (tomaculous neuropathy). Unmyelinated axons are more numerous than myelinated axons and range in diameter from 0.2 to 3 μm. Anywhere from 5 to 20 unmyelinated axons are enveloped by a single Schwann cell.

Schwann cells, regardless of their association with myelinated or unmyelinated fibers, have pale oval nuclei with an even chromatin distribution and an elongated bipolar cell body. On EM, Schwann cells can be differentiated from fibroblasts because Schwann cells have a basement membrane. Within axons there are various organelles and cytoskeletal structures, including mitochondria, vesicles, smooth endoplasmic reticulum, lysosomes, neurofilaments, and microtubules. Because protein synthesis occurs in the cell body rather than the axon itself, essential proteins and other substances synthesized in the perikaryon are transported down the axon via axoplasmic flow. A retrograde transport system serves as a feedback to the cell body. These transport systems are dependent on the microtubules and neurofilaments as well as specific proteins such as dynein and dynactin within the axons. At the distal nerve terminal, dense-cored and coated vesicles are found.

► REACTIONS TO INJURY

Although disease processes affecting nerves have different pathogenic mechanisms, these lead to two principal reactions to injury: demyelination and axonal degeneration.[3,21,24–28] Damage to Schwann cells or the myelin sheath itself can lead to demyelination. Because these diseases affect individual Schwann cells to varying degrees, the process is characteristically segmental along the length of the nerve. The disintegrating myelin is phagocytosed by Schwann cells and macrophages. Schwann cells are also stimulated to remyelinate the denuded axon. These newly remyelinated axons are thinner in total diameter and the internodes are shorter than normal—features that are best seen with teased nerve preparations. However, one can also appreciate the thinly myelinated axons on semithin sections and on EM (diameter ratio greater than 0.6). With sequential episodes of demyelination and attempted remyelination, concentric tiers of Schwann cell processes accumulate around the axons forming the so-called "onion bulbs" (Fig. 3-31). Some disease processes are associated with inclusions within Schwann cells (e.g., metachromatic leukodystrophy and certain toxic neuropathies). Other abnormalities in the myelin sheath include tomaculae (redundant folds of myelin characteristic of hereditary neuropathy with liability to pressure palsies or HNPP) and widened periodicity of compacted myelin (seen in neuropathy associated with myelin-associated glycoprotein antibodies).

Primary damage to the axon may either be due to a discrete, localized event (trauma, ischemia, etc.) or be due to an underlying abnormality of the neuronal cell body or ganglion (neuronopathy) or its axon (axonopathy). These processes lead to axonal degeneration with secondary disintegration of its myelin sheath (Fig. 3-32A). If a nerve is transected, the distal portion of the nerve undergoes an acute disintegration (termed Wallerian degeneration) characterized by breakdown of the axon and its myelin sheath into fragments forming small oval compartments (i.e., myelin ovoids). These breakdown products undergo phagocytosis by macrophages and Schwann cells. Most neuronopathies or axonopathies evolve more slowly; therefore, evidence of active axon and myelin breakdown is scant because only a few fibers are degenerating at any given time. The proximal stumps of axons that have degenerated may sprout new axons that attempt to grow along the course of the degenerated axon. Small clusters of these regenerated axons, which are small in diameter and thinly myelinated, can be recognized in cross

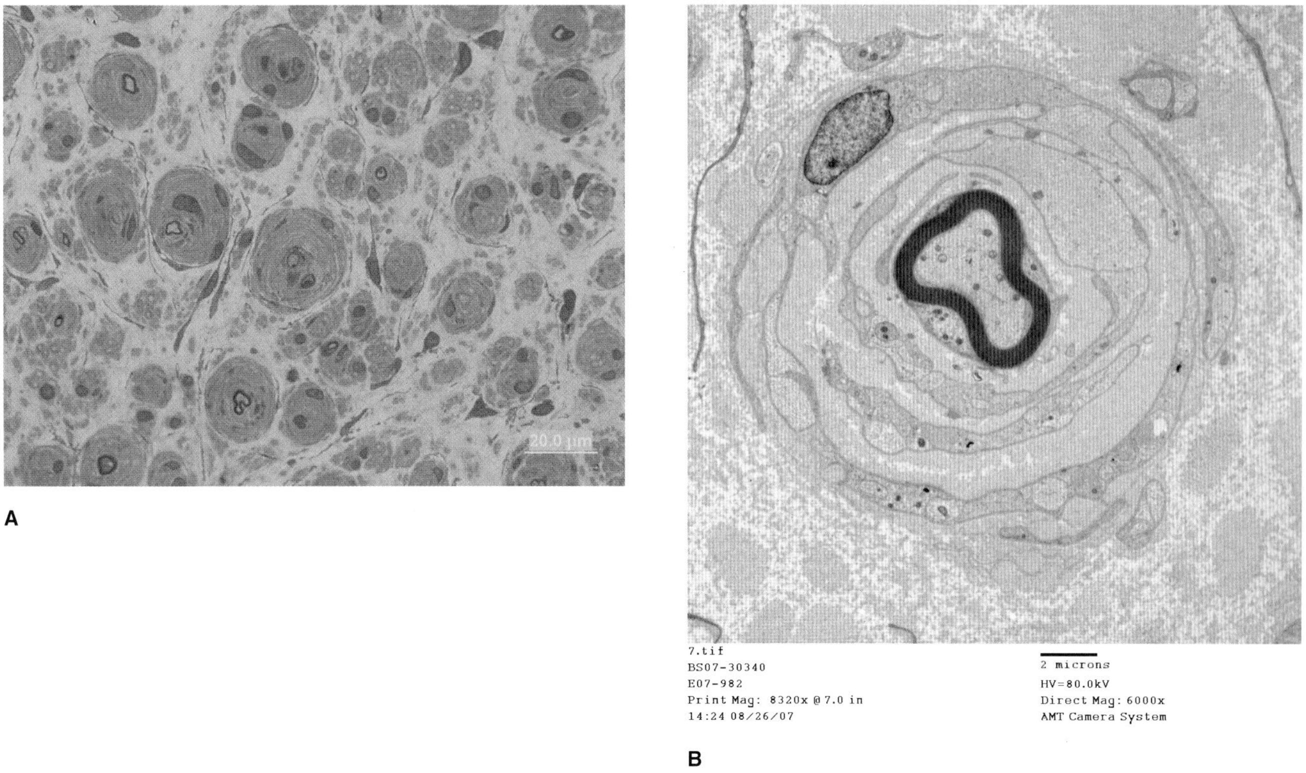

Figure 3-31. Onion bulb formation. With recurrent bouts of demyelination and remyelination, concentric layers of Schwann cell processes accumulate around the axons forming onion bulbs. Prominent onion bulbs can be seen in chronic inflammatory demyelinating neuropathy as in this case but are more typical of hereditary demyelinating neuropathies (i.e., Charcot–Marie–Tooth disease types 1, 3, and 4) on semithin section **(A)** and on electron microscopy **(B)**.

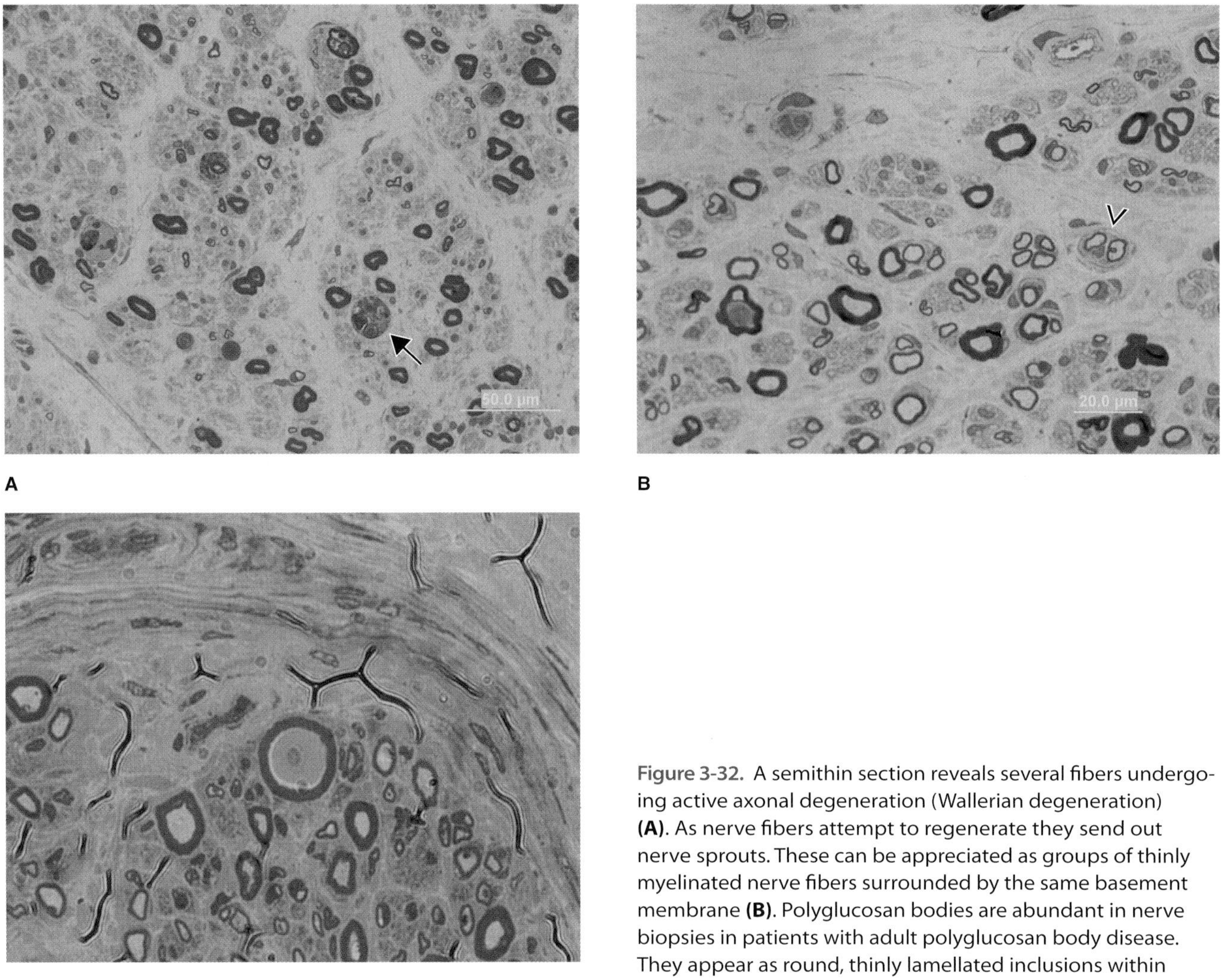

A

B

C

Figure 3-32. A semithin section reveals several fibers undergoing active axonal degeneration (Wallerian degeneration) **(A)**. As nerve fibers attempt to regenerate they send out nerve sprouts. These can be appreciated as groups of thinly myelinated nerve fibers surrounded by the same basement membrane **(B)**. Polyglucosan bodies are abundant in nerve biopsies in patients with adult polyglucosan body disease. They appear as round, thinly lamellated inclusions within axons **(C)**.

section on semithin and EM sections (Fig. 3-32B). Also, as axonal transport of essential proteins and other substances synthesized in the perikaryon is often impaired in axonopathies, axonal atrophy becomes apparent on the semithin and EM sections (G ratio less than 0.6). In contrast, enlarged axons are seen in giant axonal neuropathy and hexacarbon toxicity. Polyglucosan bodies are appreciated on semithin sections (Fig. 3-32C). These are nonspecific, and although rare polyglucosan bodies may be seen on nerve biopsies in elderly and in diabetics, they are much more abundant in patients with adult polyglucosan body disease.

In addition, nerve biopsies can reveal evidence of disease processes similar to those found in other organ systems. Amyloid deposition around blood vessels or within the endoneurium can be seen in systemic amyloidosis or in a familial amyloidotic polyneuropathy (Fig. 3-24). In systemic or isolated peripheral nerve vasculitis, there is transmural infiltration of vessel walls by inflammatory cells associated with fibrinoid necrosis of the vessel walls (Fig. 3-33). Because

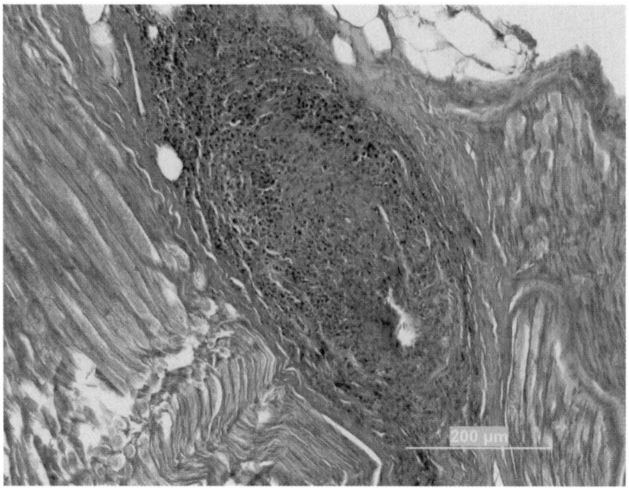

Figure 3-33. Nerve biopsy in a patient with Churg–Strauss syndrome reveals necrotizing vasculitis. Paraffin section, H&E stain.

nerve fibers course between different fascicles along the length of the nerve, patchy asymmetric loss of axons within and between fascicles is a characteristic finding of ischemic nerve injury as seen in vasculitis. Infiltration of the nerve by neoplastic or inflammatory cells can also be recognized. Leprosy is one of the most common etiologies of polyneuropathy in the world. When granulomas or diffuse inflammation of the nerve is seen, a Fite stain can be done to look for the acid-fast bacilli (Fig. 3-26).

► SKIN BIOPSY

Skin biopsies are increasingly being performed to evaluate patients with peripheral neuropathy.[20,29–41] These are most useful in patients with small fiber neuropathies in which other testing modalities provide normal or inconclusive results. Because nerve conduction studies only assess the conduction of large myelinated nerve fiber, patients with pure small fiber neuropathies will have normal nerve conduction studies. In at least a third of people with painful sensory neuropathies, intraepidermal nerve fibers density on skin biopsies represent the only objective abnormality present following extensive evaluation.[35]

The rationale behind performing most skin biopsies is to measure the density and assess the morphology of intraepidermal nerve fibers. These fibers represent the terminals of Aδ and C nociceptors, and these may be decreased in patients with small fiber neuropathies in whom nerve conduction studies and routine nerve biopsies are often normal. Skin biopsies are relatively easy to perform and are associated with a much lower risk than standard nerve biopsies. However, there are several drawbacks to skin biopsies. Importantly, these usually just confirm what you already know about the patient. That is, if a person complains of symmetric burning or tingling pain in the distal lower extremities, has normal strength and deep tendon reflexes, and has normal nerve conduction studies, then he or she likely has a small fiber neuropathy. Skin biopsies are often not useful in identifying the etiology of the neuropathy. The exception is biopsy of skin lesions in suspected cases of lepromatous neuropathy (Fig. 3-34). As stated in the previous section on nerve biopsies, we generally do not do a biopsy in order to prove that a patient has a neuropathy; rather we do so in order to identify the etiology, hopefully a treatable one. That said, assessing intraepidermal nerve fiber density and morphology may play a role in the future by defining the natural history of various neuropathies, monitoring response of the neuropathy to various therapies, and screening for the development of toxic neuropathies (e.g., during chemotherapy).[35] In addition, skin biopsies may be done to confirm a diagnosis of dermatomyositis.

Skin biopsies are usually done by performing a 3-mm punch biopsy of the skin under local anesthesia in the lower leg in an affected region. Other regions can be sampled to assess if there is a length-dependent loss of intraepidermal nerve fibers (e.g., in the dorsum of the foot, thigh, or forearm). The tissue is fixed in formalin, and then immunostaining protein gene product 9.5 (PGP 9.5) is applied to demonstrate the small intraepidermal fibers (Fig. 3-35). Morphometric methods are used to assess the number and complexity of these nerves, through parameters such as the linear density (number of fibers per millimeter of biopsy) or total length of intraepidermal nerve fibers. The morphology of the intraepidermal nerve fibers can also be assessed. Axonal swellings may be an early marker of small fiber neuropathy and may be appreciated

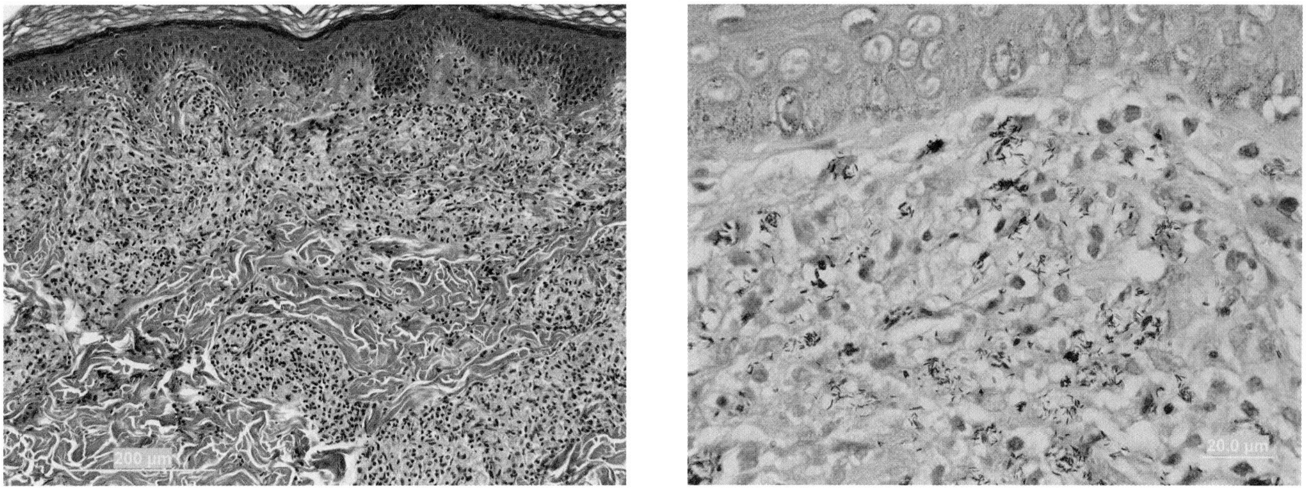

A B

Figure 3-34. Borderline leprosy. Skin biopsy demonstrates marked inflammatory cell infiltrate, H&E **(A)**. Red staining bacilli are evident on higher power with a Fite stain **(B)**

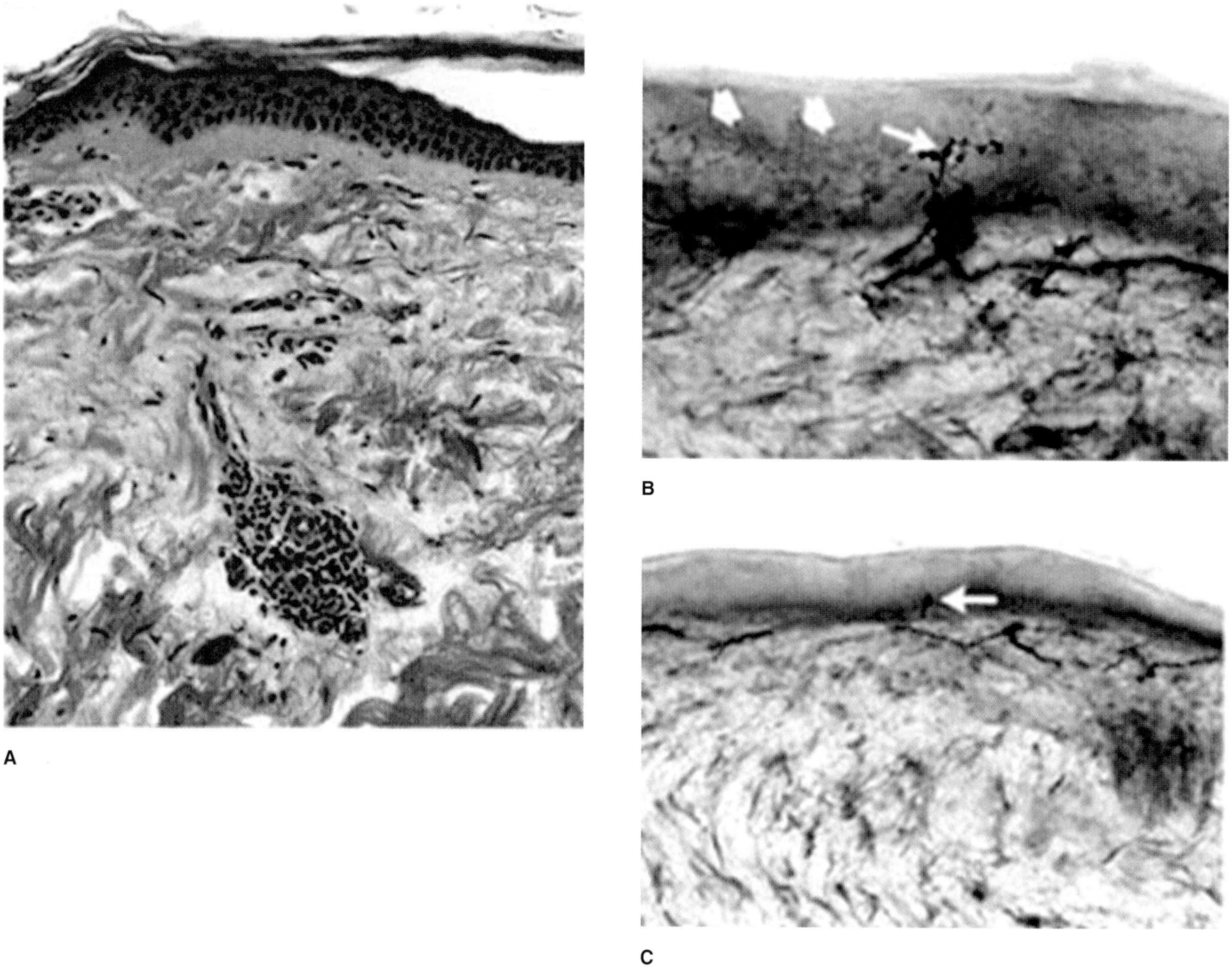

Figure 3-35. Skin biopsy in small fiber neuropathy. A specimen obtained at the time of the patient's first evaluation **(A)** shows a focal perivascular lymphocytic infiltrate (H&E, ×125). A section immunolabeled against protein gene product 9.5 reveals neural processes or axons (*thick arrows*) **(B)** showing an epidermal neurite with axonal swellings, which are abnormal (*thin arrow*). The density of nerve fibers is greater than normal (immunoperoxidase, ×500). A specimen obtained 11 months later **(C)** shows marked reduction in neurite density and axonal swelling (*arrow*) in a remaining neurite (×300). (Reproduced with permission from Drs. Thomas Smith and Lawrence Hayward, from Amato AA, Oaklander AL. Case 16–2004: A 76-year-old woman with numbness and pain in the feet and legs. *N Engl J Med.* 2004;350:2181–2189.)

before a reduction in density. However, axonal swellings can also be seen in normal individuals. Immunostaining for vasoactive intestinal polypeptide, substance P, or calcitonin gene-related proteins can be used to measure the density of sudomotor axons innervating sweat glands, piloerector nerves to hair follicles, and nerves to small arterioles. Myelin can be immunolabeled with antibodies directed against peripheral myelin protein 22 and myelin-associated glycoprotein.

▶ SUMMARY

Muscle, nerve, and skin biopsies for epidermal nerve fiber analysis can be useful in diagnosis of various neuromuscular conditions. The various histopathologic abnormalities that we mentioned are discussed in more detail in subsequent chapters with the diseases in which these appear. As with electrodiagnostic and other laboratory testing, these are only helpful in conjunction with a good *clinical* assessment and cogent differential diagnosis. Further, it is imperative that just as neuromuscular clinicians must be able to independently review and interpret results of electrodiagnostic testing, the same holds true for at least understanding biopsy reports. Whenever possible we would urge clinicians to review biopsy slides with their pathologists so that they can become more familiar with various disease processes and correlate the clinical and electrodiagnostic findings with the histopathology.

REFERENCES

1. Banker BQ, Engel AG. Basic reactions of muscle. In: Engel AG, Franzini-Armstrong C, eds. *Myology*. 3rd ed. New York, NY: McGraw-Hill; 2004:691–747.
2. Carpenter S, Karpati G. *Pathology of Skeletal Muscle*. 2nd ed. New York, NY: Oxford; 2001.
3. De Girolami U, Frosch M, Amato AA. Biopsy of nerve and muscle. In: Samuels M, Feske S, eds. *Office Practice of Neurology*. 2nd ed. Philadelphia, PA: Harcourt Health Sciences;2003:217–225.
4. Dumitru D, Amato AA. Introduction to myopathies and muscle tissue's reaction to injury. In: Dumitru D, Amato AA, Swartz MJ, eds. *Electrodiagnostic Medicine*. 2nd ed. Philadelphia, PA: Hanley & Belfus; 2002:1229–1264.
5. Engel AG. The muscle biopsy. In: Engel AG, Franzini-Armstrong C, eds. *Myology*. 3rd ed. New York, NY: McGraw-Hill; 2004: 681–690.
6. Filosto M, Tonin P, Vattemi G, et al. The role of muscle biopsy in investigating isolated muscle pain. *Neurology*. 2007;68(3): 181–186.
7. Cote AM, Jimenez L, Adelman LS, Munsat TL. Needle biopsy with the automatic Biopty instrument. *Neurology*. 1992;42: 2212–2213.
8. Edwards RH, Round JM, Jones DA. Needle biopsy of skeletal muscle: A review of 10 years experience. *Muscle Nerve*. 1983:6(9):676–683.
9. Heckmatt JZ, Moosa A, Hutson C, Maunder-Sewry CA, Dubowitz V. Diagnostic needle muscle biopsy: A practical and reliable alternative to open biopsy. *Arch Dis Child*. 1994;59:528–532.
10. Magistris MR, Kohler A, Pizzolato G, et al. Needle muscle biopsy in the investigation of neuromuscular disorders. *Muscle Nerve*. 1988;21:194–200.
11. Colling-Saltin AS. Enzyme histochemistry on skeletal muscle of the human foetus. *J Neurol Sci*. 1978;39:169–185.
12. Engel AG, Banker BQ. Ultrastructural changes in diseased muscle. In: Engel AG, Franzini-Armstrong C, eds. *Myology*. 3rd ed. New York, NY: McGraw-Hill; 2004:749–887.
13. Johnson MA, Polgar J, Weightman D, Appleton D. Data on the distribution of fiber types in thirty-six human muscles. An autopsy study. *J Neurol Sci*. 1973;18:111–129.
14. Brooke MH, Engel WK. The histographic analysis of human muscle biopsies with regard to fiber types. 1. Adult male and female. *Neurology*. 1969;19:221–233.
15. Brooke MH, Engel WK. The histographic analysis of human muscle biopsies with regard to fiber types. 2. Diseases of the upper and lower motor neuron. *Neurology*. 1969;19:378–393.
16. Brooke MH, Engel WK. The histographic analysis of human muscle biopsies with regard to fiber types. 3. Myotonias, myasthenia gravis, and hypokalemic periodic paralysis. *Neurology*. 1969;19:469–477.
17. Brooke MH, Engel WK. The histographic analysis of human muscle biopsies with regard to fiber types. 4. Children's biopsies. *Neurology*. 1969;19:591–605.
18. Metafora S, Felsani A, Cotrufo GF, et al. Neural control of gene expression in skeletal muscle fibers: The nature of the lesion in the muscular protein-synthesis machinery following denervation. *Proc R Soc Lond B Biol Sci*. 1980;209:239–255.
19. Bischoff R. Control of satellite cell proliferation. *Adv Exp Med Biol*. 1990;280:147–158.
20. Hilton DA, Jacob J, Househam L, Tengah C. Complications following sural and peroneal nerve biopsies. *J Neurol Neurosurg Psychiatry*. 2007;78:1271–1272.
21. Lacomis D. Clinical utility of peripheral nerve biopsy. *Curr Neurol Neurosci Rep*. 2005;5(1):41–47.
22. Ruth A, Schulmeyer FJ, Roesch M, Woertgen C, Brawanski A. Diagnostic and therapeutic value due to suspected diagnosis, longterm complications, and indication for sural nerve biopsy. *Clin Neurol Neurosurg*. 2005;107(3):214–217.
23. Schweikert K, Fuhr P, Probst A, Tolnay M, Renaud S, Steck AJ. Contribution of nerve biopsy to unclassified neuropathy. *Eur Neurol*. 2007;57(2):86–90.
24. Bouche P, Vallat JM. *Neuropathies Périphériques*. Paris: Doin; 1992.
25. Dyck PJ, Dyck PJB, Engelstad J. Pathologic alterations of nerves. In: Dyck PJ, Thomas PK, eds. *Peripheral Neuropathy*. 4th ed. Philadelphia, PA: WB Saunders; 2005:733–829.
26. Midroni G, Bilbao JM. *Biopsy Diagnosis of Peripheral Neuropathy*. Boston, MA: Butterworth-Heinemann; 1995.
27. Richardson EP Jr, De Girolami U. *Pathology of the Peripheral Nerve*. Philadelphia, PA: WB Saunders; 1995.
28. Ferreire G, Denef JF, Rodriguez J, Guzzetta F. Morphometric studies of normal sural nerves in children. *Muscle Nerve* 1985;8:697–704.
29. Amato AA, Oaklander AL. Case 16–2004: A 76-year-old woman with numbness and pain in the feet and legs. *N Engl J Med*. 2004;350:2181–2189.
30. Herrman DN, Griffin JW, Hauer P, Cornblath DR, McArthur JC. Intraepidermal nerve fiber density, sural nerve morphometry and electrodiagnosis in peripheral neuropathies. *Neurology*, 1999;53:1634–1640.
31. Holland NR, Stocks NR, Hauer P, Cornblath DR, Griffin JW, McArthur JC. Intraepidermal nerve fiber density in patients with painful sensory neuropathy. *Neurology*. 1997;48:708–711.
32. Holland NR, Crawford TO, Hauer P, Cornblath DR, Griffin JW, McArthur JC. Small-fiber sensory neuropathies: Clinical course and neuropathology of idiopathic cases. *Ann Neurol*. 1998; 44: 47–59.
33. McArthur JC, Stocks EA, Hauer P, Cornblath DR, Griffin JW. Intraepidermal nerve fiber density: Normative reference range and diagnostic efficiency. *Arch Neurol*. 1998;55:1513–1520.
34. McCarthy BG, Hseih ST, Stocks A, et al. Cutaneous innervation in sensory neuropathies: valuation by skin biopsy. *Neurology*. 1995;45:1845–1855.
35. Periquet MI, Novak V, Collins MP, et al. Painful sensory neuropathy: Prospective evaluation of painful feet using electrodiagnosis and skin biopsy. *Neurology*. 1999;53: 1641–1647.
36. Smith AG, Ramchandran P, Tripp S, Singleton JR. Epidermal nerve innervation in impaired glucose tolerance and diabetes-associated neuropathy. *Neurology*. 2001;57;1701–1704.
37. Sommer C, Lauria G. Skin biopsy in the management of peripheral neuropathy. *Lancet Neurol*. 2007;6:632–642.
38. Tobkin K, Guiliani MJ, Lacomis D. Comparison of different modalities for detection of small-fiber neuropathy. *Clin Neurophys*. 1999;110:1909–1912.
39. Walk D, Wendelschafer-Crabb G, Davey C, Kennedy WR. Concordance between epidermal nerve fiber density and sensory examination in patients with symptoms of idiopathic small fiber neuropathy. *J Neurol Sci*. 2007;255(1–2):23–26.
40. Wendelschafer-Crabb G, Kennedy WR, Walk D. Morphological features of nerves in skin biopsies. *J Neurol Sci*. 2006;242 (1–2):15–21.
41. England JD, Gronseth GS, Franklin G, et al. Evaluation of distal symmetric polyneuropathy: The role of autonomic testing, nerve biopsy, and skin biopsy (an evidence-based review). *Muscle Nerve*. 2009;39(1):106–115.

CHAPTER 4

Principles of Immunomodulating Treatment

▶ INTRODUCTION

The ideal of every patient and physician is to identify a diagnosis whose natural history is self-limited, or if not, a diagnosis for which an effective treatment can be administered. Autoimmunity is believed to be the contributing, if not causal, mechanism of a significant number of neuromuscular disorders.[1] Accordingly, patients with proven or suspected autoimmune neuromuscular disorders become candidates for treatments that modulate or suppress immune-mediated nerve, neuromuscular junction, or muscle dysfunction or injury. Familiarity with drugs or other interventions that suppress or modulate the patient's immune system is therefore a prerequisite for anyone practicing neuromuscular medicine.

In this book, we will define immunomodulation as any therapy that affects in any way the native activities of a patient's immune system in an attempt to mitigate disease. We will define immunosuppression as a subcategory of immunomodulation in which a patient's immunologic response is impaired by one of the three recognized mechanisms.[2,3] One mechanism, as occurs with drugs such as azathioprine, cyclophosphamide, mycophenolate, and methotrexate, curtails B-cell and T-cell proliferation by cell cycle interruption. Another mechanism, as exemplified by drugs such as the calcineurin inhibitors (e.g., cyclosporine and tacrolimus) and corticosteroids, is impairment of T-cell activation. A final mechanism of immunosuppression is accomplished by monoclonal antibodies–directed cell surface antigens, rituximab being the most notable example. Conversely, we will consider interventions such as intravenous immunoglobulin (IVIg) or plasma exchange (PLEX) to be immunomodulating, not immunosuppressive.

The authors strongly endorse the concept of evidence-based medicine. At the same time, we recognize that evidence-based medicine applies to populations and that strict adherence to evidence guidance is not always in the best interests of the individual patients we are responsible for. In neuromuscular medicine, there are numerous examples of treatments that are universally considered to be efficacious yet remain of unproven benefit by "evidence-based" standards.[4] Corticosteroids in myasthenia gravis (MG) is one notable example, discovered by innovative effort by individual clinicians. Because of the accepted efficacy of this and other historically identified empiric treatments, it is unlikely that a number of currently accepted treatments will ever be validated by large prospective studies.

Our position is also supported by personal witness of unequivocal benefit to individual patients, who respond to treatments demonstrated to be ineffective to larger populations with the same disease. Rituximab in MuSK-positive MG is such an example.[5] Accordingly, this chapter will describe, and in some cases endorse, the off-label uses of immunomodulating treatments for various neuromuscular diseases even in the absence of evidence-based support. We do so cautiously as we recognize that these idiosyncratic responses may be harmful as well as helpful. Ultimately, each physician needs, along with their patient, to determine whether the potential benefits of immunomodulating treatment, of proven or unproven benefit, exceed the probability and magnitude of potential risk.

This chapter will approach immunomodulating treatment of presumed immune-mediated disorders by focusing on the treatments, rather than the disorders themselves which will be the subject matter of subsequent chapters. A summary of these agents, and the disorders for which they may or may not be effective are summarized in Table 4-1. Details regarding dosing, side effect profiles, and recommended screening procedures are summarized in Table 4-2.

▶ GENERAL CONSIDERATIONS

Before initiating immunomodulating therapy, it is critical to consider the probability and magnitude of both the potential risk to an individual patient, as well as the potential benefit. There is a consensus that patients who receive immunomodulating treatment are at an increased risk for both infection and malignancy.[6] There is also a consensus that the risk is probably dependent on numerous variables including the genetics and comorbidities of the individual patient, the agent or agents used, as well as cumulative dose and duration of treatment. The following section will review some of these considerations facing clinicians and their patients who are contemplating immunomodulating treatment. On discussing risk with patients, we find it useful to utilize the World Health Organization guidelines which define risk as very common >1/10, common >1/100, uncommon >1/1,000, rare >1/10,000, and very rare >1/100,000.[7]

In consideration of immunomodulating treatment, it is important to be armed with knowledge relevant to a number of key issues in order to make rational treatment decisions. Of primary importance is the identification of an objective

▶ TABLE 4-1. **IMMUNOMODULATING DRUGS IN NM DISORDERS—CURRENT USAGE**

Treatment	Disorders with Evidence-Based Efficacy	Disorders with Evidence Based or Other Reports of Inefficacy	Disorders with Supportive But Inconclusive Studies	Disorders with Anecdotal Reports of Benefit
Alemtuzumab				CIDP [32–34,73] VN/NSVN[56,94] IBM[281]
Azathioprine		DM/PM[55,78,282] MMN[55]	MG [37–42]	CIDP[34] DRPLN[50] VN/NSVN[46,47,56,94] Sarcoidosis[48,83] MMN[54] IS[51–54] LEMS[49]
Corticosteroids		MMN[77] GBS[304] IBM[79]	MG[43,59–61,63,86,284–289] CIDP[34,59,65–68,71–73,74,311–313] MADSAM[69,70] VN/NSVN[46,47,56,94] Sarcoidosis[48,83] DM/PM[45,55,78]	BPN[84] DRPLN[50,241,290] IMNM[207–209] IS[51–54]
Chlorambucil				Sarcoidosis[48,83] DM/PM[202]
Cyclophosphamide			MG[104–109] VN/NSVN[46,47,56,91–94,291] MMN[54,77] CIDP[95–101]	MMN[102] DRPLN[50] Sarcoidosis[48,83] IS[51–54] DADS[103] DM/PM[45,291,292]
Cyclosporine		MMN[54]	MG[36,111–116] CIDP[34,73,118–125]	CIDP[34,73] VN/NSVN[46,47,56,94] Sarcoidosis[48,84] MMN[54] DM/PM[45,55,127–135,293,294] LEMS[126] IS[136]
Eculizumab		DM/PM[55,138]		MG[137,231]
Etanercept			DM/PM[45,148,295–298]	MG[147] CIDP[139–143] Sarcoidosis[48,83,144–146]
Infliximab		DM/PM[55,295–297,299–301]		VN/NSVN[46,47,56,94] Sarcoidosis[48,83,144]
Interferon β 1a		MMN[54,302]		CIDP[34,73,151–161] MMN[54]
IVIg[116,162,303]	GBS (adult and pediatric) [305] CIDP[64,165,195,196,237,305–311] MMN[15,166,314–320] LEMS[29,321] DM[55,193,302,322–330] MG[168–174,176–186] SPS[331]	ALS[16] IBM[332–335] DADS[336–340] LMNS[14]	DLRPN[50,341–349] MADSAM[69,70]	MFS[240,350] PN-SS[351–357] PN-IgA/IgG[337–339,358] PN-EGP[359,360] PN-Sulfatide[339,361] Polymyositis[321,325,327–329] DADS[336–339] CN[362] PN-IBD[363] PN-CTD[364,465] PN- Sarcoidosis[283] BPN[366–368] VN/NSVN[46,47,56,94] IMNM[207–209] IS[51–54]

(continued)

▶ TABLE 4-1. (CONTINUED)

Treatment	Disorders with Evidence-Based Efficacy	Disorders with Evidence Based or Other Reports of Inefficacy	Disorders with Supportive But Inconclusive Studies	Disorders with Anecdotal Reports of Benefit
Methotrexate		MMN[54] CIDP[34,125,204–206]	DM/PM[1,45,55,78,127,198–203]	VN/NSVN[46,47,56,94] Sarcoidosis[48] MMN[54] IMNM[207–209] MG[2,210]
Mycophenolate		MMN[54]	MG[213–223,226] CIDP[34,73,125,221,224–229]	VN/NSVN[46,47,56,94] Sarcoidosis[48,83,144] IMNM[207,208] IS[51–54]
Plasma exchange[233,234]	GBS[197] CIDP[233,237,238] MG[169,170,172,175,180,183,184,187–192,235,236] PN-IgA/IgG[239]	MMN[15,77] DM/PM[45,55]	LEMS[49]	DRPLN[50,241] VN/NSVN[46,47,56,94] MFS[240] IS[51–54]
Rituximab	MG[242–248] SPS[266–268]	DADS[369]	MG[249–250] DADS[252] LEMS[49] DM/PM[269] VN/NSVN[46,47,56,79–81,94]	CIDP[125,254–265] MMN[54] IMNM[207,208,270] IS[51–54]
Tacrolimus			PM/DM[269,293] MG[110,116,223,267–279]	CIDP[34] VN/NSVN[46,47,56,94] CIDP[280]

ALS, amyotrophic lateral sclerosis; BPN, brachial plexus neuritis; CIDP, chronic inflammatory demyelinating polyradiculoneuropathy; CANOMAD, chronic ataxic neuropathy, ophthalmoplegia, monoclonal IgM protein , cold agglutinins, and disialosyl antibodies; CN, cryoglobulinemic neuropathy; DADS, distal acquired demyelinating sensory neuropathy (associated with IgM monoclonal proteins and myelin-associated glycoprotein autoantibodies); DLRPN, diabetic lumbosacral radiculoplexus neuropathy; DM, dermatomyositis; GBS, Guillain–Barré syndrome; IMNM, immune-mediated necrotizing myopathy; IS, Isaac's syndrome; LEMS, Lambert–Eaton myasthenic syndrome; LMNS, lower motor neuron syndromes; MADSAM, multifocal acquired demyelinating sensory and motor neuropathy (a.k.a. Lewis–Sumner syndrome); MFS, Miller Fisher syndrome; MG, autoimmune myasthenia gravis; MMN, multifocal motor neuropathy; PM, polymyositis; PN-CTD, peripheral neuropathy associated with connective tissue disease; PN-IBD, peripheral neuropathy associated with inflammatory bowel disease; PN-IgA/IgG, peripheral neuropathy associated with IgA/IgG monoclonal proteins; PN-EGP, peripheral neuropathy associated with eosinophilic granulomatosis with polyangiitis (formerly Churg–Strauss syndrome); PN-SS, peripheral neuropathy associated with Sjögren syndrome neuropathy; SPS, stiff person syndrome; VN/NSVN, vasculitic and nonsystemic vasculitic neuropathy.

parameter to measure. A pretreatment baseline should be established in order to determine whether treatment is effective or not in the future. The ideal parameter(s) chosen should be not only quantifiable and reproducible, it (they) should correlate with meaningful improvements in patient comfort and function.

In neuromuscular disease, measurements of strength are the most commonly utilized. We have found manual muscle strength testing and handheld dynamometry (e.g., microFET2®) to be helpful in this regard, along with quantitative bedside assessments of sensation (e.g., timed vibration or the Rydel-Seiffer® tuning fork). There are many functional or symptomatic scales that have been developed for specific diseases, e.g. ALS, myasthenia, and peripheral neuropathy, that also facilitate determination of treatment response.[8–13] Unfortunately in neuromuscular disease, other biomarkers such as imaging, electromyography and nerve conduction study data, and measurement of serologic markers are not always accurate or practical means of monitoring treatment response.

A master clinician understands the natural history of the disease they are treating as well as the properties of the agents they are using. The latency between treatment and response is dependent on at least two parameters, the pharmacology of the immunomodulating agents used and the pathophysiology of the disease. For example, morbidity created by disorders that impede ion channel function, demyelinate axons without otherwise injuring them, or that injure relatively easily repairable components of the neuromuscular system such as ACh receptors may be expected to respond to an effective treatment relatively rapidly, within days to weeks in many cases. Conversely, disorders that require axon regrowth may require months before return of function becomes evident depending on the number of axons injured, the distance between the site of injury and the muscle(s) that require(s) reinnervation. Lastly, disorders that lead to significant destruction of motor or sensory cell bodies are limited in their ability to recover as their regeneration is unlikely, even if an effective treatment is initiated.

▶ TABLE 4-2. IMMUNOSUPPRESSIVE THERAPY FOR NEUROMUSCULAR DISORDERS

Therapy	Route	Dose	Side Effects	Monitor
Prednisone	Oral	0.75–1.5 mg/kg/day to start	Hypertension, increased appetite, fluid and weight gain, insomnia, hyperglycemia, hypokalemia, cataracts, gastric irritation, osteoporosis, infection, aseptic femoral necrosis, myopathy, ecchymosis, change in body habitus and facial appearance	Weight, blood pressure, serum glucose/potassium, cataract formation
Methylprednisolone	Intravenous	1 g in 100 mL/normal saline over 1–2 hours, daily or every other day for 3–6 doses	Arrhythmia, flushing, dysgeusia, anxiety, insomnia, fluid and weight gain, hyperglycemia, hypokalemia, infection	Heart rate, blood pressure, serum glucose/potassium
Azathioprine	Oral	2–3 mg/kg/day; single AM dose	Flu-like illness, hepatotoxicity, pancreatitis, leukopenia, macrocytosis, neoplasia, infection, teratogenicity	Blood count, liver enzymes
Methotrexate	Oral	7.5–25 mg weekly, single or divided doses; 1-2 day a week dosing	Hepatotoxicity, pulmonary fibrosis, infection, neoplasia, infertility, leukopenia, alopecia, GI irritation with nausea/diarrhea, stomatitis, teratogenicity	Liver enzymes, blood count, chest x-ray baseline and yearly
	Subcutaneously	20–50 mg weekly; 1 day a week dosing	Same as oral	Same as p.o.
Cyclophosphamide	Oral Intravenous	1.5–2 mg/kg/day; single AM dose 0.5–1.0 g/m^2 per month × 6–12 months	Bone marrow suppression, infertility, hemorrhagic cystitis, alopecia, infections, neoplasia, teratogenicity	Blood count, urinalysis
Cyclosporine	Oral	4–6 mg/kg/day, split into two daily doses	Nephrotoxicity, hypertension, infection, hepatotoxicity, hirsutism, tremor, gum hyperplasia, teratogenicity	Blood pressure, creatinine/BUN, liver enzymes, cyclosporine levels
Tacrolimus	Oral	0.1–0.2 mg/kg/day in two divided doses	Nephrotoxicity, hypertension, infection, hepatotoxicity, hirsutism, tremor, gum hyperplasia, teratogenicity, hyperglycemia	Blood pressure, creatinine/BUN, liver enzymes, tacrolimus levels
Mycophenolate mofetil	Oral	Adults (1 gBID to 1.5 g BID) Children (600 mg/m^2/dose BID (no more than 1 g/day in patients with renal failure)	Bone marrow suppression, hypertension, tremor, diarrhea, nausea, vomiting, headache, sinusitis, confusion, amblyopia, cough, teratogenicity, infection, neoplasia, PML	Blood count
Intravenous Immunoglobulin	Intravenous	2 g/kg over 2–5 days; then 1 g/kg every 4–8 weeks as needed	Hypotension, arrhythmia, diaphoresis, flushing, nephrotoxicity, headache, aseptic meningitis, anaphylaxis, stroke	Heart rate, blood pressure, creatinine/BUN Some check B-cell count prior to subsequent courses (but this may not be warranted)

PML, progressive multifocal leukoencephalopathy.

Furthermore, it is important to be familiar with the duration of treatment benefit as well as the latency between therapeutic intervention and clinical response. Without an appreciation of both, at least three potential risks may be encountered. A clinician may give up on a treatment before it has had a chance to work, and by doing so, initiate a second, potentially unnecessary and harmful agent. Conversely, a clinician may be overly optimistic, waiting too long for an ineffective agent to work, thus delaying exposure to an additional, potentially beneficial treatment. In addition, a clinician may unnecessarily procrastinate by waiting too long to initiate subsequent maintenance doses, allowing potentially avoidable relapses to occur and by doing so, eroding a patient's confidence in their physician.

A particularly vexing problem in this age of evidence-based medicine is the patient with a suspected or proven autoimmune disorder for which no known proven treatments exist. In these cases, a diagnostic and potentially therapeutic trial may be undertaken. IVIg is frequently used for this purpose both for its relatively rapid onset of action, its efficacy in many autoimmune diseases, and in consideration of its relative safety. For example, although current evidence does not support the routine use of IVIg in lower motor neuron syndromes, some of these patients are thought to represent cases of multifocal motor neuropathy (MMN) without demonstrable biomarkers such as elevated GM1 autoantibody titres or conduction block.[14,15] In this and other comparable situations, we follow the lead of others by typically providing a 3-month therapeutic trial of IVIg.[14,16] Although this practice may be considered somewhat arbitrary in its duration, it represents in our mind a reasonable compromise between a sufficient interval to detect benefit in this demyelinating neuropathy and the waste of an expensive resource. In the case of an MMN suspect, unequivocal stabilization would provide sufficient proof of treatment efficacy as this would differ from the inexorable progression of motor neuron disease which is the primary differential diagnostic consideration.[14]

Immunomodulating treatment strategies vary in consideration with the treatment modality employed, individual disease characteristics, and individual patient context. There are general principles however, that include the recognition of maximal achievable benefit with the goal of avoiding excessive treatment. If disease remission can be achieved, with the potential in that particular disorder for a durable, treatment-free response, an attempt should be made to wean by reducing the amount and/or frequency of administration. For example, it is not uncommon for patients with vasculitic neuropathies who respond to immunosuppression to eventually be successfully weaned from treatment after 2–3 years and enjoy years of subsequent treatment-free stability. The goal with any patient, is to ensure, through clinical or when relevant other means, continued patient improvement or stabilization. At the same time, the goal is to also limit potential adverse effects and costs of chronic treatment while at the same time achieve and sustain the best potential outcome.

These differing treatment strategies are illustrated in the following examples. Corticosteroids in MG or inflammatory myopathies or IVIg in MMN are often initiated at high "induction" doses and then gradually weaned in an attempt to identify the smallest dose or longest interval between treatments that will achieve remission or maintain an acceptable level of morbidity. Conversely, with IVIg in Guillain–Barré syndrome (GBS) or rituximab in MG, a singular prescribed course is initially delivered regardless of initial response and repeated in the future only with initial response and subsequent relapse.

▶ RISK CONSIDERATIONS WITH IMMUNOMODULATING TREATMENTS

INFECTIOUS DISEASE

Pneumocystis Jirovecii

Pneumocystis jirovecii, formerly known as *Pneumocystis carinii* (PCP), is a fungal interstitial pneumonia that occurs predominantly in individuals who are immunosuppressed as a result of their disease or its treatment.[17] It is widely accepted that 70–90% of patients who acquire PCP have received corticosteroid treatment.[18] PCP prophylaxis advocates justify its use in immunosuppressed individuals due to the potential morbidity and mortality associated infection. The mortality risk is estimated to be 30–50%, even if recognized and treated.[18]

The onset of PCP may be subacute or indolent. Typical symptoms are dyspnea on exertion, nonproductive cough, fever, and tachycardia. Diagnosis is supported by imaging evidence of bilateral pulmonary infiltrates extending outward from the perihilar regions and an elevated serum LDH. Confirmation typically requires bronchoalveolar lavage.

Prophylaxis is preferentially achieved with trimethoprim–sulfamethoxazole, 160–800 mg/day or double strength three times a week.[19] Either regimen is felt to be 90% successful in preventing PCP. In those intolerant of sulfa, atovaquone, dapsone, and pentamidine represent alternatives. For those who favor PCP prophylaxis, current recommendations suggest it should be introduced if prednisone is utilized at a dose greater than 20 mg/day for a duration that exceeds 4 weeks.

PCP prophylaxis in neuromuscular patients treated with immunomodulating agents is not practiced universally. The evidence basis for PCP prophylaxis is largely derived from cancer and pulmonary patient populations.[18] In addition, there is a paucity of information to guide clinicians regarding adjusted risk based on the number and types of agents utilized, their doses, and the duration of exposure. Although the severity of PCP infection is unquestioned, its frequency in neuromuscular patients treated with immunomodulating agents is less well known. Although many disciplines such as rheumatology and infectious disease seem to favor its use, neurologists appear to be in general less sanguine about prophylactic necessity. For example, a recent poll neuromuscular specialists posted on Rick's Real Neuromuscular Friends indicated that 53% of 45 respondents do not provide routine PCP prophylaxis in this population.[20] Many have never seen a case of PCP despite having treated many patients chronically with one or more immunomodulating agents generating a more conservative perspective than suggested above.

Tuberculosis

The risk of tuberculosis reactivation is considered to be approximately three to six times greater in patients receiving tumor necrosis factor (TNF) inhibitors and corticosteroids.[21] It becomes prudent therefore to ascertain the risk of latent tuberculosis infection (LTBI) in any individual in whom immunomodulating treatment is considered. Screening would include determining risk of prior, chest x-ray, and in those who are at risk, either tuberculin skin testing (TST) or an interferon (IFN) gamma release assay (IGRA). TST is thought to be 98% sensitive in detecting LTBI. Its limitations are that it may not detect infection in the first 8 weeks following exposure, may be falsely negative in individuals already immunocompromised, or may be falsely positive in individuals who have received prior BCG vaccination. IGRAs are complementary diagnostic tools for LTBI. They are in vitro blood tests of cell-mediated immune response to *Mycobacterium tuberculosis* and measure T-cell release of IFN-gamma following stimulation by antigens specific to *M. tuberculosis*. The two available IGRAs are QuantiFERON-TB Gold In-Tube and the T-SPOT.TB. They are the preferred means to confirm LTBI in individuals with prior BCG exposure. The IGRAs appear to be somewhat more specific and less sensitive for predicting future active TB than the tuberculin skin test but the differences are modest. Like TST, IGRA false negatives are more likely to occur in immunosuppressed individuals. Both IGRAs and the TST have high negative predictive values for development of future infection.[21]

Like all clinical decisions, prophylactic treatment of patients suspected of LBTI needs to consider the relative benefits and risks. Currently, someone with suspected LBTI who is going to receive immunosuppressant treatment with corticosteroids, TNF-α inhibitors and probably other agents, is recommended to receive prophylactic treatment with isoniazid (with pyridoxine), rifampin, or a combination of both. Isoniazid is typically prescribed as 300 mg daily for 9 months or 900 mg twice a week for 6 months. Rifampin alone is dosed at 600 mg/day for 4 months. When both drugs are used together, 600 mg of rifampin and 300 mg of isoniazid are given daily for 3 months.[21] Other considerations are the risk of isoniazid hepatotoxicity which increases with age and exposure to other hepatotoxic agents and the numerous drug interactions that occur with rifampin use.

Progressive Multifocal Leukoencephalopathy

Progressive multifocal leukoencephalopathy (PML) is a demyelinating central nervous system disorder caused by infection with the John Cunningham (JC) virus. The JC virus is ubiquitous, found in 50–60% of the normal population and is typically sequestered in peripheral organs.[22] PML is a disorder seen almost exclusively in the immunosuppressed. Even in this population, the virus rarely gains access to the central nervous system.

To date, PML has been associated with two agents employed in immune-mediated neuromuscular disorders, rituximab and mycophenolate mofetil (MMF).[23] Infliximab, etanercept, and alemtuzumab, have also been reported as PML risk factors as have other currently available monoclonal antibodies that may be employed in the treatment of neuromuscular disease in the future.[24] Undoubtedly, it will be described in association with other immunomodulating agents relevant to neuromuscular disease in the future. The risk for PML appears to be predominantly in those who harbor the JC virus prior to the introduction of immunosuppressant treatment.

Surveillance and treatment paradigms have been developed for PML in multiple sclerosis patients exposed to natalizumab.[22] Presumably as the risk of developing PML with the immunosuppressant drugs described in this chapter is thought to be very rare, we are unaware of any recommendations for JC virus surveillance and prophylaxis for any agents described in this chapter. As anticipated, recognition of PML in any patient receiving immunosuppressant drugs warrants drug discontinuation in virtually any clinical context.

Strongyloidiasis

Stongyloidiasis is a parasite that is endemic in warm moist tropical and subtropical climates such as Eastern Europe, South and Southeast Asia, Central America, South America, and sub-Saharan Africa.[25–27] It is transmitted via skin penetration by infective filariform larvae following exposure to water or soil contaminated by human or canine fecal material. The larvae are hematogenously carried to the lungs, regurgitated, and then swallowed where they mature into adults in the intestines.[25] The reproductive cycle of the nematode and resultant reinfection may continue indefinitely. The autoinfected human host frequently remains asymptomatic or experiences mild nonspecific skin and gastrointestinal symptoms.[25,26] This equilibrium may persist indefinitely.

Immunosuppression however, particularly with corticosteroids, may result in multiorgan dissemination and hyperinfection.[25,26] Control of parasitic infections requires Th2 cytokine, eosinophilic, and IgE influence, all of which are suppressed by steroids and other immunomodulating agents.[25,26] With hyperinfection, mortality is estimated to be 60–85%.[27] For this reason, parasitic and serologic surveillance is recommended for anyone at increased risk prior to immunomodulating treatment. The absence of hypereosinophilia occurs frequently in infected individuals and does not represent a sensitive screening test. Ideally, patients at risk should undergo three negative surveillance stool specimens and an ELISA screening test for IgG *Strongyloides stercoralis* antibodies available through the Centers for Disease Control before treatment is begun.[25,26] The ELISA test is thought to be 80–100% sensitive and highly specific in immunocompetent individuals. Its sensitivity drops significantly in immunosuppressed individuals. A negative test needs to be interpreted cautiously in individuals already exposed to immunomodulating treatment.[25] If infected, ivermectin, thiabendazole, and albendazole are the most commonly used therapeutic agents.[26,27] One suggested regimen for strongyloidiasis prophylaxis would be ivermectin 200 μg/kg/day for 2 days, repeated within 2 weeks.[26]

VACCINES

Questions regarding vaccination of patients in whom immunomodulating treatment is being considered or is already being received are very relevant to the practice of neuromuscular medicine. Current recommendations hold that ideally, patients should be vaccinated against influenza, pneumococcus, tetanus, hepatitis A and perhaps B prior to initiation of immunosuppression.[28] Once immunosuppression has commenced, there appears to be a consensus that vaccines containing dead virus can be utilized without undue risk but that live-virus vaccines should be avoided.[6]

PREGNANCY AND CHILDREN

Management of immunomodulating treatment in women of child-bearing age is difficult. Current evidence holds that use of corticosteroids or IVIg provides no additional risk for mother or child during pregnancy.[7,29] We are very reticent to use other immunomodulating agents in childhood unless patient morbidity provides no other options. If corticosteroids are used before full growth is achieved, it is recommended that linear growth be tested regularly and growth hormone treatment considered if necessary.[7]

CANCER

Patients who receive immunosuppressive therapy are believed to be at increased risk of developing malignancy.[28] This risk is attributed to oncogenic infectious agents, reduced immune surveillance of cells having undergone mutation in relationship to age or environmental factors, or direct effects on oncogenes.[30] Notable oncogenic organisms whose proliferation may be aided by immunosuppression include Epstein–Barr virus, human herpesvirus 8, human papillomavirus, hepatitis B and C, and helicobacter. The malignancies most commonly associated with immunosuppression include lymphoproliferative disorders, Kaposi's sarcoma, as well as anogenital, liver, and stomach cancer.[28] Data pertaining to the relative risk of developing these malignancies, indexed to the numbers, types, and length of exposure to immunosuppressant medications are lacking although it is widely accepted that both increased dose and duration of exposure are relevant.[30] Of interest, available data suggests that cancer risk rapidly dissipates following discontinuation of immunomodulating treatment.[28] The pragmatic benefit of this knowledge is uncertain given the presumption that discontinuation of an effective immunosuppressive agent is unlikely unless cancer develops. Recommendations regarding rational, evidence-based cancer surveillance protocols for patients on immunomodulating treatments are elusive and are beyond the scope of this text. Discussion of this risk should nonetheless be part of the informed consent process. Consideration of dose reduction and potentially discontinuation is recommended in those who achieve complete disease remission.

There also appears to be an increased risk of skin cancers in patients receiving immunosuppressant drugs. The incidence of squamous cell carcinoma is believed to be increased by 14–82 fold and malignant melanoma increased by a factor of 2.4 in the solid organ transplant population.[31] We routinely advise patients on immunosuppressant drugs of the increased skin cancer risk and recommend limiting sun exposure, ample use of sun-blocking agents, and routine skin surveillance.

▶ INDIVIDUAL TREATMENTS MODALITIES

In the following section, individual immunomodulating treatments commonly used in neuromuscular disease will be discussed. Consideration of mechanisms of action, specific disorders in which individual agents are often used, adverse effects and management strategies will be addressed for each modality. For more detailed management strategies, the reader is referred to the relevant chapter on the disease in question.

ALEMTUZUMAB

Mechanism of Action

Alemtuzumab is a monoclonal antibody directed against the CD52 antigen found on the cell surface of mature lymphocytes. It is used primarily in the treatment of chronic lymphocytic leukemia, cutaneous and other T-cell lymphomas. There has been limited experience with its use in neuromuscular disorders.

Uses

Seven chronic inflammatory demyelinating polyneuropathy (CIDP) patients who have received alemtuzumab have been reported to demonstrate some degree of efficacy.[32,33] An open-label multicenter trial of alemtuzumab in CIDP is underway.[34]

Adverse Effects

Some patients receiving alemtuzumab have been reported to develop autoimmune disease, most notably Graves disease and hemolytic anemia.[34]

Management Considerations

One reported protocol consists of five daily intravenous infusions of 30 mg with repeated courses as required.[34]

AZATHIOPRINE

Mechanism of Action

Azathioprine is a purine analog that acts as a cytotoxic immunosuppressive agent.[35] Its main active metabolite, 6-mercaptopurine, is a purine antagonist.[36] It is a cell-cycle–specific inhibitor, exerting its actions mainly in the resting (G1) and DNA synthesis (S) phases of the cell cycle through suppression of GTPase Rac1 activation.[2] Although its primary effects are directed at T cells, it is efficacious in T-cell–dependent antibody-mediated disorders such as MG.[1] In addition to reducing numbers of circulating T cells, it also reduces levels of B-cell–derived immunoglobulins and interleukin-2 (IL-2).

Uses

Azathioprine is a commonly used maintenance, "steroid-sparing" therapy in MG. Several trials have demonstrated the efficacy of azathioprine alone or in combination with prednisone.[37–42] Improvement is noted in 70–90% of patients with myasthenia treated with azathioprine, including some patients who are steroid resistant.[43] We commonly initiate azathioprine (or other steroid-sparing agent) along with corticosteroids in any myasthenic patient with generalized disease in whom we anticipate the need for long-term immunomodulating treatment. We do so in the hope of facilitating steroid weaning, thereby limiting risk of long-term steroid side effects. By starting early, we take advantage of the short-term benefits of corticosteroids, recognizing the delayed therapeutic latency (3–15 months) of azathioprine which may require up to 2 years to achieve full effect.[1,44]

Azathioprine is also used a second-line agent in a number of presumed immune-mediated neuromuscular diseases, either as an adjunct to steroids, as a long-term maintenance agent. On occasion, it may become a first-line agent when more typical first-line agents (e.g., corticosteroids, IVIg, or PLEX) have failed. For the most part, the use of azathioprine in nonmyasthenic NM diseases is based on expert opinion or small case series. It has been used in dermatomyositis, polymyositis, CIDP, MMN, Lambert–Eaton myasthenic syndrome (LEMS), distal acquired demyelinating sensory neuropathy (DADS) vasculitic neuropathy, diabetic lumbosacral radiculoplexus neuropathy, Isaac's syndrome, and sarcoidosis.[34,35,45–56] We would advocate for its use in dermatomyositis, polymyositis, CIDP, LEMS, and sarcoid neuropathy in a patient with significant morbidity, who responds to first-line treatment, but who experiences unacceptable side effects or other impediments to long-term treatment with more conventional first-line treatments for these disorders.

Adverse Effects

Side effects have been reported in 35–42% of individuals. Fortunately, they are often mild and tolerable. They typically, although not invariably, develop within days to weeks of drug exposure. Many individuals tolerate the drug without any apparent side effects for protracted periods of time, which along with its potential effectiveness, make it an attractive agent. [35,40] A systemic reaction characterized by fever, abdominal pain, nausea, vomiting, and anorexia occurs in 12% of patients requiring discontinuation of the drug. As mentioned, this reaction generally occurs within the first few weeks of therapy and resolves within a few days of discontinuing the azathioprine. Rechallenge with azathioprine may be successful but usually results in the recurrence of the systemic reaction. Other uncommon but major complications of azathioprine are bone marrow suppression, hepatic toxicity, pancreatitis, teratogenicity, risk of opportunistic infection and oncogenicity including increased risk of skin cancer.[35,40]

Management Considerations

Azathioprine is available in 50 mg tablets without a parenteral analog. We typically begin with one tablet a day and escalate slowly to a maintenance dose of 2–3 mg/kg/day, typically 2.5 mg/kg/day. Prior to beginning azathioprine, we typically screen for thiopurine methyltransferase (TPMT) deficiency. Patients who are heterozygous for the TPMT mutation may be able to tolerate azathioprine at lower dosages but those who are homozygous should not receive drug. They cannot metabolize it and may experience severe bone marrow toxicity. Fortunately, the majority of patients who develop adverse hematologic responses in response to azathioprine recover fully once the drug is discontinued.

In patients receiving azathioprine, complete blood count (CBC) and liver function tests are monitored every 2 weeks until the patient is on a stable dose of azathioprine and then every 3–6 months for 2 years. After that, with stable blood counts, yearly surveillance is likely to be sufficient. If the white blood count falls below 4,000/mm^3, the dose should be decreased. Azathioprine is held if the white blood count declines to 2,500/mm^3 or the absolute neutrophil count falls to 1,000/mm^3. Leukopenia can develop as early as 1 week or as late as 2 years after initiating azathioprine. As in most drugs with potential hepatotoxic effects, azathioprine should be discontinued if transaminases increase more than two to three times the baseline values. In the treatment of patients with myositis, it is important to determine whether transaminase elevation is due to liver damage from drug or muscle injury from disease. Accordingly, in these situations, we follow glutamyl transpeptidase levels (GGT), an enzyme present in liver but not muscle, in addition to AST and ALT for this reason. Liver toxicity from azathioprine generally develops within the first several months of treatment or increase in dosage. Leukopenia generally reverses in 1 month and hepatotoxicity can take several months to resolve.

An elevated mean corpuscular volume is an anticipated effect of azathioprine therapy and is used by some clinicians as an indicator of a biologic response. Allopurinol should be avoided in patients who require azathioprine because it interferes with azathioprine metabolism, increasing drug levels, and increasing the risk of bone marrow and liver toxicity.

CORTICOSTEROIDS

Mechanism of Action

Glucocorticoid effects are mediated through both genomic, nuclear glucocorticoid receptors as well as nongenomic cell surface receptors.[57,58] They are one of the most versatile immunomodulating agents available in that they affect both cell-mediated and antibody-mediated autoimmunity.[1] Corticosteroids largely affect T-cell function by producing T-cell apoptosis, suppressing the transcription of proinflammatory cytokines and impairing dendritic cell maturation.[36] Specifically, glucocorticoids increase the rate of lipocortin synthesis which promotes anti-inflammatory effects by inhibition of phospholipase A2 as well as the proinflammatory cytokines IL-1, IL-2, the IL-2 receptor, INF gamma, and TNF.

Uses

The use of corticosteroids in autoimmune MG deserves special consideration. The recognition that corticosteroids were beneficial to patients with MG was historically delayed by the initial disease worsening that occurs in approximately 30% of patients receiving high-dose steroids, typically beginning between week 1–3 and lasting approximately 1 week.[43,59–62] The mechanism of the worsening appears to be unique to disorders of neuromuscular transmission, apparently secondary to weak neuromuscular blocking properties of the drug supported by the demonstration of decremental responses to slow repetitive stimulation.[61]

Fortunately, the benefits of corticosteroids in MG became subsequently recognized. They remain a mainstay of MG treatment despite the lack of evidence-based support for its use. Corticosteroids, typically prednisone, are the first-line drug in anyone whose disease severity requires immunomodulating therapy unless other confounding clinical variables coexist.[43] Its efficacy in MG appears to be universally accepted, making it unlikely that enrollment in a placebo-controlled trial would ever succeed.

Seventy-five percent of myasthenics are estimated to improve with corticosteroid use, 30% achieving remission and 45% marked improvement.[36] Improvement may become evident within 2 weeks of initiation of high dose (0.75–1.5 mg/kg) daily dosing and is typically well established by 6–8 weeks. Absence of a significant response within 4 weeks suggests treatment failure and should prompt consideration of alternative or additional treatments. There have been reports of myasthenics who appear resistant to both the adverse and beneficial effects of prednisone who respond well to prednisolone.[36]

In patients in crisis who are intubated, parenteral methylprednisolone may be prescribed at doses of up to 1 g/day for up to 7 days before tapering to a 60–100 mg/day prednisone equivalent. In these patients, the risk of crisis provoked by steroids becomes largely irrelevant.[63] In someone with significant morbidity from generalized disease, who we do not feel is in imminent danger of crisis, and in whom we are confident that adequate monitoring can occur, we may initiate high-dose prednisone, typically at 1–1.5 mg/kg up to 100 mg/day. In others whose morbidity warrants immunomodulating treatment, but where neither disease severity or risk of crisis warrants initial high-dose treatment, we utilize the so-called "start low, go slow" approach beginning at 10 or 20 mg of prednisone per day and gradually increasing by 5–10 mg/day every week or two until the target dose of 50–100 mg/day is reached.

Corticosteroids are used in numerous other presumed immune-mediated neuromuscular disorders including a number of neuropathy syndromes. The best evidence for efficacy exists in classic CIDP with a phenotype of generalized symmetric weakness, sensory signs and symptoms, and areflexia.[34,59,64–68] Steroids also appear to be effective for the presumed CIDP variant, multifocal acquired demyelinating sensory and motor neuropathy (MADSAM), (a.k.a. Lewis–Sumner syndrome).[65,69,70] Steroids have less apparent efficacy with other presumed CIDP variants, particularly when they are pure sensory or pure motor.[65] Although prednisone is the most commonly used glucocorticoid for CIDP, successful intravenous methylprednisolone and oral dexamethasone regimens have been reported as well.[71,72]

The weight of existing evidence suggests that steroids provide no benefit and may be harmful in the aggregate in GBS, MMN, and DADS associated with IgM monoclonal proteins, or other neuropathies associated with monoclonal gammopathy of unknown significance.[65,73–77]

Corticosteroids are also considered to be effective in some but not all inflammatory myopathies.[45,59] They are commonly used as a first-line treatment based on expert opinion in dermatomyositis, polymyositis, and immune-mediated necrotizing myopathy/myositis but are considered ineffective in inclusion body myositis.[56,78,79]

There is little doubt that immunomodulating treatment favorably alters the natural history of the systemic vasculitides. Corticosteroids, often with concomitant cyclophosphamide or rituximab are the backbones of treatment for these disorders.[47,56,80–82] There is considerable support for the use of corticosteroids in the treatment of sarcoidosis and sarcoid neuropathy but no evidence-based confirmation.[83,84] There is a dearth of evidence in support of corticosteroid use in brachial plexus neuritis.[84] We are of the opinion that steroids may benefit the painful aspects of this disorder if prescribed early but they appear to have a limited, if any, benefit in altering the natural history of the disease. Corticosteroids have been used with anecdotal reports or reports based on expert opinion of benefit in stiff person syndrome and diabetic lumbosacral radiculoplexus neuropathy.[85]

Adverse Effects

It is estimated that at least 30% of patients will experience corticosteroid-induced side effects, dependent upon dose and duration of therapy.[36] Once a desired therapeutic effect is achieved, an attempt is made to wean to the lowest effective maintenance dose with 20 mg/day considered an acceptable balance between the benefits and drawbacks of long-term steroid side effects.[36] Adverse effects of corticosteroids are largely dose-dependent and include diabetes, hypertension, peptic ulcer disease, osteopenia, cataracts, glaucoma, opportunistic infections, dyslipidemia, hypokalemia, increased appetite and weight gain, insomnia, and myopathy.[59,62] Steroid psychosis and aseptic necrosis appear to be adverse effects that are idiosyncratic in nature. Interventions intended to prophylax against these complications will be addressed in the management considerations section below.

Management Considerations

Corticosteroids are frequently administered in a single daily morning dose to parallel the normal circadian peak of endogenous cortisol production.[1,59] Therapeutically, this strategy has been demonstrated to have some advantage in patients with rheumatoid arthritis although interpretation may be somewhat confounded by relief of morning stiffness, a notable source of morbidity in this disease.[7]

Once maximal efficacy has been achieved, we attempt to wean to the smallest effective maintenance dose and typically do so in an every other day format.[1,59,86] We have utilized two different strategies. One is to begin the weaning process by initially doubling the induction dose on odd days and alternating this with zero on even days while beginning to reduce the aggregate dose. For example, a patient with an induction dose of 60 mg/day would be switched to 110 mg alternating with zero on any every other day basis. The alternative strategy is to initiate the weaning process by subtracting from the odd day dosage while maintaining the even dosage, for example, 60 mg on even days, 50 mg on odd days.

The speed of weaning proceeds based on individual patient context. For example, development of significant steroid side effects such as myopathy will accelerate the weaning pace whereas any indication of disease exacerbation may put the weaning process on hold. As a general guideline, we reduce the dose by 10 mg every 2 weeks. With the first regimen, this would mean 100 mg alternating with zero. With the second regimen this would mean 60 mg alternating with 40 mg. Once a dose of 20 mg every other day is reached, we taper more slowly, typically in increments of 2 mg every 2–4 weeks based on clinical response and the potential development of signs and symptoms of potential adrenal insufficiency.

Tuberculosis, strongyloidiasis, and herpes zoster are the three infectious agents we are aware of where corticosteroids may fulminantly exacerbate pre-existing, indolent infection. Consideration may be given to shingles vaccination prior to steroid initiation in individuals. It is estimated that it is safe to administer steroids or other immunomodulating agents 2 weeks or more after administration of this or any other live virus.[28] We routinely question patients for potential exposure to tuberculosis and when in doubt perform PPD, chest x-ray, and IGRA testing. If there is suggestion for indolent TB infection, and immunomodulating treatment is medically necessary, we initiate isoniazid and pyridoxine treatment concomitantly unless otherwise contraindicated. If the patient comes from an area where strongyloidiasis is endemic, we consider baseline serologic testing and stool analysis.

Patients on long-term corticosteroids should receive baseline screening and periodic monitoring of intraocular pressure, blood pressure, blood sugar, lipids, and bone density. In particular, glucocorticoids facilitate osteopenia by interfering with bone formation through apoptosis of osteocytes and enhancing bone resorption through inhibition of osteoprotegerin, an endogenous antiresorptive cytokine.[87] In any patient who will be receiving corticosteroids for more than 3 months, it is prudent to obtain a bone density and initiate daily treatment with 2,000 IU of vitamin D3 and 1,000 mg of calcium, promote exercise and suggest no more than modest alcohol intake.[87–89] In men >50, women who are postmenopausal, or anyone with a T score of −1.5 or below, initiation of a bisphosphonate such as alendronate at a dose of 10 mg daily or 70 mg weekly, or 35 mg three times a week is recommended.[87,90]

We do not routinely recommend gastric protection in patients using chronic corticosteroids unless they are symptomatic or at increased risk for gastritis because of concomitant use of nonsteroidal anti-inflammatory agents. In these situations, prophylactic treatment with a proton pump inhibitor, misoprostol, or a cyclooxygenase 2 inhibitor is utilized.[7] In addition, patients are instructed to start a low-sodium, low-carbohydrate, high-protein diet to prevent excessive weight gain and in the case of a high-protein diet, to theoretically reduce the risk of steroid myopathy. Patients are also encouraged to slowly begin an aerobic exercise program as it is hypothesized that both osteopenia and steroid myopathy are enhanced by immobility. Lastly, augmentation of corticosteroid dosing should be considered perioperatively in order to avoid risk of adrenal insufficiency in any patient who has been receiving these drugs for more than a month.[7]

CYCLOPHOSPHAMIDE

Mechanism of Action

Cyclophosphamide is a DNA-alkylating drug and nonspecific cell cycle inhibitor, with more pronounced effects on B cells than on T cells.[2]

Uses

Within the realm of neuromuscular diseases, cyclophosphamide use is probably best established in the treatment of neuropathy. It is commonly recognized as a mainstay of treatment in systemic vasculitic neuropathy, usually in conjunction with corticosteroids and has been reported to be of benefit in nonsystemic vasculitic neuropathy as well.[45,46,91–94] In our experience and that of others, it can be an effective treatment in refractory CIDP patients.[95–101] There are anecdotal reports of beneficial effect in DADS neuropathy and MMN as well.[102,103]

Cyclophosphamide may benefit patients with MG including those with MuSK autoantibodies.[104–109] In view of its risk profile, it is typically used in the MG population only when other less-toxic agents have proven unsatisfactory.[2] A protocol that utilizes high-dose cyclophosphamide to "reboot" the bone marrow has been suggested in individuals who have failed attempts at other less-toxic regimens.[107] Because of the significant side effects described below, most clinicians avoid cyclophosphamide for MG if at all possible. Cyclophosphamide may be considered in patients with severe generalized MG refractory to other modes of immunotherapy. We have used it in refractory cases of polymyositis and dermatomyositis as well.

Adverse Effects

Cyclophosphamide has a substantial side effect profile that includes frequent nausea and vomiting with administration. Serious side effects include opportunistic infection, hemorrhagic cystitis, bone marrow depression, sterility, teratogenicity, alopecia, and late development of malignancy, particularly lymphoma and bladder cancer. The incidence of malignancy associated with cyclophosphamide use appears to increase when the cumulative dose exceeds 85 g.[1]

Management Considerations

Cyclophosphamide may be administered either orally or intravenously. The oral dose is 2–2.5 mg/kg/day typically administered as single dose each morning. The intravenous dose is 1 g/m^2 monthly for 6 consecutive months. The latter is preferred as it is thought to be less toxic and as the adverse hematologic effects are easier to time and monitor. The therapeutic latency between administration and manifest benefit is relatively short and is estimated to be 2–6 months, dependent on both drug effect and end organ healing.[44]

Patients receiving intravenous cyclophosphamide should have a baseline CBC and platelet count and urinalysis done and at minimum, a repeat CBC prior to each subsequent infusion to ensure a safe neutrophil level. Like azathioprine, repeat cyclosporine infusions are held if the WBC count and absolute neutrophil count which typically nadirs between 1–2 weeks post infusion does not reestablish itself to >2,500/mm^3 or >1,000/mm^3 respectively prior to the next dose. It is frequently recommended that cyclophosphamide recipients have yearly urine cytologic surveillance.

CYCLOSPORINE

Mechanism of Action

In the cytoplasm, cyclosporine binds to its immunophilin, cyclophilin. The cyclosporine–cyclophilin complex binds to and blocks the function of the enzyme calcineurin, eventually inhibiting T-cell activation and reducing production of the proinflammatory cytokine IL-2.[2,110]

Uses

Cyclosporine has been demonstrated to be effective in the treatment of patients with MG.[111–116] The therapeutic latency is typically 1–3 months following treatment initiation.[44] In psoriasis, the time of onset of action has been reported to be 6 weeks.[117] Mean time to maximum improvement is approximately 7 months. Cyclosporine also appears to have a steroid-sparing effect. As many as 95% of patients are able to discontinue or decrease their corticosteroid dose.

There are a number of reports that describe cyclosporine as beneficial in CIDP patients.[34,73,118–125] Like many reports of immunomodulating therapy in neuromuscular disorders, interpretation is confounded by its use in patients who have used other agents either concomitantly or previously. Cyclosporine may benefit patients with vasculitic neuropathy, both systemic and nonsystemic, sarcoid neuropathy, LEMS, dermatomyositis, and polymyositis.[45,48,56,94,126–136] Its effectiveness in MMN is suspect.[55] It is used by most clinicians as a third-line drug in patients unresponsive to other modalities.

Adverse Effects

Renal toxicity occurs in approximately a quarter of patients. The need to monitor creatinine and trough cyclosporine levels frequently has limited the enthusiasm of some clinicians for its use. Patients receiving cyclosporine or any calcineurin inhibitor may also develop a calcineurin inhibition syndrome that includes prominent and at times debilitating tremor requiring dose reduction. Cyclosporine is used in MG primarily in patients who are refractory to prednisone and azathioprine. There is a general perception that brand name drugs, for example, Neoral® or Sandimmune®, are preferable to their generic counterparts.

Management Considerations

Initially a total dose of 3.0–4.0 mg/kg/day in two divided doses is used and gradually increased to a maximum dose of 6.0 mg/kg/day as necessary. The cyclosporine dose is initially being titrated to maintain trough serum cyclosporine levels of 100–200 ng/mL. Blood pressure, electrolytes and renal function, and trough cyclosporine levels need to be monitored on a monthly basis. The dose is lowered as necessary to keep the creatinine level stable while maintaining the trough level within therapeutic range. Any upward trend of creatinine levels should promote a dose reduction. After patients achieve maximum improvement, the dose is reduced over several months to the minimum dose necessary to maintain the therapeutic response. Patients need to be informed of the numerous drugs that can aggravate renal toxicity including nonsteroidal anti-inflammatory agents and drugs that may raise blood pressure or affect serum potassium levels.

ECULIZUMAB

Mechanism of Action

Eculizumab is a humanized monoclonal antibody which acts by blocking the formation of terminal complement complex by specifically preventing the enzymatic cleavage of complement 5 (C5).[137]

Its labeled indications include paroxysmal nocturnal hemoglobinuria and atypical hemolytic uremic syndrome.

Uses

Eculizumab has been used infrequently in the treatment of autoimmune neuromuscular disease. Dermatomyositis, polymyositis, and myasthenia are the most notable examples.[55,137,138] In a prospective, placebo-controlled trial of myasthenic patients refractory to other agents, eculizumab demonstrated clinically meaningful improvements in the treatment group and a larger phase 3 clinical trial is underway.[137]

Adverse Effects

The most common adverse effects reported in the prospective study of eculizumab and MG were nausea, back pain, nasopharyngitis, and headache.[137] Renal insufficiency, anemia, leukopenia, dyspepsia, diarrhea, tachycardia, peripheral edema, fatigue, and both hypo- and hypertension have been reported. There is also an increased risk of meningococcal meningitis.

Management Considerations

In MG, one described protocol is a 600-mg eculizumab infusion weekly for 4 weeks followed by a 900 mg maintenance infusion every 2 weeks for an additional six doses.[137] Patients should receive meningococcal vaccination prior to its administration.

ETANERCEPT

Mechanism of Action

As the inflammatory response is dependent on inflammatory cytokines, and as TNF-α represents one of the major proinflammatory cytokines, it stands to reason that etanercept and other TNF-α inhibitors would be studied in the treatment of autoimmune neuromuscular disorders. Its labeled uses include rheumatoid arthritis, inflammatory spondyloarthropathy, and plaque psoriasis.

Uses

There is one report of etanercept benefitting patients with CIDP.[139] Conversely, there are reports of patients developing neuropathy with features characteristic of CIDP in association with the use of TNF antagonists.[140–143] Etanercept has also been suggested as a potential treatment in sarcoidosis but it has been reported to potentially cause sarcoidosis as well.[48,83,144–146] A clinical trial of etanercept in MG reported modest benefits in five out of eight patients.[147] Two patients experienced worsening however, and at least one patient has been reported to develop MG while receiving etanercept for rheumatoid arthritis.[146] A small randomized trial suggested a steroid-sparing benefit for etanercept in dermatomyositis.[148] It is our current perspective that etanercept should be used cautiously if at all in CIDP, MG, and sarcoid neuropathy.

Adverse Effects

In the etanercept study in refractory dermatomyositis patients, the six serious adverse events occurred in three participants comprising pregnancy and miscarriage in a partner; hospitalization for a urinary tract infection and fever of unknown origin; postherpetic neuralgia and two admissions for psychosis. Five participants in the etanercept-treated group compared to one in the placebo group had worsening of their skin disease.[148]

Other adverse effects other than the development of sarcoidosis that have been reported include anaphylaxis and other hypersensitivity reactions, positive antinuclear antibody titers with rare lupus-like syndromes, autoimmune hepatitis, rare central and peripheral nervous system demyelinating diseases including optic neuritis, transverse myelitis, multiple sclerosis, GBS and other demyelinating neuropathies, seizures or seizure exacerbation, heart failure or decreased left ventricular function, rare cases of pancytopenia and aplastic anemia, reactivation of infections notably hepatitis B, fungus, and tuberculosis. It is believed that the risk of these opportunistic infections is increased with concomitant use of corticosteroids or other agents. In addition, lymphoma has been reported in children and adolescent patients receiving TNF-blocking agents, including etanercept. Skin cancers, notably melanoma, nonmelanoma skin cancer, and Merkel cell carcinoma may develop in adults.

Management Considerations

Etanercept is typically administered subcutaneously in a dose of 25 or 50 mg once or twice weekly. Etanercept's therapeutic latency in psoriasis is estimated to be 6.6 and 9.5 weeks for high-dose and low-dose regimens respectively and is estimated at 2–6 months in MG.[44,117] Surveillance for the numerous potential adverse effects listed above should be undertaken.

INFLIXIMAB

Mechanism of Action

Infliximab is another TNF-α inhibitor that has been used sparingly in the treatment of immune-mediated neuromuscular disorders. Again, its potential mechanism of action is to suppress the effects of the proinflammatory cytokine TNF. Infliximab is approved for the treatment of inflammatory bowel disease psoriatic and rheumatoid arthritis, plaque psoriasis, and inflammatory spondyloarthropathy.

Uses

Infliximab has been reported to have a modest, suggested benefit in dermatomyositis and associated interstitial lung disease.[149] Its use has been reported in both sarcoid and vasculitic neuropathy with uncertain benefit.[48,56] We are aware of a single report describing infliximab's use in myasthenia.[150] Infliximab is one of the fastest acting immunomodulating agents. Its time of action in psoriasis is estimated to be 3.5 weeks.[117]

Adverse Effects

The most frequently occurring adverse effects have been reported to be headache, nausea, diarrhea, abdominal pain, increased transaminases, development or increased titres of antinuclear and double stranded DNA antibodies, abscess particularly in those with Crohn's disease, upper respiratory tract infections, and an infusion-related reaction. Warnings concerning risk of malignancy, myelosuppression, and opportunistic infection with agents such as hepatitis B and tuberculosis are identical to etanercept. Like etanercept, the development of CIDP has been described to occur in concert with infliximab use.[143]

Management Considerations

A typical regimen for infliximab infusion is 5 mg/kg at 0, 2, and 6 weeks, followed by 5 mg/kg every 8 weeks thereafter. In patients who initially respond but appear to develop tolerance, an increase to 10 mg/kg is permitted. In the absence of therapeutic effect, treatment is discontinued by 14 weeks.

INTERFERON α AND β

Mechanism of Action

INF β is a naturally occurring cytokine that downregulates inflammatory responses. Its biologic actions are copied by the recombinant protein INF β1a. INF α, bioengineered as INF α2a, is also a naturally occurring cytokine which upregulates the inflammatory response and it has been used primarily for the treatment of hepatitis C. Not surprisingly, it has been reported to cause autoimmune disease.[151,152] Paradoxically, it has also been used to treat patients with autoimmune diseases, notably CIDP.[125,153,154]

Uses

In neuromuscular disease, INF β1 a has been utilized primarily in the treatment of CIDP.[34,73,155–160] Although there are occasional case reports suggesting a beneficial effect, the weight of experience would not favor its use. In addition, in at least one case of concomitant multiple sclerosis and CIDP, the neuropathy worsened in response to INF β1 a.[161] With INF α, beneficial effects in CIDP are once again difficult to ascertain because of confounding considerations such as monoclonal proteins, use of other agents concomitantly, or the tendency to study patients who have been historically resistant to other treatments. Although benefit has been reported in occasional patients, at times dramatically, the use of either INF cannot be currently endorsed in CIDP.[125,153,154]

Adverse Effects

INF β1 a is well tolerated. Potential side effects include minor alterations of liver function and white cell counts. With subcutaneous preparations, skin reactions occur but serious side effects are uncommon. With INF α2 a, minor side effects such as fatigue, fever, malaise and myalgia, and arthralgia occur frequently.[34]

Management Considerations

INF β1 a is typically given at a dose of 22–44 ug via subcutaneous injection three times a week. INF α2 a is also delivered subcutaneously three times a week, typically at a dose of 3 million IU.[34]

INTRAVENOUS IMMUNOGLOBULIN

Mechanism of Action

IVIg is a blood product collected from thousands of donors composed of 95% IgG and less than 2.5% IgA. In addition, CD4, CD8, HLA molecules, and other plasma components are typically included.[16] IVIg's half-life is estimated at 18–33 days but some of its beneficial effects seem to extend beyond this period.[16,162] There is heterogeneity in different IVIg products pertaining to IgA and sodium content, type of sugar, pH and osmolality, and viral inactivation strategies employed.[162]

There have been multiple proposed IVIg mechanisms of action, one or more of which may be relevant depending on the pathophysiology of the treated disease.[163,164] Anti-idiotype antibodies contained within IVIg may react with the Fc or antigen-binding regions of pathologic autoantibodies and neutralize their effects. IVIg including nonimmunoglobulin components may beneficially interfere with T-cell function in a number of ways. It may restore the balance between T cells releasing proinflammatory Th1 and anti-inflammatory Th2 cytokines. It may cause T-cell apoptosis, interfere with T-cell interaction with antigen-presenting cells, and interrupt T-cell migration through the blood–nerve barrier. Interference with B-cell function including production of autoantibodies, activation of complement, formation of membrane attack complex, and macrophage function are other proposed mechanisms of action.[16,162]

Uses

In GBS, IVIg is typically administered as five daily doses of 0.4 mg/kg of ideal body weight, initiated as soon as possible, and preferably within the first 2 weeks of symptoms. There is currently no evidence-based support for repeat administration although we would consider this if a patient demonstrated unequivocal improvement in response to the initial 2 g/kg regimen, and then subsequently relapsed. Some neuromuscular clinicians advocate waiting for a specified threshold of morbidity such as compromised ambulation to occur before initiating treatment. Our practice is to be more aggressive, as we are not confident in our ability to predict the natural history in any individual patient while at the same time adhering to the premise that nerve injury is easier to prevent than heal.

In CIDP, we frequently use IVIg as our first-line treatment beginning with single 5-day infusion totaling 2 g/kg of IBW. If there is no response after 1 month, we will prescribe two additional monthly IVIg courses and then disband if no significant benefit occurs. If there is a meaningful response, we will continue to observe until the benefit plateaus. As rare CIDP patients have a monophasic course, we offer no further treatment unless relapse occurs in a patient who normalizes after a single 5-day infusion.[165] If the patient improves partially but incompletely, we then initiate a maintenance program. Three commonly used protocols are 0.5 g/kg every 2 weeks, 1 g/kg every 3 weeks, or 2 g/kg every month. In CIDP patients requiring maintenance IVIg treatment, we attempt to minimize the dose, and maximize the interval between doses attempting to sustain the maximal degree of achievable improvement. As the symptoms in relapsing CIDP may return insidiously allowing time for successful intervention to take place, we often discontinue treatment in individuals in whom we can achieve a drug-free remission.

Our use of IVIg in MMN differs somewhat from CIDP. The monophasic course seen in some CIDP patients does not seem to occur with the same frequency in MMN. Although spontaneous remission in individual nerve injury has been reported, we are unaware of reported self-limited cases with protracted remission. In our experience, relapses may be abrupt and severe. Reversal of deficits may be difficult if treatment is delayed, presumably due to transition to axon loss that appears to occur frequently in untreated patients.[166,167,15] The long-term natural history of untreated cases appears unfavorable.[15] As a result, we typically maintain patients on chronic treatment indefinitely in the hope of preventing these unpredictable events.[15]

We use IVIg in myasthenia predominantly in two situations, in crisis or in preparation for thymectomy in patients who we feel that improvement in their strength will reduce risk of postoperative complications.[168] In general, our experience, like others, suggests that PLEX is somewhat superior to IVIg in the management of myasthenic crises.[169] We acknowledge however, that the preponderance of literature views IVIg and PLEX to be of equivalent efficacy in this context.[168–192]

IVIg has also been demonstrated to be efficacious in the treatment of dermatomyositis. A double-blinded, placebo-controlled study demonstrated significant efficacy in patients who were already utilizing prednisone. All eight of the patients initially randomized to IVIg demonstrated significant improvement in strength and neuromuscular symptoms as did 9 out of /12 patients subsequent to crossover.[193] The tendency to use IVIg preferably is in consideration of the relative ease of use comparatively and reduced side effect profile for IVIg.[172] In general, we attempt to avoid both IVIg and PLEX in chronic disorders like myasthenia, dermatomyositis, and polymyositis unless a satisfactory response cannot be achieved by oral agents. Our position is in consideration of patient lifestyle, cost, and safety. If we use these agents as maintenance therapy in these diseases, we ascribe to a regimen similar to that described in CIDP above. We rarely employ IVIg for those disorders listed in the *disorders with anecdotal reports of benefit* column in Table 4-1.

Adverse Effects

Minor infusion-related symptoms such as chills, nausea, myalgia, headache, and vasomotor disturbances are fairly common with IVIg infusion. In an attempt to avoid this reaction, we typically pretreat our patients with 650 mg of acetaminophen and 25 mg of diphenhydramine orally. If an allergic reaction is experienced, we add 100 mg of intravenous hydrocortisone to the pretreatment regimen prior to every infusion.

Serious side effects from IVIg are rare and include thromboembolic disease such as stroke and myocardial infarction, renal failure, aseptic meningitis, congestive heart failure, and anaphylactic reactions.[16,162] The incidence of serious side effects has been reported at 4.5% although this has not been our experience.[194] Thromboembolic risk may be higher in those with atherosclerotic cardiovascular risk factors or in those with monoclonal proteins or other reasons for increased blood viscosity. Aseptic meningitis has been reported to occur in up to 10% of patients although this also has not been our experience.[16] It does not appear to be related to a particular IVIg formulation(s), occurs more frequently in migraineurs, and does not appear to be preventable with steroid pretreatment. Rechallenging patients who have previously experienced IVIg-induced aseptic meningitis should probably be avoided unless there are particularly strong indications for its use. Rechallenge appears to have a greater success in patients without a history of migraine.[16] As IVIg represents a pooled blood product, a theoretical risk of infection continues to exist. Historically, one case of transmitted hepatitis C was reported in 1994. Subsequent exposure of all IVIg products to solvent detergent of 10% caprylate have seemingly eliminated this and other viral risks.[16]

Anaphylaxis has been reported in patients deficient in IgA. The initial suggestion that this risk exists from IgG autoantibodies directed at IgA autoantibodies has been refuted by safe infusion in IgA deficient, IgG versus IgA autoantibody-carrying patients. Recent evidence suggests that IgE versus IgA is the more likely causative pathophysiology of this reaction. As the incidence of anaphylaxis in patients receiving IVIg is extremely uncommon, screening for IgA deficiency is not recommended as a routine practice prior to IVIg exposure.[16,162]

Other consequences of IVIg treatment of note include elevation of serum inflammatory markers such as erythrocyte sedimentation rates which may exceed 100 mm/h which may confound patient management. Following IVIg infusion, determination of a patient's actual immunity toward certain diseases may also be confounded.[16] Antibodies detected in a patient's serum may represent those passively transferred rather than one's generated by the patient's own immune system.

Management Considerations

The standard induction dose of IVIg is 2 g/kg typically delivered in 1 g/kg doses on two consecutive days in stable outpatients or 0.4 g/kg doses on 5 consecutive days on intolerant or fragile patients or those who will be hospitalized for that period of time. Increasingly, recommended dosing is based on IBW. For men greater than or equal to 60 in in height, this figure is calculated by the formula 50 kg + (2.3 × height in inches −60). If the height is less than 60 in, 50 kg is used as the IBW. For women the formula is identical other than 46 kg is substituted for 50 kg, both as the initial number of the formula, and as the fallback IBW if patient height is less than 5 ft.

The therapeutic onset for IVIg effect in MG is estimated to be 1–2 weeks.[162] As suggested above, the onset latency for IVIg may be equally fast if the damaged structure is an ion channel but may be more protracted if myelin, myofiber, or particularly axonal regeneration is required. The duration of effect for IVIg is variable between both disease and patient. As a general rule, IVIg half-life predicts a 4–6 weeks' benefit with responses of up to 60 days reported.[170] In consideration of the half-life of the agent wishing to neither overtreat nor allow relapse, we begin maintenance treatment at 4-week intervals. IVIg may also be successfully delivered subcutaneously, notably in CIDP.[195,196]

Subsequent dosing, as described above, is dependent on clinical context, taking into consideration the specific disease and its natural history as well as disease pathophysiology. Knowing what the likely outcome is in any given disease and the time it takes to for that improvement to become evident is critical to rational decision making. For example, the majority of outcome improvements in GBS have been measured at a month or more after treatment. Initiating IVIg after PLEX, or a second course of IVIg within the first month due to the perception that the patient has not improved sufficiently, cannot be routinely supported, based either on clinical experience or clinical trials.[197]

METHOTREXATE

Mechanism of Action

Methotrexate, which also mainly affects the G1 and S phases of the cell cycle, is a folate antagonist that can inhibit de novo synthesis of both purines and pyrimidines.[2] It is a selective inhibitor of both dihydrofolate reductase and lymphocyte proliferation. As a structural analog of folic acid, it affects adenosine-mediated inflammatory mediators resulting in apoptosis and clonal deletion of T-cell lines. It also acts to decreases the production of proinflammatory cytokines IL-1 and IL-6.

Uses

In neuromuscular disease, methotrexate is probably used with the greatest frequency in the treatment of dermato- and polymyositis.[1,45,55,78,127,198–203] It is our suspicion that this is based on the frequency with which these disorders are treated by rheumatologists who are perhaps more comfortable with its use than neurologists, rheumatologists not as frequently involved in the treatment of other neuromuscular conditions.

There are reports of methotrexate being utilized as a second or third treatment in CIDP, systemic and nonsystemic vasculitic neuropathy, sarcoidosis, MMN, myasthenia, and immune-mediated necrotizing myopathy.[2,34,46–48,54,56,94,125,204–210] One advantage of methotrexate is its relatively short onset latency in comparison to other immunomodulating agents.

Although reported in reference to the treatment of psoriasis, its beneficial effects have been measured to occur with a mean time (in 25% of treated individuals) of 3.2 weeks with high doses and 9.9 weeks with low doses.[117]

Adverse Effects

Potential side effects of methotrexate therapy include hepatotoxicity which is relatively uncommon, interstitial pneumonitis, which presents with dyspnea, fever, and dry cough and potentially leads to pulmonary fibrosis, infection, neoplasia, infertility, bone marrow suppression with leukopenia, alopecia, gastric irritation with nausea, vomiting and diarrhea, fatigue, rash, dizziness, ulcerative stomatitis, and teratogenicity.[211] Like most immunosuppressant medications, the exact incidence of neoplasia and its causal relationship to methotrexate is difficult to quantitate.[2]

Management Considerations

Methotrexate is typically initiated orally at 7.5 mg/week or lower in the context of renal insufficiency. It can be given in a single dose or in divided doses. One regimen is three divided doses administered 12 hours apart, often Saturday morning and evening and Sunday morning so that any side effects might have a chance to dissipate before the work week begins. The total dose may be gradually escalated dependent on the development of beneficial or adverse effect to a maximal dose of 25 mg/week. All patients are concomitantly treated with folate, at least 5 mg/week. Methotrexate can also be delivered subcutaneously once weekly at a dose of 20–50 mg.

Hepatic enzymes, platelet, and white blood cell counts should be monitored closely. In patients with pulmonary symptoms, methotrexate should be held until an infectious cause and pulmonary fibrosis can be excluded. Chest imaging, pulmonary function testing, and pulmonary consultation are recommended in symptomatic patients.

MYCOPHENOLATE MOFETIL

Mechanism of Action

MMF (Cellcept) inhibits lymphocytic purine synthesis by selectively inhibiting the enzyme inosine-5′-monophosphate dehydrogenase. Like azathioprine, it acts predominantly on the G1 and S phases of the cell cycle.[2] Its use results in T-cell and B-cell depletion.[212]

Uses

Within the spectrum of neuromuscular disorders, mycophenolate has been most diligently studied in MG.[213–223] Initial open-label studies suggested notable benefit in an estimated 75% of treated individuals, primarily as an adjunctive therapy.[216,218,221] Subsequent prospective studies have not been as supportive.[213,214] Mycophenolate remains a frequently utilized "steroid-sparing" agent in the treatment of MG as many neuromuscular clinicians feel that it is an effective agent, an impression supported by a study reported in a retrospective 2010 analysis of 102 patients. There is also the perception that the negative studies were flawed due to their relatively short periods of observation.[222]

There have been eight studies suggesting a benefit for mycophenolate in the treatment of CIDP.[221,224–229] Interpretation of these studies is confounded by the numerous other treatment variables that many of these patients were exposed to. There have been case reports or case series suggesting benefit of mycophenolate treatment in systemic and nonsystemic vasculitic neuropathy, sarcoid neuropathy and myositis, immune-mediated necrotizing myopathy, and Isaac's syndrome.[45–48,51–54,56,94,207,208]

Adverse Effects

MMF is usually well tolerated and has little or no renal or liver toxicity. The major side effect is diarrhea. Starting slowly and increasing the dose slowly may diminish the risk and severity of this troublesome side effect. Less common side effects include abdominal discomfort, nausea, peripheral edema, fever, and leukopenia. Measurement of drug levels is not done routinely. Adverse hematologic effects may be more common in doses of greater than 2,000 mg/day. In view of the relatively short experience with this agent, long-term safety for mycophenolate is still in question. Malignancy rates do not appear higher in the transplant population; however, there are rare reports of lymphoma or lymphoproliferative disorders developing in MG patients.[219,230] Progressive multifocal encephalopathy has been reported in a patient receiving mycophenolate for systemic lupus erythematosus and organ transplantation.[231]

Management Considerations

MMF, available in 500 mg tablets, is typically dosed at 1,000 mg twice a day. Starting at 500 mg daily or twice a day and gradually increasing the dose may diminish the incidence and severity of diarrhea. The maximal recommended dose is 1,500 mg BID. Patients who do not respond to a daily dose of 2,000 mg but respond to higher doses are relatively uncommon in our experience. Improvement has been noted in MG with a mean therapeutic latency of 9–11 weeks with a maximal effect noted by 6 months in most patients. Occasionally, the full effect may not become manifest before a year.[231] Mycophenolate is excreted through the kidneys; therefore, the dose should be decreased (no more than 1 g/day total dose) in patients with renal insufficiency.

Mycophenolic acid or mycophenolate sodium (Myfortic®) is an alternative preparation that comes in 180 and

360 mg enteric-coated tablets. As a result, it has the potential for less gastrointestinal side effects. Unlike MMF, it is not available for parenteral use. The daily dose is 720–1,440 mg/day in two divided doses.

PLASMA EXCHANGE

Mechanism of Action

Therapeutic PLEX reduces the titer of circulating antibodies within the blood stream through filtration.[232]

Uses

The most established uses for PLEX in NM disease is in GBS, CIDP, and MG.[169,170,172,175,183,184,187–192,197,233–236] Once again, because of cost, safety, and logistical considerations, PLEX is used primarily in initial induction treatment, not in chronic maintenance therapy. In MG, it is used primarily in patients in crisis or in those with moderate weakness prior to thymectomy in order to maximize their perioperative strength and minimize risk of postoperative complications. The American Academy of Neurology was unable to endorse the use of PLEX as treatment for MG in its evidence-based guideline.[233] In the mind of many neuromuscular clinicians however, including ourselves, it is as effective if not more effective than IVIg in the treatment of MG crisis.[4,231]

There are reports that provide convincing support for the use of PLEX in association with IgA and IgG monoclonal protein of uncertain significance.[233,239] There are individual or small case series that suggest potential benefit in diabetic radiculoplexus neuropathy, systemic and nonsystemic vasculitic neuropathy, Miller Fisher, stiff person and Isaac's syndrome.[46,47,51–54,56,232,240,241]

There are reports suggesting that PLEX is both effective and ineffective for LEMS and inflammatory myopathies.[49,55,232] PLEX appears to have no role in the treatment of MMN and DADS neuropathy.[15,55,77,233]

Adverse Effects

PLEX has several limitations. It has limited availability and like IVIg, cost is an issue. Many of the risks related to PLEX are related to the need for large bore catheters that need to be placed in central veins in a significant portion of individuals. Potential complications include symptoms related to alkalosis, pneumothorax, hypotension particularly in GBS patients prone to dysautonomia, sepsis, and pulmonary embolism.[233]

Management Considerations

The standard PLEX protocol is to exchange a volume of 200–250 mL/kg/day (2–3 L) for 5 days typically spread out over a 7–10-day period of time. In MG, improvement is noticeable after two to four exchanges.[232] The durability of the effect is usually a few weeks.

RITUXIMAB

Mechanism of Action

Rituximab is a monoclonal antibody directed against CD20 B cells, developed for the treatment of B-cell lymphomas. It produces B-cell depletion, postulated to occur via complement-mediated cytotoxicity, antibody-dependent cell-mediated cytotoxicity, and induction of apoptosis.[2] It also reduces T-lymphocyte activation and decreases cytokine production.[36]

Uses

There are an increasing number of reports suggesting that both AChR and MuSK MG respond favorably.[242–248] Other reports are somewhat more circumspect.[249–251]

In consideration of rituximab's efficacy in lymphoproliferative disorders, it is rational to consider its use in neuromuscular conditions associated with monoclonal proteins. DADS, an acquired, demyelinating sensory predominant neuropathy is one such disorder. It is frequently associated with an IgM kappa monoclonal protein, and frequently associated with myelin-associated glycoprotein autoantibodies. Initial reports were optimistic but subsequent, randomized, placebo-controlled trials found no benefit.[252] Others have reported disease worsening following rituximab exposure.[253] Our experience is that most patients do not respond, with rare patients responding dramatically in a manner that contrasts significantly with the natural history of this disorder. Whether the response is durable in these uncommon patients is uncertain.

There are a handful of case reports and small case series describing a benefit of rituximab in CIDP.[125,254–265] Again these are difficult to interpret as the majority of the cases are confounded by the use of other agents, the presence of monoclonal proteins or concurrent diseases like lymphoma.

There were also initial optimistic reports of rituximab in MMN but our experience and that of others has been disappointing.[55] The use of rituximab has also been reported in vasculitic neuropathy and stiff person syndrome but convincing evidence of its efficacy in these and other immune-mediated neuromuscular diseases remains lacking.[34,46,47,56,207,208,265–268]

Although a large randomized, placebo-controlled trial of rituximab showed no benefit in adults and children with polymyositis and dermatomyositis, there were many methodologic issues in regard to trial design that may have impeded the detection of efficacy.[269] We and others have used rituximab in myositis patients (non-IBM) and have found it particularly effective in patients with immune-mediated necrotizing myopathy.[270]

Adverse Effects

Rituximab is well tolerated by the majority of patients. Pruritus, nausea, vomiting, dizziness, headache, angina, cardiac dysrhythmia, anemia, leukopenia, and thrombocytopenia have been reported. Myelosuppression, PML, and lymphoma are uncommon but potential risks.[23]

Management Considerations

There are a number of dosing regimens utilized for rituximab. Our experience has been with 375 mg/m^2 infused weekly for 4 consecutive weeks. Pretreatment with 650 mg of acetaminophen and 25 mg of diphenhydramine by mouth is suggested although the drug is well tolerated by most individuals. The therapeutic latency for rituximab in myasthenics appears to be about a month but is undoubtedly longer for some disorders.[44] We have seen patients respond for 12–24 months before reinfusion is required. Our approach has been to wait at least 6 months before reinfusing and then only if initial improvement and then subsequent clinical deterioration takes place.

TACROLIMUS

Mechanism of Action

Tacrolimus binds to the FK506-binding protein (FKB), forming the tacrolimus–FKB complex, which also binds to and blocks calcineurin. Although cyclosporine and tacrolimus bind to different target molecules, both drugs inhibit T-cell activation in the same manner and as calcineurin inhibitors, reduce production of the proinflammatory cytokine IL-2.[2,110] As is the case with cyclosporine, these are two immunomodulating drugs developed for and used by the organ transplant community.

Uses

Tacrolimus, like cyclosporine, has been undoubtedly used most frequently in MG within the spectrum of neuromuscular disease.[110,116,223,271–279] It has been used either as monotherapy, or more commonly in conjunction with thymectomy or other therapies. Both favorable and equivocal results are reported.[271,273] We are aware of reported benefit in dermatomyositis/polymyositis and case reports of suggesting benefit in CIDP and vasculitic neuropathy.[56,280] Its use has been suggested in both Isaac's syndrome and LEMS without convincing literature support to our knowledge.[136]

Adverse Effects

Tacrolimus has similar toxicities to cyclosporine. It tends to be less nephrotoxic but more inclined to cause hyperglycemia.[44] Sirolimus has less renal toxicity than tacrolimus or cyclosporine. In view of this, our anecdotal experience with it in couple of patients with refractory MG has demonstrated no apparent benefit.

Management Considerations

Tacrolimus has been prescribed for myasthenic patients at a dosage of 0.1 mg/kg/day in two divided doses, and subsequently adjusted for plasma drug concentrations between 7 and 8 mg/mL.[116] Tacrolimus has been reported to benefit some who have failed to respond or become refractory to the effects of cyclosporine.

REFERENCES

1. Drachman DB. Immunotherapy in neuromuscular disorders: Current and future strategies. *Muscle Nerve*. 1996;19: 1239–1251.
2. Sathasivam S. Steroids and immunosuppressant drugs in myasthenia gravis. *Nat Clin Pract Neurol*. 2008;4(6):317–327.
3. Taylor AL, Christopher CJ, Bradley JA. Immunosuppressive agents in solid organ transplantation: Mechanisms of action and therapeutic efficacy. *Crit Rev Oncol Hematol*. 2005;56:23–46.
4. Khatri BO, McQuillen MP, Kaminski M, et al. Evidence-based guideline update: Plasmapheresis in neurologic disorders. *Neurology*. 2011;77:e101–e103.
5. Keung B, Robeson KR, DiCapua DB, et al. Long-term benefit of rituximab in MuSK autoantibody myasthenia gravis patients. *J Neurol Neurosurg Psychiatry*. 2013;84(12):1407–1409.
6. Rahier KF, Moutschen M, Van Gompel A, et al. Vaccinations in patients with immune-mediated inflammatory diseases. *Rheumatology*. 2010;49:1815–1827.
7. Hoes JN, Hacobs JW, Boers M, et al. EULAR evidence-based recommendations on the management of systemic glucocorticoid therapy in rheumatic diseases. *Ann Rheum Dis*. 2007;66:1560–1567.
8. Sharshar T, Chevret S, Mazighi M, et al. Validity and reliability of two muscle strength scores commonly used as endpoints in assessing treatment of myasthenia gravis. *J Neurol*. 2000;247:286–290.
9. Cederbaum J, Stambler N, Malta E, et al. The ALSFRS-R: A revised ALS functional rating scale that incorporates assessments of respiratory function. *J Neurol Sci*. 1999;169:13–21.
10. Dyck PJ, Davies JL, Litchy WJ, O'Brien PC. Longitudinal assessment of diabetic polyneuropathy using a composite score in the Rochester Diabetic Neuropathy Study Cohort. *Neurology*. 1997;49:229–239.
11. Gajdos P, Sharshar T, Chevret S. Standards of measurements in myasthenia gravis. *Ann N Y Acad Sci*. 2003;998:445–452.
12. Barohn RJ, McIntire D, Herbelin L, Wolfe GI, Nations S, Bryan WW. Reliability testing of the quantitative myasthenia gravis score. *Ann N Y Acad Sci*. 1998;841:769–772.
13. Bedlack RS, Simel DL, Bosworth H, Samsa G, Tucker-Lipscomb B, Sanders DB. Quantitative myasthenia gravis score: Assessment of responsiveness and longitudinal validity. *Neurology*. 2005;64(11):1968–1970.
14. Simon NG, Ayer G, Lomen-Hoerth C. Is IVIg therapy warranted in progressive lower motor neuron syndromes without conduction block? *Neurology*. 2013;81(24): 2116–2020.
15. Nobile-Orazio E, Cappellari A, Priori A. Multifocal motor neuropathy: Current concepts and controversies. *Muscle Nerve*. 2005;31:663–680.
16. Ruzhansky K, Brannagan TH III. Intravenous immunoglobulin for treatment of neuromuscular disease. *Neurol Clin Pract*. 2013;440–446.
17. Thomas CF, Limper AH. Pneumocystis pneumonia. *N Engl J Med*. 2004;350:2487–2498.

18. Kelly DM, Cronin S. PCP prophylaxis with use of corticosteroids by neurologists. *Pract Neurol.* 2014;14:74–76.
19. Neumann S, Krause SW, Maschmeyer G, Schiel X, von Lilienfeld-Toal M. Primary prophylaxis of bacterial infections and Pneumocystis jirovecii pneumonia in patients with hematological malignancies and solid tumors. *Ann Hematol.* 2013;92:433–442.
20. www.rrnmf.com. Accessed on March 24, 2012.
21. Horsburgh CR Jr, Rubin EJ. Latent tuberculosis infection in the United States. *N Engl J Med.* 2011;364:1441–1448.
22. Wingerchuk DM, Carter JL. Multiple sclerosis: Current and emerging disease-modifying therapies and treatment strategies. *Mayo Clin Proc.* 2014;89(2):225–240.
23. Zaheer F, Berger JR. Treatment-related progressive multifocal leukoencephalopathy: Current understanding and future steps. *Ther Adv Drug Safe.* 2012;3(5):227–239.
24. Takao M. Targeted therapy and progressive multifocal leukoencephalopathy (PML): PML in the era of monoclonal antibody therapies. *Brain Nerve.* 2013;65(11):1363–1374.
25. Basile A, Simzar S, Bentow J, et al. Disseminated Strongyloides stercoralis: Hyperinfection during medical immunosuppression. *J Am Acad Derm.* 2010;63(5):896–902.
26. Santiago M, Leitão B. Prevention of strongyloides hyperinfection syndrome: A rheumatological point of view. *Eur J Intern Med.* 2009;20(8):744–788.
27. Iriemenam NC, Sanyaolu AO, Oyibo WA, Fagbenro-Beyioku AF. Strongyloides stercoralis and the immune response. *Parasitol Int.* 2010;59:9–14.
28. Riminton DS, Hartung HP, Reddel SW. Managing the risks of immunosuppression. *Curr Opin Neurol.* 2011;24:217–223.
29. Ringel I, Zettl UK. Intravenous immunoglobulin therapy in neurological disease during pregnancy. *J Neurol.* 2006;253 (suppl 5):v70–v74.
30. Gutierrez-Dalmau A, Campistol JM. Immunosuppressive therapy and malignancy in organ transplant recipients: A systematic review. *Drugs.* 2007;67(8):1167–1198.
31. Dahlke E, Murray CA, Kitchen J, Chan AW. Systematic review of melanoma incidence and prognosis in solid organ transplant recipients. *Transplant Res.* 2014;3:10.
32. Hirst C, Raasch S, Llewelyn G, Robertson N. Remission of chronic inflammatory demyelinating polyneuropathy after alemtuzumab. *J Neurol Neurosurg Psychiatry.* 2006;77(6):800–802.
33. Marsh EA, Hirst CL, Llewelyn JG, et al. Alemtuzumab in the treatment of IVIG-dependent chronic inflammatory demyelinating polyneuropathy. *J Neurol.* 2010;257(6):913–919.
34. Mahdi-Rogers M, van Doorn PA, Hughes RA. Immunomodulatory treatment other than corticosteroids, immunoglobulin and plasma exchange for chronic inflammatory demyelinating polyradiculoneuropathy. *Cochrane Database Syst Rev.* 2013;6: CD003280.
35. Kissel JT, Levy RJ, Mendell JR, Griggs RC. Azathioprine toxicity in neuromuscular disease. *Neurology.* 1986;36:35–39.
36. Sanders DB, Evoli A. Immunosuppressive therapies in myasthenia gravis. *Autoimmunity.* 2010;43(5–6):428–435.
37. Gajdos P, Elkharrat D, Chevret S, Chastang C. A randomized clinical trial comparing prednisone and azathioprine in myasthenia gravis. Results of the second interim analysis. *J Neurol Neurosurg Psychiatry.* 1993;56:1157–1163.
38. Bromberg MB, Wald JJ, Forshew DA, Feldman EL, Albers JW. Randomized trial of azathioprine or prednisone for initial immunosuppressive treatment of myasthenia. *J Neurol Sci.* 1997;150:59–62.
39. Palace J, Newsom-Davis J, Lecky B. A randomized double-blind trial of prednisolone alone or with azathioprine in myasthenia gravis. *Neurology.* 1998;50:1778–1783.
40. Hohlfeld R, Michels M, Heininger K, Besinger U, Toyka KV. Azathioprine toxicity during long-term immunosuppression of generalized myasthenia gravis. *Neurology.* 1988;38:258–261.
41. Myasthenia Gravis Clinical Study Group. A randomized clinical trial comparing prednisone and azathioprine in myasthenia gravis. Results of the second interim analysis. *J Neurol Neurosurg Psychiatry.* 1993;56:1157–1163.
42. Herrllinger U, Weller M, Dichgans J, Melms A. Association of primary central nervous system lymphoma with long-term azathioprine therapy for myasthenia gravis. *Ann Neurol.* 2000;47:682–683.
43. Sanders DB, Scoppetta C. The treatment of patients with myasthenia gravis. *Neurol Clin.* 1994;12:342–368.
44. Silvestri NJ, Wolfe GI. Treatment-refractory myasthenia gravis. *J Clin Neuromuscul Dis.* 2014;15(4):167–178.
45. Amato AA, Greenberg SA. Inflammatory myopathies. *Continuum (Minneap Minn).* 2013;19(6 Muscle Disease):1615–3163.
46. Collins MP, Periquet MI, Mendell JR, Sahenk Z, Nagaraja HN, Kissel JT. Nonsystemic vasculitic neuropathy: Insights from a clinical cohort. *Neurology.* 2003;61:623–630.
47. Collins MP, Dyck PJ, Gronseth GS, et al. Peripheral Nerve Society: Guideline on the classification, diagnosis, investigation, and immunosuppressive therapy of non-systemic vasculitic neuropathy: Executive summary. *J Periph Nerv Syst.* 2010; 15: 176–184.
48. Lacomis D. Neurosarcoidosis. *Curr Neuropharmacol.* 2011;9: 429–436.
49. Maddison P. Treatment in Lambert-Eaton myasthenic syndrome. *Ann N Y Acad Sci.* 2012;1275:78–84.
50. Krendel DA, Costigan DA, Hopkins LC. Successful treatment of neuropathies in patients with diabetes mellitus. *Arch Neurol.* 1995;52:1053–1061.
51. Alessi G, De Reuck J, De Bleecker J, Vancayzeele S. Successful immunoglobulin treatment in a patient with neuromyotonia. *Clin Neurol Neurosurg.* 2000;102:173–175.
52. Ishii A, Hayashi A, Ohkoshi N, et al. Clinical evaluation of plasma exchange and high dose intravenous immunoglobulin in a patient with Isaacs' syndrome. *J Neurol Neurosurg Psychiatry.* 1994;57:840–842.
53. Van den Berg JS, van Engelen BG, Boerman RH, de Baets MH. Acquired neuromyotonia: Superiority of plasma exchange over high-dose intravenous immunoglobulin [letter]. *J Neurol.* 1999;246:623–625.
54. Jinka M, Chaudhry V. Treatment of multifocal motor neuropathy. *Curr Treat Opinions Neurol.* 2014;16(2):269.
55. Gordon PA, Winer JB, Hoogendijk JE, Choy EH. Immunosuppressant and immunomodulatory treatment for dermatomyositis and polymyositis. *Cochrane Database Syst Rev.* 2012;8:CD003643.
56. Gwathney KG, Burns TM, Collins MP, Dyck PJ. Vasculitic neuropathy. *Lancet Neurol.* 2014;13:67–82.
57. Gomes JA, Stevens RD, Lewin JJ III, Mirski MA, Bhardwaj A. Glucocorticoid therapy in neurologic critical care. *Crit Care Med.* 2005;33:1214–1224.
58. McDaneld LM, Fields JD, Bourdette DN, Bhardwaj A. Immunomodulatory therapies in neurologic critical care. *Neurocrit Care.* 2010;12(1):132–143.

59. Bromberg MB, Carter O. Corticosteroid use in the treatment of neuromuscular disorders: Empirical and evidence-based data. *Muscle Nerve*. 2004;30:20–37.
60. Johns TR. Long-term corticosteroid treatment of myasthenia gravis. *Ann N Y Acad Sci*. 1987;505:568–583.
61. Miller RG, Milner-Brown HS, Mirka A. Prednisone-induced worsening of neuromuscular function in myasthenia gravis. *Neurology*. 1986;36:729–732.
62. Panegyres PK, Squire M, Newsom-Davis J. Acute myopathy associated with large parenteral dose of corticosteroid in myasthenia gravis. *J Neurol Neurosurg Psychiatry*. 1993;56:702–704.
63. Lindberg C, Andersen O, Lefvert AK. Treatment of myasthenia gravis with methylprednisolone pulse: A double-blind study. *Acta Neurol Scand*. 1998;97:370–373.
64. Eftimov F, Winer JB, Vermeulen M, de Haan R, van Schaik IN. Intravenous immunoglobulin for chronic inflammatory demyelinating polyradiculoneuropathy. *Cochrane Database Syst Rev* 2013;12:CD001797.
65. Nobile-Orazio E. Chronic inflammatory demyelinating polyradiculoneuropathy and variants: Where we are and where we should go. *J Peripher Nerve Syst*. 2014;19(1):2–13.
66. Hughes RA, Mehndiratta MM. Corticosteroids for chronic inflammatory demyelinating polyradiculoneuropathy. *Cochrane Database Syst Rev*. 2012;8:CD002062.
67. Dyck PJ, Lais AC, Ohta M, Bastron JA, Okazaki H, Groover RV. Chronic inflammatory polyradiculoneuropathy. *Mayo Clin Proc*. 1975;50:621–637.
68. Dyck PJ, O'Brien P, Swanson C, Low P, Daube J. Combined azathioprine and prednisone in chronic inflammatory demyelinating polyneuropathy. *Neurology*. 1985;35:1173–1176.
69. Lewis RA, Sumner AJ, Brown MJ, Asbury AK. Multifocal demyelinating neuropathy with persistent conduction block. *Neurology*. 1982;32:958–964.
70. Viala K, Renie´ L, Maisonobe T, et al. Follow-up study and response to treatment in 23 patients with Lewis-Sumner syndrome. *Brain*. 2004;127:2010–2017.
71. Börü ÜT, Erdoğan H, Alp R, et al. Treatment of chronic inflammatory demyelinating polyneuropathy with high dose intravenous methylprednisolone monthly for five years: 10-year follow up. *Clin Neurol Neurosurg*. 2014;118:89–93.
72. van Schaik IN, Eftimov F, van Doorn PA, et al. Pulsed high-dose dexamethasone versus standard prednisolone treatment for chronic inflammatory demyelinating polyradiculoneuropathy (PREDICT study): A double-blind, randomised, controlled trial. *Lancet Neurol*. 2010;9(3):245–253.
73. Joint Task Force of the EFNS and the PNS. European Federation of Neurological Societies/Peripheral Nerve Society Guideline on management of chronic inflammatory demyelinating polyradiculoneuropathy: Report of a Joint Task Force of the European Federation of Neurological Societies and the Peripheral Nerve Society – First Revision. *J Peripher Nerv Syst*. 2010;15:1–9.
74. Katz JS, Saperstein DS, Gronseth G, Amato AA, Barohn RJ. Distal acquired demyelinating symmetric neuropathy. *Neurology*. 2000;54:615–620.
75. Hughes RA, Newsom-Davis JM, Perkin GD, Pierce JM. Controlled trial of prednisolone in acute polyneuropathy. *Lancet*. 1978;2:750–753.
76. Hughes RA. Ineffectiveness of high-dose intravenous methylprednisolone in Guillain-Barré syndrome. *Lancet*. 1991;338:1142.
77. Feldman EL, Bromberg MB, Albers JW, Pestronk A. Immunosuppressive treatment in multifocal motor neuropathy. *Ann Neurol*. 1991;30:397–401.
78. Joffe MM, Love LA, Leff RL, et al. Drug therapy of the idiopathic inflammatory myopathies: Predictors of response to prednisone, azathioprine, and methotrexate and a comparison of their efficacy. *Am J Med*. 1993;94(4):379–387.
79. Lotz BP, Engel AG, Nishino H, Stevens JC, Litchy WJ. Inclusion body myositis. Observations in 40 patients. *Brain*. 1989;112:727–747.
80. Miloslavsky EM, Specks U, Merkel PA, et al. Clinical outcomes of remission induction therapy for severe antineutrophil cytoplasmic antibody-associated vasculitis. *Arth Rheum*. 2013;65(9):2441–2449.
81. Jones RB, Tervaert JW, Hauser T, et al. Rituximab versus cyclophosphamide in ANCA-associated renal vasculitis. *N Engl J Med*. 2010;363:211–220.
82. Stone JH, Merkel PA, Spiera R, et al. Rituximab versus cyclophosphamide for ANCA-associated vasculitis. *N Engl J Med*. 2010;363:221–232.
83. Burns TM, Dyck PJ, Aksamit AJ, Dyck PJ. The natural history and long-term outcome of 57 limb sarcoidosis neuropathy cases. *J Neurol Sci*. 2006;244(1–2):77–87.
84. van Eijk JJ, van Alfen N, Berrevoets M, van der Wilt GJ, Pillen S, van Engelen BG. Evaluation of prednisolone treatment in the acute phase of neuralgic amyotrophy: An observational study. *J Neurol Neurosurg Psychiatry*. 2009;80(10):1120–1124.
85. Dalakas MC. Advances in the pathogenesis and treatment of patients with stiff person syndrome. *Curr Neurol Neurosci Rep*. 2008;8(1):48–55.
86. Howard FM, Duane DD, Lambert EH, Daube JR. Alternate-day prednisone: Preliminary report of a double-blind controlled study. *Ann N Y Acad Sci*. 1976;274:596–697.
87. Rothman MS, West SG, McDermott MT. Osteoporosis for the practicing neurologists. *Neurol Clin Pract*. 2014;4:34–43.
88. Adachi JD, Bensen WG, Brown J, et al. Intermittent etidronate therapy to prevent corticosteroid-induced osteoporosis. *N Engl J Med*. 1997;337:382–387.
89. Pereira RM, Carvalho JF, Paula AP, et al. Guidelines for the prevention and treatment of glucocorticoid-induced osteoporosis. *Rev Bras Rheumatol*. 2012;52(4):580–593.
90. Saag KG, Emkey R, Schnitzer TJ, et al. Alendronate for the prevention and treatment of glucocorticoid-induced osteoporosis. *N Engl J Med*. 1998;339:292–292.
91. Adu D, Pall A, Luqmani RA, et al. Controlled trial of pulse versus continuous prednisolone and cyclophosphamide in the treatment of vasculitis. *Q J Med*. 1997;90:401–409.
92. Guillevin L, Cordier JF, Lhote F, et al. A prospective, multicenter, randomized trial comparing steroids and pulse cyclophosphamide versus steroids and oral cyclophosphamide in the treatment of generalized Wegener's granulomatosis. *Arthritis Rheum*. 1997;40:2187–2198.
93. Gorson KC. Therapy for vasculitic neuropathies. *Curr Opinion Treat Neurology*. 2006;8(2):105–117.
94. Vrancken AF, Hughes RA, Said G, Wokke JH, Notermans NC. Immunosuppressive treatment for non-systemic vasculitic neuropathy. *Cochrane Database Syst Rev*. 2007;(1):CD006050.
95. Dalakas MC, Engel WK. Chronic relapsing (dysimmune) polyneuropathy: Pathogenesis and treatment. *Ann Neurol*. 1981;9(suppl):134–145.

96. McCombe PA, Pollard JD, McLeod JG. Chronic inflammatory demyelinating polyradiculoneuropathy. A clinical and electrophysiological study of 92 cases. *Brain*. 1987;110(6):1617–1630.
97. Bouchard C, Lacroix C, Planté V, et al. Clinicopathologic findings and prognosis of chronic inflammatory demyelinating polyneuropathy. *Neurology*. 1999;52(3):498–503.
98. Brannagan TH, Pradhan A, Heiman-Patterson T, et al. High-dose cyclophosphamide without stem-cell rescue for refractory CIDP. *Neurology*. 2002;58(12):1856–1858.
99. Good JL, Chehrenama M, Mayer RF, Koski CL. Pulse cyclophosphamide therapy in chronic inflammatory demyelinating polyneuropathy. *Neurology*. 1998;51(6):1735–1738.
100. Gladstone DE, Prestrud AA, Brannagan TH 3rd. High-dose cyclophosphamide results in long-term disease remission with restoration of a normal quality of life in patients with severe refractory chronic inflammatory demyelinating polyneuropathy. *J Peripher Nerv Syst*. 2005;10(1):11–6.
101. Prineas JW, McLeod JG. Chronic relapsing polyneuritis. *J Neurol Sci*. 1976;27(4):427–458.
102. Pestronk A, Cornblath DR, Ilyas A, et al. A treatable multifocal motor neuropathy with antibodies to GM1 ganglioside. *Ann Neurol*. 1988;24:73–78.
103. Leitch MM, Sherman WH, Brannagan TH 3rd. Distal acquired demyelinating symmetric polyneuropathy progressing to classic chronic inflammatory demyelinating polyneuropathy and response to fludarabine and cyclophosphamide. *Muscle Nerve*. 2013;47(2):292–296.
104. Lewis RA, Lisak RP. "Rebooting" the immune system with cyclophosphamide: Taking risks for a "cure"? *Ann Neurol*. 2003;53:7–9.
105. Lin PT, Martin BA, Winacker AB, So YT. High-dose cyclophosphamide in refractory myasthenia with MuSK antibodies. *Muscle Nerve*. 2006;33:433–435.
106. DeFeo LG, Schottlender J, Martelli NA, Molfino NA. Use of intravenous pulsed cyclophosphamide in severe, generalized myasthenia gravis. *Muscle Nerve*. 2002;26:32–36.
107. Drachman DB, Jones RJ, Brodsky RA. Treatment of refractory myasthenia: "Rebooting" with high-dose cyclophosphamide. *Ann Neurol*. 2003;53:29–34.
108. Nagappa M, Netravathi M, Taly AB, Sinha S, Bindu PS, Mahadevan A. Long-term efficacy and limitations of cyclophosphamide in myasthenia gravis. *J Clin Neurosci*. 2014;21(11):1909–1914.
109. El-Salem K, Yassin A, Al-Hayk K, Yahya S, Al-Shorafat D, Dahbour SS. Treatment of MuSK-associated myasthenia gravis. *Curr Treat Options Neurol*. 2014;16(4):283.
110. Benatar M, Sanders D. The importance of studying history: Lessons learnt from a trial of tacrolimus in myasthenia gravis. *J Neurol Neurosurg Psychiatry*. 2011;82:945.
111. Ciafaloni E, Nikhar NK, Massey JM, Sanders DB. Retrospective analysis of the use of cyclosporine in myasthenia gravis. *Neurology*. 2000;55:448–450.
112. Sanders DB, Ciafaloni E, Nikhar NK, Massey JM. Retrospective analysis of the use of cyclosporine in myasthenia [abstract]. *Neurology*. 2000;54(suppl 3):A394.
113. Tindall RS, Rollins JA, Phillips JT, Greenlee RG, Wells L, Belendiuk G. Preliminary results of a double-blind, randomized, placebo-controlled trial of cyclosporine in myasthenia gravis. *N Engl J Med*. 1987;316:719–724.
114. Tindall RS, Phillips JT, Rollins JA, Wells L, Hall K. A clinical therapeutic trial of cyclosporine in myasthenia gravis. *Ann N Y Acad Sci*. 1993;681:539–551.
115. Kurokawa T, Nishiyama T, Yamamoto R, Kishida H, Hakii Y, Kuroiwa Y. Anti-MuSK antibody positive myasthenia gravis with HIV infection successfully treated with cyclosporin: A case report. *Rinsho Shinkeigaku*. 2008;48(9):666–669.
116. Ponseti JM, Azem J, Fort JM, et al. Long-term results of tacrolimus in cyclosporine- and prednisone-dependent myasthenia gravis. *Neurology*. 2005;64:1641–1643.
117. Nast A, Sporbeck B, Rosumeck S, et al. Which antipsoriatic drug has the fastest onset of action? Systematic review on the rapidity of the onset of action. *J Invest Dermatol*. 2013;133:1963–1970.
118. Hefter H, Sprenger KB, Arendt G, Hafner D. Treatment of chronic relapsing inflammatory demyelinating polyneuropathy by cyclosporin A and plasma exchange. A case report. *J Neurol*. 1990;237(5):320–233.
119. Kolkin S, Nahman NS Jr, Mendell JR. Chronic nephrotoxicity complicating cyclosporine treatment of chronic inflammatory demyelinating polyradiculoneuropathy. *Neurology*. 1987;37(1):147–149.
120. Hodgkinson SJ, Pollard JD, McLeod JG. Cyclosporin A in the treatment of chronic demyelinating polyradiculoneuropathy. *J Neurol Neurosurg Psychiatry*. 1990;53(4):327–330.
121. Barnett MH, Pollard JD, Davies L, McLeod JG. Cyclosporin A in resistant chronic inflammatory demyelinating polyradiculoneuropathy. *Muscle Nerve*. 1998;21(4):454–460.
122. Mahattanakul W, Crawford TO, Griffin JW, Goldstein JM, Cornblath DR. Treatment of chronic inflammatory demyelinating polyneuropathy with cyclosporin-A. *J Neurol Neurosurg Psychiatry*. 1996;60(2):185–187.
123. Matsuda M, Hoshi K, Gono T, Morita H, Ikeda S. Cyclosporin A in treatment of refractory patients with chronic inflammatory demyelinating polyradiculoneuropathy. *J Neurol Sci*. 2004;224(1–2):29–35.
124. Odaka M, Tatsumoto M, Susuki K, Hirata K, Yuki N. Intractable chronic inflammatory demyelinating polyneuropathy treated successfully with ciclosporin. *J Neurol Neurosurg Psychiatry*. 2005;76(8):1115–1120.
125. Cocito D, Grimaldi S, Paolasso I, et al. Italian Network for CIDP Register. Immunosuppressive treatment in refractory chronic inflammatory demyelinating polyradiculoneuropathy. A nationwide retrospective analysis. *Eur J Neurol*. 2011;18(12):1417–1421.
126. Sanders DB. Lambert-Eaton myasthenic syndrome: Diagnosis and treatment. *Ann N Y Acad Sci*. 2003;998:500–508.
127. Vencovsky J, Jarosova K, Machacek S, et al. Cyclosporine A versus methotrexate in the treatment of polymyositis and dermatomyositis. *Scand J Rheumatol*. 2000;29(2):95–102.
128. Borleffs JC. Cyclosporine as monotherapy for polymyositis? *Transplant Proc*. 1988;20(3 suppl 4):333–334.
129. Correia O, Polonia J, Nunes JP, Resende C, Delgado L. Severe acute form of adult dermatomyositis treated with cyclosporine. *Int J Dermatol*. 1992;31(7):517–519.
130. Girardin E, Dayer JM, Paunier L. Cyclosporine for juvenile dermatomyositis. *J Pediatr*. 1988;112(1):165–166.
131. Heckmatt J, Hasson N, Saunders C, et al. Cyclosporin in juvenile dermatomyositis. *Lancet*. 1989;1(8646):1063–1066.
132. Jones DW, Snaith ML, Isenberg DA. Cyclosporine treatment for intractable polymyositis. *Arthritis Rheum*. 1987;30(8):959–960.
133. Lueck CJ, Trend P, Swash M. Cyclosporin in the management of polymyositis and dermatomyositis. *J Neurol Neurosurg Psychiatry*. 1991;54(11):1007–1008.

134. Mehregan DR, Su WP. Cyclosporine treatment for dermatomyositis/polymyositis. *Cutis*. 1993;51(1):59–61.
135. Pistoia V, Buoncompagni A, Scribanis R, et al. Cyclosporin A in the treatment of juvenile chronic arthritis and childhood polymyositis-dermatomyositis. Results of a preliminary study. *Clin Exp Rheumatol*. 1993;11(2):203–208.
136. van Sonderen A, Wirtz PW, Verschuuren JJ, Titulaer MJ. Paraneoplastic syndromes of the neuromuscular junction: Therapeutic options in myasthenia gravis, Lambert-Eaton myasthenic syndrome, and neuromyotonia. *Curr Treat Options Neurol*. 2013;15(2):224–239.
137. Howard JF Jr, Barohn RJ, Cutter GR, et al. A randomized, double-blind, placebo-controlled phase II study of eculizumab in patients with refractory generalized myasthenia gravis. *Muscle Nerve*. 2013;48(1):76–84.
138. Takada K, Bookbinder S, Furie R, et al. A pilot study of eculizumab in patients with dermatomyositis. *Arthritis Rheum*. 2002;46(suppl):S489.
139. Chin RL, Sherman WH, Sander HW, Hays AP, Latov N. Etanercept (Enbrel) therapy for chronic inflammatory demyelinating polyneuropathy. *J Neurol Sci*. 2003;210(1–2):19–21.
140. Alshekhlee A, Basiri K, Miles JD, Ahmad SA, Katirji B. Chronic inflammatory demyelinating polyneuropathy associated with tumor necrosis factor-alpha antagonists. *Muscle Nerve*. 2010;41(5):723–727.
141. Hamon MA, Nicolas G, Deviere F, Letournel F, Dubas F. Demyelinating neuropathy during anti-TNF alpha treatment with a review of the literature. *Rev Neurol*. 2007;163(12):1232–1235.
142. Lozeron P, Denier C, Lacroix C, Adams D. Long-term course of demyelinating neuropathies occurring during tumor necrosis factor-blocker therapy. *Arch Neurol*. 2009;66(4):490–497.
143. Richez C, Blanco P, Lagueny A, Schaeverbeke T, Dehais J. Neuropathy resembling CIDP in patients receiving tumor necrosis factor-alpha blockers. *Neurology*. 2005;64(8):1468–1470.
144. Moravan M, Segal BM. Treatment of CNS sarcoidosis with infliximab and mycophenolate mofetil. *Neurology*. 2009;72(4):337–340.
145. Baughman RP, Lower EE, Bradley DA, Raymond LA, Kaufman A. Etanercept for refractory ocular sarcoidosis: Results of a double-blind randomized trial. *Chest*. 2005;128(2):1062.
146. Thongpooswan S, Abrudescu A. Lung sarcoidosis in etanercept treated rheumatoid arthritis patient: A case report and review of the literature. *Case Rep Rheumatol*. 2014;2014:358567.
147. Rowin J, Meriggioli MN, Tüzün E, Leurgans S, Christadoss P. Etanercept treatment in corticosteroid-dependent myasthenia gravis. *Neurology*. 2004;63:2390–2392.
148. The Muscle Study Group. A randomized, pilot trial of etanercept in dermatomyositis. *Ann Neurol*. 2011;70:427–436.
149. Chen D, Wang XB, Zhou Y, Zhu XC. Efficacy of infliximab in the treatment for dermatomyositis with acute interstitial pneumonia: A study of fourteen cases and literature review. *Rheumatol Int*. 2013;33(10):2455–2458.
150. Kakoulidou M, Bjelak S, Pirskanen R, Lefvert AK. A clinical and immunological study of a myasthenia gravis patient treated with infliximab. *Acta Neurol Scand*. 2007;115(4):279–283.
151. Marzo ME, Tintoré M, Fabregues O, Montalbán X, Codina A. Chronic inflammatory demyelinating polyradiculoneuropathy during treatment with interferon alpha. *J Neurol Neurosurg Psychiatry*. 1998;65(4):604.
152. Meriggioli MN, Rowin J. Chronic inflammatory demyelinating polyneuropathy after treatment with interferon-alpha. *Muscle Nerve*. 2000;23(3):433–435.
153. Gorson KC, Allam G, Simovic D, Ropper AH. Improvement following interferon-alpha 2A in chronic inflammatory demyelinating polyneuropathy. *Neurology*. 1997;48(3):777–780.
154. Pavesi G, Cattaneo L, Marbini A, Gemignani F, Mancia D. Long-term efficacy of interferon-alpha in chronic inflammatory demyelinating polyneuropathy. *J Neurol*. 2002;249(6):777–779.
155. Choudhary PP, Thompson N, Hughes RA. Improvement following interferon beta in chronic inflammatory demyelinating polyradiculoneuropathy. *Neurology*. 1995;242(4):252–253.
156. Radziwill AJ, Kuntzer T, Fuhr P, Steck AJ. Long term follow up in chronic inflammatory demyelinating polyneuropathy (CIDP) under interferon beta-1a (IFN-b1 a) and intravenous immunoglobulin (IVIg). *J Neurol Neurosurg Psychiatry*. 2001;70:273.
157. Kuntzer T, Radziwill AJ, Lettry-Trouillat R, et al. Interferon-beta 1a in chronic inflammatory demyelinating polyneuropathy. *Neurology*. 1999;53(6):1364–1365.
158. Martina IS, van Doorn PA, Schmitz PI, Meulstee J, van der Meché FG. Chronic motor neuropathies: Response to interferon-beta 1a after failure of conventional therapies. *J Neurol Neurosurg Psychiatry*. 1999;66(2):197–201.
159. Vallat JM, Hahn AF, Léger JM, et al. Interferon beta-1a as an investigational treatment for CIDP. *Neurology*. 2003;60(8 suppl 3):S23–S28.
160. Hadden RD, Sharrack B, Bensa S, Soudain SE, Hughes RA. Randomized trial of interferon beta-1a in chronic inflammatory demyelinating polyradiculoneuropathy. *Neurology*. 1999;53(1):57–61.
161. Matsuse D, Ochi H, Tashiro K, et al. Exacerbation of chronic inflammatory demyelinating polyradiculoneuropathy during interferon beta-1b therapy in a patient with childhood-onset multiple sclerosis. *Intern Med*. 2005;44(1):68–72.
162. Donofrio PD, Berger A, Brannagan TH III, et al. Consensus statement: The use of intravenous immunoglobulin in the treatment of neuromuscular conditions, report of the ad hoc committee of the AANEM. *Muscle Nerve*. 2009;40:890–900.
163. Dwyer JM. Manipulating the immune system with immune globulin. *N Engl J Med*. 1992;326(2):107–116.
164. Gelfand EW. Intravenous immune globulin in autoimmune and inflammatory diseases. *N Engl J Med*. 2012;367:2015–2025.
165. Querol L, Rojas R, Casasnovas C, et al. Long-term outcome in chronic inflammatory demyelinating polyneuropathy patients treated with intravenous immunoglobulin: A retrospective study. *Muscle Nerve*. 2013;48:879–876.
166. Nobile-Orazio E, Meucci N, Barbieri S, Carpo M, Scarlato G. High dose intravenous immunoglobulin therapy in multifocal motor neuropathy. *Neurology*. 1993;43:537–544.
167. O'Leary CP, Mann AC, Lough J, Willison HJ. Muscle hypertrophy in multifocal motor neuropathy is associated with continuous motor unit activity. *Muscle Nerve*. 1997;20:479–485.
168. Huang CS, Hsu HS, Kao KP, Huang MH, Huang BS. Intravenous immunoglobulin in the preparation of thymectomy for myasthenia gravis. *Acta Neurol Scand*. 2003;108:136–138.
169. Stricker RB, Kwiatkowski BJ, Habis JA, Kiprov DD. Myasthenic crisis: Response to plasmapheresis following failure of intravenous gamma-globulin. *Arch Neurol*. 1993;50:837–840.
170. Barth D, Nabavi NM, Ng E, New P, Bril V. Comparison of IVIg and PLEX in patients with myasthenia gravis. *Neurology*. 2011;76:2017–2023.

171. Zinman L, Ny E, Bril V. IV Immunoglobulin in patients with myasthenia gravis: A randomized controlled trial. *Neurology.* 2007;68:837–841.
172. Gajdos P, Chevret S, Clair B, Tranchant C, Chastang C. Clinical trial of plasma exchange and high-dose intravenous immunoglobulin in myasthenia gravis. Myasthenia Gravis Clinical Study Group. *Ann Neurol.* 1997;41:789–796.
173. Gajdos P, Tranchant C, Clair B, et al. Treatment of myasthenia gravis exacerbation with intravenous immunoglobulin: A randomized double-blind clinical trial. *Arch Neurol.* 2005;62:1689–1693.
174. Gajdos P, Chevret S, Toyka K. Intravenous immunoglobulin for myasthenia gravis. *Cochrane Database Syst Rev.* 2006;19: CD002277.
175. Gajdos P, Chevret S, Toyka K. Plasma exchange for myasthenia gravis. *Cochrane Database Syst Rev.* 2002;4:CD002275.
176. Achiron A, Barak Y, Miron S, Sarova-Pinhas I. Immunoglobulin treatment in refractory myasthenia gravis. *Muscle Nerve.* 2000;23:551–555.
177. Cosi V, Lombardi M, Piccolo G, Erbetta A. Treatment of myasthenia gravis with high-dose intravenous immunoglobulin. *Acta Neurol Scand.* 1991;84:81–84.
178. Jongen JL, van Doorn PA, van der Meche FG. High-dose intravenous immunoglobulin therapy for myasthenia gravis. *J Neurol.* 1998;245:26–31.
179. Howard JF. Intravenous immunoglobulin for the treatment of acquired myasthenia gravis. *Neurol.* 1998;51(suppl 5):S30–S36.
180. Qureshi AI, Choudhry MA, Akbar MS, et al. Plasma exchange versus intravenous immunoglobulin treatment in myasthenic crisis. *Neurology.* 1999;52:629–632.
181. Shibata-Hamaguchi A, Samuraki M, Furui E, et al. Long-term effect of intravenous immunoglobulin on anti-MuSK antibody-positive myasthenia gravis. *Acta Neurol Scand.* 2007; 116:406–408.
182. Takahashi H, Kawaguchi N, Nemoto Y, Hattori T. High-dose intravenous immunoglobulin for the treatment of MuSK antibody-positive seronegative myasthenia gravis. *J Neurol Sci.* 2006;247:239.
183. Ronager J, Ravnborg M, Hermansen I, Vorstrup S. Immunoglobulin treatment versus plasma exchange in patients with chronic moderate to severe myasthenia gravis. *Artif Organs.* 2001;25:967–973.
184. Bril V, Barnett-Tapia C, Barth D, Katzberg HD. IVIG and PLEX in the treatment of myasthenia gravis. *Ann N Y Acad Sci.* 2012;1275(1):1–6.
185. Herrmann DN, Carney PR, Wald JJ. Juvenile myasthenia gravis: Treatment with immune globulin and thymectomy. *Pediatr Neurol.* 1998;18:63–66.
186. Selcen D, Dabrowski ER, Michon AM, Nigro MA. High-dose immunoglobulin therapy in juvenile myasthenia gravis. *Pediatr Neurol.* 2000;22:40–43.
187. Pinching AJ, Peters DK, Newsom-Davis J. Remission of myasthenia gravis following plasma-exchange. *Lancet.* 1976; 2:1373–1376.
188. Antozzi C, Gemma M, Regi B, et al. A short plasma exchange protocol is effective in severe myasthenia gravis. *J Neurol.* 1991;238:103–107.
189. Mandawat A, Mandawat A, Kaminski H, Shaker Z, Alawi AA, Alshekhlee A. Outcome of plasmapheresis in myasthenia gravis: Delayed therapy is not favorable. *Muscle Nerve.* 2011;43;578–584.
190. Howard JF. The treatment of myasthenia gravis with plasma exchange. *Semin Neurol.* 1982;2:273–279.
191. Guptill JT, Oakley D, Kuchibhatla M, et al. A retrospective study of complications of therapeutic plasma exchange in myasthenia. *Muscle Nerve.* 2013;47:170–176.
192. Dau PC, Lindstrom JM, Cassel CK, Denys EH, Shev EE, Spitler LE. Plasmapheresis and immunosuppressive drug therapy in myasthenia gravis. *N Engl J Med.* 1977;297:1134–1140.
193. Dalakas M, Illa I, Dambrosia J, et al. A controlled trial of high-dose intravenous immune globulin infusions as treatment for dermatomyositis. *N Engl J Med.* 1993;329:1993–2000.
194. Brannagan TH 3rd, Nagle KJ, Lange DJ, Rowland LP. Complications of intravenous immune globulin treatment in neurologic disease. *Neurology.* 1996;47:674–677.
195. Lazzaro C, Lopiano L, Cocito D. Subcutaneous vs intravenous administration of immunoglobulin in chronic inflammatory demyelinating polyneuropathy: An Italian cost-minimization analysis. *Neurol Sci.* 2014;35(7):1023–1034.
196. Markvardsen LH, Harbo T, Sindrup SH, Christiansen I, Andersen H, Jakobsen J; The Danish CIDP and MMN Study Group. Subcutaneous immunoglobulin preserves muscle strength in chronic inflammatory demyelinating polyneuropathy. *Eur J Neurol.* 2014;21(12):1465–1470.
197. Plasma Exchange/Sandoglobulin Guillain-Barre Syndrome Trial Group. Randomized trial of plasma exchange, intravenous immunoglobulin, and combined treatments in Guillain-Barré syndrome. *Lancet.* 1997;349:225–230.
198. Metzger AL, Bohan A, Goldberg LS, Bluestone R, Pearson CM. Polymyositis and dermatomyositis: Combined methotrexate and corticosteroid therapy. *Ann Intern Med.* 1974;81(2): 182–189.
199. Sokoloff MC, Goldberg LS, Pearson CM. Treatment of corticosteroid-resistant polymyositis with methotrexate. *Lancet.* 1971;1(7688):14–16.
200. Miller LC, Sisson BA, Tucker LB, DeNardo BA, Schaller JG. Methotrexate treatment of recalcitrant childhood dermatomyositis. *Arthritis Rheum.* 1992; 35(10):1143–1149.
201. Villalba L, Hicks JE, Adams EM, et al. Treatment of refractory myositis: A randomized crossover study of two new cytotoxic regimens. *Arthritis Rheum.* 1998;41(3):392–399.
202. Cagnoli M, Marchesoni A, Tosi S. Combined steroid, methotrexate and chlorambucil therapy for steroid-resistant dermatomyositis. *Clin Exp Rheumatol.* 1991;9(6):658–659.
203. Giannini M, Callen JP. Treatment of dermatomyositis with methotrexate and prednisone. *Arch Dermatol.* 1979; 115(10):1251–1252.
204. Mahdi-Rogers M; For the Randomised Methotrexate Chronic Inflammatory Demyelinating polyradiculoneuropathy (RMC) Trial Group. A pilot randomised controlled trial of methotrexate for CIDP: Lessons for future trials. *J Peripher Nerv Syst.* 2008;13(2):176.
205. Fialho D, Chan YC, Allen DC, Reilly MM, Hughes RA. Treatment of chronic inflammatory demyelinating polyradiculoneuropathy with methotrexate. *J Neurol Neurosurg Psychiatry.* 2006;77(4):544–547.
206. Díaz-Manera J, Rojas-García R, Gallardo E, Illa I. Response to methotrexate in a chronic inflammatory demyelinating polyradiculoneuropathy patient. *Muscle Nerve.* 2009;39(3):386–388.
207. Christopher-Stine L, Casciola-Rosen LA, Hong G, Chung T, Corse AM, Mammen AL. A novel autoantibody recognizing 200-kd and 100-kd proteins is associated with an

immune-mediated necrotizing myopathy. *Arth Rheum*. 2010; 62(9):2757–2766.
208. Grable-Esposito P, Katzberg HD, Greenberg SA, Srinivasan J, Katz J, Amato AA. Immune-mediated necrotizing myopathy associated with statins. *Muscle Nerve*. 2010;41:185–190.
209. Mohassel P, Mammen AL. Statin-associated autoimmune myopathy and anti-HMGCR autoantibodies. *Muscle Nerve*. 2013;48:477–483.
210. Pasnoor M, He J, Herbelin L, Dimachkie M, Barohn RJ; Muscle Study Group. Phase II trial of methotrexate in myasthenia gravis. *Ann N Y Acad Sci*. 2012;1275(1):23–28.
211. Visser K, van der Heijde DM. Risk and management of liver toxicity during methotrexate treatment in rheumatoid and psoriatic arthritis: A systematic review of the literature. *Clin Exp Rheumatol*. 2009;27:1017–1025.
212. Graves D, Vernino S. Immunotherapies in neurologic disease. *Med Clin North Am*. 2012;96(3):497–523.
213. The Muscle Study Group. A trial of mycophenolate mofetil with prednisone as initial immunotherapy in myasthenia gravis. *Neurology*. 2008;71:394–399.
214. Sanders DB, Hart IK, Mantegazza R, et al. An international, phase III, randomized trial of mycophenolate mofetil in myasthenia gravis. *Neurology*. 2008;71:400–406.
215. Meriggioli MN, Rowin J, Richman JG, Leurgans S. Mycophenolate mofetil for myasthenia gravis: A double-blind, placebo-controlled pilot study. *Ann N Y Acad Sci*. 2003;998:494–499.
216. Meriggioli MN, Ciafaloni E, Al-Hayk KA, et al. Mycophenolate mofetil for myasthenia gravis: An analysis of efficacy, safety, and tolerability. *Neurology*. 2003;61:1438–1440.
217. Sanders D, McDermott M, Thornton C, Tawil A, Barohn R; The Muscle Study Group. A trial of mycophenolate mofetil (MMF) with prednisone as initial immunotherapy in myasthenia gravis (MG) [abstract]. *Neurology*. 2007;68:A107.
218. Ciafaloni E, Massey JM, Tucker-Lipscomb B, Sanders DB. Mycophenolate mofetil for myasthenia gravis: An open-label pilot study. *Neurology*. 2001;56:97–99.
219. Vernino S, Salomao DR, Habermann TM, O'Neill BP. Primary CNS lymphoma complicating treatment of myasthenia gravis with mycophenolate mofetil. *Neurology*. 2005;65:639–641.
220. Hauser RA, Malek AR, Rosen R. Successful treatment of a patient with severe refractory myasthenia gravis using mycophenolate mofetil. *Neurology*. 1998;51:912–913.
221. Chaudhry V, Cornblath DR, Griffin JW, O'Brien R, Drachman DB. Mycophenolate mofetil: A safe and promising immunosuppressant in neuromuscular diseases. *Neurology*. 2001;56:94–96.
222. Hehir MK, Burns TM, Alpers J, Conaway MR, Sawa M, Sanders DB. Mycophenolate mofetil in AChR-antibody-positive myasthenia gravis: Outcomes in 102 patients. *Muscle Nerve*. 2010; 41(5):593–598.
223. Schneider-Gold C, Hartung HP, Gold R. Mycophenolate mofetil and tacrolimus: New therapeutic options in neuroimmunological diseases. *Muscle Nerve*. 2006;34(3):284–291.
224. Gorson KC, Amato AA, Ropper AH. Efficacy of mycophenolate mofetil in patients with chronic immune demyelinating polyneuropathy. *Neurology*. 2004;63(4):715–717.
225. Radziwill AJ, Schweikert K, Kuntzer T, Fuhr P, Steck AJ. Mycophenolate mofetil for chronic inflammatory demyelinating polyradiculoneuropathy: An open label study. *Eur J Neurol*. 2006;56(1):37–38.
226. Mowzoon N, Sussman A, Bradley WG. Mycophenolate (CellCept) treatment of myasthenia gravis, chronic inflammatory polyneuropathy and inclusion body myositis. *J Neurol Sci*. 2001;185(2):119–122.
227. Benedetti L, Grandis M, Nobbio L, et al. Mycophenolate mofetil in dysimmune neuropathies: A preliminary study. *Muscle Nerve*. 2004;29(5):748–749.
228. Bedi G, Brown A, Tong T, Sharma KR. Chronic inflammatory demyelinating polyneuropathy responsive to mycophenolate mofetil therapy. *J Neurol Neurosurg Psychiatry*. 2010; 81(6):634–636.
229. Umapathi T, Hughes R. Mycophenolate in treatment resistant inflammatory neuropathies. *Eur J Neurol*. 2002;9(6):683–685.
230. Dubal DB, Mueller S, Ruben BS, Engstrom JW, Josephson SA. T-cell lymphoproliferative disorder following mycophenolate treatment for myasthenia gravis. *Muscle Nerve*. 2009; 39(6):849–850.
231. Silvestri NJ, Wolfe GI. Myasthenia gravis. *Semin Neurol*. 2012; 32(3):215–226.
232. Sorgun MH, Erdogan S, Bay M, et al. Therapeutic plasma exchange in treatment of neuroimmunologic disorders: Review of 92 cases. *Transfus Apher Sci*. 2013;49(2):174–180.
233. Cortese I, Chaudhry V, So YT, Cantor F, Cornblath DR, Rae-Grant A. Evidence-based guideline update: Plasmapheresis in neurologic disorders. *Neurology*. 2011;76:294–300.
234. NIH Consensus DevelopmentConference. The utility of therapeutic plasmapheresis for neurological disorders. NIH Consensus Development. *JAMA*. 1986;256:1333–1337.
235. Yeh JH, Chiu HC. Plasmapheresis in myasthenia gravis. A comparative study of daily versus alternately daily schedule. *Acta Neurol Scand*. 1999;99:147–151.
236. Mahalati K, Dawson RB, Collins JO, Mayer RF. Predictable recovery for myasthenia gravis crisis with plasma exchange: 36 cases and review of current management. *J Clin Apher*. 1999;14:1–8.
237. Dyck PJ, Litchy WJ, Kratz KM, et al. Plasma exchange versus immune globulin infusion trial in chronic inflammatory demyelinating polyradiculoneuropathy. *Ann Neurol*. 1994; 36:838–845.
238. Mehndiratta MM, Hughes RA. Plasma exchange for chronic inflammatory demyelinating polyradiculoneuropathy. *Cochrane Database Syst Rev*. 2012;9:CD003906.
239. Dyck PJ, Low PA, Windebank AJ, et al. Plasma exchange in polyneuropathy associated with monoclonal gammopathy of undetermined significance. *N Engl J Med*. 1991;325(21):1482–1486.
240. Bai HX, Wang ZL, Tan LM, Xiao B, Goldstein JM, Yang L. The effectiveness of immunomodulating treatment on Miller Fisher syndrome: A retrospective analysis of 65 Chinese patients. *J Peripher Nerv Syst*. 2013;18(2):195–196.
241. Thaisetthawatkul P, Dyck PJ. Treatment of diabetic and nondiabetic lumbosacral radiculoplexus neuropathy. *Curr Treat Options Neurol*. 2010;12(2):95–99.
242. Baek WS, Bashey A, Sheean GL. Complete remission induced by rituximab in refractory, seronegative, muscle-specific kinase positive myasthenia gravis. *J Neurol Neurosurg Psychiatry*. 2007;78:771.
243. Díaz-Manera J, Martínez-Hernandez E, Querol L, et al. Long-lasting treatment effect of rituximab in MuSK myasthenia. *Neurology*. 2012;78:189–193.
244. Hain B, Jordan K, Deschauer M, Zierz S. Successful treatment of MuSK antibody-positive myasthenia gravis with rituximab. *Muscle Nerve*. 2006;33(4):575–580.

245. Nowak RJ, Dicapua DB, Zebardast N, Goldstein JM. Response of patients with refractory myasthenia gravis to rituximab: A retrospective study. *Ther Adv Neurol Disord*. 2011;4:259–266.
246. Collongues N, Casez O, Lacour A, et al. Rituximab in refractory and non-refractory myasthenia: A retrospective multicenter study. *Muscle Nerve*. 2012;46:687–691.
247. Steiglbauer K, Topakian R, Schäffer G, Aichner FT. Rituximab for myasthenia gravis: Three case reports and review of the literature. *J Neurol Sci*. 2009;280:120–122.
248. Blum S, Gillis D, Brown H, et al. Use and monitoring of low-dose rituximab in myasthenia gravis. *J Neurol Neurosurg Psychiatry*. 2011;82:659–663.
249. Kuntzer T, Carota A, Novy J, Cavassini M, Du Pasquier RA. Rituximab is successful in an HIV positive patient with MuSK myasthenia. *Neurology*. 2011;76:757–758.
250. Maddison P, McConville J, Farrugia ME, et al. The use of rituximab in myasthenia gravis and Lambert-Eaton myasthenic syndrome. *J Neurol Neurosurg Psychiatry*. 2011;82:671–673.
251. Gajra A, Vajpayee N, Grethlein SJ. Response of myasthenia gravis to rituximab in a patient with non-Hodgkin lymphoma. *Am J Hematol*. 2004;77(2):196–197.
252. Souayah N, Noopur R, Tick-Chong PS. Beneficial effects of Rituximab in patients with anti-MAG (myelin-associated glycoprotein) neuropathy: Case reports. *Immunopharmacol Immunotoxicol*. 2013;35(5):622–624.
253. Stork AC, Notermans NC, Vrancken AF, Cornblath DR, van der Pol WL. Rapid worsening of IgM anti-MAG demyelinating polyneuropathy during rituximab treatment. *J Peripher Nerv Syst*. 2013;18(2):189–191.
254. Gorson KC, Natarajan N, Ropper AH, Weinstein R. Rituximab treatment in patients with IVIg-dependent immune polyneuropathy: A prospective pilot trial. *Muscle Nerve*. 2007;35(1):66–69.
255. D'Amico A, Catteruccia M, De Benedetti F, et al. Rituximab in a childhood-onset idiopathic refractory chronic inflammatory demyelinating polyneuropathy. *Eur J Paediatr Neurol*. 2012;16(3):301–303.
256. Knecht H, Baumberger M, Tobòn A, Steck A. Sustained remission of CIDP associated with Evans syndrome. *Neurology*. 2004; 63(4):730–732.
257. Sadnicka A, Reilly MM, Mummery C, Brandner S, Hirsch N, Lunn MP. Rituximab in the treatment of three coexistent neurological autoimmune diseases: Chronic inflammatory demyelinating polyradiculoneuropathy, Morvan syndrome and myasthenia gravis. *J Neurol Neurosurg Psychiatry*. 2011;82(2): 230–232.
258. Münch C, Anagnostou P, Meyer R, Haas J. Rituximab in chronic inflammatory demyelinating polyneuropathy associated with diabetes mellitus. *J Neurol Sci*. 2007;256(1–2):100–102.
259. Kilidireas C, Anagnostopoulos A, Karandreas N, Mouselimi L, Dimopoulos MA. Rituximab therapy in monoclonal IgM-related neuropathies. *Leuk Lymphoma*. 2006;47(5):859–864.
260. Bodley-Scott DD. Chronic inflammatory demyelinating polyradiculoneuropathy responding to rituximab. *Pract Neurol*. 2005;5(4):242–245.
261. Briani C, Zara G, Zambello R, Trentin L, Rana M, Zaja F. Rituximab-responsive CIDP. *Eur J Neurol*. 2004;11(11):788.
262. Benedetti L, Briani C, Franciotta D, et al. Rituximab in patients with chronic inflammatory demyelinating polyradiculoneuropathy: A report of 13 cases and review of the literature. *J Neurol Neurosurg Psychiatry*. 2011;82(3):306–308.
263. Benedetti L, Franciotta D, Beronio A, Cadenotti L, Gobbi M, Mancardi GL, et al. Rituximab efficacy in CIDP associated with idiopathic thrombocytopenic purpura. *Muscle Nerve*. 2008;38(2):1076–1077.
264. Lunn MP. Rituximab usage in CIDP: A retrospective e-mail based data collection. *J Peripher Nerv Syst*. 2009;(14):92.
265. Kasamon YL, Nguyen TN, Chan JA, Nascimento AF. EBV-associated lymphoma and chronic inflammatory demyelinating polyneuropathy in an adult without overt immunodeficiency. *Am J Hematol*. 2002;69(4):289–293.
266. Baker MR, Das M, Isaacs J, Fawcdett PR, Bates D. Treatment of stiff person syndrome with rituximab. *J Neurol Neurosurg Psychiatry*. 2005;76:999–1001.
267. Dupond JL, Essalmi L, Gil H, Meaux-Ruault N, Hafsaoui C. Rituximab treatment of stiff-person syndrome in a patient with thymoma, diabetes mellitus and autoimmune thyroiditis. *J Clin Neurosci*. 2010;17(3):389–391.
268. Katoh N, Matsuda M, Ishii W, Morita H, Ikeda S. Successful treatment with rituximab in a patient with stiff-person syndrome complicated by dysthyroid ophthalmopathy. *Intern Med*. 2010;49(3):237–241.
269. Oddis CV, Reed AM, Aggarwal R, et al. Rituximab in the treatment of refractory adult and juvenile dermatomyositis and adult polymyositis: A randomized, placebo-phase trial. *Arthritis Rheum*. 2013;65:314–324.
270. Valiyil R, Casciola-Rosen L, Hong G, Mammen A, Christopher-Stine L. Rituximab therapy for myopathy associated with anti-signal recognition particle antibodies: A case series. *Arthritis Care Res (Hoboken)*. 2010;62(9):1328–1334.
271. Yoshikawa H, Kiuchi T, Saida T, Takamori M. Randomised double blind, placebo controlled study of tacrolimus in myasthenia gravis. *J Neurol Neurosurg Psychiatry*. 2011;82:970–977.
272. Ponseti JM, Gamez J, Azem J, et al. Post-thymectomy combined treatment of prednisone and tacrolimus versus prednisone alone for the consolidation of complete stable remission in patients with myasthenia gravis: A non-randomized, non-controlled study. *Curr Med Res Opin*. 2007;23:1269–1278.
273. Ponseti JM, Gamez J, Azem J, López-Cano M, Vilallonga R, Armengol M. Tacrolimus for myasthenia gravis: A clinical study of 212 patients. *Ann N Y Acad Sci*. 2008;1132:254–263.
274. Nagane Y, Utsugisawa K, Obara D, Kondoh R, Terayama Y. Efficacy of low-dose FK506 in the treatment of myasthenia gravis–a randomized pilot study. *Eur Neurol*. 2005;53:146–150.
275. Evoli A, Di Schino C, Marsili F, Punzi C. Successful treatment of myasthenia gravis with tacrolimus. *Muscle Nerve*. 2002;25(1):111–114.
276. Konishi T, Yoshiyama Y, Takamori M, Yagi K, Mukai E, Saida T. Japanese FK506 MG Study Group. Clinical study of FK506 in patients with myasthenia gravis. *Muscle Nerve*. 2003;28(5):570–574.
277. Sanders DB, Aarli JA, Cutter GR, Jaretzki A III, Kaminski HJ, Phillips LH II. Long-term results of tacrolimus in cyclosporine- and prednisone-dependent myasthenia gravis [comment]. *Neurology*. 2006; 66(6):954–955.
278. Tada M, Shimohata T, Tada M, et al. Long-term therapeutic efficacy and safety of low-dose tacrolimus (FK506) for myasthenia gravis. *J Neurol Sci*. 2006;247(1):17–20.
279. Wakata N, Saito T, Tanaka S, Hirano T, Oka K. Tacrolimus hydrate (FK506): Therapeutic effects and selection of responders in the treatment of myasthenia gravis. *Clin Neurol Neurosurg*. 2003;106(1):5–8.

280. Ahlmén J, Andersen O, Hallgren G, Peilot B. Positive effects of tacrolimus in a case of CIDP. *Transplant Proc.* 1998;30(8): 4194.
281. Dalakas MC, Rakocevic G, Schmidt J, et al. Effect of Alemtuzumab (CAMPATH 1-H) in patients with inclusion-body myositis. *Brain.* 2009;132(Pt 6):1536–1544.
282. Bunch TW, Worthington JW, Combs JJ, Ilstrup DM, Engel AG. Azathioprine with prednisone for polymyositis. A controlled, clinical trial. *Ann Intern Med.* 1980;92(3):365–369.
283. Heaney D, Geddes JF, Nagendren K, Swash M. Sarcoid polyneuropathy responsive to intravenous immunoglobulin. *Muscle Nerve.* 2004;29:447–450.
284. Agius MA. Treatment of ocular myasthenia gravis with corticosteroids: Yes. *Arch Neurol.* 2000;57:750–751.
285. Pascuzzi RM, Coslett HB, Johns TR. Long-term corticosteroid treatment of myasthenia gravis: Report of 116 patients. *Ann Neurol.* 1984;15:291–298.
286. Schneider-Gold C, Gajdos P, Toyka KV, Hohlfeld RR. Corticosteroids for myasthenia gravis. *Cochrane Database Syst Rev.* 2005;2:CD002828.
287. Bae JS, Go SM, Kin BJ. Clinical predictors of steroid-induced exacerbation in myasthenia gravis. *J Clin Neurosci.* 2006;13:1006–2010.
288. Arsura EL, Brunner NG, Namba T, Grob D. High-dose intravenous methylprednisolone in myasthenia gravis. *Arch Neurol.* 1985;42:1149–1153.
289. Mann JD, Johns TR, Campa JF. Long-term administration of corticosteroids in myasthenia gravis. *Neurology.* 1976;26: 729–740.
290. Dyck PJ, O'Brien P, Bosch P, et al. The multi-center double-blind controlled trial of IV methylprednisolone in diabetic lumbosacral radiculoplexus neuropathy. *Neurology.* 2006;66(suppl 2):A191.
291. Kono DH, Klashman DJ, Gilbert RC. Successful IV pulse cyclophosphamide in refractory PM in 3 patients with SLE. *J Rheumatol.* 1990;17(7):982–983.
292. Leroy JP, Drosos AA, Yiannopoulos DI, Youinou P, Moutsopoulos HM. Intravenous pulse cyclophosphamide therapy in myositis and Sjogren's syndrome. *Arthritis Rheum.* 1990;33(10):1579–1581.
293. Daniel MG, Malcangi G, Palmieri C, et al. Cyclosporin A and intravenous immunoglobulin treatment in polymyositis/dermatomyositis. *Ann Rheum Dis.* 2002;61:37–41.
294. Goei The HS, Jacobs P, et al. Cyclosporine in the treatment of intractable polymyositis. *Arthritis Rheum.* 1985;28(12): 1436–1437.
295. Hengstman GJ, van den Hoogen FH, Barrera P, et al. Successful treatment of dermatomyositis and polymyositis with anti-tumor-necrosis-factor-alpha: Preliminary observations. *Eur Neurol.* 2003;50(1):10–15.
296. Hengstman GJ, van den Hoogen FH, van Engelen BG. Treatment of dermatomyositis and polymyositis with anti-tumor necrosis factor-alpha: Long-term follow-up. *Eur Neurol.* 2004;52(1):61–63.
297. Efthimiou P, Schwartzman S, Kagen LJ. Possible role for tumour necrosis factor inhibitors in the treatment of resistant dermatomyositis and polymyositis: A retrospective study of eight patients. *Ann Rheum Dis.* 2006;65(9):1233–1236.
298. Sprott H, Glatzel M, Michel BA. Treatment of myositis with etanercept (Enbrel), a recombinant human soluble fusion protein of TNF-alpha type II receptor and IgG1. *Rheumatology (Oxford).* 2004;43(4):524–526.
299. Coyle K, Pokrovnichka A, French K, Joe G, Shrader J, Swan L, et al. A randomized, double-blind, placebo controlled trial of infliximab in patients with polymyositis and dermatomyositis. *Arth Rheum* 2008;58(suppl); Abstract No: 2058.
300. Riley P, McCann LJ, Maillard SM, Woo P, Murray KJ, Pilkington CA. Effectiveness of infliximab in the treatment of refractory juvenile dermatomyositis with calcinosis. *Rheumatology (Oxford).* 2008;47(6):877–880.
301. Labioche I, Liozon E, Weschler B, Loustaud-Ratti V, Soria P, Vidal E. Refractory polymyositis responding to infliximab: Extended follow-up. *Rheumatology (Oxford).* 2004;43(4): 531–532.
302. Radziwill AJ, Botez SA, Novy J, Kuntzer T. Interferon beta-1a as adjunctive treatment for multifocal motor neuropathy: An open label trial. *J Peripher Nerv Syst.* 2009;14(3):201–202.
303. Patwa HS, Chaudhry H. Katzberg H, Rae-Grant AD, So YT. Evidence-based guideline: Intravenous immunoglobulin in the treatment of neuromuscular disorders: Report of the Therapeutics and Technology Assessment Subcommittee of the American Academy of Neurology. *Neurology.* 2012;78:1009–1015.
304. Hughes RA, Raphael JC, Swan AV, van Doorn PA. Intravenous immunoglobulin for Guillain-Barré syndrome. *Cochrane Database Syst Rev.* 2006(1):CD002063.
305. Hughes RA, Donofrio PD, Bril V, et al.; ICE Group. Intravenous immune globulin (10% caprylate-chromatography purified) for the treatment of chronic inflammatory demyelinating polyradiculoneuropathy (ICE study): A randomized placebo-controlled trial. *Lancet Neurol.* 2008;7:115–116.
306. Hahn AF, Bolton CF, Zochodne DW, Feasby TE. Intravenous immunoglobulin treatment in chronic inflammatory demyelinating polyneuropathy: A double blind, placebo controlled, cross over study. *Brain.* 1996;119:1067–1077.
307. Hughes RA, Bensa S, Willison HJ, et al. Randomized controlled trial of intravenous gammaglobulin vs oral prednisolone in chronic inflammatory demyelinating polyradiculoneuropathy. *Ann Neurol.* 2001;50:195–201.
308. Mendell JR, Barohn RJ, Freimer ML, et al. Randomized controlled trial of IVIG in untreated chronic inflammatory demyelinating polyradiculoneuropathy. *Neurology.* 2001;56: 445–449.
309. Vermulen M, van Doorn PA, Brand A, Strengers PF, Jennekens FG, Bussch HF. Intravenous immunoglobulin treatment in patients with chronic inflammatory demyelinating polyneuropathy. *J Neurol Neurosurg Psychiatry.* 1993;56:36–39.
310. Van Schaik I, Winer JB, De Haan R, Vermeulen M. Intravenous immunoglobulins for chronic inflammatory demyelinating polyradiculoneuropathy. *Cochrane Database Syst Rev.* 2002;(2):CD001797.
311. Viala K, Maisonobe T, Stojkovic T, et al. A current view of the diagnosis, clinical variants, response to treatment and prognosis of chronic inflammatory demyelinating polyradiculoneuropathy. *J Peripher Nerv Syst.* 2010;15(1):50–56.
312. Mehndiratta MM, Hughes RA . Corticosteroids for chronic inflammatory demyelinating polyradiculoneuropathy. *Cochrane Database Syst Rev.* 2012;8:CD002062.
313. Eftimov F, Vermeulen M, van Doorn PA, Brusse E, van Schaik IN; PREDICT Study Group. Long-term remission of CIDP after pulsed high-dose dexamethasone or short term prednisolone treatment. *Neurology.* 2012;78:1079–1084.
314. Azulay JP, Blin O, Pouget J, et al. Intravenous immunoglobulin treatment in patients with motor neuron syndromes associated

with anti-GM1 antibodies: A double-blind, placebo-controlled study. *Neurology*. 1994;44:429–432.
315. Federico P, Zochodne DW, Hahn AF, Brown WF, Feasby TE. Multifocal motor neuropathy improved by IVIG: Randomized, double-blind, placebo-controlled study. *Neurology*. 2000;55:1256–1262.
316. Leger JM, Chassande B, Musset L, Meininger V, Bouche P, Baumann N. Intravenous immunoglobulin therapy in multifocal motor neuropathy: A double-blind, placebo-controlled study. *Brain*. 2001;124:145–153.
317. van Schaik IN, van den Berg LH, de Haan R, Vermeulen M. Intravenous immunoglobulin for multifocal motor neuropathy. *Cochrane Database Syst Rev*. 2005;18:CD004429.
318. Joint Task Force of the EFNS and the PNS. European Federation of Neurological Societies/Peripheral Nerve Society Guideline on management of multifocal motor neuropathy. Report of a joint task force of the European Federation of Neurological Societies and the Peripheral Nerve Society. *J Peripher Nerv Syst*. 2006;11:1–8.
319. Van den Berg LH, Franssen H, Wokke JH. Improvement of multifocal motor neuropathy during long-term weekly treatment with human immunoglobulin. *Neurology*. 1995;45: 987–988.
320. Joint Task Force of the EFNS and the PNS. European Federation of Neurological Societies/Peripheral Nerve Society Guideline on management of multifocal motor neuropathy. Report of a Joint Task Force of the European Federation of Neurological Societies and the Peripheral Nerve Society – first revision. *J Peripher Nerv Syst*. 2010;15:295–301.
321. Bain PG, Motomura M, Newsom-Davis J, et al. Effects of intravenous immunoglobulin on muscle weakness and calcium-channel autoantibodies in the Lambert-Eaton myasthenic syndrome. *Neurology*. 1996;47:678–683.
322. Cherin P, Herson S, Weschsler B, et al. Efficacy of intravenous gammaglobulin therapy in chronic refractory polymyositis and dermatomyositis; an open study with 20 adult patients. *Am J Med*. 1991;91:162–168.
323. Dalakas MC. Intravenous immune globulin for dermatomyositis. *N Engl J Med*. 1994;330:1392–1393.
324. Kuwano Y, Ihn H, Yazawa N, et al. Successful treatment of dermatomyositis with high-dose intravenous immunoglobulin. *Acta Derm Venereol*. 2006;86:158–159.
325. Mastaglia FL, Phillips BA, Zilko PJ. Immunoglobulin therapy in inflammatory myopathies. *J Neurol Neurosurg Psychiatry*. 1998;63:107–110.
326. Williams L, Chang PY, Park E, Gorson KC, Bayer-Zwirello L. Successful treatment of dermatomyositis during pregnancy with intravenous immunoglobulin monotherapy. *Obstet Gynecol*. 2007;109(Pt 2):561–563.
327. Cherin P, Piette JC, Wechsler B, et al. Intravenous gamma globulin as first line therapy in polymyositis and dermatomyositis: An open study in 11 adult patients. *J Rheumatol*. 1994;21:1092–1097.
328. Cherin P, Pelletier S, Teixeira A, et al. Results and longterm followup of intravenous immunoglobulin infusions in chronic, refractory polymyositis: An open study with thirty five adult patients. *Arthritis Rheum*. 2002;46:467–474.
329. Genevay S, Saudan-Kister A, Guerne PA. Intravenous gammaglobulins in refractory polymyositis: Lower dose for maintenancetreatmentiseffective. *AnnRheumDis*. 2001;60:635–636.
330. Wang DX, Shu XM, Tian XL, et al. Intravenous immunoglobulin therapy in adult patients with polymyositis/dermatomyositis: A systematic literature review. *Clin Rheumatol*. 2012;31(5):801–806.
331. Dalakas MC, Fujii M, Li M, Lufti B, Kyhos J, McElroy B. High-dose intravenous immune globulin for stiff-person syndrome. *N Engl J Med*. 2001;345:1870–1876.
332. Dalakas M, Koffman B, Fujii M, Spector S, Sivakumar K, Cupler E. A controlled study of intravenous immunoglobulin combined with prednisone in the treatment of IBM. *Neurology*. 2001;56:323–327.
333. Dalakas MC, Sonies B, Dambrosia J, Sekul E, Cupler E, Sivakumar K. Treatment of inclusion body myositis with IVIG: A double-blind placebo controlled study. *Neurology*. 1997;48:712–716.
334. Walter MC, Lochmuller H, Toepfer M, et al. High-dose immunoglobulin therapy in sporadic inclusion body myositis: A double blind placebo-controlled study. *J Neurol*. 2000;247:22–28.
335. Mukunda BN, Kumar PD, Smith HR. Long-lasting effectiveness of intravenous immunoglobulin in a patient with inclusion-body myositis. *Ann Intern Med*. 2001;134:1156.
336. Dalakas MC, Quarles RH, Farrer RG, et al. A controlled study of intravenous immunoglobulin in demyelinating neuropathy with IgM gammopathy. *Ann Neurol*. 1996;40:792–795.
337. Comi G, Roveri L, Swan A, et al. A randomised controlled trial of intravenous immunoglobulin in IgM paraprotein associated demyelinating neuropathy. *J Neurol*. 2002;249:1370–1377.
338. Gorson KC, Ropper AH, Weinberg DH, Weinstein R. Efficacy of intravenous immunoglobulin in patients with IgG monoclonal gammopathy and polyneuropathy. *Arch Neurol*. 2002;59:766–772.
339. Kornberg AJ, Pestronk A. Antibody-associated polyneuropathy syndromes: Principles and treatment. *Semin Neurol*. 2003;23:181–189.
340. Joint Task Force of the EFNS and the PNS. European Federation of Neurological Societies/Peripheral Nerve Society Guideline on management of paraproteinemic demyelinating neuropathies. Report of a Joint Task Force of the European Federation of Neurological Societies and the Peripheral Nerve Society—first revision. *J Peripher Nerv Syst*. 2010;15:185–195.
341. Courtney AE, McDonnell GV, Patterson VH. Human immunoglobulin for diabetic amyotrophy—a promising prospect? *Postgrad Med*. 2001;77:326–328.
342. Fernandes Filho JA, Nathan BM, Palmert MR, Katieji B. Diabetic amyotrophy in an adolescent responsive to intravenous immunoglobulin. *Muscle Nerve*. 2005;32:818–820.
343. Morlii T, Fujita H, Toyoshima I, Sageshima M, Ito S. Efficacy of immunoglobulin and prednisolone in diabetic amyotrophy. *Endocr J*. 2003;50:831–832.
344. Ogawa T, Taguchi T, Tanaka Y, Ikeguchi K, Nakano I. Intravenous immunoglobulin therapy for diabetic amyotrophy. *Intern Med*. 2001;40:349–352.
345. Said G, Goulon-Goeau C, Lacroix C, Moulonguet A. Nerve biopsy findings in different patterns of proximal diabetic neuropathy. *Ann Neurol*. 1994;35:559–569.
346. Pascoe MK, Low PA, Windebank AJ, Litchy WJ. Subacute diabetic proximal neuropathy. *Mayo Clin Proc*. 1997;72: 1123–1132.
347. Romdenne P, Mukendi R, Stasse P, Indekeu P, Buysschaert M, Colin IM. An unusual neuropathy in a diabetic patient:

Evidence for intravenous immunoglobulin induced effective therapy. *Diabetes Metab*. 2001;27:155–158.
348. Wada Y, Yanagihara C, Nishimura Y, Oka N. A case of diabetic amyotrophy with severe atrophy and weakness of shoulder girdle muscles showing good response to intravenous immune globulin. *Diabetes Res Clin Pract*. 2007;75:107–110.
349. Zochodne DW, Isaac D, Jones C. Failure of immunotherapy to prevent, arrest or reverse lumbosacral plexopathy. *Acta Neurol Scand*. 2003;107:299.
350. Mori M, Kuwabara S, Fukutake T, Hattori T. Intravenous immunoglobulin therapy for Miller Fisher syndrome. *Neurology*. 2007;68:1144–1146.
351. Kizawa M, Mori K, Iijima M, Koike H, Hattori N, Sobue G. Intravenous immunoglobulin treatment in painful sensory neuropathy without sensory ataxia associated with Sjogren's syndrome. *J Neurol Neurosurg Psychiatry*. 2006;77:967–969.
352. Molina JA, BenitoLeon J, Bermejo F, Jimenez FJ, Olivan J. Intravenous immunoglobulin therapy in sensory neuropathy associated with Sjogren's syndrome. *J Neurol Neurosurg Psychiatry*. 1996;60:699.
353. Pascual J, Cid C, Berciano J. High-dose i.v. immunoglobulin for peripheral neuropathy associated with Sjogren's syndrome. *Neurology*. 1998;51:650–651.
354. Taguchi Y, Takashima S, Takata M, Dougu N, Asaoka E, Inoue H. High-dose intravenous immunoglobulin in the treatment of sensory ataxic neuropathy with Sjogren's syndrome: A case report. *No To Shinkei*. 2004;56:421–424.
355. Takahashi Y, Takata T, Hoshino M, Sakurai M, Kanazawa I. Benefit of IVIG for long-standing ataxic sensory neuronopathy with Sjögren's syndrome. *Neurology*. 2003;60:503–505.
356. Wolfe GI, Nations SP, Burns DK, Herbelin LL, Barohn RJ. Benefit of IVIG for long-standing ataxic sensory neuronopathy with Sjögren's syndrome. *Neurology*. 2003;61:873.
357. Burns TM, Quijano-Roy S, Jones HR. Benefit of IVIG for long-standing ataxic sensory neuronopathy with Sjögren's syndrome. *Neurology*. 2003;61:873.
358. Ponsford S, Willison H, Veitch J, Morris R, Thomas PK. Long-term clinical and neurophysiological follow-up of patients with peripheral neuropathy associated with benign monoclonal gammopathy. *Muscle Nerve*. 2000;23:164–174.
359. Levy Y, Uziel Y, Zandman GG, et al. Intravenous immunoglobulin in peripheral neuropathy associated with vasculitis. *Ann Rheum Dis*. 2003;62:1221–1223.
360. Tsurikisawa N, Taniguchi M, Saito H, et al. Treatment of Churg-Strauss syndrome with high-dose intravenous immunoglobulin. *Ann Allergy Asthma Immunol*. 2004;92:80–87.
361. Carpo M, Meucci N, Allaria S, et al. Anti-sulfatide IgM antibodies in peripheral neuropathy. *J Neurol Sci*. 2000;176:144–150.
362. Kuhl V, Vogt T, Anghelescu I. Intravenous immunoglobulin and prednisolone treatment of cryoglobulinemic polyneuropathy. *Nervenarzt*. 2001;72:445–448.
363. Gondim FA, Brannagan TH III, Sander HW, Chin RL, Latov N. Peripheral neuropathy in patients with inflammatory bowel disease. *Brain*. 2005;128:867–879.
364. Nobuhara Y, Saito M, Goto R, et al. Chronic progressive sensory ataxic neuropathy associated with limited systemic sclerosis. *J Neurol Sci*. 2006;241:103–106.
365. Lesprit P, Mouloud F, Bierling P, et al. Prolonged remission of SLE-associated polyradiculoneuropathy after a single course of intravenous immunoglobulin. *Scand J Rheumatol*. 1996;25: 177–179.
366. Nakajima M, Fujioka S, Ohno H, Iwamoto K. Partial but rapid recovery from paralysis after immunomodulation during early stage of neuralgic amyotrophy. *Eur Neurol*. 2006;55:227–229.
367. Takakura, Y, Murai H, Furaya H, Ochi H, Kira J. A case of brachial diplegia accompanied with Sjögren's syndrome presenting good response to immunotherapies in the early course of the disease. *Rinsho Shinkeigaku*. 2005;45:346–350.
368. Tsao BE, Avery R, Shield RW. Neuralgic amyotrophy precipitated by Epstein-Barr virus. *Neurology*. 2004;62:1234–1235.
369. Léger JM, Viala K, Nicolas G, et al. Placebo-controlled trial of rituximab in IgM anti-myelin associated glycoprotein neuropathy. *Neurology*. 2013;80:2217–2225.

CHAPTER 5

The Rehabilitation of Neuromuscular Diseases

Sabrina Paganoni and Erik Ensrud

Rehabilitation is the process of assisting a person to maximize function and quality of life. Therefore, rehabilitation matters to people with neuromuscular diseases because it enables them to reach their fullest potential despite the presence of a disability. Too often, patients are told "there is nothing we can do" for their neuromuscular conditions. At times this judgment is not expressed explicitly, but transpires from nonverbal cues during patient encounters. Such attitudes cast a dark shadow on the therapeutic alliance between the physician and the patient and lead to disengagement and lower quality of care. On the contrary, here we will argue that "there is always something we can do" for our patients. While there are no life-prolonging treatments for many neuromuscular disorders, interventions are often available that can assist people in continuing to function independently and safely, both in their vocational and personal lives, manage their symptoms, and live fulfilling lives in spite of the presence of a physical impairment. In this chapter, we will look at neuromuscular diseases from a rehabilitation perspective. We will first review the role of exercise, orthoses, mobility aids, adaptive equipment, and environmental modifications with respect to their impact on function and quality of life. We will then develop a rehabilitation framework to address common neuromuscular problems such as axial weakness, spinal deformities, proximal upper and lower limb weakness, hand weakness, foot drop, falls, foot abnormalities, joint contractures, spasticity, pain, ptosis, dysphagia, and dysarthria.

Rehabilitation is sometimes overlooked because it is not clear who is in charge of it and when it should begin. It is commonly accepted that the multifaceted rehabilitation needs of neuromuscular patients are best served by a multidisciplinary team that may include neurologists, physiatrists, nurses, physical therapists (PTs), orthotists, occupational therapists (OTs), speech and language pathologists (SLPs), nutritionists, respiratory therapists, psychologists, palliative care experts, pain medicine specialists, vocational consultants, recreational therapists, and social workers. Receiving care in a multidisciplinary clinic has been suggested to benefit people with certain neuromuscular diseases [i.e., amyotrophic lateral sclerosis (ALS)] by optimizing health care delivery and, possibly, prolonging survival and enhancing quality of life.[1] But what is the role of each member of the multidisciplinary team and who is responsible for advocating for the patient and for coordinating care among the different rehabilitation professionals? Neuromuscular specialists periodically assess the patients' functional status in a neuromuscular clinic. We therefore argue that the neuromuscular specialist, most often a neurologist or a physiatrist, is ideally positioned to lead the rehabilitation efforts while leveraging the expertise of the different team members. This may seem like a daunting and time-consuming task. However, most of what is required is simply adequate knowledge of the available tools and effective communication. A clear understanding of the role and capabilities of each team member is essential for proper referrals and results in higher quality of care and a time-efficient practice.

Neuromuscular specialists most commonly refer patients to PTs, OTs, and SLPs. While there is some overlap between the skill sets of PTs and OTs, PTs specialize in gait assessment and training, biomechanics, core stability, balance, and functional mobility such as transfers.[2] PTs also specialize in teaching stretching techniques and developing aerobic conditioning and strengthening exercise programs. OTs assist people to participate in the everyday activities (occupations) they need and want to do. They focus on proper posture and ergonomics related to upper limb functional activities such as feeding, grooming, dressing, and using a telephone or a computer. Both types of therapists utilize active and passive therapeutic exercises, physical modalities (such as heat, cold, and electrical stimulation), and manual techniques (such as massage, joint mobilization, and myofascial release techniques) to address pain and impairments in strength, flexibility, balance, posture, and endurance. They may work in close contact with orthotists if orthoses (i.e., braces) are indicated and they may recommend splints, assistive devices, adaptive equipment, and/or home modifications. Some PTs and OTs specialize in assistive technology, such as systems to allow access to computers and environmental controls (e.g., lights, television, etc.) for people with motor impairment.

SLPs manage disorders of speech, language, cognition, communication, and swallowing. Some SLPs specialize in augmentative and alternative communication (AAC) technology to provide systems to supplement or replace natural speech. As an example, people with ALS may utilize voice banking to digitally record words and phrases while still able to do so, for later inclusion in a communication device. Some AAC systems incorporate computer access capabilities and options for environmental controls, both of which can generally be mounted on a wheelchair. When dysphagia is suspected, SLPs utilize clinical oral motor assessments as well as instrumental measures [i.e., fiberoptic endoscopic evaluation of swallowing (FEES) and modified barium swallow (MBS) study] for proper assessment of the swallowing impairment and to recommend diet modifications and compensatory strategies. They may also work with dieticians to optimize meal planning. Depending on the individual patient's needs, additional healthcare professionals such as respiratory therapists, psychologists, palliative care experts, pain medicine specialists, vocational consultants, recreational therapists, and social workers might provide additional expertise to address specific rehabilitation needs.

While diagnostic procedures are often complex and energy consuming in neuromuscular medicine, it is best to start thinking "functionally" early on. The International Classification of Functioning, Disability and Health (ICF) model defines impairments as deficits within the performance of an organ or body system. For example, foot drop is an impairment caused by the weakness of a group of muscles that can result from neurogenic causes or, less frequently, other neuromuscular disorders, such as myopathy or disorders of neuromuscular transmission. Activity limitation in the ICF model refers to deficient performance of basic functional tasks, such as slowed walking speed, whereas participation restriction refers to the consequent inability to fulfill a role within the home or community environment, such as self-care activities and shopping.[3] Rehabilitative interventions might target impairments, activity limitations, and/or participation restrictions.[4] Different strategies (and different outcome measures) need to be considered depending on the goal of therapy. As an example, the therapy directed toward an impairment, such as exercise and bracing to target impaired range of motion (ROM) in a weak hand, might have great functional impact even if the actual degree of improvement in ROM is small. In this example, after intervention, the person might be able to perform a previously limited activity, such as typing on a computer, and as a result be able to participate in social activities which were previously restricted. Of note, similar rehabilitation strategies can often be utilized regardless of the exact etiology.

Rehabilitation should ideally start at the first patient encounter. Certainly, rehabilitation should begin before maladaptive patterns develop. As an example, it is common experience that it is much easier to prevent, rather than treat, contractures. This notion becomes especially important in rapidly progressive diseases such as ALS and requires forward thinking on the part of the rehabilitation team. We cannot emphasize enough how crucial early intervention is for people with progressive neuromuscular weakness. For instance, even in the early stages of the disease, before the onset of severe weakness, therapists can educate patients on energy conservation techniques such as pacing, taking rest breaks, and using bracing and adaptive equipment when performing demanding activities, perhaps on an intermittent basis. Such interventions might help reduce fatigue, a highly prevalent symptom in many neuromuscular diseases.[5–7] Further, early focus on biomechanics, ergonomics, stretching, and bracing helps people to remain as functional as possible and can help to delay or even prevent many of the negative sequelae of impaired strength.

Rehabilitation should be approached in a problem-oriented fashion, focusing on what the person needs most at any particular time in the course of his/her disease in order to maintain maximal function and quality of life. Thus rehabilitation may include management of one or more impairments (e.g., impairment in strength, ROM, and tone), activity limitations (limitations with walking, standing, transferring, self-feeding, toileting, dressing, grooming, and bathing), and participation restrictions (such as participation in sports and leisure activities). Importantly, rehabilitation needs may change over time. Clinicians need to be aware of the disease's natural history and resource availability in order to anticipate needs and recommend interventions at appropriate times. In addition, rehabilitation strategies should be attentive to the person's environment and his or her family and support systems. Environmental modifications and family training are therefore integral to the rehabilitation process.

Given the multitude of functional challenges that many people with neuromuscular diseases may experience, it is best to approach them systematically by making a list of issues or a "rehabilitation assessment and plan" (rehabilitation A&P) that should be included in clinic notes alongside the medical A&P and reviewed at every follow-up visit. Developing a rehabilitation A&P requires consideration of the person's disease in relation to the changes in functional status that it creates. An individual with a generalized neuromuscular condition such as ALS or muscular dystrophy may present with weakness in multiple muscle groups which the clinician carefully records with periodic manual muscle testing performed at every follow-up visit. But what is the resulting activity limitation, and what can we do about it? If a person with ALS develops hand weakness, how does this impact his or her ability to carry out desired activities of daily living (ADLs), such as dressing and grooming, or instrumental ADLs (more complex tasks such as care of children or use of telephones and other communication devices)? Can we suggest any strategies to compensate for or adapt to the hand weakness? Is abnormal muscle tone a limitation at this time? Is the patient at risk of developing finger contractures? Can the work environment be modified to allow him or her to continue to work despite the hand weakness? Can the caregivers be trained to help with ROM exercises? Which healthcare professionals might provide optimal expertise to address this problem at this time (OTs, vocational consultants, and so on)? Can the person benefit from assistive devices to maintain independence with feeding, dressing and toileting? If the hand weakness prevents him or her from comfortably using telephones and computers, which assistive technology system can we recommend? Clearly, the extent and treatment goals of the rehabilitation A&P may differ substantially depending on the underlying pathologic process. Impairments may be limited to one domain or involve multiple systems, may be static or progressive, and may be impacted by comorbidities, such as pre-existing musculoskeletal abnormalities, and environmental limitations. Rehabilitation goals may include restoration of function for some patients. When restoration of neurologic function is not achievable, teaching adaptive or compensatory techniques may allow the person to maintain independence and prevent negative sequelae of muscle weakness such as contractures and pain. Palliative care might be needed in some neuromuscular diseases and might be viewed as the end of the rehabilitation spectrum.

In people with progressive disorders such as ALS, hereditary neuropathies, and muscular dystrophies, it is crucial to frequently reassess rehabilitation strategies and modify them with changes in disease status. As an example, if a person with ALS, Charcot-Marie-Tooth (CMT), or a distal myopathy develops ankle dorsiflexion weakness, an ankle-foot orthosis (AFO) may be prescribed to improve gait efficiency, conserve energy, and reduce fall risk. A few gait training sessions with a PT are important to successfully learn to ambulate with a brace. Later in the course of the disease, when the individual loses the ability to ambulate, a PT should provide recommendations for a customized wheelchair. A few therapy sessions might also be indicated for the patient and his or her caregiver to provide training on stretching and ROM exercises to prevent contracture formation. If the person then develops pain or is uncomfortable when sitting in the wheelchair, wheelchair evaluation should be performed and adjustments made accordingly.

Rather than writing generic therapy prescriptions, it is best to address specific problems (e.g., gait training, transfer training, wheelchair evaluation, etc.) and periodically reassess needs. Working in close contact with therapists who are familiar with neuromuscular diseases will help ensure that therapy sessions are focused on what the individual really needs at that specific time. Of note, insurance carriers limit the number of therapy sessions for which people are eligible in a given period of time. Continued skilled therapy services (i.e., performed by a skilled health care professional such as a PT) to maintain current functional status have traditionally been denied in chronic conditions because there was no expectation for the person to "improve" (a concept known as "improvement standard"). A recent settlement in the class action "Improvement Standard" lawsuit (*Jimmo vs. Kathleen Sebelius*) upheld the right of patients to continue to receive reasonable and necessary care to maintain their condition and prevent or slow decline. The type of care covered under this settlement, however, refers only to skilled care and not to maintenance programs that can be performed by the patient or with the assistance of nontherapists, including unskilled caregivers. At this time of significant changes in the American health care system, the practical impact of this settlement on the rehabilitation of people with progressive neuromuscular diseases remains to be determined. Coverage for durable medical equipment (DME) might also be limited. Loaner programs and support from patient advocacy organizations might help ease the financial burden and allow people to try different models of the same type of device before buying expensive material that they might not want or be able to use effectively. Of note, once patients are enrolled in hospice, most, if not all DME, must be paid out of pocket. Therefore, it is important to know the natural history of the disease and purchase equipment accordingly.

We will now review the tools that the rehabilitation team can use to assist people to maximize function and quality of life. We will then suggest a practical approach to address the rehabilitation problems that are most frequently encountered in neuromuscular medicine. However, one should keep in mind that rehabilitation science is in constant development and the clinical problems posed by particular patients might be unique and require creative thinking on the therapists' part. Therefore, the approach suggested here should not be viewed as a "fix-all recipe" but rather as a platform for discussion. Most importantly, with this chapter, we want to draw attention on the importance of periodic functional assessments and the need to think of rehabilitation as a fundamental part of neuromuscular medicine practice.

▶ REHABILITATION TOOLS AND STRATEGIES FOR THEIR USE

EXERCISE

It is not infrequent for people with neuromuscular diseases to inquire about exercise. Physical activity and exercise are an integral part of the premorbid lifestyle for many neuromuscular patients. Therefore, patients often ask whether exercise is safe, whether it can help slow down their disease, and what type of exercise is recommended for their particular condition. It is not easy to answer these questions. Strictly speaking, these are questions that cannot be answered based on the currently available evidence. Unfortunately, there is a paucity of literature on the topic of exercise in neuromuscular disorders.[8]

Exercise studies in neuromuscular medicine are limited in both quantity and quality. Limitations in the available studies include small sample size, heterogeneous patient population, uncontrolled and nonrandomized design, short-term training, variable exercise protocols, and outcome measures. Some investigators have attempted to circumvent difficulties in recruiting a nonexercising control group with similar disease characteristics by asking the subjects to exercise only one side of the body, with the contralateral side serving as control. A nonexercised limb, however, is not an appropriate control due to the phenomenon of cross-education. Unilateral training induces strength gains not only in the trained limb, but also in the homologous muscles of the contralateral limb.[9] Therefore, comparisons should be made between training and nontraining patients. A recent Cochrane review on exercise training for myopathies

▶ TABLE 5-1. TYPES OF EXERCISE RELEVANT TO PATIENTS WITH NEUROMUSCULAR DISEASES

Type of Exercise	Description	Benefits
Flexibility	Stretching Range-of-motion (ROM)	Part of the standard of care for the prevention and management of contractures Might help to manage pain and spasticity
Resistance/strengthening	Repeated muscle actions against resistance: – isometric – concentric – *avoid* eccentric	*Potential* role in: – strengthening weak muscles – reversing disuse weakness – delaying onset of functional impairment More disease-specific research needed
Aerobic	Dynamic activity using large muscle groups	*Potential* role in: – improving aerobic capacity – improving mood, quality of life, sleep, functional independence – preventing chronic diseases and maintaining bone density More disease-specific research needed
Balance	Balance training using different modalities	*Potential* role in: – fall risk reduction More disease-specific research needed

identified only three high-quality randomized clinical trials.[8] Additional evidence mostly comes from observational or uncontrolled trials and recommendations have been primarily based on the consensus of the expert review panel.[10] The types of exercise that are relevant to people with neuromuscular disorders are flexibility, resistance, aerobic, and balance exercises (Table 5-1).

FLEXIBILITY TRAINING

Flexibility training involves stretching and ROM exercises. The potential benefits of this type of exercise include prevention and treatment of spasticity and contractures, as well as the pain that often accompanies them. Because many people with neuromuscular diseases are at risk for the development of these complications, flexibility training is often incorporated into the standard of care.[11]

Neuromuscular specialists are ideally positioned to advocate the early initiation of flexibility training. Supervision from a PT is often needed to initiate a correct stretching program. PTs may then periodically reassess progress, guide program modifications, or suggest further treatment modalities such as positioning, splinting, bracing, orthoses, and standing devices. Stretching, however, should not be limited to therapy sessions and should be done daily for any specific joint or muscle group that is at risk for contracture development. Stretching can be done at home, school, or work, as well as in the clinic.[11] It is important for people to understand that stretching can be safely performed outside of the clinic environment either independently or with caregiver assistance, and that consistency produces the best results. In this respect, caregiver involvement is essential. When individuals cannot perform active stretching due to significant weakness, active-assisted and/or passive techniques may be implemented with caregiver's help.

AEROBIC AND STRENGTHENING EXERCISE

In comparison with data from people with neuromuscular diseases, the quality of the evidence on the beneficial effects of aerobic and strengthening exercise in the able-bodied population is excellent. In healthy individuals, moderate-intensity physical activity significantly improves overall health. In addition, it is related to improving the outcomes of several chronic diseases, such as heart disease, stroke, and type 2 diabetes. Based on this evidence, the American College of Sports Medicine (ACSM) declared that "Exercise is medicine™" inviting physicians to write exercise prescriptions to promote physical activity and exercise as standard parts of disease prevention and medical treatment.[12]

Here we define aerobic exercise training, or cardiorespiratory fitness training, as an activity that uses large muscle groups, that can be maintained continuously, and that is rhythmical and aerobic in nature such as walking, hiking, running, cycling, and swimming. Guidelines for aerobic training for the general population were published in 2008 by the US Department of Health and Human Services. The Physical Activity Guidelines for Americans state that adults aged 18 to 64 should do 150 minutes a week of moderate-intensity or 75 minutes a week of vigorous-intensity aerobic physical activity, in bouts of at least 10 minutes and preferably spread throughout the week. The same guidelines state that older adults (aged 65 and older) and individuals with disabilities should follow the same guidelines, but, if this is not possible due to limiting health conditions, they should be as physically active as their abilities allow and avoid inactivity.

The same guidelines also recommend performing muscle-strengthening activities that involve all major muscle groups 2 or more days per week. Strength training is defined as an activity performed to improve muscle strength and endurance and is typically carried out by making repeated muscle actions against resistance.[13] Strength training includes different types of muscle actions: isometric (i.e., performed at a constant muscle length with no joint movement, as in wall squat hold and plank exercises), concentric (i.e., the muscle generates force while shortening, as when lifting a dumbbell towards the body), and eccentric (i.e., the muscle generates force while lengthening, as when lowering a weight away from the body or landing back on the ground after jumping). For healthy adults, the ACSM recommends one set of about 10 exercises to condition all major muscle groups, 2 to 3 days per week. Healthy adults should complete at least one set of 8 to 12 repetitions per exercise at loads of at least 45% to 50% of the one-repetition maximum (1RM) (which is the maximal load that can be lifted throughout the full ROM once).[13,14]

But how can we translate these general guidelines into exercise recommendations for people with neuromuscular diseases? We will first review the available studies and then draw offer some general recommendations, at all times being mindful of the overarching principle of *primum non nocere*. When evaluating studies of the outcome of exercise in different patient populations, one should keep in mind that slowing the rate of functional impairment is a positive result in progressive neuromuscular diseases, while actual gain of strength or aerobic capacity might be a goal only in selected conditions. Additional factors that need to be considered are the presence of comorbidities (such as heart and restrictive lung disease in certain neuromuscular conditions), the specific disorder, rate of progression, and expected natural history.

In the available studies, primary outcome measures have mostly been limited to effects at the impairment level: aerobic capacity and measures of muscle strength. Ideally, the primary outcomes of exercise studies should also include measures of function such as improvement in the ability to walk, perform ADLs, and participate in work, sports, and recreational activities, as these are the outcomes that really matter to patients. Secondary outcomes for exercise training have included measured of pain or fatigue, quality of life, and mood. These secondary outcome measures are very important to consider as well, given the high prevalence of these problems in many neuromuscular diseases.[5–7,15,16]

Exercise Studies in ALS

Preclinical evidence gathered in the transgenic mutant SOD1 mouse model of ALS has suggested a potential benefit from moderate endurance exercise with delay in disease onset and survival.[17–19] In these mice, however, high-intensity endurance training was shown to hasten the decrease in motor performance and death.[19,20] In humans, a study by Drory et al. suggested that a regular moderate exercise program (30 minutes or less daily) might have a positive effect on disability in people with ALS.[21] The study included 25 ALS subjects who were randomized to perform a moderate daily program of activities as opposed to avoiding any physical activity beyond their usual daily requirements. At 3 months from the initiation of the study, subjects who performed regular exercise showed less deterioration on the ALS Functional Rating Scale (ALS-FRS) and the Ashworth spasticity scale.[21] At 6 months, there was no significant difference between the groups, although a trend towards less deterioration was observed in the treated group.[21] Bello-Haas et al. have recently analyzed strength training in a randomized trial which included 27 ALS subjects.[22] The study involved 6 months of training, three times a week, following an individualized program. The resistance exercise group had significantly better function, as measured by total ALS-FRS scores, and quality of life, without adverse effects as compared with subjects receiving usual care.[22] These studies suggest that moderate exercise might be safe for people with ALS, but are too small to draw definitive conclusions. Additional research is ongoing to confirm these findings and determine whether exercise might actually improve function in this population.

Exercise Studies in People with Charcot-Marie-Tooth Disease

There is only one randomized clinical trial on the effect of strength training in CMT disease. In this study, 29 CMT subjects were randomized to 24 weeks of progressive resistance exercise of their lower limbs which was performed three times a week.[23] Subjects in the training arm reported a moderate increase in knee torque without adverse effects.[23] Other small studies reported moderate strength gains in CMT patients compared to their baseline values.[24,25] Positive effects of aerobic exercise on fatigue have also been reported in this patient population.[24]

Exercise Studies in the Dystrophinopathies

Preclinical studies in the *mdx* mouse model of Duchenne muscular dystrophy have led clinicians to advise against exercise in the dystrophinopathies. Dystrophin is an important structural protein and animal studies have demonstrated contraction-induced muscle injury in dystrophinopathy, especially after eccentric exercise.[26–29] In humans, the few available studies have been small and have provided conflicting results precluding any definitive conclusions.[28,30] High-resistance strength training and eccentric exercise are universally considered inappropriate across the lifespan owing to concerns about contraction-induced muscle-fiber injury.[11] However, sub-maximum aerobic exercise is recommended by some clinicians, especially early in the course of the disease, in order to avoid disuse atrophy and other secondary complications of inactivity.[11] Most clinicians advise boys with dystrophinopathy who are ambulatory or in the early nonambulatory stage to participate in regular gentle functional strengthening and recreation-based activities in the community. In this respect, low-impact activities such as swimming appear most beneficial.[11] The optimal level of exercise for people with dystrophinopathy is the subject of current research protocols.[31–33]

Exercise Studies in FSHD

There is only one randomized clinical trial of strength training versus no training in adults with facioscapulohumeral muscular dystrophy (FSHD). The trial involved 65 participants and lasted 52 weeks.[34,35] The strength program in this study appeared to be safe, with only limited positive effects on muscle strength and volume. A study of 12 weeks of aerobic cycling showed a significant increase in aerobic capacity compared to baseline in eight subjects with FSHD with no signs of muscle damage.[36] Altogether, these studies suggest that "normal" participation in sports and work appears not to be harmful.[8] On the other hand, there is insufficient ground for general prescription of exercise programs in FSHD.[8,37]

Exercise Studies in Myotonic Dystrophy

One randomized clinical trial compared the effect of 24 weeks of strength training versus no training in adults with myotonic dystrophy.[23] Neither strength gains nor muscle damage was demonstrated in the exercise group compared to controls. A study of 12 weeks of aerobic training showed that participants with myotonic dystrophy type I improved their aerobic capacity compared to their baseline without any adverse effects.[38] Based on the available evidence, it may be inferred that moderate resistance and endurance exercise is probably safe in individuals with myotonic dystrophy, but there is still insufficient evidence of benefit.[8]

Exercise Studies in the Inflammatory Myopathies

Until the early 1990s, patients with polymyositis (PM) and dermatomyositis (DM) were discouraged from exercising out of concern that it might exacerbate muscle inflammation. More recent work, however, suggests that moderate-intensity aerobic exercise does not result in worsening muscle damage, at least as assessed by creatine kinase (CK) levels, and might in fact improve aerobic capacity.[39–42] The first randomized controlled study of aerobic exercise in adult PM/DM included 14 patients with chronic disease, defined as subjects with proximal muscle weakness due to PM/DM for at least 6 months and stable drug therapy over the 3 months prior to initiation of the program. After 6 weeks of training (bicycle exercise and step aerobics) there was an increase in oxygen uptake in the exercise group compared with the sedentary controls.[39] The same training paradigm was later reported to be safe and to result in improved aerobic capacity in a longer prospective nonrandomized study of 6 months of exercise.[43] A few open-label studies also supported the safety of resistance training in recent-onset disease, reporting unchanged CK levels after short-term exercise periods.[44,45] Analysis of CK levels is the most commonly used marker for muscle inflammation in exercise studies in myositis patients. However, CK levels do not always correspond to muscle function or disease activity. Alexanderson et al. investigated MRI scans of the thighs in 7 out of 11 patients with recent-onset myositis participating in a 12-week resistance exercise program.[44] In the follow-up MRI scans, after 12 weeks of exercise, none of the cases had additional areas of increased signal as compared to the first scan, supporting the safety of the exercise protocol.[44]

Little is known about the role of exercise in inclusion body myositis (IBM). A home exercise program consisting of 15 minutes of progressive strength training and a 15-minute walk performed 5 days a week for 12 weeks did not result in adverse effects on histopathology or significant change in serum CK level, but did not improve muscle strength.[46] More recent work by Johnson et al. showed that a combined 12-week resistance and aerobic exercise program resulted in improved aerobic capacity in seven IBM patients compared to their baseline.[47]

Exercise Studies in the Mitochondrial Myopathies

People with mitochondrial myopathies suffer from exercise intolerance due to their impaired oxidative capacity and physical deconditioning. Cejudo et al. recently reported a randomized clinical trial of combined aerobic and resistance exercise analyzing the effects of 12 weeks of training in 20 people with mitochondrial myopathy (cycle exercise and upper-body weight lifting performed 3 days a week).[48] Training increased aerobic capacity and resulted in improved muscle strength.[48] These results are in agreement with numerous other studies supporting the notion that moderate endurance exercise increases aerobic capacity in patients with mitochondrial myopathies.[49–52] A recent study of 12 weeks of resistance exercise strength training in a group of mitochondrial myopathy patients carrying a single, large-scale deletion of mtDNA resulted in strength gains.[53] Whether or not these results are applicable to other types of mitochondrial myopathy remains to be determined.

AEROBIC TRAINING IN McARDLE DISEASE

Patients with McArdle disease are susceptible to exertional cramps and rhabdomyolysis. In the past, because of the risk of rhabdomyolysis, many people with McArdle disease have been advised to avoid exercise. However, physical inactivity may worsen exercise intolerance by further reducing the limited oxidative capacity caused by blocked glycogenolysis.[54] Haller et al. examined the effect of a 14-week regimen of aerobic training on a cycle ergometer (30 to 40 minutes a day, 4 days a week) in eight subjects with McArdle disease.[54] They reported significant increases in exercise capacity with no adverse effects, in agreement with other small, nonrandomized studies supporting the use of moderate-intensity aerobic exercise for these patients.[55,56] The consensus is to advise individuals with McArdle disease to engage in regular, moderate aerobic activities to prevent deconditioning.[57] On the other hand, intense aerobic or strengthening exercises are contraindicated. Furthermore, any bout of moderate exercise should be preceded by 5 to 15 minutes of low-level "warm up" exercise. This promotes the transition to a "second wind" in which exercise capacity is increased because of increased mobilization and delivery of extramuscular fuels.[58]

BALANCE TRAINING

Many patients with neuromuscular diseases exhibit impaired balance due to a combination of sensory neuropathy, muscle weakness, and/or spasticity and are therefore at risk for falls. Whether balance training reduces this risk has not been well studied. A few small recent studies performed in patients with diabetic neuropathy suggest that balance training might result in improved balance and trunk proprioception.[59–64] Further research is needed to determine whether these early promising results are applicable to other patient populations and whether training might result in increased independence and lower risk of falls.

ADAPTIVE SPORTS

Physical activity should be viewed as a way of improving quality of life and not just a tedious set of exercises. Many people enjoy participation in sports and other recreational activities more than individual training. Previously, it had been thought that having a disability would preclude people from sports participation. Fortunately, over the last several decades, many different groups and organizations have developed adaptive sports for a variety of patient populations. Virtually any sport can be adapted to different levels of disability (Fig. 5-1). It is important to work with organizations and therapists that have extensive experience in adaptive sports to ensure that the level of modification is safe and appropriate for the individual patient's diagnosis and clinical status. The benefits of participation in adaptive sports include engagement with peers, accomplishment of goals that were thought to be out of reach, and improved mood, confidence, and self-esteem. In addition, sports can offer opportunities for people to maintain mobility in an integrated environment. Participation in adaptive sports may be especially important in the pediatric population, as kids enjoy learning through play and recreation.

GENERAL RECOMMENDATIONS FOR EXERCISE IN NEUROMUSCULAR DISEASES

While research is limited as reviewed above, recommendations for general exercise programs for people with neuromuscular diseases have been developed by several consensus panels and are summarized in Table 5-2.[10,11,65,66] Obviously, the level of training and expected outcomes depend on the diagnosis, disease severity, and rate of progression. As an example, people who are recovering from a single episode of neuralgic amyotrophy or Guillain–Barré syndrome are expected to improve their strength over time and exercise can potentially help their recovery, although this assumption is based solely on the known benefits of exercise in the healthy population rather than patients with disease. For patients with slowly progressive disease, exercise might help avoid secondary disuse or deconditioning weakness. On the other hand, some patients with rapidly progressive neuromuscular diseases might already be using their muscles at a maximal level while performing their daily activities. One should keep in mind that there is great variability in muscle strength among different muscle groups in individuals with different types and stages of neuromuscular disorders. Depending on the degree of weakness, some muscles may already be overworked. These specific muscles may need to rest and not perform additional resistance exercises. It should be noted, however, that additional research is needed before clearly defined exercise protocols can be prescribed in any specific disease population. Until then, one can be guided by the important principle of safety while drawing from the currently available studies. With regards to safety, the consensus is to allow sub-maximum aerobic training (either structured exercise or as part of recreational activities) for most patients in order to avoid deconditioning which would compound the existing weakness. In addition, when leg weakness is present, it is important to choose a mode of exercise with minimal risk of injury from falling such as recumbent stationary bike as opposed to treadmill.

Resistance exercise programs might be added as long as one is careful to avoid overwork weakness. Muscles that do not have antigravity strength should not be exercised. Repeated eccentric muscle actions should be avoided. Eccentric muscle actions result in high force production. In healthy adults, they provide an important training stimulus leading to muscle hypertrophy.[13,67] However, eccentric muscle activities are more likely to result in microdamage at the muscle level. The concern is that, in individuals with underlying muscle disease, this may result in long-lasting or irreversible muscle damage, as suggested by some preclinical studies in the mouse model of Duchenne muscular dystrophy.[29]

With any type of exercise program, it is important to pay attention to clinical signs of overwork such as excessive postexercise fatigue, pain, weakness, and delayed-onset muscle soreness, and modify physical activity accordingly.

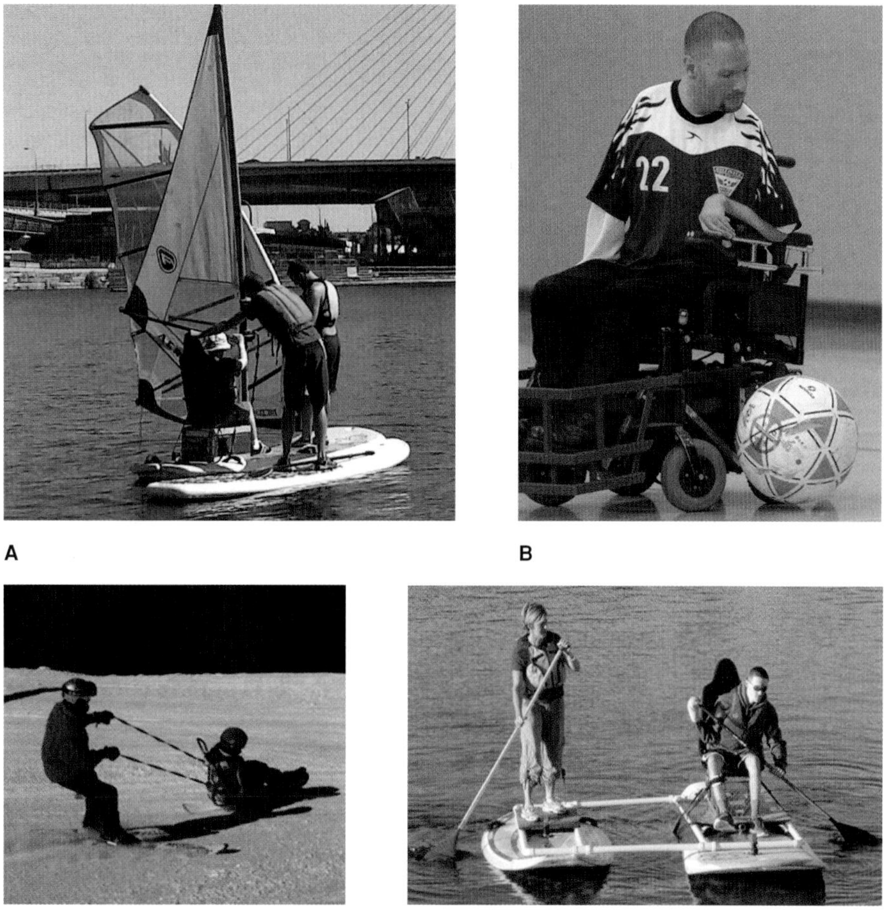

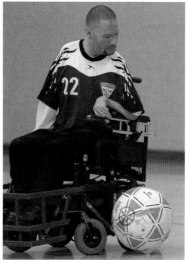

Figure 5-1. Adaptive sports. **(A)** Windsurfing can be adapted to athletes with different disabilities, including wheelchair users. The athlete sits in a high back chair and controls the back sail on a tandem board that can plane at speeds over 32.19 km/h (20 mph). Athletic trainers control the front sail and help keep the board balanced. (Used with permission of Ross Lilley, AccesSportAmerica.) **(B)** Power soccer: athletes who use power wheelchairs for mobility can participate in power soccer. A footguard is attached to the front of their power chair. This guard is for protection and is also used by the athletes to kick, dribble, and block the ball. In competition, chairs are restricted to a top speed of 10 km/h (6.2 mph). (Used with permission of Scot Goodman, Scot Goodman Photography.) **(C)** Adaptive skiing: skiing can be performed with a variety of adaptive equipment to be suitable for athletes with different disabilities. In this photo, a power wheelchair user sits in a chair on a bi-ski and is guided down the slope by a trainer. (Used with permission of Paul Martino, Adaptive Ski Program, New Mexico.) **(D)** Paddling: this set-up enables athletes to stand up or sit down paddle with the direction and support of a trainer next to them. (Used with permission of Ross Lilley, AccesSportAmerica.)

ORTHOSES

Orthoses (braces) are devices worn on a person's body to improve function, provide comfort, conserve energy, and prevent deformity. Orthoses can be prefabricated or custom made. Therapists and orthotists with experience with neuromuscular diseases can provide invaluable input as to the best orthosis to suit the individual patient's needs. Importantly, they can help adjust the orthosis as the status of a patient's functional needs change with time. Patient tolerability varies greatly; therefore, patient feedback on the comfort and fit of the device is paramount.

Cervical Orthoses

Several types of cervical orthoses, or collars, are available to support the neck. For mild weakness, a soft foam collar may be tried first as it is comfortable to wear and well tolerated.

▶ TABLE 5-2. **GENERAL EXERCISE RECOMMENDATIONS FOR PATIENTS WITH NEUROMUSCULAR DISEASES**

Type of Exercise and Potential Benefits	Practical Considerations
Flexibility training is safe and helps prevent contracture formation; it might help with pain and spasticity management	1. Encourage regular stretching and ROM exercises early on in the course of disease. 2. May need periodic supervision and training by a physical therapist (PT). 3. Caregiver participation is essential when muscle weakness prevents the patient from performing program independently.
Moderate, sub-maximum aerobic exercise is *probably* safe for most patients, and *might* help prevent deconditioning and loss of cardiopulmonary fitness	1. Select a mode of exercise with minimal risk of injury from falling (e.g., recumbent stationary bike as opposed to treadmill). 2. Be aware of exercise contraindications such as associated cardiopulmonary disease. 3. A practical approach is to begin with bouts of 10 minutes of exercise 2–3 times a week and progress as tolerated. 4. A practical way to determine if the exercise intensity is appropriate is to ask the patient to talk while exercising. If the patient cannot talk comfortably during exercise, the program is too vigorous.
Moderate resistance exercise *may* help maintain or improve strength in muscles with an initial Medical Research Council (MRC) grade 3/5 or better	1. Avoid high-resistance exercise. Choose loads that correspond to 20%–40% of a one-repetition maximum. A practical approach is to find a weight that the patient can lift comfortably 20 times. Then ask the patient to perform 2–3 sets of 10 repetitions each with that weight. Progression to heavier loads depends on the patient's diagnosis and severity of disease. 2. Do not exercise muscles that do not have antigravity strength. A PT might help identify what muscles can be safely exercised. 3. Avoid eccentric exercise.
For all types of exercise, the level of training depends on the diagnosis, stage, and severity of disease	1. Monitor for signs of overexertion. Excessive postexercise fatigue, muscle pain, or myoglobinuria are indicators that the patient is overworking and that the exercise program needs to be modified. 2. Postexercise fatigue should not interfere with daily activities. If a patient has fatigue or pain that lasts longer than 30 minutes after exercise, he/she is probably overworking.

Some people with head drop use a baseball cap attached to straps around the trunk (or "baseball-cap orthosis"[68]). For moderate to severe weakness, collars with an open air design such as the Headmaster™ or similar models are generally well accepted and provide more support than soft collars. Other types of collar, such as the traditional Philadelphia, Aspen, or Miami-J collars provide more stability. However, these collars are often poorly tolerated due to discomfort at points of contact and a sense of warmth and confinement.

Thoracolumbosacral Orthoses

The primary goal of thoracolumbosacral orthoses (TLSOs) or lumbosacral orthoses (LSOs) in patients with neuromuscular diseases is comfort. In prepubertal children at risk for neuromuscular scoliosis, TLSOs may be utilized to provide support to the spinal column during growth, although the brace cannot prevent curve progression. Molded seating supports can also be used to provide additional comfort and stability when seating. TLSO/LSOs might be helpful in adult patients as well to provide proprioceptive input, improve alignment, and ease back pain.

Upper Limb Orthoses

Many different upper limb orthoses exist. Some orthoses are used to compensate for weakness and improve function, whereas others are prescribed to allow for proper positioning, provide comfort, and prevent or treat joint contractures.

Shoulder support systems are used in neuromuscular patients with proximal weakness who experience shoulder subluxation and/or pain, as can be seen in some muscular dystrophies and motor neuron disorders. Support systems are used to approximate the head of the humerus in the glenoid fossa, with the goal of providing comfort and pain relief. It is important, however, to choose an appropriate orthosis. Single-strap hemislings position the arm close to the body in adduction, internal rotation, and elbow flexion and, with prolonged use, might promote contracture development. On the other hand, axilla roll slings ("Bobath" slings) and humeral cuff slings help to reduce shoulder subluxation without immobilizing the arm in flexion.[69] Therapists can also recommend adjustments to seating systems and arm rests for individuals who use wheelchairs for further arm support.

The balanced forearm orthosis is a functional orthosis for people with shoulder abduction weakness designed to increase independence in performing daily activities. The orthosis supports the weight of the arm against gravity while allowing for independent horizontal movement. It can be placed on a desk or mounted on a wheelchair and is used for tasks such as self-feeding and grooming.

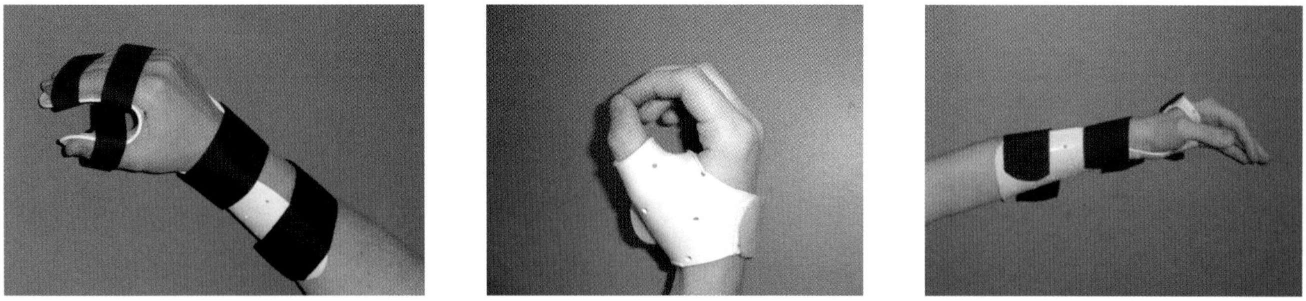

A B C

Figure 5-2. Hand splints. **(A)** Resting hand splint. **(B)** Opponens splint. **(C)** Cock-up splint. (Used with permission of Julie MacLean, Occupational Therapy Department, Massachusetts General Hospital, Boston, MA.)

Splints are hand orthoses for people with intrinsic hand muscle weakness (Fig. 5-2). They can be purchased off the shelf or can be custom made by orthotists and OTs. Resting hand splints are used during the day or at night to maintain muscle length in patients at risk of finger flexion contractures (Fig. 5-2A). Anticlaw splints can reduce claw hand deformity and improve grasp by limiting metacarpophalangeal (MCP) extension. Dynamic finger extension splints are used in individuals with finger extension weakness who still have adequate finger flexor strength. This splint extends the MCP joints so that extended fingers can flex and grasp objects. The opponens splint helps patients with prehension difficulties due to thumb weakness by keeping the thumb in an abducted and opposed position (Fig. 5-2B). The volar cock-up splint supports the wrist in 20 to 30 degrees of extension and is used in people whose wrist extension weakness prevents them from grasping (Fig. 5-2C). The tenodesis orthosis (wrist-driven prehension orthosis) allows an individual with finger flexor weakness to create a three-jaw chuck pinch using wrist extension. Splints to correct single digit deformities are also available.

Lower Limb Orthoses

The most common type of orthotic device prescribed by neuromuscular specialists is the AFO (Fig. 5-3). AFOs are used by patients with ankle dorsiflexion weakness to promote clearing of the toes and foot during the swing phase of gait, thus leading to a safer and more efficient ambulation. They are also used to prevent the development of ankle plantar flexion contractures. It is important, however, to carefully select candidates for bracing as an inappropriate brace might actually impair function. When patients need AFOs, it is best for them to be evaluated in brace clinics where PTs and orthotists work in close contact to provide customized AFOs and modify them as needed. Brace customization and modification is essential to ensure the best possible fit, patient comfort and compliance, as well as maximize functional outcomes. A few sessions of gait training with a skilled therapist are also needed to optimize braced gait. Last but not the least, patients should be instructed to perform skin checks on a regular basis and skin evaluation should be part of routine follow-up care. If skin redness, pain, or callouses develop, the brace should be promptly examined and adjusted by the orthotist. AFOs must be used with shoes which are deep and wide enough to accommodate them. They fit quite well in sneakers although they might be used with other types of shoes as well. It is best to always use shoes with the same heel height in order not to alter gait biomechanics while wearing a brace. Shoes should be in good condition as worn out shoes may affect the gait pattern and lead to reduced brace effectiveness. Some people do not want to wear ankle braces despite medical recommendation. In these circumstances, the use of footwear that crosses the ankle and is snug, such as lace-up boots, high-top sneakers, or even cowboy boots, can help provide at least some support to the ankle.

AFOs come in many different models and can be modified to suit different clinical needs (Fig. 5-3). They are generally made of either plastic or carbon fiber, with the latter being a lighter-weight option. For people with mild foot drop, dorsiflexion assist orthoses may suffice (Fig. 5-3A). These braces are lightweight and incorporate a spring that generates a dorsiflexion assist moment. Another option for mild foot drop is the posterior leaf spring (PLS) AFO (Fig. 5-3B and C). This is an orthosis with medial and lateral trim lines placed posterior to the malleoli. These braces are somewhat flexible and allow some plantar flexion to occur during heel strike. Because of their flexibility, they might not be the best choice for patients with increased tone. Hinged (articulated) AFOs include an ankle joint and are appropriate for patients with moderate weakness of ankle dorsiflexion (Fig. 5-3D). Transferring from sit to stand and negotiating stairs is easier with a hinged AFO than with a solid model, but good quadriceps strength is needed to use them. A plantar flexion stop can be incorporated into the design of a hinged AFO to prevent plantar flexion beyond a certain angle, which might be useful when spasticity is a problem. Solid AFOs provide immobilization of the ankle-foot complex and are therefore used for people with significant distal weakness and resulting medial and lateral instability of the ankle (Fig. 5-3E). However, because of the fixed ankle position, sit-to-stand transfers and climbing stairs and

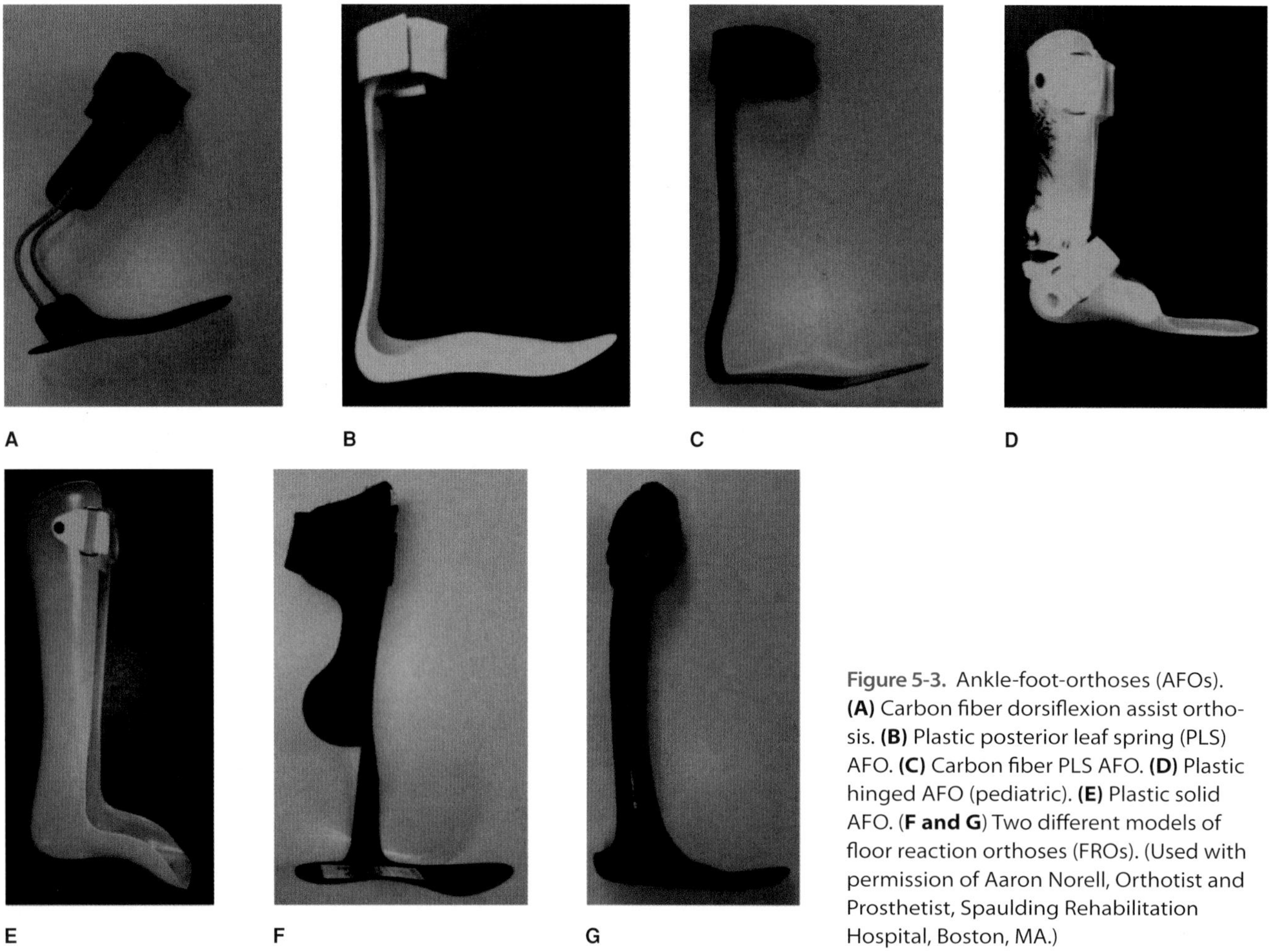

Figure 5-3. Ankle-foot-orthoses (AFOs). **(A)** Carbon fiber dorsiflexion assist orthosis. **(B)** Plastic posterior leaf spring (PLS) AFO. **(C)** Carbon fiber PLS AFO. **(D)** Plastic hinged AFO (pediatric). **(E)** Plastic solid AFO. (**F and G**) Two different models of floor reaction orthoses (FROs). (Used with permission of Aaron Norell, Orthotist and Prosthetist, Spaulding Rehabilitation Hospital, Boston, MA.)

inclines are difficult. The angle at the ankle of a solid AFO can be set in a few degrees of plantar flexion. This modification enhances knee stability and may be useful in patients with quadriceps weakness and knee buckling. Addition of an anterior (pretibial shell) might also help to counter the tendency to knee buckling. On the other hand, setting the angle in a few degrees of dorsiflexion can help limit hyperextension at the knee (genu recurvatum). If the AFO is set in dorsiflexion, the patient must have sufficient quadriceps control to compensate for the increased knee flexion moment during the loading phase of gait. Another option for people with foot drop and/or mild quadriceps weakness is to use floor reaction orthoses (FROs) (such as the Toe-OFF® braces) (Fig. 5-3F and G). FROs use ground reaction forces to offer a "push" at toe off as the orthosis dynamically unloads stored energy to assist with propulsion. This action assists with impaired ankle plantar flexion strength, which is often underdiagnosed. In addition, FROs help create a knee extension moment which may help people with weak quadriceps and a tendency to knee buckling. For patients with spasticity, additional features might be built into the AFOs including a tone-reducing foot plate, toe extensor pads, foam toe separators, metatarsal pads, sustentaculum tali lift, or a plantar flexion stop.

In addition to improving gait efficiency, AFOs can also be used at night to help to prevent or minimize progressive equinus contractures in patients with significant ankle dorsiflexion weakness or increased lower extremity tone. Nighttime AFOs can be either resting AFOs (static braces that keep the ankle aligned in a neutral position) or dynamic AFOs (which provide a low-load prolonged-duration stretch to the gastrocnemius–soleus complex) (Fig. 5-4).

In individuals with quadriceps weakness, a different type of brace that might be tried to provide knee stability is the knee-ankle-foot orthosis (KAFO) (Fig. 5-5). Many KAFOs are too heavy for practical use by individuals with progressive neuromuscular weakness. However, they have been successfully used in polio patients and may assist with ambulation in selected patients with other neuromuscular conditions such as IBM.

MOBILITY AIDS

In people with gait impairment, mobility aids are prescribed to maximize function and promote independence to the highest level possible. One should aim to prescribe the least restrictive device or piece of equipment without

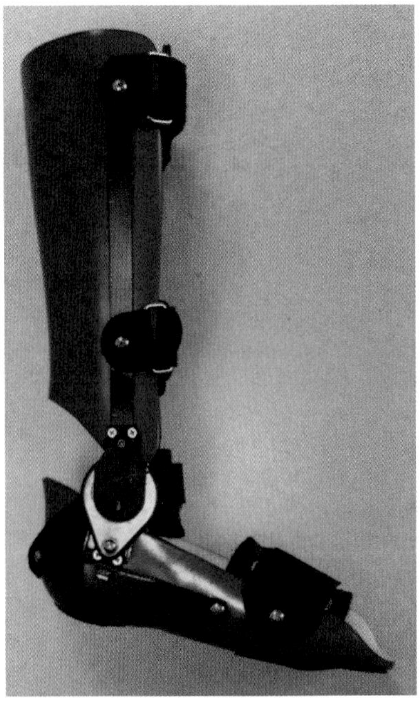

Figure 5-4. Nonambulatory AFO. This AFO provides low-load prolonged-duration stretch to the gastrocnemius–soleus complex. It might be used, especially at night, to help prevent or treat ankle plantar flexion contractures (Used with permission of Aaron Norell, Orthotist and Prosthetist, Spaulding Rehabilitation Hospital, Boston, MA.)

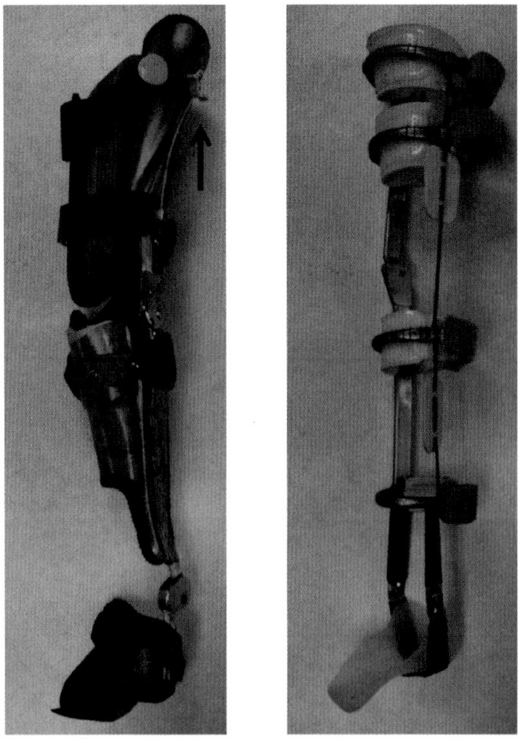

A B

Figure 5-5. Knee-ankle-foot-orthoses (KAFOs). **(A)** Trigger lock KAFO. **(B)** Stance control KAFO. With traditional KAFOs the user needs to manually lock the knee joint and walk with a straight leg. Different systems are available to lock the knee such as a trigger (*arrow* in Panel A) or drop lock mechanism. Stance control KAFOs **(B)** allow for free knee flexion during swing phase while also providing knee stability in stance phase with no need to manually lock the knee joint (Used with permission of Aaron Norell, Orthotist and Prosthetist, Spaulding Rehabilitation Hospital, Boston, MA.)

compromising safety. If the individual has a progressive disorder, it is important to address current problems as well as anticipate and plan for future needs. Most aids, particularly those classified as DME, require a written prescription, and often a letter of medical necessity, signed by the physician. Reimbursement coverage varies greatly. Therefore, it is important to work with therapists and social workers who have experience with neuromuscular disorders to allow for proper planning.

Canes, Crutches, and Walkers

Mobility aids such as canes, crutches, and walkers are prescribed to neuromuscular patients with lower limb weakness and/or balance problems to increase patient safety and promote independent ambulation (Fig. 5-6). These assistive devices widen the base of support and offload a weak limb. The decision as to what walking aid to prescribe depends on the degree of weakness/imbalance in the lower limbs, as well as strength in the trunk and upper extremities, grip strength, tone and ROM, and sensory problems. Patients are best served when they work with a PT to choose the most appropriate walking aid. A few sessions of gait training with the new device are recommended in order to maximize its use.

Canes provide the least amount of support and are usually recommended for people with only mild lower extremity impairment. The use of a cane also requires good upper limb strength. The total length of a cane should equal the distance from the upper border of the greater trochanter to the bottom of the heel of the shoe. The patient should be able to stand with the cane with the elbow flexed at 20 degrees and both shoulders level. A cane is generally carried in the hand opposite to the most affected leg. They can be used on stairs. One should lead with the stronger limb on flat ground and when ascending stairs, and with the more affected limb when descending stairs ("up with the good and down with the bad"). Patients might need to negotiate stairs on an angle and one step at a time depending on the degree of leg weakness. Canes come in a variety of styles and sizes of hand grips. Offset canes have a flat handle which can be built up allowing for better grip. This is beneficial for people with hand muscle weakness. Quad canes provide greater stability than traditional straight canes, but are heavier to lift, which limits their use in individuals with generalized progressive weakness (Fig. 5-6A).

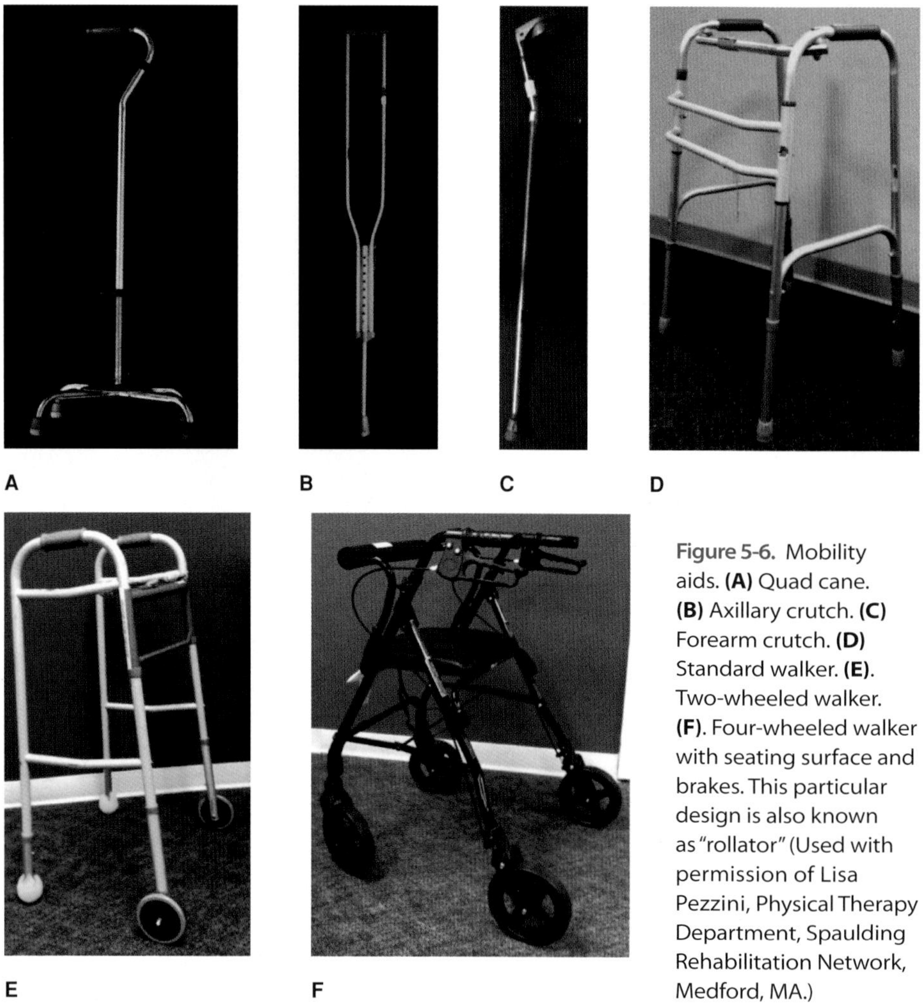

Figure 5-6. Mobility aids. **(A)** Quad cane. **(B)** Axillary crutch. **(C)** Forearm crutch. **(D)** Standard walker. **(E)**. Two-wheeled walker. **(F)**. Four-wheeled walker with seating surface and brakes. This particular design is also known as "rollator" (Used with permission of Lisa Pezzini, Physical Therapy Department, Spaulding Rehabilitation Network, Medford, MA.)

There are three types of crutches: axillary (Fig. 5-6B), forearm (also known as Canadian or Lofstrand crutches) (Fig. 5-6C), and platform. Their use requires a high degree of upper body strength, coordination, and energy. Lofstrand crutches have a forearm cuff, which can free hands for use during standing. Platform crutches are useful when clinical conditions of the forearm, wrist, or hand prevent safe or comfortable weight bearing, such as in the presence of a wrist fracture or weakness of grasp.

Walkers provide the maximum stability because of their wide base of support. However, they are bulky and may be cumbersome in confined spaces. Various types of walkers are available: standard (Fig. 5-6D), two-wheeled (Fig. 5-6E), four-wheeled (Fig. 5-6F), and with seating surfaces (Fig. 5-6F). Having a seat surface available increases the patient's independence if endurance is a problem. They may also be fitted with a shopping basket or a food tray. Standard walkers need to be lifted which can fatigue the upper limbs. Wheeled walkers do not need to be lifted and are preferred in people with generalized weakness as long as they can safely maneuver them. Four-wheeled walkers should be equipped with brakes for safety. Push-down brakes secure a walker when the patient loads his or her weight on the walker and are preferred over squeeze brakes for patients with hand weakness.

Wheelchairs

In people with significant lower limb weakness and/or imbalance, the use of a wheelchair might be indicated in order to maximize functional independence. A face-to-face mobility examination by a physician documenting inability to maintain functional ambulation and mobility-related ADLs in the home environment is required in order for patients to have wheelchairs reimbursed by Medicare, either manual or power depending on whichever is appropriate. Coverage by private insurance companies is based on their policy for DME and requires a letter of medical necessity and a prescription from the treating physician. Some insurance companies do cover equipment used only for mobility in the community with adequate justification. There is a wide range of choices in wheelchairs. PTs with a special expertise in wheelchairs often run wheelchair clinics. It is important to work with therapists who have experience with neuromuscular disorders to ensure that the optimal wheelchair is chosen for the individual patient's needs. When making decisions about wheelchairs, one should keep in mind that, at present, Medicare and most private insurers limit reimbursement to only one wheelchair every few years (generally every 5 years). Therefore, expected disease progression and future needs must be kept in mind. Of note, some patient organizations maintain loaner closets that are available to patients so that they may try and borrow different pieces of equipment.

Power scooters should be recommended with caution to people with neuromuscular diseases. Good upper limb and trunk strength are needed to drive them. In addition, they cannot be modified for disease progression or to accommodate other equipment such as mounted trays or electronic equipment. Power scooters are considered power mobility devices. Therefore, reimbursement for a scooter precludes reimbursement for a power wheelchair, which the patient might need later on in the course of his/her disease. However, they might be an option for those who can borrow or afford to purchase them. In these circumstances, they may be useful for outdoor use and energy conservation when one needs to walk long distances. Because of their long wheel base and wide turning radius it may be difficult to use them indoors.

Standard manual wheelchairs can be operated by the user alone as long as he/she has sufficient upper body function and stamina. These chairs are customized to best fit the person's needs. Multiple features of the chair need to be chosen correctly such as the weight as well as the seating characteristics. Upper body strength and endurance are impaired for many people with neuromuscular diseases. Therefore, manual wheelchairs should be of the lightweight or ultra-lightweight variety in order to enable the individual to propel the wheelchair independently. Additional chair features such as the type of cushion, type of armrest, back and footrest height need to be individualized to allow for optimal comfort, support, safety, and function. If significant disease progression is expected, manual wheelchairs are not a long-term solution. However, having a back-up manual wheelchair is important as it might be needed if the power chair needs repairs or when traveling if transport of the power chair is not an option. The need to accommodate growth is an additional consideration when prescribing wheelchairs for pediatric patients.

Transport or companion wheelchairs are lightweight chairs that are designed for ease of use and transport. They must be pushed by a caregiver. They fold to fit into a car's trunk and are generally used for traveling. Since they are relatively inexpensive, many families purchase one as a back-up chair.

Power-assist wheelchairs are sometimes used by individuals who have a slowly progressive disease to reduce the effort required to self-propel a manual wheelchair. Power-assist wheels have an electrical motor attached to the hub which provides assistance to manually propelled use. However, they are rather heavy and are not indicated for people with rapidly progressing weakness.

When manual wheelchair use is no longer possible due to generalized weakness or the need to use a ventilator or other equipment, power wheelchairs are prescribed. Transitioning to a power wheelchair is often challenging, both psychologically and logistically. The patient and caregivers need to adjust to disease progression and might need to have additional home and vehicle modifications as power wheelchairs do not fit into narrow doorways and standard cars. It is paramount to work closely with a wheelchair clinic with experience with neuromuscular disorders to ensure that the power wheelchair components are suitable for the individual's current and expected future needs. Proper seating and positioning are essential to ensure a comfortable and functional sitting posture and to prevent secondary injuries such as skin breakdown and back pain. Of note, wheelchair assessment and adjustment may be necessary as disease progresses if pain, skin problems, or poor posture are noted. Simple wheelchair modifications may significantly improve comfort and skin management. One can choose among multiple options for head and neck support, trunk support, pressure relief, seatbelts, trays, BiPAP or vent holder, and drive controls. Pressure relief allows periodic redistribution of body mass to prevent skin breakdown and is accomplished using the tilt-in-space and recline functionalities. These functions are also beneficial in minimizing dependent edema that is commonplace in these patients and for improved comfort for those who choose to sleep in their chairs. Pressure mapping might be offered to supplement clinical impression when assessing the appropriateness of the seating system. Mapping is accomplished by using a thin mat with pressure sensors that can be placed over the chair cushion to analyze interface pressures. This can also be helpful to verify if pressure relief maneuvers are performed adequately. Multiple drive controls are available to allow users with different degrees of weakness to control the power wheelchair (Fig. 5-7). Most people use a joystick to control the wheelchair, at least initially, but may then need to progress to alternative control modes such as using a head array, lip/tongue mini joystick, foot joystick, sip and puff, single switch scanning, or other methods (Fig. 5-7). The wheelchair drive control can be adapted to integrate access to AAC devices, environmental systems, and computers within a single control interface.

Some power chairs have standing capabilities. An alternative option to allow periodic standing is the use of static standing frames. Potential benefits of standing include improved bone health through weight-bearing, prevention of lower body contractures, and facilitation of social interactions and activities located on high counters and desks.

ADAPTIVE EQUIPMENT AND ENVIRONMENTAL MODIFICATIONS FOR DAILY LIVING

Activities of daily living include basic ADLs (such as eating, grooming, bathing, dressing, and toileting) and instrumental ADLs (IADLs) which consist of more complex tasks such

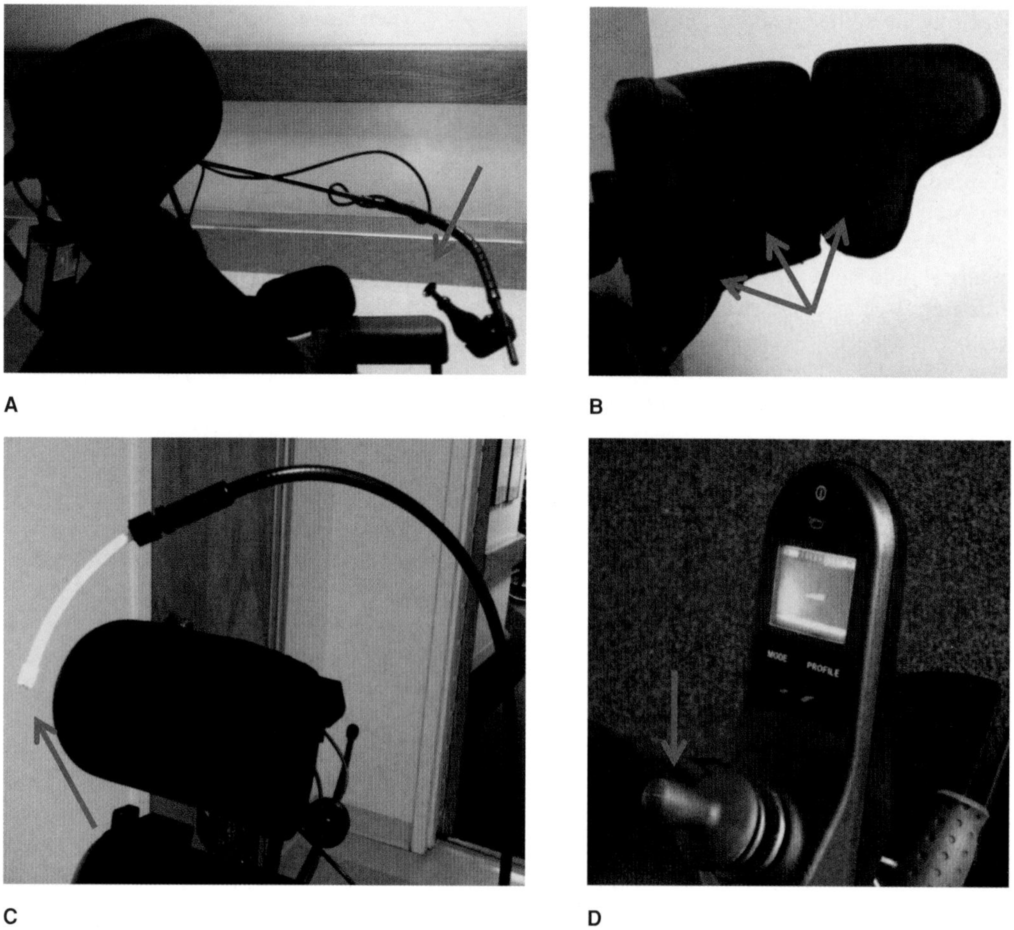

Figure 5-7. Power wheelchair drive controls. **(A)** The mini joystick (*arrow*) allows the individual to drive the wheelchair by using the lips or the tongue. **(B)** The head array is operated by coming in contact with proximity sensors located in each panel of the head array (*arrows*). **(C)** Sip and puff: this device allows wheelchair control by sipping and puffing on a straw located near the mouth (*arrow*). **(D)** The joystick (*arrow*) is used by people with at least some preserved hand/finger movements (Used with permission of Michelle Kerr, Physical Therapy Department, Spaulding Rehabilitation Hospital, Boston, MA.)

as working, driving, shopping, homemaking, and childcare. A diverse array of devices and equipment is available to enhance the independence of people with muscle weakness in their daily living. However, not all devices fit an individual person's needs and preferences, which may change over time. Therefore, the expertise of physical and OTs is often needed to help patients navigate through the different options. One should also be mindful that the cost of many of these devices is not covered by insurance.

Self-Feeding and Meal Preparation

Eating utensils can be modified to facilitate holding in the presence of hand weakness. Increasing the diameter of the handle on spoons, forks, and knives (as well as other daily tools such as writing instruments and grooming tools) improves grip (Fig. 5-8A). One can either purchase large-handled tools or cover regular utensil handles with cylindrical foam (Fig. 5-8A). Bendable utensils are also available. A spoon might be bent so that it faces the user to compensate for weakness of wrist flexion and supination. Rocker knives (or using a pizza cutter instead of a knife) make it easier to cut food (Fig. 5-8A). One can also use a cutting board with nails driven through it to hold food for chopping. When the patient's grip strength is severe enough to prevent him/her from holding any eating utensils, one can use a "universal" cuff which is a strap that one wears around the palm of the hand (Fig. 5-8B–D). The cuff has a pocket that can hold a variety of tools (Fig. 5-8B–D). Light-weight drinking cups, straw holders, and long straws to decrease the distance between hand and mouth assist with drinking (Fig. 5-8A). Using scoop dishes and plate guards helps prevent the food from falling off the side of a plate (Fig. 5-8A). Nonslip matting or using plates with suction bottoms keeps the plate from moving around on a table. Adaptive tools to open jars and cans are available. Reachers and grabbers help people get items from

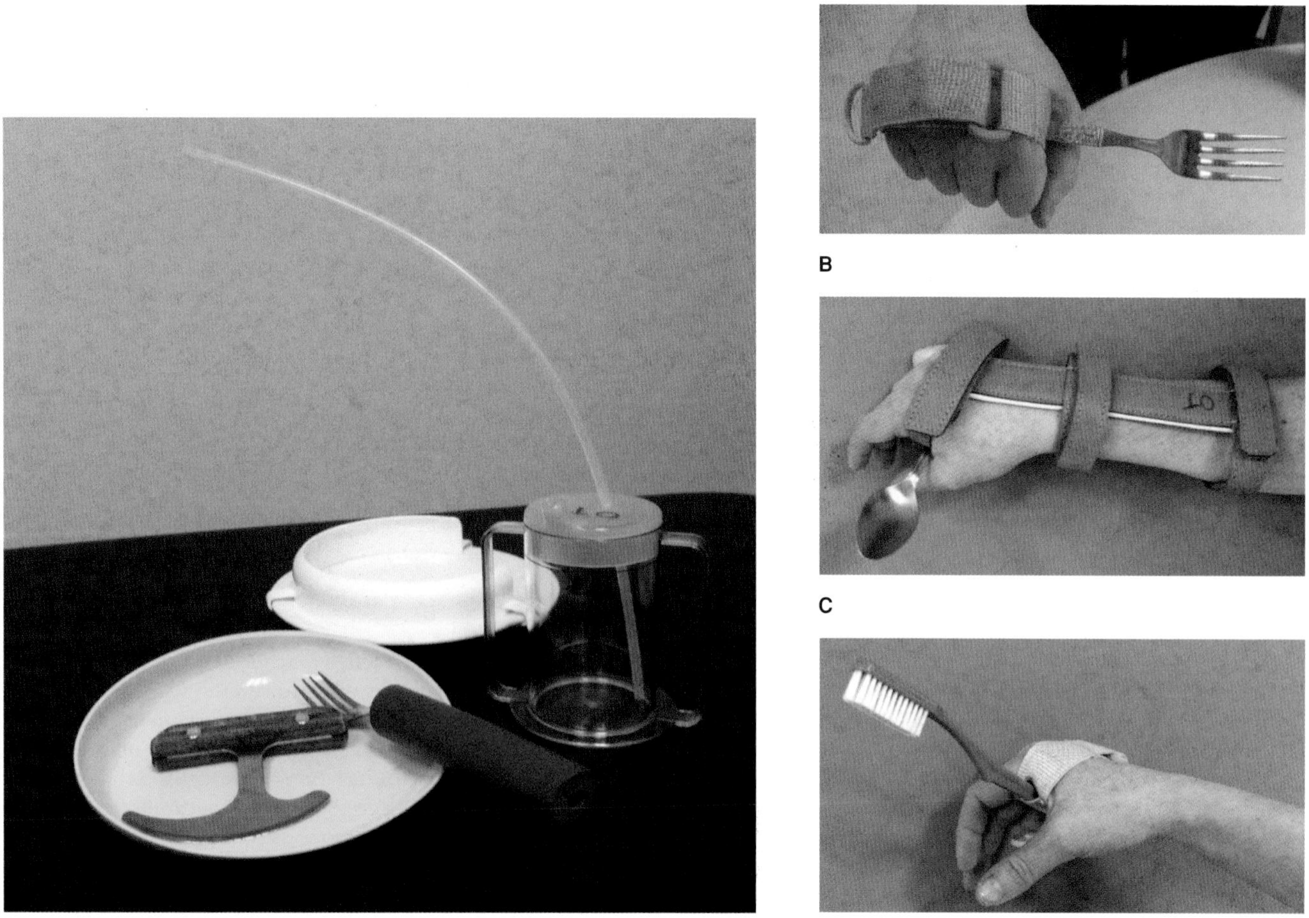

A B C D

Figure 5-8. Adaptive equipment for eating and self-care. **(A)** Multiple adaptive tools are available to aid individuals with feeding themselves. Pictured here are a scoop plate (*yellow*), a rocker knife, a fork whose handle has been enlarged by soft foam tubing, a plate guard which has been attached to a regular plate (*white*), and a long straw. (**B–D**) The universal cuff is designed to provide individuals with little to no finger control the ability to hold objects. Once centered over the palm, the device contains a pocket that can hold different types of tools including silverware, toothbrushes, brushes, and writing tools. In C, the universal cuff has been modified to provide support to a weak wrist (Used with permission of Julie MacLean, Occupational Therapy Department, Massachusetts General Hospital, Boston, MA.)

an upper cupboard and pick up objects from the floor (Fig. 5-9A and C). A mobile arm support, attached to either a table or a wheelchair, can compensate for proximal arm weakness: it will hold up the arm against gravity and help bring food to the mouth. This set-up can also be used for other activities such as turning the pages of a book and grooming.

Dressing

Buttons, zippers, snaps, and shoelaces are notoriously difficult for people with hand weakness and impaired dexterity. One can try button and snap hooks (Fig. 5-9D), zipper pulls, and shoes with either Velcro closure or elastic shoelaces. Velcro can also be sewn behind buttons for easier fastening. Using sock aids and long-handled shoe horns reduces the need for bending forward when donning and doffing socks and shoes (Fig. 5-9A and B). Dressing sticks with mechanical graspers allow patients to compensate for upper limb weakness when putting on a sweater or shirt (Fig. 5-9A). In addition to adaptive tools, OTs can suggest compensatory strategies for dressing and undressing. As an example, it is easier to don over-the-head shirts with the weaker side first, then the head, and finally the stronger side (the reverse sequence is used when doffing the shirt).

Self-Care, Bathing, and Toileting

A strap-fitted hairbrush, long-handled comb, electric toothbrush, and shaver can facilitate grooming. Cylindrical foam can be applied to the handle of multiple bath tools to facilitate grip. Pump soaps are easier to use than slippery bar soap and long-handled sponges can help with bathing (Fig. 5-9E). Transfers in the bathroom may be difficult for people with neuromuscular weakness and may pose a great danger with

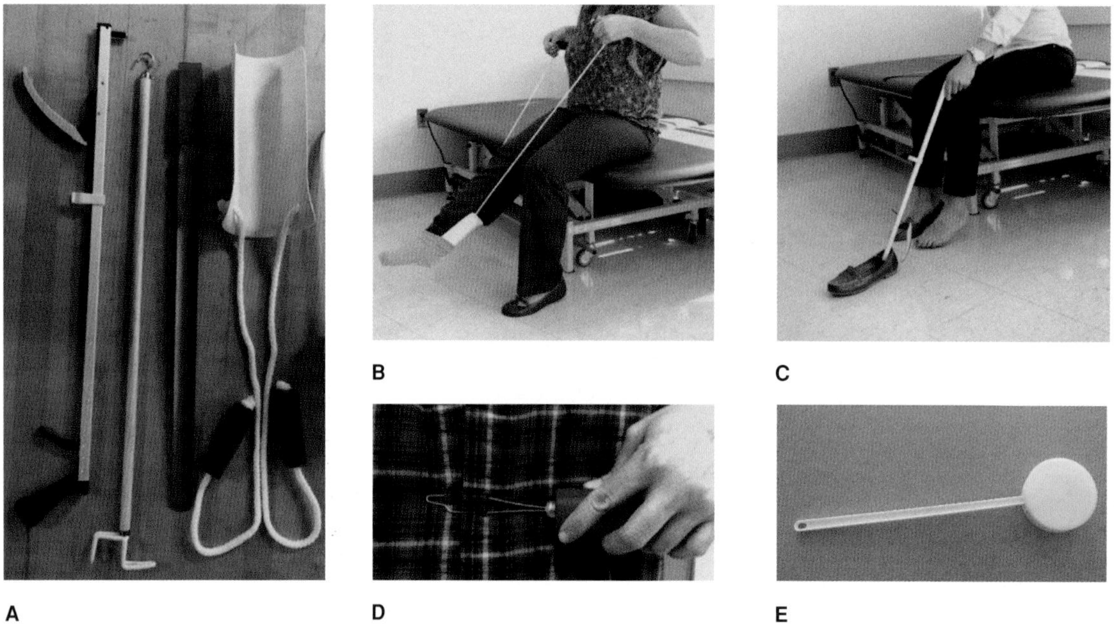

Figure 5-9. Adaptive equipment for dressing and bathing. Panel **(A)** shows, from the left, a reacher, a dressing stick, a long-handled shoe horn, and a sock aid. Panel **(B)** shows how to use a sock aid: after pulling the sock over the form and inserting the foot into the form, the individual pulls the loop handle to bring the sock up over the foot. In panel **(C)**, the reacher is used for picking up out-of-reach items. It includes a magnetic tip to pick up metal objects, and a clip for storing the reacher on a walker or wheelchair. **(D)** The button hook is a tool used to facilitate the closing of apparel that uses buttons as fasteners. The hook end is inserted through the buttonhole to capture the button by the shank and draw it through the opening. **(E)** Long-handled sponge for bathing. (Used with permission of Julie MacLean, Occupational Therapy Department, Massachusetts General Hospital, Boston, MA.)

regards to risk of falling. Installing nonskid surfaces on the floor or in the bathtub/shower and using appropriate transfer equipment may help prevent falls. People with leg weakness or imbalance may find it hard to step over the tub. A transfer tub bench is a padded board placed across the tub that provides level transfer surface. Some people need to sit in the shower for safety. A shower seat and a long-handled hose make showering easier. Grab bars are used for safe entering and exiting, but need to be installed appropriately. It is important to educate patients on the fact that regular towel racks are not safe alternatives to grab bars as they cannot support body weight. Suction grab bars are not a viable alternative either for similar reasons. For people who use wheelchairs for mobility, a roll-in shower stall and rolling shower chair are ideal. Some shower chairs can also be used as a commode or over the toilet. People who have problems with sit-to-stand transfers might benefit from a raised toilet seat. For people with balance problems or leg weakness, use of the bathroom at night can be especially dangerous. Having night lights and, if needed, a bedside commode may help minimize fall risk.

Transfers

The ability to transfer allows the transition from one position or surface to another, such as from sitting to standing, from the bed to a chair, and so forth. Transfers are taken for granted by able-bodied individuals as they are an effortless activity that is performed every day countless of times. Transfers, however, are often burdensome for neuromuscular patients and their caregivers and yet they are a necessary part of daily living. Difficulties with transfers may prevent patients from getting out of bed or leaving their homes, and may hamper their ability to participate in social events, attend doctor appointments, and enjoy outdoor activities. Therefore, transfer training and prescription of proper transfer aids are an essential component of the rehabilitation process. Importantly, transfer training must focus not only on efficiency but also on safety.

Bed mobility includes both repositioning while in bed and getting in and out of the bed. This can be facilitated by step stools, powered hospital beds, and overhead trapezes. To get up from a chair, one can place firm cushions or blocks under the seat so that the hips are higher than the knees to facilitate sit-to-stand transfers. Swivel cushions are lightweight seats that swivel in both directions and make getting in and out of a car easier. A gait (transfer) belt allows the caregiver to provide safe lifting assistance to the patient. These belts are positioned around the patient's waist and hips and prevent traction on the patient's shoulders which may be painful. They also ease caregiver burden and potential musculoskeletal strain when assisting the patient, which are important considerations as caregiver's ability to function is often integral to patients' ability to continue to live in their home. There are also self-powered hydropneumatic lifting cushions (which are portable and relatively inexpensive), as well as more expensive powered recliner lift chairs that enable a person to rise to a standing position by activating an electric control. Lift chairs can also be installed in cars or vans for ease of transfer in and out of vehicles. As lower limb weakness progresses, different techniques can be used to transfer patients, such as stand pivot and squat pivot transfers with caregiver's assistance. A pivot disc can be used to assist with stand pivot transfers if the patient is able to stand but cannot step and turn. The patient's feet are placed on the disc. The patient stands and the disc is rotated. The patient is then lowered to the new surface (such as a chair or the bed). A sliding board can be used for patients who are unable to stand. The patient can use the board independently if he/she has preserved upper body strength. Otherwise, the board can be used with the assistance of a caregiver. Finally, mechanical lifts allow for safe lifting of people who do not have the preserved strength to transfer independently. For individuals with intact cognition, the ability to direct a caregiver and provide instruction through the transfer enables a sense of autonomy despite requiring physical assistance with care.

Leisure Activities

The inability to enjoy leisure activities such as reading and writing can greatly lower quality of life. For book management, placing a book on an easel and using a page turning device that clips to the hand allows independence with reading for some patients. Automatic page turners that are activated by a switch are also commercially available. To facilitate grip, foam cylinders can be placed around writing instruments. There are also pen holders which hold the pen and allow writing as the patient moves the device. For television, telephone, and computer use, numerous options are available (reviewed below). Many adaptations exist for other leisure activities such as gardening, golfing, and fishing.

Driving

Driving is an activity symbolic of independence and control for many people, and one that is difficult to give up simply due to disability. However, it might be difficult for some neuromuscular patients to drive, especially for those with progressive weakness. Adaptive driving agencies and, in some centers, OTs can perform driving safety assessments to test the motor and cognitive skills necessary for driving. Results are used to make recommendations for vehicle modifications. Available modifications include left-foot accelerators for patients with right leg weakness and hand controls for patients with preserved upper body strength. Once the proper vehicle modifications have been identified, it is necessary to take adaptive driving lessons and a road test before the adaptations can be installed. This process is generally not covered by insurance and can be quite expensive; however, some nonprofit organizations offer grant support to defray the costs of modifications. In some states, vocational rehabilitation programs may also be available to provide this type of support.

Environmental Modifications

Environmental modifications at home, at school, and in the workplace might be necessary to optimize the independence and safety of some individuals. Such modifications can range from simple changes such as furniture rearrangement to extensive (and expensive) remodeling. Physical and OTs can provide home, workplace, and school evaluations and formulate recommendations for improved accessibility, function, and safety. Regional ADA centers can also be available to provide guidance regarding how to make both private and public facilities compliant with specifications under the Americans with Disabilities Act (www.adata.org).

For wheelchair users, ramps may be needed to enter the home if there are steps. Ramps can be portable or permanent and can be rented or purchased. Narrow doorways often require widening to accommodate a wheelchair or a walker. The height of counters, sinks, light switches, and other reachable items might require modifications for accessibility from a seated position. If an individual has difficulties negotiating stairs or is a wheelchair user and his/her bedroom is on an upper floor, it may be necessary to accommodate for ground floor living space unless one can install an elevator or stair lift. When considering a stair lift for wheelchair use, one must keep in mind that the individual will need to transfer in and out of the stair lift and leave a second wheelchair on the upper floor. Bedroom modifications are often needed to address problems with sleeping which are common among people with neuromuscular diseases. Hospital beds are used to elevate the head to reduce aspiration risk and help manage orthopnea. In addition, they allow repositioning and, in conjunction with special mattresses or mattress overlays, they can help alleviate the discomfort and risk of skin breakdown associated with limited mobility. Bathrooms are generally the smallest room in the home and often require the most modifications to accommodate patients with neuromuscular weakness. Walk-in or roll-in shower stalls, grab bars, and other adaptive equipment for toileting and bathing (described above) are examples of bathroom modifications.

Environmental control systems can be used to control appliances, lighting and heating systems, televisions, and telephones via a portable hand-held keypad or the computer, even for individuals with very severe motor weakness. Keyboards can be modified depending on the person's motor control. As an example, the keys can be expanded to accommodate excessive movements for people with ataxia or can be reduced in size for those with minimal active finger movements. Eye gaze sensing technology enables people with severe limb weakness to access computers and environmental control systems by sensing movement from the reflection of the eye. Head movement tracking and voice-activated systems are also available.

Power wheelchairs frequently do not fit into standard vehicles and may require a modified van for transportation. Many individuals do not have the financial means to purchase a modified van and thus utilize a back-up transport wheelchair to visit friends or travel to doctor appointments, for example. Alternatively, many power wheelchair users prefer to utilize accessible public transportation if it is available in their community.

A REHABILITATION APPROACH FOR COMMON NEUROMUSCULAR COMPLAINTS

After reviewing the basics of a variety of rehabilitation strategies such as exercise and the use of assistive devices, we will now suggest how to approach some of the most commonly encountered clinical problems in neuromuscular medicine from a rehabilitation perspective. Our goal is to describe how to leverage the expertise of multiple team members and integrate the different tools described above with the overarching goal of promoting patient safety, independent function, comfort, and quality of life. As each patient's set of needs, expectations, environment, and support systems are unique, the approach suggested here will need to be tailored to suit each individual and modified to adapt to changes in disease status. Thus, rather than suggesting a fixed and exhaustive solution for each clinical problem, we will propose a framework that can be used as a reference to design a customized rehabilitation plan.

AXIAL WEAKNESS AND SPINAL DEFORMITIES

Axial weakness may result in different clinical presentations including head drop (head ptosis), bent spine (camptocormia), and neuromuscular scoliosis, depending on the underlying process.

Head drop and bent spine are caused by neck extensor and paraspinal muscle weakness, respectively. In contrast with other skeletal disorders of the spine such as kyphosis, the deformity is not fixed (unless secondary contractures occur) and is corrected by passive extension or lying in the supine position. Functional consequences of these conditions might include difficulty walking, maintaining balance, conversing eye to eye, reading, and even difficulties swallowing, speaking, and breathing. Patients commonly experience pain in the nuchal region with head drop, and back pain from camptocormia, presumably due to protracted stretching of pain-sensitive spinal or paraspinal tissues. Typically, this pain is relieved by support.

Treatment is directed towards the primary pathology if possible, as in cases of head drop due to myasthenia gravis. In progressive diseases such as ALS, one can offer supportive measures to promote good postural alignment and partially correct the deformity. Early implementation of supportive measures is important to prevent secondary complications such as contractures of the neck/back in a fixed flexed posture. We have seen individuals with ALS whose dysphagia or dyspnea improved when proper neck alignment was obtained by using an appropriate cervical orthosis. Orthoses that can be used include neck collars and baseball cap orthoses. It is important for the orthosis to provide enough support, which may require customization by an experienced PT/orthotist. These braces may be used intermittently even early on in the disease for energy conservation purposes when performing certain demanding activities. Thoracic-lumbar-sacral orthoses (TLSOs) may be used to support the spine in cases of camptocormia, but are often poorly tolerated. Orthotists may be able to adapt and customize TLSOs for improved comfort (de Seze, 2008).[70] Stretching, physical modalities, and medications may be needed to prevent/treat neck and back pain.

Neuromuscular scoliosis is a sagittal deformity of the spine due to either neurogenic or myogenic disorders. It is especially common in progressive neuromuscular diseases that begin in childhood such as spinal muscular atrophy (SMA) and Duchenne muscular dystrophy.[71–73] Weakness in the trunk and paraspinal muscles leads to collapse of the developing spine into what is generally a long C-shaped curve with the apex in the thoracolumbar region.[72] Scoliosis causes discomfort and pain and, if severe, creates difficulties with seating, positioning, and breathing. TLSOs and molded seating systems may be utilized to provide support to the spinal column, but these interventions cannot prevent curve progression.[74] Spine development needs to be monitored periodically in consultation with orthopedic surgery.[11,73] In Duchenne muscular dystrophy, prolonged ambulation is associated with a reduced risk of developing scoliosis while steroid use slows curve progression.[75,76] The decision to perform surgical correction, generally spine fusion with instrumentation, depends on many factors including the patient's age, curvature progression, mobility status, and pulmonary function. Oftentimes, spine fusion is performed around the onset of puberty in anticipation of curve progression. Careful preoperative evaluation is needed due to the increased operative risks in neuromuscular patients. Benefits of spine surgery include improved sitting balance and quality of life as well as prevention of back pain.[77] Whether the correction of spinal deformities slows the rate of ventilatory decline remains controversial.[11]

PROXIMAL UPPER LIMB WEAKNESS

Proximal upper limb weakness can be seen in multiple neuromuscular disorders and can cause difficulties with a variety of activities such as carrying objects, reaching overhead, and washing one's hair. As described above, adaptive equipment is available to help with many activities of daily living including reachers, dressing sticks with mechanical graspers, and long-handled combs and brushes. A mobile arm support, attached to either a table or a wheelchair, can compensate for impaired shoulder abduction by holding up the arm against gravity. This set-up enables self-feeding for many patients and provides support for other activities such as grooming.

It is important to remember that chronic weakness of the shoulder girdle may lead to decreased ROM and pain. Other factors that are implicated in shoulder pain in neuromuscular patients are compensatory abnormal movement patterns, static positioning, spasticity, traction during inappropriately performed transfers, and contractures.[78] In a recent retrospective study of 193 ALS patients, 23% reported experiencing shoulder pain at some time during the course of their illness.[79] Thus, attention to complaints of shoulder stiffness and pain should be part of routine ALS care.

While very little evidence is available to guide management of shoulder problems in neuromuscular patients, experience suggests that a proactive ROM program can often prevent the development of shoulder pain. We generally recommend beginning a daily shoulder stretching program early on in the course of progressive neuromuscular disease that is likely to affect the shoulder girdle. Patients and their caregivers can be instructed on a simple, small set of ROM exercises which can be performed independently at home. If the individual is too weak to lift the shoulder overhead, stretching can be performed while lying down or with the assistance of a caregiver.

Once shoulder pain develops, a careful examination can identify the pain generator and guide treatment. Treatment strategies are highly individualized and include activity modification, stretching, physical modalities [heat, cold, massage, transcutaneous electrical nerve stimulation (TENS)], nonsteroidal anti-inflammatory and analgesic medications and, in selected cases, steroid injections.[80–83] Surgical intervention is rarely indicated in progressive neuromuscular conditions. Individuals with significant shoulder weakness are also at risk of developing shoulder subluxation. Early use of shoulder support slings can help approximate the head of the humerus in the glenoid fossa, thus preventing/treating shoulder subluxation and resulting pain[69]. Simple modifications such as adjusting the seating system or the arm rests of the wheelchair provide additional comfort and pain relief.

Weakness of the thoracoscapular muscles may result in winging of the scapula. This may be seen within the context of nerve injury as in trauma to the long thoracic or the spinal accessory nerves. In these circumstances, clinical observation is generally attempted first for most patients, but bracing and surgical treatment may be considered.[84] A number of myopathies can also result in scapular winging due to generalized weakness of the shoulder girdle musculature. In some patients, particularly in FSHD, the specific pattern of weakness may result in impaired shoulder ROM. Specifically, in FSHD, there is early selective weakness of the thoracoscapular muscles with relative preservation of the deltoid. When shoulder abduction is attempted using the deltoid, the scapula rotates and lifts off the chest wall impeding the movement. Scapular retraction orthoses may be tried to stabilize the shoulder blade, but they are generally considered too uncomfortable for prolonged use. Surgical scapular fixation techniques have also been proposed for people with FSHD with the goals of both improving the ability to elevate the arm at the shoulder and to improve arm strength by allowing improved scapular fixation. There have been no randomized trials of surgical versus nonsurgical treatment in muscular dystrophy patients with scapular winging. Nevertheless, case reports and case series suggest that operative interventions can produce functional benefits in selected FSHD patients.[85] However, these potential benefits have to be balanced against the need for postoperative immobilization, rehabilitation, and complications. Therefore, the decision to perform surgery is highly individualized. Surgical expertise is probably a critical factor in the success of these operations.[85]

HAND WEAKNESS

Hand weakness is seen in many neuromuscular diseases. Early symptoms of hand weakness include difficulties in opening jars and cans and turning doorknobs. In more severe cases, handwriting, cutting food, using a telephone, and a multitude of other activities of daily living become affected.

OTs have special expertise in managing problems with upper limb functional activities secondary to hand weakness. In a cohort of 102 consecutive patients with neuromuscular diseases attending an outpatient clinic, 43% of patients were considered to potentially benefit from occupational therapy.[86] The type of OT intervention, though, was entirely based on the clinical expertise of the therapist, given the lack of research on occupational therapy specifically designed for neuromuscular disorders.

Two small studies reported some functional benefits in terms of performance and satisfaction with ADLs after 12 weeks of a hand exercise program using a silicone-based putty in 5 subjects with myotonic dystrophy and 12 subjects with Welander distal myopathy, respectively.[87] OTs can recommend adaptive equipment and braces to assist with many of the functional tasks described above. Some neuromuscular conditions are characterized by specific patterns of hand weakness. As an example, IBM typically affects the flexors of the distal phalanges, while radial neuropathy may affect finger extension. Therefore, hand orthoses most often need to be custom made to be tailored to the specific pattern of muscle weakness. Other OT interventions that might be indicated for individuals with hand weakness include ROM programs and resting hand splints to prevent contracture formation, ergonomic evaluation, and environmental modifications to maximize function at home, at school, or in the workplace, as well as driving safety assessment. Hand massage, positioning, and compression gloves may be used to manage edema secondary to limited hand function.

PROXIMAL LOWER LIMB WEAKNESS

Hip girdle and proximal leg weakness are seen in a variety of neuromuscular conditions, especially in myogenic disorders. Proximal lower limb weakness results in difficulties with transfers and gait, impaired activities of daily living, and increased risk of falling. It may also result in musculoskeletal pain when muscles are abnormally activated and overworked to compensate for the impaired posture and gait.

Proximal weakness makes it difficult to stand from sitting, negotiate stairs, and get in and out of a car. Adaptive equipment such as lifting cushions, stair lifts, and swivel seats have been described above. A variety of assistive devices is also available to enhance people's independence with lower body dressing, toileting, bathing, etc. For people with mild quadriceps weakness, floor reaction orthoses provide a knee extension moment which might help to stabilize the knee (Fig. 5-3). KAFOs have been used in some polio and Duchenne patients to stabilize the knee in the setting of quadriceps weakness (Fig. 5-5).[88–90] With traditional KAFOs, however, the patient needs to walk with a locked knee which is difficult when significant hip girdle weakness is present. In addition, the weight of the KAFO often limits its practical application in neuromuscular patients. Newer stance control orthoses allow for free knee flexion during swing phase while also providing knee stability in stance phase. These braces have been trialed in patients with IBM and might have a role early in the course of the disease.[91] Further research is needed to clarify their role in patients with muscle disorders.

Lower limb muscle imbalance and abnormal gait may lead to low back and hip pain. Weakness of the hip girdle extensors results in hyperlordosis as a compensatory posture to maintain the center of gravity during ambulation. While this posture has an effective function during gait, it may also exacerbate low back pain. It is important to pay attention to symptoms of pain which may become quite disabling for the patient. Depending on the underlying neuromuscular disorder and pain generator, different interventions might be appropriate. In the absence of evidence-based guidelines, the treatment depends on the experience of the PT, physiatrist, and pain specialist. LSOs might be used for support in cases of back pain. Physical modalities such as cold, heat, massage, and TENS might be tried for comfort. An ergonomic evaluation might reveal a number of problems with the patient's work station and biomechanics that can be fixed with simple environmental and behavioral modifications. As an example, using a foot rest under one foot while standing at the kitchen counter may help ease low back pain. Gentle stretching and physical activity such as aquatic therapy might be indicated in some circumstances. If greater trochanteric pain syndrome is present, anti-inflammatory medications or steroid injections may be considered.

As weakness progresses, patients may lose the ability to ambulate. People who spend many hours a day in a wheelchair or in bed are at risk for developing hip and knee flexion contractures. These contractures are associated with further functional decline, pain, and difficulties with dressing and personal hygiene. It is important to be mindful of this potential complication and to be proactive in recommending proper positioning, braces, and ROM exercises to prevent contracture formation.

FOOT DROP

Foot drop results from weakness of the tibialis anterior and/or weakness of the long extensors of the toes (extensor hallucis longus and extensor digitorum longus) and is due to a variety of etiologies. As a consequence, either the front of the foot or the whole foot contacts or scuffs the ground during swing-through of the leg, which can have a profound effect on gait. Tripping and falling are a major associated risk. Patients may use compensatory movement patterns, such as vaulting, circumduction, hip hiking, or a steppage gait, which result in increased energy expenditure and overwork of other muscles utilized to support the abnormal pattern.[92] Further, chronic weakness of dorsiflexion may result in reduced ankle ROM and shortening and contracture of the Achilles tendon. Many of the conditions which cause weakness of the ankle dorsiflexors also weaken muscles of eversion and inversion leading to further risk of contracture development. The exact contribution and severity may differ among conditions.

Traditional rehabilitation interventions for foot drop and its sequelae include stretching and strengthening exercises, orthotic and assistive devices, and surgery. Unfortunately, there is very limited evidence to aid in the clinical decision-making process.[93] Thus, the rehabilitation of foot drop is generally guided by clinician's experience. While evidence-based recommendations cannot be made due to the lack of research, the following commonly accepted interventions should be considered based on the limited available evidence and knowledge derived from other patient populations.

Stretching is used to maintain passive ROM and prevent contracture formation. One should aim at stretching both the gastrocnemius and the soleus muscles. The former is best stretched when the knee is in an extended position while the latter can be isolated with the knee in flexion. Gait analysis of people with CMT showed that the hip flexors compensated for distal weakness and that hip flexor fatigue was a limiting factor in walking duration in these subjects.[94,95] This study suggests that strengthening proximal muscles might be used as a rehabilitation tool to improve gait function in people with foot drop.

Energy expenditure during gait increases in many patients with neuromuscular diseases.[96,97] Orthoses are used to splint the joint in a functional position with the goal of promoting a more efficient and safer gait. Studies in polio survivors showed that the energy cost of walking was decreased by wearing an orthosis.[88,89] Studies in people with CMT and FSHD suggested that use of an orthotic device resulted in improvement of walking performance and balance.[94,98,99] Gait evaluation in a brace clinic and gait training by a PT are indicated when an orthosis is being considered to ensure that the appropriate device is selected and to educate patients on its optimal use.

There has been some debate as to whether prolonged use of an orthotic device might lead to disuse atrophy. In a nonrandomized trial of 26 people with recent-onset foot drop secondary to peroneal neuropathy or L5 radiculopathy, ankle dorsiflexion strength was measured at baseline and after 6 weeks of either AFO use or no intervention.[100] All subjects had significant recovery of strength with no difference between the group that used the AFO and the group that did not, suggesting that the orthosis did not influence restoration of strength.[100] However, research on this topic is lacking in people with progressive neuromuscular diseases. In practice, we monitor gait and fall risk periodically and recommend orthoses based on clinical grounds. In cases of mild foot drop and when recovery is eventually expected, as in Guillain–Barré syndrome, one can use the AFO when walking in the community and "practice" ambulation without the brace at home as long as it is safe to do so. In rapidly progressive disease such as ALS, on the other hand, diurnal use of the brace for safety might be more appropriate.

As weakness progresses, ambulation might become unsafe even with the use of a brace, and assistive devices such as a cane, a walker, or eventually a wheelchair become necessary. Prevention and treatment of contractures resulting from chronic foot drop are described below.

FALLS

People with neuromuscular diseases may be at risk of falling due to weakness, abnormal tone, and impaired sensation and balance. Early in the course of the disease, simple strategies such as behavior modification and energy conservation techniques may suffice. As an example, people can be instructed to take rest breaks to avoid fatigue, use carts instead of carrying luggage or other objects, and negotiate stairs on an angle and one step at a time.

Oftentimes patients do not to realize that some of their usual activities might be unsafe. Simple modifications might actually allow them to continue to function independently. A home safety evaluation by a PT can identify areas for improvement such as removing carpeting, sharp edges, and using appropriate footwear and night lights. Additional environmental modifications such as installing grab bars might be indicated. PTs and OTs can also educate patients and their caregivers on safe transfer techniques.

There is insufficient evidence that exercise results in lower fall rate in neuromuscular patients.[59–64] On the other hand, the benefits of exercise for fall prevention have been well documented in other patient populations.[101–104] If indicated, lower limb orthoses (AFOs) and spasticity management may make ambulation more efficient, although evidence is lacking on the exact impact of these interventions on the risk of falling in neuromuscular patients.

As the disease progresses, mobility aids such as canes, walkers, and wheelchairs may become necessary. Some patients choose to delay the use of mobility aids as much as possible because these tools are often perceived to signify loss of independence. It is important to remember, however, that the primary objective of using assistive devices is to actually preserve independent function. Thus, as an example, the use of a cane, perhaps on an intermittent basis even early on in the disease, may enable people to enjoy activities that would otherwise be restricted. Developing a strong therapeutic alliance with therapists and orthotists who have experience with neuromuscular diseases may assist patients to learn about and become familiar with different pieces of equipment that are available to enhance their independence. Mobility aids also help minimize falls. Falling and the potential occurrence of a bone fracture do have a significant and potentially long-lasting impact on independence in people with neuromuscular diseases. This problem is compounded by the loss of bone mass seen in many of these patients.[105] The prevalence of fractures in a cohort of boys with Duchenne muscular dystrophy attending four neuromuscular clinics was 20%, with some individuals experiencing permanent loss of independent ambulation after the fracture.[106] Falling was the most frequent cause of fractures in this study. Therefore, attention to safety and fall prevention is a crucial component of any rehabilitation program.

FOOT ABNORMALITIES

Peripheral neuropathies leading to intrinsic foot muscle weakness, such as CMT, are associated with bony and soft tissue abnormalities of the feet. These deformities include pes cavus (high-arched feet), pes equinus (excessive plantar flexion), and hammer toes (when the small toes have fixed flexion of the proximal interphalangeal joints with hyperextension of the metatarsophalangeal and distal interphalangeal joints). Functional consequences include pain, callous formation, skin breakdown, and difficulty walking. Many patients complain of and may actually present with frequent ankle sprains as a result of the foot deformity and underlying muscle weakness. Nonoperative treatment includes shoe modifications to improve comfort (such as using low-heeled shoes with a deep toe box, cushioned footwear, custom-molded shoe inserts, and pads to protect the toes) as well as braces (which can range from a simple Velcro-strap ankle brace for active patients with mild ankle instability to an AFO for people with foot drop). Surgical intervention may ultimately be required in some people to correct the deformities and promote ankle stability.

JOINT CONTRACTURES

Many people with neuromuscular diseases are at risk for the development of contractures defined as limitations of full passive ROM in a joint. Causes of contractures in neuromuscular diseases include decreased ability to actively move a limb, static positioning for prolonged periods of time, agonist–antagonist muscle imbalance, spasticity, and fibrotic muscle changes. Contractures are especially common in patients with progressive diseases such as muscular dystrophies. Importantly, contractures compound existing muscle weakness and can lead to pain, limit mobility, positioning, and hygiene, and further hamper the quality of life.

Neuromuscular specialists play an important role in identifying the joints at risk for each particular patient. A commonly seen contracture site in neuromuscular diseases is the ankle in people with an imbalance between dorsiflexion and plantar flexion strength and/or tone (ankle plantar flexion contracture). Hips and knees are also at significant risk of contractures, especially in patients who spend most of their days in wheelchairs. People with hand weakness may experience wrist and finger flexion contractures. When patients are unable to raise their arms overhead, shoulder contractures may develop. Some neuromuscular diseases such as Emery–Dreifuss muscular dystrophy (EDMD) are characterized by early contracture formation, even at a stage of relatively preserved muscle strength. In EDMD, contractures of the elbow flexors and limitation of neck and trunk flexion are typical.

While the evidence supporting interventions to improve ROM in neuromuscular diseases is limited, generally accepted approaches for the prevention and treatment of contractures include stretching exercises, splinting, serial casting, and surgical correction for advanced fixed deformities.[93,107,108]

Daily standing and walking is important to prevent lower limb contracture formation.[107] As weakness progresses, daily upright weight bearing can be accomplished using standing frames or power wheelchairs with standing features.[107] While daily periods of standing are recommended by some practitioners, especially in the pediatric neuromuscular population, equipment cost and poor tolerance by some patients limit the implementation of standing programs.[11] In addition, further research is needed to determine the exact benefits of standing programs and to develop evidence-based guidelines for their use.

Early initiation of stretching and ROM programs is universally recommended for contracture prevention.[107,109] The optimal stretching regimen for people with neuromuscular diseases, however, has not been studied. One can draw from the available evidence in other populations and adjust the program to the individual patient. In healthy subjects, stretching is generally recommended one to two times per day, on most days of the week, and preferably after warm-up of the involved muscle through heat or gentle exercise. The muscle is taken to its maximal length across the affected joint until resistance is felt while stabilizing the joints that are not being moved.[2] The position is held for at least 10 seconds and then repeated several times.[2] Heat and ultrasound may enhance the effect of stretching and positioning. Patients and their caregivers can be instructed on a simple set of ROM exercises which can be performed independently at home. Ideally, such program can become part of a regular morning and evening routine. Positioning can be a useful adjunct for preventing contracture formation. As an example, lying in the prone position when possible provides an effective stretch to the hip flexors.

Bracing is another commonly used modality to prevent and manage contractures. Resting splints allow the joint to rest in a neutral position and can be used throughout the day or at night depending on the clinical scenario. In addition, one can use dynamic splints which provide low-load prolonged-duration stretch. Dynamic splinting in neuromuscular patients is most often used at the level of the ankle and at night. Unfortunately, there is no evidence to guide the timing to initiate splinting, the wear time, or the type of device.[108] A study in Duchenne muscular dystrophy showed a decrease in ankle contractures with the use of a night splint compared to intermittent stretching.[110]

When a contracture is present, one method to improve ROM is to perform serial casting. With this approach, a series of casts with incrementally increasing angles of stretch is applied over a few weeks to gradually improve ROM. At the end of the program, the final cast can be bivalved to create a night splint for long-term maintenance of the ROM. Studies in Duchenne muscular dystrophy and CMT have shown that this approach results in increased ankle ROM.[108,111,112]

Finally, surgical procedures for correction of fixed contractures might be considered. In some conditions, surgery may be performed to improve function. As an example, surgical procedures, such as tendon lengthening, tendon transfer, and tenotomy, have been used in Duchenne muscular dystrophy to prolong ambulation. At present, however, there is no consensus on whether surgery to correct contractures results in prolonged ability to walk in Duchenne patients. Therefore, the decision to perform surgery and its timing are strictly individualized.[11] Corrective surgery might also be performed in some patients as a palliative measure for comfort and positioning.[11]

SPASTICITY

Spasticity is a velocity-dependent increase in muscle tone. From a patient's perspective, spasticity is experienced as an inability to run or walk normally, often associated with leg dragging, loss of control or coordination, stiffness, spasms, pain, loss of fine dexterity, and fatigability. Spasticity generally has a negative impact on a variety of activities. However, in some cases, it may actually be of some functional benefit. As an example, increased tone in lower limb extensor muscles can assist weakened legs, allow standing during transfers, and facilitate bed mobility. Treatment, therefore, must be highly individualized.

Nonpharmacologic treatment options for spasticity are limited, but can be offered as an adjunct. A regular stretching and ROM program is important as part of a contracture prevention program. Anti-spasticity features can be incorporated into AFOs as described above. Physical modalities that have been tried to reduce spasticity include the application of superficial heat and cold, massage, TENS, ultrasound, and acupuncture. The effects of these interventions, however, are generally short lived.[113] One randomized controlled trial of moderate intensity, endurance-type exercise in 25 participants with ALS showed promising positive effects on spasticity as measured by the Ashworth scale, but the trial was too small to draw definitive conclusions.[21,114] Pharmacologic agents for spasticity include oral medications, intrathecal baclofen, and botulinum toxin injections. These have been described in Chapter 7, Table 7-3. Finally, surgical interventions such as tendon release may be considered as a palliative measure in nonambulatory individuals to facilitate hygiene or relieve discomfort.

PAIN

Some neuromuscular diseases, such as small fiber neuropathy, directly involve pain pathways. Many others, as ALS, are traditionally considered "painless" conditions. However, this could not be further from the truth as secondary painful musculoskeletal syndromes often arise in people with neuromuscular weakness. High prevalence of pain has been documented in multiple neuromuscular populations including postpolio syndrome, FSHD, and myotonic dystrophy.[115–117] Pain is reported by ALS patients even in the early stages of their disease.[118] In a study by Engel et al., the prevalence of chronic pain among youths with a variety of muscular dystrophies was a staggering 55%.[119] Thus, a comprehensive rehabilitation plan for people with neuromuscular disorders must address pain.

The etiology of chronic pain in neuromuscular diseases is generally multifactorial, with contribution from both neuropathic and musculoskeletal pain generators. Primary sites of pain are the lower limbs and the back.[117,119] The first step in managing pain is to obtain a careful history and perform thorough neurologic and musculoskeletal examinations because treatment strategies vary depending on the main pain source. Importantly, soft tissue and bone problems can "mimic" neurogenic causes of pain (as further reviewed in Chapter 36). As an example, hip and thigh pain may be due to radiculopathy, hip osteoarthritis, or trochanteric bursitis, conditions which obviously warrant completely different therapeutic approaches. Foot pain can be due to neuropathy or radiculopathy, but also due to contractures, joint deformities, plantar fasciitis, and Morton's neuromas. Hand pain may be caused by median neuropathy at the wrist, osteoarthritis or De Quervain tenosynovitis, just to name a few. We have seen ALS patients with finger flexor tenosynovitis whose pain was greatly relieved by simple local steroid injections. A careful examination can help differentiate among these conditions. If needed, referral to physiatrists or orthopedic surgeons might help assess the cause of pain and institute proper treatment. PTs having experience with neuromuscular diseases can help manage these and additional sources of pain such as trigger points, brace problems, improper transfer techniques, and poor positioning in bed or in the wheelchair. In wheelchair users, back pain can often be relieved by providing adequate lumbar support and good cushioning. Some features of power wheelchairs can help with pain management. Power elevation leg rests can help maintain hamstring length and ease back pain, while tilting the wheelchair relieves pain from gluteal pressure. Leg discomfort can also be associated with dependent edema secondary to limited mobility. Leg elevation, massage, and use of compression stockings may provide some relief. For people with advanced weakness, positioning in bed is an important issue that should not be overlooked. Bed should be fitted with pressure relief over bony prominences to avoid pain and pressure ulcers. Foam wedges can be used to facilitate proper positioning.

Medications to treat neuropathic pain have been described in Chapter 22. Musculoskeletal pain typically responds to nonsteroidal anti-inflammatory medications (NSAIDs), particularly if there is evidence of an inflammatory process such as arthritis or bursitis. As-needed or standing doses of acetaminophen may be used along with an NSAID or if NSAIDs are contraindicated. Physiatrists and PTs can help recommend other strategies to alleviate pain such as stretching, bracing, manual therapy, topical heat and ice (given alone or sequentially, as in contrast therapy), TENS, ultrasound, and iontophoresis. These physical modalities can be effective either alone or as an adjunct to pharmacologic treatment. Involvement of specialists from a pain clinic might be needed in more severe cases.

PTOSIS

Neuromuscular causes of ptosis (specifically, blepharoptosis) include Guillain–Barré and Miller-Fisher syndromes, neuromuscular junction diseases, and certain myopathies [e.g., oculopharyngeal muscular dystrophy (OPMD), mitochondrial myopathies, and myotonic dystrophy (Table 1-8). In addition to cosmetic concerns, ptosis may limit vision and interfere with driving, working, reading, and other ADLs. It may also result in neck discomfort because patients tend to compensate for ptosis by keeping a chin-up head posture. Treatment of ptosis revolves around management of the underlying disorder when disease-modifying treatments are available. In the case of the myopathies causing ptosis, no such therapies exist. Unfortunately, rehabilitation options for ptosis are very limited. Eyelid taping or eyelid prostheses (crutches) may be tried.[120] Eyelid crutches consist of attachments to glasses that hold the eyes open. Surgery is another option and different surgical techniques have been used, including silicone sling surgery which allows for adjustments for progressive ptosis. However, candidate selection is crucial. People with weak orbicularis oculi preventing complete closure of the eyelids are at risk for exposure keratopathy postoperatively.[121–123] In addition, ptosis may recur (recurrence rate among OPMD patients was 13% in a surgical series from Quebec).[124]

DYSPHAGIA

Dysphagia refers to difficulty in eating as a result of disruption in the swallowing process. Many neuromuscular diseases can cause dysphagia including motor neuron disorders, neuromuscular junction diseases, Guillain–Barré syndrome, and certain myopathies (most commonly, inflammatory myopathies, OPMD, myofibrillar myopathies, some mitochondrial disorders, myotonic dystrophy, and late stages of Duchenne and other muscular dystrophies).

Symptoms of dysphagia include coughing and/or difficulty breathing during or after meals, episodes of choking, multiple swallows per bolus, increased secretions, frequent throat clearing, wet vocal quality (suggesting pooling of secretions), and feeling that food is "stuck" in the throat. If palatal weakness is present, the patient may also experience nasal regurgitation.

Dysphagia can be classified as either oropharyngeal or esophageal. Neuromuscular disorders generally cause the former, due to disruption of oral and/or pharyngeal processes. In the oral and pharyngeal phases of swallowing, food is chewed, pushed to the pharynx under voluntary control, and then to the esophagus. During the process, posterior tongue movement and hyolaryngeal elevation are critical to achieve full airway closure (via epiglottal deflection) and esophageal opening. Pharyngeal contractions are required to move food toward the esophagus, and the nasopharynx must close to prevent food from entering the nasal passages. Approximation of the vocal folds and tilting of the arytenoids also help to prevent aspiration. In the esophageal phase of swallowing, peristalsis moves the bolus through the esophagus and then into the stomach. Esophageal dysphagia is most commonly caused by mechanical causes or motility disorders, although some neuromuscular conditions such as the inflammatory myopathies can affect the esophagus as well.

In oropharyngeal dysphagia, the type most commonly seen in neuromuscular disorders, managing liquids may be more difficult than solids, at least initially. This occurs because oropharyngeal muscle weakness results in slowing of the initial phases of swallowing. This process is outpaced by the rapidity of the liquid bolus which tends to reach the laryngeal vestibule before laryngeal protection mechanisms can be activated. Meals may require a long time to complete and become a fatiguing rather than pleasant experience. The sialorrhea (drooling) seen in some neuromuscular diseases such as ALS may be the result of decreased swallow frequency due to muscle weakness rather than an increase in salivation. Importantly, dysphagia may lead to aspiration and malnutrition, a negative prognostic factor in some conditions such as ALS.[125–127]

Speech pathologists can provide an objective measurement of dysphagia by using clinical assessments as well as instrumental measures (i.e., MBS or FEES). Clinical bedside assessment consists of observing the swallowing function using a variety of food consistencies (liquid, nectar, puree, solid). Time to consume meals may provide evidence of changes in swallowing function, especially the oral phase. MBS utilizes videofluoroscopy to visualize a contrast substance, barium sulfate, which is mixed with different food consistencies and swallowed. MBS is a sensitive technique for identifying oropharyngeal dysphagia as it allows tracing each bolus through the oral and pharyngeal phases as the person swallows.[128] The presence of penetration or aspiration into the larynx can be detected by MBS, thus helping gauge the risk of aspiration pneumonia. During the MBS examination, the clinician is also able to try strategies to see if aspiration and penetration can be minimized or eliminated. Dysphagia can also be assessed endoscopically by FEES. This technique involves feeding a nasally inserted camera into the pharynx and positioning it just above the epiglottis to allow visualization of the pharyngeal phase of swallowing.

When dysphagia is present within the context of a treatable condition such as Guillain–Barré syndrome, myasthenia gravis, or PM/DM, treatment is directed toward the underlying pathologic process. From a rehabilitation perspective, there is no evidence that exercise improves swallowing function. While waiting for dysphagia to improve or resolve, or in progressive diseases such as ALS and most myopathies, dysphagia management revolves around modification of food and fluid consistency to make them easier to chew and swallow. As an example, soft, moist foods are easier to swallow than dry, crumbly, or chewy foods. Foods that are smooth, single consistency (like pudding) are easier to manipulate in the mouth than mixed textured foods, such as dry cereal with milk. Thicker liquids (fruit nectar, smoothies) are easier to handle than water. Commercial thickeners are available to modify the consistency of liquids to the desired level. Thickening a liquid can help to slow a bolus down enough for the pharyngeal responses to occur in a timely fashion, helping to prevent aspiration. Chilling liquids or adding carbonation might provide sensory stimulation during swallowing or improve swallowing in myasthenia by rendering neuromuscular transmission more efficient. As an example, chilled, carbonated water might be easier to swallow than room-temperature plain water. A modified diet might be recommended, ranging from soft diet (tender and moist foods), to mechanical diet (ground meats, well-cooked veggies, and soft fruits that require very little chewing), to pureed (when all foods are blended to a smooth liquid consistency). Behavioral strategies that may help to prolong people's ability to continue to have *per os* intake in spite of dysphagia include taking small bites and sips, alternating bites of solid food with sips of liquid to ensure adequate clearing, sitting upright, avoid talking, paying increased attention to each individual swallow. Performing a chin tuck may facilitate safe swallowing by adding protection to the airway made vulnerable because of pharyngeal weakness, but all strategies need to be carefully considered. There is not a prescribed regimen that is appropriate for all patients with dysphagia. If malnutrition is a concern, one can try eating smaller meals with high-calorie snacks at scheduled times, choosing calorie-dense foods or high-calorie supplements. Because of difficulties managing liquids, special attention must be paid to the individual's hydration status. Gelatin and ice pops might help boost water intake. Additional strategies to promote *per os* intake, as long as it is safe, and avoid malnutrition include addressing problems with self-feeding and managing secretions. Periodic monitoring of swallowing function and nutritional status by a speech pathologist and/or dietitian helps to determine when oral intake becomes inadequate, too effortful or fatiguing, and/or compromises safety.

Alternative routes for nutrition include nasogastric tubes (generally utilized short-term) and percutaneous endoscopic gastrostomy (PEG) or radiologically inserted gastrostomy (RIG) tubes for long-term use. Enteral nutrition using either one of these methods is considered in the presence of severe bulbar symptoms, aspiration, weight loss >10%, dehydration, declining respiratory function, and diminished quality of life due to difficulties with eating/choking. In ALS, the risk of PEG placement increases when functional vital capacity falls below 50% and PEG is probably effective in prolonging survival.[129] Therefore, early intervention is advocated by many, although there is no evidence to support specific timing of PEG insertion in ALS.[129,130] Some people with progressive neuromuscular disorders choose to continue to consume limited amounts of preferred foods orally for pleasure. One should discuss the associated aspiration risks to enable the patient to make informed decisions regarding this approach.

In selected neuromuscular conditions, cricopharyngeal myotomy has been tried to alleviate dysphagia symptoms. With this procedure, the cricopharyngeal muscle, which is the major contributor to the upper esophageal sphincter (UES), is severed. This procedure might be considered in people with abnormal pharyngoesophageal junction, but adequate laryngeal/pharyngeal function, to ease the transfer of the swallowed bolus to the esophagus. Case series have reported benefits in patients with OPMD and IBM, although potential benefits have to be weighed against surgical risks.[131–136] In a series of 139 patients treated for dysphagia secondary to myopathy, complications were recorded in 16 patients, which ultimately resulted in four deaths.[132] Another method to target dysfunction at the UES is to inject the cricopharyngeal muscle with botulinum toxin. This technique was recently reported to improve dysphagia symptoms in a subset of people with motor neuron disease. Selection of appropriate candidates for the procedure was crucial as improvement was seen only in people with isolated UES hyperactivity based on videofluoroscopic or EMG assessment.[137] No improvement was seen in patients with concurrent lower motor neuron involvement of oropharyngeal muscles.[137]

DYSARTHRIA

Dysarthria is a collective name for speech disorders that impact the speed, strength, range, timing, and/or accuracy of speech movements and thus may impact the overall intelligibility of speech. Neuromuscular disorders affecting the motor neurons, the neuromuscular junction, and some myopathies can result in dysarthria. Upper motor neuron disease causes spastic dysarthria which is characterized by slow rate, harshness, and a strained-strangled vocal quality. There may be bursts of loudness and unanticipated stops. Lower motor neuron disease results in flaccid dysarthria, which presents as a weak, breathy, monopitch, and hypernasal voice. There may be imprecise articulation, but rate is generally normal. Motor neuron diseases such as ALS often present with mixed spastic-flaccid dysarthria. Dysarthria resulting from neuromuscular junction or muscle pathology typically resembles flaccid dysarthria.

When dysarthria is seen within the context of a treatable neuromuscular condition such as myasthenia gravis, treatment is directed toward the underlying pathology. On the other hand, when disease-modifying treatments are not available, referral to speech pathologists is very valuable in the evaluation and management of dysarthria. Many clinicians use intelligibility to track changes in functional speech as disease progresses. Speaking rate is another useful means of evaluating speech production as changes in speaking rate precede reduction in intelligibility in progressive neuromuscular diseases such as ALS.[138,139] These factors should be taken into account when deciding the optimal timing for referral to an SLP and when considering introduction of AAC devices.

Oral motor exercises are not likely to help in progressive neuromuscular disorders. A possible exception is myotonic dystrophy. In myotonic dystrophy, both muscle weakness and myotonia may contribute to impaired articulation. Warm-up exercises may improve fluency of speech and decrease the myotonic component of dysarthria without producing fatigue.[140]

In most chronic neuromuscular conditions, speech interventions revolve on techniques for compensation and adaptation to promote independence with communication. Reducing ambient noise, minimizing the distance between patient and listeners, and speaking face-to-face in a well lit room are the first steps to make communication as easy and effortless as possible. In restaurants, choosing a table near a wall might help reduce distractions. Compensatory techniques to prolong verbal communication include slowing speech rate, using alternative words, spelling, and repeating and over-articulating. It is also important to develop personalized communication strategies between patient and caregivers such as shared strategies for understanding gestures and a system for confirming understanding.

A fatiguing aspect of speech production for people with concurrent weakness of the muscles of breathing is the need to develop sufficient respiratory support to speak loudly. As an example, people with ALS may have difficulties calling their caregiver in an adjacent room. The use of alerting systems such as buzzers and baby monitors can help. Similarly, it is important for people with severe dysarthria to have a plan to call for help in case of emergency.

As dysarthria progresses, AAC devices may be needed to enhance the person's ability to communicate. Such systems may be used to augment natural speech or to replace it. There is a wide range of options in devices for communication. One should keep in mind that more complex technology is not necessarily better. The choice of device is affected not only by the current degree of impairment but also by the expected disease progression and patient preferences. Low-technology devices include communication boards with manual writing and letter/word/picture boards which can be used with a trained communication partner if the patient does not have functional hand use. High-technology options (defined here as anything that needs a plug or a battery) include portable voice amplifiers which allow the amplification of diminished voice volume. Message banking allows patients to record words and phrases while still intelligible and play them back when they are no longer able to say the messages themselves. These messages can be a wonderful addition to a high-tech system that has voice output capability. Text-to-speech devices are also available: messages are typed on a keyboard and displayed on small monitor while a speech synthesizer provides speech output. For people who are unable to use a keyboard, some speech-generating devices have the option of an on-screen keyboard with selection made by a switch using a scanning technique. Many people use computerized voice synthesizers on personal computers and tablets. Selection of information can be manual, by eye gaze, or by head movement tracking technology. Many of these assistive technology devices can be mounted on the person's wheelchair. Finally, brain–computer interfaces (BCIs) are an active area of research with promise for use in severe dysarthria or anarthria in people who also have severe motor impairment. BCIs transform signals originating in the brain into commands that translate into the movement of a cursor or a switch. Brain activity is captured by using either scalp recordings of electroencephalographic changes or direct recordings from the motor cortex.[141–143]

FINAL CONSIDERATIONS

The rehabilitation team is uniquely positioned to positively affect the quality of life of neuromuscular patients. It is well known that the degree of weakness and physical impairment does not directly correlate with satisfaction with life.[144–147] Interestingly, both caregivers and health care professionals tend to underestimate the quality of life of neuromuscular patients.[144] Rather, in individuals with neuromuscular diseases, quality of life correlates with social interactions, ability to direct care, feelings of hope, and alleviation of manageable disease-related symptoms, all of which are factors that can benefit from a comprehensive rehabilitation plan.[148]

▶ ACKNOWLEDGMENTS

This chapter is dedicated to the memory of Lisa Krivickas, MD, exceptional mentor, ALS clinician and researcher. We would also like to thank the following colleagues for their helpful comments and suggestions during the drafting of this chapter: Patricia Andres, DPT, MS; Jonathan Bean, MD, MS, MPH; Cheri Blauwet, MD; Amy Swartz Ellrodt, PT, DPT; Elizabeth Hansen, PT, DPT; Michelle Kerr, PT/ATP; Julie MacLean, OTR/L; Paige Nalipinski, MA, CCC, SLP; Aaron Norell, CO, BOCP; Lisa Pezzini, PT.

REFERENCES

1. Miller RG, Jackson CE, Kasarskis EJ, et al. Practice parameter update: the care of the patient with amyotrophic lateral sclerosis: multidisciplinary care, symptom management, and cognitive/behavioral impairment (an evidence-based review): report of the Quality Standards Subcommittee of the American Academy of Neurology. *Neurology*. 2009;73:1227–1233.
2. Johnson LB, Florence JM, Abresch RT. Physical therapy evaluation and management in neuromuscular diseases. *Phys Med Rehabil Clin N Am*. 2012;23:633–651.
3. Jette AM. Toward a common language for function, disability, and health. *Phys Ther*. 2006;86:726–734.
4. Holt NE, Percac-Lima S, Kurlinski LA, et al. The Boston Rehabilitative Impairment Study of the Elderly: a description of methods. *Arch Phys Med Rehabil*. 2013;94:347–355.
5. Boentert M, Dziewas R, Heidbreder A, et al. Fatigue, reduced sleep quality and restless legs syndrome in Charcot-Marie-Tooth disease: a web-based survey. *J Neurol*. 2010;257:646–652.
6. Atassi N, Cook A, Pineda CM, Yerramilli-Rao P, Pulley D, Cudkowicz M. Depression in amyotrophic lateral sclerosis. *Amyotroph Lateral Scler*. 2011;12:109–112.
7. Heatwole C, Bode R, Johnson N, et al. Patient-reported impact of symptoms in myotonic dystrophy type 1 (PRISM-1). *Neurology*. 2012;79:348–357.
8. Voet NB, van der Kooi EL, Riphagen, II, Lindeman E, van Engelen BG, Geurts A. Strength training and aerobic exercise training for muscle disease. *Cochrane Database Syst Rev*. 2010;(1)CD003907.
9. Zhou S. Chronic neural adaptations to unilateral exercise: mechanisms of cross education. *Exerc Sport Sci Rev*. 2000;28:177–184.
10. Fowler WM Jr. Role of physical activity and exercise training in neuromuscular diseases. *Am J Phys Med Rehabil*. 2002; 81:S187–195.
11. Bushby K, Finkel R, Birnkrant DJ, et al. Diagnosis and management of Duchenne muscular dystrophy, part 2: implementation of multidisciplinary care. *Lancet Neurol*. 2010;9:177–189.

12. Phillips EM, Kennedy MA. The exercise prescription: a tool to improve physical activity. *PM R*. 2012;4:818–825.
13. Micheo W, Baerga L, Miranda G. Basic principles regarding strength, flexibility, and stability exercises. *PM R*. 2012;4: 805–811.
14. Kraemer WJ, Ratamess NA, French DN. Resistance training for health and performance. *Curr Sports Med Rep*. 2002;1: 165–171.
15. Mancuso M, Angelini C, Bertini E, et al. Fatigue and exercise intolerance in mitochondrial diseases. Literature revision and experience of the Italian Network of mitochondrial diseases. *Neuromuscul Disord*. 2012;22(Suppl 3):S226–S229.
16. Angelini C, Tasca E. Fatigue in muscular dystrophies. *Neuromuscul Disord*. 2012;22(Suppl 3):S214–S220.
17. Kirkinezos IG, Hernandez D, Bradley WG, Moraes CT. Regular exercise is beneficial to a mouse model of amyotrophic lateral sclerosis. *Ann Neurol*. 2003;53:804–807.
18. Veldink JH, Bar PR, Joosten EA, Otten M, Wokke JH, van den Berg LH. Sexual differences in onset of disease and response to exercise in a transgenic model of ALS. *Neuromuscul Disord*. 2003;13:737–743.
19. Carreras I, Yuruker S, Aytan N, et al. Moderate exercise delays the motor performance decline in a transgenic model of ALS. *Brain Res*. 2010;1313:192–201.
20. Mahoney DJ, Rodriguez C, Devries M, Yasuda N, Tarnopolsky MA. Effects of high-intensity endurance exercise training in the G93 A mouse model of amyotrophic lateral sclerosis. *Muscle Nerve*. 2004;29:656–662.
21. Drory VE, Goltsman E, Reznik JG, Mosek A, Korczyn AD. The value of muscle exercise in patients with amyotrophic lateral sclerosis. *J Neurol Sci*. 2001;191:133–137.
22. Bello-Haas VD, Florence JM, Kloos AD, et al. A randomized controlled trial of resistance exercise in individuals with ALS. *Neurology*. 2007;68:2003–2007.
23. Lindeman E, Leffers P, Spaans F, et al. Strength training in patients with myotonic dystrophy and hereditary motor and sensory neuropathy: a randomized clinical trial. *Arch Phys Med Rehabil*. 1995;76:612–620.
24. El Mhandi L, Millet GY, Calmels P, et al. Benefits of interval-training on fatigue and functional capacities in Charcot-Marie-Tooth disease. *Muscle Nerve*. 2008;37:601–610.
25. Chetlin RD, Gutmann L, Tarnopolsky M, Ullrich IH, Yeater RA. Resistance training effectiveness in patients with Charcot-Marie-Tooth disease: recommendations for exercise prescription. *Arch Phys Med Rehabil*. 2004;85:1217–1223.
26. Petrof BJ. The molecular basis of activity-induced muscle injury in Duchenne muscular dystrophy. *Mol Cell Biochem*. 1998;179:111–123.
27. Allen DG, Zhang BT, Whitehead NP. Stretch-induced membrane damage in muscle: comparison of wild-type and mdx mice. *Adv Exp Med Biol*. 2010;682:297–313.
28. Markert CD, Case LE, Carter GT, Furlong PA, Grange RW. Exercise and Duchenne muscular dystrophy: where we have been and where we need to go. *Muscle Nerve*. 2012;45: 746–751.
29. Moens P, Baatsen PH, Marechal G. Increased susceptibility of EDL muscles from mdx mice to damage induced by contractions with stretch. *J Muscle Res Cell Motil*. 1993;14:446–451.
30. Markert CD, Ambrosio F, Call JA, Grange RW. Exercise and Duchenne muscular dystrophy: toward evidence-based exercise prescription. *Muscle Nerve*. 2011;43:464–478.
31. Sveen ML, Jeppesen TD, Hauerslev S, Kober L, Krag TO, Vissing J. Endurance training improves fitness and strength in patients with Becker muscular dystrophy. *Brain*. 2008;131: 2824–2831.
32. Sveen ML, Andersen SP, Ingelsrud LH, et al. Resistance training in patients with limb-girdle and becker muscular dystrophies. *Muscle Nerve*. 2013;47:163–169.
33. Jansen M, de Groot IJ, van Alfen N, Geurts A. Physical training in boys with Duchenne Muscular Dystrophy: The protocol of the No Use is Disuse study. *BMC Pediatr*. 2010;10:55.
34. van der Kooi EL, Kalkman JS, Lindeman E, et al. Effects of training and albuterol on pain and fatigue in facioscapulohumeral muscular dystrophy. *J Neurol*. 2007;254:931–940.
35. van der Kooi EL, Vogels OJ, van Asseldonk RJ, et al. Strength training and albuterol in facioscapulohumeral muscular dystrophy. *Neurology*. 2004;63:702–708.
36. Olsen DB, Orngreen MC, Vissing J. Aerobic training improves exercise performance in facioscapulohumeral muscular dystrophy. *Neurology*. 2005;64:1064–1066.
37. Pandya S, King WM, Tawil R. Facioscapulohumeral dystrophy. *Phys Ther*. 2008;88:105–113.
38. Orngreen MC, Olsen DB, Vissing J. Aerobic training in patients with myotonic dystrophy type 1. *Ann Neurol*. 2005;57: 754–757.
39. Wiesinger GF, Quittan M, Aringer M, et al. Improvement of physical fitness and muscle strength in polymyositis/dermatomyositis patients by a training programme. *Br J Rheumatol*. 1998;37:196–200.
40. Habers GE, Takken T. Safety and efficacy of exercise training in patients with an idiopathic inflammatory myopathy–a systematic review. *Rheumatology (Oxford)*. 2011;50:2113–2124.
41. Alexanderson H. Exercise in inflammatory myopathies, including inclusion body myositis. *Curr Rheumatol Rep*. 2012;14: 244–251.
42. Alexanderson H, Lundberg IE. Exercise as a therapeutic modality in patients with idiopathic inflammatory myopathies. *Curr Opin Rheumatol*. 2012;24:201–207.
43. Wiesinger GF, Quittan M, Graninger M, et al. Benefit of 6 months long-term physical training in polymyositis/dermatomyositis patients. *Br J Rheumatol*. 1998;37:1338–1342.
44. Alexanderson H, Stenstrom CH, Jenner G, Lundberg I. The safety of a resistive home exercise program in patients with recent onset active polymyositis or dermatomyositis. *Scand J Rheumatol*. 2000;29:295–301.
45. Alexanderson H, Dastmalchi M, Esbjornsson-Liljedahl M, Opava CH, Lundberg IE. Benefits of intensive resistance training in patients with chronic polymyositis or dermatomyositis. *Arthritis Rheum*. 2007;57:768–777.
46. Arnardottir S, Alexanderson H, Lundberg IE, Borg K. Sporadic inclusion body myositis: Pilot study on the effects of a home exercise program on muscle function, histopathology and inflammatory reaction. *J Rehabil Med*. 2003;35:31–35.
47. Johnson LG, Collier KE, Edwards DJ, et al. Improvement in aerobic capacity after an exercise program in sporadic inclusion body myositis. *J Clin Neuromuscul Dis*. 2009;10:178–184.
48. Cejudo P, Bautista J, Montemayor T, et al. Exercise training in mitochondrial myopathy: A randomized controlled trial. *Muscle Nerve*. 2005;32:342–350.
49. Taivassalo T, De Stefano N, Argov Z, et al. Effects of aerobic training in patients with mitochondrial myopathies. *Neurology*. 1998;50:1055–1060.

50. Taivassalo T, Gardner JL, Taylor RW, et al. Endurance training and detraining in mitochondrial myopathies due to single large-scale mtDNA deletions. *Brain.* 2006;129:3391–3401.
51. Taivassalo T, Shoubridge EA, Chen J, et al. Aerobic conditioning in patients with mitochondrial myopathies: Physiological, biochemical, and genetic effects. *Ann Neurol.* 2001;50:133–141.
52. Siciliano G, Simoncini C, Lo Gerfo A, Orsucci D, Ricci G, Mancuso M. Effects of aerobic training on exercise-related oxidative stress in mitochondrial myopathies. *Neuromuscul Disord.* 2012;22(Suppl 3):S172–S177.
53. Murphy JL, Blakely EL, Schaefer AM, et al. Resistance training in patients with single, large-scale deletions of mitochondrial DNA. *Brain.* 2008;131:2832–2840.
54. Haller RG, Wyrick P, Taivassalo T, Vissing J. Aerobic conditioning: an effective therapy in McArdle's disease. *Ann Neurol.* 2006;59:922–928.
55. Mate-Munoz JL, Moran M, Perez M, et al. Favorable responses to acute and chronic exercise in McArdle patients. *Clin J Sport Med.* 2007;17:297–303.
56. Quinlivan R, Vissing J, Hilton-Jones D, Buckley J. Physical training for McArdle disease. *Cochrane Database Syst Rev.* 2011;(12):CD007931.
57. Lucia A, Quinlivan R, Wakelin A, Martin MA, Andreu AL. The 'McArdle paradox': exercise is a good advice for the exercise intolerant. *Br J Sports Med.* 2013;47(12):728–729.
58. Haller RG. Treatment of McArdle disease. *Arch Neurol.* 2000; 57:923–924.
59. Nardone A, Godi M, Artuso A, Schieppati M. Balance rehabilitation by moving platform and exercises in patients with neuropathy or vestibular deficit. *Arch Phys Med Rehabil.* 2010;91: 1869–1877.
60. Kruse RL, Lemaster JW, Madsen RW. Fall and balance outcomes after an intervention to promote leg strength, balance, and walking in people with diabetic peripheral neuropathy: "feet first" randomized controlled trial. *Phys Ther.* 2010;90: 1568–1579.
61. Song CH, Petrofsky JS, Lee SW, Lee KJ, Yim JE. Effects of an exercise program on balance and trunk proprioception in older adults with diabetic neuropathies. *Diabetes Technol Ther.* 2011;13:803–811.
62. Richardson JK, Sandman D, Vela S. A focused exercise regimen improves clinical measures of balance in patients with peripheral neuropathy. *Arch Phys Med Rehabil.* 2001;82: 205–209.
63. Akbari M, Jafari H, Moshashaee A, Forugh B. Do diabetic neuropathy patients benefit from balance training? *J Rehabil Res Dev.* 2012;49:333–338.
64. Tofthagen C, Visovsky C, Berry DL. Strength and balance training for adults with peripheral neuropathy and high risk of fall: current evidence and implications for future research. *Oncol Nurs Forum.* 2012;39:E416–E424.
65. Cup EH, Pieterse AJ, Ten Broek-Pastoor JM, et al. Exercise therapy and other types of physical therapy for patients with neuromuscular diseases: a systematic review. *Arch Phys Med Rehabil.* 2007;88:1452–1464.
66. Abresch RT, Carter GT, Han JJ, McDonald CM. Exercise in neuromuscular diseases. *Phys Med Rehabil Clin N Am.* 2012;23:653–673.
67. Rivera-Brown AM, Frontera WR. Principles of exercise physiology: responses to acute exercise and long-term adaptations to training. *PM R.* 2012;4:797–804.
68. Fast A, Thomas MA. The "baseball cap orthosis": a simple solution for dropped head syndrome. *Am J Phys Med Rehabil.* 2008;87:71–73.
69. Zorowitz RD, Idank D, Ikai T, Hughes MB, Johnston MV. Shoulder subluxation after stroke: A comparison of four supports. *Arch Phys Med Rehabil.* 1995;76:763–771.
70. de Seze MP, Creuze A, de Seze M, Mazaux JM. An orthosis and physiotherapy programme for camptocormia: a prospective case study. *J Rehabil Med.* 2008;40:761–765.
71. Wilkins KE, Gibson DA. The patterns of spinal deformity in Duchenne muscular dystrophy. *J Bone Joint Surg Am.* 1976;58: 24–32.
72. Kouwenhoven JW, Van Ommeren PM, Pruijs HE, Castelein RM. Spinal decompensation in neuromuscular disease. *Spine (Phila Pa 1976).* 2006;31:E188–E191.
73. Sucato DJ. Spine deformity in spinal muscular atrophy. *J Bone Joint Surg Am.* 2007;89(Suppl 1):148–154.
74. Colbert AP, Craig C. Scoliosis management in Duchenne muscular dystrophy: prospective study of modified Jewett hyperextension brace. *Arch Phys Med Rehabil.* 1987;68:302–304.
75. Kinali M, Messina S, Mercuri E, et al. Management of scoliosis in Duchenne muscular dystrophy: A large 10-year retrospective study. *Dev Med Child Neurol.* 2006;48:513–518.
76. Alman BA, Raza SN, Biggar WD. Steroid treatment and the development of scoliosis in males with duchenne muscular dystrophy. *J Bone Joint Surg Am.* 2004;86-A:519–524.
77. Granata C, Merlini L, Cervellati S, et al. Long-term results of spine surgery in Duchenne muscular dystrophy. *Neuromuscul Disord.* 1996;6:61–68.
78. Robinson CM, Seah KT, Chee YH, Hindle P, Murray IR. Frozen shoulder. *J Bone Joint Surg Br.* 2012;94:1–9.
79. Ho DT, Ruthazer R, Russell JA. Shoulder pain in amyotrophic lateral sclerosis. *J Clin Neuromuscul Dis.* 2011;13:53–55.
80. Green S, Buchbinder R, Hetrick S. Acupuncture for shoulder pain. *Cochrane Database Syst Rev.* 2005;(2):CD005319.
81. Green S, Buchbinder R, Hetrick S. Physiotherapy interventions for shoulder pain. *Cochrane Database Syst Rev.* 2003;(2):CD004258.
82. Gaujoux-Viala C, Dougados M, Gossec L. Efficacy and safety of steroid injections for shoulder and elbow tendonitis: a meta-analysis of randomised controlled trials. *Ann Rheum Dis.* 2009;68:1843–1849.
83. Bloom JE, Rischin A, Johnston RV, Buchbinder R. Image-guided versus blind glucocorticoid injection for shoulder pain. *Cochrane Database Syst Rev.* 2012;8:CD009147.
84. Meininger AK, Figuerres BF, Goldberg BA. Scapular winging: an update. *J Am Acad Orthop Surg.* 2011;19:453–462.
85. Orrell RW, Copeland S, Rose MR. Scapular fixation in muscular dystrophy. *Cochrane Database Syst Rev* 2010;(1): CD003278.
86. Cup EH, Pieterse AJ, Knuijt S, et al. Referral of patients with neuromuscular disease to occupational therapy, physical therapy and speech therapy: usual practice versus multidisciplinary advice. *Disabil Rehabil.* 2007;29:717–726.
87. Aldehag AS, Jonsson H, Ansved T. Effects of a hand training programme in five patients with myotonic dystrophy type 1. *Occup Ther Int.* 2005;12:14–27.
88. Brehm MA, Beelen A, Doorenbosch CA, Harlaar J, Nollet F. Effect of carbon-composite knee-ankle-foot orthoses on walking efficiency and gait in former polio patients. *J Rehabil Med.* 2007;39:651–657.

89. Hachisuka K, Makino K, Wada F, Saeki S, Yoshimoto N. Oxygen consumption, oxygen cost and physiological cost index in polio survivors: a comparison of walking without orthosis, with an ordinary or a carbon-fibre reinforced plastic knee-ankle-foot orthosis. *J Rehabil Med*. 2007;39:646–650.
90. Bakker JP, De Groot IJ, De Jong BA, Van Tol-De Jager MA, Lankhorst GJ. Prescription pattern for orthoses in The Netherlands: use and experience in the ambulatory phase of Duchenne muscular dystrophy. *Disabil Rehabil*. 1997;19:318–325.
91. Bernhardt K, Oh T, Kaufman K. Stance control orthosis trial in patients with inclusion body myositis. *Prosthet Orthot Int*. 2011;35:39–44.
92. Waters RL, Mulroy S. The energy expenditure of normal and pathologic gait. *Gait Posture*. 1999;9:207–231.
93. Sackley C, Disler PB, Turner-Stokes L, Wade DT, Brittle N, Hoppitt T. Rehabilitation interventions for foot drop in neuromuscular disease. *Cochrane Database Syst Rev*. 2009;(3):CD003908.
94. Ramdharry GM, Day BL, Reilly MM, Marsden JF. Foot drop splints improve proximal as well as distal leg control during gait in Charcot-Marie-Tooth disease. *Muscle Nerve*. 2012;46:512–519.
95. Ramdharry GM, Day BL, Reilly MM, Marsden JF. Hip flexor fatigue limits walking in Charcot-Marie-Tooth disease. *Muscle Nerve*. 2009;40:103–111.
96. Menotti F, Felici F, Damiani A, Mangiola F, Vannicelli R, Macaluso A. Charcot-Marie-Tooth 1 A patients with low level of impairment have a higher energy cost of walking than healthy individuals. *Neuromuscul Disord*. 2011;21:52–57.
97. McCrory MA, Kim HR, Wright NC, Lovelady CA, Aitkens S, Kilmer DD. Energy expenditure, physical activity, and body composition of ambulatory adults with hereditary neuromuscular disease. *Am J Clin Nutr*. 1998;67:1162–1169.
98. Aprile I, Bordieri C, Gilardi A, et al. Balance and walking involvement in facioscapulohumeral dystrophy: a pilot study on the effects of custom lower limb orthoses. *Eur J Phys Rehabil Med*. 2013;49(2):169–178.
99. Bean J, Walsh A, Frontera W. Brace modification improves aerobic performance in Charcot-Marie-Tooth disease: a single-subject design. *Am J Phys Med Rehabil*. 2001;80:578–582.
100. Geboers JF, Janssen-Potten YJ, Seelen HA, Spaans F, Drost MR. Evaluation of effect of ankle-foot orthosis use on strength restoration of paretic dorsiflexors. *Arch Phys Med Rehabil*. 2001;82:856–860.
101. Sinaki M, Brey RH, Hughes CA, Larson DR, Kaufman KR. Significant reduction in risk of falls and back pain in osteoporotic-kyphotic women through a Spinal Proprioceptive Extension Exercise Dynamic (SPEED) program. *Mayo Clin Proc*. 2005;80:849–855.
102. Sinaki M. Exercise for patients with osteoporosis: management of vertebral compression fractures and trunk strengthening for fall prevention. *PM R*. 2012;4:882–888.
103. Cameron ID, Gillespie LD, Robertson MC, et al. Interventions for preventing falls in older people in care facilities and hospitals. *Cochrane Database Syst Rev*. 2012;12:CD005465.
104. Moyer VA. Prevention of falls in community-dwelling older adults: U.S. Preventive Services Task Force recommendation statement. *Ann Intern Med*. 2012;157:197–204.
105. Joyce NC, Hache LP, Clemens PR. Bone health and associated metabolic complications in neuromuscular diseases. *Phys Med Rehabil Clin N Am*. 2012;23:773–799.
106. McDonald DG, Kinali M, Gallagher AC, et al. Fracture prevalence in Duchenne muscular dystrophy. *Dev Med Child Neurol*. 2002;44:695–698.
107. Skalsky AJ, McDonald CM. Prevention and management of limb contractures in neuromuscular diseases. *Phys Med Rehabil Clin N Am*. 2012;23:675–687.
108. Rose KJ, Burns J, Wheeler DM, North KN. Interventions for increasing ankle range of motion in patients with neuromuscular disease. *Cochrane Database Syst Rev*. 2010;(2):CD006973.
109. Scott OM, Hyde SA, Goddard C, Dubowitz V. Prevention of deformity in Duchenne muscular dystrophy. A prospective study of passive stretching and splintage. *Physiotherapy*. 1981;67:177–180.
110. Hyde SA, FlLytrup I, Glent S, et al. A randomized comparative study of two methods for controlling Tendo Achilles contracture in Duchenne muscular dystrophy. *Neuromuscul Disord*. 2000;10:257–263.
111. Main M, Mercuri E, Haliloglu G, Baker R, Kinali M, Muntoni F. Serial casting of the ankles in Duchenne muscular dystrophy: can it be an alternative to surgery? *Neuromuscul Disord*. 2007;17:227–230.
112. Glanzman AM, Flickinger JM, Dholakia KH, Bonnemann CG, Finkel RS. Serial casting for the management of ankle contracture in Duchenne muscular dystrophy. *Pediatr Phys Ther*. 2011;23:275–279.
113. Gracies JM. Physical modalities other than stretch in spastic hypertonia. *Phys Med Rehabil Clin N Am*. 2001;12:769–792, vi.
114. Ashworth NL, Satkunam LE, Deforge D. Treatment for spasticity in amyotrophic lateral sclerosis/motor neuron disease. *Cochrane Database Syst Rev*. 2012;2:CD004156.
115. Carter GT, Jensen MP, Hoffman AJ, Stoelb BL, Abresch RT, McDonald CM. Pain in myotonic muscular dystrophy, type 1. *Arch Phys Med Rehabil*. 2008;89:2382.
116. Stoelb BL, Carter GT, Abresch RT, Purekal S, McDonald CM, Jensen MP. Pain in persons with postpolio syndrome: frequency, intensity, and impact. *Arch Phys Med Rehabil*. 2008;89:1933–1940.
117. Jensen MP, Hoffman AJ, Stoelb BL, Abresch RT, Carter GT, McDonald CM. Chronic pain in persons with myotonic dystrophy and facioscapulohumeral dystrophy. *Arch Phys Med Rehabil*. 2008;89:320–328.
118. Rivera I, Ajroud-Driss S, Casey P, et al. Prevalence and characteristics of pain in early and late stages of ALS. *Amyotroph Lateral Scler Frontotemporal Degener*. 2013;14(5–6):369–372.
119. Engel JM, Kartin D, Carter GT, Jensen MP, Jaffe KM. Pain in youths with neuromuscular disease. *Am J Hosp Palliat Care*. 2009;26:405–412.
120. Moss HL. Prosthesis for blepharoptosis and blepharospasm. *J Am Optom Assoc*. 1982;53:661–667.
121. Wong VA, Beckingsale PS, Oley CA, Sullivan TJ. Management of myogenic ptosis. *Ophthalmology*. 2002;109:1023–1031.
122. van Sorge AJ, Devogelaere T, Sotodeh M, Wubbels R, Paridaens D. Exposure keratopathy following silicone frontalis suspension in adult neuro- and myogenic ptosis. *Acta Ophthalmol*. 2012;90:188–192.
123. Kang DH, Koo SH, Ahn DS, Park SH, Yoon ES. Correction of blepharoptosis in oculopharyngeal muscular dystrophy. *Ann Plast Surg*. 2002;49:419–423.
124. Rodrigue D, Molgat YM. Surgical correction of blepharoptosis in oculopharyngeal muscular dystrophy. *Neuromuscul Disord*. 1997;7(Suppl 1):S82–S84.

125. Marin B, Desport JC, Kajeu P, et al. Alteration of nutritional status at diagnosis is a prognostic factor for survival of amyotrophic lateral sclerosis patients. *J Neurol Neurosurg Psychiatry.* 2011;82:628–634.
126. Paganoni S, Deng J, Jaffa M, Cudkowicz ME, Wills AM. Body mass index, not dyslipidemia, is an independent predictor of survival in amyotrophic lateral sclerosis. *Muscle Nerve.* 2011;44:20–24.
127. Desport JC, Preux PM, Truong TC, Vallat JM, Sautereau D, Couratier P. Nutritional status is a prognostic factor for survival in ALS patients. *Neurology.* 1999;53:1059–1063.
128. Briani C, Marcon M, Ermani M, et al. Radiological evidence of subclinical dysphagia in motor neuron disease. *J Neurol.* 1998;245:211–216.
129. Miller RG, Jackson CE, Kasarskis EJ, et al. Practice parameter update: the care of the patient with amyotrophic lateral sclerosis: drug, nutritional, and respiratory therapies (an evidence-based review): report of the Quality Standards Subcommittee of the American Academy of Neurology. *Neurology.* 2009;73: 1218–1226.
130. Braun MM, Osecheck M, Joyce NC. Nutrition assessment and management in amyotrophic lateral sclerosis. *Phys Med Rehabil Clin N Am.* 2012;23:751–771.
131. Brouillette D, Martel E, Chen LQ, Duranceau A. Pitfalls and complications of cricopharyngeal myotomy. *Chest Surg Clin N Am.* 1997;7:457–475; discussion 476.
132. Brigand C, Ferraro P, Martin J, Duranceau A. Risk factors in patients undergoing cricopharyngeal myotomy. *Br J Surg.* 2007;94:978–983.
133. Oh TH, Brumfield KA, Hoskin TL, Stolp KA, Murray JA, Bassford JR. Dysphagia in inflammatory myopathy: clinical characteristics, treatment strategies, and outcome in 62 patients. *Mayo Clin Proc.* 2007;82:441–447.
134. Oh TH, Brumfield KA, Hoskin TL, Kasperbauer JL, Basford JR. Dysphagia in inclusion body myositis: Clinical features, management, and clinical outcome. *Am J Phys Med Rehabil.* 2008;87:883–889.
135. Pellerin HG, Nicole PC, Trepanier CA, Lessard MR. Postoperative complications in patients with oculopharyngeal muscular dystrophy: a retrospective study. *Can J Anaesth.* 2007;54:361–365.
136. Gomez-Torres A, Abrante Jimenez A, Rivas Infante E, Menoyo Bueno A, Tirado Zamora I, Esteban Ortega F. Cricopharyngeal myotomy in the treatment of oculopharyngeal muscular dystrophy. *Acta Otorrinolaringol Esp.* 2012;63:465–469.
137. Restivo DA, Casabona A, Nicotra A, et al. ALS dysphagia pathophysiology: differential botulinum toxin response. *Neurology.* 2013;80:616–620.
138. Yunusova Y, Green JR, Greenwood L, Wang J, Pattee GL, Zinman L. Tongue movements and their acoustic consequences in amyotrophic lateral sclerosis. *Folia Phoniatr Logop.* 2012;64:94–102.
139. Yunusova Y, Green JR, Lindstrom MJ, Ball LJ, Pattee GL, Zinman L. Kinematics of disease progression in bulbar ALS. *J Commun Disord.* 2010;43:6–20.
140. de Swart BJ, van Engelen BG, Maassen BA. Warming up improves speech production in patients with adult onset myotonic dystrophy. *J Commun Disord.* 2007;40:185–195.
141. Simeral JD, Kim SP, Black MJ, Donoghue JP, Hochberg LR. Neural control of cursor trajectory and click by a human with tetraplegia 1000 days after implant of an intracortical microelectrode array. *J Neural Eng.* 2011;8:025027.
142. Hochberg LR, Bacher D, Jarosiewicz B, et al. Reach and grasp by people with tetraplegia using a neurally controlled robotic arm. *Nature*, 2012;485:372–375.
143. Collinger JL, Wodlinger B, Downey JE, et al. High-performance neuroprosthetic control by an individual with tetraplegia. *Lancet.* 2013;381:557–564.
144. Bach JR, Campagnolo DI, Hoeman S. Life satisfaction of individuals with Duchenne muscular dystrophy using long-term mechanical ventilatory support. *Am J Phys Med Rehabil.* 1991;70:129–135.
145. Paul RH, Nash JM, Cohen RA, Gilchrist JM, Goldstein JM. Quality of life and well-being of patients with myasthenia gravis. *Muscle Nerve.* 2001;24:512–516.
146. Simmons Z, Bremer BA, Robbins RA, Walsh SM, Fischer S. Quality of life in ALS depends on factors other than strength and physical function. *Neurology.* 2000;55:388–392.
147. Robbins RA, Simmons Z, Bremer BA, Walsh SM, Fischer S. Quality of life in ALS is maintained as physical function declines. *Neurology.* 2001;56:442–444.
148. Bromberg MB. Quality of life in amyotrophic lateral sclerosis. *Phys Med Rehabil Clin N Am.* 2008;19:591–605, x–xi.

SECTION II

SPECIFIC DISORDERS

CHAPTER 6

Amyotrophic Lateral Sclerosis

The motor neuron diseases (MNDs) are categorized by their pathological affinity for the voluntary motor system including anterior horn cells, certain motor cranial nerve nuclei, and corticospinal/bulbar tracts. Amyotrophic lateral sclerosis (ALS), also known as Lou Gehrig disease, is the most notorious of these disorders. The boundaries of what is and what is not ALS, particularly in the context of early diagnosis of individual patients, remain imprecise. In this Chapter, in an attempt to distinguish ALS from other MNDs, we consider ALS to be a disorder that has the following characteristics: (1) the clinical manifestations are dominated by signs attributable to voluntary motor system dysfunction, (2) the disease progresses rapidly both within and between different body regions, (3) that life expectancy is <5 years from clinical onset in the vast majority of cases, (4) and that no other etiology can be identified.

Despite its characterization as a motor system degeneration, ALS is best conceptualized as a multisystem disorder.[1] This perspective is reinforced by both a clinical and pathological overlap between ALS and frontotemporal lobar degeneration (FTLD) (pathological) and frontotemporal dementia (clinical).[2] Consequently, ALS is more correctly considered as a disorder in which dysfunction of the voluntary motor system involvement is the dominant source of morbidity (in the majority of cases) but in which involvement of other neurological systems at times clinically, and more commonly pathologically, develops.

The uncertain etiology of sporadic ALS (sALS) and the increasingly complex biology of ALS contribute to a lack of coherence in ALS nosology. This confusion applies to both historical and contemporary perspectives. In 1849 and 1850, respectively, Duchenne and Aran described progressive muscular atrophy (PMA), a disorder they believed to be of muscular origin. PMA has been long recognized however, to result from anterior horn cell degeneration.[3] In 1860, Duchenne first described a syndrome of progressive dysphagia and dysarthria and coined the term progressive bulbar palsy (PBP).[3] In 1874, Charcot and Cruveilhier recognized that corticospinal tracts and anterior horn cells were often affected concomitantly. Their description serves as the basis for our current construct of ALS.[3] In the next year, Erb described primary lateral sclerosis (PLS), a progressive disorder of corticospinal tracts, without (at least initially) evidence of muscle atrophy, fasciculation, or weakness.[3] ALS, PMA, PBP, and PLS are accepted by most, but not all neurologists as interrelated entities. PMA and PLS are clinically defined by the type of motor neuron affected. PBP on the other hand, is defined by site of disease onset, regardless of the type of motor neuron involved. Although survival in PMA and particularly PLS will on average exceed that of ALS, there is considerable overlap.[4–10] Survival in ALS does not differ significantly between different disease categories as described by the El Escorial criteria (EEC) (see below) including the original EEC-suspected category that is synonymous with PMA, that is an exclusively lower motor neuron (LMN) presentation.[9] Many patients with these initially limited MND (PBP, PMA, and PLS) phenotypes evolve into ALS. Unfortunately, phenotypic classification does not provide a mechanism by which to predict the natural history of disease in an individual patient. Patients with prolonged (>5 years) survival have a similar distribution of phenotypes as do patients with typical natural histories.[11] Individual patients fulfilling ALS criteria may have indolent courses whereas patients with PMA may progress rapidly with approximately a third of PMA patients dying within 3 years of symptom onset.[8,12]

Recognizing the pragmatic limitations imposed by the imprecise MND boundaries, Lord Brain, in his text of 1962, proposed the "lumped" concept of MND, presumably to acknowledge and circumvent uncertainties of the split classification. To this day, MND serves as a synonym for ALS and other forms of MND within the United Kingdom.[3] Arguably, it represents the most intellectually honest means to classify these disorders until a biological basis to justify lumping or splitting becomes available.

There have been three international consensus conferences that have attempted to provide an ALS classification scheme that is both accurate and clinically pragmatic. The first of these met in El Escorial, Spain in 1990. As there were no recognized effective treatments at that time, the primary goal was to define ALS with a high degree of sensitivity and specificity for research purposes. The proceedings of this meeting led to the subsequent publication of the EEC (Table 6-1).[13] Shortly thereafter, Riluzole was reported to alter the natural history of the disease, the first (and to this date only) drug treatment shown to do so.[14] In response to this, with promise of other effective treatments, and in recognition that the stringency of the EEC would hamper enrollment into clinical trials, a subsequent meeting was held in Airlie House, Virginia in 1998.[15] The purpose of this convocation was to modify the EEC in order to allow earlier diagnosis without reducing diagnostic specificity thus facilitating for earlier and expedited clinical trial enrollment.

▶ TABLE 6-1. **EL ESCORIAL CRITERIA—MODIFIED**[13,15]

Clinically definite ALS	Defined on clinical evidence alone by the presence of UMN, as well as LMN signs, in three regions.
Clinically probable ALS	Defined on clinical evidence alone by UMN and LMN signs in at least two regions, with some UMN signs necessarily rostral to (above) the LMN signs.
Clinically probable, laboratory-supported ALS	Defined when clinical signs of UMN and LMN dysfunction are in one region, or when clinical UMN signs alone are present in one region—coupled with LMN signs defined by EMG criteria in at least two limbs, with proper application of neuroimaging and clinical laboratory protocols to exclude other causes.
Clinically possible ALS	Defined when clinical signs of UMN and LMN dysfunction are found together in only one region or UMN signs are found alone in two or more regions, or LMN signs are found rostral to UMN signs (in absence of EMG evidence of more widespread LMN disease).
Clinically suspected ALS	Defined by a pure LMN syndrome in which other causes of LMN disease have been adequately considered and excluded by ancillary testing (this category has been deleted from the revised EEC).

ALS, amyotrophic lateral sclerosis; UMN, upper motor neuron; LMN, lower motor neuron; EEC, El Escorial criteria.

Unfortunately, the Airlie House revision of the EEC may not have resulted in earlier participation in clinical trials.[9] Despite the virtual universal acceptance of EEC and its Airlie House modifications as the "gold standard" for ALS diagnosis, they may continue to sacrifice sensitivity for specificity.[16] Patients with early MNDs are frequently restricted from participation in clinical trials at a time in their disease when they are presumably most likely to be treatment responsive. Studies suggest that only 56% of patients clinically thought to have ALS will fulfill definite or probable Airlie House diagnostic criteria at the time of diagnosis.[9] In addition, it has been recognized that the EEC classification at diagnosis, for example, definite, probable, possible, or suspected, does not correlate with clinical course and survival.[9] Furthermore, up to 10% of a clinically defined ALS population will die without achieving either of these levels of diagnostic certainty.[9] In support of this, postmortem examination of patients who would not fulfill definite or probable ALS diagnostic criteria because of phenotypes restricted to upper motor neuron (UMN) or LMN findings will have pathological confirmation of ALS.[17,18] The diagnosis of probable or definite ALS via EEC is dependent upon either clinical or lab demonstration of both UMN and LMN findings in two or three body regions (cranial, cervical, thoracic, lumbosacral) respectively. The reliable demonstration of UMN findings can be difficult and subjective, particularly in the thoracic and cranial regions. In addition, there is no reliable surrogate marker for UMN involvement as there is for lower motor disease (EMG). For these reasons, the early diagnosis of ALS via EEC/Airlie House criteria remains problematic.

In an attempt to improve sensitivity without sacrificing specificity in ALS diagnosis, a third consensus conference of experts convened in Awaji Island, Japan in 2006.[19,20] The premise of conference participants was that fasciculation potentials, particularly when "complex or unstable," represented an adequate surrogate for fibrillation potentials and positive waves as a marker of ongoing denervation. In an attempt to maintain adequate disease specificity, the authors dictated that these unstable and complex fasciculation potentials had to occur in the context of two additional features: (1) the patient had clinical features suggesting ALS, and (2) fasciculation potentials had to occur in muscles concomitantly with chronic motor unit action potential (MUAP) changes. Subsequent studies supported the Awaji hypothesis by suggesting that diagnostic sensitivity increased from 28% to 60% in comparison to EEC while maintaining the same specificity of 96%.[21,22]

Although marketed as an evidence-based document, none of the citations supporting the widespread application of the Awaji criteria have offered convincing evidence that patients achieving an early diagnosis of ALS utilizing these criteria evolve into definite ALS as determined by existing gold standards of either a typical clinical course or postmortem confirmation. In addition, the proponents imply that the demonstration of "unstable" fasciculation potentials provides a reliable means to distinguish ALS from less malignant causes of fasciculation potentials.[19,20] In a separate manuscript however, one of the authors of the Awaji manuscript refute the contention that "benign" and "malignant" fasciculation potentials can be reliably distinguished from one another.[23] We are in agreement with all three sets of criteria that consider both a clinically weak muscle and a strong muscle that electrodiagnostically displays both ongoing and chronic changes of denervation to be equivalent in defining the anatomical extent of the disease. We, like others, remain unconvinced that fasciculation potentials, unstable or otherwise, should be accepted as a surrogate marker of ongoing denervation in the absence of other EDX abnormalities.[24]

Aran first reported the occurrence of ALS in multiple family members in 1848. Nonetheless, the concept of familial ALS (fALS) was dismissed by Charcot and largely ignored until the discovery of the first ALS gene mutation in the early 1990s (Table 6-2). At least 5–10% of ALS cases associated with 13 currently recognized gene mutations occur as a result of a single gene (Mendelian) mutation.[25] In addition, it seems likely that genetic influence confers disease susceptibility in some portion of sporadic cases. It has been reported

▶ TABLE 6-2. **FAMILIAL ALS**[25,27,30,42,43]

Name	Locus/Protein	(% fALS) (% sALS)	Phenotype
Dominant Inheritance			
ALS1	21q22.1 SOD1/superoxide dismutase	(20%) (2–7%)	Adult onset—any ALS phenotype FTD uncommon (Table 6-3)
ALS3	18q21 unknown		Average age onset 45—usually leg onset
ALS4	9q34 SETX/senataxin		Juvenile onset, slow progression HSP phenotype with eventual LMN signs—no bulbar involvement Ataxia with oculomotor apraxia 2 Distal SMA
ALS6	16q11.2 FUS-TLS/fusion in sarcoma/translated in liposarcoma	(4–6%) (1%)	Average age of onset 45, LMN-D ±FTD, PD
ALS7	20p13 unknown		Adult onset
ALS8	20q13.3 VAPB/vesicle-associated membrane protein	unknown (0%)	Adult onset, slowly progressive, LMN-D phenotype
ALS9	14q11.2 ANG/angiogenin	(<2%) (<1%)	Adult onset, LMN-D ↑ incidence bulbar onset ± rapid progression ± FTD, PD
ALS10	1p36.2 TDP-43/TAR DNA binding	(4–6%) (1.5%)	ALS ± FTD PSP, PD, chorea
ALS11	6q21 FIG4/polyphosphoinositide phosphatase		High % bulbar onset CMT4J
ALS12	10p15-p14 OPTN/optineurin	(1.2%) (3.5%)	UMN-D, lower extremities, slow progression
ALS13	12q24 ATXN2/ataxin 2		ALS Spinocerebellar ataxia type 2
Not designated	9q21–22 C9ORF72	(24%) (12%)	ALS ± FTD
Not designated	9p13.3 VCP/valosin-containing protein	(<1%)	Typical ALS ± FTD Association with inclusion body myopathy, Paget disease, dementia
Not designated	3p11.2 CHMP2B/chromatin-modifying protein 2B		LMN-D or ALS phenotype ± FTD
Recessive Inheritance			
ALS2	2q33.1 alsin		Juvenile onset—UMN-D
ALS5	15q15.1q21.1 unknown		Juvenile onset
ALS12	10p15-p14 OPTN	(1.2%) (3.5%)	UMN-D, lower extremities
X-linked Inheritance			
ALS15	XP11.21 UBQLN2/ubiquilin 2	(<1%)	ALS ± FTD Rare bulbar presentations

FTD, frontotemporal lobar dysfunction; LMN-D, lower motor neuron dominant; PD, Parkinson disease; PSP, progressive supranuclear palsy; UMN-D, upper motor neuron dominant.

that there is an approximate eightfold increased lifetime risk of developing ALS in siblings or progeny of apparent sALS patients.[26]

fALS, like sALS displays phenotypic heterogeneity. Other than for an earlier average age of onset, there are no distinguishing features that allow clinical distinction between inherited and sporadic cases. The full spectrum of phenotypic heterogeneity of ALS is evident even within different point mutations of the same fALS (SOD1) gene (Table 6-3). fALS may occur with juvenile or adult onset, slow or fast progression, limb or bulbar onset, UMN or LMN predominance, and in the presence or absence of frontotemporal dysfunction.[27–30] Not only do all of these different phenotypic variations occur in both fALS and sALS, they seem to occur with similar prevalence rates. As in sALS, fALS patients may never fulfill the clinical

▶ TABLE 6-3. PHENOTYPIC VARIABILITY OF SOD MUTATIONS IN FALS[25,27,28,66]

Phenotype	SOD1 Mutation
Lower motor neuron predominant	A4 V, L84 V, D101 N
Upper motor neuron predominant	D90 A
Slow progression	G37 R (18 years), G41 D (11 years), G93 C, L144 S, L144 F
Fast progression	A4 T (1.5 years), N86 S (homozygous 5 months), L106 V (1.2 years), V148 G (2 years)
Late onset	G85 R, H46 R
Early onset	G37 R, L38 V
Female predominant	G41 D
Bulbar onset	V148I
High penetrance	D90 A homozygotes, A4 V
Low penetrance	I113 T
Posterior column involvement	E100G

SOD1, superoxide dismutase.

EEC requirements for probable or definite ALS during the patient's lifetime.

As alluded to previously, the historical conceptualization of ALS, either inherited or sporadic, is that of a degenerative disorder of anterior horn cells and pyramidal tracts. This construct is confounded by the recognition that both the clinical manifestations and pathology of ALS may affect extrapyramidal, cerebellar, and particularly, cognitive systems.[1,2] It has been estimated that anywhere from 10% to 75% of ALS patients will have subtle or overt abnormalities in executive function, behavior, and/or language if carefully sought for, implicating frontotemporal lobar dysfunction (FTD).[2,27,31,32] Estimates of overt dementia range from 15% to 40%.[2] Conversely, if patients with FTD are carefully examined, it has been suggested that 14% will have signs of definite ALS and additional 36% signs of possible disease.[33] MND may precede, occur concurrently, or follow the onset of FTD.[34] In this chapter, we will use the acronym FTD to represent frontotemporal dysfunction without necessarily implicating overt blown dementia. The intent of this departure from consensus criteria nomenclature is that it allows us to consider the full spectrum of frontotemporal deficits, not only those fulfilling the Neary diagnostic criteria for dementia.[2,35,36]

Estimates of FTD prevalence however, originate in large part from Western cultures where prolonged survival and the use of tracheostomy-assisted mechanical ventilation (TAMV) occur infrequently. Experiences in cultures where long-term ALS survivors are more prevalent, related to increased utilization of TAMV, suggest that the occurrence of dementia increases over time in ALS patients. This further supports the concept of ALS as a multisystem disorder.[37,38] ALS with dementia or involvement of other neurological systems is designated as ALS plus by the EEC.[13,39] Frontotemporal dysfunction in fALS is increasingly recognized but has not been as well described as in sALS. This may reflect ascertainment bias as FTD has been estimated to occur less in those with SOD1 mutations, the most historically prevalent genotype of fALS prior to the recognition of the C9ORF72 mutation.[2,40]

Although the focus of this chapter is ALS, the strong association with FTD and FTLD justifies a few comments relevant to the epidemiology of the latter disorder. In addition to ALS, FTLD may occur in association with cortical basal ganglionic degeneration, progressive supranuclear palsy, or other neurodegenerative conditions. In approximately 10% of cases, it is associated with an apparent autosomal dominant mode of transmission.[41] The genes most commonly related to heritable FTD that have been identified to date include microtubule-associated protein tau (MAPT) and progranulin (PGRN). MND occurs uncommonly with these mutations. Like fALS however, the locus for many fFTD cases remains unidentified.[41]

FTD co-associates with a number of fALS genotypes. Recently, hexanucleotide repeat mutations of the C9ORF72 gene have been identified as the most common cause of fALS and/or frontotemporal dementia, representing 12% of fFTD, 3% of apparent sFTD, 24% of fALS, and 4% of apparent sALS in North America.[42] In Finland, the impact of this mutation is even greater with 46% of fALS and 21% of apparent sALS cases resulting from chromosome 9 open reading frame 72 (C9ORF72) gene expansion.[43] Other mutations that are less frequent causes of FTD, but more common causes of ALS with or without FTD occur in the chromatin-modifying protein 2B (CHMP2B), fused in sarcoma (FUS), TAR DNA-binding protein (TARDBP), polyphosphoinositide phosphatase (FIG4), ubiquilin 2, and valosin-containing protein (VCP) genes.[25,44] As mentioned, FTD is recognized infrequently with SOD1.[40]

Within the general population, MNDs are uncommon. The incidence of ALS averages 1.8/100,000 across all studies. This incidence appears to be increasing both within and outside the boundaries of an aging population.[1] The average age of onset is 56 years for sporadic disease and 46 years for most dominantly inherited forms of the disease.[25,27] Teenagers and the elderly may be afflicted. Although it is widely believed that environmental factors must play at least some role in ALS pathogenesis, epidemiologic studies have failed to identify any reproducible risks other than age, gender, increased body mass index, and potentially cigarette smoking.[45–49] The historical inability to identify environmental risks may be related in part to methodology.[48,49,51] Although ALS has been reproducibly shown to occur 1.5 times more frequently in men, this ratio diminishes with advancing age and may not be true for bulbar-onset disease which seems particularly prevalent in older women.[49–52] There have been nests of apparent increased incidence. The ALS–Parkinsons–Dementia complex formerly endemic in Guam and other Western Pacific regions is the most notable example.[53] The neuronal inclusions in this disorder contain tau however, not the ubiquitin characteristic of typical (non-SOD1) ALS, suggesting that Guamanian ALS may be a different disorder. Otherwise, neither ethnicity, geography, nor occupation has been reproducibly demonstrated to alter risk.

The majority of ALS patients succumb within 2 to 5 years from symptom onset without ventilatory and nutritional support.[9,52,54] The range extends however from less than 1 year to more than 10 years without TAMV. It is estimated that a quarter of individuals will survive more than 5 years.[12,52] A vital capacity of less than 50% of predicted is associated with the need for hospice, death, or need for mechanical ventilation within 6 months.[55] Progression seems to follow a linear course, although the abrupt loss of a critical function may provide the appearance of stepwise deterioration.[54] Patients with PBP are said to have a shorter average life expectancy, although many lead protracted existences if aspiration risk is minimized and ventilation preserved or supported.[54] Young males seem to live longer on average.[54] Rilutek, participation in a multidisciplinary clinic, noninvasive positive pressure breathing, and possibly percutaneous gastrostomy are interventions that have modest benefits in prolonging life expectancy.[56]

► CLINICAL FEATURES

ALS is characterized by painless, progressive muscle weakness and atrophy (Fig. 6-1). The site of onset, the relative predominance of UMN or LMN signs, and the rate of progression are variable. Patients typically present when functional difficulties cause them to acknowledge their deficit. These initial deficits are frequently asymmetric and sometimes monomelic depending on patient vigilance. In instances where the patients do not seek early medical attention, or their physicians do not recognize the significance of the problem, the patients may not be diagnosed until their disorder is fairly advanced, months or even a year or more after onset. The initial deficits may be initially limited in distribution but should affect more than one nerve and nerve root distribution in limb-onset cases. Less commonly, the initial symptoms may be cramps, dysarthria, dysphonia or dysphagia, or related to impaired ventilation. Occasionally, the initial clinical manifestations may be head drop or bent spine syndromes related to paraspinal muscle weakness (Fig. 6-2). In this latter circumstance, the patient may actually present with back pain due to the disordered posture caused by inadequate spine support.

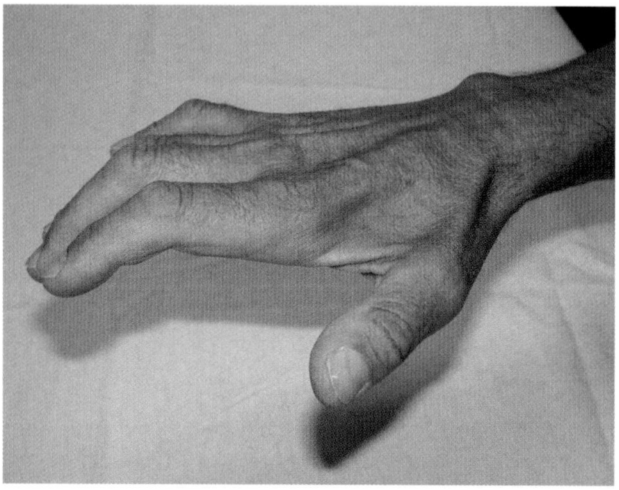

Figure 6-1. Hand atrophy in amyotrophic lateral sclerosis.

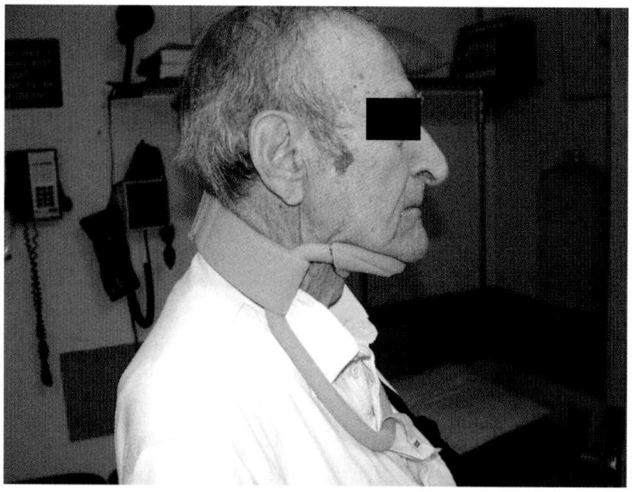

Figure 6-2. Head drop with cervical collar in amyotrophic lateral sclerosis.

Fasciculations are more commonly recognized by the examining physician than by patients. On occasion, they may be the initial manifestation of MND, particularly in those who have a pre-existing awareness of their potential significance. Patients presenting with a chief complaint of fasciculations without weakness, atrophy, or abnormal EMGs rarely have or evolve into ALS.[57] In our experience, benign fasciculations are described more than seen, tend to occur most frequently in the calf muscles, and when observed are typically repetitive in the same location in any given muscle at any specific point in time. Conversely, fasciculations that are continuous and multifocal both within and between muscles, even in the absence of weakness, are ominous. This uncommon pattern of visible frequent and multifocal fasciculations without weakness is rarely seen in other circumstances other than MND, anticholinesterase overmedication being one notable exception. Lastly, the absence of fasciculations in patients with painless weakness does not preclude the diagnosis of ALS, particularly in those with excessive subcutaneous tissue.[58] An increased frequency of muscle cramping is also common in MND. In our experience, provocation of cramps in muscles (with the exception of the calves) during manual muscle testing is seen with some frequency in ALS patients is uncommon in other disorders.

As previously alluded to, the definite clinical diagnosis of ALS is dependent on the demonstration of both LMN and UMN signs, which progress both within and between different body regions. Frequently ALS may be dominated by LMN, or less frequently UMN signs. This may occur at onset or in some patients throughout their entire disease course. Signs of LMN involvement include muscle weakness, atrophy out of proportion to disuse, attenuation or loss of deep tendon reflexes, cramps, and fasciculations.[59] When LMN weakness impairs coordination, it does so to an extent proportionate to the degree of weakness.[59] LMN features in cranial musculature in ALS are most frequently and convincingly manifest in the tongue. Atrophy is noted by the crenated, as opposed to the normal rounded edges, and fasciculations best noted with the tongue lying quietly on the floor of the mouth (Fig. 6-3). Tongue strength is best tested by pushing against the bulge in the cheek created by the patient "pocketing" their tongue on either side. Weakness of neck flexion and extension are common in ALS. Weakness of facial (e.g., eye closure) and jaw opening and closing muscles occur but are typically less evident. Ptosis and ophthalmoparesis are notable for their absence.

UMN manifestations are more diverse and, at times, more subjective than their LMN counterparts. The elicitation of Babinski signs, sustained clonus, pathologically hyperactive deep tendon reflexes, and spasticity are objective and universally accepted manifestations of UMN pathology. Unfortunately, they are not overt in a significant percentage of ALS cases, thus confounding and delaying the clinical diagnosis. Other presumptive signs of corticospinal tract pathology include reflex spread (e.g., finger flexion with percussion of the brachioradialis tendon, hip flexion with percussion of the Achilles tendon), synkinesis (coactivation of muscles not required to accomplish a requested movement), Hoffman signs, and preservation of reflexes in a wasted and weak extremity. The latter is arguably the most prevalent of the subjective UMN sign demonstrable in ALS patients.[52] In cranial innervated muscles, unequivocal UMN signs may be difficult to demonstrate. Increased emotional lability (pseudobulbar affect) and spastic dysarthria are perhaps the most frequently occurring UMN signs in this region but are more subjective than objective. Forced yawning is nonspecific. Exaggerated gag or jaw reflexes are more objective but do not occur with particularly great frequency. Arguably, slowness of attempted rapid blinking or tongue movements, in the absence of weakness, implicates central nervous system (CNS) pathology and provides support for UMN involvement in someone whose presentation is otherwise dominated by LMN signs. The same may be said for synkinesis, for example, the concomitant movement of the jaw with requested, rapid side-to-side tongue movements.

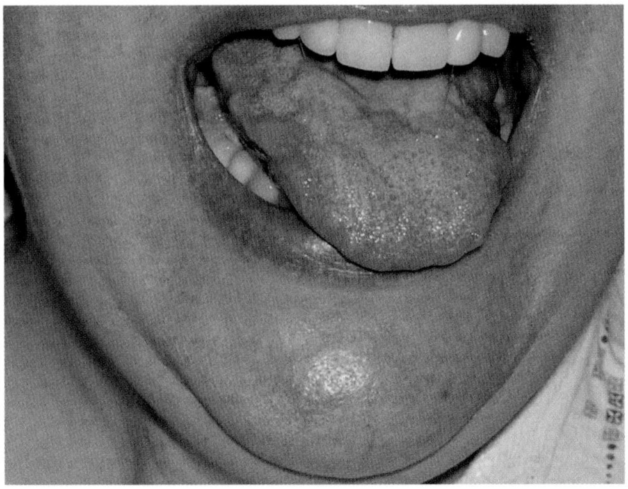

Figure 6-3. Tongue atrophy in amyotrophic lateral sclerosis.

Coordination is impaired early with UMN involvement in a manner disproportionate to the degree of weakness.[59] There is frequently a "UMN stickiness" resulting in delayed activation of requested movements associated with the normal or near-normal strength. Often, muscles not required for an attempted motion are inappropriately (synkinetically) activated. For example, contralateral foot tapping may occur with requested unilateral foot-tapping movements. With UMN disease, foot dorsiflexion strength may be normal but delayed in initiation and preceded by great toe dorsiflexion. UMN signs may be transient in ALS, as they may develop and then disappear as LMN-induced weakness evolves and trumps UMN manifestations. For example, a Babinski sign may be lost as the extensor hallucis muscle weakens.

Recognizing the value of the EEC and the Airlie House revision, we find it helpful to categorize our patients both by onset site and phenotype. Onset sites include bulbar, upper limb, lower limb, or rarely truncal or ventilatory locations. Phenotypic categories include PMA, lower motor neuron dominant (LMN-D) ALS, ALS, upper motor neuron dominant (UMN-D) ALS, and PLS. We define PMA as muscle weakness and atrophy associated with hypo- or areflexia in involved segments. LMN-D is applied to individuals with dominant LMN features associated with suggestive, but not definite UMN signs as listed above. Typically, these are individuals mentioned above whose deep tendon reflexes are either preserved or mildly increased in the involved body regions. UMN-D disease is defined by the absence of LMN signs clinically but with unequivocal signs of denervation on EMG that are not readily explained by an alternative mechanism. PLS is defined as a progressive UMN syndrome occurring without an alternative explanation without either clinical or electrodiagnostic evidence of LMN disease.

In most series, ALS is the most common presentation of MND, although even in these patients, the morbidity appears to stem primarily from LMN disease.[9,59–62] In probability, most classifications consider LMN-D to represent ALS.[52] In approximately two-thirds of cases, the initial site of involvement is in a limb, typically distally and asymmetrically located in a hand or foot.[8,9,52,58,59] Initial weakness may occur in proximal muscles as well. A definite diagnosis cannot be made until combined UMN and LMN signs spread over a period of months, both within and outside the initially affected body region. A diagnosis of ALS meeting EEC definite or probable criteria, allowing clinical trial eligibility, is obtained in only 31–56% of cases at the time of the initial examination.[9] Despite diagnostic limitations imposed by EEC, the combination of UMN and LMN findings confined to multiple segments in one limb is sinister when unassociated with pain or sensory symptoms.

It is estimated that PMA phenotype represents anywhere between 2% and 10% of MND patients.[7,8,22,52,61] This variation is undoubtedly based on whether deep tendon reflex preservation in a weak limb is or is not considered to lie within the boundaries of PMA.[7] A LMN-D presentation is estimated to occur in 7%, 26%, 29%, and 18% respectively in those whose disease begins in the bulbar, cervical, thoracic, and lumbosacral regions.[9] These statistics may be biased however, by the ease or difficulty in identifying UMN or LMN signs in any given region. For example, UMN findings in the thoracic region may be underrepresented due to the insensitive clinical means of detection. Of those who do not manifest UMN signs at onset, 22% will develop them and 90% will evolve into EEC probable or definite disease.[9] Even in the patients who fail to develop UMN features during life, the pathological features of ALS will be identified on postmortem examination.[17,18,63–65]

Other observations, supporting the concept that PMA and ALS exist as a continuum include the documentation that these disorders have overlapping natural histories. Although PMA and LMN-D patients live longer on average than patients classified as having ALS, individual patients in any of these categories may have malignant courses.[7,8,12] On average, symmetric presentations and individuals who continue to have monomelic involvement after prolong periods of observation tend to have the more indolent courses.[7,8] As would be expected, those whose measurements of ventilatory or limb strength decline precipitously have life expectancies that parallel ALS despite an absence or paucity of UMN signs.[7,8] Additional arguments in support of PMA and LMN-D as part of the ALS spectrum include the recognition that PMA phenotypes occur in at least five different SOD1 fALS genotypes. The A4 V SOD1 mutation, a rapidly progressive PMA phenotype, represents the most common SOD mutation in North America and represents the most dramatic example of this phenomenon.[62,66] FTD prevalence is estimated at 17% in PMA patients, providing further support for a common biology in the two syndromes.[67]

At times, slowly progressive forms of LMN-predominant ALS may remain confined to both upper extremities over protracted periods, producing a syndrome that has been described as flail arm, bibrachial amyotrophic diplegia (BAD), or "man-in-the-barrel" syndrome.[68,69] This disorder more commonly affects the shoulder girdles initially in comparison to the more common LMN-D forms of ALS which are more likely to begin distally and progress more rapidly. A similar more indolent syndrome, referred to a lower extremity amyotrophic diplegia (LAD) may affect both lower extremities, rendering the individual paraparetic for protracted periods before spreading to other regions.[69] In our opinion, both BAD and LAD are best conceptualized as PMA variants.

Between 25% and 40% of individuals present with "bulbar-onset" disease, that is, dysarthria or less commonly dysphagia.[9,70] As in limb-onset ALS, PBP may be dominated by UMN characteristics, LMN characteristics, or both. As with limb-onset cases, unequivocal UMN and LMN signs occurring concomitantly in cranial innervated muscles, even in the absence of limb involvement, are ominous. As in PMA and PLS, fALS may have a PBP presentation. This PBP presentation more commonly occurs in women than in men. Life expectancy in PBP has been repeatedly demonstrated to be on average less than in limb-onset disease particularly if there is an associated language-dominant FTD.[71] This prognosis does not necessarily apply to individual patients as mortality may be related more to the importance of the functions jeopardized early in the course (breathing and swallowing) than a reflection of the biology of the disease.[72] In some individuals with sporadic PBP, signs and symptoms may remain confined to the "bulbar" musculature for considerable time, affecting the physicians' confidence in the accuracy of their diagnosis, particularly with a UMN-D presentation. Some reports suggest both the prevalence and severity of FTD are increased in bulbar as opposed to limbonset cases whereas others do not. FTD has been reported to occur in as many as 48% of PBP cases if carefully sought for.[73–76] One report suggests that there is an increased incidence of language-dominant FTD in patients with bulbar-onset disease.[71]

ALS beginning as an UMN exclusive (PLS) or dominant (UMN-D) process is less common than phenotypes dominated by LMN or bulbar dysfunction.[77–81] Approximately 2–5% of ALS cases begin with a PLS phenotype.[78] The average age of onset in virtually every series is about 50 years, approximately 10 years younger than typical ALS.[78] Three-quarters of PLS cases involve the legs, initially creating an inability to effectively run or hop. In most cases, the onset is asymmetric and at times may be hemiparetic, referred to as the Mills variant.[78] In approximately 15% of cases, PLS affects the bulbar muscles initially. In 10% of cases, the upper extremities are the first region to become symptomatic.[5,6] It is commonly held that ALS spares the anterior horn of the sacral segments. As a result, it is commonly held that genitourinary symptoms do not occur in this disease. In our experience, PLS is an exception to this rule as urinary urgency and urgency incontinence may occur. Presumably this results from detrusor–sphincter dyssynergia. To further cement the biological relationship between PLS and ALS, PLS patients also appear susceptible to frontotemporal dysfunction and FTLD.[81,82]

The distinction between PLS from UMN-D ALS is based on whether LMN signs are absent (PLS) or present.[4,5] In the aforementioned reports, the authors defined the threshold for LMN involvement by EMG as abnormalities in more than two muscles (minimal number of muscles studied not defined). These abnormalities could include fibrillation potentials/positive waves, fasciculation potentials, or evidence of mild MUAP enlargement consistent with denervation and reinnervation. Presumably, these limits were defined so as to not exclude patients with minor EMG abnormalities secondary to a separate, unrelated, neurogenic injury. It has been suggested that focal weakness, bulbar symptoms at onset, or later development of weight loss and declining ventilatory function predict transition to ALS.[5]

The natural history of PLS is more favorable than PMA or ALS. In nine reported series, mean disease duration ranged between 7 and 14 years.[80] The majority (80%) of individuals with PLS who evolve into ALS do so within the first 4 years of their disorder.[5] Conversely, development of LMN features, either clinically or electrodiagnostically, may not develop until 20 or more years after the initial symptoms at which time the distinction between ALS and PLS becomes moot. The natural history of patients who do not have clinical or electrodiagnostic evidence of LMN involvement during the first 4 years of their illness is statistically superior to those who do. ALS may not be initially considered in the differential diagnosis when the initial manifestations are dominated by UMN features. Presumably, this results from the relative rarity of this condition in comparison to the other more common causes of progressive UMN disease. Typically, PLS is considered, and appropriately diagnosed, only after imaging, CSF and other investigations fail to provide an alternative explanation for a patient's worsening spasticity.

In up to 2.7% of cases, ALS may initially present with symptoms attributable to ventilatory muscle weakness.[83,84] These may escape initial detection due to their sometimes protean clinical manifestations including disordered sleep, early morning headache, fatigue, or altered sensorium. Involvement of ventilatory muscles may not be recognized until the more classic manifestations of dyspnea on exertion or orthopnea occur. It is not rare for patients to notice dyspnea for the first time after meals or while bending over to tie their shoes which restrict movement of weak diaphragms. On occasion, ALS may be first recognized in an individual who cannot be weaned from the ventilator following elective intubation. Paradoxical abdominal movements or a drop in vital capacity of more than 10% in the supine position indicates diaphragmatic weakness in patients with a suspected neuromuscular cause of ventilatory symptoms.

ALS and frontotemporal dysfunction represent overlapping disorders which exist in a continuum.[2,31–34] This association is important for a number of reasons including insight into a potential common biology. In addition, a reduced life expectancy in ALS patients with concomitant frontotemporal dysfunction has been suggested.[2,71,85] Alternative management strategies may be required when ALS and FTD coexist.[2] Both ALS and FTD may occur on either a sporadic or hereditary basis. Although it has been previously suggested that FTD may be more prevalent in patients with familial disease, others feel that the prevalence of cognitive impairment is similar in both sALS and fALS.[86] Both ALS and FTD may exist as individual disorders or develop collectively, either on a clinically evident or strictly a pathological basis. In the latter circumstance, the second disorder may or may not become clinically manifest during the lifetime of the patient.

It is estimated that 15% of patients who present with apparent sporadic FTD will have ALS and another 30% will have features suggestive of MND.[33] Conversely, 30–50% of ALS patients in most series and up to 75% in some who undergo careful testing will be identified as having some alteration in behavior, executive function, or language.[2,31,72,74,85] Estimates of dementia fulfilling Neary criteria are estimated between 15% and 41% in ALS patients.[2,29,76,87] ALS and FTD may precede the development of the other, or both may present concomitantly.[33] On occasion, patients with FTD and ALS will be found to have concomitant Parkinsonism as well.[33] The concurrence of ALS, a movement disorder, and dementia should raise the consideration of one of the known genetic causes of this triad (see above) (Table 6-2).

Minor cognitive and behavioral changes in MND patients may be overlooked for a number of reasons. They may be subtle and therefore escape detection unless appropriate screening instruments are utilized. The detection of these changes may also be obscured by the patient's writing and speaking difficulties. Behavioral changes, when recognized, may be misattributed to known consequences of ALS such as hypercapnia, depression, or pseudobulbar affect.

A nomenclature for frontotemporal dysfunction, with or without ALS, has been established and continues to evolve.[2] Patients may have a behavioral syndrome characterized by apathy, altered social and interpersonal conduct, emotional blunting, and loss of insight.[87] Alternatively, the primary deficit may be one of expressive language with speech that is dysgrammatical, associated with paraphasic errors and word-finding difficulties. Frontotemporal dysfunction may also manifest as a semantic, predominantly receptive language disorder in which the significance of words and objects lose meaning. Executive dysfunction, which is the loss of the ability to plan and organize tasks by maintenance of attention or the ability to shift sets to accomplish a goal-directed task, represents a significant component of frontotemporal dysfunction as well. Executive dysfunction has been estimated to occur in anywhere between 22% and 35% of ALS patients who do not fulfill the criteria for overt dementia.[2,34,88]

Tests of verbal fluency provide a sensitive screening method for FTD patients with cognitive impairment.[2,74]

Normal values are 8 and 13 respectively for number of words generated in 1 minute beginning with the letter D and names of animals.[2,74] Another strategy that may be even more sensitive for detecting set-shifting difficulties is to ask the patient to provide a word beginning with a specific letter alternating with a different category, for example, men's first names. Normative values for this task are seven or more pairs in 1 minute. Perseveration may be readily detected if two consecutive responses belonging to the same category are provided. A potentially useful screening test in individuals with unintelligible speech is "antisaccade" testing (the ability to look in the opposite direction in response to a lateralized visual stimulus). A patient should make no more than two errors in 10 attempts to be considered normal. There are numerous standardized tests that can be efficiently administered during a routine clinic visit. It should be pointed out that the mini-mental state examination is not a particularly sensitive test for detection of early frontotemporal dysfunction. The authors prefer the Montréal cognitive assessment (MOCA) as their standardized screening instrument of choice due to its availability, ease of use, and ability to assess frontotemporal function.[89] Behavioral abnormalities are best assessed by specific behavioral inventories.

▶ DIAGNOSIS AND DIFFERENTIAL DIAGNOSIS

sALS remains a clinical diagnosis supported by the exclusion of potentially mimicking disorders for which testing exists. In cases where the clinical diagnosis of ALS is indisputable, it can be argued that the predominant goal of testing is to validate the credibility of the diagnosis in the eyes of the patient and their family. There are a number of suggested algorithms for the evaluation of the ALS suspect based on differential diagnostic considerations.[59,100,132] It is our practice to perform limited "routine" testing in ALS suspects. It is our opinion that testing should be done on a case-by-case basis as the differential diagnostic emphasis differs depending on whether it is a UMN-D, LMN-D, or bulbar-onset phenotype (Table 6-4). Disorders that are dominated by LMN features provide the largest number of differential diagnostic considerations.

▶ TABLE 6-4. ANCILLARY TESTING IN SUSPECTED ALS PATIENTS

Tests That Should Be Considered in Any and All Suspected ALS Patients

1. EDX with multipoint motor nerve stimulation for potential conduction block, repetitive stimulation
2. Pulmonary function tests
3. Routine labs including CBC, liver function testing, calcium, TSH, urinalysis, CRP, or ESR

Tests That Could Be Considered in Selected Patients With UMN-Dominant Syndromes

1. MR imaging of brain, cervical, and/or thoracic spinal cord
2. Serum copper and ceruloplasmin
3. Serum HIV and HTLV-1 serology
4. Serum long-chain fatty acid ratios
5. HSP mutational analysis
6. CSF examination
7. fALS mutational analysis

Tests That Could Be Considered in Selected Patients With Combined UMN and LMN

1. DNA testing for selected HSP and dSMA phenotypes that may combine UMN and LMN features
2. MR imaging of brain, cervical, and/or thoracic spinal cord
3. Serum copper and ceruloplasmin
4. Serum HIV and HTLV-1 serology
5. Nerve biopsy, skin biopsy, fibroblast cultures, or genetic testing for polyglucosan disease
6. Hexosaminidase levels
7. fALS mutational analysis
8. Serum Lyme serology

Tests That Could Be Considered in Selected Patients With LMN-Dominant Syndromes

1. Serum CK levels
2. Serum immunofixation
3. Serum Lyme serology
4. GM1 antibodies
5. Voltage-gated calcium channel antibodies
6. Acetylcholine receptor and MuSK antibodies
7. Survival motor neuron gene mutational analysis (SMA I–IV)
8. Kennedy disease mutational analysis
9. CSF examination
10. Muscle biopsy
11. Single fiber EMG
12. fALS mutational analysis

Tests That Could Be Considered in Selected Patients With Bulbar-Onset Disease

1. CK
2. Acetylcholine receptor antibodies
3. Muscle biopsy
4. Single fiber EMG
5. Kennedy disease mutational analysis
6. MR brain
7. fALS mutational analysis

EDX, electrodiagnosis; CBC, complete blood count; TSH, thyroid-stimulating hormone; CRP, c-reactive protein; ESR, erythrocyte sedimentation rate; MR, magnetic resonance; HIV, human immunodeficiency virus; HTLV-1, human T lymphocytic virus; HSP, hereditary spastic paraplegia; CSF, cerebrospinal fluid; fALS, familial ALS; CK, creatine kinase; MuSK, muscle specific kinase; EMG, electromyography; dSMA, distal spinal muscular atrophy.

Multifocal motor neuropathy (MMN) is the most common LMN-D ALS mimic in most series (discussed in detail in Chapter 14).[133–138] It is distinguished from ALS by clinical, EDX, and serological means, and in some cases by response to diagnostic trials of IVIG. Potentially distinguishing clinical features include a slower rate of progression, motor deficits occurring in nerve rather than segmental (myotomal) distribution, and absence of cranial nerve and overt UMN signs.[137] Nonetheless, preservation or slight exaggeration of deep tendon reflexes in an affected limb may serve as a confounding variable.[137] The most characteristic laboratory feature is motor nerve conduction block but this can be elusive if located in very proximal or distal nerve segments. Antibodies directed at the GM1 ganglioside have been found in high titer in between 30% and 80% of these patients.[138,139] In adults with sporadic multifocal or diffuse LMN syndromes, we routinely do more extensive motor conductions looking for conduction block and order GM1 antibody screens. In addition, we consider MR imaging of the brachial or lumbosacral plexus in selected cases in an attempt to demonstrate swelling or increased signal of nerve elements which may occur in a third of MMN cases.[137] In selected cases, we have felt compelled to offer a 3-month trial of IVIG when the diagnosis remains uncertain.

Serological tests for disorders of neuromuscular transmission, typically acetylcholine receptor binding, and if negative, muscle-specific kinase antibodies should be considered in any patient with painless weakness. These tests are particularly relevant in bulbar-onset cases without atrophy or fasciculations. In cases presenting with a limb-girdle pattern of weakness, associated with diminished deep tendon reflexes and/or evidence of cholinergic dysautonomia, we would obtain voltage-gated calcium channel antibodies as one means as both a sensitive and specific test for Lambert–Eaton myasthenic syndrome. EDX remains a valuable adjunct in any suspected disorder of neuromuscular transmission evaluation. Edrophonium testing remains useful in selected suspected myasthenia cases.

Kennedy disease should be considered in males with bulbar symptoms and/or proximal weakness.[140–143] Like many MNDs, cramps, fasciculations, and atrophy are common. As with other spinal muscular atrophies, tremor may occur. There is an EDX evidence of sensory involvement which may or may not be evident clinically. Creatine kinase (CK) levels are frequently elevated in the two to five times the upper limits of normal range, similar to ALS. Features of impaired androgen effect such as gynecomastia occur. Needle EMG is dominated by features of chronic denervation and reinnervation with a relative paucity of ongoing denervation in most cases. The diagnosis is suspected when sensory nerve action potentials (SNAP) amplitudes are reduced on nerve conduction studies in a patient with proximal symmetric weakness and a predominantly chronic MND pattern with EDX. It is confirmed by identifying the characteristic trinucleotide repeats originating from the androgen receptor gene on the X chromosome.

Inclusion body myositis (IBM) and ALS typically affect individuals in the same age range. Both occur with a slightly greater incidence in males. Both are disorders that commonly demonstrate asymmetric limb weakness and atrophy. In addition, both frequently cause dysphagia, have similar levels of CK elevation, and may have fibrillation potentials and large MUAPs on EMG.[92] However, fasciculations and fasciculation potentials are not features of IBM. In addition, the large, polyphasic MUAPs seen on EMG are frequently intermixed with myopathic units in IBM. The course in IBM is typically more indolent than ALS and the pattern of weakness usually distinctive from the segmental pattern and regional spread of ALS. Quadriceps and finger/wrist flexors are typically the most severely affected. Weakness of facial and upper esophageal muscles, neck flexors, and foot dorsiflexors are common. Unlike most myopathies, asymmetric and relatively focal patterns of weakness are common. We have observed distal interphalangeal joint (DIP) flexion weakness in the thumb with relative sparing of DIP flexion of the contiguous digits. The forearm muscles are atrophic in IBM while the hand intrinsic muscles have preserved bulk (see Chapter 33). The diagnosis of IBM is typically confirmed by distinctive muscle biopsy features although most patients with ALS do not need a biopsy to exclude IBM if attentive clinical and EDX examinations are done.

Slowly progressive LMN syndromes are not uncommon in neuromuscular clinics and may be very difficult to distinguish from PMA or LMN-D ALS at onset as it their protracted course that provides the primary means of discrimination.[10,134–136] In a manner similar to PLS, 4 years has been suggested as the statute of limitations to distinguish the "benign" focal forms of MND from LMN forms of ALS.[122] The benign focal forms of MND have been referred to by a wide variety of names, the most notable of which is Hirayama disease. The classic phenotype is of a sporadic disorder presenting as slowly progressive wasting and weakness of one hand in a teenage or young adult male of Pacific-rim heritage.[144,145] The weakness often progresses within the C7–T1 segments for number of years and then arrests. It may or may not affect the opposite upper extremity in a similar distribution. Brachioradialis sparing is a notable clinical feature. Like MMN, deep tendon reflexes may be preserved in an affected extremity, although this may reflect the preferential C8–T1 segmental involvement with anatomic sparing of the C5–C7 segments where the most readily elicitable deep tendon reflexes reside. There is phenotypic heterogeneity in these slowly progressive LMN syndromes. There are cases with simultaneous involvement of the arms.[146] Not all cases occur in those of oriental descent.[147] Lower extremity syndromes exist as well which have a predilection for the posterior compartment of the leg and have been described as benign calf amyotrophy.[148] The younger age of onset, the initial involvement of distal rather than proximal upper extremity muscles, and a frequent signal change within the cervical spinal cord with MR imaging serve to distinguish the symmetrical form of Hirayama disease from the bibrachial amyotrophic diplegic variant of PMA. The differential diagnosis of

LMN-dominant forms of ALS also includes benign fasciculation syndrome. This has been previously addressed in the *Clinical Features* section.

The distal forms of spinal muscular atrophy (dSMA or hereditary motor neuropathy) would be uncommonly confused with ALS. They may be inherited in either a dominant or recessive manner. The potential resemblance to ALS originates from the occasional occurrence of UMN features, vocal cord paralysis, facial, and diaphragmatic weakness in some cases in addition to the characteristic LMN features.[149,150] One such genotype, SETX, has been characterized as both a fALS and dSMA because of the potential coexistence of UMN features.[150] To further confuse matters, the authors have had the personal experience of a SETX patient with a hereditary spastic paraparesis (HSP) phenotype. Other dSMA genotypes in which pyramidal signs may occur are mutations of the Berardinelli–Seip congenital lipodystrophy 2 (BSCL2), heat-shock protein B1 (HSPB1), and dynactin (DCTN1) (in which facial weakness may occur) genes, and an as of yet unidentified gene in a Jordanian cohort. dSMA associated with diaphragmatic palsy occurs in infants associated with mutations of the immunoglobulin mu–binding protein 2 (IGHMBP2 gene) or in dSMA4 whose gene has yet to be identified. Distal spinal muscular atrophy associated with vocal cord paralysis results from mutations in either the DCTN1 or transient receptor vallanoid 4 gene (TRPV4). Distal spinal muscular atrophy beginning in the upper extremities is associated with the glycyl-tRNA synthetase (GARS) as well as with BSCL2 gene mutations.[150]

The dSMA phenotype closely resembles and overlaps with Charcot–Marie–Tooth (CMT) disease, both being characterized by slow progression, frequent foot deformities, and a distal symmetric pattern of weakness. The difference is based largely on the presence or absence of clinical and EDX sensory loss.[150] The distinction is semantic in some cases as mutations in certain genes may produce a dSMA or CMT. Mutations in HSPB1 may result in dSMA1 or 2, or CMT2F. Mutations in HSPB8 may result in dSMA1 or 2, or CMT2L. Distal spinal muscular atrophy type 5 is also allelic with CMT2D when caused by the GARS mutation. To further confound the semiology of these diseases, FIG4 mutations may produce both fALS and CMT4J phenotypes.[150] In view of the cost of genetic testing and lack of commercial availability for many dSMA genotypes, the diagnosis of dSMA is typically based on clinical and EDX criteria. The reader is referred to the SMA chapter for further details.

On occasion, patients who have received radiation therapy may develop a delayed disorder that mimics MND.[132,151] The disorder typically begins within a few years of radiation exposure, progresses for a period of time, and then seemingly stabilizes. In the majority of cases, the syndrome occurs in patients who have received pelvic radiation, particularly for testicular tumors. This syndrome has been presumed to have an anterior horn cell localization as the weakness usually affects both lower extremities, fasciculations are common, with sensory signs and symptoms occurs infrequently. Sphincter involvement may or may not occur. Radiation-induced plexopathy or polyradiculopathy have been suggested as alternative localizations although no single locus need be mutually exclusive. The syndrome does not appear to be solely related to the total amount of radiation delivered, or the radiation per dose, which has led to hypothesis of potential synergistic pathologies such as infectious or genetic influences.[151] Diagnosis in a typical case involves the appropriate timing, deficits that remain confined to the radiation field, potentially supported by the demonstration of myokymic discharges within affected muscles.

We have rarely seen cases of a head and neck cancer presenting as a painless, progressive bulbar syndrome mimicking bulbar ALS. MR imaging of the soft tissues of the head and neck should be considered in an atypical bulbar presentation of ALS, for example, one associated with unilateral involvement of the tongue.

The differential diagnosis of PLS or UMN-D ALS phenotypes are predominantly structural and hereditary disorders, less commonly selected infectious and acquired metabolic diseases. Hereditary spastic paraparesis (HSP) and cervical spondylitic myelopathy arguably deserve the greatest consideration.[79,132,152] HSP is usually readily recognized by its slow rate of progression and a phenotype which is typically a symmetric spastic paraparesis. The upper extremities may be hyperreflexic but usually display normal strength, tone, and coordination. Bulbar involvement would be distinctly uncommon.[79,132,152] Pes cavus and minor proprioceptive deficits in the toes may occur and offer other discriminating features.[152] As with most heritable disorders, the absence of other obviously affected family member does not exclude an HSP diagnosis. The diagnosis of HSP is also rendered more difficult in complicated forms of the disease where other neurological systems, particularly the LMNs, may be involved.[153] LMN involvement has been reported in the SPG9, 10, 14, 15, 17, 20, 22, 26, 30, 38, and 41 genotypes.[152] Again, in view of the cost of genetic testing and lack of commercial availability for many HSP genotypes, the diagnosis of HSP is typically made clinically with exclusion of other causes of UMN disease. The reader is referred to the chapter on hereditary spastic paraparesis for more detailed information.

Cervical spondylitic myelopathy is usually dominated by UMN features. LMN features including hand atrophy may occur but multisegmental atrophy, weakness, fasciculations, and/or evidence of active denervation should be cautiously attributed to spinal cord compression.[132,154,155] Predomiantly LMN syndromes should be cautiously attributed to ALS. We have had the unfortunate experience of evaluating many cases of ALS with painless weakness associated with MR imaging evidence of spondylosis that have in retrospect undergone needless surgery.[156] Nonetheless, imaging of the spinal cord should be included in any MND phenotype with prominent UMN signs and no compelling "bulbar" involvement.

There are a number of other disorders that should receive some consideration in the differential diagnosis of

UMN-D or PLS presentations of MND. Primary progressive MS may present as a progressive UMN syndrome that would be addressed by MR imaging of the spinal cord and CSF examination. Dopa-responsive dystonia and stiff person syndrome may resemble progressive UMN disorders. The former diagnosis is supported by response to low-dose dopa and the latter by demonstration of antibodies against glutamic acid decarboxylase (GAD) or amphiphysin. A slowly progressive myelopathy in an young adult female may be the presenting manifestation of adrenoleukodystrophy. Usually, there are concomitant cognitive changes. Diagnosis is made by an elevated C26:C22 long-chain fatty acid ratio or by gene analysis. Retroviral infection, particularly with HTLV-1, may present as a progressive myelopathy and serological testing should be considered in symptomatic individuals at risk in residents of endemic areas or in individuals at risk by exposure through transfusion, recreational drug use, or sexual behavior.

A progressive UMN and LMN phenotype unassociated with involvement of other neurological or organ systems is almost always ALS. An ALS phenotype has been reported in association with copper deficiency.[157] The individuals reported had asymmetric foot drop as one of the initial manifestations of a progressive UMN and LMN disorder. Retrospectively, there were clinical clues that could have raised suspicion of copper deficiency in these patients. Patients with suspected ALS who have large fiber sensory loss, malabsorptive risk including prior bariatric surgery, excess zinc absorption, or concomitant anemia or cytopenia should be screened for serum copper, ceruloplasmin, and zinc levels if any of the aforementioned features are present.

Most of the other discretionary tests listed in Table 6-4 are infrequently utilized by us in the evaluation of ALS suspects. Although an ALS phenotype rarely if ever occurs in association with Lyme disease, it is a frequent inquiry on the part of our patients who live in an endemic area such as ours.[158] For this reason, it is our practice to obtain an ELISA screening test on many of our patients. We would not recommend this in areas where Lyme disease is uncommon. In view of the uncertain associations and rarity of occurrence, we reserve other testing for situations in which clinical context heightens index of suspicion. This would include testing for HIV, occult neoplasia or lymphoproliferative disorders (with or without) paraneoplastic antibodies, hexosaminidase A deficiency, thyrotoxicosis, heavy metal toxicity, polyglucosan disease, and dural venous malformations.[132,159–170] Hexosaminidase A deficiency might be considered in a young person with MND and a concomitant spinocerebellar, dystonic or bipolar syndrome. Polyglucosan disease is a phenotypic variant of glycogen storage disease type IV with phenotypic manifestations that may include distal sensory loss, a neurogenic bladder, cerebellar dysfunction, and cognitive decline.

In the absence of genetic confirmation, ALS remains a clinical diagnosis supported by the absence of evidence of other, potentially mimicking diseases. At the time of initial evaluation, ALS may be suspected but the clinical features may not have developed sufficiently to allow a physician to feel confident in confiding their suspicions with their patient. The physician may feel conflicted as to when to have this conversation. To do so prematurely hazards the possibility of being wrong. In addition, patients may lack confidence in someone who confronts them with a diagnosis of this magnitude without the appearance of due diligence. Balanced against this is the patients' need for answers. Perceived "foot dragging" and uncertainty may have equally deleterious effects on their trust in their physician. Disclosing the suspected diagnosis as early in the course as possible, following exclusion of reasonable differential diagnostic considerations, subsequent to demonstration of progression both within and outside of initially affected regions, would seem to be a reasonable approach. Many neurologists will not wait for a patient to fulfill EEC for definite or probable ALS before disclosing their suspicions. In view of the implications of an ALS diagnosis, considering the lack of a confirmatory test, and wishing to instill trust, patients are frequently counseled to seek a second opinion from a knowledgeable source.

► LABORATORY FEATURES

With the exception of identification of known pathological mutations in known fALS genes in symptomatic patients, there are no laboratory tests that currently provide disease confirmation. Testing in ALS is done for three general reasons. The first potential goal is to identify either UMN or particularly LMN involvement when it is not obvious clinically, in a patient with either an LMN- or UMN-dominant phenotype. A second diagnostic strategy is to attempt to exclude other disorders that fall within the ALS differential diagnosis. Finally, testing may be performed in an attempt to aid in disease management and prognostication, for example, forced vital capacity measurements to identify the appropriate time to discuss positive airway pressure support, percutaneous gastrostomy placement, or end-of-life decision making.

EMG and nerve conduction studies are recommended in virtually all suspected ALS patients, even when the diagnosis is clinically unequivocal. The implications of the ALS diagnosis are such that both patient and clinician wish to be as certain as possible. EMG has the capability of confirming the existence, distribution, and relative duration of LMN degeneration in support of an ALS diagnosis.[90] In addition, EDX may identify features more consistent with an alternative diagnosis as described below. The specific goals of the test are to:

1. Identify EDX abnormalities in clinically unaffected muscles to confirm a pattern consistent with ALS, that is, ongoing denervation (fibrillation potentials and sharp waves) coupled with changes implying subacute or chronic denervation and reinnervation

(a reduced number of large MUAPs, MUAP instability) demonstrable in multiple muscles innervated by multiple segments (≥2 segments in limb muscles, ≥1 muscle in cranial or thoracic muscles) in more than one body region.[91] Fasciculation potentials are a common and supportive but not required EEC electrodiagnostic requirement. As discussed above, we do not believe that convincing evidence has been provided to consider fasciculation potentials as a surrogate for fibrillation potentials and positive waves as a marker of ongoing denervation as proposed by the Awaji criteria.
2. Identify features that might implicate an ALS mimic or as the EEC refers to, an ALS-related disorder. Examples of this would include abnormal sensory conductions (Kennedy syndrome), a large decremental response (>20%) to 2 to 5 Hz repetitive stimulation without evidence of chronic denervation (myasthenia, Lambert–Eaton myasthenic syndrome), motor nerve conduction block or other demyelinating features (MMN), or EMG evidence of both small and large motor units with fibrillation potentials that might suggest inclusion body myositis in the appropriate clinical context.[92]
3. Offer insight into the rate of progression and prognosis, that is, active denervation without chronic denervation and reinnervation, motor unit variability, and a rapid decline in motor unit estimation being electrodiagnostic indicators of a more rapidly progressive course.[90]

Muscle biopsy can also serve as a surrogate for EMG to confirm LMN involvement by demonstrating a pattern of denervation atrophy characterized by scattered atrophic fibers of both fiber types that are angulated in appearance, and by small groups of atrophic fibers (Fig. 6-4). Muscle biopsy

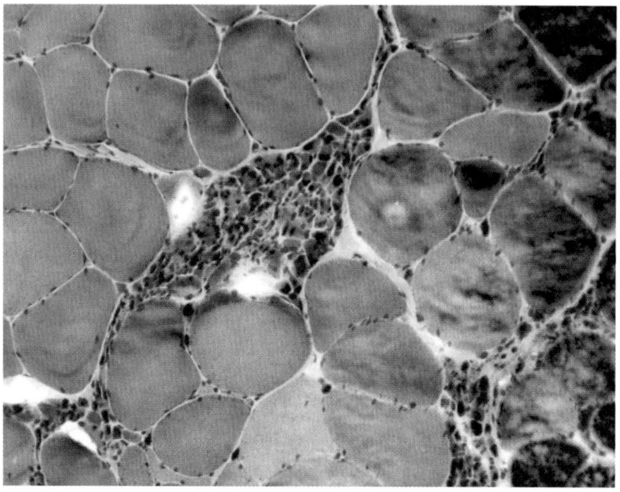

Figure 6-4. Muscle biopsy demonstrating small fiber-type grouped atrophy consistent with neurogenic atrophy and ALS (modified Gomori trichrome).

is not routinely employed in ALS as it is both more invasive and less capable of demonstrating the multifocal or diffuse neurogenic features than EMG.

Unfortunately, there are no widely available and reliable surrogates for the detection of subclinical UMN involvement. A test of this nature would be an invaluable tool in patients with PMA or LMN-D presentations. Central motor conduction velocity obtained through transcranial magnetic stimulation, magnetic resonance spectroscopy, and diffusion tensor imaging are some of the methodologies utilized that have been applied with the hope of identifying subclinical cortical spinal, or cortical bulbar tract pathology.[19,93–96] Single photon emission computerized tomography or positron emission tomography has also been used to demonstrate extra motor CNS involvement through reduced blood flow or overt atrophy in a frontotemporal lobar pattern (Fig. 6-5). All of these tests are utilized more for research than for clinical purposes as both their availability and accuracy are currently limited.

The majority of laboratory tests are done in an attempt to exclude other ALS differential diagnostic considerations or to monitor disease progress. CK levels are elevated in the serum of approximately 23–75% of ALS patients.[97,98] It is important to recognize this so as to not confuse an MND with a myopathy in a patient with painless weakness. Serum CK determination may be of value in the appropriate context. For example, an elevated CK value would favor ALS over myasthenia gravis in a patient presenting with bulbar symptoms. Tests of "pulmonary function" are done routinely. Their role is to aid in determination of prognosis and in timing of management decisions. For example, a declining vital capacity may suggest the need for positive airway pressure assistance, percutaneous gastrostomy, or initiation of end-of-life decision making discussions.

There have been significant additions to our knowledge regarding ALS-causing genes and an increased number of commercially available tests for fALS since the first edition of this book.[99] There are now at least 13 different disease-causing gene mutations.[25,43,44] The genotype for approximately half of fALS cases can now be identified. The six genes for which commercial testing is currently available include superoxide dismutase (ALS1), FUS/translated in liposarcoma (TLS) (ALS6), angiogenin (ANG) (ALS9), TAR DNA-binding protein 43 (TDP-43) (ALS10), polyphosphoinositide phosphatase (FIG4) (ALS11), and recently, the most common recognized cause of fALS, the C9ORF72 hexanucleotide expansion.

fALS mutations display varying and often incomplete penetrance.[25,27] As a result, a small percentage of patients with apparent sALS will have heritable disease. Recognizing this, we refrain from offering genetic testing to recently diagnosed individuals with apparent sporadic disease. This is in keeping with European recommendations and the results of a recent survey of North American ALS clinicians and researchers.[100,101] Although potentially viewed by some as being overly paternalistic, we feel that delivering the diagnosis of

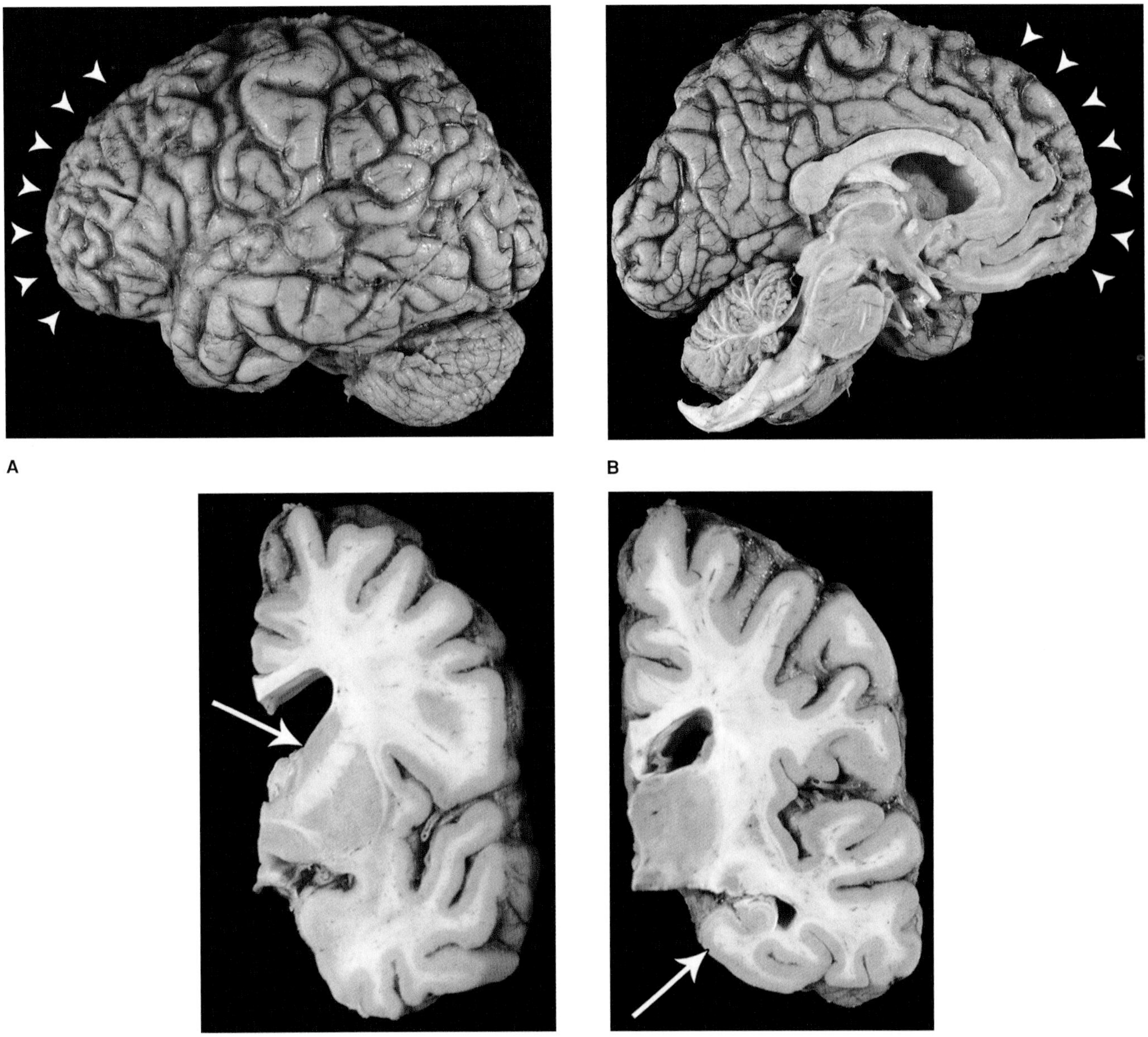

A B C D

Figure 6-5. Preferential frontal atrophy (*arrowheads*) with lateral (**A**) and parasagittal (**B**) views of the cerebrum with associated enlargement of the frontal horn and caudate flattening (*arrow*) (**C**) and relative hippocampal spraing (*arrow*) (**D**) with coronal views.

ALS is difficult enough without introducing the anxiety that other family members may be at risk in the absence of any intervention that can favorably alter the natural history of the disease. Should the patient inquire about the possibility of heritable disease, we provide them with a candid explanation of heritable risk. Should they request genetic testing under these circumstances, we will provide it but only after adequate genetic counseling that includes potential risks and benefits of testing results not only to the patient but other family members at risk. We do not routinely order genetic testing in a symptomatic individual with an affected first-degree relative who has already been genotyped.

If genetic testing is to be done, we order the most prevalent mutations first, SOD1 and C9ORF72. We reserve testing for less common mutations only if testing for these two genotypes is negative. If testing is performed in asymptomatic individuals, adequate genetic counseling is mandatory with a clear understanding of the implications of both a positive and a negative test result. Ideally, other family members at risk whose genetic status may be revealed by testing of the proband would be involved in the decision making as well.

One focus of current ALS research is the attempt to identify a biomarker or pattern of biomarkers that would provide a gold standard for diagnosis and potentially identify those at risk for ALS. This would provide the opportunity for early therapeutic intervention, offer insight into disease pathogenesis, and clarify nosology by defining whether MND represents one or more diseases.[102–106]

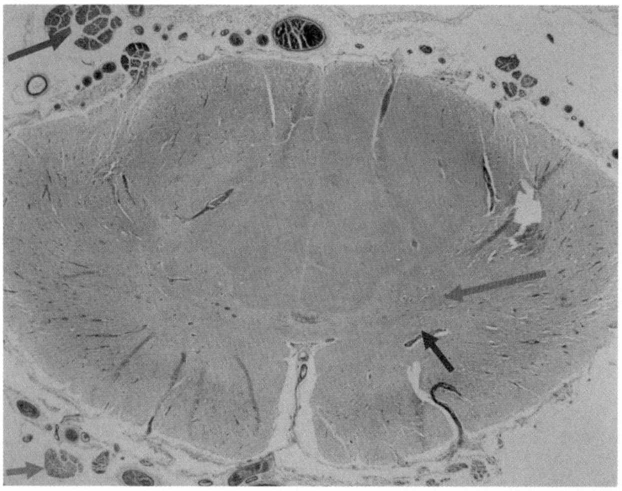

Figure 6-6. Thoracic spinal cord in a patient with amyotrophic lateral sclerosis, demonstrating reduced numbers of anterior horn cells (*red arrow*), normal complement of neurons in intermediolateral cell column (*green arrow*), atrophy of ventral root (*orange arrow*), and normal dorsal root (*blue arrow*). (Luxol fast blue/hematoxylin and eosin.)

▶ HISTOPATHOLOGY

The histopathology of ALS will be discussed from both histological and immunohistochemical perspectives. The light microscopic features of ALS in muscle are described above as they represent a potential diagnostic tool during life. The pertinent findings in the CNS however, are available on a postmortem basis only (Fig. 6-6). They consist of myelinated fiber loss in the corticospinal and corticobulbar pathways as well as loss of motor neurons within the anterior horns of the spinal cord and the motor cranial nerve nuclei at risk. As a result, ventral roots become atrophic while dorsal roots are spared. The anterior horn cell loss occurs within virtually all levels of the spinal cord with cell preservation of the intermediolateral cell columns. There is selective sparing of the third, fourth, and sixth cranial nerves as well as Onuf nucleus within the anterior horn of sacral segments 2 to 4.

As with the majority of neurodegenerative disease, the immunohistochemical signature of ALS with or without concomitant dementia is the presence of cytoplasmic inclusions representing aggregates of misfolded proteins. In familial cases of ALS associated with SOD1 gene mutations, the inclusions consist of misfolded SOD1 protein. In the majority of sALS cases, the majority of fALS genotypes not associated with SOD1 mutations, and more than half FTLD patients without ALS, these inclusions are labeled with antibodies to ubiquitin but not SOD1. These ubiquitinated inclusions (UI) are found within the cytoplasm of relevant neurons and glial cells within the primary motor cortex, brainstem motor nuclei, spinal cord, and associated white matter tracts as well as the cingulate gyrus and dentate nuclei of the cerebellum.[39,107,108] In patients with FTLD, these inclusions are found in the neocortex and hippocampus as well.[107]

Although UI are not unique to ALS or FTLD, their location and composition may be. In 2006, it was first recognized that these UI stain with TDP-43 in virtually all sALS cases and 80% of FTLD cases associated with UI.[107] UI in ALS also contain the proteins ubiquilin 2 and optineurin whose genes, when mutated, are fALS related if not causative.[109,110] Ubiquitinated inclusions that occur in neurodegenerative disorders other than ALS/FTD stain for other proteins such as tau or α-synuclein rather than TDP-43. TDP-43 is a DNA/RNA binding protein translated from a gene locus on chromosome 1. TDP-43 normally shuttles between the nucleus and cytoplasm of cells although is primarily nuclear in its location.[111] In ALS, either sporadic or non-SOD1 fALS, TDP-43 incorporated into UI is mislocalized to the cytoplasm of motor neurons (Fig. 6-7). Although TDP-43 is found in UI in the majority of FTLD patients, 20% remain TDP-43 negative.[107] In 2009, the FUS gene/protein, also related to DNA repair and RNA microprocessing, was found to colocalize to UI in non–TDP-43 FTLD cases.[25,30,107] Like TDP-43, FUS pathology in FTLD is also concentrated in the frontotemporal neocortex and hippocampus but may affect the striatum, thalamus, and brainstem as well.[103] Like mutations in the TDP-43 gene, mutations in the FUS gene may result in either an ALS and/or FTD phenotype. In addition, ubiquilin 2 pathology is prominent in the hippocampus of ALS patients with (but not without) dementia.[109]

As anticipated, the pathology and clinical phenotype do not always perfectly coincide, the latter often underestimating the former. For example, in patients with sporadic FTLD, UI/TDP-43 (+) inclusions may be found in motor neurons in the absence of any premortem

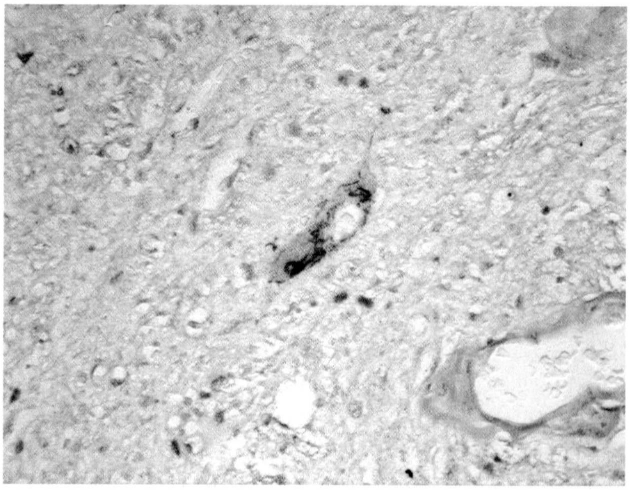

Figure 6-7. TDP-43 (+) skein in a motor neuron (lumbar) in a sporadic patient with amyotrophic lateral sclerosis (40× magnification—rabbit polyclonal antibody to human TDP-43, dilution 1:400). (Reproduced with permission from Michael Strong, MD and Robert Hammond, MD.)

evidence of MND. In addition, TDP-43 (+) inclusions are identified postmortem in the distribution characteristic of ALS as described above in patients with restricted PMA, LMN-D, and FTD/PLS phenotypes during life.[112,113] These pathological observations further cement the relationship between ALS and these phenotypically overlapping disorders.

TDP-43 (+) inclusions also occur in heritable as well as sporadic forms of FTD. Specifically they have been demonstrated in mutations of the VCP, PGRN, and TARDBP genes as well as the recently discovered C9ORF72 gene on chromosome 9. Their staining patterns appear to be identical in appearance to the TDP-43 staining pattern seen with sALS and sFTD with UI.[42,43,107] These associations add further support for a biological link between ALS and FTD in both their sporadic and familial forms.

One additional histological finding in ALS is the Bunina body. These are dense granular intracytoplasmic inclusions that stain for cystatin C, transferrin, and peripherin that are less commonly identified UI. They may be identified within the cytoplasm of motor neurons, are thought to be specific for ALS, and appear distinctive from but not necessary independent of TDP-43 aggregates.[114,115]

The vast majority of demented ALS patients will be found to have FTLD on gross inspection. Occasionally, either the patient's phenotype, or their pathology will suggest Alzheimer disease. The association is currently considered to be coincidental and not related. The immunohistochemistry of patients with prominent memory loss is typically that of a TDP-43 proteinopathy and patients with memory loss are often found to have seemingly unrelated hippocampal sclerosis with limited plaque and tangle formation.

The histology of FTLD typically consists of linear spongiosus in the first and second layer of the cortex with prominent neuronal loss in the anterior cingulate and superior frontal gyri regardless of the makeup of the associated cytoplasmic inclusions. These spongiform changes seem to segregate demented from nondemented ALS patients. The immunohistochemical properties of cytoplasmic inclusions in FTLD are varied. In greater than half of all FTLD patients, and virtually all patients with sALS, these inclusions will immunostain with ubiquitin. In approximately 40% of FTLD, the cases, the inclusions will stain for tau.[41] In patients whose inclusions stain for tau, the phenotype will not include MND but may incorporate cortical basal degeneration or progressive supranuclear palsy in addition to their FTD.

▶ PATHOGENESIS

The cause(s) of sALS remains unknown. Current hypotheses regarding disease mechanisms in sALS include oxidative damage, accumulation of toxic intracellular protein aggregates, mitochondrial dysfunction, defective axonal transport, growth factor deficiency, and/or glutamate excitotoxicity.[116] These pathophysiological mechanisms may work in series or in parallel with eventual confluence. Although our knowledge of disease pathogenesis has increased, the elements of ALS biology that contribute to disease initiation, disease propagation, or represent consequence of disease remain uncertain.

It is attractive to hypothesize that ALS is a consequence of environmental exposure and genetic risk. As previously mentioned, there is considerable phenotypic and pathological overlap between sALS and fALS. Consequently, a significant proportion of ALS research in recent years has focused on disease mechanisms in familial disease with the hope that they are relevant to sporadic disease. The recognition that specific gene mutations such as TARDNP, UBQLN2, and C9ORF72 may result in both fALS and apparent sALS, and that their protein products (TDP-43 and ubiquilin 2) can be found within neuronal inclusions in sporadic as well as familial forms of the disease lends support for this construct. Unfortunately, as described above, epidemiologic studies have failed to reproducibly identify an environmental culprit. Ultimately, the biology of ALS will have to account for the identical phenotypic heterogeneity of sporadic and familial disease, the semiselective vulnerability of motor neurons, and the tendency for the disease to spread in a regional fashion.[117] In that regard, one attractive hypothesis holds that misfolded protein aggregates in one cell can proselytize the normal analogous proteins of a neighboring cell to undergo the same pathological process, thus explaining the observed patterns of regional disease spread.[118,119]

Currently, we can only speculate as to whether ALS is a disease of singular cause capable of phenotypic diversity or the final common expression of different insults that prey upon the selected vulnerability of motor neurons. Working from the premise that sALS and fALS must share at least in part a common biology, and recognizing that similar phenotypes result from differing gene mutations, the latter paradigm that differing etiologies and disease mechanisms converge to produce a common phenotype would represent the most logical conclusion.

Since the first edition of this text, knowledge relevant to fALS knowledge has expanded at a rapid pace. As mentioned, it is the hope that insight gained from the pathophysiology of fALS will be relevant to sporadic disease as well. There are now 166 known pathological mutations of the superoxide dismutase (SOD1) gene.[25,120] In addition, mutations in at least 12 additional genes are thought to be causative of fALS.[25] These mutations along with a summary of their phenotypes are outlined in Table 6-2. In addition, there are 89 other ALS disease-related genes listed on the ALS online genetic database at the time of this writing, a resource for information relevant to both disease-causing and disease-related mutations.[121]

Currently, mutations of the SOD1 gene (ALS1) and C9ORF72 are the most common causes of fALS and constitute approximately 40–45% of cases.[25,42,43] Mutations of the C9ORF72 associated with a hexanucleotide repeat mechanism may be the most significant cause of ALS and

FTD found to date.[42,43] Less frequent causes of fALS stem from mutations of the FUS/TLS (ALS6) and TAR DNA-binding protein (TARDBP) (TDP-43) (ALS10) genes, each representing approximately 4–6% of fALS cases. Uncommon causes of fALS include mutations of the alsin (ALS2), senataxin (SETX)(ALS4), SPG11 (ALS5), vesicle-associated membrane protein–associated protein B (VAPB) (ALS8), angiogenin (ANG) (ALS9), phosphoinositide phosphatase (FIG4) (ALS11), optineurin (OPTN) (ALS12), ataxin 2 (ATXN2) (ALS13), ubiquilin (UBQLN2) (ALS15), and VCP genes.[25,28,29,42–44,62,99,107,109–111,122–128] The genes for ALS3 and ALS7 have yet to be identified.

The majority of fALS genotypes are transmitted dominantly. ALS2 and ALS5 are inherited recessively and ubiquilin 2 mutations are transmitted in an X-linked fashion. Optineurin seems unique in that both dominant and recessive inheritance patterns have been described. The penetrance of fALS is variable. SOD1 mutations were initially thought to be highly penetrant based on a bias originating from the original studies that involved a few large families in which penetrance was understandably high. In reality, less than 50% of identified ALS families have more than two identified family members.[25] Currently, penetrance is estimated to be approximately 80% in SOD1 mutations by age 85. In the highly penetrant A4 V mutation, the most prevalent SOD1 mutation in North America, 90% of individuals are clinically affected by age 70. Conversely, the I113 T mutation appears to be expressed in less than 10% of patients harboring the mutation.[25] This knowledge serves to blur the boundaries between sporadic disease and reinforce that a small percentage of apparent sALS patients will have heritable disease.

Further complicating our understanding of gene expression is the fact that the onset of symptoms in individuals with the same mutation may vary widely and that mutations in the same locus may behave differently in different populations. In the case of the D90 A CuZn SOD homozygotes, onset may vary from 20 to 94 years of age.[25,62] This locus behaves as a recessive trait in Scandinavia where heterozygotes are asymptomatic. In North America except in those of Scandinavian descent, D90 A behaves as a dominant disorder with heterozygotes developing ALS.

The mechanisms by which the aforementioned mutations initiate and/or propagate MND and FTD remain enigmatic. A common theme in ALS is the presence of inclusions within motor neurons consisting of misfolded proteins with the implication that these inclusions confer a toxic gain of function.[129] Alternatively, ALS could represent a loss of function of proteins migrating from their normal nuclear location to a pathological cytoplasmic position. As previously mentioned however, the makeup of the inclusions found in ALS is variable, with SOD1 inclusions being absent of TDP-43 staining, implicating more than one toxic mechanism.[130] Although potential mechanisms remain unknown, common themes are emerging. Ubiquilin 2 is a constituent of the ubiquitin proteasome system responsible for protein degradation which may confer a toxic gain of function when mutated.[44,109] Mutations of the TDP43, FUS, ANG, SETX, and C9ORF72 all appear to adversely affect RNA metabolism.[25,42,43,107] For example, RNA generated by pathogenic expansions of the C9ORF72 gene is hypothesized to sequester normal RNA and proteins resulting in disruption of normal transcription.[42,43] TDP-43 and FUS are both trapped into stress granules that may further hinder RNA metabolism.[131] The ataxin 2 gene, large expansions of which cause the spinocerebellar ataxia type 2 phenotype, appears to be a potent modifier of TDP-43 toxicity.[122–124] The mechanism of action for optineurin mutations in the genesis of ALS is uncertain.[25,110,125]

► MANAGEMENT

Once the diagnosis has been shared with the patient and their family, we organize their management into three domains: (1) education and psychosocial support, (2) disease-specific treatment including consideration of clinical trials, and (3) supportive care for the patient and their disease, ideally provided in a multidisciplinary setting.

In the Internet age, information is readily available to patients and their families. It is the responsibility of any physician caring for an ALS patient to direct them toward reputable educational resources. To that end, the websites provided by the Muscular Dystrophy Association (www.mda.org), the ALS Association (www.alsa.org), and the Motor Neuron Disease Association (www.mndassociation.org) are recommended. Unfortunately, there are websites, for reasons altruistic or otherwise, that provide false hope or false information. www.alsuntangled.com is a web-based resource developed by ALS clinician researchers to help patients and their families sort through this potentially confusing terrain.[171]

In part due to the paucity of effective treatments, many patients with ALS seek advice from their physicians regarding alternative, "natural treatments" for their disorder. There is no clear correct response. A dogmatic response on the part of a physician in opposition to this approach runs the risk of losing the patient. Conversely, the physician has a responsibility to dispel what seems to be a generally held perception that "natural" is synonymous with safe. It may be helpful to emphasize to a patient that any substance that is biologically active enough to be beneficial is also biologically active enough to be harmful. "Natural" substances do not benefit from the same underlying science or undergo the same scrutiny and quality control as do pharmaceuticals and pose additional risk for those reasons alone.

In many locations, support groups are available for patients and their families as a potential resource that some but not all patients and caregivers find valuable. As the disease progresses, preferentially while the patient remains capable of communicating effectively, it is the neurologist's duty to discuss with the patient their preferences regarding decisions that will inevitably have to be made. By doing so, the neurologist provides the patient with some semblance of control of their disease and provides respect for their autonomy regarding these difficult issues.

Patients and families frequently inquire about the potential genetic consequences of the disease. As discussed earlier, we are candid in disclosing that the possibility fALS cannot be entirely excluded in any apparent sALS patient. Fortunately, with adequate family history, it is possible to reassure the patient and biological relatives of the low statistical likelihood of heritable disease in the majority of cases.

There are no known treatments that can reverse or arrest disease progression in ALS. In 1994, Rilutek was identified as the first and only disease-specific treatment to date that favorably altered the natural history of the disease.[14] Its modest benefit results in 10% slowing of disease progression by approximately 10% at its customary dose of 50 mg bid. Unfortunately, this benefit is imperceptible to the patient who neither feels nor functions better. It is an expensive drug that is usually well tolerated although some experience upper gastrointestinal side effects and increased fatigue. Reversible hepatotoxicity may occur with an associated requirement for monitoring of liver function tests. Balancing the benefits of Rilutek with its potentially significant financial burden consideration is a candid conversation that should take place with patients and their families.

There have been numerous failed ALS therapeutic trials. Current clinical trials, likely to have been completed by the time of publication, involve ceftriaxone, dexpramipexole, a combination of creatinine and tamoxifen, a combination of anakinra and riluzole, NP001, and neural-derived stem cells. Trials utilizing arimoclomol and intrathecal delivery of ISIS 333611 are available for those with fALS and identified SOD1 mutations. Patients and clinicians can be kept abreast of clinical trial availability and enrollment status through websites.[172,173] Patients should be encouraged to participate in these. Not all patients will be eligible. Patients who do not meet EEC probable or definite disease criteria including those with exclusive bulbar disease, age <18 or >80, or vital capacities less than 60% of predicted are typically excluded from enrollment.

Optimal management of the patients with ALS and their families is time-consuming and requires knowledge and resources that undoubtedly surpass the capabilities of any single healthcare worker. For this reason, although potentially emotionally and physically exhausting for the patient, the multidisciplinary clinic provides a useful ALS care model. Studies have demonstrated that participation in a multidisciplinary clinic improves both quality and duration of life.[55] The goals of the clinic are to anticipate and resolve problems that adversely affect the patient's ability to function, their safety, and their comfort. During the clinic, multiple parameters including the patient's psychosocial well-being, the presence or absence of pain, their sleep quality, "bulbar" functions, fine motor skills, ventilation, and mobility and ambulation are assessed.

The revised ALS functional rating scale (ALSFRS-R) is a validated 48-point assessment tool that can be acquired both in person and over the phone. Twelve points are signed to each of four domains assessing ventilation, bulbar function, fine motor skills, and mobility. The rate of disease progression and prognosis can be estimated, a decline of less than or greater than 0.5 points per month separating slow from fast progression.[174,175]

In addition to the ALSFRS-R, we routinely monitor quantitative strength using handheld dynamometers as outlined in Chapter 1 as well as measurements of ventilatory function. Although at times helpful in reinforcing the initial diagnosis, tests of ventilatory function have the greatest utility in monitoring the disease course. Declining ventilatory muscle strength not only speaks to prognosis and helps to time discussions pertaining to end-of-life decision making, it has management implications regarding the initiation of noninvasive positive airway pressure and percutaneous gastrostomy tube insertion. The most commonly used measurements are forced vital capacity, and maximal inspiratory and expiratory pressures. A drop in forced vital capacities in the supine in comparison to the sitting position of more than 10% of the predicted value suggests a disproportionate degree of diaphragmatic weakness.

Since the first edition of this book, a revised version of the ALS practice parameter endorsed by both the American Academy of Neurology and the American Association of Neuromuscular and Electrodiagnostic Medicine has been published.[176,177] As an evidence-based document, it cannot adequately address all management decisions pertaining to ALS, it is nonetheless a helpful guideline for the practicing neurologist. Other management reviews attempt to fill the gaps by providing experienced, expert opinion.[178] Symptomatic management of poor sleep (due to immobility, depression, urinary frequency, sleep disordered breathing), pain (immobility, joint contractures, cramps, and spasticity), sialorrhea, impaired clearance of viscous secretions, laryngospasm, impaired communication, dysphagia, impaired performance of ADLs, and disordered bowel and bladder function are typically addressed with durable medical equipment or pharmacologic treatment. These interventions are outlined in (Table 6-5). It also behooves the neurologist to become familiar with the topography and limitations of the patient's residence and if necessary, to arrange for a home safety evaluation to identify areas of home modification that would benefit the patient.

There are a number of potential interventions that are often met with resistance by patients despite their potential to enhance the quality of their lives as well as maintenance of their independence. In an attempt to overcome patient reluctance, we often utilize two strategies as well as to maintain their independence. We often introduce these concepts prior to their actual need to give the patient and

▶ TABLE 6-5. **SYMPTOMATIC MANAGEMENT OF MND/ALS[176–178]**

Symptom, Management Issue	Potential Treatments	Symptom, Management Issue	Potential Treatments
Sialorrhea	Glycopyrrolate	**Mobility issues**	
	Tricyclic antidepressants	Tripping from foot drop	Ankle–foot orthoses
	Robinul	Falling secondary to	Canes
	Botulinum toxin	Quadriceps	Crutches
	Atropine	Weakness	Walker
	Salivary gland radiation		Wheelchair, manual or power
	Scopolamine patch	Bed mobility	Hospital bed with side rails and/ or trapeze
	Chorda tympani section		
Secretion clearance	Tracheostomy	Bathroom safety and functionality	Stall shower
	Cough-assist devices		Shower chair
	Home suction		Transfer bench
	Expectorants (e.g., guaifenesin)		Toilet seat extension
	Beta blockers		Shower and toilet bars
	Nebulized n-acetylcysteine and albuterol	House accessibility	Stair lift
	Secretion mobilization vests		Lift chair or chair lift
Pseudobulbar affect	Dextromethorphan hydrobromide and quinidine sulfate		Hoyer lift
			Elevators
	Tricyclic antidepressants		Ramps
	Selective serotonin reuptake inhibitors	Improved ADLs	Velcro for buttons and shoelaces
			Elastic shoelaces
			Long-handled grippers
Depression	Tricyclic antidepressants		Foam collars for pens and utensils
	Selective serotonin reuptake inhibitors	**Dysphagia—malnutrition**	Neck positioning
			Change in food consistency
	Stimulants		Percutaneous gastrostomy
Laryngospasm	Antihistamines	**Constipation**	Bulk
	H_2 receptor blockers		Fiber
	Antacids		Stool softeners/cathartics
	Proton pump inhibitors		Hydration
	Sublingual lorazepam drops	**Urinary urgency**	Tolterodine
Neck drop	Cervical collar	**Cramps**	Quinine sulfate[a]
	Hi back wheelchair with supports		Gabapentin
Communication	Augmentative communication devices		Tizanidine
			Baclofen
	Pad and pencil or erasable slates		Benzodiazepines
Hypoventilation	Positive pressure ventilators, e.g., BiPAP		Phenytoin
			Carbamazepine
	Negative pressure ventilators, e.g., Cuirass		Mexiletine
			Primrose oil
	TAMV	**Safety**	Brewer's yeast
			Lifeline
	Morphine sulfate		Phone auto dialer
	Benzodiazepines		Home safety evaluation
Contractures	Night splints	**Spasticity**	Tizanidine, dantrolene
	Botulinum toxin		Baclofen oral or intrathecal
	Range of motion exercises		Botulinum toxin

[a]Not FDA approved for this purpose.

their family a chance to adjust. Additionally, we emphasize the importance of compliance with the use of durable medical equipment and other intervention, the goals of fall prevention and maintenance of independence.

Percutaneous gastrostomy, noninvasive positive pressure ventilation (NIPPV), and mechanical gait aids are commonly recommended but are perceived as threatening by patients. All should be introduced as measures to improve the quality of life rather than duration of life, even though the latter is probably achieved with NIPPV and may be accomplished with gastrostomy feeding. There are no absolute criteria to determine optimal percutaneous gastrostomy timing. Loss of weight of >10% of baseline weight, doubling of eating time, demonstration of laryngeal penetration or aspiration, or recurrent coughing or choking during eating are the most common indicators utilized to prompt gastrostomy tube recommendation. We attempt to place percutaneous gastrostomy before the forced vital capacity falls below 50% of predicted to limit risk associated with the procedure.

NIPPV is typically recommended when the patient is symptomatic from shortness of breath, when disturbed sleep is attributed to hypoventilation, when symptoms attributable to hypercapnia such as morning headache or confusion occur, or when forced vital capacity decreases to less than 50% of predicted. Initial use occurs at night when hypoventilation is most likely to occur. Initial settings include an inspiratory pressure of 8 cm of water, an expiratory pressure of 4 cm of water, and a backup rate of 8 breaths per minute. A minimum of 6 hours of nocturnal use is encouraged. NIPPV appears to have the most dramatic effects on disease survival of any treatment options available. Although it is suspected that early use of NIPPV is beneficial in prolonging life expectancy, third-party payers typically require a forced vital capacity of <50% of predicted, a negative inspiratory force of less than 60 mm Hg, or evidence of carbon dioxide retention before reimbursement for NIPPV is authorized. This is problematic in patients who are symptomatic but who have yet to fulfill the aforementioned diagnostic criteria. Diaphragmatic pacing represents a newer ventilatory support modality. Although FDA approved for patients with significant but not severe ventilatory muscle weakness, the extent of its benefit(s) await ongoing study.

It is the responsibility of every physician caring for patients with ALS to participate in one or more discussions concerning end-of-life decisions, particularly regarding TAMV. Ideally, the patient should be given the autonomy to make these decisions at a time that they can still communicate effectively and before any ventilatory crisis might occur. Ideally, this discussion would occur at a time of the patient's choosing but may need to be initiated by the physician in some cases. In the spirit of full disclosure, the physician should inform the patient of the distasteful but realistic aspects of TAMV including considerations of cost, location of care, caretaker burden, life-expectancy even with TAMV, and potential development of future dementia.

The majority of patients with ALS in the US decline TAMV consideration although some relent at the time of crisis. Cultural values regarding quality of life, the fear of being a burden, and the associated costs of long-term care, which are typically not covered by third-party payers, represent the most likely reasons why patients decline.[37,38] Most patients choose to receive their terminal care at home. Hospice services either at home or in hospice facilities provide an invaluable resource. Many, if not all, patients fear that their death will involve physical suffering. Some may be intrepid enough to broach the subject, some may not. Providing patients with the reassurance that adequate palliation will be provided to avert physical discomfort is another important responsibility to fulfill. A frank discussion about the logistics and limits of how this will be accomplished is often appreciated by the patient, family, and caregivers. Typically, neurologists, through hospice nurses, provide for adequate treatment of pain, anxiety, dyspnea, nausea, and any other distressing symptom. This goal is usually achieved often with drugs such as morphine and lorazepam without suppressing ventilatory drive. Even if the latter were to occur, it is ethically acceptable under the principle of double effect as long as the primary intent is to relieve suffering. Fortunately, the vast majority of ALS patients appear to die peacefully and comfortably.

The role of exercise pertaining to its effect on both the disease progression and the preservation of function is a near universal inquiry by ALS patients. Studies done to date favorably report on the benefits of exercise done in moderation.[179] We recommend low-level conditioning and nonfatiguing exercise that is safe, for their patients. For example, a rowing machine or exercise bicycle would be preferable to a treadmill for a patient with lower extremity weakness or spasticity.

In patients with presumed fALS and asymptomatic family members at risk, we encourage participation in research studies that are currently being conducted at the University of Miami. Dr. Michael Benatar and colleagues offer patients the opportunity to participate in fALS-specific therapeutic trials, and provide both groups the opportunity for counseling and genotyping at no cost. Contact information is Fals@med.miami.edu.

▶ SUMMARY

HIV and cancer are disorders that were uniformly fatal within many of our professional lifetimes. Now, in many instances, these are disorders that are controllable and at times curable. For patients with ALS, their families, and their physicians, it is important to realize that similar outcomes may be realized for ALS in the foreseeable future. Until that hope is realized, neurologists caring for patients with ALS are obligated to help maintain the quality of their patients' life to the extent possible. When that is no longer feasible, they have an obligation to support the quality and dignity of their patients' death as well.

REFERENCES

1. Strong MJ. The evidence for ALS as a multisystems disorder of limited phenotypic expression. *Can J Neurol Sci.* 2001;28: 283–298.
2. Strong MJ, Grace GM, Freedman M, et al. Consensus criteria for the diagnosis of frontotemporal cognitive and behavioral syndromes in amyotrophic lateral sclerosis. *Amyotroph Lateral Scler.* 2009;10:131–146.
3. Swash M, Desai J. Motor neuron disease: classification and nomenclature. *Amyotroph Lateral Scler Other Motor Neuron Disord.* 2000;1:105–112.

4. Gordon PH, Cheng B, Katz IB, et al. The natural history of primary lateral sclerosis. *Neurology*. 2006;66:647–653.
5. Gordon PH, Cheng B, Katz IB, Mitsumoto H, Rowland LP. Clinical features that distinguish PLS, upper motor neuron dominant ALS, and typical ALS. *Neurology*. 2009;72:1948–1952.
6. Tartaglia MC, Rowe A, Findlater K, Orange JB, Grace G, Strong MJ. Differentiation between primary lateral sclerosis and amyotrophic lateral sclerosis. *Arch Neurol*. 2007;64:232–236.
7. Kim WK, Liu X, Sandner J, et al. Study of 962 patients indicates progressive muscular atrophy is a form of ALS. *Neurology*. 2009;73:1686–1692.
8. Visser J. Van den Berg-Vos RM, Frannsen H, et al. Disease course and prognostic factors of progressive muscular atrophy. *Arch Neurol*. 2007;64:522–528.
9. Traynor BJ, Codd MB, Corr B, Forde C, Frost E, Hardiman OM. Clinical features of amyotrophic lateral sclerosis according to the El Escorial and Airlie House diagnostic criteria. *Arch Neurol*. 2000;57(8):1171–1176.
10. Rowland LR. Progressive muscular atrophy and other lower motor neuron syndromes of adults. *Muscle Nerve*. 2010; 41:161–165.
11. Mateen FJ, Carone M, Sorenson EJ. Patients who survive 5 years or more with ALS in Olmstead County, 1925–2004. *J Neurol Neurosurg Psychiatry*. 2010;81:1144–1146.
12. Mortara P, Chio A, Rosso MG, Leone M, Schiffer D. Motor neuron disease in the province of Turin, Italy, 1966–1980: survival analysis in an unselected population. *J Neurol Sci*. 1984;66:165–173.
13. Brooks BR. El Escorial World Federation of Neurology criteria for the diagnosis of amyotrophic lateral sclerosis. *J Neurol Sci*. 1994;124(suppl):96–107.
14. Bensimon G, Lacomblez L, Meininger V. A controlled trial of riluzole in amyotrophic lateral sclerosis. *N Engl J Med*. 1994; 330:585–591.
15. Brooks BR, Miller RG, Swash M, Munsat TL; World Federation of Neurology Research Group on Motor Neuron Diseases. El Escorial revisited: revised criteria for the diagnosis of amyotrophic lateral sclerosis. *Amyotroph Lateral Scler*. 2000;1:293–300.
16. Ross MA, Miller RG, Berchert L, et al. Toward earlier diagnosis of amyotrophic lateral sclerosis. *Neurology*. 1998;50:768–772.
17. Chaudhuri KR, Crump SJ, Al-Sarraj S, Anderson V, Cavanagh J, Leigh PN. The validation of El Escorial criteria for the diagnosis of amyotrophic lateral sclerosis: a clinicopathological study. *J Neurol Sci*. 1995;129(suppl):11–12.
18. Ince PG, Evans J, Knopp M, et al. Corticospinal tract degeneration in the progressive muscular atrophy variant of ALS. *Neurology*. 2003;60:1252–1258.
19. Carvalho MD, Dengler R, Eisen A, et al. Electrodiagnostic criteria for diagnosis of ALS. *Clin Neurophysiol*. 2008;119: 497–503.
20. Carvalho MD, Swash M. Awaji diagnostic algorithm increases sensitivity of El Escorial criteria for ALS diagnosis. *Amyotroph Lateral Scler*. 2009;10:53–57.
21. Douglass CP, Kandler RH, Shaw PJ, McDermott CJ. An evaluation of neurophysiological criteria used in the diagnosis of motor neuron disease. *J Neurol Neurosurg Psychiatry*. 2010;81:646–649.
22. Chen A, Weimer L, Brannagan T, Colin M, et al. Experience with the Awaji Island modifications to the ALS diagnostic criteria. *Muscle Nerve*. 2010;42:831–832.
23. Mills KR. Characteristics of fasciculations in amyotrophic lateral sclerosis and the benign fasciculation syndrome. *Brain*. 2010;133:3458–3469.
24. Benatar M, Tandan R. The Awaji criteria for the diagnosis of amyotrophic lateral sclerosis; have we put the cart before the horse? *Muscle Nerve*. 2011;43:461–463.
25. Andersen P, Al-Chalabi A. Clinical genetics of amyotrophic lateral sclerosis: what do we really know? *Nat Rev Neurol*. 2011; 7:603–615.
26. Hanby MF, Scott KM, Scotton W, et al. The risk to relative of patients with sporadic amyotrophic lateral sclerosis. *Brain*. 2011;134:3454–3457.
27. Donkervoort S, Siddique T. Amyotrophic lateral sclerosis overview. http://www.ncbi.nlm.nih.gov/books/NBK1450/.
28. Andersen PM, Forsgren L, Binzer M, et al. Autosomal recessive adult-onset amyotrophic lateral sclerosis associated with homozygosity for Asp90Ala CuZn-superoxide dismutase mutation: a clinical and genealogical study of 36 patients. *Brain*. 1996;119:1153–1172.
29. Hand C, Rouleau GA. Familial amyotrophic lateral sclerosis. *Muscle Nerve*. 2002;25:135–159.
30. http://www.ncbi.nlm.nih.gov/omim/?term=familial+als
31. Murphy J, Henry R, Lagmore S, Kramer JH, Miller BL, Lomen-Hoerth C. Continuum of frontal lobe impairment in amyotrophic lateral sclerosis. *Arch Neurol*. 2007;64:530–534.
32. Strong MJ, Lomen-Hoerth C, Caselli RJ, Bigio EH, Yang W. Cognitive impairment, frontotemporal dementia and the motor neuron diseases. *Ann Neurol*. 2003;54(5):S20–S23.
33. Lomen-Hoerth C, Anderson T, Miller BM. The overlap of amyotrophic lateral sclerosis and frontotemporal dementia. *Neurology*. 2002;59:1077–1079.
34. Murphy J, Henry R, Lomen-Hoerth C. Establishing subtypes of the continuum of frontal lobe impairment in amyotrophic lateral sclerosis. *Arch Neurol*. 2007;64:330–334.
35. Neary DF, Snowden JS, Gustafson L, et al. Frontotemporal lobar degeneration: a consensus on clinical diagnostic criteria. *Neurology*. 1998;51:1546–1554.
36. Wilson CM, Grace GN, Munoz DG, He BP, Strong MJ. Cognitive impairment in sporadic ALS: a pathologic continuum underlying a multisystem disorder. *Neurology*. 2001;57:651–657.
37. Yamguchi M, Hayashi H, Hiraoka K. Ventilatory support in Japan: a new life with ALS and a positive approach to living with the disease. *Amyotrophic Lateral Sclerosis & Other Motor Neuron Disorders*. 2001;2(4):209–211.
38. Tagami M, Kimura F, Nakajima H et al. Tracheostomy and invasive ventilation in Japanese ALS patients: decision-making and survival analysis: 1990–2010. *J Neurol Sci*. 2014;344 (1–2):158–164.
39. McCluskey LR, Elman LB, Martinez-Lage M, et al. Amyotrophic lateral sclerosis-plus syndrome with TAR DNA binding protein 43 pathology. *Arch Neurol*. 2009;66(1):121–124.
40. Wicks P, Abrahams S, Papps B, et al. SOD1 and cognitive dysfunction in familial amyotrophic lateral sclerosis. *J Neurol*. 2009;256(2):234–241.
41. Goldman JS, Rademakers R, Huey ED, et al. An algorithm for genetic testing of frontotemporal lobar degeneration. *Neurology*. 2011;76:475–483.
42. DeJesus-Hernandez M, Mackenzie IR, Boeve BF, et al. Expanded GGGGCC hexanucleotide repeat in noncoding region of C9ORF72 causes chromosome 9p-linked FTD and ALS. *Neuron*. 2011;72(2):245–256.

43. Renton AE, Majounie E, Waite A, et al. A hexanucleotide repeat expansion in C9ORF72 is the cause of chromosome 9p21-linked ALS-FTD. *Neuron*. 2011;72(2):257–268.
44. Deng HX, Chen W, Hong ST, et al. Mutations in UBQLN2 cause dominant X-linked juvenile and adult-onset ALS and ALS/dementia. *Nature*. 2011;477:211–215.
45. Armon C. Smoking may be considered an established risk factor for sporadic ALS. *Neurology*. 2009;73:1693–1698.
46. Weisskopf MG, Ascherio A. Cigarettes and amyotrophic lateral sclerosis: only smoke or also fire? *Ann Neurol*. 2009;65(4):361–362.
47. Gallo V, Bueno-de-Mesquita HB, Vermeulen R, et al. Smoking and risk of amyotrophic lateral sclerosis: analysis of the EPIC cohort. *Ann Neurol*. 2009;65:378–385.
48. Nelson LM, Maguire V, Longstreth WT Jr, Matkin C. Population-based case control study of amyotrophic lateral sclerosis in western Washington State I. Cigarette smoking and alcohol consumption. *Am J Epidemol*. 2000;151:156–163.
49. Nelson LM, Matkin C, Longstreth WT Jr, Maguire V. Population-based case control study of amyotrophic lateral sclerosis in western Washington State II Diet. *Am J Epidemol*. 2000;151:164–173.
50. Worm PM. The epidemiology of motor neuron diseases: a review of recent studies. *J Neurol Sci*. 2001;191:3–9.
51. Cashman NR, Cudkowicz ME, Davidson MC, Pioro EP, Rosenfeld J; The ALS patient care database. Gender effects on duration and onset age of amyotrophic lateral sclerosis. *Amyotroph Lateral Scler Other Motor Neuron Disord*. 2001;2:41–42.
52. Chancellor AM, Slattery JM, Fraser H, Swingler RJ, Holloway SM, Warlow CP. Prognosis of adult-onset motor neuron disease: a prospective study based on the Scottish Motor Neuron Disease Register. *J Neurol*. 1993;240:339–346.
53. Bradley WG, Mash DC. Beyond Guam: the cyanobacteria/BMAA hypothesis of the cause of ALS and other neurodegenerative diseases. *Amyotroph Lateral Scler*. 2009;(10 suppl 2):7–20.
54. Magnus T, Beck M, Geiss R, Puls I, Naumann M, Toyka KV. Disease progression in amyotrophic lateral sclerosis: predictors of survival. *Muscle Nerve*. 2002;25:709–714.
55. Albert SA, Whitaker A, Rabkin JG, et al. Medical and supportive care among people with ALS in the months before death or tracheostomy. *J Pain Symptom Manage*. 2009;38:546–553.
56. Traynor BJ, Alexander M, Corr B, Frost E, Hardiman O. Effect of a multidisciplinary amyotrophic lateral sclerosis (ALS) clinic on ALS survival: a population based study, 1996–2000. *J Neurol Neurosurg Psychiatry*. 2003;74(9):1258–1261.
57. Blexrud MD, Windebank AJ, Daube JR. Long-term follow-up of 121 patients with benign fasciculations. *Ann Neurol*. 1993;34:622–625.
58. Norris F, Shepherd R, Denys E, et al. Onset, natural history and outcome in idiopathic adult motor neuron disease. *J Neurol Sci*. 1993;118:48–55.
59. Mitsumoto H. Diagnosis and progression of ALS. *Neurology*. 1997;48(suppl):S2–S8.
60. Kent-Braun JA, Walker CH, Weiner MW, Miller RG. Upper and lower motor neuron function and muscle weakness in amyotrophic lateral sclerosis. *Neurology*. 1996;46:A470.
61. Haverkamp LJ, Appel V, Appel SH. Natural history of amyotrophic lateral sclerosis in a database population. Validation of a scoring system and a model for survival prediction. *Brain*. 1995;118:707–719.
62. Andersen PM. Amyotrophic lateral sclerosis associated with mutations in the CuZn superoxide dismutase gene. *Curr Neurol Neurosci Rep*. 2006;6:37–46.
63. Brownell B, Oppenheimer DR, Hughes JR. Central nervous system in motor neuron disease. *J Neurol Neurosurg Psychiatry*. 1970;33:338–357.
64. Iwanaga K, Hayashi S, Oyake M, et al. Neuropathology of sporadic amyotrophic lateral sclerosis of long duration. *J Neurol Sci*. 1997;146:139–143.
65. Lawyer T, Netsky MG. ALS, clinico-anatomic study of 53 cases. *Arch Neurol Psychiatry*. 1953;69:171–192.
66. Cudkowicz ME, McKenna-Yasek D, Chen C, Hedley-Whyte ET, Brown RH. Limited corticospinal tract involvement in amyotrophic lateral sclerosis subjects with the A4 V mutation in the copper/zinc superoxide dismutase gene. *Ann Neurol*. 1998;43:703–710.
67. Raaphorst J, de Visser M, van Tol MJ, et al. Cognitive dysfunction and lower motor neuron disease: executive and memory deficits and progressive muscular atrophy. *J Neurol Neurosurg Psychiatry*. 2011;82:170–175.
68. Katz JS, Wolfe GI, Andersson PB, et al. Brachial amyotrophic diplegia. *Neurology*. 1999;53:1071–1076.
69. Wijesekera LC, Mathers S, Talman P, et al. Natural history and clinical features of the flail arm and flail leg ALS variants. *Neurology*. 2009;72:1087–1094.
70. Pouget JY, Robert D, Sangla I, et al. Quantitative assessment of bulbar function in ALS using an objective speech evaluation. *Neurology*. 1996;46:A470.
71. Coon EA, Sorenson EJ, Whitwell JL, Knopman DS, Josephs KA. Predicting survival and frontotemporal dementia with motor neuron disease. *Neurology*. 2011;76:1886–1893.
72. Turner MR, Scaber J, Goodfellow JA, Lord ME, Marsden R, Talbot K. Diagnostic and prognosis in bulbar-onset amyotrophic lateral sclerosis. *J Neurol Sci*. 2010;294:81–85.
73. Portet F, Cadihac C, Touchon J, Camu W. Cognitive impairment in motor neuron disease with bulbar onset. *Amyotroph Lateral Scler Other Motor Neuron Disord*. 2001;2(1):23–29.
74. Lomen-Hoerth C, Murphy J, Langmore S, Kramer JH, Olney RK, Miller B. Are amyotrophic lateral sclerosis patients cognitively normal? *Neurology*. 2003;60:1094–1097.
75. Strong MJ, Grace GM, Orange JB, Leeper HA, Menon RS, Aere C. A prospective study of cognitive impairment in ALS. *Neurology*. 1999;53:1655–1670.
76. Ringholz GM, Appel SH, Bradshaw M, Cooke NA, Mosnik DM, Schulz PE. Prevalence and patterns of cognitive impairment in sporadic ALS. *Neurology*. 2005;65:586–590.
77. Le Forestier N, Maisonobe T, Piquard A, et al. Does primary lateral sclerosis exist? A study of 20 patients and a review of the literature. *Brain*. 2001;124:1989–1999.
78. Pringle CE, Hudson AJ, Munoz DG, Kiernan JA, Brown WF, Ebers GC. Primary lateral sclerosis. Clinical features, neuropathology and diagnostic criteria. *Brain*. 1992;115:495–520.
79. Strong MJ. Primary lateral sclerosis, hereditary spastic paraplegia and amyotrophic lateral sclerosis: discrete entities or spectrum? *Amyotroph Lateral Scler Other Motor Neuron Disord*. 2005;6(1):8–16.
80. Singer MA, Statland JM, Wolfe GI, Barohn RJ. Primary lateral sclerosis. *Muscle Nerve*. 2007;35:291–302.
81. Caselli RJ, Smith BE, Osborn D. Primary lateral sclerosis: a neuropsychological study. *Neurology*. 1995;45:2005–2009.

82. Josephs KA, Dickson DW. Frontotemporal lobar degeneration with upper motor neuron disease/primary lateral sclerosis. *Neurology*. 2007;69:1800–1801.
83. Chen R, Grand'Maison F, Strong MJ, Ramsay DA, Bolton CF. Motor neuron disease presenting as acute respiratory failure: a clinical and pathological study. *J Neurol Neurosurg Psychiatry*. 1996;60:455–458.
84. Shoesmith CL, Findlater K, Rowe A, Strong MJ. Prognosis of amyotrophic lateral sclerosis with respiratory onset. *J Neurol Neurosurg Psychiatry*. 2007;78:629–631.
85. Elamin M, Phukan J, Bede P, et al. Executive dysfunction is a negative prognostic indicator in patients with ALS without dementia. *Neurology*. 2011;76:1263–1269.
86. Wheaton MW, Salamone AR, Mosnik DM, et al. Cognitive impairment in familial ALS. *Neurology*. 2007;69:1411–1417.
87. Witgert M, Salamone AR, Strutt AM, et al. Frontal lobe mediated behavioral dysfunction in amyotrophic lateral sclerosis. *Eur J Neurol*. 2010;17:103–110.
88. Massman PJ, Sims J, Cooke N, Haverkamp LJ, Appel V, Appel SH. Prevalence and correlates of neuropsychological deficits in amyotrophic lateral sclerosis. *J Neurol Neurosurg Psychiatry*. 1996;61:450–455.
89. http://www.mocatest.org/pdf_files/test/MoCA-Test-English_7_1.pdf
90. Daube JR. Electrodiagnostic studies in amyotrophic lateral sclerosis and other motor neuron disorders. *Muscle Nerve*. 2000;23:1488–1502.
91. Makki AA, Benatar M. The electromyographic diagnosis of amyotrophic lateral sclerosis: does the evidence support the El Escorial criteria? *Muscle Nerve*. 2007;35:614–619.
92. Dabby R, Lange DJ, Trojaborg W, et al. Inclusion body myositis mimicking motor neuron disease. *Arch Neurol*. 2001;58:1253–1256.
93. Agosta F, Chiò A, Cosottini M, et al. The present and the future of neuroimaging in amyotrophic lateral sclerosis. *Am J Neuroradiol*. 2010;31:1769–1777.
94. Wang S, Melhem ER, Poptani H, Woo JH. Neuroimaging in amyotrophic lateral sclerosis. *Neurotherapeutics*. 2011;8:63–71.
95. Mitsumoto H, Uluğ AM, Pullman SL, et al. Quantitative objective markers for upper and lower motor neuron dysfunction in ALS. *Neurology*. 2007;68:1402–1410.
96. van der Graff MM, Sage CA, Caan MW, et al. Upper and extra-motoneuron involvement in early motoneuron disease: a diffusion tensor imaging study. *Brain*. 2011;134:1211–1228.
97. Felice KJ, North WA. Creatine kinase values in amyotrophic lateral sclerosis. *J Neurol Sci*. 1998;160:S30–S32.
98. Chahin N, Sorenson EJ. Serum creatine kinase levels in spinal bulbar muscular atrophy and amyotrophic lateral sclerosis. *Muscle Nerve*. 2009;40:126–129.
99. Daoud H, Valdamanis PN, Gros-Louis F, et al. Resequencing of 29 candidate genes in patients with familial and sporadic amyotrophic lateral sclerosis. *Arch Neurol*. 2011;68(5):587–593.
100. Andersen PM, Borasio GD, Dengler R, et al. EFNS task force on management of amyotrophic lateral sclerosis: guidelines for diagnosis and clinical care of patients and relatives. *Eur J Neurol*. 2005;12:921–938.
101. Russell JA, Power B. Genetic testing in apparent sporadic ALS patients: surveyed opinions of the Northeastern ALS Consortium (NEALS) membership. Annual Meeting of the American Academy of Neurology. Honolulu, Hawaii, April 9–16, 2011.
102. Wagner KR. The need for biomarkers in amyotrophic lateral sclerosis drug development. *Neurology*. 2009;72:11–12.
103. Mitchell RM, Freeman WM, Randazzo WT, et al. A CSF biomarker panel for identification of patients with amyotrophic lateral sclerosis. *Neurology*. 2009;72:14–19.
104. Cudkowicz M, Swash M. CSF markers in amyotrophic lateral sclerosis: has the time come? *Neurology*. 2010;74:949–950.
105. Turner MR, Kiernan MC, Leigh PN, Talbot K. Biomarkers in amyotrophic lateral sclerosis. *Lancet Neurol*. 2009;8:94–109.
106. Bowser R, Lacomis D. Applying proteomics to the diagnosis and treatment of ALS and related diseases. *Muscle Nerve*. 2009;40:753–762.
107. Mackenzie IRA, Rademakers R, Neumann M. TDP-43 and FUS in amyotrophic lateral sclerosis and frontotemporal dementia. *Lancet Neurol*. 2010;9:995–1007.
108. Hodges JR, Davies RR, Xuereb JH, et al. Clinicopathological correlates and frontotemporal dementia. *Ann Neurol*. 2004:56(3):399–406.
109. Daoud H, Rouleau GA. A role for ubiquilin2 mutations in neurodegeneration. *Nat Rev Neurol*. 2011;7:599–600.
110. Del Bo R, Tiloca C, Pensato V, et al. Novel optineurin mutations in patients with familial and sporadic amyotrophic lateral sclerosis. *J Neurol Neurosurg Psychiatry*. 2011;82:1239–1243.
111. Arai T, Hasegawa M, Akiyama H, et al. TDP-43 is a component of ubiquitin-positive tau-negative inclusions in frontotemporal lobar degeneration and amyotrophic lateral sclerosis. *Biochem Biophys Res Commun*. 2006;351:602–611.
112. Geser F, Stein B, Partain M, et al. Motor neuron disease clinically limited to the lower motor neuron is a diffuse TDP-43 proteinopathy. *Acta Neuropathol*. 2011;121:509–517.
113. Kobayashi Z, Tsuchiya K, Arai T, et al. Clinicopathological characteristics of FTLD-TDP showing corticospinal tract degeneration but lacking lower motor neuron loss. *J Neurol Sci*. 2010;298:70–77.
114. Mizuno Y, Fujita Y, Takatama M, Okamoto K. Peripherin partially localizes in Bunina bodies in amyotrophic lateral sclerosis. *J Neurol Sci*. 2011;302:14–18.
115. Mori F, Tanji K, Miki Y, Kakita A, Takahashi H, Wakabayashi K. Relationship between Bunina bodies and TDP-43 inclusions in spinal anterior horn in amyotrophic lateral sclerosis. *Neuropathol Appl Neurobiol*. 2010;36:345–352.
116. Rothstein JR. Current hypotheses for the underlying biology of amyotrophic lateral sclerosis. *Ann Neurol*. 2009;65(suppl):S3–S9.
117. Ravits JM, LaSpada AR. ALS motor phenotype heterogeneity, focality, and spread: deconstructing motor neuron degeneration. *Neurology*. 2009;73:805–811.
118. Kuwabara S, Yokota T. Propagation: prion-like mechanisms can explain spreading of motor neuronal death in amyotrophic lateral sclerosis? *J Neurol Neurosurg Psychiatry*. 2011;82(11):1181–1182.
119. Fujimura-Kiyono C, Kimura F, Ishida S, et al. Onset and spreading patterns of lower motor neuron involvements predict survival in sporadic amyotrophic lateral sclerosis. *J Neurol Neurosurg Psychiatry*. 2011;82(11):1244–1249.
120. Siddique T, Figlewicz DA, Pericak-Vance MA, et al. Linkage of a gene causing familial amyotrophic lateral sclerosis to chromosome 21 and evidence of genetic-locus heterogeneity. *N Engl J Med*. 1991;324:1381–1384.
121. http://alsod.iop.kcl.ac.uk/

122. Van Damme P, Veldink JH, van Blitterswijk M, et al. Expanded ATXN2 CAG repeat size in ALS identifies genetic overlap between ALS and SCA2. *Neurology*. 2011;76:2066–2072.
123. Fischbeck KH, Pulst SM. Amyotrophic lateral sclerosis and spinocerebellar ataxia 2. *Neurology*. 2011;76:2050–2051.
124. Daoud H, Belzil V, Martins S, et al. Association of long ATXN2 CAG repeat sizes with increased risk of amyotrophic lateral sclerosis. *Arch Neurol*. 2011;68(6):739–742.
125. Maruyama H, Morino H, Ito H, et al. Mutations of optineurin in amyotrophic lateral sclerosis. *Nature*. 2010;465:223–227.
126. Valdmanis PN, Rouleau GA. Genetics of familial amyotrophic lateral sclerosis. *Neurology*. 2008;70:144–152.
127. Pasinelli P, Brown RH. Molecular biology of amyotrophic lateral sclerosis: insights from genetics. *Nat Genet*. 2006;7:710–723.
128. Shaw CE, Al-Chalabi A. Susceptibility genes in sporadic ALS: separating the wheat from the chaff by international collaboration. *Neurology*. 2006;67:738–739.
129. Neumann M, Kwong LK, Sampathu DM, Trojanowski JQ, Lee VM. TDP 43 proteinopathy in frontotemporal lobar degeneration and amyotrophic lateral sclerosis: protein misfolding diseases without amyloidosis. *Arch Neurol*. 2007;64(10):1388–1394.
130. Okamoto Y, Ihara M, Urushitani M, et al. An autopsy case of SOD-1 related ALS with TDP-43 positive inclusions. *Neurology*. 2011;77:1993–1995.
131. Burati E. TDP-43 and FUS in ALS/FTLD: will common pathways fit all? *Neurology*. 2011;77:1588–1589.
132. Rowland LP. Diagnosis of amyotrophic lateral sclerosis. *J Neurol Sci*. 1998;160(suppl 1):S6–S24.
133. Traynor BJ, Codd MB, Corr B, Forde C, Frost E, Hardiman O. Amyotrophic lateral sclerosis mimic syndromes: a population-based study. *Arch Neurol*. 2000;57:109–113.
134. Visser J, van den Berg-Vos RM, Franssen H, et al. Mimic syndromes in sporadic cases of progressive spinal muscular atrophy. *Neurology*. 2002;58:1593–1596.
135. Van den Berg-Vos RM, van den Berg LH, Visser J, de Visser M, Franssen H, Wokke JH. The spectrum of lower motor neuron syndromes. *J Neurol*. 2003;250:1279–1292.
136. Van den Berg-Vos RM, Visser J, Kalmihn S, et al. A long-term prospective study of the natural course of sporadic adult-onset lower motor neuron syndromes. *Arch Neurol*. 2009;66(6):751–757.
137. Nobile-Orazio E, Cappellari A, Priori A. Multifocal motor neuropathy: current concepts and controversies. *Muscle Nerve*. 2005;31:663–680.
138. Cats EA, Jacobs BC, Yuki N, et al. Multifocal motor neuropathy: association of anti-GM1 IgM antibodies with clinical features. *Neurology*. 2010;75:1961–1967.
139. Gooch CL, Amato AA. Are anti-ganglioside antibodies of clinical value in multifocal motor neuropathy? *Neurology*. 2010;75:1950–1951.
140. Finsterer J. Perspectives of Kennedy disease. *J Neurol Sci*. 2010;198:1–10.
141. Rhodes LE, Freeman BK, Auh S, et al. Clinical features of spinal and bulbar muscular atrophy. *Brain*. 2009;132:3242–3251.
142. Kennedy WR, Alter M, Sung JH. Proximal bulbar and spinal muscular atrophy of late onset. A sex-linked recessive trait. *Neurology*. 1968;18(7):671–680.
143. Parboosingh JS, Figlewicz DA, Krizus A, et al. Spinobulbar muscular atrophy can mimic ALS: the importance of genetic testing in male patients with atypical ALS. *Neurology*. 1997;49:568–572.
144. Sobue I, Saito N, Iida M, Ando K. Juvenile type of distal and segmental muscular atrophy of upper extremities. *Ann Neurol*. 1978;3:429–432.
145. Hirayama K, Tohocura Y, Tsubaki T. Juvenile muscular atrophy of unilateral extremity: a new clinical entity. *Psychiatry Neurol Jpn*. 1959;61:2190–2197.
146. Pradhan S. Bilaterally symmetric form of Hirayama disease. *Neurology*. 2009;72:2083–2089.
147. Patel DR, Knepper L, Jones HR Jr. Late-onset monomelic amyotrophy in a Caucasian woman. *Muscle Nerve*. 2008;37(1):115–119.
148. Felice KJ, Whitaker CH, Grunnet ML. Benign calf amyotrophy. *Arch Neurol*. 2003;60:1415–1420.
149. Irobi J, De Jonghe P, Timmerman V. Molecular genetics of distal hereditary motor neuropathies. *Human Mol Genet*. 2004;13:R195–R202.
150. Rossor AM, Kalmar B, Greensmith L, Reilly MM. The distal hereditary motor neuropathies. *J Neurol Neurosurg Psychiatry*. 2012;83:6–14.
151. Ésik O, Vönöczky K, Lengyel Z, Sáfrány G, Trón L. Characteristics of radiogenic lower motor neuron disease, a possible link with a possible viral infection. *Spinal Cord*. 2004;42(2):99–105.
152. Fink JF. Hereditary spastic paraplegia. *Curr Neurol Neurosci Rep*. 2006;6:65–76.
153. Meyer T, Schwan A, Dullinger JS, et al. Early-onset ALS with long-term survival associated with spastin gene mutation. *Neurology*. 2005;65:141–143.
154. Mathews JA. Wasting of the small hand muscles in upper- and mid-cervical cord lesions. *QJM*. 1998;91:691–700.
155. Stark AJ, Kennard C, Swash MA. Hand wasting in spondylotic high cord compression: an electromyographic study. *Ann Neurol*. 1981;9(1):58–62.
156. Srinivasan J, Scala S, Jones HR, Saleh F, Russell JA. Inappropriate surgeries resulting from misdiagnosis of early amyotrophic lateral sclerosis. *Muscle Nerve*. 2006;34(3):359–360.
157. Weihl CC, Lopate G. Motor neuron disease associated with copper deficiency. *Muscle Nerve*. 2006;34:789–793.
158. Quereshi M, Bedlack RS, Cudkowicz ME. Lyme serology in amyotrophic lateral sclerosis. *Muscle Nerve*. 2009;40:626–628.
159. Henning F, Hewlett RH. Brachial amyotrophic diplegia (segmental proximal spinal muscular atrophy) associated with HIV infection. *J Neurol Neurosurg Psychiatry*. 2008;79:1392–1394.
160. Verma A, Berger JR. ALS syndrome in patients with HIV-1 infection. *J Neurol Sci*. 2006;240:59–64.
161. Drory VE, Birnbaum M, Peleg L, Goldman B, Korczyn AD. Hexosaminidase A deficiency is an uncommon cause of a syndrome mimicking amyotrophic lateral sclerosis. *Muscle Nerve*. 2003;28:109–112.
162. Jackson CE, Amato AA, Bryan WW, Wolfe GI, Sakhaee K, Barohn RJ. Primary hyperparathyroidism in ALS: is there are relation? *Neurology*. 1998;50:1795–1799.
163. Stitch O, Kleer B, Rauer S. Absence of paraneoplastic antineuronal antibodies in sera of 145 patients with motor neuron disease. *J Neurol Neurosurg Psychiatry*. 2007;78:883–885.
164. Moulignier A, Moulonguet A, Pialoux G, Rozenbaum W. Reversible ALS-like disorder in HIV infection. *Neurology*. 2001;57:1995–2001.
165. Johnson WG. The clinical spectrum of hexosaminidase deficiency diseases. *Neurology*. 1981;31:1453–1456.
166. Younger DS. Motor neuron disease or malignancy. *Muscle Nerve*. 2000;23(5):658–660.

167. Gordon PH, Rowland LP, Younger DS, et al. Lymphoproliferative disorders and motor neuron disease: an update. *Neurology*. 1997;48:1671–1678.
168. Verma A, Berger JR. Primary lateral sclerosis with HIV-1 infection. *Neurology*. 2008;70(7):575–577.
169. Atkinson JL, Miller GM, Krauss WF, et al. Clinical and radiographic features of dural arteriovenous fistula, a treatable cause of myelopathy. *Mayo Clin Proc*. 2001;76:1120–1130.
170. Armon C, Daube JR. Electrophysiological signs of arteriovenous malformations of the spinal cord. *J Neurol Neurosurg Psychiatry*. 1989;52:1176–1181.
171. www.alsuntangled.com
172. https://www.clinicaltrials.gov/ct2/results?term=als&Search=Search
173. http://www.alsconsortium.org/search.ph
174. Kimura F, Fujimura C, Ishida H, et al. Progression rate of ALSFRS-R at time of diagnosis predict survival time in ALS. *Neurology*. 2006;66:265–267.
175. Gordon PH, Cheung YK. Progression rate of ALSFRS-R at time of diagnosis predict survival time in ALS. *Neurology*. 2006;67:1314–1315.
176. Miller RG, Jackson CE, Karsarskis EJ, et al. Practice Parameter update: the care of the patient with amyotrophic lateral sclerosis: drug, nutritional, and respiratory therapies (an evidence-based review): report of the Quality Standards Subcommittee of the American Academy of Neurology. *Neurology*. 2009;73:1218–1226.
177. Miller RG, Jackson CE, Karsarskis EJ, et al. Practice parameter update: the care of the patient with amyotrophic lateral sclerosis: multidisciplinary care, symptom management, and cognitive/behavioral impairment (an evidence-based review): report of the Quality Standards Subcommittee of the American Academy of Neurology. *Neurology*. 2009;73:1227–1233.
178. Simmons Z. Management strategies for patients with amyotrophic lateral sclerosis from diagnosis through death. *Neurologist*. 2005;11:257–270.
179. Dal Bello-Haas V, Florence JM, Kloos D, et al. A randomized controlled trial of resistance exercise in individuals with ALS. *Neurology*. 2007;68:2003–2007.

CHAPTER 7

Hereditary Spastic Paraparesis

The diagnosis of hereditary spastic paraparesis (HSP) is based on the identification of a phenotype characterized as a slowly progressive, symmetric, spastic paraparesis in which the morbidity is largely related to impaired leg control rather than weakness, with or without recognition of other family members. The prevalence of dominantly inherited HSP, at least in Ireland, is estimated at $1.27/10^5$.[1] Like many of the disorders discussed in this text, the nosology of HSP is confounded by insights generated by molecular biology. The HSP phenotype is now recognized to result from mutations involving at least 50 different genetic loci and 18 identified genes (Table 7-1).[2] Despite the potential precision that a classification system based solely on gene location and gene product would provide, it remains an impractical bedside tool. Due to current limitations of genetic testing, a pragmatic classification system requires at least some consideration of clinical features. This chapter will attempt to provide a classification hybrid that addresses both clinical and genetic considerations (Table 7-1).

The concept of a hereditary disorder manifesting as spasticity of the lower extremities was initially championed by Seeligmüller, Strumpell, and Lorrain in the last quarter of the 19th century. It was envisioned as a singular entity with phenotypic variation.[3] The classification system still utilized today was initially promoted by Anita Harding in 1981.[4] She proposed a dominantly inherited HSP dichotomy in which type I was considered to reflect an early-onset phenotype with predominant, if not exclusive, upper motor neuron (UMN) features. In contrast, type II HSP referred to those with late onset in which weakness and presumed lower motor neuron (LMN) involvement overshadowed the UMN signs. In 1983, her classification system was expanded to encompass complicated as well as uncomplicated forms of the syndrome.[5] Uncomplicated HSP still refers to a syndrome of spastic paraparesis in which cavus foot deformities and mild vibratory sense loss may occur as the only other associated features. Complicated HSP is defined by involvement of additional neurological and occasionally nonneurological systems as described below (Table 7-1).

In 1996, the nosology of HSP became at the same time both enhanced and complicated with discovery of the first disease producing mutation.[3] The HSPs are currently genotypically catalogued by a numerical system based on the order of individual gene discovery. Each number is prefaced by the acronym SPG which stands for spastic paraplegia gene (Table 7-1). Unlike other classification systems, subheadings distinguishing dominant from other inheritance patterns are not utilized.

▶ CLINICAL FEATURES

In virtually every case, the presenting symptoms relate to lower extremity spasticity which has a symmetric or near symmetric distribution. Symptom onset is typically recognized in the second or third decade but may become manifest as early as the first or as late as the seventh decade of life. Patients lose the ability to run or hop early in their course due to increased extensor tone in the lower extremities. Consequently the ability to fully flex the hip and the knee is impaired resulting in reduced stride length and difficulty running. Patients will describe dragging and stiffness of the legs and a tendency to trip on uneven ground. When observed, the legs may be noted to scissor or cross over each other due to increased adductor tone (Fig. 7-1). Circumduction (a rotational rather than linear advancement of the legs) is common in a compensatory attempt to avoid tripping. This risk results from a leg that is tonically extended at the hip and knee and from a tonic foot posture of inversion and plantar flexion (equinovarus posture). High-arched feet and hammer toe deformity are common but not invariable features of the illness. They are more likely to occur with disease onset in childhood at a time when the metatarsals remain malleable and vulnerable to the imbalance of forces produced by disproportionate involvement of specific muscle groups (Fig. 7-2).

HSP morbidity results in large part from the increased lower extremity extensor tone impairing lower extremity coordination. Lower motor neuron involvement may occur but is typically overshadowed by spasticity. If weakness occurs, it typically does so in a UMN pattern, with hip flexors, knee flexors, and foot dorsiflexors being typically weaker than their respective antagonists. Hyperreflexia of the lower extremities is universal, almost always accompanied by extensor plantar responses. Hyperreflexia of the upper extremities with Hoffman's signs and reflex spread is common as well. Significant loss of upper extremity function associated with weakness, increased tone, or impaired coordination occurs infrequently in most genotypes and should lead to consideration of an alternative diagnosis.

Mild posterior column involvement may occur with vibratory sense loss and occasionally position sense loss in the toes. Rarely is it severe enough to produce significant sensory ataxia. A strikingly positive Romberg sign should once again lead to consideration of an alternative diagnosis.

▶ **TABLE 7-1. HEREDITARY SPASTIC PARAPARESIS** [2,3]

Name	Locus/Gene	Inheritance	Type	Associated Features	Testing
SPG3A	14q11–q21/alastin	AD	U	Usual childhood onset minimal progression mimicking CP +/− distal amyotrophy	Available
SPG4	2p22 Spastin	AD	U/C	Onset any age 40% of AD cases +/− late cognitive, ataxia, seizures, LMN	Available
SPG6	15q11.1 NIPA1	AD	U	Late adolescent—early adult onset	Available
SPG8	8q23–q24 Strumpellin	AD	U	Typical	Available
SPG9	10q23.3–q24.2	AD	C	Cataracts, GERD, motor neuronopathy	None
SPG10	12q13/kinesin heavy chain	AD	U/C	+/− distal muscle atrophy	Available
SPG12	19q13	AD	U	Typical	None
SPG13	2q24–q34 Chaperonin 60	AD	U	Late adolescent—early adult	Research
SPG17	11q12–q14 BSCL2/seipin	AD	C	Silver syndrome amyotrophy of hands	Available
SPG19	9q33–q34	AD	U	Typical	Research
SPG29	1p31.1–p21.1	AD	C	Hearing loss Hiatal hernia Intractable vomiting	None
SPG31	2p12 REEP1	AD	U/C	+/− peripheral neuropathy	Available
SPG33	10q24.2/ZFYVE2	AD	U	Typical	Available
SPG36	12q23–q24	AD	C	Onset 20–30 years Peripheral neuropathy	No
SPG37	8p21.1–q13.3	AD	U	Typical	No
SPG38	4p16–p15	AD	C	Amyotrophy of hands	No
SPG40	unknown	AD	U	Adult onset	No
SPG41	11p14.1–p11.2	AD	C	Amyotrophy of hands	No
SPG42	3q24–q26/acetyl CoA transporter	AD	U	Onset decade 1–5	No
SPG5A	8p/CYPB1	AR	U/C	Axonal neuropathy Distal amyotrophy White matter changes	Available
SPG7	16q/paraplegin	AR	U/C	Ragged red fibers, dysarthria, dysphagia, optic atrophy, axonal neuropathy, cerebral and cerebellar atrophy	Available
SPG11	15q/spatacsin	AR	U/C	Juvenile onset, thin corpus callosum, MR, RPD Upper extremity weakness, nystagmus, dysarthria, dementia, distal amyotrophy 50% of AR cases	Available
SPG14	3q27–28	AR	C	Distal amyotrophy, MR	No
SPG15	14q/spastizin	AR	C	Pigmentary maculopathy, distal amyotrophy, dysarthria, MR	Commercial
SPG18	8p12–p11.21	AR	C	MR, thin corpus callosum	No
SPG20	13q/spastin	AR	C	"Troyer syndrome," distal amyotrophy	Available
SPG21	15q21–q22/maspardin	AR	C	Dementia, cerebellar and extrapyramidal signs, thin corpus callosum, white matter abnormalities, "Mast syndrome"	Research
SPG23	1q24–q32	AR	C	Vitiligo, premature graying, characteristic facies, "Lison syndrome"	No
SPG24	13q14	AR	C	Spastic dysarthria, pseudobulbar	No
SPG25	6q23–q21.4	AR	C	Peripheral neuropathy	No
SPG26	12p11.1–12q14	AR	C	Onset childhood, dysarthria, distal amyotrophy, mild MR	No
SPG27	10q22.1–q24.1	AR	U/C	Ataxia, dysarthria, MR, peripheral neuropathy, facial dysmorphism, short stature	No

▶ TABLE 7-1. **(CONTINUED)**

Name	Locus/Gene	Inheritance	Type	Associated Features	Testing
SPG28	14q21.3–q22.3	AR	U	Childhood onset	No
SPG29	14q	AR	U	Childhood onset	No
SPG30	2q37.3	AR	C	Distal amyotrophy, saccadic pursuit, peripheral neuropathy, cerebellar signs	No
SPG32	14q12–q21	AR	C	Mild MR, cerebellar atrophy, brainstem dysraphia	No
SPG35	16q21–q23/fatty acid 2 hydroxylase	AR	C	Childhood onset, extrapyramidal, dysarthria, dementia, seizures, white matter changes, brain iron deposition	Research
SPG39	19p13	AR	C	Distal amyotrophy	Research
SPG43	19p13.11–q12	AR	C	Hand wasting, dysarthria	No
SPG44	1q41/gap junction protein connexin 47	AR	C	Pelizaeus-Merzbacher, nystagmus, psychomotor delay, ataxia, dysarthria, CNS hypomyelination	No
SPG45	10q24.3–q25.1	AR	C	MR, contractures, optic atrophy, pendular nystagmus	No
SPG46	9p21.2–q21.12	AR	C	Dementia, cataract, ataxia thin corpus callosum	No
SPG47	1p13.2–1p12	AR	C	MR, seizures, thin corpus callosum, white matter changes	No
SPG48	7p22.1	AR	U	Late onset	Research
SPOAN syndrome	11q23	AR	C	Optic atrophy, peripheral neuropathy	No
None	5p15.31–14.1/chaperonin containing t-complex peptide 1	AR	C	Mutilating sensory neuropathy	Research
SPG1	Xq28 L1CAM	XL	C	Hydrocephalus, mental retardation, aphasia, adducted thumbs	Available
SPG2	Xq28	XL	C	White matter changes, peripheral neuropathy	Available
SPG16	Xq11.2–q23	XL	U/C	Aphasia, visual loss, mental retardation, nystagmus, GU dysfunction	No
SPG22	Xq21	XL	C	Mental retardation, ataxia, dysarthria, abnormal facies	Research
SPG34	Xq24-q25/unknown	XL	U	Typical	No
SPG	unknown	MT	C	Peripheral neuropathy, cardiomyopathy, dementia	Research

U, uncomplicated; C, complicated; CP, cerebral palsy; REEP1, receptor expression enhancing protein 1; XL, X-linked; MT, mitochondrial; RPD, retinal pigmentary degeneration; MR, mental retardation; LMN, lower motor neuron.

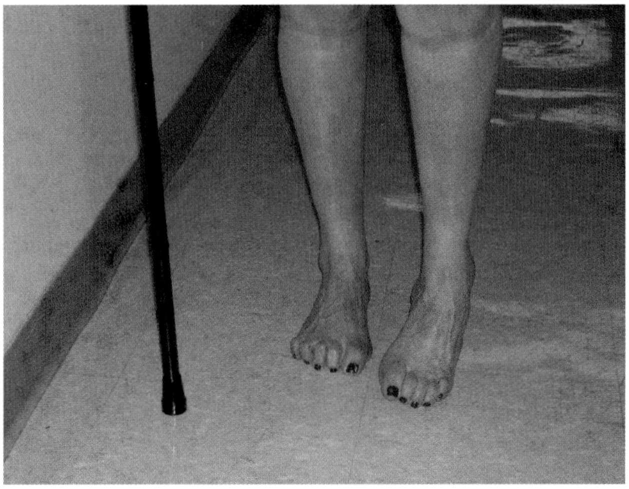

Figure 7-1. Circumducting leg with equinovarus foot posturing in HSP.

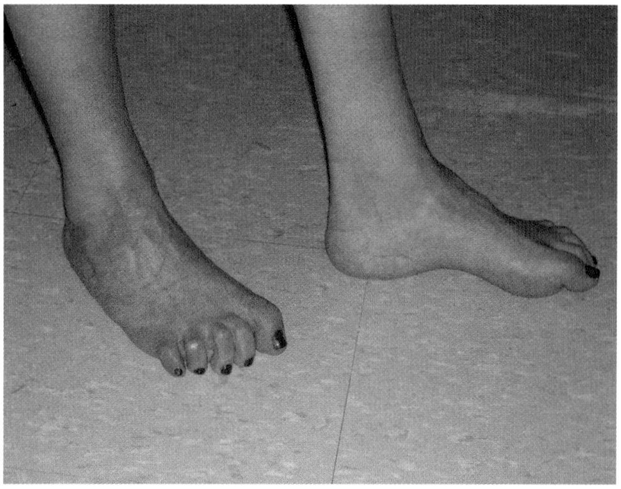

Figure 7-2. Hammer toes and cavus deformity in HSP.

Urinary frequency, urgency, and urgency incontinence are common symptoms even in uncomplicated disease. Rectal urgency and incontinence and sexual dysfunction are uncommon.

There is a wide range of associated neurological and non-neurological symptoms that can occur in complicated forms of the disease. Recognition of these additional features may aid in the identification of a specific genotype (Table 7-1). Some of the more common associated features are amyotrophy of distal limb muscles that may result from either a motor neuronopathy (SPG3A, 4, 5, 9, 10, 11, 14, 15, 17, 20, 26, 30, 38, 39, 43, 41) or peripheral neuropathy (SPG2, 5, 25, 27, 30, 31, 36, the SPOAN syndrome, and the one recognized mitochondrial mutation producing a SPG phenotype).[2,6] Distal amyotrophy may initially affect either the hands or feet, hand-wasting and spastic paraparesis being referred to as Silver syndrome.[7,8] Ataxia, nystagmus, dysarthria, and other features of cerebellar dysfunction occur less frequently (SPG21). Extrapyramidal manifestations are relatively uncommon as well (SPG21, 35).[2,6,9,10] Cognitive changes may manifest as either mental retardation or dementia (SPG4, 11, 14, 15, 18, 21, 26, 27, 32, 35, 44, 45, 46, 47). A thin corpus callosum is a relatively common feature (SPG11, 18, 21, 35, 46, 47).[2,6,10,11] Seizures, deafness, cataracts, ichthyosis, ophthalmoparesis, ocular apraxia, retinal pigmentary degeneration, and optic atrophy with visual loss are some of the other potential associated features.[2,6,12]

A uniform age of symptom onset and rate of disease progression are characteristic of uncomplicated HSP genotypes but exceptions to this general rule are not uncommon. The reasons for variations of disease onset and severity of affliction, both within and between families of the same genotype are not understood.[13] This variability does not appear to correlate directly with the mechanism of mutation, at least within the SPG4 genotype.[14] For the most part, individual families will remain segregated into either uncomplicated or complicated phenotypes but occasional families will have members with both.

▶ DIFFERENTIAL DIAGNOSIS

The differential diagnosis of HSP includes any disorder that results in UMN dysfunction of the lower extremities (Table 7-2). In our opinion, the disorder that is most likely to mimic HSP is PLS or UMN dominant ALS, either on a sporadic or inherited basis.[15–18] Slow progression, symmetry, cavus foot deformity, and loss of vibration perception in the toes favors a HSP diagnosis although these clues are relative and clinical distinction may be difficult in many cases.[19] Rapid progression, notable asymmetry, or impaired upper extremity or bulbar function would favor a PLS/UMN-D ALS diagnosis. The family history needs to be interpreted with caution as ALS like HSP may be hereditary, and as absence of other affected family members by no means precludes heritable disease.[18] The difficulty in distinguishing between HSP and ALS was recently emphasized to us in the case of a woman in her mid-30s with 20 years of seemingly sporadic, slowly progressive, spastic paraparesis, and cavus foot deformity suggesting HSP in whom a pathological mutation in a familial ALS gene (senataxin) was identified in both her and her asymptomatic father.

The differential diagnosis of HSP includes another category of heritable neuromuscular disease, distal spinal muscular atrophy/hereditary motor neuropathy. The latter, although dominated by LMN features, may include UMN features as well providing phenotypic and at times genotypic overlap between these two disease categories (Table 8-1).

Most metabolic or structural myelopathies affect sensory pathways more than HSP typically does. None-the-less, the differential diagnosis of HSP includes metabolic and structural disorders in which sensory signs or symptoms are limited. In consideration of its chronicity and frequency, cervical spondylotic myelopathy is a common differential diagnostic consideration. As emphasized in Chapter 6, we urge caution in attributing spastic paraparesis to cervical canal stenosis in the absence of significant spinal cord compression or abnormal cord signal at the level of compression.

▶ **TABLE 7-2. DIFFERENTIAL DIAGNOSIS OF HSP: TESTING CONSIDERATIONS**

Disease	Test(s)
ALS/PLS	EMG Genetic testing
Compressive myelopathy	Imaging (MR, myelographic) thoracic, cervical spine
Dural venous malformation	MR imaging, angiography, cervical, thoracic spine
Multiple sclerosis	MRI imaging brain, cervical, thoracic spine, CSF evaluation
Neuromyelitis optica	Aquaphorin autoantibodies
Retroviral infection	HIV and HTLV1 serology
Sarcoidosis	CSF evaluation Chest imaging Gallium scan
Metabolic myelopathy	Vitamin B12 Copper and ceruloplasmin
Adrenoleukodystrophy	C26–C22 long chain fatty acid ratio
Spinocerebellar degeneration	Genetic testing
Dopa-responsive dystonia	Response to l-dopa

Other myelopathic considerations in which imaging may be abnormal include dural venous fistulas, spinal forms of multiple sclerosis, and other inflammatory disorders including such as acute disseminated encephalomyelitis, neuromyelitis optica, HIV or HTLV1 inflection, and sarcoidosis. The chronological course in these latter disorders would characteristically progress at a different and usually faster pace than HSP.

Adrenoleukodystrophy and adrenomyeloneuropathy are X-linked disorders that require consideration in young men and young adult woman. Arguably, the latter cohort provides the greatest difficultly as adrenoleukodystrophy frequently presents as a slowly progressive spastic paraparesis in young adult women. Young males typically have a more severe and multisystem phenotype producing varying combinations of adrenal insufficiency, myelopathy, neuropathy, and cognitive decline. Other leukodystrophies may be considered in the differential diagnosis of complicated forms of the disease.

Vitamin B12 and copper deficiency may affect pyramidal tracts although tend to manifest primarily as posterior column myelopathies with predominant sensory loss. Other inherited disorders with prominent myelopathic features include Friedreich ataxia and spinocerebellar ataxia type III (Machado–Joseph disease). Both are more typically clinically dominated by posterior column and/spinocerebellar ataxia respectively rather than by spasticity.

Cerebral palsy is a differential diagnostic consideration in early-onset cases of HSP. This is particularly true for SPG3A associated with mutations of the atlastin gene.[20,21] Dopa-responsive dystonia may manifest itself as a progressive, spastic gait disorder of childhood. Low-dose therapy with levodopa would serve both a diagnostic and a therapeutic purpose in this disorder.

▶ LABORATORY FEATURES

Genetic testing in suspected HSP patients is emblematic of the practical problems that exist with genetic testing in general. Of more than 50 suspected recognized gene loci, 25 genes have been identified, with commercially available testing available for 14.[2,6,22,23] Of these, 19 are inherited in a dominant fashion, 27 recessively, with 5 that are X-linked and one associated with a mitochondrial genome mutation. Negative genetic testing excludes neither HSP in general or in some cases, the genotype that is being tested for. Commercially utilized methodologies may not detect certain mutational mechanisms, thus providing the opportunity for a false-negative test. For example, partial deletions of the SPAST gene (SPG4 locus) may not be detected by some commercial laboratories.[24]

Genetic testing in HSP has the highest yield in genotypes with dominantly inherited mutation patterns. Approximately 75% of patients with dominant inheritance patterns can be currently genotyped. These are the patients however, in which a confident clinical diagnosis is the easiest to establish. Facilitating genetic analysis is the knowledge that 60% of dominantly inherited cases are attributable to four HSP types, SPG3A, 4, 6, and 31. In view of the cost considerations, we would favor initial testing for the latter three genes in suspected dominant, adult-onset cases, if genetic testing is to be performed at all. As the SPG3A (atlastin) mutation frequently manifests in childhood, we would initially avoid this test in adults as well as other infrequently occurring HSP mutations.[21]

The primary problem related to genetic testing occurs in apparent sporadic or recessive cases, those in which a diagnosis of HSP is the most difficult to establish clinically. Somewhere between a quarter and a half of cases with recessive inheritance patterns may be currently genotyped.[2] SPG11 is thought to be responsible for approximately 50% of recessively inherited cases.[2] In our opinion, this should be the first gene tested in any recessive or sporadic case with a thin corpus callosum if genotyping is performed. SPG7 is thought to be the second most common AR genotype representing ≤6% of these cases.[25,26]

It is important that the clinician be aware of additional nuances of HSP genetic testing. It is estimated that approximately 10–20% of apparent sporadic cases will be found to have a gene mutation more typically associated with either a dominant or recessive inheritance pattern with SPG4 and 7 being the most commonly recognized examples of this.[17,25] Incomplete penetrance does occur in HSP, providing at least one reason for the aforementioned observation. Although anticipation is not a well-described phenomenon in HSP, particularly in uncomplicated forms, it has been reported to occur in SPG4.[6]

We strongly support the conceptual value of diagnostic confirmation of potential heritable diseases if detailed pedigree analysis is nondiagnostic. We recognize however, both the technical and financial limitations that influence routine genetic testing. This includes consideration that commercially available genetic testing is typically expensive and is commonly inadequately reimbursed by third party payers. This may create a financial burden to either the patient or the healthcare system. In view of this, and in consideration that the natural history of the disease is unlikely to be favorably altered by the knowledge of genotype, we do not routinely obtain genetic testing in HSP suspects. This practice will undoubtedly change as whole exome sequencing and the ability to distinguish benign polymorphisms from pathogenic mutations evolves.

If genotypic confirmation of the HSP diagnosis cannot be accomplished, other diagnostic testing such as imaging may be undertaken in an attempt to address other differential diagnostic considerations. Tests that may be considered are summarized in Table 7-2. Imaging in HSP is typically normal in uncomplicated cases, although atrophy of the thoracic spinal cord has been reported.[3] MR imaging of the brain may identify some of the features associated with complicated forms of HSP, including atrophy of the corpus callosum, hydrocephalus, or white matter changes. This would be of more value in identifying the type of HSP rather than establishing the initial diagnosis.

▶ HISTOPATHOLOGY

HSP appears to be a "dying back myelopathy." Affected individuals will have degeneration of both the crossed and uncrossed corticospinal tracts, most notable in the lumbosacral and thoracic segments of the spinal cord. This degeneration becomes less apparent in the cervical regions. Conversely, degeneration of the posterior columns is most evident in the fasciculus gracilis in their most centrifugal locations, that is, at the cervical–medullary junction.[3] Spinocerebellar pathways are involved in some cases to a far lesser extent. Decreased numbers of anterior horn cells and/or cortical motor neurons have been reported.

In a manner similar to the clinical overlap described above, certain HSP genotypes may have TDP-43 positive inclusions, a marker more typically associated with ALS.[27]

▶ PATHOGENESIS

The multiple HSP genotypes suggest that there is a final common pathway by which mutations of different proteins coalesce into an identical or near-identical phenotype. Although the functions of certain HSP-related proteins are understood, the means by which they induce a fairly uniform phenotype remains unknown.[2,3,28] The function of spastin (SPG4) is related to microtubule dynamics. The kinesin 5A gene (SPG10) has a role in axonal transport. Three SPG genes, paraplegin, chaperonin 60, receptor expression enhancing protein 1, and mitochondrial ATPase 6 (SPG7, 13, 31) code for mitochondrial proteins. L1 cell adhesion molecule (SPG1) plays a role in corticospinal tract development. Mutations of the proteolipid protein and the gap junction protein gamma 2 genes (SPG2, 42) result in abnormalities of myelination. The morphology of the endoplasmic reticulum is altered in mutations of the atlastin, spastin and receptor expression enhancing protein 1 genes (SPG3A, 4, 31). Disturbances of membrane trafficking, protein accumulation, and endoplasmic reticulum stress response are associated with abnormalities of strumpellin and seipin gene function (SPG8, 17).

A recurrent theme throughout this text is the increasing recognition that neuromuscular disorders historically classified as different diseases are allelic. Although this phenomenon is not as prevalent as in spinal muscular atrophy, it is relevant to HSP as well (Table 8-1). SPG3A and hereditary sensory neuropathy type I result from mutations in the atlastin gene.[28] SPG17 is allelic with both hereditary motor neuropathy type V and Charcot–Marie–Tooth disease type II.[6]

▶ MANAGEMENT

HSP management is supportive. The goal is to maintain comfort and to the extent possible, safe and independent patient mobility. There are a number of different interventions that attempt to reduce spasticity including oral tizanidine, lioresal, dantrolene, or benzodiazepines, intrathecal baclofen, or the intramuscular injection of botulinum toxin (Table 7-3). In extreme cases, surgical release of tendons may be considered in nonambulatory patients to facilitate hygiene or improve patient comfort. The treatment of spasticity requires considerable clinical judgment. The aforementioned agents rarely produce the optimally desired beneficial effect and may create unwanted side effects. Improved ambulation, comfort, and range of motion are the desired effects. Sedation, confusion, and unmasking underlying muscle weakness that may actually add to fall risk and detract from safe mobility are to be avoided. Although spasticity hinders gait, it may also paradoxically reduce fall risk. In an individual who also has considerable underlying weakness, the increased tone of extensor muscles may represent the major source of antigravity resistance. Suppression of this tone may deprive individuals of their ability to stand.

To improve tolerance, oral antispasticity drugs are typically initiated at very low doses and then titrated upward (Table 7-3). Baclofen and tizanidine are preferred as first-line agents by most. Rapid withdrawal of these agents may lead to unwanted CNS side effects, including confusion and psychosis. Dantrolene is used less frequently because of risks associated with hepatotoxicity. Benzodiazepines have less well-developed antispasticity properties and are frequently used as an adjunct rather than as a primary antispasticity treatment.

Intrathecal baclofen delivered by a programmable pump is an option if oral drugs do not provide the desired effect. The theoretical benefit is to deliver the drug directly to the afflicted end organ in small titratable doses in order to avoid the side effects commonly associated with the larger oral doses required. Intrathecal baclofen may allow certain patients who are spastic to remain ambulatory longer than their natural history would otherwise allow. A more realistic goal is to diminish refractory painful spasms or to diminish lower extremity tone to facilitate hygiene.

Injection of botulinum toxin into spastic muscles provides an alternative means to diminish muscle tone.[29] Although attractive in concept because of the ability to affect only selected muscles, identification of the best dose and obtaining reimbursement for the relatively large volumes often required provide significant obstacles to its use. Many payers limit reimbursement to 400 units per session, which may be inadequate to achieve the desired goals. The effect of botulinum toxin is greatest when the toxin is delivered in proximity to the motor point. Identification of the most severely affected muscles and delivery of the lowest effective doses are the two major principles used. Repeat injections are typically required at approximately 3-month intervals.

Urinary urgency from detrusor overactivity is a common source of morbidity in HSP patients. There are a number of pharmacological agents that may ameliorate but rarely resolve this problem. The antispasticity agents, baclofen and tizanidine, may provide some relief. The mechanism of action of baclofen is thought to be as a presynaptic agonist of GABA-B receptors that is thought to have an inhibitory effect on activity

▶ TABLE 7-3. **TREATMENT OPTIONS FOR SPASTICITY (LISTED IN APPROXIMATE ORDER OF USE)**

Drug	Initial Dose	Maximal Dose	Common or Significant Side Effects
Baclofen	5 mg po TID	20 mg po QID	Constipation, nausea, emesis, ↓ muscle tone, dizziness, headache, somnolence, coma, seizure, and abrupt withdrawal syndrome
Tizanidine	4 mg po daily	12 mg po TID	Hypotension, xerostomia, asthenia, dizziness, and sedation
Botulinum toxin type A	Varies with product—1 unit/kg	Total dose per treatment averages 250–400 units	↓ muscle tone and allergy
Benzodiazepines (e.g., diazepam)	2 mg po, IM or IV daily	15 mg po QID	Sedation, ataxia, hypotension, fatigue, respiratory depression, and withdrawal symptoms
Dantrolene	25 mg po daily	100 mg po QID	Lightheadedness, constipation, diarrhea, asthenia, headache, sedation, diplopia, visual, CHF and arrhythmia, myelosuppression, and hepatotoxicity
Intrathecal baclofen	50 μg test dose adults, 25 μg children, increase dose by 10–30%/day in adults, 5–15 μg in children titrated to response	2000 μg/day	Pump failure, catheter fracture, CNS infection, CSF leak with intracranial hypotension, and complications of baclofen
Rhizotomy	NA	NA	CSF leak with intracranial hypotension, excessive

CHF, congestive heart failure; CSF, cerebrospinal fluid; NA, not applicable; CNS, central nervous system.

of the descending bulbosacral tracts in the spinal cord. Tizanidine is an alpha adrenergic agent thought to produce presynaptic inhibition of motor neurons, potentially by reducing glutamate release, again at the spinal cord level. Typically however, the first-line treatments are muscarinic anticholinergic agents which counteract detrusor hyperreflexia mediated through parasympathetic nerve fibers traveling via the S2–4 roots and the pelvic nerve. Frequently used agents include oxybutynin, tolterodine, and trospium. Newer agents include darifenacin and solifenacin. Tricyclic antidepressants may also be utilized for their anticholinergic properties. Other, less frequently used therapies with uncertain benefit include botulinum toxin injections into the detrusor, intravesicular delivery of certain drugs including capsaicin, and S2–4 ventral root stimulation coupled with analogous dorsal rhizotomies.

Durable medical equipment and home modification can provide substantial benefit to individual patients. The reader is referred to Chapter 5 for more details. Ankle–foot orthoses are of great benefit to individual patients to prevent falls due to tripping. Ideally, they should be custom fitted to improve comfort, particularly in consideration of associated cavus foot deformities. A skilled physical therapist is an invaluable tool to decide whether a cane, Lofstran or Canadian crutches, a walker, or a wheelchair is the best solution for an individual patient. The Dashaway® walker is particularly helpful in these patients in that it diminishes the risk of falling backward more so than traditional walker designs. Power chairs and scooters may benefit some patients. Reimbursement may be problematic as payers typically require documentation that a patient is unable to propel themselves in a manual chair prior to authorization. Most HSP patients do not have this limitation. Patients who require forms of power mobility who also have trunk, upper extremity, or bulbar weakness are better served by a power chair because of the trunk support, ability to operate with a joystick control, and the ability to mount other equipment that may be beneficial to the patient. HSP patients are one group of patients where scooters, often preferred by the patient over power chairs, may be recommended.

Many patients resent the symbolism of durable medical equipment, viewing it as a "setback" and a constant reminder of their impaired condition. It may be effective to promote durable medical equipment to them as an opportunity. Specifically, it may allow them to maintain their independent mobility while minimizing the risk of falls and the potential of severe injury, the quickest and most likely threat to their independence. In patients who live in multiple-story dwellings who require access to more than one floor, stair lifts provide a safe and energy-sparing option. Patients motivated to perform daily stretching exercises claim to enjoy considerable benefit from doing so.

Like all chronic diseases, HSP patients may benefit from the resources provided by support organizations. Examples include:

- National Institute of Neurological Disorders and Stroke
- Hereditary Spastic Paraplegia Foundation, Inc., 209 Park Rd., Chelmsford MA 01824. (Phone: 703–495–9261; e-mail: community@sp-foundation.org; sp-foundation.org.)
- National Ataxia Foundation, 2600 Fernbrook Lane Suite 119, Minneapolis MN 55447. (Phone: 763–553–0020; fax: 763–553–0167, e-mail: naf@ataxia. org; www.ataxia.org.)

Genetic counseling in HSP is challenging. Although phenotypic homogeneity within families is the norm, exceptions do exist. Prenatal testing is available for certain HSP genotypes.[6] HSP does not typically reduce life expectancy, the penetrance of many HSP genotypes is quite variable, and anticipation in HSP is not recognized to be a significant issue. For these reasons, we find it difficult to recommend prenatal testing in view of the risk to the fetus associated with amniocentesis or chorionic villous sampling.

▶ SUMMARY

HSP is a heritable disorder in which >50 currently recognized gene loci correlate with a fairly homogeneous phenotypic syndrome dominated by spastic paraparesis. It is a disorder that offers the opportunity to understand how semi-selective vulnerability of a single component of the nervous system can occur as a result of seemingly disparate pathophysiologies. Like other heritable disorders in which the molecular biology is providing new insights into disease mechanisms, the nosology of the HSP will undoubtedly be revised as the overlapping genetics of different heritable disorders is increasingly clarified.

REFERENCES

1. McMonagle P, Webb S, Hutchinson M. The prevalence of "pure" autosomal dominant hereditary spastic paraplegia in the island of Ireland. *J Neurol Neurosurg Psychiatry.* 2002;72:43–46.
2. Fink JK. Hereditary spastic paraplegia. In: Rimoin DL, Connor JM, Pyeritz RE, Korf BR, eds. *Emery and Rimoin's Principles and Practice of Medical Genetics.* 6th ed. Philadelphia, PA: Churchill Livingstone Elsevier; 2011.
3. Fink JK. Hereditary spastic paraplegia. *Curr Neurol Neurosci Rep.* 2006;6:65–76.
4. Harding AE. Hereditary "pure" spastic paraplegia: A clinical and genetic study of 22 families. *J Neurol Neurosurg Psychiatry.* 1981;44:871–883.
5. Harding AE. Classification of the hereditary ataxias and paraplegias. *Lancet.* 1983;1:1151–1155.
6. Fink JK. Hereditary spastic paraplegia overview. 2009. www.genetests.org.
7. Orlacchio A, Patrono C, Gaudiello F, et al. Silver syndrome variant of hereditary spastic paraplegia: a locus to 4p and allelism with SPG4. *Neurology.* 2008;70:1959–1966.
8. Rowland LP, Bird TD. Silver syndrome: the complexity of complicated hereditary spastic paraplegia. *Neurology.* 2008;70:1948–1949.
9. Simpson MA, Cross H, Proukakis C, et al. Maspardin is mutated in Mast syndrome, a complicated form of hereditary spastic paraplegia associated with dementia. *Am J Hum Genet.* 2003;73:1147–1156.
10. Edvardson S, Hama H, Shaag A, et al. Mutations in the fatty acid 2-hydroxylase gene are associated with leukodystrophy with spastic paraparesis and dystonia. *Am J Hum Genet.* 2008;83:643–648.
11. Lossos A, Stevanin G, Meiner V, et al. Hereditary spastic paraplegia with thin corpus callosum: reduction of the SPG11 interval and evidence for further genetic heterogeneity. *Arch Neurol.* 2006;63:756–760.
12. Dick KJ, Eckhardt M, Paisan-Ruiz C, et al. Mutation of FA2H underlies a complicated form of hereditary spastic paraplegia (SPG35). *Hum Mutat.* 2010;31:E1251–E1260.
13. Fink JK, Heiman-Patterson T, Bird T, et al. Hereditary spastic paraplegia advances in genetic research. *Neurology.* 1996;46:1507–1514
14. Yip AG, Durr A, Marchuk DA, et al. Meta-analysis of age at onset in spastin-associated hereditary spastic paraplegia provides no evidence for a correlation with mutational class. *J Med Genet.* 2003;40:e106.
15. Meyer T, Schwan A, Dullinger JS, et al. Early-onset ALS with long-term survival associated with spastin gene mutation. *Neurology.* 2005;65:141–143.
16. Strong MJ, Gordin PH. Primary lateral sclerosis, hereditary spastic paraplegia and amyotrophic lateral sclerosis: Discrete entities or spectrum? *Amyotroph Lateral Scler Other Motor Neuron Disord.* 2005;6(1):8–16.
17. Brugman F, Wokke JHJ, Scheffer H, Versteeg MH, Sistermans EA, van den Berg LH. Spastin mutations in sporadic adult-onset upper motor neuron syndromes. *Ann Neurol.* 2005;58(6):865–869.
18. Brugman F, Wokke JHJ, Vianney de Jong JM, Franssen H, Faber CG, Van den Berg LH. Primary lateral sclerosis as a phenotypic manifestation of familial ALS. *Neurology.* 2005;64(10):1778–1779.
19. Brugman F, Veldink JH, Franssen H, et al. Differentiation of hereditary spastic paraparesis from primary lateral sclerosis in sporadic adult-onset upper motor neuron syndromes. *Arch Neurol.* 2009;66(4):509–514.
20. Rainier S, Sher C, Reish O, Thomas D, Fink JK. De novo occurrence of novel SPG3A/alastin mutation presenting as cerebral palsy. *Arch Neurol.* 2006;63:445–447.
21. Namekawa M, Ribai P, Nelson I, et al. SPG3 A is the most frequent cause of hereditary spastic paraplegia with onset before age 10 years. *Neurology.* 2006;66(1):112–114.
22. Fink JK, Rainer S. Hereditary spastic paraplegia: Spastin phenotype and function. *Arch Neurol.* 2004;61:830–833.
23. www.athenadiagnostics.com/content/test-catalog/
24. Beetz C, Nygrem AO, Schickel J, et al. High frequency of partial SPAST deletions in autosomal dominant hereditary spastic paraplegia. *Neurology.* 2006;67:1926–1930.
25. Brugman F, Scheffer H, Wokke JHJ. Paraplegin mutations in apparently sporadic adult-onset upper motor neuron syndromes. *Neurology.* 2008;71:1500–1505.
26. Elleuch N, Depienne C, Benomar A, et al. Mutation analysis of the paraplegin gene (SPG7) in patients with hereditary spastic paraplegia. *Neurology.* 2006;66(5):654–659.
27. Martinez-Lage M, Molina-Porcel L, Falcone D, et al. TDP-43 pathology in a case of hereditary spastic paraplegia with a NIPA1/SPG6 mutation. *Acta Neuropathol.* 2012;124(2):285–291.
28. Timmerman V, Clowes VE, Reid E. Overlapping molecular pathological themes link Charcot-Marie-Tooth neuropathies and hereditary spastic paraplegia. *Exp Neurol.* 2013;246:14–25.
29. Comella CL, Pullman SL. Botulinum toxins in neurological disease. *Muscle Nerve.* 2004;29:628–644.

CHAPTER 8

Spinal Muscular Atrophies

The spinal muscular atrophies (SMAs) have been historically conceptualized as hereditary disorders preferentially affecting anterior horn cells and selected motor cranial nerve nuclei.[1] As in all disorders caused or influenced by genetics, molecular biology has served to confound as much as clarify the nosology. We have become very aware that the historical boundaries of hereditary neuromuscular disease are inaccurate. Part of this confusion arises from phenotypic overlap. For example, although lower motor neuron (LMN) morbidity dominates most SMA phenotypes, upper motor neuron (UMN) features may occur in some forms of distal SMA. Conversely, hereditary spastic paraplegia is a predominantly UMN disorder but may have notable LMN features in some genotypes. Even more damaging to the historical nosology of hereditary neuromuscular disease is the discovery that mutations of a single gene may produce variable phenotypes that have been historically represented as two or more diseases (Table 8-1).

In this chapter, we will discuss the SMAs related to mutations of the survival motor neuron (SMN) gene, the non-SMN infantile forms of the disease, the rare childhood bulbar forms of motor neuron disease (MND), Hirayama disease, Kennedy disease, the distal SMAs, the scapuloperoneal forms of SMA, and the uncommon SMA phenotypes that occur in association with multisystem disorders (Tables 8-2 and 8-3).[2–6] We emphasize this predominantly phenotypic classification as this remains, for the most part, the most practical means by which these disorders are recognized if not diagnosed.

▶ SURVIVAL MOTOR NEURON-RELATED SMAS

The history of SMA dates to the independent descriptions of children with progressive weakness by Werdnig and Hoffman in the last decade of the 19th century.[7,8] Ironically, their cases would be classified today as SMA II rather than the more severe infantile form (SMA I) that bears their eponym. The molecular genetic era in SMA began in earnest in 1990 when a gene locus 5q13 was linked to the majority of childhood onset SMA cases.[9] In 1995, deficiency of the survival motor neuron protein type 1 (SMN 1) was identified in approximately 95% of cases as the primary cause of the disease.[10]

SMA related to mutations of the SMN 1 is currently classified into five types, SMA I–IV with SMA III subdivided into SMA IIIa and SMA IIIb.[11] SMA I–III represent the traditional infantile, intermediate, and juvenile forms of the disease. SMA IV is the adult form of the disease which is less frequently associated with SMN mutations than other forms.[12] The childhood SMAs have been historically distinguished from one another, by age of onset and the milestones achieved rather than by significant phenotypic differences. SMN-related SMAs are recessively inherited. They do not differ significantly by phenotype, only by severity which is in turn related to contributions of the SMN 2 gene as will be described subsequently. They can be considered as a continuum of a single disorder.[13] Progression and life expectancy correlate with age of onset which in turn correlates with the genetic signature as described below. Age of onset and clinical course tend to be similar in siblings.[13]

CLINICAL FEATURES

Werdnig–Hoffman disease or SMA I is the most common form of MND and the prototype of these disorders. Its incidence is estimated to occur in a range of four to ten $\times 10^5$ live births, depending on the geographic cohort studied.[13] Clinical manifestations are evident within the first 6 months of life. Affected infants are hypotonic with a symmetric, generalized, or proximally predominant pattern of weakness. The legs are usually affected to a greater degree than the arms (Fig. 8-1). As in most MNDs, facial weakness is mild and extraocular muscles are spared. Fasciculations are seen in the tongue but rarely in limb muscles, presumably due to the ample subcutaneous tissue of neonates. Manual tremor, characteristic of SMA II and SMA III, occurs uncommonly. Deep tendon reflexes are typically absent. Abdominal breathing, and bulbar symptoms such as a weak cry, poor suck and feeding, and impaired secretion clearance are commonplace. The characteristic appearance includes pectus excavatum with a diminished anterior–posterior diameter of the chest, a bell-shaped chest, and a protuberant abdomen. These features are due to the relative diaphragmatic sparing in comparison to external intercostals early in the disease course. Mild contractures may occur, but arthrogryposis is not part of the classic phenotype. There is no intellectual impairment. Children with SMA I never develop the capability of independent sitting. Without mechanical ventilation, the large majority die in the first two years of life usually as a direct or indirect consequence of bulbar and/or ventilatory muscle weakness. Eight percent of individuals will survive to 10 years of age. A 20-year lifespan is unexpected.[14]

▶ **TABLE 8-1. SMA MUTATIONS ALLELIC WITH OTHER NEUROMUSCULAR PHENOTYPES**

Locus (Gene)	SMA	ALS	CMT	HSP	Other
20q13.32 (VAPB)	SMA IV Finkel type	fALS 8			
12q24.3 (heat-shock protein 8)	HMN IIA		CMT 2L		Desmin-related myopathy
7q11.23 (heat-shock protein B1)	HMN IIB		CMT 2F		
7p14,3 (GARS)	HMN VA		CMT 2D		
11q12.3 (BSCL2)	HMN VA (Silver syndrome)		CMT 2D	SPG17	
4p16–p15	Silver syndrome			SPG38	
2p22–23 (spastin)	Silver syndrome			SPG4	
6q21 (FIG4)		ALS 11	CMT 4J		
12q24.1 (TRPV4)	Scapuloperoneal SMA or dSMA or severe congenital form of SMA		CMT 2C		
17p11.2 (PMP22)	Scapuloperoneal SMA		HNPP		
9q34 (senataxin)	HMN with UMN signs	ALS4		May look phenotypically identical to HSP	
2p13.1 (dynactin)	HMN VII	AR form of ALS1			
1q22 (lamin A/C)	SMA IV		CMT 2B1		Emery–Dreifuss MD, LGMD 1B, congenital MD
14q32.31 (dynein)	HMN I or SMA-lower leg predominant		CMT 2O		This is allelic SMA-LED (lower leg predominant)

VAPB, vesicle-associated membrane protein-associated protein B; HMN, hereditary motor neuropathy; GARS, glycyl-tRNA synthetase; dSMA, distal spinal muscular atrophy; BSCL2, Berardinelli-Seip congenital lipodystrophy; FIG4, polyphosphoinositide phosphatase; PMP22, peripheral myelin protein; LMNA, lamin A/C.

SMA II or the intermediate form of childhood SMA typically manifests between 6 and 18 months of age.[15] The disorder is clinically defined by milestone acquisition, that is, a child who sits independently but never walks. Postural hand tremor is the only significant phenotypic variance from Werdnig–Hoffman disease. Tongue fasciculations, areflexia, manual tremor, and a symmetric, proximally predominant pattern of weakness characterize the SMA II phenotype. Symptoms related to impaired bulbar function are less of an issue than in SMA I. Approximately 98% of these individuals survive to the age of 5 years and two-thirds to the age of 25 years. In view of the more protracted course and the ability to sit, patients with SMA II and SMA III patients commonly acquire kyphoscoliosis and joint contractures.

SMA III is also referred to as the Kugelberg–Welander disease or the juvenile-onset SMA.[15] It differs clinically from the intermediate form by age of onset, life expectancy, and milestones achieved. SMA IIIa is distinguished from SMA IIIb predominantly by age of onset, the former defined by symptom onset between 18 months and 3 years and the latter with symptom between 3 and 21 years. Afflicted individuals develop the ability to stand and walk which are subsequently lost in childhood, adolescence, or adulthood. Initial symptoms are referable to weakness of proximal leg muscles in the vast majority of cases. For example, the patient depicted in Figure 8-2, is now 30 and still capable of standing, became aware of his problem at age 14 when the crouched position of a hockey goalie became difficult to maintain. In SMA IIIa, 70% of patients are capable of walking 10 years after symptom onset and 20% at 40 years. In SMA IIIb, almost all patients walk at 10 years and 60% of patients remain ambulatory 40 years after symptom onset.[15] Life expectancy in SMA IIIb extends into the sixth decade and may be normal in many individuals. Like SMA II, hand tremor, areflexia, and tongue fasciculations, are commonplace in SMA III. Presumably related to the older age of these patients, and the diminished proportion of subcutaneous tissue, limb fasciculations are more evident in SMA III than in SMA I and SMA II.[14]

Recessively or dominantly inherited adult-onset SMA or SMA IV is uncommon.[16,17] Even though X-linked spinobulbar muscular atrophy is an adult-onset disorder manifesting with the same proximally predominant, symmetric pattern of weakness, it has both distinctive clinical and genetic features and will not be considered as SMA IV in this text.

SMA IV patients do not typically become aware of weakness until age 21 years or older.[18] As with other SMAs, initial symptoms are typically referable to proximal lower extremity muscles. Hip flexors and extensors and knee extensors are usually the most severely affected muscles. The shoulder

▶ TABLE 8-2. **SMA CLASSIFICATION—PROXIMAL OR GENERALIZED WEAKNESS**

Category	Eponym	Acronym	Gene/Locus	Weakness Pattern	Other Features
Infantile onset	Werdnig–Hoffman	SMA I	SMN	Proximally predominant bulbar	Ventilatory failure
		SMARD 1 HMN VI dSMA I	IGMHBP 2	Generalized severe	Ventilatory failure
		SMA 0	UBE 1	Generalized severe	Arthrogryposis facial diplegia
			VRK 1	Generalized severe	Pontocerebellar hypoplasia Microcephaly, mental retardation, nystagmus, arthrogryposis
			SCO 2	Generalized severe	Cardiomyopathy, lactic acidosis
			GLE 1	Generalized severe	Arthrogryposis facial deformities
Childhood onset		SMA II	SMN	Proximally predominant	Hand tremor
Juvenile onset	Kugelberg–Welander	SMA III	SMN	Proximally predominant	Tongue fasciculations hand tremor
Childhood bulbar syndromes	Fazio Londe		C20ORF54	Generalized with multiple cranial neuropathies	Ventilatory weakness, ataxia, UMN signs, optic atrophy, retinal pigmentary degeneration, seizures, dysautonomia
	Brown–Vialetto–Von Laere		C20ORF54	Generalized with multiple cranial neuropathies	Same as Fazio Londe with addition of *sensorineural hearing loss*
Adult onset	Kennedy disease	SBMA	Androgen receptor	Proximal bulbar	Gynecomastia tremor
		SMA IV	SMN	Proximally predominant	Tongue fasciculations, hand tremor, +/− calf hypertrophy
	Finkel type	fALS8	VAPB	Proximally predominant	
	Finnish type		unknown	Generalized legs > arms prox > distal	Cramps and fasciculations
	Okinawa type		3q13.1	Proximally predominant	Cramps and fasciculations, sensory loss
	SMA-LED		14q32.31 Dynein	Proximal lower extremities	Allelic to CMT2O (also in Table 8-1)
			LMNA	Proximally predominant	Cardiomyopathy

SMN, survival motor neuron; IGMHBP2, immunoglobulin mu binding protein 2; UBE1, ubiquitin activating enzyme 1; VRK1, vaccinia-related kinase 1; SCO2, cytochrome c oxidase 2; GLE1, S. Cerevisiae homolog like; C20ORF54, chromosome 20 open reading frame 54; VAPB, vesicle-associated membrane protein-associated protein B; LMNA, lamin A/C.
Adapted with permission from Darras BT. Non-5q spinal muscular atrophies: the alphanumeric soup thickens. *Neurology*. 2011;77(4):312–314.

abductors and elbow extensors are the most affected muscles of the arms. Tongue and limb fasciculations, hand tremor, and, in some cases, calf hypertrophy occur.[18] The latter can be confounding, particularly in males, as myopathies are a more common cause of proximal weakness in this age group. Life expectancy is normal.[18]

DIFFERENTIAL DIAGNOSIS

The differential diagnosis of SMA I is the differential diagnosis of the floppy infant (Table 8-3).[19] The majority of hypotonic neonates have a central nervous system disorder. Clinical clues implicating a potential but less common neuromuscular cause of a floppy infant include preservation of alertness, depressed or absent deep tendon reflexes, the pattern of weakness, and fasciculations if present. At least two other forms of non-SMN infantile SMA are known to exist. Recessively inherited spinal muscular atrophy with respiratory distress type 1 (SMARD1) and X-linked infantile SMA with arthrogryposis will be described subsequently.[20–22] Neonatal or congenital myasthenia, congenital muscular dystrophy, neonatal myotonic dystrophy, infantile Pompe disease, severe nemaline, myotubular or other congenital myopathies, infantile botulism, and rare hypomyelinating neuropathies are the major neuromuscular considerations in a hypotonic infant.

SMN-related SMA II–IV need to be distinguished from dominantly inherited SMAs including the Finkel type associated with mutations of the VAPB (fALS8), a disorder linked to the 14q32 locus, mutations of the lamin A/C gene (LMNA) and a disorder described in two Finnish families in which the gene has yet to be identified.[23–26] The differential also includes a wide variety of myopathic disorders, including certain muscular dystrophies (dystrophinopathies, limb-girdle, myotonic, congenital and Emery-Dreifuss), congenital myopathies; mitochondrial disorders; and lipid and glycogen storage disorders. Chronic inflammatory demyelinating

▶ TABLE 8-3. **SMA CLASSIFICATION—DISTAL OR ASYMMETRIC WEAKNESS**

Category	Harding Categorization	Gene/Locus	Phenotype	Other Features
dSMA	dHMN I	HSPB1 HSPB8 GARS DYNC1H1 7q34	AD Juvenile onset Distal LEs	+/− UMN
	dHMN IIB	HSPB1	AD	+/− UMN
	dHMN IIA	HSPB8	Adult onset	
	dHMN II	BSCL2	Distal LEs	+/− UMN
	dHMN IIC	HSBP3		
	dHMN III	11q13	AR Childhood onset Distal predominant	
	dHMN IV	PLEKHG5	AR Childhood onset Distal predominant	Diaphragmatic Paralysis Scapular winging
	dHMN VA	GARS	AD onset in hands	
	dHMN VB	BSCL2	AD onset in hands	+/− UMN
	dHMN VI	IGHMBP2	Infantile	Ventilatory distress
	dHMN VIIB	DCTN1 TRPV4	AD distal LEs	Vocal cord paralysis
	dHMN VIIA	2q14		
	None (fALS4)	SETX	AD distal LEs	UMN
	None	ATP7A	X-linked distal LEs	
	None (jerash)	9p21.1	AR distal LEs	UMN
Benign focal amyotrophy	None			Abnormal cervical spine imaging
Scapuloperoneal	None	PMP22 TRPV4	Scapuloperoneal	

HSPB1, heat-shock protein 1; HSPB8, heat-shock protein 1; GARS, glycyl-tRNA synthetase; DYNC1H1, dynein; BSCL2, Berardinelli-Seip congenital lipodystrophy; HSBP3, heat-shock protein 8; PLEKHG5, pleckstin homology domain-contain protein, family G, member 5; IGHMBP2 - IGMHBP2, immunoglobulin mu binding protein 2; DCTN1, dynactin; TRPV4, transient receptor potential cation channel, subfamily 5, member 4; SETX, senataxin; ATP7 A, ATPase Cu (2+) transporting alpha peptide; PMP22, peripheral myelin protein.
Adapted with permission from Rossor AM, Kalmar B, Greensmith L, Reilly MM. The distal hereditary neuropathies. *J Neurol Neurosurg Psychiatry.* 2012;83:6–14.

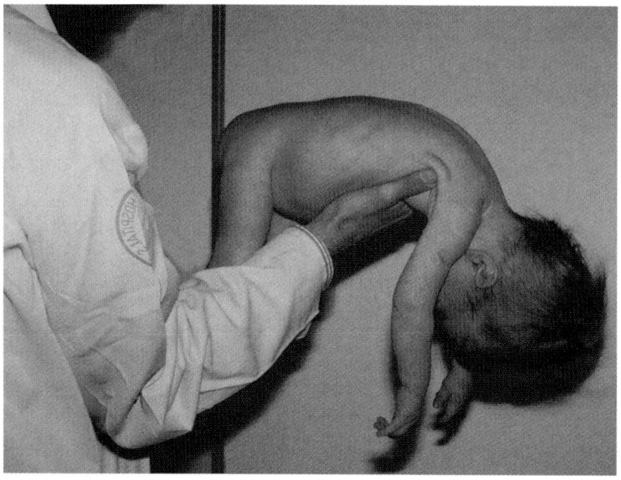

Figure 8-1. Hypotonic SMA I patient. (Used with permission of Dr. Basil Darras, Boston's Children's Hospital.)

polyradiculoneuropathy would be the primary neuropathic consideration. Congenital myasthenic syndromes should also be considered.

LABORATORY FEATURES

In Werdnig–Hoffman disease, creatine kinase (CK) is elevated, typically less than five times the upper limits of normal. In a patient with an SMA I–IV phenotype the most expeditious means to confirm the diagnosis is through SMN 1-targeted mutation analysis which identifies the exon 7 deletion, this is the genetic defect in the majority of SMA I–III, and some SMA IV cases.[10,27,28] This test will identify a mutation in approximately 95% of childhood and adolescence patients with an SMA phenotype and is felt to be nearly 100% specific.[16,29,30] In the remaining patients, sequence analysis may be performed to identify other mutations.

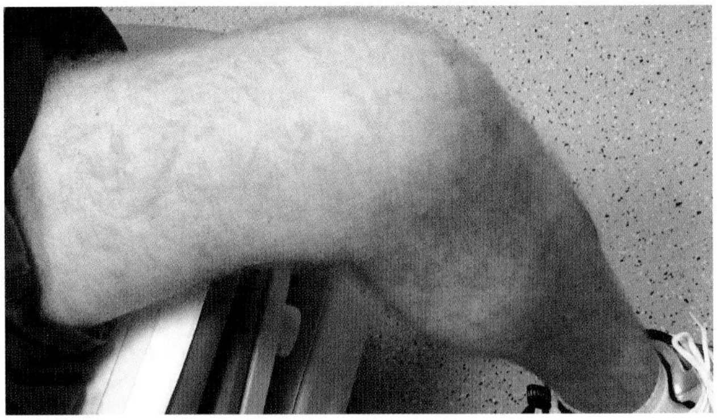

Figure 8-2. A 32-year-old male with SMA IIIb.

Patients with recessively inherited SMA IV are associated with homozygous SMN 1 deletions infrequently.[16,29,30] Analysis of the vesicle-associated membrane protein-associated protein B (VAPB) gene on chromosome 20, allelic to familial ALS type 8, may provide diagnostic confirmation in some patients with dominantly inherited SMA IV. Asymptomatic adults with SMN 1 genotypes have been described.[14,30,31,32] Although SMN mutations are highly specific for SMA, a phenotype suggesting congenital axonal neuropathy with sensory involvement has been described.[33–35]

Carrier detection and prenatal testing for SMA I–III are available through gene dosage analysis although the results need to be interpreted cautiously. A mutation detected in only one parent is reassuring but does not guarantee healthy children. Although 98% of SMA children have parents who are each heterozygotes for the SMN 1 mutation, an SMA child born of only one identified heterozygote parent can occur. This can result from either a spontaneous mutation of the child's second allele, through germline mosaicism in the seemingly normal parent or from false paternity. Interpretation of carrier testing is also complicated by consideration that both SMN 1 copies may exist on a single chromosome in 4% of individuals.[32]

ELECTRODIAGNOSIS

Historically, electrodiagnosis (EDX) was the major diagnostic tool used to support the clinical diagnosis of childhood SMA. This has been supplanted by genetic testing in the majority of cases. EMG is primarily used in individuals with a SMA phenotype without a detectable SMN mutation or in individuals who have neuromuscular disorders originating from muscle, neuromuscular junction or nerve that may resemble the SMA phenotype. With SMA or other anterior horn cell diseases, the electromyographer would anticipate a characteristic pattern of abnormal parameters. These would include low-amplitude compound muscle action potentials (CMAPs), normal sensory nerve action potential, and widespread evidence of both ongoing denervation (spontaneous discharge of fibrillation potentials and positive waves) and chronic partial denervation, and reinnervation (reduced numbers of motor unit potentials of increased amplitude and duration with muscle activation). Fasciculation potentials may or may not be identified in part because of the necessary brevity of the needle examination in many children.

EDX has a limited role in the determination of SMA prognosis. The density and geographic distribution of fibrillation potentials in comparison to changes of chronic partial denervation and reinnervation is related to the rapidity with which these disorders progress. Although pragmatically difficult to apply to the pediatric patient, motor unit instability and the rate of decline of motor unit number estimation may also provide prognostic insight.[36–38]

HISTOPATHOLOGY

The SMN-related SMAs are attributed to anterior horn cell pathology. This observation dates back to the original writings of Werdnig and Hoffman. In SMA, swelling of motor neurons laden with phosphorylated neurofilaments and glial bundles within ventral roots are common. The ubiquitinated inclusions of ALS are not seen.[39]

As with EDX, the role of muscle biopsy in SMA has greatly diminished. For all intents and purposes, EDX will arrive at the same conclusion provided by the arguably more invasive muscle biopsy. EDX has the additional advantage of more readily demonstrating the geographic distribution of these findings. In SMA I, the biopsy will demonstrate sheets of rounded, atrophic fibers of both types. Hypertrophic fibers are intermixed and are exclusively type I (Fig. 8-3). Type grouping is uncommon. In SMA II, the biopsy may

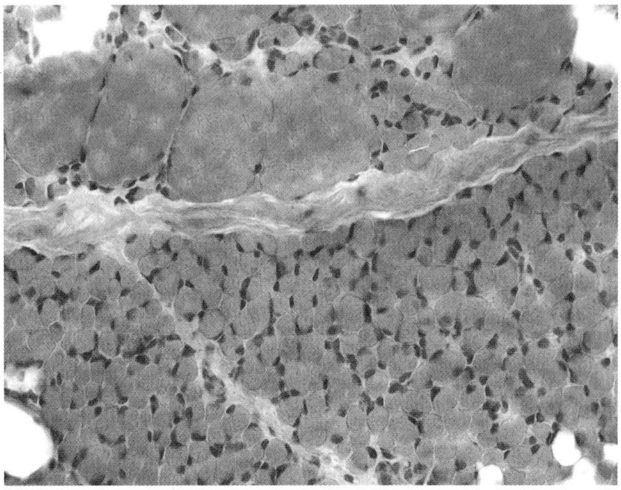

Figure 8-3. Muscle biopsy of SMA patient demonstrating complete fascicles of sheets of round, atrophic muscle fibers and a few preserved normal-sized myofibers (hematoxylin and eosin stain). (Used with permission of Dr. Umberto DiGirolami of Brigham and Women's Hospital, Boston, MA.)

be similar to SMA I or may differ because of the presence of hypertrophic type II fibers and/or the presence of type grouping. In SMA III, type grouping and group atrophy of both fiber types are common. In addition, as with many chronic neurogenic disorders, "pseudomyopathic" features such as fiber splitting, increased endomysial connective tissue, and an increased number of internal nuclei may be seen.

PATHOGENESIS

SMN-related SMA is caused by a loss of function effect due to deficiency of the SMN 1 protein caused in most cases by large deletions of exon 7 or 8 or truncation of the SMN 1 gene.[17] The SMN proteins are found in both the nucleus and cytoplasm of all cells where they have RNA processing functions. The SMN 1 protein appears to interact with a number of cytoplasmic proteins to facilitate the formation, nuclear importation, and regeneration of nuclear spliceosomal RNA.[40] The SMN 1 protein is also found to traffic in motor axons and may play a role in disordered axonal transport through its influence on β-actin mRNA.[17]

The severity of the SMA phenotype is related in part to the number of copies of the similar, but unstable and significantly less effective than the allelic protein, SMN 2.[40,41,42] The SMN 2 gene is identical to SMN 1 with the exception that exon 7 is excluded. SMA 0 is typically associated with one copy of the SMN 2 gene, SMA I with two copies, SMA IIIa with three or four copies and SMA IIIb invariably with four, and recessively inherited SMA IV with anywhere between four and eight gene copies.[11] Individuals homozygous for the SMN 1 mutation with five copies of the SMN 2 gene have been reported to be asymptomatic.[14,30,31,32] SMN 2 gene copy number is not the sole determinant of phenotypic severity. There are other complex genetic influences that are not as yet fully understood. Although 95% of affected individuals have homozygous mutations, 5% have more complex compound heterozygotic mutations with a typical deletion in one allele with a subtle intragenic defect on the other.[43] Prognostication based on SMN 2 gene copy number in SMN homozygotes should proceed cautiously. There are no known clinical consequences from mutations of the SMN 2 gene alone.

Unlike SMA 0–III, the SMA IV phenotype may be inherited in either dominant or recessive fashion. Autosomal-dominant inheritance, referred to as the Finkel type, is estimated to occur in approximately 30% of these patients.[44] This phenotype is associated with a mutation of the VAPB gene. Autosomal-dominant SMA IV is allelic to ALS 8 as some families with VAPB mutations will have UMN in addition to the more characteristic LMN findings.

MANAGEMENT

In the past decade, a number of pharmacological agents have been utilized in an attempt to increase SMN protein levels. Aminoglycosides, quinazoline derivatives and drugs that can inhibit the enzyme histone deacetylase have been used in animal models and in some cases in humans. Although valproic acid, sodium butyrate, phenylbutyrate, and trichstatin A can activate the SMN 2 promoter in vivo, no agent has demonstrated clinical benefit to date. Current strategies include the use of antisense oligonucleotides in an attempt to incorporate exon 7 into the SMN 2 gene or viral vectors to transfect the entire SMN 1 gene into the DNA of afflicted individuals. Mouse models utilizing gene therapy as well as intrathecal embryonic stem cell transplants have shown considerable promise.[17]

In 2007, guidelines for the care of the SMA patients were published based on expert consensus.[18] Readers are referred to this document for further detail. In summary, physicians are urged to provide parents, and when applicable the patient, information related to the natural history of the disease, genetic implications, and the role and availability of clinical trials. Like ALS, a multidisciplinary clinic with representation from disciplines that are familiar with the management of the nutritional, psychosocial, mobility/orthopedic, and ventilatory consequences of the disease in this age group is the recommended care model. The development of kyphoscoliosis is a common problem in children who become wheelchair bound. Spine stabilization is commonly recommended in individuals whose curves exceed 50 degrees and whose vital capacities exceed 40% of the predicted normal value. The goals of this intervention are patient comfort, ease of patient management, and potential stabilization of restrictive pulmonary deficits.[45] Tracheostomy assisted long-term mechanical ventilation, and percutaneous gastrostomy feeding tube insertion are decisions with enormous emotional and financial consequence to the parents of an affected child. Noninvasive positive pressure ventilation may provide an improved quality and duration of life in child with symptoms of ventilatory insufficiency until a decision regarding tracheostomy is required.

One genetic issue of particular importance in SMA and other heritable pediatric neuromuscular disease is the role of presymptomatic testing in siblings of affected children. The current ethical perspective, at least in the United States, is that no child should undergo presymptomatic genetic testing until they are of the age to make this decision themselves, unless a treatment that makes a meaningful difference in the natural history of the child's disease exists.

▶ NON-SMN-RELATED SMAS OF INFANCY AND CHILDHOOD

Infantile SMA with arthrogryposis, previously referred to by some as SMA 0 is an X-linked disorder associated with a mutation of the ubiquitin-activating enzyme 1 gene (UBE1) (Xp11.23). Its phenotype is very similar to SMN 1 with the exception that contractures are present at birth or early in development.[17,46]

SMARD1 is also referred to as hereditary motor neuropathy (HMN) type VI or distal SMA type I as the pattern of weakness typically affects distal more than proximal muscles.[15,17,46] Its onset is in infancy and as the name implies, is associated with compromise of ventilatory muscles, particularly the diaphragm. Understandably, without mechanical ventilation, life expectancy is limited to months in most cases. It is a recessively inherited disorder resulting from a mutation of the immunoglobulin mu binding protein 2 gene (IGHMPP2) at locus 11q13.2–q13.4.

Recessively inherited SMA may occur in association with pontocerebellar hypoplasia.[15,17,46] The phenotype of this congenital or infantile onset disorder may include microcephaly, mental retardation, nystagmus, upper limb ataxia, or in some cases arthrogryposis. It occurs as a result of mutations of the vaccinia-related kinase 1 gene (VRK1) located at locus 14q32. Recessively inherited SMA may also result from abnormal mitochondrial function due to mutations of the cytochrome oxidase 2 (SCO2) gene on locus 22q13. In addition to clinical features suggestive of SMA I, an associated cardiomyopathy with lactic acidosis may occur.[17] There is also a lethal arthrogryposis with anterior horn cell disorder (LAAHD) associated with severe facial deformities resulting from mutations of the GLE1 gene at locus 9q34.11.[46]

▶ CHILDHOOD BULBAR SMA

The syndromes of Fazio Londe and Brown–Vialetto–Van Laere (BVVLS) historically describe two bulbar syndromes, clinically distinguished from one another by the sensorineural hearing loss that occurs in the latter. Disease onset is typically within the first two decades of life. In BVVLS, the hearing loss typically precedes the development of bulbar and limb weakness.[47] These disorders are complex with involvement of multiple neurologic systems which typically include LMN weakness of the limbs and ventilatory muscles. Less common UMN signs, as well as ataxia, optic atrophy, retinal pigmentary degeneration, seizures, and dysautonomia occur. The brainstem syndrome is dominated by involvement of cranial nerves VII, IX, and XII which are more commonly affected than III, V, or VI. The disorders are usually inherited in a recessive manner and are linked to a mutation at the C20ORF54 locus.[48] The clinical course is usually progressive and fatal within years of onset. A singular case has been reported in which treatment with a low fat diet, riboflavin, carnitine, 3-hydroxybutyrate, and glycine seemed to have provided temporary clinical stabilization.[49]

▶ X-LINKED BULBOSPINAL MUSCULAR ATROPHY (KENNEDY DISEASE)

In 1968, Kennedy and colleagues described a unique X-linked form of bulbospinal muscular atrophy (SBMA) affecting middle-aged men.[50] In 1986, the genetic defect was identified on the proximal aspect of the long arm of the X chromosome by Fishbeck and colleagues.[51] In 2001, LaSpada and colleagues identified a trinucleotide repeat mutation on exon 1 of the androgen receptor (AR) gene.[52]

The prevalence of SBMA is low, estimated at 3.3×10^5 although may vary geographically. There appear to be clusters of increased prevalence in Japan and the Vasa region of Western Finland.[53]

CLINICAL FEATURES

SBMA is a X-linked, adult-onset form of SMA.[50,54] Males identify symptoms of bulbar or proximal weakness at a median onset of 41–44 years.[55,56] The average age of diagnosis in one series was 47 years although this may not be reproducible in the general population.[56] The initial symptoms however, are typically nonspecific and often begin in younger males. These include muscle cramping associated with elevated serum CK levels, tremor, gynecomastia, and/or fatigue.[55,57] Their significance is commonly overlooked at this age in the absence of disease suspicion prompted by other affected family members.

As the name implies, the clinical manifestations are largely referable to the lower cranial nerve motor nuclei and the anterior horn cells of the spinal cord. Like most disorders, there is some degree of phenotypic heterogeneity. The classic pattern is for proximally predominant and symmetric limb weakness. There are notable exceptions including distal weakness and asymmetric limb weakness that may occur in more than a half of patients.[53,56,58] The weakness is insidiously progressive although rapidly progressive weakness has been reported.[59] Hyporeflexia or areflexia is the norm.

Approximately 10% of the time, the initial symptoms pertain to involvement of brainstem motor nuclei with difficulty in swallowing, chewing, or speaking.[54] A dropped jaw may occur as well.[57] The tongue is frequently fasciculating and wasted with scalloped margins and a deep midline furrow in some cases. Facial weakness is common although tends to occur later in the disease. Perioral fasciculations are common. Like all adult-onset MNDs, extraocular movements are clinically unaffected. Breathing difficulty is uncommon but may occur late in the disease.[17] Unlike the majority of MNDs, there is often an associated, but frequently asymptomatic, sensory neuropathy/neuronopathy detected during the performance of the clinical examination or more commonly, nerve conduction studies. Postural tremor of the limbs or perioral tremor are commonplace and on occasion, may be the presenting manifestation.[53]

The median age of wheelchair dependency is 61 years or approximately 15 years after the onset of weakness. Only a third of affected individuals will be wheel chair dependent 20 years following symptom onset.[53] Life expectancy may be minimally compromised with an average life expectancy of 71.[53]

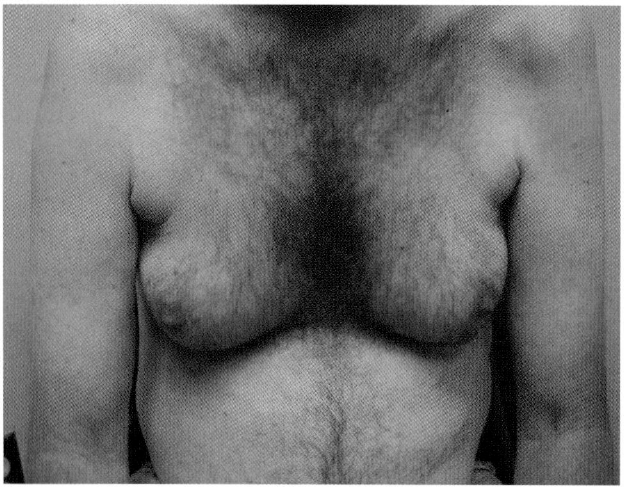

Figure 8-4. Gynecomastia in SBMA disease. (Used with permission of Paul E. Barkhaus, MD.)

Approximately half of the women who are heterozygous for the Kennedy disease mutation will be minimally symptomatic. The phenotype is similar to those experienced by young affected men with cramps, tremor, CK elevation, and perioral fasciculations.[60] The penetrance of SBMA is incomplete as not all males with the mutation will become symptomatic.[53]

The effects of Kennedy disease are not restricted to the neuromuscular system as a mutation of the AR gene would imply.[52] Affected males suffer the consequences of androgen insensitivity, including gynecomastia (Fig. 8-4), impotence, testicular atrophy, and potential infertility. There is an increased incidence of diabetes mellitus and hypertension. Hyperlipidemia and abnormal liver function are thought to occur in this population as well.[61]

DIFFERENTIAL DIAGNOSIS

Kennedy disease may be misdiagnosed as ALS.[54] DNA mutational analysis for X-linked SBMA should be at least considered in any male with suspected LMN-dominant ALS. Rapid progression and UMN signs would favor ALS whereas insidious progression, tremor, sensory neuropathy, and signs of androgen insensitivity would favor SBMA. Less frequently occurring LMN disorders such as progressive muscular atrophy, certain genotypes of fALS such as ALS 8, and SMA IV would be more difficult to clinically separate and may require careful pedigree analysis or genetic testing in order to do so. There is a proximal form of hereditary sensory motor neuropathy with locus at 3q13.1 reported in Okinawa, associated with optineurin neuronal inclusions, that may mimic the neurogenic pattern of SBMA limb weakness.[46,62] It lacks bulbar involvement however, and progresses in a fashion reminiscent of ALS. In view of its predilection to produce a limb-girdle and bulbar pattern of weakness, disorders of neuromuscular transmission such as the Lambert–Eaton myasthenic syndrome, congenital and acquired myasthenia gravis should be considered.[62,63] In view of its propensity to affect older individuals and cause symptomatic dysphagia as well as quadriceps weakness, inclusion body myositis, and to a lesser extent oculopharyngeal muscular dystrophy deserve consideration. The differential diagnosis of bulbar-onset SBMA should include syringobulbia, familial amyloidosis associated with gelsolin mutations, Tangier's disease, and facial-onset sensory motor neuropathy (FOSMN). The latter typically begins with facial sensory symptoms but may evolve to include limb-girdle weakness thus potentially mimicking SBMA.[64] A single case of an SBMA phenotype has been reported in an individual with elevated estrogen levels.[65]

LABORATORY FEATURES

Serum CK levels may be normal in approximately 10% of patients or as high as 8,000 IU/L. The use of cholesterol lowering agents may represent a confounding variable in interpreting elevated CK levels in this population.[56,59,66] As previously implied, SBMA is consideration in young males with elevated CK even if muscle weakness is not yet evident. Oligo- or azospermia, elevated levels of testosterone, progesterone, estradiol, follicle stimulating hormone, or luteinizing hormone may occur.[53] The incidence of glucose intolerance is increased. Cerebrospinal fluid is normal. The DNA mutational analysis for Kennedy disease is highly sensitive and specific although is not fully penetrant.[59] MR imaging of muscle has a limited role demonstrating fatty infiltration of affected muscles on T1-weighted images. The pattern is however nonspecific, and does not allow distinction from many other neuromuscular diseases.

ELECTRODIAGNOSIS

In Kennedy disease, EDX has a greater role than in childhood SMAs. In the SMN-related SMAs, the clinical diagnosis is commonly suspected prior to electrodiagnostic testing leading directly to genetic testing. In contrast, as neurogenic causes of proximal symmetric weakness in adults are uncommon, SBMA may not be considered until after the EMG is performed and demonstrates a predominantly chronic, neurogenic pattern.

The electrodiagnostic findings in Kennedy disease are similar to any other MND with at least two exceptions. Unlike most MNDs, there is involvement of the sensory system in SBMA manifested by absent or low-amplitude SNAPs and H reflexes.[58] Greater than 95% of individuals will have involvement of at least one sensory nerve. Upper extremity sensory conductions seem just as likely as lower extremity sensory conductions to be abnormal in a manner consistent with a dorsal root ganglionopathy. In addition, the denervation on needle examination in Kennedy disease is typically dominated by chronic features (reduced numbers of enlarged MUAPs) with a paucity of the markers of ongoing denervation (fibrillation potentials and positive waves) that characterize the more rapidly progressive MNDs.

HISTOPATHOLOGY

In Kennedy disease, the muscle biopsy changes of neurogenic atrophy are typical, including angulated atrophic fibers of both types, and pyknotic nuclear clumps. For some reason, fiber-type grouping is unusual.[53] In addition, like many chronic neurogenic disorders, "pseudomyopathic" features including increased numbers of central nuclei, regenerating fibers, and necrotic fibers are seen. Occasionally, inflammatory cells may be seen. Animal modeling would suggest that these findings may be related to a separate myopathic disease component that may precede motor neuron degeneration.[61] Sural nerve biopsy predictably identifies loss of myelinated fibers.[59] On postmortem examination, there is loss of brainstem and spinal motor nuclei as well as dorsal root ganglion cells. Inclusions formed by the accumulation of the mutated AR are noted. Inclusions are also found through numerous regions of the central nervous system including the basal ganglia.[53] The ubiquitintated inclusions of ALS are not seen.

PATHOGENESIS

Kennedy disease was the first trinucleotide repeat disorder to be described.[52] SBMA results from an expansion of the cytosine-adenine-guanine (CAG) trinucleotide sequence in the first exon of the AR gene on the X chromosome. Normal males will have 21–37 repeats whereas affected males will have 40–62. A normal repeat number will remain stable in subsequent generations whereas progeny of individuals with 38 or 39 repeats may develop disease from gene expansion. The number of repeats correlates inversely with onset age of limb weakness but not necessarily with disease severity, rate of progression, cramps, CK levels, tremor, or endocrine abnormalities.[53,55,67] Expansion of the repeat size and anticipation appears to occur in SBMA resulting in earlier disease onset in subsequent generations. The majority of cases appear to be genetically transmitted; spontaneous mutations are thought to occur rarely. Approximately 30% of diagnosed individuals in one series had no other identifiable family members.[56]

The unstable polyglutamine CAG expansion appears to be pathogenic through a toxic gain of function. The expanded AR protein appears to misfold and aggregate in the nuclei of motor neurons and dorsal root ganglia.[53,68] Although the nuclear presence of this misfolded AR protein is a disease prerequisite, it would not appear to be the sole mechanism of toxicity as the burden of protein accumulation does not appear to correlate with the extent of toxicity.[53] The presence of the normal AR ligands, testosterone and dihydrotestosterone, are necessary for the phenotype to develop. Disease expression is also dependent on AR binding to DNA. This concept is supported by observations of the rare female homozygotes, or in mouse models in which homozygous females and mutant castrated males where little if any disease develops.[53,56] The actual mechanism(s) by which the misfolded protein and synergistic effects of androgens are toxic to motor neurons and dorsal root ganglia are not fully understood. There is evidence to support attenuation of transcriptional activity of the AR with a resultant decrease in histone acetylation, mitochondrial dysfunction, and caspase-dependent apoptotic contributions.[53,61] In addition, there is evidence-impaired axonal transport with disordered function of dynactin, a protein whose gene when mutated may produce a distal SMA phenotype.[61]

MANAGEMENT

Treatment for SBMA remains largely symptomatic. Cramps may respond to nightly stretching and medications such as valproate, mexiletine gabapentin, tizanidine, baclofen, magnesium, or carbamazepine although in our experience, none of these are particularly effective. Quinine remains in our estimation the most effective drug for cramps but is approved by the FDA solely for the treatment of malaria. Tremor is rarely severe enough to warrant treatment but may respond to propranolol or primidone. Gynecomastia, if problematic, may be treated with hormonal therapy, castration, or surgical reduction. Durable medical equipment to facilitate safe mobility is a mainstay of treatment in the latter stages of the disease. Percutaneous gastrostomy and noninvasive positive pressure (rare) ventilation are important interventions in patients where impaired swallowing and breathing become severe enough to compromise the patient's health or quality of life. The criteria for initiation are similar to that described in the ALS chapter.

As the development of SBMA is testosterone dependent, therapeutic strategies have understandably been directed at the androgenic system. Unfortunately, testosterone replacement provides no benefit. Leuprorelin, an LHRH-agonist that reduces testosterone release, and prevents nuclear relocation of mutated AR, has been shown to have a therapeutic effect on animal models of the disease.[69] A single trial in humans had modest chemical and clinical results.[53,70] There are other experimental constructs that appear to have beneficial effects on animal disease models. AR coregulators such as ARA 70 hold promise as they inhibit the distribution and aggravation of the abnormal AR protein. Histone deacetylase inhibitors, such as sodium butyrate, may inhibit some of the adverse effects of the accumulated, mutated AR. Heat-shock protein (HSP) inducers may serve to help facilitate degradation of misfolded AR.

▶ BENIGN FOCAL AMYOTROPHIES (HIRAYAMA DISEASE, JUVENILE SEGMENTAL SPINAL MUSCULAR ATROPHY)

In 1959, Hirayama described a slowly progressive, focal motor neuron disorder affecting the upper extremities.[71] It has been referred to by a variety of names including monomelic amyotrophy and juvenile segmental spinal muscular atrophy (JSSMA).[71] JSSMA implies a genetic mechanism however, and there is no currently known genetic cause. Although there have been occasional reports of more than one first-degree family member involved, the majority of cases appear to be sporadic. The survival motor neuron genes 1 and 2 have been excluded from consideration. The construct of monomelic amyotrophy is also flawed. With Hirayama disease and other related phenotypes, bilateral involvement is not rare. For these reasons, we concur with Felice that the classification of these disorders as benign focal amyotrophies (BFAs) represents the most cogent nosology due to their tendency to produce regional patterns of weakness that are indolent and commonly plateau after an initial period of progression.[72]

CLINICAL FEATURES

Hirayama disease typically becomes symptomatic between ages 15 and 25 years, with a range of 2–30 years.[73,74] Males are affected in 60–88% of cases.[75] The typical phenotype is atrophy and weakness that develops insidiously in C7–T1 hand and forearm muscles unilaterally, typically in the dominant extremity (Fig. 8-5). Preserved brachioradialis bulk in contrast to the atrophied medial flexor compartment muscles is a notable observation in many cases. Over the course of months to years, the weakness may spread gradually to more proximal arm muscles. In 30–40% of cases, there is clinical weakness of the opposite limb, with an even higher percentage having

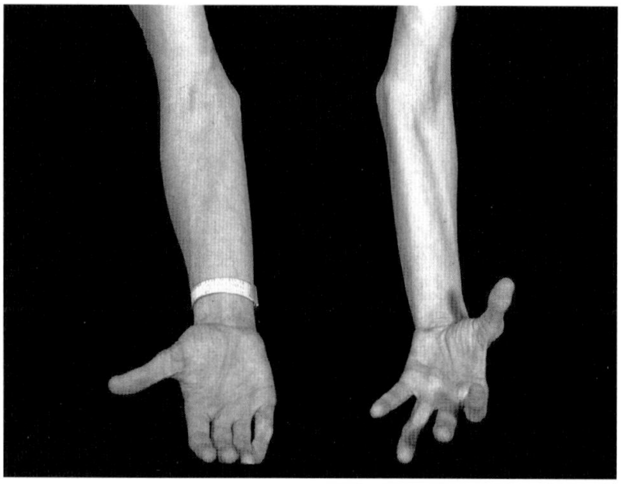

Figure 8-5. Asymmetric forearm and hand atrophy in Hirayama disease.

electrodiagnostic evidence of bilateral involvement.[74,75] In 75% of cases, disease progression arrests within 5 years.[75] Unlike most non-ALS anterior horn cell diseases, reflexes in the involved limb may be spared although neither overt pyramidal nor bulbar involvement occurs.[72] This may represent a reflection of the C8–T1 segmental involvement which provides no adequate deep tendon reflex for testing. One observation that ties BFA to SMA is the common occurrence of tremor in both. In BFA however, the tremor may occur with or be potentially caused by "contraction fasciculations" of involved muscles.[76] Fasciculations are not commonly observed in muscles at rest. Although a significant decline in affected limb function in the cold is common with all MNDs, "cold paresis" is particularly emphasized in this population.[74,77] Hyperhidrosis of the involved limb(s) has been described.

BFA has been described less frequently in Western populations. Not all patients with BFA adhere precisely to the phenotype originally described by Hirayama. Precise boundaries are difficult without a reliable biological marker. A bilateral symmetric form of the disease has been described and in one large series represented 10% of cases although even in these cases the disease evolved asymmetrically.[77] There are lower extremity analogs that are similar in every way except topography. The first of these was described in an Indian population in 1981 where most affected individuals had weakness distributed throughout the affected lower limb although preferential quadriceps involvement did occur.[68,78,79] A syndrome of benign calf amyotrophy represents another phenotype and in our experience, is more common in North Americans than is the Hirayama phenotype. Like Hirayama, it may be either unilateral or bilateral in approximately half of affected individuals and appears to have a similar male predominance.[72]

DIFFERENTIAL DIAGNOSIS

In our experience, focal limb-onset presentations of MND are often attributed to the more commonly occurring compressive mononeuropathies or cervical radiculopathy. If the patient has coincident evidence of cervical spondylosis on imaging or electrodiagnostic evidence of ulnar nerve slowing at the elbow or prolonged median distal latencies, unnecessary surgical intervention may take place.[80] A practical rule of thumb is that painless weakness in the absence sensory symptoms rarely represents a surgically correctable condition although the Hirayama phenotype provides one possible exception. Another possible exception to this is true thoracic outlet syndrome. In this rare disorder, the inevitable sensory involvement may be masked by the insidiously progressive nature of the disorder so that chronic hand atrophy and weakness becomes the predominant clinical problem. In our experience with this disorder, first rib resection may alleviate associated discomfort and prevent further progression but is unlikely to restore meaningful hand bulk or strength.

In keeping with the purely motor nature of this disorder, the differential diagnosis of Hirayama disease would include other MNDs, particularly progressive muscular atrophy, multifocal motor neuropathy, or perhaps even polio if an accurate onset history cannot be obtained.[81] Pathology of the spinal cord itself, for example, syringomyelia, should be considered. In our experience, surgically amenable spinal cord or nerve root disese is an uncommon cause of painless limb weakness without sensory signs or symptoms. As one potential exception to this general rule, a condition referred to as cervical spondylitic amyotrophy may produce a syndrome of hand amyotrophy presumed to represent central, cervical cord ischemia provoked by spondylytic compression at a more rostral level.[82]

LABORATORY FEATURES

As will be described in the pathophysiology section, many consider Hirayama disease to represent a compressive/ischemic myelopathy. Imaging of the cervical spine in flexion may demonstrate forward movement of the posterior cervical dura mater and ligaments resulting in flattening of the spinal cord against the C5–C6 vertebral bodies in approximately 90% of cases.[83] The posterior cervical subarachnoid space tends to be obliterated and a crescent shaped posterior epidural space that enhances with contrast is seen. The latter has been attributed to engorgement of the epidural venous plexus.[75] These changes seem to be most pronounced in younger individuals in the progressive stages of their disease and dissipate with a course that seems to parallel the natural history of the disease.[76] The patient may be left with an atrophic lower cervical cord with increased T2 signal in the anterior horn.[75–77]

Like all MNDs, modest elevations of serum CK levels are seen but apparently, only in a minority of cases.[74] Spinal fluid is normal or demonstrates a mild increase in protein content.[76]

ELECTRODIAGNOSIS

The electrodiagnostic features of Hirayama disease are no different than any other motor disease, other than for a relative restriction in their distribution. The abnormalities are typically more widespread than would be predicted on a clinical basis.[84] Electromyographic findings in the opposite, asymptomatic hand for example occur in approximately 90% of cases.[74,76] One would expect reduced recruitment of enlarged MUAPs in the majority of patients and abnormal spontaneous activity occurring in a smaller percentage.[74] Unlike thoracic outlet syndrome and ALS, the ulnar CMAP amplitude recording from the ADM is often more severely reduced than the median CMAP recording from the APB.[75,85] This suggests that the C8 segment is more severely affected than the T1 segment. This observation is consistent with the compressive mechanism described below which occurs maximally at C5–C6. Relevant sensory conductions, in particular the ulnar and medial antebrachial cutaneous SNAPs should be spared. In addition, there should be no suggestion of demyelinating features on motor nerve conductions.

HISTOPATHOLOGY

Muscle biopsies are not routinely performed for Hirayama disease. When performed, they have demonstrated the anticipated findings of a chronic denervating disorder, i.e., fiber-type grouping, and small groups of angular, atrophic fibers.[74,76] The opportunity to study the pathological findings of the cervical spinal cord in Hirayama disease are limited but in a solitary report, reduced numbers of anterior horn cells from C5 to T1, most severely seen at the C7–C8 levels, and degeneration of some of the remaining motor neurons was seen. In addition, mild associated central necrosis and gliosis was seen. These changes have been postulated to represent an ischemic mechanism, perhaps secondary to epidural venous congestion.[86]

PATHOPHYSIOLOGY

The proposed ischemic changes in the cervical spinal cord in the single autopsied case of Hirayama disease led to the hypothesis of a compressive mechanism.[86] In 2000, Hirayama reported the results of dynamic imaging in 73 patients and 20 controls.[76]

Ninety-four percent of patients had significant forward displacement and flattening of the posterior surface of the cervical cord during neck flexion. Presumptively this compromised the cord blood supply, with preferential susceptibility of the anterior horn to ischemia. Other observations from this study that were consistent with clinical observations were the frequent asymmetric flattening of the cord, and the lesser degrees of cord distortion in older patients in whom progression had stopped.[86] It has been hypothesized that the typical onset age of Hirayama disease, the arrest of disease progression, and the resultant reduction of posterior dural compression as affected individuals age, are related to accelerated growth that can occur in young men of this age.[76] In further support of the proposed mechanism, there have been reports of young individuals who engage in repetitive head rocking activities who develop the clinical and imaging features of the disease.[87] Although the compressive/ischemic mechanism of BFA has convincing support and appears to be largely accepted, there has been historical controversy as to the validity of the hypothesis.[88,89]

MANAGEMENT

The management of BFA is largely symptomatic. Tendon transfer has been utilized in an attempt to improve hand function.[90] Techniques have been utilized to restore hand bulk and appearance if not function.[91] The use of cervical collars has been associated with the observation that the arrest of disease progression occurs earlier than suggested by the normal natural history.[76] Cervical fusion with duraplasty has been utilized with unclear influence on the natural history of the disease.[92]

▶ DISTAL SPINAL MUSCULAR ATROPHY

We, along with other authors, consider distal spinal muscular atrophy (dSMA) and HMN to be synonymous.[46,93] Presumably, the duplication of terms is based on differing schools of thought about disease pathophysiology. dSMA suggests that the disease begins in the anterior horn, whereas HMN implies initial pathology of the motor axon. To the best of our knowledge, neither motor nerve nor spinal cord pathology has been reported to provide conclusive support for either position. We would speculate that those who support the HMN nomenclature do so because of the length-dependent phenotype in most cases that resembles Charcot–Marie–Tooth (CMT) disease, and sensory nerve biopsy evidence of axon loss in some but not all cases.[94,95] In addition, as described below, molecular biological knowledge of these disorders identifies that at least some cases are related to mutations of genes that code for axon transport proteins. Conversely, we hypothesize that the support for dSMA as a motor neuronopathy is based on normal sensory conductions, normal sensory nerve biopsies in some cases, and an electrodiagnostic and muscle biopsy pattern that is identical to other MNDs.[94] In addition, we suspect that the non–length-dependent pattern of proximal weakness that exists in most SMAs, that would be more consistent with anterior horn cell pathology, has been extrapolated to the nosology of distal forms of the disease as well.

The initial seminal work on the nosology of these disorders was introduced by Harding and Thomas in 1980.[96] It was based on inheritance pattern and phenotype. Currently, the most pragmatic classifications include a hybrid of clinical and genetic considerations.[93]

CLINICAL FEATURES

The dSMAs are conceptualized as slowly progressive disorders that produce symmetric or near symmetric weakness and atrophy of distal muscles.[93,96,97] Like CMT, dorsiflexion of the toes and feet and foot eversion are usually the initially and the most severely involved functions. It is not rare however for the posterior compartment of the leg to be preferentially affected.[93] In many cases, the hands will eventually become involved. Unlike CMT, there is neither clinical nor electrophysiological evidence of sensory involvement. Fasciculations are uncommonly recognized.

There is however, considerable phenotypic variability. Although the majority of currently recognized genotypes produce the aforementioned leg onset disease pattern, other mutations can produce a phenotype that begins in the hands, that involves the vocal cords or diaphragms, or one that produces pyramidal tract findings in addition to LMN features. The combination of an LMN disorder beginning in the hands and UMN features in the legs has been referred to as the eponym, Silver syndrome.[98–100] Like CMT, foot deformities such as pes cavus and hammer toes are common and kyphoscoliosis is estimated to occur in 25% of cases (Table 8-3).

There is also heterogeneity in the age of onset and inheritance pattern. Most patients become symptomatic in the second or third decade but dHMN VI can begin at birth or in the first year of life. Inheritance in dSMA is dominant in approximately 30% of cases with recessive, X-linked, or seemingly sporadic representing the remainder.[68,101]

Harding's original classification included seven categories.[93,96] Types I and II were distinguished only by onset age, type I being juvenile and type II being adult. In both cases, the phenotype was the classic pattern of distal symmetric leg weakness and inheritance was autosomal dominant. Type III disease represents this same classic phenotype inherited in a recessive fashion. Type IV is similar to type III with the addition of diaphragmatic weakness. Type V disease is dominantly inherited and characterized by upper limb predominance. Type VI is a specific recessively inherited disorder associated to date with a single gene mutation that results in a severe form with ventilatory distress, typically beginning within the first year of life. Type VII disease is dominantly inherited and associated with vocal cord paralysis and facial weakness. Individuals with the uncommon mutations that cause dHMN VII may develop frontal temporal dementia as well. X-linked forms of the disease, dSMAs associated with pyramidal tract features, and a congenital form were not considered in the initial Harding classification scheme (Table 8-3).[93,96]

Although certain mutations may produce more than one of the aforementioned phenotypic pattern, there is a reasonable phenotype/genotype correlation within the boundaries of dSMA (Table 8-3). Having said that, a number of these genes may produce phenotypes that have been historically designated as other diseases, most notably CMT (Table 8-1).

DIFFERENTIAL DIAGNOSIS

The distal SMAs are frequently diagnosed as CMT. Other than for the presence or absence of sensory involvement, the disorders may be phenotypically identical. That many of the dSMAs are allelic with forms of CMT cast doubt on whether distal SMA and axonal forms of CMT disease will be considered different disorders in the future. The distal SMAs may be readily confused with a number of the distal myopathy genotypes which may present with slowly progressive symmetric weakness of foot plantar or dorsiflexion. The childhood forms of dSMA will need to be distinguished from the more commonly occurring SMN-related disorders. As we alluded, there is both genetic and phenotypic overlap between the distal SMA, ALS, and hereditary spastic paraparesis.

LABORATORY FEATURES

Other than genetic testing, blood work has little relevance in dSMA. CK measurements are rarely reported but appear to normal or mildly elevated.[94,101] There are currently nine recognized genetic loci for dSMA that produce approximately 20% of clinically recognized cases.[93] Currently, genetic testing is available for a limited number of dSMA mutations including HSP 8, transient receptor potential cation channel (TRPV4), senataxin (SETX), and dynactin (DCTN1). As the diagnostic yield is low, as the cost is high, and as knowledge derived from successful genotyping has limited relevance to patient management decisions, we rarely if ever pursue this option. There is a potential role for MR imaging in dSMA. A pattern of muscle atrophy believed to be unique to the TRPV4 mutation has been described.[102]

ELECTRODIAGNOSIS

Sensory nerve conductions are by definition normal in this disorder, at least in the majority of cases early in the disease course. CMAP amplitudes may be reduced or absent. Conduction velocities and motor latencies are preserved in a manner proportionate to the degree of axon loss. Needle electromyography demonstrates largely findings of chronic denervation and reinnervation in a distribution that extends well beyond the recognized pattern of weakness.[8]

HISTOPATHOLOGY

Muscle biopsy is rarely performed on these patients unless EDX studies do not adequately distinguish between a nerve and muscle disease. If performed, a neurogenic pattern is seen with angulated atrophy, fiber-type grouping, and group atrophy. Sensory nerve biopsy results, as previously mentioned may be either normal or show axon loss.[94,95] As previously mentioned, we are unaware of any pathological reports of either motor nerve or spinal cord in this disorder.[93]

PATHOGENESIS

There are nine gene mutations that are currently known to produce a dSMA phenotype. These genes are however responsible for only 20% of cases.[93] The proteins associated with dSMA loci have diverse functions including protein folding, axonal transport, cation-channel function, and RNA metabolism. The dHMN VII phenotype secondary to the dynactin gene mutation lends strong support to the axonal transport hypothesis as dynactin is a microtubular motor protein responsible for retrograde axonal transport.[103]

MANAGEMENT

The therapy for this disorder remains symptomatic. Patients will frequently benefit from ankle foot orthoses to prevent tripping or night splints to prevent contracture if the hands are involved. Durable equipment is a helpful means by which to preserve safe and independent ambulation. Only a minority of cases will require a wheelchair. Patients with ventilatory weakness may benefit from positive airway pressure devices and patients with vocal cord paralysis may benefit from procedures that may improve vocal cord functionality.

▶ SCAPULOPERONEAL SMA (DAVIDENKOW DISEASE)

Other than the childhood bulbar syndromes, the neurogenic scapuloperoneal syndromes undoubtedly represent the least common SMA phenotype. As will be described below, classifying this syndrome as an SMA may be erroneous. This disorder bears the eponym Davidenkow syndrome after the individual who initially described it in 1939.[104]

CLINICAL FEATURES

Recognition typically occurs in late childhood or early adulthood. Asymmetric weakness of the shoulder girdles and foot dorsiflexors are the usual initial manifestations. Weakness may progress to a more generalized pattern over a period of years.

Twelve of Davidenkow's original 13 patients had a familial disorder with apparent-dominant inheritance.[104] Sporadic cases have been described as well.[102] Neurogenic scapuloperoneal syndrome has been classified as an SMA even though distal sensory loss was common in Davidenkow's original series. Despite the frequent occurrence of foot deformities and sensory loss, he eschewed any relationship to CMT although others have not shared his conviction.[106]

DIFFERENTIAL DIAGNOSIS

Most scapuloperoneal syndromes are myopathic. Recognized myopathies that may present in this pattern include facioscapulohumeral dystrophy, scapuloperoneal myopathy, Emery–Dreifuss dystrophy, Pompe disease, myofibrillar myopathy, congenital myopathy, and inclusion body myopathy with Paget disease and frontotemporal dementia (IBMPFD).[107,108]

LABORATORY FEATURES

CK is likely to be normal in most if not all cases. Genetic testing for the PMP22 gene mutation may be considered if the patient or other family members has features suggesting CMT or hereditary liability to pressure palsy (HNPP).

ELECTRODIAGNOSIS

EDX in neurogenic scapuloperoneal syndromes may identify features consistent with SMA rather than features suggestive of the more common "myopathic" forms of this phenotype. Although there are limited electrodiagnostic reports in this disorder, abnormal sensory nerve conductions may occur.[105,109]

HISTOPATHOLOGY

Nerve pathology demonstrates axon loss with secondary demyelinating features. To the best of our knowledge the histological hallmarks of HNPP, tomaculae, have not been demonstrated in any individual with a scapuloperoneal phenotype.

PATHOGENESIS

In our opinion, although the construct of a neurogenic scapuloperoneal is valid and useful, both its classification and causation remain unclear.[105] In keeping with Davidenkow's original (ignored) observations, the disorder appears in many cases to be a nerve disease, not an MND, and allelic to HNPP.[109] The phenotype has also been linked to mutations of the TRPV4 gene which also may cause a dSMA phenotype.[110,111]

MANAGEMENT

Again, management is supportive and symptomatic. Ankle foot orthoses aid walking and prevent tripping. Scapular fixation braces may be utilized in attempt at improved scapular stabilization and improved antigravity use of the arms. Although to the best of our knowledge, it has not been used in neurogenic causes of the scapuloperoneal syndrome, scapular arthrodesis represents potential intervention worthy of consideration in selected cases.

▶SUMMARY

The SMAs are lower motor neuron disorders that are phenotypically and genetically heterogeneous. With the insights provided by molecular biology, it is safe to predict that future nosology of what has been historically considered SMA will be revised considerably. More importantly, molecular biological insights into disease pathogenesis provide the hope of future treatment that is both rational and effective. Until then, supportive care by committed clinicians remains of paramount importance.

REFERENCES

1. Byers RK, Banker BQ. Infantile muscular atrophy. *Arch Neurol.* 1961;5:140–164.
2. Barth PG. Pontocerebellar hypoplasias. An overview of a group of inherited neurodegenerative disorders with fetal onset. *Brain Dev.* 1993;15:411–422.
3. Chou SM. Controversy over Werdnig-Hoffman disease and multiple system atrophy. *Curr Opin Neurol.* 1993;6:861–864.
4. Chou SM, Gilbert EF, Chum RW, et al. Infantile olivopontocerebellar atrophy with spinal muscular atrophy (infantile OPCA + SMA). *Clin Neuropathol.* 1990;9:21–32.
5. Gorgen-Pauly U, Sperner J, Reiss I, Gehl HB, Reusche E. Familial pontocerebellar hypoplasia type I with anterior horn cell disease. *Eur J Paediatr Neurol.* 1999;3:33–38.
6. Ryan MM, Cooke-Yarborough CM, Procopis PG, Ouvrier RA. Anterior horn cell disease and olivopontocerebellar hypoplasia. *Pediatr Neurol.* 2000;23:180–184.
7. Hoffman J. Ueber chronische spinale muskelatrophie im kindersalter auf familiarer basis. *Dtsch Z Nervenheilkd.* 1892;3:427–470.
8. Werdnig G. Zwei fruhinfantile hereditare falle von progressiver muskelatrophie unter dem bilde der dystropine, ager auf neurotischer grundlage. *Arch Psychiatr.* 1891;22:437–481.
9. Brzustowicz LM, Lehner T, Castilla LH, et al. Genetic mapping of chronic childhood-onset spinal muscular atrophy to chromosome 5q11.2–13.3. *Nature.* 1990;344:540–541.
10. Lefebvre S, Burglen L, Reboullet S, et al. Identification and characterization of a spinal muscular atrophy-determining gene. *Cell.* 1995;80:155–165.
11. Kolb SJ, Kissel JT. Spinal muscular atrophy: a timely review. *Arch Neurol.* 2011;68(8):979–984.
12. Claremont O, Burlet P, Lefebvre S, Bürglen L, Munnich A, Melki J. SMN gene deletions in adult-onset spinal muscular atrophy. *Lancet.* 1995;346:1712–1713.
13. Munsat TL. Workshop report: International SMA collaboration. *Neuromuscul Disord.* 1991;1:81.
14. Bertini E, Burghes A, Bushby K, et al. 134th ENMC international workshop: Outcome measures and treatment of spinal muscular atrophy 11–13 February 2005, Naarden, The Netherlands. *Neuromuscul Disord.* 2005;15:802–816.
15. Zerres K, Rudnik-Schoneborn S, Forrest E, Lusakowska A, Borkowska J, Hausmanowa-Petrusewicz I. A collaborative study on the natural history of childhood and juvenile onset proximal spinal muscular atrophy (type II and III SA): 569 patients. *J Neurol Sci.* 1997;146:67–72.
16. Brahe C, Servidei S, Zappata S, Riccdi E, Tonali P, Neri G. Genetic homogeneity between childhood-onset and adult-onset autosomal recessive spinal muscular atrophy. *Lancet.* 1995;346:741–742.
17. Wee CD, Kong L, Sumner CJ. The genetics of spinal muscular atrophies. *Curr Opin Neurol.* 2010;23:450–458.
18. Wang CH, Finkel RS, Bertini ES, et al. Consensus statement for standard of care in spinal muscular atrophy. *J Child Neurol.* 2007;22(8):1027–1049.

19. David WS, Jones HR Jr. Electromyography and biopsy correlation with suggested protocol for evaluation of the floppy infant. *Muscle Nerve*. 1994;17(4):424–430.
20. Grohmann K, Varon R, Stolz P, et al. Infantile spinal muscular atrophy with respiratory distress type 1 (SMARD1). *Ann Neurol*. 2003;54:719–724.
21. Grohmann K, Schuelke M, Diers A, et al. Mutations in the gene encoding immunoglobulin mu-binding protein 2 cause spinal muscular atrophy with respiratory distress type 1. *Nat Genet*. 2001;29:75–77.
22. Kobayashi H, Baumback L, Matise TC, Schiavi A, Greenberg F, Hoffman EP. A gene for a severe lethal form of X-linked arthrogryposis (X-linked infantile spinal muscular atrophy) maps to human chromosome Xp11.3-q11.2. *Hum Mol Genet*. 1995;4:1213–1216.
23. Harms MB, Allred P, Gardner R Jr, et al. Dominant spinal muscular atrophy with lower extremity predominance: linkage to 14q32. *Neurology*. 2010;75:539–546.
24. Jokela M, Penttilä S, Huovinen S, et al. Late-onset lower motor neuronopathy. *Neurology*. 2011;77:334–340.
25. Nishimura AL, Mitne-Neto M, Silva HC, et al. A mutation in the vesicle-trafficking protein VAPB causes late-onset spinal muscular atrophy and amyotrophic lateral sclerosis. *Am J Hum Genet*. 2004;75:822–831.
26. Rudnik-Schoneborn S, Borzenhart E, Eggermann T, et al. Mutations of the LMNA gene can mimic autosomal dominant proximal muscular atrophy. *Neurogenetics*. 2007;8:137–142.
27. Feldkotter M, Schwarzer V, Wirth R, Wienker TF, Wirth B. Quantitative analyses of SMN1 and SMN2 based on real-time lightCycler PCR: fast and highly reliable carrier testing and prediction of severity of spinal muscular atrophy. *Am J Hum Genet*. 2002;70(2):358–368.
28. Rodrigues NR, Owen N, Talbot K, Ignatius J, Dubowitz V, Davies KE. Deletions in the survival motor neuron gene on 5q13 in autosomal recessive spinal muscular atrophy. *Hum Mol Genet*. 1995;4:631–634.
29. Figlewicz DA, Orrell RW. The genetics of motor neuron disease. *ALS Other Motor Neuron Dis*. 2003;4:225–231.
30. Hahnen E, Forkert R, Marke C, et al. Molecular analysis of candidate genes of 5q13 in autosomal recessive spinal muscular atrophy: evidence of homozygous deletions of the SMN gene in unaffected individuals. *Hum Mol Genet*. 1995;4:1927–1933.
31. Prior TW, Swoboda KJ, Scott HD, Hejmanowski AQ. Homozygous SMN1 deletions in unaffected family members and modification of the phenotype by SMN2. *Am J Med Genet A*. 2004;130A(3):307–310.
32. Prior TW, Russman BS. Spinal muscular atrophy. www.genetests.org
33. Hergersberg M, Glatzel M, Capone A, et al. Deletions in spinal muscular atrophy gene repair in a newborn with neuropathy and extreme generalized muscular weakness. *Eur J Paediatr Neurol*. 2000;4:35–38.
34. Korinthenberg R, Sauer M, Ketelsen UP, et al. Congenital axonal neuropathy caused by deletions in the spinal muscular atrophy region. *Ann Neurol*. 1997;42:364–368.
35. MacLeod MJ, Taylor JE, Lunt PW, Mathew CG, Robb SA. Prenatal onset spinal muscular atrophy. *Eur J Paediatr Neurol*. 1999;3:65–72.
36. Daube JR. Electrophysiologic studies in diagnosis and prognosis of motor neuron diseases. *Neurol Clin*. 1985;3:473–493.
37. Olney RK, Yuen EC, Engstrom JW. The rate of change in motor unit number estimates predicts survival in patients with amyotrophic lateral sclerosis. *Neurology*. 1999;52(suppl 2):A3.
38. Armon C, Brandstater ME. Motor unit number estimate-based rates of progression of ALS predict patient survival. *Muscle Nerve*. 1999;22(11):1571–1575.
39. Urbanits S, Budka H. Spinal pathology in spinal muscular atrophy in comparison with amyotrophic lateral sclerosis. *Wien Med Wochenschr*. 1996;146(9–10):199–200.
40. Nicole S, Diaz CC, Frugier T, Melki J. Spinal muscular atrophy: recent advances and future prospects. *Muscle Nerve*. 2002;26:4–13.
41. Elsheikh B, Prior T, Zhang X, et al. An analysis of disease severity based on SMN2 copy number in adults with spinal muscular atrophy. *Muscle Nerve*. 2009;40:652–656.
42. Brahe C. Copies of the survival motor remaining gene in spinal muscular atrophy: the more, the better. *Neuromuscul Disord*. 2000;10:274–275.
43. Fraidakis MJ, Drunat S, Maisonobe T, et al. Genotype-phenotype relationship in two SMA III patients with novel mutations in the Tudor domain. *Neurology*. 2012;78:551–556.
44. Finkel N. A forma pseudomiopatica tardia da atrofia muscular progressiva heredo-familial. *Arq Neuropsiquiatr*. 1962;20:307–322.
45. Russman BS. Spinal muscular atrophy. *Med Neurol*. www.medlink.com.
46. Darras BT. Non-5q spinal muscular atrophies: the alphanumeric soup thickens. *Neurology*. 2011;77:312–314.
47. http://omim.org/entry/211530
48. Green P, Wiseman M, Crow YJ, et al. Brown-Vialetto-Van Laere syndrome, a ponto-bulbar palsy with deafness, is caused by mutations in C20ORF54. *Am J Hum Genet*. 2010;86:485–489.
49. Bosch AM, Abeling NG, Ijlst L, et al. Brown-Vialetto-Van Laere and Fazio Londe syndrome is associated with a riboflavin transporter defect mimicking mild MADD: a new inborn error of metabolism with potential treatment. *J Inherit Metab Dis*. 2011;34(1):159–164.
50. Kennedy WR, Alter M, Sung JH. Progressive proximal bulbar and spinal muscular atrophy of late onset. A sex-linked recessive trait. *Neurology*. 1968;18(7):671–680.
51. Fishbeck KH, Ionasescu V, Ritter AW, et al. Localization of the gene for X-linked spinal muscular atrophy. *Neurology*. 1986;36:1595–1598.
52. LaSpada AR, Wilson EM, Lubahn DB, Harding AE, Fishbeck KH. Androgen receptor gene mutations in X-linked spinal and bulbar muscular atrophy. *Nature*. 1991;352(6330):77–79.
53. Finsterer J. Perspectives of Kennedy's disease. *J Neurol Sci*. 2010;298:1–10.
54. Parboosingh JS, Figlewicz DA, Krizus A, et al. Spinobulbar muscular atrophy can mimic ALS: the importance of genetic testing in male patients with atypical ALS. *Neurology*. 1997;49:568–572.
55. Atsuta N, Watanabe H, Ito M, et al. Natural history of spinal and bulbar muscular atrophy (SBMA): a study of 223 Japanese patients. *Brain*. 2006;129:1446–1455.
56. Rhodes LE, Freeman BK, Auh S, et al. Clinical features of spinal and bulbar muscular atrophy. *Brain*. 2009;132:3242–3251.
57. Sumner CJ, Fischbeck KH. Jaw drop in Kennedy's disease. *Neurology*. 2002;59:1471–1472.
58. Ferrante MA, Wilbourn AJ. The characteristic electrodiagnostic features of Kennedy's disease. *Muscle Nerve*. 1997;20:323–329.

59. Amato AA, Prior TW, Barohn FJ, Snyder P, Papp A, Mendell JR. Kennedy's disease: A clinicopathologic correlation with mutations in the androgen receptor gene. *Neurology.* 1993;43:791–794.
60. Schmidt BJ, Greenberg CR, Allingham-Hawkins DJ, Spriggs EL. Expression of X-linked bulbospinal muscular atrophy (Kennedy disease) in two homozygous women. *Neurology.* 2002;59:770–772.
61. Katsuno M, Banno H, Suzuki K, Adachi H, Tanaka F, Sobue G. Molecular pathophysiology and disease-modifying therapies for spinal and bulbar muscular atrophy. *Arch Neurol.* 2012;69(4):436–440.
62. Nakagawa M. Optinurin inclusions in proximal hereditary motor and sensory neuropathy (HMSN-P): familial amyotrophic lateral sclerosis with sensory neuronopathy? *J Neurol Neurosurg Psychiatry.* 2011;82:1299.
63. Burns TM, Russell JA, LaChance DH, Jones HR. Oculobulbar involvement is typical with Lambert-Eaton myasthenic syndrome. *Ann Neurol.* 2003;53(2):270–273.
64. Isoardo G, Troni W. Sporadic bulbospinal muscle atrophy with facial-onset sensory neuropathy. *Muscle Nerve.* 2008;37:659–662.
65. Luo JJ. Hyperestrogenemia simulating kennedy disease. *J Clin Neuromuscular Dis.* 2007;9(2):291–296.
66. Chahin N, Sorenson EJ. Serum creatine kinase levels in spinal bulbar muscular atrophy and amyotrophic lateral sclerosis. *Muscle Nerve.* 2009;40:126–129.
67. Igarashi S, Tanno Y, Onodera O, et al. Strong correlation between the number of CAG repeats in androgen receptor genes and the clinical onset of features of spinal and bulbar muscular atrophy. *Neurology.* 1992;42:2300–2302.
68. Van Den Berg-Vos RM, Van Den Berg LH, Visser J, de Visser M, Franssen H, Wokke JH. The spectrum of lower motor neuron syndromes. *J Neurol.* 2003;250:1279–1292.
69. Katsuno M, Adachi H, Doyu M, et al. Leuprorelin rescues polyglutamine-dependent phenotypes in a transgenic mouse model of spinal and bulbar muscular atrophy. *Nat Med.* 2003; 9:768–773.
70. Banno H, Katsuno M, Suzuki K, et al. Phase 2 trial of leuprorelin in patients with spinal and bulbar muscular atrophy. *Ann Neurol.* 2009;65:140–150.
71. Hirayama K, Toyokura Y, Tsubaki T. Juvenile muscular atrophy of unilateral upper extremity: a new clinical entity. *Psychiatr Neurol Jpn.* 1959;61:2190–2197.
72. Felice KJ, Whitaker CH, Grunnet ML. Benign calf amyotrophy: clinicopathologic study of 8 patients. *Arch Neurol.* 2003;60:1415–1420.
73. Hirayama K, Tsubaki T, Toyokura Y, Okinaka S. Juvenile muscular atrophy of unilateral upper extremity. *Neurology.* 1963;13:373–380.
74. Sobue I, Saito N, Iida M, Ando K. Juvenile type of distal and segmental muscular atrophy of upper extremities. *Ann Neurol.* 1978;3:429–432.
75. Huang YC, Ro LS, Chang HS, et al. A clinical study of Hirayama disease in Taiwan. *Muscle Nerve.* 2008;37:576–582.
76. Hirayama K. Juvenile muscular atrophy of distal upper extremity (Hirayama disease). *Intern Med.* 2000;39(4):283–290.
77. Pradhan S. Bilaterally symmetric form of Hirayama disease. *Neurology.* 2009;72:2083–2089
78. Gourie-Devi M, Suresh TG, Shankar SK. Monomelic amyotrophy. *Arch Neurol.* 1984;41:388–394.
79. Prabhakar S, Chopra JS, Banerjee AK, Rana PV. Wasted leg syndrome: a clinical electrophysiological and histopathological study. *Clin Neurol Neurosurg.* 1981;83:19–28.
80. Saleh F, Russell JA, Jones HR, Arle K, Srinivasan J. Prevalence of surgical procedures in early ALS. *Muscle Nerve.* 2006;34(3): 359–360.
81. McMillan HJ, Darras BT, Kang PB, Saleh F, Jones HR. Pediatric monomelic amyotrophy: evidence for poliomyelitis in vulnerable populations. *Muscle Nerve.* 2009;40:860–863.
82. Mathews JA. Wasting of the small hand muscles in upper and mid-cervical cord lesions. *QJM.* 1998;91:691–700.
83. Hirayama K, Tokumaru Y. Cervical dural sac and spinal cord in juvenile muscular atrophy of distal upper extremity. *Neurology.* 2000;54:1922–1926.
84. Van den Berg-Vos RM, Visser J, Franssen H, et al. Sporadic lower motor neuron disease with adult onset: classification of subtypes. *Brain.* 2003;126:1036–1047.
85. Lyu RK, Huang YC, Wu YR, et al. Electrophysiological features of Hirayama disease. *Muscle Nerve.* 2011;44:185–190.
86. Hirayama K, Tomonaga M, Kitano K, Yamada T, Kojima S, Arai K. Focal cervical poliopathy causing juvenile muscular atrophy of distal upper extremity: a pathological study. *J Neurol Neurosurg Psychiat.* 1987;50:285–290.
87. Jeannet PY, Kuntzer T, Deonna T, Roulet-Perez E. Hirayama disease associated with a severe rhythmic movement disorder involving neck flexions. *Neurology.* 2005;64:1478–1479,
88. Pradhan S, Gupta RK. Juvenile asymmetric segmental spinal muscular atrophy (Hirayama disease). *Acta Neurol Scand.* 2003;107:74–75.
89. Willeit J, Kiechl S, Kiechl-Kohlendorfer U, Golaszewski S, Peer S, Poewe W. Juvenile asymmetric segmental spinal muscular atrophy (Hirayama disease): three cases without evidence of "flexion myelopathy". *Acta Neurol Scand.* 2001;104:320–322.
90. Chiba S, Yonekura K, Nonaka M, Imai T, Matumoto H, Wada T. Advanced Hirayama disease with successful improvement of activities of daily living by operative reconstruction. *Intern Med.* 2004;43(1):79–81.
91. Puwanant A, Evangelisti SM, Griggs RC. Treating the chief complaint: hand rejuvenation for Hirayama disease. *Neurology.* 2011;77:190–191.
92. Konno S, Goto S, Murakami M, Mochizuki M, Motegi H, Moriya H. Juvenile amyotrophy of the distal upper extremity: pathologic findings of the dura mater and surgical management. *Spine (Phila Pa 1976).* 1997;22(5):486–492.
93. Rossor AM, Kalmar B, Greensmith L, Reilly MM. The distal hereditary neuropathies. *J Neurol Neurosurg Psychiatry.* 2012; 83:6–14.
94. McLeod JG, Prineas JW. Distal type of chronic spinal muscular atrophy. Clinical, electrophysiological and pathological studies. *Brain.* 1971;94:703–714.
95. Frequin ST, Gabreels FJ, Gabreels-Festen AA, Joosten EM. Sensory axonopathy in hereditary distal spinal muscular atrophy. *Clin Neurol Neurosurg.* 1991;93(4):323–326.
96. Harding AE, Thomas PK. Genetic aspects of hereditary motor and sensory neuropathy (type I and II). *J Med Genet.* 1980;17:329–336.
97. Irobi J, De Jonghe P, Timmerman V. Molecular genetics of distal hereditary motor neuropathies. *Hum Mol Genet.* 2004;13(2):195–202.
98. Rohkamm B, Reilly MM, Lochmüller H, et al. Further evidence for genetic heterogeneity of distal HMN type V, CMT2

with predominant hand involvement and Silver syndrome. *J Neurol Sci.* 2007;263:100–106.

99. Timmerman V, Clowes VE, Reid E. Overlapping molecular pathological themes link Charcot-Marie-Tooth neuropathies and hereditary spastic paraplegias. *Exp Neurol.* 2012;246: 14–25.
100. Orlacchio A, Patrano C, Gaudiello F, et al. Silver syndrome variant of hereditary spastic paraplegia. *Neurology.* 2008;70: 1959–1966.
101. Takata RI, Speck Martins CE, Passosbeuno MR, et al. A new locus for recessive spinal muscular atrophy at Xq13.1-q21. *J Med Genet.* 2004;41:224–229.
102. Astrea G, Brisca G, Fiorillo C, et al. Muscle MRI in TRPV4-related congenital distal SMA. *Neurology.* 2012;78(5):364–365.
103. Puls I, Oh SJ, Sumner CJ, et al. Distal spinal and bulbar muscular atrophy caused by dynactin mutation. *Ann Neurol.* 2005;57:687–694.
104. Dawidenkow S. Uber die scapuloperoneale amyotrophie (Die Familie Z). *Z Ges Neurol Psychiatr.* 1929;122:628–650.
105. Hyser CL, Kissel JT, Warmolts JR, Mendell JR. Scapuloperoneal neuropathy: a distinct clinicopathologic entity. *J Neurol Sci.* 1988;87(1):91–102.
106. Harding AE, Thomas PK. Distal and scapuloperoneal distributions of muscle involvement occurring within a family with type I hereditary motor and sensory neuropathy. *J Neurol.* 1980;224(1):17–23.
107. Barohn RJ, Watts GD, Amato AA. A case of late-onset proximal and distal muscle weakness. *Neurology.* 2009;73(19):1592–1597.
108. Selcen D. Myofibrillar myopathies. *Neuromuscul Disord.* 2011; 21:161–171.
109. Verma A. Neuropathic scapuloperoneal syndrome (Davidenkow's syndrome) with chromosome 17p11.2 deletion. *Muscle Nerve.* 2005;32(5):668–671.
110. Isozumi K, DeLong R, Kaplan J, et al. Linkage of scapuloperoneal spinal muscular atrophy to chromosome 12q24.1-q24.31. *Hum Mol Genet.* 1996;5(9):1377–1382.
111. Dai J, Cho TJ, Unger S, et al. TRPV4-pathy, a novel channelopathy affecting diverse systems. *J Hum Genet.* 2010;55(7):400–402.

CHAPTER 9

Other Motor Neuron Disorders

The previous three chapters discussed motor neuron diseases (MNDs) that are inherited or degenerative in etiology. This chapter will focus on the less common (of this era), largely acquired motor neuron syndromes including the acute and delayed effects of poliomyelitis and other neurotropic viral infections. In addition, other less common causes of lower motor neuron (LMN) disease such as the potential association with malignancy and radiation exposure will be discussed.

► POLIOVIRUS AND OTHER INFECTIOUS CAUSES OF MOTOR NEURON DISEASE

Technically, poliomyelitis implies inflammation of spinal cord grey matter regardless of cause resulting in a phenotype of acute flaccid paralysis (AFP). In this chapter, in order to avoid confusion, we will refer to poliomyelitis as the myelopathy associated with infection with the three strains of the poliovirus, distinguishing it from other infectious myelopathies that may also be dominated by LMN weakness. Other infectious myelopathies or myeloradiculopathies with signs and symptoms of notable sensory or long-tract involvement will not be addressed.

Poliomyelitis dates to antiquity. Endemic polio continues to occur in countries where vaccination programs and public health measures are suboptimal. In these cultures, individuals are likely to be exposed early in life. Cases occur more randomly than in epidemic disease and paralytic disease tends to be less severe in this population typically affected at an earlier age. Epidemic polio is a disorder of considerable historical interest. Epidemics tended to occur in the summer and early fall when people were more likely to be in contact with common water sources and each other. Individuals were typically exposed at an older age frequently resulting in more severe disease.

The Salk vaccine, a killed injectable product, became available in 1955. In the early 1960s, the live, attenuated oral vaccine (Sabin) was introduced providing two notable advantages, ease of delivery and long-term immunity. The disadvantage, however, was the potential for infection in vaccinated individuals, or those coming in contact with the vaccinated individuals who were themselves inadequately immunized. People in the latter category most at risk were those who had emigrated from countries without adequate vaccination programs, those whose religious or cultural beliefs opposed vaccination, or those whose immunity had lapsed from the exclusive use of the Salk vaccine. Since 2000, no cases of AFP from the polio virus have been reported in the United States coincident with withdrawal of Sabin vaccine usage.[1]

Although poliomyelitis is a disease of largely historical interest in the United States as a public health menace, it continues to have relevance on a number of levels. It is one of the earliest and best models of selective neuronal vulnerability from environmental cause. The development and distribution of effective polio vaccines represents one of the most notable triumphs of translational medicine in the 20th century. The relevance of poliomyelitis persists as well in that survivors of the paralytic polio epidemics of the late 1940s and early 1950s continue to populate neurology clinics.[1]

CLINICAL FEATURES

Poliomyelitis may occur as a monophasic or biphasic disease. The initial symptoms ("minor illness") are nonspecific, lasting 1–2 days. The symptoms are predominantly constitutional or gastrointestinal in nature consisting of some combination of fever, malaise, pharyngitis, headache, nausea, vomiting, and/or abdominal cramping. In the majority of individuals who are infected, the illness is self-limited and ends at this point. In individuals who fall victim to the "major illness", symptoms may occur immediately or after a delay of up to 10 days. The major illness is defined by any central nervous system (CNS) involvement including aseptic meningitis, encephalitis, or any paralytic component affecting bulbar, trunk, ventilatory, or limb musculature. Stiff neck, back pain, and fever are prominent.

Encephalitis occurs with or without a paralytic component in less than 5% of cases.[2] The manifestations may include tremulousness, obtundation, agitation, autonomic dysfunction (hypertension, hypotension, tachycardia, arrhythmias, excessive sweating), and/or upper motor neuron signs.

Although poliomyelitis is best known for its paralytic manifestations, weakness develops in 2% or less of infected individuals. The paresis typically evolves over the course of a few days. In individuals destined to develop paralytic disease, prominent myalgias, cramping, and fasciculations precede paralysis by 48 hours or less. The paresis is typically asymmetric and is confined to the limbs and trunk in half of the cases (Fig. 9-1). There is preferential involvement of the lower extremities and proximal muscles but these tendencies are relative and of limited value in the evaluation of an individual

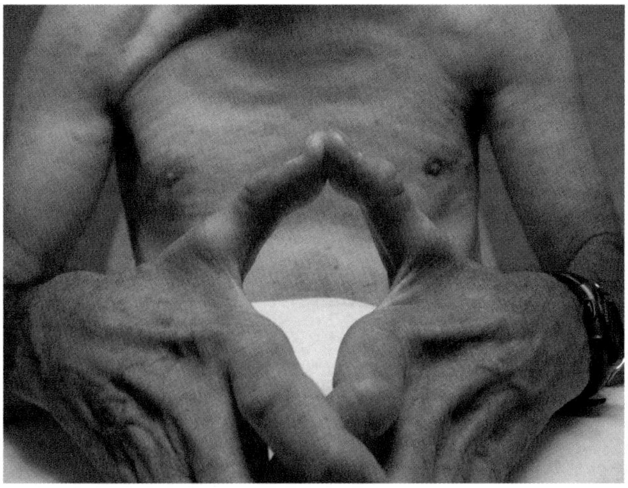

Figure 9-1. Asymmetric pectoralis and severe intrinsic hand muscle wasting in a 67-year-old who contracted polio in 1955 affecting only cervical segments.

case. About 10–15% of cases have weakness limited to bulbar muscles; the majority of these occur in children. A similar percentage is afflicted with both spinal and bulbar weakness. The most frequently affected cranial nerves are the 7th, 9th, and 10th.[2] In adults, bulbar weakness is invariably accompanied by limb weakness. Ventilatory failure is more common in this latter group. Affected limbs are paretic if not plegic with deep tendon reflexes diminished or absent. As in virtually all disorders with a predilection for anterior horn cells, the 3rd, 4th, and 6th cranial nerves are inexplicably spared. Sensory signs and symptoms are atypical although poliomyelitis may rarely result in a transverse myelitis phenotype.[3,4]

The natural history of AFP from the polio virus is variable, dependent in large part on the severity and extent of the initial illness. Less than 10% of individuals will die from the acute illness, typically due to the complications of ventilatory failure or immobility. Those who survive typically regain strength. Patients with mild weakness typically regain most, if not all, of their strength presumably due to the effectiveness of reinnervation through collateral sprouting of unaffected, neighboring neurons or through recovery of reversibly injured anterior horn cells.[5] The majority of this recovery takes place over the course of the first 3–6 months and plateaus by 2 years. Patients with severe initial weakness typically are left with residual atrophy and weakness. A chronic persistent form of poliomyelitis can occur in children who are immunosuppressed and have received modified live vaccination. It typically begins a few months after vaccination and is invariably lethal.[6,7]

DIAGNOSIS AND DIFFERENTIAL DIAGNOSIS

Differential diagnostic considerations for AFP are listed in Table 9-1. Other nonpolio enterovirus species and neurotropic viral agents are also capable of producing paralytic disease (Table 9-2).[8-10] The most common culprits are enterovirus 71 and the flaviviruses, including Japanese encephalitis, dengue, tick-borne encephalitis, and West

► TABLE 9-1. DIFFERENTIAL DIAGNOSIS OF ACUTE FLACCID PARALYSIS POLIO VIRUS INFECTIONS

Disorder	Clinical Features	Diagnosis
Other viral causes of poliomyelitis	May be indistinguishable from polio with viral prodrome, followed by aseptic meningitis and acute, asymmetric limb, and bulbar paralysis, ± encephalitic component	Cultures of throat, stool, or CSF PCR and reverse transcriptase PCR for other viruses causing AFP (Table 9-2) Increased T2 signal of anterior horns with spinal MRI
Guillain–Barré syndrome	Acute onset of motor > sensory signs and symptoms affecting limbs and cranial nerves—dysautonomia	Elevated CSF protein without pleocytosis Electrodiagnostic (EDX) pattern of acquired demyelinating neuropathy
Transverse myelitis	Acute-onset paraparesis or quadriparesis with sensory level—back pain	↑ signal, swelling on spinal cord MR imaging
Botulism	Cranial nerve including extraocular muscle weakness, generalized weakness, and symptoms of cholinergic dysautonomia occurring in appropriate clinical context	EDX findings of a presynaptic disorder of neuromuscular transmission Toxin isolation or organism culture from wound, stool, or ingested food
Rabies	Pain, weakness, and sensory symptoms in the bitten limb in 20% of individuals who are affected	Clinical diagnosis in context of appropriate exposure
Porphyria	Prodrome of abdominal pain, encephalopathy including psychosis, followed by acute, proximally predominant motor > sensory neuropathy	Family history (variable) Increased products of heme synthesis in urine
Spinal epidural abscess	Back pain Rapidly progressive paraparesis/quadriparesis with sensory level	Imaging of spine Blood cultures
Hypokalemia and hypophosphatemia	Rapidly progressive, symmetric, and generalized weakness	Potassium <2 mEq/L Phosphorus <1 mg/dL

▶ **TABLE 9-2. OTHER VIRAL AGENTS CAUSING POLIOMYELITIS**

West Nile virus
Japanese encephalitis virus
Tick-borne encephalitis
Enterovirus 71
Rabies virus

Nile virus (WNV).[10,11] With the decline in poliomyelitis, Japanese encephalitis and WNV appear to be the most common causes of infectious AFP in southeast Asia and North America respectively.[11] "Dumb" rabies may present uncommonly as a paralytic illness.[12]

This list is not exhaustive and other viral agents that are more typically associated with encephalitis may occasionally produce an AFP phenotype. Agents such as herpes simplex virus type-2, varicella zoster virus, cytomegalovirus, Epstein–Barr virus, and Coxsackie A & B viruses may produce weakness but typically affect other aspects of the spinal cord in addition to the anterior horns producing concomitant sensory involvement. Paresis caused by nonpolio agents is typically less severe than that produced by polio viruses, though West Nile infection is a notable exception.[12]

Other notable infectious agents have less certain associations with MND phenotypes. HIV-infected patients have been uncommonly reported with different MND phenotypes resembling amyotrophic lateral sclerosis (ALS) including the bibrachial amyotrophic diplegia form of progressive muscular atrophy, but the significance of these associations remains unclear.[13] The pace of progression would be unlikely to be as acute as with poliomyelitis. Importantly, MND is an unlikely phenotypic presentation of Lyme disease.[14]

The differential diagnosis of AFP includes other disorders that present with acute weakness occurring in either a regional or generalized pattern, particularly in the absence of sensory symptoms. Of these, the Guillain–Barré syndrome (GBS) is the most common and notable. Porphyria may produce an acute generalized neuropathy. Disorders of neuromuscular transmission need to be considered, particularly botulism in consideration of its acuity. Severe hypokalemia (<2 mEq/L), hyperkalemia (>7 mEq/L), and hypophosphatemia (<1 mEq/L) are potential causes of acute generalized weakness. In the appropriate context, and in view of their acuity, tick paralysis, intoxication from marine toxins, reptile and insect envenomations, and vasculitic neuropathy need to be considered. In many but not all cases, sensory signs and symptoms will serve as distinguishing features from poliomyelitis and other causes of AFP.

LABORATORY FEATURES

The evaluation of the patient with AFP ideally begins with magnetic resonance (MR) imaging of the relevant aspects of the neuraxis. The findings in poliomyelitis are indistinguishable from other viral myelopathies.[15,16] Hyperintense T2 signal abnormalities which may extend longitudinally over a number of segments are centered in the ventral horns on axial images. Additional findings may include T1 signal abnormalities indicated of hemorrhagic necrosis, short-lived enhancement with gadolinium, and cord expansion due to swelling. Routine blood work has a very limited role in the evaluation of a suspected polio patient. Like all anterior horn cell diseases, mild elevations of serum creatine kinase (CK) values are common.

The value of electrodiagnosis in cases of AFP is largely to identify a motor neuron pattern and to distinguish it from an acute neuropathy pattern. As the most common differential diagnostic consideration is GBS, it is particularly important to look for demyelinating features such as prolonged distal and F wave/H reflex latencies [in the setting of normal compound muscle action potential (CMAP) amplitudes], waveform dispersion, and conduction block, none of which would not be expected in anterior horn cell diseases. Although interpretation of sensory nerve conduction study results may be difficult in the first week of an illness, reduction in sensory nerve action potential (SNAP) amplitudes is not expected in polio but would be the norm in GBS and other neuropathies. The acute motor axonal neuropathy variant of GBS is a notable exception to this rule.

The electrodiagnostic (EDX) findings in poliomyelitis would include reduced CMAP amplitudes in weak muscles, reduced recruitment of initially normal-appearing motor unit potentials, and within 3 weeks, evidence of ongoing denervation in the form of positive waves and fibrillation potentials occurring in a multifocal, segmental distribution including the paraspinal musculature. The EDX features of postpolio muscular atrophy will be addressed in the postpolio section.

Examination of the cerebrospinal fluid (CSF) is integral to the diagnosis and differential diagnosis of poliomyelitis although may be initially negative in 10% of cases. Within 2 weeks of onset, however, a pleocytosis develops. Initially, there may be a neutrophilic predominance, but 50–200 lymphocytes/mm^3 represent the typical pattern. These cells typically dissipate within 2 weeks. There is a gradual increase in the CSF protein level to a peak of 300 mg/dl or less, which then resolves within 2 months. This pattern is similar with all of the viral agents that may produce a poliomyelitis syndrome. Hypoglycorracchia would be a rare finding.

CSF viral cultures are rarely positive in poliomyelitis. Currently, the gold standard for viral identification in the CNS is the polymerase chain reaction (PCR) for DNA viruses and reverse transcription PCR for RNA viruses.[10] CSF antibody levels may be helpful, as the presence of IgM antibodies that cannot cross the blood–brain barrier implies production within the CNS. A four-fold rise in serum antibody levels comparing chronic to acute serum or viral culture obtained from stool or throat provide diagnostic confirmation but are of limited value in acute diagnosis. The virus will be shed from the saliva for weeks and from the stool for months following infection aiding diagnosis in cases where the patient is not seen acutely. Unfortunately, identification of a specific viral agent remains elusive in the majority of AFP cases.

HISTOPATHOLOGY

The original pathologic studies of the CNS in acute poliomyelitis were made by Bodian, at times within days of disease onset.[5] The earliest pathologic changes were in motor neurons consisting of dissolution of the cytoplasmic Nissl substance (chromatolysis) occurring in the absence of inflammation. Although neuronal loss appeared independent of inflammation suggesting an apoptotic mechanism of cell death, the presence of inflammation in the anterior horn or neuronophagia was described as a poor prognostic indicator.

The macroscopic spinal cord pathology can include pial inflammation, vascular dilatation, and petechial hemorrhages.[17] In addition to the anterior horn cells, particularly of the cervical and lumbar regions, poliomyelitis may affect neurons of the intermediate, intermediolateral, and posterior horns of the spinal cord; the dorsal root ganglia; the precentral motor cortex; hypothalamus; thalamus; cerebellar roof nuclei and vermis; nucleus ambiguous; nuclei of the facial, hypoglossal, vestibular, and trigeminal nerves; as well as the reticular formation of the brainstem.[5] Other than for hyperplasia of lymphatic tissues, the pathology of poliomyelitis is largely confined to the CNS.[18]

PATHOGENESIS

There are three known serotypes of the poliovirus. Type 1 is most frequently associated with paralytic disease. Poliomyelitis is typically contracted through fecal–oral transmission, infection often initiated within families by infants not adequately toilet trained. The incubation period is typically 6–20 days. The virus replicates in the oropharyngeal and intestinal mucosa, amplifies in lymphatic tissue, and typically goes through two viremic phases, the second of which may result in CNS disease. The exact mechanism of CNS invasion is unclear but either a disrupted blood–brain barrier or entry through neuromuscular junctions with retrograde axonal transport has been suggested. This provides a potential explanation for why AFP is more common and severe in older individuals whose fast axonal transport mechanisms are better established.[19]

Susceptibility to poliomyelitis is conferred by the presence of the poliovirus receptor (PVR) or CV155 that allows viral entry into motor neurons.[20] CV155 is a protein belonging to an immunoglobulin-like class of proteins known as nectins that promote cell surface adhesion. The PVR normally exists only in primates but transgenic mice expressing this gene are disease susceptible and have provided an animal model that has offered valuable insights into disease pathogenesis. For example, the CV155 protein expresses itself embryologically in transgenic mouse neurons destined to become anterior horn cells suggesting a potential mechanism for the selective vulnerability of motor neurons. Genetic susceptibility to paralytic polio (PP) has been suspected but never proven.

TREATMENT

The best current treatment for poliomyelitis is prevention. The peak incidence of AFP from the polio virus occurred in the United States in 1952 with more than 20,000 new victims. Subsequent to the introduction of vaccine programs, the annual incidence fell to approximately 10 cases a year, the majority of which were felt to be vaccine-related. Since the moratorium on the modified-live virus (Sabin) vaccine in 2000, no new cases in the United States have occurred.

There are no known antiviral agents effective against the polio virus. Strategies to alter the structure of the PVR to prevent viral access to motor neurons has been theoretically proposed. We are aware of anecdotal reports of intravenous immune globulin (IVIG) being utilized in AFP due to WNV and in postpolio syndrome (PPS) but not in acute poliomyelitis.[21,22]

The treatments for polio and other causes of AFP remain largely symptomatic. Acute care measures include monitoring of, and if needed, support for hypoventilation and dysautonomia. Prevention of pressure injury to skin and nerve is of great importance as is attention to adequate nutrition particularly in patients with bulbar disease. Treatment of the sequelae of polio involves consideration of durable equipment needs and orthopedic procedures and is addressed in Chapter 5.

▶ WEST NILE VIRUS

The WNV has been recognized as a human pathogen since 1937. The first documented cases in humans in the United States were in 1999. WNV has supplanted poliovirus as the most common viral cause of AFP in adults in this country. It is a mosquito-borne pathogen belonging to the *Flavivirus* family, all members of which have been reported to cause an AFP syndrome.

CLINICAL FEATURES

Like poliomyelitis, most individuals who are infected remain asymptomatic or develop minimal symptoms. A minor, flu-like illness develops in approximately 20% of patients. Those who become symptomatic do so suddenly with combination of fever, malaise, anorexia, nausea, emesis, diarrhea, headache, photosensitivity, neck pain and stiffness, myalgia, rash, and/or lymphadenopathy.[23,24]

Meningoencephalitis and/or AFP develops in approximately 1 out of 150 infected individuals. Meningoencephalitis is the more common phenotype. Most, but not all, patients with AFP have concomitant meningeal or encephalitic signs and symptoms. There is at least a suggestion that the elderly and immunocompromised, particularly those with T cell deficiencies, are most at risk.[24,25]

The clinical spectrum of meningoencephalitis is quite broad and may include high fever, nuchal rigidity, seizures, and cognitive impairment including confusion, memory loss, and aphasia. Movement disorders are a common feature of WNV encephalitis and may have either hyperkinetic manifestations such as tremor or myoclonus or a hypokinetic syndrome with Parkinsonism. Stiff-person syndrome has been reported.[26] In addition, patients with WNV infection are more prone to develop systemic manifestations than poliomyelitis. Chorioretinitis is reported to occur in 75% of patients with meningoencephalitis. Hepatitis, pancreatitis, rhabdomyolysis, and myocarditis may occur.[24]

AFP as a consequence of WNV infection is a well-established concept.[23,25,27–32] Like polio, the phenotype is that of an acute onset of asymmetric flaccid weakness which usually develops over a 3- to 8-day period.[23] Unlike polio, older individuals appear to be at the greatest risk with the mean age of affected individuals being 55 years. The facial nerve is affected frequently which could prompt confusion with GBS or Lyme polyradiculopathy. Ventilatory muscle involvement with the need for mechanical breathing support occurs. As in AFP secondary to poliomyelitis, the outcome is variable with residual deficits being commonplace. Fatality rates in patients with WNV meningoencephalitis average 9% and are reported to be as high as 14%, invariably affecting those greater than 50 years of age.[24,33] It is estimated that only a third of individuals affected with meningoencephalitis will be fully recovered 1 year after their illness.[24]

DIAGNOSIS AND DIFFERENTIAL DIAGNOSIS

The diagnosis of West Nile should be considered in any case of AFP of acute to subacute onset, particularly if associated with features of meningitis and/or encephalitis. The majority of cases will be seasonal and related to periods of mosquito activity. Nonetheless, the diversity of transmission mechanisms described below, that are not seasonally dependent, allow for potential WNV infection in patients at risk at any time of year. The differential diagnosis of AFP secondary to WNV is identical to that described in the poliomyelitis section.

LABORATORY FEATURES

Imaging has a supportive role in diagnosis. High-resolution MR imaging of the spine may demonstrate increased signal in the ventral horns or ventral roots in West Nile patients with AFP.[25,34,35] Leptomeningeal, ventral root, and cauda equina enhancement, as well as increased signal in the basal ganglia, mesial temporal lobes, brainstem, cerebellum, and thalami have been described with MR imaging in patients with WNV infection.[33,36–38]

The earliest reports of WNV patients with AFP, based on EDX data, suggested polyneuropathy as the likely cause of patient weakness. This is no longer felt to be the case. Subsequent reports of AFP associated with WNV infection describe an EDX pattern identical to poliomyelitis.[25] Sensory nerve conductions are normal. CMAP amplitudes are normal or reduced without demyelinating features. Needle examination reveals evidence of reduced recruitment of normal-appearing motor unit action potentials (MUAPs) if done acutely. Within 1–3 weeks, fibrillation potentials and positive waves develop in a generalized pattern that includes clinically unaffected as well as clinically weak muscles.[25]

Routine laboratory studies have limited utility in suspected WNV infection. Like poliomyelitis, patients with AFP secondary to WNV infection can be anticipated to have modest elevations of serum CK levels. The CSF examination in cases of meningoencephalitis and/or AFP should include enzyme-linked immunosorbent assays for IgM and IgG antibodies for the WNV. WNV reverse transcriptase PCR and viral culture should be utilized as well due to their specificity. Unfortunately, both suffer from inadequate diagnostic sensitivity and cannot be relied upon to exclude the diagnosis. The preliminary CSF results typically include a pleocytosis of between 5 and 500 cells/mm^3 in 96% of cases. Initially, there may be a sizeable proportion of neutrophils, but transition to lymphocytic predominance occurs. CSF protein levels are normal in 7% of cases, elevated to $<$100 mg/dl in 63% of cases, and elevated to $>$100 mg/dl in 26% of all meningoencephalitis cases but in 47% of cases with a predominantly encephalitic phenotype.[39]

The Centers for Disease Control and Prevention provide diagnostic criteria for both probable and confirmed meningoencephalitis due to WNV which presumably extrapolate to an AFP syndrome as well. A probable diagnosis requires the appropriate clinical syndrome, occurring at the appropriate time of year associated with a singular serum determination of IgM antibodies to WNV detected by antibody capture enzyme-linked immunosorbent assay. A definite diagnosis requires the identical clinical context with more complex serologic confirmation provided through one of four potential testing methods. These options include either a four-fold increase in serum antibody concentration (usually over a 4-week interval), isolation of WNV antigen or genomic sequences usually through reverse transcription PCR, detection of virus-specific IgM antibodies in CSF, or serum IgG antibodies in addition to IgM.[24,36,40] These testing paradigms are not mutually exclusive and can be used in a complementary fashion. One unfortunate issue related to WNV serologic testing is the recognition that the latency between infection and seroconversion may be up to 8 days.[41]

HISTOPATHOLOGY

The histopathology of WNV meningoencephalitis is characterized by perivascular and leptomeningeal chronic inflammation, the formation of microglial nodules, neuronal necrosis within gray matter, and neuronophagia with a predilection for the temporal lobes, basal ganglia, and brainstem. In individuals with AFP, similar findings are noted in the spinal cord, particularly in the lumbar region. The predominant inflammatory cells are CD3+ T lymphocytes and CD68+ macrophages.[33,36,42]

PATHOGENESIS

WNV is primarily transmitted to humans by mosquitoes. Most cases occur in August and September in temperate climates when mosquitoes become more likely to feed on humans than birds. Transmission also occurs through blood transfusion, organ transplantation, dialysis, occupational exposure, breast feeding, eating or handling infected birds, and via the transplacental route.[24,33,36] The risk associated with transfusion is related to an imperfect ability to screen donated blood products.

In addition to humans, other mammals and birds are also susceptible, the latter providing undoubtedly the largest reservoir as well as the probable mechanism for rapid geographic spread. To that point, although the initial United States cases were reported in New York City, the major outbreaks in USA have occurred in the Midwest. Human epidemics are usually preceded by large kills of infected birds.

In a manner similar to poliomyelitis, viral replication occurs in skin and lymph nodes with two viremic stages. Also similar is the need for blood–brain barrier to be rendered permeable in order to serve as a portal for CNS inoculation. All flaviviruses, including WNV, gain access to targeted cells through receptor-mediated endocytosis and fusion from within acidic endosomes. The cell entry process of flaviviruses is mediated by the viral E glycoprotein.[43] Both the frequency and severity of CNS disease appear to be related to loss of function of the chemokine receptor CCR5 whose normal function is to regulate trafficking of lymphocytes to the infected brain in viral diseases such as HIV and WNV.[24] The WNV infects astrocytes as well as neurons. One theory of motor neuron death in WNV is similar to the one proposed for ALS. Specifically, it has been suggested that anterior horn cells fall victim to excitotoxicity promoted by the impaired reuptake of glutamate resulting from damaged astrocytes.[24]

TREATMENT

There are no antiviral agents proven to be effective against WNV. Vaccines are in development but are not currently available. IVIG, particularly the product obtained in populations where WNV is endemic, has been reported to have anecdotal success in case reports but no support from controlled trials has been provided to date.[22] Similar reports with mixed results in response to interferon α-2b have also been published.[10,44–47] The symptomatic and supportive treatment of WNV patients experiencing AFP is identical to poliomyelitis both in the acute care and rehabilitation settings.

► POSTPOLIO SYNDROME/POSTPOLIO PROGRESSIVE MUSCULAR ATROPHY (PPMA)

Post-polio syndrome (PPS) was first suggested as a specific entity by Cornil and Lépine in 1875 who described the clinical and postmortem features of an individual who developed progressive weakness following a remote episode of poliomyelitis.[48] This concept received no more than cursory attention until 1981 when an international symposium of experts was convened in Chicago in response to the slowly progressive weakness experienced by the large numbers of people affected by the epidemics of the early 1940s and early 1950s with convincing evidence of slowly progressive weakness after a protracted period of disease stability.[49] This has been referred to by the more specific name of PPMA which will be preferentially used in this chapter.

A number of controversies remain. The clinical boundaries of what is attributable to direct and indirect effects of "old polio" remain incompletely defined. Some symptoms attributed to PPS are not readily explained by the known pathology of the disease. They can be nonspecific and potentially attributable to other disorders prevalent in an aging population. Even with the more readily conceptualized signs and symptoms of PPMA such as fatigue, progressive atrophy, and weakness, no consensus exists to explain the mechanism of new weakness or the latency between the initial illness once thought to be self-limited and the onset of PPMA.

CLINICAL FEATURES

PPMA has been estimated to occur in between 22 and 85% of individuals previously affected with paralytic polio with the largest survey suggesting a prevalence of 50%.[50–52] The latency between the acute illness and the onset of PPMA has been reported to range between 8 and 71 years with an average interval of 35 years.[53–55] Risk factors for PPMA appear to be related primarily to the severity of the acute illness which in turn proportionate to the age of disease onset. An additional risk factor appears to be the degree of recovery from the acute illness. Patients who are more successful in regaining strength after acute illness seem less susceptible to PPMA than those of similar age and whose initial recovery is more successful.[56] Finally, excessive exercise

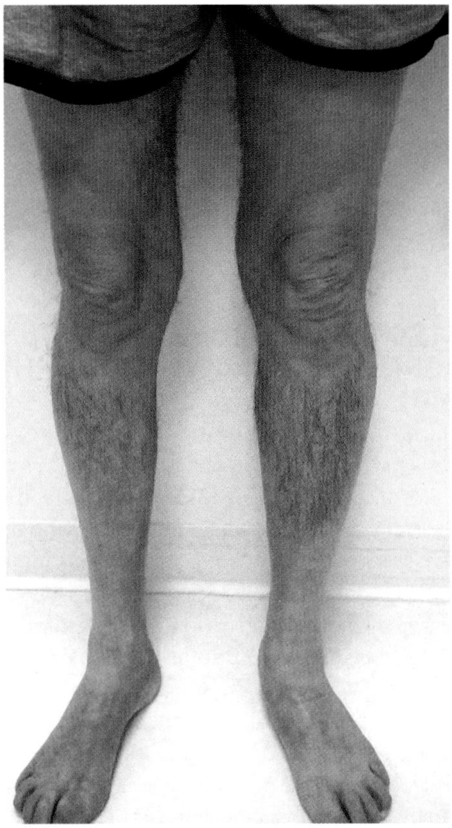

Figure 9-2. Right > left leg atrophy in a patient with childhood poliomyelitis with 2 years of insidiously progressive leg weakness due to PPMA.

following recovery from the acute illness is a purported risk factor and is concordant with contemporary thinking regarding PPMA pathogenesis (see below).[56,57]

PPMA tends to affect muscles that were the most severely affected at the time of the acute illness (Fig. 9-2). Less frequently, PPMA may affect muscles, even patients, thought to have been clinically unaffected at the time of initial illness.[5] This theory is supported by the knowledge that 50–60% loss of motor neurons must occur before weakness is typically detected. Progressive atrophy and weakness in PPMA can affect virtually any limb, trunk, cranial or ventilatory muscle group. As with all MNDs, clinical involvement of extraocular muscles does not occur in either acute poliomyelitis or PPMA.

As mentioned, the progression in PPMA is insidiously slow. The decline in ventilatory function as been estimated to occur at an annual rate of 2%.[58] Limb muscle strength has been estimated to deteriorate at an annual rate of 1%.[49,59] One study when conducted for only 5 years failed to detect progression which became apparent only after the same cohort was observed for a lengthier period of time.[60,61]

The most common symptoms attributed to PPMA are fatigue, arthralgias, and myalgias; these are estimated to occur in greater than 80%, 70%, and 70% of patients respectively.[62] The more objective sign of PPMA, progressive weakness, is estimated to occur in 70–90% of patients in previously afflicted muscles and in 50–60% of patients in previously unaffected muscles.[62] Dysphagia is the most common bulbar symptom in PPMA patients, developing in approximately 30% of patients.[62] New symptoms attributable to ventilatory insufficiency occur in approximately 40% of patients, typically in those who had ventilatory problems during their acute illness.[62]

Some symptoms that patients with PPMA experience are readily understood. Fatigue has many potential causes directly or indirectly related to the initial illness including declining strength, development of sleep apnea or reactive depression, or declining ventilation. The latter may be the result of PPMA affecting ventilatory muscles or chest wall restriction due to kyphoscoliosis. Both obstructive and central sleep apnea are prevalent in the PPMA cohort.[63] Sleep-disordered breathing occurs most commonly in patients with previous bulbar polio.[64] Hypopharyngeal muscles, normally relaxed during rapid eye movement (REM) sleep, may further weaken as a consequence of the late effects of polio and contribute to airway obstruction. Both aging and reduced exercise capacity related to the acute illness predispose to deconditioning and weight gain which undoubtedly play a role in sleep-disordered breathing as well. Central sleep apnea is likely to represent an adverse late effect on neurons within the breathing center in the brainstem reticular formation.

Other symptoms such as depression, anxiety, and nonspecific pain occur frequently in the postpolio cohort and are less readily attributable to direct effects of prior poliomyelitis.[5] Arthralgias and myalgias are estimated to occur in approximately 40–80% of PPMA patients.[65] Musculoskeletal complaints are readily understandable. Joint pains are likely related to accelerated degenerative joint disease resulting from years of imbalanced forces brought to bear on joints resulting from weakness of stabilizing muscle groups. Adhesive capsulitis secondary to joint immobility is another logical cause of joint discomfort. Myalgias are equally understandable in muscles overworked in their attempts to accomplish the same amount of work with a diminishing number of motor units. Cold intolerance is also readily attributable to declining muscle mass and muscle activity in addition to the effects of advancing age. Acrocyanosis may occur and is presumably due to loss of neurons within the intermediolateral cell column during the acute illness.

Other symptoms are more difficult to attribute to the known pathology of polio.[5,61] Impaired concentration and the ability to process information with the usual speed are complaints sometimes voiced by postpolio patients. This may result as an indirect effect of impaired sleep patterns or CO_2 retention. Alternatively, physicians should be cognizant that adverse psychological effects can result from late polio. Patients' sense of well-being can be seriously undermined by their realization that their muscles are weakening and that they may be losing control of a disease with which they had formerly believed that they had achieved an equilibrium.

DIAGNOSIS AND DIFFERENTIAL DIAGNOSIS

The diagnostic criteria for PPMA are straightforward. They include a history of illness consistent with acute poliomyelitis, chronologically related evidence of motor neuron loss identified either clinically or electrodiagnostically, and a history supportive of at least partial recovery of strength and function in the months following the acute illness. As mentioned, a hiatus between initial illness and subsequent development of fatigue and progressive weakness measured in years is required. Signs and symptoms of PPMA have been reported to begin as early as 8 years after the initial illness or as late as 71 years, with an average of 35 years. Lastly, other rational differential diagnostic considerations must be excluded.[59]

The most relevant exclusionary considerations in PPMA are other MNDs, particularly ALS. With the increased prevalence of PPMA in the 1970s, it was proposed that new weakness in paralytic polio patients might represent ALS, implying that prior polio represented an ALS risk factor.[59] Longitudinal observations in PPMA patients that include slow rates of progression and absence of upper motor neuron (UMN) features have put this hypothesis to rest. Nonetheless, poliomyelitis is not ALS protective and prior PP victims developing ALS have been reported, and have raised the secondary question as to whether ALS in these patients represents reactivation of the poliovirus.[66,67] At least one postmortem study suggests that this is not the case.[66]

Identification of ALS in a prior polio victim may be challenging. Arguably, an accelerated rate of progression atypical of PPMA is the most distinctive clue. UMN findings are understandably unlikely to develop in previously atrophic and weak limbs. Their development in previously unaffected limbs represents the other major clinically distinguishing tool.[67] Fasciculations may occur in both ALS and PPMA although they are less common in the latter.[5] There are differences between the serologic, EDX, and pathologic profiles in ALS and PPMA patients but these are relative and not pathognomonic.[67] These will be discussed in the laboratory section below.

Any disorder that may produce painless weakness must be considered in a prior polio victim who is getting weaker and evaluated for if the pattern of weakness or rate of progression is atypical for PPMA. These are outlined in detail in the differential diagnosis of ALS in Chapter 6 and include disorders of muscle such as inclusion body myositis (IBM), disorders of neuromuscular transmission such as myasthenia, other MNDs such as benign focal amyotrophy and Kennedy disease, and multifocal motor neuropathy.

In view of the nonspecific nature of many complaints offered by aging PPMA patients such as fatigue, it is prudent to consider and address other common systemic causes of these symptoms by performance of a careful general examination and relevant testing before attributing these symptoms to PPMA. In addition, patients with prior PP are likely to be at greater risk of compressive mononeuropathies and monoradiculopathies than an age-matched population, suggesting a need for a greater index of suspicion for these potentially treatable disorders in this population.

LABORATORY FEATURES

There are two potential goals of laboratory testing in patients with prior paralytic polio, to identify those who have developed PPMA, and to distinguish PPMA from other disorders that might mimic it. Regarding identification of PPMA, there are no definite serologic, EDX, or pathologic means by which to distinguish patients with prior paralytic polio who have transitioned into PPMA from those who have not.[68] There are conflicting opinions as to whether an elevated level of serum CK discriminates between these two groups.[69,70] EDX evidence of ongoing denervation appears to occur with equal prevalence in both symptomatic and asymptomatic patients with PP.[68,71] The same holds true for muscle biopsy where the pathologic hallmark of acute denervation, angulated and atrophic muscle fibers seen either individually or in groups, is evident in both groups.[71] Identification of PPMA is therefore made largely on clinical grounds.

There is an EDX distinction between PPMA and ALS but it is largely quantitative rather than qualitative. Large MUAPs may occur in both disorders but in view of the rate of disease progression and limitations of reinnervation in ALS, are unlikely to exceed 8 mV in amplitude in this disorder. This information is of limited value; however, as there are no MUAP characteristics that confirm ALS in a patient with prior PP.[67] In addition, the absence of extremely large MUAPs in the 15–25-mV range do not preclude a diagnosis of PPMA.[67] Features of active denervation and unstable neuromuscular transmission such as fibrillation potentials, MUAP variability, decremental responses to slow repetitive stimulation, and increased jitter measurements although more prevalent in ALS, occur in PPMA as well.[67] The presence and degree of elevated serum CK levels also appear to be a poor discriminator between patients with PPMA and ALS.[70] We do not routinely recommend routine muscle biopsy in PPMA patients. When performed, there are characteristics that would aid in distinguishing between PPMA and ALS. Atrophic fibers that are angular in their morphology are seen in both disorders as is type grouping, although large groups are not typical of ALS.[67] (Fig. 9-3) CSF biomarkers have been suggested as a potential mechanism to identify PPMA patients.[72]

HISTOPATHOLOGY

Muscle biopsy in PPMA invariably demonstrates evidence of denervation and reinnervation. Type grouping of both

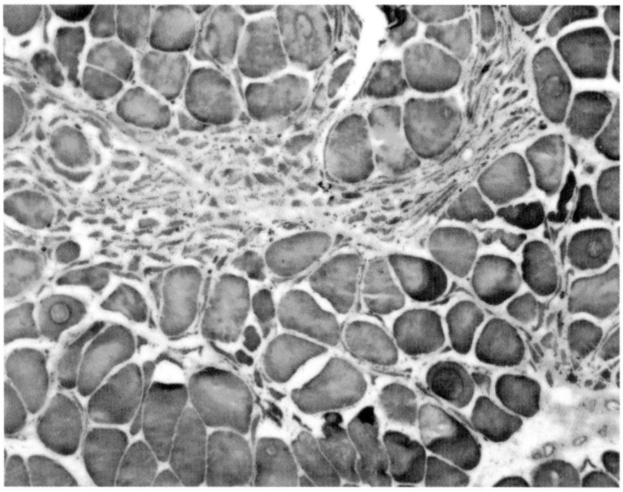

Figure 9-3. Quadriceps muscle biopsy [modified Gömöri trichrome at low (40X) power] demonstrating large group atrophy from patient in Figure 9-2.

type 1 and type 2 fibers occur. Group size may be extremely large with as many as 200 fibers of the same group bunched together.[5,67] Other neurogenic features such as pyknotic nuclear clumping, grouped atrophy, and isolated angular, atrophic fibers may be seen.[49] Like all chronic denervating diseases, "myopathic" features such rare pockets of endomysial inflammation, increased internal nuclei, and myofiber vacuolization are occasionally evident.[5,73] The spinal cord pathology of patients with PPMA demonstrates the fairly nonspecific findings of perivascular lymphocytic infiltrates, neuronal atrophy, and gliosis proportionate to the degree of neuronal loss.[5]

PATHOGENESIS

Differing opinions persist as to the cause of delayed and slowly progressive weakness in patients with prior AFP from poliomyelitis. The three most popular theories are an increased risk of premature death of enlarged motor units, persistent poliovirus infection, and an immune mediated mechanism.[62] In our opinion, the enlarged motor unit theory is the most credible. Observations suggest that the largest motor units, those associated with large fiber-type grouping and the most extensive collateral reinnervation, are the motor units most susceptible to premature failure and death.[68] It is logical to believe that the demands placed on these enlarged motor units over time, or with excessive exercise as mentioned above, would predispose them to a premature demise. It is also logical to believe that loss of these larger motor units would lead to a more notable loss in strength than would loss of a normal motor unit during the normal aging process.

There is evidence that poliovirus and other picornaviruses may persist in the CNS of animals.[19] The evidence that this occurs in humans and is the mechanism behind PPMS is limited. Perhaps the most convincing evidence comes from a study that detected the poliovirus genome through PCR technology in over half of the PPMA patients but in none of their controls.[74] The majority of studies, however, have been negative or inconclusive in this regard.[62] To the best of our knowledge, there has been no unequivocal pathologic evidence of the poliovirus genome or evidence of persistent infection in PPMA patients.[5,66] The support for a potential autoimmune mechanism stems in large part from pathologic evidence identifying inflammation in the absence of an infectious agent.[62] Oligoclonal bands and inflammatory cytokines in the CSF have been inconsistently reported.[61]

TREATMENT

The management of PPMA is largely supportive. A high index of suspicion is required to identify issues not directly related to the late effects of polio that may have specific and effective treatments. Much of the morbidity of PPMA is related to impaired mobility that may benefit from bracing, durable medical equipment, or the judicious use of orthopedic procedures. The reader is referred to Chapter 5 for more detailed information. Symptomatic treatment of bulbar and ventilatory symptomatology follows the principles outlined in Chapter 6. Secretion clearance issues may be improved upon by hydration, expectorants, suction, oscillating vests, and cough-assist devices. Swallowing issues may be addressed by attention to the consistencies and size of food ingested, head position during swallowing, and eventually by the provision of percutaneous gastrostomy. Ventilatory issues, particularly at night, may benefit from positive airway pressure, usually delivered noninvasively (BiPAP) but occasionally delivered through tracheostomy-assisted mechanical ventilation. Diaphragmatic pacing, recently approved by the FDA for selected ALS patients, provides a theoretical but unproven benefit for PPMA patients as well.

► MND AND MALIGNANCY

Malignancy can adversely affect the nervous system through numerous mechanisms. Although relatively uncommon and often controversial, a number of neuromuscular syndromes, usually but not always dominated by LMN features, have been associated with malignancy and its treatments.[75] These include ALS and all of its subtypes including PMA and PLS, neurolymphomatosis, paraneoplastic motor neuropathy, multifocal motor neuropathy, subacute motor neuronopathy, GBS, and stiff-person syndrome (SPS).[76-80] Although LMN syndromes have been described in association with both solid tumors and hematologic malignancies, perusal of existing literature would suggest that the most frequent association and widest phenotypic diversity occur with lymphoma.[75–77,79,80–83]

The motor neuron disorders described in this chapter, particularly those related to neoplasia, are rare in comparison to the more common degenerative or hereditary disorders. Practical guidelines that would help neurologists to decide when and how to look for underlying malignancy in ALS patients would be helpful. It has been historically suggested that the presence of a monoclonal protein in the serum or urine, a CSF protein value of >75 mg/dL or oligoclonal banding in the spinal fluid should prompt a search for lymphoma in an MND patient.[75] This strategy is no longer frequently employed by most specialists as its ability to identify a treatable condition is minute.[77] Alternatively, knowledge of the phenotypes and behaviors of these uncommon syndromes and the features that distinguish them from more common MNDs provide another means to identify patients who would be most likely to benefit from a more intense search for an underlying tumor.

RADIATION MYELOPATHY

Radiation therapy was first recognized in 1948 as an uncommon cause of an acquired LMN disorder. There are numerous case reports or reviews describing this syndrome.[53,80,84–94] Radiation-induced motor neuron disease (RIMND) occurs most commonly in association with prophylactic radiation of lower thoracic and lumbar fields for testicular tumors.[80,91] The phenotype may be more representative of the selective vulnerability of motor neurons or ventral roots in the lumbosacral region, rather than the focus of radiation, as RIMND confined to the lower extremities has been described in individuals receiving whole neuraxis radiation.[89] Its incidence appears to increase with radiation dosage, most reported cases having occurred in individuals receiving 40 Gy or more.[91] The authors' perception is that RIMND occurs or is reported less frequently now in comparison to the past which may reflect dose reduction, refinement in radiotherapy technique, or recognition that the concept is no longer novel.[88] The syndrome may also affect other body regions after radiation of the neck, thorax, or abdomen, but is distinctly uncommon, with neurologic injury being more commonly myelopathic in these conditions.[92,93]

Clinical onset is typically delayed for months or more, commonly years following treatment.[80] The disease often progresses for a period of time within the distribution of affected nerve elements, only to plateau and stabilize in many cases.[80,91] Painless weakness is the predominant symptom. It is often monomelic at onset, evolving into an asymmetric, paraparetic distribution affecting multiple nerve and nerve root distributions. It is, commonly associated with amyotrophy, cramps and fasciculations lending clinical support to an anterior horn localization. The presence of radiation dermatitis probably increases the likelihood that the neurologic syndrome in the appropriate topographic area is causally related. Sensory and genitourinary involvement is notable for its absence in most but not all reports. When present however, sensory symptoms typically represent a delayed and minor component, often with preserved SNAPs in the symptomatic distribution.[91]

The diagnosis of RIMND is based predominantly on a typical phenotype occurring in the appropriate clinical context, coupled with the exclusion of other nonradiation induced motor neuron syndromes. Localization to motor neurons (or ventral roots/motor nerves) is presumed through combination of clinical and EDX assessment. CSF examination may be normal or demonstrate a mild elevation in protein.[88,89,91]

The EDX features of RIMND are similar to other MNDs. Sensory conductions in involved segments are normal, supporting an anterior horn cell, ventral root, or motor nerve localization.[84] CMAPs are reduced proportionate to the degree of involvement of the analogous spinal cord segment. Needle electromyography demonstrates the usual features of both ongoing denervation (fibrillation potentials and positive waves) and chronic denervation and reinnervation (reduced recruitment of MUAPs that are increased in amplitude and duration). The demonstration of myokymic discharges on EMG has been described in some but not all cases.[86,91]

The implication that RIMND is an anterior horn cell disease is also supported by in vitro studies suggesting disproportionate vulnerability of anterior cells to radiation.[86] Others have argued that RIMND is more properly termed a polyradiculopathy based on imaging and pathologic evidence. Ventral root enhancement on MRI has been reported in some but not all cases.[91] Rare reports of autopsied cases support this conclusion, demonstrating thickening, nodularity, and hemorrhagic discoloration in nerve roots but no abnormalities within the spinal cord.[91] Conversely, others have reported chromatolysis of anterior horn cell.

Regarding the mechanism, it has been hypothesized that radiation may allow for reactivation of a latent virus with predilection for anterior cells, analogous to poliomyelitis. To the best of our knowledge, there is no data to support this theory.[89] The pathologic demonstration of hyalization of blood vessels in response to radiation, particularly in nerve roots, suggests a chronic ischemic mechanism.[91] Selective vulnerability of Schwann cells to radiation as demonstrated in vitro may potentially contribute to disease pathogenesis.[95] Chemotherapy does not appear to play a role.[91]

There is no recognized effective treatment for RIMND. In view of the consideration that vaso-occlusive disease is the basis of nerve injury, attempted treatments have included anticoagulants, and hyperbaric oxygen in addition to immunomodulating agents such as corticosteroids and d-penicillamine.

PARANEOPLASTIC MND

Paraneoplasia is estimated to cause no more than 1% of neurologic syndromes occurring in patients with malignancy.[78] In general, paraneoplastic syndromes are more common in solid tumors than in hematologic malignancies and are more likely to affect the central rather than the peripheral nervous system. One apparent exception to this generalization is an LMN syndrome. Although rare, and historically controversial, MND appears to be the most common paraneoplastic manifestation of lymphoma affecting the peripheral neuromuscular system.[75,82] Conversely, lymphoma appears to be the tumor most commonly associated with a paraneoplastic LMN syndrome.[82] Although paraneoplastic syndromes associated with lymphoma and CNS disorders may be commonly associated with Ma or Tr antibodies, LMN syndromes occurring in association with lymphoma have yet to be associated with a reproducible, paraneoplastic antibody.[82]

Paraneoplastic LMN syndromes may occur in isolation as described above or may represent one component of a multisystem paraneoplastic syndrome. This usually occurs within the context of encephalomyelitis (PEM), often associated with the Hu antibody in CSF and/or serum. In one series, 20% of 71 patients with anti-Hu (+) PEM patients had a recognized LMN component.[96] In further support of the existence of a paraneoplastic LMN syndrome is the knowledge that these Hu antibodies cross react with malignancy and with motor neurons.[83] Although the majority of reported cases of paraneoplastic MNDs preferentially affected LMNs, other motor neuron syndromes (e.g., ALS, PLS, and SPS) have been described as paraneoplastic syndromes as well.[75,78,79] A relationship between ALS and cancer has been long debated.[97] This association has been particularly emphasized in lymphoproliferative disorders. Currently the association is considered coincidental although a prevalence of cancer of up to 8–10% in an ALS population has been reported.[98,99] The SPS phenotype frequently overlaps with PLS with the exception of a more typically indolent course in PLS. These paraneoplastic PLS/SPS cases may be associated with breast cancer or lymphoma and amphiphysin antibodies.[79,100]

Paraneoplastic MNDs may respond to successful treatment of the underlying neoplasm in some cases.[80] Insufficient evidence exists to adequately predict treatment responsiveness in these rare syndromes.

SUBACUTE MOTOR NEURONOPATHY

Subacute motor neuronopathy (SMN) is another presumed MND associated with Hodgkin's or non-Hodgkin's lymphoma and/or their treatments.[101] Although first described in single case reports, the most comprehensive description was provided by a review of 10 cases in 1979. Eighty percent of these cases had been radiated. Most, but not all, had received differing chemotherapy regimens as well. Subacute motor neuronopathy appears to differ from RIMND in three notable ways, the type of underlying malignancy, the phenotype, and the natural history.

Like RIMND, the pattern of weakness in subacute motor neuronopathy is notable for its asymmetry. Unlike RIMND, the distribution appears to be more generalized. It may begin in the arms and frequently affects the upper extremities and neck muscles in addition to the legs. At least one of the originally described cases had prominent UMN signs suggesting ALS, although on autopsy, these clinical findings were likely explicable by the demonstration of superimposed progressive multifocal leukoencephalopathy.[101] Differing natural histories also distinguish subacute motor neuronopathy from RIMND. Subacute motor neuronopathy is characterized by a period of initial progression followed by stabilization. After months or years, significant improvement and even normalization of patient strength may occur.

CSF analysis in subacute motor neuronopathy may either be normal or demonstrate a modest elevation in protein levels. Reported EDX patterns are typical of MND. Nerve biopsy results, when reported, are normal further supporting an anterior or nerve root localization. Muscle biopsy in reported cases uniformly describe the neurogenic features of angular atrophy in individual fibers and/or in small groups. The pathologic findings in autopsied cases have not been uniform which is understandable in view of the complex nature of the described cases with their associated confounding variables. In both cases in which autopsied findings were described however, the construct of an MND was supported by significant cell loss in the anterior horns with associated ventral root atrophy. Remaining motor neurons often demonstrated angular atrophy of anterior horn cells, and clumped Nissl substance or eosinophilic staining within them. As SMN patients are immunosuppressed, there is increased theoretical vulnerability of infection from organisms with tropism for anterior horns. For this reason, it is important to note reported absence of microgliosis or any evidence of inflammation or superimposed infection in anterior horns in SMN patients.[101]

OTHER LMN SYNDROMES ASSOCIATED WITH MALIGNANCY

There are a number of neuromuscular syndromes that typically affect the peripheral nerve, root, or plexus rather than the anterior horn cell that are usually readily distinguishable from MND based on clinical or EDX patterns. On certain occasions, these other syndromes may have LMN predominance making the distinction more difficult. For sake of completeness, these disorders will be briefly mentioned here. GBS appears to occur more frequently in certain malignancies, particularly lymphoma.[78] In one of its forms, acute motor axonal neuropathy, there is little or no sensory involvement which could confound the distinction from an MND. Neurolymphomatosis, that is, infiltration of peripheral nerve by lymphoma, is predominantly associated with non-Hodgkin lymphoma. Typically, there is associated pain and sensory loss. The phenotype is variable extending from a progressive mononeuropathy to regional neuropathy syndromes such as a radiculoplexopathy to a more generalized polyneuropathy that undoubtedly represents a confluent, multifocal neuropathy.[76,102–104] Polyradiculopathy may occur from neoplastic meningitis from both solid tumors, lymphoma and leukemia. It may also occur as a result of certain infections with predilection for nerve roots such as varicella zoster or cytomegalovirus in immunosuppressed individuals. It has also been suggested that the syndrome of multifocal motor neuropathy may occur in patients with lymphoma.[105]

▶SUMMARY

This chapter addresses the MNDs that are neither inherited nor degenerative in etiology. Although poliomyelitis, the most notorious of these disorders, is hopefully a disorder of largely historical domestic interest, neurologists and physiatrists remain responsible for the care of many of the disease's victims. In addition, other less prevalent virions have the same apparent affinity for anterior horn cells and the capability of producing an identical or near-identical syndrome of AFP. Consequently, neurologists should remain aware of both the acute and the chronic features of these "other MNDs" of infectious and noninfectious etiology.

REFERENCES

1. Alexander LN, Seward JF, Santibanez TA, et al. Vaccine policy changes and epidemiology of poliomyelitis in the United States. *JAMA*. 2004;292:1696–1701.
2. Jerath A, Reddy C, Jerath N, Johnson RT. Poliomyelitis. 2009 www.medlink.com.
3. Plum F. Sensory loss with poliomyelitis. *Neurology*. 1956;6: 166–172.
4. Foley KM, Beresford RH. Acute poliomyelitis beginning as transverse myelopathy. *Arch Neurol*. 1974;30:182–183.
5. Dalakas MC. Pathogenetic mechanisms of post-polio syndrome: morphological, electrophysiological, virological, and immunological correlations. *Ann N Y Acad Sci*. 1995;753:167–185.
6. Wyatt HV. Poliomyelitis in hypogammaglobulinemics. *J Infect Dis*. 1973;128:802–806.
7. Wright PF, Hatch MH, Kasselberg AG, Lowry SP, Wadlington WB, Karzon DT. Vaccine-associated poliomyelitis in a child with sex-linked agammaglobulinemia. *J Pediatr*. 1977;91: 408–412.
8. Mehrabi Z, Shahmahmoodi S, Eshraghian MR, et al. Molecular detection of different types of non-polio enteroviruses in acute flaccid paralysis cases and healthy children, a pilot study. *J Clin Virology*. 2011;50(2):181–182.
9. Dias AP, Tavares FN, Costa EV, da Silva EE. Evaluation of a protocol for rapid diagnosis of enterovirus associated with acute flaccid paralysis cases. *J Clin Virology*. 2009;46(4):337–340.
10. Kincaid O, Lipton HL. Viral myelitis: An update. *Curr Neurol Neurosci Rep*. 2006;6(6):469–474.
11. Johnson RT, Cornblath DR. Poliomyelitis and flavivirus. *Ann Neurol*. 2003;53(6):691–692.
12. Ghosh JB, Roy M, Lahiri K, Bala AK, Roy M. Acute flaccid paralysis due to rabies. *J Pediatr Neurosci*. 2009;4(1):33–35.
13. Verma A, Berger JR. ALS syndrome in patients with HIV-1 infection. *J Neurol Sci*. 2006;240:59–64.
14. Quereshi M, Bedlack RS, Cudkowicz ME. Lyme serology in amyotrophic lateral sclerosis. *Muscle Nerve*. 2009;40:626–628.
15. Kornreich L, Dagan I, Gunebaqum M. MRI in acute poliomyelitis. *Neuroradiology*. 1996;38:371–372.
16. Haq A, Wasay M. Magnetic resonance imaging in poliomyelitis. *Arch Neurol*. 2006;63(5):778.
17. Jubelt B, Gallez-Hawkins G, Narayan O, Johnson RT. Pathogenesis of human poliovirus infection in mice. I. Clinical and pathological studies. *J Neuropathol Exp Neurol*. 1980;39: 138–148.
18. Erb IH. Pathology of poliomyelitis. *Can Med Assoc J*. 1931;25 (5):547–551.
19. Ford DJ, Ropka SL, Collins GH, Jubelt B. The neuropathology observed in wild-type mice inoculated with human poliovirus mirrors human paralytic poliomyelitis. *Microb Pathog*. 2002;33:97–107.
20. Fuchs A, Cella M, Giurisato E, Shaw AS, Colonna M. Cutting edge: CD96 (tactile) promotes NK cell-target cell adhesion by interacting with the poliovirus receptor (CD155). *J Immun*. 2004;172:3994–3998.
21. Koopman FS, Uegaki K, Gilhus NE, Beelen A, de Visser M, Nollet F. Treatment for post-polio syndrome. *Cochrane Database Syst Rev*. 2011;(2):CD007818.
22. Walid MS, Mahmoud FA. Successful treatment with intravenous immunoglobulin of acute flaccid paralysis caused by West Nile virus. *Perm J*. 2009;13(3):43–46.
23. Jeha LE, Sila CA, Lederman RJ, Prayson RA, Isada CM, Gordon SM. West Nile virus infection: A new acute paralytic illness. *Neurology*. 2003;61:55–59.
24. Lanska DJ. West Nile virus. http://www.medlink.com 2011.
25. Al-Shekhlee A, Katirji B. Electrodiagnostic features of acute paralytic poliomyelitis associated with West Nile virus infection. *Muscle Nerve*. 2004;29:376–380.
26. Hassin-Baer S, Kirson ED, Shulman L, et al. Stiff-person syndrome following West Nile fever. *Arch Neurol*. 2004;61:938–941.
27. Flaherty ML, Wijdicks EF, Stevens JC, et al. Clinical and electrophysiologic patterns of flaccid paralysis due to West Nile virus. *Mayo Clin Proc*. 2003;78:1245–1248.
28. Leis AA, Stokic DS, Webb RM, Slavinski SA, Fratkin J. Clinical spectrum of muscle weakness in human West Nile virus infection. *Muscle Nerve*. 2003;28:302–308.
29. Sejvar JJ, Haddad MB, Tierney BC, et al. Neurologic manifestations and outcome of West Nile virus infection. *JAMA*. 2003;290:511–515.
30. Sejvar JJ. West Nile virus and "poliomyelitis". *Neurology*. 2004; 63:206–207.
31. Leis AA, Stokic DS, Polk JL, Dostrow V, Winkelmann M. A poliomyelitis-like syndrome from West Nile virus infection. *N Engl J Med*. 2002;347(16):1278–1279.
32. Glass JD, Samuels O, Rich MM. Poliomyelitis due to West Nile virus. *N Engl J Med*. 2002;347(16):1280–1281.
33. Kelley TW, Prayson RA, Isada CM. Spinal cord disease in West Nile virus infection. *N Engl J Med*. 2003;348:564–566.
34. Li J, Loeb JA, Shy ME, et al. Asymmetric flaccid paralysis: A neuromuscular presentation of West Nile virus infection. *Ann Neurol*. 2003;53:703–710.
35. Park M, Hui JS, Bartt RE. Acute anterior radiculitis associated with West Nile virus infection. *J Neurol Neurosurg Psychiatry*. 2003;74:823–825.

36. Roos KL. Fever and asymmetrical weakness in the summer: Evidence of a West Nile virus-associated poliomyelitis-like illness. *Mayo Clin Proc.* 2003;78(19):1205–1206.
37. Watson NK, Schneck MJ, Bartt RE, Ouff SA, Hayden MK, Beavis KG. Focal neurologic deficit as a frequent manifestation of West Nile virus infection. *Neurology.* 2003;60(Suppl1):A96–A97.
38. Petropoulou KA, Gordon SM, Prayson RA, Ruggierri PM. West Nile virus meningoencephalitis: MR imaging finding. *AJNR Am J Neuroradiol.* 2005;26(8):1986–1995.
39. Tyler KL, Pape J, Goody RJ, Corkill M, Kleinschmidt-DeMaster BK. CSF findings in 250 patients with serologically confirmed West Nile virus meningitis and encephalitis. *Neurology.* 2006;66(3):361–365.
40. Centers for Disease Control and Prevention. *Epidemic/epizootic West Nile virus in the United States: Guidelines for Surveillance, Prevention, and Control.* Fort Collins, CO: U.S. Department of Health and Human Services; 2003.
41. Roos KL. West Nile encephalitis and myelitis. *Curr Opin Neurol.* 2004;17(3):343–346.
42. Doron SI, Dashe JF, Adelman LS, Brown WF, Werner BG, Hadley S. Histopathologically proven poliomyelitis with quadriplegia and loss of brainstem function due to West Nile virus infection. *CID.* 2003;37:e74–e77.
43. Smit JM, Moesker B, Rodenhuis-Zybert I, Wilschut J. Flavivirus cell entry and membrane fusion. *Viruses.* 2011;3(2):160–171.
44. Chan-Tack KM, Forrest G. Failure of interferon alpha-2b in a patient with West Nile virus meningoencephalitis and acute flaccid paralysis. *Scand J Infect Dis.* 2005;37(11–12):944–946.
45. Anderson JF, Rahal JJ. Efficacy of interferon alpha-2b and ribavirin against West Nile virus in vitro. *Emerg Infect Dis.* 2002;8(1):107–108.
46. Lewis M, Amsden JR. Successful treatment of West Nile virus infection after approximately 3 weeks into the disease course. *Pharmacotherapy.* 2007;27(3):455–458.
47. Hayes EB, Sejvar JJ, Zaki SR, Lanciotti RS, Bode AV, Campbell GL. Virology, pathology, and clinical manifestations of West Nile virus disease. *Emerg Infect Dis.* 2005;11:1174–1179.
48. Cornil V, Lépine R. Sur un cas de paralysie générale spinale antérieure subaigue, suivi d'autopsie. *Gaz Med (Paries).* 1875;4:127–129.
49. Dalakas MC, Elder G, Hallett M, et al. A long-term follow-sup study of patients with post-poliomyelitis neuromuscular symptoms. *N Engl J Med.* 1986;314:959–963.
50. Codd MB, Mulder DW, Kurland LT, Berard CM, O'Fallon WM. Poliomyelitis in Rochester, Minnesota, 1935–1955: Epidemiology and long-term sequelae. A preliminary report. In: Halstead LS, Wiechers DO, eds. *Late Effects of Poliomyelitis.* Miami, FL: Symposia Foundation; 1985:121–134.
51. Windebank AJ, Litchy WJ, Daube JR, Kurland LT, Codd MB, Iverson R. Late effects of paralytic poliomyelitis in Olmsted County, Minnesota. *Neurology.* 1991;41:501–507.
52. Bruno RL. Post-polio sequelae: Research and treatment in the second decade. *Orthopedics.* 1991;14(11):1185–1193.
53. Mathis S, Dumas P, Neau JP, Gil R. Pure motor neuropathy, an uncommon complication of radiotherapy: Report of 3 cases and review of the literature. *Rev Med Interne.* 2007;28(6):377–387.
54. Halstead LS, Diechers DL, Rossi CD. Late effects of poliomyelitis: A national survey. In: Halstead LS, Wiechers DO, eds. *Late Effects of Poliomyelitis.* Miami, FL: Symposia Foundation; 1985:11–33.
55. Jubelt B, Cashman NR. Neurological manifestations of the post-polio syndrome. *Crit Rev Neurobiol.* 1987;3:199–220.
56. Klingman J, Chui H, Corgiat M, Perry J. Functional recovery; a major risk factor for the development of postpoliomyelitis muscular atrophy. *Arch Neurol.* 1998;45:645–647.
57. Trojan DA, Cashman NR, Shapiro S, Tansey CM, Esdaile JM. Predictive factors for post-poliomyelitis syndrome. *Arch Phys Med Rehabil.* 1994;75:770–777.
58. Bach JR, Alba AS, Bodofsky E, Curran FJ, Schulteiss M. Glossopharyngeal breathing and noninvasive aids in the management of post-polio respiratory insufficiency. *Birth Defects Orig Artic Ser.* 1987;23(4):99–113.
59. Mulder DW, Rosenbaum RA, Layton DD Jr. Late progression of poliomyelitis or forme fruste amyotrophic lateral sclerosis? *Mayo Clin Proc.* 1972;47:756–761.
60. Sorenson EJ, Daube JR, Windebank AJ. A 15-yr follow up of neuromuscular function in patients with prior poliomyelitis. *Neurology.* 2005;64:1079–1072.
61. Windebank AJ, Litchy WJ, Daube JR, Iverson R. Lack of progression of neurologic deficit in survivors of paralytic polio: A five-year prospective population-based study. *Neurology.* 1996;46:80–84.
62. Ramachandran TS, Ramachandran A, Johnson RT. Post-polio syndrome http://www.medlink.com 2011.
63. Guilleminault C, Motta J. Sleep apnea syndrome as a long-term sequela of poliomyelitis. In: Guilleminault C, ed. *Sleep Apnea Syndromes.* New York: Alan R Liss; 1978:309–315.
64. Siegel H, McCutchen C, Dalakas M, et al. Physiologic events initiating REM sleep in patients with the postpolio syndrome. *Neurology.* 1999;52:516–522.
65. Gawne AC, Halstead LS. Post-polio syndrome: Pathophysiology and clinical management. *Crit Rev Phys Rehabil Med.* 1995;7:147–188.
66. Roos RP, Viola MV, Wollmann R, Hatch MH, Antel JP. Amyotrophic lateral sclerosis with antecedent poliomyelitis. *Arch Neurol.* 1980;37:312–313.
67. Salajegheh M, Bryan WW, Dalakas MC. The challenge of diagnosing ALS in patients with prior poliomyelitis. *Neurology.* 2006;67:1078–1079.
68. Cashman NR, Maselli R, Wollmann RL, Roos R, Simon R, Antel JP. Late denervation in patients with antecedent paralytic poliomyelitis. *N Engl J Medi.* 1987;317(1):7–12.
69. Windebank AJ, Litchy WJ, Daube JR, Kurland LT, Codd MB, Iverson R. Late effects of paralytic poliomyelitis in Olmsted County, Minnesota. *Neurology.* 1991;41:501–507.
70. Nelson KR. Creatine kinase and fibrillation potentials in patients with late sequelae of polio. *Muscle Nerve.* 1990;13(8):722–725.
71. Ravits J, Hallett M, Baker M, Nilsson J, Dalakas MC. Clinical and electromyographic studies of postpoliomyelitis muscular atrophy. *Muscle Nerve.* 1990;13:667–674.
72. Gonzalez H, Ottervald J, Nilsson KC, et al. Identification of novel candidate protein biomarkers for the post-polio syndrome: Implications for diagnosis, neurodegeneration and neuroinflammation. *J Proteomics.* 2009;71(6):670–681.
73. Semino-Mora C, Dalakas MC. Rimmed vacuoles with beta-amyloid and ubiquitinated filamentous deposits in the muscles of patients with long-standing denervation (postpoliomyelitis muscular atrophy): similarities with inclusion body myositis. *Hum Pathol.* 1998;29(10):1128–1133.
74. Julien J, Leparc-Goffart I, Lina B, et al. Postpolio syndrome: Poliovirus persistence is involved in the pathogenesis. *J Neurol.* 1999;246(6):472–476.

75. Younger DS, Rowland LP, Latov N, et al. Lymphoma, motor neuron diseases, and amyotrophic lateral sclerosis. *Ann Neurol.* 1991;29:78–86.
76. Kelly JJ, Karcher DS. Lymphoma and peripheral neuropathy: A clinical review. *Muscle Nerve.* 2005;31:301–313.
77. Gordon PH, Rowland LP, Younger DS, et al. Lymphoproliferative disorders and motor neuron disease: An update. *Neurology.* 1997;48:1671–1678.
78. Rudnicki SA, Dalmau J. Paraneoplastic syndromes of the spinal cord, nerve, and muscle. *Muscle Nerve.* 2000;23:1800–1818.
79. Forsyth PA, Dalmau J, Graus F, Cwik V, Rosenblum MK, Posner JB. Motor neuron syndromes in cancer patients. *Ann Neurol.* 1997;41:722–730.
80. Rowland LP. Diagnosis of amyotrophic lateral sclerosis. *J Neurol Sci.* 1998;160(Suppl 1):S6–S24.
81. Stern BV, Baehring JM, Kleopa KA, Hochberg FH. Multifocal motor neuropathy with conduction block associated with metastatic lymphoma of the nervous system. *J Neurooncol.* 2006;78(1):81–84.
82. Briani C, Vitaliani R, Grisold W, Spectrum of paraneoplastic disease associated with lymphoma. *Neurology.* 2011;76:705–710.
83. Younger DS. Motor neuron disease and malignancy. *Muscle Nerve.* 2000;23:658–660.
84. Van den Berg-Vos RM, Van den Berg LH, Visser J, de Visser M, Franssen H, Wokke JH. The spectrum of lower motor neuron syndromes. *J Neurol.* 2003;250:1279–1292.
85. Greenfield MM, Stark FM. Post-irradiation neuropathy. *AJR Am Roentgenol.* 1948;60:617–622.
86. Lamy C, Mas JL, Varet B, Ziegler M, de Recondo J. Postradiation lower motor neuron syndrome presenting as monomelic amyotrophy. *J Neurol Neurosurg Psychiatry.* 1991;347:648–649.
87. Walton JN, Tomlinson BE, Pearce GW. Subacute "poliomyelitis" and Hodgkin's disease. *J Neurol Sci.* 1068;6:435–445.
88. Tallaksen CM, Jetne V, Fosså S. Postradiation lower motor neuron syndrome: A case report and brief literature review. *Acta Oncologica.* 1997;36(3):345–347.
89. Sadowsky CH, Sachs E, Ochoa J. Post-radiation motor neuron syndrome. *Arch Neurol.* 1976;33:786–786.
90. Horowitz SL, Stewart JD. Lower motor neuron syndrome following radiotherapy. *Can J Neurol Sci.* 1983;10:56–58.
91. Bowen J, Gregory R, Squier M, Donaghy M. The post-irradiation lower motor neuron syndrome neuronopathy or radiculopathy? *Brain.* 1996;119:1429–1439.
92. Malapert D, Brugieres P, Degos JD. Motor neuron syndrome in arms after radiation treatment. *J Neurol Neurosurg Psychiatry.* 1991;54:1123–1124.
93. Shapiro BE, Bordorf G, Schwann L, Preston DC. Delayed radiation-induced bulbar palsy. *Neurology.* 1996;46:1604–1606.
94. DeCarolis P, Montagna P, Cipulli M, Baldrati A, d'Alessandro R, Sacquegna T. Isolated lower motorneuron involvement following radiotherapy. *J Neurol Neurosurg Psychiatry.* 1986;49:718–719.
95. Cavanagh JB. Effects of x-radiation on the proliferation of cells in peripheral nerve during wallerian degeration in the rat. *Br J Radiol.* 1968;41:275–281.
96. Dalmau J, Graus F, Rosenblum, Posner JB. Anti-Hu associated paraneoplastic encephalomyelitis/sensory neuronopathy. A clinical study of 71 patients. *Medicine.* 1992;71:59–72.
97. Rowland LP. Paraneoplastic primary lateral sclerosis and amyotrophic lateral sclerosis. *Ann Neurol.* 1997;41(6):703–705.
98. Norris FR Jr, Engel WK. Carcinomatous amyotrophic lateral sclerosis. In: Brain WR, Norris FH Jr, eds. *The Remote Effects of Cancer on the Nervous System.* New York: Grune and Statton; 1965:24–34.
99. Gubbay SS, Kahana E, Zilber N, Cooper G, Pintov S, Leibowitz Y. Amyotrophic lateral sclerosis. A study of its presentation and prognosis. *J Neurol.* 1985;232:295–300.
100. McKeon A, Robinson MT, McEvoy KM, et al. Stiff-man syndrome and variants: Clinical course, treatments, and outcomes. *Arch Neurol.* 2012;69(2):230–238.
101. Schold SC, Cho ES, Somasundaram M, Posner JV. Subacute motor neuronopathy: A remote effect of lymphoma. *Ann Neurol.* 1979;5:271–287.
102. Viala K, Béhin A, Maisonobe T, et al. Neuropathy in lymphoma: A relationship between the pattern of neuropathy, type of lymphoma and prognosis. *J Neurol Neurosurg Psychiatry.* 2008;79:778–782.
103. Walk D, Handelsman A, Beckmann E, Kozloff M, Shapiro C. Mononeuropathy multiplex due to infiltration of lymphoma in hematologic remission. 1998;21:823–826.
104. Diaz-Arrastia R, Younger DS, Hair L, et al. Neurolymphomatosis: A clinicopathologic syndrome re-emerges. *Neurology.* 1992;42:1136–1141.
105. Noguchi M, Mori K, Yamazaki S, Suda K, Sato N, Oshimi K. Multifocal motor neuropathy caused by a B-cell lymphoma producing a monoclonal IgM autoantibody against peripheral nerve myelin glycolipids GM1 and GD1B. *Br J Haemotol.* 2003;123:600–605.

CHAPTER 10

Disorders of Motor Nerve Hyperactivity

Complaints referable to muscle such as pain, spasm, stiffness, fatigue and/or abnormal movements within a muscle are commonplace in the practice of medicine. As the cause is often elusive, both patients and physicians may become frustrated as many with these complaints will remain undiagnosed despite thorough investigation. There are many sources for this diagnostic elusiveness. With the exception of cramps and fasciculations, the disorders described in this chapter are uncommon. In addition, most of the disorders that will be described have nonspecific and overlapping clinical features. Successful diagnosis requires a heightened index of clinical suspicion, detailed knowledge concerning each disorder's phenotypic characteristics, and awareness of the serologic and electrodiagnostic (EDX) features of each syndrome.

Motor nerve hyperactivity disorders frequently result in reduced exercise intolerance and impaired mobility. They originate from numerous central and neuromuscular system localizations. This chapter will restrict itself to disorders thought to originate from motor nerves and the upper motor neurons that control them. Cramps, fasciculations, tetany, tetanus, the cramp–fasciculation syndrome (CFS), Isaacs syndrome (IS), Satoyoshi syndrome, stiff person syndrome (SPS) and hyperekplexia will all be discussed. As the differential diagnosis of many of these disorders overlaps, the majority of the differential diagnostic considerations will be primarily emphasized in the first section devoted to muscle cramping.

Historical writings on motor nerve hyperactivity disorders have been potentially confusing. Different names have been used for the same syndrome. Nomenclature to describe clinical observations has overlapped with that used to describe frequently associated electromyographic waveforms. In an attempt to avoid this, and as neurologists deeply appreciative of history and those who created it, we will be preferentially referring to these syndromes by their eponyms whenever appropriate. We will also follow the suggestion of Gutmann et al.[1] by using a single term (e.g., fasciculations, myokymia) to refer to clinically observed phenomenon and refer to EDX waveforms as potentials or discharges (e.g., fasciculations potentials, myokymic discharges).

▶ CRAMPS, FASCICULATIONS, AND THE CRAMP–FASCICULATION SYNDROME

CLINICAL FEATURES

Cramps refer to a sudden, involuntary, and painful shortening of an entire muscle belly accompanied by a squeezing sensation and visible, palpable muscle induration. As cramps tend to incorporate multiple if not all the motor units in one or more muscles, they typically generate sufficient force to induce abnormal posturing of relevant joints. Cramps are characteristically relieved by massage or stretching. They have a tendency to recur if the muscle is prematurely returned to its unstretched position. They will spontaneously remit within minutes in most cases.

Cramps occur commonly. Their prevalence in a "normal" population is estimated at 35% in one study and in 95% of young, healthy people who recently initiated exercise in another.[2,3] Their prevalence is increased in the elderly, in pregnant females, and subsequent to exercise in those who have recently begun unaccustomed activity. Cramps are a considerable source of morbidity for afflicted individuals, particularly if nocturnal. In the majority of cases however, they are unassociated with serious disease and considered benign. Benign cramps are most prevalent in the calf. Familial cramp syndromes have been reported.

Pathologic cramps as a symptom of an underlying neuromuscular disease occur less frequently. Although potentially representative of nerve or nerve root diseases, their most notorious if not frequent association is with the motor neuron diseases (MND). Cramps may represent an early symptom in amyotrophic lateral sclerosis (ALS) X-linked bulbospinal atrophy or multifocal motor neuropathy.[4,5] In MND, they are frequently mentioned in passing and represent a minor component of the illness in most but may represent a significant source of morbidity in some. Like fasciculations, they tend to dissipate as the disease progresses.

In general, benign cramps occur at rest or following exercise. In our experience, cramping provoked by manual muscle testing occurs with some regularity in MND patients. Exertional cramping during protracted or intense exercise is more typically associated with metabolic muscle disease and has been reported as an uncommon phenotype of Becker muscular dystrophy.[6]

Fasciculations, unlike cramps, represent the discreet, random contraction of the muscle fibers in an individual motor unit. Unlike cramps, the patient may not be aware of them. As fasciculations represent activation of a single motor unit, movement at a relevant joint is uncommon. In our experience, if movement at a joint if occurs, it tends to be seen in situations where reinnervated and enlarged motor units act on a small joint, for example, the first dorsal interosseous on the metacarpophalangeal joint of the index finger. Fasciculations, when occurring in isolation, are typically benign. Characteristics of benign fasciculations are their tendency to occur repetitively for seconds at a single site, in a single muscle.[6] Fasciculations occurring in multiple locations in one muscle or multiple muscles simultaneously is disconcerting as is the concomitant finding of weakness, atrophy or hyperreflexia.

Cramps and fasciculations occurring in concert are also a cause for concern and increase the likelihood of an underlying neuromuscular disease, particularly when not localized to a singular muscle like the calf. This association may suggest CFS in which patients experience myalgias, cramps, stiffness, myokymia, and fasciculations that occur in some combination. The symptoms of CFS are frequently provoked by exercise and promote exercise intolerance. Eight of nine initially reported cases were considered vocationally disabled.[7] In our estimation, CFS may be conceptualized as a limited expression of IS with which it may share not only clinical but serologic and/or electrophysiologic features.[8,9] Further support for the association is provided by the observation that some patients with CFS have features of an encephalopathy analogous to Morvan syndrome, an IS variant.[10]

DIAGNOSIS AND DIFFERENTIAL DIAGNOSIS

Muscle cramps remain a largely clinical diagnosis dependent for the most part on patient description. Differential diagnostic strategies are twofold: (1) to distinguish cramps from other causes of unwanted muscle contraction and pain and (2) to identify an underlying cause for the cramping. Cramps represent one of many potential causes of myalgia or muscle pain.

The differential diagnosis of cramps includes disorders originating from the central nervous system (CNS) and other neuromuscular locations. Although the mechanism of unwanted muscle activation is not fully understood in many of the following disorders, it may be accurate to conceptualize neural disorders of involuntary muscle contraction as positive events resulting from a lower threshold for nerve activation or prolonged depolarization. In contrast, myopathies producing unwanted muscle contraction may be considered as a negative phenomenon, that is, a failure of muscle relaxation after voluntary activation. Myopathies capable of producing involuntary muscle contraction, myalgia or/and stiffness will be covered more extensively in later chapters of this text but will be briefly mentioned here for completeness.

Myotonia may be considered as the prototypic disorder of failed muscle relaxation. Myotonia differs from benign cramps in that it is typically painless and provoked by muscle activation. Myotonia is characterized by a completely different EDX signature, that is, myotonic as opposed to cramp discharges demonstrable with needle electromyography.

As described above, metabolic myopathies may produce unwanted muscle contraction, induration and myalgia by physiologic contracture. These inherited defects result in most cases from impaired glycogen or lipid metabolism, leading to muscle energy failure, and resulting in painful muscle shortening. Intense or protracted exercise is typically required to deplete readily available muscle fuel sources and provoke contractures. Physiologic contractures are also distinguished from cramps by their EDX signature of electrical silence which is also a feature of rippling muscle and Brody diseases.

Rippling muscle disease (RMD) is clinically defined by observation of wave-like rippling of muscles, typically provoked by muscle stretch or percussion. Patients may complain of muscle stiffness and muscle hypertrophy may be observed on examination.[11] RMD can be inherited in an autosomal dominant fashion caused by mutations of the caveolin-3 gene. The reader is referred to Chapter 27 for further discussion regarding the evaluation of the numerous phenotypes associated with mutations of this gene, including LGMD1 C. RMD may occur as an autoimmune disorder as well with clinical, EDX and serologic manifestations that overlap with other motor nerve hyperactivity disorders. This belief is based upon an apparent association with myasthenia gravis, thymoma and detection of autoantibodies such as acetylcholine receptor binding (AChRB), voltage-gated potassium channel (VGKC) or neuronal ganglionic acetylcholine receptor (NGAChR).[10–12] Unlike disorders of motor nerve hyperactivity, the EDX signature of rippling muscles is electrical silence. The EDX examination, however, may identify features of an underlying myopathy.[10,11] Patients with RMS typically have a 3–25-fold increase in their serum CK levels.[11]

Brody disease is another rare inherited myopathy producing physiologic contractures through disruption of calcium reuptake within the sarcoplasmic reticulum of muscle.[13–17] It results from a mutation in the in the fast-twitch skeletal muscle sarcoplasmic reticulum Ca–ATPase gene (*SERCA1*) in some but not all cases.[17,18] Its morbidity stems from impaired muscle relaxation that is exercise-induced, associated with stiffness affecting muscle of the limbs and face. A more detailed description may be found in the chapter describing the nondystrophic myotonias. Cold may aggravate the symptoms of Brody disease as it may aggravate the stiffness associated with myotonic disorders.

Malignant hyperthermia and neuroleptic malignant syndrome are other disorders resulting in unwanted muscle rigidity, typically recognized by associated signs and symptoms and the context in which they occur. Malignant hyperthermia is an inherited disorder and like Brody disease represents disordered sarcoplasmic reticulum function. The neuroleptic malignant syndrome appears to be related to dopaminergic receptor dysfunction, presumably within the CNS.

The palmaris brevis syndrome is characterized by a spontaneous, irregular, nonpainful contraction of the palmaris brevis muscle resulting in "wrinkling" motions of the palm.[19] It has been associated with C8-T1 radiculopathy, pathology of the deep branch of the ulnar nerve in Guyon canal, and occupational risk. The EDX features of the palmaris brevis syndrome have been reported as spontaneous rapid discharges of single MUAPs of normal morphology and myokymic discharges associated with normal motor and sensory conduction studies.

Focal dystonias such as writer's cramp produce unwanted muscle contraction and are uncomfortable although are typically not as painful as cramps. They are most readily identified by the characteristic activities that provoke them.

The characteristic features of all of these disorders are involuntary muscle contraction and the stiffness that may accompany it. Many of these disorders are accompanied by discomfort or pain. The differential diagnosis of disorders that are dominated by generalized or focal myalgias, unassociated with unwanted muscle contraction, stiffness and movement is far more extensive and exceeds the scope of this book. The reader is referred to an excellent review article on cramps for a comprehensive list of these conditions.[2]

The differential diagnosis of cramps also has to take into consideration whether the cramps are primary or secondary in their etiology. The latter is defined by their association with another underlying illness. Primary cramping occurs with the greatest frequency in calf and intrinsic foot muscles and as previously mentioned in older individuals, often at rest (particularly at night) or following unaccustomed exercise.[2] Volume depletion is generally considered a benign cause of cramping that may be related in turn to exercise, hemodialysis, emesis, diarrhea, and diuretic use.

Secondary cramping (Table 10-1) associates with a variety of toxic or metabolic disturbances and the MNDs. These associated conditions are identified through careful history taking, and by clinical, EDX, and judicious laboratory assessment. Metabolic conditions associated with cramping include hypoadrenalism, hypothyroidism, pregnancy, uremia, and cirrhosis. Cramps may also be hereditary in nature, either related or unrelated to a definable disease. Cramps may be provoked by a number of medications (Table 10-1). Finally, cramps and fasciculations are most commonly associated with disorders of anterior horn cells and to a lesser extent neuropathy and radiculopathy.[2]

TABLE 10-1. CAUSES OF MUSCLE CRAMPING, FASCICULATION, STIFFNESS[1]

By localization
- Spinal cord
  - Stiff-person syndrome
  - Tetanus
  - Demyelination (e.g., multiple sclerosis)
- Anterior horn cell diseases
  - ALS
  - X-linked bulbospinal muscular atrophy
  - Post-polio muscular atrophy
- Radiculopathy
  - Compressive—discogenic/spondylotic, tumor
  - Tumor infiltration
  - Nonstructural (e.g., diabetes mellitus, sarcoidosis, infection, radiation-induced)
- Nerve
  - Multifocal motor neuropathy
  - Cramp fasciculation syndrome
  - Tetany
  - Palmaris brevis syndrome
- Muscle
  - Brody disease
  - Myotonic disorders
  - Metabolic muscle diseases (glycogen storage, lipid storage, mitochondrial)
  - Dystrophinopathy
- Uncertain
  - Satoyoshi syndrome

By etiology
- Benign
  - Advanced age
  - Post-exercise
  - Pregnancy
- Metabolic
  - Hypothyroidism
  - Hypoadrenalism
  - Uremia
  - Cirrhosis
  - Dialysis
  - Dehydration with electrolyte loss
- Medication (common)
  - Diuretics
  - Cholesterol-lowering agents
  - β-adrenergic agonists
  - H2 receptor blockers
  - Nifedipine
  - Ethanol

LABORATORY FEATURES

The EDX evaluation of patients with suspected cramps is done primarily to exclude secondary causes of cramping such as MND or to identify other forms of spontaneous discharges that might suggest an alternative cause of motor nerve hyperactivity. The EDX signature of cramping is the cramp discharge, an involuntary, often irregular and "sputtering" discharge of multiple, normal appearing motor unit action potentials (MUAPs). Cramp discharges begin abruptly and fire at a collective frequency of up to 150 Hz.[20] Cramp discharges are most commonly encountered in normal individuals during activation of the gastrocnemius muscle. They are usually readily identifiable by both their morphologic characteristics and firing pattern. The discharges are made up of multiple, normal MUAPs. Like the cramp itself, the number of MUAPs contributing to the cramp discharge builds up and then dissipates. Fasciculation potentials may be recognizable both at the initial and terminal portions of cramp potentials.

In SPS and tetanus, the MUAP is typically less dense and more continuous without the aforementioned crescendo decrescendo pattern. A more commonly occurring potential EDX mimic of cramp potentials is normal, voluntarily activated MUAPs in patients who have an underlying tremor or are experiencing respiratory alkalosis related to anxiety or hyperventilation. MUAPs in this situation are also normal but differ as they are voluntarily activated and discharge in clusters. Once again, the similarities are based on waveform morphology, not firing pattern. End-plate potentials are the waveform most likely to be confused with cramp discharges based upon firing pattern. They discharge with the same sputtering pattern as cramp discharges but their waveform morphology is readily distinguishable.

The EDX signatures of other disorders of muscle induration and stiffness when symptomatic are typically distinctive. They include the electrical silence of the muscle diseases as described above, the myotonic discharges seen in the myotonic disorders, and the myokymic, grouped and neuromyotonic discharges characteristic of IS.

In a patient with true cramps, it would be reasonable to obtain blood for thyroid stimulating hormone (TSH), creatinine, magnesium, and calcium as well as to assess for orthostatic hypotension and serum potassium as screening tests for adrenal insufficiency. Genetic testing for familial forms of MND (ALS, pediatric and adult spinal muscular atrophy) may be considered if warranted by clinical and EDX context. An elevation in serum CK in a patient with cramping may be more confounding than helpful. If cramps are persistent, an elevation of serum CK may occur and may take 3–8 days to normalize.[21] This is important to recognize so as to not assume CK elevations in this setting implicate an underlying MND.

Fasciculation potentials are readily recognized electromyographically by their morphology and firing pattern. They are MUAPs that fire individually in a random fashion unlike those that are voluntarily activated (Fig. 10-1). Consecutive fasciculation potentials usually represent different motor units. Like fasciculations, the distinction between benign and pathologic fasciculation potentials is in a large part determined by the clinical and electrophysiologic company that they keep. Attempts to assign pathologic significance to fasciculation potentials based on their morphology has been described, but in our opinion is of more academic than pragmatic clinical interest.[22–24] Unlike many of the other

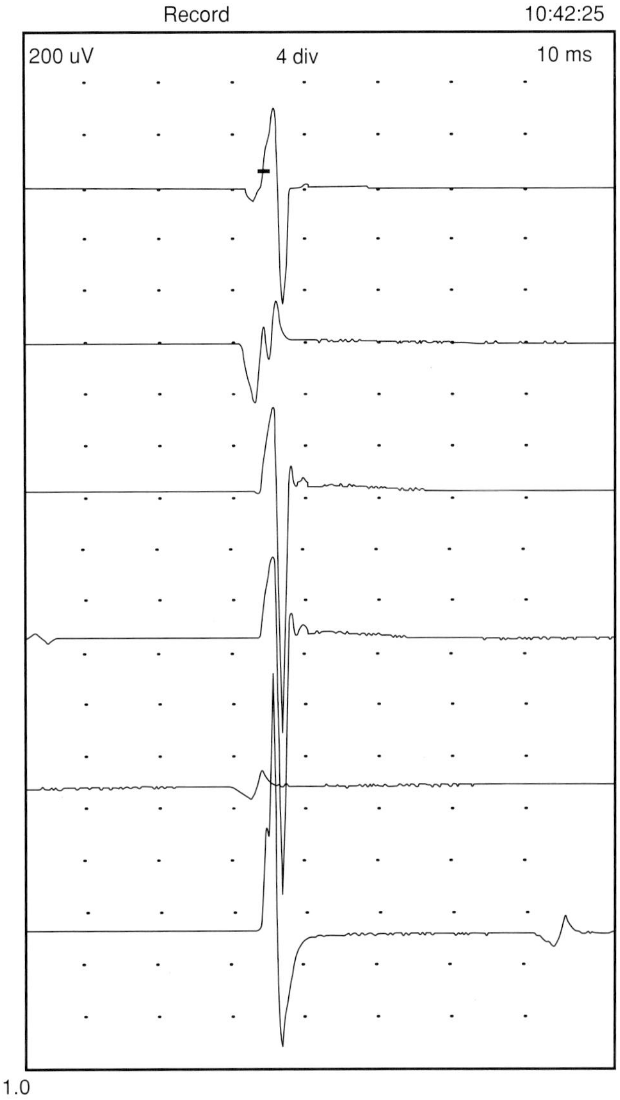

Figure 10-1. Fasciculation potential—single, random, and spontaneous discharges of normal appearing but differing motor unit action potentials.

disorders described in this chapter, fasciculations occurring in isolation do not appear to have an autoimmune etiology. In one study, no patient with benign fasciculations had autoantibodies directed against either the VGKC or NGAChR that may be found in other disorders of motor nerve hyperactivity described in this chapter.[10] Unless there is clinical or EDX suspicion of a secondary cause for fasciculations, no blood work is required.

The EDX findings in CFS include fasciculation potentials, cramp discharges, multiplets and even neuromyotonic discharges.[9] In addition, repetitive stimulation of peripheral nerves may produce afterdischarges in some cases in a manner similar to IS although the specificity of these afterdischarges has been called into question (Fig. 10-2).[8,25] Other EDX abnormalities including myokymic and complex repetitive discharges; fibrillation potentials and positive waves;

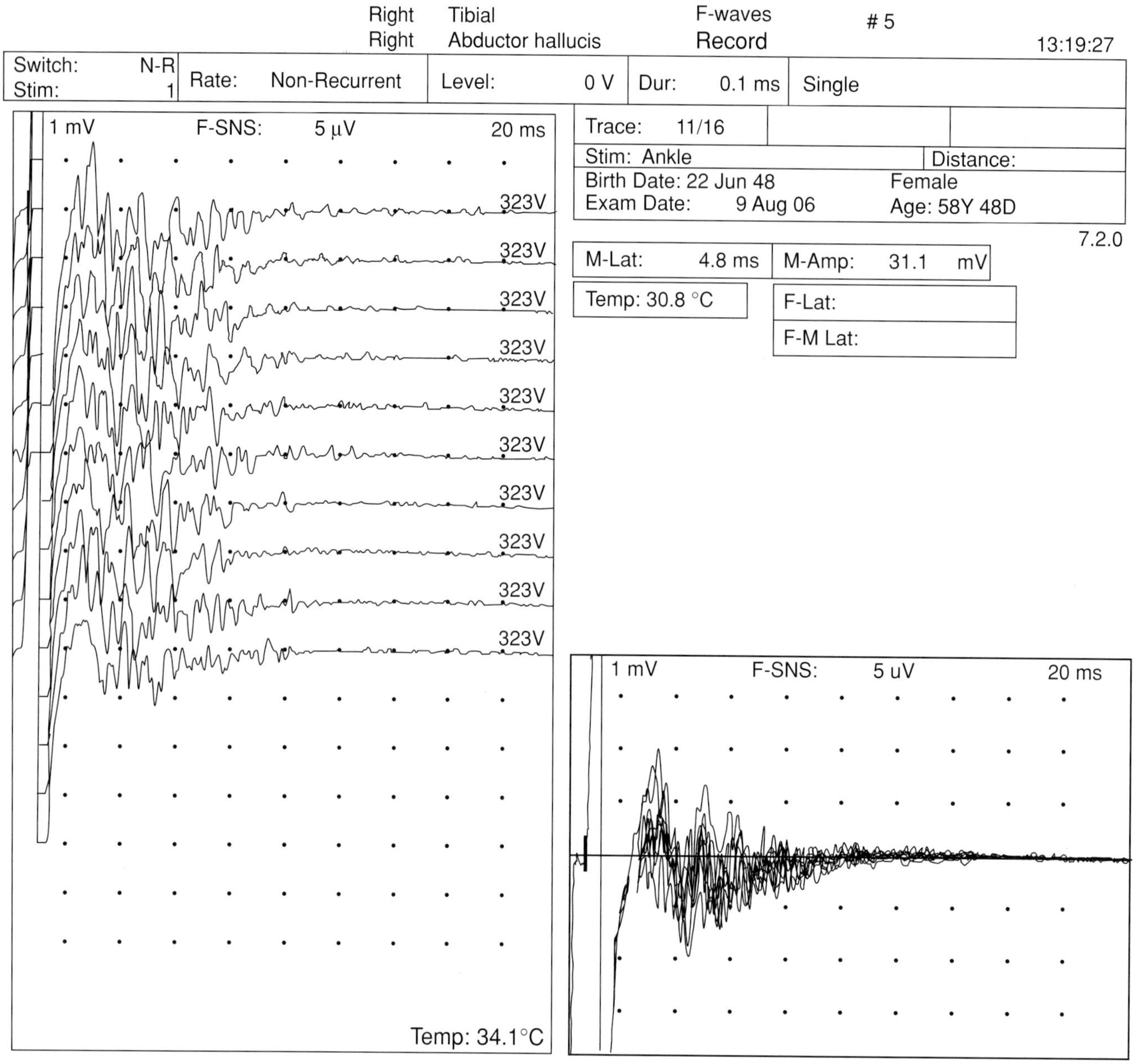

Figure 10-2. Rastered CMAPs from the tibial nerve in response to single stimuli resulting in repetitive afterdischarges. (Used with permission of Steven Vernino, MD, and Alpa Shah, MD, UT Southwestern Medical Center, Dallas, TX.)

and morphological changes of MUAPs suggesting chronic partial denervation and reinnervation are typically notable for their absence.[7,26] Patients with CFS may possess circulating VGKC (16%) or neuronal ganglionic NGAChR (6%) antibodies.[9,10,27–29]

In patients with complaints of cramps and/or fasciculations, it is our tendency to be conservative in our testing unless there are historical or examination features of concern. A family history suggestive of neuromuscular disease, visible fasciculations or other adventitious movements of muscle such as myokymia or muscle weakness/atrophy would be indications for EDX testing. We would reserve autoantibody testing for patients who complain of muscle stiffness in the absence of apparent extrapyramidal disease, particularly if associated with either clinical or EDX evidence of motor nerve hyperactivity such as widespread cramps or cramp potentials, fasciculations or fasciculation potentials, myokymia or myokymia discharges, spontaneously discharging high-frequency multiplets or neuromyotonic discharges.

HISTOPATHOLOGY

Patients with CFS may have features of neurogenic atrophy with muscle biopsy.[7] As neurogenic atrophy can be accurately and less invasively be predicted by electromyographic examination, and as muscle biopsy rarely identifies the etiology of the neurogenic condition, muscle biopsy is uncommonly performed in these patients.

PATHOGENESIS

The weight of experimental evidence supports a neurogenic origin for both cramps and fasciculations.[2] Specifically, the generator appears to be located within distal nerve terminals. There are a number of lines of evidence to support this. Cramps can be provoked in normal humans by repetitive stimulation of motor nerves distal to a complete, pharmacologically induced nerve block.[30] Cramps are often preceded and followed by fasciculation potentials implicating a shared generator. The waveform morphology of cramp potentials is that of MUAP. This does not preclude a CNS generator but diminishes the likelihood of a muscle or neuromuscular generator. Cramps may seemingly occur in a single muscle at any given time, sparing other muscles in the same myotome, making a CNS generator unlikely.

Even though cramps occur more commonly in patients who are pregnant or who exercise, no measurable metabolic differences have been identified in either group compared to those who do not experience cramping.[2] Cramping has been precipitated by infusion of hypotonic fluids implicating fluid or solute movement between extracellular and intracellular compartments as the causative mechanism.[2]

TREATMENT

Evidence to guide clinicians in the prevention and treatment of cramps is limited and may be reviewed in an American Academy of Neurology (AAN) evidence-based publication.[31] Prevention of cramping related to exertion and fluid loss can be attempted with the prophylactic use of salt tablets, hydration, and routine or pre-/post-exercise stretching. Successful prevention of cramps occurring under other circumstances may be achieved with the avoidance of offending drugs or when necessary, by using prophylactic medication.[2,31] Typically, these agents are dispensed preferentially at night, as sleep interruption is usually the most bothersome source of morbidity. Medications that have been used for this purpose are reviewed in Table 10-2. Of these, only quinine sulfate has achieved level A support as an efficacious treatment.[31]

Unfortunately, the FDA considers the use of quinine to be associated with unacceptable risk for any condition except malaria.[32] The incidence of serious side effects with quinine is estimated at 2–4%.[31] The official position of the AAN regarding quinidine, which can still be prescribed as Qualquin®, is that "select patients can be considered for an individual therapeutic trial once potential side effects are taken into account."[31] The AAN suggests that quinine be utilized in the setting of significant cramp morbidity and failure of other agents. Unfortunately, other agents possess only anecdotal or equivocal efficacy (Table 10-2).

The traditional approach to the treatment of symptomatic cramps if related to dehydration or exercise includes intravenous saline (not dextrose) solutions with electrolyte replacement.[2,31] An acute cramp can usually be aborted by stretching the involved muscle(s) although this will not necessarily prevent recurrence.

In our experience, patients who are psychologically troubled by an apparent benign fasciculation syndrome are reassured by providing them with a copy of the notable Mayo Clinic manuscript describing what is almost always a benign natural history.[33] Patients with CFS typically respond to treatment with anticonvulsants such as carbamazepine or phenytoin, again demonstrating similarities to IS.

▶ ISAACS SYNDROME OR NEUROMYOTONIA

This syndrome was first described by Denny-Brown in 1948.[34] Its eponym, IS, originates from the description of two patients by Isaacs in 1961 manifesting as progressive muscle stiffness associated with continuous muscle fiber activity.[35] IS or acquired neuromyotonia as it is commonly referred to, has also been referred to as the syndrome of continuous muscle fiber activity, normocalcemic tetany, armadillo disease, quantal squander, or generalized or undulating myokymia. Like many clinical syndromes associated with ion channel dysfunction, it may occur as either an autoimmune or a hereditary disorder. Autoimmune IS is the more common form of the disease, with or without an associated neoplasm (Table 10-3).[9,10,36,37]

CLINICAL FEATURES

IS may affect individuals of any age including neonates but is most commonly a disorder of adolescents and young adults.[38] The cardinal clinical feature is muscle stiffness, typically provoked by use, resulting from motor nerve hyperactivity and the associated involuntary and undesired muscle contraction.[2,9,27,35,36,41,42] A very characteristic feature is the adventitious movements that are observed in muscles, notably continuous muscle undulation or rippling (myokymia) and intermittent, focal muscle twitching (fasciculations).

The stiffness of IS has been referred to as pseudomyotonia. The use of this term is discouraged by the American Association of Neuromuscular and Electrodiagnostic Medicine and is considered ambiguous by many neuromuscular experts. Nonetheless, it is a term that is difficult to ignore in this context as pseudomyotonia has been used by many IS authors to describe a clinical phenomenon that mimics clinical myotonia. Pseudo-myotonia is distinguished from myotonia as pseudo-myotonic stiffness does not typically diminish with repetitive muscle use or during sleep and although provoked

▶ **TABLE 10-2. DRUGS UTILIZED IN THE TREATMENT OF CRAMPS**[2,31,192]

Drug	Dosage Range	Comments	Common or Serious Adverse Effects/Monitoring
Drugs where adequate trials have been performed suggesting efficacy			
Quinine sulfate	324 mg qhs	Level A support for efficacy FDA warning against off-label use of quinine products (cramps) "Should be avoided for routine use in the management of muscle cramps because of the potential of toxicity, but in select patients they can be considered for an individual therapeutic trial once potential side effects are taken into account."	1. Cinchonism (visual, auditory and GI symptoms, headache, fever) 2. Prolonged QT interval 3. Thrombotic thrombocytopenic purpura
Vitamin B complex	Including 30 mg pyridoxine	Level C support for efficacy	Lightheadedness Nausea Dyspepsia
Naftidrofuryl	300 mg bid	Level C support for efficacy	Not available in the United States
Diltiazem	30 mg qhs	Level C support for efficacy in frequency but not severity	No side effects reported at this dose
Drugs where trials have been performed suggesting inefficacy			
Gabapentin	3600 mg/day	Class 1 study	Lightheadedness Drowsiness Limb swelling
Vitamin E	800 U qhs	No benefit suggested	
Magnesium citrate	900 mg	Class 2 study—no benefit suggested	Diarrhea Lightheadedness Nausea Dyspepsia
Magnesium sulfate	300 mg	Class 2 study—no benefit suggested	Diarrhea Lightheadedness Nausea Dyspepsia
Drugs utilized without benefit of adequate trials			
Baclofen	20–80 mg day	No adequate trials	
Levetiracetam	500–1500 mg bid	Benefit in cramp frequency and severity in open label trial of ALS patients	
Verapamil	120 mg qhs	Benefit in cramp frequency in unblended elderly population	
Carbamazepine	200 mg bid–tid	Anecdotal benefit	Leukopenia Transaminitis Hyponatremia Vestibular symptoms
Phenytoin	300 qhs	Anecdotal benefit	Vestibular symptoms
Tocainide	200–400 mg bid	Anecdotal benefit	
Calcium	0.5–1 g qd	Anecdotal benefit	
Amitriptyline	25–100 mg qhs	Anecdotal benefit	Sedation Sicca symptoms Urinary retention
Benadryl	50 mg qhs	Anecdotal benefit	Sedation Sicca symptoms Urinary retention
Botulinum toxin	Varies	Reported benefit when injected locally	Local or distant weakness
Creatinine	12 mg prior to dialysis	Reported benefit in dialysis patients	No adverse effects reported

by muscle activation, is not provoked by muscle percussion.[36] Most importantly, unlike true myotonia, the unwanted muscle contractions of pseudo-myotonia are not associated with myotonic discharges. The involuntary contraction of pseudo-myotonia is associated with the spontaneous discharge of MUAPs in the form of one or more of the following: fasciculation potentials, myokymic discharges or erratic bursts known as multiplets. "Pseudomyotonia" often results in abnormal posturing mimicking the joint positioning of tetany such as carpopedal spasm, plantar flexion of the foot at the ankle,

TABLE 10-3. NEUROMYOTONIA/NEUROMYOTONIC DISCHARGES—SECONDARY CAUSES[74,191]

By localization
- Neuronopathies
  - ALS
- Neuropathies
  - Charcot–Marie Tooth disease
  - Guillain–Barré syndrome
  - Chronic inflammatory demyelinating polyneuropathy
  - Isaacs syndrome
- Disorders of neuromuscular transmission
  - Myasthenia gravis

By etiology
- Radiation
  - Brain
  - Head and neck
- Neoplasia
  - Small-cell carcinoma of the lung
  - Thymoma
  - Hodgkin disease
- Drugs
  - Penicillamine
- Immune mediated
  - Primary systemic sclerosis
  - Bone marrow transplantation
- Familial
  - Autosomal dominant neuromyotonia
- Amyloidosis

enhanced spinal curvature, facial grimacing, and flexion of the elbows, wrists, hips, and knee.[39,40]

In contrast to the SPS, adventitious movements are highly characteristic and these movements as well as muscle stiffness tends to be more generalized at onset, affecting the limb as well as trunk muscles. From an EDX standpoint, distal muscles are more likely than proximal muscles to display abnormal spontaneous discharges.[43] In addition to the continuous muscle fiber activity, muscle hypertrophy, hyperhidrosis, and weight loss are frequent concomitants, all of which may result from excessive muscular activity.[10] Symptoms of dysautonomia occur in as many as 93% of patients with concomitant CNS involvement (see below).[9,36,44]

The signs and symptoms of IS may be generalized or focal in distribution. In addition to the limbs and trunk, the tongue, face, and pharynx may be involved resulting in difficulty in speaking (hoarseness or dysarthria) and swallowing. Dyspnea, believed to result from stiffness of chest wall muscles, was a prominent symptom in Isaacs' initial cases.[35] Ocular neuromyotonia has been implicated as a cause of intermittent, spasmodic diplopia, occurring either spontaneously or in response to sustained eccentric gaze.[45–47] Ocular neuromyotonia may occur either as a component of the IS or as an isolated event following parasellar radiation. Involuntary finger flexion has also been described as an isolated manifestation of this syndrome.[48,49]

The physical examination of the IS patient may include observations of stiff posture with slight trunk flexion, shoulder elevation and abduction, and elbow flexion.[40] Widespread fasciculations and myokymia are seen and appear as continuous undulating or quivering of the underlying muscles.[50] These adventitious movements may be particularly prominent in the facial, pectoral, and calf muscles and may be provoked by muscle contraction. Pseudomyotonia, like myotonia may be demonstrable as delayed relaxation of eye or hand opening following forceful eye closure or a strong grip. Length-dependent sensory loss, weakness and reflex loss are indicative of axonal polyneuropathy which occurs in approximately a third of cases.[51–53] Diminished or lost deep tendon reflexes provide another distinguishing feature from the SPS. Muscle hypertrophy may be focal or generalized.[54] The trapezius muscles may appear particularly prominent when the patient is viewed from the front.[35] Chvostek and Trousseau signs may be appreciated despite normal calcium levels.[55,56]

IS may occur in association with other neurologic manifestations. Morvan syndrome, the most notable example of this, refers to CNS involvement occurring with peripheral neuromuscular hyperexcitability.[44] The encephalopathy of Morvan syndrome manifests as confusion, agitation, insomnia, amnesia, and hallucinations.[9,35,57,58] Seizures occur in approximately a third of cases.[44] To clarify terms, the phenotype of limbic encephalitis is considered synonymous with the CNS component of Morvan syndrome, the difference in the two disorders being the absence of peripheral manifestations (neuromyotonia) in limbic encephalitis.[59] Morvan syndrome occurs almost exclusively in males.[37,44] Despite its responsiveness to immunomodulating treatment in some cases, the natural history is variable. Cases associated with thymoma frequently have an unsatisfactory outcome.

Nonspecific complaints of numbness and paresthesia may represent either an axonal peripheral neuropathy that occurs with some frequency or persistent depolarization of sensory nerves.[44,51] The latter concept is supported by microneurographic recordings demonstrating the same spontaneous activity of sensory axons that occurs in their motor counterparts.[55] Neuropathic pain syndromes also appear linked to Morvan syndrome, with both overlapping clinical and serologic profiles.[44]

DIAGNOSIS AND DIFFERENTIAL DIAGNOSIS

The diagnosis of IS is established by the clinical features, supported by the characteristic EDX findings, and in many cases, the presence of autoantibodies. The differential diagnosis of IS needs to be considered in three domains: disorders that mimic the clinical phenotype, disorders that appear to occur at increased frequency in patients with either IS or Morvan syndrome and disorders that share the EDX features of the disorder (Table 10-3).

The differential diagnosis of IS consists largely of the other disorders discussed in this chapter, as well as those previously summarized in the cramps and fasciculations section. Causes of muscle stiffness that originate from the extrapyramidal system are beyond the scope of this book. The differential diagnosis of each of the EDX features that may be seen in IS patients (fasciculation potentials, cramp, myokymic and neuromyotonic discharges, multiplets) can be found in appropriate tables in Chapter 2.

It is somewhat difficult and artificial to distinguish diseases occurring at increased frequency in IS secondary causes of IS and secondary causes of neuromyotonic discharges. Myasthenia gravis has been reported to occur in 9% of patients with neuromyotonia. The vast majority of patients with myasthenia and neuromyotonia will have the traditional binding autoantibodies in their serum directed against the nicotinic acetylcholine receptor.[10] Neoplasms, particularly thymoma, may be found in as many as 40% of patients. Small cell carcinoma of the lung, Hodgkin lymphoma, and rarely plasmacytoma, ovarian, renal, bladder, and thyroid cancers occur as comorbidities in both IS and Morvan syndrome.[9,10,44,51,52,60–64] Like other paraneoplastic disorders, IS may precede the recognition of lung cancer by years.[27]

Neuromyotonic discharges do not occur as a universal feature of IS nor are they unique to this disorder. They can occur as a consequence of radiation injury to affected nerves.[45,46] Neuromyotonic discharges have been reported as an association with certain neuropathies, particularly those with strong demyelinating characteristics such as Charcot–Marie–Tooth disease, Guillain–Barré syndrome, and chronic inflammatory demyelinating polyradiculoneuropathy. They have been rarely described in association with ALS, amyloidosis, and rattlesnake envenomation as well as disorders also felt to have autoimmune mechanisms such as primary systemic sclerosis, systemic lupus, celiac disease, bone marrow transplantation, graft versus host disease, and penicillamine therapy.[9,36,40,55–76] Autosomal dominant heritable neuromyotonia has been described.[76]

LABORATORY FEATURES

An autoimmune basis for Isaacs and Morvan syndromes is strongly supported by the recognition that VGKC antibodies occur in both the serum and cerebrospinal fluid (CSF) in many of these patients.[9,27,44,77,78] These autoantibodies have been demonstrated in 54% of IS patients and 79% of Morvan syndrome patients.[10,44] Although these antibodies appear to be most closely associated with these two disorders, they may occur with many other neurologic phenotypes including limbic encephalitis.[79,80] Other neuronal and often paraneoplastic antibodies (notably NGAChR, CRMP-5, amphiphysin, and antinuclear neuronal type 4 have been identified in a small portion of the Isaacs and Morvan syndrome patients.[10] Patients may have other markers of autoimmunity including increased protein, immunoglobulins, and oligoclonal bands within the CSF.[9] Serum abnormalities including elevated CK levels in IS and hyponatremia in Morvan syndrome .[44,51,80]

Motor and sensory nerve conduction studies (NCS) are often normal in patients with the idiopathic or familial form of IS although may indicate a concomitant polyneuropathy in some patients.[9,40,42,55,56,81–83] If one looks closely however, repetitive afterdischarges are often evident following standard motor conduction and F-wave studies similar to what may be identified in organophosphate poisoning (Fig. 10-2).[76,84] Microneurographic recordings demonstrate afterdischarges in sensory as well as motor nerve fibers.[54]

Multiple potential types of abnormal EDX spontaneous activity characterize IS.[9,43,75,82,85,86] Neuromyotonic, myokymic or cramps discharges, fasciculation or fibrillation potentials and positive sharp waves may occur individually or in combination.[9,43] One of the most characteristic EDX signatures of IS are spontaneous bursts of grouped MUAPs known as multiplets.[43] These are similar in appearance to myokymic discharges but are distinguished by their random rather than semi-rhythmic discharge pattern and by their faster intraburst frequency. Myokymic discharges typically have slower intrabursts discharge frequencies. The discharge frequency is always <150 Hz and is more typically in the 40–80 Hz range.[87] Although there is some overlap, the intraburst discharge frequency of multiplets is typically higher and overlaps with the neuromyotonic discharge range, reaching 350 Hz in some cases.[43]

Neuromyotonic discharges, the EDX signature of IS, is a term that was presumably coined to recognize both their neural origin and their association with the clinical phenomenon of pseudomyotonia.[1] As previously mentioned, they are neither a particularly sensitive or specific for Isaacs syndrome. They may be found in any muscle including those of the face and extraocular muscles.[26,86] These discharges are provoked by needle movement or muscle contraction. They represent high-frequency discharges of single MUAPs that occur at random intervals with intradischarge frequencies of greater than 150 Hz and up to 500 Hz or intraspike intervals in the 2–5 ms range.[87] They cannot sustain themselves at these frequencies and rapidly dissipate in a decrescendo pattern.[87] It is this decrescendo pattern that distinguishes them from multiplets. They begin and end abruptly with a duration measured in seconds (Fig. 10-3). The resultant sound has been described as "pinging" or likened to the scream of a Formula 1 engine.

Myokymic discharges are seen at a greater frequency in IS than neuromyotonic discharges.[40] Their distinction from neuromyotonic discharges may be artificial in that each individual burst of discharges are felt to originate from motor nerve and are constituted from individual MUAPs.[1] Myokymic discharges are considered different from neuromyotonic discharges by their intraburst frequency as described above, by their firing pattern, and by the diseases they associate with. They are defined and recognized as spontaneously firing grouped discharges that occur in a repetitive, semi-rhythmic pattern

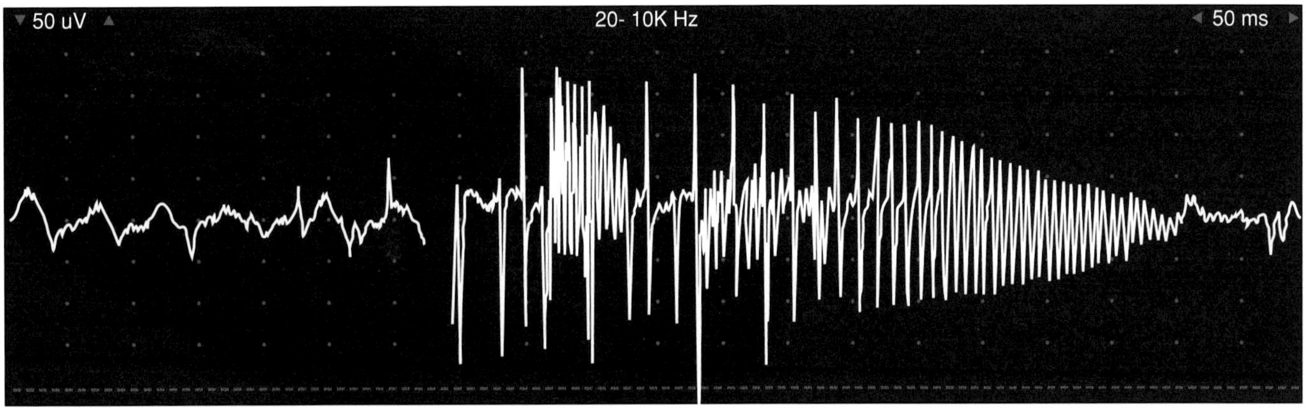

Figure 10-3. Neuromyotonic discharge—abrupt onset, high frequency and high pitched, and rapidly dissipating. (Used with permission of Devon Rubin, MD, Mayo Clinic, Jacksonville, FL.)

with intervening periods of electrical silence (Fig. 10-4), thus differing from the singular decrescendo burst of a neuromyotonic discharge. Their intradischarge frequency is considerably slower than neuromyotonic discharges.[26] The associated sound has been likened to troops marching in unison.

The EDX of IS as described in the literature focuses on abnormal spontaneous activity. In part, this is because the abnormal spontaneous discharges may obscure the visualization of voluntarily activated MUAPs. MUAP analysis may also be confounded by the coexistence of either peripheral neuropathy or myasthenia. MUAPs in IS may be normal or may fire in multiplets, in a manner reminiscent of tetany.[23]

MR imaging of the brain in Morvan syndrome is typically normal whereas positron emission tomography (PET) scanning routinely demonstrates focal or generalized hypometabolism.[44] Elevated CSF protein levels, lymphocytic pleocytosis, and/or oligoclonal banding are found in approximately half of Morvan syndrome patients.[44] Imaging of the chest is recommended to address the potential for thymoma, lung cancer, or lymphoma.

HISTOPATHOLOGY

Neither nerve nor muscle biopsy are routinely performed in suspected IS cases. If performed, sural nerve biopsies may be normal or reveal evidence of a concomitant neuropathy with a reduction in myelinated fibers numbers or evidence of demyelination.[55] Grouped atrophy and fiber-type grouping that may be demonstrable on muscle biopsy is also consistent with a peripheral neuropathy.[56,88–90] Histopathologic evidence of an inflammatory myopathy has been reported.[51]

PATHOGENESIS

IS is a disorder that appears to originate from terminal nerve twigs or the neuromuscular junction.[36] Neuromyotonic discharges are abolished by curare or botulinum toxin and persist following general or spinal anesthesia, and in most cases, proximal nerve block.[9,36,91] In some cases however,

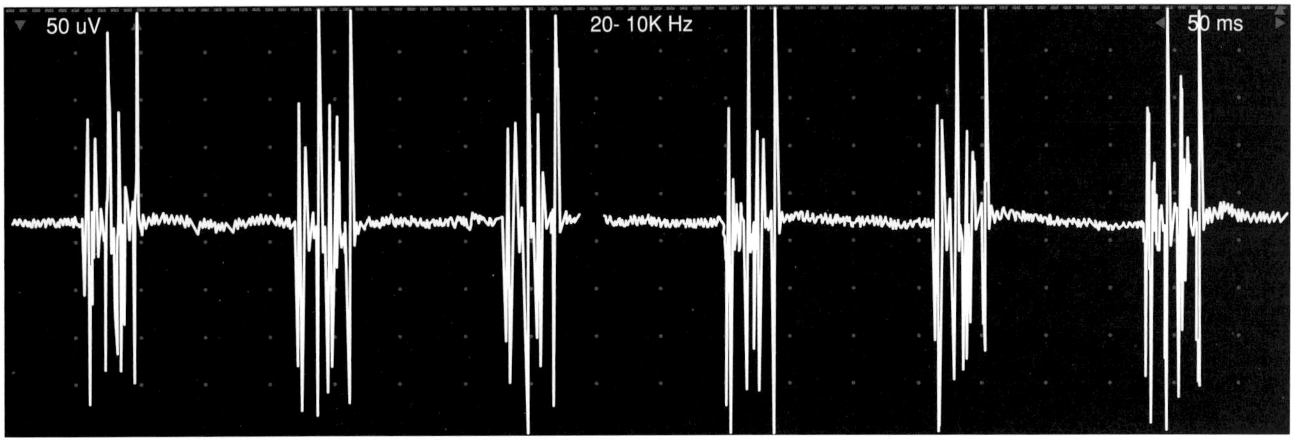

Figure 10-4. Myokymic discharges—semirhythmic-grouped discharges. (Used with permission of Devon Rubin, MD, Mayo Clinic, Jacksonville, FL.)

discharges appear to originate from more proximal aspects of nerve.[36,83,86,90,92,93] These observations would be consistent with the presumed autoimmune mechanisms described below as antibodies would have the greatest access to nerve at terminal twigs and roots where the blood–nerve barrier is least well established. The observation that neuromyotonic discharges have been reported to occur in both acquired and hereditary demyelinating neuropathies begs the question as to whether ephaptic transmission may facilitate the generation of these discharges. Conversely, the prevalence of axonopathy in IS provokes the syllogistic question as to whether the axonopathy promotes or results from the peripheral nerve hyperexcitability of neuromyotonia.[51]

The demonstration of VGKC antibodies in the serum and CSF of IS patients in 1995 and reinforced in numerous subsequent publications have provided both incontrovertible evidence of autoimmunity and a potential pathophysiological explanation for peripheral nerve hyperexcitability.[9,36,78,80,94] Blocking these ion channels, localized to the juxtaparanodal region of both PNS and CNS axons reduces the hyperpolarizing effect of channel activation, preventing the nerve action potential from dissipating and leading to retrograde depolarization of certain terminal twigs and reactivation of other terminal twigs belonging to the same motor unit.[36,59,95]

Initial experiments demonstrated that divalent VGKC antibodies appeared to accelerate and degrade potassium channels by a cross-linking mechanism independent of complement.[96] Subsequent observations however, have shown that VGKC autoantibodies do not appear to directly adversely affect potassium channels although do reduce potassium channel current amplitude after prolonged exposure.[59] Other more specific target antigens that indirectly influence potassium channel function in Isaacs and Morvan syndrome patients have been sought for and found. These include contactin-associated protein-like 2 (CASPR2), leucine-rich glioma inactivated (LGi1), and contactin-2 antigens.[44,80,97] These have been referred to as VGKC-complex proteins.[80] CASPR2 appears to concentrate VGKC in the juxtaparanodal regions of both peripheral and CNS axons. CASPR2 autoantibodies may lead to potassium channel dysfunction through impaired clustering and appears to be the principle antigenic target in neuromyotonia.[97] LGl1 on the other hand appears to be the principle antigenic target in limbic encephalitis. That it localizes to specific brain regions in experimental animals may well explain the selected vulnerability of certain neuronal populations and the nature of the characteristic clinical manifestations of Morvan syndrome.[44]

Support for the clinical observations of paresthesias, sensory neuropathy, or neuropathic pain syndromes in IS patients comes from passive transfer experiments that have demonstrated increased quantal content and repetitive firing of dorsal root ganglia cells in mice injected with sera from patients with IS.[78]

TREATMENT

Various forms of immunotherapy have partial efficacy in patients with IS. There is no standard algorithm. As a general rule, treatment protocols couple symptomatic treatment with immunosuppression. Plasma exchange (PLEX) and intravenous immunoglobulin (IVIG) are generally considered to have a faster onset of action than oral immunomodulating drugs. Although either may be effective, there is a general consensus that PLEX is the more effective of the two in IS. Azathioprine or corticosteroid treatment are usually utilized in addition in an attempt to avoid the inconvenience and cost associated with maintenance IVIG or PLEX.[9,81,98–102] Rituximab may be a reasonable option in refractory cases of Isaacs syndrome; this may be more cost-effective than frequent maintenance courses of IVIG or PLEX, but one needs to consider the small but consequential risk of infection, including progressive multifocal leukoencephalopathy.

Symptomatic treatment with antiepileptic medications that block sodium channels such as phenytoin or carbamazepine or decrease neuronal excitability through other mechanisms (e.g., baclofen, mexiletine, valproic acid, and gabapentin) may provide some measure of symptomatic relief.[9,76,82,84,89] As in other autoimmune diseases, patients may seemingly enter a period of protracted remission following treatment, require prolonged maintenance therapy, or succumb if treatments are ineffective or complications of the disease ensue.

▶ TETANUS

CLINICAL FEATURES

Despite their entirely different causes and mechanisms, both tetanus and tetany are derived from the Greek word for spasm, that is, tetanos. Like the SPS, tetanus is a disorder of sustained muscle rigidity with superimposed painful spasms. The natural history of tetanus consists of an incubation period varying from a few days to weeks with a mean of 8 days.[103] A shorter duration between exposure and symptom onset portends the development of severe disease with intense spasms and bulbar symptoms. Once begun, the clinical manifestations tend to progress for 10-14 days. If the patient avoids secondary complications of the illness and survives, recovery typically begins approximately a month after symptom onset and is often complete. However, the mortality rate may be as high as 30% particularly in neonates, in older patients with co-morbidities, and in locations where supportive medical care may be limited.[104]

The clinical manifestations of tetanus are dependent upon the inoculation site (if identifiable), the extent of toxin spread, and the patient's premorbid immunization status.[103,104] Tetanus may begin and remain local in proximity to the wound site producing "local" or "cephalic" tetanus. This is a somewhat artificial distinction as the majority of these patients will progress to a generalized form of the disease. If the disease remains localized, for example, as monomelic rigidity, the diagnosis may be difficult. Cephalic tetanus may mimic one or more cranial nerve palsies, the effects of which may include laryngospasm with associated breathing and phonation difficulties, dysphagia, as well as impaired extraocular movement and pupillary function. Evidence of muscle overactivity provides a helpful clue as to the cause of these symptoms which more commonly occurs with diseases that produce muscle weakness.

In generalized tetanus, the initial symptoms that typically precede the development of the more recognizable spasms are nonspecific, including irritability, akathisia, diaphoresis, and tachycardia.[105] The most distinctive symptom of tetanus is painful muscle spasms that more often than not begin either near the wound or in the masseter or facial muscles. The former, trismus or lockjaw is the disease's most notorious manifestation. Trismus may be provoked by tactile stimulation of the posterior pharyngeal wall, a reflex thought to represent both a sensitive and a specific bedside test. Involvement of muscles innervated by the facial nerve may produce a characteristic facial posture known as risus sardonicus, resulting from contraction of muscles that straighten the normal bowed appearance of the upper lip (Fig. 10-5).

Paraspinal and abdominal muscles are the next groups that are most commonly affected and may contribute to ventilatory insufficiency or mimic an abdominal emergency. In severe cases, violent stimulus-induced spasms may produce opisthotonus, a dramatic overarching of the back along with a fisted posture of the hands (Fig. 10-6). If the limbs are involved, proximal more than distal muscles are typically involved, severe generalized cases or local involvement in proximity to the wound site representing potential exceptions. Spasms are often triggered by an emotional or sensory stimuli, or by attempted patient movement.[103,104]

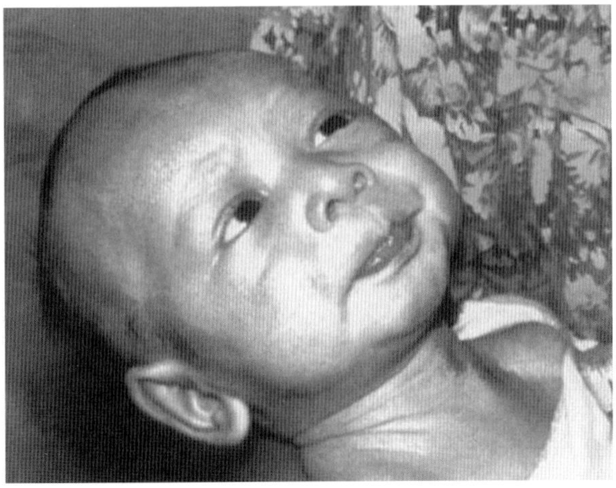

Figure 10-5. Risus sardonicus in infantile tetanus. (Used with permission of the Immunization Action Coalition, St. Paul, MN.)

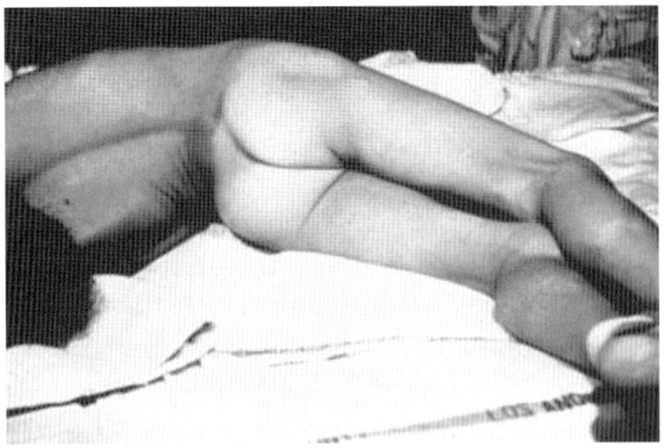

Figure 10-6. Opisthotonus. (Used with permission of the Immunization Action Coalition, St. Paul, MN.)

Dysautonomia, primarily expressing itself through excessive adrenergic influence, manifests as hypertensive crises, arrhythmia, and hyperhidrosis.[103,104] Prominent sialorrhea may contribute to airway compromise. Fever occurs commonly. Alteration of consciousness represents an effect of hypoxia. The sensorium otherwise, if accessible, remains clear. The offending tetanus toxin (tetanospasmin) does not cause permanent neurologic injury. Complete recovery may occur if the patient can be spared from hypoxic and other secondary consequences of the disease.

Uncommonly, tetanus may result from anaerobic infection of the middle ear or paranasal sinuses.[103,104] This may result in "local" tetanus, producing trismus as well as motor cranial nerve dysfunction as described, potentially including ophthalmoparesis. Tetanus may also proliferate in the uterus and represents a feared complication of parturition or abortion in nonhygienic facilities.

Neonatal tetanus is predominantly a disease of underdeveloped countries.[103,104] It typically originates from an umbilical stump infection in a child born of an unimmunized mother. Local customs that include application of substances to the umbilical stump that unknowingly harbor spores may contribute to risk of the disease. Symptom onset is typically within the first 2 weeks of life, manifesting as a poorly feeding infant with prominent muscle twitching. Changes in cranial musculature provide valuable clues. The jaw may clamp tight on a finger placed in the mouth. The upper lip stiffens, the eyelids are closed tightly, and the forehead is continuously wrinkled. Mortality in neonatal tetanus is high. Neonatal tetanus accounted for two-thirds of the 300,000 deaths attributed to tetanus worldwide in the year 2000.[105]

DIAGNOSIS AND DIFFERENTIAL DIAGNOSIS

Tetanus is diagnosed by the characteristic clinical manifestations including trismus and reflex spasms occurring in an inadequately immunized individual, chronologically associated with a potentially responsible source of infection. Eliciting trismus by a provocative, tactile pharyngeal stimulus, referred to as the spatular test, is felt to be a sensitive screening mechanism. It is estimated that *Clostridium tetani* can be cultured from wounds in a third of cases if deep necrotic tissue is harvested. There are no effective bioassays for the tetanus toxin either in blood or in the CSF.

Despite multiple attempts, there is no EDX pattern that has adequate specificity or sensitivity to confirm a diagnosis of tetanus. Silent periods and single fiber evaluations attempting to identify disordered neuromuscular transmission have been attempted without success. The most common EDX of tetanus is the continuous and simultaneous firing of normal MUAPs in symptomatic agonist and antagonist muscles. This pattern is nonspecific and can be seen in other disorders such as the SPS.

The differential diagnosis of trismus includes dental infection and paraneoplastic brainstem encephalitis. Trismus and painful spasms are not typical of most dystonias. Drug-induced dystonias have to be considered in cephalic tetanus as they may affect ocular movements. A chronologic relationship to drug exposure and a prompt and dramatic response to anticholinergic drugs provide diagnostic clues. Rabies needs to be considered in the differential diagnosis of cephalic tetanus when dysphagia is part of the symptom complex. Patients with rabies are frequently encephalopathic, have dysautonomic symptoms that are more likely to be cholinergic in nature (sialorrhea), do not tend to have continuous muscular rigidity, and have a CSF pleocytosis if tested.

Other extrapyramidal disorders in which dystonia is a prominent feature may resemble generalized tetanus but are typically chronic and result in distorted postures that are recognizably different from those of the disorders described above, for example, torticollis. Meningoencephalitis may be associated with fever, nuchal and paraspinal rigidity. Associated seizures may further contribute to tonic and phasic increases in the trunk and limb tone. SPS is characterized by the same axial rigidity and superimposed spasm as tetanus but is typically more insidious in onset and typically lacks the prominent cephalic involvement of tetanus. Neuroleptic malignant syndrome produces profound muscular rigidity and significant dysautonomia. Exposure to an offending drug, fever, altered mental status, and absence of spasm are potential distinguishing features from tetanus. Peritonitis and localized tetanus affecting the abdominal wall may be confused for each other. Spasticity is never acute, although spasms and involuntary jerking of the extremities may occur. The pattern of increased muscle tone is usually distinctive, affecting flexors in the upper extremities and extensors in the lower extremities preferentially. The limbs are affected more so than the trunk and head in contrast to tetanus. Strychnine is a CNS glycine antagonist, which is used primarily as rat poison. It impedes postsynaptic inhibition of motor neurons in the spinal cord. The phenotype is almost identical to tetanus other than the absence of trismus and the onset that occurs within minutes to hours of exposure. The diagnosis is dependent on a history of exposure in addition to the expected clinical manifestations. Reflex spasms are superimposed upon tonic rigidity affecting upper extremity flexors, lower extremity extensors, and facial muscles resulting in risus sardonicus.

LABORATORY FEATURES

As mentioned above, *C. tetani* can be cultured in approximately a third of infected wounds. No other organism-specific diagnostic test available as toxin assays are not available in either serum or CSF.

Regarding differential diagnostic considerations, strychnine assays can be performed by specialized laboratories. CSF examination should be obtained if possible if meningoencephalitis is considered. Elevated levels of CSF protein and immunoglobulins may occur in some cases of tetanus but are nonspecific and of little clinical value. Testing for glutamic acid decarboxylase (GAD) autoantibodies is reasonable if there is any suspicion for SPS. Like the SPS, electromyographic evaluation may reveal MUAP activation occurring involuntarily and simultaneously in agonist and antagonist muscles. Secondary complications such as inappropriate secretion of antidiuretic hormone and rhabdomyolysis requires monitoring of serum sodium, CK, and creatinine.

PATHOGENESIS

Tetanus results from wounds, often penetrating, that are contaminated by spores of the organism *C. tetani*, a gram-positive anaerobic rod. In underdeveloped countries, septic abortion, infected umbilical stumps, burns, intramuscular injections, and compound fractures provide common portals of entry. In developed countries, the organism is commonly introduced by contaminated puncture wounds sustained through recreational drug use or in areas where fecal debris from animals is prevalent such as farms.

Outside of the human body, the organism is resilient, surviving exposure to certain disinfectants and boiling for short periods of time. The spores may remain viable for decades. They thrive particularly in warm, moist soil contaminated by animal fecal material. Germination and proliferation occurs under optimal conditions, including those provided by wounds with tissue necrosis, foreign bodies, tissue ischemia, or co-infection with other organisms.

Under anaerobic conditions, the spores will germinate and release two exotoxins: tetanospasmin and tetanolysin. The role of the latter in disease expression is unknown. There are three known mechanisms by which tetanospasmin may adversely affect the nervous system. Localized tetanus is thought to occur as a consequence of direct binding to peripheral nerve terminals proximate to the wound site. Generalized disease results from retrograde transport of toxin into the CNS via motor nerves. Within the CNS, the toxin migrates transynaptically into GABAergic (brainstem) and glycinergic (spinal cord) inhibitory interneurons. Tetanospasmin blocks neurotransmitter release by cleaving synaptobrevin [vesicle-associated membrane protein (VAMP)], a protein essential for vesicle docking at synaptic membrane release sites.[106,107] Hematogenous dissemination of toxin may contribute to generalized disease by adversely affecting neuromuscular transmission through a presynaptic effect, similar but of far lesser magnitude to botulism.[108,109] It is hypothesized that this lower motor neuron effect, typically overshadowed by CNS hyperactivity, may be particularly relevant to cranial nerve dysfunction. Glycine inhibition is also believed to have an adverse effect on preganglionic sympathetic neurons translating to increased plasma catecholamine levels and heightened sympathetic activity.

The early involvement of cranial muscles is presumptively due to their shorter length and early arrival of neurotoxin to brainstem via this retrograde transport mechanism. Cranial, trunk, and limb muscles are usually affected in that order presumably due to the relationship of nerve length and retrograde neurotoxin transport. Recovery from tetanus is dependent on the genesis of new presynaptic nerve terminals of inhibitory interneurons.[103,110]

TREATMENT

The primary treatment strategy for tetanus is prevention. Tetanus is an uncommon illness due to the existence of effective vaccination programs. During a 2-year period in the United States in the 1990s, only 124 cases were reported.[104] To further amplify the efficacy of prevention, a vaccination program for pregnant women with tetanus toxoid in India reduced the annual number of cases of neonatal tetanus from 9313 to 653 over a 21-year period of time.[111] Although vaccination is extremely effective, rare individuals may develop tetanus even with a complete and up-to-date tetanus vaccination program and demonstration of pre-existing tetanus antibodies.[112] In countries where vaccination programs and medical access are limited, neonatal tetanus is more prevalent. In developed countries, the incidence of tetanus is higher in older individuals. Waning immunity from remote immunization may play a significant role in this observation.[103]

Vaccination against tetanus can be delivered either passively (tetanus toxoid) or actively (tetanus-specific immunoglobulin). The former, developed in the 1940s, is the preferred vaccination method. Primary vaccination for infants consists of five doses of tetanus toxoid delivered at 2, 4, and 6 months of age, as well as at 15–18 months and 4–6 years. The fifth dose is not required if the fourth was received after age 4. Typically, tetanus toxoid is combined with pertussis and diphtheria vaccines for the first five doses. Following these initial five doses, pertussis is deleted and tetanus toxoid/diphtheria boosters are recommended at 10-year intervals.

Primary vaccination is indicated in adults when their childhood vaccination history is uncertain or in a bone marrow transplant is planned.[104] It consists of three injections, the first two of which are separated by a minimum of 4 weeks, and the last dose done 6–12 months subsequent to the second. In individuals who have received a "clean" wound, vaccination is considered adequate if previously vaccinated and if a tetanus booster has been received within 10 years. In the setting of a "dirty" wound, a booster within 5 years would be considered with adequate primary vaccination. In a patient who has been wounded, whose tetanus immunization has "expired" or their immune status compromised by HIV infection, dialysis, chronic chloroquine exposure (and potentially other immunosuppressant agents), both primary vaccination with tetanus toxoid and human tetanus immunoglobulin (250 units intramuscularly) should be administered at different sites.

With the development of symptomatic tetanus, the goals are to: (1) limit further production of tetanospasmin by wound debridement and antimicrobial therapy, (2) neutralize if possible, the effects of existing, unbound toxin by active immunization, (3) provide symptomatic treatment of painful spasms, impaired ventilation, and swallowing; and (4) treat symptoms referable to dysautonomia. Patients with tetanus without obvious wounds should have orifices examined, such as the external ear or rectum, with removal of foreign bodies if relevant. Patients with tetanus should be considered for early lumbar puncture if indicated, and particularly prophylactic intubation and enteral feeding tube placement as both are frequently required and become technically difficult once rigidity and spasms begin in earnest.

Elimination of the toxin source involves removal of any foreign body, debridement of any necrotic tissue, and delivery of antibiotics with anaerobic efficacy. The latter is recommended despite absence of proven efficacy. Metronidazole, penicillin, third-generation cephalosporins, clindamycin, or erythromycin are typically administered and may reduce the need for muscle relaxants and sedatives. Penicillin G is given in doses ranging from 10–12 million units per day. Metronidazole appears to be equally effective and may be preferential in view of penicillin's stimulatory effect on the cortex. The customary dose is 500 mg IV q6h for 7–10 days.

Conversely, neutralization of unbound circulating toxin has documented efficacy in shortening disease duration and improving recovery rates.[104] Human tetanus immune globulin should be administered at a dose of 500 units intramuscularly as soon as possible, ideally before the wound is manipulated. The addition of intrathecal (1000 units) to intramuscular administration appears to result in even better outcomes.[113] Equine-derived tetanus immune globulin may be used if human-derived immune globulin is not available. Infection with *C. tetani* does not stimulate active immunity by the host.

Treatment of symptomatic spasms is important for patient comfort, to improve ventilation and to prevent thermal and mechanical injury from excessive and sustained muscular contraction. Treatment should be titrated to patient response. Like the SPS, exceedingly high doses may be both required and tolerated. Benzodiazepines (lorazepam—up to 80 mg a day, diazepam—up to 500 mg a day, or midazolam) with preservation of consciousness. Neuromuscular blocking agents, and/or baclofen are commonly used. Vecuronium at a dose of 6–8 mg/h is preferred over pancuronium, as the latter has catecholamine reuptake-blocking properties that may contribute to autonomic instability. Baclofen may be administered orally or intrathecally. The initial intrathecal dose is 40–200 μg followed by a continuous infusion of 20 μg/h.[114,115] Meticulous catheter care is required to minimize the risk of meningitis from prolonged intrathecal catheter placement. Labetalol (0.25–1.0 mg/min), morphine (0.5–1.0 mg/kg/h), magnesium sulfate, atropine, clonidine, and epidural bupivacaine have all been used with some degree of reported benefit for hyperadrenergic and other autonomic manifestations.[110] As with all illnesses associated with protracted recovery periods, vigorous supportive care including tracheostomy is frequently required to minimize the risk of secondary complications to which these patients are susceptible.

► TETANY

CLINICAL FEATURES

Tetany is a disorder of nerve hyperexcitability provoked by hypocalcemia with or without vitamin D deficiency, hypomagnesemia or alkalosis. The syndrome has both motor and sensory features and is characterized by the development of paresthesias which initially occur in the digits and in a circumoral distribution. The paresthesias may in some cases have a lateralized preponderance and may spread to the proximal extremities. Paresthesias are followed by manifestations of motor nerve hyperactivity manifesting as spasmodic muscle contraction resulting in characteristic patterns of extremity posturing. The most characteristic of these is "carpal spasm" consisting of a "fisted" posture with the thumb adducted against the palm covered by fingers that are flexed at the metacarpophalangeal joints, extended at the proximal interphalangeal joints and adducted against each other. In more severe cases, the wrists and elbows may assume a flexed posture as well. In the lower extremities, the pedal portion of carpal pedal spasm, the tendency is for the toes to flex and the ankle to assume the equinovarus posture, that is, plantar flexed and inverted. Unlike tetanus, the effects of tetany are more pronounced in limb as opposed to cranial and axial muscles and influence sensory as well as motor function due to their peripheral nerve effects. In severe cases however, laryngospasm may occur and trunk muscles may be affected potentially resulting in opisthotonus.[1]

Carpal spasm may be elicited in patients at risk by inflating a blood pressure cuff to greater than systolic blood pressure for ≤3 minutes (Trousseau sign). Spasm of facial muscles may be provoked in these patients by digital percussion of the facial nerve at the angle of the jaw (Chvostek sign).

DIAGNOSIS AND DIFFERENTIAL DIAGNOSIS

Tetany is diagnosed by recognition of the characteristic pattern of paresthesias, typical hand-and-foot postures, and a positive response to the provocative maneuvers described above. The diagnosis is further supported by identification of reduced serum levels of ionized calcium or magnesium. Cases of normocalcemic, normomagnesemic tetany do however occur.[116] Cases in which reduced ionized calcium has been detected in arterial but not venous blood have been described as well.

The differential diagnosis of tetany once again includes any disorder that produces cramps or cramp-like painful muscle contractions. Diagnostic considerations should include consideration of drug-induced tetany, typically resulting from alterations in magnesium homeostasis. Potential offenders include proton pump inhibitors, diuretics, epidermal growth factor receptor modulators, some antimicrobials and chemotherapeutic agents, and of particular interest to neuromuscular clinicians, calcineurin inhibitors such as tacrolimus and certain monoclonal antibodies including bevacizumab.[117–119]

LABORATORY FEATURES

All patients with unwanted muscle contractions should have ionized calcium, 25 hydroxy-vitamin D and magnesium levels assessed in their serum. Tetany induced by hyperventilation will be associated with an arterial blood gas pattern consistent with acute respiratory alkalosis (i.e., a reduced PCO2 and elevated pH). The EDX signature of tetany is grouped discharges that may occur spontaneously (myokymic discharges) or in response to voluntary activation (multiplets).

PATHOGENESIS

The effects of tetany are believed to result from a neural generator.[120] Concomitant sensory and motor symptoms support this. The neural hyperexcitability of tetany is thought to result from the effects of hypocalcemia or hypomagnesemia on sodium channels.[119] Reduction in serum calcium or magnesium levels are thought to result in preferential and enhanced sodium channel opening resulting in prolonged nerve depolarization and hyperexcitability. Calcineurin inhibitors are thought to promote hypomagnesemia by inhibition of the transient receptor ion channel (magnesium) 6 (TRPM6) channel that is responsible for the renal tubular reabsorption of magnesium. In addition, there is a potential direct effect of calcineurin inhibitors on the muscle. These drugs inhibit calmodulin-mediated calcium uptake in muscle, potentially augmenting unwanted muscle contraction through prolonged sodium channel activation at this level as well.[118]

TREATMENT

The treatment of tetany involves recognition and correction of hypocalcemia and/or hypomagnesemia if detectable. With symptomatic hypocalcemia, the goal is to elevate the corrected serum calcium to >7.0 mg/dl. This can be accomplished by infusions of calcium gluconate at doses of 15–20 meq/kg delivered over 4–6 hours. Conditions causing chronic hypocalcemia can be managed with 1–3 g of elemental calcium replacement a day. In the case of acute symptomatic hypomagnesemia, magnesium sulfate can be delivered either intramuscularly or intravenously. The intravenous dose is typically a bolus of 4–6 g followed by 2–3 g per hour as required. Vitamin D deficiency is treated with oral replacement. Vitamin D2 is the most economic way to accomplish this at daily doses of 25,000 to 150,000 IU. If hyperventilation is the cause, breathing into a paper bag will address this problem acutely. Addressing the underlying cause of hyperventilation is important if a patient is repeatedly symptomatic. Drugs that potentially cause symptomatic hypomagnesemia should be removed if possible with consideration of patient comorbidities.

► SATOYOSHI SYNDROME

CLINICAL FEATURES

Satoyoshi syndrome is a rare, presumed autoimmune disorder, predominantly affecting individuals in the first two decades of life.[1,121–125] Females are affected twice as frequently as males. Satoyoshi syndrome occurs worldwide but appears to have the greatest prevalence in Japan.[122] It is characterized by painful muscle spasms of the extremities, typically beginning in the legs, but progressing to involve the entire body including the trunk, neck, and masticatory muscles. In Japan, it has been also referred to as "komura-gaeri" (calf-spasm) disease.[125] The spasms, like those of IS are commonly provoked by movement, persist during sleep and interfere with gait.[122,125] Unlike IS adventitious muscle movements such as myokymia and fasciculations are not described.[123,124] The spasms commonly distort posture, typically last for a few minutes and recur after short intervals. Although these paroxysms may be the sole manifestation of Satoyoshi syndrome, the syndrome is best conceptualized as a multisystem disorder associated with alopecia, diarrhea, and short stature. Short stature may occur as a result of impaired nutrition and/or endocrine abnormalities that may include amenorrhea as well as growth retardation.[123,127] The amenorrhea, at least in some cases, is a consequence of hypergonadotropic hypogonadism and primary ovarian failure.[32] Bony deformities may occur in Satoyoshi syndrome. They have been hypothesized to result from the influence of repeated forceful muscle spasm on developing bone.[122] Life expectancy is reduced attributed predominantly to nutritional deficiency.[122,125]

DIAGNOSIS AND DIFFERENTIAL DIAGNOSIS

Satoyoshi syndrome remains a clinical diagnosis, suspected when movement-related painful muscle spasms develop in children and adolescents, accompanied by alopecia, diarrhea, short stature, and in post-pubescent females, amenorrhea. The laboratory abnormalities and responsiveness to immunomodulating treatment described below provide diagnostic support.

LABORATORY FEATURES

Lab testing results may reflect malnutrition or malabsorption. Consistent with this conclusion are duodenal imaging abnormalities felt to be consistent with chronic inflammatory change. Endoscopy may demonstrate atrophic gastric mucosa and multiple ulcerations.[125,126] X-rays may reveal osteolytic lesions of the epiphysis and metaphysis of bone.[122] Serum CK levels may be elevated.[125,126,128] The serum IgE level has been elevated in at least two cases.[127,128] In post-pubescent females, levels of sex hormones may be reduced and gonadotropin levels elevated.[122] Although a number of circulating autoantibodies including those directed at the acetylcholine receptor and GAD enzyme have been anecdotally reported, there has been no consistent pattern identified to date.[126,128] Despite the presence of acetylcholine receptor antibodies in some cases, we are unaware of any reports of Satoyoshi syndrome associated with thymic abnormality. As titers of GAD autoantibodies are frequently elevated in high titers in the SPS, the significance of low-level titers of these antibodies in Satoyoshi syndrome awaits further clarification. Routine EDX studies done in Satoyoshi syndrome patients when muscles are quiescent are normal. Surface EMG recordings during involuntary muscle contraction reveals high amplitude, synchronous motor unit discharges that are pervasive throughout the entire muscle belly.[128]

HISTOPATHOLOGY

Inflammatory changes within the mucosa have been demonstrated with duodenal biopsy.[125]

PATHOGENESIS

Satoyoshi syndrome is suspected to have an autoimmune mechanism. Other autoimmune diseases such as myasthenia, idiopathic thrombocytopenia, and immune-mediated nephropathies appear to occur with increased frequency in Satoyoshi syndrome.[125] As previously mentioned, a nonspecific pattern of autoantibodies may be identified in the serum of Satoyoshi syndrome patients. A single report has described a circulating antibody reacting to a 90-kDa protein found in the brain, stomach, and duodenum but not the uterus.[125]

The pathophysiology of muscle contraction in Satoyoshi syndrome is unknown. It appears to differ from cramps in that surface EMG recordings of motor unit discharges are synchronous, not random, and occur in uniform rather than a migrating pattern throughout the muscle belly.

TREATMENT

In view of its rarity, there is no standardized approach to the treatment of Satoyoshi syndrome. A variety of agents have been used unsuccessfully for the treatment of spasms. Botulinum toxin may be locally effective (e.g., masticatory spasm) but is impractical for widespread application. Carbamazepine was effective in at least one case whereas baclofen provided no benefit.[122] Case reports suggest that immunomodulation may favorably alter the natural history of the disease in some but not all cases. Significantly beneficial responses to muscle spasms, alopecia and gastrointestinal symptoms have been reported with tacrolimus, methotrexate, corticosteroids, and IVIG.[122,125,126] Conversely, both corticosteroids and IVIG have been reported to be ineffective.[122,126,128–130] Appropriate hormonal replacement may be considered.

▶ STIFF-PERSON SYNDROME

CLINICAL FEATURES

Moersch and Woltman described the stiff-man syndrome in 1956 based on their experience with 14 patients afflicted with a syndrome of fluctuating but progressive muscle rigidity and spasm that preferentially affected the axial muscles.[131] For multiple reasons including its greater prevalence in women, this disorder is now commonly referred to as the SPS.[132–134]

Unlike most of the other most of the disorders considered in this chapter, SPS is a CNS disorder, best conceptualized in our minds as a encephalomyelopathy in which the myelopathic features predominate in most cases.[132,135,136] Like other autoimmune and paraneoplastic disorders, the onset is often acute–subacute although it may go undiagnosed for years.[137] SPS affects women twice as frequently as men with a median onset of 35–40 years of age.[137,138] The best estimate of prevalence is less than 1×10^6.[134] In view of its rarity and the often protean nature of its onset symptoms, for example, low back pain, the diagnosis may be delayed by an average of 6 years following symptom onset.[132,134]

In the classic form of the disease, the initial symptom is typically painful muscle stiffness in the lumbosacral and abdominal regions.[135,136,139,140] One of the key features of SPS is the propensity for agonist and antagonist muscles to be affected simultaneously. As the disease progresses, there is a propensity for the muscle rigidity to spread to involve the proximal muscles of the lower extremities. Eventually, any muscle under voluntary control may be affected. Limb involvement may be symmetric or asymmetric. Falls constitute a significant risk and source of morbidity. Fear of falling is a significant source of anxiety for these patients.

At onset, paroxysmal muscle spasms are the norm. They usually become more persistent as the disease worsens if left untreated. These spasms, superimposed upon baseline muscle stiffness, may begin abruptly, last for seconds to minutes as individual events, and may recur in clusters that may persist for hours.[134,141–143] They are often provoked or intensified by movement, by tactile, emotional, or auditory stimuli, or by cold weather or intercurrent infection.[144] The spasms may be powerful enough to break bones, dislocate joints, or incite rhabdomyolysis. The spasms may be so dramatic as to mimic the opisthotonic posturing of tetanus.[134,145] Unlike IS, spasms are typically diminished if not alleviated by general anesthesia, benzodiazepines, and sleep.[135] The paroxysms of SPS may be associated with adrenergic symptoms of dysautonomia including diaphoresis, hypertension, tachycardia, tachypnea, and pupillary dilatation.[133] Rarely, the dysautonomia may result in sudden death.[134,146,147]

Like many clinical syndromes, the clinical manifestations of SPS may be heterogeneous.[148] Focal presentations have been referred to as "stiff-limb" syndrome.[137,148–152] Focal onset SPS may or may not progress to more generalized disorder. If the phenotype remains focal, SPS may not be readily suspected. Cervical involvement may result in restricted head movement. Thoracoabdominal rigidity may result in symptoms whose mechanism may not be initially recognized as being related to restricted muscle movement including ventilatory insufficiency (dyspnea on exertion, orthopnea, exercise intolerance, inability to swim underwater) and impaired gastric distention (early satiety). Facial involvement resulting in facial masking has been described in some cases, leading to the erroneous diagnosis of Parkinson disease.[132] Dysphagia, dysarthria, and disordered ocular motility have been rarely described without overt encephalitis.[147] Whether these represent limited forms of brainstem encephalitis is uncertain. Alternatively, myasthenia should be considered with the development of oculobulbar symptoms in SPS.[134]

Although the phenotype of SPS is typically dominated by myelopathic signs and symptoms, many patients have signs and symptoms suggesting cerebral involvement as well. Dysphoria, anxiety, phobias, and depression are common. These affective symptoms if coupled with unusual postures and movements such as pelvic thrusting may lead to an erroneous diagnosis of hysteria. In one series, 8% of individuals were given an initial psychogenic diagnosis.[137] Most have attributed these affective and behavioral symptoms to represent understandable reactions of the patient to their illness.[153] Given our current knowledge regarding the pathogenesis of this disease and its potential to affect the brain as well as the spinal cord, it is rational to hypothesize that these symptoms represent an encephalitic component in at least some cases.[138]

Although rare, the existence of a progressive encephalomyelitis with rigidity and myoclonus variant of this disease (PERM) or "jerking stiff-man syndrome" lends further support for this hypothesis.[134,135,148,149–151] In this syndrome, progressive rigidity progresses within weeks to years to include cognitive impairment. Associated features include myoclonus, nystagmus, opsoclonus, impaired ocular motility, dysarthria, and dysphagia. Seizures may occur in up to 10% of cases.[160] Other encephalopathic manifestations of SPS have been described including a subacute cerebellar syndrome, brainstem encephalitis, temporal lobe epilepsy, dystonia, and retinopathy.[135] Of these, the cerebellar syndrome appears to be the most prevalent. It is characterized by prominent ataxia, dysarthria, and eye movement abnormalities superimposed on muscle stiffness and spasms.[136] Peripheral neuropathy and motor neuronopathy have also been reported to occur as part of the PERM complex.[137] The course of PERM is relentless. Death may occur within weeks to months of brain involvement.

The clinical examination of the "typical" SPS patient often reveals accentuation of the normal lumbar lordosis with resultant restriction of spine mobility. As a result, a patient's lower back may fail to flatten and contact the bed when lying supine. Their ability to touch their toes may be severely restricted similar to an spondyloarthropathy patient. In SPS however, the lumbar lordotic curve is increased rather than decreased both in the upright and attempted flexed positions. Although nonspecific, the paraspinal muscles in SPS are typically indurated to palpation. As a result, the patient's flexibility, mobility, and ambulation are hampered. The patient's gait may be described as stiff, robotic, and spastic in nature. In addition to abnormal axial postures, other abnormal postures during spasms may include extension and slight abduction of the leg, inversion and plantar flexion of the foot that may be mistaken as foot drop, or pronation and extension of the upper extremity.[134,136] Deep tendon reflexes are commonly increased and sustained ankle clonus and Babinski signs may occur.[137] A triple flexion response in response to lower extremity stimulation may be observed.[134] The head retraction reflex is a bedside test that can be utilized in an SPS suspect.[20] It is positive in 50% or more of SPS or PERM patients but is nonspecific and may occur in other CNS disorders of hyperexcitability as well. A positive response is contraction of neck muscles, with or without head movement, in response to a gentle tap to the glabella, bridge of the nose, lip or cheek in a patient whose eyes are closed.

DIAGNOSIS AND DIFFERENTIAL DIAGNOSIS

The diagnosis of SPS is typically arrived at by recognition of the clinical features, coupled with a typical antibody profile, electrophysiologic support when necessary, and benzodiazepine responsiveness. The latter provides both diagnostic and therapeutic benefits.[134] In typical cases, signs and symptoms of either lower motor neuron, sensory, or cognitive involvement should dissuade the clinician from the diagnosis. Some have suggested that pyramidal and extrapyramidal features are atypical in SPS [134], although that has not been our experience or the experience of others.[137,146] A number of our cases have been referred by neurosurgeons for myelopathic phenotypes associated with negative spinal cord imaging.

The diagnosis of SPS is confirmed, in the appropriate clinical context, by the demonstration of GAD-65 or amphiphysin autoantibodies in significant titres the serum or CSF. GAD-65 autoantibodies in SPS, unlike diabetes, are typically found in high titers. They also differ from diabetes in that they are typically directed toward the amino terminus of the molecule.[135,161,162] In patients who are GAD-65 seronegative, other less specific markers of autoimmunity including oligoclonal banding in the CSF and the presence of other serum autoantibodies offer diagnostic support. Many have described the value of EMG in demonstrating involuntary activation of MUAPs simultaneously in agonist/antagonist muscle pairs. In our experience, we have not found this to be either sensitive or specific enough to utilize as a major determinant in the decision to initiate immunomodulating treatment in a patient with suspected SPS who is seronegative. Other testing, particularly spinal cord imaging and CSF analysis, may be required to exclude the other differential diagnostic considerations listed below.

The differential diagnosis of SPS includes many of the other disorders listed in this chapter particularly IS, chronic tetanus, Brody syndrome, Satoyoshi syndrome, and in children, hyperekplexia. Other compressive and noncompressive myelopathies including primary lateral sclerosis, primary progressive MS, neuromyelitis optica, and retroviral infection with HTLV-1 bear some resemblance to SPS. Extrapyramidal disorders, particularly those with dystonia should be considered as well. In individuals who develop symptoms of intracranial disease in addition to their stiffness, Morvan syndrome and other autoimmune often paraneoplastic causes of limbic encephalitis including those associated with Hu, Ri, VGKC, and n-methyl d-aspartic acid (NMDA) receptor autoantibodies should be considered. Although patients with SPS may be mislabeled as psychogenic, the opposite misdiagnosis may occur as well as psychogenic patients with muscle pain and unusual postures may be considered to have SPS.[138]

Other autoimmune disorders may associate with SPS with an increased frequency. SPS is thought to be paraneoplastic in 5% of individuals.[132,134] Patients with paraneoplastic SPS may have a preferential involvement of the upper extremities and cranial nerves.[132,134] Malignancies reported in SPS include breast cancer and small-cell carcinoma of the lung, and less commonly Hodgkin disease, thymoma, colon, and ovarian cancer. The majority of these occur in GAD-65 seronegative patients.[65,134,135,163–165]

Other nonparaneoplastic autoimmune disorders both within and outside of the nervous system associate with SPS. This is particularly true in those who possess GAD antibodies. These comorbidities may include encephalomyelitis with seizures, cerebellitis, myasthenia gravis, hypo- and hyperthyroidism, pernicious anemia, celiac disease, adrenal insufficiency, systemic lupus erythematosus, rheumatoid arthritis, ovarian failure, and vitiligo.[132,134,165,166] Diabetes mellitus is particularly prevalent and may exist in up to 70% of patients with SPS.[160]

The decision regarding potential evaluation for underlying malignancy should probably depend on the context of the individual patient. The presence of amphiphysin antibodies, a strong family history of breast or ovarian cancer or smoking, and predominant upper extremity or cranial nerve involvement are features that will increase the diagnostic yield of identifying an underlying malignancy.[60,134,164] In an environment where neither cost nor availability are considerations, 18 F fluorodeoxyglucose positron emission tomography (FDG PET) scanning would represent the presumed screening method of choice to search for an occult malignancy.

LABORATORY FEATURES

The association of GAD autoantibodies and SPS was first reported in 1988.[167] Antibodies directed against the 65KD isoform of GAD (GAD-65) may be found in high titer in 85% of SPS patients as opposed to the other isoform, GAD-67 for which autoantibodies are present in less than 50% of affected individuals.[135,136,167,168] If only patients with the classic phenotype are considered, the prevalence of anti-GAD antibodies in SPS may exceed 90%.[148] GAD-65 autoantibodies in high titre typically designated as >20 nmol/L are found in only 1% of normal individuals and 5% of patients with other neurologic diseases.[138] GAD-65 autoantibodies are also demonstrable in the CSF in 75% of cases.[135,169] They are present in the CSF in lower titer than in serum but with a 10-fold increase when indexed against serum implicating intrathecal synthesis.[135] Patients with the rare PERM phenotype may be seropositive or seronegative. In addition to GAD-65, autoantibodies directed against the glycine receptor alpha-1 subunit (GLRA1) and the NMDA receptors have been reported in this illness.[155]

Although commonly assayed by immunocytochemical technique, the greatest sensitivity in GAD-65 autoantibody detection is achieved with radioimmunoassay.[135] GAD autoantibodies are not specific for SPS and are found in approximately 5% of individuals with other neurologic disorders. These include individuals with cerebellar ataxia, palatal myoclonus, limbic encephalitis, localization-related epilepsy, and ceroid lipofuscinosis.[134,135,138] GAD-65 autoantibody titers do not correlate with disease severity, duration, or treatment responsiveness.[170]

Paraneoplastic SPS is more commonly associated with autoantibodies directed against amphiphysin than GAD-65.[135,136,145,163,164] Amphiphysin antibodies are found in approximately 5% of SPS cases, almost always in women. There is a considerable overlap between paraneoplastic SPS and amphiphysin-positive SPS but they are not synonymous. Amphiphysin autoantibodies may occur in other non-SPS paraneoplastic syndromes including limbic encephalitis, cerebellar degeneration, and sensory neuronopathy.[136] Conversely, paraneoplastic SPS may rarely associate with other autoantibodies. GAD-65 autoantibodies may occur rarely in individuals with SPS who have an underlying malignancy such as renal cancer or thymoma.[135,152,169–171] The encephalomyelitic form of SPS with opsoclonus may have anti-Ri antibodies, often associated with adenocarcinoma of the lung. There have been individual case reports linking paraneoplastic SPS with gephyrin (GHPN) autoantibodies.[136,172,173] Amphiphysin and GAD-65 autoantibodies virtually never coexist.

Oligoclonal bands in the CSF are common in SPS.[174] Their presence may provide valuable support for the diagnosis of SPS in an individual who does not possess the more specific biomarkers of anti-GAD or amphiphysin antibodies in either serum or their CSF. Other organ-specific autobodies may be found in SPS including anti-thyroid, anti-intrinsic factor, anti-nuclear, anti-RNP, and anti-gliadin.[135] Routine testing for these less specific autoantibodies is not generally recommended as they are more likely representative of an underlying autoimmune diathesis than indicative of SPS.

Regarding EDX evaluation of the SPS patient, routine nerve conduction studies are normal. Needle electromyography of symptomatic muscles will reveal MUAPs with normal morphology and firing rates. The only difference between SPS and normal patients is that these MUAPs fire involuntarily and simultaneously in both agonist and antagonist muscle groups. This pattern must be interpreted with caution however, as spontaneously firing MUAPs in a single muscle is commonplace in a normal, tense individual. In addition, it is possible for a normal individual to consciously activate agonist and antagonist and feign this pattern of abnormality should they be incented to do so. In our opinion, the greatest value of EDX in a suspected SPS patient is to exclude the waveforms that characterize other disorders that should be considered in the SPS differential diagnosis.

A number of other electrophysiologic techniques, not routinely applied in clinical settings, may demonstrate abnormalities consistent with known SPS pathophysiology.[134,135] In keeping with the lack of CNS inhibition that occurs in this disease, hyperexcitability of the reflex arc in SPS can be demonstrated. Vibration-induced inhibition of

H reflexes is a GABAergic phenomenon that may be suppressed in SPS. Enhancement of exteroceptive reflexes appears to be specific for SPS. This phenomenon involves the demonstration of prolonged, tonic activity in multiple muscles not typically activated by a brief train of suprathreshold electrical stimuli to peripheral sensory nerve. With the blink reflex, it may be possible to demonstrate a contralateral R1 response. Excessive muscle activation in response to auditory stimuli (startle response) both in degree and in distribution can be recorded in SPS.[134] The electrical analogue of the head retraction reflex described in the clinical section is one example of this where discharges from the trapezius muscles can be obtained by electrical stimulation of a trigeminal nerve branch.[173,175]

MR imaging of the brain and spinal cord in SPS patients is usually normal.[136,176] Specifically, SPS patients with cerebellar syndromes do not demonstrate cerebellar atrophy.[136] MR spectroscopy however, may demonstrate a significant regional decrease in GABA levels in the motor cortices in these patients.[136,176,177]

HISTOPATHOLOGY

Histologic findings in SPS are limited and inconsistent, thus suggesting a predominantly physiologic rather than histologic pathogenesis.[131,134,178–180] Postmortem examination may reveal loss of anterior horn cells, interneurons, and small alpha and gamma motor neurons within the spinal cord or cerebellum but these findings are inconsistent.[138] More overt pathology is seen in PERM where perivascular inflammation in the cord, brain, and brainstem may be identified.[134,154,173–182]

PATHOGENESIS

Current consensus holds that SPS is an autoimmune disease, related to circulating autoantibodies to proteins involved in gamma amino butyric acid (GABA) neurotransmission, resulting in impaired GABAergic inhibition of α-motor neurons within the brain and spinal cord. The exact pathogenic mechanisms, specifically whether these autoantibodies are causal, remains unknown.[138]

l-Glutamic acid decarboxylase (GAD) is an enzyme that catalyzes the decarboxylation of glutamate to gaba-Aminobutyric acid (GABA). GAD is widely prevalent in the cytosol, specifically the inner surface of synaptic vesicles of GABA secreting neurons within the CNS.[138] GABA is the major inhibitory neurotransmitter within the forebrain whereas both GABA and glycine serve in this capacity within the spinal cord. There are other proteins relevant to SPS and CNS, which causes neuromuscular hyperexcitability.[183] Amphiphysin is another cytosolic presynaptic protein that is responsible for the retrieval of the vesicular protein following GABA exocytosis.[135] GABA-receptor-associated protein (GABARAP) is a postsynaptic protein that stabilizes and surface expression of GABA-A receptors as well as modulating their conductance.[136] Approximately 65–70% of GAD-65 seropositive SPS patients will have antibodies that react with this protein.[135,136] These antibodies inhibit the surface expression and impair the stability of GABA-A receptors.[136] Gephyrin is a postsynaptic protein responsible for the clustering of glycine receptors in the spinal cord and GABA-A receptors within the brain, essential for their proper functioning.[136] Accordingly, knockout of the GHPN gene in mice results in an SPS phenotype.

The exact roles of the autoantibodies remain however, uncertain. GAD-65 specific autoantibodies harvested from SPS patients inhibit GAD activity and GABA synthesis in vitro.[182] They are presumed to adversely affect inhibitory GABA interneurons in the spinal gray matter and cortex, leading to continuous tonic firing of α-motor neurons.[134,184,185] Given the logic of this hypothesis, the high prevalence of GAD-65 autoantibodies in high-titer in SPS patients, and their apparent intrathecal synthesis, it is tempting to suggest that GAD-65 have a direct pathogenic role. Inhibition of GABA synthesis and interference with GABA vesicle exocytosis are proposed mechanisms.[135]

There are however, conflicting observations. As GAD-65, as well as amphiphysin and GHPN, are cytosolic proteins, it is unlikely to be recognized by the immune system unless GAD were to migrate to the cell surface. In addition, neither infants with transient autoantibodies transferred from mothers with GAD65 seropositive SPS, nor mice who have received passively transferred GAD-65 autoantibodies develop disease.[135]

Paraneoplastic SPS occurs primarily in individuals with autoantibodies directed against amphiphysin, or rarely in patients with GAD-65, Ri, or GHPN autoantibodies.[134,135,163,164] A causal relationship between amphiphysin autoantibodies and SPS is supported by the production of a similar clinical response in animals to whom these autoantibodies have been passively transferred.[135] Response to immune-modulating treatment in some cases offers further support for the autoimmune hypothesis in amphiphysin-associated SPS. As one other potential paraneoplastic association in SPS, GAD-65 is a protein also expressed in thymic tissue, providing a potential pathogenic link between SPS and thymic pathology.[137]

Autoimmunity may not represent an isolated disease mechanism in SPS. There may be an additional genetic predisposition based on major histocompatibility genotype. The DQβ1*0201 allele is present in approximately 70% of patients and along with the DRβ1 allele is closely associated with SPS.[136] This is also a prevalent allele in patients with diabetes without SPS. Conversely, the presence of the DQB1*0602 allele seems to be protective.[135]

TREATMENT

The treatment of SPS involves the use of both symptomatic agents to enhance GABAergic influences and immunomodulating treatments aimed at the presumed autoimmune basis of the disease.[135,136] In the case of paraneoplastic SPS, treatment and if possible eradication of the underlying tumor represent the initial therapeutic goal. Patients are typically treatment responsive although complete eradication of symptoms is the exception rather than the rule. A significant portion of affected individuals remain dependent on others for at least some activities of daily living.[136]

Benzodiazepines have been the historical mainstay of symptomatic treatment. Patients require and are tolerant of large doses, with a median daily diazepam dose of 40 mg required to provide efficacy without excessive side effect. Although many SPS patients tolerate doses of benzodiazepines that normal patients would not, unwanted CNS side effects still represent a limitation of this therapy. Antispasticity drugs provide a second line of symptomatic treatment. Baclofen, tizanidine, and dantrolene have been used with some success although our experience has not been as rewarding as suggested in the literature.[136] Baclofen can also be used intrathecally and has been shown to have some benefit in controlled trials but is associated with the potential risk of significant complication.[136,185] A number of anticonvulsants with mechanisms of action that augment GABA effect have been tried with anecdotal report of benefit including gabapentin, valproic acid, levetiracetam, vigabatrin, and tiagabine. Botulinum toxin may benefit individual patients as well but is limited by its cost, and the need for large doses to adequately address large axial muscle groups.

Of the immunomodulating agents, only IVIG and rituximab have been studied in clinical trials in SPS. To the best of our knowledge, the rituximab trial conducted at the NIH is yet to be published. The rituximab trial was prompted by its relevant mechanism of action as well as by case reports of beneficial and protracted responses to rituximab.[186–188] The IVIG trial involved 16 patients and reported improved morbidity and reduction in GAD autoantibody titers with treatment.[189]

There have been many reports describing anecdotal responses to other immunomodulating therapies but a limited evidence basis by which to judge efficacy. In general, efforts to assess treatment efficacy in SPS are hampered not only by the rarity of the condition but by the lack of adequate parameters by which to measure it. PLEX has benefited some patients. Corticosteroids are less attractive than in other diseases, in view of the high concordance of diabetes. Azathioprine, methotrexate, and mycophenolate have been tried. Anecdotally, we have been impressed that corticosteroids and mycophenolate have modest benefit with clinical improvement upon exposure and demonstration of worsening that is chronologically related to drug withdrawal after the patient has experienced long periods of drug-related stability. As in other paraneoplastic syndromes, successful treatment of the underlying malignancy may lessen the morbidity of the associated SPS. As paraneoplastic SPS is uncommon the theoretical concern that immunomodulating agents might promote growth of an occult cancer by reducing immune surveillance is of less concern than in disorders such as the Lambert–Eaton myasthenic syndrome.

▶ HYPEREKPLEXIA

CLINICAL FEATURES

Hyperekplexia originates from the Greek ekplexis meaning surprise, an apt description for the exaggerated startle response that characterizes the syndrome. It is characterized by nonepileptic, paroxysmal rigidity and hyperreflexia in response to external, often auditory stimuli. The startle response frequently includes eye blinking and trunk flexion similar to a salaam attack in West syndrome. Voluntary movement is typically precluded during the spasm. Hyperekplexia is typically a newborn disorder but often persists to some degree during adult life. Affected adults often experience drop attacks as their major manifestation. Occasionally, onset may be delayed. In neonates, it may be provoked by handling. Child care such as changing a diaper may be impaired do to the inability to passively abduct the legs. The spasms tend to disappear during sleep but may occur at night during arousals. The examination of the hyperekplectic individual may reveal an exaggerated head retraction response as is described above in the SPS. Gentle tapping of the tip of the nose will elicit a startle response in affected babies. The severity of hyperekplexia varies and in extreme cases, it can result in neonatal cardiac arrest and death.[190]

DIAGNOSIS AND DIFFERENTIAL DIAGNOSIS

The diagnosis of hyperekplexia is based on the appropriate clinical syndrome beginning in infancy, associated with normal electroencephalography, supported by family history, and confirmed when possible by genotyping. Of the disorders described in this chapter, hyperekplexia bears the closest resemblance to the SPS or childhood tetanus. At one time, hyperekplexia was referred to as stiff-baby syndrome. Undoubtedly the most prevalent and difficult differential diagnostic consideration from a clinical perspective in infancy is infantile spasms associated with the West syndrome. Consciousness is not altered in most hyperekplexia attacks as it is in the seizures of infantile spasm but this may not be clinically apparent in infancy. Mutations of the rho guanine nuclear exchange factor 9 (ARHGEF9) gene described below are an exception, resulting in hyperekplexia coupled with an early infantile epileptic encephalopathy. Cerebral palsy or other causes of spastic quadriplegia, a tic disorder or adverse reaction to neuroleptics are other differential diagnostic considerations. As it may also produce stimulus-related falls, cataplexy may be confused with hyperekplexia in the absence of a detailed history.

LABORATORY FEATURES

Genetic testing is available from research laboratories for all of the five currently recognized genotypes. Electroencephalography is recommended to address the possibility of infantile spasms. EMG has little or no role in the evaluation of suspected patients.

HISTOPATHOLOGY

There is limited pathologic data in hyperekplexia. Rare autopsy and muscle biopsy reports identify no pathologic findings.[191]

PATHOGENESIS

There are currently five known gene mutations that result in a hyperekplexia phenotype.[192] Of these, mutations of the glycine receptor alpha-1subunit (GLRA-1) accounts for 80% of cases. Other responsible mutations include the glycine receptor beta subunit (GLRB), the GHPN, and solute carrier family 6 (SLC6A5) genes. The latter encodes a presynaptic glycine transporter. Mutations of the rho guanine nuclear exchange factor 9 (ARHGEF9) gene alter the synthesis of the protein collybistin whose function is to interact with the protein GHPN whose function in CNS inhibition will be described below.

Like SPS, hyperekplexia is presumed to have a CNS localization. The startle response is thought to originate from an established neural network within the pontomedullary reticular formation with the response becoming manifest when normal inhibitory influences are lacking.

TREATMENT

There have been no studies addressing therapeutic intervention in hyperekplexia. Clonazepam has been reported to have a beneficial effect. Phenytoin, carbamazepine, piracetam, clobazam, vigabatrin, phenobarbital, 5-hydroxytryptophan, and diazepam have been used anecdotally with uncertain benefit. Positioning a child in a flexed, fetal position may abort a spasm.

▶ SUMMARY

With the exception of cramps and fasciculations, the disorders described in this chapter are uncommon. Most of these disorders have, to some extent, overlapping clinical features. Successful diagnosis requires a heightened index of clinical suspicion, detailed knowledge concerning each disorder's phenotypic characteristics, and awareness of the serologic and EDX features of each syndrome. Many of these disorders appear to have an autoimmune pathogenesis, some of which are in turn related to underlying malignancies. No singular treatment paradigm exists for any of these disorders. In many cases, both immunomodulating therapies and symptomatic measures will provide relief from disease morbidity.

REFERENCES

1. Gutmann L, Libell D, Gutmann L. When is myokymia neuromyotonia? *Muscle Nerve*. 2001;24:151–153.
2. Miller TM, Layzer RB. Muscle cramps. *Muscle Nerve*. 2005; 32:431–442.
3. Norris FH Jr, Gasteiger EL, Chatfield PO. An electromyographic study of induced and spontaneous muscle cramps. *Electroencephalogr Clin Neurophysiol*. 1957;9(suppl):139–147.
4. Atsuta N, Watanabe H, Ito M, et al. Natural history of spinal and bulbar muscular atrophy (SBMA): a study of 223 Japanese patients. *Brain*. 2006;129:1446–1455.
5. Sperfeld AD, Karitzky J, Brummer D, et al. X-linked bulbospinal neuronopathy. *Arch Neurol*. 202;59:1921–1926.
6. Gospe SM, Lazaro RP, Lava NS, Grootscholten PM, Scott MO, Fischbeck KH. Familial X-linked myalgia and cramps. *Neurology*. 1989;39:1277–1280.
7. Tahmoush AJ, Alonso RJ, Tahmoush GP, Heiman-Patterson TD. Cramp–fasciculation syndrome. *Neurology*. 1991;41:1021–1024.
8. Masland RL. Cramp-fasciculation syndrome. *Neurology*. 1992; 42:466.
9. Newsom-Davis J, Mills KR. Immunological associations of acquired neuromyotonia (Isaacs' Syndrome). *Brain*. 1993;116: 453–469.
10. Vernino S, Lennon VA. Ion channel and striational antibodies define a continuum of autoimmune neuromuscular hyperexcitability. *Muscle Nerve*. 2002;26:702–707.
11. George JS, Harikrishnan S, Ali I, Baresi R, Hanemann CO. Acquired rippling muscle disease in association with myasthenia gravis. *J Neurol Neurosurg Psychiatry*. 2010;81(1):125–126.
12. Lo HP, Bertini E, Mirabella M, et al. Mosaic caveolin-3 expression in acquired rippling muscle disease without evidence of myasthenia gravis or acetylcholine receptor autoantibodies. *Neuromuscul Disord*. 2011;21(3):194–203.
13. Brody IA. Muscle contracture induced by exercise. A syndrome attributable to decreased relaxing factor. *N Engl J Med*. 1969;281:187–192.
14. Benders AA, Veerkamp JH, Oosterhof A, et al. Ca2+ homeostasis in Brody's disease. A study in skeletal muscle and cultured muscle cells and the effects of dantrolene an verapamil. *J Clin Invest*. 1994;94:741–748.
15. Karpati G, Charuk J, Carpenter S, Jablecki C, Holland P. Myopathy caused by a deficiency of Ca2+-adenosine triphosphatase in sarcoplasmic reticulum (Brody's disease). *Ann Neurol*. 1986;20:38–49.
16. Danon MJ, Karpati G, Charuk J, Holland P. Sarcoplasmic reticulum adenosine triphosphatase deficiency with probable autosomal dominant inheritance. *Neurology*. 1988;38(5):812–815.
17. Voermans NC, Laasn AE, Oosterhof A, et al. Brody syndrome: a clinically heterogeneous entity distinct from Brody disease. *Neuromuscul Disord*. 2012;22(11):944–954.
18. Odermatt A, Taschner PE, Khanna VK, et al. Mutations in the gene-encoding SERCA1, the fast-twitch skeletal muscle sarcoplasmic reticulum Ca2-ATPase, are associated with Brody disease. *Nat Genet*. 1996;14:191–194.
19. Liguori R, Donadio V, DiStasi V, Cianchi C, Montagna P. Palmaris brevis spasm: an occupational syndrome. *Neurology*. 2003;60:1705–1707.
20. Rowland LP. Cramps, spasms and muscle stiffness. *Rev Neurol (Paris)*. 1985;141:261–273.

21. Katirji B, Al-Jaberi MM. Creatine kinase revisited. *J Clin Neuromuscul Dis*. 2001;2:158–163.
22. Carvalho MD, Swash M. Fasciculation potentials: a study of amyotrophic lateral sclerosis and other neurogenic disorders. *Muscle Nerve*. 1998;21:336–344.
23. Daube JR, Rubin DI. Needle electromyography. *Muscle Nerve*. 2009;39:244–270.
24. Mills KR. Characteristics of fasciculations in amyotrophic lateral sclerosis and the benign fasciculation syndrome. *Brain*. 2010;133:3458–3469.
25. Verdru P, Leenders J, Van Hees J. Cramp-fasciculation syndrome. *Neurology*. 1992;42:1846–1847.
26. Eisen A. Electromyography in disorders of muscle tone. *Can J Neurol Sci*. 1987;14:501–505.
27. Hart IK, Maddison P, Newsom-Davis J, Vincent A, Mills KR. Phenotypic variants of autoimmune peripheral nerve hyperexcitability. *Brain*. 2002;125:1887–1895.
28. Vincent A, Lang B, Kleopa KA. Autoimmune channelopathies and related neurological disorders. *Neuron*. 2006;52:123–138.
29. Vernino S, Auger RG, Emslie-Smith AM, Harper CM, Lennon VA. Myasthenia thymoma, presynaptic antibodies, and a continuum of neuromuscular hyperexcitability. *Neurology*. 1999;53:1233–1239.
30. Lambert E. Electromyography in amyotrophic lateral sclerosis. In: Norris FH, Kurland LT, eds. *Motor Neuron Diseases; Research on Amyotrophic Lateral Sclerosis and Related Disorders*. New York, NY: Grune & Stratton; 1968:135–153.
31. Katzberg HD, Khan AH, So YT. Assessment: symptomatic treatment for muscle cramps (an evidence based review). *Neurology*. 2010;74:691–696.
32. Food and Drug Administration, Department of Health and Human Services. Drug products containing quinine; enforcement action dates. Federal Register 2006;71:75557–75560.
33. Blexrud MD, Windebank AJ, Daube JR. Long-term follow-up of 121 patients with benign fasciculations. *Ann Neurol*. 1993; 34:622–625.
34. Denny-Brown D, Foley JM. Myokymia and the benign fasciculation of muscle cramps. *Trans Assoc Am Physicians*. 1948;61:88–96.
35. Isaacs H. A syndrome of continuous muscle fiber activity. *J Neurol Neurosurg Psychiatry*. 1961;24:319–325.
36. Vincent A. Understanding neuromyotonia. *Muscle Nerve*. 2000;23:655–657.
37. Kleopa KA, Barchi RL. Genetic disorders of neuromuscular ion channels. *Muscle Nerve*. 2002;26:299–325.
38. Balck JT, Garcia-Mullin R, Good E, et al. Muscle rigidity in a new born due to continuous peripheral nerve excitability. *Arch Neurol*. 1972;27:413–425.
39. Mertens HG, Zschocke S. Neuromyotonie. *Klin Wochenschrift*. 1965;43:917–925.
40. Jamieson PW, Katirji MG. Idiopathic generalized myokymia. *Muscle Nerve*. 1994;17:42–51.
41. Isaacs H, Frere G. Syndrome of continuous muscle fiber activity. *S Afr Med J*. 1974;48:1601–1607.
42. Isaacs H. Continuous muscle fiber activity in an Indian male with additional evidence of terminal motor fiber activity. *J Neurol Neurosurg Psychiatry*. 1967;30:126–133.
43. Maddison P, Mills KR, Newsom-Davis J. Clinical electrophysiological characterization of the acquired neuromyotonia phenotype of autoimmune peripheral nerve hyperexcitability. *Muscle Nerve*. 2006;33(6):801–808.
44. Irani SR, Pettingill P, Kleopa KA, et al. Morvan syndrome: clinical and serological observations in 29 cases. *Ann Neurol*. 2012;72:241–255.
45. Barroso L, Hoyt W. Episodic exotropia from lateral rectus neuromyotonia-appearance and remission after radiation therapy for a thalamic glioma. *J Pediatr Ophthalmol Strabismus*. 1993;30:56–57.
46. Lessell S, Lessell IM, Rizzo JF. Ocular neuromyotonia after radiation therapy. *Am J Ophthalmol*. 1986;102:766–770.
47. Yuruten B, Ilhan S. Ocular neuromyotonia: a case report. *Clin Neurol Neurosurg*. 2003;105(2):140–142.
48. Miwa H, Kajimoto Y, Takagi R, Hironishi M, Kondo T. Isolated finger flexion caused by continuous muscle fiber activity. *No To Shinkei*. 2002;54(6):271–273.
49. Modarres H, Samuel M, Schon F. Isolated finger flexion: a novel form of focal neuromyotonia. *J Neurol Neurosurg Psychiatry*. 2000;69:110–113.
50. Lublin FD, Tsairis P, Streletz LJ, et al. Myokymia and impaired muscular relaxation with continuous motor unit activity. *J Neurol Neurosurg Psychiatry*. 1979;42:557–562.
51. Rubio-Agusti I, Perez-Miralles F, Sevilla T, et al. Peripheral nerve hyperexcitability; a clinical and immunologic study of 38 patients. *Neurology*. 2011;76:172–178.
52. Waerness E. Neuromyotonia and bronchial carcinoma. *Electromyogr Clin Neurophysiol*. 1974;14:527–535.
53. Zisfein J, Sivak M, Aron AM, et al. Isaacs' syndrome with muscle hypertrophy reversed by phenytoin therapy. *J Neurol Neurosurg Psychiatry*. 1983;40:241–242.
54. Weiss N, Behin A, Psimaras D, Delattre J-Y. Post-irradiation neuromyotonia of spinal accessory nerves. *Neurology*. 2011;76:1188–1190.
55. Lance JW, Burke D, Pollard J. Hyperexcitability of motor and sensory neurons in neuromyotonia. *Ann Neurol*. 1979;5:523–532.
56. Oda K, Fukushima N, Shibasaki H, et al. Hypoxia-sensitive hyperexcitability of the intramuscular nerve axons in Isaacs' syndrome. *Ann Neurol*. 1989;25:140–145.
57. Barber PA, Andersson NE, Vincent A. Morvan's syndrome associated with voltage-gated K channel antibodies. *Neurology*. 2000;54:771–772.
58. Lee EK, Maselli RA, Ellis WG, Agius MA. Morvan's fibrillary chorea: a paraneoplastic manifestation of thymoma. *J Neurol Neurosurg Psychiatry*. 1998;65:857–862.
59. Kleopa KA, Elman LB, Lang B, Vincent A, Scherer SS. Neuromyotonia and limbic encephalitis sera target mature Shaker-type K+ channels: subunit specificity correlates with clinical manifestations. *Brain*. 2006;129:1570–1584.
60. Rosin L, De Camilli P, Butler M, et al. Stiff-man syndrome in a woman with breast cancer: an uncommon central nervous system paraneoplastic syndrome. *Neurology*. 1998;50:94–98.
61. Caress JB, Abend WK, Preston DC, Logigian EL. A case of Hodgkin's lymphoma producing neuromyotonia. *Neurology*. 1997;49:258–259.
62. Garcia-Merino A, Cabello A, Mora JS, et al. Continuous muscle fiber activity, peripheral neuropathy, and thymoma. *Ann Neurol*. 1991;29:215–218.
63. Partanen VS, Soininen H, Saksa M, et al. Electromyographic and nerve conduction findings in a patient with neuromyotonia, normocalcemic tetany, and small-cell lung cancer. *Acta Neurol Scand*. 1980;61:216–226.
64. Issa SS, Herskovitz S, Lipton RB. Acquired neuromyotonia as a paraneoplastic manifestation of ovarian cancer. *Neurology*. 2011;76:100–101.
65. Evoli A, Lo Monaco M, Marra R, Lino MM, Batocchi AP, Tonali PA. Multiple paraneoplastic diseases associated with thymoma. *Neuromuscul Disord*. 1999;9:601–603.

66. Perini M, Ghezzi A, Basso PF, et al. Association of neuromyotonia with peripheral neuropathy, myasthenia and thymoma: a case report. *Ital J Neurol Sci*. 1994;15:307–310.
67. Aarli JA. Neuromyotonia and rippling muscles. Two infrequent concomitants to myasthenia gravis with thymoma. *Acta Neurol Scand*. 1997;96:342.
68. Heidenreich F, Vincent A. Antibodies to ion-channel proteins in thymoma with myasthenia, neuromyotonia, and peripheral neuropathy. *Neurology*. 1998;50:1483–1485.
69. Martinellli P, Patuelli A, Minardi C, Cau A, Riviera AM, Dal Posso F. Neuromyotonia, peripheral neuropathy and myasthenia gravis. *Muscle Nerve*. 1996;19:505–510.
70. Odabasi Z, Joy JL, Claussen GC, Herrera GA, Oh SJ. Issacs' syndrome associated with chronic inflammatory demyelinating polyneuropathy. *Muscle Nerve*. 1996;19:210–215.
71. Hahn AF, Parkes AW, Bolton CW, et al. Neuromyotonia in hereditary motor neuropathy. *J Neurol Neurosurg Psychiatry*. 1991;54:230–235.
72. Reeback J, Benton S, Swash M, et al. Penicillamine-induced neuromyotonia. *Br Med J*. 1979;2:1464–1465.
73. Vasilescu C, Alexianu M, Dan A. Neuronal type of Charcot–Marie–Tooth disease with a syndrome of continuous motor unit activity. *J Neurol Sci*. 1984;63:11–25.
74. Welch LK, Appenzeller O, Bicknell JM. Peripheral neuropathy with myokymia, sustained muscular contraction, and continuous motor unit activity. *Neurology*. 1972;22:161–169.
75. Gutmann L, Gutmann L. Myokymia and neuromyotonia 2004. *J Neurol*. 2004;251(2):138–142.
76. Auger RG, Daube JR, Gomez MR, et al. Hereditary form of sustained muscle activity of peripheral nerve origin causing generalized myokymia and muscle stiffness. *Ann Neurol*. 1985;15:13–21.
77. Hart IK, Waters C, Vincent A, et al. Autoantibodies detected to expressed K+ channels are implicated in neuromyotonia. *Ann Neurol*. 1997;41:238–256.
78. Shilito P, Molenaar PC, Vincent A, et al. Acquired neuromyotonia: evidence for autoantibodies directed against K+ channels of peripheral nerves. *Ann Neurol*. 1995;38:714–722.
79. Tan KM, Lennon VA, Klein CJ, Boeve EF, Pittock SJ. Clinical spectrum of voltage-gated potassium channel autoimmunity. *Neurology*. 2008;70:1883–1890.
80. Lee R, Buckley C, Irani SR, Vincent A. Autoantibody testing in encephalopathies. *Pract Neurol*. 2012;12:4–13.
81. Bady B, Chauplannaz G, Vial C. Autoimmune aetiology for acquired neuromyotonia. *Lancet*. 1991;338:1330.
82. Brown TJ. Isaacs' syndrome. *Arch Phys Med Rehabil*. 1984;65:27–29.
83. Lutschg J, Jerusalem F, Ludin H, et al. The syndrome of "continuous muscle fiber activity". *Arch Neurol*. 1978;35:198–205.
84. Dhand UK. Issacs's syndrome: clinical and electro-physiological response to gabapentin. *Muscle Nerve*. 2006;34:646–650.
85. Hughes RC, Matthews WB. Pseudo-myotonia and myokymia. *J Neurol Neurosurg Psychiatry*. 1969;32:11–14.
86. Arimura K, Sonoda Y, Watanabe O, et al. Issacs' syndrome as a potassium channelopathy of the nerve. *Muscle Nerve Suppl*. 2002;11:S55–S58.
87. Daube JR. Myokymia and neuromyotonia. *Muscle Nerve*. 2001;24:1711–1712.
88. Barron SA, Heffner RR. Continuous muscle fiber activity: a case with unusual clinical features. *Arch Neurol*. 1979;36:520–521.
89. Isaacs H, Heffron JJ. The syndrome of "continuous muscle fiber activity: cured: further studies. *J Neurol Neurosurg Psychiatry*. 1974;37:1231–1235.
90. Jackson DL, Satya-Murti S, Davis L, et al. Isaacs syndrome with laryngeal involvement: an unusual presentation of myokymia. *Neurology*. 1979;29:1612–1615.
91. Deymeer F, Emre Öge A, Serdaroglu P, Yazici JK, Özdemir C, Baslo A. The use of botulinum toxin in localizing neuromyotonia to the terminal branches of the peripheral nerve. *Muscle Nerve*. 1998;21:643–646.
92. Irani PF, Purohit AV, Wadia NH. The syndrome of continuous muscle fiber activity. *Acta Neurol Scand*. 1977;55:273–288.
93. Sakai T, Hosokawa S, Shibasaki H, et al. Syndrome of continuous muscle-fiber activity: increased CSF GABA and effect of dantrolene. *Neurology*. 1983;33:495–498.
94. Hart IK. Acquired neuromyotonia: a new autoantibody-mediated neuronal potassium channelopathy. *Am J Med Sci*. 2000;319:209–216.
95. Ruff RL. Upsetting the balance among membrane channels can produce hyperexcitablity or inexcitability. *Neurology*. 2007;69:2036–2037.
96. Wallis WE, Van Poznak A, Plum F. Generalized muscular stiffness, fasciculations, and myokymia of peripheral nerve origin. *Arch Neurol*. 1970;22:430–439.
97. Lancaster E, Huijbers MG, Bar C, et al. Investigations of Caspr2, an autoantigen of encephalitis and neuromyotonia. *Ann Neurol*. 2011;69:303–311.
98. Sinha S, Newsom-Davis J, Mills K, Byrne N, Lang B, Vincent A. Autoimmune aetiology for acquired neuromyotonia (Isaacs' syndrome). *Lancet*. 1991;338:75–77.
99. Alessi G, De Reuck J, De Bleecker J, Vancayzeele S. Successful immunoglobulin treatment in a patient with neuromyotonia. *Clin Neurol Neurosurg*. 2000;102:173–175.
100. Ho WK, Wilson JD. Hypothermia, hyperhidrosis, myokymia and increased urinary excretion of catecholamines associated with a thymoma. *Med J Aust*. 1993;158:787–788.
101. Ishii A, Hayashi A, Ohkoshi N, et al. Clinical evaluation of plasma exchange and high dose intravenous immunoglobulin in a patient with Isaacs' syndrome. *J Neurol Neurosurg Psychiatry*. 1994;57:840–842.
102. Van den Berg JS, van Engelen BG, Boerman RH, de Baets MH. Acquired neuromyotonia: superiority of plasma exchange over high-dose intravenous immunoglobulin [letter]. *J Neurol*. 1999;246:623–625.
103. Roos KL. Tetanus. *Semin Neurol*. 1991;11(3):205–214.
104. Srikiatkhachorn A, Hemachudha T, Johnson RT. Tetanus. *Medlink Neurology*. 2011. www.medlink.com
105. Vandelaer J, Birmingham M, Gasse F, et al. Tetanus in developing countries: an update on the maternal and neonatal tetanus elimination initiative. *Vaccine*. 2003;21:3442.
106. Schiavo G, Benfata F, Poulain B, et al. Tetanus and botulinum toxin-B neurotoxins block neurotransmitter release by proteolytic cleavage of synaptobrevin. *Nature*. 1992;359:832–835.
107. Link E, Edelman L, Chou JH, et al. Tetanus toxin action: inhibition of neurotransmitter release linked to synaptobrevin proteolysis. *Biochem Biophys Res Commun*. 1992;189:1017–1023.
108. Price DL, Griffin JW. Tetanus toxin: retrograde axonal transport of systemically administered toxin. *Neurosci Lett*. 1977;4:61–65.
109. Montecucco C, Schiavo G. Structure and function of tetanus and botulinum neurotoxins. *Q Rev Biophys*. 1995;28:423–472.
110. Sexton DJ, Westerman EL. Tetanus. UpToDate Online. 2006;14:3.
111. Verma R, Khanna P. Tetanus toxoid vaccine: elimination of neonatal tetanus in selected states of India. *Hum Vaccin Immunother*. 2012;8(10):1439–1442. [Epub ahead of print]

112. Berger SA, Cherubin CE, Nelson S, Levine L. Tetanus despite preexisting antitetanus antibody. *JAMA*. 1978;240:769–770.
113. Kabura L, Ilibagiza D, Menten J, Van den Ende J. Intrathecal versus intramuscular administration of human antitetanus immunoglobulin or equine tetanus antitoxin in the treatment of tetanus: a meta-analysis. *Trop Med Int Health*. 2006;11:1075–1081.
114. Engrand N, Guerot E, Rouamba A, Vilain GA. The efficacy of intrathecal baclofen in severe tetanus. *Anesthesiology*. 1999;90:1773–1776.
115. Santos ML, Mota-Miranda A, Alves-Pereira A, Gomes A, Correia J, Marçal N. Intrathecal baclofen for the treatment of tetanus. *Clin Infect Dis*. 2004;38:321–328.
116. Sehgal V, Vijayan S, Yasmin S, Srirangalingam U, Pati J, Drake WM. Normocalcaemic tetany. *Clin Med*. 2011;11(6):594–595.
117. Anwikar SR, Bandekar MS, Patel TK, Patel PB, Kshirsagar NA. Tetany: possible adverse effect of bevacizumab. *Indian J Cancer*. 2011;48(1):31–33.
118. Lameris AL, Monnens LA, Bindels RJ, Hoenderop JG. Drug-induced alterations in Mg2 +homoeostasis. *Clin Sci (Lond)*. 2012;123(1):1–14.
119. Aiyangar A, Chowdhary P, Rao K, Kiran K. Normocalcaemic, normomagnesaemic tetany with tacrolimus. *Nephrology*. 2011;16(8):784–785.
120. Brick JF, Gutmann L, McComas CF. Calcium effect on generation and amplification of myokymic discharges. *Neurology*. 1982;32;618–622.
121. Satoyoshi E, Yamada K. Recurrent muscle spasms of central origin. A report of two cases. *Arch Neurol*. 1967;16:254–264.
122. Heger S, Kuester RM, Volk R, Stephani U, Sippell WG. Satoyoshi syndrome: a rare multisystemic disorder requiring systemic and symptomatic treatment. *Brain Dev*. 2006;28(5):300–304.
123. Satoyoshi E. A syndrome of progressive muscle spasm, alopecia, and diarrhea. *Neurology*. 1978;28:458–471.
124. Ikeda K, Satoyoshi E, Kinoshita M, Wakata N, Iwasaki Y. Satoyoshi's syndrome in an adult: a review of the literature of adult onset cases. *Intern Med*. 1998;37:784–787.
125. Matsuura E, Matsuyama W, Sameshima T, Arimura K. Satoyoshi syndrome has antibody against brain and gastrointestinal tissue. *Muscle Nerve*. 2007;36:400–403.
126. Endo K, Yamamoto T, Nakamura K, et al. Improvement of Satoyoshi syndrome with tacrolimus and corticosteroids. *Neurology*. 2003;600:2014–2015.
127. Uddin AB, Walters AS, Ali A, Brannan T. A unilateral presentation of 'Satoyoshi syndrome'. *Parkinsonism Relat Disord*. 2002;8(3):211–213.
128. Drost G, Verrips A, Hooijkass H, Zwarts M. Glutamic acid decarboxylase antibodies in Satoyoshi syndrome. *Ann Neurol*. 2004;55(3):450–451.
129. Cecchin CR, Felix TM, Magalhaes RB, Furlanetto TW. Satoyoshi syndrome in a Caucasian girl improved with glucocorticoids – a clinical report. *Am J Med Genet*. 2003;118A:52–54.
130. Arita J, Hamano S, Nara T, Maekawa K. Intravenous gammaglobulin therapy of Satoyoshi syndrome. *Brain Dev*. 1996;18:409–411
131. Moersch FP, Woltman HW. Progressive fluctuating rigidity and spasm (stiff-man syndrome): report of a case and some observations in 13 other cases. *Mayo Clin Proc*. 1956;31:421–427.
132. Dalakas M, Fujii M, Li M, McElroy B. The clinical spectrum of anti-GAD antibody-positive patients with stiff-person syndrome. *Neurology*. 2000;55:1531–1535.
133. Shannon KM. Stiff-person syndrome. *Medlink Neurol*. 2006;1–17. www.medlink.com.
134. Espay AJ, Chen R. Rigidity and spasms from autoimmune encephalomyelopathies: stiff-person syndrome. *Muscle Nerve*. 2006;34:677–690.
135. Rakocevic G, Floeter MK. Autoimmune stiff person syndrome and related myelopathies: understanding of electrophysiological and immunological processes. *Muscle Nerve*. 2012;45:623–634.
136. Dalakas MC. Advances in the pathogenesis and treatment of patients with stiff person syndrome. *Curr Neurol Neurosci Rep*. 2008;8:48–55.
137. McKeon A, Robinson MT, McEvoy KM, et al. Stiff-man syndrome and variants. *Arch Neurol*. 2012;69(2):230–238.
138. Alexopoulos H, Dalakas MC. A critical update on the immunopathogenesis of stiff-person syndrome. *Eur J Clin Invest*. 2010; 40(11)1018–1025.
139. Jog MS, Lambert CD, Lang AE. Stiff-person syndrome. *Can J Neurol Sci*. 1992;19:383–388.
140. McEvoy KM. Stiff-man syndrome. *Mayo Clin Proc*. 1991;66: 300–304.
141. Olafson RA, Mulder DW, Howard FM. "Stiff-man" syndrome: a review of the literature, report of three additional cases and discussion of pathophysiology and therapy. *Mayo Clin Proc*. 1964;39:31–144.
142. Gordon EE, Januszko DM, Kaufman L. A critical survey of stiff-man syndrome. *Am J Med*. 1967;42:582–589.
143. Miller F, Korsvik. Baclofen in the treatment of stiff-man syncrome. *Ann Neurol*. 1981;9:51–52.
144. Folli F. Stiff-man syndrome, 40 years later. *J Neurol Neurosurg Psychiatry*. 1998;65:618.
145. Petzold GC, Marcucci M, Butler MH, et al. Rhabdomyolysis and paraneoplastic stiff-man syndrome with amphiphysin autoimmunity. *Ann Neurol*. 2004;55:286–290.
146. Mitosumoto H, Schwartzman MJ, Estes ML, et al. Sudden death and paroxysmal autonomic dysfunction in stiff-man syndrome. *J Neurol*. 1991;238:91–96.
147. Hadavi S, Noyce AJ, Leslie RD, Giovannoni G. Stiff person syndrome. *Pract Neurol*. 2011;11:272–282.
148. Barker RA, Revesz T, Thom M, Marsden CD, Brown P. Review of 23 patients affected by the stiff man syndrome: clinical subdivision into stiff trunk(man) syndrome, stiff limb syndrome, and progressive encephalomyelitis with rigidity. *J Neurol Neurosurg Psychiatry*. 1998;65:633–640.
149. Brown P, Marsden CD. The stiffman and stiffman-plus syndromes. *J Neurol*. 1999;246:648–652.
150. Saiz A, Graus F, Valldeoriola F, Valls-Sole J, Tolosa E. Stiff-leg syndrome: a focal form of stiff-man syndrome. *Ann Neurol*. 1998;43:400–403.
151. Souza-Lima CF, Ferraz HB, Braz CA, Araujo AM, Manzano GM. Marked improvement in a stiff-limb patient treated with intravenous immunoglobulin. *Mov Disord*. 2000;15:358–359.
152. Silverman IE. Paraneoplastic stiff-person syndrome. *J Neurol Neurosurg Psychiatry*. 1999;67(1):126–127
153. Ameli R, Snow J, Rakocevic G, Dalakas MC. A neuropsychological assessment of phobias in patients with stiff person syndrome. *Neurology*. 2005;64:1961–1963.
154. Warren JD, Scott G, Blumbergs PC, Thompson PD. Pathological evidence of encephalomyelitis in the stiff man syndrome with anti-GAD antibodies. *J Clin Neurosci*. 2002;9:328–329.
155. Turner MR, Irani SR, Leite MI, Nithi K, Vincent A, Ansorge O. Progressive encephalomyelitis with rigidity and myoclonus:

glycine and NMDA receptor antibodies. *Neurology*. 2011;77:439–443.

156. Whiteley AM, Swash M, Urich H. Progressive encephalomyelitis with rigidity. Its relation to subacute myoclonic spinal neuronitis and to the stiff-man syndrome. *Brain*. 1976;99:27–42.
157. Howell DA, Lees AJ, Toghill PJ. Spinal internuncial neurones in progressive encephalomyelitis with rigidity. *J Neurol Neurosurg Psychiatry*. 1979;42:773–785.
158. Kasperek S, Zebrowski S. Stiff-man syndrome and encephalomyelitis. *Arch Neurol*. 1971;24:22–30.
159. Leigh PN, Rothwell JC, Traub M, Marsden CD. A patients with reflex myoclonus and muscle rigidity: "Jerking stiff-man syndrome". *J Neurol Neurosurg Psychiatry*. 1980;43:1125–1131.
160. Lorish TR, Thorsteinsson G, Howard FM. Stiff-man syndrome updated. *Mayo Clin Proc*. 1989;64:629–636.
161. Baekkeskov S, Aanstoot HJ, Christgau S, et al. Identification of the 64 K autoantigenin insulin-dependent diabetes as the GABA-synthesizing enzyme glutamic acid decarboxylase. *Nature*. 1990;347:151–156.
162. Verge CF, Stenger D, Bonifacio E, et al. Combined use of autoantibodies (IA-2 autoantibody, GAD autoantibody, insulin autoantibody, cytoplasmic islet cell antibodies) in type 1 diabetes: combinatorial Islet Autoantibody Workshop. *Diabetes*. 1998;47:1857–1866.
163. De Camilli P, Thomas A, Cofiell R, et al. The synaptic vesicle-associated protein amphiphysin is the 128 kD autoantigen of stiff-man syndrome with breast cancer. *J Exp Med*. 1993;178:2219–2223.
164. Folli F, Solimena M, Cofiell R, et al. Autoantibodies to a 128-kd synaptic protein in three women with the stiff-man syndrome and breast cancer. *N Engl J Med*. 1993;328:546–551.
165. Grimaldi LM, Martino G, Braaghi S, et al. Heterogeneity of autoantibodies in stiff-man syndrome. *Ann Neurol*. 1993;34:57–64.
166. Amato AA, Cornmann EW, Kissel JT. Treatment of stiff-man syndrome with intravenous immunoglobulin. *Neurology*. 1994;44:1652–1654.
167. Solimena M, Folli F, Denis-Donini S, et al. Autoantibodies to glutamic acid decarboxylase in a patient with stiff-man syndrome, epilepsy, and type I diabetes mellitus. *N Engl J Med*. 1988;318:1012–1020.
168. Solimena M, Folli F, Aparisi R, Pozza G, De Camilli P. Autoantibodies to GABA-ergic and pancreatic beta cells in stiff-man syndrome. *N Engl J Med*. 1990;322:1555–1560.
169. Rakocevic G, Faju R, Dalakas MC. Anti-glutamic acid decarboxylase antibodies in the serum and cerebrospinal fluid of patients with stiff-person syndrome: correlation with clinical severity. *Arch Neurol*. 2004;61:902–904.
170. Thomas S, Critchley P, Lawden M, et al. Stiff person syndrome with eye movement abnormality, myasthenia gravis, and thymoma. *J Neurol Neurosurg Psychiatry*. 2005;76:141–142.
171. McHugh JC, Murray B, Renganathan R, Connolly S, Lynch T. GAD antibody positive paraneoplastic stiff person syndrome in a patient with renal cell carcinoma. *Mov Disord*. 2007;22:1343–1346.
172. Feng G, Tintrup H, Kirsch J, et al. Dual requirement for gephyrin in glycine receptor clustering and molybdoenzyme activity. *Science*. 1998;282:1321–1324.
173. McCabe DJ, Turner NC, CChao D, et al. Paraneoplastic stiff-person syndrome: with metastatic adenocarcinoma and anti-Ri antibodies. *Neurology*. 2004;62:1402–1404.
174. Meinck HM, Thompson PD. Stiff man syndrome and related conditions. *Mov Disord*. 2002;17:853–866.
175. Berger C, Meinck HM. Head retraction reflex in stiff-man syndrome and related disorders. *Mov Disord*. 2003;18:906–911.
176. Levy LM, Levy-Reis I, Fujii M, Dalakas MC. Brain gamma-aminobutyric acid changes in stiff-person syndrome. *Arch Neurol*. 2005;62:970–974.
177. Levy LM, Dalakas MC, Floeter MK. The stiff-person syndrome: an autoimmune disorder affecting neurotransmission of gamma-aminobutyric acid. *Ann Intern Med*. 1999;131:522–530.
178. Asher R. A woman with the stiff-man syndrome. *Br Med J*. 1958;14:265–266.
179. Cohen L. Stiff-man syndrome. Two patients treated with diazepam. *JAMA*. 1966;195:222–224.
180. Trethowan WH, Allsop JL, Turner B. The "stiff-man" syndrome. A report of two further cases. *Arch Neurol*. 1960;3:448–456.
181. Holmoy T, Skorstad G, Hestvik AL, Alvik KM, Vartdal F. Protective and detrimental immunity: lessons from stiff person syndrome and multiple sclerosis. *Acta Neurol Scand Suppl*. 2009;(189):22–26.
182. Thompson PD. The stiff-man syndrome and related disorders. *Parkinsonism Relat Disord*. 2001;8:147–153.
183. Dinkel K, Meinck HM, Jury KM, Karges W, Richter W. Inhibition of gamma –aminobutyric acid synthesis by glutamic acid decarboxylase autoantibodies in stiff-mann syndrome. *Ann Neurol*. 1998;44:194–201.
184. Ishida K, Mitoma H, Song SY, et al. Selective suppression of cerebellar GABAergic transmission by an autoantibody to glutamic acid decarboxylase. *Ann Neurol*. 1999;46:263–267.
185. Silbert PL, Masumoto JY, McManis PG, Stolp-Smith KA, Elliott BA, McEvoy KM. Intrathecal baclofen therapy in stiff-man syndrome: a double-blind, placebo-controlled trial. *Neurology*. 1995;45:1893–1897.
186. Baker MR, Das M, Isaacs J, Fawcdett PR, Bates D. Treatment of stiff person syndrome with rituximab. *J Neurol Neurosurg Psychiatry*. 2005;76:999–1001.
187. Dupond JL, Essalmi L, Gil H, Meaux-Ruault N, Hafsaoui C. Rituximab treatment of stiff-person syndrome in a patient with thymoma, diabetes mellitus and autoimmune thyroiditis. *J Clin Neurosci*. 2010;17(3):389–391.
188. Katoh N, Matsuda M, Ishii W, Morita H, Ikeda S. Successful treatment with rituximab in a patient with stiff-person syndrome complicated by dysthyroid ophthalmopathy. *Intern Med*. 2010;49(3):237–241.
189. Dalakas MC, Fujii M, Li M, Lufti B, Kyhos J, McElroy B. High-dose intravenous immune globulin for stiff-person syndrome. *N Engl J Med*. 2001;345:1870–1876.
190. Panayiotopoulas CP. Hyperekplexia. *Medlink Neurol*. 2007. www.medlink.com.
191. Lerman-Sagie T, Watemberg M, Vinkler C, Fishof J, Leshinsky-Silver E, Lev D. Familial hyperekplexia and refractory status epilepticus: a new autosomal recessive syndrome. *J Child Neurol*. 2004;19:522–525.
192. Tijssen MAJ, Rees MI. Hyperekplexia. http://www.ncbi.nlm.nih.gov/books/NBK1260/

CHAPTER 11

Charcot–Marie–Tooth Disease and Related Disorders

Hereditary neuropathies may account for as many as 50% of previously undiagnosed peripheral neuropathies referred to large neuromuscular centers. Charcot–Marie–Tooth (CMT) disease is the most common type of hereditary neuropathy, but, rather than one disease, CMT is a syndrome of several genetically distinct disorders (Table 11-1). In this chapter, we discuss CMT and related neuropathies. In the subsequent chapters, we will review other less common hereditary neuropathies (Chapters 12, 16, and 30).

The various subtypes of CMT are classified according to the nerve conduction velocities (NCVs), presumed pathology (e.g., demyelinating or axonal), mode of inheritance (autosomal-dominant, autosomal recessive, or X-linked), age of onset (e.g., infancy or childhood/adulthood), and the specific mutated gene (Table 11-1).[1–8] Updated information including recent mutations causing CMT can be found on the Internet: http://www.molgen.ua.ac.be/CMTMutations/DataSource/MutByGene.cfm. Type 1 CMT or CMT1 refers to inherited demyelinating motor and sensory neuropathies, whereas the axonal motor and sensory neuropathies are classified as CMT2. Both CMT1 and CMT2 usually begin in childhood or early adult life; however, onset later in life can occur, particularly in CMT2. CMT1 is associated with autosomal-dominant or X-linked inheritance, while CMT2 can be autosomal-dominant, autosomal-recessive, or X-linked. Most patients with different subtypes of CMT1 looked phenotypically indistinguishable from each other and subtypes of CMT2 and X-linked CMT. Some authorities advocate for classifying as CMT1 (dominant, recessive, or X-linked) and CMT2 (dominant, recessive, or X-linked) along with dominant-intermediate and recessive intermediate subtypes. However, reports of CMT3 and CMT4 remain in the literature so we will still discuss these. CMT3 is an autosomal-dominant neuropathy that appears in infancy and is associated with severe demyelination or hypomyelination. CMT4 is an autosomal-recessive motor and sensory neuropathy that typically begins in childhood or early adult life. Unfortunately, classification of these neuropathies is not straightforward. Mutations of the same gene can lead to neuropathies associated with nerve conduction studies (NCS) and histopathology that may reflect either a primary demyelinating or an axonal process, an autosomal-dominant or recessive inheritance, and a clinical phenotype with overlap between CMT and hereditary sensory and autonomic neuropathy (HSAN), hereditary motor neuropathy (distal spinal muscular atrophy), and hereditary spastic paraplegia (HSP) (Fig. 11-1). The causal mutated genes have many different functions (Table 11-2, Fig. 11-2). There are no specific medical therapies for any of the CMTs, but physical and occupational therapy can be beneficial as can bracing (e.g., ankle–foot orthotics for foot drop) and other orthotic devices.

▶ CMT TYPE 1 (CMT1)

CLINICAL FEATURES

CMT1 is the most common form of hereditary neuropathy, with the ratio of CMT1:CMT2 being approximately 2:1. Individuals with CMT1 usually present in the first to third decades with distal leg weakness, although patients may remain asymptomatic even late in life. There is an early predilection for the anterior compartment (peroneal muscle group), resulting in progressive foot drop. This leads to poor clearance of the toes when walking particularly on uneven surfaces. People with CMT1 often present with frequent tripping, falling, and recurrent ankle sprains. Affected individuals generally do not complain numbness or tingling, which can be helpful in distinguishing CMT from acquired forms of neuropathy.

Although people with CMT1 usually do not complain of sensory loss, reduced sensation to all modalities is apparent on examination. Muscle stretch reflexes are unobtainable or reduced throughout. There is often atrophy of the muscles below the knee (particularly the anterior compartment), leading to the appearance of the so-called inverted champagne bottle legs. However, rare individuals have asymmetric pseudohypertrophy of the calves.[9] Most will have pes cavus, equinovarus, or hammertoe deformities (Fig. 11-3), which lead to aching in the feet. Rather than having a heel strike while ambulating, affected people land flat-footed or on their toes and thus use a steppage gait to help prevent tripping. Approximately two-thirds of individuals with CMT1 also have distal weakness and atrophy of the arms. Claw–hand deformities of the hands may develop in the most severely affected. Mild-to-moderate proximal weakness can develop over time as well, which can lead to diagnostic confusion with chronic inflammatory demyelinating polyneuropathy (CIDP). In addition, some individuals manifest with phrenic nerve involvement leading to respiratory weakness.[10] Rarely, patients with hypertrophy of nerve roots can be severe enough such that it leads to compression of the spinal cord

▶ TABLE 11-1. **CLASSIFICATION OF CHARCOT–MARIE–TOOTH DISEASE AND RELATED NEUROPATHIES**

Name	Inheritance	Gene Location	Gene
CMT1			
CMT1A	AD	17p11.2	*PMP22* (usually duplication of gene)
CMT1B	AD	1q21–23	*MPZ*
CMT1C	AD	16p13.1–p12.3	*LITAF*
CMT1D	AD	10q21.1–22.1	*ERG2*
CMT1E (with deafness)	AD	17p11.2	Point mutations in *PMP22*
CMT1F	AD	8p13–21	*NEFL/NFL*
CMT1G	AD	14q32.33	*IFN2*
CMT1X	X-linked dominant	Xq13	*GJB1*
HNPP	AD	17p11.2	*PMP22*
		1q21–23	*MPZ*
CMT2			
CMT2A1	AD	1p36.2	*KIF1B*
CMT2A2 (allelic to HMSN VI with optic atrophy)	AD	1p36.2	*MFN2*
CMT2B	AD	3q13–q22	*RAB7*
CMT2B1 (allelic to LGMD1B)	AR	1q21.2	*LMNA*
CMT2B2	AD	19q13	*MED25*
CMT2C (with vocal cord and diaphragm paralysis)	AD	12q23–24	*TRPV4*
CMT2D (allelic to distal SMA5)	AD	7p14	*GARS*
CMT2E (allelic to CMT1F)	AD	8p21	*NEFL*
CMT2F	AD	7q11–q21	*HSPB1*
CMT2G	AD	12q12–q13	?
CMT2H (allelic to CMT2K and CMT4A)	AD	8q21.3	*GDAP1*
CMT2I and 2J (allelic to CMT1B)	AD	1q22	*MPZ*
CMT2K (allelic to CMT2H and CMT4A)	AD/AR	8q13–q21	*GDAP1*
CMT2L (allelic to distal hereditary motor neuropathy type 2)	AD	12q24	*HSPB8*
CMT2M	AD	19p13.2	*DYN2*
CMT2N	AD	16q22.1	*AARS*
CMT2O	AD	14q32.31	*DYNC1HI*
CMT2P	AD/AR	9 q33	*LRSAM1*
CMR2	AR		*DNAJB2*
CMT2X	X-linked	Xq22.3	*PRPSI*
CMT2X	X-linked	Xp22.11	*PDGK3*
DI-CMT			
DI-CMTA	AD	10q24.1–q25.1	?
DI-CMTB	AD	19p12–p13.2	*DYN2*
DI-CMTC	AD	1p34–p35	*YARS*
RI-CMT	AR	1p36.31	*PLEKHG5*
CMT3 (Dejerine–Sottas disease, congenital hypomyelinating neuropathy)	AD	17p11.2	*PMP22*
	AD	1q21–23	*MPZ*
	AR	10q21.1–22.1	*ERG2*
	AR	19q13	*PRX*
CMT4			
CMT4A (allelic to CMT2H and 2K)	AR	8q13–21.1	*GDAP1*
CMT4B1	AR	11q23	*MTMR2*
CMT4B2	AR	11p15	*MTMR13*
CMT4C	AR	5q23–33	*SH3TC2*
CMT4D (HMSN-Lom)	AR	8q24	*NDRG1*
CMT4E (congenital hypomyelinating neuropathy)	AR		Probably includes *PMP22*, *MPZ*, and *ERG2*
CMT4F	AR	19q13.1–13.3	*PRX*
CMT4G (CMT-Russe type)	AR	10q23.2	*HK1*

(*continued*)

► **TABLE 11-1. (CONTINUED)**

Name	Inheritance	Gene Location	Gene
CMT4H	AR	12q12–q13	*FGD4*
CMT4J	AR	6q21	*FIG4*
Other hereditary neuropathies			
HNA	AD	17q24	*SEPT9*
HMSN-P	AD	3q13–q14	*TFG*

CMT, Charcot–Marie–Tooth; DI-CMT, dominant intermediate CMT; HNNP, hereditary neuropathy with liability to pressure palsies; HNA, hereditary neuralgic amyotrophy; SMA, spinal muscular atrophy; LGMD, limb girdle muscular dystrophy; HMSN-P, hereditary motor and sensory neuropathy-proximal; AD, autosomal dominant; AR, autosomal recessive; Genes: AARS, alanyl-trRNA synthetase; BSCL2, Berardinelli–Seip congenital lipodystrophy type 2; DNM2, dynamin 2; DYNCH1H1, cytoplasmic dynein 1 heavy chain 1; EGR2, early-growth response 2; GARS, glycyl-tRNA synthetase; GDAP1, ganglioside-induced differentiation-associated protein 1; GJB1, gap junction B1/connexin-32; HSJ1 (or DNAJB2), heat-shock protein J1 (or DnaJ Hsp40); HSPB1 (or HSP27), heat-shock 27-kDa protein 1; HSPB8 (or HSP22), heat-shock 22-kDa protein 8; HK6, hexokinase 6; IFN2, inverted formin 2; LITAF, lipopolysaccharide-induced tumor necrosis factor-alpha factor; LMNA, lamin A/C nuclear envelope protein; LSRAM1, leucine-rich repeat and sterile alpha motif containing 1; MED25, mediator complex subunit; MFN2, mitofusin 2; MTMR2, myotubularin-related protein 2; SBF2, SET-binding factor 2; SH3TC2, SH3 domain and tetratricopeptide repeat domain 2; NDRG1, N-myc downstream-regulated gene 1; NEFL, neurofilament light chain; NGF, nerve growth factor; MPZ, myelin protein zero; PLEKHG5, pleckstrin homology domain-containing protein; PMP22, peripheral myelin protein 22; PDK3, pyruvate dehydrogenase kinase isoenzyme 3; PRSP1, phosphoribosyl pyrophosphate synthetase 1;PRX, periaxin; RAB7, small GTPase late endosomal protein RAB7; TRPV4, transient receptor potential cation channel subfamily V, member 4;YARS, tyrosyl-tRNA synthetase.

or cauda equina (see Fig. 24-14 in Chapter 24). Hypertrophy of the nerves, especially posterior to the ear and arm regions, may be visualized and palpated. Approximately one-third of patients with CMT1 have an essential tremor (Roussy–Levy syndrome). Some individuals who are affected also develop deafness or Adie's pupils. Further, one subtype, CMT1G, is associated with focal segmental glomerulosclerosis. It is important to examine family members of patients with possible CMT. Although there may be no family history of CMT, careful examination of the family may demonstrate other members with features of the neuropathy. This can be important in clarifying a diagnosis and in providing genetic counseling.

► **TABLE 11-2. PATHOGENIC TARGETS INVOLVED IN INHERITED NEUROPATHIES**

Myelin structure and function (PMP22, MPZ, CX32, PRX, MMTR2, MMTR13/SBF2, IFN2)
Axonal structure (NGF, NEFL, FGD4)
Axonal transport (DYM2, DYNC1 H, NFL, RAB7, WNK1, KIF1B, NDRG1, SH3TC2)
Golgi body formation (FAM134B)
Endoplasmic reticulum formation (ATL1, ALT2, ATL3)
Sphingolipid metabolism (SPTLC1, SPTLC2)
Nuclear structure (LMNA)
DNA transcription (ERG2, LITAF, MED25)
RNA translation (GARS, YARS, AARS, BCL2)
DNA methylation (DNMT1)
Protein degradation chaperones and stress regulation (LITAF, BAG3, HSPB1, HSP27, HSJ1)
Mitochondrial DNA maintenance (see Chapter 30)
Mitochondrial fission or fusion (MFN2, GDAP1)
Ion channels (TRPV4, SCN9A, SCN10A, SCN11A, HINT1)

LABORATORY FEATURES

Cerebrospinal fluid (CSF) protein levels may be elevated. Besides genetic testing, NCS are the most important laboratory tests in the evaluation of people suspected of having CMT. The NCS are invaluable in determining if patients have a demyelinating or axonal neuropathy and, if demyelinating, if it is uniform or multifocal, which is useful in distinguishing CMT from CIDP.[2,11,13] Uniform slowing of NCVs is suggestive of a hereditary demyelinating neuropathy, while multifocal slowing is more typical of CIDP. At birth and in infancy, NCVs may be normal or only minimally slowed in children with CMT1. However, the NCVs rapidly decline, and, by 3–5 years of age, the nadir in NCV slowing is achieved and remains stable throughout the rest of the person's life. However, the compound muscle action potential (CMAP) amplitudes continue to diminish over time, reflecting ongoing loss of axons. Distal motor latencies at birth are commonly borderline abnormal. These latencies continue to increase until approximately the age of 10 years, at which time there is little further prolongation of the distal latencies. A detailed discussion of specific nerve conduction abnormalities in CMT1 follows.

Motor NCS

Motor NCVs by definition are slowed to less than 38 m/s in the upper extremities, but in most cases the NCVs are in the 20–25 m/s range.[2,7,11–13] Patients with point mutations in peripheral myelin protein 22 (*PMP22*) and myelin protein zero (*MPZ*) genes can have even slower conduction velocities (CVs) approaching that seen in CMT3 (10 m/s or less).[14,15] As will be discussed in the subsequent section, some people with *MPZ* mutations have only slightly slow or normal NCVs and thus by NCV criteria can be

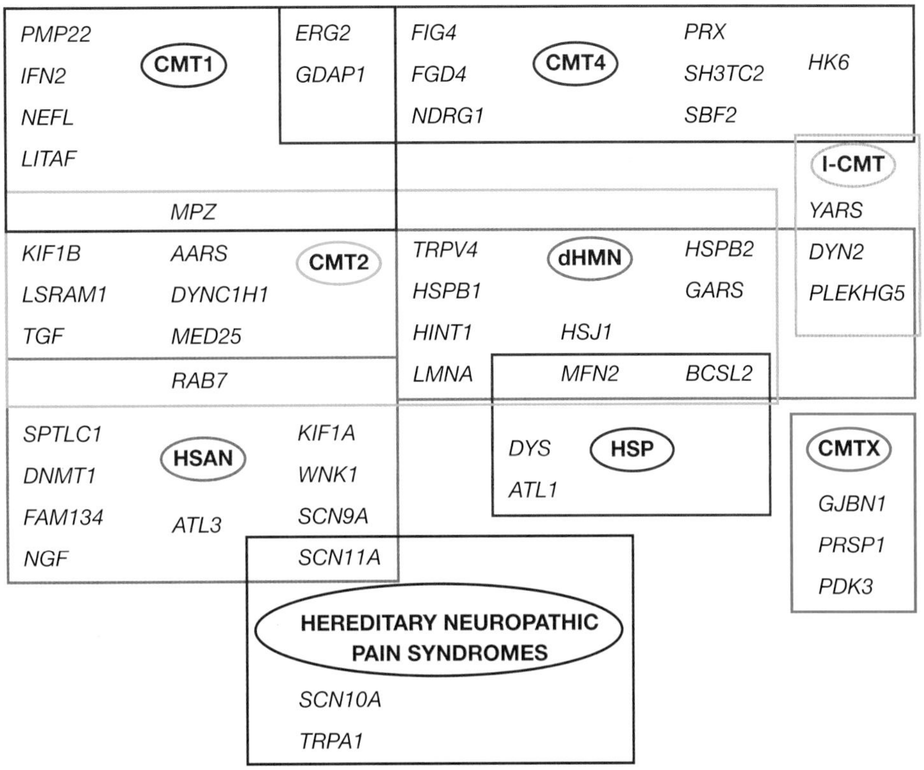

Figure 11-1. The overlap of CMT, HSAN, dHMN, HSP, episodic pain syndrome, and related disorders. Diseases: CMT, Charcot–Marie–Tooth disease (CMT1, demyelinating, autosomal dominant; CMT2, axonal, autosomal dominant or recessive; CMT4, demyelinating, autosomal recessive; CMTX, X-linked; I-CMT, intermediate CMT); dHMN, distal hereditary motor neuropathies; HSN, hereditary sensory neuropathies; HSP, hereditary spastic paraplegia. Genes: AARS, alanyl-trRNA synthetase; ATL, atlastin; BSCL2, Berardinelli–Seip congenital lipodystrophy type 2; DNM2, dynamin 2; DNMT1, DNA methyltransferase 1; DYNCH1H1, cytoplasmic dynein 1 heavy chain 1; DYS, dystonin; EGR2, early-growth response 2; FAM134B, family with sequence similarity 134, member B; GARS, glycyl-tRNA synthetase; GDAP1, ganglioside-induced differentiation-associated protein 1; GJB1, gap junction B1/connexin-32; HSJ1 (or DNAJB2), heat-shock protein J1 (or DNAJ Hsp40); HSPB1 (or HSP27), heat-shock 27-kDa protein 1; HSPB8 (or HSP22), heat-shock 22-kDa protein 8; HK6, hexokinase 6; HINT1, histidine triad nucleotide binding protein 1; IFN2, inverted formin 2; LITAF, lipopolysaccharide-induced tumor necrosis factor-alpha factor; LMNA, lamin A/C nuclear envelope protein; LSRAM1, leucine-rich repeat and sterile alpha motif containing 1; MED25, mediator complex subunit; MFN2, mitofusin 2; MTMR2, myotubularin-related protein 2; SBF2, SET-binding factor 2; SH3TC2, SH3 domain and tetratricopeptide repeat domain 2; NDRG1, N-myc downstream-regulated gene 1; NEFL, neurofilament light chain; NGF, nerve growth factor; MPZ, myelin protein zero; PLEKHG5, pleckstrin homology domain-containing protein; PMP22, peripheral myelin protein 22; PDK3, pyruvate dehydrogenase kinase isoenzyme 3; PRSP1, phosphoribosyl pyrophosphate synthetase 1; PRX, periaxin; RAB7, small GTPase late endosomal protein RAB7; SPTLC1, serine palmitoyltransferase long chain base 1; TRPA1, transient receptor potential A 1; TRPV4, transient receptor potential cation channel subfamily V, member 4; YARS, tyrosyl-tRNA synthetase; WNK1, protein kinase, lysine-deficient 1.

classified as having CMT2.[12,16] Demyelination is generally uniform; therefore, patients with CMT1 do not usually demonstrate conduction block or temporal dispersion on NCS.[13,17] However, there are well-documented cases of genetically proven CMT1A with nonuniform slowing and CVs over 42 m/s and thus might mimic an acquired neuropathy.[9] Temporal dispersion of nerve conduction and irregularity of conduction slowing have been reported in CMT1C.[18] In addition, mutations in MPZ, ERG2, GJB1, FIG4, SH3TC2 also cause hereditary neuropathies with acquired demyelinating features.

Distal motor latencies are usually markedly prolonged. The CMAPs may be absent when recordings are attempted from severely atrophic muscles. It is useful in people with wasted foot intrinsics to perform motor NCS in the lower limb by recording from the tibialis anterior muscle. F-waves are usually absent but, when obtainable, the latencies are extremely prolonged.

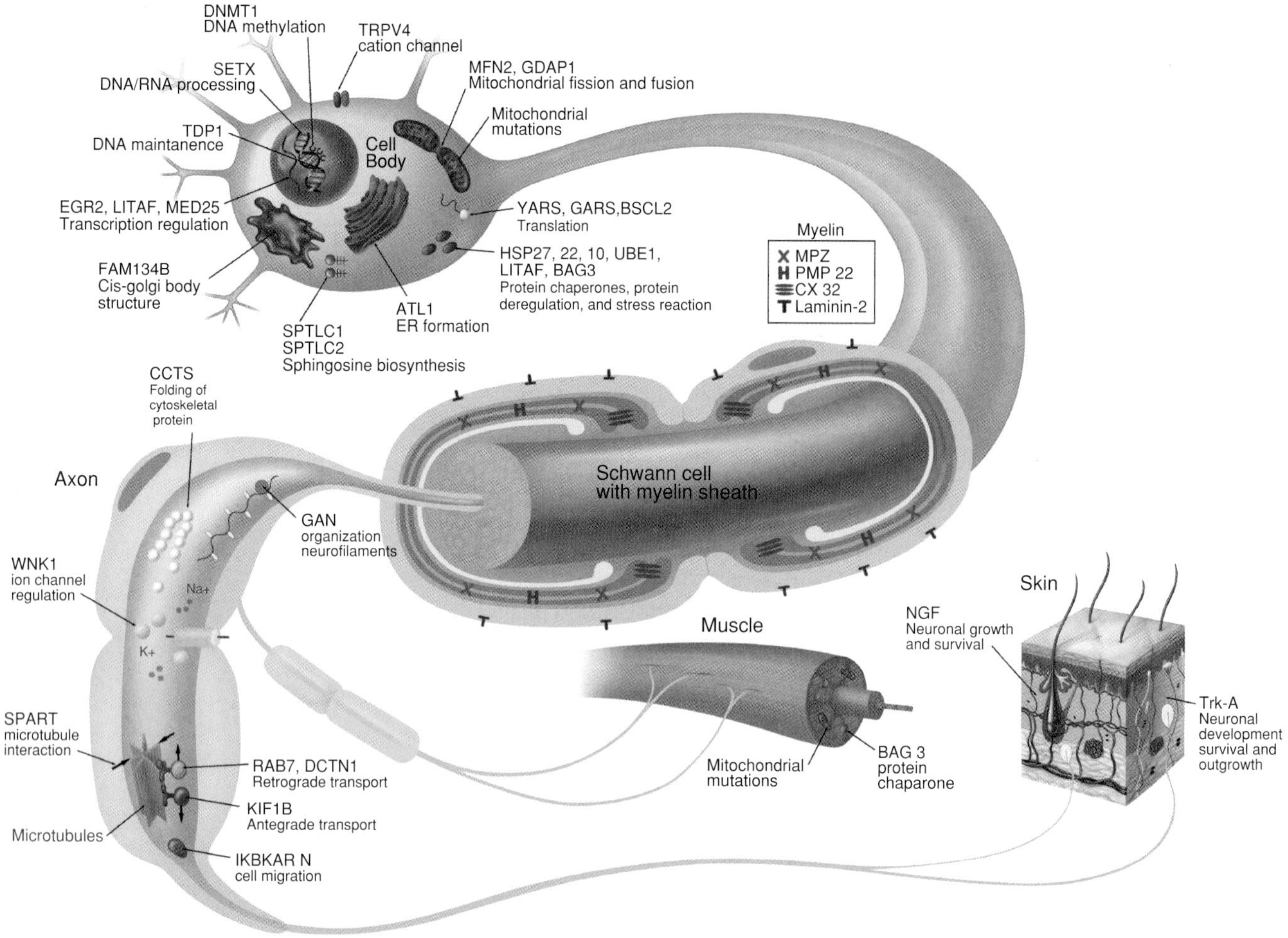

Figure 11-2. Molecular targets of inherited neuropathies demonstrate the diverse pathogenesis of these different neuropathies.

There is no correlation between the NCVs and the clinical severity of the neuropathy.[19] The NCVs are quite slow in childhood, even when there are minimal clinical deficits. Further, asymptomatic adults can have prolonged distal motor latencies and slow NCV. It is apparent that weakness and loss of function are more related to the degree of axon loss, rather than the extent of demyelination and slowing of nerve conduction.

Motor Nerve Unit Estimates

Motor nerve unit estimates can assess motor unit loss in CMT and may better reflect axonal loss than CMAP amplitude in view of reinnervation which to a certain extent may camouflage the extent of axon loss.[20]

Sensory NCS

The sensory nerve action potentials (SNAPs) are usually unobtainable or very low in amplitude.[21–29] When recordable, the distal latencies are very prolonged and NCVs are markedly slow.

Evoked Potentials

Somatosensory evoked potentials have demonstrated slowing of central conduction in CMT1. Visual-evoked potentials also reveal similar slowing in the optic pathways.

Needle Electromyography

Electromyography (EMG) reveals positive sharp waves and fibrillation potentials along with reduced recruitment of long-duration, high-amplitude, and polyphasic motor unit action potentials (MUAPs) in the distal legs and lesser in the arms.[24] Evidence of active denervation and reinnervation may also be found in some of the proximal muscles.

HISTOPATHOLOGY

We do not perform nerve biopsies on people suspected of having CMT1, as the diagnosis can usually be made by less invasive testing (e.g., NCS and genetic studies). Nevertheless, nerve biopsies, when done are strikingly abnormal.[7,12,25,26] The enlarged gross appearance of the peripheral nerves led to the

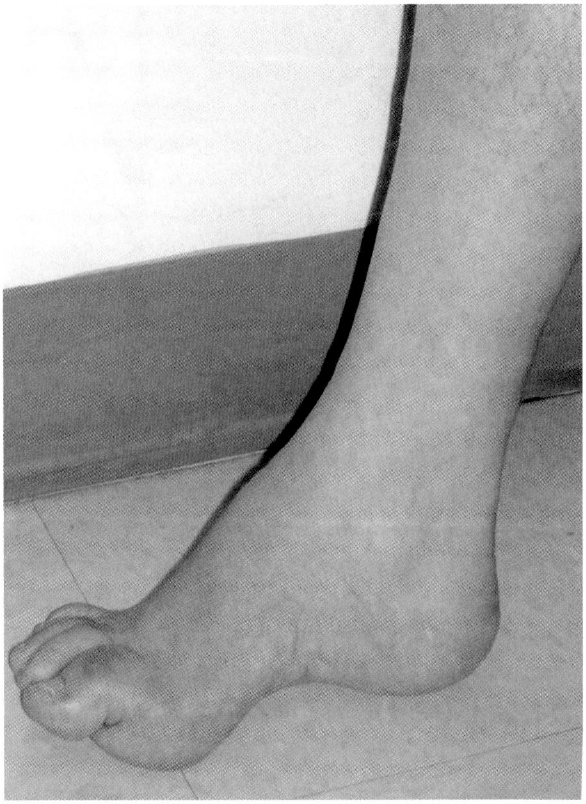

Figure 11-3. CMT1. Note the high arch (pes cavus) of the foot and hammertoes of a patient with CMT1.

early designation of CMT1 as a hypertrophic neuropathy. Light microscopy reveals reduction of myelinated nerve fibers with a predilection for the loss of the large-diameter fibers.[24,25] The diameters of the axons are also decreased; on the whole there is an increase in the density of neurofilaments within these atrophic axons. Early in life, the peripheral nerves may appear normally myelinated, but over time axons become thinly myelinated. Recurrent demyelination and remyelination lead to reduced internodal length, while Schwann cell proliferation results in the formation of the so-called onion bulbs (Fig. 11-4). In patients with CMT1B, occasionally biopsies reveal tomacula, uncompacted myelin, and focally folded or widened myelin sheaths (Fig. 11-5).[4,14,27] Demyelination, neuronal loss, and axonal atrophy are slightly more prominent distally. Autopsy studies demonstrate the loss of myelinated fibers in the posterior columns in the spinal cord.

MOLECULAR GENETICS AND PATHOGENESIS

CMT1 is a genetically heterogeneous disorder (Tables 11-1 and 11-2 and Figs. 11-1 and 11-2).[1–8] In addition, there is phenotypic heterogeneity associated with mutations in specific genes. CMT1A (*PMP22* duplication) is by far the most common form of CMT1, representing 70% of cases, while 20% have CMT1B, and 10% have one of the other subtypes.

CMT1A

Approximately 85% of people with CMT1A have a 1.5-megabase (MB) duplication within chromosome 17p11.2–12 where the *PMP22* gene lies.[28,29] Thus, these individuals carry three copies of the *PMP22* rather than two. In contrast, inheritance of the chromosome with the deleted segment results in affected individuals having only one copy of the *PMP22* gene and leads to hereditary neuropathy with liability to pressure palsies (HNPP). Although these disorders are inherited in an autosomal-dominant fashion, de

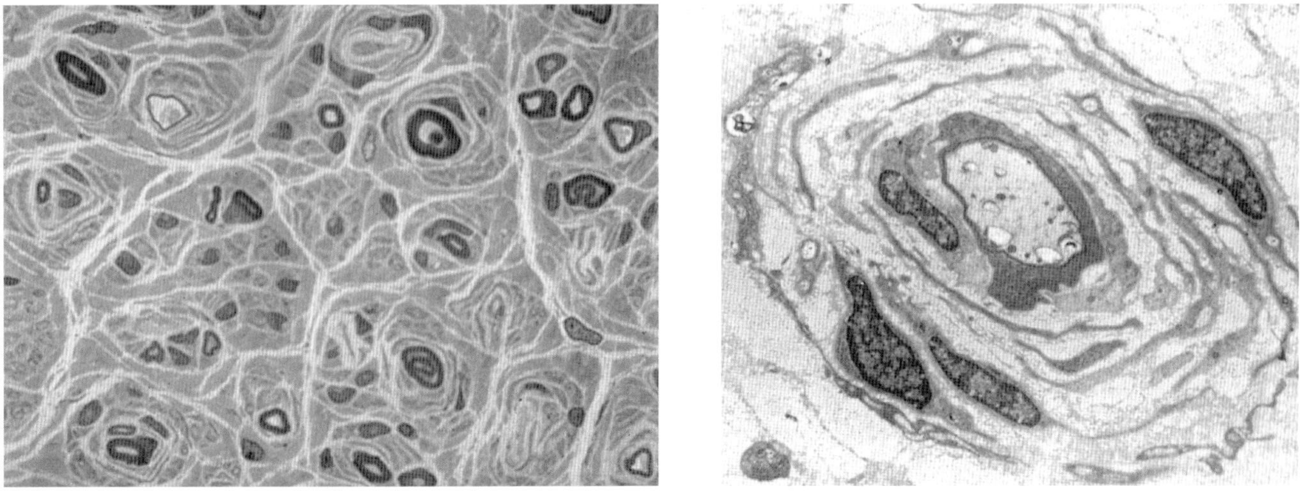

A B

Figure 11-4. CMT1. Nerve biopsy demonstrates a reduction of myelinated nerve fibers, thinly myelinated fibers, and onion-bulb formations (**A**, semithin section). Electron microscopy reveals proliferation of Schwann cell processes surrounding demyelinated fiber forming a so-called onion bulb **(B)**. (Reproduced with permission from www.neuropathologyweb.org/chapter12.)

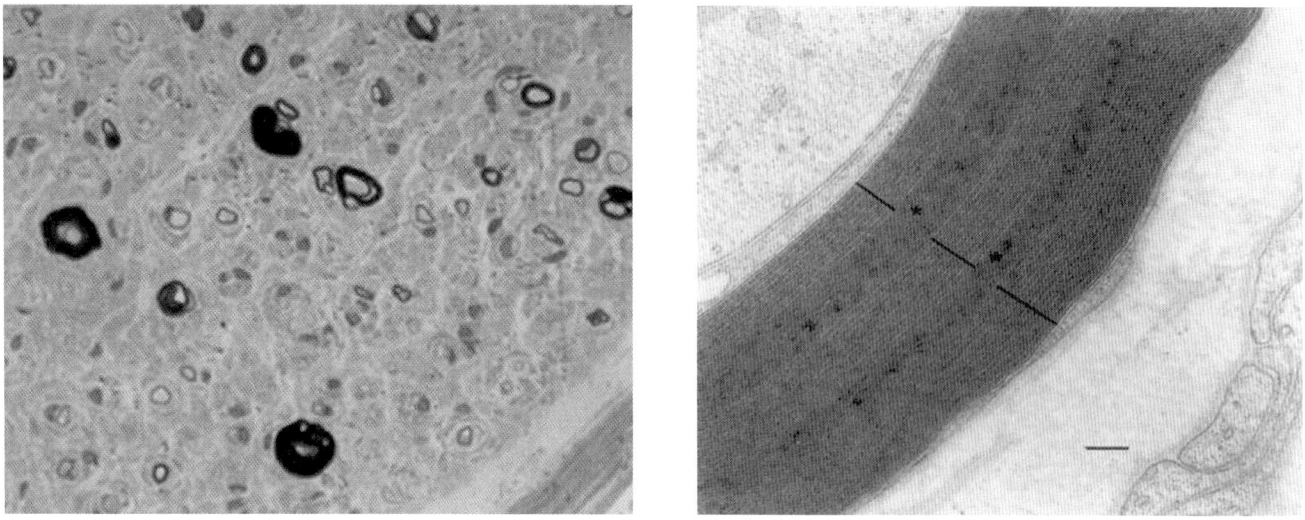

A B

Figure 11-5. CMT1B. Semithin section reveals rarefaction of myelinated fibers, foldings of myelin, and onion-bulb proliferations of Schwann cells **(A)**. Note the alternate disposition of normal (*stars*) and uncompacted myelin lamellae (*lines*), Scale bar = 0.2 μm **(B)**. (Reproduced with permission from Vallat JM, Magy L, Lagrange E, et al. Diagnostic value of ultrastructural nerve examination in Charcot–Marie–Tooth disease: Two CMT1B cases with pseudo-recessive inheritance, *Acta Neuropathol.* 2007;113(4):443–449.)

novo mutations do occur. Most de novo duplications are paternally inherited and are believed to arise due to unequal crossover during meiosis. De novo mutations of maternal origin are probably caused by intrachromosomal rearrangement.[30] In keeping with this abnormal dosage effect of *PMP22*, people affected with trisomy 17p (thus, containing three copies of the *PMP22*) also have a demyelinating sensorimotor polyneuropathy.[31]

Some individuals with CMT1A have point mutations in *PMP22*.[32] These individuals can more closely resemble Dejerine–Sottas (CMT3) phenotypically, in which they are more severely affected at an earlier age, demonstrate slower NCVs (<10 m/s), and have more prominent histopathology than those with the classic duplication.[15] Other individuals present with a milder phenotype with pressure-induced palsies (e.g., HNPP as discussed in a subsequent section).

The pathogenic basis for CMT1A is likely due to a toxic gain of function of the PMP22 protein. This protein accounts for 2–5% of myelin protein and is expressed in compact portions of the peripheral myelin sheath. An increased expression of PMP22 mRNA and the protein itself in the myelin sheaths has been demonstrated on nerve biopsies in CMT1A; however, late in the course PMP22 expression actually decreases.[33–36] The exact function of PMP22 in the peripheral nerves is not known, but it may be important in maintaining the structural integrity of myelin, acting as an adhesion molecule, or regulating the cell cycle. Regeneration-associated remyelination is delayed in nerve xenografts implanted from individuals with CMT1A into mice.[37] Further, PMP22 must also be essential for maintaining the integrity of the axon itself, as there is evidence of axonal atrophy on nerve biopsies in people with CMT1A.

CMT1B

Approximately 20% of people with CMT1 have CMT1B, which is caused by mutations in the *MPZ* gene located on chromosome 1q22–23 that encodes for myelin protein zero.[38–40] CMT1B is for the most part clinically, electrophysiologically, and histologically indistinguishable from CMT1A. However, patients with *MPZ* mutations are more likely to have more "axonal" physiology on NCS than those patients with *PMP22* mutations. Also, CMT associated with Adies' pupils is more common in patients with *MPZ* mutations. MPZ is an integral myelin protein and accounts for more than half of the myelin protein in peripheral nerves. It is a member of the immunoglobulin superfamily and consists of an extracellular immunoglobulin-like domain, a transmembrane domain, and a cytoplasmic domain.[1] MPZ localizes to the tight compact regions of myelin, where it may play a role in maintaining tight compaction by forming links between adjacent myelin layers. Nerve biopsies in people with CMT1B reveal abnormalities similar to that noted in CMT1A. However, occasionally tomaculae and uncompacted myelin are apparent, which are not typically seen on nerve biopsy in CMT1A.[4,14,41] Immunohistochemistry and ultrastructural studies on nerve biopsy specimens may demonstrate decreased expression of MPZ protein.[42] Some mutations in the *MPZ* gene have been associated with a severe demyelinating CMT3 phenotype, while others are associated with NCS suggestive of an axonopathy or CMT2. The specific location of the mutations in the *MPZ* gene and how these affect the function of the myelin protein probably account for the phenotypic heterogeneity.

CMT1C

This rare neuropathy is caused by mutations in the *LITAF* gene (lipopolysaccharide-induced tumor necrosis factor-alpha factor) located on chromosome 16p13.1–p12.3.[18,43,44] In a large study of 968 unrelated cases of CMT1, the percentage of patients with LITAF mutations was only 0.6%.[44] *LITAF*, also known as *SIMPLE* (small integral membrane protein of the lysosome/late endosome), encodes a protein that is expressed on Schwann cells and may play a role in protein degradation pathways.[45]

CMT1D

Mutations in the early growth response 2 (*ERG2*) gene on chromosome 10q21.1–q22.1 are responsible for CMT1D.[46] ERG2 is believed to be a transcription factor that binds DNA through three zinc finger domains and likely has an important action in regulating myelin genes in Schwann cells. CMT1D accounts for <1% of molecular-defined cases of CMT1.

CMT1E

This refers to kinships with CMT1 associated with deafness. It has been demonstrated to be allelic to CMT1A and caused by point mutations in *PMP22*.[5]

CMT1F

CMT1F is caused by mutations in the neurofilament light chain (*NEFL* or *NFL*) gene located on chromosome 8p13–21.[47,48] It is usually associated with low-amplitude CMAPs and normal or only slightly slow NCVs and thus is often categorized as an axonal form of CMT (CMT2E). However, some cases have been reported with motor NCVs in the mid-twenties and thus have been classified as a CMT1F.

CMT1G

CMT1G is associated with focal segmental glomerulosclerosis (FSGS) and is caused by mutations in the gene that codes for inverted formin 2 (*INF2*).[49,50] Mutations in this gene are also a major cause of isolated FSGS. Approximately one-third of patients have sensorineural hearing loss as well. Some affected individuals have intellectual disabilities and abnormalities in the white matter and ventricular dilatation on brain MRI. Formin 2 interacts with Rho-GTPase CDC42 and myelin and lymphocyte protein (MAL) and is felt to be important in the essential steps of myelination and myelin maintenance.

▶ HEREDITARY NEUROPATHY WITH LIABILITY TO PRESSURE PALSIES

Because HNPP is associated with mutations affecting *PMP22* and less commonly *MPZ*, we discuss it here before moving on to CMT2.

CLINICAL FEATURES

HNPP or tomaculous neuropathy is inherited in an autosomal-dominant manner.[21,51–61] The neuropathy usually manifests within the second or third decade, although some affected individuals present earlier and others remain asymptomatic their entire life. People usually describe painless numbness and weakness in the distribution of a single peripheral nerve, although multiple mononeuropathies and cranial neuropathies can occur. Symptomatic mononeuropathy or multiple mononeuropathies are often precipitated by trivial compression of nerve(s), as it can occur with wearing a backpack, leaning on the elbows, or crossing one's legs for even a short period of time. These pressure-related mononeuropathies usually resolve, although it may take several weeks or months. The most commonly affected sites are the median nerve at the wrist (carpal tunnel syndrome), ulnar nerve at the elbow (cubital tunnel syndrome), radial nerve in the arm (spiral groove insult), and peroneal nerve at the fibular head. In addition, the brachial plexus can be involved after carrying a heavy shoulder bag or backpack. Further, some individuals who are affected manifest with a progressive or relapsing, generalized, and symmetric sensorimotor peripheral neuropathy that resembles CMT or even CIDP.[21,51,54] On examination, there is decreased sensation to all modalities, particularly large fiber functions. Muscle stretch reflexes are usually reduced throughout, but these can be normal. Pes cavus deformities and hammertoes are often evident, as seen in CMT.

LABORATORY FEATURES

Although the clinical symptoms and signs are typically focal, NCS often reveal diffuse abnormalities.[21,51–64] Sensory and motor NCS usually demonstrate moderately prolonged distal latencies and slightly slow NCVs with normal or reduced amplitudes. Slowing of NCVs, conduction block, and temporal dispersion are accentuated across typical sites of entrapment or compression (i.e., the carpal and cubital tunnel, Guyon's canal, and across the fibular head). In addition, there also appears to be a distal accentuation of nerve conduction slowing, irrespective of possible compression.[51,52,59] However, this length-dependent slowing has not been appreciated by all.[60,61] NCS may also be abnormal in asymptomatic family members who carry the mutation. Findings of widespread conduction slowing superimposed on the focal demyelinating lesions that correlate with the mononeuropathies, whether clinically evident or not, are a clue to this disorder.

HISTOPATHOLGY

Nerve biopsies demonstrate focal globular thickening of the myelin sheath, which is best appreciated on teased fiber preparations.[51,56,62,65] The thickened myelin resembles as a

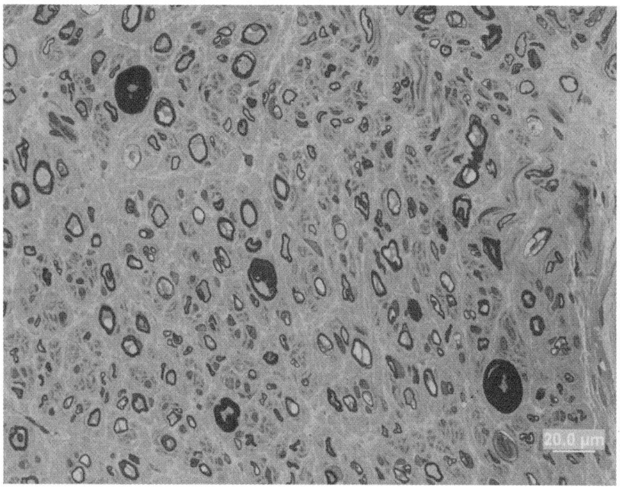

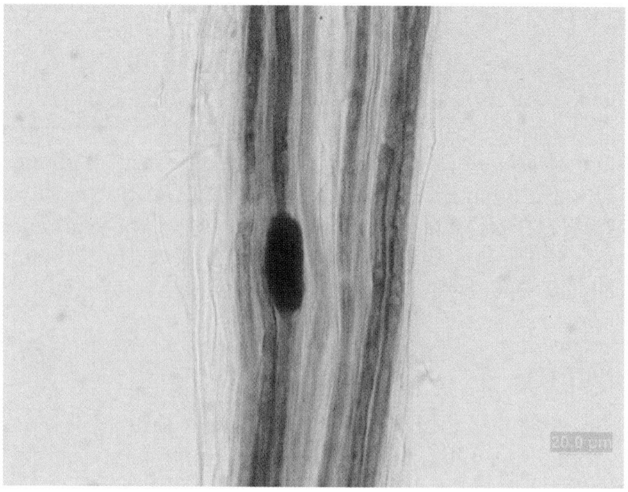

A B

Figure 11-6. HNPP nerve biopsy. Transverse section of toluidine blue-stained epon-embedded sural nerve from a patient with HNPP reveals scattered thinly myelinated nerve fibers and fibers with redundant myelin swellings **(A)**. Teased fiber preparation demonstrates a sausage-shaped myelin swelling or tomacula **(B)**.

sausage, hence the name tomaculous neuropathy (Latin: sausage) (Fig. 11-6). These tomaculae represent redundant loops of myelin. In addition, nerve biopsies reveal a reduction in large myelinated fibers, segmental demyelination and remyelination, and axonal atrophy and degeneration similar to but not as severe as that seen in CMT1.

MOLECULAR GENETICS AND PATHOGENESIS

Approximately 85% of cases of HNPP are caused by an inverse of the mutation that is responsible for most cases of CMT1A.[21,51,66] While CMT1A is usually associated with a 1.5-MB duplication in chromosome 17p11.2, an extra copy of the *PMP22* gene, HNPP is caused by inheritance of the chromosome with the corresponding 1.5-MB deletion of this segment and thus have only one copy of the PMP22 gene. De novo deletions are usually paternally inherited and arise due to unequal crossing-over during meiosis, while rare de novo mutations are of female origin and the result of intrachromosomal rearrangements.[30] In addition, as with CMT1A, mutations within the *PMP22* gene itself can cause HNPP.[67] Why some point mutations in the *PMP22* gene result in a CMT1A clinical phenotype and other are associated with a HNPP phenotype is not known. It is speculated that mutations causing CMT1A produce a gain of function of the PMP22 protein, while mutations causing HNPP cause a loss of function of the PMP22 protein. Nerve biopsies demonstrate an underexpression of PMP22 mRNA and the protein[33,35] that inversely correlate with the mean diameter of the axons and clinical severity.[68] Normal expression of PMP22 protein appears important for proper axonal development.

▶ CMT TYPE 2 (CMT2)

CLINICAL FEATURES

CMT2 refers to the "axonal" hereditary motor and sensory neuropathies. Most of these are associated with autosomal-dominant inheritance, but they can be inherited in an autosomal-recessive or X-linked manner. The prevalence of CMT2 is about half that of CMT1. There are many well-defined subtypes based on the clinical features and genetic localization (Table 11-1).[7,23–25,69–125] CMT2A2 caused by mitofusin 2 mutations is the most common subtype accounting for approximately one-third of CMT2 cases overall.[74–76] The different subtypes can be difficult to distinguish from one another and even from CMT1; however, there are clinical features that may be helpful. CMT2 tends to present later in life compared to CMT1. Individuals who are affected usually become symptomatic by the second decade but some remain asymptomatic into late adult life while others present in the first decade of life.[73,78] People with CMT2 tend to have less severe involvement of the intrinsic hand muscles than that appreciated in CMT1. In contrast, CMT2 is more likely to have profound atrophy and weakness of the posterior compartments (gastrocnemius and soleus) of the distal legs in addition to the anterior compartment involvement (peroneal and anterior tibial) compared to CMT1. Generalized areflexia is rare in CMT2, while it is rather common in CMT1. Ankle reflexes are usually absent in both types. Individuals with CMT2 are less likely to have a tremor (Roussy–Levy syndrome) than people with CMT1. Although patients generally do not complain of sensory loss or paresthesia, 50–70% of those with CMT2 have significant reductions in light touch, pain, joint position, and vibration sense on examination. While pes cavus and hammertoe deformities may be seen in CMT2, these are less frequent than in CMT1.

There are some features that also help distinguish the different subtypes of CMT2. For example, optic atrophy, hearing loss, pyramidal tract, and subcortical white matter abnormalities on brain magnetic resonance imaging findings are sometimes seen in CMT2A2, which was previously reported as hereditary motor and sensory neuropathy type 6 (HMSN VI) and overlaps with the HSPs.[79,80] Severe mutilating neuropathic ulcerations similar to those typically seen in HSAN type 1 (HSAN1) sometimes complicate CMT2B.[81–84]

CMT2B1 is actually inherited in an autosomal recessive fashion and early cases were reported in North Africa and the Middle East, where consanguineous marriages are not uncommon.[85–88] The age of onset has ranged from 6 to 27 years in these small series, and the course of the neuropathy is variable. The neuropathy can progress rapidly with severe distal and proximal weakness of the arms and legs evolving in a few years, while other affected individuals have only mild weakness two decades after the onset of symptoms.

CMT2C is associated with vocal cord paralysis and diaphragmatic weakness, in addition to limb involvement.[3,89–92] The age of onset and symptoms are variable, and it can begin in infancy when it may manifest with breathing difficulties and stridor. Laryngeal weakness is more often insidious in onset and presents as progressive hoarseness. In addition, the phrenic nerves may be affected, leading to diaphragm weakness, reduced ventilatory function, and orthopnea. Some people will require tracheostomy and mechanical ventilation. Severe atrophy of the distal limbs is common. Individuals who are affected can develop proximal weakness as well. There is mild sensory loss to all modalities and deep tendon reflexes are reduced. Pes cavus can be appreciated in some patients, but such foot deformities are not as common as seen in CMT1, CMT2A, or CMT2B. Similar cases have been reported in the literature as hereditary distal spinal muscular atrophy with vocal cord paralysis.[90,93]

CMT2D is another genetically distinct autosomal-dominant form of CMT2.[94–98] The hands are more severely affected than the distal legs. Selected wasting of the first interosseus muscles is often appreciated. Onset of weakness is usually appreciated in the late teens (range between the ages of 12 and 36 years), and the neuropathy has a slowly progressive course. Distal hypesthesia to all sensory modalities and areflexia are appreciated. Pes cavus, hammertoes, and scoliosis are variably present. Enlarged palpable nerves are not appreciated. This disorder is allelic to distal spinal muscular atrophy type 5.[95–97]

CMT2E is a rare neuropathy usually manifested in the second or third decade of life with progressive distal leg weakness.[47,48,99] Some patients develop deafness. Sensory loss, pes cavus, and areflexia are also often appreciated on examination.

CMT2F was reported in a Russian family with symmetric weakness and atrophy of the distal legs greater than the arms, with onset age 15–25 years.[100,101]

CMT2G was described in a large Spanish kinship with typical CMT2 phenotype, with an age at onset being 9–76 (mean 29) years. Most patients developed symptoms in the second decade of life.[102]

CMT2H, CMT2K, and CMT4A are allelic disorders caused by mutations in *GDAP1*. Affected individuals may have vocal cord paralysis. They can have axonal or demyelinating abnormalities on NCS. We discuss this more in the CMT4A section.

CMT2I is associated with late-onset axonal neuropathy, Adie's pupil, and hearing loss. It is caused by mutations in *MPZ* that are more typically associated with demyelinating neurophysiology (CMT1B).

CMT2J, a late-onset neuropathy (usually fifth or sixth decade) associated with hearing loss and pupillary abnormalities (Adie's pupil), is also allelic to CMT1B and caused is by mutations in *MPZ*.

CMT2L was reported in a large Chinese family.[103] Onset of the disease was between 15 and 33 years of age with symmetric weakness of the distal lower limbs, mild-to-moderate sensory impairment including pain and touch, and absent muscle stretch reflexes.

CMT2M is more commonly classified as dominant intermediate CMT type B (CMTDIB) because NCVs are usually in the intermediate range. It is allelic to a form of centronuclear myopathy.[104–106]

CMT2N is associated with an age of onset ranging from early childhood to sixth decade of variable severity.[107–109] Sensorineural hearing loss may be seen in some individuals. NCVs are in the intermediate range.

CMT2O presents in childhood with delayed motor milestones and abnormal gait.[110] Some affected individuals have paresthesia and neuropathic pain, while some have learning disabilities.

CMT2P is associated with a relatively mild, very slowly progressive axonal neuropathy with age of onset in the second or third decade of life.[111,112]

LABORATORY FEATURES

The similarities between the CMT1 and CMT2 make it difficult to definitely distinguish between these neuropathies on clinical grounds alone; thus, NCS are invaluable. It is usually not difficult to differentiate CMT2 from the more common chronic idiopathic axonal neuropathy. Although there is electrophysiological evidence of motor involvement in chronic idiopathic axonal neuropathy, sensory symptoms predominate the clinical picture in this neuropathy, while motor signs and symptoms are the major clinical features in CMT2.[113]

NCS can help distinguish CMT1 from CMT2 [7,11,24,70,71]; however, these do not help ascertain the various subtypes of CMT2. Sensory NCS reveal reduced or absent SNAP amplitudes in both the upper and lower limbs. CVs are normal or only slightly reduced. Likewise, the distal sensory latencies are either normal or only mildly prolonged. The motor NCS demonstrate reduced CMAP amplitudes, particularly in the legs, except in CMT2D in which the distal arms are affected more than the legs. Distal motor latencies are normal or only mildly prolonged. NCVs are normal or only slightly slow, usually greater than 37 m/s in the upper extremities. However, cases of CMT2E have been reported with motor NCVs in the mid-twenties and thus may be classified as a subtype of CMT1.[48,114] Some have had slowing of NCVs in an intermediate range and are designated as having dominant intermediate CMT. Needle EMG reveals fasciculation and fibrillation potentials, particularly in distal extremity muscles. A few patients with CMT2 have been reported to have continuous MUAP firing resembling neuromyotonia; these discharges are abolished with peripheral neuromuscular blockade.[115,116] The MUAPs can be increased in amplitude and duration with a higher-than-normal number of polyphasic potentials. Recruitment is reduced in weak muscles as well.

HISTOPATHOLOGY

Nerve biopsies in CMT2 demonstrate a generalized reduction in myelinated fibers, particularly the large myelinated fibers.[83,117] Axonal atrophy, wallerian degeneration, and small clusters of thinly myelinated fibers representing regenerating axons can be appreciated. As opposed to CMT1, onion bulbs are not a prominent feature in CMT2. Abnormal accumulations of mitochondria may be appreciated on electron microscopy (EM) in CMT2A2. Some forms such as CMT2E are associated with giant axons and accumulation of disorganized neurofilaments.[47]

MOLECULAR GENETICS AND PATHOGENESIS

CMT2 is a genetically heterogeneous group of disorders (Table 11-1).[1,3–8]

CMT2A1 is caused by mutations in a microtubule motor kinesin-like protein gene, *KIF1B*, located on chromosome 1p36.2.[118,119] The kinesin superfamily is involved in axonal transport and likely impairment of this function leads to axon degeneration. Subsequent to the discovery of mutations in the *KIF1B* gene, missense mutations in the mitochondrial fusion protein mitofusin 2 gene, *MFN2*, also located on chromosome 1p36.2, were found.[120] The majority of patients with CMT2A have *MFN2* mutations (CMT2A2), which account for one-third of CMT2 cases overall.[75,77] Mitofusin 2 localizes to the outer mitochondrial membrane, where it regulates the mitochondrial network architecture by fusion of mitochondria. Mitochondria undergo a dynamically regulated balance between fusion and fission reactions of their tubular and branched membrane network in order to maximize cell functions, such as equilibrating mitochondrial gene products to overcome acquired somatic mutations of mitochondrial DNA and establishing a uniform membrane potential at the mitochondrial double membrane and regulation of apoptosis.[120] Mutations in *MFN2* lead to abnormal mitochondrial trafficking, which may explain the length-dependent severity of the associated neuropathy.[77,121]

CMT2B (3q13–q22) is caused by mutations in a small GTPase late endosomal protein encoded by the *RAB7* gene.[83,122] Mutations in this gene also cause a form of HSAN1 (see below). The encoded protein serves as a guanine-nucleotide exchange factor for the Rho family of GTPase enzymes (RhoGTPases). Rho guanine-nucleotide exchange factors regulate the activity of small RhoGTP-ase by catalyzing the exchange of bound GDP by GTP. In turn, RhoGTPases play a pivotal role in regulating the actin cytoskeleton by their ability to influence cell polarity, microtubule dynamics, membrane-transport pathways, and transcription-factor activity, as well as RhoGTPases in neuronal morphogenesis, including cell migration, axonal growth and guidance, dendrite elaboration and plasticity, and synapse formation.[83]

CMT2B1 is usually caused by homozygous mutations in the *LMNA* gene located on chromosome 1q21.[85–88] This gene encodes for the nuclear envelop protein, lamin A/C. This gene is also mutated in patients with LGMD (limb girdle muscular dystrophy) 1B and EDMD2 (Emery Dreifuss 2) (see Chapter 24). CMT2B2 is caused by mutations in *MED25* on chromosome 19q13 that encodes for mediator of RNA polymerase II transcription subunit 25. The encoded protein is essential in the assembly of a functional preinitiation complex with RNA polymerase II and other transcription factors. Both CMT2B1 and CMT2B2 are inherited in an autosomal-recessive rather than autosomal-dominant manner.

CMT2C is caused by mutations in the transient receptor potential cation channel, subfamily V, member 4 gene (*TRPV4*).[9–93] CMT2C is allelic to some forms of distal HMN and scapuloperoneal spinal muscular atrophy. How a mutation in this cation channel that mediates calcium influx causes neuropathy is not exactly known.

CMT2D and distal spinal muscular atrophy type 5 are allelic disorders caused by mutations in the glycyl-tRNA synthetase (*GARS*) gene on chromosome 7p14.[94–98] Glycyl-tRNA synthetase is a member of the family of aminoacyl-tRNA synthetases, responsible for charging tRNAs with their cognate amino acids. The pathogenic mechanism by which mutations in this gene lead to CMT2D/distal spinal muscular atrophy type 5 is not completely understood.

CMT2E is allelic with CMT1F and is caused by mutations in the *NEFL* gene located on chromosome 8p13–21.[47,48,99,114] Neurofilaments are important for proper organization, function, and regeneration of axons as well as for axonal transport. Furthermore, neurofilament light chain encoded by *NEFL* plays a major role in regulating the expression and function of other neurofilament proteins.

CMT2F is caused by mutations in the *HSPB1* gene located on chromosome 7q11–q21 that encodes for 27-kDa small heat-shock or HSP27.[100,101] Mutations in this gene are also responsible for some patients categorized as having distal spinal muscular atrophy.[101]

CMT2G has been localized to chromosome 12q12–q13, but the gene has not been identified.[102]

CMT2H is caused by mutations in the gene that encodes for ganglioside-induced differentiation-associated protein 1 (*GDAP1*) and is allelic to CMT2K and CMT4A, which is discussed in a separate section.

CMT2I refers to late-onset cases with mutations in *MPZ* gene (CMT1B) but in which the neurophysiology and nerve biopsies look more axonal and thus can be classified as a form of CMT2.[16,124] Likewise, CMT2J, which is associated with hearing loss and Adie's pupil, is also associated with mutations in *MPZ* gene.

CMT2K refers to early-onset neuropathy (usually before the age of 2 years), which is caused by mutations in *GDAP1* gene located on chromosome 8q13–q21. This is allelic to CMT2K and CMT4A.[88] Some individuals who are affected have vocal cord paralysis. The mechanism by which this causes axonal degeneration is not known.

CMT2L is caused by mutations in the *HSPB8* gene located on chromosome 12q2 that encodes for small heat-shock protein 22-kDa protein 8 (HSP22).[103,125] Mutations in this gene are also responsible for distal hereditary motor neuropathy type 2. HSP22 forms homodimers and larger oligomers with other HSPs. The mutation may lead to an increased tendency to form cytoplasmic protein aggregates.[125]

CMT2M is allelic to CMTDIB and is caused by mutations in the *DNM2* gene on chromosome 19p13.2. This gene encodes for dynamin 2 that belongs to a subfamily of GTP-binding proteins.[104–106] Dynamins are associated with microtubules and bind proteins that bind actin and other cytoskeletal proteins.

CMT2N is caused by mutations in alanyl-tRNA synthetase (*AARS*) on chromosome 16q22.1.[107–109] AARS catalyzes the attachment of alanyl to the appropriate tRNA.

CMT2O is caused by heterozygous mutation in the dynein, cytoplasmic 1, heavy chain 1 (*DYNC1H1*) gene on chromosome 14q32.[110] Dyneins are a group of microtubule-activated ATPases that have a role in retrograde axonal transport and organelle movement.

CMT2P is caused by mutations in the ubiquitin ligase *LRSAM1* gene (leucine-rich repeat and sterile alpha motif containing 1) located on chromosome 9q33. Inheritance was autosomal recessive in one family [111] and autosomal dominant [112] in another. The encoded protein regulates cell adhesion molecules, has ubiquitin ligase activity, and plays a role in receptor endocytosis, but the exact mechanism by which it caused neuropathy is unknown.

Mutations in the gene that encodes DNAJB2 *(HSJ1)* is another rare cause of autosomal-recessive CMT2 and dHMN (no specific CMT2 or dHMN number have been assigned to this neuropathy as yet).[126,127] Mutations in other genes (*HSPB1, HSPB8, BSCL2, GARS, DYNC1H1, TRPV4, HINT1, PLEKHG5*) can be associated with either dHMN or CMT phenotypes, and disparate phenotypes can be seen even within the same family.

▶ DOMINANT INTERMEDIATE CMT

Dominant intermediate CMT (DI-CMT) disease refers to forms of CMT in which the CVs show only mild slowing (>38 m/s) in the upper extremities) and in which there are both demyelinating and axonal features on nerve biopsies. The clinical features are for the most part similar to what was described previously in CMT1 and CMT2 sections. Different chromosomal loci have been linked with three autosomal-dominant, "intermediate" types of CMT: DI-CMTA (10q24.1–q25.1), DI-CMTB (19p12–p13.2), and DI-CMTC (1p34–p35). The causal gene for DI-CMTA has not been found. Mutations in dynamin 2 (*DYN2*) gene have been found in DI-CMTB.[104–106] Of note, mutations in the same gene have been found in adult-onset centronuclear myopathy. *DYN2* mutations should be considered in those with a classical mild to moderately severe phenotype, particularly when seen in combination with neutropenia or cataracts.[105] Dynamin 2 belongs to the family of large GTPases and is important in endocytosis, membrane trafficking, actin assembly, and centrosome cohesion.[106] DI-CMTC is caused by mutations in the *YARS* gene that encodes for tyrosyl-tRNA synthetase.[128,129] Tyrosyl-tRNA synthetase appears to be localized to axon terminals and probably plays a role in protein biosynthesis.

▶ RECESSIVE INTERMEDIATE CMT

Mutations in the pleckstrin homology domain-containing protein, family G, member 5 (*PLEKHG5*) gene on chromosome 1p36.31 leads to an intermediate form of autosomal-recessive CMT disease.[130–132] Mutations in this gene also cause autosomal-recessive distal spinal muscular atrophy type 4. The encoded protein activates the nuclear factor kappa B signaling pathway. Affected individuals developed distal weakness and atrophy that were worse in the legs and associated with foot deformities, areflexia, and moderately slow NCVs. The age at onset was variable. Nerve biopsies demonstrated a loss of large myelinated fibers and thinly myelinated fibers.

▶ CMT TYPE 3 (DEJÉRINE–SOTTAS DISEASE, CONGENITAL HYPOMYELINATING NEUROPATHY)

CLINICAL FEATURES

CMT3 was originally described by Dejérine and Sottas as a hereditary demyelinating sensorimotor polyneuropathy presenting in infancy or early childhood.[7,133–144] Although initially CMT3 was believed to be an autosomal-recessive disorder because of a lack of family history,[11,134] most cases are due to spontaneous mutations in the *PMP22*, *MPZ*, or *ERG2* genes. Further, most cases of the so-called congenital hypomyelination neuropathy[138,139]also represent a severe form of CMT3.[140]

CMT3 usually manifests as generalized weakness at birth or in early childhood. Affected infants can be hypotonic and often have distal contractures (arthrogryposis multiplex). Ventilatory distress and swallowing difficulties can develop in severe cases, leading to death in several months. In less severe cases, infants may appear normal at birth, but motor milestones are delayed. Some children achieve independent ambulation, although it may take several years. Distal muscles are affected more than proximal muscles. Weakness can progress and render some ambulatory patients to a wheelchair.

The peripheral nerves may be visible or palpably enlarged. There is a reduction in all sensory modalities, particularly those conveyed by large myelinated fibers (i.e., vibration and proprioception) and generalized areflexia. Sensory ataxia of the limbs and trunk can be profound. Sensorineural hearing and abnormal pupillary reaction to light can be detected in some children. Skeletal deformities (e.g., pes cavus and kyphoscoliosis) are common.

LABORATORY FEATURES

CSF protein levels are usually elevated. Motor NCVs are markedly slow, typically 5–10 m/s or less; the distal motor latencies are markedly increased; and the amplitudes are reduced.[2,23,138,141,142] Sensory responses are usually unobtainable. Needle EMG demonstrates increased insertional activity with variable degrees of positive sharp waves and fibrillation potentials, and reduced recruitment of MUAPs.[144] In milder cases of CMT3 in which reinnervation can occur, large-amplitude, long-duration, polyphasic MUAPs are apparent. However, in severe cases, the MUAPs can appear small and almost "myopathic" in appearance.

HISTOPATHOLOGY

Nerve biopsies in CMT3 are markedly abnormal.[140,145–147] One can see hypomyelination with redundant basal lamina or classical onion bulbs as well as amyelination. There is an increase in the size of nerve fasciculi with a reduction in the numbers of myelinated fibers, while unmyelinated nerve fibers are less affected.

The most common histopathological abnormality is hypomyelination with basal lamina onion bulbs. There is marked loss of myelinated nerve fibers, with the remaining axons surrounded by onion bulbs composed of multiple layers of basement membranes, with only one or two thin Schwann cell lamella in the outer ring. These abnormalities are typically found in cases of infantile or early-onset neuropathy. Although some of the infants have respiratory and swallowing problems, nearly all survive. However, affected children rarely achieve independent ambulation and most are wheelchair dependent.

Occasionally, nerve biopsies reveal hypomyelination, with classical onion bulbs composed of concentrically arranged thin Schwann cell lamellae, enclosing nearly all the fibers. This histopathological appearance is associated with a more benign neuropathy. Affected children can appear normal at birth but subsequently fail to meet normal motor milestones. They usually are eventually able to ambulate but may require assistance over time.

Other cases are associated with a marked reduction of nerve fibers with the remaining fibers having minimal myelin. Onion bulbs are not apparent. These so-called congenital amyelinating neuropathies are the most severe form of CMT3 and are usually lethal.

MOLECULAR GENETICS AND PATHOGENESIS

CMT3 is a genetically heterogeneous disorder. As previously discussed, CMT3 was initially felt to be an autosomal-recessive disorder. However, de novo heterozygous point mutations have been discovered in the genes for *PMP22, MPZ,* and *ERG2*, which are also genes responsible for autosomal-dominant CMT1.[2,7,46,136,148] Further, a CMT3 phenotype was described in a child with four copies of the *PMP22* gene as a result of both parents having the typical CMT1A duplication of 17p22.[28] Thus, there exists a wide spectrum of clinical, electrophysiolgical, and histological phenotypes associated with mutations in *PMP22, MPZ,* and the *ERG2* genes. Some individuals who are affected have a mild CMT1 phenotype with only asymptomatic slowing of NCV, while others manifest with severe congenital amyelinating neuropathy, resulting in severe generalized weakness and death in infancy. The severity of CMT is probably related to the exact locations of the mutations in the *PMP22, MPZ,* and the *ERG2* genes and how these mutations specifically affect the function of the myelin proteins or how these interact with one another and the axons.

► CMT TYPE 4

CLINICAL FEATURES

This subgroup of CMT is characterized by a severe, childhood-onset, sensorimotor polyneuropathy that is usually inherited in an autosomal-recessive fashion. The electrophysiological and histological features can have demyelinating or axonal features.[7,8,149]

CMT4A was initially reported in Tunisian families but has subsequently been reported elsewhere.[88,150–157] As previously mentioned it is allelic to CMT2H and CMT2K. Distal weakness is usually noted within the first 2 years of life. Motor development is generally delayed, and progressive weakness involving the proximal muscles is apparent by the end of the first decade. Some individuals who are affected become wheelchair dependent by the third decade of life. Vocal cord paresis and diaphragm paralysis can occur.[151,158] Mild sensory loss and areflexia are evident on clinical examination, as are scoliosis, pes cavus, and other skeletal deformities.

CMT4B is characterized clinically by distal greater than proximal weakness affecting the legs more than the arms and histologically by the abundance of focally folded myelin sheaths on nerve biopsy.[159–161] Weakness is usually apparent at birth or within the first year of life but may not be apparent until the third decade. Motor milestones are often delayed but children do generally become ambulatory. Weakness is slowly progressive and the ability to ambulate without a wheelchair may be lost over time. Sensation is reduced, particularly large fiber function, and muscle stretch reflexes are generally unobtainable. Some people develop scoliosis.

CMT4C was initially described in two Algerian kinships, but has been reported now elsewhere.[162] The main clinical features are delay in walking until 18–24 months, deformities in the feet and spine by 5 years of age, and distal greater than proximal leg and arm weakness. Reduced sensation primarily affects large fiber modalities and is evident prominently in patients with severe motor weakness. Some patients develop sensorineural hearing loss. Muscle stretch reflexes are reduced or absent. Hypertrophy of the nerves may be appreciated.

CMT4D is probably allelic to hereditary motor and sensory neuropathy with deafness—Lom (HMSN-Lom) (discussed in a subsequent section).

CMT4E is another name for congenital hypomyelinating neuropathy and most of these cases have mutations in *PMP22, MPZ,* and the *ERG2* genes. So, we feel that these are better classified as CMT3, which is discussed previously.

CMT4F is an autosomal-recessive neuropathy that otherwise resembles CMT3 clinically and electrophysiologically.[163–165] Individuals who are affected manifest in early childhood, with weakness leading to developmental motor delay, sensory loss, and areflexia. Pes cavus and kyphoscoliosis are common.

CMT4G, also known as CMT-Russe type, has been reported in several gypsy kinships. Distal lower extremity weakness develops in the first two decades of life followed by distal upper extremity weakness.[166,167]

CMT4H presents in the first 2 years of life with severe weakness and resembles CMT3 clinically and electrophysiologically.[168,169]

CMT4J manifests in childhood or early adulthood with severe and often rapidly progressive motor weakness. Weakness can be quite asymmetric and resemble motor neuron disease, but the NCS features suggest a demyelinating polyneuropathy in addition to severe axonal loss.[170–172]

LABORATORY FEATURES

CSF protein is reportedly normal in CMT4A and CMT4C but has been elevated in some reported cases of CMT4B. NCS are markedly abnormal in the various subtypes of CMT4.[150,159,160,173] SNAPs are generally unobtainable, while CMAPs are usually reduced in amplitude. In CMT4A, the CVs can range from being quite slow (<20 m/s) to being normal. Thus, electrophysiologically, CMT4A can appear to be a primary demyelinating neuropathy in some patients and an axonal neuropathy in others.[88,150–157] Motor NCVs are often less than 10 m/s in CMT4B.[159–161] In CMT4C, motor NCVs are slightly faster (ranging from 14 to 32 m/s, mean 24 m/s in the median nerve).[161] CMT4F is associated with marked slowing of motor NCVs.[174]

HISTOPATHOLOGY

In CMT4A, nerve biopsies reveal a marked reduction of myelinated nerve fibers, severe hypomyelination, and basal lamina onion bulbs (Figs. 11-7 and 11-8).[150,152–157] Hypomyelination, loss of myelinated nerve fibers, basal lamina onion bulbs, and numerous fibers with excessively folded myelin sheaths are features of CMT4B.[27,159,160] Some have characterized these focal myelin thickenings as tomacula,[159] while others have advocated that these are histologically distinct from tomacula.[160] In CMT4C, there is a marked reduction of large-diameter myelinated nerve fibers with relative sparing of small- and intermediate-diameter fibers.[162] The remaining axons are thinly myelinated and surrounded by Schwann cell proliferation forming classic onion bulbs. CMT4F is characterized by severe axonal loss, with remaining axons being hypomyelinated and associated with onion bulbs (Fig. 11-9).[163–165] In addition, occasional tomacula formation with focal myelin thickening, abnormalities of the paranodal myelin loops, and focal absence of paranodal septate-like junctions between the terminal loops and the axon are appreciated in CMT4F.[174]

MOLECULAR GENETICS AND PATHOGENESIS

CMT4A is caused by mutations in the ganglioside-induced differentiation-associated protein 1 gene (*GDAP1*) located on chromosome 8q13–q21.[88,150–158,176] Both neurons and Schwann cells express GDAP1, which may explain why mutations may be associated with electrophysiological and histopathological features of either an axonal or a demyelinating neuropathy.[177,178] The GDAP1 protein is located in the mitochondrial outer membrane and helps regulate the mitochondrial network, which when abnormal leads to CMT.

CMT4B with focally folded myelin sheaths appears to be genetically heterogeneic.[173,175,179,180] Focally folded myelin

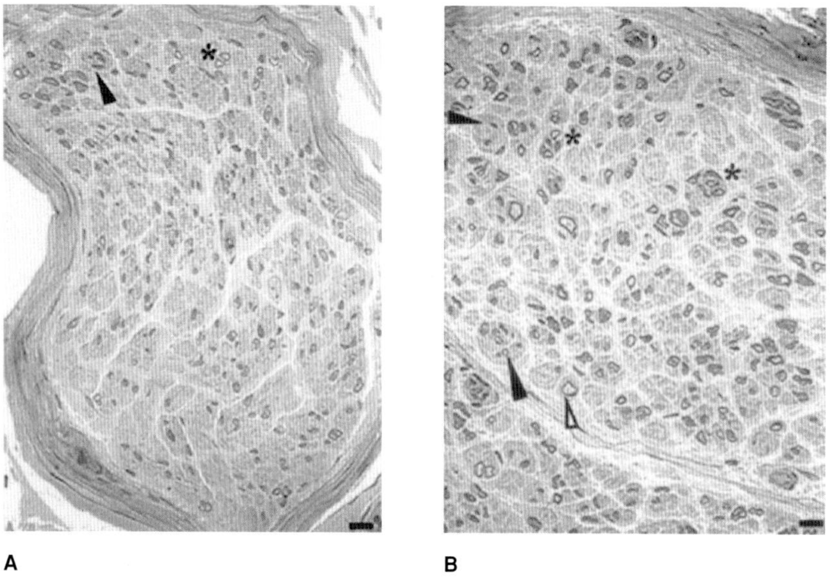

Figure 11-7. CMT4A. Semithin transverse section through sural nerve from two patients **(A and B)**, showing a pronounced depletion of myelinated fibers. Remaining fibers are of very small size, sometimes assembled in regenerative clusters*. Note the proliferation of Schwann cells in circular fashion forming onion bulbs, particularly around cluster (*black arrowhead*). Some fibers are thinly myelinated (*open arrowheads*). Scale bar = 10 μm. (Reproduced with permission from Sevilla T, Cuesta A, Chumillas MJ, et al. Clinical, electrophysiological and morphological findings of Charcot–Marie–Tooth neuropathy with vocal cord palsy and mutations in the GDAP1 gene. *Brain*. 2003;126(Pt 9):2023–2033.)

sheaths are not specific for CMT4B, as these have also been described in patients with point mutations in the *MPZ* gene, which is the causative gene in CMT1B.[181] CMT4B1 is caused by mutations in the myotubularin-related protein 2 (*MTMR2*) gene located on chromosome 11q23 [179,180] The MTMR2 protein is a dual specificity phosphatase, and its deficiency may lead to the phosphorylation of an as-yet-unknown substrate that results in Schwann cell proliferation and abnormal myelinogenesis.[179] Of note, a related member of this same protein family, MTM1, is responsible for

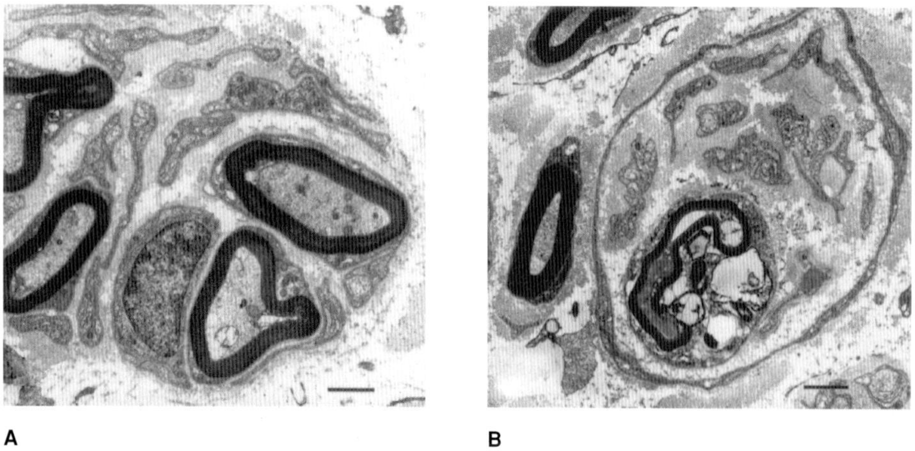

Figure 11-8. CMT4A. Electron microscopy. **(A)** A cluster of small myelinated fibers is surrounded by a concentric array of Schwann cell processes with which numerous unmyelinated axons are associated. **(B)** A myelinated fiber undergoing active axonal degeneration along with several groups of unmyelinated fibers fully encircled by a single Schwann cell. Scale bars = 2 μm. (Reproduced with permission from Sevilla T, Cuesta A, Chumillas MJ, et al. Clinical, electrophysiological and morphological findings of Charcot–Marie–Tooth neuropathy with vocal cord palsy and mutations in the GDAP1 gene. *Brain*. 2003;126(Pt 9):2023–2033.)

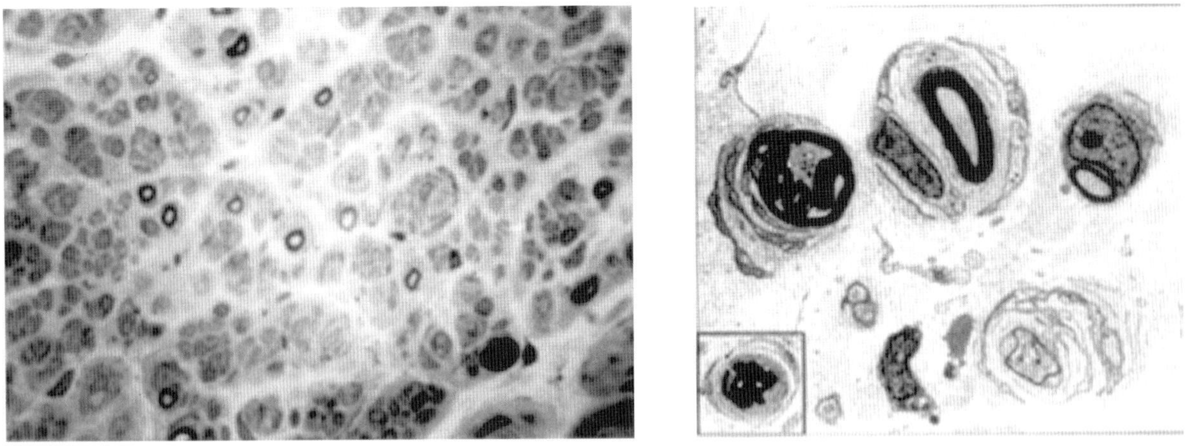

A B

Figure 11-9. CMT4F. **(A)** Light microscopy. Cross semithin–epon section of the sural nerve. Loss of myelinated fibers of all diameters, small onion-bulb structures, and tomacula. **(B)** Electron microscopy. Onion-bulb formations, fiber with focally folded myelin. *Inset*: A naked axon with myelin infoldings surrounded by an onion bulb of mixed type. (Reproduced with permission from Kabzinska D, Drac H, Sherman DL, et al. Charcot–Marie–Tooth type 4 F disease caused by S399fsx410 mutation in the PRX gene. *Neurology*. 2006;66(5):745–747.)

X-linked myotubular myopathy (see Chapter 27). Mutations in *MTMR2* may lead to malfunction of neural membrane recycling, membrane trafficking, and/or endocytic or exocytotic processes, combined with altered axon–Schwann cell interactions.[182] Studies suggest that the loss of MTMR2 protein decreases Schwann cells proliferation and survival and may impair the first stages of myelination of the peripheral nervous system.[183]

CMT4B2 is caused by mutation in the myotubularin-related 13 gene (*MTMR13*), also known as SET-binding factor 2 (SBF2) on chromosome 11p15.[161,184] This protein is a member of the pseudophosphatase branch of myotubularins and bears striking homology to MTMR2. Myotubularin-related proteins have been suggested to work in phosphoinositide-mediated signaling events, which may also convey control of myelination.

CMT4C is caused by mutations in *SH3TC2* located on chromosome 5q23–33 that encodes a protein called SH3 domain and tetratricopeptide repeats 2.[162]

CMT4D is better known as HSMN-Lom and is discussed in the next section.

CMT4E is another name for congenital hypomyelinating neuropathy, but most of these cases have mutations in *PMP22, MPZ,* or *ERG2* genes.

CMT4F is caused by mutations in the gene that encodes for periaxin (*PRX*) located on chromosome 19q13.13–q13.2.[163,165,174] Periaxin normally localizes to the Schmidt–Lanterman incisures and paranodal membranes and is thought to be important in myelin–axon interactions and maintenance of normal myelin structure.

CMT4G has been linked to mutations in the hexokinase 1 gene (*HK1*) located on chromosome 10q23.2.[166,167] Hexokinase 1 catalyzes the first step in glucose metabolism, using ATP for the phosphorylation of glucose to glucose-6-phosphate. Mutations in *HK1* can also cause hemolytic anemia. The mechanisms by which mutations in this gene cause neuropathy are not known.

CMT4H is caused by mutations in the *FGD4* gene located on chromosome 12p11.21–q13.11 that encodes for FYVE, RhoGEF, and PH domain-containing protein 4 also known as frabin.[169,169] frabin is a GDP/GTP nucleotide exchange factor and may have a role in mediating actin cytoskeleton changes during cell migration, morphogenesis-polarization, and division. Mutations in *FGD4* may lead to impaired Rho GTPase signaling.

CMT4J is caused by mutations in the *FIG4* gene located on chromosome 6q21 that encodes for FIG4 homolog, CAC1 phosphatase domain containing *Saccharomyces cerevisiae*.[170–172] This enzyme is a phosphoinositide phosphatase and is felt to regulate intracellular membrane trafficking by recruiting effector proteins to the surface of specific organelles. However, the mechanism by which neuropathy is caused is not understood.

▶ HMSN-LOM/CMT4D

CLINICAL FEATURES

HMSN-Lom or CMT4D is a rare autosomal-recessive demyelinating neuropathy that was initially recognized in Bulgarian gypsies from the town of Lom [123,186]; however, not all affected people are of gypsy ancestry.[187] Individuals who are affected develop distal leg weakness in the first decade of life, which progresses to involve the hands by the second decade of life. Subsequently, hearing loss is generally noted in the third decade. Reduced sensation to all modalities and hyporeflexia are appreciated on examination. Pes cavus, hammer toes, clawing of the hands, and scoliosis are also common.

LABORATORY FEATURES

NCS reveal a demyelinating sensorimotor polyneuropathy.[123,186] Sensory studies are generally unobtainable, but when SNAPs are present, the distal latencies are prolonged and the NCVs are slow. Motor NCS are remarkable for markedly prolonged distal latencies and slow NCVs (ranging from 9 to 20 m/s) in the arms and legs. Active denervation changes are appreciated on needle EMG. Brainstem auditory–evoked potentials reveal both peripheral and central slowing of auditory conduction. Subcortical white matter abnormalities may be appreciated on magnetic resonance imaging of the brain.[187]

HISTOPATHOLOGY

Sural nerve biopsies reveal a loss of large and small myelinated nerve fibers with relative preservation of unmyelinated axons. Remaining axons are thinly myelinated, and onion-bulb formations may also be evident.

MOLECULAR GENETICS AND PATHOGENESIS

HMSN-Lom is caused by mutations in the N-myc downstream-regulated gene 1 (*NDRG1*) located on chromosome 8q24.[123] NDRG1 may function as a signaling protein shuttling between the cytoplasm and nucleus; it may have a role in growth arrest and cell differentiation.[123]

▶ X-LINKED CMT

CMT1X

Clinical Features

CMT1X is an X-linked dominant disorder with clinical features similar to CMT1, except that the neuropathy is much more severe in men than in women.[7,12,188–192] CMT1X accounts for approximately 12% of the overall CMT cases. Men usually present in the first two decades of life with atrophy and weakness of the distal arms and legs, areflexia, pes cavus, hammertoes, and claw-hand deformities. Some patients have disproportionate involve of hand intrinsic muscles with the abductor policis brevis being more involved than the first dorsal interossei, so-called "split hand syndrome". Most do not complain of a sensory disturbance, although reduced sensation to all modalities can be demonstrated on examination. As opposed to men, obligate women carriers are frequently asymptomatic, and if they manifest with symptoms the, onset is usually after the second decade of life. The neuropathy is also typically less severe in affected women. Rarely, patients with CMT1X can present with transient CNS symptoms and marked white matter lesions on magnetic resonance imaging scans.[193–195]

Laboratory Features

NCS reveal features of both demyelination and axonal degeneration, which are more severe in men compared to women.[2,12,188,189,191,192,196–199] SNAPs are reduced in amplitude or absent in the majority of patients but, when obtainable, the distal latencies are prolonged and CVs are slow. Peroneal CMAPs are absent in as many as two-thirds of patients, while median and ulnar CMAPs are often reduced in amplitude.[189,191] Distal motor latencies are prolonged in men more than in women with CMT1X.[189]

In men, motor NCVs in the arms and legs are moderately slow (median nerve 31 +/− 6 m/s; peroneal nerve 31.0 +/− 3.9 m/s).[191] NCVs in men with CMT1X are approximately 10 m/s faster than that usually seen in autosomal-dominant forms of CMT1. By comparison, motor NCVs in women with CMT1X are usually only slightly slow (median nerve 44.6 +/− 8.8 m/s; peroneal nerve 33.8 +/− 8.1 m/s).[191] As previously discussed, uniform slowing of motor NCVs is the rule in CMT1 and helps distinguish hereditary from acquired forms of demyelinating polyneuropathy.[17] However, nonuniform slowing of conduction velocities between different nerves and along different segments of individual nerves resulting in temporal dispersion has been described in some cases of CMT1X, particularly in women.[198,199] Motor unit nerve estimates demonstrate a reduction in units, which correlates with clinical severity.[192]

Histopathology

Sensory nerve biopsies reveal a loss of myelinated nerve fibers, especially of large-diameter fibers, along with axonal degeneration and atrophy, and clusters of thinly myelinated regenerating fibers.[12,189,196,198] A mild degree of Schwann cell proliferation (onion bulbs) can also be seen surrounding some of the thinly myelinated fibers. A mixture of demyelination and remyelination is evident on teased fiber preparations.

Molecular Genetics and Pathogenesis

CMT1X is caused by mutations in the *GJB1* gene located on chromosome Xq13 that encodes for Gap junction beta 1 protein, also known as connexin 32.[2,7,190,192,200–202] Connexins are gap junction structural proteins, which are important in cell-to-cell communication. Connexin 32 oligomerizes into a hexameric structure on the Schwann cell lamella in the paranodal region and Schmidt–Lanterman incisures, where it forms intercellular channels. These channels allow diffusion of ions, nutrients, and other small molecules through the compact myelin to the inner most layers of the myelin sheath and the axon itself. The mutations in *GJB1* lead to demyelination and axonal degeneration.[198,203]

CMT2X

There are several forms of X-linked recessive axonal motor and sensory neuropathy or CMT2X, but only two have identified genetic causes.[204–206] Distal limb weakness, atrophy, and sensory loss develop in early childhood. Some forms are associated with optic atrophy, hearing loss, or intellectual disabilities. One form of CMT2X is caused by mutations in *PRPSI* located on chromosome Xq22.3 that encodes for phosphoribosyl pyrophosphate synthetase 1.[205] Mutations in this gene also cause Arts syndrome, an X-linked disorder characterized by mental retardation, early-onset hypotonia, ataxia, delayed motor development, hearing impairment, and optic atrophy. In addition, some patients with *PRPS1* mutations manifest with isolated X-linked sensorineural deafness.

Another form of CMT2X is caused by mutations in the pyruvate dehydrogenase kinase isoenzyme 3 gene (*PDK3*) located on Xp22.1.[206] PDK3 is an enzyme located in the mitochondrial matrix that assists in regulating the pyruvate dehydrogenase complex, by reversible phosphorylation.

▶ MISCELLANEOUS HEREDITARY MOTOR AND SENSORY NEUROPATHIES

PROXIMAL HEREDITARY MOTOR AND SENSORY NEUROPATHY/NEURONOPATHY (HMSN-P)

Clinical Features

Proximal hereditary motor and sensory neuropathy/neuronopathy resembles Kennedy disease (see Chapter 8), except that it is inherited in an autosomal-dominant fashion rather than being an X-linked disorder.[207] Muscle cramps are often the earliest symptoms. Affected individuals usually develop progressive proximal muscle atrophy, weakness, and fasciculations in the legs worse than in the arms after the age of 30 years (mean 45 +/− 6 years) and typically become nonambulatory 5–20 years after onset of symptoms. Facial muscles are also slightly weak, but neck flexors and extensors remain relatively strong. The tongue may be slightly weak, but dysphagia and dysarthria are not common. Nevertheless, bulbar and respiratory muscle weakness can develop late in the course of the disease. Some patients complain of mild dysesthesias in the distal legs and hands. Decreased sensation to all modalities, particularly vibratory perception and proprioception, is evident on examination. As in Kennedy disease, muscle stretch reflexes are diminished or absent, neurogenic tremor is common, and there is an association with type 2 diabetes mellitus.

Laboratory Features

Serum creatine kinase (CK) levels are often mildly elevated. SNAPs are reduced in amplitude or unobtainable as in Kennedy disease. CMAP amplitudes can be moderately decreased, while the distal latencies and NCVs are relatively preserved. Needle EMG reveals diffuse fasciculation and fibrillation potentials and decreased recruitment of long-duration, large-amplitude, polyphasic MUAPs.

Histopathology

Nerve biopsies show a loss of large and small myelinated nerve fibers with preservation of unmyelinated nerve fibers.[207] An autopsy demonstrated only a few remaining atrophic anterior horn cells along with significant loss off neurons in the spinal roots, cauda equina, and dorsal root ganglia.[207]

Molecular Genetics and Pathogenesis

This disorder is caused by heterozygous mutations in the TRK-fused gene (*TFG*) gene, which is located on chromosome 3p14.1–q13 (Table 11-1).[207,208] The encoded protein plays a role in the normal dynamic function of the endoplasmic reticulum and its associated microtubules. Mutations in *TFG* are also responsible for autosomal-recessive familial spastic paraplegia type 57.

HEREDITARY NEURALGIC AMYOTROPHY

Clinical Features

Hereditary neuralgic amyotrophy (HNA) is an autosomal-dominant disorder, characterized by recurrent attacks of pain, weakness, and sensory loss in the distribution of the brachial plexus often beginning in childhood.[209] These attacks are similar to those seen with idiopathic brachial plexitis (Parsonage–Turner syndrome), and most patients fully or at least partially recover over several weeks or months. Varying degrees of hypotelorism, epicanthal folds, cleft palate, syndactyly, micrognathia, and facial asymmetry are seen in some patients. HNA can be distinguished from brachial plexopathy that can occur in HNPP because of the lack of severe pain in HNPP. Further, unlike HNPP, the neuropathy in HNA is restricted to the brachial plexus and is axonal in nature.

Laboratory Features

The electrodiagnostic findings are typically of classic brachial plexitis.[209] Amplitudes of SNAPs and CMAPs of the affected trunks, cords, divisions, and individual nerves are reduced, while the distal latencies and CVs relatively preserved. Needle EMG reveals fibrillation and positive sharp waves in affected muscle groups along with decreased recruitment of MUAPs. Following reinnervation, especially after recurrent attacks of paresis, large polyphasic MUAPs become evident. NCS and EMG of the unaffected arm and the lower limbs are normal. The electrophysiological studies in HNA reflect an axonal process localized to the brachial plexus, while HNPP is a generalized or multifocal process, which is demyelinating in nature.

Histopathology

Sural nerve biopsies should be normal in patients with HNA. Although tomaculae have been reported in some patients,[56] these were most likely cases of HNPP rather than HNA.

Molecular Genetics and Pathogenesis

HNA appears to be genetically heterogeneous. Some forms of HNA are caused by mutations in the gene encoding for septin 9 (*SEPT9*) located on chromosome 17q25.[210] Septins may be important in formation of the neuronal cytoskeleton and have a role in cell division.

SCAPULOPERONEAL NEUROPATHY

Clinical Features

A scapuloperoneal distribution of weakness can be seen in several different myopathic and neurogenic disorders, including scapuloperoneal muscular dystrophy (some cases of which have also been termed myofibrillar myopathy - see Chapter 27), a scapuloperoneal neuropathy (Davidenkow syndrome), and a pure motor neuropathy/spinal muscular atrophy form.[92,93,210–219] In regard to scapuloperoneal neuropathy or motor neuropathy, symptoms usually develop insidiously in the second or third decade of life. The early symptoms are related to progressive foot drop, with individuals complaining of tripping easily and recurrent ankle sprains similar to CMT. Gradually, proximal weakness of the legs and shoulder girdle arises. Examination reveals muscle wasting about the shoulder girdle (pectoralis, serratus anterior, rhomboids, supraspinatus, infraspinatus, trapezius, deltoid, and brachioradialis) muscles as well as the anterior compartment (peroneal innervated) muscles of the legs. Distal musculature of the arms is relatively spared. The unusual muscle distribution of proximal upper limb and distal lower limb muscles is the clinical distinguishing characteristic of the scapuloperoneal syndromes. Sensation may be normal or reduced. Muscle stretch reflexes may be normal or reduced and the plantar responses are flexor. Pes cavus and hammertoes are commonly appreciated.

Laboratory Features

Median and ulnar CMAPs and NCS are typically normal in the arms; however, peroneal CMAPs are usually reduced in amplitude with the preservation of distal latency and CV. The SNAPs may be reduced in amplitude in the legs and arms, but individuals with scapuloperoneal motor neuropathy or spinal muscular atrophy (SMA) have normal sensory studies. The needle EMG examination reveals reduced recruitment of large-amplitude, long-duration, polyphasic MUAPs in weak muscle groups.

Histopathology

Sural and superficial peroneal nerve biopsies demonstrate axonal degeneration. Autopsies have demonstrated degeneration of the anterior horn cells. Muscle biopsy demonstrates small angulated fibers, grouped atrophy, and fiber-type grouping, which can help distinguish the neuropathy from cases of scapuloperoneal myopathy.

Molecular Genetics and Pathogenesis

The pathogenic basis for the different forms of scapulperoneal neuropathy or SMA is heterogeneous. Some cases appear to be inherited in an autosomal-dominant or autosomal-recessive pattern. One individual with Davidenkow syndrome was found to have the monochromosomic 17p11.2 deletion, which often is associated with HNPP.[219] More commonly, another autosomal-dominant form of scapuloperoneal neuropathy or SMA and congenital distal SMA are caused by heterozygous mutations in the *TRPV4* gene and is allelic disorders to CMT2C.[92,93,218]

HEREDITARY NEUROPATHY WITH NEUROMYOTONIA

There are a few reports of patients with a hereditary motor or sensorimotor polyneuropathy with neuromyotonia.[115,220,221] Patients manifest with distal weakness and impaired relaxation (action myotonia). Most have few sensory symptoms and signs, however sural nerve biopsy has revealed a loss of myelinated nerve fibers in some. NCS usually reveal low amplitude CMAPs while EMG demonstrates neuromyotonic discharges. Mutations in the histidine triad nucleotide binding protein 1 gene (*HINT1*) are the cause, but the pathogenic mechanism by which these mutations cause neuropathy are unknown.

HEREDITARY SENSORY AND AUTONOMIC NEUROPATHIES

HSANs constitute a rare group of hereditary neuropathy in which sensory and autonomic dysfunction predominate over motor function loss, unlike CMT in which motor findings are most prominent (Table 11-3).[7,82,222,223] Nevertheless, affected individuals can develop motor weakness and thus can overlap with CMT (Fig. 11-1). There are no specific medical therapies available to treat these neuropathies, other than prevention and treatment of mutilating skin and bone lesions. Affected individuals are advised to utilize a night light to limit risk of nocturnal falls, to avoid walking in their bare feet, and to inspect their feet frequently for foreign bodies in order to minimize risk of infection and the subsequent morbidity that delayed detection of an infection may cause.

HSAN Type 1

Clinical Features

The HSAN1 is the most common of the HSANs and is inherited in an autosomal-dominant fashion. HSAN1 usually presents in the second to fourth decades and this later age

▶ TABLE 11-3. **HEREDITARY SENSORY AND AUTONOMIC NEUROPATHIES**

Type	Inheritance	Chromosome	Gene	Onset	Clinical Features	Neurophysiology	Pathology
HSAN1A	AD	9q22	*SPTLC1*	Second to fourth decades	Loss of pain and temperature sensation; autonomic functions relatively spared (except for reduced sweating); arthropathies and foot ulcers are common; distal weakness may develop	Normal or only mildly reduced CMAPs and SNAPs amplitudes; near nerve recordings: reduced amplitudes of Aδ and C-fibers; abnormal QST (particularly temperature perception); SSR: absent	Distal greater than proximal loss of small myelinated and unmyelinated fibers more than large myelinated fibers
HSAN1B	AD	3p24–p22	*RAB7*	Second decade +	Same as HSAN1A with prominent distal weakness	As above	As above
HSAN1C	AD	14q24.3	*SPTLC2*	Second decade +	Same as HSAN1A	As above	As above
HSAN1D	AD	14q22.1	*ATL1*	Second decade +	Spasticity (allelic to SPG30)	As above	As above
HSAN1E	AD	19p13.2	DNA methyltransferase 1	Second decade +	Early hearing loss and dementia	As above	As above
HSAN2A	AR	12p13.33	*WNK1*	Infancy to early childhood	Severe loss of sensation to all modalities (particularly touch-pressure/vibration); mutilation of hands and feet; impaired sweating, impotence, and bladder function	Absent SNAPs; normal or only mildly reduced CMAPs amplitudes; abnormal QST (particularly vibratory perception)	Virtual absence of large myelinated fibers; mild loss of small myelinated and unmyelinated fibers
HSAN2B	AR	5p15.1	*FAM134B*				
HSAN2C	AR	2q37	*KIF1A*				
HSAN2D	AD	2q24.3	*SCN9 A*				
HSAN3A	AR	9q21	*IKAP*	Infancy	Severe autonomic dysfunction (labile BP, sweating, and temperature); decreased pain–temperature sensation more than touch/vibration; absence of fungiform papillae and taste; increased mortality; contractures seen with *DYS* mutations	Decreased SNAP amplitudes; mild slowing of CMAP velocities; abnormal QST; normal SSR	Marked reduction of small myelinated and unmyelinated fibers and to a lesser extent large myelinated fibers; loss of neurons in sympathetic ganglia
HSAN3B	AR	6912.1	*DYS*				
HSAN4	AR	3q	*trkA/NGF* receptor	Infancy	Absence of pain and temperature sensation; episodic fevers, postural hypotension, and anhidrosis; self-mutilation; mental retardation	Mildly reduced amplitudes and slow CVs of SNAPs and to a lesser extent of CMAPs; abnormal QST (particularly temperature perception); SSR: intact	Virtual absence of small myelinated and unmyelinated fibers and a moderate loss of large myelinated fibers
HSAN5	AR	1p11.2–p13.2 2q24.3	*NGFB* *SCN9A*	Infancy	Congenital indifference to painful stimuli despite intact sensation to all modalities and normal deep tendon reflexes	Normal SNAPs, CMAPs, QST, and SSR	Normal nerve biopsies or only mild loss of small myelinated and unmyelinated fibers
HSAN6 or 3C	AR	6.p12	*DYS*				
HSAN7	AD	3p22.2	*SCN11A*		Congenital Insensitivity to pain		

HSAN, hereditary sensory and autonomic neuropathy; AD, autosomal dominant; AR, autosomal recessive; TrkA/NGF, tyrosine kinase A/nerve growth factor; SPTLC1, serine palmitoyltransferase long chain base 1; IKAP, I_kB kinase complex-associated protein; DNMT1, DNA methyltransferase 1; DYS, dystonin; FAM134B, family with sequence similarity 134, member B; KIF1 A, kinesin family 1 A; WNK1, protein kinase, lysine-deficient 1; SNAP, sensory nerve action potential; CMAP, compound muscle action potential; QST, quantitative sensory testing; SSR, sympathetic skin response.

of onset is helpful in distinguishing it from other subtypes of HSANs, which typically manifest in infancy or childhood.[7,222–225] HSAN1 is slowly progressive and predominantly affects the small myelinated and unmyelinated nerve fibers, resulting in the loss of pain and temperature sensation in the feet and hands. This can lead to the development of deep dermal ulcerations, recurrent osteomyelitis, Charcot joints, bone loss, gross foot and hand deformities, and amputated digits. Although most people with HSAN1 do not complain of numbness, they often describe burning, aching, or lancinating pains. Autonomic neuropathy is not a prominent feature, but bladder dysfunction and reduced sweating in the feet may occur.

On examination, there is reduced sensation to all modalities, particularly to pin prick and temperature. Mild-to-moderate distal arm and leg weakness develop over time. However, some individuals develop severe distal extremity weakness early in the course.[225] Muscle stretch reflexes are usually absent at the ankles but may be normal or reduced elsewhere. As with CMT, pes cavus and hammertoe deformities can be seen.

Laboratory Features

CSF examination is usually normal. Increased levels of IgA in the serum may be seen. Sensory NCS reveal normal or only mildly reduced amplitudes with normal distal latencies and NCVs.[225,226] Reduced amplitudes of Aδ and C potentials reflecting the loss of small myelinated and unmyelinated nerve fibers can be appreciated on near-nerve recordings. Motor NCS are relatively spared; however, reduced amplitudes and slowing of conduction can develop over time. Needle EMG can demonstrate positive sharp waves and fibrillation potentials, with large MUAPs suggesting chronic reinnervation. Sympathetic skin responses are often unobtainable.[226]

Histopathology

Peripheral nerve biopsies demonstrate reduced density of all fiber sizes with a preferential loss of small myelinated and unmyelinated fibers (Fig. 11-10).[225] Muscle biopsies demonstrate features of neurogenic atrophy due to motor nerve involvement. Autopsy studies have revealed degeneration of dorsal root ganglia neurons and of the posterior columns, suggesting a primary sensory neuronopathy or ganglionopathy.

Molecular Genetics and Pathogenesis

HSAN1-like neuropathy is genetically heterogeneous.[227–239]

HSAN1A is the most common subtype and is caused by mutations in the serine palmitolytransferase long chain base 1 (*SPTLC1*) gene that is located on chromosome 9q22.[227–229] Serine palmitolytransferase catalyzes the rate-limiting, regulatory step in the biosynthesis of sphingolipids, and the autosomal-dominant inheritance suggests that the mutations either cause a gain of function of the enzyme or result in dominant-negative inhibition.[228] Mutations in *SPTLC1* in lymphoblast cell lines cause an increase in the de novo synthesis of ceramide (a sphingolipid) that appears to trigger apoptotic cell death.[229]

HSAN1B associated with cough and gastroesophageal reflux in a large Australian family is caused by mutations in *RAB7* located on 3p22–p24 and is allelic to CMT2B.[232,233]

HSAN1C is caused by mutations in *SPTLC2*.[230,231]

HSAN1D is caused by mutations in the gene that encodes for atlastin 1 (*ATL1*).[234] In addition to features of HSAN1, affected individuals may have spasticity of their lower extremities. In this regard, mutations in *ATL1* are also responsible for early-onset HSP (SPG30).

Recently, whole genome sequencing has also revealed mutations in *ATL3* as a cause of HSAN as well.[235–236]

HSAN1E is caused by mutations in the DNA methyltransferase 1 gene (*DNMT1*) that is associated with an autosomal-dominant inheritance of sensory neuropathy with sensorineural hearing loss and early-onset dementia.[237–239] The neurological deficits began between the second and fourth decades and were progressive, with death occurring in the fifth and sixth decades. DNA methyltransferase adds methyl groups to DNA which effects gene expression, but how this causes neuropathy is unclear.

HSAN Type 2

Clinical Features

HSAN2 is an autosomal-recessive disorder that manifests at birth or early childhood, with severe sensory loss to all modalities and areflexia.[26,240–244] Unlike HSAN1, patients with HSAN2 do not complain of lancinating pains. Autonomic dysfunction manifests with impaired sweating, bladder dysfunction, and impotence. However, postural hypotension is not common. Muscle strength is relatively normal. Scoliosis may be present. The severe sensory loss leads to pressure ulcers, Charcot joints, osteomyelitis, and bone resorption, and amputation of digits in the hands and feet can occur (Fig. 11-11).

Laboratory Features

Sensory NCS usually absent, while the CMAPs are normal or have slightly reduced amplitudes.[26,241,244] Needle EMG can reveal positive sharp waves, fibrillation potentials, and a reduced recruitment of large, polyphasic MUAPs, particularly in the distal legs.

Histopathology

Nerve biopsies demonstrate a virtual absence of all myelinated fibers with less severe diminution of unmyelinated fibers (Fig. 11-12).

Molecular Genetics and Pathogenesis

HSAN2A is caused by mutations in the protein kinase, lysine-deficient 1 gene, *PRKWNK1*, now better known as just *WNK1*, which is located on chromosome 12p13.33.[243,245] This protein may play a role in the development and/or maintenance of peripheral sensory neurons or their supporting Schwann cells.

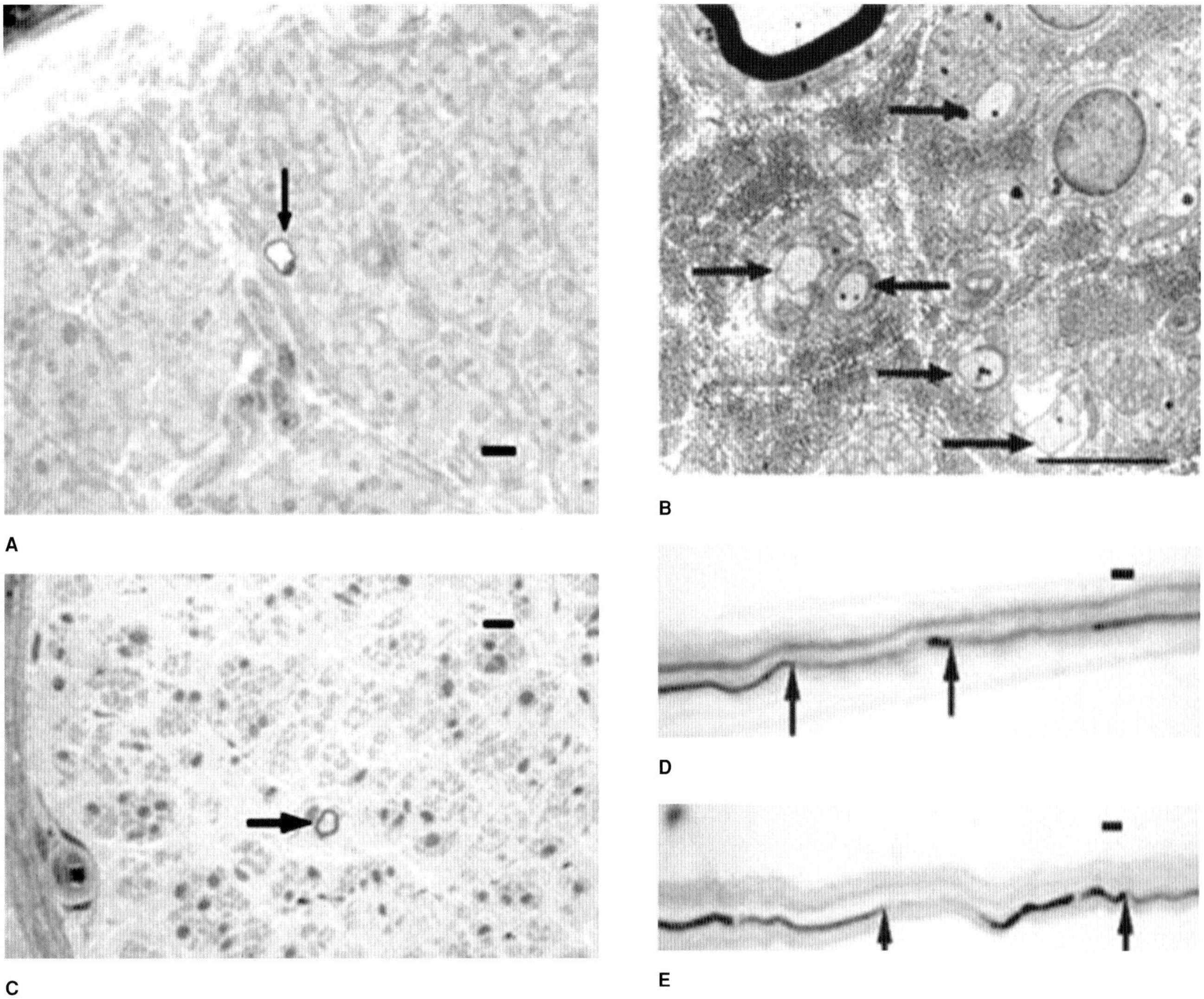

Figure 11-10. Hereditary sensory and autonomic neuropathy type 1. A 1-μm stained resin section **(A)** and electron micrograph **(B)** of a sural nerve biopsy. The single myelinated fiber in **(A)** (*arrow*) is visible at the top of **(B)**; many more unmyelinated axons (*arrows*) remain than myelinated axons. Scale bar = 10 μm **(A)** and 5 μm **(B)**. A 1-μm stained resin section **(C)** and teased fiber preparation of the sural nerve biopsy from another patient with HSNA1 **(D and E)**. There are around 50 myelinated fibers in the whole biopsy. At least two of them appear to have internodes that seem to be demyelinating in a segmental pattern (between *arrows* **D and E**). Scale bar = 10 μm **(C)** and 20 μm **(D and E)**. (Reproduced with permission from Houlden H, King R, Blake J, et al. Clinical, pathological and genetic characterization of hereditary sensory and autonomic neuropathy type 1 (HSAN I). *Brain*. 2006;129(Pt 2):411–425.)

HSAN2B is caused by mutations in the *FAM134B* (family with sequence similarity 134, member B; KIF1 A, kinesin family 1 A) gene on chromosome 5p15.1.[246–248] This protein is expressed on the Golgi complex, but how it causes HSAN is unclear.

HSAN2C is caused by homozygous or compound heterozygous mutation in the kinesin, heavy chain member 1A gene (*KIF1A*) on chromosome 2q37.[249,250] Mutations in the *KIF1A* can also cause HSP type 30. The encoded protein interacts with *WNK1* and is involved in the anterograde transport of synaptic-vesicle precursors along axons.[249]

HSAN2D is caused by mutations in *SCN9A* that encodes Na(v)1.7 sodium channels.[251] Additional symptoms in affected patients included hyposmia, hearing loss, bone dysplasia, and hypogeusia. Interestingly, mutations in *SCN9A* have also been associated with a congenital indifference to pain (HSAN4 or 5), hereditary small fiber polyneuropathy, erythromelagia, and paroxysmal extreme pain disorder (discussed at the end of the chapter).[252]

HSAN3 (Riley–Day Syndrome; Familial Dysautonomia)

Clinical Features

HSAN3 is a rare autosomal-recessive disorder that manifests in infancy with feeding difficulties due to poor suck, crying

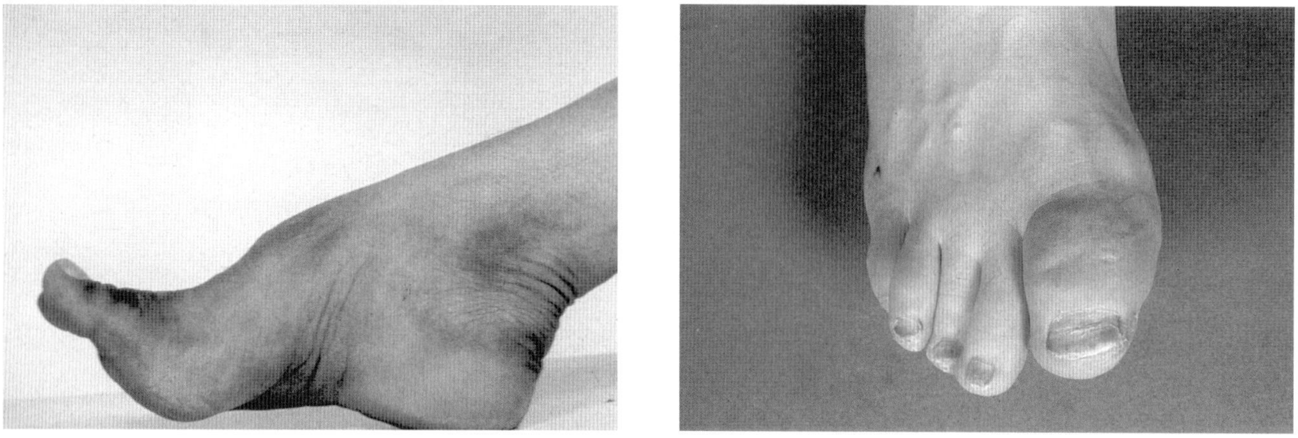

A B

Figure 11-11. Hereditary sensory and autonomic neuropathy type 2. Foot deformities such as pes cavus are common **(A)**. Because of the severe lack of sensation, these patients are prone to developing neurogenic arthropathies **(B)**. (Reproduced with permission from Amato AA, Dumitru D. Hereditary neuropathies. In: Dumitru D, Amato AA, Swartz MJ, eds. *Electrodiagnostic Medicine*. 2nd ed. Philadelphia, PA: Hanley & Belfus; 2002:889–936.)

without tears (alacrima), blotchy skin, unexplained fluctuations in body temperature and blood pressure, and repeated vomiting.[135,253–255] Other autonomic features include esophageal and gastrointestinal dysmotility, excessive sweating, tonic pupils, and postural hypotension. Recurrent pulmonary infections are common. Developmental delay and seizures may also occur, although intelligence is normal. Most patients are of Ashkenazi Jewish heritage in whom the incidence of the disease is 1:3700 live births and carrier frequency is 1:32.[256] HSAN3 is associated with an increased mortality, with a 30-year survival of approximately 50%.[256] However, there have been a few cases with clinical features of HSAN3 and contractures (clubbed feet and clenched hands) and a more severe lethal course.[257] These affected infants were found to have a different gene than more common form of HSAN3.

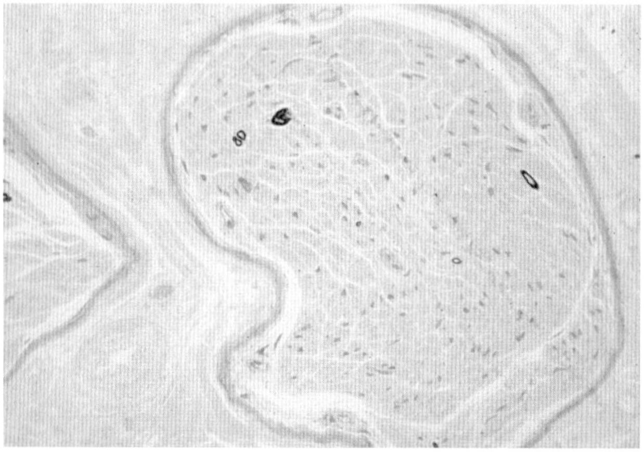

Figure 11-12. Hereditary sensory and autonomic neuropathy type 2. Sural nerve biopsy reveals a severe loss of myelinated and unmyelinated nerve fibers. Semithin, epoxy resin. (Reproduced with permission from Amato AA, Dumitru D. Hereditary neuropathies. In: Dumitru D, Amato AA, Swartz MJ, eds. *Electrodiagnostic Medicine*. 2nd ed. Philadelphia, PA: Hanley & Belfus; 2002:889–936.)

Examination reveals reduced pain and temperature perception and, to a lesser extent, a reduction in proprioception and vibration. Of note, there is an absence of fungiform papillae of the tongue and impaired taste sensation. Muscle strength is usually normal. Muscle stretch reflexes are reduced or absent. Corneal reflexes are also often absent. Mutilation and amputations of the distal extremities are not usually seen in HSAN3, but occasional Charcot joints occur. Short stature and scoliosis are common.

Laboratory Features

SNAPs have only slightly reduced amplitudes and slow CVs, while CMAPs are normal. Sympathetic skin responses are preserved, but quantitative sensory testing reveals impaired heat, cold, and vibratory perception.[135]

Histopathology

Autopsy studies have demonstrated a loss of neurons within the cervical and thoracic sympathetic ganglia as well as in the dorsal root ganglia and trigeminal sensory nucleus. Sural nerve biopsies reveal a marked reduction of unmyelinated fibers (5–15% of normal) and a less severe reduction in the number of large myelinated fibers (15–50% of normal).

Molecular Genetics and Pathogenesis

HSAN3A is caused by mutations in the $I_K B$ kinase complex-associated protein (*IKAP*) gene located on chromosome 9q31.[256–260] The IKAP protein may activate genes important in the development of sensory and autonomic neurons. Importantly, carrier detection and prenatal diagnosis can be made. HSAN3B (also reported as HSAN6) is associated with contractures and poorer prognosis is caused by mutations in the gene that encodes dystonin (*DYS*).[257]

HSAN4 (Congenital Insensitivity to Pain with Anhidrosis)

Clinical Features

HSAN4 is an extremely rare autosomal-recessive disorder that manifests in infancy or childhood with an insensitivity to pain, self-mutilation, anhidrosis, and reduced mentation.[135,261] Individuals who are affected become extremely poikilothermic and are at risk of hyperthermia due to their inability to sweat in hot temperatures. In addition, they can develop severe postural hypotension. Sensory examination demonstrates a prominent loss of pain and temperature perception, while vibratory sensation and proprioception are less severely affected. Motor strength and reflexes are preserved.

Laboratory Features

NCS reveal normal or only slightly reduced SNAP and CMAP amplitudes and CVs. Quantitative sensory testing reveals markedly abnormal heat and cold perception and to a lesser extent vibratory perception.[135] Unlike HSAN3, sympathetic skin responses are unobtainable in HSAN4.[135,262]

Histopathology

As expected on the basis of the clinical examination, sural nerve biopsies reveal a virtual absence of unmyelinated and small myelinated fibers and to a lesser extent a reduction of large fibers to 45–65% of normal.[135,263]

Molecular Genetics and Pathogenesis

HSAN4 is caused by mutations in the tyrosine kinase A–nerve growth factor receptor gene (*trkA/NGF*) located on chromosome 3q.[264–266] However, no mutations in this gene have been identified in some individuals with a similar phenotype, suggesting genetic heterogeneity of HSAN4. Tyrosine kinase receptors are ligands for neurotrophins. In this regard, NGF, a neurotrophin, binds to trkA receptors, which are highly expressed on dorsal root ganglia and sympathetic neurons. Once bound to the receptor, the trkA–NGF complex is internalized into the nucleus of the neuron, where it regulates the expression of genes important for neuronal maturation, growth, and survival. Mutations in the trkA/NGF receptor results in a loss of function of this receptor–ligand complex, which in turn leads to degeneration of sympathetic ganglion neurons and nociceptive sensory neurons derived from the neural crest.[264,266]

HSAN5 (Congenital Indifference to Pain)

Clinical Features

HSAN5 is similar to HSAN4 is that affected individuals have a congenital insensitivity or indifference to pain. Those with HSAN5 do not appear to recognize or react to painful stimuli (i.e., withdrawal) from birth despite having normal sensitivity to other sensory modalities, normal strength, and muscle stretch reflexes.[185,267–270] There is no obvious dysautonomia.

Laboratory Features

Motor and sensory NCS, quantitative sensory testing, and autonomic testing are all usually normal.

Histopathology

Reports of sural nerve biopsies have yielded mixed results. Some have reported normal densities of myelinated and unmyelinated nerve fibers,[185] while other studies have described a mild reduction of small myelinated and unmyelinated fibers.[267–270]

Molecular Genetics and Pathogenesis

Mutations in the *NGFB* gene on chromosome 1p11.2–p13.2 were identified in one family classified as having HSAN5.[269,270] Some could argue that this family actually represents a more benign subtype of HSAN4 because the nerve biopsies were abnormal although neurophysiological testing was normal. In this regard, it is interesting that NGFB binds to trkA, which is mutated in HSAN4 (see "HSAN Type 4" section).

Mutations in *SCN9A* aside from causing HSAN2D also can cause HSAN with congenital indifference to pain.[271–273] In addition, some patients with congenital insensitivity to pain have been found to be caused by mutations in *SCN11A*, which encodes the voltage-gated sodium channel Nav1.9; some have classified this as HSAN7.[274]

▶ ERYTRHOMELAGIA

CLINICAL FEATURES

Erythromelalgia is a rare disorder characterized by episodic erythema, intense burning pain and warmth of the hands or feet.[252,275–278] It can occur in an inherited condition (autosomal dominant) or may be acquired. The acquired or secondary form can occurs in association with myeloproliferative diseases, neuropathies, and autoimmune diseases. Onset of symptoms can begin or may begin spontaneously at any age in the hereditary form.

LABORATORY FEATURES

NCS, quantitative sensory testing, and sudomotor testing may be normal or abnormal.[276]

HISTOPATHOLOGICAL FEATURES

Skin biopsies may reveal reduced epidermal nerve fiber density. In addition, perivascular inflammation and edema, fibrosis or arterioles, thickening of arteriolar basement membranes, and smooth muscle hyperplasia may be observed.[276]

MOLECULAR GENETICS AND PATHOGENESIS

Autosomal-dominant hereditary erythromelalgia is caused by mutations in the *SCN9A* gene that encodes the Nav1.7 channel.[252,277–279] As previously discussed, mutations in this gene also cause HSAN2D or a form of HSAN4. The Nav1.7 sodium channel is preferentially expressed in most nociceptive dorsal root ganglion neurons and in sympathetic neurons and plays an important role in nociception and vasomotor regulation. Some mutations produced a hyperpolarized voltage-dependence of activation, slower kinetics of deactivation, and impaired steady-state slow inactivation while others do not.

▶ TREATMENT

This is a very difficult to treat disorder. Some patients respond to lidocaine-like medications (e.g., lidoderm patches, mexilitine) and antiepileptic medication (e.g., gabapentin) but many are refractory and require opiates.[278,280]

▶ OTHER SODIUM CHANNELOPATHIES NEUROPATHIES

Paroxysmal extreme pain disorder (formerly known as familial rectal pain) is an autosomal-dominant disorder characterized by severe episodes of perineal and rectal, ocular, and mandibular pain that is often associated with dysautonomia including flushing, lacrimation, rhinorrhea, bradycardia, and apnea.[252,281,282] Interestingly, it is also caused by mutations in *SCN9A* which again encodes the Nav1.7 channel.

Familial episodic pain syndrome type 1 is an autosomal-dominant disorder associated with severe episodes of pain, predominantly in the chest and arms, but occasionally involving the abdomen and legs.[252,283] The onset is usually in infancy. The episodes of pain typically lasts about 60–90 minutes, can be triggered by hunger and cold, and are typically refractory to standard pain medications. The neurological examination, NCS, and IENF densities are usually normal. This disorder is caused by mutations in *TRPA*, which encodes the transient receptor potential A1 channel.

Familial episodic pain syndrome type 2 is an autosomal-dominant disorder characterized by adult-onset of paroxysmal pain mainly affecting the distal lower extremities (summary by Faber et al., 2012). Caused by mutations in *SCNA10A* encoding the Nav1.8 channel.[284]

Familial episodic pain syndrome type 3 is yet another autosomal-dominant disorder associated with paroxysmal pain affecting distal hands and feet that has been reported in two Chinese kindreds and was found to be caused by a mutation in *SCN11A* that encodes the Nav1.9 channel.[285]

Interestingly, approximately 30% of patients in one series with otherwise idiopathic **painful, small fiber neuropathy** had missense substitutions in *SCN9A*.[286,287] This is an overestimate as some of the sequence changes reported have subsequently been found to be benign sequence changes.[7,252] Nonetheless, mutations in *SCN9A* are a cause of small fiber neuropathy and have been reported in other series of patients.[288,289] Symptoms and signs are similar to idiopathic small fiber polyneuropathy discussed in detail in Chapter 22. Affected individuals however tended to be younger than the older patients who more typically develop small fiber polyneuropathy. Na(v)1.7 is expressed in the sensory dorsal root ganglion and sympathetic ganglion neurons and their small diameter peripheral axons. Some mutations impair slow inactivation can produce DRG neuron hyperexcitability that contributes to pain.[287–294]

Rare patients with otherwise idiopathic small fiber neuropathy also have been found to have mutations in *SCN10A* that encodes for a different sodium channel, Nav1.8.[252,284294,295] This sodium channel is preferentially expressed in small diameter dorsal root neurons. Mutations have been demonstrated to shift activation in a hyperpolarizing direction, thus rendering neurons hyperexcitability.

▶ APPROACH TO GENETIC TESTING

Some argue (especially insurance companies) that most patients do not need genetic testing as there are no specific medical therapies available for any of the subtypes of CMT. However, we feel that genetic testing can aid in prognosis and genetic counseling, help in avoiding of unnecessary and invasive tests (e.g., nerve biopsies), and perhaps unnecessary trials of potentially harmful treatments and (e.g., immunosuppressive agents, intravenous immunoglobulin) when there is diagnostic doubt (e.g., possible CIDP). One good argument for genetic testing and following up carefully phenotyped patients is to learn more about the natural history of all types of CMT including the rare types so that we can provide a more accurate prediction of the natural history of disease in individual patients in the future.[296]

The diagnostic approach to patients with a possible hereditary neuropathy can be daunting given the large number a causal genes and phenotypic variability even within a genotype. Fortunately, useful guidelines are available to help direct which genetic tests should be ordered on the basis of inheritance pattern, age of onset, severity, and motor NCVs.[296–299] A large study and proposed diagnostic algorithms from Dr. Shy's group based on the results of genetic testing on their very large cohort of presumed CMT patients (787 patients of which 527 were genotyped) is particularly helpful.[299] Importantly, approximately 92% of the 527 genetically defined CMT patients in their cohort had mutations in one of only four genes (*PMP22, MPZ, GJB1,* and *MFN2*).[299]

For patients who undergo genetic testing, they proposed that patients with a classical CMT phenotype with slow NCVs (between 16 and 35 m/s), initially should be screened for *PMP22* duplications as this is the most common mutation.[299] If this is negative then patients should next be screened for *GJB1* mutations (CMT1X), or if there is clear male-to-male transmission, *MPZ* (CMT1B). Only if these targets are negative would they suggest screening for point mutations in *PMP22, LITAF/SIMPLE,* and *EGR2*.

Those with severely slow NCV (≤15 m/s) and who begin to walk after 15 months of age should have testing for both the *PMP22* duplication and *MPZ* mutations.[299] Affected individuals with such severely slow NCVs who walk before 15 months of age should be tested only for the *PMP22* duplication. If no *PMP22* duplication or *MPZ* mutations are found, they next suggest sequencing *PMP22*.

Individuals with intermediate MNCVs (between 35 and 45 m/s) usually have CMT1X or CMT1B. For patients with no male-to-male transmission, intermediate conductions, and a classical phenotype, the authors recommend first screening for *GJB1* mutations.[299] If this testing is negative, testing should proceed to *MPZ* mutations. Alternatively, if there is male-to-male transmission, patients should be first screened for *DNM2* mutations as seen in CMT1B. As no patients with CMT1A had intermediate conduction velocities, testing for a *PMP22* duplication would not be warranted. If testing for *MPZ* and *GJB1* is negative, patients could be screened for mutations in the less common dominant intermediate forms of CMT including *DNM2* (DI-CMTB) and *YARS* (DI-CMTC). *DYN2* mutations should also be considered those with cataracts and neutropenia.

In severe childhood onset CMT2 screening should begin with testing of *MFN2* gene as this is the most common cause of CMT2.[299] If this is negative, testing for *MPZ* and *GJB1*would be reasonable. Sequencing *MPZ* and *GJB1* also would be the initial genes to screen for late-onset CMT2; if there was male-to-male transmission in the pedigree only *MPZ* screening is necessary.

Genetic testing for the much rarer forms of hereditary neuropathy (e.g., HSAN) is likewise based on age of onset, inheritance pattern, and the clinical phenotype as discussed in this chapter.

Some of the above may be moot in the next several years and next generation, whome exome, and whole genome sequencing become more widely available and cheaper.[300] The down side of exome sequencing is that only exons are sequenced so mutations in promoter regions or intron segments important in RNA splicing may be missed. This technique may be particularly useful in identifying novel CMT-associated genes, particularly in CMT2 in which only about 30% of cases can be genotyped at present. The additional problem, particularly with novel genes or in previously unreported sequence changes in genes known to cause a neuropathy is whether or not the alteration is truly a disease-causing mutation or a benign polymorphism.

▶ SUMMARY

As one can see, there is marked variability in clinical phenotype associated with mutations in individual genes and the same clinical phenotype can be caused by mutation in various genes associated with CMT. Further, there is much overlap of CMT with distal motor neuropathies and HSAN. A practical approach to diagnosis is based on clinical and electrodiagnostic features. Clear autosomal-dominant, autosomal-recessive, or X-linked pattern of inheritance combined with data from NCS (e.g., demyelinating, axonal, or intermediate physiology) are helpful in directing which genes one should preferentially check for mutations. Unfortunately, there are no specific medical treatments available at this time but genetic counseling and supportive therapies (e.g., physical and occupational therapy, bracing) are important and certainly can improve function and quality of life (see Chapter 4).

REFERENCES

1. Harding AE. From the syndrome of Charcot, Marie, and Tooth to disorders of peripheral myelin proteins. *Brain.* 1995;118:809–818.
2. Lewis RA, Sumner AJ, Shy ME. Electrophysiological features of inherited demyelinating neuropathies: A reappraisal in the era of molecular diagnosis. *Muscle Nerve.* 2000;23:1472–1487.
3. Mendell JR. Charcot–Marie–Tooth neuropathies and related disorders. *Semin Neurol.* 1998;18:41–47.
4. Ouvrier RA. Correlation between the histopathologic, genotypic, and phenotypic features of hereditary peripheral neuropathies in children. *J Child Neurol.* 1996;11:133–146.
5. Boerkoel CF, Takashima H, Garcia C, et al. Charcot–Marie–Tooth disease and related neuropathies: Mutation distribution and genotype–phenotype correlation. *Ann Neurol.* 2002;51(2):190–201.
6. Pleasure DE. Genetics of Charcot–Marie–Tooth disease [Editorial]. *Arch Neurol.* 2003;60(4):481–482.
7. Klein CJ, Duan X, Shy ME. Inherited neuropathies: Clinical overview and update. *Muscle Nerve.* 2013;48(4):604–622.
8. Tazir M, Bellatache M, Nouioua S, Vallat JM. Autosomal recessive Charcot-Marie-Tooth disease: From genes to phenotypes. *J Peripher Nerv Syst.* 2013;18(2):113–129.
9. Krampitz DE, Wolfe GI, Fleckenstein JL, Barohn RJ. Charcot–Marie–Tooth type 1 A presenting as calf hypertrophy and muscle cramps. *Neurology.* 1998;51:1508–1509.
10. Carger GT, Kilmer DD, Bonekat WH, Lieberman JS, Fowler WM Jr. Evaluation of phrenic nerve and pulmonary function in hereditary motor and sensory neuropathy, type I. *Muscle Nerve.* 1992;15:459–462.
11. Harding AE, Thomas PK. The clinical features of hereditary motor and sensory neuropathy type I and II. *Brain.* 1980;103:259–280.
12. Hattori N, Yamamoto M, Yoshihara T, et al.; Study Group for Hereditary Neuropathy in Japan. Demyelinating and axonal features of Charcot–Marie–Tooth disease with mutations of myelin-related proteins (PMP22, MPZ and Cx32): A clinicopathological study of 205 Japanese patients. *Brain.* 2003;126(Pt 1):134–151.

13. Kaku DA, Parry GJ, Malamut R, Lupski JR, Garcia CA. Uniform slowing of conduction velocities in Charcot–Marie–Tooth polyneuropathy type 1. *Neurology*. 1993;43:2664–2667.
14. Bird TD, Kraft GH, Lipe GH, Kenney KL, Sumi SM. Clinical and pathological phenotype of the original family with Charcot–Marie–Tooth type 1B: A 20-year study. *Ann Neurol.* 1997;41:463–469.
15. Gabreëls-Festen AA, Bolhuis PA, Hoogendijk JE, Vaentijn LJ, Eshuis EJ, Gabreëls FJ. Charcot–Marie–Tooth disease type 1 A: Morphological phenotype of the 17p duplication versus PMP22 point mutations. *Acta Neuropathol (Berl).* 1995;90: 645–649.
16. Santoro L, Manganelli F, Di Maria E, et al. A novel mutation of myelin protein zero associated with an axonal form of Charcot–Marie–Tooth disease. *J Neurol Neurosurg Psychiatry.* 2004;75(2):262–265.
17. Lewis RA, Sumner AJ. The electrodiagnostic distinctions between chronic familial and acquired demyelinating neuropathies. *Neurology*. 1982;32:592–596.
18. Bennett CL, Shirk AJ, Huynh HM, et al. SIMPLE mutation in demyelinating neuropathy and distribution in sciatic nerve. *Ann Neurol*. 2004;55(5):713–720.
19. Dyck PJ, Lambert EH, Mulder DW. Charcot–Marie–Tooth disease: Nerve conduction and clinical studies of a large kinship. *Neurology*. 1963;13:1–11.
20. Lewis RA, Li J, Fuerst DR, Shy ME, Krajewski K. Motor unit number estimate of distal and proximal muscles in Charcot–Marie–Tooth disease. *Muscle Nerve*. 2003;28(2):161–167.
21. Amato AA, Barohn RJ. Hereditary liability to pressure palsies: Association with central nervous system demyelination. *Muscle Nerve*. 1996;19:770–773.
22. Combarros O, Calleja J, Figols J, Cabello A, Berciano J. Dominantly inherited motor and sensory neuropathy type I: Genetic, clinical, electrophysiological and pathological features in four families. *J Neurol Sci*. 1983;61:181–191.
23. Dyck PJ, Lambert EH. Lower motor and primary sensory neuron diseases with peroneal muscular atrophy. *Arch Neurol.* 1968;18:603–618.
24. Buchthal F, Behse F. Peroneal muscular atrophy (PMA) and related disorders: I. Clinical manifestations as related to biopsy findings, nerve conduction and electromyography. *Brain*. 1977;100:41–66.
25. Behse F, Buchthal F. Peroneal muscular atrophy (PMA) and related disorders: II. Histological findings in sural nerves. *Brain*. 1977;100:67–85.
26. Dyck PJ. Histologic measurements and fine structure of biopsied sural nerve: Normal and in peroneal muscular atrophy, hypertrophic neuropathy, and congenital sensory neuropathy. *Mayo Clin Proc*. 1966;41:742–774.
27. Kochanski A, Drac H, Kabzinska D, Hausmanowa-Petrusewicz I. A novel mutation, Thr65Ala, in the MPZ gene in a patient with Charcot–Marie–Tooth type 1B disease with focally folded myelin. *Neuromuscul Disord*. 2004;14(3):229–232.
28. Lupski JR, deOca-Luna RM, Slaugenhaupt S, et al. DNA duplication associated with Charcot–Marie–Tooth disease type 1 A. *Cell*. 1991;66:219–232.
29. Raemakears P, Timmerman V, Nellis E, et al. Duplication in chromosome 17p11.2 in Charcot–Marie–Tooth disease type 1 a (CMT1 a). The HMSN Collaborative Group. *Neuromuscul Disord*. 1991;1:93–97.
30. Lopes J, Ravise N, Vandenberghe A, et al. Fine mapping of de novo CMT1 A and HNPP rearrangements within CMT1 A-REPS evidences two distinct sex-dependent mechanisms and candidate sequences involved in recombination. *Hum Mol Genet*. 1998;7:141–148.
31. Chance PF, Bird TD, Matsunami N, et al. Trisomy 17p associated with Charcot–Marie–Tooth neuropathy type 1 A phenotype: Evidence for gene dosage as a mechanism in CMT1 A. *Neurology*. 1992;42:2295–2299.
32. Roa BB, Garcia CA, Suter U, et al. Evidence for Charcot–Marie–Tooth disease type 1 A association with point mutation in the PMP22 gene. *N Engl J Med*. 1993;5:189–194.
33. Gabriel JM, Erne B, Pareyson D, Sghirlanzoni A, Taroni F, Steck AJ. Gene dosage effects in hereditary peripheral neuropathy. Expression of peripheral myelin protein 22 in Charcot–Marie–Tooth disease type 1 A and hereditary neuropathy with liability to pressure palsies nerve biopsies. *Neurology*. 1997;49:1635–1640.
34. Hanemann CO, Stoll G, D'Urso D, et al. Peripheral myelin protein-22 expression in Charcot-Marie Tooth disease type 1 A sural nerve biopsies. *J Neurosci Res*. 1994;37:654–659.
35. Vallat JM, Sindou P, Preux PM, et al. Ultrastructural PMP22 expression in inherited demyelinating neuropathies. *Ann Neurol.* 1996;39:813–817.
36. Yoshikawa H, Nishimura T, Nakatsuji Y, et al. Elevated expression of messenger RNA for peripheral myelin protein 22 in biopsied peripheral nerves of patients with Charcot–Marie–Tooth disease type 1 A. *Ann Neurol*. 1994;35:445–450.
37. Sahenk Z, Chen L, Mendell JR. Effects of PMP22 duplication and deletion on the axonal cytoskeleton. *Ann Neurol.* 1999;45:16–24.
38. Hayasaka K, Himoro M, Sato W, et al. Charcot–Marie–Tooth neuropathy type 1B is associated with mutations of the myelin P0 gene. *Nat Genet*. 1993;5:31–34.
39. Kulkens T, Bulhuis PA, Wolterman RA, et al. Deletion of serine 34 codon from the major peripheral myelin protein P0 gene in Charcot–Marie–Tooth disease type 1B. *Nat Genet*. 1993;5:35–39.
40. Su Y, Brooks DG, Li L, et al. Myelin protein zero gene mutated in Charcot–Marie–Tooth type 1B. *Proc Natl Acad Sci USA*. 1993;90:10856–10860.
41. Vallat JM, Magy L, Lagrange E, et al. Diagnostic value of ultrastructural nerve examination in Charcot–Marie–Tooth disease: Two CMT 1B cases with pseudo-recessive inheritance. *Acta Neuropathol (Berl)*. 2007;113(4):443–449.
42. Sindou P, Vallat JM, Chapon F, et al. Ultrastructural protein zero expression in Charcot–Marie–Tooth type 1B disease. *Muscle Nerve*. 1999;22:99–104.
43. Street VA, Bennett CL, Goldy JD, et al. Mutation of a putative protein degradation gene LITAF/SIMPLE in Charcot–Marie–Tooth disease 1 C. *Neurology*. 2003;60(1):22–26.
44. Latour P, Gonnaud PM, Ollagnon E, et al. SIMPLE mutation analysis in dominant demyelinating Charcot–Marie–Tooth disease: Three novel mutations. *J Peripher Nerv Syst*. 2006;11(2):148–155.
45. Shirk AJ, Anderson SK, Hashemi SH, Chance PF, Bennett CL. SIMPLE interacts with NEDD4 and TSG101: Evidence for a role in lysosomal sorting and implications for Charcot–Marie–Tooth disease. *J Neurosci Res*. 2005;82(1):43–50.
46. Warner LE, Mancias P, Butler IJ, et al. Mutations in the early growth response 2 (ERG2) gene are associated with hereditary myelinopathies. *Nat Genet*. 1998;18:382–384.
47. Fabrizi GM, Cavallaro T, Angiari C, et al. Giant axon and neurofilament accumulation in Charcot–Marie–Tooth disease type 2E. *Neurology*. 2004;62(8):1429–1431.

48. Zuchner S, Vorgerd M, Sindern E, Schroder JM. The novel neurofilament light (NEFL) mutation Glu397Lys is associated with a clinically and morphologically heterogeneous type of Charcot–Marie–Tooth neuropathy. *Neuromuscul Disord.* 2004;14(2):147–157.
49. Mademan I, Deconinck T, Dinopoulos A, et al. De novo INF2 mutations expand the genetic spectrum of hereditary neuropathy with glomerulopathy. *Neurology.* 2013;81(22):1953–1958.
50. Boyer O, Nevo F, Plaisier E, et al. INF2 mutations in Charcot-Marie-Tooth disease with glomerulopathy. *N Engl J Med.* 2011;365:2377–2388.
51. Amato AA, Gronseth G, Callerame K, Kagan-Hallet KS, Bryan W, Barohn RJ. Tomaculous neuropathy: A clinical and electrophysiological study in patients with and without 1.5 Mb deletions in chromosome 17p11.2. *Muscle Nerve.* 1996;19:16–22.
52. Andersson PB, Yuen E, Parko K, So YT. Electrodiagnostic features of hereditary neuropathy with liability to pressure palsies. *Neurology.* 2000;54:40–44.
53. Hirota N, Kaji R, Yoshikawa H, et al. Hereditary neuropathy with liability to pressure palsies: Distinguishing clinical and electrophysiological features among patients with multiple entrapment neuropathy. *J Neurol Sci* 1996;139:187–189.
54. Le Forestier N, LeGuern E, Coullin P, et al. Recurrent polyradiculoneuropathy with the 17p11.2 deletion. *Muscle Nerve* 1997;20:1184–1186.
55. Lenssen PPA, Gabreels-Festen AAWM, Valentijn LJ, et al. Hereditary neuropathy with liability to pressure palsies. Phenotypic differences between patients with the common deletion and a PMP22 frame shift mutation. *Brain.* 1998;121:1451–1458.
56. Madrid R, Bradley WG. The pathology of neuropathies with focal thickening of the myelin sheath (Tomaculous neuropathy). *J Neurol Sci.* 1975;25:415–448.
57. Mouton P, Tardieu S, Goudier R, et al. Spectrum of clinical and electrophysiologic features in HNPP patients with the 17p11.2 deletion. *Neurology.* 1999;52:1440–1446.
58. Verhagen WIM, Gabreels-Festen AAWM, van Wensen PJM, et al. Hereditary neuropathy with liability to pressure palsies: A clinical, electrophysiological, and morphological study. *J Neurol Sci.* 1993;116:176–184.
59. Hong YH, Kim M, Kim HJ, Sung JJ, Kim SH, Lee KW. Clinical and electrophysiologic features of HNPP patients with 17p11.2 deletion. *Acta Neurol Scand.* 2003;108(5):352–358.
60. Li J, Krajewski K, Shy ME, Lewis RA. Hereditary neuropathy with liability to pressure palsy: The electrophysiology fits the name. *Neurology.* 2002;58(12):1769–1773.
61. Li J, Krajewski K, Lewis RA, Shy ME. Loss-of-function phenotype of hereditary neuropathy with liability to pressure palsies. *Muscle Nerve.* 2004;29(2):205–210.
62. Behse F, Buchthal F, Carlsen F, et al. Hereditary neuropathy with liability to pressure palsies. *Brain.* 1972;95:777–794.
63. Joy JL, Oh SJ. Tomaculous neuropathy presenting as acute recurrent polyneuropathy. *Ann Neurol.* 1989;26:98–100.
64. Stögbauer F, Young P, Kerschensteiner M, Ringelsein EB, Assman G, Funke H. Recurrent brachial plexus palsies as the only clinical expression of neuropathy with liability to pressure palsies associated with a de novo deletion of peripheral myelin protein-22 gene. *Muscle Nerve.* 1998;21:1199–1201.
65. Bosch EP, Chui HC, Martin MA, et al. Brachial plexus involvement in familial pressure-sensitive neuropathy: Electrophysiological and morphological findings. *Ann Neurol.* 1980;8:620–624.
66. Chance PF, Alderson MK, Leppig KA, et al. DNA deletion associated with hereditary neuropathy with liability to pressure palsies. *Cell.* 1993;72:143–151.
67. Sahenk Z, Chen L, Freimer M. A novel PMP22 point mutation causing HNPP phenotype. Studies on nerve xenografts. *Neurology.* 1998;51:702–707.
68. Schenone A, Nobbio L, Caponnetto C, et al. Correlation between PMP-22 messenger RNA expression and phenotype in hereditary neuropathy with liability to pressure palsies. *Ann Neurol.* 1997;42:866–872.
69. Berciano J, Combarros O, Figols J, et al. Hereditary motor and sensory neuropathy type II. *Brain.* 1986;109:897–914.
70. Bouche' P, Gherardi R, Cathala HP, et al. Peroneal muscular atrophy: Part 1. Clinical and electrophysiological study. *J Neurol Sci.* 1983;61:389–399.
71. Dyck PJ, Lambert EH. Lower motor and primary sensory neuron disease with peroneal muscular atrophy. *Arch Neurol.* 1968;18:619–625.
72. Teunissen LL, Notermans NC, Franssen H, Van Engelen BG, Baas F, Wokke JH. Disease course of Charcot–Marie–Tooth disease type 2: A 5-year follow-up study. *Arch Neurol.* 2003;60(6):823–828.
73. Bienfait HM, Verhamme C, van Schaik IN, et al. Comparison of CMT1 A and CMT2: Similarities and differences. *J Neurol.* 2006;253(12):1572–1580.
74. Bienfait HME, Baas F, Koelman JHTM, et al. Phenotype of Charcot–Marie–Tooth disease Type 2. *Neurology.* 2007;68:1658–1667.
75. Lawson VH, Graham BV, Flanigan KM. Clinical and electrophysiologic features of CMT2 A with mutations in the mitofusin 2 gene. *Neurology.* 2005;65(2):197–204.
76. Verhoeven K, Claeys KG, Zuchner S, et al. MFN2 mutation distribution and genotype/phenotype correlation in Charcot–Marie–Tooth type 2. *Brain.* 2006;129(Pt 8):2093–2102.
77. Loiseau D, Chevrollier A, Verny C, et al. Mitochondrial coupling in Charcot–Marie–Tooth Type 2 A disease. *Ann Neurol.* 2007;61:315–323.
78. Gabreëls-Festen AAWM, Joosten EMG, Gabreëls FJM, et al. Hereditary motor and sensory neuropathy of neuronal type with onset in early childhood. *Brain.* 1991;114:1855–1870.
79. Chung KW, Kim SB, Park KD, et al. Early onset severe and late-onset mild Charcot–Marie–Tooth disease with mitofusin 2 (MFN2) mutations. *Brain.* 2006;129:2103–2118.
80. Zuchner S, De Jonghe P, Jordanova A, et al. Axonal neuropathy with optic atrophy is caused by mutations in mitofusin 2. *Ann Neurol.* 2006;59(2):276–281.
81. De Jonghe P, Timmerman V, Fitzpatrick D, Spoelders P, Martin J-J, Van Broeckhoven C. Mutilating neuropathic ulcerations in a chromosome 3q13–q22 linked Charcot–Marie–Tooth disease type 2B family. *J Neurol Neurosurg Psychiatry.* 1997;62:570–573.
82. Auer-Grumbach M, De Jonghe P, Verhoeven K, et al. Autosomal dominant inherited neuropathies with prominent sensory loss and mutilations: A review. *Arch Neurol.* 2003;60(3):329–334.
83. Verhoeven K, De Jonghe P, Coen K, et al. Mutations in the small GTP-ase late endosomal protein RAB7 cause Charcot–Marie–Tooth type 2B neuropathy. *Am J Hum Genet.* 2003;72:722–727.
84. Meggouh F, Bienfait HM, Weterman MA, de Visser M, Baas F. Charcot–Marie–Tooth disease due to a de novo mutation of the RAB7 gene. *Neurology.* 2006;67(8):1476–1478.

85. De Sandre-Giovannoli A, Chaouch M, Kozlov S, et al. Homozygous defects in LMNA, encoding lamin A/C nuclear-envelope proteins, cause autosomal recessive axonal neuropathy in human (Charcot–Marie–Tooth disorder type 2) and mouse. *Am J Hum Genet.* 2002;70(3):726–736. Erratum in *Am J Hum Genet.* 2002;70(4):1075.
86. Chaouch M, Allal Y, De Sandre-Giovannoli A, et al. The phenotypic manifestations of autosomal recessive axonal Charcot–Marie–Tooth due to a mutation in Lamin A/C gene. *Neuromuscul Dis.* 2003;13(1):60–67.
87. Tazir M, Azzedine H, Assami S, et al. Phenotypic variability in autosomal recessive axonal Charcot–Marie–Tooth disease due to the R298 C mutation in lamin A/C. *Brain.* 2004;127 (Pt 1):154–163.
88. Bouhouche A, Birouk N, Azzedine H, et al. Autosomal recessive axonal Charcot–Marie–Tooth disease (ARCMT2): Phenotype–genotype correlations in 13 Moroccan families. *Brain.* 2007;130(Pt 4):1062–1075.
89. Dyck PJ, Litchey WJ, Minnerath S, et al. Hereditary motor and sensory neuropathy with diaphragm and vocal cord paresis. *Ann Neurol.* 1994:35:608–615.
90. Pridmore C, Baraister M, Brett EM, Harding AE. Distal spinal muscular atrophy with vocal cord paralysis. *J Med Genet.* 1992;29:197–199.
91. Klein CJ, Cunningham JM, Atkinson EJ, et al. The gene for HMSN2 C maps to 12q23–24: A region of neuromuscular disorders. *Neurology.* 2003;60:1151–1156.
92. Echaniz-Laguna A, Dubourg O, et al. Phenotypic spectrum and incidence of TRPV4 mutations in patients with inherited axonal neuropathy. *Neurology.* 2014;82(21):1919–1926.
93. Deng H-X, Klein CJ, Yan J, et al. Scapuloperoneal spinal muscular atrophy and CMT2 C are allelic disorders caused by alterations in TRPV4. *Nat Genet.* 2010;42:165–169.
94. Ionasescu V, Searby C, Shefield VC, Roklina T, Nishimura D, Ionasescu R. Autosomal dominant Charcot–Marie–Tooth axonal neuropathy mapped on chromosome 7p (CMT2D). *Hum Mol Genet.* 1996;5:1373–1375.
95. Sambuughin N, Sivakumar K, Selenge B, et al. Autosomal dominant distal spinal muscular atrophy type V (dsSMA-V) and Charcot–Marie–Tooth disease type 2D (CMT2D) segregate within a large kindred and map to a refined region on chromosome 7p15. *J Neurol Sci.* 1998;161:23–28.
96. Antonellis A, Ellsworth RE, Sambuughin N, et al. Glycyl tRNA synthetase mutations in Charcot–Marie–Tooth disease type 2D and distal spinal muscular atrophy type V. *Am J Hum Genet.* 2003;72:1293–1299.
97. Sivakumar K, Kyriakides T, Puls I, et al. Phenotypic spectrum of disorders associated with glycyl-tRNA synthetase mutations. *Brain.* 2005;128(Pt 10):2304–2314.
98. James PA, Cader MZ, Muntoni F, Childs AM, Crow YJ, Talbot K. Severe childhood SMA and axonal CMT due to anticodon binding domain mutations in the GARS gene. *Neurology.* 2006;67(9):1710–1712. Erratum in *Neurology.* 2007;68(9): 711.
99. Jordanova A, De Jonghe P, Boerkoel CF, et al. Mutations in the neurofilament light chain gene (NEFL) cause early onset severe Charcot–Marie–Tooth disease. *Brain.* 2003;126:590–597.
100. Ismailov SM, Fedotov VP, Dadali EL, et al. A new locus for autosomal dominant Charcot–Marie–Tooth disease type 2 (CMT2 F) maps to chromosome 7q11–q21. *Eur J Hum Genet.* 2001;9:646–650.
101. Evgrafov OV, Mersiyanova I, Irobi J, et al. Mutant small heat-shock protein 27 causes axonal Charcot–Marie–Tooth disease and distal hereditary motor neuropathy. *Nat Genet.* 2004;36(6):602–606.
102. Nelis E, Berciano J, Verpoorten N, et al. Autosomal dominant axonal Charcot–Marie–Tooth disease type 2 (CMT2G) maps to chromosome 12q12–q13.3. *J Med Genet.* 2004;41(3):193–197.
103. Tang BS, Zhao GH, Luo W, et al. Small heat-shock protein 22 mutated in autosomal dominant Charcot–Marie–Tooth disease type 2 L. *Hum Genet.* 2005;116(3):222–224.
104. Zuchner S, Noureddine M, Kennerson M, et al. Mutations in the pleckstrin homology domain of dynamin 2 cause dominant intermediate Charcot–Marie–Tooth disease. *Nat Genet.* 2005;37(3):289–294.
105. Claeys KG, Züchner S, Kennerson M. Phenotypic spectrum of dynamin 2 mutations in Charcot-Marie-Tooth neuropathy. *Brain.* 2009;132(Pt 7):1741–1752.
106. Fischer D, Herasse M, Bitoun M, et al. Characterization of the muscle involvement in dynamin 2-related centronuclear myopathy. *Brain.* 2006;129(Pt 6):1463–1469.
107. Latour P, Thauvin-Robinet C, Baudelet-Mery C, et al. A major determinant for binding and aminoacylation of tRNA-Ala in cytoplasmic alanyl-tRNA synthetase is mutated in dominant axonal Charcot-Marie-Tooth Disease. *Am J Hum Genet.* 2010;86:77–82.
108. Lin K-P, Soong B-W, Yang C-C, et al. The mutational spectrum in a cohort of Charcot-Marie-Tooth disease type 2 among the Han Chinese in Taiwan. *PLoS One.* 2011;6:e29393.
109. McLaughlin HM, Sakaguchi R, Giblin W, et al. A recurrent loss-of-function alanyl-tRNA synthetase (AARS) mutation in patients with Charcot-Marie-Tooth disease type 2 N (CMT2 N). *Hum Mutat.* 2012;33:244–253.
110. Weedon MN, Hastings R, Caswell R, et al. Exome sequencing identifies a DYNC1H1 mutation in a large pedigree with dominant axonal Charcot-Marie-Tooth disease. *Am J Hum Genet.* 2011;89:308–312.
111. Guernsey DL, Jiang H, Bedard K et al. Mutation in the gene encoding ubiquitin ligase LRSAM1 in patients with Charcot-Marie-Tooth disease. *PLoS Genet.* 2010;6:1–7.
112. Weterman MA, Sorrentino V, Kasher PR, et al. A frameshift mutation in LRSAM1 is responsible for a dominant hereditary polyneuropathy. *Hum Mol Genet.* 2011;21:358–370.
113. Teunissen LL, Notermans NC, Fransen H, et al. Difference between hereditary motor and sensory neuropathy type 2 and chronic idiopathic axonal neuropathy. A clinical and electrophysiological study. *Brain.* 1997;120:955–962.
114. Fabrizi GM, Cavallaro T, Angiari C, et al. Charcot–Marie–Tooth disease type 2E, a disorder of the cytoskeleton. *Brain.* 2007;130(Pt 2):394–403.
115. Hahn AF, Parkes AW, Bolton CF, et al. Neuromyotonia in hereditary motor neuropathy. *J Neurol Neurosurg Psychiatry.* 1991;54:230–235.
116. Vasilescu C, Marilena A, Dan A. Neuronal type of Charcot–Marie–Tooth disease with a syndrome of continuous motor unit activity. *J Neurol Sci.* 1984;63:11–25.
117. Schroder JM. Neuropathology of Charcot–Marie–Tooth and related disorders. *Neuromol Med.* 2006;8(1–2):23–42.
118. Zhao C, Takita J, Tanaka Y, et al. Charcot–Marie–Tooth disease type 2 A caused by mutation in a microtubule motor KIF1B-beta. *Cell.* 2001;105(5):587–597. Erratum in *Cell.* 2001;106(1): 127.

119. Ben Othame K, Middleton LT, Loprest LJ. Localization of a gene (CMT2 A) for autosomal dominant Charcot–Marie–Tooth type 2 to chromosome 1p and evidence for genetic heterogeneity. *Genomics*. 1993;17:370–375.
120. Zuchner S, Mersiyanova IV, Muglia M, et al. Mutations in the mitochondrial GTPase mitofusin 2 cause Charcot–Marie–Tooth neuropathy type 2 A. *Nat Genet*. 2004;36(5):449–451.
121. Baloh RH, Schmidt RE, Pestronk A, Milbrandt J. Altered axonal mitochondrial transport in the pathogenesis of Charcot–Marie–Tooth disease from mitofusin 2 mutations. *J Neurosci*. 2007;27(2):422–430.
122. Kwon JM, Eliott JL, Yee W, et al. Assignment of a second Charcot–Marie–Tooth type II locus to chromosome 3q. *Am J Hum Genet*. 1995;57:853–858.
123. Kalaydjieva L, Gresham D, Gooding R, et al. N-myc downstream-regulated gene 1 is mutated in hereditary motor and sensory neuropathy—Lom. *Am J Hum Genet*. 2000;67:47–58.
124. Auer-Grumbach M, Strasser-Fuchs S, Robl T, Windpassinger C, Wagner K. Late onset Charcot–Marie–Tooth 2 syndrome caused by two novel mutations in the MPZ gene. *Neurology*. 2003;61(10):1435–1437.
125. Fontaine JM, Sun X, Hoppe AD, et al. Abnormal small heat shock protein interactions involving neuropathy-associated HSP22 (HSPB8) mutants. *FASEB J*. 2006;20(12):2168–2170.
126. Blumen SC, Astord S, Robin V, et al. A rare recessive distal hereditary motor neuropathy with HSJ1 chaperone mutation. *Annals Neurol*. 2012;71:509–519.
127. Gess B, Michaela Auer-Grumbach M, Schirmacher A, et al. HSJ1-related hereditary neuropathies: Novel mutations and extended clinical spectrum. *Neurology*. 2014;83:1726–1732.
128. Jordanova A, Thomas FP, Guergueltcheva V, et al. Dominant intermediate Charcot–Marie–Tooth type C maps to chromosome 1p34–p35. *Am J Hum Genet*. 2003;73(6):1423–1430.
129. Jordanova A, Irobi J, Thomas FP, et al. Disrupted function and axonal distribution of mutant tyrosyl-tRNA synthetase in dominant intermediate Charcot–Marie–Tooth neuropathy. *Nat Genet*. 2006;38:197–202.
130. Azzedine H, Zavadakova P, Plante-Bordeneuve V, et al. PLEKHG5 deficiency leads to an intermediate form of autosomal-recessive Charcot-Marie-Tooth disease. *Hum Molec Genet*. 2013;22:4224–4232.
131. Kim HJ, Hong YB, Park JM, et al. Mutations in the PLEKHG5 gene is relevant with autosomal recessive intermediate Charcot-Marie-Tooth disease. *Orphanet J Rare Dis*. 2013;8:104.
132. Maystadt I, Rezsohazy R, Barkats M, et al. The nuclear factor kappa-beta-activator gene PLEKHG5 is mutated in a form of autosomal recessive lower motor neuron disease with childhood onset. *Am J Hum Genet*. 2007;81:67–76.
133. Déjérine J, Sottas J. Sur la névrite: Interstitielle, hypertrophique et progressive de l'enfance. *CR Soc Biol (France)*. 1893;45:63–96.
134. Harding AE, Thomas PK. Autosomal recessive forms of hereditary motor and sensory neuropathy. *J Neurol Neurosurg Psychiatry*. 1980;43:669–678.
135. Hilz MJ, Stemper B, Axelrod FB. Sympathetic skin response differentiates hereditary sensory autonomic neuropathies III and IV. *Neurology*. 1999;52:1652–1657.
136. Roa BB, Dyck PJ, Marks HG, et al. Dejerine–Sottas syndrome associated with point mutation in the peripheral myelin protein 22 (PMP22) gene. *Nat Genet*. 1993;5:269–273.
137. Timmerman V, De Jonghe P, Ceuterick C, et al. Novel missense mutation in the early growth response 2 gene associated with Dejerine–Sottas syndrome phenotype. *Neurology*. 1999;52:1827–1832.
138. Dyck PJ, Lambert EH, Sanders K, et al. Severe hypomyelination and marked abnormality of conduction in Dejerine-Sottas hypertrophic neuropathy: Myelin thickness and compound action potential of sural nerve in vitro. *Mayo Clin Proc*. 1971;46:432–436.
139. Guzzetta F, Ferriere G, Lyon G. Congenital hypomyelination polyneuropathy: Pathological findings compared with polyneuropathies starting later in life. *Brain*. 1982;105:395–416.
140. Gabreëls-Festen AAWM, Gabreëls FJM, Jennekens FGI, Janssen-van Kempen TW. The status of HMSN type III. *Neuromuscul Disord*. 1994;4:63–69.
141. Andermann F, Lloyd-Smith DL, Mavor H, et al. Observations on hypertrophic neuropathy of Dejerine and Sottas. *Neurology*. 1962;12:712–724.
142. Joostens E, Gabreëls F, Gabreëls-Festen A, et al. Electron microscopic heterogeneity of onion-bulb neuropathies of the Dejerine–Sottas type. *Acta Neuropathol*. 1974;27:105–118.
143. Kennedy WR, Shung JH, Berry JF. A case of congenital hypomyelination neuropathy. *Arch Neurol*. 1977;34:337–345.
144. Harati Y, Butler IJ. Congenital hypomyelinating neuropathy. *J Neurol Neurosurg Psychiatry*. 1985;48:1269–1276.
145. Dyck PJ, Gomez MR. Segmental demyelination in Dejerine–Sottas disease: Light, phase-contrast, and electron microscopic studies. *Mayo Clin Proc*. 1968;43:280–296.
146. Dyck PJ, Ellefson RD, Lais AC, et al. Histologic and lipid studies of sural nerves in inherited hypertrophic neuropathy: Preliminary report of a lipid abnormality in nerve and liver in Dejerine–Sottas disease. *Mayo Clin Proc*. 1970;45:286–327.
147. Towfighi J. Congenital hypomyelination neuropathy: Glial bundles in cranial and spinal nerve roots. *Ann Neurol*. 1981;10:570–573.
148. Ionasescu V, Searby C, Ionasescu R, Chatkupt S, Patel N, Koenigsberger R. Dejerine–Sottas neuropathy in mother and son with the same point mutation of PMP22 gene. *Muscle Nerve*. 1997;20:97–99.
149. Nicholson G, Ouvrier R. GDAP1 mutations in CMT4: Axonal and demyelinating phenotypes? The exception "proves the rule". *Neurology*. 2002;59(12):1835–1836.
150. Ben Othame K, Hentani F, Lennon F, et al. Linkage of a locus (CMT4 A) for autosomal recessive Charcot–Marie–Tooth disease to chromosome 8q. *Hum Mol Genet*. 1993;2:1625–1628.
151. Stojkovic T, Latour P, Viet G, et al. Vocal cord and diaphragm paralysis, as clinical features of a French family with autosomal recessive Charcot–Marie–Tooth disease, associated with a new mutation in the GDAP1 gene. *Neuromuscul Disord*. 2004;14(4):261–264.
152. Ammar N, Nelis E, Merlini L, et al. Identification of novel GDAP1 mutations causing autosomal recessive Charcot–Marie–Tooth disease. *Neuromuscul Disord*. 2003;13(9):720–728.
153. Sevilla T, Cuesta A, Chumillas MJ, et al. Clinical, electrophysiological and morphological findings of Charcot–Marie–Tooth neuropathy with vocal cord palsy and mutations in the GDAP1 gene. *Brain*. 2003;126(Pt 9):2023–2033.
154. Birouk N, Azzedine H, Dubourg O, et al. Phenotypical features of a Moroccan family with autosomal recessive Charcot–Marie–Tooth disease associated with the S194X mutation in the GDAP1 gene. *Arch Neurol*. 2003;60(4):598–604.
155. Boerkoel CF, Takashima H, Nakagawa M, et al. CMT4 A: Identification of a Hispanic GDAP1 founder mutation. *Ann Neurol*. 2003;53(3):400–405.

156. Senderek J, Bergmann C, Ramaekers VT, et al. Mutations in the ganglioside-induced differentiation-associated protein-1 (GDAP1) gene in intermediate type autosomal recessive Charcot–Marie–Tooth neuropathy. *Brain.* 2003;126(Pt 3):642–649.
157. Nelis E, Erdem S, Van Den Bergh PY, et al. Mutations in GDAP1: Autosomal recessive CMT with demyelination and axonopathy. *Neurology.* 2002;59(12):1865–1872.
158. Cuesta A, Pedrola L, Sevilla T, et al. The gene encoding ganglioside-induced differentiation-associated protein-1 is mutated in Charcot–Marie–Tooth type 4 A disease. *Nat Genet.* 2002;1:22–25.
159. Gabreëls-Festen AAWM, Joosten EMG, Gabreëls FJM, et al. Congenital demyelinating motor and sensory neuropathy with focally folded myelin sheaths. *Brain.* 1990;113:1629–1643.
160. Schenone A, Abbruzzese M, Uccelli A, et al. Hereditary motor and sensory neuropathy with myelin outfoldings: Clinical, genetic, and neuropathological study of three cases. *J Neurol Sci.* 1994;122:20–27.
161. Senderek J, Bergmann C, Weber S, et al. Mutation of the SBF2 gene, encoding a novel member of the myotubularin family, in Charcot–Marie–Tooth neuropathy type 4 B2/11p15. *Hum Mol Genet.* 2003;12(3):349–356.
162. Senderek J, Bergmann C, Stendel C, et al. Mutations in a gene encoding a novel SH3/TPR domain protein cause autosomal recessive Charcot-Marie-Tooth type 4 C neuropathy. *Am J Hum Genet.* 2003;73:1106–1119.
163. Boerkoel CF, Takashima H, Stankiewicz P, et al. Periaxin mutations cause recessive Dejerine–Sottas neuropathy. *Am J Hum Genet.* 2001;68:325–333.
164. Delague V, Bariel C, Tuffery S, et al. Mapping of a new locus for autosomal recessive demyelinating Charcot–Marie–Tooth disease to 19q13.1–13.3 in a large consanguineous Lebanese family: Exclusion of MAG as a candidate gene. *Am J Hum Genet.* 2000;67:236–243.
165. Kabzinska D, Drac H, Sherman DL, et al. Charcot–Marie–Tooth type 4 F disease caused by S399fsx410 mutation in the PRX gene. *Neurology.* 2006;66(5):745–747.
166. Rogers T, Chandler D, Angelicheva D, et al. A novel locus for autosomal recessive peripheral neuropathy in the EGR2 region on 10q23. *Am J Hum Genet.* 2000;67:664–671.
167. Sevilla T, Martinez-Rubio D, Marquez C, et al. Genetics of the Charcot-Marie-Tooth disease in the Spanish Gypsy population: The hereditary motor and sensory neuropathy-Russe in depth. *Clin Genet.* 2013;83:565–570.
168. Delague V, Jacquier A, Hamadouche T, et al. Mutations in FGD4 encoding the Rho GDP/GTP exchange factor FRABIN cause autosomal recessive Charcot-Marie-Tooth type 4 H. *Am J Hum Genet.* 2007;81(1):1–16.
169. Stendel C, Roos A, Deconinck T, et al. Peripheral nerve demyelination caused by a mutant Rho GTPase guanine nucleotide exchange factor, frabin/FGD4. *Am J Hum Genet.* 2007;81(1):158–164.
170. Chow CY, Zhang Y, Dowling JJ, et al. Mutation of FIG4 causes neurodegeneration in the pale tremor mouse and patients with CMT4 J. *Nature.* 2007;448:68–72.
171. Zhang X, Chow CY, Sahenk Z, et al. Mutation of FIG4 causes a rapidly progressive, asymmetric neuronal degeneration. *Brain.* 2008;131:1990–2001.
172. Lenk GM, Ferguson CJ, Chow CY, et al. Pathogenic mechanism of the FIG4 mutation responsible for Charcot-Marie-Tooth disease CMT4 J. *PLoS Genet.* 2011;7:e1002104.
173. Gambardella A, Bolino A, Muglia M, et al. Genetic heterogeneity in autosomal recessive hereditary motor and sensory neuropathy with focally folded myelin sheaths (CMT4B). *Neurology.* 1998;50:799–801.
174. Takashima H, Boerkoel CF, De Jonghe P, et al. Periaxin mutations cause a broad spectrum of demyelinating neuropathies. *Ann Neurol.* 2002;51(6):709–715.
175. Sander SA, Ouvrier RA, McLeod JG, Nicholson GA, Pollard JS. Clinical syndromes associated with tomacula or myelin swellings in sural nerve biopsies. *J Neurol Neurosurg Psychiatry.* 2000;68:483–488.
176. Baxter RV, Ben Othmane K, Rochelle JM, et al. Ganglioside-induced differentiation-associated protein-1 is mutant in Charcot–Marie–Tooth disease type 4 A/8q21. *Nat Genet.* 2002;1: 21–22.
177. Niemann A, Ruegg M, La Padula V, Schenone A, Suter U. Ganglioside-induced differentiation associated protein 1 is a regulator of the mitochondrial network: New implications for Charcot–Marie–Tooth disease. *J Cell Biol.* 2005;170(7):1067–1078.
178. Pedrola L, Espert A, Wu X, Claramunt R, Shy ME, Palau F. GDAP1, the protein causing Charcot–Marie–Tooth disease type 4 A, is expressed in neurons and is associated with mitochondria. *Hum Mol Genet.* 2005;14(8):1087–1094.
179. Bolino A, Muglia M, Conforti FL, et al. Charcot–Marie–Tooth type 4B is caused by mutations in the gene encoding myotubularin-related protein-2. *Nat Genet.* 2000;25:17–19.
180. Nelis E, Erdem S, Tan E, et al. A novel homozygous missense mutation in the myotubularin-related protein 2 gene associated with recessive Charcot–Marie–Tooth disease with irregularly folded myelin sheaths. *Neuromuscul Disord.* 2002;12(9):869–873.
181. Nakagawa M, Suehara M, Saito A, et al. A novel MPZ gene mutation in dominantly inherited neuropathy with focally folded myelin sheaths. *Neurology.* 1999;52:1271–1275.
182. Berger P, Bonneick S, Willi S, Wymann M, Suter U. Loss of phosphatase activity in myotubularin-related protein 2 is associated with Charcot–Marie–Tooth disease type 4B1. *Hum Mol Genet.* 2002;11(13):1569–1579.
183. Chojnowski A, Ravise N, Bachelin C, et al. Silencing of the Charcot–Marie–Tooth associated MTMR2 gene decreases proliferation and enhances cell death in primary cultures of Schwann cells. *Neurobiol Dis.* 2007;26:323–331.
184. Azzedine H, Bolino A, Taieb T, et al. Mutations in MTMR13, a new pseudophosphatase homologue of MTMR2 and Sbf1, in two families with an autosomal recessive demyelinating form of Charcot–Marie–Tooth disease associated with early-onset glaucoma. *Am J Hum Genet.* 2003;72(5):1141–1153.
185. Landrieu P, Said G, Alaire C. Dominantly transmitted congenital indifference to pain. *Ann Neurol.* 1990;27:574–578.
186. Ishpekova BA, Christova LG, Alexandrov AS, Thomas PK. The electrophysiological profile of hereditary motor and sensory neuropathy—Lom. *J Neurol Neurosurg Psychiatry.* 2005;76(6):875–878.
187. Echaniz-Laguna A, Degos B, Bonnet C, et al. NDRG1-linked Charcot–Marie–Tooth disease (CMT4D) with central nervous system involvement. *Neuromuscul Disord.* 2007;17(2):163–168.
188. Gutierrez A, England JD, Sumner AJ, et al. Unusual electrophysiological findings in X-linked dominant Charcot–Marie–Tooth disease. *Muscle Nerve.* 2000;23:182–188.
189. Hahn AF, Brown WF, Koopman WJ, Feasby TE. X-linked dominant hereditary motor and sensory neuropathy. *Brain.* 1990;113:1511–1525.

190. Lewis RA. The challenge of CMTX and connexin 32 mutations. *Muscle Nerve*. 2000;23:147–149.
191. Nicholson G, Nash J. Intermediate nerve conduction velocities define X-linked Charcot–Marie–Tooth neuropathy families. *Neurology*. 1993;43:2555–2564.
192. Shy ME, Siskind C, Swan ER, et al. CMT1X phenotypes represent loss of GJB1 gene function. *Neurology*. 2007;68(11):849–855.
193. Hanemann CO, Bergmann C, Senderek J, Zerres K, Sperfeld AD. Transient, recurrent, white matter lesions in X-linked Charcot–Marie–Tooth disease with novel connexin 32 mutation. *Arch Neurol*. 2003;60(4):605–609.
194. Schelhaas HJ, Van Engelen BG, Gabreels-Festen AA, et al. Transient cerebral white matter lesions in a patient with connexin 32 missense mutation. *Neurology*. 2002;59(12):2007–2008.
195. Paulson HL, Garbern JY, Hoban TF, et al. Transient central nervous system white matter abnormality in X-linked Charcot–Marie–Tooth disease. *Ann Neurol*. 2002;52(4):429–434.
196. Birouk N, LeGuern E, Maisonobe T, et al. X-linked mutations Charcot–Marie–Tooth disease with connexin-32 mutations: Clinical and electrophysiological study. *Neurology*. 1998;50:1074–1082.
197. Nicholson G, Yeung L, Corbett A. Efficient neurophysiologic selection of X-linked Charcot–Marie–Tooth families. Ten novel mutations. *Neurology*. 1998;51:1412–1416.
198. Tabaraud F, LaGrange E, Sindou P, Vandenberghe A, Levy N, Vallat JM. Demyelinating X-linked Charcot–Marie–Tooth disease: Unusual electrophysiological findings. *Muscle Nerve*. 1999;22:1442–1447.
199. Dubourg O, Tardieu S, Birouk N, et al. Clinical, electrophysiological and molecular genetic characteristics of 93 patients with X-linked Charcot–Marie–Tooth disease. *Brain*. 2001;124:1958–1967.
200. Bergoffen J, Scherer SS, Wang S, et al. Connexin mutations in X-linked Charcot–Marie–Tooth disease. *Am J Hum Genet*. 1993;262:2039–2042.
201. Fairweather N, Bell C, Cochrane S, et al. Mutation in the connexin 32 gene in X-linked dominant Charcot–Marie–Tooth neuropathy. *Hum Mol Genet*. 1994;3:355–358.
202. Ionasescu V, Searby C, Ionasescu R. Point mutations of connexin 32 (GJB1) gene in X-linked dominant Charcot–Marie–Tooth neuropathy. *Hum Mol Genet*. 1994;3:355–358.
203. Sahenk Z, Chen L. Abnormalities in the axonal cytoskeleton induced by a connexin-32 mutation in nerve xenografts. *J Neurosci Res*. 1998;51:174–184.
204. Priest JM, Fischbeck KH, Nouri N, Keats BJ. A locus for axonal motor-sensory neuropathy with deafness and mental retardation maps to Xq24–q26. *Genomics*. 1995;29:409–412.
205. Kim H-J, Sohn K-M, Shy ME, et al. Mutations in PRPS1, which encodes the phosphoribosyl pyrophosphate synthetase enzyme critical for nucleotide biosynthesis, cause hereditary peripheral neuropathy with hearing loss and optic neuropathy (CMT5X). *Am J Hum Genet*. 2007;81:552–558.
206. Kennerson ML, Yiu EM, Chuang DT, et al. A new locus for X-linked dominant Charcot-Marie-Tooth disease (CMTX6) is caused by mutations in the pyruvate dehydrogenase kinase isoenzyme 3 (PDK3) gene. *Hum Mol Genet*. 2013;22(7):1404–1416.
207. Takashima H, Nakagawa M, Nakahara K, et al. A new type of hereditary motor and sensory neuropathy linked to chromosome 3. *Ann Neurol*. 1997;41:771–780.
208. Ishiura H, Sako W, Yoshida M, et al. The TRK-fused gene is mutated in hereditary motor and sensory neuropathy with proximal dominant involvement. *Am J Hum Genet*. 2012;91:320–329.
209. Chance PF, Lensch MW, Lipe H, Brown RH Sr, Brown RH Jr, Bird TD. Hereditary neuralgic amyotrophy and hereditary neuropathy with liability to pressure palsies: Two distinct genetic disorders. *Neurology*. 1994;44:2253–2257.
210. Kuhlenbaumer G, Hannibal MC, Nelis E, et al. Mutations in SEPT9 cause hereditary neuralgic amyotrophy. *Nat Genet*. 2005;37:1044–1046.
211. Davidenkow S. Scapuloperoneal amyotrophy. *Arch Neurol*. 1939;41:694.
212. Emery ES, Fenichel GM, Eng G. A spinal muscular atrophy with scapuloperoneal distribution. *Arch Neurol*. 1968;18:129–133.
213. Ricker K, Mertens HG, Schimrig K. The neurogenic scapuloperoneal syndrome. *Eur Neurol*. 1968;1:257–274.
214. Mercelis R, Demeester J, Martin JJ. Neurogenic scapuloperoneal syndrome in childhood. *J Neurol Neurosurg Psychiatry*. 1980;43:888–896.
215. Harding AE, Thomas PK. Distal and scapuloperoneal distribution of muscle involvement occurring within a family with type 1 hereditary motor and sensory neuropathy. *J Neurol*. 1980;224:17–23.
216. Hyser CL, Kissel JT, Warmolts JR, Mendell JR. Scapuloperoneal neuropathy: A distinct clinicopathologic entity. *J Neurol Sci*. 1988;87:91–102.
217. Tandan R, Verma A, Mohire M. Adult onset autosomal recessive neurogenic scapuloperoneal syndrome. *J Neurol Sci*. 1989;94:201–209.
218. Isozumi K, DeLong R, Kaplan J, et al. Linkage of scapuloperoneal spinal muscular atrophy to chromosome 12q24.1–q24.31. *Hum Mol Genet*. 1996;5:1377–1382.
219. Verma A. Neuropathic scapuloperoneal syndrome (Davidenkow's syndrome) with chromosome 17p11.2 deletion. *Muscle Nerve*. 2005;32(5):668–671.
220. Zhao H, Race V, Matthijs G, et al. Exome sequencing reveals HINT1 mutations as a cause of distal hereditary motor neuropathy. *Eur J Hum Genet*. 2014;22(6):847–850.
221. Zimoń M, Baets J, Almeida-Souza L, et al. Loss-of-function mutations in HINT1 cause axonal neuropathy with neuromyotonia. *Nat Genet*. 2012;44(10):1080–1083.
222. Davidson G, Murphy S, Polke J, et al. Frequency of mutations in the genes associated with hereditary sensory and autonomic neuropathy in a UK cohort. *J Neurol*. 2012;259(8): 1673–1685.
223. Rotthier A, Baets J, De Vriendt E, et al. Genes for hereditary sensory and autonomic neuropathies: A genotype-phenotype correlation. *Brain*. 2009;132(Pt 10):2699–2711.
224. Denny-Brown D. Hereditary sensory radicular neuropathy. *J Neurol Neurosurg Psychiatry*. 1951;14:237–252.
225. Houlden H, King R, Blake J, et al. Clinical, pathological and genetic characterization of hereditary sensory and autonomic neuropathy type 1 (HSAN I). *Brain*. 2006;129(Pt 2): 411–425.
226. Shivji ZM, Ashby P. Sympathetic skin responses in hereditary sensory and autonomic neuropathy and familial amyloid neuropathy are different. *Muscle Nerve*. 1999;22:1283–1286.
227. Bejaoui K, McKenna-Yasek D, Hosler BA, et al. Confirmation of linkage of type 1 hereditary sensory neuropathy to human chromosome 9q22. *Neurology*. 1999;52:510–515.
228. Bejaoui K, Wu C, Scheffler MD, et al. SPTLC1 is mutated in hereditary sensory neuropathy, type 1. *Nat Genet*. 2001:27:261–262.

229. Dawkins JL, Hulme DJ, Brambhatt SB, Auer-Grumbach M, Nicholson GA. Mutations in SPTLC1, encoding serine palmitoyl transferase long chain base subunit-1, cause hereditary sensory neuropathy type 1. *Nat Genet*. 2001:27:309–312.
230. Rotthier A, Auer-Grumbach M, Janssens K, et al. Mutations in the SPTLC2 subunit of serine palmitoyltransferase cause hereditary sensory and autonomic neuropathy type I. *Am J Hum Genet*. 2010;87:513–522.
231. Murphy SM, Ernst D, Wei Y, et al. Hereditary sensory and autonomic neuropathy type 1 (HSANI) caused by a novel mutation in SPTLC2. *Neurology*. 2013;80(23):2106–2011.
232. Kok C, Kennerson ML, Spring PJ, Ing AJ, Pollard JD, Nicholson GA. A locus for hereditary sensory neuropathy with cough and gastroesophageal reflux on chromosome 3p22–p24. *Am J Hum Genet*. 2003;73(3):632–637.
233. Houlden H, King RH, Muddle JR, et al. A novel RAB7 mutation associated with ulcero-mutilating neuropathy. *Ann Neurol*. 2004;56(4):586–590.
234. Guelly C, Zhu P-P, Leonardis L, et al. Targeted high throughput sequencing identifies mutations in atlastin-1 as a cause of hereditary sensory neuropathy type I. *Am J Hum Genet*. 2011;88:99–105.
235. Fischer D, Schabhüttl M, Wieland T, Windhager R, Strom TM, Auer-Grumbach M. A novel missense mutation confirms ATL3 as a gene for hereditary sensory neuropathy type 1. *Brain*. 2014;137(Pt 7):e286.
236. Kornak U, Mademan I, Schinke M, et al. Sensory neuropathy with bone destruction due to a mutation in the membrane-shaping atlastin GTPase 3. *Brain*. 2014;137(Pt 3):683–692.
237. Wright A, Dyck PJ. Hereditary sensory neuropathy with sensorineural deafness and early-onset dementia. *Neurology*. 1995;45:560–562.
238. Klein CJ, Botuyan MV, Wu Y, et al. Mutations in DNMT1 cause hereditary sensory neuropathy with dementia and hearing loss. *Nat Genet*. 2011;43:595–600.
239. Klein CJ, Bird T, Ertekin-Taner N, et al. DNMT1 mutation hot spot causes varied phenotypes of HSAN1 with dementia and hearing loss. *Neurology*. 2013;80(9):824–828.
240. Nukada H, Pollock M, Haas LF. The clinical spectrum and morphology of type II hereditary sensory neuropathy. *Brain*. 1982;105:647–665.
241. Schoene WC, Asbury AK, Astrom KE, et al. Hereditary sensory neuropathy. *J Neurol Sci*. 1970;11:463–487.
242. Winkelmann RK, Lambert EH, Hayles AB. Congenital absence of pain. *Arch Dermatol*. 1962;85:325–338.
243. Loggia ML, Bushnell MC, Tétreault M, et al. Carriers of recessive WNK1/HSN2 mutations for hereditary sensory and autonomic neuropathy type 2 (HSAN2) are more sensitive to thermal stimuli. *J Neurosci*. 2009;29:2162–2166.
244. Ohta M, Ellefson RD, Lambert EH, et al. Hereditary sensory neuropathy, Type II. *Arch Neurol*. 1973;29:23–37.
245. Lafreniere RG, MacDonald ML, Dube MP, et al. Study of Canadian Genetic Isolates. Identification of a novel gene (HSN2) causing hereditary sensory and autonomic neuropathy type II through the Study of Canadian genetic isolates. *Am J Hum Genet*. 2004;74(5):1064–1073.
246. Kurth I, Pamminger T, Hennings JC, et al. Mutations in FAM134B, encoding a newly identified Golgi protein, cause severe sensory and autonomic neuropathy. *Nat Genet*. 2009;41:1179–1181.
247. Ilgaz Aydinlar E, Rolfs A, Serteser M, Parman Y. Mutation in FAM134B causing hereditary sensory neuropathy with spasticity in a Turkish family. *Muscle Nerve*. 2014;49(5):774–775.
248. Rivière JB, Verlaan DJ, Shekarabi M, et al. A mutation in the HSN2 gene causes sensory neuropathy type II in a Lebanese family. *Ann Neurol*. 2004;56:572–575.
249. Riviere J-B, Ramalingam S, Lavastre V, et al. KIF1 A, an axonal transporter of synaptic vesicles, is mutated in hereditary sensory and autonomic neuropathy type 2. *Am J Hum Genet*. 2011;89:219–230.
250. Shekarabi M, Girard N, Rivière JB, et al. Mutations in the nervous system—Specific HSN2 exon of WNK1 cause hereditary sensory neuropathy type II. *J Clin Invest*. 2008;118:2496–2505.
251. Yuan J, Matsuura E, Higuchi Y, et al. Hereditary sensory and autonomic neuropathy type IID caused by an SCN9 A mutation. *Neurology*. 2013;80:1641–1649.
252. Bennett DL, Woods CG. Painful and painless channelopathies. *Lancet Neurol*. 2014;13(6):587–599.
253. Aguayo AJ, Nair CPV, Bray GM. Peripheral nerve abnormalities in the Riley–Day syndrome. *Arch Neurol*. 1971;24:106–116.
254. Brown JC. Nerve conduction in familial dysautonomia (Riley–Day syndrome). *J Am Med Assoc*. 1967;201:200–202.
255. Brown WJ, Beauchemin JA, Linde LM. A neuropathological study of familial dysautonomia (Riley–Day syndrome) in siblings. *J Neurol Neurosurg Psychiatry*. 1964;27:131–139.
256. Blumenfeld A, Slaugenhaupt SA, Liebert CB, et al. Precise genetic mapping and haplotype analysis of familial dysautonomia gene on human chromosome 9q31. *Am J Hum Genet*. 1999;64:1110–1118.
257. Edvardson S, Cinnamon Y, Jalas C, et al. Hereditary sensory autonomic neuropathy caused by a mutation in dystonin. *Ann Neurol*. 2012;71(4):569–572.
258. Anderson SL, Coli R, Daly IW, et al. Familial dysautonomia is caused by mutations of the IKAP gene. *Am J Hum Genet*. 2001;68:753–758.
259. Eng CM, Slaugenhaupt SA, Blumenfeld A, et al. Prenatal diagnosis of familial dysautonomia by analysis of linked CA-repeat polymorphisms on chromosome 9q31–33. *Am J Med Genet*. 1995;59:349–355.
260. Slaugenhaupt SA, Blumenfeld A, Gil SP, et al. Tissue-specific expression of a splicing mutation in the IKBKAP gene causes familial dysautonomia. *Am J Hum Genet*. 2001;68:598–605.
261. Swanson AG, Buchan GC, Alvord EC. Anatomic changes in congenital insensitivity to pain: Absence of small primary sensory neurons in ganglia, roots, and Lissauer's tract. *Arch Neurol*. 1965;12:12–19.
262. Shorer Z, Moses SW, Hershkovitz E, Pinsk V, Levy J. Neurophysiologic studies in congenital insensitivity to pain with anhidrosis. *Pediatr Neurol*. 2001;25(5):397–400.
263. Goebel HH, Veit S, Dyck PJ. Confirmation of virtual unmyelinated fiber absence in hereditary sensory neuropathy type IV. *J Neuropathol Exp Neurol*. 1980;39:670–675.
264. Greco A, Villa R, Tubino B, Romano L, Penso D, Pierotti MA. A novel NTRK1 mutation associated with congenital insensitivity to pain with anhidrosis. *Am J Hum Genet*. 1999;64:1207–1210.
265. Indo Y, Tsuruta M, Hayashida Y, et al. Mutations in the trkA/NGF receptor gene in patients with congenital insensitivity to pain with anhidrosis. *Nat Genet*. 1996;13:485–488.
266. Indo Y. Molecular basis of congenital insensitivity to pain with anhidrosis (CIPA): Mutations and polymorphisms in TRKA (NTRK1) gene encoding the receptor tyrosine kinase for nerve growth factor. *Hum Mutat*. 2001;18(6):462–471.

267. Dyck PJ, Mellinger JF, Reagan TJ, et al. Not "indifference to pain" but varieties of hereditary sensory and autonomic neuropathy. *Brain.* 1983;106:373–390.
268. Low PA, Burke WJ, McLeod JG. Congenital sensory neuropathy with selective loss of small myelinated nerve fibers. *Ann Neurol.* 1978;3:179–182.
269. Einarsdottir E, Carlsson A, Minde J, et al. A mutation in the nerve growth factor beta gene (NGFB) causes loss of pain perception. *Hum Mol Genet.* 2004;13(8):799–805.
270. Houlden H, King RH, Hashemi-Nejad A, et al. A novel TRK A (NTRK1) mutation associated with hereditary sensory and autonomic neuropathy type V. *Ann Neurol.* 2001;49(4):521–525.
271. Cox JJ, Reimann F, Nicholas AK, et al. An SCN9 A channelopathy causes congenital inability to experience pain. *Nature.* 2006;444:894–898.
272. Goldberg YP, MacFarlane J, MacDonald ML, et al. Loss-of-function mutations in the Nav1.7 gene underlie congenital indiff erence to pain in multiple human populations. *Clin Genet.* 2007;71:311–319.
273. Ahmad S, Dahllund L, Eriksson AB, et al. A stop codon mutation in SCN9 A causes lack of pain sensation. *Hum Mol Genet.* 2007;16:2114–2121.
274. Leipold E, Liebmann L, Korenke GC, et al. A de novo gain-of-function mutation in SCN11 A causes loss of pain perception. *Nat Genet.* 2013;45:1399–1404.
275. Kalgaard OM, Seem E, Kvernebo K. Erythromelalgia: A clinical study of 87 cases. *J Intern Med.* 1997;242(3):191–197.
276. Davis MD, Weenig RH, Genebriera J, Wendelschafer-Crabb G, Kennedy WR, Sandroni P. Histopathologic findings in primary erythromelalgia are nonspecific: Special studies show a decrease in small nerve fiber density. *J Am Acad Dermatol.* 2006; 55(3):519–522.
277. Yang Y, Wang Y, Li S, et al. Mutations in SCN9 A, encoding a sodium channel alpha subunit, in patients with primary erythermalgia. *J Med Genet.* 2004;41(3):171–174.
278. Lampert A, Dib-Hajj SD, Tyrrell L, Waxman SG. Size matters: Erythromelalgia mutation S241 T in Nav1.7 alters channel gating. *J Biol Chem.* 2006;281(47):36029–36035.
279. Michiels JJ, te Morsche RH, Jansen JB, Drenth JP. Autosomal dominant erythermalgia associated with a novel mutation in the voltage-gated sodium channel alpha subunit Nav1.7. *Arch Neurol.* 2005;62(10):1587–1590.
280. McGraw T, Kosek P. Erythromelalgia pain managed with gabapentin. *J Anesthesiol.* 1997;86(4):988–990.
281. Fertleman CR, Ferrie CD, Aicardi J, et al. Paroxysmal extreme pain disorder (previously familial rectal pain syndrome). *Neurology.* 2007;69:586–595.
282. Choi JS, Boralevi F, Brissaud O, et al. Paroxysmal extreme pain disorder: A molecular lesion of peripheral neurons. *Nat Rev Neurol.* 2011;7:51–55.
283. Kremeyer B, Lopera F, Cox JJ, et al. A gain-of-function mutation in TRPA1 causes familial episodic pain syndrome. *Neuron.* 2010;66:671–80.
284. Faber CG, Lauria G, Merkies ISJ, et al. Gain-of-function Nav1.8 mutations in painful neuropathy. *Proc Nat Acad Sci.* 2012;109:19444–19449.
285. Zhang XY, Wen J, Yang W, et al. Gain-of-function mutations in SCN11 A cause familial episodic pain. *Am J Hum Genet.* 2013;93:957–966.
286. Faber CG, Hoeijmakers JG, Ahn HS, et al. Gain of function Nav1.7 mutations in idiopathic small fiber neuropathy. *Ann Neurol.* 2012;71:26–39.
287. Persson AK, Liu S, Faber CG, Merkies IS, Black JA, Waxman SG. Neuropathy-associated Nav1.7 variant I228M impairs integrity of dorsal root ganglion neuron axons. *Ann Neurol.* 2013;73:140–145.
288. Han C, Hoeijmakers JG, Liu S, et al. Functional profiles of SCN9 A variants in dorsal root ganglion neurons and superior cervical ganglion neurons correlate with autonomic symptoms in small fibre neuropathy. *Brain.* 2012;135:2613–2628.
289. Han C, Hoeijmakers JG, Ahn HS, et al. Nav1.7-related small fiber neuropathy: Impaired slow-inactivation and DRG neuron hyperexcitability. *Neurology.* 2012;78:1635–1643.
290. Ahn HS, Vasylyev DV, Estacion M, et al. Differential effect of D623 N variant and wild-type Na(v)1.7 sodium channels on resting potential and interspike membrane potential of dorsal root ganglion neurons. *Brain Res.* 2013;1529:165–177.
291. Fertleman CR, Baker MD, Parker KA, et al. SCN9 A mutations in paroxysmal extreme pain disorder: Allelic variants underlie distinct channel defects and phenotypes. *Neuron.* 2006;52:767–774.
292. Estacion M, Dib-Hajj SD, Benke PJ, et al. NaV1.7 gain-of-function mutations as a continuum: A1632E displays physiological changes associated with erythromelalgia and paroxysmal extreme pain disorder mutations and produces symptoms of both disorders. *J Neurosci.* 2008;28:11079–11088.
293. Dib-Hajj SD, Estacion M, Jarecki BW, et al. Paroxysmal extreme pain disorder M1627K mutation in human Nav1.7 renders DRG neurons hyperexcitable. *Mol Pain.* 2008;4:37.
294. Cheng X, Dib-Hajj SD, Tyrrell L, et al. Mutations at opposite ends of the DIII/S4-S5 linker of sodium channel Nav1.7 produce distinct pain disorders. *Mol Pain.* 2010;6:24.
295. Huang J, Yang Y, Zhao P, et al. Small-fiber neuropathy Nav1.8 mutation shifts activation to hyperpolarized potentials and increases excitability of dorsal root ganglion neurons. *J Neurosci.* 2013;33:14087–14097.
296. Han C, Vasylyev D, Macala LJ, et al. The G1662 S NaV1.8 mutation in small fibre neuropathy: Impaired inactivation underlying DRG neuron hyperexcitability. *J Neurol Neurosurg Psychiatry.* 2014;85(5):499–505.
297. Amato AA. Reilly MM. The death panel for Charcot-Marie-Tooth panels. *Neurol.* 2011;69:1–5.
298. England JD, Gronseth GS, Franklin G, et al. Evaluation of distal symmetric polyneuropathy: The role of laboratory and genetic testing (an evidence-based review). *Muscle Nerve.* 2009;39:116–125.
299. Saporta AS, Sottile SL, Miller LJ, Feely SM, Siskind CE, Shy ME. Charcot-Marie-Tooth disease subtypes and genetic testing strategies. *Ann Neurol.* 2011;69:22–33.
300. Klein CJ, Middha S, Duan X, et al. Application of whole exome sequencing in undiagnosed inherited polyneuropathies. *J Neurol Neurosurg Psychiatry.* 2014;85(11):1265–1272.

CHAPTER 12

Other Hereditary Neuropathies

In Chapter 11, we reviewed Charcot–Marie–Tooth syndrome and related hereditary neuropathies. Here we discuss some of the more rare types of hereditary neuropathies (Table 12-1). Familial amyloid polyneuropathy is discussed in Chapter 16 (Neuropathies Associated with Systemic Disease).

▶ NEUROPATHIES ASSOCIATED WITH LYSOSOMAL STORAGE DISORDERS

The lysosomal storage disorders are associated with abnormal accumulation of lysosomal products (e.g., sphingolipids, mucolipids, etc.) within neurons, leading to dysmyelination and axonal degeneration of both central and peripheral nerves (Table 12-1). Usually, the central nervous system (CNS) manifestations overshadow the peripheral neuropathy in most of these disorders. However, some patients present with peripheral neuropathy, which can be associated with significant disability.

METACHROMATIC LEUKODYSTROPHY

Clinical Features

There are three characteristic forms of metachromatic leukodystrophy (MLD) defined by age of onset: (1) late infantile, (2) juvenile, and (3) adult onset.[1–14] Most patients have the late infantile–onset MLD variant and develop progressive generalized weakness, decline in mental functions, dysarthria, and worsening gait between 1 and 2 years of age. Children become quadriparetic, spastic, and cortically blind and often develop seizures. On examination, generalized muscle weakness, hypotonia, hyporeflexia, and extensor plantar responses are appreciated. Most children die within 5–6 years after onset of symptoms.

The juvenile form of MLD typically presents later in childhood or adolescence but is associated with clinical features similar to the late infantile form of the disease. Patients with adult-onset MLD usually develop slowly progressive dementia, psychosis, spasticity, ataxia, extrapyramidal signs, visual impairment, and incontinence in the third or fourth decade of life.[15]

Laboratory Features

Magnetic resonance imaging (MRI) of the brain often demonstrates increased signal on T2-weighted images in the subcortical white matter (Fig. 12-1).

The diagnosis is suggested by demonstrating decreased arylsulfatase A activity in urine, from leukocytes, or from cultured fibroblasts and can be confirmed with genetic testing. Prenatal diagnosis can be made by amniocentesis. Cerebral spinal fluid (CSF) protein is usually markedly elevated in the 100–300 mg/dL range. Motor nerve conduction studies (NCS) reveal mild to moderately reduced amplitudes, prolonged distal latencies, and marked slowing of conduction velocities (NCVs) that range from 10 to 20 m/s in the legs and 20 to 40 m/s in the arms.[1,2,4,5,7–12,15–17] Conduction block is not seen, but occasionally temporal dispersion is appreciated.[11] Sensory NCS are often unobtainable, but when recordable the sensory nerve action potentials (SNAPs) are reduced in amplitude with slightly to moderately prolonged latencies and slow NCVs. Visual, brainstem, and somatosensory-evoked potentials are delayed.

Histopathology

Autopsy studies reveal degeneration of myelin in the CNS and peripheral nerves (Fig. 12-2).[3,6,10,12] Nerve biopsies are not routinely performed but can also demonstrate a decrease in myelinated fibers with evidence of demyelination and remyelination (Fig. 12-3A). The characteristic abnormality is accumulation of metachromatically staining inclusions in cytoplasm of Schwann cells (Fig. 12-3B). On electron microscopy (EM), these inclusions appear as lamellated bodies within Schwann cells (Fig. 12-3C).

Molecular Genetics and Pathogenesis

MLD is an autosomal-recessive disorder caused by mutations in the arylsulfatase A (*ARSA*) or the prosaposin (*PSAP*) genes.[18] Arylsulfatase A gene and prosaposin are both enzymes required for metabolizing galactosylsulfatide (cerebroside sulfatase), a glycolipid, present in myelin membranes. Deficiency of arylsulfatase A or the proteolytic product of prosaposin results in the accumulation of sulfatides (inclusions) in Schwann cells and oligodendrocytes resulting in dysmyelination.

▶ TABLE 12-1. **RARE HEREDITARY NEUROPATHIES**

Hereditary Disorders of Lipid Metabolism
Metachromatic leukodystrophy
Krabbe disease (globoid cell leukodystrophy)
Fabry disease
Adrenoleukodystrophy/adrenomyeloneuropathy
Refsum disease
Tangier disease
Cerebrotendinous xanthomatosis
Hereditary Ataxias With Neuropathy
Friedreich ataxia
Vitamin E deficiency
Spinocerebellar ataxia
Abetalipoproteinemia (Bassen–Kornzweig disease)
Ataxia-telangiectasia
Oculomotor apraxia type 1
Oculomotor apraxia type 2
Cockayne syndrome
Porphyria
Acute intermittent porphyria (AIP)
Hereditary coproporphyria (HCP)
Variegate porphyria (VP)
Others
Giant axonal neuropathy
Polyglucosan body neuropathy
Familial amyloid polyneuropathy

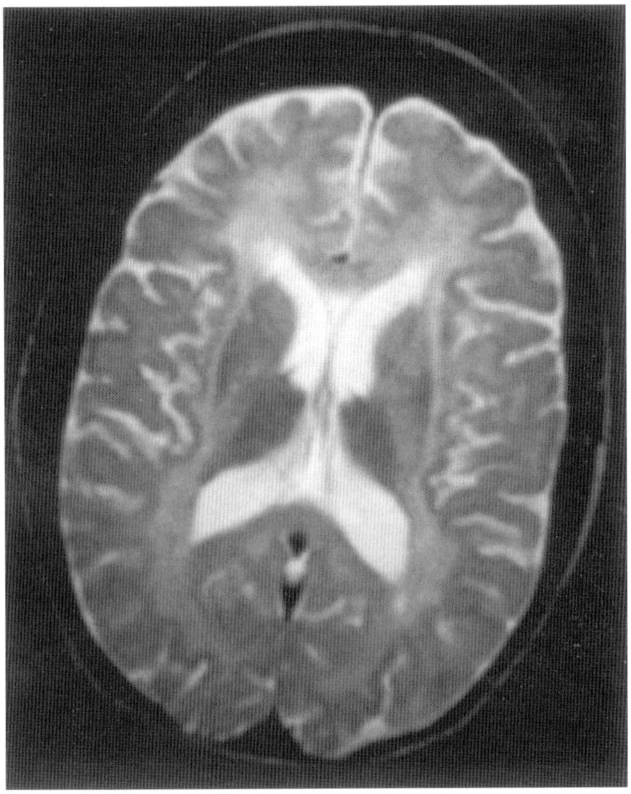

Figure 12-1. MRI of brain in a patient with MLD demonstrates widespread white matter disease on T2-weighted image. (Reproduced with permission from www.uiowa.edu/~c064s01/nr287.htm.)

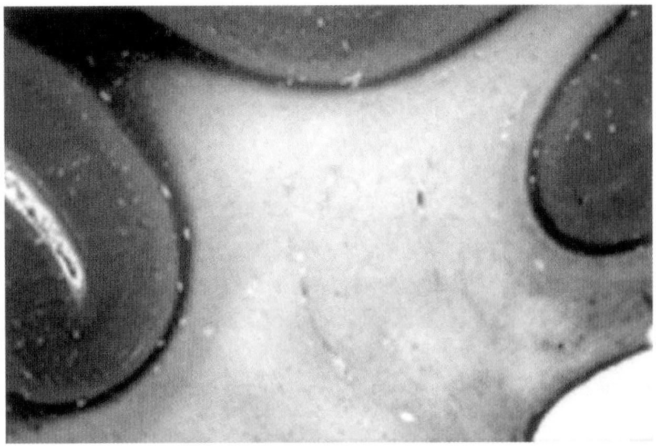

Figure 12-2. MLD pathology. Lysosomal storage of sulfatides kills oligodendrocytes and Schwann cells. Sulfatides discharged from dying cells are picked up by histiocytes. The white matter shows diffuse loss of myelin, which spares the subcortical fibers. (Reproduced with permission from www.neuropathologyweb.org/chapter 10/chapter 10.)

Treatment

No specific medications are helpful, but bone marrow transplantation may be beneficial in some patients.[19]

KRABBE DISEASE (GLOBOID CELL LEUKODYSTROPHY)

Clinical Features

Krabbe disease is another autosomal-recessive myelinopathy, affecting both the CNS and the peripheral nervous system (PNS). As with MLD, Krabbe typically presents early in infancy or less frequently, in adulthood.[20–32] Krabbe disease usually manifests between 3 and 8 months of age. Infants who are affected often appear normal at birth but later become extremely irritable and appear hypersensitive to various stimuli which may provoke opisthotonos.[24] They develop feeding difficulties, recurrent vomiting, and often generalized tonic–clonic seizures. Progressive weakness and spasticity, blindness, and deafness ensue. Muscle stretch reflexes initially may be pathologically brisk but become hypoactive as concurrent polyneuropathy worsens. Plantar responses are extensor. Death generally occurs by the age of 2 years.

Less commonly, Krabbe disease presents later in childhood or adult life with progressive dementia, spastic paraparesis or hemiparesis, cerebellar ataxia, cortical blindness, and optic atrophy.[27,31–36] Although peripheral neuropathy is common, it is overshadowed by the CNS abnormalities. Pes cavus and scoliosis may be seen.

Laboratory Features

Diagnosis is made by demonstrating decreased β-galactosidase activity in leukocytes or cultured fibroblasts and can be

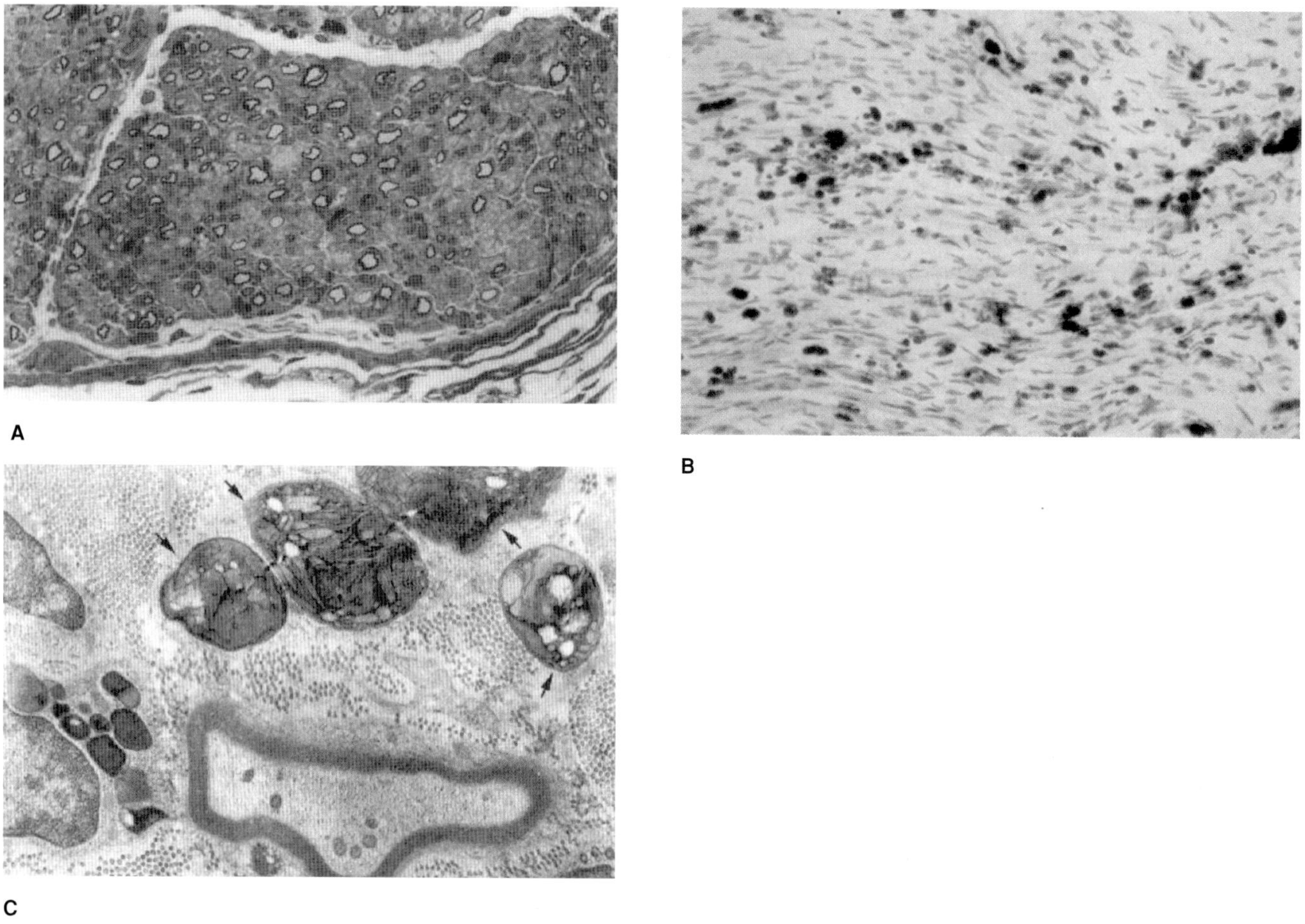

Figure 12-3. **(A)** Diffuse hypomyelination involving both large- and small-diameter fibers. Toluidine blue stain; original magnification, ×240. (Reproduced with permission from Bindu PS, Mahadevan A, Taly AB, Christopher R, Gayathri N, Shankar SK. Peripheral neuropathy in metachromatic leucodystrophy. A study of 40 cases from south India. *J Neurol Neurosurg Psychiatry* 2005;76(12):1698–1701.) **(B)** Nerve biopsy stained with cresyl violet demonstrating dense metachromatic deposits within Schwann cells obscuring the nerve fibers in the endoneurium. With acid cresyl violet, these take on a brown color (brown metachromasia), hence the term metachromatic leukodystrophy. (Reproduced with permission from www.neuropathologyweb.org/chapter10/chapter 10.) **(C)** Electron micrograph showing tuff stone inclusion bodies composed of stacks of lamellar discs and plates (*arrows*), enclosed within a membrane in the endoneurium. Original magnification, ×10,000. (Reproduced with permission from Bindu PS, Mahadevan A, Taly AB, Christopher R, Gayathri N, Shankar SK. Peripheral neuropathy in metachromatic leucodystrophy. A study of 40 cases from south India. *J Neurol Neurosurg Psychiatry*. 2005;76(12):1698–1701.)

confirmed by genetic testing. Chorionic villi can be biopsied for prenatal diagnosis. Approximately 50% of the individuals affected have increased CSF protein concentrations.[27,31] MRI of the brain reveals evidence of demyelination involving the corticospinal tracts and optic radiations as well as demyelination or atrophy of the posterior part of the corpus callosum.[31,33,34] Motor NCS demonstrate mild to moderately reduced compound muscle action potential (CMAP) amplitudes, moderately prolonged distal latencies, moderately slow NCV, and delayed or absent F-waves.[20–25,27,28,30–34,36] Sensory NCS reveal absent responses or SNAPs with markedly reduced amplitudes and mildly prolonged distal latencies and slow CV.

Histopathology

Moderate cortical atrophy, loss of CNS white matter, gliosis, and globoid cells (macrophages filled with galactocerebroside) are appreciated on autopsy. Nerve biopsies also demonstrate a loss of myelinated fibers and segmental demyelination or hypomyelination, and macrophages filled with galactocerebroside.[21,27,31–34,36,37] The abnormal inclusions within macrophages stain with periodic acid Schiff (indicating glycogen), faintly with Sudan black (indicating lipid), and with acid phosphate (suggesting that these are within lysosomes). Unlike MLD, the inclusions in Krabbe disease are not metachromatic. On EM, electron-dense granules and tubular crystalloid inclusions are evident in the cytoplasm of these histiocytes.

Molecular Genetics and Pathogenesis

Krabbe disease is autosomal recessive caused by mutations in the β-galactosidase gene (*GALC*) located on chromosome 14q24.3-q32.1.[31,33,34] β-Galactosidase metabolizes galactocerebroside to ceramide and galactose as well as catalyzes the hydrolysis of psychosine. The abnormal accumulation of galactocerebroside and psychosine leads to the degeneration of Schwann cells and oligodendrocytes.

Treatment

There is no proven effective therapy for Krabbe disease, although bone marrow and hematopoietic stem cell transplantation may prove to be useful treatments.[19,38,39]

FABRY DISEASE

Clinical Features

Fabry disease (angiokeratoma corporis diffusum) is an X-linked disorder that usually affects males in childhood or adolescence.[13,40–52] Individuals who are affected typically present with burning or lancinating dysesthesia in the hands and feet. Angiokeratomas, which appear as reddish purple maculopapular lesions, are characteristically found around the umbilicus, scrotum, inguinal region, and perineum (Fig. 12-4). In addition, tiny red angiectasia may be visualized in the nailbeds, oral mucosa, and conjunctiva. The major cause of morbidity and mortality is related to accumulation of ceramide trihexoside in walls of blood vessels leading to hypertension, renal failure, coronary artery disease, strokes, and death by the fifth decade of life. Occasionally, women develop a mild painful sensory neuropathy but only rarely do they have significant atherosclerotic disease.

Laboratory Features

A decrease in α-galactosidase activity can be demonstrated in leukocytes or cultured fibroblasts. Diagnosis can be confirmed by genetic testing. Prenatal diagnosis can be made by amniocentesis. NCS are usually normal but mildly decreased amplitudes of motor, and sensory NCS may be seen.[40–47] Quantitative sensory testing reveals impaired temperature perception indicative of small fiber dysfunction.[44,45,47,49,50]

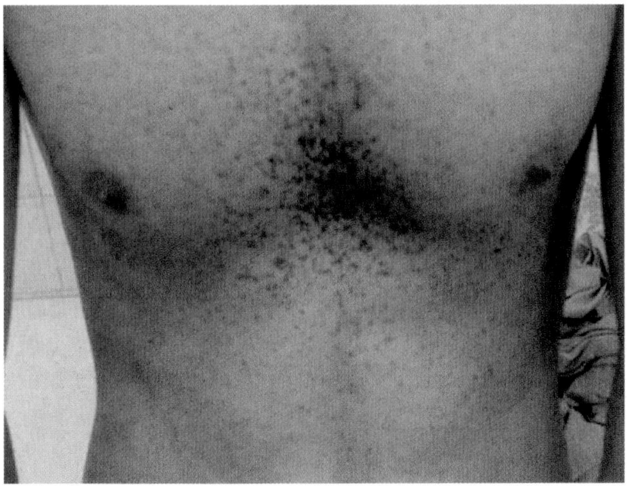

Figure 12-4. Fabry disease. Anterior chest with multiple, tiny, red, and hyperkeratotic papules. (Reproduced with permission from Sodaifi M, Aghaei S, Monabati A. Cutaneous variant of angiokeratoma corporis diffusum associated with angiokeratoma circumscriptum. *Dermatol Online J.* 2004;10(1):20.)

Histopathology

Nerve biopsies are not routinely done, but they can reveal a marked reduction of small myelinated and unmyelinated nerve fibers (Fig. 12-5). Glycolipid granules may be appreciated in ganglion cells of the peripheral and sympathetic nervous systems and in perineurial cells.[42,43] Reduced epidermal nerve fiber density may also be seen on skin biopsies.[46,48–50]

Molecular Genetics and Pathogenesis

Fabry disease is caused by mutations in the α-galactosidase gene (*GLA*) located on chromosome Xq21–22. Decreased α-galactosidase enzyme activity leads to the accumulation of ceramide trihexoside in nerves and blood vessels.

Treatment

Enzyme replacement therapy with agalactosidose-beta may improve the neuropathy if patients are treated early prior to irreversible nerve fiber loss.[50,51,53,54]

► PEROXISOMAL DISORDERS

Peroxisomes are organelles within the cytoplasm that contain enzymes essential in fatty acid oxidation (distinct from mitochondrial enzymes associated with β-oxidation), bile acid and cholesterol synthesis, and amino acid metabolism. These disorders are the result of mutations in genes encoding for structural proteins or specific peroxisomal enzymes.

ADRENOLEUKODYSTROPHY/ ADRENOMYELONEUROPATHY

Clinical Features

Adrenoleukodystrophy (ALD) and adrenomyeloneuropathy (AMN) are allelic X-linked dominant disorders. ALD is more common and manifests in young males as progressive dementia, optic atrophy, cortical blindness, hearing loss, seizures, and spasticity.[13,55–62] At least 90% of patients with ALD also have adrenal insufficiency. The onset of symptoms in ALD is usually between the age of 4 and 8 years, and death usually occurs within 2 years of onset of symptoms. Less commonly, ALD develops in adolescence or young adult life and progresses at a slower rate. Affected individuals may be misdiagnosed as having multiple sclerosis. Later-onset cases may also present with psychiatric symptoms leading to misdiagnosis as schizophrenia.

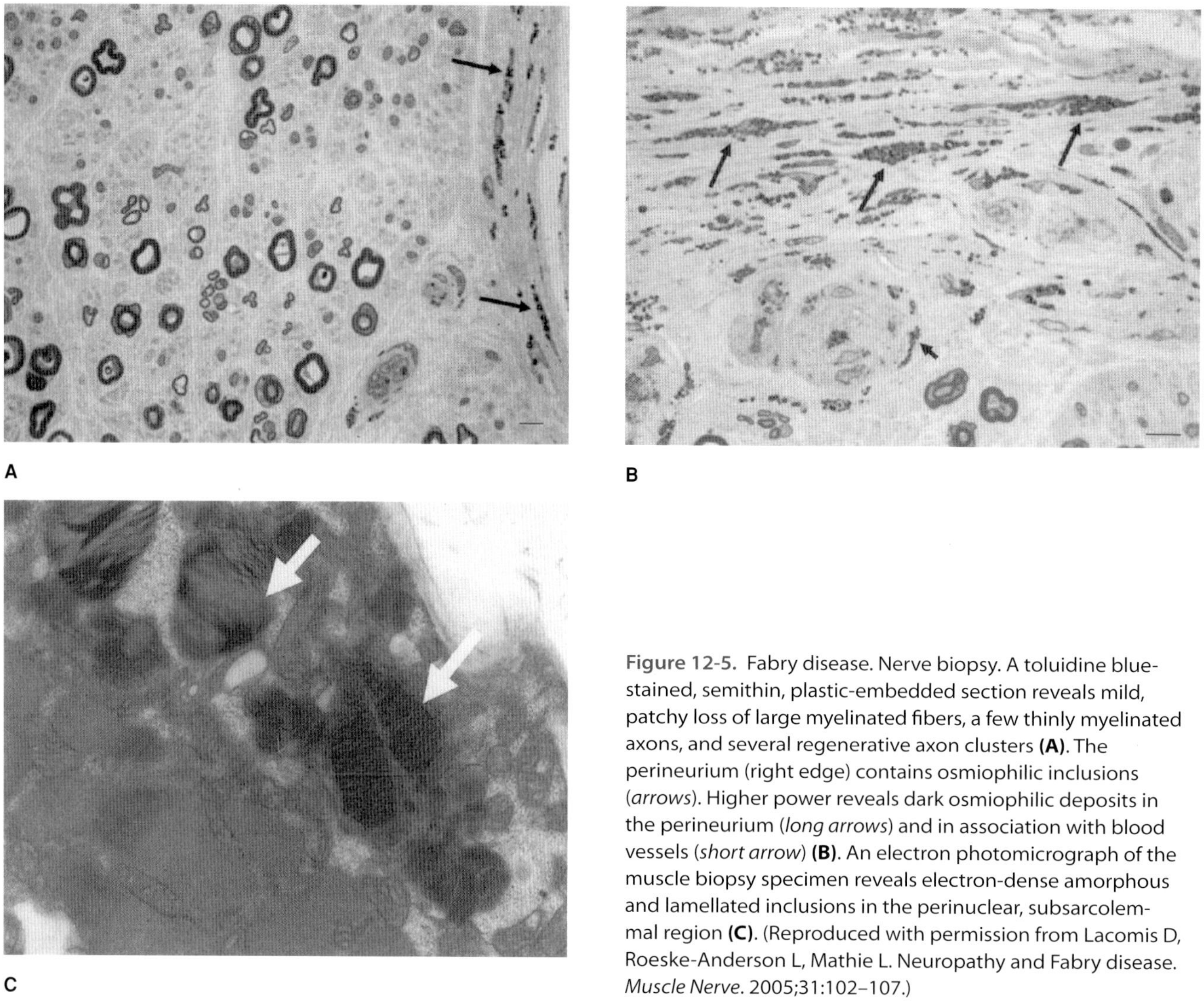

Figure 12-5. Fabry disease. Nerve biopsy. A toluidine blue-stained, semithin, plastic-embedded section reveals mild, patchy loss of large myelinated fibers, a few thinly myelinated axons, and several regenerative axon clusters **(A)**. The perineurium (right edge) contains osmiophilic inclusions (*arrows*). Higher power reveals dark osmiophilic deposits in the perineurium (*long arrows*) and in association with blood vessels (*short arrow*) **(B)**. An electron photomicrograph of the muscle biopsy specimen reveals electron-dense amorphous and lamellated inclusions in the perinuclear, subsarcolemmal region **(C)**. (Reproduced with permission from Lacomis D, Roeske-Anderson L, Mathie L. Neuropathy and Fabry disease. *Muscle Nerve.* 2005;31:102–107.)

Approximately 30% of cases present with the AMN phenotype and usually manifests in the third to fifth decade of life.[58,61,63] Individuals affected develop progressive spastic paraplegia along with a mild to moderate peripheral neuropathy. Muscle stretch reflexes may be normal or reduced. Progressive dementia indicative of cerebral involvement can develop in some patients later in the course of the disease. Adrenal insufficiency is evident in approximately two-thirds of patients. Rare patients present with an adult-onset spinocerebellar ataxia or only with adrenal insufficiency.

Although these are X-linked disorders, women occasionally develop symptoms. Manifesting women carriers usually develop a myelopathy later in life (average age in late thirties) and again are often misdiagnosed with multiple sclerosis or familial spastic paraparesis.[58]

Laboratory Features

Diagnosis is made on finding that very long-chain fatty acid (VLCFA) levels (C24, C25, and C26) are increased in the serum.[61,64] The ratio of hexacosanoic acid to docosanoic or erucic acid (C26:C22) and tetracosanoic acid to docosanoic acid (C24:C22) are increased in both ALD and AMN. VLCFA levels can be assessed in neonates and can be used to screen for the disease shortly after birth. Because VLCFA levels are similar in ALD and AMN, these are not helpful in predicting the clinical phenotype. As many as 85% of obligate female carriers also have elevated VLCFA levels. Some, but not all, individuals have laboratory evidence of adrenal insufficiency. Diagnosis is confirmed by genetic testing.

MRI scans reveal confluent subcortical white matter demyelination in ALD, preferentially in the posterior parietal–occipital regions (Fig. 12-6).[60] MRI abnormalities of the cerebral white matter also develop later in the course in nearly half of patients with AMD but are not uniformly present in late-onset cases.

NCS are usually normal in ALD. However, AMN is usually associated with a sensorimotor polyneuropathy. Typically, sensory and motor NCS reveal slightly reduced amplitudes, prolonged distal latencies, and slight slow CVs,

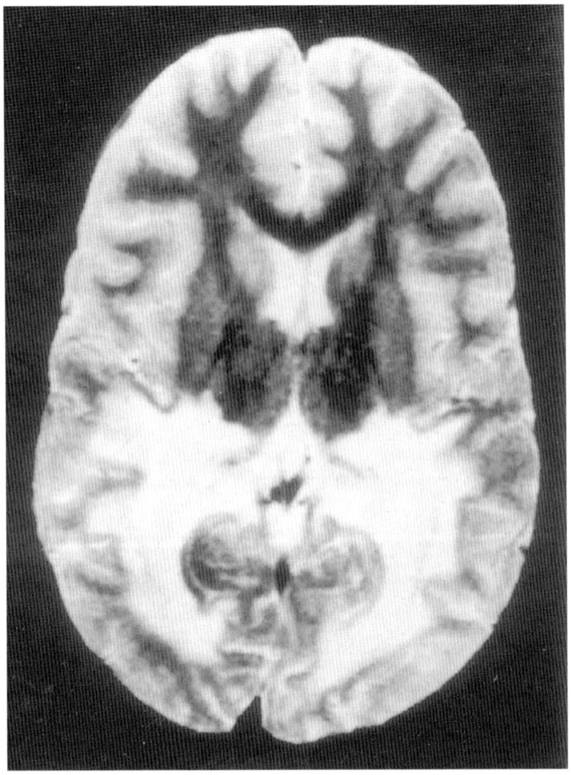

Figure 12-6. Cerebral T2-weighted MRI of an 8-year-old boy with impaired visual acuity and seizures due to adrenoleukodystrophy. (Reproduced with permission from van Geel BM, Assies J, Wanders RJA, Barth PG. X-linked adrenoleukodystrophy: clinical presentation, diagnosis, and therapy. *J Neurol Neurosurg Psychiatry*. 1997;63(1):4–14.)

suggesting a primary axonopathy with secondary demyelination.[55,56,59,62,63,65,66] Occasionally, patients fulfill electrophysiological criteria for a primary demyelination.[67] Somatosensory and visual-evoked potentials demonstrate evidence of central slowing.[57,59]

Histopathology

We do not perform nerve biopsies routinely, but they can demonstrate a loss of myelinated and unmyelinated nerve fibers. On EM, lamellar inclusions are evident in the cytoplasm of Schwann cells (Fig. 12-7). Autopsies in ALD demonstrate demyelination and perivascular inflammation, particularly in the parietal and occipital regions.[58] The spinal cord displays bilateral, usually symmetrical, long tract degeneration, particularly of the gracile tract in a dying-back pattern.[67]

Molecular Genetics and Pathogenesis

ALD and AMN are caused by mutations in the peroxisomal transmembrane adenosine triphosphate-binding cassette transporter gene (*ABCD1*), located on chromosome Xq28.[58,61] The ABC transporter protein is part of peroxins family of proteins, which are involved in the transport, biogenesis, and

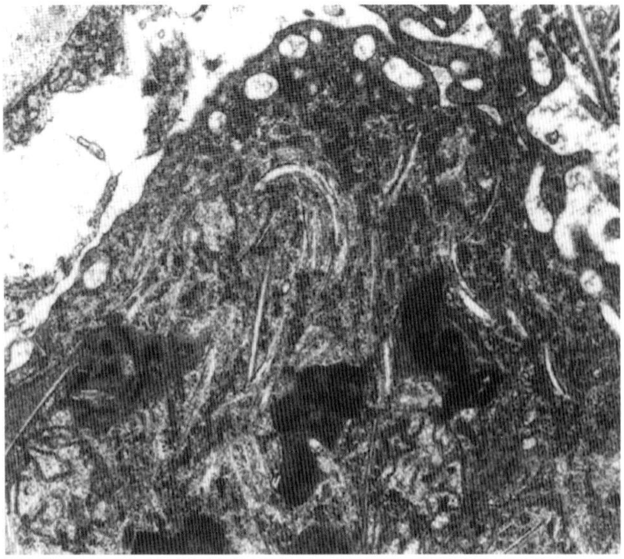

Figure 12-7. Adrenoleukodystrophy. Characteristic cellular inclusions (trilamellar membranes containing VLCFA cholesterol esters) are seen with the electron microscope in adrenal cortical cells, white matter histiocytes, Leydig cells, and Schwann cells. (Reproduced with permission from www.neuropathologyweb.org/chapter10/chapter 10.)

proliferation of peroxisomes.[68] There is no clear genotype–phenotype correlation associated with any specific mutation, and phenotypic heterogeneity can be found even within the family members who carry the same genetic mutation. Mutations in the gene cause impaired transport of VLCFA or VLCFA CoA synthetase into peroxisomes, thus decreasing β-oxidization of VLCFA; but how this leads to dysmyelination and axonal degeneration is not known.

Treatment

Adrenal insufficiency is managed by replacement therapy. There is however no proven effective therapy for the neurologic manifestations of ALD and AMN.[58] Diets low in VLCFAs and supplemented with Lorenzo oil (erucic and oleic acids) reduce the levels of VLCFAs and increase the levels of C22 in serum, fibroblasts, and liver; however, such changes have not been consistently noted in the brain.[69] Rare reports suggest clinical and MRI improvement in individual patients treated with Lorenzo oil, but several large open-label trials of Lorenzo oil failed to demonstrate significant efficacy.[61,70,71] Bone marrow transplantation has also been suggested in patients with early ALD or AMN.[19,61]

REFSUM DISEASE (HMSN IV)

Clinical Features

Refsum disease is a peroxisomal disorder associated with impaired α-oxidation of phytanic acid. The disease can manifest in infancy to early adulthood with the classic tetrad of (1) peripheral neuropathy, (2) retinitis pigmentosa (often the earliest symptom which manifests as night blindness), (3) cerebellar ataxia, and (4) elevated CSF protein concentration.[72–77] Patients with Refsum disease may also develop sensorineural hearing loss, cardiac conduction abnormalities, ichthyosis, and anosmia. Some or all of these clinical findings are usually manifest in the majority of patients by the end of the second decade. Infantile Refsum disease falls within the clinical spectrum of Zellweger syndrome and neonatal ALD, albeit much milder in severity.

Although not typically a presenting manifestation, most individuals who are affected develop distal numbness and paresthesia in the legs by their twenties. The distal legs become atrophic and weak and patients develop progressive foot drop. Subsequently, the proximal leg and arm muscles may become weak. Interestingly, the neuropathy can have a fluctuating course. On examination, a length-dependent loss of vibration, proprioception, and light touch is appreciated. Hypertrophic nerves may be palpated. Muscle stretch reflexes are reduced or absent throughout.

Laboratory Features

Serum phytanic acid levels are elevated, usually greater than 200 μmol/L, as may the CSF protein concentration. Other abnormalities include an increased phytanic acid/pristanic acid ratio, elevated pipecolic acid concentration, and reduced phytanoyl-CoA hydroxylase enzyme activity. Genetic testing can be done to confirm the disorder. Sensory NCS reveal reduced amplitudes and prolonged latencies/slow CVs.[76] Motor NCS demonstrate normal or moderately reduced amplitudes, mildly or moderately prolonged distal latencies, and mild to marked slowing of CV to the 10–30 m/s range.[72,74,75]

Histopathology

Nerve biopsies demonstrate a loss of myelinated nerve fibers, with remaining axons often thinly myelinated and associated with onion-bulb formation.

Molecular Genetics and Pathogenesis

Refsum disease is autosomal recessive and can be caused by mutations in two different genes.[78] Classical Refsum disease with childhood or early adult onset is caused by mutations in the gene that encodes for phytanoyl-CoA α-hydroxylase (*PHYX*) located on chromosome 10p13 in 90% of affected individuals.[79,80] This peroxisomal enzyme helps catalyze α-oxidation of phytanic acid. The defect leads to the accumulation of phytanic acid in various organs including the CNS and PNS, leading to neuronal degeneration. Less common, mutations in the gene that encodes for peroxin 7 receptor protein (*PRX 7*) located on chromosome 6q22–24 are responsible for Refsum disease.[78,81,82] Mutations in the *PEX7* gene that encodes for the peroxisome-targeting signal type 2 receptor are seen in less than 10% of individuals. Mutations in PEX7 also cause rhizomelic chondrodysplasia punctata type 1, a severe peroxisomal disorder.

Treatment

Refsum disease is treated by removing phytanic precursors (phytols: fish oils, dairy products, and ruminant fats) from the diet. In addition to the noticed clinical improvement, the NCS also improve with appropriate dietary restrictions as well as with plasma exchange.[72–75]

TANGIER DISEASE

Clinical Features

Tangier disease is a rare autosomal-recessive disorder associated with a deficiency of high-density lipoprotein. The first reported patients came from Tangier island located in Chesapeake Bay—thus the name. Tangier disease may present as (1) an asymmetric mononeuropathy multiplex, (2) a slowly progressive symmetric polyneuropathy predominantly in the legs, or (3) a pseudosyringomyelia appearance in which there is dissociation between loss of pain/temperature and position/vibration in the arms.[83–92] Deposition of cholesterol esters within the tonsils leads to their swollen, yellowish-orange appearance. In addition, splenomegaly and lymphadenopathy may be apparent.

Laboratory Features

Serum high-density lipoprotein cholesterol levels are markedly reduced while triacylglycerol levels are increased. Genetic testing is available to confirm the diagnosis. Motor and sensory NCS can be normal or associated with moderately reduced amplitudes, prolonged distal latencies, partial conduction block, and slow CVs.[84–88,90,91] The asymmetric nature of the polyneuropathy and demyelinating features including conduction block may mimic Lewis–Sumner syndrome (e.g., multifocal acquired demyelinating sensory and motor neuropathy or MADSAMN—see Chapter 14).[90,91]

Histopathology

Nerve biopsies are not required for the diagnosis, but studies have reported they reveal axonal degeneration with demyelination, remyelination, and redundant myelin folds (i.e., tomacula).[83,92–94] EM demonstrates abnormal accumulation of lipid in Schwann cells, particularly those encompassing unmyelinated and small myelinated nerve (Fig. 12-8).[83,92] There appears to be preferential involvement of noncompacted myelin region of the paranode for lipid storage in the myelinated Schwann cells.

Molecular Genetics and Pathogenesis

Tangier disease is caused by mutations in the ATP-binding cassette-1 gene (*ABCA1*) located in chromosome 9q22–31.[95,96] The pathogenic basis of the peripheral neuropathy is unknown but may be similar to ALD/AMN, which are also caused by mutations involving the ABC transporter superfamily.

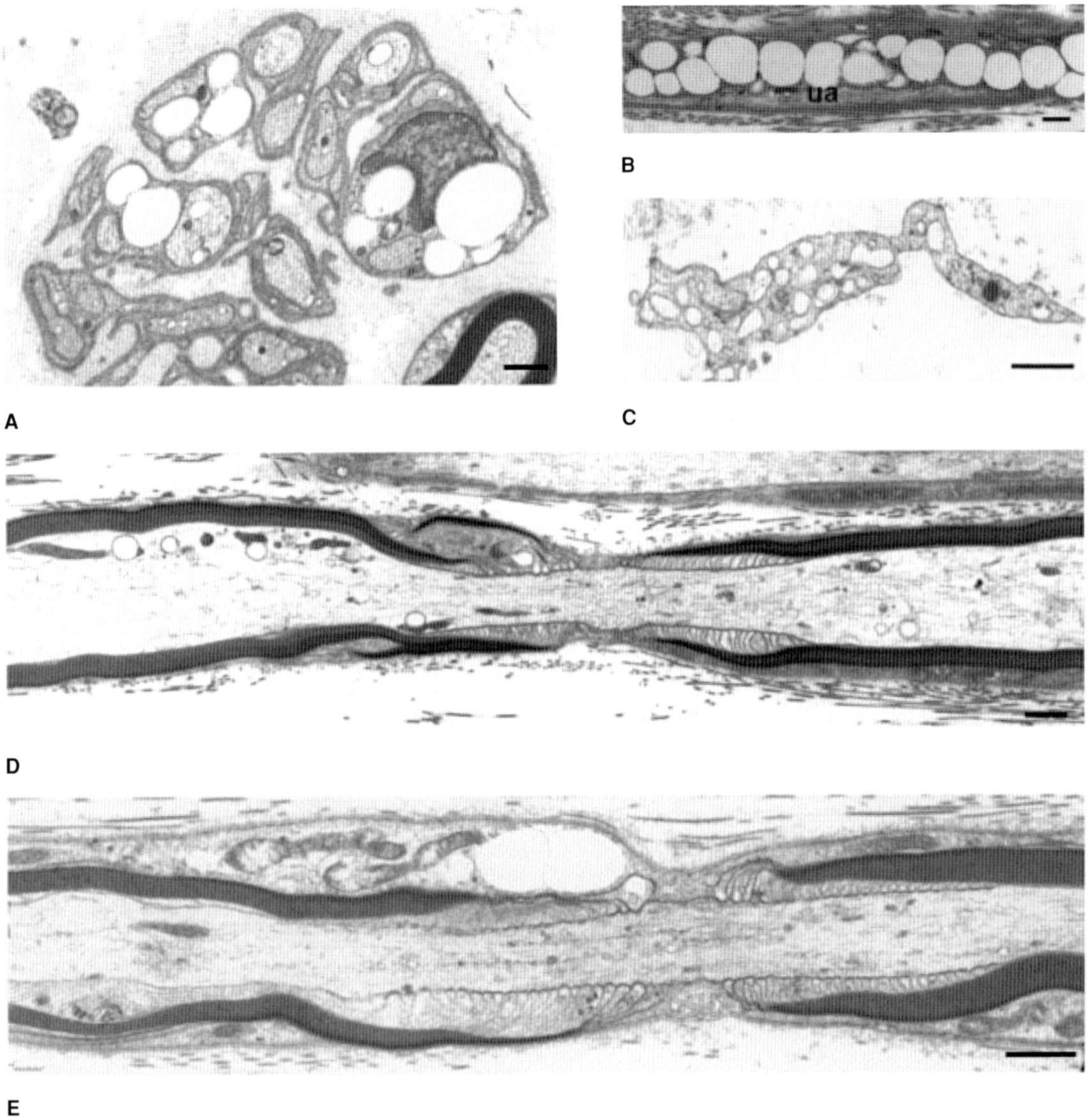

Figure 12-8. Tangier disease. Electron micrographs. **(A)** Transverse section showing multiple electron-lucent vacuoles in the cytoplasm of unmyelinated Schwann cells. **(B)** Longitudinal section showing linearly arranged vacuoles in Schwann cell cytoplasm of an unmyelinated axon (ua). **(C)** Multiple vacuoles in a fibroblast. **(D)** Small vacuoles in the disrupted paranodal myelin terminal loops. **(E)** Large vacuoles in the paranodal abaxonal Schwann cell cytoplasm. Bar = 1 μm. (Reproduced with permission from Cai Z, Blumbergs PC, Cash K, et al. Paranodal pathology in Tangier disease with remitting-relapsing multifocal neuropathy. *J Clin Neurosci.* 2006;13(4):492–497.)

Treatment

There is no specific treatment.

CEREBROTENDINOUS XANTHOMATOSIS (CHOLESTANOLOSIS)

Clinical Features

Cerebrotendinous xanthomatosis is a rare autosomal-recessive disorder that usually presents after the second decade with progressive dementia, spasticity, ataxia, and a mild sensory neuropathy.[97–104] The name of the disorder arises because of the common occurrence of xanthomas on tendons and the skin. Cataracts are another frequent complication. Most individuals who are affected die in the fourth decade of life because of complications from premature atherosclerosis.

Laboratory Features

Serum level of cholestanol is increased. Genetic testing can be performed to confirm the diagnosis. NCS are variable, depending on the presence and the degree of severity of peripheral neuropathy.[97,99,100,103] Motor and sensory may be normal or reveal absent amplitudes, with slightly prolonged distal latencies, and mildly slow CVs suggestive of an axonal sensorimotor polyneuropathy.

Histopathology

Nerve biopsies reveal a loss of myelinated nerve fibers with variable degrees of demyelination and onion-bulb formation. Lipid inclusions are evident in Schwann cells.

Molecular Genetics and Pathogenesis

This disorder is caused by mutations in the sterol 27 hydroxylase gene located on chromosome 2, which results in impaired metabolism of cholestanol, the 5α-dihydro derivative of cholesterol.[105] Cholestanol accumulates in body tissues, including peripheral nerves, thereby resulting in the associated clinical features.

Treatment

Early treatment with chenodeoxycholic acid may lead to a decrease in serum cholestanol and diminished excretion of bile alcohols in urine accompanied by clinical improvement.[98] Motor and sensory NCS improved in one patient following plasma exchange and treatment with chenodeoxycholic acid.[99]

▶ HEREDITARY ATAXIAS

The hereditary ataxias are a group of progressive neurodegenerative disorders characterized by varying degrees of degeneration of the cerebral cortex, basal ganglia, cerebellum, brainstem, corticospinal tracts, spinocerebellar tracts, motor neurons, and peripheral nerves (Table 12-1). The associated peripheral neuropathy with some of these disorders is usually overshadowed by the CNS abnormalities. However, the neuropathy can be quite prominent in Friedreich ataxia (FA) and an inherited form of vitamin E deficiency.

FRIEDREICH ATAXIA

Clinical Features

FA usually presents between 2 and 16 years of age with gait ataxia (63%), generalized clumsiness (25%), difficulty ambulating (4%), scoliosis (5%), tremor (1%), and cardiomyopathy (2%).[106–113] However, several genetically confirmed late-onset cases have been described.[108,114,115] FA is the most common form of autosomal-recessive ataxia. Dysarthria, optic atrophy, pigmentary retinopathy, nystagmus, reduced hearing, ataxia, pyramidal and lower motor neuron weakness, distal limb atrophy, scoliosis, and pes cavus are evident on examination. In addition, reduced vibratory sensation and proprioception associated with diminished muscle stretch reflexes are seen, often associated with extensor plantar responses.[108,114,115] Rarely, affected individuals have retained reflexes.[116] Some patients develop dementia. FA is a progressive disorder and most patients are wheelchair dependent with 15 years of onset of symptoms. There is increased mortality with the mean age of death in the mid to late thirties.

Laboratory Features

Genetic testing is available for diagnosis. MRI of the brain is usually normal, but the cervical spinal cord is often atrophic.[114–116] Electrocardiogram reveals nonspecific abnormalities (e.g., nonspecific ST and T-wave changes, low-voltage QRS complexes, deep Q-waves, and conduction defects) in at least 30% of patients. Echocardiogram reveals increased thickness of the interventricular septum in approximately two-thirds of affected individuals; later in the course a dilated cardiomyopathy may develop. Sensory NCS are associated with absent or reduced amplitudes.[106–108,111,112,114,117] H-reflexes are absent. Motor NCS are less affected[107,108,118]; however, central motor conduction may be slow on magnetic stimulation studies.[119,120] Somatosensory-evoked potentials demonstrate reduced or absent cortical potentials and slowing of central conduction.[118,121,122]

Histopathology

Sural nerve biopsies reveal a loss of large myelinated fibers.[122] On autopsy, the posterior columns are markedly atrophied and the dorsal roots are considerably decreased in size compared to the ventral roots.

Molecular Genetics and Pathogenesis

FA is autosomal recessive, usually caused by expanding GAA trinucleotide repeat mutation within the first intron of the frataxin gene (*FXN*) located on chromosome 9q13.[123,124] The normal gene contains 40 or fewer copies of the GAA triplet repeats, while patients with FA usually have 100 to more than 1,700 repeats. Approximately 2% of cases are caused by point mutations within the frataxin gene.[125] The mutations result in low or absent levels of frataxin, a mitochondrial protein of unclear function. Frataxin is speculated to have a role in iron metabolism, protection against free radical toxicity, or mitochondrial DNA replication.[125]

Treatment

There is no medical treatment for FA. However, patients may benefit from speech, occupational, and physical therapy. Cardiac function needs to be monitored and treated appropriately.

VITAMIN E DEFICIENCY

Clinical Features

Vitamin E or α-tocopherol is a lipid-soluble vitamin present in the lipid bilayer of cell membranes.[122,126–132] Vitamin E deficiency can arise due to (1) deficient fat absorption (e.g., cystic fibrosis, chronic cholestasis, short-bowel syndrome, and intestinal lymphangiectasia), (2) deficient fat transport (abetalipoproteinemia, hypobetalipoproteinemia, normotriglyceridemic abetalipoproteinemia, and chylomicron retention disease), or (3) secondary to mutations in α-tocopherol transfer protein.

The clinical manifestations of hereditary and secondary vitamin E deficiency resemble those seen in FA. Onset in the hereditary cases is usually between the ages of 5 and 10 years. Affected individuals manifest with slowly progressive ataxia, dysarthria, reduced vibratory perception and proprioception, diminished or absent muscle stretch reflexes with extensor plantar responses, and generalized weakness. Pes cavus deformities and scoliosis are common. Ophthalmoplegia, optic neuropathy, and retinitis pigmentosa are seen in acquired cases of vitamin E deficiency but are not typically present in the hereditary form.

Laboratory Features

Serum vitamin E levels are reduced. Patients deficient in vitamin E secondary to malabsorption of fat also have low serum levels of cholesterol, triglycerides, very low-density lipoproteins (VLDLs), vitamin A, and vitamin C. These levels are normal in patients with hereditary vitamin E deficiency in which there is isolated vitamin E deficiency. Hereditary cases can be confirmed with genetic testing. Sensory NCS reveal absent potentials or low amplitudes.[122,127,128,130,131] Motor conduction studies are usually normal, although slightly prolonged distal latencies and slow NCVs may be found.[122,128] Somatosensory-evoked potentials may be unobtainable but, when recordable, demonstrate slowing of central conduction and reduced amplitudes.

Histopathology

Autopsies and nerve biopsies demonstrate a marked loss of dorsal root ganglion cells, large-diameter myelinated fibers, and degeneration of the dorsal columns and reductions in the cells of the gracile and cuneate nuclei. Vacuoles may be evident in the myelin sheath, and the Schmidt–Lanterman incisures may appear disrupted.

Molecular Genetics and Pathogenesis

Isolated vitamin E deficiency is inherited in an autosomal-recessive manner and is caused by mutations in the α-tocopherol transfer protein gene (*TTPA*) located on chromosome 8q13.[126,129] As a result, there is reduced incorporation of vitamin E into serum VLDLs.[132] Although absorption of vitamin E in the intestines and incorporation into chylomicrons are normal, recycling of vitamin E is dependent on α-tocopherol transfer protein into VLDL. Thus, vitamin E is rapidly eliminated and levels are diminished in the CNS and PNS.

Vitamin E may have antioxidant properties and may assist in modulating against glutamate excitotoxicity. The dorsal root ganglia and the posterior column nuclei have the lowest concentrations of vitamin E in the nervous system and might therefore be particularly sensitive to diminishing concentrations of vitamin E and its possible neuroprotective effects.

Treatment

Early treatment may stabilize or improve neurologic function. Patients are started on vitamin E 400 mg twice a day, and the dosage is gradually increased up to 100 mg/kg per day until vitamin E levels normalize.[128]

ABETALIPOPROTEINEMIA (BASSEN–KORNZWEIG DISEASE)

Clinical Features

Abetalipoproteinemia or Bassen–Kornzweig disease is characterized by the combination of ataxia, retinitis pigmentosa, steatorrhea, and loss of sensation in the distal arms and legs.[133–136] Affected individuals usually present with ataxia and vision loss at night within the first two decades of life. The ataxia is progressive and leads to the loss of independent ambulation by the fourth or fifth decades of life. On physical examination, patients are often short in stature and have pes cavus and hammer toes. Reduction in vibration sensation and proprioception is apparent along with sensory ataxia. Muscle stretch reflexes are reduced or absent. Mild distal muscle atrophy and weakness may be appreciated. Ophthalmoparesis may be observed in some patients.

Laboratory Features

Acanthocytes are seen on blood smear. Total serum cholesterol, low-density lipoproteins and VLDLs, and chylomicrons are reduced, as are serum concentrations of the fat-soluble vitamins A, E, and K. The electrophysiological abnormalities are very similar to those found in FA and vitamin E deficiency.[137–139] The sensory SNAPs are absent or reveal reduced amplitudes with minimal slowing of conduction and normal or borderline distal sensory latencies. The CMAP amplitudes are normal or only slightly reduced, while distal latencies and CVs are preserved or only mildly slow. Central conduction slowing may be appreciated on somatosensory and visual-evoked potential studies.[138,140] Brainstem auditory-evoked responses are characteristically normal, which is the only distinguishing electrophysiological feature between this disorder and FA.

Histopathology

Nerve biopsies demonstrate axonal degeneration with a loss of large-diameter myelinated fibers as well as demyelination and remyelination on teased nerve fiber analysis. Degeneration of the posterior columns and the ventral spinocerebellar tracts has been appreciated on autopsies.

Molecular Genetics and Pathogenesis

This is an autosomal-recessive disorder caused by mutations in the *MTTP* gene that encodes for microsomal triglyceride transfer protein large subunit. This protein is important in lipoprotein assembly and absorption of fat-soluble vitamins from the intestinal tract. This most likely leads to decreased vitamin E, leading to the neurologic deficits in this disorder.

Treatment

Patients should be treated by replacing fat-soluble vitamins, in particular vitamin E.

ATAXIA-TELANGIECTASIA

Clinical Features

Ataxia-telangiectasia is characterized by childhood onset (usually in first 5 years of life) of cerebellar ataxia, oculocutaneous telangiectasia, oculomotor dyspraxia, and frequent sinopulmonary infections.[109,141,142] Motor milestones are delayed, but mental functioning is well preserved. Affected children develop choreoathetotic movements and dysarthric speech within the first decade. Sensory examination reveals a marked loss of proprioception and vibration sense and muscle stretch reflexes are reduced or absent. Distal motor weakness may become apparent over time.

Laboratory Features

Variable immune deficiency with reduced levels of IgA and IgG can be seen along with an increase in serum α-fetoprotein (AFP) levels. The electrophysiological abnormalities are similar to those found in FA with absent or reduced amplitudes of the SNAPs, with only a mild reduction in the NCVs or prolongation in the distal sensory latencies.[109,141] Similar but less striking abnormalities can be seen on motor NCS. Genetic testing is done to confirm the diagnosis.

Histopathology

Sural nerve biopsies reveal a loss of large myelinated nerve fibers.

Molecular Genetics and Pathogenesis

The disorder is inherited in an autosomal-recessive manner and is caused by mutations in the ataxia telangiectasia mutated (*ATM*) gene located on chromosome 11q23, which encodes for phosphatidylinositol-3 kinase.[142,143] This enzyme is important in signal transduction, meiotic recombination, and cell-cycle regulation, and the mutations in the ATM gene result in impaired DNA repair. Cytogenetic testing reveals a 6–10-fold increase in chromosome breakage following ionizing irradiation. Further, there is increased spontaneous breakage and specific translocations involving the T-cell receptor genes on chromosome 7 and 14.

Treatment

There is no specific treatment.

ATAXIA WITH OCULOMOTOR APRAXIA TYPE 1

Clinical Features

Ataxia with oculomotor apraxia type 1 (AOA1) was initially described in Japanese patients and characterized by early-onset, slowly progressive cerebellar ataxia, mental retardation (though some have normal intellect), choreoathetosis, followed by oculomotor apraxia and an axonal motor peripheral neuropathy.[144–147] Typically, patients present with gait imbalance between the ages of 2 and 10 years, followed by slurred, then poor coordination of the arms with mild intention tremor. Oculomotor apraxia develops a few years after the onset of ataxia and progresses to external ophthalmoplegia. Progressive generalized weakness and areflexia evolve with loss of ambulation usually occurring about 7–10 years after onset.

Laboratory Features

MRI scans demonstrated cerebellar atrophy.[144–147] Electrodiagnostic studies reveal evidence of an axonal sensorimotor polyneuropathy.[144–147] Serum concentration of AFP is usually elevated. In addition, hypoalbuminemia and hypercholesterolemia become evident, particularly during the later stages of the disease. Diagnosis is confirmed by genetic testing.

Histopathology

Sural nerve biopsy is not routinely done but has revealed severe loss of small and large myelinated fibers with preservation of the unmyelinated nerve fibers.[144]

Molecular Genetics and Pathogenesis

AOA1 is caused by mutations in the *APTX* gene that encodes for aprataxin, which is involved in DNA single-strand break repair.[145] The mechanism by which defects in aprataxin result in central and peripheral nerve damage is not at all clear.

Treatment

There is no specific treatment.

ATAXIA WITH OCULOMOTOR APRAXIA TYPE 2

Clinical Features

Ataxia with oculomotor apraxia type 2 (AOA2) is characterized by progressive cerebellar atrophy, choreoathetosis, and axonal sensorimotor polyneuropathy, and oculomotor apraxia (the later in approximately 60% of affected individuals) with an onset between the ages of 3 and 30 years.[148–155]

Laboratory Features

There is usually elevated serum concentration of AFP. Electrodiagnostic studies reveal features of a mixed demyelinating, and axonal sensorimotor neuropathy. Diagnosis is made by genetic testing.

Histopathology

Sural nerve biopsy has reportedly showed severe depletion of large and small myelinated fibers.[151] Autopsy studies have demonstrated a marked loss of Purkinje cells in the cerebellar cortex, loss of neurons in the dentate nucleus, chromatolysis of the oculomotor and raphe nuclei in the brainstem, severe demyelination of the gracilis and cuneatus funiculi, and degeneration of the Clarke columns with gliosis in the spinal cord.[151]

Molecular Genetics and Pathogenesis

AOA2 is caused by mutations in *SETX*, the gene that encodes the protein senataxin. Mutations in this gene are also responsible for the dominant juvenile form of familial amyotrophic lateral sclerosis type 4. Senataxin may modulate neurite growth through fibroblast growth factor 8 signaling.[155] However, the exact mechanism by which defects in senataxin result in central and peripheral nerve damage is not known.

Treatment

There is no specific treatment.

COCKAYNE SYNDROME

Clinical Features

Cockayne syndrome is a rare disorder caused by defects in DNA repair and is associated with various systemic abnormalities, including central and PNS dysmyelination.[156–162] Most children appear normal at birth, but by the end of the first year of their life they are noted to have reduced growth rates and signs of aging. Between 4 and 10 years of age, they develop progeric facial appearance, cognitive decline, ataxia, areflexia, hearing loss, photosensitivity, pigmentary retinopathy, and dwarfism.

Laboratory Features

Motor and sensory NCS may demonstrate moderate to marked reduction in NCVs and prolonged distal latencies.[156,157,161,162]

Histopathology

Nerve biopsies reveal segmental demyelination and inclusions within Schwann cell.[144,163]

Molecular Genetics and Pathogenesis

Cockayne syndrome is an autosomal-recessive disorder that can be caused by mutations in two different genes that encode for DNA excision repair proteins: *ERCC6* (65% of individuals) and *ERCC8* (35% of individuals). Defects in these transcription factors that interact with RNA polymerase II result in impaired transcription initiation, nucleotide excision, and DNA repair.[165] The inability to properly excise and repair spontaneous DNA mutations results in accelerated signs of aging and increased risk of malignancy.

Treatment

There is no specific treatment.

► MISCELLANEOUS HEREDITARY NEUROPATHIES

GIANT AXONAL NEUROPATHY

Clinical Features

Giant axonal neuropathy presents in the first decade of life with progressive gait difficulty.[146–173] Children who are affected appear to have a normal birth and meet early motor milestones. However, around the age of 2 years they begin to exhibit signs of imbalance. By about 4 years of age, signs of a sensorimotor polyneuropathy and cerebellar ataxia are evident. Cognitive impair ensues. Sensory examination reveals a decrease in all sensory modalities in a length-dependent distribution along with mild distal muscle atrophy and weakness. Muscle stretch reflexes are usually absent in the legs and reduced in the arms, while extensor plantar responses are appreciated. Truncal and limb ataxias are evident. Patients have characteristic curly or kinky hair.

Laboratory Features

NCS reveal absent or reduced amplitudes of SNAPs and CMAPs with normal or slightly prolonged distal latencies and mildly slow CVs.[172,174–176] Diagnosis is confirmed by genetic testing (see below).

Histopathology

Nerve biopsies demonstrate loss of myelinated axons with segmental demyelination and, notably, giant axonal swellings (Fig. 12-9).[166–172] On EM, these axonal swellings consist of abnormal accumulations of densely packed intermediate-sized neurofilaments that are most prominent distally and in the paranodal regions. Similar giant axons occur in toxic neuropathies caused by exposure to *n*-hexane, methyl *n*-butyl ketone, acrylamide, carbon disulfide, 2,5-hexanedione, and triorthocresyl (tri-*o*-cresyl) phosphate.

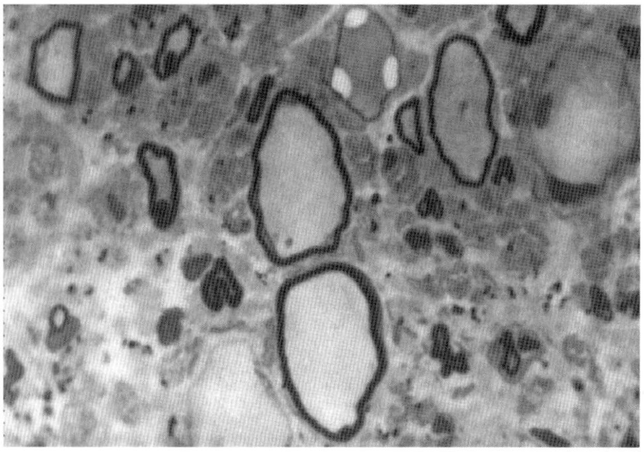

Figure 12-9. Giant axonal neuropathy. Semithin section of the sural nerve showing a giant axon filled with masses of neurofilaments. (Reproduced with permission from Demir E, Bomont P, Erdem S, et al. Giant axonal neuropathy: clinical and genetic study in six cases. *J Neurol Neurosurg Psychiatry*. 2005;76(6):825–832.)

Molecular Genetics and Pathogenesis

Giant axonal neuropathy is caused by mutations in the gigaxonin gene (*GAN*) located on chromosome 16q24.[177] Gigaxonin is a cytoskeletal protein, which may be important in actin–cytoskeletal interactions.

Treatment

There is no specific treatment.

INFANTILE NEUROAXONAL DYSTROPHY

Clinical Features

Infantile neuroaxonal dystrophy presents in the first or second year of life, with progressive psychomotor regression, visual loss, generalized hypotonia, and weakness.[178–181] Those children who eventually ambulate usually lose the ability to walk independently over time due to progressive weakness, spasticity, and ataxia. Some affected children develop complex partial or generalized tonic–clonic seizures. Muscle stretch reflexes are usually reduced. Optic atrophy is apparent on funduscopic examination.

Laboratory Features

MRI scans reveal cerebellar and cerebral atrophy, hyperintensity on T2-weighted images in the periventricular white matter and dentate nuclei, and hypointense T2 images in the globus pallidus and substantia nigra.[179] The optic chiasm is often thin. Motor and sensory NCS may reveal decreased amplitudes and mild to moderate slowing of CV.[178–181] EMG demonstrates active denervation and features of a motor neuron disease. Visual-evoked potentials are unobtainable or have prolonged latencies.

Histopathology

Axonal swellings with spheroid bodies can be found on biopsies of peripheral nerves, muscle, skin, and conjunctiva.[178–181]

Molecular Genetics and Pathogenesis

Mutations in the gene, *NAGA*, which encodes for the lysosomal enzyme, α-*N*-acetyl-galactosamine, has been identified in some[181] but not all patients with infantile neuroaxonal dystrophy.[179]

Treatment

There is no specific treatment.

ADULT POLYGLUCOSAN BODY DISEASE

Clinical Features

Adult polyglucosan body disease (APBD) is allelic to glycogen storage disease type IV [glycogen branching enzyme (GBE) deficiency] that typically manifests as a myopathy and is discussed in Chapter 29. In contrast, APBD usually presents in adults as progressive upper and lower motor neuron loss, sensory nerve involvement, cerebellar ataxia, neurogenic bladder, and dementia.[182–192] Occasionally, polyglucosan body neuropathy manifests in children. There is a predilection for APBD in the Ashkenazi population.

Laboratory Features

The serum CK may be normal or slightly elevated. An axonal sensorimotor neuropathy is apparent on NCS while the EMG abnormalities reflect a superimposed polyradiculopathy.[182,185,187] APBD may be diagnosed by demonstrating a reduction of GBE activity in leukocytes or cultured skin fibroblasts. MRI of the brain reveals hyperintense white matter abnormalities on T2- and fluid-attenuated inversion recovery sequences predominantly in the periventricular regions, the posterior limb of the internal capsule, the external capsule, the pyramidal tracts, and medial lemniscus of the pons and medulla (Fig. 12-10).[182]

Histopathology

Routine light and EM reveals deposition of varying amounts of finely granular and filamentous polysaccharide (polyglucosan bodies) in the CNS, peripheral nerves (axons and Schwann cells), and skin (Figs. 12-11 and 12-12).[182,183,186,185,191] These polyglucosan bodies are PAS positive and diastase resistant, suggesting the accumulation of polysaccharides other than glycogen. They are not specific for this disorder and can be seen occasionally in nerve biopsies from patients with other diseases. This polysaccharide resembles amylopectin in that it has longer than normal peripheral chains and few branch

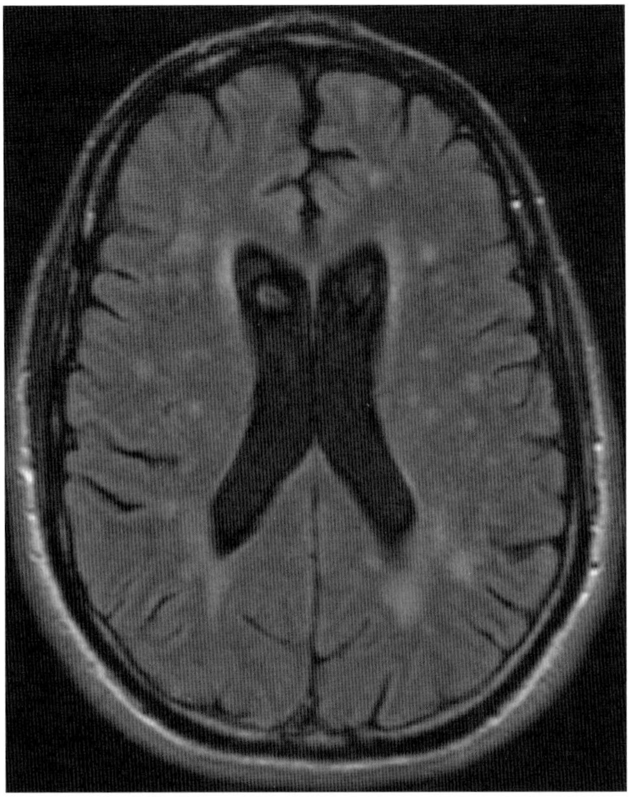

Figure 12-10. MRI of brain in a patient with adult polyglucosan body disease reveals scattered hyperintense white matter abnormalities fluid-attenuated inversion recovery sequences.

points. Autopsy studies have demonstrated abnormal polysaccharide material in the motor neurons in the brainstem and spinal cord.[183,186]

Molecular Genetics and Pathogenesis

Polyglucosan body neuropathy is inherited in an autosomal-recessive manner and is caused by mutations in the glycogen branching enzyme gene (*GBE1*).[182,188,190,192] The mechanism by which the abnormal accumulation of polysaccharide results in nerve damage is not known.

Treatment

There is no specific treatment.

PORPHYRIA

Clinical Features

Porphyria is actually a group of inherited disorders caused by defects in heme biosynthesis. There are three forms of porphyria that are associated with peripheral neuropathy as well as CNS abnormalities: acute intermittent porphyria (AIP), hereditary coproporphyria (HCP), and variegate porphyria (VP) (Fig. 12-13).[13,193–202] The acute neurologic manifestations are quite similar; however, a photosensitive rash is seen with HCP and VP but not in AIP. Attacks of porphyria can be precipitated by certain drugs (usually those metabolized by the P450 system), hormonal changes (e.g., pregnancy and luteal phase of the menstrual cycle), and dietary restrictions.

An acute attack of porphyria is often heralded by acute abdominal pain. Subsequently, patients may develop agitation, hallucinations, or seizures. Several days later, back and leg pain followed by weakness can occur and may mimic Guillian–Barré syndrome. Motor involvement can be asymmetric and can preferentially involve either proximal or distal muscles, and either the arms or legs. Cranial nerves can also be affected, leading to facial weakness and dysphagia. Sensory impairment may be difficult to determine if the patient is encephalopathic. Muscle stretch reflexes are often reduced. Autonomic dysfunction manifested by signs of sympathetic overactivity (e.g., pupillary dilatation, tachycardia, and hypertension) is common. Constipation, urinary retention, and incontinence can also be seen. Recovery is usually good, provided treatment is instituted rapidly to prevent excessive amounts of axonal damage.

Laboratory Features

The CSF protein can be normal or mildly elevated. Liver function tests and blood counts are usually normal. Some patients are hyponatremic due to inappropriate secretion of antidiuretic hormone. The urine may appear brownish in color secondary to the high concentration of porphyrin metabolites. The diagnosis is made by evaluating the urine or stool for the accumulating intermediary precursors of heme (i.e., δ-aminolevulinic acid, porphobilinogen, uroporphobilinogen, coproporphyrinogen, and protoporphyrinogen).[196] The reduced activity of specific enzymes can also be measured in erythrocytes and leukocytes. Genetic testing is available to confirm the specific defect.

Sensory NCS usually demonstrate normal NCVs and distal sensory latencies, but the amplitudes may be slightly reduced, although not to the same degree as the CMAPs are reduced.[195,196,198,199,201–206] Motor NCVs are only mildly reduced or normal, and distal motor latencies are normal or only slightly prolonged. The primary abnormality on NCS is the marked reduction in CMAP amplitudes. Needle EMG demonstrates primarily a reduced recruitment, fibrillation potentials, and positive sharp waves.

Histopathology

Axonal degeneration is apparent on nerve biopsies.

Molecular Genetics and Pathogenesis

The porphyrias are inherited in an autosomal-dominant fashion.[196] AIP is associated with porphobilinogen deaminase deficiency, HCP is caused by defects in coproporphyrin oxidase, and VP is associated with protoporphyrinogen oxidase (Fig. 12-13). The pathogenesis of the neuropathy is not

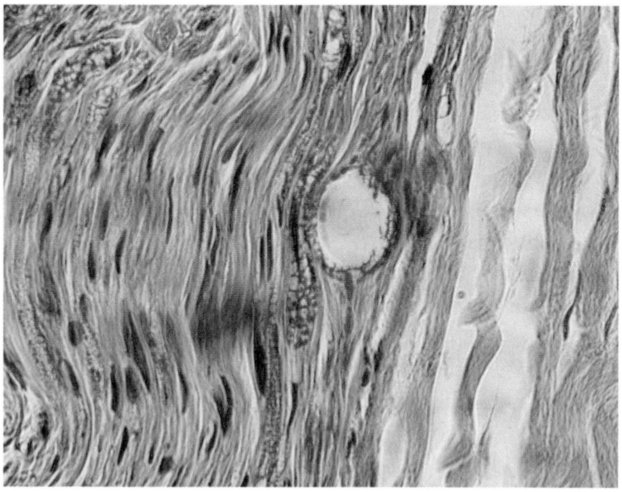

A

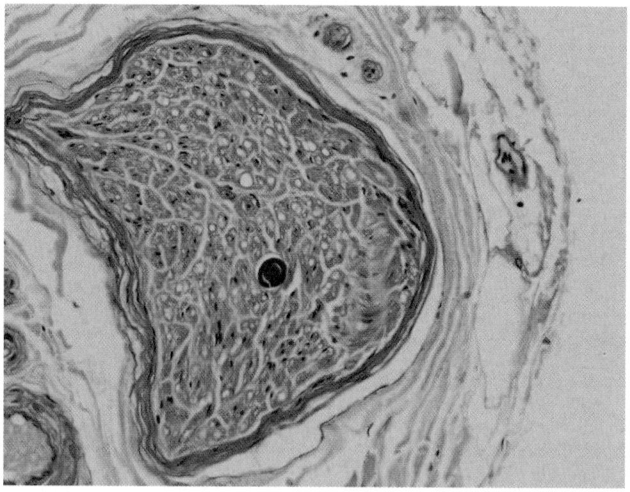

B

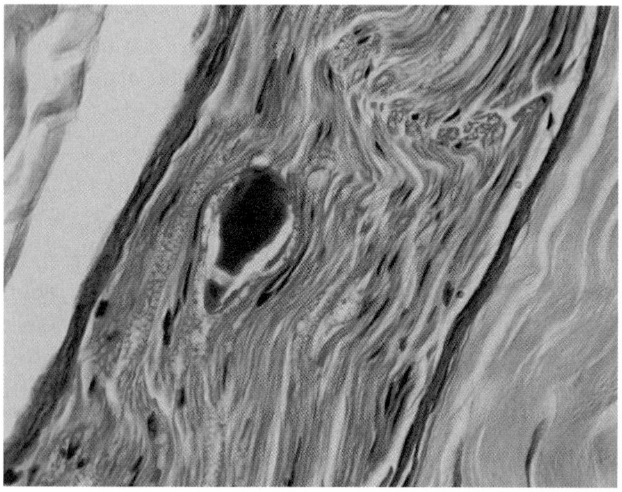

C

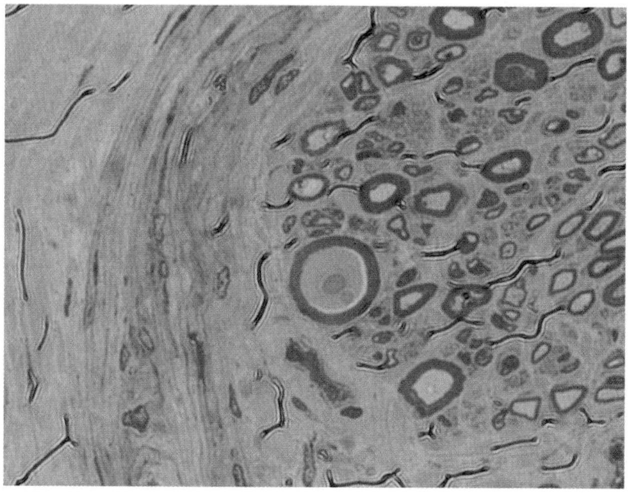

D

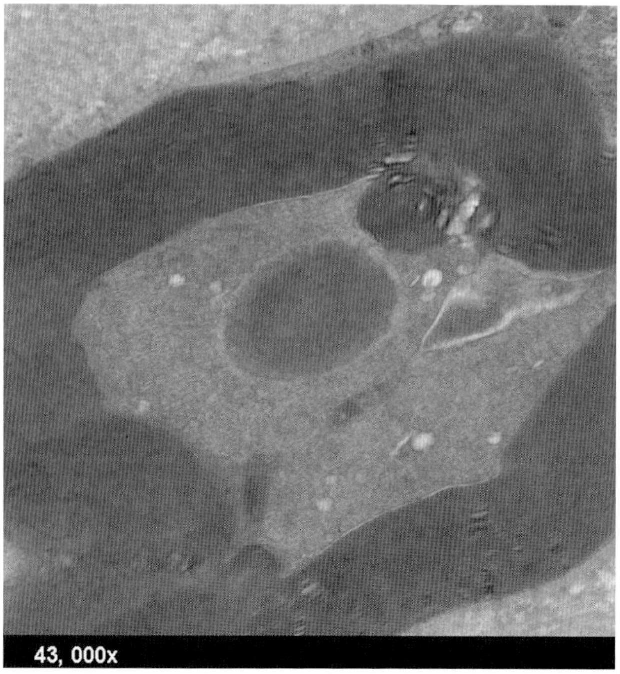

E

Figure 12-11. Adult polyglucosan body disease. Sural nerve biopsy demonstrates polyglucosan bodies within the axons in polyglucosan body neuropathy as seen trichrome stain **(A)**, PAS in cross-section **(B)**, PAS in longitudinal section **(C)**, on semithin section **(D)**, and electron microscopy **(E)**.

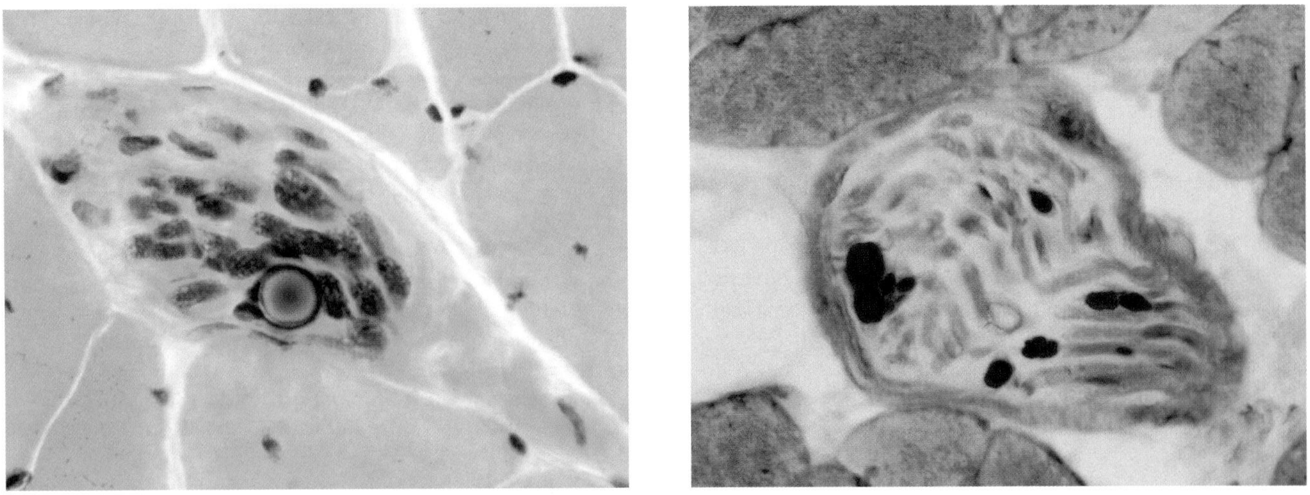

A B

Figure 12-12. Polyglucosan bodies can also be appreciated in nerve twigs on muscle biopsy, modified Gomori trichrome **(A)** and PAS **(B)**.

completely understood. The biochemical alterations in heme production may affect production of energy via effects on oxidative phosphorylation in the mitochondria. The inability to detoxify various drugs in the liver may have secondary toxic effects on the nervous system. Finally, some recent studies suggest that porphyrin precursor neurotoxicity may arise due to activation of transcription factors pivotal in regulating cell survival.[207,208]

Treatment

Patients should be treated with hematin and glucose to reduce the accumulation of heme precursors. Intravenous glucose is started at a rate of 10–20 g/h. If there is no improvement within 24 hours, intravenous hematin 2–5 mg/kg per day for 3–14 days should be given. This hematin dose can be infused over a 30–60-minute period. Drugs that can precipitate the acute porphyric attack should be avoided.

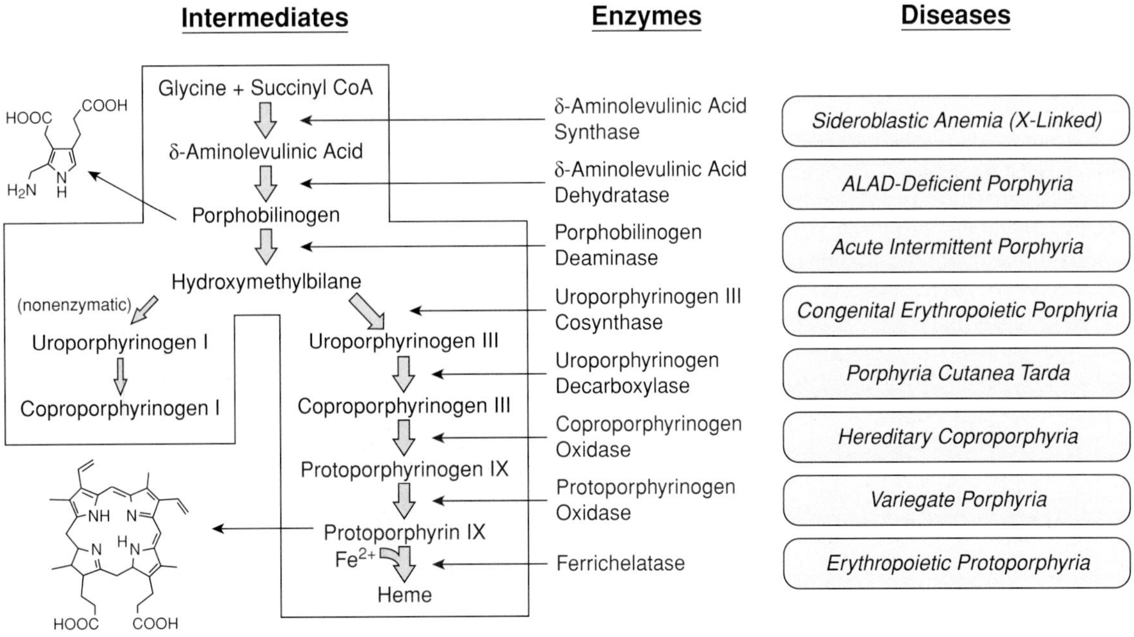

Figure 12-13. Porphyria pathway. Schematic representation of hepatic heme synthesis pathway. Defects in specific enzymes at various intermediate steps (boxes) controlling the synthesis of heme can lead to different clinical forms of porphyria. All of the noted diseases (boxes) have the potential to result in a neuropathy except porphyria cutanea tarda.

▶ SUMMARY

These hereditary neuropathies are uncommon but need to be considered in the right clinical context. Because of the hereditary nature of these neuropathies, some of which are quite devastating, diagnosis is important particularly for genetic counseling. With the exception of Fabry disease in which enzyme replacement therapy is available and perhaps ALD/AMN in which patients may be treated with Lorenzo oil, most of these disorders can only be treated symptomatically.

REFERENCES

1. Clark JR, Miller RG, Vidgoff JM. Juvenile-onset metachromatic leukodystrophy: biochemical and electrophysiologic studies. *Neurology*. 1979;29:346–353.
2. Cruz Martinez A, Ferrer MT, Fueyo E, Galdos L. Peripheral neuropathy detected on electrophysiological study as first manifestation of metachromatic leukodystrophy in infancy. *J Neurol Neurosurg Psychiatry*. 1975;38:169–174.
3. Dayan AD. Peripheral neuropathy of metachromatic leukodystrophy: observations on segmental demyelination and remyelination and the intracellular distribution of sulphatide. *J Neurol Neurosurg Psychiatry*. 1967;30:311–318.
4. Fullerton PM. Peripheral nerve conduction in metachromatic leukodystrophy (Sulphatide lipodosis). *J Neurol Neurosurg Psychiatry*. 1964;27:100–105.
5. Hahn AF, Gordon BA, Feleki V, Gilbert JJ. A variant form of metachromatic leukodystrophy without arylsulfatase deficiency. *Ann Neurol*. 1982;12:33–36.
6. Martin JJ, Ceuterick C, Mercelis R, Joris C. Pathology of peripheral nerves in metachromatic leukodystrophy: a comparative study of ten cases. *J Neurol Sci*. 1982;53:95–112.
7. Shapiro LJ, Aleck KA, Kaback MM, et al. Metachromatic leukodystrophy without arylsulfatase deficiency. *Pediatr Res*. 1979;13:1179–1181.
8. Yudell A, Gomez MR, Lambert EH, Dockerty MB. The neuropathy of sulfatide lipidosis (metachromatic leukodystrophy). *Neurology*. 1967;17:103–111.
9. Cameron CL, Kang PB, Burns TM, Darras BT, Jones HR Jr. Multifocal slowing of nerve conduction in metachromatic leukodystrophy. *Muscle Nerve*. 2004;29(4):531–536.
10. Coulter-Mackie MB, Applegarth DA, Toone JR, Gagnier L, Anzarut AR, Hendson G. Isolated peripheral neuropathy in atypical metachromatic leukodystrophy: a recurrent mutation. *Can J Neurol Sci*. 2002;29:159–163.
11. Comabella M, Waye JS, Raguer N, et al. Late-onset metachromatic leukodystrophy clinically presenting as isolated peripheral neuropathy: Compound heterozygosity for the IVS2+1G->A mutation and a newly identified missense mutation (Thr408Ile) in a Spanish family. *Ann Neurol*. 2001;50:108–112.
12. Bindu PS, Mahadevan A, Taly AB, Christopher R, Gayathri N, Shankar SK. Peripheral neuropathy in metachromatic leucodystrophy. A study of 40 cases from south India. *J Neurol Neurosurg Psychiatry*. 2005;76:1698–1701.
13. Kararizou E, Karandreas N, Davaki P, Davou R, Vassilopoulos D. Polyneuropathies in teenagers: a clinicopathological study of 45 cases. *Neuromuscul Disord*. 2006;16:304–307.
14. MacFaul R, Cavanagh N, Lake BD, Stephens R, Whitfield AE. Metachromatic leukodystrophy: review of 38 cases. *J Neurol Neurosurg Psychiatry*. 1982;57:168–175.
15. Wulff CH, Trojaborg W. Adult metachromatic leukodystrophy: neurophysiologic findings. *Neurology*. 1985;35:1776–1778.
16. Pilz H, Hopf HC. A preclinical case of late adult metachromatic leukodystrophy? *J Neurol Neurosurg Psychiatry*. 1972;35:360–364.
17. Thomas PK, King RH, Kocen RS, Brett EM. Comparative ultrastructural observations on peripheral nerve abnormalities in the late infantile, juvenile and late onset forms of metachromatic leukodystrophy. *Acta Neuropathol (Berl)*. 1977;39:237–245.
18. Gieselmann V, Zlotogora J, Harris A, Wenger DA, Morris CP. Molecular genetics of metachromatic leukodystrophy. *Hum Mutat*. 1994;4:233–242.
19. Krivit W, Peters C, Shapiro EG. Bone marrow transplantation as effective therapy of central nervous system disease in globoid cell leukodystrophy, metachromatic leukodystrophy, adrenoleukodystrophy, mannosidosis, fucosidosis, aspartylglucosaminuria, Hurler, Maroteau–Lamy, Sly syndromes, and Gaucher disease type III. *Curr Opin Neurol*. 1999;12:167–176.
20. Darras BT, Kwan ES, Gilmore HE, Ehrenberg BL, Rabe EF. Globoid cell leukodystrophy: cranial computed tomography and evoked potentials. *J Child Neurol*. 1986;1:126–130.
21. Dunn HG, Lake BD, Dolman CL, Wilson J. The neuropathy of Krabbe's infantile cerebral sclerosis. *Brain*. 1969;92:329–344.
22. Dunn HG, Dolman CL, Farrell DF, Tischler B, Hasinoff C, Woolf LI. Krabbe's leukodystrophy without globoid cells. *Neurology*. 1976;26:1035–1041.
23. Gutmann L, Hogan G, Chou SM. The peripheral neuropathy of Krabbe's (globoid) leukodystrophy. *Electroencephalogr Clin Neurophysiol*. 1969;27:715–716.
24. Hagberg B. The clinical diagnosis of Krabbe's infantile leukodystrophy. *Acta Paediatr*. 1963;52:213.
25. Hogan GR, Gutmann L, Chou SM. The peripheral neuropathy of Krabbe's (globoid) leukodystrophy. *Neurology*. 1969;19:1094–1100.
26. Lieberman JS, Oshtory M, Taylor RG, Dreyfus PM. Perinatal neuropathy as an early manifestation of Krabbe's leukodystrophy. *Arch Neurol*. 1980;37:446–447.
27. Loonen MC, Van Diggelsen OP, Janse HC, Kleijer WJ, Arts WF. Late-onset globoid cell leukodystrophy (Krabbe's disease). Clinical and genetic delineation of two forms and their relation to the early infantile form. *Neuropediatrics*. 1985;16:137–142.
28. Thomas PK, Halpern JP, King RH, Patrick D. Galactosylceramide lipidosis: novel presentation as a slowly progressive spinocerebellar degeneration. *Ann Neurol*. 1984;16:618–620.
29. Korn-Lubetzki I, Dor-Wollman T, Soffer D, Raas-Rothschild A, Hurvitz H, Nevo Y. Early peripheral nervous system manifestations of infantile Krabbe disease. *Pediatr Neurol*. 2006;28:115–118.
30. Siddiqi ZA, Sanders DB, Massey JM. Peripheral neuropathy in Krabbe disease: electrodiagnostic findings. *Neurology*. 2006;67:263–267.
31. Debs R, Froissart R, Aubourg P, et al. Krabbe disease in adults: phenotypic and genotypic update from a series of 11 cases and a review. *J Inherit Metab Dis*. 2013;36:859–868.

32. Malandrini A, D'Eramo C, Palmeri S, et al. Peripheral neuropathy in late-onset Krabbe disease: Report of three cases. *Neurol Sci.* 2013;34:79–83.
33. Marks HG, Scavina MT, Kolodny EH, Palmieri M, Childs J. Krabbe's disease presenting as a peripheral neuropathy. *Muscle Nerve.* 1997;20:1024–1028.
34. Sato JI, Tokumoto H, Kurohara K, et al. Adult-onset Krabbe disease with homozygous T1853 C mutation in the galactocerebroside gene. Unusual MRI findings of corticospinal tract demyelination. *Neurology.* 1997;49:1392–1399.
35. Jardim LB, Giugliani R, Pires RF, et al. Protracted course of Krabbe disease in an adult patient bearing a novel mutation. *Hum Mol Genet.* 1999;56:1014–1017.
36. Sabatelli M, Quaranta L, Madia F, et al. Peripheral neuropathy with hypomyelinating features in adult-onset Krabbe's disease. *Neuromuscul Disord.* 2002;12:386–391.
37. Matsumoto R, Oka N, Nagahama Y, Akiguchi I, Kimura J. Peripheral neuropathy in late-onset Krabbe's disease: histochemical and ultrastructural findings. *Acta Neuropathol (Berl).* 1996;92:635–639.
38. Krivit W, Shapiro EG, Peters C, et al. Hematopoietic stem cell transplantation in globoid-cell leukodystrophy. *N Engl J Med.* 1998;338:1119–1126.
39. Siddiqi ZA, Sanders DB, Massey JM. Peripheral neuropathy in Krabbe disease: effect of hematopoietic stem cell transplantation. *Neurology.* 2006;67:268–272.
40. Fukuhara N, Suzuki M, Fujita N, et al. Fabry's disease on the mechanism of the peripheral nerve involvement. *Acta Neuropathol (Berl).* 1975;33:9–21.
41. Kocen RS, Thomas PK. Peripheral nerve involvement in Fabry's disease. *Arch Neurol.* 1970;22:81–88.
42. Ohnishi A, Dyck PJ. Loss of small peripheral sensory neurons in Fabry's disease. *Arch Neurol.* 1974;31:120–127.
43. Sheth KJ, Swick HM. Peripheral nerve conduction in Fabry's disease. *Ann Neurol.* 1980;7:319–323.
44. Lacomis D, Roeske-Anderson L, Mathie L. Neuropathy and Fabry's disease. *Muscle Nerve.* 2005;31:102–107.
45. Dutsch M, Marthol H, Stemper B, Brys M, Haendl T, Hilz MJ. Small fiber dysfunction predominates in Fabry neuropathy. *J Clin Neurophysiol.* 2002;19(6):575–586.
46. Scott LJ, Griffin JW, Luciano C, et al. Quantitative analysis of epidermal innervation in Fabry disease. *Neurology.* 1999;52:1249–1254.
47. Luciano CA, Russell JW, Banerjee TK, et al. Physiological characterization of neuropathy in Fabry's disease. *Muscle Nerve.* 2002;26:622–629.
48. Toyooka K. Fabry disease. *Handb Clin Neurol.* 2013;115:629–642.
49. Üçeyler N, Kahn AK, Kramer D, et al. Impaired small fiber conduction in patients with Fabry disease: a neurophysiological case-control study. *BMC Neurol.* 2013;13:47.
50. Üçeyler N, He L, Schönfeld D, et al. Small fibers in Fabry disease: baseline and follow-up data under enzyme replacement therapy. *J Peripher Nerv Syst.* 2011;16:304–314.
51. Bersano A, Lanfranconi S, Valcarenghi C, Bresolin N, Micieli G, Baron P. Neurological features of Fabry disease: Clinical, pathophysiological aspects and therapy. *Acta Neurol Scand.* 2012;126:77–97.
52. Liguori R, Di Stasi V, Bugiardini E, et al. Small fiber neuropathy in female patients with Fabry disease. *Muscle Nerve.* 2010;41:409–412.
53. Hilz MJ, Brys M, Marthol H, Stemper B, Dutsch M. Enzyme replacement therapy improves function of C-, Adelta-, and Abeta-nerve fibers in Fabry neuropathy. *Neurology.* 2004;62:1066–1072.
54. Schiffmann R, Floeter MK, Dambrosia JM, et al. Enzyme replacement therapy improves peripheral nerve and sweat function in Fabry disease. *Muscle Nerve.* 2003;28:703–710.
55. Aubourg P, Scotto J, Rocchiccioli F, Feldmann-Pautrat D, Robain O. Neonatal adrenoleukodystrophy. *J Neurol Neurosurg Psychiatry.* 1986;49:77–86.
56. Griffin JW, Goren E, Schaumburg H, Engel WK, Loriaux L. Adrenomyeloneuropathy: A probable variant of adrenoleukodystrophy. *Neurology.* 1977;27:1107–1113.
57. Martin JJ, Lowenthal A, Ceuterick C, Gacoms H. Adrenomyeloneuropathy: A report on two families. *J Neurol.* 1982;226:221–232.
58. Moser HW. Adrenoleukodystrophy: phenotype, genetics, pathophysiology, and therapy. *Brain.* 1997;120:1485–1508.
59. Vercruyssen A, Martin JJ, Mercelis R. Neurophysiologic studies in adrenomyeloneuropathy: a report of five cases. *J Neurol Sci.* 1982;56:327–336.
60. van Geel BM, Assies J, Wanders RJ, Barth PG. X linked adrenoleukodystrophy: clinical presentation, diagnosis, and therapy. *J Neurol Neurosurg Psychiatry.* 1997;63:4–14.
61. Moser H, Dubey P, Fatemi A. Progress in X-linked adrenoleukodystrophy. *Curr Opin Neurol.* 2004;17:263–269.
62. Engelen M, van der Kooi AJ, Kemp S, et al. X-linked adrenomyeloneuropathy due to a novel missense mutation in the ABCD1 start codon presenting as demyelinating neuropathy. *J Peripher Nerv Syst.* 2011;16:353–355.
63. Chaudhry V, Moser HW, Cornblath DR. Nerve conduction studies in adrenomyeloneuropathy. *J Neurol Neurosurg Psychiatry.* 1996;61(2):181–185.
64. Moser AB, Kreiter N, Bezman L, et al. Plasma very long chain fatty acids in 3000 peroxisomal disease patients and 29000 controls. *Ann Neurol.* 1999;45:100–110.
65. Toifl K, Mamoli B, Waldhauser F. A combination of spastic paraparesis, polyneuropathy and adrenocortical insufficiency—a childhood form of adrenomyeloneuropathy? *J Neurol.* 1981;225:47–55.
66. van Geel BM, Koelman JH, Barth PG, Ongerboer de Visser BW. Peripheral nerve abnormalities in adrenomyeloneuropathy: a clinical and electrodiagnostic study. *Neurology.* 1996;46:112–118.
67. Powers JM, DeCiero DP, Cox C, et al. The dorsal root ganglia in adrenomyeloneuropathy: neuronal atrophy and abnormal mitochondria. *J Neuropathol Exp Neurol.* 2001;60:493–501.
68. Baumgartner MR, Poll-The BT, Verhoeven NM, et al. Clinical approach to inherited peroxisomal disorders. *Ann Neurol.* 1998;44:720–730.
69. Poulos A, Gibson R, Sharp P, Beckman K, Grattan-Smith P. Very long chain fatty acids in X-linked adrenoleukodystrophy brain after treatment with Lorenzo's oil. *Ann Neurol.* 1994;36:741–746.
70. Aubourg P, Adamsbaum C, Lavallard-Rousseau MC, et al. A two year trial of oleic acid and erucic acids (Lorenzo's oil) as treatment for adrenomyeloneuropathy. *N Engl J Med.* 1993;329:745–752.
71. Van Geel B. Progression of abnormalities in adrenomyeloneuropathy and neurologically asymptomatic X-linked adrenole-

ukodystrophy despite treatment with "Lorenzo's oil". *J Neurol Neurosurg Psychiatry*. 1999;67:290–299.
72. Eldjarn L, Try K, Stokke O, et al. Dietary effects on serum-phytanic acid levels and on clinical manifestations in heredopathia atactica polyneuritiformis. *Lancet*. 1966;1:691–693.
73. Gibberd FB, Billimoria JD, Page NG, Retsas S. Heredopathia atactica polyneuritiformis (Refsum's disease) treated by diet and plasma exchange. *Lancet*. 1979;1:575–578.
74. Refsum S. Heredopathia atactica polyneuritiformis: phytanic acid storage disease, Refsum's disease: a biochemically well-defined disease with specific dietary treatment. *Arch Neurol*. 1981;38:605–606.
75. Steinberg D, Mize CE, Herndon JH, Fales HM, Engel WK, Vroom FQ. Phytanic acid in patients with Refsum's syndrome and response to dietary treatment. *Arch Intern Med*. 1970;125:75–87.
76. Tuck RR, McLeod JG. Retinitis pigmentosa, ataxia, and peripheral neuropathy. *J Neurol Neurosurg Psychiatry*. 1983;46:206–213.
77. Verny C, Prundean A, Nicolas G, et al. Refsum's disease may mimic familial Guillain Barre syndrome. *Neuromuscul Disord*. 2006;16:805–808.
78. Jansen GA, Waterham HR, Wanders RJ. Molecular basis of Refsum disease: sequence variations in phytanoyl-CoA hydroxylase (PHYH) and the PTS2 receptor (PEX7). *Hum Mol Genet*. 2004;23:209–218.
79. Jansen GA, Ofman R, Ferndinandusse S, et al. Refsum's disease is caused by mutations in the phytanoyl-CoA hydroxylase gene. *Nat Genet*. 1997;17:190–193.
80. Wierzbicki AS, Lloyd MD, Schofield CJ, Feher MD, Gibberd FB. Refsum's disease: a peroxisomal disorder affecting phytanic acid alpha-oxidation. *J Neurochem*. 2002;80:727–735.
81. Jansen GA, Hogenhout EM, Ferdinandusse S, et al. Human phytanoyl-CoA hydroxylase: resolution of the gene structure and the molecular basis of Refsum's disease. *Hum Mol Genet*. 2000;9:1195–1200.
82. van den Brink DM, Brites P, Haasjes J, et al. Identification of PEX7 as the second gene involved in Refsum disease. *Am J Hum Genet*. 2003;72:471–477.
83. Dyck PJ, Ellefson RD, Yao JK, Herbert PN. Adult-onset of Tangier disease: 1. Morphometric and pathologic studies suggesting delayed degradation of neutral lipids after fiber degeneration. *J Neuropathol Exp Neurol*. 1978;37:119–137.
84. Engel WK, Dorman JD, Levy RI, Fredrickson DS. Neuropathy in Tangier disease. *Arch Neurol*. 1967;17:1–9.
85. Gibbels E, Schaefer HE, Runne U, Schröder JM, Haupt WF, Assmann G. Severe polyneuropathy in Tangier's disease mimicking syringomyelia or leprosy. *J Neurol*. 1985;232:283–294.
86. Haas LF, Austad WI, Bergin JD. Tangier disease. *Brain*. 1974;97:351–354.
87. Kocen RS, LLoyd JK, Lascelles PT, Fosbrooke AS, Willims D. Familial alipoprotein deficiency (Tangier disease) with neurological abnormalities. *Lancet*. 1967;1:1341–1345.
88. Kocen RS, King RH, Thomas PK, Haas LF. Nerve biopsy findings in two cases of Tangier disease. *Acta Neuropathol (Berl)*. 1973;26:317–326.
89. Pollock M, Nukada H, Frith RW, Simcock JP, Allpress S. Peripheral neuropathy in Tangier disease. *Brain*. 1983;106:911–928.
90. Zyss J, Béhin A, Couvert P, et al. Clinical and electrophysiological characteristics of neuropathy associated with Tangier disease. *J Neurol*. 2012;259:1222–1226.
91. Théaudin M, Couvert P, Fournier E, et al. Lewis-Sumner syndrome and Tangier disease. *Arch Neurol*. 2008;65:968–970.
92. Cai Z, Blumbergs PC, Cash K, et al. Paranodal pathology in Tangier disease with remitting-relapsing multifocal neuropathy. *J Clin Neurosci*. 2006;13:492–497.
93. Hager H, Zimmermann P. Licht- und electronenmikroskopische sowie cytometrische untersuchungern an peripheren nerven bei morbus Tangier. *Acta Neuropathol (Berl)*. 1979;45:53–59.
94. Zuchner S, Sperfeld AD, Senderek J, Sellhaus B, Hanemann CO, Schroder JM. A novel nonsense mutation in the ABC1 gene causes a severe syringomyelia-like phenotype of Tangier disease. *Brain*. 2003;126(Pt 4):920–927.
95. Bodzioch M, Orso E, Klucken J, et al. The gene encoding ATP-binding cassette transporter 1 is mutated in Tangier disease. *Nat Genet*. 1999;22:347–351.
96. Rust S, Rosier M, Funke H, et al. Tangier disease is caused by mutations in the gene encoding ATP-binding cassette transporter 1. *Nat Genet*. 1999;22:352–355.
97. Argov Z, Soffer D, Eisenberg S, Zimmerman Y. Chronic demyelinating peripheral neuropathy in cerebrotendinous xanthomatosis. *Ann Neurol*. 1986;20:89–91.
98. Berginer VM, Salen G, Shefer S. Long-term treatment of cerebrotendinous xanthomatosis with chenodeoxycholic acid. *N Engl J Med*. 1984;311:1649–1653.
99. Donaghy M, King RH, McKeran RO, Schwartz MS, Thomas PK. Cerebrotendinous xanthomatosis: clinical, electrophysiological and nerve biopsy findings, and response to treatment with chenodeoxycholic acid. *J Neurol*. 1990;237:216–219.
100. Katz DA, Scheinberg L, Horoupian DS, Salen G. Peripheral neuropathy in cerebrotendinous xanthomatosis. *Arch Neurol*. 1985;42:1008–1010.
101. Ohnishi A, Yamashita Y, Goto I, Kuroiwa Y, Murakami S, Ikeda M. De- and remyelination and onion bulb in cerebrotendinous xanthomatosis. *Acta Neuropathol (Berl)*. 1979;45:43–45.
102. Philippart M, van Bogaert L. Cholestanolosis (cerebrotendinous xanthomatosis). *Arch Neurol*. 1969;21:603–610.
103. Salen G, Berginer B, Shore V, et al. Increased concentrations of cholestanol and apolipoprotein B in the cerebrospinal fluid of patients with cerebrotendinous xanthomatosis. *N Engl J Med*. 1987;316:1233–1238.
104. Kuritzky A, Berginer VM, Korczyn AD. Peripheral neuropathy in cerebrotendinous xanthomatosis. *Neurology*. 1979;29:880–881.
105. Leitersdorf E, Safadi R, Meiner V, et al. Cerebrotendinous xanthomatosis in the Israeli Druze: molecular genetics and phenotype characteristics. *Am J Hum Genet*. 1994;55:907–915.
106. Ackroyd RS, Finnegan JA, Green SH. Friedreich's ataxia. *Arch Dis Child*. 1984;59:217–221.
107. Caruso G, Santoro L, Perretti A, et al. Friedreich's ataxia: electrophysiological and histologic findings in patients and relatives. *Muscle Nerve*. 1987;10:503–515.
108. Cruz Martinez A, Anciones B, Palau F. GAA trinucleotide repeat expansion in variant Friedreich's ataxia families. *Muscle Nerve*. 1997;20:1121–1126.
109. Dunn H. Nerve conduction studies in children with Friedreich's ataxia and ataxia telangiectasia. *Dev Med Child Neurol*. 1973;15:324–337.
110. Harding AE. Friedreich's ataxia: a clinical and genetic study of 90 families with an analysis of early diagnostic criteria and intrafamilial clustering of clinical features. *Brain*. 1981;104:589–620.
111. McLeod JG. An electrophysiological and pathological study of peripheral nerves in Friedreich's ataxia. *J Neurol Sci*. 1971;12:333–349.

112. Santoro L, Perretti A, Crisci C, et al. Electrophysiological and histological follow-up study in 15 Friedreich's ataxia patients. *Muscle Nerve*. 1990;13:536–540.
113. Salih MA, Ahlesten G, Stalberg E, et al. Friedreich's ataxia in 13 children: presentation and evolution with neurophysiologic, electrocardiographic, and echocardiographic features. *J Child Neurol*. 1990;5:321–326.
114. Klockgether T, Chamberlain S, Wüller U, et al. Late-onset Friedreich's ataxia. Molecular genetics, clinical neurophysiology, and magnetic resonance imaging. *Arch Neurol*. 1993;50:803–806.
115. Ragno M, De Michele G, Cavalcanti F, et al. Broadened Friedreich's ataxia phenotype after gene cloning. Minimal GAA expansion causes late-onset spastic ataxia. *Neurology*. 1997;49:1617–1620.
116. Klockgether T, Zühlke C, Schulz JB, et al. Friedreich's ataxia with retained tendon reflexes: molecular genetics, clinical neurophysiology, and magnetic resonance imaging. *Neurology*. 1996;46:118–121.
117. Caruso G, Santoro L, Perretti A, et al. Friedreich's ataxia: electrophysiological and histological findings. *Acta Neurol Scand*. 1983;67:26–40.
118. Pedersen L, Trojaborg W. Visual, auditory and somatosensory pathway involvement in hereditary cerebellar ataxia, Friedreich's ataxia and familial spastic paraplegia. *Electroencephalogr Clin Neurophysiol*. 1981;52:283–297.
119. Claus D, Harding AE, Hess CW, Mills KR, Murray NM, Thomas PK. Central conduction in degenerative ataxic disorders: a magnetic stimulation study. *J Neurol Neurosurg Psychiatry*. 1988;51:790–795.
120. Cruz Martinez A, Anciones B. Central motor conduction to upper and lower limbs after magnetic stimulation of the brain and peripheral nerve abnormalities in 20 patients with Friedreich's ataxia. *Acta Neurol Scand*. 1992;85:323–326.
121. Jones SJ, Baraister M, Halliday AM. Peripheral and central somatosensory nerve conduction studies in Friedreich's ataxia. *J Neurol Neurosurg Psychiatry*. 1980;43:495–503.
122. Zouri M, Feki M, Ben Hamida C, et al. Electrophysiology and nerve biopsy: comparative study in Friedreich's ataxia and Friedreich's ataxia phenotype with vitamin E deficiency. *Neuromuscul Disord*. 1998;8:416–425.
123. Campuzano V, Montermini L, Molto MD, et al. Friedreich's ataxia: autosomal recessive disease caused by intronic GAA triplet repeat expansion. *Science*. 1996;27:1423–1427.
124. Gray JV, Johnson KJ. Waiting for frataxin. *Nat Genet*. 1997;16: 323–325.
125. Pandolfo M. Molecular pathogenesis of Friedreich's ataxia. *Arch Neurol*. 1999;56:1201–1208.
126. Gotoda T, Arita M, Arai H, et al. Adult-onset spinocerebellar dysfunction caused by a mutation in the gene for the alpha-tocopherol transfer protein. *N Engl J Med*. 1995;333:1313–1318.
127. Guggenheim MA, Ringel SP, Silverman A, Grabert BE. Progressive neuromuscular disease in children with chronic cholestasis and vitamin E deficiency: diagnosis and treatment with alpha tocopherol. *J Pediatr*. 1982;100:51–58.
128. Jackson CE, Amato AA, Barohn RJ. Isolated vitamin E deficiency. *Muscle Nerve*. 1996;19:1161–1165.
129. Ouachi K, Arita M, Kayden H, et al. Ataxia with isolated vitamin E deficiency is caused by mutations in the alpha-tocopherol transfer protein. *Nat Genet*. 1995;9:141–145.
130. Krendel DA, Gilchrist JM, Johnson AO, Bossen EH. Isolated deficiency of vitamin E with progressive neurologic deterioration. *Neurology*. 1987;37:538–540.
131. Werlin SL, Harb JM, Swick H, Blank E. Neuromuscular dysfunction and ultrastructural pathology in children with chronic cholestasis and vitamin E deficiency. *Ann Neurol*. 1983;13:291–296.
132. Traber MG, Sokol RJ, Burton GW, et al. Impaired ability of patients with familial isolated vitamin E deficiency to incorporate alpha-tocopherol into lipoproteins secreted by the liver. *J Clin Invest*. 1990;85:397–407.
133. Kott E, Delpre G, Kadish U, Dziatelovsky M, Sandbank U. Abetalipoproteinemia (Bassen-Kornzweig syndrome). *Acta Neuropathol (Berl)*. 1977;37:255–258.
134. Muller DP, Lloyd JK. Effect of large oral doses of vitamin E on the neurological sequelae of patients with abetalipoproteinemia. *Ann N Y Acad Sci*. 1982;393:133–144.
135. Schwartz JF, Rowland LP, Eder H, et al. Bassen-Kornzweig syndrome: deficiency of serum b-lipoprotein. *Neurology*. 1963;8:438–454.
136. Sobrevilla LA, Goodman JL, Kane CA. Demyelinating central nervous system disease, macular atrophy and acanthocytosis (Bassen–Kornzweig syndrome). *Am J Med*. 1964;37:821–828.
137. Brin MF, Pedley TA, Lovelace RE, et al. Electrophysiologic features of abetalipoproteinemia: functional consequences of vitamin E deficiency. *Neurology*. 1986;36:669–673.
138. Lowry NJ, Taylor MJ, Bellknapp W, et al. Electrophysiological studies in five cases of abetalipoproteinemia. *Can J Neurol Sci*. 1984;11:60–63.
139. Miller RG, Davis CJ, Illingworth DR, Bradley W. The neuropathy of abetalipoproteinemia. *Neurology*. 1980;30:1286–1291.
140. Fagan ER, Taylor MJ. Longitudinal multimodal evoked potentials studies in abetalipoproteinemia. *Can J Neurol Sci*. 1987;14:617–621.
141. Martinez AC, Barrio M, Gutierrez AM, López. Abnormalities in sensory and mixed evoked potentials in ataxiatelangiectasia. *J Neurol Neurosurg Psychiatry*. 1977;40:44–49.
142. Woods GG. DNA repair disorders. *Arch Dis Child*. 1998;78: 78–184.
143. Savitsky L, Bar-Shira A, Gilad S, et al. A single ataxia telangiectasia gene product similar to PI-3 kinase. *Science*. 1995;268: 1749–1753.
144. Le Ber I, Moreira MC, Rivaud-Péchoux S, et al. Cerebellar ataxia with oculomotor apraxia type 1: clinical and genetic studies. *Brain*. 2003;126:2761–2772.
145. Castellotti B, Mariotti C, Rimoldi M, et al. Ataxia with oculomotor apraxia type1 (AOA1): novel and recurrent aprataxin mutations, coenzyme Q10 analyses, and clinical findings in Italian patients. *Neurogenetics*. 2011;12:193–201.
146. Amouri R, Moreira M, Zouari M, et al. Aprataxin gene mutations in Tunisian families. *Neurology*. 2004;63:928–929.
147. Barbot C, Coutinho P, Chorão R, et al. Recessive ataxia with ocular apraxia: review of 22 Portuguese patients. *Arch Neurol*. 2001;58:201–205.
148. Vantaggiato C, Cantoni O, Guidarelli A, et al. Novel SETX variants in a patient with ataxia, neuropathy, and oculomotor apraxia are associated with normal sensitivity to oxidative DNA damaging agents. *Brain Dev*. 2014;36(8):682–689.
149. Fogel BL, Perlman S. Clinical features and molecular genetics of autosomal recessive cerebellar ataxias. *Lancet Neurol*. 2007;6:245–257.
150. Le Ber I, Brice A, Dürr A. New autosomal recessive cerebellar ataxias with oculomotor apraxia. *Curr Neurol Neurosci Rep*. 2005;5:411–417.

151. Criscuolo C, Chessa L, Di Giandomenico S, et al. Ataxia with oculomotor apraxia type 2: a clinical, pathologic, and genetic study. *Neurology*. 2006;66:1207–1210.
152. Gazulla J, Benavente I, López-Fraile IP, et al. Sensory neuronopathy in ataxia with oculomotor apraxia type 2. *J Neurol Sci*. 2010;298:118–120.
153. Nanetti L, Cavalieri S, Pensato V, et al. SETX mutations are a frequent genetic cause of juvenile and adult onset cerebellar ataxia with neuropathy and elevated serum alpha-fetoprotein. *Orphanet J Rare Dis*. 2013;8:123.
154. Moreira MC, Klur A, Watanabe M, et al. Senataxin, the ortholog of a yeast RNA helicase, is mutant in ataxia-ocular apraxia 2. *Nat Genet*. 2004;36:225–227.
155. Vantaggiato C, Bondioni S, Airoldi G, et al. Senataxin modulates neurite growth through fibroblast growth factor 8 signalling. *Brain*. 2011;134:1808–1828.
156. Grunnet ML, Zimmerman AW, Lewis RA. Ultrastructure and electrodiagnosis of peripheral neuropathy in Cockayne's syndrome. *Neurology*. 1983;33:1606–1609.
157. Ohnishi A, Mitsudome A, Murai Y. Primary segmental demyelination in the sural nerve in Cockayne's syndrome. *Muscle Nerve*. 1987;10:163–167.
158. Sugarman GI, Landing BH, Reed WB. Cockayne syndrome: clinical study of two patients and neuropathologic findings in one. *Clin Pediatr*. 1977;16:225–232.
159. Rapin I, Lindenbaum Y, Dickson DW, Kraemer KH, Robbins JH. Cockayne syndrome and xeroderma pigmentosum. *Neurology*. 2000;55:1442–1449.
160. Moosa A, Dubowitz V. Peripheral neuropathy in Cockayne's syndrome. *J Neurol Neurosurg Psychiatry* 1970;45:674.
161. Lewis RA, Grunnet ML, Zimmerman W. Peripheral nerve demyelination in Cockayne's syndrome. *Muscle Nerve*. 1982; 5:557.
162. Vos A, Gabreels-Festen A, Joosten E, Gabreëls F, Renier W, Mullaart R. The neuropathy of Cockayne syndrome. *Acta Neuropathol (Berl)*. 1983;61:153–156.
163. Roy S, Srivastava RN, Gupta PC, Mayekar G. Ultrastructure of peripheral nerve in Cockayne's syndrome. *Acta Neuropathol (Berl)*. 1973;24:345–349.
164. Smits MG, Gabreels FJ, Renier WO, et al. Peripheral and central myelinopathy in Cockayne's syndrome. Report of 3 siblings. *Neuropediatrics*. 1982;13:161–167.
165. Tatin D. RNA polymerase II elongation complexes containing the Cockayne syndrome group b protein interact with a molecular complex containing transcription factor IIH components xeroderma pigmentosum B and p62. *J Biochem (Tokyo)*. 1998;273:27794–27799.
166. Asbury AK, Gale MK, Cox SC, Baringer JR, Berg BO. Giant axonal neuropathy—a unique case with segmental neurofilamentous masses. *Acta Neuropathol (Berl)*. 1972;20:237–247.
167. Igisu H, Ohta M, Tabira T, Hosokawa S, Goto I. Giant axonal neuropathy. *Neurology*. 1975;25:717–725.
168. Koch T, Schultz P, Williams R, Lampert P. Giant axonal neuropathy: a childhood disorder of microfilaments. *Ann Neurol*. 1977;1:438–451.
169. Kumar K, Barre P, Nigro M, Jones MZ. Giant axonal neuropathy: clinical, electrophysiologic, and neuropathologic features in two siblings. *J Child Neurol*. 1990;5:229–234.
170. Mohri I, Taniike M, Yoshikawa H, Higashiyama M, Itami S, Okada S. A case of giant axonal neuropathy showing focal aggregation and hypophosphorylation of intermediate filaments. *Brain Dev*. 1998;20:594–597.
171. Prineas JW, Ouvrier RA, Wright RG, Walsh JC, McLeod JG. Giant axonal neuropathy—a generalized disorder of cytoplasmic microfilament formation. *J Neuropathol Exp Neurol*. 1976;35:458–470.
172. Demir E, Bomont P, Erdem S, et al. Giant axonal neuropathy: clinical and genetic study in six cases. *J Neurol Neurosurg Psychiatry*. 2005;76(6):825–832.
173. Ouvrier RA, Prineas J, Walsh JC, Reye RD, McLeod JG. Giant axonal neuropathy—a third case. *Proc Aust Assoc Neurol*. 1974;11:137–144.
174. Berg BO, Rosenberg SH, Asbury AK. Giant axonal neuropathy. *Pediatrics*. 1972;49:894–899.
175. Carpenter S, Karpati G, Andermann F, Gold R. Giant axonal neuropathy. *Arch Neurol*. 1974;31:312–316.
176. Mizuno Y, Otsuka S, Takano Y, et al. Giant axonal neuropathy. *Arch Neurol*. 1979;36:107–108.
177. Bomont P, Cavalier P, Bondeau F, et al. The gene encoding gigaxonin, a member of the cytoskeletal BTB/Kelch repeat family is mutated in giant axonal neuropathy. *Nat Genet*. 2000; 26:370–374.
178. Aicardi J, Castelein P. Infantile neuroaxonal dystrophy. *Brain*. 1979;102:727–748.
179. Nardocci N, Zorzi G, Farina L, et al. Infantile neuroaxonal dystrophy. Clinical spectrum and diagnostic criteria. *Neurology*. 1999;52:1472–1478.
180. Raemakers VT, Lake BD, Harding B, et al. Diagnostic difficulties in infantile neuroaxonal dystrophy. A clinicopathological study of eight cases. *Neuropediatrics*. 1987;18:170–175.
181. Schindler D, Bishop DF, Wolfe DE, et al. Neuroaxonal dystrophy due to lysosomal α-N-acetyl-galactosaminase deficiency. *N Engl J Med*. 1989;320:1735–1740.
182. Mochel F, Schiffmann R, Steenweg ME, et al. Adult polyglucosan body disease: natural history and key magnetic resonance imaging findings. *Ann Neurol*. 2012;72:433–441.
183. Robitaille Y, Carpenter S, Karpati G, DiMauro SD. A distinct form of adult polyglucosan body disease with massive involvement of central and peripheral neuronal processes and astrocytes: a report of four cases and a review of the occurrence of polyglucosan bodies in other conditions such as Lafora's disease and normal ageing. *Brain*. 1980;103:315–336.
184. Klein CJ, Boes CJ, Chapin JE, et al. Adult polyglucosan body disease: case description of an expanding genetic and clinical syndrome. *Muscle Nerve*. 2004;29:323–328.
185. Cafferty MS, Lovelace RE, Hays AP, Servidei S, Dimauro S, Rowland LP. Polyglucosan body disease. *Muscle Nerve*. 1991;14:102–107.
186. Sindern E, Ziemssen F, Ziemssen T, et al. Adult polyglucosan body disease: a postmortem correlation study. *Neurology*. 2003;61:263–265.
187. Vucic S, Pamphlett R, Wills EJ, Yiannikas C. Polyglucosan body disease myopathy: an unusual presentation. *Muscle Nerve*. 2007;35:536–539.
188. Massa R, Bruno C, Martorana A, de Stefano N, van Diggelen OP, Federico A. Adult polyglucosan body disease: proton magnetic resonance spectroscopy of the brain and novel mutation in the GBE1 gene. *Muscle Nerve*. 2008;37:530–536.
189. Bruno C, Servidei S, Shanske S, et al. Glycogen branching enzyme deficiency in adult polyglucosan body disease. *Ann Neurol*. 1993;33:88–93.

190. Bruno C, van Diggelen OP, Cassandrini D, et al. Clinical and genetic heterogeneity of branching enzyme deficiency (glycogenosis type IV). *Neurology*. 2004;63:1053–1058.
191. McMaster KR, Powers JM, Hennigar GR, Wohltmann HJ, Farr GH Jr. Nervous system involvement in type IV glycogenosis. *Arch Neurol*. 1979;103:105–111.
192. Lossos A, Meiner Z, Barash V, et al. Adult polyglucosan body disease in Ashkenazi Jewish patients carrying the Tyr329 Ser mutation in the glycogen-branching enzyme gene. *Ann Neurol*. 1998;44:867–872.
193. Bonkowsky HL, Schady W. Neurologic manifestations of acute porphyria. *Semin Liver Dis*. 1982;2:108–124.
194. Ridley A. The neuropathy of acute intermittent porphyria. *Q J Med*. 1969;38:307–333.
195. Wenger S, Meisinger V, Brucke T, Deecke L. Acute porphyric neuropathy during pregnancy—effect of hematin therapy. *Eur Neurol*. 1998;39:187–188.
196. Albers JW, Fink JK. Porphyric neuropathy. *Muscle Nerve*. 2004;30(4):410–422.
197. King PH, Petersen NE, Rakhra R, Schreiber WE. Porphyria presenting with bilateral radial motor neuropathy: evidence of a novel gene mutation. *Neurology*. 2002;58:1118–1121.
198. Kochar DK, Poonia A, Kumawat BL, Shubhakaran, Gupta BK. Study of motor and sensory nerve conduction velocities, late responses (F-wave and H-reflex) and somatosensory evoked potential in latent phase of intermittent acute porphyria. *Electromyogr Clin Neurophysiol*. 2000;40(2):73–79.
199. Muley SA, Midani HA, Rank JM, Carithers R, Parry GJ. Neuropathy in erythropoietic protoporphyrias. *Neurology*. 1998;51(1):262–265.
200. Marcelis R, Hassoun A, Verstraeten L, De Bock R, Martin JJ. Porphyric neuropathy and hereditary delta-aminolevulinic acid dehydratase deficiency in adults. *J Neurosci*. 1990;95:39–47.
201. Hengstman GJ, de Laat KF, Jacobs B, van Engelen BG. Sensorimotor axonal polyneuropathy without hepatic failure in erythropoietic protoporphyria. *J Clin Neuromuscul Dis*. 2009;11:72–76.
202. Lin CS, Park SB, Krishnan AV. Porphyric neuropathy. *Handb Clin Neurol*. 2013;115:613-627.
203. Albers JW, Robertson WC, Daube JR. Electrodiagnostic findings in acute porphyric neuropathy. *Muscle Nerve*. 1978;1:292–296.
204. Anzil AP, Dozic S. Peripheral nerve changes in porphyric neuropathy: findings in a sural nerve biopsy. *Acta Neuropathol (Berl)*. 1978;42:121–126.
205. Bosch EP, Pierach CA, Bossenmaier I, Cardinal R, Thorson M. Effect of hematin in porphyric neuropathy. *Neurology*. 1977;27:1053–1056.
206. Flugel KA, Druschky KF. Electromyogram and nerve conduction in patients with acute intermittent porphyria. *J Neurol*. 1977;214:267–279.
207. Wilson GN. Tales from the neural genome: the lessons of homozygous porphyria. *Arch Neurol*. 2004;61:1650–1651.
208. Solis C, Martinez-Bermejo A, Naidich TP, et al. Acute intermittent porphyria: studies of the severe homozygous dominant disease provides insights into the neurologic attacks in acute porphyrias. *Arch Neurol*. 2004;61:1764–1770.

CHAPTER 13

Guillain–Barré Syndrome and Related Disorders

Landry described a condition characterized by acute ascending paralysis in 1859. Later, Guillain, Barré, and Strohl noted the areflexia and the albuminocytologic dissociation in the cerebral spinal fluid (CSF) associated with this neuropathy.[1] The contributions of Landry and Strohl have been neglected, and the neuropathy has been most commonly referred to as Guillain–Barré syndrome (GBS). In 1949, Haymaker and Kernohan detailed the histopathologic features seen in 50 fatal cases of GBS. The earliest features noted were edema of the proximal nerves and the subsequent degeneration of the myelin sheaths within the first week of the illness. They did not appreciate inflammatory cell infiltrate until later in the course of the illness.[2] However, another group reported prominent perivascular inflammation in the spinal roots, dorsal root ganglia, cranial nerves, and randomly along the whole length of peripheral nerves, along with segmental demyelination adjacent to the areas of inflammation, in 19 autopsy cases of GBS.[3] Thus, the term acute inflammatory demyelinating polyradiculoneuropathy (AIDP), which is quite descriptive of the disease process, has been historically used synonymously with GBS.[4–7] It is now appreciated that GBS is not a single disorder but again a syndrome of several types of acute immune-mediated polyneuropathies (Table 13-1).[8–11] In addition to AIDP, there are two axonal forms of GBS: acute motor–sensory axonal neuropathy (AMSAN) and acute motor axonal neuropathy (AMAN). Further, some disorders that appear clinically different from AIDP (e.g., the Miller Fisher syndrome [MFS] and acute autonomic neuropathy) may share similar pathogenesis and can be considered variants of GBS.

▶ ACUTE INFLAMMATORY DEMYELINATING POLYRADICULONEUROPATHY

EPIDEMIOLOGY AND ANTECEDENT ILLNESS

AIDP is the most common cause of acute generalized weakness, with an annual incidence ranging from 0.9 to 4 per 100,000 population.[7,10–13] The neuropathy can occur at any age, with a peak age of onset of approximately 38–40 years. There may be a slight male predominance.

Approximately 60–70% of patients with AIDP have a history of a recent infection a few weeks prior to the onset of the neuropathy.[7,10,11] A control study of 154 patients with GBS revealed serologic evidence of recent *Campylobacter jejuni* (32%), cytomegalovirus (13%), Epstein–Barr virus (10%), and *Mycoplasma pneumoniae* (5%) infection.[14] The serologic signatures of these infections were more prevalent than in the control population. Other studies have also reported that 15–45% of patients with AIDP have serologic evidence of recent *Campylobacter* enteritis.[15–22] The relationship between *C. jejuni* infection and the different variants of GBS (AIDP, AMSAN, and AMAN) has been the subject of many reports and is discussed in detail in the pathogenesis sections of these disorders. Other infectious agents associated with GBS include influenza, hepatitis A, B, C, and E, and human immunodeficiency virus (HIV).[7,10,20,23,24] In HIV infection, AIDP usually occurs at the time of seroconversion or early in the course of the disease.

Vaccinations, most notably for swine flu, have been associated with GBS.[25,26] Slightly increased risks of GBS have been associated with seasonal flu (influenza) vaccination. Most studies [27–31], but not all [32,33], have seen a slightly increased risk of GBS following H1N1 vaccination. No significant increased risk of GBS was found with meningococcus [34] and hepatitis [35] vaccinations, while one study of human papilloma virus (PPV4) revealed no increase in risk of GBS compared to other vaccinations.[36]

Other disorders have been associated with a possible increased risk of GBS, including other autoimmune disorders (i.e., systemic lupus erythematosus), lymphoma, organ rejection or graft versus host disease following solid organ and bone marrow transplantation, and perhaps recent surgery.[10] Certain immunomodulating agents, such as tumor-necrosis alpha blockers, may increase the risk of developing GBS.[37]

CLINICAL FEATURES

AIDP usually presents with numbness and tingling in the feet that gradually progresses up the legs and then into the arms (Table 13-2).[7,10,11,38] Numbness and paresthesia can also involve the face and trunk. Severe, aching, prickly, or burning neuritic pain sensations in the back and limbs are present in at least half the patients and may be particularly common in children. Large fiber modalities (touch, vibration, and

▶ TABLE 13-1. **GUILLAIN–BARRE SYNDROME AND RELATED DISODERS**

Acute inflammatory demyelinating polyradiculoneuropathy (AIDP)
Acute motor and sensory axonal neuropathy (AMSAN)
Acute motor axonal neuropathy (AMAN)
Other GBS variants
Miller Fisher syndrome
Idiopathic cranial polyneuropathy
Pharyngeal–cervical–brachial
Paraparetic GBS
Acute sensory neuronopathy/ganglionopathy
Acute small fiber neuropathy
Acute autonomic neuropathy

GBS, Guillain–Barré syndrome.

position sense) are more severely affected than small fiber functions (pain and temperature perception). Although initial symptoms are typically sensory in nature, progressive muscle weakness quickly becomes the dominant feature in most cases. Progressive weakness typically accompanies the sensory disturbance. The severity can range from mild distal weakness to complete quadriplegia and need for mechanical ventilation. Weakness is usually first noted in the legs and ascends to the arms, trunk, head, and neck. Ropper reported that 56% had onset of weakness in the legs, 12% in the arms, and 32% simultaneously in the arms and legs.[7,10] Occasionally, there is a descending presentation with onset in the cranial nerves, with subsequent progression to the arms and legs. Mild facial weakness is also often apparent in at least half of the patients during the course of the illness. Ophthalmoparesis and ptosis develop in 5–15% of patients. The bowel and bladder are usually spared, although these may become involved in particularly severe disease states. Muscle stretch reflexes progressively diminish and frequently become unobtainable in keeping with the multifocal demyelination and desynchronization of impulse transmission. Autonomic instability is common in AIDP with hypotension or hypertension and occasionally cardiac arrhythmias. Progressive reversible leukoencephalopathy syndrome (PRES) has also been associated with GBS and may rarely be the initial disease manifestation.[39–45]

The neuropathy usually progresses over the course of 2–4 weeks. Approximately 50% of patients reach their nadir by 2 weeks, 80% by 3 weeks, and 90% by 4 weeks.[7,10] Progression of symptoms and signs for over 8 weeks excludes GBS and suggests the diagnosis of chronic inflammatory demyelinating polyneuropathy (CIDP). Subacute onset with progression of the disease over 4–8 weeks has been termed subacute inflammatory demyelinating polyneuropathy. Patients with subacute inflammatory demyelinating polyneuropathy may have a monophasic illness like AIDP or may behave like CIDP and continue to progress unless treated with immunosuppressive or immunomodulating agents.

▶ TABLE 13-2. **DIAGNOSTIC FEATURES OF ACUTE INFLAMMATORY DEMYELINATING POLYRADICULONEUROPATHY**

I. Required for diagnosis
  1. Progressive weakness of variable degree from mild paresis to complete paralysis
  2. Generalized hypo- or areflexia

II. Supportive of diagnosis
  1. Clinical features
     a. Symptom progression: Motor weakness rapidly progresses initially but ceases by 4 weeks. Nadir attained by 2 weeks in 50%, 3 weeks in 80%, and 4 weeks in 90%.
     b. Demonstration of relative limb symmetry regarding paresis.
     c. Mild to moderate sensory signs.
     d. Frequent cranial nerve involvement: Facial (cranial nerve VII) 50% and typically bilateral but asymmetric; occasional involvement of cranial nerves XII, X, and occasionally III, IV, and VI as well as XI.
     e. Recovery typically begins 2–4 weeks following plateau phase.
     f. Autonomic dysfunction can include tachycardia, other arrhythmias, postural hypotension, hypertension, and other vasomotor symptoms.
     g. A preceding gastrointestinal illness (e.g., diarrhea) or upper respiratory tract infection is common.
  2. Cerebrospinal fluid features supporting diagnosis
     a. Elevated or serial elevation of CSF protein.
     b. CSF cell counts are <10 mononuclear cell/mm^3.
  3. Electrodiagnostic medicine findings supportive of diagnosis
     a. 80% of patients have evidence of NCV slowing/conduction block at some time during disease process.
     b. Patchy reduction in NCV attaining values less than 60% of normal.
     c. Distal motor latency increase may reach three times the normal values.
     d. F-waves indicate proximal NCV slowing.
     e. About 15–20% of patients have normal NCV findings.
     f. No abnormalities on nerve conduction studies may be seen for several weeks.

III. Findings reducing possibility of diagnosis
  1. Asymmetric weakness
  2. Failure of bowel/bladder symptoms to resolve
  3. Severe bowel/bladder dysfunction at initiation of disease
  4. Greater than 50 mononuclear cells/mm^3 in CSF
  5. Well-demarcated sensory level

IV. Exclusionary criteria
  1. Diagnosis of other causes of acute neuromuscular weakness (e.g., myasthenia gravis, botulism, poliomyelitis, and toxic neuropathy)
  2. Abnormal CSF cytology suggesting carcinomatous invasion of the nerve roots

CSF, cerebral spinal fluid; NCS, nerve conduction velocity.
Reproduced with permission from Amato AA, Dumitru D. Acquired Neuropathies. In: Dumitru D, Amato AA, Swartz MJ (eds). *Electrodiagnostic Medicine*, 2nd edn. Philadelphia, PA: Hanley & Belfus, 2002.

Approximately 25–30% of patients with AIDP develop ventilatory failure. Because the immune attack of AIDP has an early predilection for the nerve roots. For this reason it is important to follow the strength of neck flexors and extensors and shoulder abductors closely. These muscle groups are innervated by cervical roots close to the phrenic nerve (C3C4), and thus, correlate well with diaphragmatic strength and impending ventilatory failure. Once the disease nadir is reached, there is a plateau phase of several days to weeks followed by gradual recovery over several months. However, 50–85% of patients have some degree of residual deficits as many as 7 years after disease onset, with 5–10% of patients having disabling motor or sensory symptoms as well as severe fatigue.[7,10,11,38,46–48]

Furthermore, perhaps as many as 5–10% of patients who initially improve will have a relapse within a few days or up to 3 weeks after completion of treatment, and there are cases of CIDP that have begun acutely. It can therefore at times be difficult to ascertain initially if a patient will behave as AIDP or will evolve into CIDP and require long-term immunotherapy.

Subtypes and variants	IgG autoantibodies to
Guillain-Barré syndrome	
Acute inflammatory demyelinating polyneuropathy	None
Facial variant: Facial diplegia and paresthesia	None
Acute motor axonal neuropathy	GM1, GD1a
More and less extensive forms	
Acute motor–sensory axonal neuropathy	GM1, GD1a
Acute motor-conduction-block neuropathy	GM1, GD1a
Pharyngeal–cervical–brachial weakness	GT1a > GQ1b >> GD1a
Miller Fisher syndrome	GQ1b, GT1a
Incomplete forms	
Acute ophthalmoparesis (without ataxia)	GQ1b, GT1a
Acute ataxic neuropathy (without ophthalmoplegia)	GQ1b, GT1a
CNS variant: Bickerstaff's brain-stem encephalitis	GQ1b, GT1a

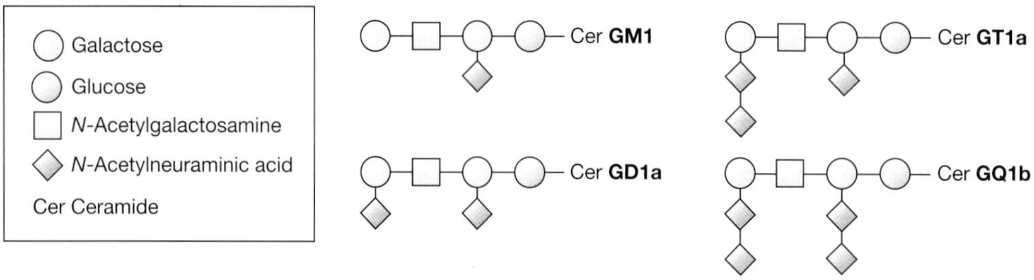

Figure 13-1. Spectrum of disorders in the Guillain–Barré syndrome and associated antiganglioside antibodies. IgG autoantibodies against GM1 or GD1a are strongly associated with acute motor axonal neuropathy, as well as the more extensive acute motor–sensory axonal neuropathy and the less extensive acute motor-conduction-block neuropathy. IgG anti-GQ1b antibodies, which cross-react with GT1a, are strongly associated with the Miller Fisher syndrome, its incomplete forms (acute ophthalmoparesis [without ataxia] and acute ataxic neuropathy [without ophthalmoplegia]), and its more extensive form, Bickerstaff's brain-stem encephalitis. Pharyngeal–cervical–brachial weakness is categorized as a localized form of acute motor axonal neuropathy or an extensive form of the Miller Fisher syndrome. Half the patients with pharyngeal–cervical–brachial weakness have IgG anti-GT1a antibodies, which often cross-react with GQ1b. IgG anti-GD1a antibodies have also been detected in a small percentage of patients. The anti-GQ1b antibody syndrome includes the Miller Fisher syndrome, acute ophthalmoparesis, acute ataxic neuropathy, Bickerstaff's brain-stem encephalitis, and pharyngeal–cervical–brachial weakness. The presence of clinical overlap also indicates that the Miller Fisher syndrome is part of a continuous spectrum with these conditions. Patients who have had the Guillain–Barré syndrome overlapped with the Miller Fisher syndrome or with its related conditions have IgG antibodies against GM1 or GD1 a as well as against GQ1b or GT1a, supporting a link between AMAN and the anti-GQ1b syndrome. CNS, central nervous system. (Reproduced with permission from Yuki N, Hartung H-P. Guillain-Barré syndrome. *N Engl J Med.* 2012;366:2294–2304.)

The diagnosis of acute-onset CIDP should be considered when a patient thought to have GBS deteriorates again after 8 weeks from onset or when there are 3 or more relapses.[49]

The mortality rate in GBS ranges from 2–5%, with patients dying as a result of respiratory distress syndrome, aspiration pneumonia, pulmonary embolism, cardiac arrhythmias, and sepsis related to secondarily acquired infections.[7,10,50] Most patients die during the recovery period and not while they are actually getting weaker.[50] Risk factors for a poor prognosis (slower and incomplete recovery) include: age greater than 50–60 years, abrupt onset of profound weakness, the need for mechanical ventilation, delay from onset of weakness to treatment, and cumulative distal compound muscle action potential (CMAP) amplitudes less than 10–20% of normal.[21,50–58]

LABORATORY FEATURES

Albuminocytologic dissociation, that is, elevated CSF protein levels accompanied by no or only a few mononuclear cells, is present in over 80% of patients after 2 weeks. However, within the first week of symptoms, CSF protein levels are normal in approximately one-third of patients. When CSF pleocytosis of more than 10 lymphocytes/mm^3 (particularly with cell counts greater than 50/mm^3) is found, AIDP-like neuropathies related to Lyme disease, recent HIV infection, or sarcoidosis need to be considered. Elevated liver function tests are common and may be attributed to viral hepatitis (A, B, C, and E), Epstein–Barr virus, or cytomegalovirus infection. Some patients develop hyponatremia due to inappropriate anti-diuretic hormone (SIADH) secretion.[59,60] Unlike the axonal forms of GBS, antiganglioside antibodies appear to be uncommon in AIDP (Fig. 13-1). However, antibodies directed against moesin, a protein expressed on peripheral nerve myelin, have been found in AIDP associated with recent CMV infection.[61] Enhancement of the nerve roots may be appreciated on magnetic resonance imaging of the spine.[62]

Various electrophysiologic criteria for demyelination have been developed to aid in the diagnosis of AIDP (Table 13-3).[8] The electrophysiologic features of demyelination include: prolonged distal latencies, slow conduction velocities, temporal dispersion, conduction block, and prolonged F-wave latencies.

MOTOR CONDUCTION STUDIES

Within the first week, motor conduction studies can be normal or show only minor abnormalities. The maximum degree of motor conduction abnormality occurs within 3–8 weeks, with 80–90% of patients with AIDP having abnormalities in at least one of the motor nerve parameters (distal CMAP latency, F-wave latency, conduction velocity, and/or conduction block) within 5 weeks of onset.[8,51,52,63–67] F-wave studies are useful because of the early predilection for the proximal nerve segments and spinal roots in AIDP.[51,52,63,68] Prolonged or absent F-waves and H-reflexes are found in 80–90% of patients during the course of AIDP.[51,52,63,69] They provided greater specificity for a demyelinating neuropathy when prolonged than when they are nonspecifically absent. Albers and colleagues found that prolonged distal latencies and diminished CMAP amplitude were the earliest electrophysiologic abnormalities.[63] Within 1 week of symptoms, the mean distal CMAP amplitudes were reduced to approximately 50% of normal and declined further over the next several weeks. Prolonged distal motor latencies and prolonged or absent F-waves were appreciated by the North American Guillain–Barré Syndrome Study Group, reported as the earliest abnormal features—findings that reflect the early predilection for involvement of the proximal spinal roots and distal motor nerve terminals in GBS.[51,52] Slowing of conduction velocities, temporal dispersion of the CMAP waveforms, and conduction block become

▶ TABLE 13-3. ELECTRODIAGNOSTIC MEDICINE CRITERIA FOR PERIPHERAL NERVE DEMYELINATION[a]

I. Conduction velocity reduced in two or more nerves
   1. If CMAP amplitude is >80% of lower limit of normal (LLN) then the NCV must be <80% of LLN
   2. If CMAP amplitude <80% of LLN, then the NCV must be <70% of LLN

II. CMAP conduction block or abnormal temporal dispersion in one or more nerves
   1. Regions to examine for these findings include
      a. Peroneal nerve between fibular head and ankle
      b. Median nerve between wrist and elbow
      c. Ulnar nerve between wrist and below elbow
   2. Partial conduction block criteria
      a. CMAP duration difference between the above noted proximal and distal sites of stimulation must be <15%, and
      b. A >50% drop in CMAP negative spike duration, or baseline-to-peak amplitude
   3. Abnormal temporal dispersion and possible conduction block
      a. CMAP duration difference between the above proximal and distal sites of stimulation is >15%, and
      b. A >20% drop in CMAP negative spike duration, or baseline-to-peak amplitude

III. Prolonged distal motor latencies (DML) in two or more nerves
   1. If CMAP amplitude is >80% of the LLN; then the DML must be >125% of the upper limit of normal (ULN)
   2. If the CMAP is <80% of the LLN, then the DML must be >150% of the ULN

IV. Prolonged minimum F-wave latency or absent F-wave
   1. F-waves performed in two or more nerves (10–15 trials)
   2. If the CMAP amplitude is >80% of the LLN, then the F-wave latency must be >120% of the ULN
   3. If the CMAP amplitude is <80% of the LLN, then the F-wave latency must be >150% of the ULN

[a]Three of the four features must be present.
Data from Cornblath DR. Electrophysiology in Guillain–Barré syndrome. *Ann Neurol.* 1990;(27suppl):S17–S20.

apparent later in the course. The motor conduction abnormalities remain at their nadir for approximately 1 month and then gradually improve over the next several weeks to months, but it may take a year or more for normalization.[63] There is no correlation between the nerve conduction velocities (NCVs) or distal motor latencies and clinical severity of the neuropathy, although distal CMAP amplitudes less than 10–20% of normal are associated with a poorer prognosis.[51–56,58]

Meulstee and colleagues applied the electrophysiologic criteria for demyelination designed by Albers et al.,[63] Barohn et al.,[70] and Asbury and Cornblath[51,52,71] to 135 patients with AIDP sequentially studied during the Dutch-GBS plasma exchange (PE) and intravenous immunoglobulin (IVIG) trials.[72] The sensitivity of the criteria for diagnosing demyelination ranged from 3–36% during the first study (performed at a median of 6 days, range 2–15 days after onset) to 13–46% during the third study (performed at a median of 34 days, range 29–49 days after onset).

SENSORY CONDUCTION STUDIES

Sensory studies in the arms can be affected more severely and earlier than the sural sensory nerve action potentials (SNAPs), resulting in a condition known as "sural sparing," a helpful diagnostic finding when present.[63] Sural sparing is not unique to GBS, however, and can be seen in other non-length-dependent neuropathy syndromes such as sensory neuronopathies. The exact explanation is multifactorial. Perhaps, entrapment sites are more prone to attack, which could account for slowing of the median SNAP across the carpal tunnel. More likely, because AIDP is a multifocal demyelinating disorder rather than a length-dependent process typical of most axonal neuropathies, the median, ulnar, or radial SNAPs may be affected prior to the sural SNAPs.

About 40–60% of patients eventually demonstrate either amplitude reduction or slow conduction velocities, with maximal abnormalities being seen after 4–6 weeks.[63,69] Reduced SNAP amplitudes can be the result of secondary axonal degeneration, conduction block, or phase cancellation related to differential demyelination and slowing of the sensory nerve fibers. Sensory conduction velocities can be slow and distal latencies prolonged. By definition, the AMAN variant of GBS is associated with normal sensory conduction studies.

Rarely, some persons may present with what appears to be pure sensory symptoms and signs, but careful evaluation usually reveals some motor nerve conduction abnormalities.[73,74] With a pure sensory presentation, other disorders (acute sensory neuronopathy or ganglionopathy) must be ruled out.[7]

NEEDLE ELECTROMYOGRAPHIC EXAMINATION

The earliest abnormality on electromyography (EMG) is a reduced recruitment of motor unit action potentials (MUAPs).[63] Positive sharp waves and fibrillation potentials may be appreciated 2–4 weeks after onset of weakness as some degree of axon loss is common even in AIDP.[75] Myokymic discharges may be seen, especially in facial muscles.

AUTONOMIC TESTING

Autonomic instability can be assessed by looking at heart rate variability with deep breathing or Valsalva maneuvers, with about 35% of patients demonstrating an abnormality.[76] Sympathetic skin response may be absent, but this has poor sensitivity.

HISTOPATHOLOGY

Nerve biopsies are not routinely performed in patients suspected of having GBS. Nonetheless, biopsies have demonstrated endoneurial and perivascular mononuclear cell infiltrate consisting of macrophages and lymphocytes may be seen on light microscopy.[7,77–79] There may be an initial preference for the nerve root region, areas where peripheral nerves are commonly entrapped (e.g., carpal and cubital tunnels), and the motor nerve terminals. The earliest pathophysiologic features are often appreciated at the nodes of Ranvier, where there is loosened paranodal myelin and subsequent demyelination of the internodal segments. Monocellular infiltrates may be appreciated in areas of segmental demyelination (Fig. 13-2). Polymorphonuclear cells, in addition to monocytes, may be associated with axonal degeneration in severe cases. During the recovery phase, remyelination is appreciated. Myelin thickness is reduced and the number of internodes is increased compared to normal peripheral nerve.

Autopsy studies of patients in China who died early in the course of their illness have shed light on the pathology of GBS, including AIDP, AMSAN, and AMAN.[80–83] In two patients who died at 7 and 9 days after onset of the neuropathy, autopsies revealed completely demyelinated peripheral nerves accompanied by extensive lymphocytic infiltrate.[82] However, in a patient who died only 3 days after symptom onset, the peripheral nerves had only scant inflammatory infiltrate and just a few of the nerves were completely demyelinated. Markers of complement activation were demonstrated on the outermost surface of the Schwann cells, and early vesicular changes in the myelin sheaths, beginning in the outer lamellae, were appreciated on electron microscopy.

PATHOGENESIS

A T-cell-mediated process may play a role, given the inflammatory cells apparent in the nerves, markers of

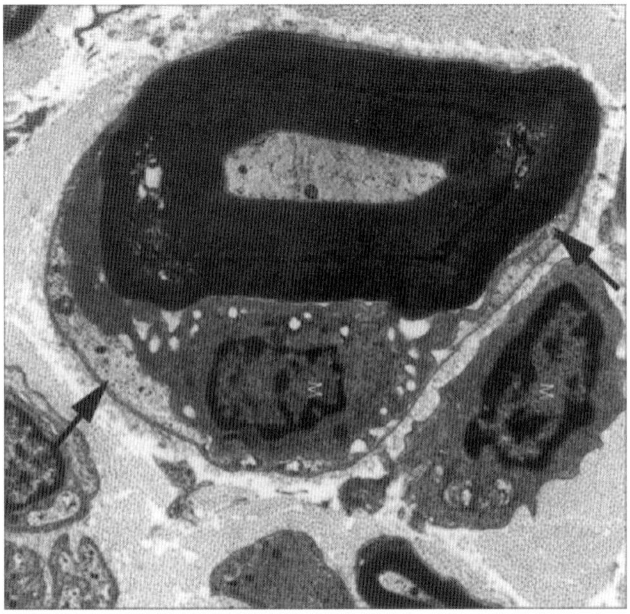

Figure 13-2. Nerve fiber from patient with AIDP. Electron micrograph shows that a macrophage (M) has invaded Schwann cell basement membrane and stripped the abaxonal Schwann cell cytoplasm (*arrows*). (Reproduced with permission from Hughes RA, Cornblath DR. Guillain–Barre syndrome. *Lancet.* 2005;366(9497):1653–1666.)

T-cell activation (e.g., soluble interleukin-2 receptor and interferon-γ) in the serum, and the resemblance to experimental allergic neuritis.[9,84–87] The humoral arm of the immune system has been implicated by the demonstration of ganglioside antibodies in many patients and the clinical improvement following plasmapheresis.[85,86] Further, injection of serum from patients with AIDP into nerves of animal models induces complement-dependent demyelination and conduction block.[88] Buchwald et al. investigated the effect of serum from 10 patients with GBS on mouse hemidiaphragm using a macro-patch-clamp technique and observed depressed presynaptic transmitter release and, in some cases, activation of postsynaptic channels.[89] The neuromuscular blockade was independent of complement, and there was no link to the presence (in six patients) or absence (in four patients) of antibodies to GM1 or GQ1b.

One study revealed that 56 out of 233 (23%) patients with GBS had circulating immunoglobulin G autoantibodies against proliferating, nonmyelinating human Schwann cells.[90] Immunofluorescence was localized at the distal tips (leading lamella) of the Schwann cell processes and of nerve-growth cones. Serum immunoreactivity was also observed in teased nerve fiber preparations. The authors speculated that the immune attack may be directed against nonmyelin proteins and epitopes possibly involved in Schwann cell–axon interaction.[90]

The nature of the epitope is not known but probably is a glycolipid. Molecular similarity between myelin epitope(s) and glycolipids expressed on *Campylobacter*, *Mycoplasma*, CMV, and other infectious agents, which precede attacks of AIDP, may be the underlying trigger for the immune attack.[11,82] Antibodies directed against these infectious agents may cross-react with specific antigens on the Schwann cell because of this molecular mimicry. These autoantibodies may bind to the Schwann cells and then activate the complement cascade, leading to lysis of myelin sheaths (Fig. 13-3).[11,82] Inflammatory cells are subsequently recruited to complete the demyelinating process.

TREATMENT

PE[53,54,91–93] and IVIG[54,94] have been proven effective treatments of AIDP (Table 13-4).[95–98] In the North American trial, PE reduced the time necessary to improve one clinical grade, time to walk unaided, time on a ventilator, and the percentages of patients improving after 1 and 6 months compared to the control group.[92] The French Plasmapheresis Group confirmed that PE was efficacious in GBS.[91] The exact mechanism is unclear, but it is likely that PE removes autoantibodies, immune complexes, complement, or other humoral factors involved in the pathogenesis of AIDP. The standard course of PE is 200–250 mL/kg of patient body weight over 10–14 days. Thus, a 70-kg patient would receive 14,000–17,500 mL (14–17.5 L) total exchange, which can be accomplished by 4–6 alternate day exchanges of 2–4 L each.

IVIG has replaced PE in most centers as the treatment of choice of AIDP. IVIG was shown to be at least as effective as PE in nonambulatory adults treated within the first 2 weeks in a prospective trial (Table 13-4).[54,94,99] Importantly, there is no added benefit of IVIG following PE, and it certainly makes no sense to give IVIG and then perform PE.[54] The dose of IVIG is 2.0 g/kg body weight infused over 2–5 days. Randomized trials are needed to decide the effect of IVIG in children, in adults with mild disease, and in adults who start treatment after more than 2 weeks.[95] IVIG may inhibit the binding of ganglioside antibodies to their respective antigens, thereby preventing complement activation and subsequent pathophysiologic effects.[100]

Treatment with IVIG or PE should begin within the first 7–10 days of symptoms. As the improvement with PE and IVIG is often not immediate (mean time to improvement of one clinical grade in the various controlled, randomized PE and IVIG studies ranged from 6 days to 27 days), there is often an impulse to augment the initial treatment attempt.[91,92,94] There is, however, no evidence that PE beyond 250 mL/kg[91,101–103] or IVIG greater than 2 g/kg are of any added benefit in patients with AIDP, who have stable deficits that are not improving as quickly as the patient and their physician would like. Further, as noted above, there is no indication for PE followed by IVIG or vice versa. Nonetheless, as many as 10% of patients treated with either PE [91,103] or IVIG [101,102] develop a relapse following initial improvement. In patients who suffer such relapses, we give additional courses of PE or IVIG.

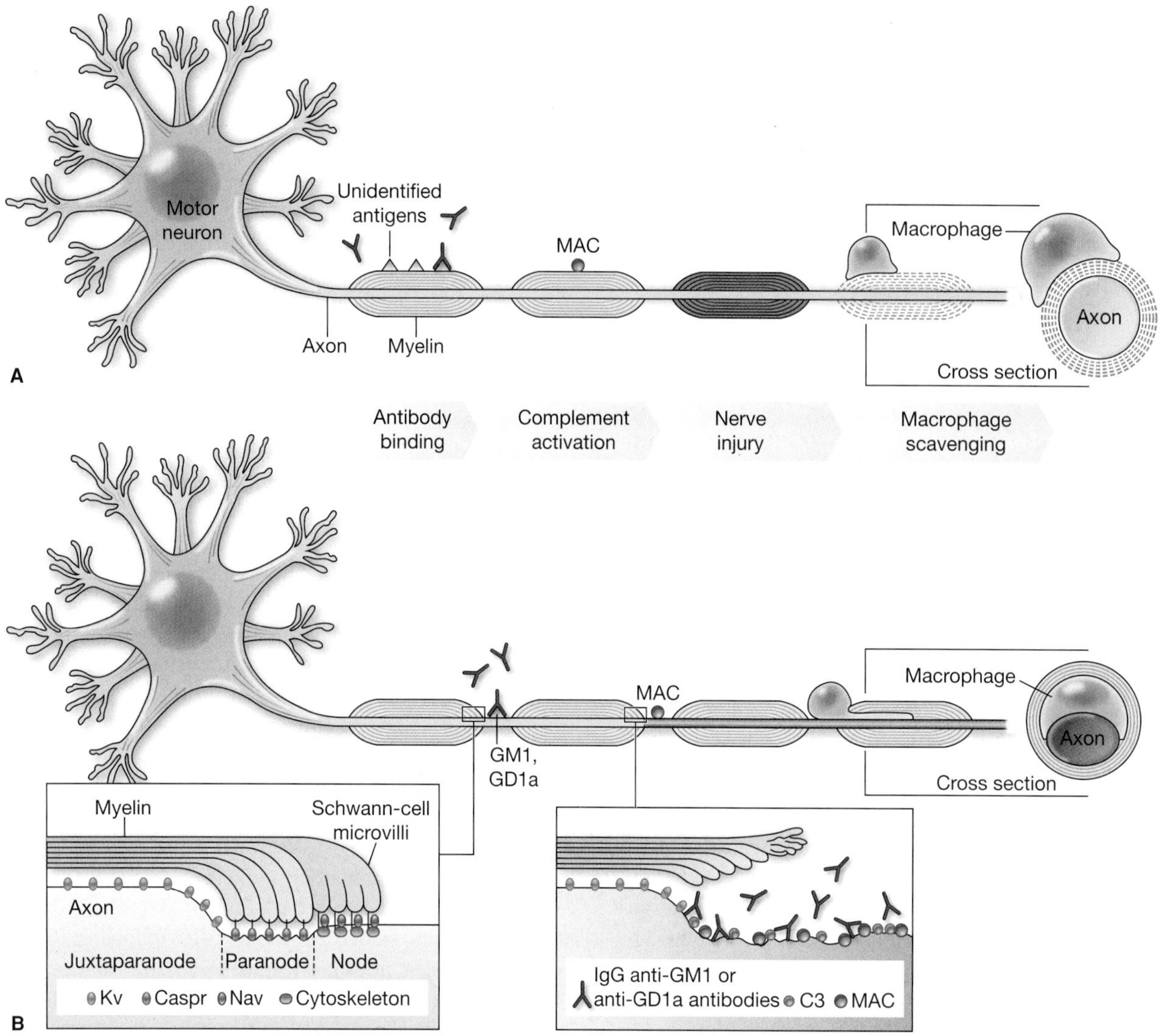

Figure 13-3. Possible Immune mechanisms in GBS. Panel A shows the immunopathogenesis of AIDP. Although autoantigens have yet to be unequivocally identified, autoantibodies may bind to myelin antigens and activate complement. This is followed by the formation of membrane-attack complex (MAC) on the outer surface of Schwann cells and the initiation of vesicular degeneration. Macrophages subsequently invade myelin and act as scavengers to remove myelin debris. Panel B shows the immunopathogenesis of acute axonal forms of GBS (AMAN and AMSAN). Myelinated axons are divided into four functional regions: the nodes of Ranvier, paranodes, juxtaparanodes, and internodes. Gangliosides GM1 and GD1a are strongly expressed at the nodes of Ranvier, where the voltage-gated sodium (Nav) channels are localized. Contactin-associated protein (Caspr) and voltage-gated potassium (Kv) channels are respectively present at the paranodes and juxtaparanodes. IgG anti-GM1 or anti-GD1a autoantibodies bind to the nodal axolemma, leading to MAC formation. This results in the disappearance of Nav clusters and the detachment of paranodal myelin, which can lead to nerve-conduction failure and muscle weakness. Axonal degeneration may follow at a later stage. Macrophages subsequently invade from the nodes into the periaxonal space, scavenging the injured axons. (Reproduced with permission from Yuki N, Hartung H-P. Guillain-Barré syndrome. *N Engl J Med.* 2012;366:2294–2304.)

Unlike CIDP, corticosteroids do not appear to be beneficial in the treatment of GBS, and some patients have done worse with steroids. A small study of 25 patients treated with IVIG and intravenous methylprednisolone[104] did better than a historical control group treated with IVIG alone.[94] However, a much larger British study of 142 patients treated with methylprednisolone or placebo (approximately half the patients in each group were also treated with PE) failed to demonstrate the efficacy of corticosteroids.[105] A double-blind, placebo-controlled randomized study of IVIG plus intravenous methylprednisolone compared to IVIG plus placebo in 233 patients with GBS revealed no significant difference between treatment with methylprednisolone and IVIG versus IVIG alone.[106]

▶ TABLE 13-4. **GUILLAIN–BARRÉ SYNDROME: PLASMAPHERESIS AND IVIG TRIALS**[54,91,92,94]

	Plasmapheresis Group	Control Group	IVIG Group
North American Trial			
Number of patients	122	123	
Time to improve one clinical grade (days)	19	40	
Time to walk unaided (all patients) (days)	53	85	
Time to walk unaided (ventilator patients) (days)	97	169	
Time on ventilator (days)	9	23	
Percentage improved at 1 month	59	39	
Percentage improved at 6 months	97	87s	
French Trial			
Number of patients	109	111	
Percentage of patients on ventilator after study (days)	18	31	
Time to wean from ventilator (days)	70	111	
Time to walk unaided (days)	28	45	
Time in hospital	21	42	
Dutch IVIG Trial			
Number of patients	73		74
% of patients improving one clinical grade after 4 weeks	34		53
Time to improve one clinical grade (days)	41		27
Time to clinical Grade 2 (days)	69		55
Ventilator dependent by week 2 (%)	42		27
Number of multiple complications	16		5
PE/Sandoglobulin Trial Group			
Number of patients	121		130
Mean change in clinical grade after 4 weeks	0.9		0.8
Time to wean from ventilator (days)	29		26
Time to walk unaided (days)	49		51
Number of patients unable to walk after 48 weeks	19 (16.7%)		21 (16.5%)

Reproduced with permission from Amato AA, Dumitru D. Acquired neuropathies. In: Dumitru D, Amato AA, Swartz MJ (eds). Electrodiagnostic Medicine, 2nd edn. Philadelphia, PA: Hanley & Belfus, 2002.

Thus, there is no strong support in the medical literature for supplemental corticosteroid use in patients with GBS.

▶ CHILDHOOD AIDP

Children with AIDP have clinical, laboratory, and electrophysiologic findings similar to affected adults.[8,79,96,107–111] An antecedent infection within 2 months of the attack is appreciated in approximately 75% of children having AIDP. Most children present with back and extremity pain. Generalized weakness, ventilatory failure, sensory loss (including sensory ataxia), and autonomic dysfunction can develop. Laboratory evaluation is remarkable for an elevated CSF protein. Sural nerve biopsies in children with GBS demonstrate similar histopathologic abnormalities as those described in adults.[79]

The clinical and electrophysiologic features as well as response to treatment are similar to what are seen in adu lts.[96,108–111] It is essential to look for ticks, particularly in children, as tick paralysis can mimic GBS.[9,112] Removal of the tick leads to improvement of strength and function.

▶ AXONAL GBS: AMSAN

CLINICAL FEATURES

Feasby and colleagues were the first to detail an axonal variant of GBS in 1986.[113] Initially, the existence of an axonal variant was met with early skepticism[55,113], however subsequent autopsy studies confirmed that AMSAN is a real entity.[80,81] Clinically and often by early electrodiagnostic studies, patients with AMSAN are indistinguishable from those with AIDP.[8,11,55,79–81,113–120] Usually, sensory symptoms begin in the hands or feet and later progress. Sensation to all modalities is reduced and areflexia is usually evident. Patients with AMSAN rapidly develop progressive and severe generalized weakness over only a few days, as opposed to progression over a couple of weeks in most patients with AIDP. Ophthalmoplegia, dysphagia, and ventilatory muscle weakness can occur. Dysautonomia including labile blood pressure and cardiac arrhythmias may complicate AMSAN as well. Recovery of strength and function is slow and often incomplete compared to AIDP.[118] Only a few children have been reported with AMSAN, and there is some suggestion that the prognosis is better than in adults.[113,120]

LABORATORY FEATURES

Albuminocytologic dissociation of the CSF protein is usually seen. Evidence of a recent infection with *C. jejuni* and antibodies directed against nerve gangliosides, particularly GM1 antibodies, are demonstrated in many patients with AMSAN.[11,81,121–123] NCS reveal markedly diminished amplitudes or absent CMAPs and SNAPs within 7–10 days of onset.[8,51,113,115–119,124,125] As discussed in the AIDP section, low-amplitude CMAPs are one of the earliest electrophysiologic abnormalities noted in AIDP; thus, low-amplitude CMAPs do not necessarily imply axonal degeneration. Distal conduction block with or without demyelination also leads to low-amplitude distal CMAPs.[55,114] Initially, it is often impossible to distinguish AIDP from AMSAN by nerve conduction studies; however, serial nerve conduction studies may be helpful.[114] Most patients with AIDP will eventually develop other features of demyelination (e.g., significantly prolonged distal latencies and F-wave latencies, slow CVs, more proximal conduction block, or temporal dispersion). The distal latencies of the CMAPs and the NCVs, when obtainable, should be normal or only mildly affected in AMSAN. Needle EMG demonstrates a markedly abnormal reduction in recruitment. Several weeks after the presentation of major motor weakness, abundant fibrillation potentials and positive sharp waves can be detected in most muscles, especially those located in the distal regions of the limbs.[122,123,126]

Antiganglioside antibodies, particularly GM1 and GD1a IgG antibodies, are found in some patients with axonal GBS (both AMSAN and AMAN) and correlate with recent *C. jejuni* infection (Fig. 13-1).[11,18,19,22,127] Serologic evidence of recent antecedent *C. jejuni* infection is evident in 15–45% of GBS patients.[7,10,11,14–19,21,22,128] Molecular mimicry between gangliosides expressed on nerve fibers and glycolipids present on *C. jejuni* may account for their association with axonal GBS and may play a role in the pathogenesis of the disorder. Gangliosides, which are proteins located on peripheral nerves, are composed of a ceramide attached to one or more sugar residues and contain sialic acid. The 4 major gangliosides in regard to GBS (i.e., GM1, GD1a, GT1a, and GQ1b) differ with regard to the number and position of their sialic acids (Fig. 13-3).[11]

HISTOPATHOLOGY

Nerve biopsy performed early in the course of the disorder may help differentiate "axonal" GBS from "pseudoaxonal" GBS that otherwise appear similar because of their clinical, laboratory, and electrophysiologic similarities. It nerve biopsies are not indicated however, in clinical practice. Nerves biopsied late in the disease course of AIDP or AMSAN may show axonal degeneration, and it can be difficult to distinguish a primary axonopathy from secondary axonal degeneration. Sensory and motor nerve biopsies in several patients with inexcitable motor and sensory conduction studies (i.e., AMSAN) revealed severe demyelination rather than primary axonal degeneration.[124,126,129–131] Nevertheless, some patients with inexcitable CMAPs and SNAPs have features that suggest a primary axonal insult.[80,81,113,116] Unlike AIDP, demyelination and lymphocytic infiltrates are absent or only minimally present on nerve biopsy or at autopsy in patients with AMSAN; rather, prominent axonal degeneration affecting the ventral and dorsal roots and the peripheral nerves is appreciated. As many as 80% of teased fibers reveal axonal degeneration, while demyelinating features are rare.[113,116] A marked loss of both myelinated and unmyelinated axons is evident. Griffin and colleagues reported that the autopsies of three patients with AMSAN who died early in the course of their illness; they found prominent axonal degeneration of the spinal roots and peripheral nerves without demyelination or significant inflammation.[81] Numerous macrophages were present in the periaxonal space of myelinated internode, as were rare intra-axonal macrophages. Similar histologic abnormalities are seen in AMAN but are not typically noted in AIDP. An autopsy on another patient with AMSAN demonstrated inflammatory cell infiltrates comprising lymphocytes and macrophages in the spinal cord.

PATHOGENESIS

The pathogenic basis of AMSAN is unknown but is most likely due to an immune-mediated attack directed against epitopes on the axon.[9,11,81,87] AMSAN often follows *C. jejuni* infection and may lead to the production of the antibodies directed against various nerve gangliosides (e.g., GM1 or GM1a) (Figs. 13-1 and 13-3).[11] These gangliosides are present on the nodal axolemma and may be the target of the immune attack due to molecular mimicry.[11,122,123] Early in the course or with mild disease, binding of the antibodies to neural epitopes may result in only physiologic conduction block. However, complement activation on nodal and later internodal axolemma and recruitment of macrophages can result in axonal degeneration.

TREATMENT

There have been no prospective treatment studies specifically for AMSAN; however, we treat patients with IVIG or PE.

▶ ACUTE MOTOR AXONAL NEUROPATHY

EPIDEMIOLOGY

McKhann and colleagues initially described this variant in patients with seasonal outbreaks of acute flaccid paralysis in northern China.[132,133] They initially named the disorder the "Chinese paralytic syndrome," but because similar cases subsequently were described throughout the world, the term "AMAN" is more appropriate.[134,135] In northern China, AMAN is the most common variant of GBS and, although it is less frequent in other areas of the world, AMAN is still quite common. In this regard, 27 of the 147 (18%) patients enrolled in the Dutch GBS trial comparing IVIG to PE were later classified as having AMAN.[94,135] An antecedent illness occurs in 30–85% of patients with AMAN—most often a gastrointestinal infection.[79,127,133,135] Consistent with this is the recognition that 67–92% of patients have had serologic evidence of a recent *C. jejuni* infection.[133,135]

CLINICAL FEATURES

AMAN occurs in children and adults, and similar to AMSAN, it begins abruptly, in this case with generalized weakness rather than sensory symptoms.[8,11,79,110,132–134,136] The distal muscles are often more severely affected than proximal limb muscles, while cranial nerve deficits and ventilatory failure requiring mechanical ventilation can be seen in up to one-third of patients.[132,133,135] Unlike AIDP and AMAN, there are no sensory signs or symptoms. However, autonomic dysfunction (e.g., cardiac arrhythmias, blood pressure fluctuations, and hyperhidrosis) may occur. Muscle stretch reflexes may be normal or absent, although some patients develop hyperactive reflexes during the recovery period.[65,133,134,137] The median time of recovery is similar to that seen in typical AIDP, and most affected individuals have a good recovery within 1 year. Residual distal limb weakness is common.[136] The mortality rate is less than 5%.[133] Second attacks of the illness have been described in northern Chinese patients, but the actual recurrence rate is not known.[133]

LABORATORY FEATURES

As with AIDP and AMSAN, albuminocytologic dissociation in the CSF is seen, and this absence of prominent CSF pleocytosis helps distinguish AMAN from poliomyelitis, which it would otherwise mimic.[132–135] Serologic evidence of recent *C. jejuni* infection and GM1 and GD1a are demonstrated in the majority of patients with AMAN (Fig. 13-1).[11,127,133,135,138]

NCS reveals low-amplitude or unobtainable CMAPs with normal SNAPs.[8,132–136,139] When CMAPs are obtained, the distal latencies and conduction velocities are normal, as are F-waves latencies when obtainable. The decreased CMAP amplitudes may be a reflection of distal conduction block, degeneration restricted to the distal motor nerve terminals, or widespread dying back axonal degeneration. Rare cases of proximal conduction block without other features of demyelination have also been reported.[65] EMG reveals fibrillation potentials and positive sharp waves and decreased recruitment of MUAPs.[132–136] Autonomic studies are relatively spared in AMAN compared to AIDP.

HISTOPATHOLOGY

The earliest histologic abnormality is lengthening of the nodal gaps. Immunocytochemistry reveals deposition of IgG and complement activation products (i.e., C3 and C5b-9) on the nodal and internodal axolemma of motor fibers rather than axonal degeneration.[82] In contrast, there is early deposition of immunoglobulin and complement on Schwann cells rather than the axons in AIDP.[82] Macrophages are recruited into the affected nodes of Ranvier and periaxonal space via complement-derived chemotropic factors.[82] The macrophages migrate through the Schwann cell basal lamina into the nodal gap, where these inflammatory cells dissect beneath the myelin sheath into the periaxonal space (Fig. 13-4). As macrophages enter the periaxonal space, the axon retracts away from the adaxonal Schwann cell. In severe cases, the axons then begin to degenerate but the innermost myelin sheath (adaxonal lamella) appears intact. Active degeneration and severe loss of large myelinated intramuscular nerve fibers can also be demonstrated on motor point biopsy.[136] An autopsy on a patient with AMAN demonstrated inflammatory cell infiltrates comprising lymphocytes and macrophages in the spinal cord.

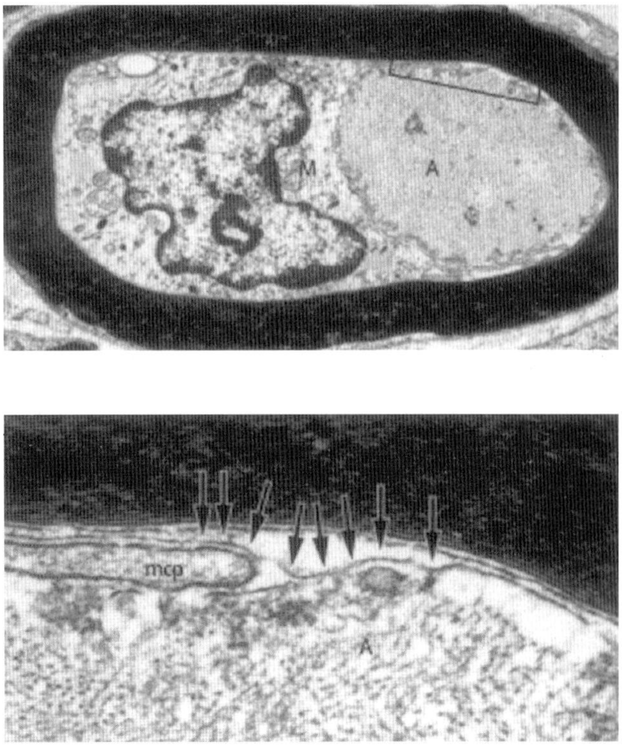

Figure 13-4. Nerve fiber from patient with AMAN. Lower panel is enlargement of box in upper panel. Electron micrograph shows macrophage (M) that has invaded the periaxonal space and axolemma (*arrows*) surrounding the axon (A); mcp, macrophage process. (Reproduced with permission from Griffin JW, Li CY, Macko C, et al. Early nodal changes in the acute motor axonal neuropathy pattern of the Guillain–Barré syndrome. *J Neurocytol.* 1996;25(1):33–51.)

PATHOGENESIS

AMAN is most likely caused by an immune-mediated attack against an unknown epitope(s) on the nodal axolemma (Figs. 13-1 and 13-3).[11] Axonal degeneration appears to develop predominantly in the motor nerve terminals, and only occasionally more proximally in the nerve roots.[139] Perhaps the antibodies are directed against GM1 or GD1a gangliosides that cross-react with the lipopolysaccharide membrane of *Campylobacter*.[82] The binding of antibodies to the nodal axolemma may decrease the sodium current or increase the potassium current, thereby resulting in conduction block.[140] Experimental studies demonstrate that GBS sera containing ganglioside antibodies cause neuronal cell lysis by targeting specific cell surface gangliosides and, secondly, that this cell lysis is complement dependent. In these studies, the GD1a cell membrane pool appeared to be more susceptible to ganglioside antibody-mediated injury than the GM1 pool. Of note, IVIG significantly decreased this complement-dependent cytotoxicity.

TREATMENT

There have not been any treatment trials devoted to AMAN, although 27 of the 147 (18%) patients enrolled in the Dutch GBS trial comparing IVIG to PE were later classified as having AMAN.[94,135] Subgroup analysis of the AMAN group suggested that the IVIG-treated patients may recover faster than PE-treated patients. However, there was no significant difference in outcome, regardless of treatment (IVIG, PE, or PE followed by IVIG) between AIDP and AMAN, in a subgroup analysis of 369 patients.[127]

▶ OTHER GBS VARIANTS

Besides AMSAN and AMAN, there are several other variants of GBS including the MFS (comprised of ataxia, areflexia, and ophthalmoplegia), idiopathic cranial polyneuropathy, pharyngeal–cervical–brachial weakness with or without ophthalmoparesis, and paraparetic weakness.[141–145] These disorders may represent oligosymptomatic or forme frustes of AIDP. Of these possible GBS variants, the MFS is best characterized. Other disorders that might be considered variants of GBS include acute sensory ganglionopathies and acute autonomic neuropathies.

▶ MILLER FISHER SYNDROME

CLINICAL FEATURES

MFS, first described in 1956, [141] is characterized by ataxia, areflexia, and ophthalmoplegia.[7,11,96,145–150] There is a spectrum between MFS and the syndrome of Bickerstaff encephalitis, which is associated with altered consciousness in addition to ataxia and, ophthalmoplegia.[146,147,151] The mean age of onset of MFS is in the early forties, but it can occur in children. There is a 2:1 male predominance. As with other forms of GBS, an antecedent infection is common, occurring in over two-thirds of the cases. Double vision is usually the earliest symptom (39%), followed by unsteadiness and incoordination due to a sensory ataxia (21%). Asymmetric oculomotor weakness may be seen, but this often progresses to complete ophthalmoplegia. Ptosis also occurs but pupillary involvement is uncommon. Other cranial nerves are also affected with facial weakness evident in 57%, dysphagia in 40%, and dysarthria in 13% patients. Approximately 50% of the patients complain of paresthesias of the face and distal limbs during the course, and areflexia is evident on examination in over 80%. Mild proximal limb weakness may develop in approximately one-third of cases, and some patients progress to develop severe generalized weakness similar to typical AIDP.[145,148–150] Recovery usually begins within about 2 weeks following the onset of symptoms, and a full return of function is usually seen within 3–5 months.

LABORATORY FEATURES

CSF protein is usually elevated without significant pleocytosis.[7,145] Serologic evidence of recent infection by *C. jejuni* and ganglioside antibodies, in particular anti-GQ1b, is evident in many patients (Fig. 13-2).[151–153] A large study of 123 patients with MFS demonstrated CSF albuminocytologic dissociation in 59% of patients during the first 3 weeks of illness, while serum GQ1b IgG antibodies were positive in 85%. While the incidence of CSF albuminocytologic dissociation increased from the first to second weeks, GQ1b IgG antibodies peaked in the first week. GQ1b IgG antibodies are also seen in Bickerstaff encephalitis.

NCS reveals reduced amplitudes of SNAPs out of proportion to any prolongation of the distal latencies or slowing of sensory conduction velocities.[8,151,154–158] CMAPs in the arms and legs are usually normal. However, mild-to-moderate reduction of facial CMAP amplitudes is evident in over 50% of patients with MFS.[155] A loss or mild delay of R1 and R2 responses may be appreciated on blink reflex testing.[149,155,159]

HISTOPATHOLOGY

Nerve biopsy and autopsy data are limited and need to be viewed cautiously, as some of the cases began with ophthalmoplegia, ataxia, and areflexia but later evolved to severe quadriparesis characteristic of more typical AIDP.[160] The brainstem appeared normal or revealed only secondary chromatolysis of the oculomotor, trochlear, or abducens nuclei. Demyelination and mild inflammatory infiltrates were noted along the course of these cranial nerves and in the sensory ganglia of peripheral nerves.

PATHOGENESIS

The pathogenic basis for the disorder is not known, although it is likely autoimmune, with preferential early attack directed against the sensory ganglia and oculomotor nerve fibers.[7,145] Recent antecedent infections (e.g., *C. jejuni*) suggest that autoantibodies directed against these infectious agents cross-react with neuronal epitopes (e.g., GQ1b) (Figs. 13-1 and 13-3).[11] In this regard, oculomotor fibers and the sensory ganglion are enriched in GQ1b and antibodies directed against this protein are detected in most patients with MFS. Immunohistochemistry studies reveal that GQ1b antibodies stain sensory neurons in the dorsal root as well as cerebellar nuclei. In mice infused with serum from patients with MFS, the GQ1b antibodies bound to neuromuscular junctions and, in a complement-dependent process, this resulted in massive quantal release of acetylcholine from nerve terminals; this lead to blockage of neuromuscular transmission.[161] The similarities between MFS and Bickerstaff encephalitis suggests that these disorders fall along a spectrum and there may be central nervous system (CNS) as well as peripheral nervous system (PNS) involvement in MFS.[146]

TREATMENT

There are no controlled treatment trials of patients with MFS. A large retrospective study of 92 patients with MFS (28 treated with IVIG, 23 treated with PE, and 41 who did not receive treatment) suggested that IVIG might have slightly hastened the improvement of the ophthalmoplegia and ataxia, while PE was of no benefit.[162] The reason for the lack of significant improvement was that the natural history of MFS is of good recovery. Nonetheless, in the absence of any controlled trials, we treat patients with IVIG.[147] In this regard, IVIG inhibits the binding of GQ1b antibodies to GQ1b, thereby preventing complement activation and subsequent pathophysiologic effects in ex vivo mouse models, suggesting that it might be beneficial.[100]

▶ IDIOPATHIC SENSORY NEURONOPATHY/ GANGLIONOPATHY

BACKGROUND

This disorder is believed to be caused by an autoimmune attack directed against the dorsal root ganglia. The differential diagnosis of sensory neuronopathy includes a paraneoplastic syndrome, which is typically associated with anti-Hu antibodies, and a sensory ganglionitis related to Sjögren syndrome. Certain medications or toxins, infectious agents, and other systemic disorders are also associated with a sensory neuronopathy. Despite extensive evaluation, many cases of sensory neuronopathy have no clear etiology, the so-called idiopathic sensory neuronopathy. The acute cases may represent a variant of GBS, although the onset can be insidiously progressive as well.

CLINICAL FEATURES

Idiopathic sensory neuronopathy is a rare disorder that usually presents in adulthood (mean age of onset 49 years, with range 18–81 years) and has a slight female predominance.[8,163–167] Symptoms can develop over a few hours or evolve more insidiously over several months or years, and the course can be monophasic with a stable or remitting deficit, chronic progressive, or chronic relapsing. Unlike typical GBS, only a few patients report a recent antecedent infection. The presenting complaint is numbness and tingling face, trunk, or limbs, which can be painful. Symptoms begin asymmetrically and in the upper limbs in nearly half of the patients, suggesting a ganglionopathy as opposed to a length-dependent process. Usually, the sensory symptoms become generalized, but they can remain asymmetric. Patients also describe clumsiness of the hands and gait instability.

On examination, marked reduction in vibration and proprioception are found, while pain and temperature sensations are less affected. Manual muscle testing is usually normal. Some muscle groups may appear weak, but this is usually secondary to impaired modulation of motor activity due to the proprioceptive defect. Most patients have sensory ataxia, which can be readily demonstrated by having the patient perform the finger–nose–finger test with their eyes open and then closed. Patients may have only mild dysmetria with their eyes open, but when their eyes are closed, they consistently miss their nose and the examiner's stationed finger. Pseudoathetoid movements of the extremities may also be appreciated. Patients exhibit a positive Romberg sign and, not surprisingly, describe more gait instability in the dark or while washing their hair with their eyes closed. Muscle stretch reflexes are decreased or absent, while plantar reflexes are flexor.

A detailed history and examination are essential to exclude a toxin-induced neuronopathy, paraneoplastic syndrome, or disorder related to a connective tissue disease (i.e., Sjögren syndrome). Importantly, the sensory neuronopathy can precede the onset of malignancy or sicca symptoms (i.e., dry eyes and mouth); therefore, these disorders should always be kept in mind. Pertinent laboratory and malignancy workup, including a careful general examination, paraneoplastic antibodies and potentially PET scanning should be ordered. We refer patients to ophthalmology for Rose Bengal stain and Schirmer's test. A lip or parotid gland biopsy is obtained in all patients suspected of having Sjögren syndrome. Subacute sensory neuronopathy has also been associated with recent Epstein–Barr virus infection.[167]

LABORATORY FEATURES

The CSF protein is normal or only slightly elevated in most patients. However, the CSF protein can be markedly elevated (reportedly as high as 300 mg/dL) when examined within a few days in cases with a hyperacute onset. Only rare patients exhibit CSF pleocytosis. MRI scan can reveal gadolinium enhancement of the posterior spinal roots or increased signal abnormalities on T2-weighted images in the posterior columns of the spinal cord.[168] Some patients have a monoclonal gammopathy (IgM, IgG, or IgA). Ganglioside antibodies, particularly GD1b antibodies, have been demonstrated in some cases of idiopathic sensory neuronopathy associated with IgM monoclonal gammopathy.[169]

Antineuronal nuclear antibodies (e.g., anti-Hu antibodies) should be assayed in all individuals with sensory neuronopathy to evaluate for a paraneoplastic syndrome. Likewise, antinuclear, SS-A, and SS-B antibodies should be ordered to look for evidence of Sjögren syndrome, which can also present with a sensory neuronopathy.

The classic NCS finding is low-amplitude or absent SNAPs.[164,165,168] When SNAPs are obtainable, the distal sensory latencies and NCVs are normal or only mildly abnormal. In contrast, motor nerve conduction studies either are normal or reveal only mild abnormalities. In addition, H-reflexes and blink reflexes may typically be unobtainable.[170] An abnormal blink reflex favors a nonparaneoplastic etiology for a sensory neuronopathy but does not exclude an underlying malignancy.[171] The masseter reflex or jaw jerk is abnormal in patients with sensory neuropathy but is usually preserved in patients with sensory neuronopathy.[170] The masseter reflex is unique amongst the stretch reflexes in that the cell bodies of the afferent limb lie in the mesencephalic nucleus within the CNS. This differs from the sensory cell bodies innervating the limbs, which reside in the dorsal root ganglia of the PNS. The afferent cell bodies lie in the Gasserian ganglia that are outside the CNS, which explains why the blink reflex can be impaired in sensory ganglionopathies.

HISTOPATHOLOGY

Sensory nerve biopsies may reveal a preferential loss of large myelinated fibers compared to small myelinated fibers or similar loss of both large- and small-diameter nerve fibers. Mild perivascular inflammation may be seen, but prominent endoneurial infiltrate is not appreciated. There is no evidence of segmental demyelination.

An autopsy performed 5 weeks after onset of idiopathic sensory neuronopathy in one man revealed widespread inflammation involving sensory and autonomic ganglia, with loss of associated neurons and Wallerian degeneration of the posterior nerve roots and dorsal columns being evident.[163] The motor neurons and roots appeared normal. Immunohistochemical analysis suggested a CD8+ T-cell-mediated cytotoxic attack against the ganglion neurons.

PATHOGENESIS

Autoimmune sensory neuronopathies are caused by an autoimmune attack directed against the dorsal root ganglia. Serum from affected patients immunostains dorsal root ganglia cells in culture and inhibits neurite growth.[172] The neuronal epitope is unknown, but the ganglioside GD1b has been hypothesized to be the target antigen.[169] GD1b localizes to neurons in the dorsal root ganglia, and antibodies directed against this ganglioside have been detected in some patients with idiopathic sensory neuronopathy.[163] Further, rabbits immunized with purified GD1b develop ataxic sensory neuropathy, with loss of the cell bodies in the dorsal root ganglia and axonal degeneration of the dorsal column of the spinal cord without demyelination or an inflammatory infiltrate.

TREATMENT

Various modes of immunotherapy have been tried, including corticosteroids, PE, and IVIG.[163,168] However, there have been no prospective, double-blinded, placebo-controlled trials. Occasionally, patients appear to improve with therapy; however, some improve spontaneously and many stabilize without treatment. In our experience, most patients have not experienced a dramatic improvement following treatment. Perhaps this is due to the inherent inability of dorsal root ganglion cells to regenerate. However, in patients seen in the acute setting or in those with a chronic progressive deficit, a trial of immunotherapy may be warranted.

▶ ACUTE SMALL FIBER SENSORY NEUROPATHY

CLINICAL FEATURES

Small fiber neuropathies typically present insidiously with slowly progressive burning pain and paresthesia in the distal lower extremities, which may later involve the proximal legs and upper extremities (see Chapter 22). Most are idiopathic in nature, but diabetes mellitus, amyloidosis, Sjögrens' syndrome, and hereditary sensory and autonomic neuropathy need to be excluded. Rarely, patients present acutely with symptoms suggestive of a small fiber neuropathy that may, or may not, be length-dependent.[173,174] An antecedent infection is common. Neurologic examination discloses normal muscle strength, length-dependent or non–length-dependent sensory loss for pain and temperature, normal proprioception, and vibration senses with normal or brisk muscle stretch reflexes. However, non–length-dependent sensory loss and burning sensation can also be seen.[174] The burning dysesthesia usually disappear within 4 months; however, the numbness and objective sensory loss tend to persist longer.

LABORATORY FEATURES

CSF examination may reveal albuminocytologic dissociation. Motor and sensory conduction studies that primarily assess large fiber function are normal. Autonomic testing may be abnormal.

HISTOPATHOLOGY

Nerve biopsies have not been reported. However, skin biopsies in some patients have shown reduced nerve fiber density, which in most cases was worse in the thigh compared to calf.[34]

PATHOGENESIS

The acute clinical presentation often follows an infection and CSF findings suggest that this may be a rare GBS variant.

TREATMENT

A trial of IVIG would seem warranted in patients who present in the acute phase of the illness.

▶ AUTOIMMUNE AUTONOMIC NEUROPATHY

CLINICAL FEATURES

Young et al. were the first to report a detailed clinical, laboratory, and histologic description of a patient with acute pandysautonomia.[175,176] Subsequently, there have been a number of small reports of idiopathic autonomic neuropathy.[8,177–193] Many of these cases are presumed to have an autoimmune basis. This is a heterogeneous neuropathy in terms of onset, the type of autonomic deficits, the presence or absence of somatic involvement, and the degree of recovery. A Mayo Clinic series of 27 cases of idiopathic autonomic neuropathy followed for a mean of 32 months found that approximately 20% of patients had selective cholinergic dysfunction, while 80% had various degrees of widespread sympathetic and parasympathetic dysfunction.[189] The most common symptom is orthostatic dizziness or lightheadedness, occurring in about 80% of patients. Gastrointestinal involvement is present in over 70%, with patients complaining of nausea, vomiting, diarrhea, constipation, ileus, or postprandial bloating. Heat intolerance and poor sweating are also present in the majority of patients. Blurred vision, dry eyes and mouth, urinary retention or incontinence, and impotence are common. Numbness, tingling, and dysesthesia of the distal extremities are evident in about 30% of patients, but muscle strength is normal. Most patients have a monophasic course similar to GBS with progression, followed by a plateau and slow recovery or a stable deficit.[189] Although some patients exhibit a complete recovery,[176,191] it tends to be incomplete in most.[189]

LABORATORY FEATURES

The CSF often reveals slightly elevated protein without pleocytosis.[189] Supine plasma norepinephrine levels are not different, but standing levels are significantly reduced, when compared to normal controls.[189] In a large study, patients with idiopathic autonomic neuropathy 18/106 (18%) had high levels of ganglionic acetylcholine receptor (AChR) autoantibodies.[193,194] The seropositive group had a significant overrepresentation of abnormal pupillary responses, sicca complex, and lower gastrointestinal tract dysautonomia. A subacute mode of onset was more common in the seropositive group. In this regard, rabbits immunized with a neuronal AChR alpha3 subunit fusion protein produce ganglionic AChR antibodies and develop autonomic failure.[195] Immunohistochemical staining of superior cervical ganglia and myenteric plexus neurons reveals intact presynaptic nerve terminals and postsynaptic neurons containing cytoplasmic AChR, but lacking surface AChR.

Routine motor and sensory NCS and EMG are usually unremarkable.[189] Quantitative sensory testing may reveal abnormalities in thermal thresholds.[183] Autonomic testing can show abnormalities.[196,197] Orthostatic hypotension and reduced variability of the heart rate on deep breathing are evident in over 60% of affected individuals.[189] An abnormal response to Valsalva maneuver (i.e., exaggerated fall in blood pressure during early phase II of the response, absent recovery of systolic and diastolic blood pressure during late phase II, or reduced or absent overshoot of systolic and diastolic pressures during phase IV) has been demonstrated in over 40% of patients. Sympathetic skin response may be absent.[179,198] Abnormal quantitative sudomotor axon reflex test scores are seen in 85% of patients.[189] Most patients have abnormal thermoregulatory sweat tests, with areas of anhidrosis in 12–97% of the body. Gastrointestinal studies may reveal hypomotility anywhere from the esophagus to the rectum.

HISTOPATHOLOGY

Nerve biopsies reveal reduced density of mainly small-diameter myelinated nerve fibers, along with stacks of empty Schwann cell profiles and collagen pockets.[176,180,182,186,189,198] Scant epineurial perivascular inflammation may be seen.

PATHOGENESIS

The disorder is suspected to be the result of an autoimmune attack directed against peripheral autonomic fibers or the ganglia.[182] A subset of patients may have antibodies directed against calcium channels, which are present on presynaptic autonomic nerve terminals.

TREATMENT

PE, prednisone, IVIG, and other immunosuppressive agents have been tried with variable success.[181,182188,189] The most important aspect of management is supportive therapy for orthostatic hypotension and bowel and bladder symptoms.[161,162] Fludrocortisone is effective at increasing plasma volume but should be administered only in the morning or in the morning and at lunch to avoid nocturnal/supine hypertension. We begin treatment at 0.1 mg/day and increase by 0.1 mg every 3–4 days until their standing time and blood pressure are controlled. Midodrine, a peripheral alpha1 adrenergic agonist, may also be effective and can be used in combination with fludrocortisone.[199,200] Midodrine is started at 2.5 mg/day and can gradually be increased to 40 mg/day in divided doses (every 2–4 hours) as necessary. Gastrointestinal hypomotility can be treated with metoclopramide, cisapride, or erythromycin. Bulking agents, laxatives, and enemas may be need in patients with constipation. Urology should be consulted in patients with neurogenic bladders. Patient may require cholinergic agonists (e.g., bethanechol), intermittent self-catheterization, or other modes of therapy.

▶ SUMMARY

GBS is an acquired immune-mediated neuropathy. It most commonly presents in the Western hemisphere as AIDP in which the immune attack is directed against myelin in peripheral nerves. Occasionally, the immune attack is directed against the axons of motor and sensory nerves (AMSAN) or just axons of motor nerves (AMAN). These axonal variants of GBS are more common in Asia but do occur worldwide. Other immune-mediated neuropathies such as MFS, acute autonomic neuropathy, acute sensory neuronopathies, and acute small fiber neuropathies may also fall into the spectrum of GBS. The natural history of most of these neuropathies is for gradual spontaneous improvement that may be facilitated with IVIG or PE.

REFERENCES

1. Guillain G, Barré JA, Strohl A. Sur un syndrome de radiculonevrite avec hyper albiminose du loquide cephalo-rachiden sas raection cellulaire. Remarques sur les catarcteres cliniques et graphiques des reflexes tendeneux. Bulletins et Memories de la Societe Medicale des Hospitaux de Paris, Masson et Cie 1916;40:1462–1470.
2. Haymaker W, Kernohan JW. The Landry–Guillain–Barré syndrome: a clinicopathologic report of fifty fatal cases and a critique of the literature. *Medicine (Baltimore).* 1949;28(1):59–141.
3. Asbury AK, Arnason BG, Adams RD. The inflammatory lesion in idiopathic polyneuritis. Its role in pathogenesis. *Medicine (Baltimore).* 1969;48(3):173–215.
4. Brown WF, Feasby TE. Sensory evoked potentials in Guillain–Barré polyneuropathy. *J Neurol Neurosurg Psychiatry.* 1984;47(3):288–291.
5. Kennedy RH, Danielson MA, Mulder DW, Kurland LT. Guillain–Barré syndrome: a 42-year epidemiologic and clinical study. *Mayo Clin Proc.* 1978;53(2):93–99.
6. Ropper AH. Severe acute Guillain–Barré syndrome. *Neurology.* 1986;36(3):429–432.
7. Ropper AH, Wijdicks EFM, Truax BT. *Guillain–Barré Syndrome.* Philadelphia, PA: FA Davis; 1991.
8. Amato AA, Dumitru D. Acquired neuropathies. In: Dumitru D, Amato AA, Swartz MJ, eds. *Electrodiagnostic Medicine.* 2nd ed. Philadelphia, PA: Hanley & Belfus, Inc.; 2002:937–1041.
9. Hughes RA, Cornblath DR. Guillain–Barre syndrome. *Lancet.* 2005;366(9497):1653–1666.
10. Ropper AH. The Guillain–Barré syndrome. *N Engl J Med.* 1992;326(17):1130–1136.
11. Yuki N, Hartung H-P. Guillain-Barré syndrome. *N Engl J Med.* 2012;366(24):2294–2304
12. Alter M. The epidemiology of Guillain–Barré syndrome. *Ann Neurol.* 1990;(27suppl):S7–S12.
13. Shui IM, Rett MD, Weintraub E, et al; Vaccine Safety Datalink Research Team. Guillain-Barré syndrome incidence in a large United States cohort (2000–2009). *Neuroepidemiology.* 2012;39(2):109–115.
14. Jacobs BC, Rothbarth PH, van der Meché FG, et al. The spectrum of antecedent infections in Guillain–Barré syndrome: a case-control study. *Neurology.* 1998;51(4):1110–1115.
15. Bolton CF. The changing concepts of Guillain–Barré syndrome. *N Engl J Med.* 1995;333(21):1415–1417.
16. Feasby TE, Hughes RAC. *Campylobacter jejuni*, antiganglio-sides antibodies, and Guillain–Barré syndrome. *Neurology.* 1998;51(2):340–342.
17. Griffin JW, Ho TW. The Guillain–Barré syndrome at 75: the *Campylobacter* connection. *Ann Neurol.* 1993;34(2):125–127.
18. Rees JH, Gregson NA, Hughes RA. Anti-ganglioside GM1 antibodies in Guillain–Barré syndrome and their relationship to *Campylobacter jejuni* infection. *Ann Neurol.* 1995;38(5):809–816.
19. Rees JH, Soudain SE, Gregson NA, Hughs RA. *Campylobacter jejuni* infection and Guillain–Barré syndrome. *N Engl J Med.* 1995;333(21):1415–1417.
20. Van Koningsveld R, Van Doorn PA, Schmitz PIM, Ang CW, Van der Meché FG. Mild forms of Guillain–Barré syndrome in an epidemiologic survey in the Netherlands. *Neurology.* 2000;54(3):620–625.
21. Visser LH, Schmitz PI, Meulstee J, van Doorn PA, van der Meché FG. Prognostic factors of Guillain–Barré syndrome after intravenous immunoglobulin or plasma exchange. *Neurology.* 1999;53:598–604.
22. Vriesendorp FJ, Mishu B, Li CY, et al. Serum antibodies to GM1, peripheral nerve myelin, and *Campylobacter jejuni* in patients with Guillain–Barré syndrome and controls: correlation and prognosis. *Ann Neurol.* 1993;34:130–135.

23. Geurtsvankessel CH, Islam Z, Mohammad QD, Jacobs BC, Endtz HP, Osterhaus AD. Hepatitis E and Guillain-Barre Syndrome. *Clin Infect Dis.* 2013;57(9):1369–1370.
24. van den Berg B, van der Eijk AA, Pas SD, et al. Guillain-Barré syndrome associated with preceding hepatitis E virus infection. *Neurology.* 82(6):491–497.
25. Kwong JC, Vasa PP, Campitelli MA, et al. Risk of Guillain-Barré syndrome after seasonal influenza vaccination and influenza health-care encounters: a self-controlled study. *Lancet Infect Dis.* 2013;13(9):769–776.
26. Galeotti F, Massari M, D'Alessandro R, et al. Risk of Guillain-Barré syndrome after 2010–2011 influenza vaccination. *Eur J Epidemiol.* 2013;28(5):433–444.
27. Dodd CN, Romio SA, Black S, et al. International collaboration to assess the risk of Guillain Barré Syndrome following Influenza A (H1N1) 2009 monovalent vaccines. *Vaccine.* 2013;31(40):4448–4458.
28. De Wals P, Deceuninck G, Toth E, et al. Risk of Guillain-Barré syndrome following H1N1 influenza vaccination in Quebec. *JAMA.* 2012;308(2):175–181.
29. Crawford NW, Cheng A, Andrews N, et al. Guillain-Barré syndrome following pandemic (H1N1) 2009 influenza A immunisation in Victoria: a self-controlled case series. *Med J Aust.* 2012;197:574–578.
30. Salmon DA, Proschan M, Forshee R, et al; H1N1 GBS Meta-Analysis Working Group. Association between Guillain-Barré syndrome and influenza A (H1N1) 2009 monovalent inactivated vaccines in the USA: a meta-analysis. *Lancet.* 2013;381 (9876):1461–1468.
31. Polakowski LL, Sandhu SK, Martin DB, et al. Chart-confirmed Guillain-Barre syndrome after 2009 H1N1 influenza vaccination among the medicare population, 2009–2010. *Am J Epidemiol.* 2013;178(6):962–973.
32. Greene SK, Rett M, Weintraub ES, et al. Risk of confirmed Guillain-Barre syndrome following receipt of monovalent inactivated influenza A (H1N1) and seasonal influenza vaccines in the Vaccine Safety Datalink Project, 2009–2010. *Am J Epidemiol.* 2012;175(11):1100–1109.
33. Greene SK, Rett MD, Vellozzi C, et al. Guillain-Barré Syndrome, influenza vaccination, and antecedent respiratory and gastrointestinal infections: a case-centered analysis in the vaccine safety datalink, 2009–2011. *PLoS One.* 2013;8(6):e67185.
34. Velentgas P, Amato AA, Bohn RL, et al. Risk of Guillain-Barré syndrome after meningococcal conjugate vaccination. *Pharmacoepidemiol Drug Saf.* 2012;21(12)1350–1358.
35. Souayah N, Yacoub HA, Khan HM, et al. Analysis of data from the CDC/FDA vaccine adverse event reporting system (1990–2009) on Guillain-Barre syndrome after hepatitis vaccination in the USA. *J Clin Neurosci.* 2012;19(8):1089–1092.
36. Ojha RP, Jackson BE, Tota JE, Offutt-Powell TN, Singh KP, Bae S. Guillain-barre syndrome following quadrivalent human papillomavirus vaccination among vaccine-eligible individuals in the United States. *Hum Vaccin Immunother.* 2013;10(1):232–237.
37. Alvarez-Lario B, Prieto-Tejedo R, Colazo-Burlato M, Macarrón-Vicente J. Severe Guillain-Barré syndrome in a patient receiving anti-TNF therapy. Consequence or coincidence. A case-based review. *Clin Rheumatol.* 2013;32(9):1407–1412.
38. González-Suárez I, Sanz-Gallego I, Rodríguez de Rivera FJ, Arpa J. Guillain-Barre´ syndrome: natural history and prognostic factors: a retrospective review of 106 cases. *BMC Neurol.* 2013;(13):95.
39. Rigamonti A, Basso F, Scaccabarozzi C, Lauria G. Posterior reversible encephalopathy syndrome as the initial manifestation of Guillain-Barré syndrome: case report and review of the literature. *J Peripher Nerv Syst.* 2012;17:356–360.
40. Abraham A, Ziv S, Drory VE. Posterior reversible encephalopathy syndrome resulting from Guillain-Barre´-like syndrome secondary to West Nile virus infection. *J Clin Neuromuscul Dis.* 2001;12:113–117.
41. Bavikatte G, Gaber T, Eshiett MU. Posterior reversible encephalopathy syndrome as a complication of Guillain-Barre´ syndrome. *J Clin Neurosci.* 2010;17:924–926.
42. Delalande S, De Se'ze J, Hurtevent JP, Stojkovic T, Hurtevent JF, Vermersch P. Cortical blindness associated with Guillain-Barre´ syndrome: a complication of dysautonomia? *Rev Neurol (Paris).* 2005;161:465–467.
43. Elahi A, Kelkar P, St Louis EK. Posterior reversible encephalopathy syndrome as the initial manifestation of Guillain-Barre´ syndrome. *Neurocrit Care.* 2004;1:465–468.
44. Exteberria A, Lonneville S, Rutgers MP, Gille MP. Posterior reversible encephalopathy syndrome as a revealing manifestation of Guillain-Barre´ syndrome. *Rev Neurol (Paris).* 2012;168: 283–286.
45. Sutter R, Mengiardi B, Lyrer P, Czaplinski A. Posterior reversible encephalopathy syndrome as the initial manifestation of a Guillain-Barre´ syndrome. *Neuromuscul Dis.* 2009;19:709–710.
46. de la Cour CD, Jacobsen J. Residual neuropathy in long-term population-based follow-up of Guillain–Barre´ syndrome. *Neurology.* 2005;64:246–253.
47. Garssen MP, Bussmann JB, Schmitz PI, et al. Physical training and fatigue, fitness, and quality of life in Guillain–Barre´ syndrome and CIDP. *Neurology.* 2004;63(12):2393–2395.
48. Merkies IS, Schitz PI, Samijn JP, van der Meche FG, van Doorn PA. Fatigue in immune-mediated polyneuropathies. European Inflammatory Neuropathy Cause and Treatment (ICANT) Group. *Neurology.* 1999;53:1648–1654.
49. Ruts L, Drenthen J, Jacobs BC, van Doorn PA; Dutch GBS Study Group. Distinguishing acute-onset CIDP from fluctuating Guillain-Barre syndrome: a prospective study. *Neurology.* 2010;74:1680–1686.
50. van den Berg B, Bunschoten C, van Doorn PA, Jacobs BC. Mortality in Guillain-Barre syndrome. *Neurology.* 2013;80: 1650–1654.
51. Cornblath DR, Mellits ED, Griffin JW, et al. Motor conduction studies in Guillain–Barré syndrome: description and prognostic value. *Ann Neurol.* 1988;23:354–359.
52. Cornblath DR. Electrophysiology in Guillain–Barré syndrome. *Ann Neurol.* 1990;(27suppl):S17–S20.
53. McKhann GM, Griffin JW, Cornblath DR, et al. Plasmapheresis and Guillain–Barré syndrome: analysis of prognostic factors and the effect of plasmapheresis. *Ann Neurol.* 1988;23:347–353.
54. Randomized trial of plasma exchange, intravenous immunoglobulin, and combined treatments in Guillain–Barré syndrome. Plasma Exchange/Sandoglobulin Guillain–Barré Syndrome Trial Group. *Lancet.* 1997;349:225–230.
55. Triggs WJ, Cros D, Gominak SC, et al. Motor nerve excitability in Guillain–Barré syndrome: the spectrum of conduction block and axonal degeneration. *Brain.* 1992;115(Pt 5):1291–1302.

56. van der Meche' FG, Meulstee J, Kleyweg RP. Axonal damage in Guillain-Barré syndrome. *Muscle Nerve.* 1991;14(10):997–1002.
57. Winer JB, Hughes RA, Greenwood RJ, Perkin GD, Healy MJ. Prognosis in Guillain-Barré syndrome. *Lancet.* 1985; 1(8439):1202–1203.
58. Winer JB, Hughes RA, Osmond C. A prospective study of acute idiopathic neuropathy. I. Clinical features and their prognostic value. *J Neurol Neurosurg Psychiatry.* 1988;51(15):605–612.
59. Ramanathan S, McMeniman J, Cabela R, Holmes-Walker DJ, Fung VS. SIADH and dysautonomia as the initial presentation of Guillain-Barré syndrome. *J Neurol Neurosurg Psychiatry.* 2012;83:344–345.
60. Hoffmann O, Reuter U, Schielke E, Weber JR. SIADH as the first symptom of Guillain-Barré syndrome. *Neurology.* 1999;53 (6):1365.
61. Sawai S, Satoh M, Mori M, et al. Membrane-organizing extension spike protein, moesin, is a possible target molecule for cytomegalovirus-related Guillain-Barré syndrome. *Neurology.* 2014;83:113–117.
62. Gorson KC, Ropper AH, Muriello A, Blair R. Prospective evaluation of MRI lumbosacral root enhancement in acute Guillain-Barré syndrome. *Neurology.* 1996;47:813–817.
63. Albers JW, Donofrio PD, McGonable TK. Sequential electrodiagnostic abnormalities in acute inflammatory demyelinating polyradiculoneuropathy. *Muscle Nerve.* 1985;8:528–539.
64. Brown WF, Feasby TE. Conduction block and denervation in Guillain-Barré polyneuropathy. *Brain.* 1984;107:219–239.
65. Capasso M, Caporale CM, Pomilio F, Gandolfi P, Lugaresi A, Uncini A. Acute motor conduction block neuropathy. Another Guillain-Barre syndrome variant. *Neurology.* 2003;61: 617–622.
66. Gordon PH, Wibourn AJ. Early electrodiagnostic findings in Guillain-Barre´ syndrome. *Arch Neurol.* 2001;58:913–917.
67. Ropper AH, Wijdicks EF, Shahani BT. Electrodiagnostic abnormalities in 113 consecutive patients with Guillain-Barré syndrome. *Arch Neurol.* 1990;47:881–887.
68. Ropper AH, Chiappa KH. Evoked potentials in Guillain-Barré syndrome. *Neurology.* 1986;36:587–590.
69. Olney RK, Aminoff MJ. Electrodiagnostic features of the Guillain-Barré syndrome: the relative sensitivity of different techniques. *Neurology.* 1990;40:471–475.
70. Barohn RJ, Kissel JT, Warmolts JR, Mendell JR. Chronic inflammatory polyradiculoneuropathy. Clinical characteristics, course, and recommendations for diagnostic criteria. *Arch Neurol.* 1989;46:878–884.
71. Asbury AK, Cornblath DR. Assessment of current diagnostic criteria for Guillain-Barré syndrome. *Ann Neurol.* 1990; (27suppl):S21–S24.
72. Meulstee J, van der Meche' FG. Electrodiagnostic criteria for polyneuropathy and demyelination: application in 135 patients with Guillain-Barré syndrome. Dutch Guillain-Barré Study Group. *J Neurol Neurosurg Psychiatry.* 1995;59(5):482–486.
73. Dawson DM, Samuels MA, Morris J. Sensory form of acute polyneuritis. *Neurology.* 1988;38:1728–1731.
74. van der Meche' FG, Meulstee J, Vermeulen M, Kievit A. Patterns of conduction failure in the Guillain-Barré syndrome. *Brain.* 1988;111(Pt 2):415–416.
75. Eisen A, Humphreys P. The Guillain-Barré syndrome. A clinical and electrodiagnostic study of 25 cases. *Arch Neurol.* 1974;30:438–443.
76. Perssons A, Solders G. R–R variations in Guillain-Barré syndrome: a test of autonomic dysfunction. *Acta Neurol Scand.* 1983;67:294–300.
77. Honavar M, Tharakan JK, Hughes RA, Leibowitz S, Winer JB. A clinico-pathological study of the Guillain-Barré syndrome: nine cases and literature review. *Brain.* 1991;114(Pt 3):1245–1269.
78. Kanda T, Hayashi H, Tanabe H, Tsubaki T, Oda M. A fulminant case of Guillain-Barré syndrome: topographic and fibre size related analysis of demyelinating changes. *J Neurol Neurosurg Psychiatry.* 1989;52(7):857–864.
79. Lu JL, Sheik KA, WU HS, et al. Physiologic–pathologic correlation in Guillain-Barré syndrome in children. *Neurology.* 2000;54(1):33–39.
80. Griffin JW, Li CY, Ho TW, et al. Guillain-Barré syndrome in northern China: the spectrum of neuropathologic changes in clinically defined cases. *Brain.* 1995;118(Pt 3):577–595.
81. Griffin JW, Li CY, Ho TW, et al. Pathology of the motor-sensory axonal Guillain-Barré syndrome. *Ann Neurol.* 1996;39(1): 17–28.
82. Hafer-Macko C, Hsieh S-T, Li CY, et al. Acute motor axonal neuropathy: an antibody mediated attack on axolemma. *Ann Neurol.* 1996:40(4):635–644.
83. Hafer-Macko CE, Sheihk KA, Li CY, et al. Immune attack on the Schwann cell surface in acute inflammatory demyelinating polyneuropathy. *Ann Neurol.* 1996;39(5):625–635.
84. Hartung H-P, Hughes RA, Taylor WA, Heininger K, Reiners K, Toyka KV. T cell activation in Guillain-Barré syndrome and in MS: elevated serum levels of soluble IL-2 receptors. *Neurology.* 1990;40:215–218.
85. Hartung H-P, Pollard JD, Harvey GK, Toyka KV. Immunopathogenesis and treatment of the Guillain-Barré syndrome. Part I. *Muscle Nerve.* 1995;18:137–153.
86. Hartung H-P, Pollard JD, Harvey GK, Toyka KV. Immunopathogenesis and treatment of the Guillain-Barré syndrome. Part II. *Muscle Nerve.* 1995;18:154–164.
87. Willison HJ. The immunobiology of Guillain-Barre´ syndromes. *J Peripher Nerv Syst.* 2005;10(2):94–112.
88. Feasby TE, Hahn AF, Gilbert JJ. Passive transfer studies in Guillain-Barré polyneuropathy. *Neurology.* 1982;32:1159–1167.
89. Buchwald B, Toyka KV, Zielasek J, Weishaupt A, Schweiger S, Dudel J. Neuromuscular blockade by IgG antibodies from patients with Guillain-Barre´ syndrome: a macro-patch-clamp study. *Ann Neurol.* 1998;44:913–922.
90. Kwa MS, van Schaik IN, De Jonge RR, et al. Autoimmunoreactivity to Schwann cells in patients with inflammatory neuropathies. *Brain.* 2003;126(Pt 2):361–375.
91. Efficiency of plasma exchange in Guillain-Barré syndrome: role of replacement fluids. French Cooperative Group on Plasma Exchange in Guillain-Barré Syndrome. *Ann Neurol.* 1987;22(6):753–761.
92. Plasmapheresis and acute Guillain-Barré syndrome. The Guillain-Barré syndrome Study Group. *Neurology.* 1985;35: 1096–1104.
93. French Cooperative Group on Plasma Exchange in Guillain-Barré Syndrome. The appropriate number of plasma exchanges in Guillain-Barré syndrome. *Ann Neurol.* 1997;41:298–306.
94. van der Meche' FGA, Schmidtz PIM. A randomized trial comparing intravenous immunoglobulin and plasma exchange in Guillain-Barré syndrome. Dutch Guillain- Barré Study Group. *N Engl J Med.* 1992;326:1123–1129.

95. Hughes RA, Wijdicks EF, Barohn R, et al; Quality Standards Subcommittee of the American Academy of Neurology. Practice parameter: immunotherapy for Guillain–Barre´ syndrome: report of the Quality Standards Subcommittee of the American Academy of Neurology. *Neurology*. 2003;61(6):736–740.
96. Hung PL, Chang WN, Huang LT, et al. A clinical and electrophysiologic survey of childhood Guillain–Barre´ syndrome. *Pediatric Neurology*. 2004;30(2):86–91.
97. Hughes RA, Swan AV, van Doorn PA. Intravenous immunoglobulin for Guillain-Barré syndrome. *Cochrane Database Syst Rev*. 2012;(7):CD002063. doi: 10.1002/14651858.CD002063
98. Raphaël JC, Chevret S, Hughes RA, Annane D. Plasma exchange for Guillain-Barré syndrome. *Cochrane Database Syst Rev*. 2012;(7):CD001798. doi: 10.1002/14651858
99. Bril V, Ilse WK, Pearse R, Dhanani A, Sutton D, Kong K. Pilot trial of immunoglobulin versus plasma exchange in patients with Guillain–Barré syndrome. *Neurology*. 1996;46(1):100–103.
100. Jacobs BC, O'Hanlon GM, Bullens RW, Veitch J, Plomp JJ, Willison HJ. Immunoglobulins inhibit pathophysiological effects of anti-GQ1b-positive sera at motor nerve terminals through inhibition of antibody binding. *Brain*. 2003;126:2220–2234.
101. Castro LH, Ropper AH. Human immune globulin infusion in Guillain–Barré syndrome: worsening during and after treatment. *Neurology*. 1993;43:1034–1036.
102. Irani DN, Cornblath DR, Chaudry V, Borel C, Hanley DF. Relapse in Guillain–Barré syndrome after treatment with human immune globulin. *Neurology*. 1993;43:1034–1036.
103. Ropper AH, Albers JW, Addison R. Limited relapse in Guillain–Barré syndrome after plasma exchange. *Arch Neurol*. 1988;45:314–315.
104. Treatment of Guillain–Barré syndrome with high-dose immune globulins combined with methylprednisolone: a pilot study. Dutch Guillain–Barré Study Group. *Ann Neurol*. 1994; 35(6):749–752.
105. Double-blind trial of intravenous methylprednisolone in Guillain–Barré syndrome. Guillain–Barré Syndrome Steroid Trial Group. *Lancet*. 1993;341(8845):586–590.
106. van Koningsveld R, Schmitz PI, Meche FG, Visser LH, Meulstee J, van Doorn PA; Dutch GBS study group. Effect of methylprednisolone when added to standard treatment with intravenous immunoglobulin for Guillain–Barre´ syndrome: randomised trial. *Lancet*. 2004;363(9404):192–196.
107. Delanoe C, Sebire G, Landrieu P, Huault G, Metral S. Acute inflammatory demyelinating polyneuropathy in children: clinical and electrodiagnostic studies. *Ann Neurol*. 1998;44:350–356.
108. Bradshaw DY, Jones HR. Guillain–Barré syndrome in children: clinical course, electrodiagnosis, and prognosis. *Muscle Nerve*. 1992;15:500–506.
109. Rantala H, Uhari M, Niemela M. Occurrence, clinical manifestations, and prognosis of Guillain–Barré in children. *Arch Dis Child*. 1991;66:706–709.
110. Tekgul H, Serdaroglu G, Tutuncuoglu S. Outcome of axonal and demyelinating forms of Guillain–Barre syndrome in children. *Pediatr Neurol*. 2003;28:295–299.
111. Devos D, Magot A, Perrier-Boeswillwald J, et al. Guillain-Barré syndrome during childhood: particular clinical and electrophysiological features. *Muscle Nerve*. 2013;48:247–251.
112. Vedanarayanan VV, Evans OB, Subramony SH. Tick paralysis in children: electrophysiology and possibility of misdiagnosis. *Neurology*. 2002;59:1088–1090.
113. Feasby TE, Gilbert JJ, Brown WF, et al. An acute axonal form of Guillain–Barré polyneuropathy. *Brain*. 1986;109:1115–1126.
114. Triggs WJ, Gominak SC, Cros DP, et al. Inexcitable motor nerves and low amplitude motor responses in the Guillain–Barré syndrome: distal conduction block or severe axonal degeneration. *Muscle Nerve*. 1991;14:892.
115. Brown WF, Feasby TE, Hahn AF. Electrophysiological changes in the acute "axonal" form of Guillain–Barré syndrome. *Muscle Nerve*. 1993;16:200–205.
116. Feasby TE, Hahn A, Brown W, Bolton CF, Gilbert JJ, Koopman WJ. Severe axonal degeneration in acute Guillain–Barré syndrome: evidence of two different mechanisms? *J Neurol Sci*. 1993;116:185–192.
117. Van der Meche FG, Meulstee J, Kleyweg RP. Axonal damage in Guillain–Barré syndrome. *Muscle Nerve*. 1991;14(10): 997–1002.
118. Miller RG, Peterson GW, Daube JR, Albers JW. Prognostic value of electrodiagnosis in Guillain–Barré syndrome. *Muscle Nerve*. 1988;11(7):769–774.
119. Wexler I. Sequence of demyelination-remyelination in Guillain–Barré disease. *J Neurol Neurosurg Psychiatry*. 1983;46: 168–174.
120. Reisin RC, Cersosimo R, Garcia Alvarez M, Massoaro M, Fejerman N. Acute "axonal" Guillain–Barré syndrome in childhood. *Muscle Nerve*. 1993;16:1310–1316.
121. Kuwabara S, Asahina M, Koga M, Mori M, Yuki N, Hattori T. Two patterns of clinical recovery in Guillain–Barré syndrome with IgG anti-GM1 antibody. *Neurology*. 1998;51(6):1656–1660.
122. Yuki N, Yoshino H, Sato S, Miyatake T. Acute axonal polyneuropathy associated with anti-GM1 antibodies following *Campylobacter* enteritis. *Neurology*. 1990;40(12):1900–1902.
123. Yuki N, Yamada M, Sato S, et al. Association of IgG anti-GD1 a antibody with severe Guillain–Barré syndrome. *Muscle Nerve*. 1993;16(6):642–647.
124. Hall SM, Hughes RC, Atkinson PF, McColl I, Gale A. Motor nerve biopsy in severe Guillain–Barré syndrome. *Ann Neurol*. 1992;31(4):441–444.
125. Yokota T, Kanda T, Hirashima F, Hirose K, Tanabe H. Is acute axonal form of Guillain–Barré syndrome a primary axonopathy? *Muscle Nerve*. 1992;15(10):1211–1213.
126. Berciano J, Coria F, Monton F, Calleja J, Figols J, Lafarga M. Axonal form of Guillain–Barré syndrome: evidence for macrophage-associated demyelination. *Muscle Nerve*. 1993; 16:744–751.
127. Hadden RDM, Cornblath DR, Hughes RAC, et al. Electrophysiological classification of Guillain–Barré syndrome: clinical associations and outcome. Plasma Exchange/Sandoglobulin Guillain-Barré Syndrome Trial Group. *Ann Neurol*. 1998;44(5):780–788.
128. Ho TW, Mishu B, Li CY, et al. Guillain–Barré syndrome in northern China: relationship to *Campylobacter jejuni* infection and antiglycolipid antibodies. *Brain*. 1995;118:597–605.
129. Bohlega S, Stigsby B, Haider A, McLean D. Guillain–Barré syndrome with severe demyelination mimicking axonopathy. *Muscle Nerve*. 1997;20:514–516.
130. Fuller GN, Jacobs JM, Lewis PD, Lane RJ. Pseudoaxonal Guillain–Barré syndrome: severe demyelination mimicking axonopathy. A case with pupillary involvement. *J Neurol Neurosurg Psychiatry*. 1992;55:1079–1083.

131. Massaro ME, Rodriguez EC, Pociecha J, et al. Nerve biopsy in children with severe Guillain–Barré syndrome and inexcitable motor nerves. *Neurology.* 1998;51(2):394–398.
132. McKhann GM, Cornblath DR, Ho TW, et al. Clinical and electrophysiological aspects of acute paralytic disease of children and young adults in northern China. *Lancet.* 1991;338(8767): 593–597.
133. McKhann GM, Cornblath DR, Griffin JW, et al. Acute motor axonal neuropathy in northern China: the spectrum of neuropathologic changes in clinically defined cases. *Brain.* 1995;118(Pt 3):577–595.
134. Jackson CE, Barohn RJ, Mendell JR. Acute paralytic syndrome in three American men. *Arch Neurol.* 1993;50:732–735.
135. Visser LH, van der Meche' FG, van Doorn PA, et al. Guillain–Barré syndrome without sensory loss (acute motor neuropathy). A subgroup with specific clinical, electrodiagnostic and laboratory features. Dutch Guillain-Barré Study Group. *Brain.* 1995;118(Pt 4):841–847.
136. Ho TW, Hsieh S-T, Nachamkin I, et al. Motor nerve terminal degeneration provides a potential mechanism for rapid recovery in acute motor axonal neuropathy after *Campylobacter* infection. *Neurology.* 1997;48(3):717–724.
137. Kuwabara S, Nakata M, Sung JY, et al. Hyperreflexia in axonal Guillain–Barre´ syndrome subsequent to *Campylobacter jejuni* enteritis. *J Neurol Sci.* 2002;199(1–2):89–92.
138. Ho TW, Willison HJ, Nachamkin I, et al. Anti-GD1 a antibody is associated with axonal but not demyelinating forms of Guillain–Barré syndrome. *Ann Neurol.* 1999;45(2):168–173.
139. Tamura N, Kuwabara S, Misawa S, et al. Time course of axonal regeneration in acute motor axonal neuropathy. *Muscle Nerve.* 2007;35(6):793–795.
140. Takigawa T, Yashuda H, Kikkawa R. Antibodies against GM1 gangliosides affect K+ and Na+ currents in isolated rat myelinated nerve fibers. *Ann Neurol.* 1995;37:436–442.
141. Fisher CM. An unusual variant of acute idiopathic polyneuritis (syndrome of ophthalmoplegia, ataxia, and areflexia). *N Engl J Med.* 1956;255:57–65.
142. Ropper AH. Unusual clinical variants and signs in Guillain–Barré syndrome. *Arch Neurol.* 1986;43:1150–1152.
143. Ropper AH. Further regional variants of acute immune polyneuropathy. *Arch Neurol.* 1994;51:671–675.
144. Wakerley BR, Yuki N. Pharyngeal-cervical-brachial variant of Guillain-Barre´ syndrome. *J Neurol Neurosurg Psychiatry.* 2014;85(3):339–344
145. Berlit P, Rakicky J. The Miller Fisher syndrome. Review of the literature. *J Clin Neuroophthalmol.* 1992;12:57–63.
146. Odaka M, Yuki N, Yamada M, et al. Bickerstaff's brainstem encephalitis: clinical features of 62 cases and a subgroup associated with Guillain–Barre syndrome. *Brain.* 2003;126(Pt 10): 2279–2290.
147. Overell J, Hsieh S, Odaka M, Yuki N, Willison H. Treatment for Fisher syndrome, Bickerstaff's brainstem encephalitis and related disorders. *Cochrane Database Syst Rev.* 2007; (1):CD004761.
148. Blau I, Casson I, Liberman A, Weiss E. The not-so-benign Miller Fisher syndrome. *Arch Neurol.* 1980;37(6):384–385.
149. Hatanaka T, Higashino H, Yasuhara A, Kobayashi Y. Miller Fisher syndrome: etiological significance of serial blink reflexes and MRI Study. *Electromyogr Clin Neurophysiol.* 1992;32(6): 317–319.
150. Shuaib A, Becker WJ. Variants of Guillain–Barré syndrome: Miller Fisher syndrome, facial diplegia, and multiple cranial nerve palsies. *Can J Neurol Sci.* 1987; 14:611–616.
151. Umapathi T, Tan EY, Kokubun N, Verma K, Yuki N. Non-demyelinating, reversible conduction failure in Fisher syndrome and related disorders. *J Neurol Neurosurg Psychiatry.* 2012;83:941–948.
152. Chiba A, Kusonoki S, Shimizu T, Kanazawa I. Serum IgG antibody to ganglioside GQ1b is a possible marker of Miller Fisher syndrome. *Ann Neurol.* 1992;312:677–679.
153. Yuki N, Sato S, Tsuji S, Ohsawa T, Miyatake T. Frequent presence of anti-GQ1b antibody in Fisher's syndrome. *Neurology.* 1993;43:414–417.
154. De Pablos C, Calleja J, Fernandez F, Berciano J. Miller Fisher syndrome: an electrophysiologic study. *Electromyogr Clin Neurophysiol.* 1988;28(1):21–25.
155. Fross RD, Daube JR. Neuropathy in the Miller Fisher syndrome: clinical and electrophysiologic findings. *Neurology.* 1987;37:1493–1498.
156. Jamal GA, McLeod WN. Electrophysiologic studies in Miller Fisher syndrome. *Neurology.* 1984;34:685–688.
157. Sauron B, Bouche P, Cathala H-P, Chain F, Castaigne P. Miller Fisher syndrome: clinical and electrophysiologic evidence of peripheral origin in 10 cases. *Neurology.* 1984;34:953–956.
158. Weiss JA, White JC. Correlation of 1 A afferent conduction with ataxia of Fisher syndrome. *Muscle Nerve.* 1986;9:327–332.
159. Dehaene I, Martin JJ, Geens K, Cras P. Guillain–Barré syndrome with ophthalmoplegia: clinicopathological study of the central and peripheral nervous systems, including the oculomotor nerves. *Neurology.* 1986;36:851–854.
160. Phillips MS, Stewart S, Anderson JR. Neuropathological findings in Miller Fisher syndrome. *J Neurol Neurosurg Psychiatry.* 1984;47:492–495.
161. Plomp JJ, Molenaar PC, O'Hanlon GM, et al. Miller Fisher anti-GQ1b antibodies: α-latrotoxin-like effects on motor end plates. *Ann Neurol.* 1999;45(2):189–199.
162. Mori M, Kuwabara S, Fukutake T, Hattori T. Intravenous immunoglobulin therapy for Miller Fisher syndrome. *Neurology.* 2007;68;1144–1146.
163. Hainfellner JA, Kristferitsch W, Lassmannn H, et al. T cell-mediated ganglionitis associated with acute sensory neuronopathy. *Ann Neurol.* 1996;39:543–547.
164. Knazan M, Bohlega S, Berry K, Eisen A. Acute sensory neuronopathy with preserved SEPs and long-latency reflexes. *Muscle Nerve.* 1990;13(5):381–384.
165. Sterman AB, Schaumburg HH, Asbury AK. The acute sensory neuronopathy syndrome: a distinct clinical entity. *Ann Neurol.* 1980;7:354–358.
166. Kuntzer T, Atoine J-C, Steck AJ. Clinical features and pathophysiological basis of sensory neuronopathies (ganglionopathies). *Muscle Nerve.* 2004;30:255–268.
167. Rubin D, Daube JR. Subacute sensory neuropathy associated with Epstein–Barr virus. *Muscle Nerve.* 1999;22:1607–1610.
168. Wada M, Kato T, Yuki N, et al. Gadolinium-enhancement of the spinal posterior roots in acute sensory ataxic neuropathy. *Neurology* 1997;49(5):1470–1471.
169. Dalakas MC. Autoimmune ataxic neuropathies (sensory ganglionopathies): are glycolipids the responsible autoantigens? *Ann Neurol.* 1996;39:419–442.
170. Auger RG. The role of the masseter reflex in the assessment of subacute sensory neuropathy. *Muscle Nerve.* 1998;21:800–801.

171. Auger RG, Windebank AJ, Lucchinetti CF, Chalk CH. Role of the blink reflex in the evaluation of sensory neuronopathy. *Neurology.* 1999;53:407–408.
172. Van Dijk GW, Wokke JH, Notermans NC, van den Berg LH, Bar PR. Indications for an immune-mediated etiology of idiopathic sensory neuronopathy. *J Neuroimmunol.* 1997;74:165–172.
173. Seneviratne U, Gunasekera S. Acute small fibre sensory neuropathy: another variant of Guillain–Barre syndrome? *J Neurol Neurosurg Psychiatry.* 2002;72:540–542.
174. Gorson KC, Herrmann DN, Thiagarajan R, et al. Non-length dependent small fiber neuropathy small neuropathy/ganglionopathy. *J Neurol Neurosurg Psychiatry.* 2008;79:163–169.
175. Young RR, Asbury AK, Adams RD, Corbett JL. Pure pandysautonomia with recovery. *Trans Am Neurol Assoc.* 1969;94: 355–357.
176. Young RR, Asbury AK, Corbett JL, Adams RD. Pure pandysautonomia with recovery. Description and discussion of diagnostic criteria. *Brain.* 1975;98:613–636.
177. Bennett JL, Mahalingam R, Wellish MC, Gilden DH. Epstein–Barr virus associated with acute autonomic neuropathy. *Ann Neurol.* 1996;40:453–455.
178. Colan RV, Snead OC 3rd, Oh SJ, Benton JW Jr. Steroid-responsive polyneuropathy with subacute onset in childhood. *J Pediatr.* 1980;97:374–377.
179. Fagius J, Westerberg CE, Olsson Y. Acute pandysautonomia and severe sensory deficit with poor recovery. A clinical, neurophysiological, and pathological study. *J Neurol Neurosurg Psychiatry.* 1983;46:725–733.
180. Feldman EL, Bromberg MB, Blaivas M, Junck L. Acute pandysautonomic neuropathy. *Neurology.* 1991;41:746–748.
181. Heafield MT, Gammage MD, Nightingale S, Williams AC. Idiopathic dysautonomia treated with intravenous immunoglobulin. *Lancet.* 1996;347:28–29.
182. Koike H, Watanabe H, Sobue G. The spectrum of immune-mediated autonomic neuropathies: insights from the clinicopathological features. *J Neurol Neurosurg Psychiatry.* 2013;84:98–106.
183. Low PA, Dyck PJ, Lambert EH, et al. Acute pandysautonomic neuropathy. *Ann Neurol.* 1983;13(4):412–417.
184. Mericle RA, Triggs WJ. Treatment of acute pandysautonomia with intravenous immunoglobulin. *J Neurol Neurosurg Psychiatry.* 1997;62:529–531.
185. McLeod JG, Tuck RR. Disorders of the autonomic nervous system: Part 1. Pathophysiology and clinical features. *Ann Neurol.* 1987;21:419–430.
186. Neville BG, Sladen GE. Acute autonomic neuropathy following herpes simplex infection. *J Neurol Neurosurg Psychiatry.* 1984;47:648–650.
187. Pavesi G, Gemignani F, Macaluso GM, et al. Acute sensory and autonomic neuropathy: possible association with coxsackie B virus infection. *J Neurol Neurosurg Psychiatry.* 1992;55(7): 613–615.
188. Smith AA, Vermeulen M, Koelman J, Wielman J, Wieling W. Unusual recovery from acute pandysautonomia after immunoglobulin therapy. *Mayo Clin Proc.* 1997;72:333–335.
189. Suarez GA, Fealey RD, Camileri M, Low PA. Idiopathic autonomic neuropathy: clinical, neurophysiologic, and follow-up studies on 27 patients. *Neurology.* 1994;44:1675–1682.
190. Taubner RW, Salanova V. Acute dysautonomia and polyneuropathy. *Arch Neurol.* 1984;41:1100–1101.
191. Venkataraman S, Alexander M, Gnanamuthu C. Postinfectious pandysautonomia with complete recovery after intravenous immunoglobulin therapy. *Neurology.* 1998;51:1764–1765.
192. Yahr MD, Frontera AT. Acute autonomic neuropathy. Its occurrence in infectious mononucleosis. *Arch Neurol.* 1975;32: 132–133.
193. Klein CM, Vernino S, Lennon VA, et al. The spectrum of autoimmune autonomic neuropathies. *Ann Neurol.* 2003;53(6): 752–758.
194. Sandroni P, Vernino S, Klein CM, et al. Idiopathic autonomic neuropathy: comparison of cases seropositive and seronegative for ganglionic acetylcholine receptor antibody. *Arch Neurol.* 2004;61(1):44–48.
195. Vernino S, Low PA, Lennon VA. Experimental autoimmune autonomic neuropathy. *J Neurophysiol.* 2003;90(3): 2053–2059.
196. McDougall AJ, McLeod JG. Autonomic neuropathy, I. Clinical features, investigation, pathophysiology, and treatment. *J Neurol Sci.* 1996;137:79–88.
197. McLeod JG, Tuck RR. Disorders of the autonomic nervous system: Part 2. Investigation and treatment. *Ann Neurol.* 1987;21:519–529.
198. Yokota T, Hayashi M, Hirashima F, Mitani M, Tanabe H, Tsukagoshi H. Dysautonomia with acute sensory motor neuropathy. A new classification of acute autonomic neuropathy. *Arch Neurol.* 1994;51:1022–1031.
199. Jankovic J, Gilden JL, Hiner BC, et al. Neurogenic orthostatic hypotension: a double-blind, placebo-controlled study with midodrine. *Am J Med.* 1993;95:34–48.
200. Low PA, Gilden JL, Freeman R, Sheng KN, McElligott MA. Efficacy of midodrine vs. placebo in neurogenic orthostatic hypotension. A randomized, double-blind multicenter study. *JAMA.* 1997;227(13):1046–1051.

CHAPTER 14

Chronic Inflammatory Demyelinating Polyradiculoneuropathy and Related Neuropathies

Like Guillain–Barré syndrome (GBS), chronic inflammatory demyelinating polyradiculoneuropathy (CIDP) is a syndrome with both classic and variant phenotypes. In the case of GBS, the classic phenotype is referred to as acute inflammatory demyelinating polyradiculoneuropathy (AIDP), a disorder characterized by areflexia, generalized and usually symmetric weakness, and sensory involvement. Likewise, the classic phenotype of CIDP, typically referred to simply as CIDP, shares many of the characteristic clinical and electrodiagnostic (EDX) features as GBS.

As the cause of CIDP is unknown and there is no universally agreed upon diagnostic gold-standard for CIDP (15 CIDP and 16 EDX-proposed diagnostic criteria paradigms to date), the classification of the chronic acquired demyelinating neuropathies remain in flux.[1,2] This chapter will address the majority of the chronic, acquired, predominantly demyelinating, and presumably inflammatory neuropathy syndromes. POEMS, with its associated CIDP-like neuropathy phenotype, will be the notable exception, discussed separately in Chapter 19.[3,4]

Current classification schemes often consider any neuropathy that fulfills the EDX criteria for CIDP to be categorized as CIDP or a CIDP variant. Multifocal motor neuropathy (MMN) is the notable exception, now being considered as a separate entity by virtually all neuromuscular experts.[5] We however, consider the CIDP spectrum to include only those disorders which have common phenotypic, EDX, cerebrospinal fluid, and therapeutic responsiveness features with the classic syndrome.[2,6,7] Included in this category are multifocal acquired demyelinating and sensory motor neuropathy (MADSAM) (a.k.a. Lewis Sumner syndrome) as well as some pure motor and pure sensory variants. Conversely, we will consider other chronic, acquired, and predominantly demyelinating neuropathy syndromes as separate entities if they differ significantly, particularly in consideration of their phenotype, natural history, and their therapeutic responsiveness profiles. We do so even if they fulfill EDX criteria for CIDP. Within this latter category, we will discuss distal acquired demyelinating sensorimotor (DADS) neuropathy, MMN, chronic immune sensory polyradiculopathy (CISP), and multifocal acquired motor axonopathy (MAMA) and attempt to distinguish them based on clinical, EDX, natural history, and response to treatment data (Table 14-1).

▶ CHRONIC INFLAMMATORY DEMYELINATING POLYRADICULONEUROPATHY

The first report of apparent CIDP, referred to as recurrent polyneuritis, is credited to Eichorst in 1890.[8] In the mid-1950s, animal models of both acute and chronic experimental allergic neuritis provided scientific support for an autoimmune pathophysiology. This concept was further cemented by a seminal report by Austin in 1958 describing steroid responsiveness in patients with relapsing polyneuritis.[9] Nonetheless, "chronic relapsing polyneuritis" was often considered to be a form of GBS in early publications until the mid 1970s.[10,11] Arguably, two developments promoted widespread neurological awareness of CIDP. The first was the availability and widespread utilization of nerve conduction studies, techniques that allowed for the noninvasive recognition of the demyelinating features that characterize this syndrome, demyelination of peripheral nerves having been previously demonstrable only by pathological means. The second seminal moment in the history of CIDP occurred with the 1975 publication by Peter Dyck, considered by many to be the patriarch of peripheral neuropathy in the United States.[12]

CLINICAL FEATURES

The prevalence of CIDP has been reported to range from 0.8 to 8.9/10^5 patients depending on the population studied. Although this may suggest different susceptibility between different geographical locations or ethnicities, this data may be heavily biased based on the diagnostic criteria utilized in different studies.[13] CIDP usually presents in adults (peak incidence at about 30–60 years of age) but it can manifest at any age including infants and children.[11,12,14–30] The relapsing

▶ TABLE 14-1. COMPARISON OF THE CHRONIC ACQUIRED IMMUNE-MEDIATED DEMYELINATING POLYNEUROPATHIES

	CIDP	DADS	MADSAM	MMN
Clinical Features				
Weakness	Symmetric proximal and distal	None or only mild symmetric distal	Asymmetric, distal > proximal, arms > legs	Asymmetric, distal > proximal, arms > legs
Sensory loss	Yes; symmetric	Yes; distal and symmetric	Yes; asymmetric	No
Reflexes	Symmetrically reduced or absent	Symmetrically reduced or absent	Asymmetrically reduced or absent	Asymmetrically reduced or absent
Electrophysiology				
CMAPs	Demyelinating features including CB	Demyelinating features excluding CB	Demyelinating features including CB	Demyelinating features including CB
SNAPs	Abnormal	Abnormal	Abnormal	Normal
Laboratory Findings				
CSF protein	Usually elevated	Usually elevated	Usually elevated	Usually normal
Monoclonal protein	Occasionally present, usually IgG or IgA	IgM usually present (most anti-MAG)	Rarely present	Rarely present
GM1 antibodies	Rarely present	Rarely present	Rarely present	Frequently present
Sensory nerve biopsies	Demyelinating/remyelinating features are common	Demyelinating/remyelinating features are common, with IgM deposition evident in paranodal regions	Demyelinating/remyelinating features are common	Demyelinating/remyelinating features are scant, if present
Treatment Response				
Prednisone	Yes	Poor	Yes	No
Plasma exchange	Yes	Poor	Not adequately studied	No
IVIg	Yes	Poor	Yes	Yes
Cyclophosphamide	Yes	Poor	Not adequately studied	Yes

CIDP, chronic inflammatory demyelinating polyneuropathy; DADS, distal acquired demyelinating symmetrical; MADSAM, multifocal acquired demyelinating sensory and motor; MMN, multifocal motor neuropathy; CMAPs, compound motor action potentials; SNAPs, sensory nerve action potentials; CB, conduction block; CSF, cerebrospinal fluid; MAG, myelin-associated glycoprotein; IVIg, intravenous immunoglobulin. Reproduced with permission from Saperstein DS, Katz JS, Amato AA, Barohn RJ. The spectrum of the acquired chronic demyelinating polyneuropathies. *Muscle Nerve*. 2001;24:311–324.

form tends to present earlier, usually in the twenties.[12,14] There is a slightly increased male prevalence, up to two-thirds of cases in some series.[12,31–33] Like GBS, CIDP may begin or relapse in association with an antecedent event that may include infection (10–30%), vaccination, surgery, trauma, or pregnancy.[12,13,15,24,25,34,35] CIDP may account for 10–33% of initially undiagnosed peripheral neuropathies in some series.[14,36,37] It is possible however, that these statistics represent a biased perspective considering that CIDP patients with their attendant morbidity are more likely to be referred to academic neuropathy clinics than are the far more abundant, indolent, length-dependent, sensory predominant, and frequently idiopathic axonopathies of the elderly.

The natural history of CIDP needs to be considered both with and without the influence of treatment. Up to 18% of CIDP patients will evolve acutely in such a manner to be initially confused with GBS.[32,38–40] Approximately 12% will evolve subacutely over a 4–8 week period, also confounding the distinction of CIDP from GBS in some cases.[41–44] These subacute cases may have a monophasic course with recovery reminiscent of GBS or have a progressive or relapsing course thereby justifying a CIDP diagnosis. In our minds subacute inflammatory demyelinating polyradiculoneuropathy represents a "holding" diagnosis until such time as categorization of GBS or CIDP can be made.

Regarding the natural history of treatment of naïve CIDP patients, the seminal paper by Peter Dyck and colleagues in 1975 describe four disease trajectories: (1) chronic monophasic (15%), (2) chronic relapsing (fluctuations of weakness or improvement over weeks or months) (34%), (3) stepwise progressive (34%), and (4) steady progressive (15%).[12] With treatment, a consensus group of experts, using a CIDP disease activity status scale, determined that a minority of patients (11%) achieved a status of "cure," defined by a stable examination off treatment for more than 5 years.[31] Half of these patients had normal examinations and the remainder had apparent mild and presumably minor clinical findings. Twenty percent of their 106 patients were considered in remission, similar to the cure group with the exception that they had not been medication-free for 5 years. Forty-four percent of patients in this series were classified as having stable active disease in which ongoing treatment was required. Another 7% improved in response to treatment which had recently been administered, precluding classification elsewhere. Finally, 18% were labeled as unstable active disease. A third of this cohort had not received treatment and two-thirds or 11% of the entire group were identified as unstable and active with treatment unresponsiveness.

Classic CIDP is a subacute to chronic, motor predominant disorder that presents with a non–length-dependent and symmetric pattern of weakness.[2,6,12–14,32,36,45,46] It is estimated that approximately half of CIDP patients present in this manner although these statistics may be biased by the inclusion of patients with DADS and CISP variants within the CIDP denominator.[33] Although distal limb muscles may be more severely affected early, significant and at times dominant involvement of proximal limb muscles is characteristic of the syndrome. This is estimated to occur in approximately 75–90% of patients, 90% of which will have a symmetric pattern.[9,11,13–16,31,47] In addition, approximately 80–94% of CIDP patients, like GBS, will have sensory symptoms and usually signs that may be the presenting or relapsing manifestation but that are usually rapidly overshadowed by the morbidity of their weakness.[13,31,47] Although the sensory symptoms are usually most pronounced in the distal extremities, they can be frequently identified as being nonlength dependent by affecting the hands before, at the same time, or soon after involvement of the feet. This is notably different from most length-dependent axonal neuropathies. Loss of large-fiber sensory modalities is typically more pronounced than their small-fiber counterparts but loss of all sensory modalities is not rare. Accordingly, dysesthesias occur in 15–50% of affected individuals.[12,15,48] When back pain occurs early in the syndrome in a manner similar to GBS, it is presumed to represent nerve root inflammation.[49] In addition, CIDP patients along with most acquired demyelinating polyneuropathies, have generalized areflexia (70%) or hyporeflexia in 97% of cases. Pathophysiologically, this is a presumptive effect of desynchronous impulse transmission associated with the temporal dispersion so frequently identified electrodiagnostically.[13,31]

Involvement of cranial nerves, phrenic nerves, and other nerves innervating intercostal and other ventilatory muscles, and the autonomic nervous system may occur in CIDP but are far less prevalent than in GBS.[13] Bifacial weakness although typically mild, occurs more commonly in our experience than the 15% reported figure.[12,14,15,31,47] Ophthalmoplegia, vestibulocochlear symptoms, and bulbar weakness are less common manifestations.[12,14–16,20,50,51] A rare presentation is neck extensor weakness leading to the dropped head syndrome.[52] Papilledema may be seen in rare patients with CIDP, but its presence should heighten consideration toward POEMS syndrome (polyneuropathy, organomegaly, endocrinopathy, monoclonal gammopathy, and skin changes).[12,53] Symptoms of dysautonomia are uncommon and typically mild when present, affecting distal postganglionic axons and producing mild, cholinergic, predominantly sudomotor dysfunction[12,15,54–56] Ventilatory failure in CIDP also occurs much less frequently than in GBS, but can occur perhaps more commonly in POEMS patients and is one source of mortality in this disease.[33,56–58] We have had one experience with a patient with typical CIDP, exquisitely treatment responsive for years, who eventually became refractory to multiple different therapies, eventually becoming "locked-in" and ventilator dependent. Postural tremor may occur in CIDP. Rarely it may be the presenting and initially dominant symptom. At times, patients seem to be ataxic in a manner disproportionate to the degree of their weakness or sensory loss, reminiscent of Miller Fisher syndrome.

Pure motor forms of CIDP are estimated to occur in 5–15% of CIDP patients, pure sensory forms in 15–35%, and notable asymmetries in 30% of patients.[32,33] These statistics have to be interpreted with caution however as different series may include patients that may represent DADS, MMN, or MADSAM neuropathies. Pure motor forms are fairly easy to identify in most cases as the characteristic EDX features of acquired demyelination are the norm. A steroid responsive, pure motor axonal form of CIDP, analogous to the acute motor axonal neuropathy (AMAN) variant of GBS, has been described.[57,59]

Pure sensory variants of CIDP are more difficult to define as they may or may not have concomitant demyelinating features on motor conduction studies which are arguably, the most reliable means by which to classify them as CIDP variants.[15,32,60–62] Some of these patients will develop significant weakness and evolve into typical CIDP.[63] Many, however will remain as pure sensory syndromes. Whether most if not all of these should be more appropriately classified as DADS neuropathy or CISP is a rhetoric question for which there is no consensus answer. Patients that have been described as sensory CIDP seem to fit into one of three categories.[33] Approximately, half will have EDX features of demyelination despite absence of any clinical evidence of motor involvement, similar if not identical to the DADS phenotype at presentation.[33,64] The second group, constitutes approximately a quarter of the pure sensory phenotype.[15] These patients have sensory signs and symptoms, coupled with abnormal sensory nerve action potential (SNAP) amplitudes, but normal motor conduction studies. These patients have been classified as CIDP, largely as a result of characteristic nerve histopathology. It is our suspicion that this group is the one more likely to have an alternative diagnosis, for example, sensory neuronopathy. The third group, representing the remaining 25% of the pure sensory CIDP phenotype, manifests as a pure sensory clinical presentation often associated with sensory ataxia, coupled with normal routine conduction studies.[15] In these cases, elevated cerebral spinal fluid (CSF) protein levels and abnormal somatosensory conductions in the face of normal SNAPs implicate a nerve root localization. As such, these patients are similar if not identical to the described CISP syndrome.[60,65–68]

As many as 3% of patients with CIDP develop evidence of central nervous system (CNS) demyelination clinically, electrophysiologically (evoked potential studies), or by magnetic resonance imaging (MRI).[69–75] Attacks of CNS demyelination can precede or follow the onset of CIDP. Like multiple sclerosis (MS), asymptomatic lesions may be detected by MRI and may represent a CIDP variant or coexisting MS.

TABLE 14-2. EUROPEAN FEDERATION OF NEUROLOGICAL SOCIETIES/PERIPHERAL NERVE SOCIETY DIAGNOSTIC CRITERIA FOR CIDP

Diagnostic Category	Definite	Probable	Possible
Required clinical criteria	Clinical criteria IA or IB and II	Clinical criteria IA or IB and II	Clinical criteria IA or IB and II
Required EDX criteria	EDX criteria I	EDX II	EDX III
Alternative means to achieve diagnostic category	Probable with 1 supportive Possible with 2 supportive	Possible with 1 supportive	

Clinical criteria:
IA Chronic progressive, stepwise or relapsing course.
Proximal and distal weakness.
Sensory involvement—4 limbs.
Reduced or absent deep tendon reflexes—4 limbs.
IB Partial sparing of reflexes
Distal weakness only.
Asymmetric or focal presentations.
Pure motor or sensory presentations.
CNS involvement.
II Exclusionary criteria—other demyelinating neuropathies (hereditary, diphtheria), MAG autoantibodies, MMN, sphincter disturbance.
EDX criteria:
I Definite: Demyelinating features in 2 or more motor nerves.
Conduction slowing <30% ULN.
Prolonged distal latencies >50% ULN.
F wave slowing (latency >20% with CMAP > 80% LLN) (latency >50% ULN with CMAP <80% LLN).
F wave absence (CMAP >20% LLN) + one other demyelinating parameter.
Conduction block (CMAP <50% LLN).
Temporal dispersion (CMAP duration >30% different between proximal and distal CMAPS) (distal CMAP duration >9 months).
II Probable: >30% CMAP amplitude reduction in proximal response in two nerves (CMAP >20% LLN) or one nerve with one other demyelinating feature in a second nerve.
III Possible: Same as **II** in a single nerve.
Supportive criteria:
Albumonocytologic dissociation.
MR imaging evidence of nerve root or plexus enhancement or hypertrophy.
Biopsy features of demyelination/remyelination in >5 (electron microscopy) or 6 (teased fibers) nerve fibers.
Improvement following immunomodulatory treatment.

Adapted with permission from Hughes RA , Bouche P, Cornblath DR, et al. European Federation of Neurological Societies/Peripheral Nerve Society guideline on management of chronic inflammatory demyelinating polyradiculoneuropathy: Report of a joint task force of the European Federation of Neurological Societies and the Peripheral Nerve Society. *Eur J Neurol*. 2006;13(4):326–332.

DIAGNOSIS AND DIFFERENTIAL DIAGNOSIS

As previously mentioned, there are 15 published diagnostic criteria for CIDP that place variable emphasis on the importance of clinical, EDX, cerebrospinal fluid, nerve root imaging, nerve biopsy features, and response to treatment data.[2,75] Of these, the criteria proposed by the European Federation of Neurological Societies (EFNS) in conjunction with the Peripheral Nerve Society (PNS) in 2006 are viewed as having the optimal balance between diagnostic sensitivity and specificity with a 97% and 92% positive and negative predictive value, respectively (Table 14-2).[2,32,45] In summary, these criteria emphasize the importance of the clinical presentation and findings. They consider the results of CSF analysis, MRI, nerve biopsy, and response to treatment to be supportive considerations (Fig. 14-1). In other words, a diagnosis of definite CIDP can be made without any supportive tests in a patient with symmetric proximal and distal weakness, sensory signs and symptoms, and generalized hypo- or areflexia if their illness progresses or relapses over a period of more than 2 months in the setting of typical EDX findings. The probable and possible diagnostic categories are also determined by a combination of clinical and EDX criteria. When available, supportive data allows escalation of the diagnostic criteria. Our beliefs parallel the ENFS/PNS criteria with the following exceptions. We are very cautious about making a CIDP diagnosis in pure sensory cases, particularly in those with a DADS phenotype, particularly if there is an IgM monoclonal protein (MCP), with or without myelin-associated glycoprotein (MAG) autoantibodies.

Accurate diagnosis is important for research purposes, both in consideration of clinical trial inclusion and in order to be able to eventually illuminate the cause(s) of this syndrome. We believe however, that in clinical practice, the most important value of accurate diagnosis is to decide who to treat and what to treat them with. Avoiding expensive and potentially harmful treatment without likely benefit while at the same time ensuring that potentially treatment responsive individuals are identified are two self-evident benefits of accurate diagnosis. In order to achieve that goal we place the greatest emphasis on the patient's phenotype and the supporting EDX data. We follow the lead of the EFNS/PNS in considering a characteristic CSF pattern, found in approximately 90% of patients, to be helpful but not diagnostically mandatory.

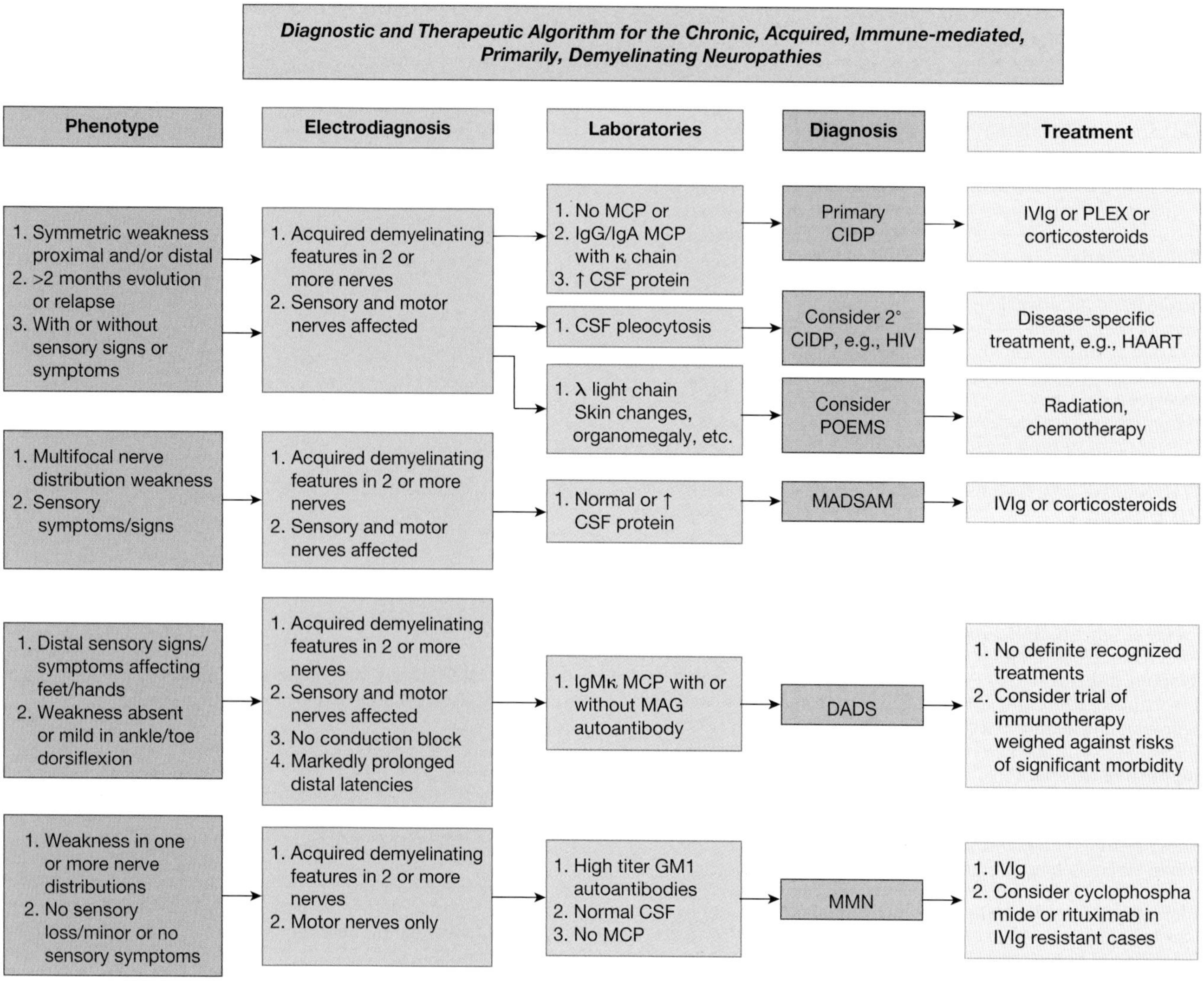

Figure 14-1. Chronic acquired demyelinating polyneuropathies. Diagnostic flow diagram: Diagnosis of chronic acquired demyelinating polyneuropathy and specific neuropathy syndrome (CIDP, MADSAM, DADS, MMN) is arrived at predominantly by phenotype coupled with EDX assessment. Other supportive testing is applied when necessary to clarify the diagnosis in atypical cases or aid in the identification of secondary causes of chronic acquired demyelinating neuropathy. Abbreviations: CIDP, chronic inflammatory demyelinating polyradiculoneuropathy; MADSAM, multifocal acquired demyelinating sensory and motor neuropathy; DADS, distal acquired demyelinating sensory neuropathy; MMN, multifocal motor neuropathy; CSF, cerebrospinal fluid; MCP, monoclonal protein; IVIg, intravenous immunoglobulin; PLEX, plasma exchange; GM1, GM1 autoantibodies; MAG, myelin associated glycoprotein; HIV, human immunodeficiency virus; POEMS, polyneuropathy, organomegaly, endocrinopathy, monoclonal protein, skin changes.

For a number of reasons, we do not routinely recommend nerve biopsy as a means to diagnose CIDP, particularly when the diagnosis is well established by clinical and EDX means. We are more apt to perform nerve biopsies in atypical cases with the primary goal of excluding alternative diagnosis.

Regarding the application of EDX to CIDP, we believe that its role is to support the diagnosis in a patient with a compatible phenotype, not to establish it in the absence of a compatible clinical picture. Our position is supported by the knowledge that an EDX pattern compatible with an acquired demyelinating neuropathy is characteristic of a number of disparate phenotypes whose natural history and response to treatment may vary considerably from classic CIDP, for example, POEMS syndrome and DADS neuropathy.[3,4,7,54,66,81] Even hereditary demyelinating neuropathies may at times have EDX patterns compatible with CIDP.[77] We do not adhere to the concept that a diagnosis of CIDP can be established by electrodiagnosis alone.

The differential diagnosis of CIDP begins in its distinction from GBS. As previously mentioned, up to 18% of individuals who will eventually develop a relapsing or progressing course justifying a CIDP diagnosis will have an initial evolution rapid enough to suspect GBS.[33,38–40] In these individuals, it would be pragmatic to initiate treatment with either intravenous immunoglobulin (IVIg) or plasma exchange (PLEX) and reserve any consideration of corticosteroids until the trajectory of the illness justifies a CIDP diagnosis.

CIDP is typically considered a primary diagnosis. In approximately a quarter of individuals, a concomitant systemic disease may be identifiable[2,14,34,45,78–82] with lymphoma and diabetes being the most prevalent in one series. (Table 14-3)[33] Not included in this table are CIDP phenotypes which have been described in association with drugs such as cyclosporine, tacrolimus, and tumor necrosis alpha blockers.[79,80,93–97] It is likely that the neuropathy in such cases is caused by the altered immune status of the patient, not to a direct toxic effect of the drug. Associations between CIDP and other disorders may represent two different diseases sharing a common pathophysiological mechanism or in the case of diabetes, a common disorder with a similar phenotype occurring coincidentally. Alternatively, and probably less commonly, CIDP might be caused by consequences of the primary systemic disease. The last consideration is the coexistence of two unrelated conditions, the second disorder being identified as a byproduct of the diagnostic scrutiny provided by the evaluation of the first.

In the early part of this century, there was considerable debate as to whether there was an increased incidence of CIDP in diabetic patients, or whether these were two disorders that might in some cases have overlapping clinical, EDX, or CSF features.[98–103] The practical consideration of this question revolves around the consideration of immunomodulating treatment in diabetics with "CIDP-like" features. Confounding this decision is the realization that nerve biopsy specimens of patients with diabetic radiculoplexopathy may have inflammatory features and may respond to immunomodulating treatment, without invoking any consideration of CIDP phenotype a demyelinating EDX signature.[104,105]

Arguably, the most confusing consideration relevant to conditions associated or perhaps causally related to CIDP is the coexistence of an MCP. That a relationship exists is supported by a reported incidence of MCPs in CIDP as 22–30% [32,33,106,107] in comparison to 10% in polyneuropathies in general which in turn, is 6–10 fold greater than in an age-matched population.[106] Confusion arises as the neuropathies associated with MCPs may share phenotypic and EDX features with CIDP, or they may not. For example, the neuropathy associated with IgM MGUS commonly fulfills EDX criteria for CIDP, even if the phenotype (DADS) is disparate in the majority of cases. In addition, patients with IgM MCPs differ in most cases from CIDP without MCPs or those associated with IgG/IgA MCPs as they have (1) a definable autoantibody in many cases (anti-MAG), (2) a differing natural history, (3) a distinctive histopathology, and (4) a different response to treatment.[14,106,108,109]

Conversely, although IgA/IgG-associated neuropathies frequently have an axonal EDX profile, they may manifest with both the clinical and EDX features of CIDP.[109] They tend to manifest more motor involvement, faster progression, less of a demyelinating EDX profile, and better treatment responsiveness than do their IgM counterparts. For these reasons, like others,[2,14,45,102,109] we do not consider the presence of an MCP, particularly if IgG or IgA, to preclude a CIDP diagnosis as have others.[12,15]

When a neuropathy coexists with an MCP, it is usually an MCP of unknown significance (MGUS). It is important to remain aware that an MCP may be representative of an underlying systemic disease which needs to be considered not only at the time that the MCP is recognized but subsequently as MGUS may evolve into lymphoma, Waldenstrom macroglobulinemia, chronic lymphocytic leukemia, multiple myeloma, POEMS syndrome, amyloidosis, heavy chain disease, or cryoglobulinemia.[109]

Most diagnostic criteria for CIDP require exclusion of other neuropathies with definable etiologies that may have overlapping features. This list has to be to some extent flexible, given the uncertainties of CIDP diagnostic boundaries as discussed above. According to the EFNS criteria, hereditary neuropathies including demyelinating CMT genotypes and Refsum disease should be considered and excluded when relevant, to the extent possible.[45] In addition, these criteria consider MMN and DADS neuropathy associated with (but not without) demonstrable MAG autoantibodies as separate disorders. We find this latter argument somewhat specious as the ability to detect MAG autoantibodies varies considerably depending on the technique used and as on the whole, DADS patients with and without MAG autoantibodies are indistinguishable.[110] It is our personal bias that amyloidosis should warrant special consideration in individuals with "CIDP-like" phenotypes with axonal EDX signatures, particularly in association with symptoms of extraneural or autonomic involvement.[90]

TABLE 14-3. MEDICAL CONDITIONS ASSOCIATED WITH CHRONIC ACQUIRED IMMUNE-MEDIATED DEMYELINATING POLYNEUROPATHY

HIV infection
Inflammatory bowel disease
Systemic lupus erythematosus
Diabetes mellitus
Monoclonal gammopathy of uncertain significance (MGUS)
Paraneoplastic
POEMS syndrome
Lymphoma
Castleman disease
Waldenstrom macroglobulinemia (usually associated with DADS phenotype)
Small cell carcinoma of the lung
Carcinoma of the pancreas
Carcinoma of the colon
Cholangiocarcinoma
Melanoma
Bone marrow and solid organ transplantations (often in setting of graft vs. host disease or rejection)
Neurotoxicity
Hepatitis B and C
Sarcoidosis
Membranous glomerulonephropathy
Organ and stem cell transplantation

LABORATORY FEATURES

Most patients (80–95%) have an elevated CSF protein (>45 mg/dL) with a mean of 135 mg/dL and levels that may exceed 1,200 mg/dL.[10–12,14,16,48] Very high CSF protein levels associated with CIDP should trigger consideration of POEMS syndrome or blockade of the spinal canal from hypertrophic nerve roots. Similar to GBS, the CSF cell count is usually normal, although up to 10% of patients have greater than five lymphocytes/mm^3. Elevated CSF cell counts should lead to the consideration of HIV infection, sarcoidosis, Lyme disease, and lymphomatous or leukemic infiltration of nerve roots. Oligoclonal bands may be demonstrated in the CSF in approximately 65% of patients.[111,112]

Blood testing in CIDP is done largely in consideration of alternative diagnoses, associated diseases, or secondary causes. As previously discussed, a monoclonal gammopathy (IgA, IgG, or IgM) is present in up to 30% of patients with CIDP.[14,47,48,63,102,107,113] A small number of patients have GM1, P_2, and particularly P_0 (20%) autoantibodies.[45,114–117] Antitubulin antibodies were reported in one study of CIDP[117] but was not seen in others.[118,119] More recently, autoantibodies directed at novel nodal and paranodal myelin and axonal antigens have been reported in small numbers of CIDP patients (see below).[127–129] Many would consider the detection of MAG autoantibodies helpful, particularly in those patients with a DADS phenotype. In our estimation however, detection of these antibodies provide little if any practical value beyond the detection of an IgM MCP in most cases.[109] We believe that autoantibody testing currently has a limited role in the evaluation of a CIDP suspect.

Otherwise, as always, we feel that the evaluation of a CIDP patient should be determined in consideration of the clinical context of the individual case. In general, we follow the recommendations of the EFNS and obtain a complete blood count, urinalysis, C reactive protein or sedimentation rate, glycosylated hemoglobin, creatinine, transaminases, serology for Lyme disease, hepatitis B and C, and antinuclear antibodies in addition to a serum and in some cases urine immunofixation.[45] In cases in which an MCP is detected, evaluation for POEMS syndrome, lymphoma, myeloma, and amyloid are undertaken as warranted.

Hypertrophy and enhancement of the nerve roots and peripheral nerves may be appreciated with MRI which has been proposed as supportive criteria for diagnosis.[45,120–122] Rarely, a myelopathy can develop secondary to the markedly enlarged nerve roots compressing the spinal cord.[123]

ELECTRODIAGNOSTIC FEATURES

Multiple nerves should be evaluated on NCS because of the multifocal nature of the disease process; some nerves can have normal conduction studies, while other nerves are abnormal. Various electrophysiological criteria for demyelination have been devised.[1,2,14,45,78,124,125] Again, our position is that EDX assessment is an integral component of the CIDP diagnosis, but that it does not determine the diagnosis independent of clinical assessment. Less than two-thirds of patients with CIDP fulfill electrophysiological criteria for demyelination, regardless of the criteria utilized.[1,33]

Motor Conduction Studies

Motor conduction studies include assessment of compound muscle action potential (CMAP) amplitudes, distal latencies, conduction velocities (CVs), F wave latencies, and waveform morphological changes such as temporal dispersion or conduction block. These are the most useful EDX tools in the evaluation of a patient with suspected CIDP.[1,2,14,45] As previously mentioned, there are at minimum 16 EDX criteria for CIDP that have been proposed. For purposes of simplicity, we will summarize those EDX criteria proposed by the EFNS/PNS which require demonstration of one or more of the following characteristic demyelinating abnormalities in at least two motor nerves (Table 14-2)[45]:

1. Prolongation of motor distal latencies by >50% of the upper limits of normal (ULN).
2. Reduction in CV to <30% of the lower limits of normal (LLN).
3. Conduction block as defined by CMAP reduction of >50%.
4. Temporal dispersion as defined by >30% increase in CMAP duration in proximal compared to distal CMAP or distal CMAP duration exceeding 9 ms.
5. 20% increase in F wave latency if CMAP >80% LLN, >50% increase in F wave latency if CMAP <80% LLN, or absence of F waves in motor nerves with CMAP >20% LLN.

We would add the following caveats to the interpretation of these criteria. We are cautious about including conduction block at common compression entrapment sites, conduction block of the tibial nerve, and absent F waves of the peroneal nerve as fulfilling the diagnostic criteria for CIDP. Although of uncertain utility, phrenic nerve conduction abnormalities in CIDP patients occur and do so with greater frequency than in MMN.[126] In addition, we would be willing to identify a conduction block with a reduction of CMAP amplitude of less than 50% if the waveform change occurs abruptly over a short segment of a nerve in a location where neither entrapment or compression are likely.

As patients' strength and function improve, repeat NCS may demonstrate evidence of improvement with increases in CMAP amplitudes and CVs along with reduction in the magnitude of conduction block.[16,127–133] In keeping with this, conduction block in motor nerves is an uncommon findings in patients with DADS neuropathy in keeping with the frequently pure sensory (clinical) nature of their phenotype, at least at onset.[106,109] Clinical improvement is primarily the result of resolving conduction block, although some may be attributed to improved ion channel function without remyelination, collateral sprouting, or regeneration of axons.

Sensory Conduction Studies

Most patients with CIDP have SNAPs that are reduced in amplitude or absent in both the upper and the lower extremities.[10,14–16,61,107,133,134] When present, SNAPs may demonstrate conduction slowing either as prolonged distal latencies and/or slow CVs. However, this "slowing" is usually not as severe as that demonstrated in motor nerves. In a study of 18 patients using the near-nerve technique, sensory conduction slowing was only moderately slow in proportion to the degree of amplitude loss.[135] A helpful feature when present is the identification of median, ulnar, or radial SNAPs abnormalities when the sural or superficial peroneal SNAPs are normal. This pattern of "sural" sparing suggests a non-length-dependent process (most axonal neuropathies are length dependent). When sensory EDX abnormalities are worse in the arms than in the legs, one needs to consider a predominantly demyelinating neuropathy or sensory ganglionopathy.

Needle Electromyography

Insertional and spontaneous activities are often normal on needle electromyography (EMG). However, fibrillation potentials are not rare as there is often some element of secondary axonal loss. Occasionally, myokymic discharges may be seen related to ephaptic transmission between demyelinated nerve fibers. The earliest and perhaps only abnormality one might see on EMG is reduced recruitment (fast-firing) motor unit action potentials (MUAPs) that otherwise appear morphologically normal.

Evoked Potential and Autonomic Studies

Rare patients have abnormal visual-evoked, brainstem auditory-evoked, and somatosensory-evoked potentials suggestive of superimposed central demyelination.[72,73] Another application of SSEPs, like H reflexes, is their utility in identifying pathology of the dorsal roots. SSEP and H reflex abnormalities occurring in the context of normal SNAPs referable to the same dermatome(s) imply pathology of the dorsal root such as believed to occur in CISP (see below)[60,65–68] Although most patients are not symptomatic, evidence of subclinical autonomic neuropathy is not uncommon.[54–56] Blood pressure and heart rate responses to tilt testing followed by the 30/15 heart rate ratio in response to deep breathing are the most frequently abnormal autonomic studies.

HISTOPATHOLOGY

Nerve biopsies in CIDP should be interpreted with the realization that a sensory nerve is being examined in a disorder that typically has a motor predominant phenotype. As a result, neither the extent nor type of abnormality identified may be fully representative of the entire disease process. Nerve biopsy is a useful, but not requisite diagnostic tool, for CIDP, arguably of greater utility in excluding other disorders than in proving the existence of CIDP.[136,137] Biopsies are particularly useful when vasculitis, lymphomatous infiltration, amyloidosis, or sarcoidosis are considered.

Nerve biopsies may reveal segmental demyelination and remyelination which may not be evident due to the multifocal nature of the process (Fig. 14-2).[12,14,70,136,138,139] Chronic demyelination and remyelination result in proliferation of surrounding Schwann cell processes known as "onion bulbs." These are the basis of hypertrophic nerves and are seen CIDP although they are not as prominent as in demyelinating forms of Charcot–Marie–Tooth disease (see Fig. 3-31). Myelinated fibers are usually reduced in number. Fibers examined in semithin sections demonstrate myelin thickness that is disproportionately thin in relationship to axon diameter indicate remyelination (Fig. 14-2C). Teased nerve fiber analysis demonstrates segmental demyelination and/or remyelination in 23–46%, axonal degeneration in 21–42%, mixed demyelinating and axonal features in 12.5%, and normal findings in 18–43.5% of nerve biopsies from studied CIDP patients.[12,14] (see Fig. 3-30).

Endoneurial and perineurial edema may also be appreciated on biopsy. Inflammatory cell infiltrate may be evident in the epineurium, perineurium, or endoneurium. It is often perivascular when detectable but often quite subtle or absent in nerve biopsy specimens (Fig. 14-2A).[12,14] Inflammatory cells are better appreciated with immunostaining for lymphocytes (Fig. 14-2B).[140,141] This inflammatory component comprises of macrophages, CD3+-activated T cells (mainly CD8+ but also CD4+ cells lymphocytes), and dendritic cells.[141,142] Of note, a similar frequency of inflammatory cell infiltrate within nerves is seen in a variety of neuropathies, raising questions concerning the pathogenic role of these cells.[140] The matrix metalloproteinases MMP-2 and MMP-9 (gelatinase A and B) are overexpressed in the peripheral nerves in patients with CIDP.[143] These enzymes are secreted by T cells and are capable of digesting basement membrane proteins, thereby facilitating the infiltration of inflammatory cells into peripheral nerves.

On electron microscopy (EM), macrophages may be noted to penetrate the basement membrane with displacement of the Schwann cell cytoplasm, lyse superficial myelin lamellae, penetrate along intraperiod lines, and engulf the disrupted myelin by endocytosis. By doing so, they disrupt the nodes of Ranvier, and by doing so, presumptively saltatory conduction.[144] Subsequently, Schwann cells are recruited to remyelinate the demyelinated internodes. The demyelinated axons diminish in diameter as much as 50% but later regain some of their diameter following remyelination.

PATHOGENESIS

There are numerous aspects of both the anatomy and physiology of peripheral nerve that are relevant to both normal

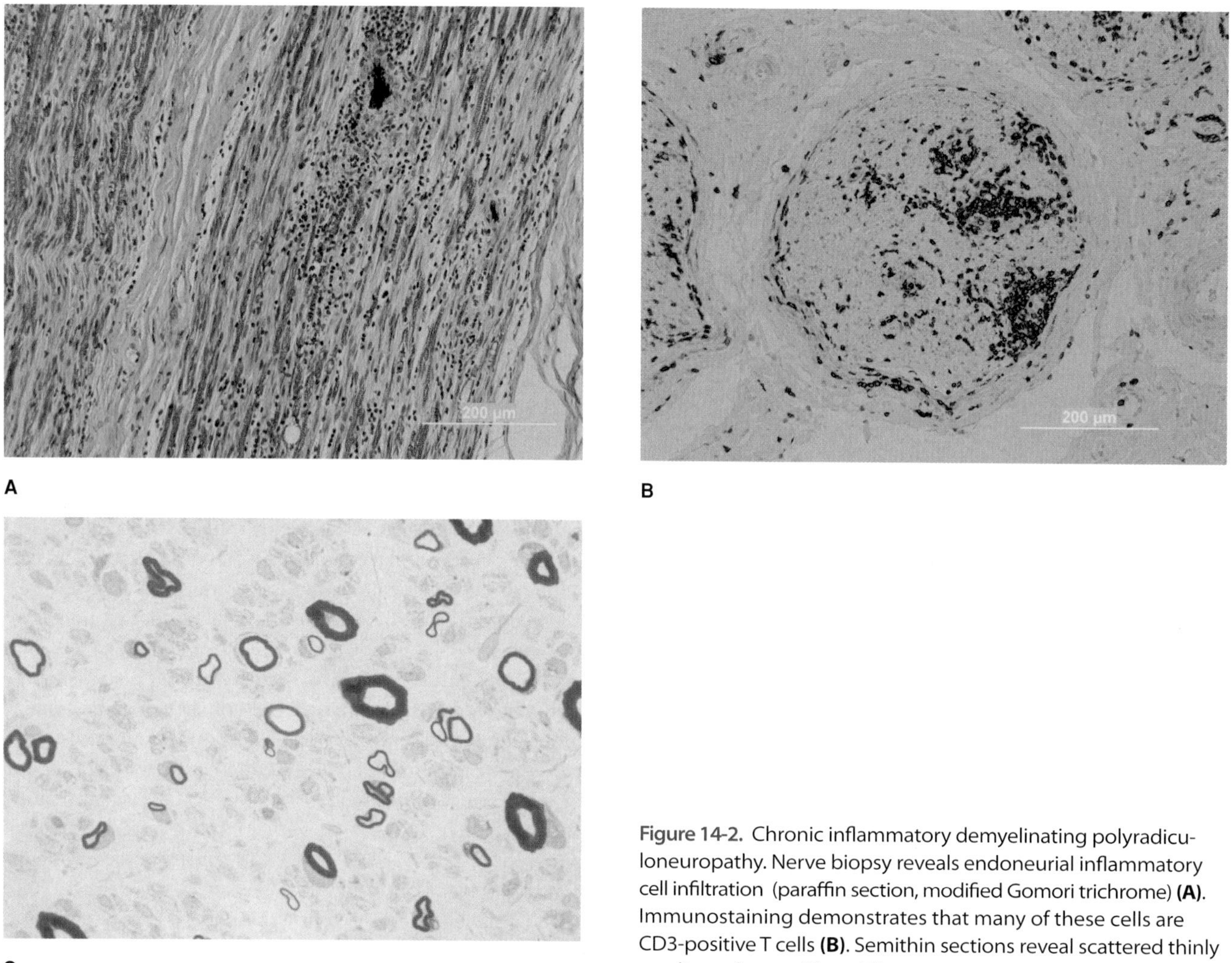

Figure 14-2. Chronic inflammatory demyelinating polyradiculoneuropathy. Nerve biopsy reveals endoneurial inflammatory cell infiltration (paraffin section, modified Gomori trichrome) **(A)**. Immunostaining demonstrates that many of these cells are CD3-positive T cells **(B)**. Semithin sections reveal scattered thinly myelinated nerve fibers **(C)**.

impulse transmission, and to the mechanisms of abnormal nerve transmission associated with the acquired, immune-mediated, and demyelinating polyneuropathies. These variables include axonal diameter which varies under normal circumstance between the node of Ranvier and the internode as well as the intervening paranode and juxtaparanode (Fig. 14-3). In addition, normal and abnormal nerve impulse transmission are related to many factors pertaining to the surrounding myelin sheath, and to the type, location, and density of the ion channels upon which action potential generation is ultimately dependent.

There are many lines of evidence that would identify CIDP as an autoimmune disorder although disease mechanisms remain poorly understood.[145] In particular, the antigen(s) to which the immune attack is targeted and specific roles of the humoral and cellular system played in the pathogenesis of CIDP remain in large part unknown. Anatomically, the pathological changes associated with CIDP are demonstrable at the root, plexus, and nerve level.[146] Autoantibodies against glycolipids such as GM1 and GD1a are logical choices as responsible pathogenic agents in CIDP as these antigenic targets are located on the nodal axolemma of motor nerves. GM1 and GD1a autoantibodies are capable of interfering with ion channel function although perhaps not at an order of magnitude sufficient to disrupt impulse transmission. In addition, these gangliosides are found as well as on the cell surface of *Campylobacter jejuni*, the precipitating agent in many cases of the AMAN variant of GBS with which these autoantibodies are so closely associated. Furthermore, GM1 and GD1 knockout mice demonstrate that these gangliosides are essential for the integrity of node/internode junctions. Paranodal loops in these animal models do not attach to the axolemma, Na channels are disrupted, and K channels are mislocated to the paranode.[145] Nonetheless, ganglioside autoantibodies have not been routinely identifiable in CIDP patients.[121]

As previously mentioned, some CIDP patients will have antibodies directed against myelin P_0, which along with PMP-22 are transmembrane components of compact myelin. These antigens are probably more relevant to hereditary than acquired demyelinating neuropathies. Current opinion does not strongly support either a pathogenic or

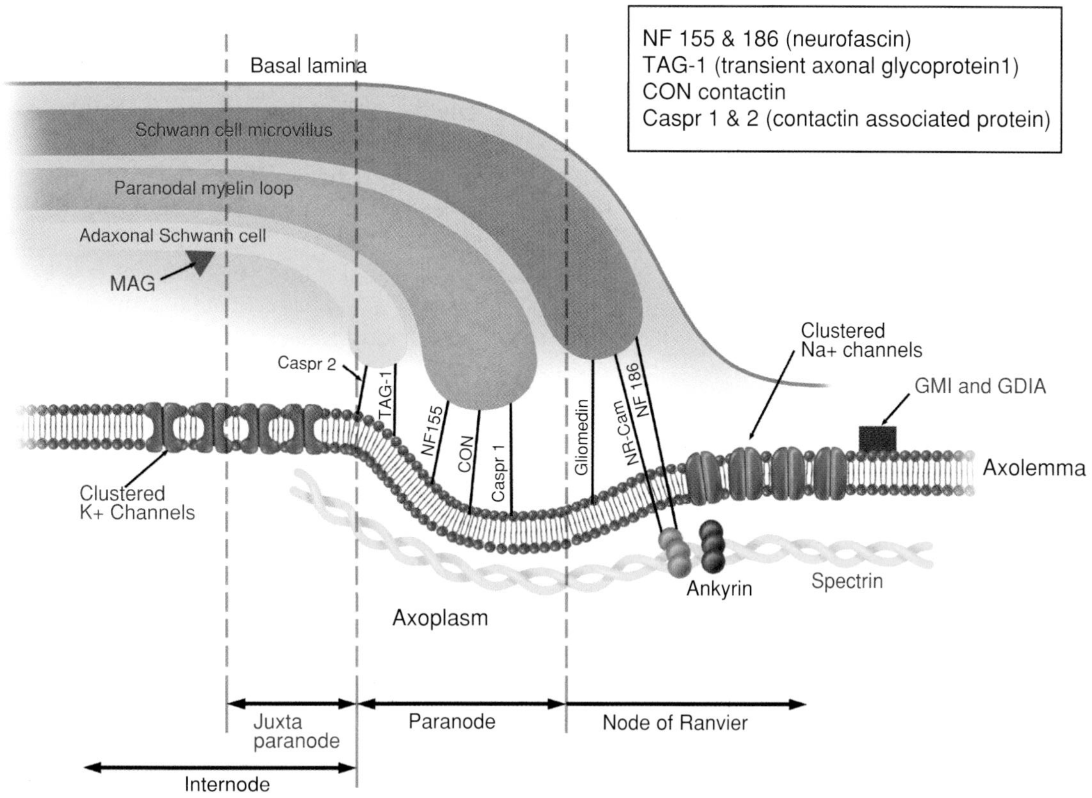

Figure 14-3. Simplified schematic of a peripheral nerve fiber (motor) node/internode junction with locations of proteins and ion channels potentially relevant to the pathogenesis of chronic, acquired, demyelinating polyneuropathies.

diagnostic role for these autoantibodies in CIDP. Recently, a small number of GBS and CIDP patients have been shown to have autoantibodies targeting novel antigens residing in nodal and paranodal regions many of which are responsible for the positioning and anchoring of ion channels in strategic locations along the axolemma.[145] Specifically, Na channels are anchored to spectrin of the axonal cytoskeleton via ankyrin-G and to gliomedin of the Schwann cell microvilli via Nr-CAM and neurofascin-186. The juxtaparanodal type 1 K channels are anchored by contactin-associated protein-2 (Caspr-2) and transient axonal glycoprotein-1 (TAG-1), the latter being an adhesion molecule that resides on the juxtaparanodal axolemma and apposing Schwann cell membranes (Fig. 14-3). Of apparent physiological importance is the separation of clustered Na channels in nodal regions from the clustered potassium channels in the juxtaparanodal regions which is dependent upon interactions between axonal Caspr and contactin which are connected to neurofascin-155 of paranodal myelin loop. Autoantibodies directed against contactin, neurofascin, Nr-CAM, and gliomedin have been described in small numbers of CIDP patients.[144,147,148]

Failure of regulatory T-cell mechanism is thought to underlie persistent or recurrent disease, differentiating CIDP from the acute inflammatory demyelinating polyneuropathy form of GBS.[45,116] CD8+ T-cell–mediated autoimmunity has been demonstrated.[142] The rapid improvement that occasionally follows PLEX or IVIg and the demonstration of immunoglobulin and complement on peripheral nerve tissues suggest a role of the humoral arm of the immune system as well.[16,149] Theoretically, autoantibodies may impair ion channel function and by doing so produce an EDX pattern suggesting rapidly reversible axon loss similar to the AMAN variant of GBS. Ion channel dysfunction may also theoretically result in EDX evidence of conduction block as well.[145]

Physiologically, conduction block is most frequently attributed to paranodal and internodal demyelination which impairs axon potential propagation.[145,146,150] Demyelination of a nerve segment produces an increased transverse capacitance and reduced resistance in the area. This causes a leakage of current and increases the time required for the longitudinal current to reach the next node of Ranvier. If the current leakage is too excessive, current may be insufficient to depolarize the next node of Ranvier, necessary for continued impulse transmission. It is this conduction block not just the slowing of velocity, which is responsible for motor weakness. Weakness may also occur as a result of axon loss, the mechanism of which in CIDP is poorly understood.

TREATMENT

Corticosteroids, PLEX, and IVIg have been demonstrated to be beneficial in randomized controlled trials in CIDP patients, both in adults and children. (Table 14-4).[7,33,128,151–156] In one study, 66%, 59%, and 62% of individuals responded to IVIg, corticosteroids, and PLEX respectively.[33] This same therapeutic equivalence between IVIg and PLEX was demonstrated in one prospective trial.[129] Another clinical trial comparing IVIg versus prednisolone for 6 weeks demonstrated no short-term differences in efficacy.[151] It is generally held that failure to respond to one of these three treatments does not predict failure with the other two.[13] In one study, half of the patients who failed corticosteroids responded to IVIg.[157] Although CIDP should be considered a chronic disease, it is also a treatable disease with one study describing 40% of patients treated largely with IVIg and/or corticosteroids becoming independent of activities of daily living achieving a modified Rankin scale of two or less.[33] Despite treatment responsiveness, it is also important to point out that not all CIDP patients require treatment, and as always, clinical judgment of potential risk versus benefit is essential.[33] Our decision to

▶ **TABLE 14-4. IMMUNOMODULATING THERAPY FOR CHRONIC ACQUIRED DEMYELINATING POLYNEUROPATHIES**

Therapy	Neuropathy Used for	Route	Dose	Side Effects	Monitor
Prednisone	CIDP, MADSAM	p.o.	1–1.5 mg/kg/d for 2–4 weeks, then switch to QOD	Hypertension, fluid and weight gain, hyperglycemia, hypokalemia, cataracts, glaucoma, gastric irritation, and osteoporosis	Weight, blood pressure, glucose, potassium, ophthalmologic examination
Methylprednisone	CIDP, MADSAM	i.v.	1 g in 100 mL/normal saline over 1–2 h, three to six doses, daily or every other day	Arrhythmia, flushing, dysgeusia, anxiety, insomnia, fluid and weight gain, hyperglycemia, and hypokalemia	Heart rate Blood pressure Glucose Potassium
Azathioprine	CIDP, MADSAM	p.o.	2–3 mg/kg/d; single AM dose	Flu-like illness, hepatotoxicity, leukopenia, macrocytosis, and neoplasia	Monthly blood count and liver enzymes × 3 months then yearly
Cyclophosphamide	CIDP, MMN, MADSAM	p.o.	1.5–2 mg/kg/d; single AM dose	Leukopenia, hemorrhagic cystitis, alopecia, infections, and neoplasia	Monthly blood count and urinalysis for duration of treatment Urine cytology
		i.v.	0.5–3 g/m^2 (max 85 mg/kg)	Same as p.o. (although more severe) and nausea/vomiting	Same
Cyclosporine	CIDP, MADSAM	p.o.	3–6 mg/kg/d; BID.	Nephrotoxicity, hypertension, hepatotoxicity, hirsutism, tremor, and gum hyperplasia	Blood pressure Trough cyclosporine level Creatinine Liver enzymes
Rituximab	MMN, DADS	i.v.	375 mg/m^2 weekly × 4 weeks or 750 mg/m^2 (up to 1 g) × 2 weeks; usually the course will need to be repeated in 6–12 months	Infusion-related symptom complex (e.g. hypotension, rash, chills, urticaria, angioedema, and bronchospasm), asthenia, headaches, nausea vomiting, dizziness, and infection	CBC
Intravenous immunoglobulin (IVIg)	CIDP, MMN, MADSAM	i.v.	0.4 g/kg/d over 5 days, or 1 g/kg/d over 2 days × 3 months; then if effective, 1 g/kg q 4–8 weeks	Hypotension, arrhythmia, diaphoresis, flushing, nephrotoxicity, headache, aseptic meningitis, and anaphylaxis	Heart rate Blood pressure, Creatinine
Plasmapheresis	CIDP, MADSAM	i.v.	Remove total of 200–250 cc/kg plasma over 7–14 days; may require periodic exchanges	Hypotension, arrhythmia, electrolyte imbalance, anemia, and coagulation disorders	Heart rate, blood pressure, blood count, electrolytes, PT/PTT, volume removed and replaced

p.o., oral; i.v., intravenous; CIDP, chronic inflammatory demyelinating polyneuropathy; MMN, multifocal motor neuropathy; MADSAM, multifocal acquired demyelinating sensory and motor neuropathy; PT, prothrombin time; PTT, partial thromboplastin time; BUN, blood urea nitrogen; Red type, strong evidence of efficacy; Blue type, possible efficacy.

treat is determined primarily by the neuropathy phenotype and by the extent that the patient's comfort and function are affected by the neuropathy. Like others, we do not consider the coexistence of an MCP, particularly if IgA/IgG as a reason to withhold treatment in a patient with a typical generalized and symmetric pattern of weakness.[14]

Corticosteroids

Anecdotal cases and small series have long shown that corticosteroids can be beneficial in both adults and children,[9,10,14,16,33,158] further supported in a randomized control trial of oral prednisone in patients with CIDP.[159] Despite this limited evidence-based support, their use is supported by a Cochrane review in view of their long-term use and general acceptance of their benefit.[155] When we treat CIDP with corticosteroids, prednisone is initiated at a dose of 1–1.5 mg/kg (up to 100 mg) per day for 2–4 weeks, with transition to alternate day treatment as outlined in Chapter 4 (e.g., either 100 mg QOD or 60 mg alternating with 50 mg every other day).[14,36] Patients remain on relatively high doses of prednisone until their strength is normalized or there is a clear plateau in clinical improvement. When weaning begins, the trajectory it takes is dependent on the contextual features of the individual case. Typically, we begin the taper after a month or two of the induction dose, particularly if there are either signs of improvement or the development of unwanted side effects. We slowly taper the prednisone by 5 mg every 2–3 weeks until the dose is 20 mg every other day. At that point, dosing is reduced no faster than 2.5 mg every week or 5 mg every 2 weeks. Using this method of treatment, the time of initial improvement ranges from several days to 5 months (mean 1.9 months), the time to maximum improvement averages 6.6 months, with significant improvement in strength and function appreciated in 95% of treated patients after 1 year.[14]

In addition to traditional oral prednisone regimens, pulsed steroids either with intravenous methylprednisolone or with oral dexamethasone have been attempted with the hope of more rapid therapeutic onset and the potential for fewer side effects.[157,160–162] One study using pulsed dexamethasone at a dose of 40 mg daily for 4 consecutive days for a total of 6 cycles (if required) demonstrated faster improvement, longer remissions, fewer relapses, and fewer side effects in comparison to a more conventional oral prednisolone regimen.[157] Another study using a very similar design was unable to demonstrate any advantage over a similar pulsed oral dexamethasone regimen in comparison to a more traditional oral prednisolone.[162] Further information regarding the use of corticosteroids including mechanism(s) of action and adverse effects can be found in Chapter 4.

Plasma Exchange

PLEX, although likely to be equally effective, is less likely to be used as a CIDP treatment in comparison to corticosteroids or IVIg.[156,163] In all probability, this is based on considerations of availability and convenience as well as safety concerns. It remains an effective option in patients who are refractory or have contraindications to IVIg and/or corticosteroids. Efficacy of PLEX was demonstrated in prospective, randomized, double-blinded, placebo-controlled trials using sham PLEX.[128,131] However, the response to PLEX is transient, usually lasting only a few weeks, and therefore repeated courses of PLEX must be given intermittently or other, augmentative immunomodulating treatments used. The characteristic regimen is to exchange approximately 200–250 mL/kg body weight five to six times over a 2-week period. This identifies another notable benefit of IVIg which is the ability to treat on consecutive days, potentially reducing length-of-stay in a potentially hospitalized population. PLEX is usually used in combination with prednisone in patients with severe generalized weakness as the combination may provide a more rapid response than prednisone alone. In addition, protracted maintenance treatment with PLEX is often inconvenient, impractical and not endorsed by the evidence-based guideline from the American Academy of Neurology.[163] In those patients who require maintenance exchanges, the strategy once again is to reduce the number and frequency of exchanges while maintaining an optimal, achievable functional and comfort level. Like IVIg, a therapeutic/diagnostic trial of PLEX may be useful in patients in whom the CIDP diagnosis is uncertain or in whom corticosteroids are optimally avoided, for example, those with diabetes, HIV, or those in whom a diagnosis of GBS is considered.[98] Once again, the relatively rapid response to PLEX allows an earlier determination of whether or not such patients could have an immune-responsive neuropathy. Further detail regarding PLEX and potential adverse effects may be found in Chapter 4.

Intravenous Immunoglobulin

IVIg has been demonstrated to be effective in CIDP treatment, as demonstrated in controlled clinical trials and supported by a Cochrane meta-analysis.[131,154,157,164–166] Three of four trials comparing IVIg against placebo and another three comparing IVIg against either steroids or PLEX-demonstrated benefit.[167] Efficacy is estimated to be as high as 82% in one study.[33] Another observer-blinded, prospective, randomized trial found no clear difference in efficacy between IVIg and PLEX.[129] Unlike PLEX, it is endorsed by the American Academy of Neurology for both the long-term as well as short-term treatment of CIDP.[168] In further comparison to corticosteroids, the INCAT group demonstrated essentially no significant difference in the short-term between IVIg and prednisolone during a 6-week period.[151] In addition, retrospective studies have demonstrated that approximately 25% of CIDP patients achieve remission and 65% clinical stability with long-term IVIg treatment.[169]

There is a strong consensus that IVIg is the treatment of choice in CIDP for a number of reasons in addition to its efficacy.[7] It is generally accepted that the long-term side effect profiles favor IVIg over corticosteroids. In addition, there are occasional individuals who achieve a durable remission, estimated at 55% after 24 weeks in one study, potentially obviating the need for protracted steroid treatment.[170] Finally, initial use of IVIg as opposed to steroids eliminates the problem by the desire to initiate rapid treatment in a patient where there is diagnostic uncertainty between CIDP and GBS.

As the effects of IVIg are often transient, repeated courses of IVIg are necessary. The treatment regimen needs to be individualized. We initiate IVIg at a dose of 2 g/kg body weight over 2–5 days monthly for at least 3 months. Subsequent dosing is dependent on clinical response with a regimen of 1 g/kg every 3 weeks demonstrated to be effective in one study.[170] As always, the strategy is to ascertain the minimally effective dose, typically 1–2 g/kg every 3–8 weeks based on individual response.[170] In patients who become refractory to IVIg, courses of PLEX may restore IVIG responsiveness.[171]

IVIg is generally well tolerated. Although it has been suggested that individuals with IgA deficiency may be at risk for anaphylaxis from IVIg,[172] we agree with others that this reaction is rare and that the risk may be overstated.[167,173,174] Other adverse effects are addressed in Chapter 4.

Other Treatment Options

Interferon-β, etanercept, rituximab, cyclophosphamide, azathioprine, mycophenolate mofetil, fludarabine, alemtuzumab, methotrexate nataluzimab, and cyclosporine have all been used in the treatment of CIDP.[152] None have demonstrated benefit according to a Cochrane review with the caveat that the studies may have been too small to identify a modest benefit.[175] In addition, as reviewed in Chapter 4 and mentioned earlier in this chapter, tumor necrosis factor alpha blockers have been associated with CIDP, prompting caution in their use in this disorder. In essentially all cases, treatments other than IVIg, PLEX, and corticosteroids are used only as secondary agents, only when an acceptable response cannot be obtained by the three primary treatments. Again details pertaining to the mechanisms of action, administration, and adverse effects of these agents can be found in Chapter 4.

Small anecdotal reports suggest a beneficial effect of azathioprine at doses of 100–300 mg/d.[15,16,176–179] A prospective, randomized, but nonblinded 9-month study of 27 patients with CIDP failed to demonstrate a benefit of azathioprine (2 mg/kg/d) when added to prednisone.[181] The dose of azathioprine may have been too small however (we go up to 3 mg/kg/d) and the duration of this study may have been too short for a beneficial effect to become evident. A beneficial response from azathioprine may require a longer than 9 month exposure to adequate doses.

A number of small series along with our own personal experience suggest that both oral and monthly pulses of intravenous cyclophosphamide can be beneficial in patients with CIDP.[10,15,16,35,180,182–186] We prefer a monthly pulsed intravenous cyclophosphamide regimen as it is associated with less risks of hemorrhagic cystitis. We use cyclophosphamide as a last resort because of its side effect profile. None-the-less, we have seen patients rendered essentially quadriplegic by their disease and refractory to multiple other therapies regain complete independence in activities of daily living after a 6-month course of 1 g/m^2/month treatment.[187]

Cyclosporine also appears effective in some patients with CIDP, even in those refractory to other modes of therapy, including prednisone, PLEX, IVIg, and cyclophosphamide.[71,180,188–194] There have been limited studies reporting improvement with methotrexate for CIDP patients, some of whom were treatment resistant.[195–197] Both α and β interferons have been administered to CIDP patients.[180,198–206] Interferon-β1 a was reported to have modest benefit in small initial studies but a double-blind, placebo-controlled, crossover study in 10 patients with CIDP failed to confirm that.[200] Interferon-α has also been suggested to have a benefit in CIDP. CIDP has been reported however, to develop in individuals taking the drug for other reasons. Neither interferon can be endorsed for CIDP use at this time.

Mycophenolate mofetil is an immunomodulating agent that selectively inhibits the proliferation of T and B lymphocytes by blocking the rate-limiting enzyme in the de novo synthesis of guanosine nucleotides. A few small studies have suggested that mycophenolate mofetil may benefit patients with CIDP.[207,208] Other reports have been less favorable.[209] There appears to be a modest benefit in approximately 20% of CIDP patients with stabilization and successful reduction in steroid or IVIg therapy.[210] The response in general appears to be infrequent and modest.[180,211–214] Rituximab has been the subject of nine reports, again with suggestive but unproven benefit.[215–223] Total lymphoid irradiation was reported to be effective in three of four patients unresponsive to prednisone or cyclophosphamide.[224] A total of eight patients have received autologous or allogenic peripheral blood stem cell transplantation with uncertain benefit to date with relapse reported in some cases where initial improvement was reported.[175]

▶ MULTIFOCAL ACQUIRED AND DEMYELINATING SENSORY AND MOTOR NEUROPATHY (LEWIS SUMNER SYNDROME)

CLINICAL FEATURES

Lewis and colleagues described the first cases of patients with multifocal demyelinating neuropathy with persistent conduction block.[225] The term MADSAM neuropathy is often used in contrast with MMN, the other notably multifocal chronic, acquired, immune-mediated demyelinating neuropathy.[226] As the name implies, the pattern of signs and symptoms in MADSAM neuropathy patients are those of a multifocal neuropathy (Table 14-1).[32,226–234] As with MMN, there is a male predominance with an average age of onset in the early fifties typically in the upper extremities.[235] At times, MADSAM may mimic a brachial plexus neuritis.[236–238] Onset in the lower extremities may occur however, and commonly develops over time without treatment in the more typical upper extremity onset cases.

Motor and sensory symptoms can be recognized to be in the distribution of discrete peripheral nerves if the patient is evaluated before the disease progresses with confluence of deficits. Some patients describe pain and paresthesias. Cranial neuropathies have been reported in approximately 30% of cases, including optic, oculomotor, trigeminal, and facial neuropathies.[235] Dysautonomia is apparently rare but has been reported.[236] Muscle stretch reflexes can be normal or reduced depending on the nerves affected. As MADSAM mimics CIDP in virtually every way except for its multifocal phenotype, we consider it to be a CIDP variant.[226,227]

LABORATORY FEATURES

Although the phenotype of MADSAM mimics MMN, both the CSF and autoantibody profile as well as the therapeutic responsiveness differ significantly. CSF protein levels, unlike MMN, are often elevated (mean level of around 70 mg/dL). Antiglycolipid autoantibodies such as GM1 commonly seen in MMN are rarely encountered.[226–233] The EDX pattern in MADSAM is that of an acquired, predominantly demyelinating neuropathy. Conduction block and/or temporal dispersion has been reported in 82% of patients, prolonged distal latencies in 23%, abnormal (typically prolonged) F responses in two-thirds, and slow CVs in 44% of patients in one or more motor nerves.[226–233,235] These demyelinating features are identical to CIDP with the understandable exception that they may be less widespread in their distribution. In contrast to MMN, the SNAPs are affected. EMG reveals decreased recruitment of MUAPs in affected muscles as a consequence of conduction block or of axon loss. If axon loss develops, fibrillation potentials and enlarged MUAPs indicative of chronic denervation and reinnervation may also be detected. Ultrasound and MRI have been utilized to detect the nerve lesions of MADSAM.[137–240]

HISTOPATHOLOGY

Sensory nerve biopsies, not routinely recommended, demonstrate many thinly myelinated nerve fibers, subperineurial and endoneurial edema, mild onion-bulb formations, and occasional inflammatory cell infiltrates.[226,228–233] Inflammatory cells are often perivascular.[231] Asymmetric loss of large myelinated nerve fibers between and within fascicles may be appreciated.[226,228,230] Findings suggestive of demyelination are reported to occur in 77% of individuals.[235]

TREATMENT

Most patients with MADSAM improve with IVIg treatment (Table 14-4).[226–233,235,236,241,242] Also, in contrast to MMN but similar to CIDP, most patients with MADSAM respond to treatment with corticosteroids.[226,227,230–233,239] Protocols are identical to those utilized for CIDP.

► DADS NEUROPATHY

CLINICAL FEATURES

DADS neuropathy was first described as a distinct syndrome in 2000 (Table 14-1).[63] Like the authors of that manuscript, we believe that the differences in phenotype, natural history, histopathology, and treatment response justify that DADS be classified differently from CIDP, even if the EDX profile is similar.[63] The DADS phentotype is distinctive. We consider it to be for all intents and purposes synonymous to the anti-MAG or IgM-associated neuropathy designations. DADS is a typically insidious disorder of middle aged to usually older individuals that often progresses very slowly, at a pace notably distinctive from CIDP in most affected individuals.[14,243] The mean age of onset has been reported as 59–67 years and the disorder appears to be more common in males.[243,244] The natural history is variable. The disorder may become incapacitating for some, largely due to loss of balance from the sensory ataxia.[244] A considerable number of patients, however, will retain the capability of walking independently without durable medical equipment, years or even a decade or more after symptom onset, a notable consideration in the risk/benefit analysis of treatment decision making. It has been reported that DADS patients with MAG autoantibodies are more likely to have a more indolent course with less disability.[244]

DADS is a disorder that is dominated by distal, symmetric sensory signs and symptoms, frequently associated with sensory ataxia.[6,243] Sensory symptoms typically begin in the feet symmetrically and eventually involve the hands.[243] Wavering or loss of balance accentuated by eye closure is the norm even early in the course. In keeping with its acquired, demyelinating pathophysiology, generalized hyporeflexia or areflexia is also typical. Despite the notable demyelinating EDX features affecting motor nerves, there is little if any motor involvement at first. If and when weakness develops, it is typically found initially in toe and foot dorsiflexors although may become more widespread in patients who have been afflicted for many years. It is important to recognize that weakness may be overestimated in some patients due to the degree of proprioceptive loss. Making sure that the patient sees the tested body part during manual muscle testing is important in this regard. Postural tremor is a common phenotypic feature.[243,235–247] Conversely, compatible with the seemingly large-fiber predominance of this disorder, pain is rarely a significant clinical feature. Similarly, involvement of cranial nerves should suggest an alternative diagnosis.

LABORATORY FEATURES

Patients with DADS neuropathy invariably fulfill EDX criteria for CIDP. Notable differences may be in the amount of slowing that occurs in DADS patients in distal as opposed to more proximal segments of nerve. Marked prolongation of distal motor latencies are a hallmark of this disorder. It has been reported by some, not all, that the terminal latency index (TLS), a parameter that directly contrasts conduction speed in the distal as opposed to more proximal segments of nerve, is affected to a greater extent than in other chronic, acquired, demyelinating neuropathy syndromes.[6] In addition, conduction blocks in motor nerves occur uncommonly with this disorder.[109,243] This is consistent with the initial absence of weakness in most cases.

Up to 85% of individuals with DADS will have a MCP.[63,248] The majority of these will be IgM kappa with an occasional patient with an IgG MCP.[6,248] In turn, up to two-thirds of the patients with DADS and IgM MCP will be found to have autoantibodies directed against MAG or a related epitope. Rarely, a patient will be found to have MAG autoantibodies without a detectable MCP. It is in this population, that is patients with a DADS phenotype, with characteristic demyelinating EDX features, who do not have a detectable MCP, in whom we find assessment of MAG autoantibodies most helpful. Our diagnostic strategy is based on the generally held perception that there are no pragmatic differences in DADS patients based on the presence or absence of anti-MAG activity. In addition, anti-MAG activity can be occasionally demonstrated in contrasting phenotypes underscoring the importance of the phenotype, not the serology in the definition of the syndrome.[249] Autoantibodies directed against glycolipids are not characteristically identified in this syndrome.

An elevation of CSF protein levels without a cellular response is characteristic of DADS patients. There appears to be no significant difference in comparison to CIDP, either the number of patients with elevated CSF protein levels, or magnitude of protein elevation.[14]

HISTOPATHOLOGY

Nerve biopsies, which should be infrequently performed, characteristically identify features suggestive of demyelination and remyelination in DADS patients.[6,243] Not unexpectedly, concomitant axon loss may occur as well.[343] A characteristic feature however is that patients with MAG autoantibodies may be shown to have binding of these autoantibodies to peripheral nerve myelin with immunohistochemical staining of nerve biopsy specimens. In addition, a characteristic separation of myelin lamella demonstrable with EM, consistent with the known function of MAG, suggests a pathogenic rather than simply a reactionary role for these autoantibodies in this disease. This finding is described in 95% of individuals with neuropathy, IgM MCP, and MAG autoantibodies.[243]

PATHOGENESIS

Myelin associated glycoprotein is a transmembrane, structural glycoprotein found in noncompact myelin on its abaxonal surface, on paranodal loops, and in Schmidt–Lanterman incisures.[145,146] As mentioned, the binding of MAG autoantibodies to myelin, the characteristic widening of myelin lamellae found in DADS patients consistent with disruption of normal MAG function, and the ability to reproduce the pathology in passive-transfer experiments utilizing human MAG autoantibodies and chickens suggests a pathogenic role for MAG autoantibodies and perhaps for the almost invariably associated IgM MCP.[146,243]

TREATMENT

Unlike classic CIDP where the majority of individuals seem responsive to immunomodulating treatment, DADS appears to be refractory to treatment in the majority of cases, with or without an IgM MCP or MAG autoantibodies. Although treatment responsiveness equivalent to CIDP has been reported[32] this appears to be by far the exception rather than the rule both in the literature and in our experience.[6,14,108,243,247,250–252] IVIg has been reported to be effective in 16% and 25% of cases,[243,253,254] PLEX in 40%,[254] and cyclophosphamide in 36%.[254] None of these benefits have been demonstrated to be either durable or achieve statistical significance.[255] Treatment of DADS with either IVIg or PLEX is currently not recommended by the guidelines provided by the AAN.[163,168] The most recent enthusiasm has been for rituximab which is a logical treatment with initially reported benefit.[256–261] A subsequent prospective, randomized trial however, demonstrated no meaningful benefit in the DADS population as a whole.[262] In addition, another study suggested rapid worsening in patients receiving the drug.[263] Our experience suggests that there are rare DADS patients who respond to rituxan. In consideration of this, and the indolent nature of the syndrome in most cases, we consider therapeutic decision making in DADS to be challenging in this disorder.

▶ MULTIFOCAL MOTOR NEUROPATHY

CLINICAL FEATURES

MMN is a presumed immune-mediated demyelinating neuropathy. A number of separate case reports from in the early to mid 80s first brought attention to a potentially reversible form of motor neuropathy, in some cases with demonstrable conduction block.[264–267] Like MADSAM, MMN typically presents with a multifocal neuropathy pattern affecting individual peripheral nerves. Unlike MADSAM, it is a typically a pure motor syndrome characterized by asymmetrical weakness, cramps, fasciculations, and in many cases eventual atrophy (Table 14-1).[264,268–285] The typical patient is a middle-aged male with a male-to-female ratio of approximately 3:1. The age of symptom onset ranges from the early 20s to late 60s with a mean of approximately 40 years of age.[286] Rarely, childhood onsets are encountered.[287] The onset is usually insidious, and the weakness typically progresses, often stepwise, over the course of several years to involve other nerve distributions and other limbs.

Like MADSAM, MMN typically commences in distal muscles of the upper extremities. Most patients present with intrinsic hand weakness, wrist drop, or in some cases foot drop illustrating that upper extremity onset is not invariable, and that leg onset cases do occur. Although mild sensory symptoms may be occasionally reported, unlike MADSAM, sensory signs and abnormal SNAPs are not typically encountered at least early in its course.

The differential diagnosis of MMN is largely those disorders that are either predominantly motor or that have a multifocal pattern of weakness. As a disorder of motor nerves with frequent monomelic onset, amytrophic lateral sclerosis (ALS) is arguably the major consideration. In one series, MMN was the most common ALS mimic[288] although MMN occurs far less commonly than its more malignant counterpart.[270,289] The cramps and fasciculations that can occur in MMN contribute to the potential confusion between the two disorders. Demonstrating a nerve rather than segmental pattern of weakness is a helpful, discriminating clinical feature in favor of MMN. Other features of MMN include weakness in the absence of atrophy and absence of overt upper motor neuron signs although neither of these features exclude ALS with certainty. Unequivocal corticospinal tract signs (i.e., clonus, spasticity, and extensor plantar responses) are not seen in MMN. Assessment of deep tendon reflexes should be interpreted with caution as suppressed reflexes can occur in lower motor neuron dominant ALS and preserved or even enhanced reflexes can occur in MMN if no nerve associated with a deep tendon reflex is affected. Other differential diagnostic considerations that may be relatively focal and purely motor include occasional cases of acquired or congenital myasthenia which may have a predilection for wrist and finger extensors in some cases and certain myopathies such as inclusion body myositis. In consideration of multifocality, MADSAM, MAMA (see below), acute brachial plexus neuropathy, and vasculitic neuropathy should be considered as well.

Although MMN is predominantly a disorder of limb weakness, a number of atypical features may occur. Abnormal vibration sense, has been reported in a fifth of patients by at least one author.[286] Muscle hypertrophy, believed to be secondary to the underlying myokymic discharges has been reported although eventual axon loss and atrophy are common. Cranial nerve involvement including ophthalmoparesis as a presenting manifestation has been reported.[290,291] Phrenic nerve involvement and ventilatory failure appear to be uncommon but potential features of the syndrome.[292,293]

As implied by its name, MMN affects two or more motor nerves. Intuitively, MMN usually starts as a mononeuropathy.[284–297] The astute neuromuscular clinician will consider MMN in cases of monofocal motor neuropathy and will search diligently for conduction block or MR evidence of focal, inflammatory nerve lesions.[294] The concern is of course, the potential attribution of a mononeuropathy to a more commonly occurring entrapment or compression syndrome with at least the potential for unnecessary surgical intervention. Clinicians should be wary of this potential trap, particularly if the mononeuropathy is pure motor, or has clinical or EDX features suggesting localization to an uncommon compression or entrapment site.

In summary, the current consensus diagnostic criteria for MMN include weakness in two or more nerves, with the demonstration of conduction block in two or more nerves, in the absence of upper motor neuron signs, and clinical and EDX sensory deficits.[282] A minimum of 50% reduction in CMAP amplitude in a proximal location is required for the designation of conduction block. There are a number of reasons as to why this standard may sacrifice sensitivity for specificity, potentially disqualifying a patient from effective treatment. First of all, criteria for conduction block do not account for the length of the segment tested. Many would consider a sudden drop in CMAP amplitude and associated reduced area under the curve to represent definitive conduction block even if it does meet the 50% criteria. In addition, conduction blocks often occur in inaccessible nerve segments, thus limiting the ability to identify them and increasing the probability of a false-negative study. Accordingly, we agree with those who recommend treatment in those with a typical phenotype, in the absence of demonstrable conduction block or antiglycolipid antibodies, where response to treatment may be equally effective in comparison to those who fulfill all diagnostic criteria.[285,298–301]

LABORATORY FEATURES

Autoantibodies directed against gangliosides or glycolipids concentrated on the axonal membranes of motor axons and Schwann cell membranes have been purported to be diagnostic biomarkers and potentially pathogenic agents in MMN.[280,283,286,302–304] The GM1 autoantibody is the most notable of these. Asialo GM1, GM2, and GD1b autoantibodies are less prevalejnt, and are therefore presumably less significant. Their prevalence of GM1 autoantibodies in this disorder is variable. Anywhere from 22% to 84% of patients with MMN will have IgM GM1 autoantibodies, the difference is often attributed to methodological differences.[286,305] In one recent series of 88 patients IgM, IgG, and IgA GM1 autoantibodies were found in 43%, 1%, and 5% of cases, respectively with IgM

GM2 autoantibodies in 6% of cases and IgM GD1b in 9%.[286,305] In this same series, the presence and higher titre of GM1 autoantibodies correlated with more severe weakness and disability, correlating as well with more severe axon loss as might be anticipated. Despite these observations suggesting a "dose-effect" relationship, the significance of these antibodies regarding their role in disease pathogenesis is still not clear.[305,306] In addition, both the limited sensitivity and specificity of GM1 autoantibodies even in high titres makes them a supportive but neither diagnostic nor exclusionary biomarker for MMN.

The other and undoubtedly more important diagnostic tool in suspected MMN, is the ability to identify persistent conduction block in motor nerve segments not usually associated with compression or entrapment.[264,272,274,276–282] There are no universally accepted criteria for defining definitive conduction block.[307] Consensus criteria for conduction block have been published and are site and nerve specific.[282] A reduction in the distal CMAP amplitude can be seen in chronic lesions due to secondary axonal loss, or at least theoretically as a consequence of distal conduction block.

Although motor conduction block has been considered the EDX hallmark of MMN, other features of demyelination (i.e., prolonged distal latencies, temporal dispersion, slow CVs, and prolonged or absent F waves) are frequently identified on motor NCS.[272,275,298,308,309] As previously mentioned, there should be no sensory conduction abnormalities including across the region where conduction block can be demonstrated in motor fibers.[276,282] Predictably, EDX evidence of demyelination is found more often in the nerves of the arms and is distributed randomly over lower arm, upper arm, and shoulder segments.[275,310] Approximately one-third of electrophysiological abnormalities are found in nerves innervating muscles considered clinically normal.[310]

Needle EMG demonstrates decreased recruitment in weak muscles.[264,275,290,304] Fibrillation potentials and positive sharp waves can be seen due to secondary axonal loss, more commonly in long-standing cases. Fasciculation potentials, complex repetitive discharges, and myokymic discharges are observed occasionally, not routinely recommended.

CSF protein is usually normal in patients with MMN, which can help differentiate the neuropathy from CIDP and MADSAM. Both MR imaging, particularly MR neurography, and ultrasound may be useful tools for demonstrating enlargement or enhancement of peripheral nerve, particularly within the brachial plexus.[309,311] Ultrasound has been reported to detect lesions in the majority of MMN cases, some of which, like EDX of conduction block, appear to be asymptomatic.[311]

HISTOPATHOLOGY

Sensory nerve biopsies in MMN are usually normal, although slight reduction of myelinated fibers or axonal degeneration has been appreciated.[276,277,280,313,314] Motor axons studied from forearm nerves, the brachial plexus and the obturator nerve may reveal thinly myelinated axons and small onion bulbs indicative of demyelination as well as evidence of axonal degeneration in the form of regenerating clusters and loss of myelinated axons.[143] Mild perivascular inflammation has been reported.[262,309]

PATHOGENESIS

Although initially considered to be a variant of CIDP, most authorities now regard MMN as a distinct entity.[13,32,284] It is tempting to hypothesize that antibodies targeting specific gangliosides are pathogenic because of the location of their target antigens which are largely sequestered on motor axons in paranodal regions.[145] In addition, it has been demonstrated that GM1 autoantibodies not only bind to GM1 but activate complement in vivo making it conceivable that IgM mediates motor nerve injury at the nodes of Ranvier. Further support for complement mediated motor nerve dysfunction triggered by IgM GM1 autoantibodies comes from the demonstration that IVIg in vitro can inhibit complement activation.[316] Nonetheless, a pathogenic role for asialo GM1, GM2, and GD1b autoantibodies has yet to be conclusively demonstrated. Further undermining a potential pathogenic role for GM1 autoantibodies is the observation that the reduction of antibody titers correlates with clinical improvement following immunotherapy in some[279,280] but not all patients.[273,317] Further, there has been no association between the presence or absence of ganglioside antibodies and response to immunotherapy in some series.[275,313,318,319] MMN patient's sera injected into rat nerve in vivo and in vitro has been demonstrated to induce conduction block in some[310,320–322] but not all studies.[323] Not all patients with MMN have detectable ganglioside antibodies. Currently, GM1 autoantibodies are considered to be a biomarker without a defined causative role.[142]

The mechanism of conduction block and the muscle weakness that follows is conceivably a consequence of ion channel dysfunction rather than demyelination. This hypothesis is extrapolated from one report of AMAN associated with GM1 autoantibodies where conduction block and slowing occurred rapidly in the absence of remyelinating electrophysiological features.[324] In that vein, GM1 autoantibodies have been demonstrated to adversely affect sodium and potassium currents in different in vitro models.[325,326] It is possible that demyelination in MMN may not be the initial pathophysiological mechanism but the consequence of a prolonged autoimmune attack.

There have been a number of potential associations with other conditions that could potentially provide insight into the cause or mechanisms of the disease. Given the known existence of the GM1 antigen on the cell surface of *C. jejuni* and the association between this organism and another motor neuropathy, the AMAN variant of GBS, it is understandable that an association between MMN and *C. jejuni* might exist. A 1996 report identified such an association in one case but a subsequent study of MMN patients found serological evidence of *C. jejuni* infection in only one in 20 patients.[327,328] MMN has been reported to complicate treatment with tumor necrosis factor alpha blockers, probably through modulation of the immune system.[329,330] MMN has also been reported to worsen during pregnancy.[331]

TREATMENT

Unlike CIDP and MADSAM, patients with MMN generally do not respond to corticosteroids or PLEX (Table 14-1).[274,276,277,280,290,317,332–335] Fortunately, MMN is typically responsive to IVIg as demonstrated in small case reports[22,220,273,275,286,290,300,319,335–357] as summarized in a Cochrane and other reviews,[339–341] and as demonstrated in a double-blinded, placebo-controlled trial.[342] Treatment is with a typical regimen of IVIg, 2 g/kg over 2–5 days with subsequent maintenance courses as necessary. Improvement is usually noted within a few days or first few weeks of treatment. Most patients need repeated infusions every 2–4 weeks. Not everyone with MMN responds to IVIg, particularly those with long-standing disease before starting treatment, those with a later age of onset and patients who have significant muscle atrophy and presumptive axon loss[213,319] We advocate three monthly courses of IVIg before concluding that a patient has failed treatment. We recognize however that the failure of IVIg to reverse well establish axon loss does not mean treatment failure and that maintenance IVIg treatment may prevent further attacks in someone who seems unresponsive, attacks that often occur unpredictably. Follow-up EDX findings imply that IVIg treatment may favorably influence the mechanisms of remyelination or reinnervation but that axon loss cannot necessarily be prevented.[273] IVIg has also been successfully used with a subcutaneous delivery system in this disease.[343,344]

Other treatments utilized in MMN are of uncertain benefit. There have been case reports of MMN patients treated with interferon-β1 A, azathioprine, cyclosporine, methotrexate, and mycophenolate mofetil with at best, equivocal results.[340,341,345] Intravenous cyclophosphamide was the first therapy noted to be useful in MMN, although no double-blinded, placebo-controlled trials have been performed.[274,276,277,280,304,318] When given in combination with IVIg it may prolong the interval between IVIg infusions.[346] We reserve cyclophosphamide for patients who fail IVIg. A typical protocol is to start with intravenous cyclophosphamide in a dose of 0.5 g/m^2/month in a single one day effusion in order to avoid severe side effects. Subsequent monthly doses are gradually increased to 0.75 g/m^2 if tolerated and then to 1 g/m^2. We attempt to limit the risk of hemorrhagic cystitis with aggressive hydration and with prescription of Mesna. Subsequent screening of urine cytology is recommended on a long-term basis. Pretreatment with ondansetron or granisetron is used to minimize or eliminate nausea. Rituximab has been used to treat a number of immune-mediated neuropathies including MMN.[196,220,304,347] Those who respond require periodic maintenance dosing.[348] Not everyone however improves in response to rituximab and some continue to decline.[220] Randomized control trials are necessary to confirm the efficacy of rituximab.

MULTIFOCAL ACQUIRED MOTOR AXONOPATHY

Rare patients have the clinical phenotype of MMN but have only axonal features on EDX studies.[300,349,350] The "MAMA" acronym has been used to describe these patients.[349] Unlike patients with MMN, most patients with MAMA lack GM1 antibodies and by definition lack demyelinating EDX features. As the causes of axon loss multifocal neuropathy is far more extensive than demyelinating etiologies, a diagnosis of MAMA should be made cautiously so as to not miss a vasculitic illness or another disorder capable of infarcting or infiltrating nerves in a multifocal pattern. Some individuals with MAMA improve with prednisone or IVIg. It is felt that this rare subgroup of patients is distinct from typical MMN and other established motor neuron disorders (e.g., ALS). The implication is that if a patient has the clinical appearance of MMN with weakness in the distribution of individual nerves rather than myotomes and no upper motor neuron abnormalities, then a therapeutic trial of immunomodulating treatment may be warranted.

▶ CHRONIC IMMUNE SENSORY POLYRADICULOPATHY

CLINICAL FEATURES

This rare entity may represent a restricted form of CIDP.[60,65–68] Patients present with an insidious onset of progressive, non-length dependent, numbness and paresthesia of the extremities, and frequently, sensory ataxia. Symptoms and signs may be asymmetric. On examination, large-fiber sensory functions are profoundly affected. Muscle stretch reflexes are reduced or absent. In contrast, muscle strength is preserved. The differential diagnosis includes a paraneoplastic sensory neuronopathy/ganglionopathy (e.g., anti-Hu syndrome), sensory ganglionopathy associated with Sjogren's syndrome or pure sensory CIDP.

LABORATORY FEATURES

As in more classic CIDP, CSF protein is usually elevated but cell count in the CSF is normal. Serology is negative for GM1, GD1b, GQ1b, antinuclear, anti-Ro, and anti-La antibodies. Routine motor and sensory NCS are normal as is needle EMG.[60,65–68] H reflexes are typically abnormal. Further, abnormal somatosensory-evoked potentials are usually evident with prolonged N13 (cervical) or N9–N13 interpeak latencies in the arms or prolonged latencies of lumbar potential and N/P 37 cortical potential with normal popliteal latency, reflecting slowing of conduction in the proximal segments of the nerves. MRI may reveal thickening and enhancement of nerve roots (Fig. 14-4).[65,67]

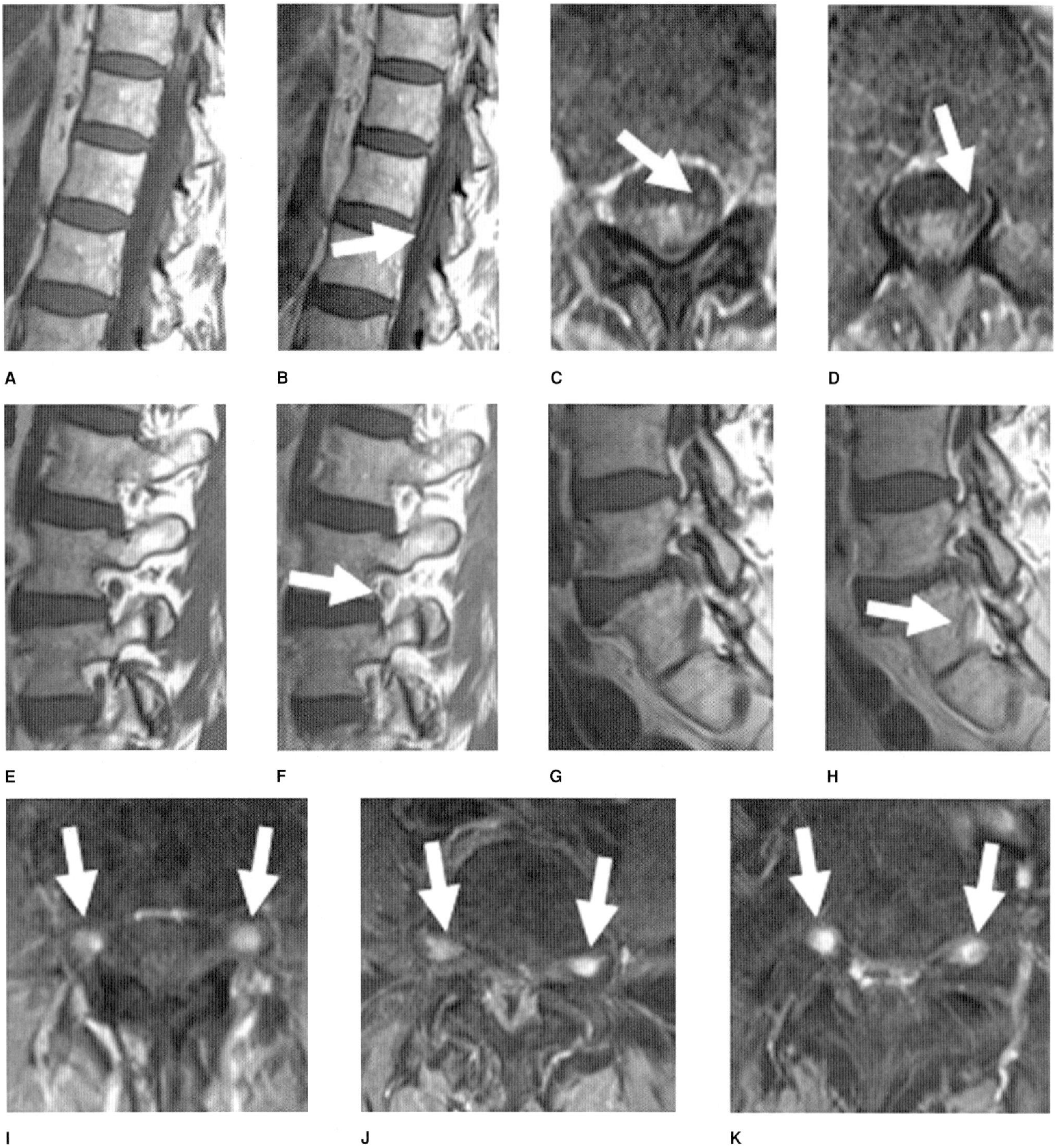

Figure 14-4. MRI of lumbosacral spine in a patient with CISP. Sagittal T1-weighted MRI with fat saturation before **(A)** and after **(B)** IV administration of gadolinium contrast shows abnormal enhancement of a left-sided nerve root at the T12–L1 vertebral level (**B**, *arrow*), also seen on axial postcontrast images (**C, D**, *arrows*). Multiple other nerve roots of the cauda equina demonstrated abnormal contrast enhancement though none were enlarged or clumped. Sagittal precontrast **(E, G)** and postcontrast **(F, H)** images of the intervertebral foramina show abnormal enhancement of right-sided dorsal root ganglia at L2–L3 (**F**, *arrow*) and L4–L5 (**H**, *arrow*). Axial postcontrast images show abnormal enhancement of the bilateral dorsal root ganglia at L2–L3 (**I**, *arrows*), L4–L5 (**J**, *arrows*), and L5–S1 (**K**, *arrows*). (Reproduced with permission from Berkowitz AL, Jha RM, Klein JP. Clinical reasoning: An 85-year-old man with paresthesias and an unsteady gait. *Neurology*. 2013;80(12):e120–e126.)

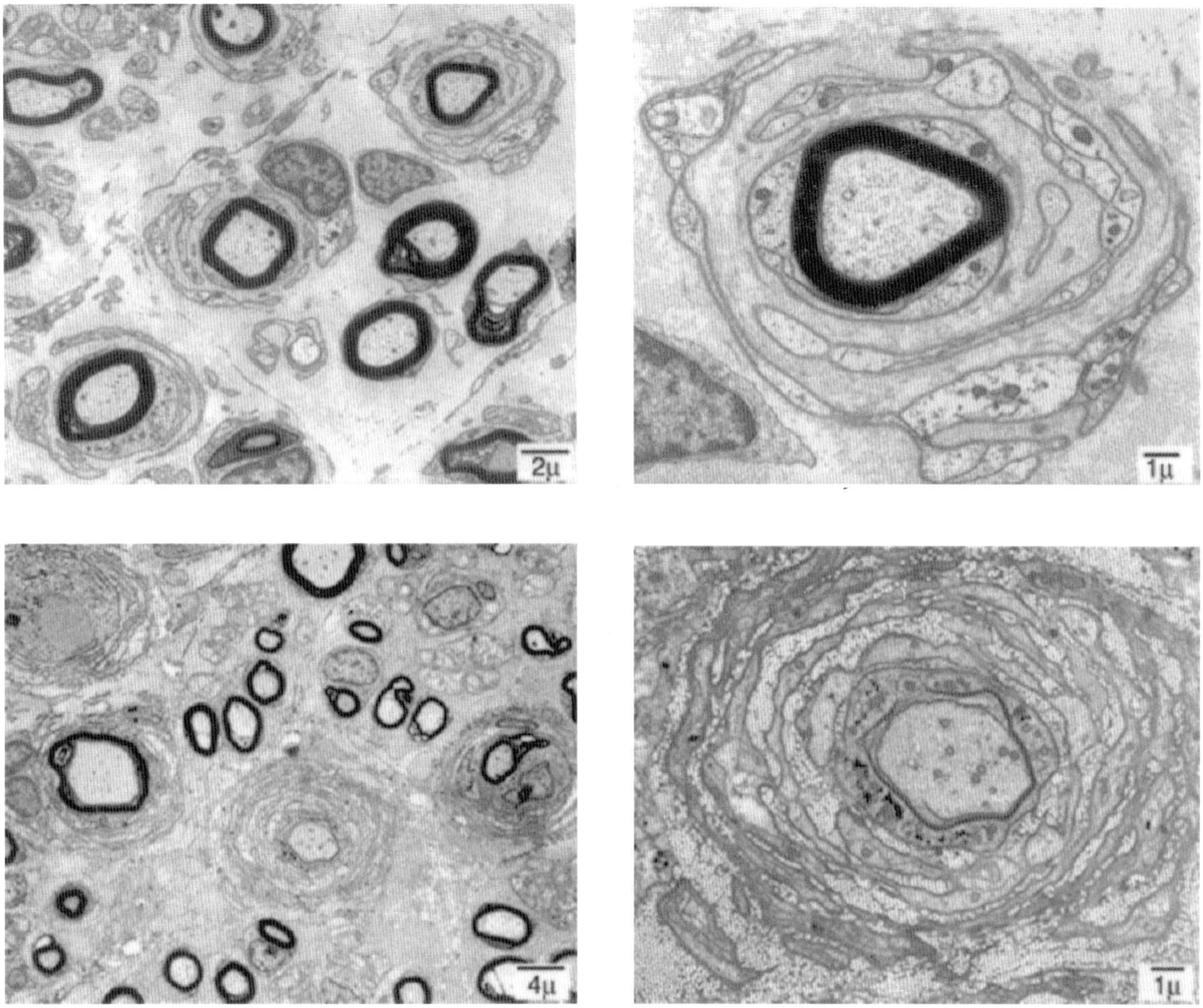

Figure 14-5. Electron micrographs from lumbar dorsal rootlet biopsies of patients with CISP reveal evidence of chronic demyelination and abortive repair. The left column (taken at low power) shows frequent onion-bulb formations associated with thinly myelinated and demyelinated profiles. The right column demonstrates two of these onion bulbs at higher power; the one on the bottom right shows an axon with only a few layers of myelin lamellae. Onion bulbs like these were very common in these two biopsies. (Reproduced with permission from Sinnreich M, Klein CJ, Daube JR, Engelstad J, Spinner RJ, Dyck PJB. Chronic immune sensory polyneuropathy. A possibly treatable sensory ataxia. *Neurology*. 2004;63(9):1662–1669.)

HISTOPATHOLOGY

Biopsies of lumbar sensory rootlets has been reported to demonstrate a decreased density of large myelinating fibers, demyelinated axons, endoneurial edema, and onion-bulb formation (Fig. 14-5).[65]

TREATMENT

Patients may respond to corticosteroids or IVIg in a manner similar to CIDP.

► IDIOPATHIC PERINEURITIS

CLINICAL FEATURES

Perineuritis is a nonspecific histological abnormality characterized by inflammation and thickening of the perineurium, found in neuropathies associated with diabetes mellitus, connective tissue diseases, ulcerative colitis, vasculitis (including cryoglobulinemia), lymphoma, and other malignancies.[351–356] However, perineuritis can occur as an isolated disorder without an apparent underlying systemic disorder.[350,357] The clinical presentation associated is variable.[22,355,357] Some patients develop sensory loss, dysesthesias, hyperpathia, and weakness in the distribution of multiple individual nerves, while others manifest with generalized symmetric motor and sensory loss indistinguishable from AIDP or CIDP. Migrating areas of sensory loss have also been described. The course of the neuropathy can be remitting and relapsing. Hypesthesia and hyperpathia are often appreciated on examination and a positive Tinel's sign may be present over involved nerves. Large-fiber sensory functions are typically less affected than small-fiber modalities. Muscle strength is usually preserved, but cases with generalized weakness, suggestive of GBS or CIDP, have been reported.[355] Muscle stretch reflexes are often normal in patients with pure sensory symptoms.

LABORATORY FEATURES

CSF, ANA, ESR, liver function tests, serum protein electrophoresis, and vasculitic profile are usually normal.[351,357] The presence of an abnormal laboratory workup should lead to the consideration of an underlying systemic disorder such as vasculitis. NCS demonstrate SNAPs that are either reduced in amplitude or absent, occurring in a multifocal or generalized pattern. Motor NCS and EMG are normal unless patients have a multifocal neuropathy or radiculoplexopathy with both motor and sensory involvement.[354,355]

HISTOPATHOLOGY

Nerve biopsies reveal the prominent thickening and fibrosis of the perineurium along with perineural infiltration with lymphocytes and macrophages.[351,355,357] Mild perivascular inflammation may be evident as well. Myelinated nerve fiber loss due to axonal degeneration is expected.

PATHOGENESIS

The pathogenic basis for the disorder is unknown but likely to be autoimmune in nature. Perineuritis may inflict damage via ischemia, impairment of nutrient or toxin flow to and from nerve fibers in the endoneurium, or by direct humoral or cellular autoimmune attack against the nerve fibers.

TREATMENT

Response to immunotherapy is variable and difficult to ascertain because the natural history of the neuropathy may be one of remissions and relapses. We have tried prednisone and IVIg in such idiopathic cases with variable success in patients with mainly sensory disturbances.

▶ SUMMARY

The acquired chronic inflammatory demyelinating polyneuropathies include CIDP, DADS, MADSAM, MMN, and possibly CISP. These neuropathies are distinguished from one another on the basis of their phenotypes, their natural histories and their treatment responsiveness, and to lesser extent by their laboratory features. They are distinguished from their far more prevalent axonal counterparts predominantly by their phenotype coupled with their EDX features. Their importance is underscored as they represent collectively, the largest group of treatable neuropathy syndromes. Accordingly, early and accurate diagnosis and prompt treatment are of paramount importance.

REFERENCES

1. Bromberg MB. Review of the evolution of electrodiagnostic criteria for chronic demyelinating polyradiculopathy. *Muscle Nerve*. 2011;43:780–794.
2. Breiner A, Brannagan TH 3rd. Comparison of sensitivity and specificity among 15 criteria for chronic inflammatory demyelinating polyneuropathy. *Muscle Nerve*. 2014;50(1):40–46.
3. Mauermann ML, Sorenson EJ, Dispenzieri A, et al. Uniform demyelination and more severe axonal loss distinguish POEMS syndrome from CIDP. *J Neurol Neurosurg Psychiatry*. 2012;83:480–486.
4. Nasu S, Misawav S, Sekiguchi Y, et al. Different neurological and physiological profiles in POEMS syndrome and chronic inflammatory demyelinating polyneuropathy. *J Neurol Neurosurg Psychiatry*. 2012;83:476–479.
5. van Schaik IN, Léger JM, Nobile-Orazio E, et al. Joint Task Force of the EFNS and the PNS. European Federation of Neurological Societies/Peripheral Nerve Society guideline on management of multifocal motor neuropathy. *J Peripher Nerv Syst*. 2010;15:295–301.
6. Saperstein DS, Katz JS, Amato AA, Barohn RJ. The spectrum of the acquired chronic demyelinating polyneuropathies. *Muscle Nerve*. 2001;24:311–324.
7. Van den Bergh PY, Hadden RD, Pouche P, et al. European Federation of Neurological Societies/Peripheral Nerve Society guideline on management of chronic inflammatory demyelinating polyradiculoneuropathy: Report of a joint task force of the European Federation of Neurological Societies and the Peripheral Nerve Society–First Revision. *J Peripher Nerv Syst*. 2010;15(1):1–9.
8. Burns TM. Chronic inflammatory demyelinating polyneuropathy. *Arch Neurol*. 2004;61(6):973–975.
9. Austin JH. Recurrent polyneuropathies and their corticosteroid treatment: With five-year observations of a placebo-controlled case treated with corticotrophin, cortisone and prednisone. *Brain*. 1958;81:157–192.
10. Prineas JW, McLeod JR. Chronic relapsing polyneuritis. *J Neurol Sci*. 1976;27:427–458.
11. Thomas PK, Lascelles RG, Hallpike JF, Hewer RL. Recurrent and chronic relapsing Guillain-Barre' polyneuritis. *Brain*. 1969;92:589–606.
12. Dyck PJ, Lais AC, Ohta M, Bastron JA, Okazaki H, Groover RV. Chronic inflammatory polyradiculoneuropathy. *Mayo Clin Proc*. 1975;50:621–637.

13. Nobile-Orazio E. Chronic inflammatory demyelinating polyradiculoneuropathy and variants: Where are we and where should we go? *J Peripher Nerv Syst*. 2014;19:2–13.
14. Barohn RJ, Kissel JT, Warmolts JR, Mendell JR. Chronic inflammatory polyradiculoneuropathy. Clinical characteristics, course, and recommendations for diagnostic criteria. *Arch Neurol*. 1989;46:878–884.
15. McCombe PA, Pollard JD, McLeod JG. Chronic inflammatory demyelinating polyradiculoneuropathy: A clinical and electrophysiological study of 92 cases. *Brain*. 1987;110:1617–1630.
16. Dalakas MC, Engel WK. Chronic relapsing (dysimmune) polyneuropathy: Pathogenesis and treatment. *Ann Neurol*. 1981;9(Suppl):134–145.
17. Simmons Z, Wald JJ, Albers JW. Chronic inflammatory demyelinating polyradiculoneuropathy in children: II. Long-term follow-up, with comparison to adults. *Muscle Nerve*. 1997;20(12):1569–1575.
18. Simmons Z, Wald JJ, Albers JW. Chronic inflammatory demyelinating polyradiculoneuropathy in children: I. Presentation, electrodiagnostic studies, and initial clinical course, with comparison to adults. *Muscle Nerve*. 1997;20(8):1008–1015.
19. Markowitz JA, Jeste SS, Kang PB. Child Neurology: Chronic inflammatory demyelinating polyradiculoneuropathy in children. *Neurology*. 2008;71:e74–e78.
20. Costello F, Lee AG, Afifi AK, Kelkar P, Kardon RH, White M. Childhood-onset chronic inflammatory demyelinating polyradiculoneuropathy with cranial nerve involvement. *J Child Neurol*. 2002;17(11):819–823. Erratum in *J Child Neurol* 2003;18(3):179.
21. Sladky JT, Brown JM, Berman PH. Chronic inflammatory demyelinating polyneuropathy of infancy: A corticosteroid responsive disorder. *Ann Neurol*. 1986;20:76–81.
22. Colan RV, Snead OC, Oh SJ, Benton JW Jr. Steroid-responsive polyneuropathy with subacute onset in childhood. *J Pediatr*. 1980;97:374–377.
23. De Vivo D, Engel WK. Remarkable recovery of a steroid-responsive recurrent polyneuropathy. *J Neurol Neurosurg Psychiatry*. 1970;33:62–69.
24. Gabreels-Festen AA, Hageman AT, Gabreels FJ, et al. Chronic inflammatory demyelinating polyneuropathy in two siblings. *J Neurol Neurosurg Psychiatry*. 1986;49:152–156.
25. Tasker W, Chutarian AM. Chronic polyneuritis of childhood. *J Pediatr*. 1969;74:699–708.
26. Uncini A, Parano E, Lange DJ, De Vivo DC, Lovelace RE. Chronic inflammatory demyelinating polyneuropathy in childhood: Clinical and electrophysiological features. *Child Nerv Syst*. 1991;7:191–196.
27. Vedanarayanan VV, Kandt RS, Lewis DV, DeLong GR. Chronic inflammatory demyelinating polyradiculoneuropathy of childhood: Treatment with high-dose intravenous immunoglobulin. *Neurology*. 1991;41:828–830.
28. Nevo Y, Topaloglu H. 88th ENMC international workshop: Childhood chronic inflammatory demyelinating polyneuropathy (including revised diagnostic criteria), Naarden, The Netherlands, December 8–10, 2000. *Neuromuscul Disord*. 2002;12(2):195–200.
29. Barisic N, Regis S, Pazanin L. Long-term follow-up of children with chronic relapsing polyneuropathy. *Pediatr Neurol*. 2002;26(4):293–297.
30. Byers RK, Taft LT. Chronic multiple peripheral neuropathy of childhood. *Pediatrics*. 1957;20:517–537.
31. Gorson KC, van Schaik IN, Merkies IS, et al. Chronic inflammatory demyelinating polyneuropathy disease activity status: Recommendations for clinical research standards and use in clinical practice. *J Peripher Nerv Syst*. 2010;15:326–333.
32. Tackenberg B, Lunemann JD, Steinbrecher A, et al. Classifications and treatment responses in chronic immune-mediated demyelinating polyneuropathy. *Neurology*. 2007;68:1622–1629.
33. Viala K, Maisonobe T, Stojkovic T, et al. A current view of the diagnosis, clinical variants and response to treatment and prognosis of chronic inflammatory demyelinating polyradiculopathy. *J Peripher Nerv Syst*. 2010;15:50–56.
34. McCombe PA, McManis PG, Frith JA, Pollard JD, McLeod JG. Chronic inflammatory demyelinating neuropathy associated with pregnancy. *Ann Neurol*. 1987;21:102–104.
35. Bouchard C, Lacroix C, Planté V, et al. Clinicopathologic findings and prognosis of chronic inflammatory demyelinating polyneuropathy. *Neurology*. 1999;52(3):498–503.
36. Mendell JR. Chronic inflammatory demyelinating polyradiculoneuropathy. *Ann Rev Med*. 1993;44:211–219.
37. Dyck PJ, Oviatt KF, Lambert EH. Intensive evaluation of referred unclassified neuropathies yields improved diagnosis. *Ann Neurol*. 1981;10:222–226.
38. Mori K, Hattori N, Sugiura M, et al. Chronic inflammatory demyelinating polyneuropathy presenting with features of GBS. *Neurology*. 2002;58:979–982.
39. Ruts L, Drenthen J, Jacobs BC, van Doom PA. Distinguishing acute-onset CIDP from fluctuating Guillain-Barré syndrome: A prospective study. *Neurology*. 2010;74:1680–1686.
40. Mygland A, Monstad P, Vedeler C. Onset and course of chronic inflammatory demyelinating polyneuropathy. *Muscle Nerve*. 2005;31(5):589–593.
41. Hughes R, Sanders E, Hall S, Atkinson P, Colchester A, Payan P. Subacute idiopathic demyelinating polyradiculoneuropathy. *Arch Neurol*. 1992;49:612–616.
42. Oh SJ, Kurokawa K, de Almeida DF, Ryan HF, Claussen GC. Subacute inflammatory demyelinating polyneuropathy. *Neurology*. 2003;61:1507–1512.
43. Ruts L, van Koningsveld R, van Doorn PA. Distinguishing acute-onset CIDP from Guillain–Barre syndrome with treatment related fluctuations. *Neurology*. 2005;65(1):138–140.
44. Rodriguez-Casero MV, Shield LK, Kornberg AJ. Subacute inflammatory demyelinating polyneuropathy in children. *Neurology*. 2005;64(10):1786–1788.
45. Hughes RA, Bouche P, Cornblath DR, et al. European Federation of Neurological Societies/Peripheral Nerve Society guideline on management of chronic inflammatory demyelinating polyradiculoneuropathy: Report of a joint task force of the European Federation of Neurological Societies and the Peripheral Nerve Society. *Eur J Neurol*. 2006;13(4):326–332.
46. Koller H, Kieser B, Jander S, Hartung HP. Chronic inflammatory demyelinating polyneuropathy. *N Engl J Med*. 2005;352:1343–1356.
47. Simmons Z, Albers JW, Bromberg MB, Feldman EL. Presentation and initial clinical course in patients with chronic inflammatory demyelinating polyradiculoneuropathy: Comparison of patients without and with monoclonal gammopathy. *Neurology*. 1993;43(11):2202–2209.
48. Gorson KC, Allam G, Ropper AH. Chronic inflammatory demyelinating polyneuropathy: Clinical features and response to treatment of 67 consecutive patients with and without monoclonal gammopathy. *Neurology*. 1997;48:321–328.

49. Boukhris S, Magy L, Khalil M, Sindou P, Vallat JM. Pain as the presenting symptom of chronic inflammatory demyelinating polyradiculoneuropathy (CIDP). *J Neurol Sci*. 2007;254(1–2):33–38.
50. Frohman EM, Tusa R, Mark AS, Cornblath DR. Vestibular dysfunction in chronic inflammatory demyelinating polyneuropathy. *Ann Neurol*. 1996;39:529–535.
51. Chalmers AC, Miller RG. Chronic inflammatory polyradiculoneuropathy with ophthalmoplegia. *J Clin Neuroophthalmol*. 1986;6(3):166–168.
52. Hoffman D, Gutmann L. The dropped head syndrome with chronic inflammatory demyelinating polyneuropathy. *Muscle Nerve*. 1994;17:808–810.
53. Nakanishi T, Sobue I, Toyokura Y, et al. The Crow-Fukase syndrome: A study of 102 cases in Japan. *Neurology*. 1984;34(6):712–720.
54. Stamboulis E, Katsaros N, Koutsis G, Iakovidou H, Giannakopoulou A, Simintzi I. Clinical and subclinical autonomic dysfunction in chronic inflammatory demyelinating polyradiculoneuropathy. *Muscle Nerve*. 2006;33(1):78–84.
55. Yamamoto K, Watarai M, Hashimoto T, Ikeda S. Chronic inflammatory demyelinating polyradiculoneuropathy with autonomic involvement. *Muscle Nerve*. 2005;31(1):108–112.
56. Figueroa JJ, Dyck PJ, Laughlin RS, et al. Autonomic dysfunction in chronic inflammatory demyelinating polyradiculoneuropathy. *Neurology*. 2012;78(10):702–708.
57. Henderson RD, Sandroni P, Wijdicks EF. Chronic inflammatory demyelinating polyneuropathy and respiratory failure. *J Neurol*. 2005;252(10):1235–1237.
58. Zivković SA, Peltier AC, Iacob T, Lacomis D. Chronic inflammatory demyelinating polyneuropathy and ventilatory failure: Report of seven new cases and review of the literature. *Acta Neurol Scand*. 2011;124(1):59–63.
59. Uncini A, Sabatelli M, Mignogna T, Lugaresi A, Liguori R, Montagna P. Chronic progressive steroid responsive axonal polyneuropathy: A CIDP variant or a primary axonal disorder? *Muscle Nerve*. 1996;19:365–371.
60. Cros D, Chiappa KH, Patel S, Gominak S. Acquired pure sensory demyelinating polyneuropathy: A chronic inflammatory polyradiculoneuropathy variant? *Ann Neurol*. 1992;32:280.
61. Oh SJ, Joy JL, Kuruoglu R. "Chronic sensory demyelinating neuropathy": Chronic inflammatory demyelinating polyneuropathy presenting as a pure sensory neuropathy. *J Neurol Neurosurg Psychiatry*. 1992;55:677–680.
62. Oh SJ, Joy JL, Sunwoo I, Kuruoglu R. A case of chronic sensory demyelinating neuropathy responding to immunotherapies. *Muscle Nerve*. 1992;15:255–256.
63. Berger AR, Herskovitz S, Kaplan J. Late motor involvement in cases presenting as "chronic sensory demyelinating polyneuropathy". *Muscle Nerve*. 1995;18(4):440–444.
64. Katz JS, Saperstein DS, Gronseth G, Amato AA, Barohn RJ. Distal acquired demyelinating symmetric (DADS) neuropathy. *Neurology*. 2000;54:615–620.
65. Sinnreich M, Klein CJ, Daube JR, Engelstad J, Spinner RJ, Dyck PJ. Chronic immune sensory polyneuropathy. A possibly treatable sensory ataxia. *Neurology*. 2004;63:1662–1669.
66. Citak KA, Dickoff DJ, Simpson DM. Progressive sensory radiculopathy responsive to corticosteroid therapy. *Muscle Nerve*. 1993;16:679–680.
67. Burton M, Anslow P, Gray W, Donaghy M. Selective hypertrophy of the caudal equina nerve foots. *J Neurol*. 2002;249:337–340.
68. Caporale CM, Staedler C, Gobbi C, Bassetti CL, Uncini A. Chronic inflammatory lumbosacral polyradiculopathy: A regional variant of CIDP. *Muscle Nerve*. 2011;44(5):833–837.
69. Feasby TE, Hahn AF, Koopman WJ, Lee DH. Central lesions in chronic inflammatory demyelinating polyneuropathy: A MRI study. *Neurology*. 1990;40:476–478.
70. Mendell JR, Kolkin S, Kissel JT, Weiss KL, Chakeres DW, Rammohan KW. Evidence for central nervous system demyelination in chronic inflammatory demyelinating polyradiculoneuropathy. *Neurology*. 1987;37:1291–1294.
71. Ormerod IEC, Waddy HM, Kermode AG, Murray NM, Thomas PK. Involvement of the central nervous system in chronic inflammatory demyelinating polyneuropathy: A clinical, electro-physiological and magnetic resonance imaging study. *J Neurol Neurosurg Psychiatry*. 1990;53:789–793.
72. Pakalnis A, Drake ME, Barohn RJ, Chakeres DW, Mendell JR. Evoked potentials in chronic inflammatory demyelinating polyneuropathy. *Arch Neurol*. 1988;45:1014–1016.
73. Rubin M, Karpati G, Carpenter S. Combined central and peripheral myelinopathy. *Neurology*. 1987;37:1287–1290.
74. Thomas PK, Walker WH, Rudge P, et al. Chronic demyelinating peripheral neuropathy associated with multifocal central nervous system demyelination. *Brain*. 1987;110:53–76.
75. Uncini A, Gallucci M, Lugaresi A, Porrini AM, Onofrj M, Gambi D. CNS involvement in chronic inflammatory demyelinating demyelinating polyneuropathy: An electrophysiological and MRI study. *Electromyogr Clin Neurophysiol*. 1991;31:365–371.
76. Koski CL. Baumgarten M, Magder LS, et al. Derivation and validation of diagnostic criteria for chronic inflammatory demyelinating polyneuropathy. [25 refs]. *J Neurol Sci*. 2009;277(1–2):1–8.
77. Ryan MM, Jones HR Jr. CMTX mimicking childhood chronic inflammatory demyelinating neuropathy with tremor. *Muscle Nerve*. 2005;31(4):528–530.
78. Cornblath DR, Asbury AK, Albers JW, Feasby TE. Research criteria for diagnosis of chronic inflammatory demyelinating polyneuropathy (CIDP). *Neurology*. 1991;41:617–618.
79. Amato AA, Collins MP. Neuropathies associated with malignancy. *Semin Neurol*. 1998;18:125–144.
80. Amato AA, Barohn RJ. Neurological complications of transplantation. In: Harati Y, Rolack LA eds. *Practical Neuroimmunology*. Boston, MA: Butterworth-Heineman; 1997:341–375.
81. Amato AA, Barohn RJ, Sahenk Z, Tushka PJ, Mendell JR. Polyneuropathy complicating bone marrow and solid organ transplantation. *Neurology*. 1993;43:1513–1518.
82. Antoine JC, Mosneir JF, Lapras J, et al. Chronic inflammatory demyelinating polyneuropathy associated with carcinoma. *J Neurol Neurosurg Psychiatry*. 1996;60:188–190.
83. Antoine JC, Mosneir JF, Honnorat J, et al. Paraneoplastic demyelinating neuropathy, subacute sensory neuropathy, and anti-Hu antibodies: Clinicopathological study of an autopsy case. *Muscle Nerve*. 1998;21:850–857.
84. Bird SJ, Brown MJ, Shy ME, Scherer S. Chronic inflammatory demyelinating polyneuropathy associated with malignant melanoma. *Neurology*. 1996;46:822–824.
85. Taylor BV, Wijdicks EF, Poterucha JJ, Weinser RH. Chronic inflammatory demyelinating polyneuropathy complicating liver transplantation. *Ann Neurol*. 1995;38:828–831.
86. Weiss MD, Luciano CA, Semino-Mora C, Dalakas MC, Quarles RH. Molecular mimicry in chronic inflammatory

demyelinating polyneuropathy and melanoma. *Neurology*. 1998;51:1738–1741.

87. Smyth S, Menkes DL. Coincident membranous glomerulonephritis and chronic inflammatory demyelinating polyradiculoneuropathy: Questioning the autoimmunity hypothesis. *Muscle Nerve*. 2008;37(1):130–135.
88. Inoue A, Tsukada N, Koh CS, Yanagisawa N. Chronic relapsing demyelinating polyneuropathy associated with hepatitis B infection. *Neurology*. 1987;37(10):1663–1666.
89. Rechthand E, Cornblath DR, Stern BJ, Meyerhoff JO. Chronic demyelinating polyneuropathy in systemic lupus erythematosus. *Neurology*. 1984;34(10):1375–1377.
90. Mathis S, Magy L, Diallo L, Boukhris S, Vallat JM. Amyloid neuropathy mimicking chronic inflammatory demyelinating polyneuropathy. *Muscle Nerve*. 2012;45(1):26–31.
91. Panjwani M, Truong LD, Eknoyan G. Membranous glomerulonephritis associated with inflammatory demyelinating peripheral neuropathies. *Clin Neurol Neurosurg*. 1996;27(2):279–283.
92. Wu AD, Russell JA, Bouthot BA: Chronic inflammatory polyneuropathy and membranous glomerulonephropathy: Report of two cases. *J Clin Neuromusc Dis*. 2001;3:70–74.
93. Erdem S, Freimer ML, O'Dorisio T, Mendell JR. Procainamide-induced chronic inflammatory demyelinating polyradiculoneuropathy. *Neurology*. 1998;50:824–825.
94. Richez C, Blanco P, Lagueny A, Schaeverbeke T, Dehais J. Neuropathy resembling CIDP in patients receiving tumor necrosis factor-alpha blockers. *Neurology*. 2005;64(8):1468–1470.
95. Alshekhlee A, Basiri K, Miles JD, Ahmad SA, Katirji B. Chronic inflammatory demyelinating polyneuropathy associated with tumor necrosis factor-alpha antagonists. *Muscle and Nerve*. 2010;41(5):723–727.
96. Hamon MA, Nicolas G, Deviere F, Letournel F, Dubas F. Demyelinating neuropathy during anti-TNF alpha treatment with a review of the literature. *Rev Neurol*. 2007;163(12):1232–1235.
97. Lozeron P, Denier C, Lacroix C, Adams D. Long-term course of demyelinating neuropathies occurring during tumor necrosis factor-blocker therapy. *Arch Neurol*. 2009;66(4):490–497.
98. Gorson KC, Ropper AH, Adelman LS, Weinberg DH. Influence of diabetes mellitus on chronic inflammatory demyelinating polyneuropathy. *Muscle Nerve*. 2000;23:37–43.
99. Haq RU, Pendlebury WW, Fries TJ, Tandan R. Chronic inflammatory demyelinating polyradiculoneuropathy in diabetic patients. *Muscle Nerve*. 2003;27(4):465–470.
100. Sharma KR, Cross J, Ayyar DR, Martinez-Arizala A, Bradley WG. Diabetic demyelinating polyneuropathy responsive to intravenous immunoglobulin therapy. *Arch Neurol*. 2002;59(5):751–757.
101. Sharma KR, Cross J, Farronay O, Ayyar DR, Shebert RT, Bradley WG. Demyelinating neuropathy in diabetes mellitus. *Arch Neurol*. 2002;59(5):758–765.
102. Jann S, Berretta S, Bramerio MA. Different types of chronic inflammatory demyelinating polyneuropathy have a different clinical course and response to treatment. *Muscle Nerve*. 2005;32: 351–356.
103. Ayyar DR, Sharma KR. Chronic inflammatory demyelinating polyradiculoneuropathy in diabetes mellitus. *Curr Diab Rep*. 2004;4:409–412.
104. Dyck PJ, Norell JE, Dyck PJ. Microvasculitis and ischemia in diabetic lumbosacral radiculoplexus neuropathy. *Neurology*. 1999;53(9):2113–2121.
105. Dyck PJ, Windebank AJ. Diabetic and non-diabetic lumbosacral radiculoplexus neuropathies: New insights into pathophysiology and treatment. *Muscle Nerve*. 2002;25(4):477–491.
106. Simmons Z. Paraproteinemia and neuropathy. *Curr Opin Neurology*. 1999;12(5):589–595.
107. Bromberg MB, Feldman EL, Albers JW. Chronic inflammatory demyelinating polyradiculoneuropathy: Comparison of patients with and without an associated monoclonal gammopathy. *Neurology*. 1992;42(6):1157–1163.
108. Dyck PJ, Low PA, Windebank AJ, et al. Plasma exchange in polyneuropathy associated with monoclonal gammopathy of undetermined significance. *N Engl J Med*. 1991;325(21): 1482–1486.
109. Hadden RD, Nobile-Orazio E. Sommer CL, et al. European Federation of Neurological Societies/Peripheral Nerve Society Guideline on management of paraproteinemic demyelinating neuropathies. Report of a Joint Task Force of the European Federation of Neurological Societies and the Peripheral Nerve Societ–first revision. *J Peripher Nerv Syst*. 2010;15:185–195.
110. Nobile-Orazio E. Update on neuropathies associated with monoclonal gammopathy of undetermined significance (2008–2010). *J Peripher Nerv Syst*. 2010;15:302–306.
111. Dalakas MC, Houff SA, Engel WK, Madden DL, Sever JL. CSF "monoclonal" bands in chronic relapsing polyneuropathy. *Neurology*. 1980;30:864–867.
112. Seguradi OG, Kruger H, Mertens HG. Clinical significance of serum and CSF findings in the Guillain–Barre syndrome and related disorders. *J Neurol*. 1986;233:202–208.
113. Simmons Z, Albers JW, Bromberg MB, Feldman EL. Long-term follow-up of patients with chronic inflammatory demyelinating polyneuropathy, with and without monoclonal gammopathy. *Brain*. 1995;118:359–368.
114. Khalili-Shirazi A, Atkinson P, Gregson N, Hughes RA. Antibody response to P_0 and P_2 myelin proteins in Guillain–Barre syndrome and chronic idiopathic demyelinating polyradiculoneuropathy. *J Neuroimmunol*. 1993;46:245–252.
115. Allen D, Giannopoulos K, Gray I, et al. Antibodies to peripheral nerve myelin proteins in chronic inflammatory demyelinating polyradiculoneuropathy. *J Peripher Nerv Syst*. 2005; 10(2):174–180.
116. Hughes RA, Allen D, Makowska A, Gregson NA. Pathogenesis of chronic inflammatory demyelinating polyradiculoneuropathy. *J Peripher Nerv Syst*. 2006;11(1):30–46.
117. Connolly AM, Pestronk A, Trotter JL, Feldman EL, Corn-blath DR, Olney RK. High-titer selective serum anti-tubulin antibodies in chronic inflammatory demyelinating polyneuropathy. *Neurology*. 1993;43:557–562.
118. Manfredini E, Nobile-Orazio E, Allaria S, Scarlato G. Anti-alpha and beta-tubulin IgM antibodies in dysimmune neuropathies. *J Neurol Sci*. 1995;133:79–84.
119. van Schaik IN, Vermeulen M, van Doorn PA, Brand A. Anti-á-tubulin antibodies have no diagnostic value in patients with chronic inflammatory demyelinating polyneuropathy. *J Neurol*. 1995;242:599–562.
120. De Silva RN, Willison HJ, Doyle D, Weir AI, Hadley DM, Thomas AM. Nerve root hypertrophy in chronic inflammatory demyelinating polyneuropathy. *Muscle Nerve*. 1994;17:168–170.
121. Mizuno K, Nagamatsu M, Hattori N, et al. Chronic inflammatory demyelinating polyradiculoneuropathy with diffuse and massive peripheral nerve hypertrophy: Distinctive clinical and magnetic resonance imaging features. *Muscle Nerve*. 1998;21:805–808.

122. Crino PB, Grossman RI, Rostami A. Magnetic resonance imaging of the cauda equina in chronic inflammatory demyelinating polyneuropathy. *Ann Neurol.* 1993;33:311–313.
123. Staff NP, Figueroa JJ, Parisi JE, Klein CJ. Hypertrophic nerves producing myelopathy in fulminant CIDP. *Neurology.* 2010;75(8):750.
124. Nicolas G, Maisonobe T, Le Forestier N, Leger JM, Bouche P. Proposed revised electrophysiological criteria for chronic inflammatory demyelinating polyradiculoneuropathy. *Muscle Nerve.* 2002;25(1):26–30.
125. Albers JW, Kelly JJ. Acquired inflammatory demyelinating polyneuropathies: Clinical and electrodiagnostic features. *Muscle Nerve.* 1989;12:435–451.
126. Macia F, Le Masson G, Rouanet-Larriviere M, et al. A prospective evaluation of phrenic nerve conduction in multifocal motor neuropathy and chronic inflammatory demyelinating polyneuropathy. *Muscle Nerve.* 2003;28(3):319–323.
127. Cruz Martinez A, Rabano J, Villoslada C, Cabello A. Chronic inflammatory demyelinating polyneuropathy as first manifestation of human immunodeficiency virus infection. *Electromyogr Clin Neurophysiol.* 1990;30:379–383.
128. Dyck PJ, Daube J, O'Brien PC, et al. Plasma exchange in chronic inflammatory demyelinating polyradiculoneuropathy. *N Engl J Med.* 1986;314:461–465.
129. Dyck PJ, Litchey WJ, Kratz KM, et al. Plasma exchange versus immune globulin infusion trial in chronic inflammatory demyelinating polyradiculoneuropathy. *Ann Neurol.* 1994; 36:838–845.
130. Grand-Masion F, Feasby TE, Hahn AF, Koopman WJ. Recurrent Guillain–Barre' syndrome. *Brain.* 1992;115:1093–1106.
131. Hahn AF, Bolton CF, Pillay N, et al. Plasma-exchange therapy in chronic inflammatory demyelinating polyneuropathy: A double-blind, sham-controlled, cross-over study. *Brain.* 1996;119:1055–1066.
132. Hahn AF, Bolton CF, Zochodne D, Feasby TE. Intravenous immunoglobulin treatment in chronic inflammatory demyelinating polyneuropathy: A double-blind, placebo-controlled, cross-over study. *Brain.* 1996;119:1067–1077.
133. van der Merche' FG, Vermeulen M, Busch HF. Chronic inflammatory demyelinating polyneuropathy: Conduction failure before and during immunoglobulin or plasma therapy. *Brain.* 1989;112:1563–1571.
134. Bragg JA, Benatar MG. Sensory nerve conduction slowing is a specific marker for CIDP. *Muscle Nerve.* 2008;38:1599–1603.
135. Krarup C, Trojaborg W. Sensory pathophysiology in chronic acquired demyelinating neuropathy. *Brain.* 1996;19:257–270.
136. Vallat JM, Tabaraud F, Magy L, et al. Diagnostic value of nerve biopsy for atypical chronic inflammatory demyelinating polyneuropathy: Evaluation of eight cases. *Muscle Nerve.* 2003;27(4):478–485.
137. Molenaar DS, Vermeulen M, de Haan R. Diagnostic value of sural nerve biopsy in chronic inflammatory demyelinating polyneuropathy. *J Neurol Neurosurg Psychiatry.* 1998;64:84–89.
138. Krendel DA, Parks HP, Anthony DC, St Clair MB, Graham DG. Sural nerve biopsy in chronic inflammatory demyelinating polyradiculoneuropathy. *Muscle Nerve.* 1989;12:257–264.
139. Bosboom WM, van den Berg LH, Franssen H, et al. Diagnostic value of sural nerve demyelination in chronic inflammatory demyelinating polyneuropathy. *Brain.* 2001;124:2427–2438.
140. Cornblath DR, Griffin DE, Welch D, Griffin JW, McArthur JC. Quantitative analysis of endoneurial T-cells in human sural nerve biopsies. *J Neuroimmunol.* 1990;26:113–116.
141. Matsummuro K, Izumo S, Umehara F, Osame M. Chronic inflammatory demyelinating polyneuropathy: Histological and immunopathological studies in biopsied sural nerves. *J Neurol Sci.* 1994;127:170–178.
142. Schneider-Hohendorf T, Schwab N, Uçeyler N, Göbel K, Sommer C, Wiendl H. CD8+ T-cell immunity in chronic inflammatory demyelinating polyradiculoneuropathy. *Neurology.* 2012;78(6):402–408.
143. Leppert D, Hughes P, Hiber S, et al. Matrix metalloproteinase upregulation in chronic inflammatory demyelinating polyneuropathy and nonsystemic vasculitic neuropathy. *Neurology.* 1999;53:62–70.
144. Querol L, Nogales-Gadea G, Rojas-Garcia R, et al. Neurofascin IgG4 antibodies in CIDP associated with disabling tremor and poor response to IVIg. *Neurology.* 2014;82:879–886.
145. Franssen H, Straver DC. Pathophysiology of immune- mediated demyelinating neuropathies – part I Neurology. *Muscle Nerve.* 2014;48:851–864.
146. Franssen H, Straver DC. Pathophysiology of immune- mediated demyelinating neuropathies – part II Neurology. *Muscle Nerve.* 2014;49:4–20.
147. Querol L, Nogales-Gadea G, Rojas-Garcia R, et al. Antibodies to contactin-1 in chronic inflammatory demyelinating polyneuropathy. *Ann Neurol.* 2013;73:370–380.
148. Willison H, Scherer SS. Ranvier revisited. *Neurology.* 2014;83:106–108.
149. Kwa MS, van Schaik IN, De Jonge RR, et al. Autoimmunoreactivity to Schwann cells in patients with inflammatory neuropathies. *Brain.* 2003;126:361–375.
150. Kaji R. Physiology of conduction block in multifocal motor neuropathy and other demyelinating neuropathies. *Muscle Nerve.* 2003;27(3):285–296.
151. Hughes R, Bensa S, Wilson H, et al. Randomized controlled trial of intravenous immunoglobulin versus oral prednisolone in chronic inflammatory demyelinating polyradiculoneuropathy. *Ann Neurol.* 2001;50:195–201.
152. Brannagan TH 3rd. Current treatments of chronic immune-mediated demyelinating polyneuropathies. *Muscle Nerve.* 2009;39(5):563–578.
153. Lunn MP, Willison HJ. Diagnosis and treatment in inflammatory neuropathies. *J Neurol Neurosurg Psychiatry.* 2009;80(3): 249–258.
154. Eftimov F, Winer JB, Vermeulen M, de Haan R, Van Schaik IN. Intravenous immunoglobulin for chronic inflammatory demyelinating polyradiculopneuropathy. *Cochrane Database Syst Rev.* 2013;12:CD001797.
155. Mehndiratta MM, Hughes RA. Corticosteroids for chronic inflammatory demyelinating polyradiculopathy. *Cochrane Database Syst Rev.* 2002;(1):CD002062.
156. Mehndiratta MM, Hughes RA, Agarwal P. Plasma exchange for chronic inflammatory demyelinating polyradiculoneuropathy. *Cochrane Database Syst Rev.* 2004;(3):CD003906.
157. Eftimov F, Vermeulen M, van Doorn PA, Brusse E, van Schaik IN; PREDICT. Long-term remission of CIDP after pulsed dexamethasone or short-term prednisolone treatment. *Neurology.* 2012;78(14):1079–1084.
158. Oh SJ. Subacute demyelinating polyneuropathy responding to corticosteroid treatment. *Arch Neurol.* 1978;35:509–516.
159. Dyck PJ, O'Brien PC, Oviatt KF, et al. Prednisone improves chronic inflammatory demyelinating polyradiculoneuropathy more than no treatment. *Ann Neurol.* 1982;11:136–141.

160. Molenaar DS, van Doorn PA, Vermuleulen M. Pulsed high dose dexamethasone treatment in chronic inflammatory demyelinating polyneuropathy: A pilot study. *J Neurol Neurosurg Psychiatry*. 1997;62:388–390.
161. Lopate G, Pestronk A, Al-Lozi M. Treatment of chronic inflammatory demyelinating polyneuropathy with high-dose intermittent intravenous methylprednisolone. *Arch Neurol*. 2005;62(2):249–254.
162. van Schaik IN, Eftimov F, van Doorn PA, et al. Pulsed high-dose dexamethasone versus standard prednisolone treatment for chronic inflammatory demyelinating polyradiculoneuropathy (PREDICT study): A double-blind, randomised, controlled trial. *Lancet Neurol*. 2010;9(3):245–253.
163. Cortese I, Chaudhry V, So YT, Cantor F, Cornblath DR, Rae-Grant A. Evidence-based guideline update: Plasmapheresis in neurologic disorders: report of the Therapeutics and Technology Assessment Subcommittee of the American Academy of Neurology. *Neurology*. 2011;76(3):294–300.
164. van Doorn PA, Brand A, Strengers PF, Meulstee J, Vermeulen M. High dose intravenous immunoglobulin treatment in chronic inflammatory demyelinating polyneuropathy. A double-blind placebo controlled crossover study. *Neurology*. 1990;40:209–212.
165. Mendell JR, Barohn RJ, Freimer ML, et al. Randomized controlled trial of IVIg in untreated chronic inflammatory demyelinating polyradiculoneuropathy. *Neurology*. 2001;56: 445–449.
166. Vermeulen M, van Doorn PA, Brand A, Strengers PF, Jennekens FG, Busch HF. Intravenous immunoglobulin treatment in patients with chronic inflammatory demyelinating polyneuropathy: A double blind, placebo controlled study. *J Neurol Neurosurg Psychiatry*. 1993;56:36–39.
167. Donofrio PD, Berger A, Brannagan TH III, et al. Consensus statement: The use of intravenous immunoglobulin in the treatment of neuromuscular conditions, report of the ad hoc committee of the AANEM. *Muscle Nerve*. 2009;40:890–900.
168. Patwa HS, Chaudhry V, Katzberg H, Rae-Grant AD, So YT. Evidence-based guideline: Intravenous immunoglobulin in the treatment of neuromuscular disorders: Report of the Therapeutics and Technology Assessment Subcommittee of the American Academy of Neurology. *Neurology*. 2012;78(13):1009–1015.
169. Querol L, Rojas-Garcia R, Casasnovas C, et al. Long-term outcome in chronic inflammatory demyelinating polyneuropathy patients treated with intravenous immunoglobulin: A retrospective study. *Muscle Nerve*. 2013;48(6):870–876.
170. Hughes RA, Donofrio P, Bril V, et al. Intravenous immune globulin (10% caprylate-chromatography purified) for the treatment of chronic inflammatory demyelinating polyradiculoneuropathy (ICE study): A randomised placebo-controlled trial. *Lancet Neurol*. 2008;7(2):136–144.
171. Berger AR, Hershkowitz S, Scelsa S. The restoration of IVIg efficacy by plasma exchange in CIDP. *Neurology*. 1995; 45:1628–1629.
172. Duhem C, Dicato MA, Ries F. Side-effects of intravenous immunoglobulins. *Clin Exp Immunol*. 1994;97(Suppl):79–83.
173. Ropper AH. Current treatments for CIDP. *Neurology*. 2003;60(suppl3):S16–S22.
174. Ruzhansky K, Brannagan TH III. Intravenous immunoglobulin for treatment of neuromuscular disease. *Neurol Clin Pract*. 2013;440–446.
175. Mahdi-Rogers M, van Doorn PA, Hughes RA. Immunomodulatory treatment other than corticosteroids, immunoglobulin and plasma exchange for chronic inflammatory demyelinating polyradiculoneuropathy. *Cochrane Database Syst Rev*. 2013;6:CD003280.
176. Cendrowski W. Treatment of polyneuropathy with azathioprine and adrenal steroids. *Acta Med Pol*. 1977;18:147–156.
177. Palmer KNV. Polyradiculoneuropathy treated with cytotoxic drugs. *Lancet*. 1966;1:265.
178. Pentland B, Adams GG, Mawdsley C. Chronic idiopathic polyneuropathy treated with azathioprine. *J Neurol Neurosurg Psychiatry*. 1982;45:866–869.
179. Walker GL. Progressive polyradiculoneuropathy: Treatment with azathioprine. *Aust N Z J Med*. 1979;9:184–187.
180. Cocito D, Grimaldi S, Paolasso I, et al. Immunosuppressive treatment in refractory chronic inflammatory demyelinating polyradiculoneuropathy. A nationwide retrospective analysis. *Eur J Neurol*. 2011;18(12):1417–1421.
181. Dyck PJ, O'Brien PC, Swanson C, Low P, Daube J.. Combined azathioprine and prednisone in chronic inflammatory demyelinating polyneuropathy. *Neurology*. 1985;35:1173–1176.
182. Good JL, Chehrenama M, Mayer RF, Koski CL. Pulsed cyclophosphamide in chronic inflammatory demyelinating polyneuropathy. *Neurology*. 1998;51:1735–1738.
183. Koski CL. Guillain–Barre syndrome and chronic inflammatory demyelinating polyneuropathy: Pathogenesis and treatment. *Semin Neurol*. 1994;14:123–130.
184. Brannagan TH, Alaedini A, Gladstone DE. High-dose cyclophosphamide without stem cell rescue for refractory multifocal motor neuropathy. *Muscle Nerve*. 2006;34(2):246–250.
185. Fowler H, Vulpe M, Markes G, Egolf C, Dau PC. Recover from chronic progressive polyneuropathy after treatment with plasma exchange and cyclophosphamide. *Lancet*. 1979;2: 1193.
186. Brannagan TH 3rd, Pradhan A, Heiman-Patterson T, et al. High-dose cyclophosphamide without stem-cell rescue for refractory CIDP. *Neurology*. 2002;58(12):1856–1858.
187. Gladstone DE, Prestrud AA, Brannagan TH 3rd. High-dose cyclophosphamide results in long-term disease remission with restoration of a normal quality of life in patients with severe refractory chronic inflammatory demyelinating polyneuropathy. *J Peripher Nerv Syst*. 2005;10(1):11–16.
188. Barnett MH, Pollard JD, Davies L, McLeod JG. Cyclosporine A in resistant chronic inflammatory demyelinating polyradiculoneuropathy. *Muscle Nerve*. 1998;21:454–460.
189. Hodgkinson SJ, Pollard JD, McLeod JG. Cyclosporine A in the treatment of chronic demyelinating polyradiculopathy. *J Neurol Neurosurg Psychiatry*. 1990;53:327–330.
190. Mahttanakul W, Crawford TO, Griffin JW, Goldstein JM, Cornblath DR. Treatment of chronic demyelinating polyneuropathy with cyclosporine-A. *J Neurol Neurosurg Psychiatry*. 1996;60:185–187.
191. Hefter H, Sprenger KB, Arendt G, Hafner D. Treatment of chronic relapsing inflammatory demyelinating polyneuropathy by cyclosporin A and plasma exchange. A case report. *J Neurol*. 1990;237(5):320–323.
192. Kolkin S, Nahman NS Jr, Mendell JR. Chronic nephrotoxicity complicating cyclosporine treatment of chronic inflammatory demyelinating polyradiculoneuropathy. *Neurology*. 1987;37(1):147–149.

193. Matsuda M, Hoshi K, Gono T, Morita H, Ikeda S. Cyclosporin A in treatment of refractory patients with chronic inflammatory demyelinating polyradiculoneuropathy. *J Neurol Sci.* 2004;224(1-2):29–35.
194. Odaka M, Tatsumoto M, Susuki K, Hirata K, Yuki N. Intractable chronic inflammatory demyelinating polyneuropathy treated successfully with ciclosporin. *J Neurol Neurosurg Psychiatry.* 2005;76(8):1115–1120.
195. Fialho D, Chan YC, Allen DC, Reilly MM, Hughes RA. Treatment of chronic inflammatory demyelinating polyradiculoneuropathy with methotrexate. *J Neurol Neurosurg Psychiatry.* 2006;77(4):544–547.
196. Mahdi-Rogers M, RMC Trial Group. Randomised Methotrexate Chronic Inflammatory Demyelinating polyradiculoneuropathy (RMC) Trial Group. A pilot randomised controlled trial of methotrexate for CIDP: Lessons for future trials. *J Periph Nerv Syst.* 2008;13(2):176.
197. RMC Trial Group. Randomised controlled trial of methotrexate for chronic inflammatory demyelinating polyradiculoneuropathy (RMC trial): A pilot, multicentre study. *Lancet Neurol.* 2009;8(2):158–164.
198. Choudhary PP, Thompson N, Hughes RA. Improvement following interferon-beta in chronic inflammatory demyelinating polyneuropathy. *J Neurol.* 1995;242:252–253.
199. Sabatelli M, Mignogna T, Tippi G, et al. Interferon alpha may benefit steroid unresponsive chronic inflammatory demyelinating polyneuropathy. *J Neurol Neurosurg Psychiatry.* 1995; 58:638–639.
200. Hadden RD, Sharrack B, Bensa S, Soudain SE, Hughes RA. Randomized trial of interferon β-1 a in chronic inflammatory demyelinating polyradiculoneuropathy. *Neurology.* 1999;53:57–61.
201. Kuntzer T, Radziwill AJ, Lettry-Trouillat R, et al. Interferon-beta1 a in chronic inflammatory demyelinating polyneuropathy. *Neurology.* 1999;53(6):1364–1365.
202. Martina IS, van Doorn PA, Schmitz PI, Meulstee J, van der Meché FG. Chronic motor neuropathies: Response to interferon-beta1 a after failure of conventional therapies. *J Neurol Neurosurg Psychiatry.* 1999;66(2):197–201.
203. Vallat JM, Hahn AF, Léger JM, et al. Interferon beta-1 a as an investigational treatment for CIDP. *Neurology.* 2003;60(8 suppl 3):S23–S28.
204. Gorson KC, Allam G, Simovic D, Ropper AH. Improvement following interferon-alpha 2 A in chronic inflammatory demyelinating polyneuropathy. *Neurology.* 1997;48(3):777–780.
205. Pavesi G, Cattaneo L, Marbini A, Gemignani F, Mancia D. Long-term efficacy of interferon-alpha in chronic inflammatory demyelinating polyneuropathy. *J Neurol.* 2002;249(6):777–779.
206. Hughes RA, Gorson KC, Cros D, et al. Intramuscular interferon beta-1 a in chronic inflammatory demyelinating polyradiculoneuropathy. *Neurology.* 2010;74(8):651–657.
207. Chaudhry V, Cornblath DR, Griffin JW, O'Brien R, Drachman DB. Mycophenolate mofetil: A safe and promising immunosuppressant in neuromuscular diseases. *Neurology.* 2001; 56:94–96.
208. Spies JM, Pollard JD. Mycophenolate mofetil is effective therapy for refractory CIDP. *J Peripher Nerv Syst.* 2003;8:61.
209. Umapathi T, Hughes R. Mycophenolate in treatment-resistant inflammatory neuropathies. *Eur J Neurol.* 2002;9:683–685.
210. Gorson KC, Amato AA, Ropper AH. Efficacy of mycophenolate mofetil in patients with Chronic immune demyelinating polyneuropathy. *Neurology.* 2004;63:715–717.
211. Radziwill AJ, Schweikert K, Kuntzer T, Fuhr P, Steck AJ. Mycophenolate mofetil for chronic inflammatory demyelinating polyradiculoneuropathy: An open-label study. *Eur Neurol.* 2006;56(1):37–38.
212. Mowzoon N, Sussman A, Bradley WG. Mycophenolate (CellCept) treatment of myasthenia gravis, chronic inflammatory polyneuropathy and inclusion body myositis. *J Neurol Sci.* 2001;185(2):119–122.
213. Benedetti L, Grandis M, Nobbio L, et al. Mycophenolate mofetil in dysimmune neuropathies: A preliminary study. *Muscle Nerve.* 2004;29(5):748–749.
214. Bedi G, Brown A, Tong T, Sharma KR. Chronic inflammatory demyelinating polyneuropathy responsive to mycophenolate mofetil therapy. *J Neurol Neurosurg Psychiatry.* 2010; 81(6):634–636.
215. Bodley-Scott D. Chronic inflammatory demyelinating polyradiculoneuropathy responding to rituximab. *Pract Neurol.* 2005;5(4):242–245.
216. Briani C, Zara G, Zambello R, Trentin L, Rana M, Zaja F. Rituximab-responsive CIDP. *Eur J Neurol.* 2004;11(11): 788.
217. Benedetti L, Franciotta D, Beronio A, et al. Rituximab efficacy in CIDP associated with idiopathic thrombocytopenic purpura. *Muscle Nerve.* 2008;38(2):1076–1077.
218. Benedetti L, Briani C, Franciotta D, et al. Rituximab in patients with chronic inflammatory demyelinating polyradiculoneuropathy: A report of 13 cases and review of the literature. *J Neurol Neurosurg Psychiatry.* 2011;82(3):306–308.
219. D'Amico A, Catteruccia M, De Benedetti F, et al. Rituximab in a childhood-onset idiopathic refractory chronic inflammatory demyelinating polyneuropathy. *Eur J Paediatr Neurol.* 2012;16(3):301–303.
220. Gorson KC, Natarajan N, Ropper AH, Weinstein R. Rituximab treatment in patients with IVIg-dependent immune polyneuropathy: A prospective pilot trial. *Muscle Nerve.* 2007;35(1): 66–69.
221. Knecht H, Baumberger M, Tobòn A, Steck A. Sustained remission of CIDP associated with Evans syndrome. *Neurology.* 2004;63(4):730–732.
222. Münch C, Anagnostou P, Meyer R, Haas J. Rituximab in chronic inflammatory demyelinating polyneuropathy associated with diabetes mellitus.*J Neurol Sci.* 2007;256(1–2):100–102.
223. Sadnicka A, Reilly MM, Mummery C, Brandner S, Hirsch N, Lunn MP. Rituximab in the treatment of three coexistent neurological autoimmune diseases: Chronic inflammatory demyelinating polyradiculoneuropathy, Morvan syndrome and myasthenia gravis. *J Neurol Neurosurg Psychiatry.* 2011; 82(2):230–232.
224. Rosenberg NL, Lacy JR, Kennaugh RC, Holters VM, Neville HE, Kotzin BL. Treatment of refractory chronic demyelinating polyneuropathy with lymphoid irradiation. *Muscle Nerve.* 1985;8:223–232.
225. Lewis RA, Sumner AJ, Brown MJ, Asbury AK. Multifocal demyelinating neuropathy with persistent conduction block. *Neurology.* 1982;32(9):958–964.
226. Saperstein DS, Amato AA, Wolfe GI, et al. Multifocal acquired demyelinating sensory and motor neuropathy. The Lewis–Sumner syndrome. *Muscle Nerve.* 1999;22:560–566.
227. Amato AA, Jackson CE, Kim JY, Worley KL. Chronic relapsing brachial plexus neuropathy with persistent conduction block. *Muscle Nerve.* 1997;20:1303–1307.

228. Gibbels E, Behse F, Haupt WF. Chronic multifocal neuropathy with persistent conduction block (Lewis–Sumner syndrome). *Clin Neuropathol.* 1993;12:343–352.
229. Gorson KC, Ropper AH, Weinberg DH. Upper limb predominant, multifocal chronic inflammatory demyelinating polyneuropathy. *Muscle Nerve.* 1999;22:758–765.
230. Nukada H, Pollock M, Haas LF. Is ischemia implicated in chronic multifocal demyelinating neuropathy? *Neurology.* 1989;39:106–110.
231. Oh SJ, Claussen GC, Dae SK. Motor and sensory demyelinating mononeuropathy multiplex (multifocal motor and sensory demyelinating neuropathy): A separate entity or a variant of chronic inflammatory demyelinating polyneuropathy. *J Peripher Nerv Syst.* 1997;2:362–369.
232. Ropper AH, Gorson KC, Weinberg DH. Focal upper limb predominant CIDP. *Neurology.* 1998;50(suppl 4):A144.
233. Viala KL, Renié T, Maisonobe A, et al. Follow-up study and response to treatment in 23 patients with Lewis–Sumner syndrome. *Brain.* 2004;127:2010–2017.
234. Oh SJ, LaGanke C, Powers R, Wolfe GI, Quinton RA, Burns DK. Multifocal motor sensory demyelinating neuropathy: Inflammatory demyelinating polyradiculoneuropathy. *Neurology.* 2005;65(10):1639–1642.
235. Rajabally YA, Chavaeda G. Lewis-Sumner syndrome of pure upper-limb onset: Diagnostic, prognostic, and therapeutic features. *Muscle Nerve.* 2009;39:206–220.
236. Tramontozzi LA III, Russell JA. Orthostatic intolerance in multifocal acquired demyelinating sensory and motor neuropathy. *J Clin Neuromusc Dis.* 2012;1:34–39.
237. Puwanant A, Herrmann DH. Multifocal acquired densory and motor neuropathy. *Neurology.* 2012;79:1742.
238. Simó M, Casasnovas C, Martínez-Yélamos S, Martínez-Mato JA. Multifocal acquired demelinating sensory and motor neuropathy presenting as idiopathic hypertrophic brachial neuropathy. *J Neurol Neurosurg Psychiatry.* 2009;80:674–675.
239. Kerasnoudis A. Ultrasonography of MADSAM neuropathy: Focal nerve enlargements at sites of existing and resolved conduction blocks. *Neuromuscul Disord.* 2012;22(11):1032.
240. Scheidl E, Böhm J, Simó M, et al. Ultrasonography of MADSAM neuropathy: Focal nerve enlargements at sites of existing and resolved conduction blocks. *Neuromuscul Disord.* 2012;22(7):627–631.
241. Bayas A, Gold R, Naumann M. Long-term treatment of Lewis–Sumner syndrome with subcutaneous immunoglobulin infusions. *J Neurol Sci.* 2013;324:53–56.
242. Attarian S, Verschueren A, Franques J, Salort-Campana E, Jouve E, Pouget J. Response to treatment in patients with Lewis-Sumner syndrome. *Muscle Nerve.* 2011;44(2):179–184.
243. Ellie E, Vital A, Steck A, Boiron JM, Vital C, Julien J. Neuropathy associated with "benign" anti-myelin-associated glycoprotein IgM gammopathy: Clinical, immunological, neurophysiological pathological findings and response to treatment in 33 cases. *J Neurol.* 1996;243(1):34–43.
244. Niermeijer JM, Fischer K, Eurelings M, Franssen H, Wokke JH, Notermans NC. Prognosis of polyneuropathy due to IgM monoclonal gammopathy: A prospective cohort study. *Neurology.* 2010;74(5):406–412.
245. Dalakas MC, Teräväinen H, Engel WK. Tremor as a feature of chronic relapsing and dysgammaglobulinemic polyneuropathies. Incidence and management. *Arch Neurol.* 1984;41(7):711–714.
246. Smith IS. The natural history of chronic demyelinating neuropathy associated with benign IgM paraproteinaemia. A clinical and neurophysiological study. *Brain.* 1994;117(Pt 5): 949–957.
247. Yeung KB, Thomas PK, King RH, et al. The clinical spectrum of peripheral neuropathies associated with benign monoclonal IgM, IgG and IgA paraproteinaemia. Comparative clinical, immunological and nerve biopsy findings. *J Neurol.* 1991;238 (7):383–391.
248. Donofrio PD. Immunotherapy of idiopathic inflammatory neuropathies.*Muscle & Nerve.* 2003;28(3):273–292.
249. Kawagashira Y, Kondo N, Atsuta N, et al. IgM MGUS anti-MAG neuropathy with predominant muscle weakness and extensive muscle atrophy. *Muscle Nerve.* 2010;42(3):433–435.
250. Kissel JT, Mendell JR. Neuropathies associated with monoclonal gammopathies. *Neuromuscul Disord.* 1996;6(1):3–18.
251. Nobile-Orazio E, Meucci N, Baldini L, Di Troia A, Scarlato G. Long-term prognosis of neuropathy associated with anti-MAG IgM M-proteins and its relationship to immune therapies. *Brain.* 2000;123(Pt 4):710–717.
252. Mygland A, Monstad P. Chronic acquired demyelinating symmetric polyneuropathy classified by pattern of weakness. *Arch Neurol.* 2003;60(2):260–264.
253. Cook D, Dalakas M, Galdi A, Biondi D, Porter H. High-dose intravenous immunoglobulin in the treatment of demyelinating neuropathy associated with monoclonal gammopathy. *Neurology.* 1990;40(2):212–214.
254. Gorson KC, Ropper AH, Weinberg DH, Weinstein R. Treatment experience in patients with anti-myelin-associated glycoprotein neuropathy. *Muscle Nerve.* 2001;24(6):778–786.
255. Lunn MP, Nobile-Orazio E. Immunotherapy for IgM anti-Myelin-Associated Glycoprotein paraprotein-associated peripheral neuropathies. *Cochrane Database Syst Rev.* 2006;(2):CD002827.
256. Niermeijer JM, Eurelings M, Lokhorst HL, et al. Rituximab for polyneuropathy with IgM monoclonal gammopathy. *J Neurol Neurosurgery Psychiatry.* 2009;80(9):1036–1039.
257. Benedetti L, Briani C, Grandis M, et al. Predictors of response to rituximab in patients with neuropathy and anti-myelin associated glycoprotein immunoglobulin M. *J Peripher Nerv Syst.* 2007;12(2):102–107.
258. Benedetti L, Briani C, Franciotta D, et al. Long-term effect of rituximab in anti-mag polyneuropathy. *Neurology.* 2008;71(21):1742–1744.
259. Renaud S, Gregor M, Fuhr P, et al. Rituximab in the treatment of polyneuropathy associated with anti-MAG antibodies. *Muscle Nerve.* 2003;27(5):611–615.
260. Dalakas MC, Rakocevic G, Salajegheh MK, et al. Placebo-controlled study of rituximab in IgM anti-myelin-associated glycoprotein antibody demyelinating polyneuropathy. *Ann Neurol.* 2009;65:286–293.
261. Souayah N, Noopur R, Tick-Chong PS. Beneficial effects of Rituximab in patients with anti-MAG (myelin-associated glycoprotein) neuropathy: Case reports. *Immunopharmacol Immunotoxicol.* 2013;35(5):622–624.
262. Léger JM, Viala K, Nicolas G, et al. Placebo-controlled trial of rituximab in IgM anti-myelin-associated glycoprotein neuropathy. *Neurology.* 2013;80(24):2217–2225.
263. Stork AC, Notermans NC, Vrancken AF, Cornblath DR, van der Pol WL. Rapid worsening of IgM anti-MAG demyelinating polyneuropathy during rituximab treatment. *J Peripher Nerv Syst.* 2013;18(2):189–191.

264. Chad DA, Hammer K, Sargent J. Slow resolution of multifocal weakness and fasciculation: A reversible motor neuron syndrome. *Neurology*. 1986;36:1260–1263.
265. Parry GJ, Holtz SJ, Ben-Zeev D, Drori JB. Gammopathy with proximal motor axonopathy simulating motor neuron disease. *Neurology*. 1986;36(2):273–276.
266. Rowland LP, Defendini R, Sherman W, et al. Macroglobulinemia with peripheral neuropathy simulating motor neuron disease. *Ann Neurol*. 1982;11(5):532–536.
267. Tucker T, Layzer RB. Subacute, reversible motor neuron disease. Abstract. *Neurology*. 1985;35(suppl1):108.
268. Auer RN, Nell RB, Lee MA. Neuropathy with onion bulb formations and pure motor manifestation. *Can J Neurol Sci*. 1989;16:194–197.
269. Van den Berg-Vos RM, Franssen H, Wokke JH, Van den Berg LH. Multifocal motor neuropathy: Long-term clinical and electrophysiological assessment of intravenous immunoglobulin maintenance treatment. *Brain*. 2002;125:1875–1886.
270. Chaudhry V. Multifocal motor neuropathy. *Semin Neurol*. 1998;18:73–81.
271. Chaudhry V, Cornblath DR, Griffin JW, Corse AM, Kuncl RW, Drachman DL. Multifocal motor neuropathy or CIDP?—Reply. *Ann Neurol*. 1993;34:750–751.
272. Chaudhry V, Corse AM, Cornblath DR, Kuncl RW, Freimer ML, Griffin JW. Multifocal motor neuropathy: Electrodiagnostic features. *Muscle Nerve*. 1994;17:198–205.
273. Chaudhry V, Corse AM, Cornblath DR, et al. Multifocal motor neuropathy: Response to human immune globulin. *Ann Neurol*. 1993;33:237–242.
274. Feldman EL, Bromberg MB, Albers JW, Pestronk A. Immunosuppressive treatment in multifocal motor neuropathy. *Ann Neurol*. 1991;30:397–401.
275. Katz JS, Wolfe GI, Bryan WW, Jackson CE, Amato AA, Barohn RJ. Electrophysiologic findings in multifocal motor neuropathy. *Neurology*. 1997;48:700–707.
276. Krarup C, Stewart JD, Sumner AJ, et al. A syndrome of asymmetric limb weakness with motor conduction block. *Neurology*. 1990;40:118–127.
277. Parry GJ, Clarke S. Multifocal acquired demyelinating neuropathy masquerading as motor neuron disease. *Muscle Nerve*. 1988;11:103–107.
278. Parry GJ, Sumner AJ. Multifocal motor neuropathy. *Neurol Clin*. 1992;10:671–684.
279. Pestronk A, Chaudhry V, Feldman EL, et al. Lower motor neuron syndromes defined by patterns of weakness, nerve conduction abnormalities, and high titers of antiglycolipid antibodies. *Ann Neurol*. 1990;27:316–326.
280. Pestronk A, Cornblath DR, Ilyas AA, et al. A treatable multifocal motor neuropathy with antibodies to GM1 gangliosides. *Ann Neurol*. 1988;24:73–78.
281. Roth G, Rohr J, Magistris MR, et al. Motor neuropathy with proximal multifocal persistent conduction block, fasciculations and myokymia. *Eur Neurol*. 1986;25:416–423.
282. Olney RK, Lewis RA, Putnam TD, Campellone JV Jr. American Association of Electrodiagnostic Medicine. Consensus criteria for the diagnosis of multifocal motor neuropathy. *Muscle Nerve*. 2003;27(1):117–121.
283. Parry GJ. Motor neuropathy with multifocal conduction block. *Semin Neurol*. 1993;13:269–275.
284. Vlam L, van der Pol WL, Cats EA, et al. Multifocal motor neuropathy. *Nat Rev Neurol*. 2011;8:48–58.
285. Slee M, Selvan A, Donaghy M. Multifocal motor neuropathy: The diagnostic spectrum and response to treatment. *Neurology*. 2007;69(17):1680–1687.
286. Cats EA, van der Pol WL, Piepers S, et al. Correlates of outcome and response to IVIg in 88 patients with multifocal motor neuropathy. *Neurology*. 2010;75(9):818–825.
287. Moroni I, Bugiani M, Ciano C, Bono R, Pareyson D. Childhood-onset multifocal motor neuropathy with conduction blocks. *Neurology*. 2006;66(6):922–924.
288. Traynor BJ, Codd MB, Corr B, Forde C, Frost E, Hardiman O. Amyotrophic lateral sclerosis mimic syndromes: A population-based study. *Arch Neurol*. 2000;57:109–113.
289. Miyashiro A, Matsui N, Shimatani Y, et al. Are multifocal motor neuropathy patients underdiagnosed? An epidemiological survey in Japan. *Muscle Nerve*. 2014;49(3):357–361.
290. Kaji R, Shibasaki H, Kimura J. Multifocal demyelinating motor neuropathy: Cranial nerve involvement and immunoglobulin therapy. *Neurology*. 1992;42:506–509.
291. Pringle CE, Belden J, Veitch JE, Brown WF. Multifocal motor neuropathy presenting as ophthalmoplegia. *Muscle Nerve*. 1997;20:347–351.
292. Boonyapisit K, Katirji B. Multifocal motor neuropathy presenting with respiratory failure. *Muscle Nerve*. 2000;23(12):1887–1890.
293. Beydoun SR, Copeland D. Bilateral phrenic neuropathy as a presenting feature of multifocal motor neuropathy with conduction block. *Muscle Nerve*. 2000;23(4):556–559.
294. Felice KJ, Goldstein JM. Monofocal motor neuropathy: Improvement with intravenous immunoglobulin. *Muscle Nerve*. 2002;25:674–678.
295. Manganelli F, Pisciotta C, Iodice R, Calandro S, Santoro L. Nine-year case history of monofocal motor neuropathy. *Muscle Nerve*. 2008;38:927–929.
296. Jafari H, Carlander B, Camu W. Monofocal motor neuropathy responsive to intravenous immunoglobulins. *Muscle Nerve*. 2000;23:1610–1611.
297. Alentorn A, Alberti MA, Montero J, Casasnovas C. Monofocal motor neuropathy with conduction block associated with adalimumab in rheumatoid athritis. *Joint Bone Spine*. 2011;78:536–537.
298. Pakiam AS, Parry GJ. Multifocal motor neuropathy without overt conduction block. *Muscle Nerve*. 1998;21:243–245.
299. Nobile-Orazio E, Cappellari A, Meucci N, et al. Multifocal motor neuropathy: Clinical and immunological features and response to IVIg in relation to the presence and degree of motor conduction block. *J Neurol Neurosurg Psychiatry*. 2002;72(6):761–766.
300. Delmont E, Azulay JP, Giorgi R, et al. Multifocal motor neuropathy with and without conduction block: A single entity? *Neurology*. 2006;67(4):592–596.
301. Chaudhry V, Swash M. Multifocal motor neuropathy: Is conduction block essential?*Neurology*. 2006;67(4):558–559.
302. Kaji R, Hirota N, Oka N, et al. Anti-GM1 antibodies and impaired blood–nerve barrier may interfere with remyelination in multifocal motor neuropathy. *Muscle Nerve*. 1994;17:108–110.
303. Kornberg AJ, Pestronk A. The clinical and diagnostic role of anti-GM_1 antibody testing. *Muscle Nerve*. 1994;17:100–104.
304. Levine TD, Pestronk A. IgM antibody-related polyneuropathies: Treatment with B-cell depletion chemotherapy using rituximab. *Neurology*. 1999;52:1701–1704.
305. Gooch CL, Amato AA. Are anti-ganglioside antibodies of clinical value in multifocal motor neuropathy? *Neurology*. 2010;75(22):1950–1951.

306. Parry GJ. Antiganglioside antibodies do not necessarily play a role in multifocal motor neuropathy. *Muscle Nerve.* 1994;17:97–99.
307. Cornblath DR, Sumner AJ, Daube J, et al. Conduction block in clinical practice. *Muscle Nerve.* 1991;14:869–871.
308. Comi G, Amadio S, Galardi G, Fazio R, Nemni R. Clinical and neurophysiological assessment of immunoglobulin therapy in five patients with multifocal motor neuropathy. *J Neurol Neurosurg Psychiatry.* 1994;57(suppl):35–37.
309. Weimer LH, Grewal RP, Lange DJ. Electrophysiologic abnormalities other than conduction block in multifocal motor neuropathy. *Muscle Nerve.* 1994;9:1089.
310. Van Asseldonk JT, Van den Berg LH, Van den Berg-Vos RM, Wieneke GH, Wokke JH, Franssen H. Demyelination and axonal loss in multifocal motor neuropathy: Distribution and relation to weakness. *Brain.* 2003;126:186–198.
311. Beekman R, van den Berg LH, Franssen H, Visser LH, van Asseldonk JT, Wokke JH. Ultrasonography shows extensive nerve enlargements in multifocal motor neuropathy. *Neurology.* 2005;65(2):305–307.
312. Zhou L, Yousem DM, Chaudhry V. Role of magnetic resonance neurography in brachial plexus lesions. *Muscle Nerve.* 2004;30(3):305–309.
313. Bouche P, Moulonguet A, Younes-Chennoufi AB, et al. Multifocal motor neuropathy with conduction block: A study of 24 patients. *J Neurol Neurosurg Psychiatry.* 1995;59:38–44.
314. Corse AM, Chaudhry V, Crawford TO, Cornblath DR, Kuncl RW, Griffin JW. Sensory nerve pathology in multifocal motor neuropathy. *Ann Neurol.* 1996;39:319–325.
315. Kaji R, Nobuyuki O, Tsuji T, et al. Pathological findings at the site of conduction block in multifocal motor neuropathy. *Ann Neurol.* 1993;33:152–158.
316. Yuki N, Watanabe H, Nakajima T, Späth PJ. IVIG blocks complement deposition mediated by anti-GM1 antibodies in multifocal motor neuropathy. *J Neurol Neurosurg Psychiatry.* 2011;82(1):87–91.
317. Nobile-Orazio E, Meucci N, Barbieri S, Carpo M, Scarlato G. High-dose intravenous immunoglobulin therapy in multifocal motor neuropathy. *Neurology.* 1993;43:537–544.
318. Tan E, Lynn DJ, Amato AA, et al. Immunosuppressive treatment of motor neuron syndromes. Attempts to distinguish a treatable disorder. *Arch Neurol.* 1994;51:194–200.
319. Markson L, Janzen D, Bril V. Response to therapy in demyelinating motor neuropathy. *Muscle Nerve.* 1998;21:1769–1771.
320. Arasaki K, Kusunoki S, Kudo N, Kanazawa I. Acute conduction block in vitro following exposure to antiganglioside sera. *Muscle Nerve.* 1993;16:587–593.
321. Roberts M, Willison HJ, Vincent A, Newsom-Davis J. Multifocal motor neuropathy human sera block distal motor nerve conduction in mice. *Ann Neurol.* 1995;38:111–118.
322. Santoro M, Uncini A, Corbo M, et al. Experimental conduction block induced by serum from a patient with anti-GM_1 antibodies. *Ann Neurol.* 1992;31:385–390.
323. Harvey GK, Toyka KV, Zielasek J, et al. Failure of anti-GM1 IgG or IgM to induce conduction block following intraneural transfer. *Muscle Nerve.* 1995;18:388–394.
324. Kuwabara S, Yuki N, Koga M, et al. IgG anti-GM1 antibody is associated with reversible conduction failure and axonal degeneration in Guillain-Barré syndrome. *Ann Neurol.* 1998;44(2):202–208.
325. Takigawa T, Yashuda H, Kikkawa R. Antibodies against GM1 gangliosides affect K+ and Na+ currents in isolated rat myelinated nerve fibers. *Ann Neurol.* 1995;37:436–442.
326. Weber F, Rüdel R, Aulkemeyer P, Brinkmeier H. Anti-GM1 antibodies can block neuronal voltage-gated sodium channels. *Muscle Nerve.* 2000;23(9):1414–1420.
327. White JR, Sachs GM, Gilchrist JM. Multifocal motor neuropathy with conduction block and Campylobacter jejuni. *Neurology.* 1996;46(2):562–563.
328. Terenghi F, Allaria S, Scarlato G, Nobile-Orazio E. Multifocal motor neuropathy and Campylobacter jejuni reactivity. *Neurology.* 2002;59(2):282–284.
329. Rodriguez-Escalera C, Belzunegui J, Lopez-Dominguez L, Gonzalez C, Figueroa M. Multifocal motor neuropathy with conduction block in a patient with rheumatoid arthritis on infliximab therapy. *Rheumatology.* 2005;44(1):132–133.
330. Tektonidou MG, Serelis J, Skopouli FN. Peripheral neuropathy in two patients with rheumatoid arthritis receiving infliximab treatment. *Clin Rheumatol.* 2007;26(2):258–260.
331. Chaudhry V, Escolar DM, Cornblath DR. Worsening of multifocal motor neuropathy during pregnancy. *Neurology.* 2002;59(1):139–141.
332. Charles N, Benott P, Vial C, Bierme T, Moreau T, Bady B. Intravenous immunoglobulin treatment in multifocal motor neuropathy. *Lancet.* 1992;340:182.
333. Donaghy M, Mills KR, Boniface SJ, et al. Pure motor demyelinating neuropathy: Deterioration after steroid treatment and improvement with intravenous immunoglobulin. *J Neurol Neurosurg Psychiatry.* 1994;57:778–783.
334. Olney RK, Pestronk A. Prednisone treatment of multifocal motor neuropathy. *Neurology.* 1992;42(Suppl 3):178.
335. Leger JM, Chassande B, Musset L, Meininger V, Bouche P, Baumann N. Intravenous immunoglobulin therapy in multifocal motor neuropathy: A double-blind, placebo-controlled study. *Brain.* 2001;124:145–153.
336. Azulay JP, Rihet P, Pouget J, et al. Long term follow up of multifocal motor neuropathy with conduction block under treatment. *J Neurol Neurosurg Psychiatry.* 1997;62:391–394.
337. Cruz Martinez A, Arpa J, Lara M. Electrophysiological improvement after intravenous immunoglobulin in motor neuropathy with multifocal conduction block. *J Neurol Neurosurg Psychiatry.* 1993;56:1236–1237.
338. Federico P, Zochodne DW, Hahn AF, Brown WF, Feasby TE. Multifocal motor neuropathy improved by IVIG: Randomized, double-blind, placebo-controlled study. *Neurology.* 2000;55:1256–1262.
339. Umapathi T, Hughes RA, Nobile-Orazio E, Leger JM. Immunosuppressant and immunomodulatory treatments for multifocal motor neuropathy. *Cochrane Database Syst Rev.* 2009;(1):CD003217.
340. van Schaik IN, Bouche P, Illa I, et al. European Federation of Neurological Societies, Peripheral Nerve Society. European Federation of Neurological Societies/Peripheral Nerve Society guideline on management of multifocal motor neuropathy. *Eur J Neurol.* 2006;13(8):802–808.
341. Jinka M, Chaudhry V. Treatment of multifocal motor neuropathy. *Curr Treat Options Neurol.* 2014;16(2):269.
342. Azulay JP, Blin O, Pouget J, et al. Intravenous immunoglobulin treatment in patients with motor neuron syndromes associated with anti-GM1 antibodies: A double-blind, placebo-controlled study. *Neurology.* 1994;44:429–432.

343. Harbo T, Andersen H, Jakobsen J. Long-term therapy with high doses of subcutaneous immunoglobulin in multifocal motor neuropathy. *Neurology*. 2010;75(15):1377–1380.
344. Eftimov F, Vermeulen M, de Haan RJ, van den Berg LH. van Schaik IN. Subcutaneous immunoglobulin therapy for multifocal motor neuropathy. *J Periph Nerv Syst*. 2009;14(2): 93–100.
345. Van den Berg-Vos RM, Van den Berg LH, Franssen H, Van Doorn PA, Merkies IS, Wokke JH. Treatment of multifocal motor neuropathy with interferon-beta1 A. *Neurology*. 2000;54(7):1518–1521.
346. Meucci N, Cappellari A, Barbieri S, Scarlato G, NobileOrazio E. Long term effect of intravenous immunoglobulins and oral cyclophosphamide in multifocal motor neuropathy. *J Neurol Neurosurg Psychiatry*. 1997;63:765–769.
347. Ruegg SJ, Fuhr P, Steck AJ. Rituximab stabilizes multifocal motor neuropathy increasingly less responsive to IVIg. *Neurology*. 2004;63(11):2178–2179.
348. Pestronk A, Florence J, Miller T, Choksi R, Al-Lozi MT, Levine TD. Treatment of IgM antibody associated polyneuropathies using rituximab. *J Neurol Neurosurg Psychiatry*. 2003;74: 485–489.
349. Katz JS, Barohn RJ, Kojan S, et al. Axonal multifocal motor neuropathy without conduction block or other features of demyelination. *Neurology*. 2002;58:615–620.
350. Sansa-Fayos G, Viguera-Martinez ML, Ribera-Perpina G, Martinez-Perez JM. Axonal multifocal motor neuropathy. A case report. *Rev Neurol*. 2005;41(7):444–446.
351. Asbury AK, Picard EH, Baringer JR. Sensory perineuritis. *Arch Neurol*. 1972;26:302–312.
352. Chad DA, Smith TW, DeGirolami U, Hammer K. Perineuritis and ulcerative colitis. *Neurology*. 1986;36:1377–1379.
353. Konishi T, Saida K, Ohnishi A, Nishitani H. Perineuritis in mononeuritis multiplex with cryoglobulinemia. *Muscle Nerve*. 1982;5:173–177.
354. Simmons Z, Albers JW, Sima AA. Perineuritis presenting as mononeuropathy multiplex. *Muscle Nerve*. 1992; 15:630–635.
355. Sorenson EJ, Sima AA, Blaivas M, Sawchuck K, Wald JJ. Clinical features of perineuritis. *Muscle Nerve*. 1997;20: 1153–1157.
356. Yamada M, Owada K, Eishi Y, Kato A, Yokota T, Furukawa T. Sensory perineuritis and non-Hodgkins T-cell lymphoma [Letter]. *Eur Neurol*. 1994;34:298–299.
357. Matthews WB, Squier MV. Sensory perineuritis. *J Neurol Neurosurg Psychiatry*. 1988;51:473–475.

CHAPTER 15

Vasculitic Neuropathies

Vasculitis is an immune-mediated disorder directed against blood vessels, which results in ischemia to end organs supplied by the affected blood vessels.[1–5] The vasculitides can be distinguished and classified based on at least three nosologic categories. They can be differentiated based on the caliber of vessel involved (i.e., small, medium, or large vessel). They can be distinguished on whether the disorder is primary [e.g., polyarteritis nodosa (PAN), microscopic polyangiitis (MPA), granulomatosis with polyangiitis (GAN, formerly known as Wegener granulomatosis), and Churg–Strauss syndrome (CSS)] or secondary to other systemic disorders (e.g., connective tissue disease, malignancy, infection, or drug reaction). Furthermore, the vasculitides can be separated based on whether they are systemic or isolated to the peripheral nervous system (PNS), and if associated with antineutrophil cytoplasmic antibodies (ANCAs) (Table 15-1).[2,3] Vasculitis is much more common in adults but can develop in children.[6]

▶ CLINICAL FEATURES

PNS vasculitis can present as (1) a mononeuropathy or multiple mononeuropathies, (2) overlapping mononeuropathies, or (3) distal symmetric polyneuropathies (Fig. 15-1).[3–8] In the first pattern, patients may present with just a mononeuropathy, but usually multiple nerves eventually become affected over time, giving a distinct asymmetric pattern of involvement in the distribution of individual nerves. With the second pattern, different nerves on both sides of the body are affected but to varying degrees, leading to a generalized, yet asymmetric, pattern of involvement. Finally, with gradual progression, somewhat uniform and generalized involvement of peripheral nerves results in what looks like a distal symmetric polyneuropathy. Approximately 60–70% of patients present with mononeuropathy or multiple mononeuropathies (multifocal neuropathy or mononeuropathy multiplex pattern), while 30–40% of patients present as a distal symmetric polyneuropathy.[7] There is a large differential diagnosis of patients with a multiple mononeuropathy (Table 15-2). For this reason, multifocal neuropathy, multiple mononeuropathies, or mononeuropathy multiplex are preferable terminologies to mononeuritis multiplex because the latter term implies a histologically defined disorder rather than a clinically defined syndrome.

Patients usually complain of burning or tingling pain in the distribution of the affected nerve(s). On examination, weakness and sensory loss are evident as well. Rare patients have purely sensory symptoms and signs.[9] Muscle stretch reflexes may be normal or diminished, depending on whether or not the involved nerve innervating is in a reflex arc. For example, involvement of the sciatic nerve would lead to a diminished ankle jerk, but a median nerve infarct would not result in a loss of a biceps or triceps reflex.

▶ LABORATORY FINDINGS

Most patients have elevated erythrocyte sedimentation rate (ESR) or C-reactive protein (CRP).[2,10] Some vasculitides are associated with ANCAs, antinuclear antibodies (ANAs), cryoglobulins, rheumatoid factor, leukocytosis, and anemia. ANCAs are of particular importance as they are 85% sensitive and 99% specific for vasculitis.[11] The ANCAs are subclassified as cytoplasmic (cANCA) or perinuclear (pANCA) based on their immunofluorescence staining pattern and antigenic target; cANCAs are directed against proteinase 3 (PR3), while pANCAs target myeloperoxidase (MPO). PR3/cANCA is associated with granulomatosis with polyangiitis, while MPO/pANCA is typically associated with MPA, CSS, and less commonly PAN. MPO/pANCA has also been seen in minocycline-induced vasculitis.

Affected nerves may appear enlarged and hypoechoic with ultrasound.[12–14] MR imaging may also be useful to identify nerve lesions.[15,16] Motor and sensory nerve conduction studies demonstrate unobtainable potentials or reduced amplitudes.[3,7,8,17–20] In particular, it is important to look for side-to-side asymmetries in amplitudes that reflect the multifocal nature of the pathology. Distal latencies are normal or slightly prolonged, while conduction velocities are normal or only mildly reduced. Conduction block or pseudoconduction block may be demonstrated in some affected nerves.[21–24] The presence of conduction block or temporal dispersion in a patient with a multifocal neuropathy pattern should suggest a disorder such as the multifocal acquired demyelinating sensory and motor (MADSAM) neuropathy variant of chronic inflammatory demyelinating polyneuropathy (CIDP). The needle electromyography (EMG) reveals denervation changes in affected muscle groups. Again, the EMG abnormalities are often also asymmetric.

▶ HISTOPATHOLOGY

The sural, superficial peroneal (sensory branch), and superficial radial sensory nerves are the most common nerves

▶ TABLE 15-1. VASCULITIDES ASSOCIATED WITH PERIPHERAL NEUROPATHY

- Primary Vasculitis
  - Large vessel vasculitis
    - Giant cell (temporal) arteritis
  - Medium and small vessel vasculitis
    - Polyarteritis nodosa
    - Churg–Strauss syndrome
    - Granulomatosis with angiitis
    - Microscopic polyangiitis
    - Nonsystemic vasculitic neuropathy
- Secondary Vasculitis
  - Vasculitis associated with connective tissue diseases
  - Vasculitis associated with Behçet disease
  - Vasculitis associated with sarcoidosis
  - Vasculitis associated with malignancies
  - Vasculitis associated with infections
  - Vasculitis associated with cryoglobulinemia
  - Vasculitis associated with hypersensitivity reaction (leukocytoclastic angiitis)—uncommonly associated with a peripheral neuropathy

that are biopsied.[1,4,5,25] Suspected vasculitis is one of the few clinical situations in which we routinely perform nerve biopsy. We usually biopsy the superficial peroneal nerve, if it is involved clinically and by nerve conduction studies (NCS). This is because the peroneus brevis muscle can also be biopsied from the same incision site, and the diagnostic yield is increased when the nerve and muscle both are biopsied (Fig. 15-2).[5,25–27] Diagnostic criteria for pathologically definite vasculitis include transmural inflammatory cell infiltration and fibrinoid necrosis of the vessel wall (Fig. 15-3).[1,4,7,19,28–31] Supportive features of acute vasculitis also include loss or fragmentation of internal elastic lamina and loss/fragmentation/separation of smooth muscles in the media (can be highlighted by elastin and antismooth muscle actin staining), vascular or perivascular hemorrhage, acute thrombosis, and leukocytoclasia. Immunocytochemistry may reveal immunoglobulin (IgM and/or IgG), complement, and membrane attack complex deposition on blood vessels.[32] Signs of repair may be seen in chronic vasculitis and include intimal

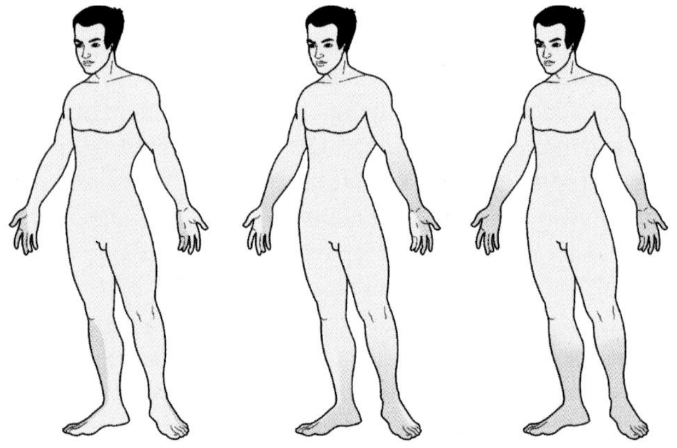

A True multiple mononeuropathy **B** Overlapping (extensive) multiple mononeuropathy **C** Distal symmetric polyneuropathy

Figure 15-1. Patterns of involvement in vasculitic neuropathy. Vasculitis can present as **(A)** a mononeuropathy or multiple mononeuropathies, **(B)** overlapping mononeuropathies, or **(C)** distal symmetric polyneuropathies.

▶ TABLE 15-2. MULTIFOCAL NEUROPATHIES/MULTIPLE MONONEUROPATHIES: DIFFERENTIAL DIAGNOSIS

- Peripheral Nerve Vasculitis
  - Polyarteritis nodosa
  - Granulomatosis with angiitis
  - Churg–Strauss syndrome
  - Microscopic polyangiitis
  - Connective tissue disorders associated with vasculitic neuropathies (e.g., SLE, RA, MCTD)
  - Nonsystemic vasculitic neuropathy
  - Remote effect of cancer
- Other Immune-Medicated Neuropathies
  - Multifocal acquired demyelinating sensory and motor neuropathy [MADSMN, asymmetric chronic inflammatory demyelinating polyradiculoneuropathy (CIDP)]
  - Multifocal motor neuropathy
  - Sensory perineuritis
  - Lumbosacral/brachial plexus neuritis
  - Postsurgical neuritis
- Granulomatous Infiltration
  - Sarcoid
  - Lymphomatoid granulomatosis
- Infectious Neuropathies
  - Leprosy
  - Herpes zoster
  - Lyme disease
  - HIV
  - CMV
  - Hepatitis B and C
- Compression Neuropathy
  - Primary compression neuropathies (e.g., traumatically induced)
  - Secondary compression neuropathies (e.g., superimposed on generalized peripheral nerve disease; e.g., diabetes mellitus and carpal/cubital tunnel syndrome)
  - Hereditary liability to pressure palsy
- Other Disorders
  - Diabetes mellitus
  - Amyloidosis
  - Neoplastic infiltration (particularly lymphoma and leukemia)
  - Peripheral nerve tumors (e.g., neurofibromatosis)
  - Atherosclerotic vascular disease (monomelic neuropathy secondary to acute large artery occlusion of AV shunts/fistulas)
  - Drug induced (e.g., interferon-α, leukotriene receptor antagonist, tumor necrosis factor-α inhibitors, leflunomide, amphetamine, sulfonamides)

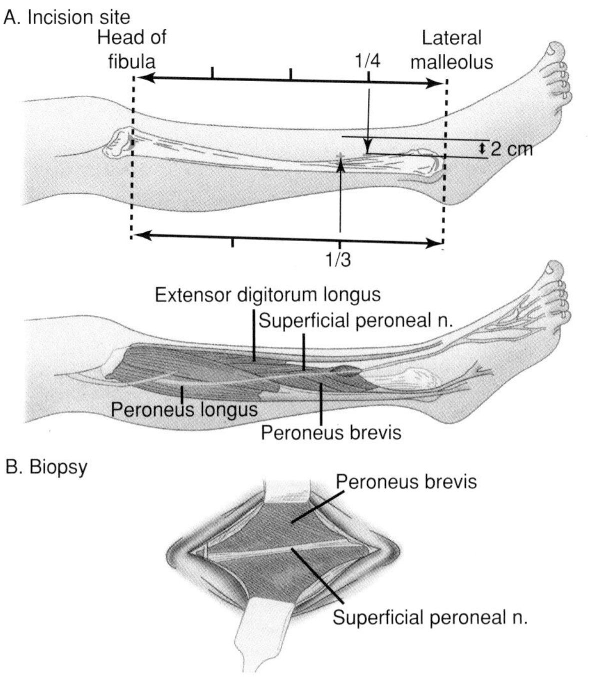

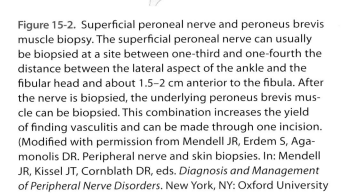

Figure 15-2. Superficial peroneal nerve and peroneus brevis muscle biopsy. The superficial peroneal nerve can usually be biopsied at a site between one-third and one-fourth the distance between the lateral aspect of the ankle and the fibular head and about 1.5–2 cm anterior to the fibula. After the nerve is biopsied, the underlying peroneus brevis muscle can be biopsied. This combination increases the yield of finding vasculitis and can be made through one incision. (Modified with permission from Mendell JR, Erdem S, Agamonolis DR. Peripheral nerve and skin biopsies. In: Mendell JR, Kissel JT, Cornblath DR, eds. *Diagnosis and Management of Peripheral Nerve Disorders*. New York, NY: Oxford University Press; 2001.)

hyperplasia, fibrosis of media, adventitial/periadventitial fibrosis, and recanalization of the lumen. Common findings are asymmetrical nerve fiber loss between and within individual nerve fascicles and active axonal degeneration. Nerve biopsies can also demonstrate immunostaining for the receptor for advanced glycosylation end products, nuclear factor-kappaB, and interleukin-6 that are expressed by CD4(+), CD8(+), and CD68(+) cells invading nerves. Immunostaining can be identified in mononuclear cells, epineurial and endoneurial vessels, and in the perineurium.[33] This data suggest that the receptor for advanced glycosylation end products pathway plays a critical proinflammatory role in vasculitic neuropathy. Matrix metalloproteinases (e.g., MMP-9) are upregulated as well and may play an important role as means for inflammatory cell invasion.[34] In addition to vasculitis, muscle biopsies may show evidence of muscle infarction (Fig. 15-4). Skin biopsies have also demonstrated reduced epidermal nerve fiber density in some cases of vasculitic neuropathy.[26,35,36]

▶ PRIMARY SYSTEMIC VASCULITIC DISORDERS AFFECTING LARGE- AND MEDIUM-SIZED VESSELS

GIANT CELL VASCULITIS

Temporal arteritis and Takayasu arteritis are the two forms of giant cell arteritis, but peripheral neuropathy only occurs in the setting of temporal arteritis.[10,37] Giant cell arteritis affects medium- and large-sized vessels, particularly the aortic arch and the internal and external carotid arteries, and the vertebral arteries. Patients may present with headaches, jaw and tongue claudication, generalized myalgias, vision loss secondary to ischemic optic neuropathy, or stroke. Approximately 14% of patients develop multifocal neuropathy/multiple mononeuropathies, radiculopathies, plexopathies, or a generalized sensorimotor peripheral neuropathy.[10] The temporal artery is often tender and a palpable cord can be felt. Ultrasound of the arteries may reveal thickening. Temporal artery biopsies reveal inflammatory infiltrate with giant cells in only two-thirds of suspected cases. Patients generally respond quite well to treatment with corticosteroids.

▶ PRIMARY SYSTEMIC VASCULITIC DISORDERS AFFECTING MEDIUM- AND SMALL-SIZED VESSELS

POLYARTERITIS NODOSA

PAN, the most common of the necrotizing vasculitides, is a systemic disorder involving small- and medium-caliber arteries in multiple organs.[1,2,4,11,28] PAN has an incidence ranging from 2 to 9 per million and usually presents between 40 and 60 years of age. The most common pattern of nerve involvement is multifocal neuropathy/multiple mononeuropathies. The sciatic nerve or its peroneal or tibial branches are the most frequently involved nerves. Cranial neuropathies and central nervous system (CNS) involvement are rare, occurring in <2% of patients.[2] Other organ systems affected include the heart, liver, kidneys, gastrointestinal that may lead to liver or renal failure, abdominal pain, and gastrointestinal bleeding. Notably, the lungs are generally spared. Myalgias and arthralgias occur in 30–70% of patients. Vasculitis involving the skin results in petechiae, livedo reticularis, subcutaneous nodules, and distal gangrene.[38] Orchitis is also a common complication. Constitutional symptoms include weight loss, fever, and loss of appetite.

Although not as commonly found as in MPA and CSS, approximately 10–20% of PAN patients have MPO/pANCA. An elevated ESR is seen in the majority of patients.[2] One-third of cases are associated with hepatitis B antigenemia,[2,38] but PAN can also complicate hepatitis C virus (HCV) and human immunodeficiency virus (HIV) infections.[2,39] Abdominal

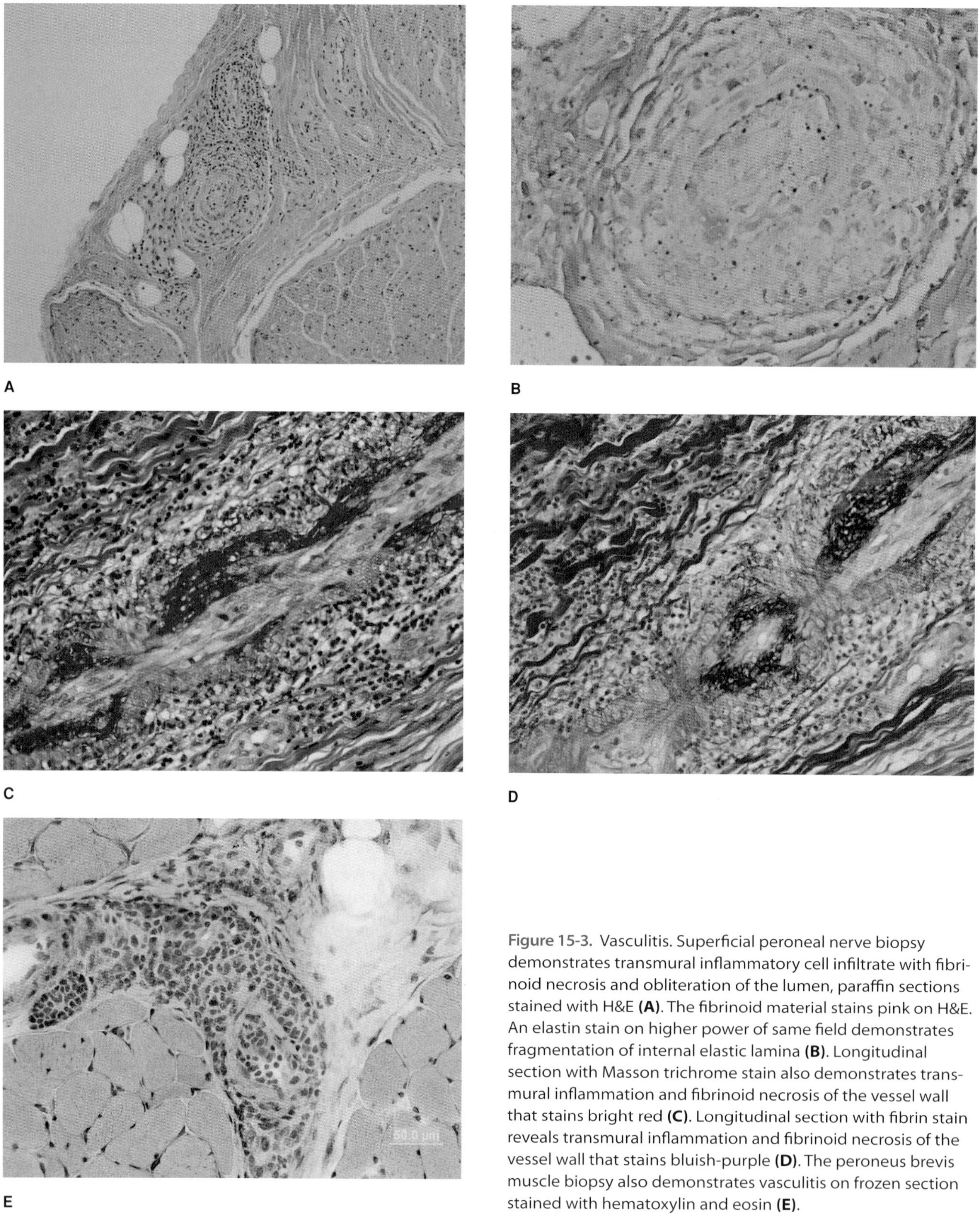

Figure 15-3. Vasculitis. Superficial peroneal nerve biopsy demonstrates transmural inflammatory cell infiltrate with fibrinoid necrosis and obliteration of the lumen, paraffin sections stained with H&E **(A)**. The fibrinoid material stains pink on H&E. An elastin stain on higher power of same field demonstrates fragmentation of internal elastic lamina **(B)**. Longitudinal section with Masson trichrome stain also demonstrates transmural inflammation and fibrinoid necrosis of the vessel wall that stains bright red **(C)**. Longitudinal section with fibrin stain reveals transmural inflammation and fibrinoid necrosis of the vessel wall that stains bluish-purple **(D)**. The peroneus brevis muscle biopsy also demonstrates vasculitis on frozen section stained with hematoxylin and eosin **(E)**.

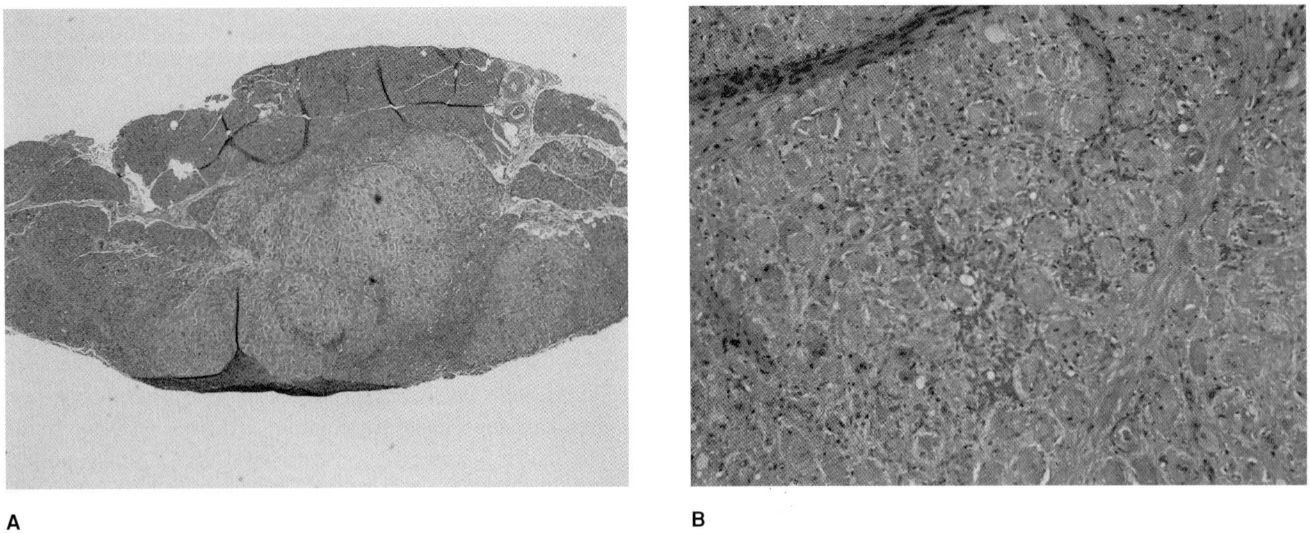

Figure 15-4. Muscle biopsy demonstrates an area of muscle infarct and some hemorrhagic conversion at low **(A)** and high power **(B)** paraffin sections stained with H&E.

angiograms can reveal a vasculitic aneurysm, a useful finding in patients with nondiagnostic biopsies.

Medium-sized arteries are usually affected; however, smaller-sized vessels can be involved in PAN.[2,4] Nerve biopsies may demonstrate transmural infiltration of CD8+ T cells, macrophages, and polymorphonuclear cells along with fibrinoid necrosis of the vessel wall. IgM, IgG, complement, and membrane attack complex deposition may be appreciated on blood vessels. Unlike CSS, granulomas and eosinophilic infiltration are not seen on nerve biopsies in PAN. The pathogenic mechanism of PAN is unknown, although a T cell–dependent process with secondary complement-mediated vascular damage has been postulated.[4]

CHURG-STRAUSS SYNDROME (ALLERGIC ANGIITIS/GRANULOMATOSIS)

CSS manifests with signs and symptoms similar to PAN except that respiratory involvement is common in CSS.[1,2,40–44] The incidence of CSS is about one-third that of PAN, but the frequency of neurological complications is about the same. In this regard, multifocal neuropathy/multiple mononeuropathies develop in as many as 75% of individuals who are affected.[2] People with CSS typically present with allergic rhinitis, nasal polyposis, sinusitis, and late-onset asthma (after the age of 35 years). Symptoms and signs of systemic vasculitis occur an average of 3 years after the onset of asthma and even longer after the onset of nasal symptoms. Anywhere from 16% to 49% of patients with CSS develop a necrotizing glomerulonephritis as opposed to an ischemic nephropathy that can complicate PAN. Several cases of CSS have been reported in patients treated with leukotriene antagonists after weaning corticosteroids.[45]

Routine laboratory workup reveals eosinophilia, leukocytosis, elevated ESR, CRP, rheumatoid factor, and serum IgG and IgE levels. One should consider CSS in any patient with a neuropathy and peripheral eosinophilia. Approximately two-thirds of individuals who are affected have MPO/pANCA.[2,11] Chest x-rays reveal that pulmonary infiltrates are present in nearly half of patients.

Nerve biopsies may demonstrate necrotizing vasculitis with CD8+ cytotoxic T lymphocytes, CD4+ cells and, to a lesser extent, eosinophilic infiltrates (Fig. 15-5).[2,42,46] In addition, intravascular and extravascular granulomas are occasionally found in and around affected blood vessels.

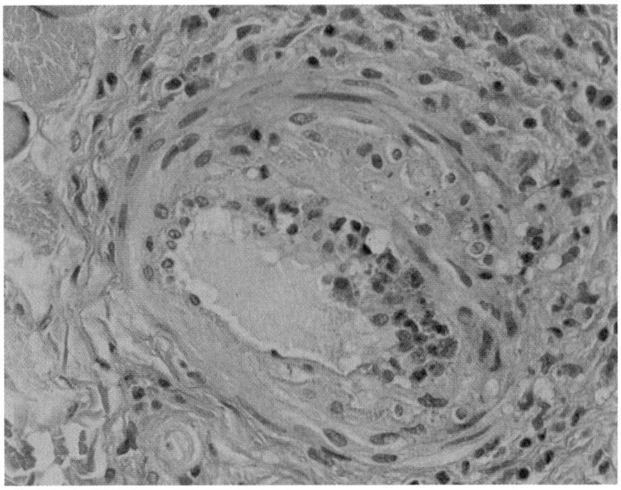

Figure 15-5. Churg–Strauss syndrome. Nerve biopsy demonstrates transmural infiltration of a vessel wall that includes eosinophils and obliteration of the lumen. Paraffin section stained with H&E.

GRANULOMATOSIS WITH POLYANGIITIS

Granulomatosis with polyangiitis (GAN) was formerly referred to as Wegener granulomatosis. The latter term is no longer recommended as Dr. Wegener was a high-ranking Nazi physician, and the facility he was assigned to in Poland was associated with unethical humane experimentation. GAN is characterized by necrotizing vasculitis and granulomas involving the upper and lower respiratory tract and kidneys (glomerulonephritis).[1,4,47–54] Early respiratory symptoms (e.g., nasal discharge, cough, hemoptysis, and dyspnea) can help distinguish this from other vasculitides. In a large prospective study of 128 patients with granulomatosis with polyangiitis, 64 patients (50%) developed CNS or PNS involvement.[47] Peripheral neuropathy occurred in 56 patients and in 9 cases the CNS was involved. Thirty-one patients had a distal symmetric polyneuropathy, while 25 had multifocal neuropathy/multiple mononeuropathies. Neuropathy is more common in patients with severe renal involvement.[51] Cranial neuropathies, particularly the second, sixth, and seventh nerves, develop in approximately 5–10% of cases as a result of extension of the nasal or paranasal granulomas rather than vasculitis.[47,53]

The majority of affected individuals have PR3/cANCAs, and this test has a specificity of 98% and sensitivity of 95%.[51] The histological appearance of the vasculitis is similar to PAN, with involvement of medium- and small-sized blood vessels. In addition, granulomatous infiltration of the respiratory tract and necrotizing glomerulonephritis are also seen. The absence of peripheral eosinophilia, eosinophilic infiltrates on biopsy, and asthma help distinguish granulomatosis with polyangiitis from CSS.

MICROSCOPIC POLYANGIITIS

MPA clinically resembles PAN and CSS, except that diffuse alveolar damage and interstitial fibrosis develop due to involvement of pulmonary capillaries.[1,2,4,42,43,55] The incidence of MPA is about one-third that of PAN. The average age of onset is 50 years and polyneuropathy complicates MPA in 14–36% of cases.[2,4,55]

Laboratory evaluation is remarkable for renal insufficiency, hematuria, and MPO/pANCA in most patients. PR3/cANCA can also occasionally be detected. As suggested by the name, MPA affects small arterioles, veins, and capillaries.[2,4] In contrast to PAN, there are few or no immune deposits on the blood vessels. Kidney biopsies reveal focal segmental thrombosis and necrotizing glomerulonephritis.

BEHÇET SYNDROME

This disorder is characterized by recurrent oral and genital ulcerations, inflammation of the eye, arthritis, thrombophlebitis, skin lesions, and vasculitic lesions of these organs involving the small- to medium-sized arteries.[56–59] The CNS complications (brainstem strokes, meningoencephalitis, and psychosis) are more common than peripheral neuropathy.

▶ SECONDARY SYSTEMIC VASCULITIDES

VASCULITIS ASSOCIATED WITH CONNECTIVE TISSUE DISEASE

Neuropathies are not uncommon in people with connective tissue diseases, although necrotizing vasculitis as the cause is infrequent (see Chapter 16). That said, secondary vasculitis can complicate rheumatoid arthritis, systemic lupus erythematosus and Sjögren syndrome, and, less frequently, systemic sclerosis.[18,60,61] The clinical, histological, and electrophysiological features are similar to PAN. In addition, vasculitis may be seen in sarcoidosis (see Chapter 16).

INFECTION-RELATED VASCULITIS

Vasculitic neuropathy can arise as a complication of a variety of infections.[39,62,63] The most common infectious agents associated with vasculitic neuropathy are HIV, hepatitis B and C, cytomegalovirus, Epstein–Barr viruses, and herpes varicella zoster (discussed in Chapter 17). Multifocal neuropathy/multiple mononeuropathies related to HIV or cytomegalovirus infection occur in up to 3% of patients with acquired immune deficiency syndrome (AIDS).[64] As previously discussed, hepatitis B and C infections are associated with PAN, a medium-sized systemic vasculitis, as well as a small vessel vasculitis associated with cryoglobulinemia. Vasculitic neuropathy may also complicate Lyme disease.

MALIGNANCY-RELATED VASCULITIS

Rarely, cancers have been associated with vasculitic neuropathy. Small cell lung cancer and lymphoma are the most common implicated malignancies, but leukemia, other myelodysplastic syndromes, and carcinomas of the kidneys, bile duct, prostate, and stomach have also been described.[65–74] However, most of the reported cases were not associated with a necrotizing vasculitis, rather only nonspecific transmural or perivascular inflammation of small blood vessels without fibrinoid necrosis was seen on biopsy. In this regard, several of the cases with "vasculitic" neuropathy associated with lung cancer and anti-Hu antibodies were reported as having vasculitis, although this disorder is not a true necrotizing vasculitis (see Chapter 19).[65] Multiple mononeuropathies or generalized neuropathy associated with lymphomas are often paraneoplastic in etiology or due to lymphomatous infiltration of the nerves. However, rare cases of vasculitic neuropathy have been reported in the setting of lymphoma.[72]

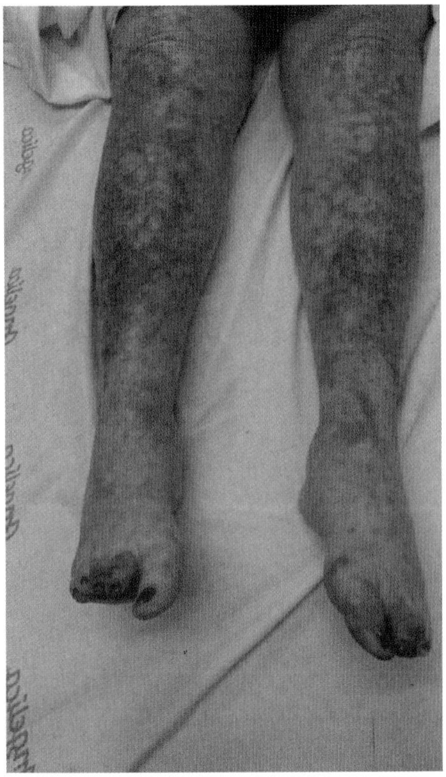

Figure 15-6. Hypersensitivity vasculitis. Severe petechial lesions are evident on bilateral lower extremities.

DRUG-INDUCED HYPERSENSITIVITY VASCULITIS

Hypersensitivity vasculitis is often secondary to drug reactions and is a self-limited process as opposed to the systemic necrotizing vasculitides.[4] Skin manifestations (e.g., petechiae) predominate the clinical picture of hypersensitivity vasculitis and neuropathy is uncommon (Fig. 15-6). Minocycline may be an exception as we and others have seen typical vasculitic neuropathy as a complication.[16,75,76] Drugs of abuse (e.g., amphetamine, cocaine, and opioids) also can cause vasculitis of the CNS or PNS.[77,78] The pathogenesis most likely relates to a complement-mediated leukocytoclastic reaction.

VASCULITIS SECONDARY TO ESSENTIAL MIXED CRYOGLOBULINEMIA

Cryoglobulins are circulating immune complexes consisting of immunoglobulins directed against polyclonal immunoglobulins. These complexes precipitate out of solution when exposed to a cool temperature but dissolve back into solution when rewarmed, thus the name cryoglobulin. There are actually three types of cryoglobulins. Type I cryoglobulins are monoclonal immunoglobulins, usually IgM, directed against polyclonal IgG. These are most commonly seen in individuals with plasma cell dyscrasias. Type II cryoglobulins are composed of a combination of monoclonal IgM and polyclonal immunoglobulins directed against polyclonal IgG. Type III cryoglobulins are a mixture of polyclonal IgM, IgG, and IgA directed against polyclonal IgG. Type II and III cryoglobulins are seen in patients with so-called mixed cryoglobulinemia and typically occur in the setting of lymphoproliferative disorders, connective tissue diseases, HIV, and hepatitis B and hepatitis C infection. Most patients with mixed cryoglobulinemia are associated with hepatitis C antigenemia. *Essential* mixed cryoglobulinemia is the term used when mixed cryoglobulinemia is found in the absence of an underlying disease. Peripheral neuropathy develops in 25–90% of patients with cryoglobulinemia of any type.[21,79–86] The neuropathy may manifest as a painful, distal, symmetric sensory or sensorimotor polyneuropathy; as multifocal/multiple mononeuropathies; or rarely as a pure small fiber neuropathy.[21]

The lack of local HCV replication in nerve biopsies suggests that that HCV-mixed cryoglobulinemia-associated neuropathy results from virus-triggered immune-mediated mechanisms rather than direct nerve infection and in situ replication.[84,87] The neuropathy may arise due to ischemia from hyperviscosity or due to vasculitis related to immune complex deposition in small epineurial blood vessels. NCS are similar to PAN. Conduction block was appreciated on motor NCS in one report.[21]

NONSYSTEMIC OR ISOLATED PNS VASCULITIS

Nearly 60% of vasculitis is restricted to peripheral nerves.[1,3,6,7,25,30,88–91] This so-called nonsystemic vasculitis or isolated PNS vasculitis is usually seen in adults, but children can also be affected.[6] The clinical, electrophysiological, and histopathological features of isolated PNS vasculitis are quite similar to PAN, except that there is no significant involvement of other organ systems. Individuals who are affected may present with multiple mononeuropathies or a generalized symmetric sensorimotor polyneuropathy. Laboratory testing may demonstrate elevated ESR or positive ANA titers. Vasculitis may be apparent on muscle biopsies,[5] but the peripheral nerves are predominantly affected. The diagnostic yield of finding vasculitis is increased by biopsying both muscle and nerve.

The vasculitis typically involves small- and medium-sized arteries of the epineurium and perineurium, and immune complex deposition on these blood vessels may be appreciated on biopsy. MMPs, in particular MMP-2 and MMP-9 (gelatinase A and B), are upregulated in the peripheral nerves in patients with nonsystemic vasculitis.[92] T cells are the predominant source of MMP-2 and MMP-9, although stromal cells of the perineurium and endoneurium may also secrete MMP. These enzymes digest the subendothelial basement membrane and thus facilitate inflammatory cells to penetrate the blood–nerve barrier.

The prognosis for isolated PNS vasculitis is much better than that for systemic vasculitic disorders. Although some patients may be managed with corticosteroids alone, the combination of corticosteroid and cyclophosphamide has been reported to more likely result in remission and improves disability.[25]

POSTSURGICAL INFLAMMATORY NEUROPATHY

Most neuropathies that occur following surgery are felt to be due to stretching or compression of nerves. However, a recent study has suggested that some of these neuropathies may be secondary to inflammation. In a study of 23 patients who developed neuropathies following a surgical procedure, 12 had no history of direct trauma to a nearby nerve and were suspected of having an autoimmune neuritis.[93] A total of 21 patients had abnormal nerve biopsies that showed increased epineurial perivascular lymphocytic inflammation (9 small, 5 moderate, and 7 large), with 15 having findings suggestive of microvasculitis. Some of these patients apparently improved upon treatment with immunotherapy, but we do not know if the natural history might be gradual improvement. This entity seems similar to idiopathic brachial plexus and lumbosacral radiculoplexus neuropathy—some of which may occur after surgeries. Fibrinoid necrosis of vessel walls is not typical, but there is transmural or perivascular inflammation.

TREATMENT OF VASCULITIC NEUROPATHY

There is a lack of randomized therapeutic trials of corticosteroids and other immunosuppressive agent therapies in vasculitic neuropathy.[1,11,30] Nonetheless, the mainstay of initial treatment of systemic vasculitis has been the combination of corticosteroids and cyclophosphamide.[2,4,11,43,94–96] Since the use of corticosteroids to treat systemic vasculitis began in the 1950s, the 5-year survival rate increased from 10% to 55% by the mid-to-late 1970s.[2] The addition of cyclophosphamide to corticosteroids further increased the 5-year survival rate to more than 80%.[2,97] We tend to be aggressive in our treatment approach because treatment failure in a disease such as PAN may be lead to a catastrophic event, such as a bowel or myocardial infarction. Hypersensitivity vasculitis and sometimes isolated PNS vasculitis may be treated with only prednisone. However, a large retrospective series suggested that the combination of corticosteroids and cyclophosphamide was more effective than corticosteroids alone as mentioned previously.[25] There is less experience with other immunotherapies in the treatment of vasculitis. Methotrexate (0.15–0.3 mg/kg per week) in combination with corticosteroids can be effective in GAN.[54,98] Azathioprine, cyclosporine, tacrolimus, chlorambucil, and intravenous immunoglobulin have been tried in refractory cases with variable success.[95,96,109–111] More recently, rituximab has gained popularity as it appears effective in ANCA-associated vasculitis and cryoglobulinemia. The current recommended treatment strategy is dependent on the type of vasculitis.

Treatment of ANCA-Associated Vasculitis (MPA, CSS, and GAN)

As mentioned, treatment of ANCA-associated vasculitis has been induction with corticosteroids and cyclophosphamide and then replacing cyclophosphamide with another second-line agent after 3–6 months as outlined in the previous section. However, there have been several reports suggesting rituximab may be beneficial[11,99–106] and two randomized clinical trials[107,108] showing that the combination of rituximab and corticosteroids is not inferior to cyclophosphamide and corticosteroids. Thus, the combination of corticosteroids (e.g., prednisone 1.0–1.5 mg/kg daily) and rituximab is increasingly recommended as the standard initial treatment of choice. Rituximab is typically given at a dosage of 375 mg per meter-squared weekly for 4 weeks.

Treatment of Vasculitis Associated with HCV-Mixed Cryoglobulinemia

Treatment of mixed cryoglobulinemia requires removal of the antigen. In patients with mixed cryoglobulinemia due to hepatitis C infection treatment with α-interferon appears to be effective.[11,13,66,83,112–121] Combination of α-interferon and ribavirin also has yield positive results though no randomized, controlled trials have been performed.[122–124] Use of high-dose corticosteroids and cyclophosphamide may allow the virus to persist and replicate, thus increasing the risk of liver failure. Methotrexate is avoided due to the risk of direct hepatotoxicity.

A short course of corticosteroids has been used to control the initial manifestations of the systemic vasculitis followed by plasma exchange and α-interferon.

Recently, there have been several reports suggesting rituximab may be beneficial in cryoglobulinemic vasculitis.[125–135] Two randomized, open-label studies comparing rituximab to standard treatment with immunosuppressive agents demonstrated a greater response rate with rituximab.[136,137] Two studies compared treatment with rituximab and antivirals (Peg-interferon-alpha/riboflavin) to antiviral alone and, again, the rituximab-treated patients seemed to do better.[138,139] On this basis, we usually initiate treatment with plasma exchange followed by the combination of rituximab and antiviral therapy.

Treatment of Non-ANCA Vasculitis (PAN and Isolated PNS Vasculitis)

We typically treat with oral prednisone 1.5 mg/kg per day (up to 100 mg per day) as a single dose in the morning in addition to cyclophosphamide. After 2–4 weeks, we switch from daily to alternate-day prednisone (i.e., 100 mg every other day). However, if a patient is diabetic, we treat with daily corticosteroids (e.g., prednisone 50 mg daily) so as not to have wide fluctuations in blood glucose. In patients with severe vasculitis, we may initiate treatment with a pulse of intravenous methylprednisolone (1 g intravenously every day for 3 days), then switch to oral corticosteroids. Patients are concurrently started on calcium and vitamin D supplementation and sometimes on a bisphosphonate to prevent and treat steroid-induced osteoporosis.

In addition, oral or intravenous cyclophosphamide is started. Oral cyclophosphamide at a dose of 1.0–2.0 mg/kg is a more potent suppressor of the immune system but is associated with more adverse side effects (e.g., hemorrhagic cystitis) than intravenous doses. Thus, we usually treat patients with monthly intravenous pulses of cyclophosphamide at a dose of 500–1,000 mg/m^2 of body surface area. Hydration is essential to minimize bladder toxicity. We also often premedicate patients with sodium 2-mercaptoethane sulfonate to reduce the incidence of bladder toxicity and with antiemetics to diminish nausea. Following intravenous pulses of cyclophosphamide, the leukocyte count drops. The nadir of the leukopenia occurs between 7 and 18 days, during which time the risk of infection is greatest. We check complete blood counts and urinalysis prior to each treatment. Urinalysis is obtained every 3–6 months after treatment because of the risk of future bladder cancer.

If patients do not respond to pulsed cyclophosphamide, oral dosing should be tried before concluding that the patient failed cyclophosphamide treatment. High-dose corticosteroids and cyclophosphamide are continued until the patient begins to improve or at least the deficit stabilizes. This usually occurs within 3–6 months. Subsequently, we discontinue cyclophosphamide and start methotrexate (7.5 mg per week). The methotrexate dose is gradually increased as necessary. At the same time, we begin to taper the prednisone by 5 mg every 2–3 weeks. In our experience, the disease may "burn itself out" and immunomodulating drugs may be successfully weaned after a year or more resulting in a prolonged drug-free remission in some cases.

Extrapolating to ANCA-associated vasculitis, rituximab might be beneficial in isolated PNS vasculitis, but we just do not have literature to support its use at this time. However, we certainly would use it in patients refractory to prednisone and cyclophosphamide and perhaps prior to cyclophosphamide use. In patients with hepatitis B–associated vasculitis, we usually treat with antiviral medications, plasma exchange, and a short course of corticosteroids. IVIG and rituximab have been used but the literature is scant; we also worry about increasing viral load with immunosuppressive agents and rituxan use.

▶ SUMMARY

There are a number of causes of systemic vasculitis that can affect peripheral nerves, and many times the vasculitis may be isolated to the peripheral nerves. Individuals who are affected may manifest with mononeuropathy, multifocal neuropathy/multiple mononeuropathies, and overlapping mononeuropathies, or even as a generalized symmetric sensorimotor polyneuropathy. It is important to take a detailed medical history for disorders that may be associated with vasculitis (e.g., connective tissue diseases, viral hepatitis, and late-onset asthma). Useful laboratory tests include assessment for eosinophilia, ANAs, MPO/pANCA, PR3/cANCA, ESR, CRP, rheumatoid factor, cryoglobulins, hepatitis serology, and urinalysis. We like to have histological confirmation of vasculitis before initiating what can turn out to be long-term immunosuppressive therapy. The diagnostic yield of a combined superficial peroneal nerve and peroneus brevis muscle biopsy, when clinically affected, is high. Most patients improve with immunotherapy.

REFERENCES

1. Burns TM, Schaublin GA, Dyck PJ. Vasculitic neuropathies. *Neurol Clin.* 2007;25:89–113.
2. Guillevin L, Lhote F, Gherardi R. Polyarteritis nodosa, microscopic polyangiitis, and Churg–Strauss syndrome: Clinical aspects, neurologic manifestations, and treatment. *Neurol Clin.* 1997;15:865–886.
3. Hawke SH, Davies L, Pamphlet R, Guo YP, Pollard JD, McLeod JG. Vasculitic neuropathy. *Brain.* 1991;114:2175–2190.
4. Kissel JT, Mendell JR. Vasculitic neuropathy. *Neurol Clin.* 1992;10:761–781.
5. Said G, Lacroix-Ciaudo C, Fujimura H, Blas C, Faux N. The peripheral neuropathy of necrotizing arteritis: A clinicopathological study. *Ann Neurol.* 1988;23:461–465.
6. Ryan MM, Tilton A, De Girolami U, Darras BT, Jones HR Jr. Paediatric mononeuritis multiplex: A report of three cases and review of the literature. *Neuromuscul Disord.* 2003;13(9):751–756.
7. Kissel JT, Slivka AP, Warmolts JR, Mendell JR. The clinical spectrum of necrotizing angiopathy of the peripheral nervous system. *Ann Neurol.* 1985;18:251–257.
8. Amato AA, Dumitru D. Acquired neuropathies. In: Dumitru D, Amato AA, Swartz MJ, eds. *Electrodiagnostic Medicine*. 2nd ed. Philadelphia, PA: Hanley & Belfus; 2002: 937–1041.
9. Seo JH, Ryan HF, Claussen GC, Thomas TD, Oh SJ. Sensory neuropathy in vasculitis. A clinical, pathologic, and electrophysiologic study. *Neurology.* 2004;63:874–878.
10. Caselli RJ, Daube JR, Hunder GG, Whisnant JP. Peripheral neuropathic syndromes in giant cell (temporal) arteritis. *Neurology.* 1988;38:685–689.
11. Collins MP. The vasculitic neuropathies: An update. *Curr Opin Neurol.* 2012;25:573–585.
12. Ito T, Kijima M, Watanabe T, Sakuta M, Nishiyama K. Ultrasonography of the tibial nerve in vasculitic neuropathy. *Muscle Nerve.* 2007;35:379–382.
13. Schmidt WA, Seifert A, Gromnica-Ihle E, Krause A, Natusch A. Ultrasound of proximal upper extremity arteries to increase the diagnostic yield in large-vessel giant cell arteritis. *Rheumatology (Oxford).* 2008;47:96–101.
14. Nodera H, Sato K, Terasawa Y, Takamatsu N, Kaji R. High-resolution sonography detects inflammatory changes in vasculitic neuropathy. *Muscle Nerve.* 2006;34:380–381.

15. Sanada M, Terada M, Suzuki E, Kashiwagi A, Yasuda H. MR angiography for the evaluation of non-systemic vasculitic neuropathy. *Acta Radiol.* 2003;44:316–318.
16. Thaisetthawatkul P, Sundell R, Robertson CE, Dyck PJ. Vasculitic neuropathy associated with minocycline use. *J Clin Neuromuscul Dis.* 2011;12:231–234.
17. Bouche P, Léger JM, Travers MA, Cathala HP, Castaigne P. Peripheral neuropathy in systemic vasculitis: Clinical and electrophysiologic study of 22 patients. *Neurology.* 1986;36:1598–1602.
18. Hietaharju A, Jaaskelainen S, Kalimo H, Hietarinta M. Peripheral neuromuscular manifestations in systemic sclerosis (scleroderma). *Muscle Nerve.* 1993;16:1204–1212.
19. Wees SJ, Sunwoo IN, Oh SJ. Sural nerve biopsy in systemic vasculitis. *Am J Med.* 1981;71:525–532.
20. Zivkovic SA, Ascherman D, Lacomis D. Vasculitic neuropathy: Electrodiagnostic findings and association with malignancies. *Acta Neurol Scand.* 2007;115(6):432–436.
21. Lippa CF, Chad DA, Smith TW, Kaplan MH, Hammer K. Neuropathy associated with cryoglobulinemia. *Muscle Nerve.* 1986;9:626–631.
22. McCluskey L, Feinberg D, Cantor C, Bird S. "Pseudo-conduction block" in vasculitic neuropathy. *Muscle Nerve.* 1999;22:1361–1366.
23. Mohamed A, Davies L, Pollard JD. Conduction block in vasculitic neuropathy. *Muscle Nerve.* 1988;21:1084–1088.
24. Ropert A, Metral S. Conduction block in neuropathies with necrotizing vasculitis. *Muscle Nerve.* 1990;13:102–105.
25. Collins MP, Periquet MI, Mendell JR, Sahenk Z, Nagaraja HN, Kissel JT. Nonsystemic vasculitic neuropathy: Insights from a clinical cohort. *Neurology.* 2003;61(5):623–630.
26. Agadi JB, Raghav G, Mahadevan A, Shankar SK. Usefulness of superficial peroneal nerve/peroneus brevis muscle biopsy in the diagnosis of vasculitic neuropathy. *J Clin Neurosci.* 2012;19:1392–1396.
27. Vrancken AF, Gathier CS, Cats EA, Notermans NC, Collins MP. The additional yield of combined nerve/muscle biopsy in vasculitic neuropathy. *Eur J Neurol.* 2011;18:49–58.
28. Kissel JT, Levy RJ, Mendell JR, Griggs RC. Azathioprine toxicity in neuromuscular disease. *Neurology.* 1986;36: 35–39.
29. Kissel JT, Riethman JL, Omerza J, Rammohan KW, Mendell JR. Peripheral nerve vasculitis: Immune characterization of the vascular lesions. *Ann Neurol.* 1989;25:291–297.
30. Panegyres PK, Blumbergs PC, Leong AS, Bourne AJ. Vasculitis of peripheral nerve and skeletal muscle: Clinicopathological correlation and immunopathic mechanism. *J Neurol Sci.* 1990;100:193–202.
31. Collins MP, Dyck PJ, Gronseth GS, et al. Peripheral Nerve Society Guideline on the classification, diagnosis, investigation, and immunosuppressive therapy of non-systemic vasculitic neuropathy: Executive summary. *J Peripher Nerv Syst.* 2010;15:176–184.
32. Collins MP, Periquet-Collins I, Sahenk Z, Kissel JT. Direct immunofluoresence in vasculitic neuropathy: Specificity of vascular immune deposits. *Muscle Nerve.* 2010;42:62–69.
33. Haslbeck KM, Bierhaus A, Erwin S, et al. Receptor for advanced glycation end product (RAGE)-mediated nuclear factor-kappaB activation in vasculitic neuropathy. *Muscle Nerve.* 2004;29(6):853–860.
34. Renaud S, Erne B, Fuhr P, et al. Matrix metalloproteinases-9 and -2 in secondary vasculitic neuropathies. *Acta Neuropathol.* 2003;105(1):37–42.
35. Chao CC, Hsieh ST, Shun CT, Hsieh SC. Skin denervation and cutaneous vasculitis in eosinophilia-associated neuropathy. *Arch Neurol.* 2007;64(7):959–965.
36. Uçeyler N, Devigili G, Toyka KV, Sommer C. Skin biopsy as an additional diagnostic tool in non-systemic vasculitic neuropathy. *Acta Neuropathol.* 2010;120:109–116.
37. Koorey DJ. Cranial arteritis: A twenty year review of cases. *Aust N Z J Med.* 1984;14:143–147.
38. Guillevin L, Lhote F, Jarrousse B, Fain O. Treatment of polyarteritis nodosa and Churg–Strauss syndrome. A meta-analysis of 3 prospective controlled trials including 182 patients over 12 years. *Ann Med Interne (Paris).* 1992;143:405–416.
39. Cacoub P, Maisonobe T, Thibault V, et al. Systemic vasculitis in patients with hepatitis C. *J Rheumatol.* 2001;28(1):109–118.
40. Chumbley LC, Harrison EG Jr, DeRemee RA. Allergic granulomatosis and angiitis (Churg–Strauss syndrome): Report and analysis of 30 cases. *Mayo Clin Proc.* 1977;52:477–484.
41. Cooper BJ, Bacal E, Patterson R. Allergic angiitis and granulomatosis. *Arch Intern Med.* 1978;138:367–371.
42. Hattori N, Ichimura M, Nagamatsu M, et al. Clinicopathological features of Churg–Strauss syndrome-associated neuropathy. *Brain.* 1999;122:427–439.
43. Hattori N, Mori K, Misu K, Koike H, Ichimura M, Sobue G. Mortality and morbidity in peripheral neuropathy associated Churg–Strauss syndrome and microscopic polyangiitis. *J Rheumatol.* 2002;29(7):1408–1414.
44. Oh SJ, Herrera GA, Spalding DM. Eosinophilic vasculitis neuropathy in the Churg–Strauss syndrome. *Arthritis Rheum.* 1986;29:1173–1175.
45. Boccagni C, Tesser F, Mittino D, et al. Churg–Strauss syndrome associated with the leukotriene antagonist montelukast. *Neurol Sci.* 2004;25(1):21–22.
46. Nagashima T, Cao B, Takeuchi N, et al. Clinicopathological studies of peripheral neuropathy in Churg–Strauss syndrome. *Neuropathology.* 2002;22(4):299–307.
47. de Groot K, Schmidt DK, Arlt AC, Gross WL, Reinhold-Keller E. Standardized neurologic evaluations of 128 patients with Wegener granulomatosis. *Arch Neurol.* 2001;58(8):1215–1221.
48. Drachman DA. Neurological complications of Wegener's granulomatosis. *Arch Neurol.* 1963;8:145–155.
49. Fauci AS, Haynes BF, Katz P, Wolff SM. Wegener's granulomatosis: Prospective clinical and therapeutic experience with 85 patients for 21 years. *Ann Intern Med.* 1983;98:76–85.
50. Hoffman GS, Kerr GS, Leavitt RY, et al. Wegener granulomatosis: An analysis of 158 patients. *Ann Intern Med.* 1992;116: 488–498.
51. Jaffe IA. Wegener's granulomatosis and ANCA syndromes. *Neurol Clin.* 1997;15:887–891.
52. Jimenez-Mendez HJ, Yablon SA. Electrodiagnostic characteristics of Wegener's granulomatosis-associated peripheral neuropathy. *Am J Phys Med Rehabil.* 1992;71:6–11.
53. Nishino H, Rubino FA, DeRemmee RA, Swanson JW, Parisi JE. Neurological involvement in Wegener's granulomatosis: An analysis of 324 consecutive patients at the Mayo Clinic. *Ann Neurol.* 1993;33:4–9.
54. Stern GM, Hoffbrand AV, Urich H. The peripheral nerves and skeletal muscle in Wegener's granulomatosis: A clinicopathological study of four cases. *Brain.* 1965;88:151–164.
55. Savage CO, Winearls CG, Evans DJ, Rees AJ, Lockwood CM. Microscopic polyarteritis: Presentation, pathology and prognosis. *Q J Med.* 1985;56:467–483.

56. Frayha RA, Afifi AK, Bergman RA, Nader S, Bahuth NB. Neurogenic muscular atrophy in Behçet's disease. *Clin Rheumatol.* 1985;4:202–211.
57. Namer IJ, Karabudak R, Zileh T, Ruacan S, Küçükali T, Kansu E. Peripheral nervous system involvement in Behçet's disease. *Eur Neurol.* 1987;26:235–240.
58. Takeuchi A, Kodama M, Takatsu M, Hashimoto T, Miyashita H. Mononeuritis multiplex in incomplete Behçet's disease: A case report and the review of the literature. *Clin Rheumatol.* 1989;8:375–380.
59. Wakayama T, Takayaniagi T, Iida M, et al. A nerve biopsy study in two cases of neuro-Behçet's syndrome. *Clin Neurol (Tokyo).* 1975;14:519–525.
60. Mawrin C, Brunn A, Rocken C, Schroder JM. Peripheral neuropathy in systemic lupus erythematosus: Pathomorphological features and distribution pattern of matrix metalloproteinases. *Acta Neuropathol.* 2003;105(4):365–372.
61. Rosenbaum R. Neuromuscular complications of connective tissue diseases. *Muscle Nerve.* 2001;24(2):154–169.
62. Gerber O, Roque C, Colye PK. Vasculitis owing to infection. *Neurol Clin.* 1997;15:903–925.
63. Kanai K, Kuwabara S, Mori M, Arai K, Yamamoto T, Hattori T. Leukocytoclastic-vasculitic neuropathy associated with chronic Epstein–Barr virus infection. *Muscle Nerve.* 2003;27(1):113–116.
64. Brannagan TH. Retroviral-associated vasculitis of the nervous system. *Neurology.* 1997;15:927–944.
65. Amato AA, Collins MP. Neuropathies associated with malignancy. *Semin Neurol.* 1998;18:125–144.
66. Naarendorp M, Kallemuchikkal U, Nuovo GJ, Gorevic PD. Longterm efficacy of interferon-alpha for extrahepatic disease associated with hepatitis C virus infection. *J Rheumatol.* 2001;28(11):2466–2473.
67. Oh SJ, Slaughter R, Harrell L. Paraneoplastic vasculitic neuropathy: A treatable neuropathy. *Muscle Nerve.* 1991;14:152–156.
68. Saif MW, Hopkins JL, Gore SD. Autoimmune phenomena in patients with myelodysplastic syndromes and chronic myelomonocytic leukemia. *Leuk Lymphoma.* 2002;43(11):2083–2092.
69. Sanche-Guerrero J, Guterre-Urena S, Vidaller A, Reyes E, Iglesias A, Alarcón-Segovia D. Vasculitis as a paraneoplastic syndrome. Report of 11 cases and review of the literature. *J Rheumatol.* 1990;17:1458–1462.
70. Torvik A, Berntzen AE. Necrotizing vasculitis without visceral involvement. Post-mortem examination of three cases with effecting of skeletal muscles and peripheral nerves. *Acta Med Scand.* 1968;184:69–77.
71. Turner MR, Warren JD, Jacobs JM, et al. Microvasculitic paraproteinaemic polyneuropathy and B-cell lymphoma. *J Peripher Nerv Syst.* 2003;8(2):100–107.
72. Vincent D, Dubas F, Haue JJ, et al. Nerve and muscle microvasculitis in peripheral neuropathy: A remote effect of cancer. *J Neurol Neurosurg Psychiatry.* 1986;49:1007–1010.
73. Younger DS, Dalmau J, Inghirami G, Sherman WH, Hays AP. Anti-Hu-associated peripheral nerve and muscle vasculitis. *Neurology.* 1994;44:181–183.
74. Fain O, Hamidou M, Cacoub P, et al. Vasculitides associated with malignancies: Analysis of sixty patients. *Arthritis Rheum.* 2007;57:1473–1480.
75. Ogawa N, Kawai H, Yamakawa I, Sanada M, Sugimoto T, Maeda K. Case of minocycline-induced vasculitic neuropathy. *Rinsho Shinkeigaku.* 2010;50:301–305.
76. Kermani TA, Ham EK, Camilleri MJ, Warrington KJ. Polyarteritis nodosa-like vasculitis in association with minocycline use: A single-center case series. *Semin Arthritis Rheum.* 2012;42:213–221.
77. Brust JCM. Vasculitis owing to substance abuse. *Neurol Clin.* 1997;15:945–957.
78. Stafford CR, Bogdanoff BM, Green L, Spector HB. Mononeuropathy multiplex as a complication of amphetamine angiitis. *Neurology.* 1975;25:570.
79. Cavaletti G, Petruccioli MG, Crespi V, Pioltelli P, Marmiroli P, Tredici G. A clinico-pathological and follow-up study of 10 cases of essential type II cryoglobulinemic neuropathy. *J Neurol Neurosurg Psychiatry.* 1990;53:886–889.
80. David WS, Peine C, Schlesinger P, Smith SA. Nonsystemic vasculitic mononeuropathy multiplex, cryoglobulinemia, and hepatitis C. *Muscle Nerve.* 1996;19:1596–1602.
81. Ferri C, La Civita L, Cirafisi C, et al. Peripheral neuropathy in mixed cryoglobulinemia: Clinical and electrophysiologic investigations. *J Rheumatol.* 1992;19:889–895.
82. Gemignani F, Pavesi G, Fiocchi A, Manganelli P, Ferraccioli G, Marbini A. Peripheral neuropathy in essential mixed cryoglobulinemia. *J Neurol Neurosurg Psychiatry.* 1992;55:116–120.
83. Khella SL, Frost S, Hermann GA, et al. Hepatitis C infection, cryoglobulinemia, and vasculitis neuropathy. Treatment with interferon alpha: Case report and literature review. *Neurology.* 1995;45:407–411.
84. Nemni R, Corbo M, Fazio R, Quattrini A, Comi G, Canal N. Cryoglobulinemic neuropathy. *Brain.* 1988;111:541–552.
85. Thomas FP, Lovelace RE, Ding Z-S, et al. Vasculitic neuropathy in patient with cryoglobulinemia and anti-MAG IgM monoclonal gammopathy. *Muscle Nerve.* 1992;15:891–898.
86. Valli G, De Vecchi A, Gaddi L, Nobile-Orazio E, Tarantino A, Barbieri S. Peripheral nervous system involvement in essential cryoglobulinemia and nephropathy. *Clin Exp Rheumatol.* 1989;7:479–483.
87. Authier FJ, Bassez G, Payan C, et al. Detection of genomic viral RNA in nerve and muscle of patients with HCV neuropathy. *Neurology.* 2003;60(5):808–812.
88. Davies L, Spies JM, Pollard JD, McLeod JG. Vasculitis confined to peripheral nerves. *Brain.* 1996;119:1441–1448.
89. Dyck PJ, Benstead TJ, Conn DL, et al. Nonsystemic vasculitic neuropathy. *Brain.* 1987;110:843–854.
90. Nicholai A, Bonetti B, Lazzarino LG, Ferrari S, Monaco S, Rizzuto N. Peripheral nerve vasculitis: A clinicopathological study. *Clin Neuropathol.* 1995;14:137–141.
91. Said G. Necrotizing peripheral nerve vasculitis. *Neurol Clin.* 1997;15:835–848.
92. Leppert D, Hughes P, Hiber S, et al. Matrix metalloproteinase upregulation in chronic inflammatory demyelinating polyneuropathy and nonsystemic vasculitic neuropathy. *Neurology.* 1999;53:62–70.
93. Staff NP, Engelstad J, Klein CJ, et al. Post-surgical inflammatory neuropathy. *Brain.* 2010;133:2866–2880.
94. Vrancken AF, Hughes RA, Said G, Wokke JH, Notermans NC. Immunosuppressive treatment for non-systemic vasculitic neuropathy. *Cochrane Database Syst Rev.* 2007;(1):CD006050.
95. Callabrese LH. Therapy of systemic vasculitis. *Neurol Clin.* 1997;15:973–991.
96. Donofrio PD. Immunotherapy of idiopathic inflammatory neuropathies. *Muscle Nerve.* 2003;28:273–292.

97. Mathew L, Talbot K, Love S, Puvanarajah S, Donaghy M. Treatment of vasculitic peripheral neuropathy: A retrospective analysis of outcome. *QJM*. 2007;100(1):41–51.
98. Langford CA, Talar-Williams C, Barron KS, Sneller MC. Use of a cyclophosphamide-induction methotrexate-maintenance regimen for the treatment of Wegener's granulomatosis: Extended follow-up and rate of relapse. *Am J Med*. 2003;114(6):463–469.
99. Jones RB, Ferraro AJ, Chaudhry AN, et al. A multicenter survey of rituximab therapy for refractory antineutrophil cytoplasmic antibody-associated vasculitis. *Arthritis Rheum*. 2009;60:2156–2168.
100. Holle JU, Dubrau C, Herlyn K, et al. Rituximab for refractory granulomatosis with polyangiitis (Wegener's granulomatosis): Comparison of efficacy in granulomatous versus vasculitic manifestations. *Ann Rheum Dis*. 2012;71:327–333.
101. Eriksson P. Nine patients with antineutrophil cytoplasmic antibody-positive vasculitis successfully treated with rituximab. *J Intern Med*. 2005;257:540–548.
102. Brihaye B, Aouba A, Pagnoux C, Cohen P, Lacassin F, Guillevin L. Adjunction of rituximab to steroids and immunosuppressants for refractory/relapsing Wegener's granulomatosis: A study on 8 patients. *Clin Exp Rheumatol*. 2007;25(1 suppl 44):S23–S27.
103. Ramos-Casals M, Garcia-Hernandez FJ, de Ramon E, et al. Off-label use of rituximab in 196 patients with severe, refractory systemic autoimmune diseases. *Clin Exp Rheumatol*. 2010;28:468–476.
104. de Menthon M, Cohen P, Pagnoux C, et al. Infliximab or rituximab for refractory Wegener's granulomatosis: Long-term follow up. A prospective randomised multicentre study on 17 patients. *Clin Exp Rheumatol*. 2011;29(1 suppl 64):S63–S71.
105. Rees F, Yazdani R, Lanyon P. Long-term follow-up of different refractory systemic vasculitides treated with rituximab. *Clin Rheumatol*. 2011;30:1241–1245.
106. Roccatello D, Sciascia S, Rossi D, et al. Long-term effects of rituximab added to cyclophosphamide in refractory patients with vasculitis. *Am J Nephrol*. 2011;34:175–180.
107. Jones RB, Tervaert JW, Hauser T, et al. Rituximab versus cyclophosphamide in ANCA-associated renal vasculitis. *N Engl J Med*. 2010;363:211–220.
108. Stone JH, Merkel PA, Spiera R, et al. Rituximab versus cyclophosphamide for ANCA-associated vasculitis. *N Engl J Med*. 2010;363:221–232.
109. Levy Y, Uziel Y, Zandman GG, et al. Intravenous immunoglobulins in peripheral neuropathy associated with vasculitis. *Ann Rheum Dis*. 2003;62(12):1221–1223.
110. Richter C, Schanbel E, Csernok E, et al. Treatment of ANCA-associated vasculitis with high-dose intravenous immunoglobulin. *Arthritis Rheum*. 1994;37:S353.
111. Guillevin L, Lhote F, Cohen P, et al. Polyarteritis nodosa related to hepatitis B virus. A prospective study with long-term observation of 41 patients. *Medicine (Baltimore)*. 1995;74:238–253.
112. Balart LA, Perillo R, Roddenberry J, et al. Hepatitis C RNA in liver of chronic hepatitis C patients before and after interferon alpha treatment. *Gastroenterology*. 1993;104:1472–1477.
113. Casato M, Lagana B, Antonelli G, Dianzani F, Bonomo L. Long-term results of therapy with interferon-alpha for type II essential mixed cryoglobulinemia. *Blood*. 1991;78:3142–3147.
114. Davis GL, Balart LA, Schiff ER, et al. Treatment of chronic hepatitis C with recombinant interferon alpha. A multicenter randomized controlled trial. *N Engl J Med*. 1989;321:1501–1506.
115. DiBisceglie AM, Martin P, Kassianides CK, et al. Recombinant interferon alpha therapy for chronic hepatitis C. A randomized, double-blind, placebo controlled trial. *N Engl J Med*. 1989;321:1501–1506.
116. Durand JM, Kaplanski G, Lefevre P, et al. Effect of interferon-α 2b on cryoglobulinemia related to hepatitis C virus infection [letter]. *J Infect Dis*. 1992;165:778–779.
117. Ghini M, Mascia MT, Gentilini M, Mussini C. Treatment of cryoglobulinemic neuropathy with α-interferon [letter]. *Neurology*. 1996;46:588–589.
118. Ferri C, Marzo E, Longombardo G, et al. Interferon-alpha in mixed cryoglobulinemia patients: A randomized, crossover-controlled trial. *Blood*. 1993;81:1132–1136.
119. Dammacco F, Sansonno D, Han JH, et al. Natural interferon-alpha versus its combination with 6-methyl-prednisolone in the therapy of type II mixed cryoglobulinemia: A long-term, randomized, controlled study. *Blood*. 1994;84:3336–3343.
120. Misiani R, Bellavita P, Fenili D, et al. Interferon alfa-2 a therapy in cryoglobulinemia associated with hepatitis C virus. *N Engl J Med*. 1994;330:751–756.
121. Lauta VM, De Sangro MA. Long-term results regarding the use of recombinant interferon alpha-2b in the treatment of II type mixed essential cryoglobulinemia. *Med Oncol*. 1995;12:223–230.
122. Saadoun D, Resche-Rigon M, Thibault V, Piette JC, Cacoub P. Antiviral therapy for hepatitis C virus-associated mixed cryoglobulinemia vasculitis: A long-term follow-up study. *Arthritis Rheum*. 2006;54:3696–3706.
123. Mazzaro C, Monti G, Saccardo F, et al. Efficacy and safety of peginterferon alfa-2b plus ribavirin for HCV-positive mixed cryoglobulinemia: A multicentre open-label study. *Clin Exp Rheumatol*. 2011;29:933–941.
124. El Khayat HR, Fouad YM, El Amin H, Rizk A. A randomized trial of 24 versus 48 weeks of peginterferon alpha-2a plus ribavirin in Egyptian patients with hepatitis C virus genotype 4 and rapid viral response. *Trop Gastroenterol*. 2012;33:112–117.
125. Lamprecht P, Lerin-Lozano C, Merz H, et al. Rituximab induces remission in refractory HCV associated cryoglobulinaemic vasculitis. *Ann Rheum Dis*. 2003;62(12):1230–1233.
126. Zaja F, De Vita S, Mazzaro C, et al. Efficacy and safety of rituximab in type II mixed cryoglobulinemia. *Blood*. 2003;101(10):3827–3834.
127. Ramos-Casals M, Stone JH, Cid MC, Bosch X. The cryoglobulinaemias. *Lancet*. 2012;379:348–360.
128. Saadoun D, Delluc A, Piette JC, Cacoub P. Treatment of hepatitis C-associated mixed cryoglobulinemia vasculitis. *Curr Opin Rheumatol*. 2008;20:23–28.
129. Pietrogrande M, De Vita S, Zignego AL, et al. Recommendations for the management of mixed cryoglobulinemia syndrome in hepatitis C virus-infected patients. *Autoimmun Rev*. 2011;10:444–454.
130. Ferri C, Cacoub P, Mazzaro C, et al. Treatment with rituximab in patients with mixed cryoglobulinemia syndrome: Results of multicenter cohort study and review of the literature. *Autoimmun Rev*. 2011;11:48–55.
131. Sansonno D, De Re V, Lauletta G, Tucci FA, Boiocchi M, Dammacco F. Monoclonal antibody treatment of mixed cryoglobulinemia resistant to interferon alpha with an anti-CD20. *Blood*. 2003;101:3818–3826.
132. Zaja F, De Vita S, Mazzaro C, et al. Efficacy and safety of rituximab in type II mixed cryoglobulinemia. *Blood*. 2003;101:3827–3834.

133. Saadoun D, Resche-Rigon M, Sene D, Perard L, Karras A, Cacoub P. Rituximab combined with Peg-interferon-ribavirin in refractory hepatitis C virus-associated cryoglobulinaemia vasculitis. *Ann Rheum Dis.* 2008;67:1431–1436.
134. Petrarca A, Rigacci L, Caini P, et al. Safety and efficacy of rituximab in patients with hepatitis C virus-related mixed cryoglobulinemia and severe liver disease. *Blood.* 2010;116:335–342.
135. Visentini M, Ludovisi S, Petrarca A, et al. A phase II, single-arm multicenter study of low-dose rituximab for refractory mixed cryoglobulinemia secondary to hepatitis C virus infection. *Autoimmun Rev.* 2011;10:714–719.
136. De Vita S, Quartuccio L, Isola M, et al. A randomized controlled trial of rituximab for the treatment of severe cryoglobulinemic vasculitis. *Arthritis Rheum.* 2012;64:843–853.
137. Sneller MC, Hu Z, Langford CA. A randomized controlled trial of rituximab following failure of antiviral therapy for hepatitis C virus-associated cryoglobulinemic vasculitis. *Arthritis Rheum.* 2012;64:835–842.
138. Dammacco F, Tucci FA, Lauletta G, et al. Pegylated interferon-alpha, ribavirin, and rituximab combined therapy of hepatitis C virus-related mixed cryoglobulinemia: A long-term study. *Blood.* 2010;116:343–353.
139. Saadoun D, Resche Rigon M, Sene D, et al. Rituximab plus Peg-interferon-alpha/ribavirin compared with Peg-interferon-alpha/ribavirin in hepatitis C-related mixed cryoglobulinemia. *Blood.* 2010;116:326–334.

CHAPTER 16

Neuropathies Associated with Systemic Disease

Neuropathies are associated with a number of systemic disorders (Table 16-1). Neuropathies related to vasculitis, infection, endocrinopathies, cancer, and medications are discussed in other chapters. The neuropathies discussed in this chapter may be directly or indirectly related to the systemic disorder (e.g., nutritional deficiency due to malabsorption in gastrointestinal disease).

▶ NEUROPATHIES ASSOCIATED WITH CONNECTIVE TISSUE DISEASES

SJÖGREN SYNDROME

Clinical Features

Sjögren syndrome is characterized by the sicca complex: xerophthalmia (dry eyes), xerostomia (dry mouth), and dryness of other mucous membranes. It is more common in women and typically presents in middle adult life. Sjögren syndrome can be complicated by central nervous system (CNS) and peripheral nervous system (PNS) involvement. The CNS manifestations can mimic transverse myelitis or multiple sclerosis. Peripheral neuropathy occurs in 2–22% of patients with Sjögren syndrome.[1–13] Furthermore, peripheral neuropathy can be the presenting feature of Sjögren syndrome and develop in patients without the typical sicca symptoms.

The most common form of peripheral neuropathy is a length-dependent axonal sensorimotor neuropathy characterized by numbness and tingling in the distal portions of the limbs.[1,2,6,7,9–11] Mild distal muscle weakness may also be seen. A pure small fiber neuropathy characterized by burning discomfort and tingling is also common.[14,15] Signs of autonomic nervous system dysfunction involving the cardiovascular system are often evident.[16,17] Necrotizing vasculitis may be responsible for as many as one-third of the cases of neuropathy associated with Sjögren syndrome.[8] Vasculitis should be suspected in patients with an asymmetric, multiple mononeuropathy pattern of involvement. Cranial neuropathies, particularly involving the trigeminal nerve, can also be seen.[18]

Sjögren syndrome is also associated with sensory neuronopathy/ganglionopathy.[1–3,7,10,19–21] Patients with sensory ganglionopathies develop progressive numbness and tingling of the limbs, trunk, and face. Although the symptoms may seem length-dependent, a careful history and examination typically uncovers a non–length-dependent pattern. Symptoms can involve the arms more than the legs, and involvement can be quite asymmetric or even unilateral. Patches of numbness may occur in unusual locations like the perioral regions, back of the head, or the trunk. The onset can be acute or insidious. Sensory examination demonstrates severe vibratory and proprioceptive loss leading to sensory ataxia. Romberg sign is noted in patients with lower limb involvement. The lack of proprioception may lead to pseudoathetotic posturing of affected arms and legs. There can also be diminished sensation in the face. Signs of autonomic neuropathy also may be appreciated: Adie pupil, anhidrosis, fixed tachycardia, and orthostatic hypotension. Muscle stretch reflexes are often reduced or absent. Muscle strength is usually normal.

Laboratory Features

Patients with neuropathy due to Sjögren syndrome may have antinuclear antibodies (ANA), SS-A/Ro, and SS-B/La antibodies in the serum, but many do not.[7] Cerebrospinal fluid is usually normal. Schirmer test and Rose-Bengal stain are useful for diagnosing keratoconjunctivitis. The diagnosis can be confirmed by parotid gland or lip biopsies demonstrating a lymphocytic invasion of salivary glands. Salivary gland biopsies can demonstrate histopathological features of Sjögren syndrome even in patients without complaints of dry mouth.[7]

Nerve conduction studies (NCS) in patients with distal sensorimotor polyneuropathy demonstrate absent or reduced amplitudes of sensory nerve action potentials (SNAPs) with normal or only mildly slow conduction velocities.[1,2,6,12] Motor conduction studies are less affected but may show slightly reduced amplitudes. Abnormal blink reflexes and cutaneous masseter inhibitory reflexes may be appreciated in patients with trigeminal neuropathy.[18]

NCS in patients with sensory neuronopathy/ganglionopathy demonstrate absent or reduced amplitudes of the SNAPs in a non–length-dependent manner such that these may be

TABLE 16-1. NEUROPATHIES ASSOCIATED WITH SYSTEMIC DISORDERS

Connective tissue disease
Sjögren syndrome or sicca complex
Rheumatoid arthritis
Systemic lupus erythematosus
Scleroderma
Mixed connective tissue disease
Sarcoidosis
Celiac disease
Inflammatory bowel disease
Ulcerative colitis
Crohn disease
Hypereosinophilic syndrome
Uremia
Primary biliary sclerosis
Liver disease
Whipple disease
Gout
Critical illness polyneuropathy
Amyloidosis
Acquired
Familial
Vasculitis
Isolated peripheral nerve vasculitis
Vasculitis associated with systemic disease
Granulomatosis with angiitis
Polyarteritis nodosa
Churg–Strauss syndrome
Microscopic polyangiitis
Infection
HIV
HTLV1
CMV
EBV
Lyme
Syphilis
Cancer
Direct tumor infiltration of nerves
Paraneoplastic

abnormal in the arms while normal in the legs.[1–3,5,12,19–21] In addition, there may be asymmetric involvement. Motor conduction studies and electromyography (EMG) are usually normal. If the trigeminal nerve is affected, blink reflexes may also be abnormal.[22] An important clinical and electrophysiological feature that can help distinguish length-dependent sensory neuropathy from a sensory neuronopathy/ganglionopathy is the preservation of the masseter reflex or jaw jerk in the latter.[23] The masseter reflex is unique amongst the stretch reflexes in that the cell bodies of the afferent limb lie in the mesencephalic nucleus within the CNS as opposed to the dorsal root ganglia where the sensory cell bodies innervating the extremities lie. Thus, the mesencephalic nucleus is often spared in ganglionopathies and so the associated masseter reflex is preserved. In contrast, the Gasserian ganglion, which is responsible for conveying sensory nerves responsible for facial sensation and the blink reflex, reside outside the CNS, and thus the blink reflex may be abnormal.

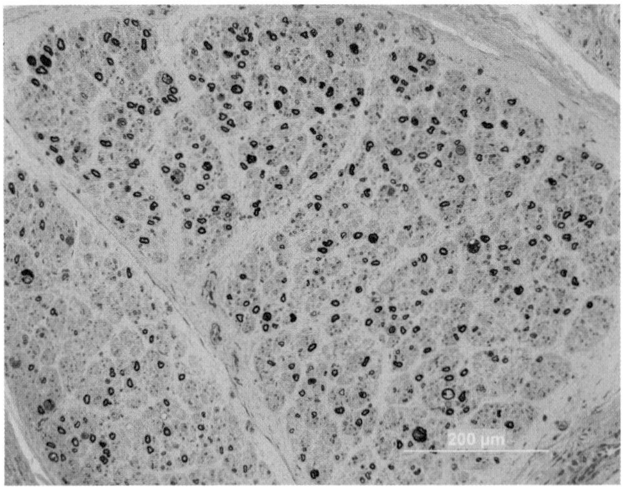

Figure 16-1. Sjögren syndrome. Sural nerve biopsy demonstrates a moderate reduction of large and small myelinated nerve fibers and evidence of axonal degeneration. Plastic section stained with toluidine blue.

Histopathology

Peripheral nerve biopsies in patients with the more common sensorimotor polyneuropathy demonstrate axonal degeneration and some degree of secondary segmental demyelination (Fig. 16-1).[1,2,6] Nonspecific perivascular inflammation involving perineurial or endoneurial blood vessels is occasionally seen. Rarely, necrotizing vasculitis is appreciated.

Biopsy of sensory nerves in patients with sensory neuronopathy/ganglionopathy may reveal a loss of large myelinated fibers and perivascular lymphocytic (CD8 T cells) inflammation involving endoneurial or perineurial vessels.[1–3] Biopsy of the dorsal root ganglion have shown lymphocytic (mainly CD8 T cells) infiltration and degeneration of cell bodies.[3]

Reduced epidermal nerve fiber density or abnormal morphology may be demonstrated on skin biopsies in a non–length-dependent manner, suggesting that patients with painful small fiber neuropathies commonly have a small fiber sensory neuronopathy/ganglionopathy rather than a "dying-back" axonopathy.[14]

Pathogenesis

The pathogenic basis of the distal sensory or sensorimotor polyneuropathy is unknown but is presumably autoimmune in nature. Some cases may caused by vasculitis. The sensory neuronopathy/ganglionopathy appears to be the result of cell-mediated autoimmune attack directed against the sensory ganglia. The specific antigen(s) and trigger of the autoimmune attack are not known.

Treatment

There are no proven therapies for the neuropathies related to Sjögren syndrome. When vasculitis is suspected, immunosuppressive agents may be beneficial. IVIG may be useful in nonvasculitic sensory and sensorimotor neuropathies, however the benefit of such therapy in sensory neuronopathy/ganglionopathy is much less clear.[3,11,19,24–26]

RHEUMATOID ARTHRITIS

Clinical Features

Peripheral neuropathy occurs in at least 50% of patients with rheumatoid arthritis (RA).[13,27–32] Vasculitic neuropathy develops in 40–50% of patients with RA, making it the third most common cause of vasculitic neuropathy following polyarteritis nodosa (PAN) and isolated peripheral nervous system vasculitis. Neuropathic symptoms usually manifest 10–15 years after manifestations of other symptoms of RA, although rarely the neuropathy can be the presenting feature. Rheumatoid vasculitis can present with multiple neuropathies or generalized symmetric pattern of involvement. In addition, the neuropathy associated with RA may be secondary to amyloid deposition.[27] Carpal tunnel syndrome is not uncommon, occurring in 10% of patients in one series.[27]

Demyelinating neuropathies (sensorimotor or pure sensory chronic inflammatory demyelinating polyneuropathy (CIDP), multifocal motor neuropathy) may develop as a complication of drugs used to treat the RA [e.g., antitumor necrosis factor-alpha (TNF-α) therapy and leflunomide].[33,34] These neuropathies may or may not improve after discontinuation of the TNF-α blocker. In cases in which the neuropathy does not get better, treatment with other immunotherapies (e.g., corticosteroids or IVIG) may be warranted.

Laboratory Features

ANA, elevated ESR, and rheumatoid factor are often detected in the serum. NCS in patients with vasculitic neuropathy demonstrate absent or reduced amplitudes of SNAPs and compound muscle action potentials (CMAPs), often in an asymmetric, non-length-dependent pattern with normal or only mildly slow conduction velocities. Those with neuropathy related to medications typically have features of demyelination.

Histopathology

Nerve biopsies often reveal thickening of the epineurial and endoneurial blood vessels as well as perivascular inflammation, perhaps related to the so-called microvasculitis (Fig. 16-2). Occasionally, there is necrotizing vasculitis with transmural inflammatory cell infiltration and fibrinoid necrosis of vessel walls. In a retrospective series of 108 patients with RA, 23 underwent sural nerve biopsies.[27] Abnormalities included perineurial thickening ($n = 5$), amyloid deposits ($n = 4$), perivascular infiltrate ($n = 4$), loss of myelin fibers ($n = 2$), and necrotizing vasculitis ($n = 1$).

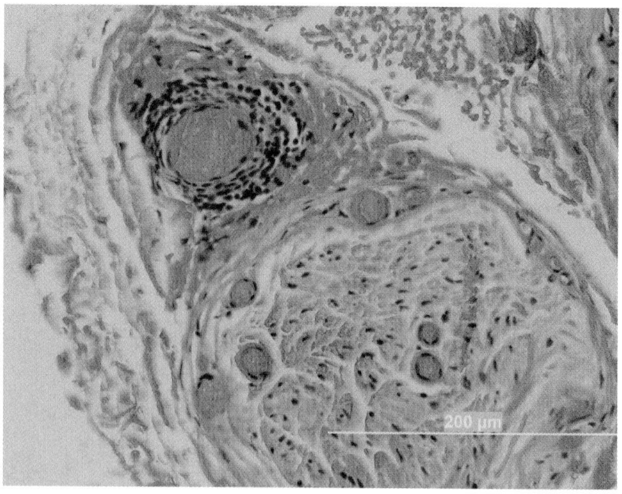

Figure 16-2. Rheumatoid arthritis. Sural nerve biopsy reveals an epineurial vessel with perivascular inflammation and scattered perineurial and endoneurial dilated capillaries with thickened walls. Paraffin section stained with Hematoxylin & Eosin (H&E).

Treatment

In most cases, the neuropathy is presumably autoimmune in nature and may respond to immunomodulating therapies. Of course, those with demyelinating polyneuropathy secondary to TNF-α blockage should first go off the medication. If the neuropathy does not improve they may need to be treated as well with IVIG or corticosteroids; they should also avoid treatment with other TNF-α blockers in the future.

SYSTEMIC LUPUS ERYTHEMATOSUS

Clinical Features

Systemic lupus erythematosus (SLE) is a common connective tissue disease with prevalence in adults of approximately 1 in 2,000. SLE can be associated with multiple organ system involvement and associated laboratory abnormalities. CNS complications are more common than peripheral neuropathies, although 2–27% of individuals with SLE clinically develop a peripheral neuropathy.[13,35–43] Most of the time the neuropathy manifests as slowly progressive sensory loss beginning in the feet. Some patients develop burning pain and paresthesia with normal reflexes and NCS suggestive of a pure small fiber neuropathy.[40,41]

Less common are mononeuropathies, cranial neuropathies, and multiple mononeuropathies. The longer the disease progresses, the more likely the multiple mononeuropathies are to fuse and overlap, creating an increasingly symmetric pattern that mimicks a length-dependent axonal sensorimotor polyneuropathy. Of 1,533 patients in a large SLE database, 207 (14%) had a peripheral neuropathy.[35] Of these, 40% were non–SLE-related. Polyneuropathy was diagnosed in 56%, multiple mononeuropathies in 9%, cranial neuropathy in 13%, and mononeuropathy in 11% of patients. Most presentations were asymmetric (59%) and distal weakness occurred in 34%. Rarely, patients manifest with generalized sensorimotor polyneuropathy meeting clinical, laboratory, electrophysiological, and histological criteria for either acute or chronic inflammatory demyelinating polyneuropathy (AIDP or CIDP).[44–46]

Laboratory Features

ANA, anti–double-stranded DNA, and anti-Ro antibodies may be demonstrated in the serum. Abnormal NCS occur in 24–56% of patients with SLE.[38,39] Most commonly, the NCS reveal a length-dependent, axonal sensory polyneuropathy.[47] However, as many as 20% of patients may have features of demyelination on NCS.[35,44–46]

Histopathology

Nerve biopsies may demonstrate endoneurial mononuclear inflammatory infiltrates and increased expression of class II antigens within nerve fascicles and on endothelial cells, suggesting an autoimmune pathogenesis.[37] Upregulation of matrix metalloproteinase-3 and matrix metalloproteinase-9 within the vessel walls has also been observed.[48] Skin biopsies may reveal decreased density of epidermal nerve fibers suggestive of a small fiber neuropathy.[40,41]

Pathogenesis

The pathogenic basis of the associated neuropathy is likely multifactorial. Neuropathy may be related to the underlying vasculopathy characteristic of SLE, which however is rare associated with histological evidence of necrotizing vasculitis. Some patients may develop neuropathy due to other systemic complications of SLE (i.e., renal failure and uremic neuropathy).

Treatment

Immunosuppressive therapy is beneficial in patients with vasculitic neuropathy. Immunosuppressive agents are less likely to be effective in patients with a generalized sensory or sensorimotor polyneuropathy without evidence of vasculitis. Patients with an AIDP- or CIDP-like neuropathy should be treated accordingly (see Chapters 13 and 14).

SYSTEMIC SCLEROSIS (SCLERODERMA)

Scleroderma is associated with progressive fibrosis of the skin, gastrointestinal tract, kidney, and lung.[13,49–53] A distal symmetric, mainly sensory, polyneuropathy complicates 5–67% of cases. Cranial mononeuropathies can also develop, most commonly affecting the trigeminal nerve, leading to numbness and dysesthesias in the face. Occasionally, seventh and ninth cranial neuropathies develop.

The CREST syndrome (calcinosis, Raynaud phenomenon, esophageal dysmotility, sclerodactyly, and telangiectasia) is considered a limited form of scleroderma. Multiple mononeuropathies have been described in a small percentage (1–2%) of patients with CREST syndrome.[54] The electrophysiological and histological features of nerve biopsies are those of an axonal sensory greater than motor polyneuropathy.

MIXED CONNECTIVE TISSUE DISEASE

Mixed connective tissue disease represents an overlap syndrome of SLE, scleroderma, and myositis. A mild distal axonal sensorimotor polyneuropathy reportedly occurs in approximately 10% of patients.[13,55] Trigeminal neuropathy is also a recognized complication of this syndrome.

▶ OTHER PRESUMABLY IMMUNE-MEDIATED NEUROPATHIES

SARCOIDOSIS

Clinical Features

Sarcoidosis, a systemic granulomatous disorder, can affect the CNS, peripheral nerves, and muscle.[56–59] The etiology is unknown. Women are more commonly affected than men. Nonspecific constitutional symptoms of fever, weight loss, arthralgias, and fatigue are usually the presenting complaints of most patients. Erythematous subcutaneous nodules about the anterior shin and enlarged peripheral lymph nodes may be noted. Granulomatous uveitis can lead to significant visual impairment and even blindness. Pulmonary involvement as well as mucosal lesions of the nose and sinuses are common.

The peripheral nervous system or CNS is involved in about 5% of patients with sarcoidosis and may be the presenting manifestation.[56–59] In the CNS, granulomas most typically involve the meninges, hypothalamus, and pituitary gland. Cranial nerves are also frequently involved. The most common cranial nerve to be involved is the seventh nerve, which can be affected bilaterally. Any cranial nerve may be affected however, particularly the second and eighth. Often the neuropathy is relapsing and remitting in nature. Some patients develop a radiculopathy or a polyradiculopathy. With a generalized root involvement, the clinical presentation can

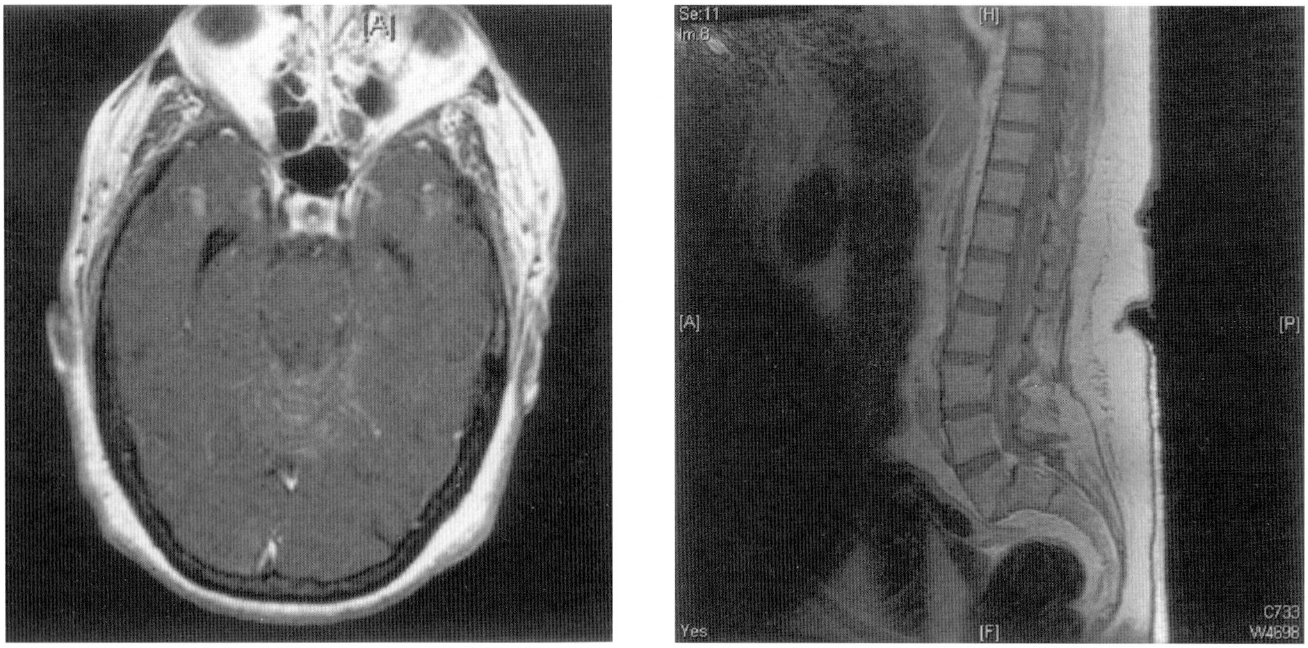

A B

Figure 16-3. Sarcoidosis. MRI scan of the brain with contrast demonstrates enhancement of the meninges around the cerebellum **(A)** and of the cauda equina **(B)** in a patient who presented with multiple cranial neuropathies and a polyradiculopathy.

mimic AIDP or CIDP. Rarely, patients may present with an acute sensory ataxia with sphincter dysfunction.[60] Patients can also present with mononeuropathies, multiple mononeuropathies, or a generalized, slowly progressive, primarily sensory greater than motor polyneuropathy.[61,62] Some have features of a pure small fiber neuropathy or a non–length-dependent neuronopathy/ganglionopathy pattern.[61–66]

Laboratory Features

Hilar adenopathy is often but not always appreciated on chest radiographs. MRI scans may demonstrate enhancement of the meninges in the brain, particularly in the posterior fossa, and of affected spinal roots in patients with radiculopathy (Fig. 16-3).[61] PET and gallium scans can also demonstrate abnormalities. CSF may reveal pleocytosis and an elevated white blood cell count.[61] Angiotensin converting enzyme (ACE) levels may be elevated in those with lung disease, but it is neither a very sensitive test nor a specific test. In patients with subclinical neuropathy, the most common finding is an absence or reduction in SNAP amplitudes in a mononeuropathy multiplex pattern.[59,67] In patients with the symmetric sensorimotor peripheral neuropathy, the SNAPs may be absent or reduced in amplitude.[59,68] Motor NCS also reveal reduced or absent CMAP amplitudes in the lower limbs, with decreased or borderline normal CMAPs in the upper limbs. Patients may also show EMG changes suggestive of a radiculopathy or polyradiculopathy.[57] Quantitative sensory testing often reveals abnormal thermal thresholds, and autonomic testing may be abnormal indicative of small fiber involvement.[64,66]

Histopathology

Nerve biopsies can reveal noncaseating granulomas infiltrating the endoneurium, perineurium, and epineurium along with lymphocytic necrotizing angiitis (Fig. 16-4).[59,62,69] There is a combination of axonal loss as well as demyelination. Muscle biopsies likewise can demonstrate noncaseating granulomas in the endomysium even in patients without an underlying myopathy.[59] Skin biopsies may reveal reduced

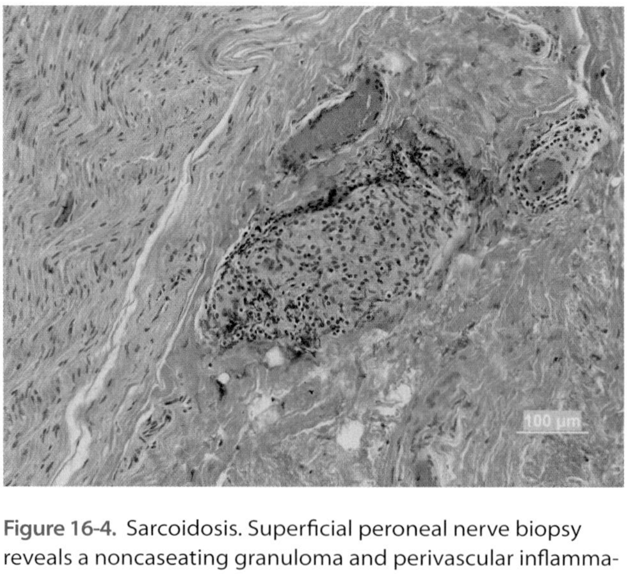

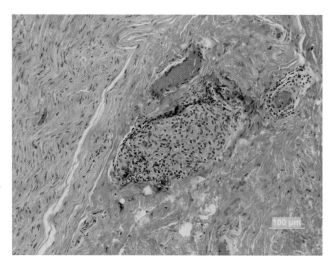

Figure 16-4. Sarcoidosis. Superficial peroneal nerve biopsy reveals a noncaseating granuloma and perivascular inflammation in the epineurium. Paraffin section stained with H&E.

intraepidermal nerve fiber density suggestive of a small fiber neuropathy in some patients.[63,65]

Pathogenesis

Sarcoidosis is an autoimmune disorder, although the etiology and pathogenic mechanism of the disorder is unclear. Neuropathies may result from invasion or direct compression by granulomas or as a result of ill-defined factors associated with inflammation such as cytokine toxicity, or ischemic damage.[62] One also needs to consider neuropathy associated with TNF-α blockade (in cases of demyelinating polyneuropathy).[33,34]

Treatment

Neurosarcoidosis, particularly of the cranial nerves, may respond well to corticosteroid treatment.[57,61] If patients are resistant to corticosteroids, other immunosuppressive/immunomodulating therapies can be tried (e.g., cyclosporine, methotrexate, IVIG, and TNF-α blockers).[70] A few patients with small fiber neuropathy have responded to IVIG as well.[71]

CELIAC DISEASE (GLUTEN-INDUCED ENTEROPATHY OR NONTROPICAL SPRUE)

Clinical Features

Intolerance to gluten, which is a protein found in wheat and wheat products, results in a malabsorption syndrome (weight loss, abdominal distention, and steatorrhea). Diagnosis of celiac disease is based on the documentation of (1) malabsorption, (2) demonstration of blunting and flattening of jejunal villi, and (3) clinical and histological improvement following the institution of a gluten-free diet.[72] A causal relationship between celiac disease and potential neurological complications remains somewhat controversial. The prevalence of neurological complications is variable and is estimated to occur in 10–40% of affected patients, with ataxia and peripheral neuropathy being the most common problems.[73–75] The neuropathy associated with celiac disease usually manifests as distal sensory loss, paresthesias, and imbalance. Generalized sensorimotor polyneuropathy, motor neuropathy, multiple mononeuropathies, autonomic neuropathy, and neuromyotonia have also been reported in association with celiac disease or antigliadin/antiendomysial antibodies.[72–85] Neurological examination often demonstrates loss of large fiber sensory modalities, mild distal muscle weakness, reduced or absent muscle stretch reflexes, and an ataxic gait. Signs of a small fiber neuropathy or autonomic neuropathy may be evident.[81,82]

Laboratory Features

Antigliadin and endomysial antibodies are often detected in the serum of patients with celiac disease but are nonspecific. NCS usually demonstrate reduced SNAP amplitudes with only mildly reduced nerve conduction velocities (NCVs) or prolonged distal latencies.[73,74,79,80,83,84] Motor conduction studies demonstrate a mild reduction in the NCVs with preservation of distal motor latencies and CMAP amplitudes. Autonomic studies may be abnormal in patients with autonomic neuropathy.[82] Rare cases with neuromyotonic discharges have been appreciated.[79]

Histopathology

Nerve biopsy may reveal a loss of large myelinated fibers.[73] Skin biopsies can demonstrate loss of epidermal nerve fibers suggestive of a small fiber neuropathy in some patients.[81] In one small series, autopsy of three patients revealed inflammation in the dorsal root ganglia with degeneration of the posterior columns of the spinal cord.[76] In another report, a loss of Purkinje cells in the cerebellum was described along with degeneration of the posterior columns and corticospinal tracts, cortical atrophy and loss of neurons in the thalamus, basal ganglia, and brainstem.[78]

Pathogenesis

The neuropathy may be secondary to malabsorption of vitamins B12 and E. However, some patients have no appreciable vitamin deficiencies. The pathogenic basis for the neuropathy in these patients is unclear but may be autoimmune in etiology.[73,83]

Treatment

Some patients may improve with gluten-free diet,[76] many others do not.[72,85] In patients with vitamin B12 or E deficiency, replacement therapy may improve or stabilize the neuropathy.

INFLAMMATORY BOWEL DISEASE

Ulcerative colitis and Crohn disease are inflammatory disorders of the bowel and are associated with various neurological abnormalities including peripheral neuropathy. Acute or chronic demyelinating neuropathies (including multifocal motor neuropathy),[86–91] generalized axonal sensory or sensorimotor polyneuropathy,[91,92] small fiber neuropathy,[91] brachial plexopathy,[89,93] multiple mononeuropathies,[89] and cranial neuropathies[89] can complicate ulcerative colitis and Crohn disease. The neuropathies in these cases may be autoimmune in nature, secondary to toxicity of treatment (e.g., metronidazole), nutritional (e.g., vitamin B12 deficiency), or idiopathic. An acute neuropathy with multifocal demyelination and conduction blocks on NCS has been reported in patients with inflammatory bowel disease treated with TNF-α blockers.[94] In addition, patients can develop weakness secondary to myasthenia gravis or myositis (including polymyositis, dermatomyositis, and granulomatous myositis).[89]

PRIMARY BILIARY CIRRHOSIS

Clinical Features

Primary biliary cirrhosis (PBC) is an autoimmune disorder directed against the biliary ducts in the liver. Peripheral neuropathy is the most common neurological complication of PBC. The neuropathy usually manifests with distal numbness and tingling.[95–99] Large fiber sensory modalities are predominantly affected, leading to reduced or absent muscle stretch reflexes. Muscle strength is typically normal but may be reduced in patients with a CIDP-like neuropathy. The neuropathy may be immune-mediated, or caused by anti–TNF-α therapy or metronidazole.[33,34,98] Myasthenia gravis, Lambert–Eaton syndrome, and myositis can also complicate PBC.

Laboratory Features

Liver function tests are elevated, and antimitochondrial antibodies can be detected in the sera of some patients with PBC. NCS demonstrates reduced or absent SNAPs. The motor conduction and needle EMG portions of the evaluation are typically normal.

Histopathology

Nerve biopsies usually reveal a loss of large myelinated fibers without evidence of segmental demyelination.

Pathogenesis

The neuropathy could have an immunological basis or may be related to unknown toxins that might be accumulating secondary to the liver failure. In addition, the neuropathy may be associated with treatments (e.g., TNF-α blockade or metronidazole).[98]

Treatment

PBC is treated with immunosuppressive therapy and ultimately liver transplantation. Whether or not transplantation affects the peripheral neuropathy has not been adequately addressed.

HYPEREOSINOPHILIC SYNDROME

The hypereosinophilic syndrome is characterized by eosinophilia associated with various skin, cardiac, hematologic, and neurological abnormalities.[100–102] Multiple mononeuropathies or a generalized, symmetric polyneuropathy occurs in 6–14% of patients. In addition, some develop an inflammatory myopathy. NCS reveal features suggestive of axonal sensorimotor peripheral neuropathy. The pathogenic basis for the neuropathy is not known but may be autoimmune in nature. The multiple organ dysfunction, including the peripheral nervous system, is believed to occur as a result of the eosinophilia or some by-products of the eosinophils.

► OTHER NEUROPATHIES ASSOCIATED WITH SYSTEMIC DISEASE

UREMIC NEUROPATHY

Clinical Features

Renal failure is associated with both CNS and peripheral nervous system complications.[103–107] At least 60% of patients with renal failure (usually with glomerular filtration rates below 12 mL/min) develop neuropathy characterized by length-dependent numbness, tingling, and allodynia. Muscle cramps in the distal legs and restless legs syndrome are also common. Reduced sensation, particularly large fiber modalities, and diminished muscle stretch reflexes are appreciated on neurological examination. Mild distal greater than proximal muscle weakness may be noted. Rarely, patients develop rapidly progressive weakness and sensory loss very similar to AIDP, which improves with an increase in renal dialysis or transplantation.[103,104,107]

Mononeuropathies can also occur, the most common of which is carpal tunnel syndrome. These neuropathies are often related to hemodialysis equipment that uses a Cuprophan membrane. This is because this membrane fails to completely remove a small β2-microglobulin, that is normally catabolized by the healthy kidney. β2-Microglobulin can deposit throughout the body, including the transverse carpal ligament. Individuals who are affected are also prone to developing ulnar neuropathy at the elbow and peroneal nerve injury about the fibular head. Damage to the brachial plexus or the peripheral nerves may also occur secondary to improper limb positioning or traction during renal transplant surgery. Ischemic monomelic neuropathy affecting the median, ulnar, and radial nerves can complicate arteriovenous shunts created in the arm for dialysis.[108]

NCS in patients with uremia reveal features of a length-dependent, primarily axonal, sensorimotor polyneuropathy.[105,106,109,110] Sensory studies are reduced in amplitude, if obtainable, distal latencies prolonged and conduction velocities slowed. Most patients have either prolonged or absent H-reflexes, and somatosensory-evoked potential studies reveal both peripheral and central slowing of conduction. Motor conduction studies reveal normal or mildly reduced amplitudes. Distal latencies and conduction velocities can be normal or reflect moderate slowing of conduction. F-waves are usually absent or demonstrate delayed latencies. The posterior tibial and peroneal motor studies are affected earlier than the median and ulnar studies.

Patients with mononeuropathies often have NCS compatible with superimposed focal demyelination or axonal loss. With ischemic monomelic neuropathy, the EMG and NCS abnormalities reveal severe axonopathy in the territory of the ischemic insult.[108] The median, radial, and ulnar SNAPs may be absent or reduced in amplitude, depending on the degree and time period of ischemia. If CMAPs are elicited, the distal motor latencies are relatively normal as are the conduction velocities. Pseudoconduction block or actual conduction block may be seen across the ischemic segments, particularly within the first week of injury before complete Wallerian degeneration of the affected nerve distal to the nerve infarct can occur. Needle EMG demonstrates a marked reduction in motor unit action potentials (MUAPs) with abundant positive sharp waves and fibrillation potentials along with decreased recruitment. The pattern of EMG abnormalities is typically length dependent, affecting distal more than proximal muscles innervated by the same peripheral nerve.

Histopathology

In uremic neuropathy, sural nerve biopsies demonstrate a loss of nerve fibers, particularly the large myelinated nerve fibers; active axonal degeneration; and segmental and paranodal demyelination.[111] At autopsy, chromatolysis of anterior horn cells and degeneration of the fasciculus gracilis have been noted in the spinal cord.

Pathogenesis

It is unclear what the primary pathophysiological mechanism of uremic neuropathy is and equally unclear whether the Schwann cell or the axon is the primary target of the essential metabolic or toxic abnormality.

Treatment

The sensorimotor polyneuropathy may be stabilized by hemodialysis and improved upon successful renal transplant, if performed prior to the loss of large numbers of axons.[106,107,112–116] Patients with carpal tunnel syndrome can be treated with surgical release. Median neuropathy at the wrist related to amyloid deposition in the form of β2-microglobulin is much less common nowadays with newer dialysis techniques currently in use. Patients with ischemic monomelic neuropathy should undergo revision of their shunt so as to allow more blood flow to the nerves. If treated early enough, the motor and sensory symptoms can resolve quickly, indicating an ischemic-induced conduction block rather than peripheral nerve infarction. Severe ischemia resulting in infarction is associated with a delayed and incomplete recovery.

CHRONIC LIVER DISEASE

Generalized sensorimotor peripheral neuropathy, characterized by numbness, tingling, and minor weakness in the distal aspects of primarily the lower limbs, commonly occurs in patients with chronic liver failure.[96,117–121] In addition, autonomic dysfunction is present in approximately 50% of patients with severe liver disease.[121] The cause of the neuropathy is quite variable. Neuropathy may be directly related to the underlying cause of the liver disease (e.g., alcoholism, viral infection, porphyria, amyloidosis, mitochondrial cytopathy), associated nutritional deficiencies, and complications of treatment such as transplantation (e.g., toxic effect of drugs or altered immunity related to immunosuppression). It is not known if hepatic failure in and of itself can cause peripheral neuropathy. Perhaps, toxins may accumulate secondary to the liver disease that could damage peripheral nerves. Electrophysiological abnormalities are thus variable and dependent on the cause of the liver failure. Most often, NCS demonstrate reduced SNAP amplitudes, while motor NCS are usually normal or show only slightly diminished amplitudes. Quantitative sensory and autonomic tests are abnormal in most patients.[96,121] Sural nerve biopsies reveal both segmental demyelination and axonal loss.

WHIPPLE DISEASE

Clinical Features

Whipple disease is characterized by abdominal pain, diarrhea, malabsorption, weight loss, arthralgias, fever, and peripheral lymphadenopathy, accompanied by enlargement of the celiac, mesenteric, and periaortic lymph nodes.[72,122–125] CNS involvement can lead to dementia, supranuclear ophthalmoparesis, convergence nystagmus, myoclonus, oromandibular myorhythmia, insomnia, hyperphagia, and polydipsia. Rarely, patients develop a sensorimotor polyneuropathy.[122–125]

Laboratory Features

The cerebrospinal fluid examination in patients with CNS involvement typically demonstrates polymorphonuclear cells and macrophages.[72] MRI scans reveal gadolinium enhancement suggestive of ependymitis/meningitis. Sensory and motor NCS may demonstrate reduced amplitudes with mild impairment of conduction velocities.[122]

Histopathology

Small bowel biopsies demonstrate PAS-positive macrophages containing the gram-positive rod-shaped bacterium, *Tropheryma whippeli*, in the mucosa. The organism can also be identified in the CNS, but there have been no reports of peripheral nerve or muscle histopathology in patients with suspected neuropathy or myopathy.

Pathogenesis

Whipple disease is caused by the actinomycete—*T. whippeli*. The pathogenic basis of the neuropathy is not known, but some symptoms of the polyneuropathy may be the result of malabsorption of necessary vitamins. Another possibility is that the neuropathy may be caused by bacterial infiltration and subsequent inflammatory involvement of the peripheral nerves.

Treatment

Whipple disease can be treated with chloramphenicol and trimethoprim-sulfamethoxazole.[72]

▶ GOUT

Some patients with gout have been reported to develop a sensorimotor peripheral neuropathy, characterized by length-dependent sensory loss or mononeuropathies at the usual sites of compression at the wrist and elbow.[126] Sensory and motor NCS may reveal reduced amplitudes with normal or only mild alterations of conduction velocities or distal latencies.

CRITICAL ILLNESS POLYNEUROPATHY

Background

The most common causes of acute generalized weakness leading to admission to a medical intensive care unit (ICU) are Guillain–Barré syndrome (GBS) and myasthenia gravis. However, weakness developing in patients who are critically ill while in the ICU is usually caused by critical illness polyneuropathy (CIP),[127–130] critical illness myopathy (CIM) (also known as acute quadriplegic myopathy),[131–137] or, much less commonly, prolonged neuromuscular blockade.[138] From a clinical and electrophysiological standpoint, it can be quite difficult to distinguish these disorders. Although a few authorities feel that CIP is more frequent than CIM,[129] most specialists and the authors' own anecdotal experiences suggest that CIM is more common than CIP.[134,136,139] In a series of 88 patients who developed weakness while in an ICU, CIM was three times as common as CIP (42% vs. 13%); prolonged neuromuscular blockade occurred in only one patient who also had CIM.[134] In patients who survive the underlying sepsis and multiorgan failure, muscle strength recovers slowly over several months.

Clinical Features

CIP can develop as a complication of sepsis and multiple organ failure.[127–130] Neuropathies are common in the subset of critically ill patients due to extensive burn surfaces.[140,141] Often, CIP presents as an inability to wean a patient from a ventilator. Concomitant encephalopathy may limit the neurological examination, in particular the sensory examination; however, generalized weakness can still be appreciated. Cranial nerves are relatively spared, although mild facial weakness can occur. Muscle stretch reflexes are absent or reduced.

Laboratory Features

Serum creatine kinase (CK) is usually normal. An elevated serum CK would point to CIM as opposed to CIP.

The electrophysiological hallmark is markedly reduced amplitudes or absent CMAPs with preserved motor conduction velocities and distal motor latencies.[128–130,142] Repetitive stimulation studies should be normal. The SNAPs are significantly diminished in amplitude or absent. Importantly, it is important to recognize that low-amplitude SNAPs do not necessarily implicate CIP as the cause of weakness. Patients may have an age-related decrease in SNAP amplitudes or the SNAPs may be abnormal secondary to an underlying coincidental condition (e.g., diabetes mellitus and uremia). In addition, lower extremity edema is common in these patients potentially obscuring SNAPs on a technical basis. Thus, the patients could still have CIM rather than CIP even if the SNAPs are abnormal. Lastly, CIP and CIM are not mutually exclusive and may occur concurrently.

Needle EMG in CIP usually reveals profuse positive sharp waves and fibrillation potentials. It is not unusual for patients with severe weakness to be unable to recruit MUAPs. When MUAPs are recruited, these are often small and polyphasic in morphology. These small units have been attributed to early reinnervation, but may occur because there is degeneration of distal motor nerve terminals without reinnervation early in the course. Thus, MUAP morphology may resemble what is commonly seen in myopathies. Most published studies fail to discuss the recruitment pattern of MUAPs. One would expect to see decreased recruitment of these small MUAPs in a neurogenic process. However, decreased recruitment can also be seen in severe myopathies when all the muscle fibers of a motor unit have degenerated. Nevertheless, if one sees early recruitment of small duration, polyphasic MUAPs, CIM is most likely.

Direct muscle stimulation may help distinguish CIP from CIM, as it bypasses the distal motor nerve and neuromuscular junction.[135,136] In a neuropathic process or prolonged neuromuscular blockade, the muscle membranes should retain its excitability and the direct muscle stimulation CMAP amplitude should be near normal compared to the low or absent nerve stimulation–evoked CMAP. In contrast, in CIM in which there is reduced muscle membrane excitability, both the nerve stimulation–evoked and the direct muscle stimulation CMAPs are reduced. The ratio of nerve stimulation–evoked CMAP to direct muscle stimulation CMAP should be close to 1:1 (greater than 0.9) in CIM and should approach zero (0.1 or less) in a CIP or neuromuscular junction disorder.[116,117]

Histopathology

Nerve biopsies demonstrate axonal degeneration.[130] On autopsies, chromatolysis of anterior horn cells, loss of dorsal root ganglion cells, and axonal degeneration of motor and sensory nerves have been observed.[130] Muscle biopsies may reveal atrophic and targetoid or core-like lesion fibers suggestive of acute neurogenic process.[130] However, these light microscopic features can be seen in myopathies. Other studies have found loss of myosin thick filaments on muscle biopsy and morphology of intramuscular nerves and those of multiple nerve roots and proximal nerves to be normal on autopsy, suggesting that these cases may all be CIM.[139]

Pathogenesis

The pathogenic basis of CIP is not known. Perhaps, circulating toxins and metabolic abnormalities associated with sepsis and multiorgan failure impair axonal transport or mitochondrial function, leading to axonal degeneration.[130] As mentioned, some have questioned the existence of CIP and suggested that most, if not all, such cases are CIM.[143]

Treatment

There is no specific therapy for critical illness neuropathy other than supportive care and treatment of the underlying sepsis and organ failure.

▶ AMYLOID POLYNEUROPATHY

Amyloid comprises 10–20 nm, nonbranching protein fibrils, which aggregate to form three-dimensional β-pleated sheets that are resistant to proteolytic decomposition.[144,145] Amyloidosis can be hereditary or acquired and is associated with systemic proteinaceous deposition in multiple organs (e.g., kidney, liver, heart, and GI tract) including peripheral nerves and muscle (Table 16-2). Familial forms of amyloidosis are inherited in an autosomal-dominant fashion and can be caused by mutations in the transthyretin (TTR), apolipoprotein A1, or gelsolin genes. In primary or AL amyloidosis, the abnormal protein deposition is composed of immunoglobulin light chains. AL amyloidosis occurs in the setting of multiple myeloma, Waldenström macroglobulinemia, lymphoma, other plasmacytomas or lymphoproliferative disorders, or in the absence of identifiable disease.[146] Approximately 10% of patients with a presumptive diagnosis of systemic AL amyloidosis actually have hereditary amyloidosis with genetic testing.[147] Secondary amyloidosis (AA) can complicate RA and other chronic inflammatory diseases and is associated with the accumulation of protein A but is not associated with a polyneuropathy.

▶ **TABLE 16-2. AMYLOID NEUROPATHY**

Acquired
Primary or AL amyloidosis
Secondary amyloidosis
Familial amyloid polyneuropathy (FAP)
Transthyretin-related amyloidosis (FAP types I and II)
Apolipoprotein A1-related amyloidosis (type III FAP or Van Allen type)
Gelsolin-related amyloidosis (FAP type IV, Finnish)

Amyloid deposits have a characteristic apple-green birefringence when stained with Congo red and observed under polarized light and bright red under rhodamine fluorescence. Amyloid is also metachromatic when stained with methyl violet or crystal violet and also stains with Alcian blue. On nerve biopsy, amyloid deposition may be demonstrated in the endoneurium, perineurium, or epineurium and around blood vessels (Fig. 16-5).[148] Chronic inflammatory cell infiltrate may be appreciated. Concomitant muscle biopsy may also reveal amyloid deposits encasing muscle fibers or around blood vessels. The appearance of the Congo red or metachromatic staining does not distinguish between the various subtypes of amyloidosis. Immunohistochemistry using antibodies directed against light chains, apolipoprotein A, gelsolin, and TTR and genetic testing is required to distinguish between the various forms of amyloidosis. Proteomic analysis of nerve tissue using laser microdissection (LMD) and mass spectrometric (MS)-based proteomic analysis can distinguish specific types of amyloid independent of clinical information.[149]

PRIMARY OR AL AMYLOIDOSIS

Clinical Features

Patients with primary (AL) amyloidosis can present with nephrotic syndrome, congestive heart failure, cardiac arrhythmia, purpura, bruises, sicca syndrome, dyspnea due to pleural effusions, gastrointestinal dysmotility (nausea/constipation/diarrhea/pain), splenomegaly, hepatomegaly, lymphadenopathy, fatigue, weight loss, myopathy, carpal tunnel syndrome, or polyneuropathy.[150,151] It is more common in men over 50 years of age, which may help distinguish AL from familial amyloidosis, which usually presents earlier in adult life. However, AL amyloidosis can develop in people in their thirties and hereditary amyloidosis can present later in life.

Polyneuropathy develops in as many as 30% of patients with AL amyloidosis and can be the presenting manifestation.[151–154] There is an early predilection for small fiber modalities resulting in painful dysesthesias and burning sensations along with diminished pain and temperature sensation and allodynia on examination. The legs are usually affected in a symmetric, length-dependent fashion; however, the trunk can be involved and as many as 20% or more present asymmetrically in a multifocal neuropathy pattern.[153] Carpal tunnel syndrome occurs in 25% of patients and may be the initial complication. Cranial nerves may be affected. The neuropathy is slowly progressive, and eventually weakness develops along with large fiber sensory loss. Generalized proximal and distal weakness can develop such that it resembles CIDP.[153] Most patients develop

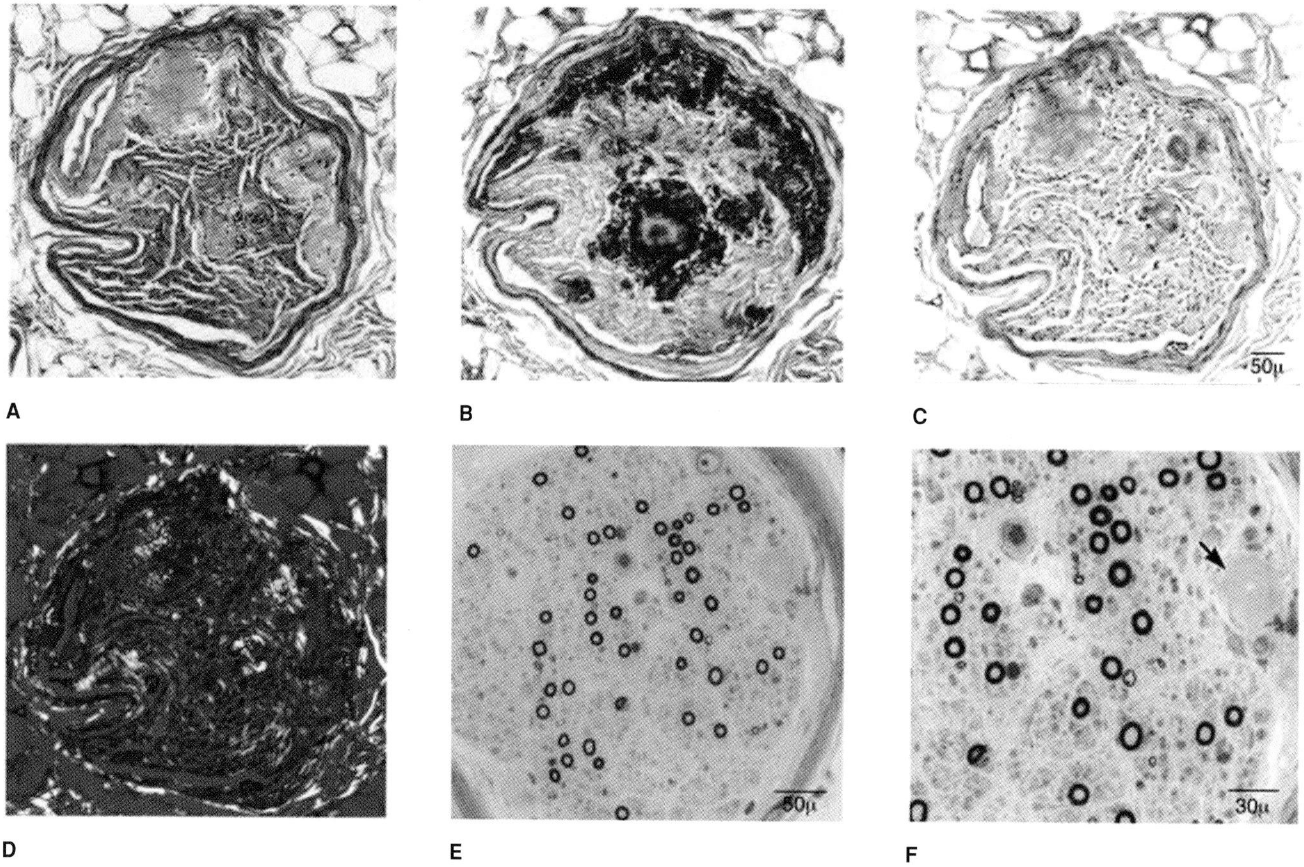

Figure 16-5. Superficial radial nerve biopsy (**A–D**, paraffin sections and **E and F**, epoxy sections). Serial paraffin cross sections show (**A**, hematoxylin and eosin stain) areas of eosinophilic amorphous deposits in the endoneurium and in the walls of endoneurial microvessels. The deposits react to lambda light chain preparations **(B)**, stain salmon-pink on Congo red stain **(C)**, and, when viewed under polarized light **(D)**, show apple-green birefringence in the areas of amorphous material. The semithin epoxy sections **(E and F)** show a moderately reduced density of myelinated fibers. Unlike the clinical symptoms and findings (that are large fiber predominant), the biopsy shows relatively more severe reduction of small myelinated fibers in comparison to large myelinated fibers. The *arrow* shows a region of amyloid infiltration of an endoneurial microvessel. These findings are diagnostic of primary amyloidosis from a lambda light chain. (Reproduced with permission from Tracy JA, Dyck PJ, Dyck PJ. Primary amyloidosis presenting as upper limb multiple mononeuropathies. *Muscle Nerve.* 2010;41(5):710–715.)

autonomic involvement with postural hypertension, syncope, impotence, bowel and bladder incontinence, constipation, and impaired sweating. Occasionally, enlarged peripheral nerves are appreciated by an astute clinician. The general physical examination can demonstrate limb edema, hoarse voice, hepatomegaly, and macroglossia. Patients generally die from their systemic illness (renal failure and cardiac disease).

Laboratory Features

The monoclonal protein can be composed of IgG, IgA, IgM, or only free light chain. Lambda (λ) is more common than κ light chain (>2:1) in AL amyloidosis, in contrast to multiple myeloma in which κ light chains are more common. Immunoelectrophoresis (IEP) or immunofixation (IFE) of the serum and urine is more sensitive in identifying monoclonal proteins than serum or urine protein electrophoresis (SPEP or UPEP); but serum-free light-chain assay is even more sensitive and thus should be performed on patients with possible amyloid neuropathy. Hypogammaglobulinemia, anemia, renal failure, proteinuria, and transaminitis due to liver involvement may be seen. The serum CK levels can also be elevated in patients with concurrent amyloid myopathy. The cerebrospinal fluid protein is often increased (with normal cell count), and thus the neuropathy may be mistaken for CIDP.[153]

Sensory nerve action amplitudes are usually reduced or absent in involved nerves. When obtainable, the distal sensory latencies can be normal or only moderately prolonged and the conduction velocities are similarly normal or moderately slow. Motor conductions are less involved than the sensory conduction but, nonetheless, are frequently abnormal. Motor NCVs can be normal or moderately reduced.[151–158] The distal motor latencies are normal or only moderately prolonged in the upper limbs and usually prolonged in the lower limbs. CMAP amplitudes are normal or only mildly reduced during the early course of the disease and not as severely affected as the SNAP. The motor and sensory conduction abnormalities are usually symmetric but can be asymmetric in patients with multifocal neuropathies.[153] Electrophysiological evidence of superimposed median neuropathy at the wrist (carpal tunnel syndrome) is common.

Needle EMG examination usually reveals positive sharp waves and fibrillation potentials along with reduced recruitment of long-duration, high-amplitude, polyphasic MUAPs in affected muscles. Myotonic discharges and myopathic MUAPs, particularly in more proximal muscles, may be seen in patients with superimposed amyloid myopathy.

Histopathology

Nerve biopsies reveal axonal degeneration and severe loss of small myelinated and unmyelinated fibers. There is a less pronounced but obvious degeneration of the large myelinated nerve fibers as well. Congo red staining reveals amyloid deposition in a globular or diffuse pattern within the perineurial, epineurial, and endoneurial connective tissue as well as in and around blood vessel walls (Fig. 16-5).[152] Amyloid deposition can also be demonstrated in the sympathetic and dorsal root ganglion. Because of the patchy, multifocal pattern of amyloid deposition, biopsies are not always diagnostic. Other sites commonly biopsied include the kidney, rectal mucosa, stomach, abdominal fat pad, salivary glands, muscle, and skin. Abdominal fat pad biopsies seem to be the most sensitive method to detect amyloid deposits and these are abnormal in 85% of patients. Immunohistochemistry is helpful in demonstrating that the amyloid is composed of λ, or less frequently κ, light chains.

Pathogenesis

The pathogenic basis for the neuropathy associated with amyloidosis is unclear and may be multifactorial. Amyloid deposition in the epineurial and endoneurial connective tissue may lead to compression of nerve fibers with focal demyelination and axonal degeneration. Deposition around blood vessels might cause ischemic damage to nerve fibers.[159] Transport of nutrients into and waste products out of the nerves may also be affected by amyloid deposition within the endoneurium and epineurium and around blood vessels.

Treatment

The prognosis of patients with primary amyloidosis is poor, with a median survival of less than 2 years. Death is generally secondary to progressive congestive heart failure or renal failure. Chemotherapy with melphalan, prednisone, colchicine that reduces the concentration of monoclonal proteins, and autologous stem cell transplantation may prolong survival and improve the neuropathy.[160–162] The severity of baseline cardiac and renal involvement, number of organs involved, and presence of autonomic neuropathy may be independent, adverse determinant of survival in these patients.[162]

▶ FAMILIAL AMYLOID POLYNEUROPATHIES

Although frequently clinically indistinguishable from primary amyloidosis, familial amyloid polyneuropathy (FAP) is phenotypically and genetically heterogeneous. It is caused by mutations in the genes for TTR (prealbumin), apolipoprotein A1, or gelsolin.[146,157,163–168] Diagnosis of familial amyloidosis is made by detection of amyloid deposition in abdominal fat pad, rectal, or nerve biopsies or with genetic testing (Fig. 16-6). Unlike, the nonhereditary forms of amyloidosis, monoclonal gammopathies are not present and the abnormal amyloid deposits do not immunostain for immunoglobulin light chains. In contrast, these amyloid deposits may stain for TTR, apolipoprotein A1, or gelsolin.

Nerve biopsies in the different forms of FAP reveal findings similar to that seen in AL amyloidosis. Amyloid deposition can be multifocal or diffuse within the endoneurium, epineurium, or perineurium, as well as around blood vessels in autonomic ganglia and in peripheral nerves.[157,165] Importantly, in approximately 50% of FAP, nerve biopsies do not demonstrate amyloid deposits perhaps secondary to sampling error.[169] As mentioned previously, immunohistochemistry and even LMD and MS-based proteomic analysis can be used to distinguish specific types of amyloid.[142]

There is a loss of myelinated nerve fibers, particularly small myelinated and unmyelinated nerve fibers. These deposits encroach upon the nerve fibers, resulting in axonal degeneration and segmental demyelination. The clinical features, histopathology, and electrophysiological studies reveal abnormalities consistent with a generalized or multifocal, predominantly axonal but occasionally demyelinating, sensorimotor polyneuropathy.[155,161–171] Cerebrospinal fluid can reveal elevated protein levels with normal cell count again mimicking CIDP. The pathogenic bases for the FAP neuropathies are likely similar to that noted with AL neuropathy.

TTR-RELATED AMYLOIDOSIS (FAP TYPES I AND II)

Clinical Features

The majority of patients with FAP have mutations in the TTR gene. There appear to be two somewhat different

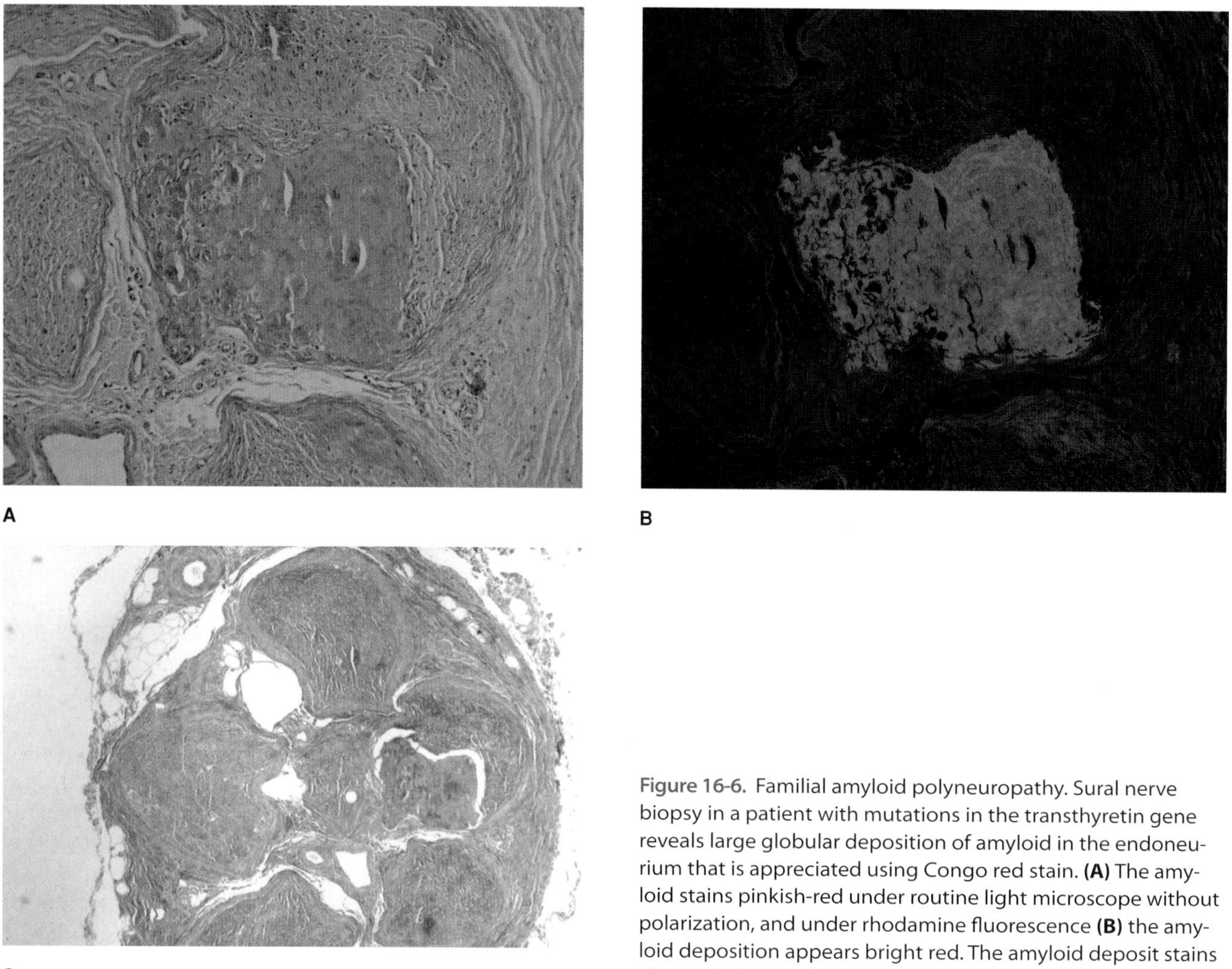

A

B

C

Figure 16-6. Familial amyloid polyneuropathy. Sural nerve biopsy in a patient with mutations in the transthyretin gene reveals large globular deposition of amyloid in the endoneurium that is appreciated using Congo red stain. **(A)** The amyloid stains pinkish-red under routine light microscope without polarization, and under rhodamine fluorescence **(B)** the amyloid deposition appears bright red. The amyloid deposit stains blue with Alcian blue **(C)**.

clinical phenotypes associated with TTR-related amyloidosis: FAP I and a less severe FAP II. FAP I was originally reported in the Portuguese,[172] but it affects multiple ethnic groups with particularly large foci in Sweden and Japan.[143,163,166–168,173–177] Patients usually develop insidious onset of numbness and painful paresthesia in the distal lower limbs in the third to fourth decade of life, although some patients develop the disorder later in life.[173,174] Pain and thermal sensation are the most common modalities affected. Carpal tunnel syndrome is uncommon. Autonomic involvement can be severe, leading to postural hypotension, constipation or persistent diarrhea, erectile dysfunction, and impaired sweating. Distal and later proximal muscle atrophy and weakness develop over time such that the patients may be mistaken for having CIDP.[155,177] Occasional cranial neuropathies, leading to pupillary changes, decreased saliva secretion, diminished facial (including corneal) sensation, dysphonia, dysphagia, and facial weakness occur. Amyloid deposition also occurs in the heart, kidneys, liver, and the corneas. Patients usually die by 10–15 years after the onset of symptoms from cardiac failure or complications from malnutrition.

A milder form of TTR-associated FAP (Type II FAP) was initially described in families in Indiana and Switzerland and is characterized by the development of carpal tunnel syndrome and later by a mild generalized sensorimotor polyneuropathy.[143,145,166] Although erectile dysfunction can be seen, severe autonomic dysfunction is unusual. As with FAP I, vitreous opacities may be appreciated. Although there can be systemic involvement, severe nephropathy or cardiomyopathy usually does not develop. Thus, most patients with FAP II have a relatively long survival, with little morbidity related to the amyloidosis. The symptoms of carpal tunnel syndrome can be relieved with surgical decompression.

Molecular Genetics and Pathogenesis

More than 100 different mutations within the *TTR* gene located on chromosome 18q11.2–12.1 have been associated with FAP types I and II.[146,166,170,175,178] A mutation involving a methionine to valine substitution at position 30 (Val30Met) in the *TTR* gene is the most common mutation associated with type I FAP, while serine substitutions at position 84 and histidine at position 58 are the most common mutations associated with FAP type II. There can be variability in the age of onset and severity even within families with the Val-30Met mutations. TTR functions as a transport protein for vitamin A and thyroxin. Over 90% of the body's TTR is synthesized in the liver. The amino acid substitutions lead to the formation of the β-pleated sheet structure of the protein and its resistance to degradation by proteases, thus its amyloidogenic properties.

Treatment

Because the liver produces much of the body's TTR, liver transplantation has been used to treat FAP related to TTR mutations. Serum TTR levels decrease after transplantation and improvement in clinical and neurophysiological features has been reported.[170,175,178,179] However, abnormal TTR can continue to be synthesized in the CNS (by the choroid plexus) and within the eyes, potentially resulting in progressive deficits from local accumulation in these areas. Oral administration of tafamidis meglumine, which prevents misfolding and deposition of mutated TTR, is under evaluation in patients with TTR FAP.[174] There is an ongoing clinical trial of diflunisal in TTR-related FAP.[180] Both of these medications are hypothesized to decrease the fibril-forming ability of mutant TTR protein.

APOLIPOPROTEIN A1-RELATED AMYLOIDOSIS (TYPE III FAP OR VAN ALLEN TYPE)

Clinical Features

FAP type III was originally described by Dr. Van Allen in a family from Iowa.[181,182] The neuropathy usually manifests as numbness and painful dysesthesias in the lower limbs in the fourth decade of life. Gradually, the symptoms progress to the distal upper limbs and proximal muscle weakness and atrophy develop. Although autonomic neuropathy is not severe, some patients develop diarrhea, constipation, or gastroparesis. Most patients die from systemic complications of amyloidosis (e.g., renal failure) 12–15 years after the onset of the neuropathy.

Molecular Genetics and Pathogenesis

FAP type III is caused by mutations leading to arginine for glycine substitution at position 26 (Arg26Gly) in the apolipoprotein A1 gene on chromosome 11q23–qter.[183] Apolipoprotein A1 is a major component of high-density lipoproteins. As with TTR mutations, the amino acid substitution probably impairs its degradation by proteases.

Treatment

There are no specific medical therapies.

GELSOLIN-RELATED AMYLOIDOSIS (FAP TYPE IV, FINNISH)

Clinical Features

FAP IV was initially described in Finland and is characterized by the combination of lattice corneal dystrophy, multiple cranial neuropathies (e.g., facial palsies and bulbar weakness), and cutis laxa.[184–188] Onset of symptoms is usually in the third decade of life. Over time, a mild generalized sensorimotor polyneuropathy develops. Autonomic dysfunction does not occur. Cutis laxa manifests as loose or hanging skin affecting the scalp and face (Fig. 16-7).

Histopathology

Autopsy studies have demonstrated a different distribution of amyloid deposition in FAP type IV than the other types of amyloidosis.[189] Histological, immunohistochemical, and electron microscopic studies reveal deposition of gelsolin amyloid, particularly in the vascular walls and perineurial sheaths. Nerve roots are more severely affected than distal nerves. The marked proximal nerve involvement with gelsolin-related angiopathy is a characteristic feature of FAP type IV. There was also preferential large fiber loss, not generally seen in other forms of amyloid neuropathy.

Molecular Genetics and Pathogenesis

Type IV amyloidosis is caused by mutations in the gelsolin gene.[190–192] Gelsolin is an actin-binding protein found in plasma, leukocytes, and other cells. The resultant mutations and amino acid substitutions lead to a charge change on the protein, which may render the molecule resistant to proteases.

Treatment

There are no specific medical therapies. However, facial plastic surgical procedures can help fix the cosmetic problems associated with cutis laxa.[184]

▶ SUMMARY

As discussed, neuropathies may complicate many different systemic disorders. It is important to distinguish neuropathies that may be directly related to the underlying disorder, caused by treatment (toxic neuropathy), or just be coincidental occurrence as management may differ according to the etiology. Thus, as discussed in Chapter 1, it is always important to take a detailed medical history and examination to

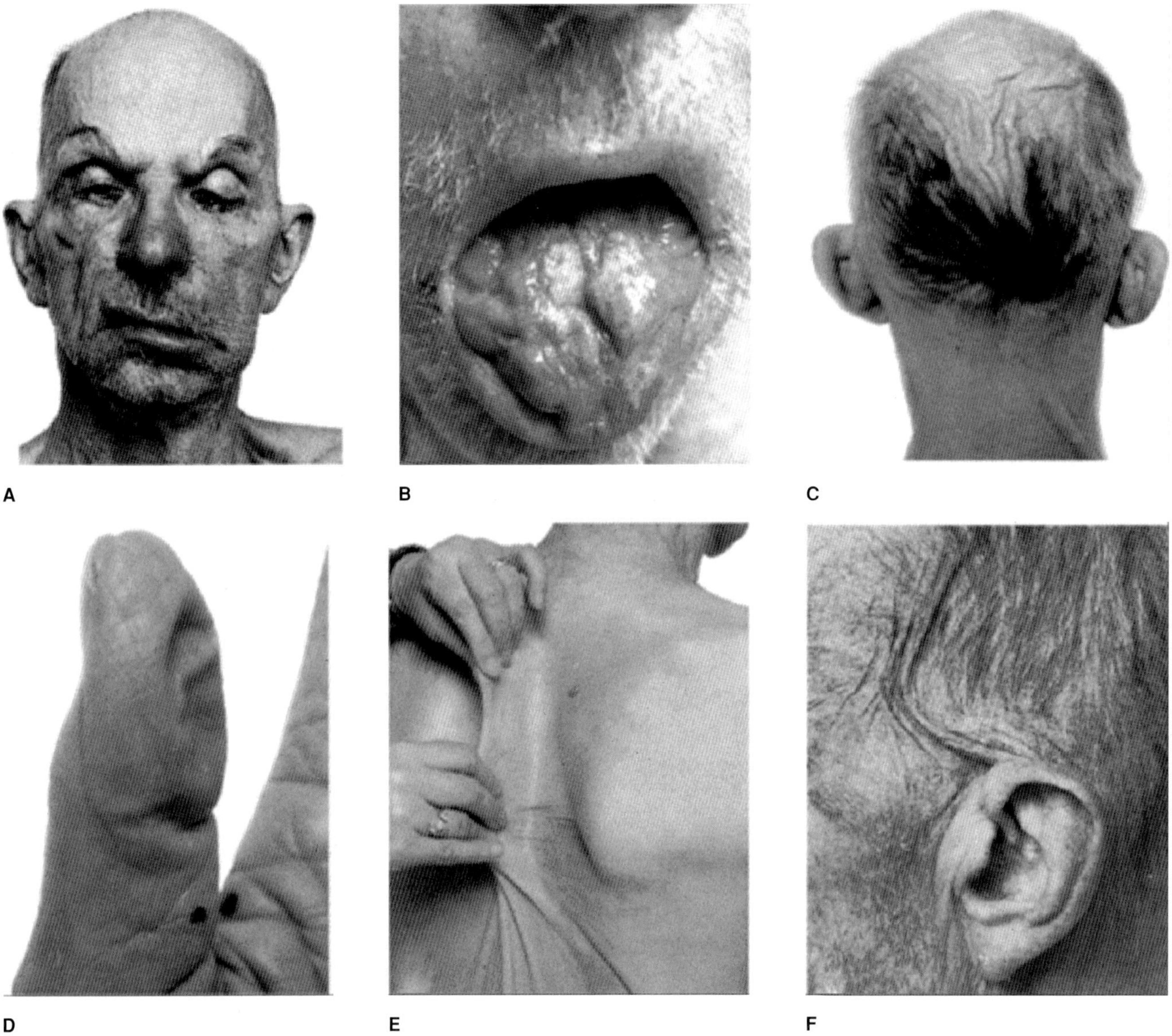

Figure 16-7. Clinical characteristics in hereditary gelsolin amyloidosis. **(A)** The drooping face of a 79-year-old male patient, after corrective facial surgery. Note also the loss of frontotemporal hair and thinning of the eyebrows. **(B)** The tongue is morel-like and macroglossic. **(C)** Drooping ears and abnormally lax, folded, and unelastic skin of the scalp with thinning of scalp hair. Cutis laxa affecting **(D)** the thumb and **(E)** the back. **(D and F)** The thumb and scalp skin retain their deformed state after pressure for 2–5 minutes. (Reproduced with permission from Kiuru-Enari S, Keski-Oja J, Haltia M. Cutis laxa in hereditary gelsolin amyloidosis. *Br J Dermatol.* 2005;152(2):250–257.)

assess for an underlying systemic disorder that may be associated with the neuropathy.

REFERENCES

1. Gemignani F, Marbini A, Pavesi G, et al. Peripheral neuropathy associated with primary Sjögren's syndrome. *J Neurol Neurosurg Psychiatry.* 1994;57:983–986.
2. Grant IA, Hunder GG, Homburger HA, Dyck PJ. Peripheral neuropathy associated with sicca complex. *Neurology.* 1997;48:855–862.
3. Griffin JW, Cornblath DR, Alexander E, et al. Ataxic sensory neuropathy and dorsal root ganglionitis associated with Sjögren's syndrome. *Ann Neurol.* 1990;27:304–315.
4. Kennett RP, Harding AE. Peripheral neuropathy associated with sicca syndrome. *J Neurol Neurosurg Psychiatry.* 1986;49:90–92.
5. Malinow K, Yannakakis GD, Glusman SM, et al. Subacute sensory neuronopathy secondary to dorsal root ganglionitis in primary Sjögren's syndrome. *Ann Neurol.* 1986;20:535–537.
6. Mellgren S, Conn DL, Steven JC, et al. Peripheral neuropathy in primary Sjögren's syndrome. *Neurology.* 1989;39:390–394.
7. Gorson KC, Ropper AH. Positive salivary gland biopsy, Sjögren syndrome, and neuropathy: Clinical implications. *Muscle Nerve.* 2003;28(5):553–560.

8. Ramos-Casals M, Anaya JM, Garcia-Carrasco M, et al. Cutaneous vasculitis in primary Sjögren syndrome: Classification and clinical significance of 52 patients. *Medicine*. 2004;83(2):96–106.
9. Mori K, Iijima M, Sugiura M, et al. Sjögren's syndrome associated painful sensory neuropathy without sensory ataxia. *J Neurol Neurosurg Psychiatry*. 2003;74(9):1320–1322.
10. Mori K, Iijima M, Koike H, et al. The wide spectrum of clinical manifestations in Sjögren's syndrome-associated neuropathy. *Brain*. 2005;128:2518–2534.
11. Font J, Ramos-Casals M, de la Red G, et al. Pure sensory neuropathy in primary Sjögren's syndrome. Long term prospective followup and review of the literature. *J Rheumatol*. 2003;30(7):1552–1557.
12. Pavlakis PP, Alexopoulos H, Kosmidis ML, et al. Peripheral neuropathies in Sjögren syndrome: A new reappraisal. *J Neurol Neurosurg Psychiatry*. 2011;82:798–802.
13. Rosenbaum R. Neuromuscular complications of connective tissue diseases. *Muscle Nerve*. 2001;24(2):154–169.
14. Chai J, Herrmann DN, Stanton M, Barbano RL, Logigian EL. Painful small-fiber neuropathy in Sjögren syndrome. *Neurology*. 2005;65:925–927.
15. Lopate G, Pestronk A, Al-Lozi M, et al. Peripheral neuropathy in an outpatient cohort of patients with Sjögren's syndrome. *Muscle Nerve*. 2006;33(5):672–676.
16. Kovacs L, Paprika D, Takacs R, et al. Cardiovascular autonomic dysfunction in primary Sjögren's syndrome. *Rheumatology*. 2004;43(1):95–99.
17. Goto H, Matsuo H, Fukudome T, Shibuya N, Ohnishi A, Nakamura H. Chronic autonomic neuropathy in a patient with primary Sjögren's syndrome. *J Neurol Neurosurg Psychiatry*. 2000;69(1):135.
18. Urban PP, Keilmann A, Teichmann EM, Hopf HC. Sensory neuropathy of the trigeminal, glossopharyngeal, and vagal nerves in Sjögren's syndrome. *J Neurol Sci*. 2001;186(1–2):59–63.
19. Asahina M, Kuwabuara S, Asahina M, Nakajima M, Hattori T. D-penicillamine treatment for chronic sensory ataxia neuropathy associated with Sjögren's syndrome. *Neurology*. 1998;51: 1451–1453.
20. Hankey GJ, Gubbay SS. Peripheral neuropathy associated with sicca syndrome. *J Neurol Neurosurg Psychiatry*. 1987;50:1085.
21. Laloux P, Brucher JM, Guerit JM, Sindic CJ, Laterre EC. Subacute sensory neuronopathy associated with Sjögren's sicca syndrome. *J Neurol*. 1988;235:352–354.
22. Auger RG, Windebank AJ, Lucchinetti CF, Chalk CH. Role of the blink reflex in the evaluation of sensory neuronopathy. *Neurology*. 1999;53:407–408.
23. Auger RG. The role of the masseter reflex in the assessment of subacute sensory neuropathy. *Muscle Nerve*. 1998;21:800–801.
24. Kizawa M, Mori K, Iijima M, Koike H, Hattori N, Sobue G. Intravenous immunoglobulin treatment in painful sensory neuropathy without sensory ataxia associated with Sjögren's syndrome. *J Neurol Neurosurg Psychiatry*. 2006;77(8):967–969.
25. Chen WH, Yeh JH, Chiu HC. Plasmapheresis in the treatment of ataxic sensory neuropathy associated with Sjögren's syndrome. *Eur Neurol*. 2001;45(4):270–274.
26. Rist S, Sellam J, Hachulla E, et al. Experience of intravenous immunoglobulin therapy in neuropathy associated with primary Sjögren's syndrome: A national multicentric retrospective study. *Arthritis Care Res*. 2011;63:1339–1344.
27. Agarwal V, Singh R, Wiclaf, et al. A clinical, electrophysiological, and pathological study of neuropathy in rheumatoid arthritis. *Clin Rheumatol*. 2008;27:841–844.
28. Bayrak AO, Durmus D, Durmaz Y, Demir I, Canturk F, Onar MK. Electrophysiological assessment of polyneuropathic involvement in rheumatoid arthritis: Relationships among demographic, clinical and laboratory findings. *Neurol Res*. 2010;32:711–714.
29. Chamberlain MA, Bruckner FE. Rheumatoid neuropathy: Clinical and electrophysiologic features. *Ann Rheum Dis*. 1970;29:609–616.
30. Peyronnard J-M, Charron L, Beaudet F, Couture F. Vasculitic neuropathy in rheumatoid disease and Sjögren's syndrome. *Neurology*. 1982;32:839–845.
31. Scott DG, Bacon PA, Tribe CR. Systemic rheumatoid vasculitis: A clinical and laboratory study of 50 cases. *Medicine*. 1981;60:288–297.
32. Weller RO, Bruckner FE, Chamberlain MA. Rheumatoid neuropathy: A histological and electrophysiological study. *J Neurol Neurosurg Psychiatry*. 1970;33:592–604.
33. Lozeron P, Denier C, Lacroix C, Adams D. Long-term course of demyelinating neuropathies occurring during tumor necrosis factor alpha blocker therapy. *Arch Neurol*. 2009;66:490–497.
34. Alshekhlee A, Basiri K, Miles JD, Ahmad SA, Katirji B. Chronic inflammatory demyelinating polyneuropathy associated with tumor necrosis factor-alpha antagonists. *Muscle Nerve*. 2010;41:723–727.
35. Florica B, Aghdassi E, Su J, Gladman DD, Urowitz MB, Fortin PR. Peripheral neuropathy in patients with systemic lupus erythematosus. *Semin Arthritis Rheum*. 2011;41:203–211.
36. Hughes RA, Cameron JS, Hass SM, Heaton J, Payan J, Teoh R. Multiple mononeuropathy as an initial presentation of systemic lupus erythematosus-nerve biopsy and response to plasma exchange. *J Neurol*. 1982;228:239–247.
37. McCombe PA, McLeod JG, Pollard JD, Guo YP, Ingall TJ. Peripheral sensorimotor and autonomic neuropathy associated with systemic lupus erythematosus. *Brain*. 1987;110: 533–549.
38. McNicholl JM, Glynn D, Mongey A-B, Hutchinson M, Bresihan B. A prospective study of neurophysiologic, neurologic, and immunologic abnormalities in systemic lupus erythematosus. *J Rheumatol*. 1994;21:1061–1066.
39. Sivri A, Hascelik Z, Celiker R, Basgoze O. Early detection of neurological involvement in systemic lupus erythematosus patients. *Electromyogr Clin Neurophysiol*. 1995;35:195–199.
40. Omdal R, Mellgren SI, Goransson L, et al. Small nerve fiber involvement in systemic lupus erythematosus: A controlled study. *Arthritis Rheum*. 2002;46(5):1228–1232.
41. Goransson LG, Tjensvoll AB, Herigstad A, Mellgren SI, Omdal R. Small-diameter nerve fiber neuropathy in systemic lupus erythematosus. *Arch Neurol*. 2006;63(3):401–404.
42. Enevoldson TP, Wiles CM. Severe vasculitic neuropathy in systemic lupus erythematosus and response to cyclophosphamide. *J Neurol Neurosurg Psychiatry*. 1991;54:468–469.
43. Kissel JT, Slivka AP, Warmolts JR, Mendell JR. The clinical spectrum of necrotizing angiopathy of the peripheral nervous system. *Ann Neurol*. 1985;18:251–257.
44. Rechtland E, Cornblath DR, Stern BJ, Meyerhoff JO. Chronic demyelinating polyneuropathy in systemic lupus erythematosus. *Neurology*. 1984;34:1375–1377.
45. Lewis M, Gibson T. Systemic lupus erythematosus with recurrent Guillain–Barré-like syndrome treated with intravenous immunoglobulins. *Lupus*. 2003;12:857–859.
46. Ait Benhaddou E, Birouk N, El Alaoui-Faris M, et al. Acute Guillain–Barré-like polyradiculoneuritis revealing acute

systemic lupus erythematosus: Two case studies and review of the literature. *Rev Neurol.* 2003;159(3):300–306.
47. Omdal R, Loseth S, Torbergsen T, Koldingsnes W, Husby G, Mellgren SI. Peripheral neuropathy in systemic lupus erythematosus—a longitudinal study. *Acta Neurol Scand.* 2001;103 (6):386–391.
48. Mawrin C, Brunn A, Rocken C, Schroder JM. Peripheral neuropathy in systemic lupus erythematosus: Pathomorphological features and distribution pattern of matrix metalloproteinases. *Acta Neuropathol (Berl).* 2003;105(4):365–372.
49. Dierckx RA, Aichner F, Gerstenbrand F, Fritsch P. Progressive systemic sclerosis and nervous system involvement. *Eur Neurol.* 1987;26:134–140.
50. Hietaharju A, Jaaskelainen S, Kalimo H, Hietarinta M. Peripheral neuromuscular manifestations in systemic sclerosis (scleroderma). *Muscle Nerve.* 1993;16:1204–1212.
51. Lecky BR, Hughes RA, Murray NM. Trigeminal sensory neuropathy: A study of 22 cases. *Brain.* 1987;110:1463–1485.
52. Lee P, Bruni J, Sukenik S. Neurological manifestations in systemic sclerosis (scleroderma). *J Rheumatol.* 1984;11:480–483.
53. Poncelet AN, Connolly MK. Peripheral neuropathy in scleroderma. *Muscle Nerve.* 2003;28:330–335.
54. Dyck PJ, Hunder GG, Dyck PJ. A case-control and nerve biopsy study of CREST multiple mononeuropathy. *Neurology.* 1997;49:1641–1645.
55. Bennet RM, Bong DM, Spargo BH. Neuropsychiatric problems in mixed connective tissue disease. *Am J Med.* 1978;65:955–962.
56. Delaney P. Neurologic manifestations of sarcoidosis. *Ann Intern Med.* 1977;87:336–345.
57. Koffman B, Junck L, Elias SB, Feit HW, Levine SR. Polyradiculopathy in sarcoidosis. *Muscle Nerve.* 1999;22:608–613.
58. Zuniga G, Ropper AH, Frank J. Sarcoid peripheral neuropathy. *Neurology.* 1991;41:1558–1561.
59. Said G, Lacroix C, Plante-Bordeneuve V, et al. Nerve granulomas and vasculitis in sarcoid peripheral neuropathy: A clinicopathological study of 11 patients. *Brain.* 2002; 125(Pt 2):264–275.
60. De Marco O, Riffaud L, Pinel JF, Edan G. Systemic sarcoidosis revealed by acute ataxic sensory polyradiculoneuropathy. *Rev Neurol.* 2003;159(11):1060–1062.
61. Burns TM, Dyck PJ, Aksamit AJ, Dyck PJ. The natural history and long-term outcome of 57 limb sarcoidosis neuropathy cases. *J Neurol Sci.* 2006;244(1–2):77–87.
62. Vital A, Lagueny A, Ferrer X, Louiset P, Canron MH, Vital C. Sarcoid neuropathy: Clinico-pathological study of 4 new cases and review of the literature. *Clin Neuropathol.* 2008;27:96–105.
63. Bakkers M, Merkies IS, Lauria G, et al. Intraepidermal nerve fiber density and its application in sarcoidosis. *Neurology.* 2009;73:1142–1148.
64. Khan S, Zhou L. Characterization of non-length-dependent small-fiber sensory neuropathy. *Muscle Nerve.* 2012;45:86–91.
65. Hoitsma E, Marziniak M, Faber CG, et al. Small fibre neuropathy in sarcoidosis. *Lancet.* 2002;359(9323):2085–2086.
66. Hoitsma E, Drent M, Verstraete E, et al. Abnormal warm and cold sensation thresholds suggestive of small-fibre neuropathy in sarcoidosis. *Clin Neurophysiol.* 2003;114(12):2326–2333.
67. Challenor YB, Felton CP, Brust JC. Peripheral nerve involvement in sarcoidosis: An electrodiagnostic study. *J Neurol Neurosurg Psychiatry.* 1984;47:1219–1222.
68. Nemni R, Galassi G, Cohen M, et al. Symmetric sarcoid polyneuropathy: Analysis of a sural nerve biopsy. *Neurology.* 1981;31:1217–1223.
69. Souayah N, Chodos A, Krivitskaya N, Efthimiou P, Lambert WC, Sharer LR. Isolated severe vasculitic neuropathy revealing sarcoidosis. *Lancet Neurol.* 2008;7:756–760.
70. Heaney D, Geddes JF, Nagendren K, Swash M. Sarcoid polyneuropathy responsive to intravenous immunoglobulin. *Muscle Nerve.* 2004;29(3):447–450.
71. Parambil JG, Tavee JO, Zhou L, Pearson KS, Culver DA. Efficacy of intravenous immunoglobulin for small fiber neuropathy associated with sarcoidosis. *Respir Med.* 2011;105:101–105.
72. Perkin GD, Murray-Lyon I. Neurology and the gastrointestinal system. *J Neurol Neurosurg Psychiatry.* 1998;65:291–300.
73. Chin RL, Sander HW, Brannagan TH, et al. Celiac neuropathy. *Neurology.* 2003;60:1581–1585.
74. Hadjivassiliou M, Grunewald R, Sharrack B, et al. Gluten ataxia in perspective: Epidemiology, genetic susceptibility and clinical characteristics. *Brain.* 2003;126(Pt 3):685–691.
75. Shen DT, Lebwohl B, Verma H, et al. Peripheral neuropathic symptoms in celiac disease and inflammatory bowel disease. *Clin Neuromuscul Dis.* 2012;13:137–145.
76. Hadjivassiliou M, Rao DG, Wharton SB, Sanders DS, Grünewald RA, Davies-Jones AG. Sensory ganglionopathy due to gluten sensitivity. *Neurology.* 2010;75:1003–1008.
77. Collin P, Maki M. Associated disorders in coeliac disease: Clinical adult coeliac disease. *Scand J Gastroenterol.* 1994;29:769–775.
78. Cooke WT, Smith WT. Neurological disorders associated with coeliac disease. *Brain.* 1966;86:686–718.
79. Hadjivassiliou M, Chattopadhyay AK, Davies-Jones GA, Gibsin A, Grunewald RA, Lobo AJ. Neuromuscular disorder as a presenting feature of coeliac disease. *J Neurol Neurosurg Psychiatry.* 1997;63:770–775.
80. Kaplan JG, Horoupian D, DeSouza T, Brin M, Schaumburg H, Pack D. Distal axonopathy associated with chronic gluten enteropathy: A treatable disorder. *Neurology.* 1988;38:642–645.
81. Brannagan TH III, Hays AP, Chin SS, et al. Small-fiber neuropathy/neuronopathy associated with celiac disease: Skin biopsy findings. *Arch Neurol.* 2005;62(10):1574–1578.
82. Gibbons CH, Freeman R. Autonomic neuropathy and coeliac disease. *J Neurol Neurosurg Psychiatry.* 2005;76(4):579–581.
83. Chin RL, Tseng VG, Green PH, Sander HW, Brannagan TH III, Latov N. Multifocal axonal polyneuropathy in celiac disease. *Neurology.* 2006;66(12):1923–1925.
84. Luostarinen L, Himanen SL, Luostarinen M, Collin P, Pirttila T. Neuromuscular and sensory disturbances in patients with well treated coeliac disease. *J Neurol Neurosurg Psychiatry.* 2003; 74(4):490–494.
85. Cicarelli G, Della Rocca G, Amboni M, et al. Clinical and neurological abnormalities in adult celiac disease. *Neurol Sci.* 2003;24(5):311–317.
86. Chad DA, Smith TW, DeGirolami U, Hammer K. Perineuritis and ulcerative colitis. *Neurology.* 1986;36:1377–1379.
87. Humbert P, Monnier G, Billerey C, Birgen C, Dupond JL. Polyneuropathy: An unusual extraintestinal manifestation if Crohn's disease. *Acta Neurol Scand.* 1989;80:301–306.
88. Konagaya Y, Konagaya M, Takayanagi T. Chronic polyneuropathy and ulcerative colitis. *Jpn J Med.* 1989;28:72–74.
89. Lossos A, Argov Z, Ackerman Z, Abramsky O. Peripheral neuropathy and folate deficiency as the first sign of Crohn's disease. *J Clin Gastroenterol.* 1991;13:442–444.
90. Zimmerman J, Steiner I, Gavish D, Argov Z. Guillain–Barré syndrome: A possible extraintestinal manifestation of ulcerative colitis? *J Clin Gastroenterol.* 1985;7:301–303.

91. Gondim FA, Brannagan TH III, Sander HW, Chin RL, Latov N. Peripheral neuropathy in patients with inflammatory bowel disease. *Brain*. 2005;128(Pt 4):867–879.
92. Nemni R, Fazio R, Corbo M, Sessa M, Comi G, Canal N. Peripheral neuropathy associated with Crohn's disease. *Neurology*. 1987;37:1414–1417.
93. Cohen MG, Webb J. Brachial neuritis with colitic arthritis [letter]. *Ann Intern Med*. 1987;106:780–781.
94. Singer OS, Otto B, Steinmetz H, Zieman U. Acute neuropathy with multiple conduction blocks after TNFα monoclonal antibody therapy. *Neurology*. 2004;63:1754.
95. Charron L, Peyronnard J-M, Marchand L. Sensory neuropathy associated with primary biliary cirrhosis. *Arch Neurol*. 1980;37:84–87.
96. Chaudhry V, Corse AM, O'Brien R, Cornblath DR, Klein AS, Thuluvath PJ. Autonomic and peripheral (sensorimotor) neuropathy in chronic liver disease: A clinical and electrophysiological study. *Hepatology*. 1999;29:1698–1703.
97. Ludwig J, Dyck PJ, LaRusso NF. Xanthomatous neuropathy of liver. *Hum Pathol*. 1982;13:1049–1051.
98. Singh S, Kumar N, Loftus EV Jr, Kane SV. Neurologic complications in patients with inflammatory bowel disease: Increasing relevance in the era of biologics. *Inflamm Bowel Dis*. 2013;19(4):864–872.
99. Sassi SB, Kallel L, Ben Romdhane S, Boubaker J, Filali A, Hentati F. Peripheral neuropathy in inflammatory bowel disease patients: A prospective cohort study. *Scand J Gastroenterol*. 2009;44:1268–1269.
100. Chusid MJ, Dale DC, West BC, Wolff SM. The hypereosinophilic syndrome: Analysis of fourteen cases with review of the literature. *Medicine*. 1975;54:1–17.
101. Dorfman LJ, Ransom BR, Forno LS, Kelts A. Neuropathy in the hypereosinophilic syndrome. *Muscle Nerve*. 1983;6:291–298.
102. Monaco S, Lucci B, Laperchia N, et al. Polyneuropathy in hypereosinophilic syndrome. *Neurology*. 1988;38:494–496.
103. Bolton CF, McKneown MJ, Chen R, Toth B, Remtulla H. Subacute uremic and diabetic polyneuropathy. *Muscle Nerve*. 1997;20:59–64.
104. Ropper AH. Accelerated neuropathy of renal failure. *Arch Neurol*. 1993;50:536–539.
105. Amato AA, Dumitru D. Acquired neuropathies. In: Dumitru D, Amato AA, Zwarts M, eds. *Electrodiagnostic Medicine*. 2nd ed. Philadelphia, PA: Hanley & Belfus, Inc; 2002:937–1041.
106. Krishnan AV, Kiernan MC. Uremic neuropathy: Clinical features and new pathophysiological insights. *Muscle Nerve*. 2007;35:273–290.
107. Ho DT, Rodig NM, Kim HB, et al. Rapid reversal of uremic neuropathy following renal transplantation in an adolescent. *Pediatr Transplant*. 2012;16(7):E296–E300.
108. Bolton CF, Driedger AA, Lindsay RM. Ischaemic neuropathy in uraemic patients caused by bovine arteriovenous shunt. *J Neurol Neurosurg Psychiatry*. 1979;42:810–814.
109. Ogura T, Makinodan A, Kubo T, Hayashida T, Hirasawa Y. Electrophysiological course of uraemic neuropathy in haemodialysis patients. *Postgrad Med J*. 2001;77(909):451–454.
110. Thomas PK, Hillinrake K, Lascelles RG, et al. The polyneuropathy of chronic renal failure. *Brain*. 1971;94:761–780.
111. Dyck PJ, Johnson WJ, Lambert EH, O'Brien PC. Segmental demyelination secondary to axonal degeneration in uremic neuropathy. *Mayo Clin Proc*. 1971;46:400–431.
112. Bolton CF, Baltzan MA, Baltzan RF. Effects of renal transplantation in uremic neuropathy. A clinical and electrophysiologic study. *N Engl J Med*. 1971;284:1170–1175.
113. Bolton CF, Lindasy RM, Linton AL. The course of uremic neuropathy during chronic hemodialysis. *Can J Neurol Sci*. 1975;2:332–333.
114. Bolton CF. Electrophysiologic changes in uremic neuropathy after successful renal transplantation. *Neurology*. 1976;26:152–161.
115. Bolton CF. Peripheral neuropathies associated with chronic renal failure. *Can J Neurol Sci*. 1980;7:89–96.
116. Oh SJ, Clements RS, Lee YW, Diethelm AG. Rapid improvement in nerve conduction velocity following renal transplantation. *Ann Neurol*. 1978;4:369–373.
117. Kardel T, Nielsen VK. Hepatic neuropathy: A clinical and electrophysiological study. *Acta Neurol Scand*. 1974;50:513–526.
118. Knill-Jones RP, Goodwill CJ, Dayan AD, Williams R. Peripheral neuropathy in chronic liver disease: Clinical, electrodiagnostic, and nerve biopsy findings. *J Neurol Neurosurg Psychiatry*. 1972;35:22–30.
119. Seneviratne KN, Peiris OA. Peripheral nerve function in chronic liver disease. *J Neurol Neurosurg Psychiatry*. 1970;33:609–614.
120. Lee JH, Jung WJ, Choi KH, Chun MH, Ha SB, Lee SK. Nerve conduction study on patients with severe liver syndrome and its change after transplantation. *Clin Transplant*. 2002;16(6):430–432.
121. McDougall AJ, Davies L, McCaughan GW. Autonomic and peripheral neuropathy in endstage liver disease and following liver transplantation. *Muscle Nerve*. 2003;28(5):595–600.
122. Cruz Martinez A, Gonzalez P, Garza E, Bescansa E, Anciones B. Electro-physiologic follow-up in Whipple's disease. *Muscle Nerve*. 1987;10:616–620.
123. Halperin JJ, Landis DM, Kleinman GM. Whipple disease of the nervous system. *Neurology*. 1982;32:612–617.
124. Gerard A, Sarrot-Reynauld F, Liozon E, et al. Neurologic presentation of Whipple disease: Report of 12 cases and review of the literature. *Medicine*. 2002;81(6):443–457.
125. Pauletti C, Pujia F, Accorinti M, et al. An atypical case of neuro-Whipple: Clinical presentation, magnetic resonance spectroscopy and follow-up. *J Neurol Sci*. 2010;297:97–100.
126. Delaney P. Gouty neuropathy. *Arch Neurol*. 1983;40:823–824.
127. Bolton CF, Gilbert JJ, Hahn AF, Sibbald WJ. Polyneuropathy in critically ill patients. *J Neurol Neurosurg Psychiatry*. 1984;47:1223–1231.
128. Bolton CF, Laverty DA, Brown JD, Witt NJ, Hahn AF, Sibbald WJ. Critically ill polyneuropathy: Electrophysiological studies and differentiation from Guillain–Barré syndrome. *J Neurol Neurosurg Psychiatry*. 1986;49:563–573.
129. Leijten FS, Harink-de Weerd JE, Poortvleit DC, de Weerd AW. The role of polyneuropathy in motor convalescence after prolonged mechanical ventilation. *JAMA*. 1995;274:1221–1225.
130. Zochodne DW, Bolton CF, Wells GA, et al. Critical illness polyneuropathy: A complication of sepsis and multiple organ failure. *Brain*. 1987;110:819–842.
131. Deconinck N, Van Parijs V, Beckers-Bleukx G, Van den Bergh P. Critical illness myopathy unrelated to corticosteroids or neuromuscular blocking agents. *Neuromuscul Disord*. 1998;8:186–192.
132. Lacomis D, Smith TW, Chad DA. Acute myopathy and neuropathy in status asthmaticus: Case report and literature review. *Muscle Nerve*. 1993;16:84–90.

133. Lacomis D, Giuliani MJ, Van Cott A, Kramer DJ. Acute myopathy of the intensive care: Clinical, electromyographic, and pathological aspects. *Ann Neurol.* 1996;40:645–654.
134. Lacomis D, Petrella JT, Giuliani MJ. Causes of neuromuscular weakness in the intensive care unit: A study of ninety-two patients. *Muscle Nerve.* 1998;21:610–617.
135. Rich MM, Teener JW, Raps EC, Schotland DL, Bird SJ. Muscle is electrically inexcitable in acute quadriplegic myopathy. *Neurology.* 1996;46:731–736.
136. Rich MM, Bird SJ, Raps EC, McClaskey LF, Teener JW. Direct muscle stimulation in acute quadriplegic myopathy. *Muscle Nerve.* 1997;20:665–673.
137. Zochodne DW, Ramsey DA, Saly V, Shelley S, Moffatt S. Acute necrotizing myopathy of the intensive care: Electrophysiological studies. *Muscle Nerve.* 1994;17:285–292.
138. Barohn RJ, Jackson CE, Rogers SJ, Ridings LW, McVey AL. Prolonged paralysis due to nondepolarizing neuromuscular blocking agents and corticosteroids. *Muscle Nerve.* 1994;17:647–654.
139. Sander HW, Golden M, Danon MJ. Quadriplegic areflexic ICU illness: Selective thick filament loss and normal nerve histology. *Muscle Nerve.* 2002;26(4):499–505.
140. Carver N, Logan A. Critical illness polyneuropathy associated with burns: A case report. *Burns.* 1989;15:179–180.
141. Marquez S, Turley JJ, Peters WJ. Neuropathy in burn patients. *Brain.* 1993;116:471–483.
142. Z'Graggen WJ, Lin CS, Howard RS, Beale RJ, Bostock H. Nerve excitability changes in critical illness polyneuropathy. *Brain.* 2006;129(Pt 9):2461–2470.
143. Mahloudji M, Teasdall RD, Adamkiewicz JJ. The genetic amyloidosis with particular reference to hereditary neuropathic amyloidosis Type II (Indiana or Rukavina type). *Medicine.* 1969;l48:1–37.
144. Kyle RA, Bayrd ED. Amyloidosis: Review of 236 cases. *Medicine.* 1975;54:271–299.
145. Rukavina JG, Block WD, Jacksone CE. Primary systemic amyloidosis: A review and an experimental genetic and clinical study of 29 cases with particular emphasis on the familial form. *Medicine.* 1956;35:239–334.
146. Adams D. Hereditary and acquired amyloid polyneuropathy. *J Neurol.* 2001;248:647–657.
147. Lachmann HJ, Chir B, Booth DR, et al. Misdiagnosis of hereditary amyloidosis as AL (primary) amyloidosis. *N Engl J Med.* 2002;346:1786–1791.
148. Rajani B, Rajani V, Prayson RA. Peripheral nerve amyloidosis in sural nerve biopsies: A clinicopathologic analysis of 13 cases. *Arch Pathol Lab Med.* 2000;124(1):114–118.
149. Klein CJ, Vrana JA, Theis JD, et al. Mass spectrometric-based proteomic analysis of amyloid neuropathy type in nerve tissue. *Arch Neurol.* 2011;68:195–199.
150. Duston MA, Skinner M, Anderson J, Cohen AS. Peripheral neuropathy as an early marker of AL amyloidosis. *Arch Intern Med.* 1989;149:358–360.
151. Kelly JJ Jr, Kyle RA, O'Brien PC, Dyck PJ. The natural history of peripheral neuropathy in primary systemic amyloidosis. *Ann Neurol.* 1979;6:1–7.
152. Kyle RA, Greipp PR. Amyloidosis (AL). Clinical and laboratory features in 229 cases. *Mayo Clin Proc.* 1983;58:665–683.
153. Vucic S, Chon PS, Cros D. Atypical presentations of amyloid neuropathy. *Muscle Nerve.* 2003;28(6):696–702.
154. Tracy JA, Dyck PJ, Dyck PJ. Primary amyloidosis presenting as upper limb multiple mononeuropathies. *Muscle Nerve.* 2010;41:710–715.
155. Mathis S, Magy L, Diallo L, Boukhris S, Vallat JM. Amyloid neuropathy mimicking chronic inflammatory demyelinating polyneuropathy. *Muscle Nerve.* 2012;45:26–31.
156. Andersson R, Blom S. Neurophysiological studies in primary hereditary amyloidosis with polyneuropathy. *Acta Med Scand.* 1972;191:233–239.
157. Dyck PJ, Lambert EH. Dissociated sensation in amyloidosis. *Arch Neurol.* 1969;20:490–507.
158. Thomas PK, King RH. Peripheral nerve changes in amyloid neuropathy. *Brain.* 1974;97:395–406.
159. Berghoff M, Kathpal M, Khan F, Skinner M, Falk R, Freeman R. Endothelial dysfunction precedes C-fiber abnormalities in primary (AL) amyloidosis. *Ann Neurol.* 2003;53(6):725–730.
160. Skinner M, Sanchorowala V, Seldin DC, et al. High dose melphalan and autologous stem-cell transplantation in patients with AL amyloidosis. An 8-year study. *Ann Intern Med.* 2004;140:85–93.
161. Dispenzieri A, Kyle RA, Lancy MG, et al. Superior survival in primary systemic amyloidosis patients undergoing peripheral blood stem cell transplantation: A case control study. *Blood.* 2004;101:3960–3963.
162. Dingli D, Tan TS, Kumar SK, et al. Stem cell transplantation in patients with autonomic neuropathy due to primary (AL) amyloidosis. *Neurology.* 2010;74:913–918.
163. Blom S, Steen L, Zetterlund B. Familial amyloidosis with polyneuropathy type I. *Acta Neurol Scand.* 1981;63:99–110.
164. Boysen G, Galassi G, Kamieniecka Z, Schlaeger J, Trojaborg W. Familial amyloidosis with cranial neuropathy and corneal lattice dystrophy. *J Neurol Neurosurg Psychiatry.* 1979;42:1020–1030.
165. Hanyu N, Ikeda S, Nakadai A, Yanagisawa N, Powell HC. Peripheral nerve pathological findings in familial amyloid polyneuropathy: A correlative study of proximal sciatic nerve and sural nerve lesions. *Ann Neurol.* 1989;25:340–350.
166. Hund E, Linke RP, Willig F, Graus A. Transthyretin-associated neuropathic amyloidosis. Pathogenesis and treatment. *Neurology.* 2001;56:431–435.
167. Luis ML. Electroneurophysiological studies in familial amyloid polyneuropathy–Portuguese type. *J Neurol Neurosurg Psychiatry.* 1978;41:847–850.
168. Sobue G, Nakao N, Murakami K, et al. Type I familial amyloid polyneuropathy. *Brain.* 1990;113:903–919.
169. Luigetti M, Conte A, Del Grande A, et al. TTR-related amyloid neuropathy: Clinical, electrophysiological and pathological findings in 15 unrelated patients. *Neurol Sci.* 2013;34(7):1057–1063.
170. Blanco-Jerez CR, Jimenez-Escrig A, Gobernado JM, et al. Transthyretin Tyr77 familial amyloid polyneuropathy: A clinicopathological study of a large kindred. *Muscle Nerve.* 1998;21:1478–1485.
171. Briemberg HR, Amato AA. Transthyretin amyloidosis presenting with multifocal demyelinating mononeuropathies. *Muscle Nerve.* 2004;29(2):318–22.
172. Anrade C. A peculiar form of peripheral neuropathy. *Brain.* 1952;75:408–426.
173. Plante-Bordeneuve V, Lalu T, Misrahi M, et al. Genotypic-phenotypic variations in a series of 65 patients with familial amyloid polyneuropathy. *Neurology.* 1998;51:708–714.

174. Planté-Bordeneuve V, Ferreira A, Lalu T, et al. Diagnostic pitfalls in sporadic transthyretin familial amyloid polyneuropathy (TTR-FAP). *Neurology*. 2007;69:693–698.
175. Planté-Bordeneuve V, Said G. Familial amyloid polyneuropathy. *Lancet Neurol*. 2011;10:1086–1097.
176. Benson MD, Kincaid JC. The molecular biology and clinical features of amyloid neuropathy. *Muscle Nerve*. 2007;36:411–423.
177. Cappellari M, Cavallaro T, Ferrarini M, et al. Variable presentations of TTR-related familial amyloid polyneuropathy in seventeen patients. *J Peripher Nerv Syst*. 2011;16:119–129.
178. Bergethon PR, Sabin TD, Lewis D, Simms RW, Cohen AS, Skinner M. Improvement in the polyneuropathy associated with familial amyloid polyneuropathy after liver transplantation. *Neurology*. 1996;47:944–951.
179. Adams D, Samule D, Goulin-Goeau C, et al. The course and prognostic factors of familial amyloid polyneuropathy after liver transplantation. *Brain*. 2000;123:1495–1504.
180. Berk JL, Suhr OB, Sekijima Y, et al. The Diflunisal Trial: Study accrual and drug tolerance. *Amyloid*. 2012;19:37–38.
181. Van Allen MW, Frolich JA, Davis JR. Inherited predisposition to generalized amyloidosis. *Neurology*. 1969;19:10–25.
182. Joy T, Wang J, Hahn A, Hegele RA. APOA1 related amyloidosis: A case report and literature review. *Clin Biochem*. 2003;36:641–645.
183. Nichols WC, Gregg RE, Brewer BH, Benson MD. A mutation in apolipoprotein A1 Iowa type of familial amyloidotic polyneuropathy. *Genomics*. 1990;8:318–323.
184. Pihlamaa T, Suominen S, Kiuru-Enari S. Familial amyloidotic polyneuropathy type IV–gelsolin amyloidosis. *Amyloid*. 2012;19:30–33.
185. Asahina A, Yokoyama T, Ueda M, et al. Hereditary gelsolin amyloidosis: A new Japanese case with cutis laxa as a diagnostic clue. *Acta Derm Venereol*. 2011;91:201–203.
186. Kiuru-Enari S, Keski-Oja J, Haltia M. Cutis laxa in hereditary gelsolin amyloidosis. *Br J Dermatol*. 2005;152:250–257.
187. Meretoja J. Familial systemic paramyloidosis with lattice dystrophy of the cornea, progressive cranial neuropathy, skin changes and various internal symptoms. *Ann Clin Res*. 1969;1:314–324.
188. Haltia M, Levy E, Meretohi J, Fernandez-Madrid I, Koivunene O, Frangione B. Gelsolin gene mutation at codon 187 in familial amyloidosis, Finnish: DNA-diagnostic assay. *Am J Med*. 1992;42:357–359.
189. Kiuru-Enari S, Somer H, Seppalainen AM, Notkola IL, Haltia M. Neuromuscular pathology in hereditary gelsolin amyloidosis. *J Neuropathol Exp Neurol*. 2002;61(6):565–571.
190. Gorevic PD, Munoz PC, Gorgone G, et al. Amyloidosis due to a mutation in the gelsolin gene in an American family with lattice corneal dystrophy type II. *N Engl J Med*. 1991;325:1780–1785.
191. Kiuru S. Gelsolin-related familial amyloidosis, Finnish type (FAF), and its variants found worldwide. *Amyloid*. 1998;5:55–66.
192. Maury CP, Liljestrom M, Boysen G, Tornroth T, de la Chapelle A, Nurmiaho-Lassila EL. Danish type gelsolin related amyloidosis: 654G-T mutation is associated with a disease pathogenetically and clinically similar to that caused by the 654G-A mutation (familial amyloidosis of the Finnish type). *J Clin Pathol*. 2000;53:95–99.

CHAPTER 17

Neuropathies Associated with Infections

Neuropathies can result directly from various bacterial and viral infections, as well as from an indirect or parainfectious autoimmune response to the infection (Table 17-1). Parainfectious neuropathies (e.g., Guillain–Barré syndrome associated with various infections and vasculitis associated with hepatitis) are discussed in detail in other chapters.

► LEPROSY (HANSEN DISEASE)

CLINICAL FEATURES

Leprosy is caused by the acid-fast bacteria *Mycobacterium leprae*. Leprosy is the most common cause of peripheral neuropathy in Southeast Asia, Africa, and South America. The main route of transmission is felt to be from person-to-person spread via nasal droplets. The bacteria is very slow growing with an incubation period that can vary between 2 and 40 years, customarily between 5 and 7 years.[1]

There is a spectrum of clinical manifestations ranging from tuberculoid leprosy at one end to lepromatous leprosy on the other end of the spectrum, with borderline leprosy in between based upon the Ridley–Joplin classification (Table 17-2).[1–5] The World Health Organization (WHO) introduced a simpler classification based on the number of skin lesions to help guide treatment: multibacillary (six more skin lesions) and paucibacillary (fewer than six skin lesions) leprosy.[1] In general, lepromatous leprosy is always multibacillary, and tuberculoid leprosy is usually paucibacillary; borderline leprosy can be either multibacillary or paucibacillary. The clinical manifestations of the disease are determined by the immunological response of the host to the infection. In tuberculoid leprosy, the cell-mediated immune response is intact.[1–5] Thus, there are focal, circumscribed inflammatory responses to the bacteria within the affected areas of skin and nerves. The resulting skin lesions appear as well-defined, scattered hypopigmented patches and plaques with raised, erythematous borders (Figs. 17-1 and 17-2). Cutaneous nerves are often affected, resulting in a loss of sensation in the center of these skin lesions. Cooler regions of the body (e.g., face and limbs) are more susceptible than warmer regions such as the groin or axilla. In addition, the ulnar nerve at the medial epicondyle, the median nerve at the distal forearm, the peroneal nerve at the fibular head, the sural nerve, the greater auricular nerve, and the superficial radial nerve at the wrist are common sites of involvement and become encased with granulomas, leading to mononeuropathy or mononeuropathy multiplex. These nerves are thickened and often palpable.

In lepromatous leprosy, cell-mediated immunity is severely impaired, leading to extensive infiltration of the bacilli and hematogenous dissemination, producing confluent and symmetrical areas of rash, anesthesia, and anhidrosis.[1–5] Neuropathies tend to be more severe in the lepromatous subtype. As in the tuberculoid form, there is a predilection for the involvement of cooler regions of the body. Infiltration of the organism in the face leads to the loss of eyebrows and eyelashes and exaggeration of the natural skin folds, leading to the so-called "leonine facies." Superficial cutaneous nerves of the ears and distal limbs are also commonly affected. A slowly progressive symmetric sensorimotor polyneuropathy gradually develops due to widespread invasion of the bacilli into the epi-, peri-, and endoneurium. Distal extremity weakness may be seen, but large fiber sensory modalities and muscle stretch reflexes are relatively spared. Involvement of nerve trunks leads to superimposed mononeuropathies, including facial neuropathy.

Neuropathies are most common in patients with borderline leprosy.[2,3,5] Patients can develop generalized symmetric sensorimotor polyneuropathies, mononeuropathies, and mononeuropathy multiplex, including multiple mononeuropathies in atypical locations, such as the brachial plexus. Borderline leprosy is associated with clinical and histological features of both the lepromatous and the tuberculoid forms of leprosy (Table 17-2 and Fig. 17-3). There is partial impairment in cellular immunity in patients with borderline leprosy, such that there is some degree of mycobacterial spread as well as an inflammatory response. The immunological state is considered unstable in patients with borderline leprosy in that the immune response and clinical manifestations can shift up and down the spectrum.

Patients with leprosy may present with isolated peripheral neuropathy without skin lesions, particularly in endemic areas.[6,7] Most cases of the so-called pure neuritic leprosy have the tuberculoid or borderline tuberculoid subtypes of the disease.

▶ TABLE 17-1. **INFECTIOUS AGENTS ASSOCIATED WITH NEUROPATHIES**

Bacterial:
Mycobacterium leprae (Leprosy)
Borrelia burdorferi (Lyme disease)
Corynebacterium diphtheriae (Diphtheria)
Viral:
Human immunodeficiency virus (HIV)
Distal symmetric polyneuropathy
Acute inflammatory demyelinating polyradiculoneuropathy
Chronic inflammatory demyelinating polyradiculoneuropathy
Other polyradiculoneuropathy
Mononeuropathy multiplex
Autonomic neuropathy
Sensory ganglionopathy
Human T-lymphocytic type 1 (HTLV-1)
Cytomegalovirus (CMV)
Hepatitis B and C
Herpes varicella-zoster (HVZ)

LABORATORY FEATURES

Sensory nerve conduction studies (NCS) are usually absent in the lower limb and are reduced in amplitude in the arms.[1,6,7] Motor NCS may demonstrate reduced amplitudes in affected nerves.[8,9] Motor conduction velocities are normal or slightly reduced; however, a few patients may demonstrate values less than 20 m/s in both the upper and the lower limb. Electromyography (EMG) reveals mild-to-moderate degrees of active denervation. The pattern of involvement on the EMG and NCS can be generalized as symmetric or reflective of a mononeuropathy or multiple mononeuropathies, as apparent from the clinical features. Ultrasound can demonstrate enlarged axons, particularly of the median nerve in distal forearm near the carpal tunnel and of the ulnar nerve just proximal to the medial epicondyle (Fig. 17-4).[10]

▶ TABLE 17-2. **CLINICAL, LABORATORY, IMMUNOLOGICAL, AND HISTOPATHOLOGICAL FEATURES OF LEPROSY**

	Tuberculous Leprosy (TT)	Mid-Borderline Leprosy (BB)	Lepromatous Leprosy (LL)
Lepromin test	Positive (>5 mm induration)	+/− (2–5 mm induration)	Negative (0–2 mm induration)
Bacterial index	0	2–4	5–6
Morphological index (MI)	Low (down to zero)	Moderate	High (up to 10)
Immunology	Cell-mediated immunity: intact; CD4 > CD8 lymphocytes; Th1 cytokines expressed: IL-2 and γ-IF	Cell-mediated immunity: unstable (can range and switch from intact to absent)	Cell-mediated immunity: absent; CD8 > CD4 lymphocytes; Th2 cytokines expressed: IL-4, IL-5, and IL-10
Skin lesions	Few localized and well-demarcated large skin lesions; erythematous macules and plaques with raised borders; centers of lesions may be hypopigmented	Size, number, and appearance of the skin lesions are intermediate between that seen in the TT and LL poles	Multiple, symmetrical small macules and papules; older lesions form plaques and nodules
Histopathology	Localized granulomas and giant cells encompassed by dense lymphocytic infiltrate extending to epidermis; Fite stain: negative for bacteria	Granulomas with epithelioid cells but no giant cells Not localized by zones of lymphocytes Lymphocytes, if present, are diffusely infiltrating Fite stain: slightly positive	Scant lymphocytes, but if present diffuse along with organism-laden foamy macrophages Fite stain: marked positive
Neuropathies	Mononeuropathy of the superficial cutaneous nerves or large nerve trunks (i.e., ulnar, median, and peroneal nerves), multiple mononeuropathies; pure neuritic leprosy may be seen	The neuropathies can range in the spectrum of that seen in TT to LL	Distal symmetric sensory and sensorimotor polyneuropathies are more common than mononeuropathy; pure neuritic leprosy is not seen
Treatment[a]	Paucibacillary Dapsone 100 mg daily Rifampin 600 mg per month Duration: 6 months		Multibacillary Dapsone 100 mg daily Rifampin 600 mg per month Clofazimine 300 mg per month and 50 mg daily Duration: 1–2 years or until skin smears is zero

The features of the borderline tuberculoid (BT) form ranges between the TT and BB forms. The features of the borderline lepromatous (BL) form ranges between that seen in BB and LL forms of leprosy.
[a]Treatment based on World Health Organization recommendations.

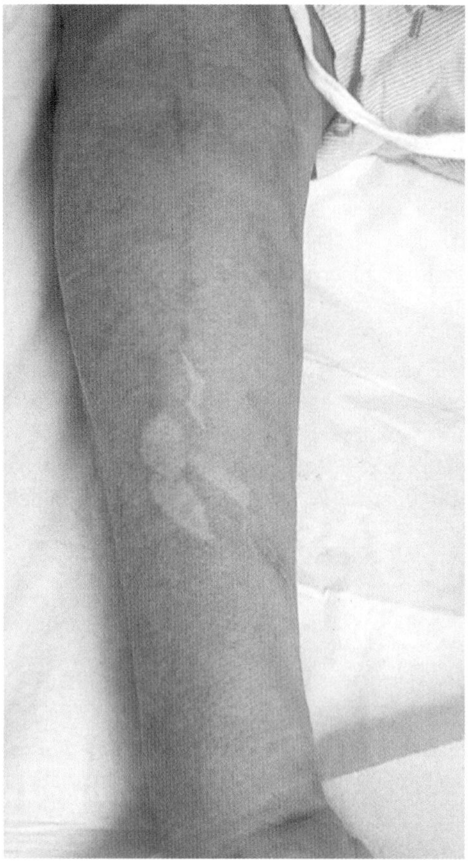

Figure 17-1. Tuberculoid leprosy. Hypopigmented skin lesions are evident on lateral aspect of forearm in a patient with tuberculoid leprosy.

HISTOPATHOLOGY

Leprosy is usually diagnosed with skin lesion biopsy and using the Fite method to stain the acid-fast bacilli red (Fig. 17-3).[3] The morphological index (MI) is the ratio of viable to non-viable organisms on skin smears. The bacteriological index (BI) is a logarithmically scaled measure of the density of bacilli in the dermis. Both the MI and BI have been used to measure treatment response.

The host's immune response to the bacilli determines the histopathology (Table 17-2).[1–5] Nerve biopsies can also be diagnostic, particularly when there are no apparent skin lesions. The tuberculoid form is characterized by granulomas formed by macrophages and T lymphocytes (CD4 T lymphocytes greater than CD8). Caseating granulomas may or may not be present. Importantly, bacilli are not seen. In contrast, with lepromatous leprosy, large number of infiltrating bacilli, CD8 greater than CD4 lymphocytes, and organism-laden, foamy macrophages with minimal granulomatous infiltration are evident (Fig. 17-5A). The bacilli are best appreciated using the Fite stain, where they can be seen as red staining rods in clusters within the endoneurium, within macrophages, or within Schwann cells (Fig. 17-5B). On electron microscopy, the bacilli appear as dense osmiophilic rods surrounded by a clear halo (Figs. 17-5C and D). Borderline leprosy can have histological features of both tuberculoid and lepromatous leprosy.

PATHOGENESIS

The clinical and pathological spectrum of the disease is dependent on the host's immune response to *M. leprae* and reflects the relative balance between the Th1 and Th2 response (Table 17-2).[1–5] The tuberculoid form defines one end of the spectrum, in which the CD4 T cells predominate. These CD4 T cells produce interleukin-2 and gamma-interferon which in turn lead to activation of macrophages. On the other extreme, the lepromatous form is dominated by CD8 cells, which produce interleukin-4, interleukin-5, and interleukin-10, thereby downregulating cell-mediated immunity and inhibiting macrophages. The borderline subtypes exhibit immune responses spanning the spectrum between the tuberculoid and lepromatous forms.

TREATMENT

Patients are treated with multiple drugs: dapsone, rifampicin, and clofazimine depending on the form of leprosy they have (Table 17-2).[1–4] The current WHO recommendations for adults with multibacillary leprosy are as follows: rifampicin (600 mg once a month), dapsone (100 mg daily), and clofazimine (300 mg once a month and 50 mg daily) for 1 to 2 years.[11] For adults with paucibacillary leprosy, the WHO recommends rifampicin (600 mg once a month) and dapsone (100 mg daily) for 6 months.[11] For adults with single skin lesion paucibacillary leprosy the recommended WHO regimen is a single dose of rifampicin: 600 mg, ofloxacin: 400 mg, and minocycline: 100 mg. Proven relapses are re-treated with multidrug regimen.

The WHO recommendations are controversial as there have been no clinical trials to support their efficacy and the relapse rate of multibacillary leprosy is high. Thus, some advocate for more aggressive treatment based in part on Ridley–Joplin classification: tuberculoid leprosy to be treated with dapsone 100 mg daily for 5 years and lepromatous leprosy to be treated with rifampin 600 mg daily for 3 years and dapsone 100 mg daily for life.[1]

Patients should be instructed on the side effects of these medications before starting treatment. Rifampicin may make the urine turn a slightly reddish color for a few hours after its intake. Clofazimine causes brownish-black discoloration and dryness of skin. However, this disappears within few months after stopping treatment. The main side effect of dapsone is allergic reaction, causing itchy

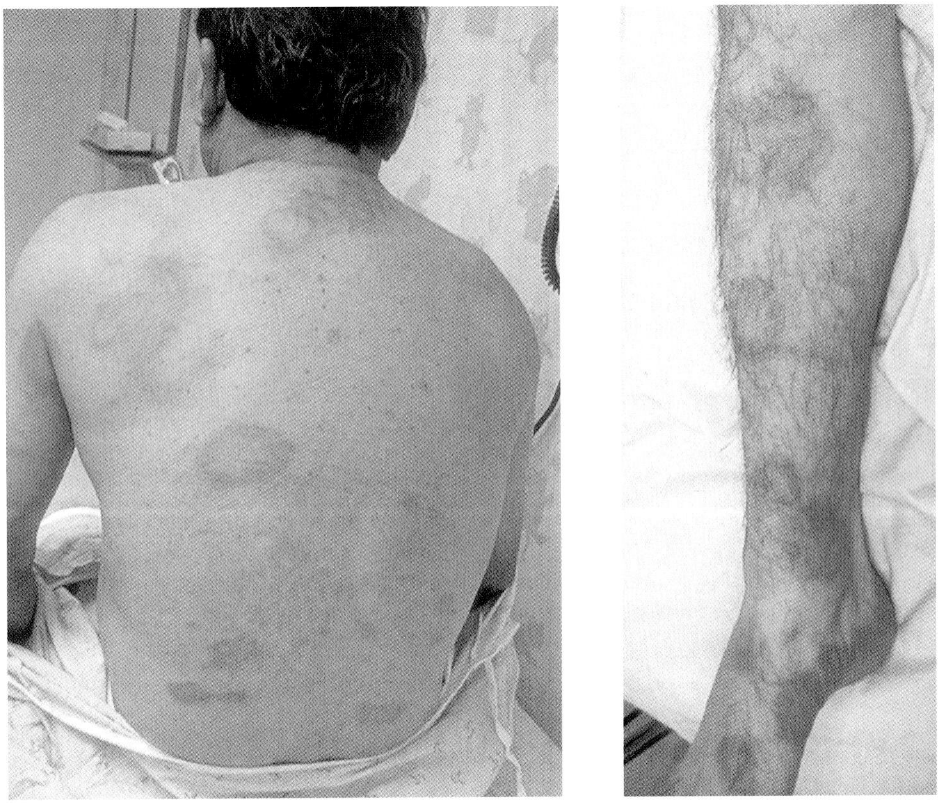

A B

Figure 17-2. Borderline leprosy. A patient with borderline leprosy has multiple skin lesions with hypopigmented center with raised erythematous borders on the back **(A)** and on the leg **(B)**. (Reproduced with permission from Amato AA, Dumitru D. Acquired neuropathies. In: Dumitru D, Amato AA, Swartz MJ, eds. *Electrodiagnostic Medicine*, 2nd ed. Philadelphia, PA: Hanley & Belfus; 2002.)

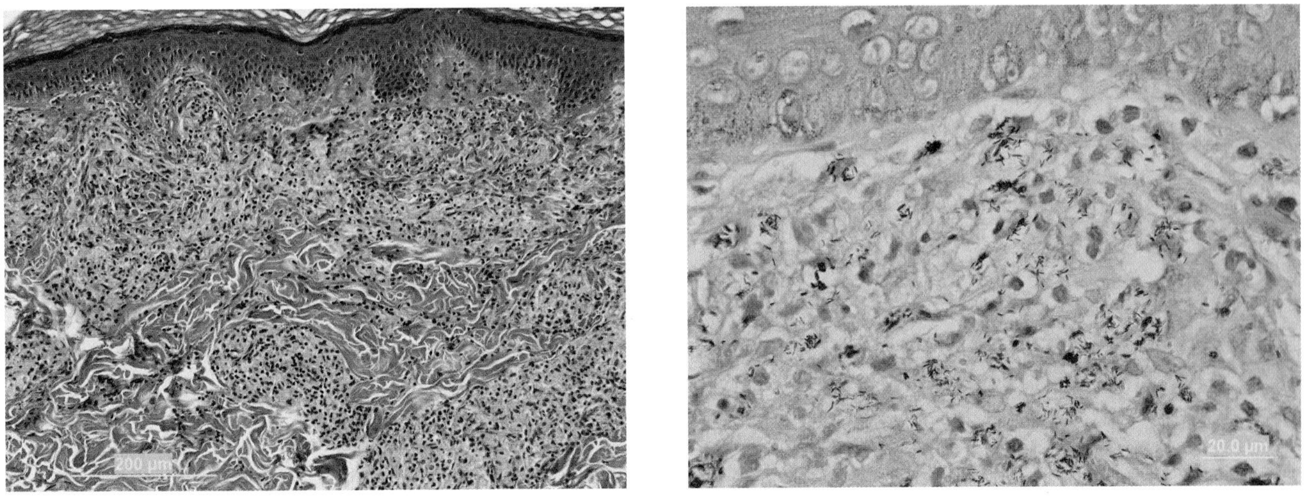

A B

Figure 17-3. Borderline leprosy. Skin biopsy demonstrates marked inflammatory cell infiltrate, H&E **(A)**. Red staining bacilli are evident on higher power with a Fite stain **(B)**.

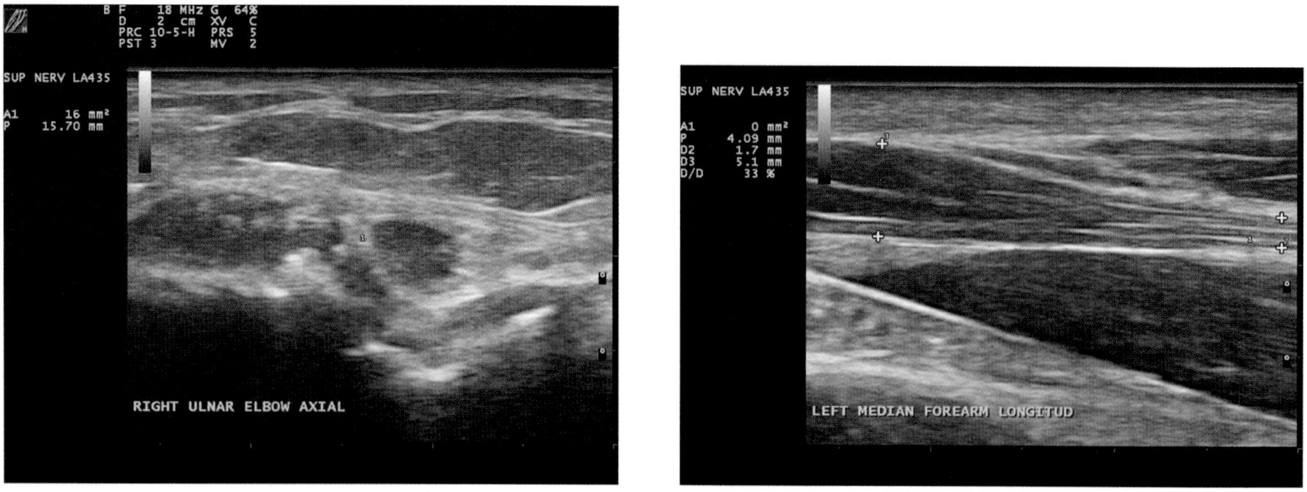

A B

Figure 17-4. Ultrasound in patient with lepromatous leprosy demonstrates swelling of the ulnar nerve at that elbow just proximal to the medial epicondyle with an area of 16 mm-squared (normal <10 mm^2) **(A)**. There was also swelling of the median nerve in the distal forearm as it approached the carpel tunnel as the diameter 1.4 mm at D2 to 5.1 mm **(B)**.

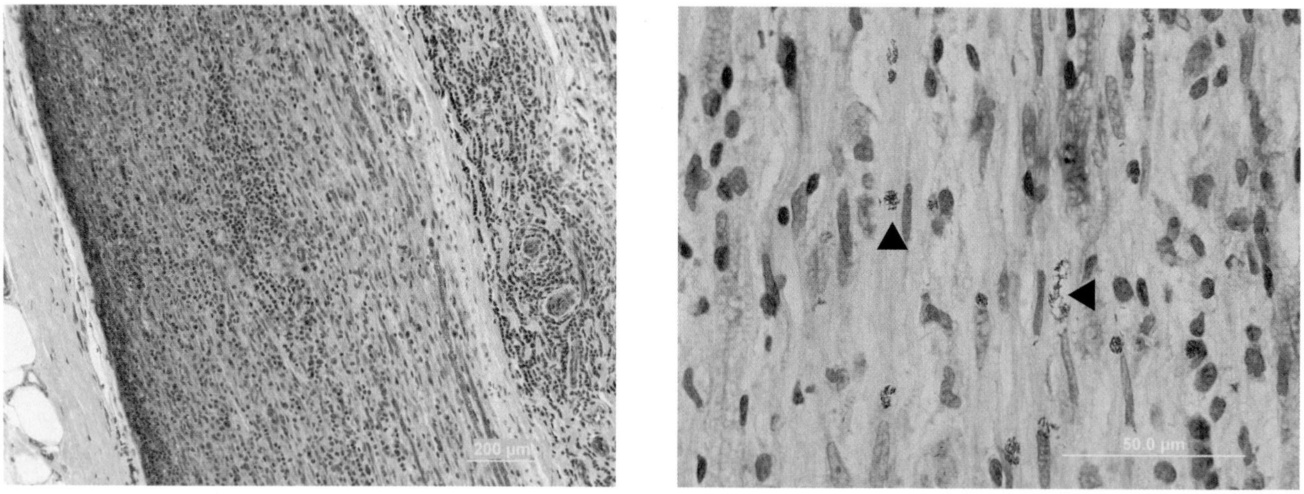

A B

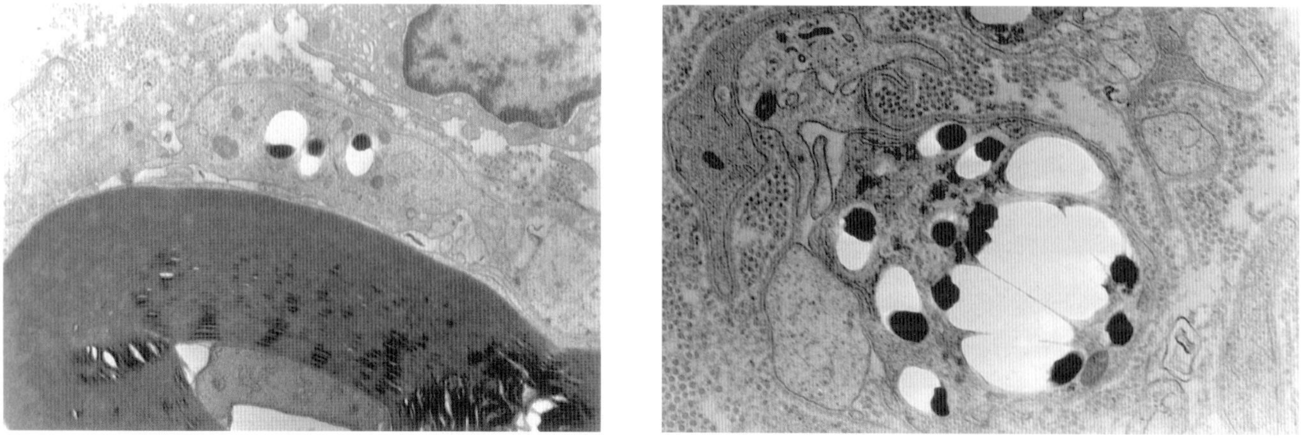

C D

Figure 17-5. Borderline leprosy. Sural nerve biopsy perivascular and diffuse endoneurial inflammation consisting of lymphocytes and macrophages, paraffin section stained with trichrome **(A)**. Fite stain reveals red staining bacilli (the so-called "red snappers") sometimes in clusters in the endoneurium and within Schwann cells **(B)**. Electron microscopy reveals electron-dense bacilli with surrounding clear halos within the cytoplasm of a Schwann cell surrounding a myelinated axon **(C)** and on higher power within a Schwann cell surrounding unmyelinated axons **(D)**.

skin rashes and exfoliative dermatitis. Patients known to be allergic to drugs containing sulfa should not be given dapsone.

Treatment is sometimes complicated by the so-called reversal reaction, particularly in borderline leprosy.[1–3] The reversal reaction can occur at any time during treatment and develops because of a shift to the tuberculoid end of the spectrum, as the result of an increase in cellular immunity during treatment. The cellular response is upregulated as evidenced by an increased release of tumor necrosis factor-alpha, gamma-interferon, and interleukin-2 with new granuloma formation. This can result in an exacerbation of the skin lesions and the neuropathy. High-dose corticosteroids blunt this adverse reaction and is often used prophylactically in high-risk patients (i.e., those with borderline leprosy) at treatment onset.

Erythema nodosum leprosum is another adverse reaction that usually occurs during treatment of patients with lepromatous leprosy.[1–3,12] Multiple erythematous, sometimes painful, subcutaneous nodules appear, and may be associated with worsening of the neuropathy. Erythema nodosum leprosum probably results from slow degradation of bacilli and release of new antigens. Subsequently, antigen–antibody complexes form and complement is activated in affected tissue. Erythema nodosum leprosum is commonly treated with corticosteroids, clofazimine, or thalidomide.

A recent review looked at 13 studies involving 445 participants treated for erythema nodosum leprosum with corticosteroids, clofazimine, thalidomide, and other agents (i.e., pentoxifylline, indomethacin, and levamisole).[12] The quality of the trials was generally poor and results could not be pooled due to the treatments being so heterogeneous. That said, clofazimine treatment was felt to be superior to prednisolone and thalidomide.[12]

Prevention of leprosy is of primary importance. It is recommended that children exposed to leprosy in the household be prophylactically treated with rifampin daily for 6 months.[2,3] Various vaccinations are available, including BCG, killed leprae, and chemically modified organisms.

▶ LYME DISEASE

CLINICAL FEATURES

Lyme disease is caused by infection with *Borrelia burgdorferi*, a spirochete, transmitted by ticks. The deer tick, *Ixodes dammini*, is responsible for the disease in most cases. Ticks acquire the spirochetes by feeding on an infected host (e.g., deer) and then transmit the spirochetes to the next host (e.g., humans) at a later feed. It takes approximately 12–24 hours of tick attachment to transfer the spirochetes.

There are three recognized stages of Lyme disease: (1) early infection with localized erythema migrans, (2) disseminated infection, and (3) late-stage infection. The localized response occurs within 1 month of a tick bite. It consists of an erythematous circular region centered around the area of the original tick bite. The erythematous area gradually expands and the center of the lesion becoming clear creating a bull's eye appearance. The rash resolves spontaneously after approximately a month. Importantly, not all patients with Lyme disease develop erythema migrans. The second stage of the illness is marked by dissemination of the spirochetes throughout the body. Patients develop systemic symptoms including fever, chills, localized adenopathy, fatigue, myalgias, headache, neck and back pain, and additional skin lesions about the body. Cardiac involvement may lead to pericarditis and heart block. Inflammatory arthritis of large and small joints may also occur.

Neurological complications may develop during the second and third stages of infection (Table 17-3).[13–22] Facial neuropathy is the most common neurological manifestation of Lyme disease and is bilateral in about half of cases, which is rare for idiopathic Bell palsy. Involvement of nerves is frequently asymmetric. Patients with Lyme disease may also manifest with multiple mononeuropathies or, more commonly in our experience, with radiculopathy or polyradiculopathy. Although often considered in the differential diagnosis of GBS, it usually does not resemble cases of GBS given the asymmetric nature and electrophysiological features (see below). Rarely, affected patients develop an inflammatory myopathy as opposed to neuropathy.[22]

The late stage of infection is characterized by further destructive inflammatory changes in the joints. The distal extremities develop a bluish discoloration of the skin (acrodermatitis chronica atrophicans). Spirochetes may be readily cultured from biopsies of these sites. Approximately 50% of patients have numbness, paresthesia, weakness, and cramps in the distal extremities, and proprioception and vibration are reduced as are muscle stretch reflexes.

LABORATORY FEATURES

Examination of the cerebrospinal fluid (CSF) should demonstrate lymphocytic pleocytosis and increased protein in

▶ **TABLE 17-3. NEUROLOGICAL DISORDERS ASSOCIATED WITH LYME DISEASE**

Encephalitis/meningitis
Myelitis
Cranial neuropathies (e.g., facial nerve palsy)
Peripheral neuropathy
Mononeuropathies
Multiple mononeuropathies
Radiculopathy
Plexopathy
Inflammatory myopathy

patients with polyradiculitis, cranial neuropathies, and central nervous system involvement. Immunofluorescent or enzyme-linked immunosorbent assay may detect antibodies directed against the spirochete in the serum and CSF. False-positive reactions are not uncommon and, therefore, Western blot analysis should be performed to confirm a positive enzyme-linked immunosorbent assay.

Electrodiagnostic studies are suggestive of a primary axonopathy. In a patient with a mononeuropathy or multiple mononeuropathies, NCS typically reveal reduced compound muscle action potential (CMAP) and sensory nerve action potential (SNAP) amplitudes.[13,17–22] Those with facial nerve palsies have reduced facial nerve CMAPs and abnormal blink reflexes.[15] The electrophysiological abnormalities are often asymmetric.[23,24] Needle EMG reveals increased insertional and spontaneous activity in the form of fibrillation potentials and positive sharp waves and decreased recruitment of neurogenic-appearing motor unit action potentials (MUAPs). Patients presenting with a radiculopathy may have normal motor and sensory NCS, but the EMG is abnormal as above.

HISTOPATHOLOGY

Nerve biopsies are not typically performed in patients with Lyme disease and symptoms of neuropathy, but can reveal perivascular infiltration of plasma cells and lymphocytes around small endoneurial, perineurial, and epineurial blood vessels without clear necrotizing vasculitis. Axonal degeneration and secondary demyelination can be seen.

PATHOGENESIS

Peripheral nerve involvement may be the result of an indirect immunological response and/or some form of vasculopathy.

TREATMENT

Recommended treatment of facial nerve palsies in adults is the combination of amoxicillin 500 mg p.o. q.i.d. plus probenecid 500 mg q.i.d. for 2–4 weeks. Patients who are allergic to penicillin can be treated with doxycycline 100 mg p.o. b.i.d. for 2–4 weeks. Children less than 4 years of age can be treated with amoxicillin 20–40 mg/kg/d in four divided doses for 2–4 weeks. If allergic to penicillin, children can be treated with erythromycin 30 mg/kg/d in four divided doses for 2–4 weeks.

Adult patients with other types of peripheral neuropathy are treated with intravenous (IV) penicillin 20–24 million units/d for 10–14 days or ceftriaxone 2 g IV q.d. for 2–4 weeks. Those allergic to penicillin should receive doxycycline 100 mg p.o. b.i.d. for 30 days. Children with Lyme neuropathy can receive IV penicillin G 250,000 U/kg/d in divided doses for 10–14 days or ceftriaxone 50–80 mg/kg/d IV for 2–4 weeks.

► DIPHTHERITIC NEUROPATHY

CLINICAL FEATURES

Diphtheria is caused by the bacteria *Corynebacterium diphtheriae*. Individuals who are infected present with "flu-like" symptoms of generalized myalgias, headache, fatigue, low-grade fever, and irritability within a week to 10 days of the exposure. A whitish membranous exudate may be appreciated in the pharynx with or without swollen or tender cervical lymph nodes. Cardiovascular involvement can manifest as cardiac arrhythmias and hypotension. About 20–70% of patients develop a peripheral neuropathy caused by a toxin released by the bacteria.[25–28] Three to four weeks after infection, patients may note decreased sensation in their throat and begin to develop dysphagia, dysarthria, or hoarseness. Around the same time, patients develop blurred vision, particularly when looking at near objects. Pupils react to light but fail to accommodate. Additional cranial nerves may also become involved. Ventilatory muscle weakness can develop due to phrenic nerve involvement. A generalized polyneuropathy may manifest 2 or 3 months following the initial infection characterized by numbness, paresthesia, and weakness of the arms and legs. Neurological examination reveals a reduction in perception of all sensory modalities. Distal greater than proximal weakness is seen. Weakness may progress over a period of weeks, such that patients are unable to ambulate. Muscle stretch reflexes are diminished or absent throughout in keeping with the demyelinating nature of the neuropathy. Rarely, bowel and bladder function are affected.

LABORATORY FEATURES

CSF protein can be elevated with or without a lymphocytic pleocytosis.[29] Sensory NCS often reveal absent SNAPs.[27] Motor NCS demonstrate markedly reduced conduction velocities (<50% of mean values) in the arms and legs.[26,27,29,30] The distal motor latencies are only mildly to moderately prolonged. The NCS become abnormal by 2 weeks following onset of neuropathic symptoms and reach their nadir by 5–8 weeks. Subsequently, there is slow and steady improvement in the NCS that lag behind clinical recovery.

HISTOPATHOLOGY

Segmental demyelination and axonal degeneration have been appreciated in the nerve roots and the more distal segments of the peripheral nerve.[25] Degeneration of dorsal root ganglia may be observed as well.

PATHOGENESIS

The bacteria release diphtheria exotoxin which binds to Schwann cells and inhibits synthesis of myelin proteins.[31]

TREATMENT

Antitoxin and antibiotics should be given within 48 hours of symptom onset. Although early treatment reduces the incidence and severity of some complications (i.e., cardiomyopathy), it does not appear to alter the natural history of the associated peripheral neuropathy. The neuropathy usually resolves after several months. Patients need to be managed with supportive care (e.g., mechanical ventilation, PE prophylaxis, physical therapy) as discussed in the chapter on GBS (Chapter 13).

▶ HUMAN IMMUNODEFICIENCY VIRUS

Human immunodeficiency virus (HIV) infection can result in a variety of neuromuscular complications (Table 17-4), including peripheral neuropathies. Approximately 20% of individuals infected with HIV develop a neuropathy which may be as a direct result of the virus itself, other associated viral infections [e.g., cytomegalovirus (CMV) infection], or neurotoxicity secondary to antiviral medications.[32–35] The neuropathy associated with antiviral medications are discussed in Chapter 20. The major presentations of peripheral neuropathy associated with HIV infection include (1) distal symmetric polyneuropathy (DSP), (2) inflammatory demyelinating polyneuropathy (including both AIDP and CIDP), (3) multiple mononeuropathies (e.g., vasculitis, CMV related), (4) polyradiculopathy (usually CMV related), (5) autonomic neuropathy, and (6) sensory ganglionitis.[36–43]

▶ **TABLE 17-4. NEUROLOGICAL COMPLICATIONS ASSOCIATED WITH HIV INFECTION**

Central nervous system
Opportunistic infections
Progressive multifocal leukoencephalopathy
HIV-associated encephalopathy (AIDS dementia)
Lymphomas and other malignancies
Subacute combined degeneration (B12 deficiency)
Vacuolar myelopathy
Peripheral nervous system disorders
Distal symmetric polyneuropathy
Motor neuronopathy
Acute and chronic inflammatory demyelinating polyradiculoneuropathy
Polyradiculoneuropathy/multiple mononeuropathies caused by other infections (e.g., cytomegalovirus, hepatitis B or C, and herpes zoster)
Autonomic neuropathy
Sensory ganglionopathy
Toxic neuropathy (antiretroviral medications)
Myopathy
Toxic myopathy (antiretroviral medications)
Inflammatory (polymyositis or inclusion body myositis)
Infectious (opportunistic infections)
Myopathy secondary to wasting/cachexia

▶ HIV-RELATED DISTAL SYMMETRIC POLYNEUROPATHY

CLINICAL FEATURES

DSP is the most common form of peripheral neuropathy associated with HIV infection and usually is seen in patients with AIDS.[32,33,35,44,45] It is characterized by numbness and painful paresthesia involving the distal legs and arms. Some patients are asymptomatic but have reduced sensation to all modalities on examination. Mild distal muscle weakness may be appreciated. Proximal leg and distal arm weakness may develop late in the course of the disease. Muscle stretch reflexes are reduced at the ankles but are relatively preserved at the knees and in the arms.

LABORATORY FEATURES

CSF examination may demonstrate an increased protein and mild lymphocytic pleocytosis in patients with HIV infection regardless of the stage of the infection and the presence or absence of peripheral neuropathy.[46,47] Vitamin B12 deficiency is noted in some[48,49] but not all patients.[50–52] NCS and EMG reveal abnormalities suggestive of a symmetric, axonal sensory greater than motor polyneuropathy.[32,34,53–56]

HISTOPATHOLOGY

Nerve biopsies are not routinely performed in HIV patients with DSP but typically reveal axonal degeneration and a loss in the total number of both myelinated and demyelinated axons (Fig. 17-6).[41,53,56–59] A reduction of cell bodies in the dorsal root ganglia may be appreciated, as well as secondary degeneration of the dorsal columns. Mild perivascular inflammation consisting of macrophages and T lymphocytes is seen along with the evidence of increased cytokine expression. Reduced density of small myelinated epidermal nerve fibers is appreciated in the epidermis with skin biopsy.[60]

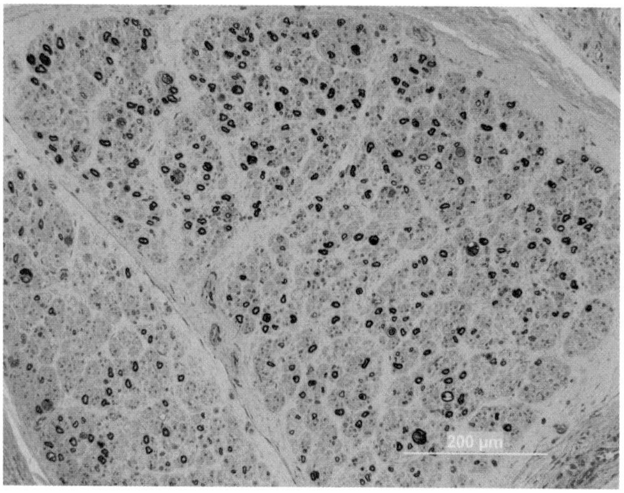

Figure 17-6. HIV neuropathy. Sural nerve biopsy in a patient with distal symmetric sensory neuropathy demonstrates a mild reduction in myelinated nerve fibers. Epoxy embedded, toluidine blue stain.

PATHOGENESIS

The pathogenic basis for DSP is unknown but is not due to actual infection of the peripheral nerves. Viral coat proteins may mediate nerve fiber damage and hyperalgesia through direct and indirect mechanisms.[45] These proteins may be directly toxic to axons. In addition, the glial and macrophage response activated by virus may indirectly damage neurons by the release of cytokines from surrounding inflammatory cells. Vitamin B12 deficiency may contribute to some cases but is not a major cause of most cases of DSP. Various antiretroviral agents (e.g., dideoxycytidine, dideoxyinosine, and stavudine) are also neurotoxic and may cause a painful sensory neuropathy.[55,61–63]

TREATMENT

The neuropathy is not responsive to treatment with antiretroviral medications and therapy is largely symptomatic. We usually initiate treatment with neuropathic pain medications (see Chapter 22, Table 22-3).

► HIV-RELATED INFLAMMATORY DEMYELINATING POLYRADICULONEUROPATHY

CLINICAL FEATURES

Both AIDP and CIDP can occur as a complication of HIV infection.[35,45,64] AIDP usually develops at the time of seroconversion, whereas CIDP can occur anytime in the course of the infection. Clinical features are indistinguishable from idiopathic AIDP or CIDP.

LABORATORY FEATURES

In addition to elevated protein levels, lymphocytic pleocytosis is evident in the CSF—a finding that helps distinguish HIV-associated polyradiculoneuropathy from idiopathic AIDP/CIDP. Motor and sensory NCS are similar to that seen in idiopathic AIDP and CIDP (Chapters 13 and 14).[30,64–66] Motor and sensory NCS may demonstrate slow conduction velocities, prolonged distal latencies and F waves, conduction block, and/or temporal dispersion.

HISTOPATHOLOGY

Nerve biopsies are not be performed routinely, but can show features identical to those found in idiopathic AIDP and CIDP.[30,57]

TREATMENT

We usually treat patients with HIV-associated AIDP or CIDP with intravenous immunoglobulin (IVIg) or plasmapheresis (PE).[30,65] Prednisone can be used in CIDP, but we try to avoid steroids and other second-line immunosuppressive agents because of the long-term implications of immunosuppression in patients with HIV.

► HIV-RELATED PROGRESSIVE POLYRADICULOPATHY (SECONDARY CMV INFECTION)

CLINICAL FEATURES

An acute, progressive lumbosacral polyradiculoneuropathy secondary to CMV infection can develop in patients with AIDS.[35,45] Patients usually present with severe radicular pain, numbness, and weakness in the legs, which is usually asymmetric. Loss of perineal sensation with bowel and bladder incontinence is common. The arms and cranial nerves may also be affected. Reduced or absent muscle stretch reflexes are appreciated on examination. Plantar responses are usually flexor but can be extensor if a superimposed CMV myelitis is also present. Patients usually have evidence of CMV infection in other parts of the body (i.e., CMV retinitis).

LABORATORY FEATURES

CSF is abnormal, demonstrating an increased protein level along with a reduced glucose concentration and, notably, a neutrophilic pleocytosis. CMV can be cultured from the CSF, blood, and urine. NCS often demonstrate an asymmetric reduction of amplitudes of the SNAPs and CMAPs with active denervation changes on EMG in muscles innervated by affected nerve roots and nerves including the paraspinals.[67,68] The axonal nature and distribution of these abnormalities are quite distinct from those found in both CIDP and DSP respectively, helping to differentiate these various disorders.

HISTOPATHOLOGY

With postmortem examination, inflammatory infiltrates associated with varying degrees of axonal loss are evident in the ventral and dorsal roots, particularly in the lumbar regions. Occasionally, the cranial nerves exiting from the brainstem may be involved in association with the myelitis. CMV inclusions may be found in endothelial cells and macrophages on nerve biopsy specimens when obtained.[69]

PATHOGENESIS

The polyradiculoneuropathy may be caused by the direct infection of neurons by CMV or ischemia secondary to associated vasculitis.

TREATMENT

The polyradiculoneuropathy may improve with ganciclovir or foscarnet, if treatment is started early.[68,70] However, the prognosis is poor, and most patients die within several weeks or months.

▶ HIV-RELATED MULTIPLE MONONEUROPATHIES

CLINICAL FEATURES

Multiple mononeuropathies can also develop in patients with HIV infection usually in the context of AIDS.[35,45] Weakness, numbness, paresthesia, and pain are evident in the distribution of affected nerves.

LABORATORY FEATURES

Elevated CSF protein and mononuclear pleocytosis may be seen. EMG and NCS demonstrate features of axon loss as seen with other forms of multiple mononeuropathies caused by vasculitis (see Chapter 15).[71]

HISTOPATHOLOGY

Nerve biopsies can reveal axonal degeneration with necrotizing vasculitis or perivascular inflammation.[72] CMV inclusions may be seen in endothelial cells and macrophages on electron microscopy.[69]

PATHOGENESIS

The pathogenic basis for this disorder is likely multifactorial. The neuropathy may be caused by vasculitis related to deposition of HIV antigen–antibody complexes in the walls of blood vessel, concomitant hepatitis B or C infection, or CMV infection.

TREATMENT

Corticosteroid treatment is indicated in vasculitis directly due to HIV infection. Multiple mononeuropathies secondary to concurrent hepatitis B or C infection can be treated with plasma exchange, antiviral agents (e.g., vidarabine), or α-interferon. Short courses of prednisone and cyclophosphamide may be necessary. If CMV is suspected, treatment with ganciclovir or foscarnet should be initiated.

▶ HIV-RELATED AUTONOMIC NEUROPATHY

CLINICAL FEATURES

An autonomic neuropathy characterized by orthostatic hypotension, impaired sweating, diarrhea, impotence, and bladder dysfunction can develop acutely or insidiously in patients with HIV infection.[73–75] Clinical features are similar to those seen with idiopathic autonomic neuropathy.

LABORATORY FEATURES

CSF can reveal pleocytosis and increased protein. Most patients have electrodiagnostic features similar to that noted in DSP. In addition, autonomic function testing is usually abnormal.[74]

PATHOGENESIS

An immune-mediated mechanism similar to that suspected in idiopathic autonomic neuropathy is likely.

TREATMENT

A trial of corticosteroids, IVIg, or PE may be tried. Symptoms of autonomic neuropathy are treated symptomatically.

▶ HIV-RELATED SENSORY NEURONOPATHY/ GANGLIONOPATHY

Dorsal root ganglionitis is a very rare complication of HIV infection, but neuronopathy can be the presenting manifestation.[76] Patients develop sensory ataxia similar to idiopathic sensory neuronopathy/ganglionopathy. Autopsies have demonstrated inflammatory cell infiltrate in the dorsal root ganglia along with the loss of cell bodies and degeneration of myelinated nerve fibers in the peripheral nerves. NCS reveal amplitudes or absence of SNAPs. Again, a trial of corticosteroids, IVIg, or PE may be considered.

▶ HUMAN T-LYMPHOCYTE TYPE 1 INFECTION

Besides the more common myelopathy (tropical spastic paraparesis), human T-lymphocyte type 1 (HTLV-1) infection is also associated with an axonal sensorimotor polyneuropathy.[77–79] The neuropathy can be seen even in patients without a myelopathy. HTLV-1 infection has also been associated with myositis. NCS demonstrate abnormalities suggestive of an axonal, sensory greater than motor, length-dependent neuropathy.[79] Sural nerve biopsy when performed can reveal axonal degeneration with secondary demyelination and inflammatory cell infiltrates. There is one report of CIDP occurring in the setting of HTLV-1 infection.[80]

▶ CYTOMEGALOVIRUS

CMV can cause an acute lumbosacral polyradiculopathy and multiple mononeuropathies in patients with HIV infection or other causes of severe immunosuppression as previously noted.

▶ EPSTEIN–BARR VIRUS

Epstein–Barr virus infection has been associated with AIDP, cranial neuropathies, mononeuropathy multiplex, brachial plexopathy, lumbosacral radiculoplexopathy, and sensory neuronopathies.[81]

▶ HEPATITIS VIRUSES

Hepatitis B and C can cause multiple mononeuropathies related to vasculitis, AIDP, or CIDP, as previously discussed (Chapters 13 and 14).

▶ HERPES VARICELLA-ZOSTER VIRUS

CLINICAL FEATURES

Peripheral neuropathy from herpes varicella-zoster (HVZ) infection is the result of reactivation of latent virus or a primary infection. Primary infection is the cause of "chicken pox." Reactivation of the virus later in life leads to dermal zoster. In patients who are immunocompromised, HVZ infection can be associated with severe disseminated zoster. Two-thirds of infections in adults are characterized by dermal zoster, in which severe pain and paresthesias develop in a dermatomal region, followed within a week or two by a vesicular rash in the same distribution. The vesicular skin lesions clear by 2 weeks. Approximately 25% of patients who are affected have continued pain (postherpetic neuralgia). In a large series of patients, zoster developed in thoracic dermatomes in nearly 50%, lumbosacral region in 18%, trigeminal distribution in the head in an additional 18%, and the cervical dermatomes in the remainder.

Weakness in muscles innervated by roots corresponding to the dermatomal distribution of skin lesions occurs in 5–30% of patients.[82–84] The weakness usually develops within the first 2 weeks of the skin eruption but can vary between several hours and a month. Unilateral phrenic nerve involvement can lead to hemidiaphragmatic paralysis.[85] When the thoracic myotomes are involved, hernias can occur through weakened abdominal wall musculature.[86,87] Muscle strength usually improves over time. Rarely, patients develop AIDP following HVZ infection.[88,89] Additional neurological manifestations of herpes zoster infection include encephalitis and angiitis leading to vascular events.

LABORATORY FEATURES

CSF protein may be elevated with or without pleocytosis. The virus is difficult to culture from the CSF, but polymerase chain reaction can be used to confirm the presence of the virus in the CSF. Sensory NCS reveal reduced or absent SNAPs in affected nerves.[90–92] Motor NCS demonstrate normal reduced CMAP amplitudes.[83,84,90,92] Positive sharp waves and fibrillation potentials and neurogenic-appearing MUAPs and recruitment can be observed on needle EMG in muscles of affected myotomes.[83,84,90,92]

HISTOPATHOLOGY

The basic pathological neural reaction is that of axonal degeneration with some degree of secondary segmental demyelination. With respect to the sensory system, severe infections can result in the destruction of dorsal root ganglion cells with the secondary loss of posterior column fibers.

PATHOGENESIS

Following initial infection, the HVZ migrates up the sensory nerves and takes residence in the sensory ganglia, where the virus appears to be insulated from the host's immune defense mechanisms. When the host becomes immunosuppressed, the virus can reactivate and replicate. HVZ travels down the sensory nerves including cutaneous nerves and result in the typical cutaneous zoster lesions. The inflammatory response in the spinal nerve may involve motor axons resulting in muscle weakness.

TREATMENT

Acyclovir helps improve the rate of healing of the skin lesions, but acyclovir neither alone nor in combination with corticosteroids reduces the frequency or severity of postherpetic neuralgia. Intravenous acyclovir should be administered in immunocompromised patients with severe infections. The treatment of postherpetic neuralgia is symptomatic. Our first-line treatment of choice is lidoderm patches applied over the regions with neuralgic pain. Gabapentin,[93] carbamazepine, topical capsaicin ointment, and tricyclic antidepressants[94] may also reduce the pain in some patients. Opioids are warranted as well in patients with refractory pain.[95]

▶ SUMMARY

Neuropathies associated with infection are not uncommon. In fact, lepromatous neuropathy may be the most common form of neuropathy, particularly in nonindustrialized nations. Further, neuropathies related to HIV infection have increased, owing to the spread of this infection and longer life span of treated individuals rendering them susceptible to the neurotoxic effects of the infection and antiretroviral infections. Lyme disease likewise needs to be considered in endemic regions. Notably, many of these neuropathies are treatable; thus, diagnosis is essential.

REFERENCES

1. Rodrigues LC, Lockwood DN. Leprosy now: epidemiology, progress, challenges, and research gaps. *Lancet Infect Dis.* 2011;11:464–470.
2. Altman D, Amato A. Lepromatous neuropathy. *J Clin Neuromuscul Dis.* 1999;1:68–73.
3. Nations SP, Katz JS, Lyde CB, Barohn RJ. Leprous neuropathy: an American perspective. *Semin Neurol.* 1998;18(1):113–124.
4. Ooi WW, Srinivasan J. Leprosy and the peripheral nervous system: basic and clinical aspects. *Muscle Nerve.* 2004;30(4):393–409.
5. Ridley DS, Jopling WH. Classification of leprosy according to immunity. A five-group system. *Int J Lepr Other Mycobact Dis.* 1966;34:255–276.
6. Rodriguez G, Sanchez W, Chaleta JG, Soto J. Primary neuritic leprosy. *J Am Acad Dermatol.* 1993;29:1050–1052.
7. Jardim MR, Chimelli L, Faria SC, et al. Clinical, electroneuromyographic and morphological studies of pure neural leprosy in a Brazilian referral centre. *Lepr Rev.* 2004;75(3):242–253.
8. McLeod JG, Hargrave JC, Walsh JC, Booth GC, Gye RS, Barron A. Nerve conduction studies in leprosy. *Int J Lepr Other Mycobact Dis.* 1975;43:21–31.
9. Amato AA, Dumitru D. Acquired neuropathies. In: Dumitru D, Amato AA, Swartz MJ, eds. *Electrodiagnostic Medicine*, 2nd ed. Philadelphia, PA: Hanley & Belfus; 2002:937–1041.
10. Bathala L, Kumar K, Pathapati R, Jain S, Visser LH. Ulnar neuropathy in hansen disease: clinical, high-resolution ultrasound and electrophysiologic correlations. *J Clin Neurophysiol.* 2012;29:190–193.
11. World Health Organization (WHO) recommended MDT regimens. http://www.who.int/lep/mdt/regimens/en
12. Van Veen NH, Lockwood DN, Van Brakel WH, Ramirez J Jr, Richardus JH. Interventions for erythema nodosum leprosum. A Cochrane review. *Lepr Rev.* 2009;80:355–372.
13. Halperin JJ, Little BW, Coyle PK, Dattwyler RJ. Lyme disease: cause of a treatable peripheral neuropathy. *Neurology.* 1987;37:1700–1706.
14. Halperin J, Luft BJ, Volkman DJ, Dattwyler RJ. Lyme neuroborreliosis. *Brain.* 1990;113:1207–1221.
15. Krishnamurthy KB, Liu GT, Logigian EL. Acute Lyme neuropathy presenting with polyradicular pain, abdominal protrusion, and cranial neuropathy. *Muscle Nerve.* 1993;16:1261–1264.
16. Logigian EL, Steere AC. Clinical and electrophysiologic findings in chronic neuropathy of Lyme disease. *Neurology.* 1992;42:303–311.
17. Oey PL, Franssen H, Bersen RA, Wokke JH. Multifocal conduction block in a patient with *Borrelia burgdorferi* infection. *Muscle Nerve.* 1991;14:375–377.
18. Scelsa SN, Hershkovitz S, Berger AR. A predominantly motor polyradiculopathy of Lyme disease. *Muscle Nerve.* 1996;19:780–783.
19. Pachner AR, Steere AC. The triad of neurologic manifestations of Lyme disease: meningitis, cranial neuritis, and radiculoneuritis. *Neurology.* 1985;35:47–53.
20. Vallat JM, Hugon J, Lubeau M, Leboutet MJ, Dumas M, Desproges-Gotteron R. Tick-bite meningoradiculoneuritis: clinical, electrophysiologic, and histologic findings in 10 cases. *Neurology.* 1987;37:749–753.
21. Wulff CH, Hansen K, Strange P, Trojaborg W. Multiple mononeuritis and radiculitis with erythema, pain, elevated CSF protein and pleocytosis (Bannwarth's syndrome). *J Neurol Neurosurg Psychiatry.* 1983;46:485–490.
22. Schoenen J, Sianard-Gainko J, Carpentier M, Reznik M. Myositis during *Borrelia burgdorferi* infection (Lyme disease). *J Neurol Neurosurg Psychiatry.* 1989;52:1002–1005.
23. Halperin JJ, Volkman DJ, Luft BJ, Dattwyler RJ. Carpal tunnel syndrome in Lyme borrelliosis. *Muscle Nerve.* 1989;12:397–400.
24. Halperin JJ, Pass HL, Anand AK, Luft BJ, Volkman DJ, Dattwyler RJ. Nervous system abnormalities in Lyme disease. *Ann N Y Acad Sci.* 1988;539:24–34.
25. Fisher CM, Adams RD. Diphtheritic polyneuritis; a pathological study. *J Neuropathol Exp Neurol.* 1956;15:243–268.
26. Kazemi B, Tahjernia AC, Zandian K. Motor nerve conduction in diphtheria and diphtheritic myocarditis. *Arch Neurol.* 1973;29:104–106.
27. Kurdi A, Abdul-Kader M. Clinical and electrophysiological studies of diphtheritic neuritis in Jordan. *J Neurol Sci.* 1979;42:243–250.
28. Solders G, Nennesmo I, Persson A. Diphtheritic neuropathy, an analysis based on muscle and nerve biopsy and repeated neurophysiological and autonomic function tests. *J Neurol Neurosurg Psychiatry.* 1989;52:876–880.
29. Créange A, Meyrignac C, Roualdes B, Degos JD, Gherardi RK. Diphtheritic neuropathy. *Muscle Nerve.* 1995;18:1460–1463.
30. Cornblath DR, McArthur JC, Kennedy PG, Witte AS, Griffin JW. Inflammatory demyelinating peripheral neuropathies associated with human T-cell lymphotropic virus type III infection. *Ann Neurol.* 1987;21:32–40.

31. Pleasure DE, Feldmann B, Prokop DJ. Diphtheria toxin inhibits the synthesis of myelin proteolipid and basic proteins by peripheral nerve in vivo. *J Neurochem*. 1973;20:81–90.
32. Floeter MK, Civetello LA, Everett CR, Dambrosia J, Luciano CA. Peripheral neuropathy in children with HIV infection. *Neurology*. 1997;49:207–212.
33. Marra CM, Boutin P, Collier AC. Screening for distal sensory peripheral neuropathy in HIV-infected persons in research and clinical settings. *Neurology*. 1998;51:1678–1681.
34. Tagliati M, Grinnell J, Godbold J, Simpson DM. Peripheral nerve function in HIV infection: clinical, electrophysiologic, and laboratory findings. *Arch Neurol*. 1999;56:84–89.
35. Robinson-Papp J, Simpson DM. Neuromuscular diseases associated with HIV-1 infection. *Muscle Nerve*. 2009;40:1043–1053.
36. Barohn RJ, Gronseth GS, LeForce BR, et al. Peripheral nervous system involvement in a large cohort of human immunodeficiency virus-infected individuals. *Arch Neurol*. 1993;50:167–171.
37. Cornblath DR, McArthur JC. Predominantly sensory neuropathy in patients with AIDS and AIDS-related complex. *Neurology*. 1988;38:794–796.
38. Dalakas MC, Pezeshkpour GH. Neuromuscular diseases associated with human immunodeficiency virus infection. *Ann Neurol*. 1988;23:S38–S48.
39. de la Monte SM, Gabuzda DH, Ho DD, et al. Peripheral neuropathy in the acquired immunodeficiency syndrome. *Ann Neurol*. 1988;23:485–492.
40. Fuller GN, Jacobs JM, Guiloff RJ. Nature and incidence of peripheral nerve syndrome in HIV infection. *J Neurol Neurosurg Psychiatry*. 1993;56:372–381.
41. Hall CD, Snyder CR, Messenheimer JA, et al. Peripheral neuropathy in a cohort of human immunodeficiency virus infected patients. Incidence and relationship to other nervous system dysfunction. *Arch Neurol*. 1991;48:1273–1274.
42. Lange DJ. AAEM minimonograph #41: neuromuscular diseases associated with HIV-1 infection. *Muscle Nerve*. 1994;17:16–30.
43. McArthur JC, Cohen BA, Selnes OA, et al. Low prevalence of neurological and neuropsychological abnormalities in otherwise healthy HIV-1-infected individuals: results from the multicenter AIDS Cohort Study. *Ann Neurol*. 1989;26:601–611.
44. Kamerman PR, Moss PJ, Weber J, Wallace VC, Rice AS, Huang W. Pathogenesis of HIV-associated sensory neuropathy: evidence from in vivo and in vitro experimental models. *J Peripher Nerv Syst*. 2012;17:19–31.
45. Simpson DM, Olney RK. Peripheral neuropathies associated with human immunodeficiency virus infection. *Neurol Clin*. 1992;10:685–711.
46. Barohn RJ, Gronseth GS, Amato AA, et al. Is there any relationship between cerebral spinal fluid and nerve conduction abnormalities in HIV positive individuals? *J Neurol Sci*. 1996;136:81–85.
47. Marshall DW, Brey RL, Butzin CA, et al. CSF changes in a longitudinal study of 124 neurologically normal HIV-1-infected U.S. Air Force personnel. *J Acquir Immune Defic Syndr*. 1991;4:777–781.
48. Beach RS, Morgan R, Wilkie F, et al. Plasma vitamin B12 level as a potential cofactor in studies of human immunodeficiency virus type 1-related cognitive changes. *Arch Neurol*. 1992;49:501–506.
49. Kieburtz KD, Giang DW, Schiffer RB, Vakil N. Abnormal vitamin B12 metabolism in human immunodeficiency virus infection: association with neurological dysfunction. *Arch Neurol*. 1991;48:312–314.
50. Dal Pan GJ, Allen RH, Glass JD, et al. Cobalamin (vitamin B12)-dependent metabolism is not altered in HIV-1-associated vacuolar myelopathy. *Ann Neurol*. 1993;34:281–282.
51. Robertson KR, Stern RA, Hall CD, et al. Vitamin B12 deficiency and nervous system disease in HIV infection. *Arch Neurol*. 1993;50:807–811.
52. Veilleux M, Paltiel O, Falutz J. Sensorimotor neuropathy and abnormal vitamin B12 metabolism in early HIV infection. *Can J Neurol Sci*. 1995;22:43–46.
53. Bailey RO, Baltch AL, Venkatesh R, Singh JK, Bishop MB. Sensory motor neuropathy associated with AIDS. *Neurology*. 1988;38:886–891.
54. Chavanet P, Solary E, Giroud M, et al. Infraclinical neuropathies related to immunodeficiency virus infection associated with higher T-helper cell count. *J Acquir Immune Defic Syndr*. 1989;2:564–569.
55. Dubinsky RM, Yarchoan R, Dalakas M, Broder S. Reversible axonal neuropathy from treatment of AIDS and related disorders with 2′,3′-dideoxycytidine (ddC). *Muscle Nerve*. 1989;12:856–860.
56. Fuller GN, Jacobs JM, Guiloff RJ. Subclinical peripheral nerve involvement in AIDS: an electrophysiological and pathological study. *J Neurol Neurosurg Psychiatry*. 1991;54:318–324.
57. Chaunu MP, Ratinahirana H, Raphael M, et al. The spectrum of the changes on 20 nerve biopsies in patients with HIV infection. *Muscle Nerve*. 1989;12:452–459.
58. Fuller GN, Jacobs JM, Guiloff RJ. Axonal atrophy in painful peripheral neuropathy in AIDS. *Acta Neuropathol*. 1990;81:198–203.
59. Rance NE, McArthur JC, Cornblath DR, Landstrom DL, Griffin JW, Price DL. Gracile tract degeneration in patients with sensory neuropathy and AIDS. *Neurology*. 1998;38:265–271.
50. Herrman DN, Griffin JW, Hauer P. Intraepidermal nerve fiber density, sural nerve morphometry and electrodiagnosis in peripheral neuropathies. *Neurology*. 1999;53:1634–1640.
61. Berger AR, Arezzo JC, Schaumburg HH, et al. 2′,3′-dideoxycytidine (ddC) toxic neuropathy: a study of 52 patients. *Neurology*. 1993;43:358–362.
62. Kieburtz KD, Seidlin M, Lambert JS, Dolin R, Reichman R, Valentine F. Extended follow-up of peripheral neuropathy in patients with AIDS and AIDS-related complex treated with dideoxyinosine. *J Acquir Immune Defic Syndr*. 1992;5:60–64.
63. Leung GP. Iatrogenic mitochondriopathies: a recent lesson from nucleoside/nucleotide reverse transcriptase inhibitors. *Adv Exp Med Biol*. 2012;942:347–369.
64. Brannagan TH III, Zhou Y. HIV-associated Guillain–Barre syndrome. *J Neurol Sci*. 2003;208(1–2):39–42.
65. Leger JM, Bouche P, Bolgert F, et al. The spectrum of polyneuropathies in patients infected with HIV. *J Neurol Neurosurg Psychiatry*. 1989;52:1369–1374.
66. Przedbroski S, Liesnard C, Voordecker P, et al. Inflammatory demyelinating polyradiculoneuropathy associated with human immunodeficiency virus infection. *J Neurol*. 1988; 235:359–361.
67. Dalakas MC, Yarchoan R, Spitzer R, Elder G, Sever JL. Treatment of human immunodeficiency virus-related polyneuropathy with 3′-azido-2′,3′-dideoxythymidine. *Ann Neurol*. 1988;23:S92–S94.

68. Miller RG, Storey JR, Greco CM. Ganciclovir in the treatment of progressive AIDS-related polyradiculopathy. *Neurology.* 1990;40:569–574.
69. Roullet E, Assuerus V, Gozlan J, et al. Cytomegalovirus multifocal neuropathy in AIDS: analysis of 15 consecutive cases. *Neurology.* 1994:44:2174–2182.
70. Kim YS, Hollander H. Polyradiculopathy due to cytomegalovirus: report of two cases in which improvement occurred after prolonged therapy and review of the literature. *Clin Infect Dis.* 1993;17:32–37.
71. Lipkin WI, Parry G, Kiprov D, Abrams D. Inflammatory neuropathy in homosexual men with lymphadenopathy. *Neurology.* 1985;35:1479–1483.
72. Said G, Lacroix-Ciaudo C, Fujimura H, Blas C, Faux N. The peripheral neuropathy of necrotizing arteritis: a clinicopathological study. *Ann Neurol.* 1988;23:461–465.
73. Cohen JA, Laudenslager M. Autonomic nervous system involvement in patients with human immunodeficiency virus infection. *Neurology.* 1989;39:1111–1112.
74. Craddock C, Pasvol G, Bull R, Protheroe A, Hopkin J. Cardiorespiratory arrest and autonomic neuropathy in AIDS. *Lancet.* 1987;2:16–18.
75. Lin-Greenberger A, Taneja-Uppal N. Dysautonomia and infection with the human immunodeficiency virus. *Ann Intern Med.* 1987;106:167.
76. Elder G, Dalakas M, Pezeshkpour G, Sever J. Ataxic neuropathy due to ganglioneuronitis after probable acute human immunodeficiency virus infection. *Lancet.* 1986;2:1275–1276.
77. Kiwaki T, Umehara F, Arimura Y, et al. The clinical and pathological features of peripheral neuropathy accompanied with HTLV-I associated myelopathy. *J Neurol Sci.* 2003;206(1):17–21.
78. Leite AC, Silva MT, Alamy AH, et al. Peripheral neuropathy in HTLV-I infected individuals without tropical spastic paraparesis/HTLV-I-associated myelopathy. *J Neurol.* 2004; 251(7):877–881.
79. Saeidi M, Sasannejad P, Foroughipour M, Shahami S, Shoeibi A. Prevalence of peripheral neuropathy in patients with HTLV-1 associated myelopathy/tropical spastic paraparesis (HAM/TSP). *Acta Neurol Belg.* 2011;111:41–44.
80. Ali A, Char G, Hanchard B. Chronic inflammatory demyelinating polyneuropathy in a patient infected with human T lymphotropic virus type I. *BMJ Case Rep.* 2009; doi: 10.1136/bcr03.2009.1680.
81. Rubin DI, Daube JR. Subacute sensory neuropathy associated with Epstein–Barr virus. *Muscle Nerve.* 1999;22:1607–1610.
82. Greenberg MK, McVey AL, Hayes T. Segmental motor involvement in herpes zoster: an EMG study. *Neurology.* 1992;42: 1122–1123.
83. Haanpää M, Häkkinen V, Nurmikko T. Motor involvement in acute herpes zoster. *Muscle Nerve.* 1997;20:1433–1438.
84. Modelli M, Scarpini C, Malandrini A, Romano C. Painful neuropathy after diffuse herpes zoster. *Muscle Nerve.* 1997; 20:229–231.
85. Dutt AK. Diaphragmatic paralysis caused by herpes zoster. *Am Rev Respir Dis.* 1970;101:755–758.
86. Glantz RH, Ristanovic RK. Abdominal muscle paralysis from herpes zoster. *J Neurol Neurosurg Psychiatry.* 1988;51: 885–886.
87. Gottschau P, Trojaborg W. Abdominal muscle paralysis associated with herpes zoster. *Acta Neurol Scand.* 1991;84:344–347.
88. Dayan AD, Ogul E, Graveson GS. Polyneuritis and herpes zoster. *J Neurol Neurosurg Psychiatry.* 1972;35:170–175.
89. Sander EA, Peters AC, Gratana JW, Hughes RA, Guillain–Barré syndrome after varicella zoster infection. *J Neurol.* 1987;234:437–439.
90. Gardner-Thorpe C, Foster JB, Barwick DD. Unusual manifestations of herpes zoster. A clinical and electrophysiological study. *J Neurol Sci.* 1976;28:427–447.
91. Rosenfeld T, Price MA. Paralysis in herpes zoster. *Aust N Z J Med.* 1985;15:712–716.
92. Sachs GM. Segmental zoster paresis: An electrophysiological study. *Muscle Nerve.* 1996;19:784–786.
93. Segal AZ, Rordorf G. Gabapentin as novel treatment for post-herpetic neuralgia. *Neurology.* 1996;46:1175–1176.
94. Max MB. Treatment of post-herpetic neuralgia: antidepressants. *Ann Neurol.* 1994;35:S50–S53.
95. Rowbotham MC. Managing post-herpetic neuralgia with opioids and local anesthetics. *Ann Neurol.* 1994;35:S46–S49.

CHAPTER 18

Neuropathies Related to Nutritional Deficiencies

Patients can develop neuropathies due to inadequate nutrition and subsequent vitamin deficiency (Table 18-1). Nutritional deficiency-related polyneuropathies are currently uncommon, especially in developed countries. However, these neuropathies do occur and are important because they are potentially treatable. Malnutrition may occur in chronic alcoholics and in patients with chronic illness, unusual diets, and obesity surgery. Some vitamin deficiencies (e.g., vitamins B12 and E) often occur because of impaired gastrointestinal absorption rather than poor dietary intake. In other cases, neuropathy may develop secondary to the effects of medications (e.g., isoniazid causing vitamin B6 deficiency). The clinical and laboratory features of most nutritional polyneuropathies are similar to those of the more common polyneuropathies. Timely and accurate diagnosis is important because patients can improve with replacement therapy.

▶ THIAMINE (VITAMIN B1) DEFICIENCY

CLINICAL FEATURES

Thiamine deficiency or beriberi is uncommon nowadays and primarily occurs as a consequence of chronic alcohol abuse, recurrent vomiting, total parenteral nutrition, inappropriately restrictive diets, and perhaps bariatric surgery.[1] The symptoms arising from insufficient dietary intake of thiamine are known as beriberi and may present in two forms: dry beriberi and wet beriberi. The difference between these two types of beriberi is simply the presence (wet beriberi) or absence (dry beriberi) of congestive heart failure and lower limb edema. Affected individuals usually present with numbness, tingling, and burning in the distal lower extremities, which subsequently spread to involve the proximal legs and upper extremities.[2] On examination, a mild-to-moderate reduction in all sensory modalities is noted in a stocking distribution along with diminished muscle stretch reflexes. Mild, predominantly distal weakness may be appreciated. Congestive heart failure with edema of the lower legs is seen in the so-called wet beriberi.

LABORATORY FEATURES

Measuring thiamine concentration in serum and urine is not very reliable.[3] Assay of erythrocyte transketolase activity and the increase in activity after adding thiamine pyrophosphate (TPP) appears to be more accurate and reliable.[4–7] Sensory nerve conduction studies (NCS) reveal reduced or absent sensory nerve action potentials (SNAPs) amplitudes with relative preservation of distal sensory latencies and conduction velocities.[2] The motor NCS may be normal or demonstrate slightly reduced amplitudes.

HISTOPATHOLOGY

Sural nerve biopsies reveal loss of primarily large myelinated axons.[1,8] Necropsy studies have demonstrated chromatolysis of the anterior horn cells and dorsal root ganglia cells along with axonal degeneration and secondary demyelination of the posterior columns.

PATHOGENESIS

Most meats and vegetables contain adequate amounts of thiamine, in particular unrefined cereal grains, wheat germ, yeast, soybean flour, and pork.[3] It is absorbed in the small intestine by both passive diffusion and active transport. Here, thiamine is converted to TPP.[3] Because stores of thiamine in the body are limited and its half-life is only 10–14 days, 1–1.5 mg daily of thiamine should be part of any routine diet else deficiency can arise.[3]

Thiamine and TPP catalyze the decarboxylation of alpha-ketoacids to coenzyme A moieties, an important process in ATP synthesis in mitochondria.[3] TPP plays a role in the formation of myelin.[9] Thiamine may also affect neuronal conduction by altering membrane sodium channel function.[10,11]

TREATMENT

Thiamine 100 mg/d should be given intravenously or intramuscularly in deficient patients. In patients with thiamine deficiency secondary to alcohol use, discontinuation of alcohol is imperative. In addition to the likely direct toxic influences on Schwann cells and peripheral nerves, ethanol is likely to impair thiamine utilization even when blood levels are normal.[12] Cardiomyopathy usually is quite responsive to thiamine replacement, although improvement in neurologic

TABLE 18-1. NUTRITIONAL DEFICIENCY ASSOCIATED WITH PERIPHERAL NEUROPATHY

Thiamine (vitamin B1) deficiency
Pyridoxine (vitamin B6) deficiency
Cobalamin (vitamin B12) deficiency
Folate deficiency
Vitamin E deficiency
Copper deficiency
Hypophosphatemia

function is more variable and less dramatic.[13] Motor deficits appear to improve more so than sensory.[14] Some improvement is expected in most patients, but this typically occurs slowly over 6–12 months. In patients with severe neuropathy permanent deficits are typical.[2]

▶ PYRIDOXINE (VITAMIN B6 DEFICIENCY)

Pyridoxine not only is neurotoxic when taken in large dosages (see Chapter 20),[15–18] but can also be associated with a sensorimotor polyneuropathy when deficient. Pyridoxine deficiency is usually associated with isoniazid and hydralazine treatment.[19–21] Pyridoxine deficiency may also result from malnutrition (e.g., chronic alcoholism) or in patients receiving chronic peritoneal dialysis.[22] The symptoms of vitamin B6 deficiency are nonspecific. Affected individuals manifest with a sensory greater than motor polyneuropathy similar to most idiopathic neuropathies. The electrophysiology studies reflect an axonal sensorimotor polyneuropathy.[19,20] Vitamin B6 levels can be measured in blood. Deficient patients should be treated with 50–100 mg/d of vitamin B6.[23,24] This should also be given prophylactically in patients being treated with isoniazid or hydralazine.[25]

▶ COBALAMIN (VITAMIN B12) DEFICIENCY

CLINICAL FEATURES

Patients with vitamin B12 deficiency can present with central nervous system (CNS) or peripheral nervous system (PNS) abnormalities with or without hematologic findings (megaloblastic anemia).[26–34] Those affected may manifest with numbness and sensory ataxia due to posterior column dysfunction and spastic weakness due to pyramidal tract insult (subacute combined degeneration). In addition, they may have altered mental status. Most patients have signs and symptoms of both CNS and PNS involvement, with reduction of vibratory perception and proprioception, positive Romberg sign, sensory ataxia, decreased or absent reflexes at the ankles, and brisk reflexes elsewhere. Plantar responses can be either extensor or flexor. Because of the myelopathy, patients may present with numbness restricted to the hands potentially mimicking carpal tunnel syndrome. A subacute onset and constant, rather than intermittent numbness would favor vitamin B12 deficiency. A positive Lhermitte's sign may be present owing to swelling in the cervical spinal cord.

LABORATORY FEATURES

Serum vitamin B12 assays are not sensitive, as many symptomatic patients may have serum vitamin B12 levels that are within the normal range.[35,36] Serum levels of the vitamin B12 metabolites, methylmalonic acid (MMA) and homocysteine (Hcy), are much more sensitive in detecting deficiency of B12.[36,37] MMA and Hcy levels are increased (i.e., evidence of B12 deficiency) in 5–10% of patients with serum vitamin B12 levels less than 300 pg/mL and in 0.1–1% of those with levels greater than 300 pg/mL.[37] We measure MMA and Hcy levels in patients with polyneuropathy who are suspected of having vitamin B12 deficiency (e.g., those with a sudden onset of symptoms, symptoms beginning in the hands, findings suggestive of myelopathy, or risk factors for vitamin B12 malabsorption). In addition, we routinely measure copper, ceruloplasmin, and zinc levels in the same group of patients as copper deficiency manifests in a virtually identical manner.

In the absence of symptomatic gastrointestinal disease, it probably is not necessary to seek a diagnosis of pernicious anemia in a patient with vitamin B12 deficiency because this information will not alter management.[38] A Schilling test can be done to diagnose pernicious anemia.[39] It is a multistep and therefore inconvenient test which is now uncommonly utilized. Anti-intrinsic factor antibodies are specific for pernicious anemia but are found in only 50% of patients.[40] The combination of elevated gastrin and antiparietal cell antibodies is more sensitive and specific for pernicious anemia.[41]

NCS reveal absent or reduced SNAP amplitudes with CMAPs amplitudes that are normal or slightly reduced. Motor and sensory distal latencies and conduction velocities are essentially normal or only mildly abnormal.[26–30,34,42] Somatosensory-evoked potentials and magnetic stimulation studies may reveal prolongation of central conduction time.[29,32] Magnetic resonance imaging (MRI) scans of the cervical cord can reveal increased signal on T2 images in the posterior columns (Fig. 18-1).[43]

HISTOPATHOLOGY

Degeneration of the posterior columns and corticospinal tracts has been found at autopsies. Nerve biopsies reveal loss of large myelinated fibers, axonal degeneration, and secondary segmental demyelination.[31,34,44]

PATHOGENESIS

Cobalamin is found in meat, fish, and dairy products but is not present in fruits, vegetables, and grains. Vitamin B12 requires a transport molecule, intrinsic factor, which is

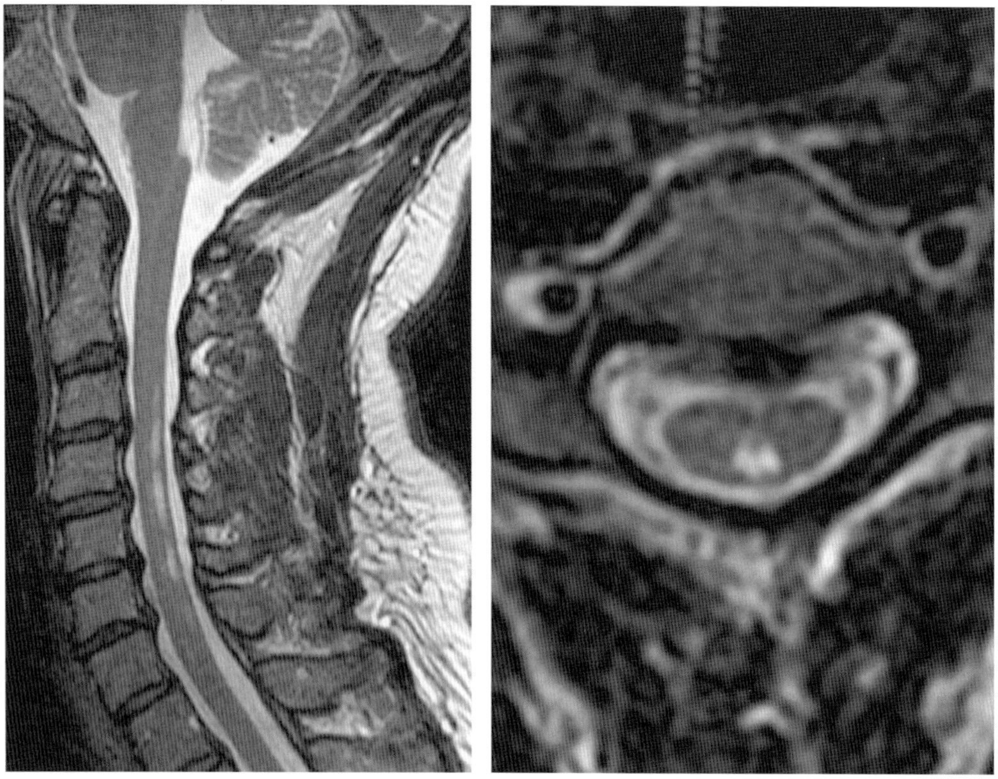

Figure 18-1. Vitamin B12 deficiency. Sagittal (*left image*) and axial (*right image*) T2 MRI in subacute combined degeneration (SCD) showing abnormal hyperintensity in the posterior columns. The patient had markedly reduced vibration and position sense and a Romberg sign; the tendon reflexes were preserved and there were no corticospinal tract or peripheral nerve signs. (Reproduced with permission from Ropper AH, Samuels MA, Klein JP, eds. *Adams and Victor's Principles of Neurology*, 10th ed. New York, NY: McGraw-Hill; 2014.)

synthesized and secreted by gastric parietal cells. Vitamin B12 deficiency can result from lack of dietary intake (strict vegetarian diet), lack of intrinsic factor (pernicious anemia with autoimmune destruction of parietal cells or gastrectomy), malabsorption syndromes (sprue or lower ileum resection), genetic defects in methionine synthetase, and bacteria (blind-loop syndrome) or bacterial or parasitic consumption prior to its absorption. Cobalamin functions as an enzyme necessary for demethylation of methyltetrahydrofolate.[45] Tetrahydrofolate, in turn, is required for the production of folate coenzymes that are necessary for DNA synthesis. The pathogenic mechanism for the neuropathy/myelopathy associated with cobalamin deficiency is not known but may be related to impairment in DNA synthesis, decreased methylation of myelin phospholipids, or buildup of methylmalonic and propionic acids that serve as abnormal substrates for fatty acid synthesis, leading to aberrant myelination.[45]

TREATMENT

We generally treat deficient patients with B12 1,000 μg IM/week for 1 month, followed by 1,000 μg IM/month thereafter. It may be possible to treat vitamin B12 deficiency with oral replacement. A randomized trial comparing treatment with 2,000-mg oral vitamin B12/day to 1,000-mg intramuscular vitamin B12/month showed similar improvements in hematologic indices, serum MMA and Hcy, and neurologic symptoms.[46] However, a minority of subjects had neurologic symptoms, and the methods by which clinical efficacy was assessed were lacking.

Approximately 2% of patients experience worsening sensory symptoms for unclear reasons during the first month of treatment.[47] The response to treatment of vitamin B12 deficiency polyneuropathy, separate from other neurologic complications of vitamin B12, has not been well studied. Patients with vitamin B12 deficiency polyneuropathy/myelopathy probably do not show an immediate response to treatment and may not respond at all.[34,48] The duration of symptoms is an important determinant of treatment response.[47,49,50]

▶ VITAMIN B12 DEFICIENCY SECONDARY TO NITROUS OXIDE INHALATION

Nitrous oxide can inactivate methylcobalamin, leading to neuropathy and subacute combine degeneration in individuals with low or borderline vitamin B12 levels, euphemistically referred to as "anesthetica paresthetica."[51–54] Physical examination, electrodiagnostic findings, and nerve biopsies are similar to that seen in B12 deficiency, as described in the previous section.

▶ FOLATE DEFICIENCY

CLINICAL FEATURES

Folate deficiency is associated with neurologic abnormalities similar to those complicating B12 deficiency.[55,56] Subacute combined degeneration of the posterior columns and corticospinal tracts, sensorimotor peripheral neuropathy, and altered mental status can develop.

LABORATORY FEATURES

Serum folate levels should be reduced. It is necessary to measure both serum folate and vitamin B12 levels to define a pure folic acid deficiency. Megaloblastic anemia may be evident on a complete blood count and smear. Sensory and motor NCS are similar to those seen with B12 deficiency.

PATHOGENESIS

Folate is found in fruit and vegetables and in liver. It is primarily absorbed in the proximal jejunum. Isolated folic acid deficiencies are extremely rare but can occur in the elderly on poor diets, alcoholics, young persons' consuming only snack foods, partial gastrectomies, duodenojejunal resections, celiac disease, and disorders of the jejunal mucosa.[55,56] Several drugs (e.g., phenytoin, phenobarbital, sulfasalazine, and colchicine) can also interfere with the optimal utilization of folic acid. The mechanism by which folic acid deficiency results in a polyneuropathy is not known; however, folic acid is required in DNA synthesis.

TREATMENT

Administration of folic acid usually results in good clinical recovery.

▶ VITAMIN E DEFICIENCY

CLINICAL FEATURES

Vitamin E or alpha-tocopherol is a lipid-soluble antioxidant vitamin that is present in the lipid bilayer constituting the cell membrane.[57,58] There is a close relationship between the metabolism of lipids and that of vitamin E. There are three major mechanisms associated with vitamin E deficiency: (1) deficient fat absorption (e.g., cystic fibrosis, chronic cholestasis, short-bowel syndrome, and intestinal lymphangiectasia), (2) deficient fat transport (abetalipoproteinemia, hypobetalipoproteinemia, normotriglyceridemic abetalipoproteinemia, and chylomicron retention disease), and (3) a genetically based abnormality of vitamin E metabolism. Patients with vitamin E deficiency usually present with progressive difficulty ambulating and impaired coordination of the hands.[59–62] Some individuals complain of weakness and sensory loss. Dysarthria can also occur.

Physical examination is remarkable for ataxia of the trunk and upper and lower extremities.[59–62] There is prominent loss of proprioception and vibratory perception. Muscle stretch reflexes are reduced or absent. Manual muscle testing can be difficult secondary to the ataxia, but there can be proximal muscle weakness, suggesting a superimposed myopathic process. Ocular examination may reveal ophthalmoplegia and retinopathy.

LABORATORY FEATURES

Vitamin E (alpha-tocopherol) levels in the serum are low. With hyperlipidemia, the vitamin E level may be normal. In such cases, the ratio of total serum vitamin E to the total serum lipid concentration is a more sensitive indicator of vitamin E deficiency.[63]

NCS reveal reduced amplitudes or absent SNAPs.[57–64] The sensory nerve conduction velocities are normal or only slightly reduced. Somatosensory-evoked potentials demonstrate normal peripheral nerve potentials with marked slowing and attenuation of central responses consistent with slowing of central conduction with loss of posterior column fibers.[65] Motor NCS are normal.

HISTOPATHOLOGY

Autopsy studies demonstrate swelling and degeneration of axons in the posterior columns and spinocerebellar tracts along with neuronal loss and lipofuscin accumulation in the gracile and cuneate nuclei.[60,66,67] Changes within the basal ganglia may be seen. Sural nerve biopsies show nonspecific abnormalities including the loss of large myelinated fibers, axonal degeneration, regenerating sprouts, occasional vacuoles in the myelin sheath, and breakup of the Schmidt–Lanterman incisures, but little in the way of primary demyelination.[68,69]

PATHOGENESIS

There are four main types of vitamin E, the most active of which is alpha-tocopherol. Vitamin E is lipid soluble and absorbed in the small intestine. Vitamin E is incorporated into chylomicrons and is transported to the liver. Here, vitamin E is incorporated into very low-density lipoproteins in a step requiring alpha-tocopherol transfer protein. Deficiency of this transfer protein is associated with hereditary vitamin E deficiency (discussed in Chapter 12). Vitamin E may serve to eliminate free radicals and stabilize cell membrane structure.[70]

Vitamin E deficiency is usually due to factors other than insufficient intake.[71] As mentioned, deficiency can result secondary to disorders of lipid malabsorption or transport. Abetalipoproteinemia is a rare autosomal-dominant disorder characterized by steatorrhea, pigmentary retinopathy, acanthocytosis, and progressive ataxia that is associated with vitamin E deficiency.[72] Cystic fibrosis can also be complicated by vitamin E deficiency secondary to malabsorption. There are also genetic forms of isolated vitamin E.[73,74] Mutations in the alpha-tocopherol transfer protein gene, *TTPA,* located on chromosome 8q13 result in loss of vitamin E.[75,76] Vitamin E deficiency may also complicate various liver and biliary disorders as well as surgical removal of parts of the intestines leading to short bowel or dumping syndrome.[64,77,78]

TREATMENT

Therapy is aimed at preventing progression, but improvement in neurologic function may occur. The specific dose of vitamin E is dependent upon the cause of deficiency.[71] In cases of isolated vitamin E deficiency, patients are treated with 1,500–6,000 international units (IU)/day in divided doses. Patients with chronic cholestasis are initially treated with 50 IU/kg/d and the dose is increased in 50 IU/kg increments up to a 200 IU/kg/d as required to obtain a normal serum tocopherol to lipid ratio. Patients with cystic fibrosis, who are receiving oral pancreatic enzyme therapy, require doses of 5–10 IU/kg/d. Those with short bowel syndrome are given 300–5,400 IU/d. Abetalipoproteinemia is treated with vitamin E 150–300 IU/kg/d and vitamin A 15,000–20,000 IU/d.

▶ POSTGASTRECTOMY/BARIATRIC SURGERY DEFICIENCIES

Polyneuropathy may complicate gastric/bariatric surgery for gastric ulcers, cancer, or morbid obesity.[14,79–82] The clinical picture is variable and may include acute or subacute sensory loss, burning feet, generalized weakness that can resemble Guillain–Barré syndrome, mononeuropathies, and radiculoplexus neuropathy.[82–86] Some cases are complicated by CNS dysfunction resembling Wernicke–Korsakoff syndrome. In the largest retrospective series, 71 out of 435 (16%) of patients who underwent bariatric surgery developed some type of peripheral neuropathy. The neuropathy is associated with malnutrition and the rapidity of weight loss and usually develops within the first 1½ years following weight loss surgery.[79,82,86] The latency between surgery and symptoms ranges from a few months to years in patients following total or partial gastrectomy for ulcer or cancer.[14,87]

Weight reduction surgical procedures include gastrojejunostomy, gastric stapling, vertical banded gastroplasty, and gastrectomy with Roux-en-Y anastomosis. Although thiamine deficiency seems to be a factor (given the frequent co-occurrence of the Wernicke–Korsakoff syndrome), there is not good documentation of thiamine deficiency in the reported cases. In some cases, one or more vitamin deficiencies are identified.[88] In many cases, no specific deficiency is identified. Electrodiagnostic studies most commonly reveal evidence of a length-dependent, axonal, sensory greater than motor polyneuropathy.

HISTOPATHOLOGY

Sural nerve biopsies when obtained may reveal active axonal degeneration and mild perivascular, endoneurial, and epineurial infiltrate.

PATHOGENESIS

The basis of the neuropathies is unclear but likely to result from multiple nutritional deficiencies.

TREATMENT

Patients should be treated with parenteral vitamin supplementation and, on occasion, reversal of the surgical bypass.[82,88,89] Patients with protracted vomiting after weight reduction surgery should receive total parenteral nutrition and vitamins. Patients can recover if started on treatment early, though some will have persistent sensory loss and weakness. The duration and severity of deficits before identification and treatment of neuropathy are important predictors of final outcome.

▶ COPPER DEFICIENCY

CLINICAL FEATURES

Copper deficiency is associated with an unusual myeloneuropathy, neutropenia, and sometimes pancytopenia.[82,90–100] The clinical phenotype is similar to vitamin B12 deficiency. Most patients manifest with numbness and tingling in the legs, weakness, spasticity, and gait difficulties. Large-fiber sensory function is impaired, reflexes are brisk, and plantar responses are extensor. In some cases, light touch and pinprick sensation are affected and NCS indicate sensorimotor axonal polyneuropathy in addition to myelopathy.[91,93] A severe motor axonopathy can also be seen.[94] The weakness and sensory loss in some cases is primarily due to a myelopathy.[95] Demyelinating lesions may be appreciated on brain MRI, and some patients have ocular dysmetria indicating brain involvement.[95]

LABORATORY FEATURES

Besides low–serum-copper levels, some cases are associated with high levels of zinc. Microcytic anemia and neutropenia[90,93–98,101,102] and occasionally pancytopenia[91] are also seen. Bone marrow biopsy may reveal abnormalities of a myelodysplastic syndrome. Cerebrospinal fluid may be normal or show mildly elevated protein or immunoglobulin synthesis rate.[91,94,95,97] MRI may demonstrate abnormal T2-weighted signal in the dorsal columns.[90,94,95,97,98]

NCS may reveal features of a sensorimotor axonal polyneuropathy.[91,93,97,98] Somatosensory-evoked potentials demonstrate impaired conduction in the central pathway in those with myelopathy.[97,98]

HISTOPATHOLOGY

Sural nerve biopsies may show evidence of axonal degeneration.[97,98]

PATHOGENESIS

Copper is absorbed in the stomach and proximal jejunum accounting for why deficiency may complicate gastric surgery.[90,93,103] The reason that zinc can lead to copper deficiency is that it upregulates the production of metallothionein in the gut, which in turn reduces copper absorption.[104,105] Interestingly, some denture creams contain a large amount of zinc and can lead to hypocupremia and neurologic disease.[96] Copper deficiency may also result from malnutrition, prematurity, total parenteral nutrition, and copper chelating agents.[101,103]

TREATMENT

The myeloneuropathy may improve with oral or intravenous copper replacement quickly[90,92,93] but benefits may not be seen for months or years.[91,95,97] and some patients do not improve at all.[94] In contrast to the variable clinical improvement, the pancytopenia usually normalizes with copper replacement therapy.[97]

HYPOPHOSPHATEMIA

Hyperalimentation with inadequate phosphate supplementation can lead to hypophosphatemia and the development of a subacute and severe sensorimotor peripheral neuropathy, which can clinically resemble Guillain–Barré syndrome.[106,107] Typically, serum phosphate levels need to be below 1 mg/dL for this to occur. Paresthesias are initially noted in the feet and ascend to involve the upper limbs and remainder of the body. Impaired ambulation secondary to both weakness and sensory ataxia occurs over the course of hours to days. Generalized weakness, ataxia, depressed muscle stretch reflexes, and reduced perception of all sensory modalities are appreciated on examination. Weakness may also involve the ventilatory muscles requiring mechanical assistance. NCS reveal an absence of SNAPs, reduced CMAP amplitudes, and slow conduction velocities. Correction of the hypophosphatemia results in clinical and electrophysiologic improvement.

▶ ALCOHOLIC NEUROPATHY

CLINICAL FEATURES

Alcoholics can develop a generalized axonal sensorimotor polyneuropathy.[12,108–112] Usually the neuropathy is slowly progressive, although some cases with acute or subacute presentation resembling Guillain–Barré syndrome have been reported.[113,114] Unlike Guillain–Barré syndrome, CSF protein in alcohol-related acute axonal polyneuropathy is usually normal or only slightly elevated. Most cases are preceded by prominent weight loss for 2–3 months. Most patients manifest with an insidious onset of numbness, paresthesia, and burning pain suggestive of a small fiber polyneuropathy. It is estimated that the equivalent of 10 oz of 86 proof-distilled spirits were 3 L of beer a day for 3 or more years, which is the threshold for alcoholic neuropathy. It has also been hypothesized that the lead content of wine may also contribute to the pathogenesis of alcoholic neuropathy.[12]

Examination demonstrates a reduction of all sensory modalities in a glove and stocking distribution, worse in the lower compared to upper limbs. Muscle stretches are reduced or absent. Mild distal leg weakness may be appreciated, but proximal leg and arm strength is usually normal. An occasional patient presents with symptoms and signs suggestive of a myopathy as opposed to neuropathy. NCS reveal features suggestive of a generalized axonal sensory or sensorimotor polyneuropathy.[12,108–110,112]

HISTOPATHOLOGY

Nerve biopsies may reveal loss of large- and small-caliber myelinated fibers along with Wallerian degeneration and secondary segmental demyelination.[112,114]

PATHOGENESIS

The exact etiology of peripheral nerve insult in alcoholism is unknown but may in part be related to both a nutritional deficiency (e.g., vitamin B group and folate) and a direct toxic effect of alcohol on peripheral nerves.[12]

TREATMENT

Abstaining from alcohol and consuming an optimal diet can result in an improvement of the peripheral neuropathy.[114]

▶ SUMMARY

Nutritional neuropathies are not particularly common. However, because they can be treatable with correction of the deficit, it is important to be vigilant for signs and symptoms that would suggest a nutritional deficiency. In particular, those patients with gastrointestinal disease or history of gastric bypass may be particularly vulnerable.

REFERENCES

1. Ohnishi A, Tsuji S, Igisu H, et al. Beriberi neuropathy. Morphometric study of sural nerve. *J Neurol Sci.* 1980;45:177–190.
2. Hong CZ. Electrodiagnostic findings of persisting polyneuropathies due to previous nutritional deficiency in former prisoners of war. *Electromyogr Clin Neurophysiol.* 1986;26:351–363.
3. McCormick DB, Greene HL. Vitamins. In: Burtis CA, Ash-wood ER, eds. *Tierz Textbook of Clinical Chemistry.* Philadelphia, PA: Saunders; 1999:999–1028.
4. Brin M, Tai M, Ostashever AS, Kalinsky H. The effect of thiamine deficiency on the activity of erythrocyte hemolysate transketolase. *J Nutr.* 1960;71:273–281.
5. Brin M. Erythrocyte transketolase in early thiamine deficiency. *Ann N Y Acad Sci.* 1962;98:528–541.
6. Jeyasingham MD, Pratt OE, Burns A, Shaw GK, Thomson AD, Marsh A. The activation of red blood cell transketolase in groups of patients especially at risk from thiamin deficiency. *Psychol Med.* 1987;17:311–318.
7. Jeyasingham MD, Pratt OE, Shaw GK, Thomson AD. Changes in the activation of red blood cell transketolase of alcoholic patients during treatment. *Alcohol.* 1987;22:259–365.
8. Takahashi K, Nakamura H. Axonal degeneration in beriberi neuropathy. *Arch Neurol.* 1976;33:836–841.
9. Collins RC, Lonergan ET. Transketolase and myelin. *N Engl J Med.* 1971;285:751–752.
10. Cooper JR, Pincus JH. The role of thiamin in nervous tissue. *Neurochem Res.* 1979;4:223–229.
11. Schoffeniels E. Thiamine phosphorylated derivatives and bioelectrogenesis. *Arch Int Physiol Biochim.* 1983;91:233–242.
12. Mellion M, Gilchrist JM, de la Monte S. Alcohol- related peripheral neuropathy: nutritional, toxic, or both? *Muscle Nerve.* 2011;43:309–316.
13. Jolliffe N. The diagnosis, treatment and prevention of vitamin B1 deficiency. *Bull N Y Acad Med.* 1939;15:469–478.
14. Koike H, Misu K, Hattori N, et al. Postgastrectomy polyneuropathy with thiamine deficiency. *J Neurol Neurosurg Psychiatry.* 2001;71:357–362.
15. Albin RL, Albers JW, Greenberg HS, et al. Acute sensory neuropathy-neuronopathy from pyridoxine overdose. *Neurology.* 1987;37:1729–1732.
16. Dalton K, Dalton MJ. Characteristics of pyridoxine overdose neuropathy syndrome. *Acta Neurol Scand.* 1987;76:8–11.
17. Parry GJ, Bredesen DE. Sensory neuropathy with low dose pyridoxine. *Neurology.* 1985;35:1466–1468.
18. Schaumburg H, Kaplan J, Windsbank A, et al. Sensory neuropathy from pyridoxine abuse. A new megavitamin syndrome. *N Engl J Med.* 1983;309:445–448.
19. Gammon GD, Burge FW, King G. Neural toxicity in tuberculous patients treated with isoniazid (isonicotinic acid hydrazide). *AMA Arch Neurol Psychiatry.* 1953;70:64–69.
20. Lubing HN. Peripheral neuropathy in tuberculosis patients treated with isoniazid. *Am Rev Tuberc.* 1953;68:458–461.
21. Selikoff IJ, Robitzek EH, Ornstein CG. Treatment of pulmonary tuberculosis with hydrazide derivatives of nicotinic acid. *J Am Med Assoc.* 1952;150(10):973–980.
22. Moriwaki K, Kanno Y, Nakamoto H, Okada H, Suzuki H. Vitamin B6 deficiency in elderly patients on chronic peritoneal dialysis. *Adv Perit Dial.* 2000;16:308–312.
23. Ruffin JM, Smith DT. Treatment of pellagra with special reference to the use of nicotinic acid. *South Med J.* 1939;32:40–47.
24. Sebrel WH, Butler RE. Riboflavin deficiency in man (ariboflavinosis). *Public Health Rep.* 1939;54:2121–2131.
25. Marcus R, Coulston AN. Water-soluble vitamins. In: Gilman AG, Goodman LS, Rall TW, Murad F, eds. *Goodman and Gilman's the Pharmacological Basis of Therapeutics*, 7th ed. New York, NY: Macmillan Publishing Company; 1985:1551–1572.
26. Fine EJ, Hallett M. Neurophysiological study of subacute combined degeneration. *J Neurol Sci.* 1980;45:331–336.
27. Fine EJ, Soria E, Paroski MW, Petryk D, Thomasula L. The neurophysiological profile of vitamin B_{12} deficiency. *Muscle Nerve.* 1990;13:158–164.
28. Hahn AF, Gilbert JJ, Brown WF. A study of the sural nerve in pernicious anemia. *Can J Neurol Sci.* 1976;3:217.
29. Hemmer B, Glocker FX, Schumacher M, Deuschl G, Lucking CH. Subacute combined degeneration: clinical, electrophysiological, and magnetic resonance imaging findings. *J Neurol Neurosurg Psychiatry.* 1998;65:822–827.
30. Kayser-Gatchalian MC, Neundorfer B. Peripheral neuropathy with vitamin B_{12} deficiency. *J Neurol.* 1977;214:183–193.
31. Kosik KS, Mullins TF, Bradley WG, Tempelis LD, Cretella AJ. Coma and axonal degeneration in vitamin B12 deficiency. *Arch Neurol.* 1980;37:590–592.
32. Krumholz A, Weiss HD, Goldstein PJ, Harris KC. Evoked responses in vitamin B12 deficiency. *Ann Neurol.* 1981;9:407–409.
33. Lockner D, Reizenstein P, Wennberg A, Widén L. Peripheral nerve function in pernicious anemia before and after treatment. *Acta Haematol.* 1969;41:257–263.
34. McCombe PA, McLeod JG. The peripheral neuropathy of vitamin B12 deficiency. *J Neurol Sci.* 1984;66:117–126.
35. Carmel R. Current concepts in cobalamin deficiency. *Annu Rev Med.* 2000;51:357–375.
36. Savage DG, Lindenbaum J, Stabler SP, Allen RH. Sensitivity of serum methylmalonic acid and total homocysteine determinations for diagnosing cobalamin and folate deficiencies. *Am J Med.* 1994;96:239–246.
37. Lindenbaum J, Savage DG, Stabler SP, Allen RH. Diagnosis of cobalamin deficiency: II. Relative sensitivities of serum cobalamin, methylmalonic acid, and total homocysteine concentrations. *Am J Hematol.* 1990;34:99–107.
38. Stabler SP. Screening the older population for cobalamin (vitamin B12) deficiency. *J Am Geriatr Soc.* 1995;43:1290–1297.
39. Swain R. An update of vitamin B12 metabolism and deficiency states. *J Fam Pract.* 1995;41:595–600.

40. Chanarin I. *The Megaloblastic Anemias*. 2nd ed. Oxford, England: Blackwell Scientific Publications; 1979.
41. Metz J, Bell AH, Flicker L, et al. The significance of subnormal serum vitamin B12 concentration in older people: a case control study. *J Am Geriatr Soc*. 1996;44:1355–1361.
42. Saperstein DS, Wolfe GI, Nations SP, Herbelin LL, Barohn RJ. Electrodiagnostic features of cobalamin deficiency polyneuropathy. *Muscle Nerve*. 2002;26:574.
43. Bou-Haidar P, Peduto AJ, Karunaratne N. Differential diagnosis of T2 hyperintense spinal cord lesions: part B. *J Med Imaging Radiat Oncol*. 2009;53:152–159.
44. Abarbanel JM, Frishers S, Osimani A. Vitamin B12 deficiency neuropathy: sural nerve biopsy study. *Isr J Med Sci*. 1986;22:909–911.
45. Green R, Kinsella LJ. Current concepts in the diagnosis of cobalamin deficiency. *Neurology*. 1995;45:1435–1440.
46. Kuzminski AM, Del Giacco EJ, Allen RH, Stabler SP, Lindenbaum J. Effective treatment of cobalamin deficiency with oral cobalamin. *Blood*. 1998;92:1191–1198.
47. Healton EB, Savage DG, Brust JC, Garrett TJ, Lindenbaum J. Neurologic aspects of cobalamin deficiency. *Medicine (Baltimore)*. 1991;70:229–245.
48. Saperstein DS, Wolfe GI, Gronseth GS, et al. Challenges in the identification of cobalamin-deficiency polyneuropathy. *Arch Neurol*. 2003;60:1296–1301.
49. Hyland HH, Farquharson RF. Subacute combined degeneration of the spinal cord in pernicious anemia. *Arch Neurol Psychiatry*. 1936;36:1166–1205.
50. Ungley CC. Subacute combined degeneration of the cord: I. Response to liver extracts. II. Trials with vitamin B12. *Brain*. 1949;72:382–427.
51. Heyer EJ, Simpson DM, Bodis-Wollner I, Diamond SP. Nitrous oxide: clinical and electrophysiologic investigation of neurologic complications. *Neurology*. 1986;36:1618–1622.
52. Layzer RB, Fishman RA, Schafer JA. Neuropathy following abuse of nitrous oxide. *Neurology*. 1978;28:504–506.
53. Sahenk Z, Mendell JR, Couri D, Nachtman J. Polyneuropathy from inhalation of N_2O cartridges through a whipped-cream dispenser. *Neurology*. 1978;28:485–487.
54. Vishnubhakat SM, Beresford HR. Reversible myeloneuropathy of nitrous oxide abuse: serial electrophysiological studies. *Muscle Nerve*. 1991;14:22–26.
55. Enk C, Hougaard K, Hippe E. Reversible dementia and neuropathy associated with folate deficiency 16 years after partial gastrectomy. *Scand J Haematol*. 1980;25:63–66.
56. Fehling C, Jagerstad M, Linstrand K, et al. Folate deficiency and neurological disease. *Arch Neurol*. 1974;30:263–265.
57. Guggenheim MA, Ringel SP, Silverman A, Grabert BE. Progressive neuromuscular disease in children with chronic cholestasis and vitamin E deficiency: diagnosis and treatment with alpha tocopherol. *J Pediatr*. 1982;100:51–58.
58. Harding AE. Vitamin E and the nervous system. *Crit Rev Neurobiol*. 1987;3(1):89–103.
59. Bertoni JM, Abraham FA, Falls HF, Itabashi HH. Small bowel resection with vitamin E deficiency and progressive spinocerebellar syndrome. *Neurology*. 1984;34:1046–1052.
60. Rosenblum JL, Keating JP, Prensky AL, Nelson JS. A progressive neurologic syndrome in children with chronic liver disease. *N Engl J Med*. 1981;304:503–508.
61. Ko HY, Park-Ko I. Electrophysiologic recovery after vitamin E-deficient neuropathy. *Arch Phys Med Rehab*. 1999;80:964–967.
62. Brin M, Pedley TA, Lovelace RE, et al. Electrophysiologic features of abetalipoproteinemia: functional consequences of vitamin E deficiency. *Neurology*. 1986;36:669–673.
63. Sokol RJ, Heubi JE, Iannaccone ST, Bove KE, Balistreri WF. Vitamin E deficiency with normal serum vitamin E concentrations in children with chronic cholestasis. *N Engl J Med*. 1984;310:1209–1212.
64. Satya-Murti S, Howard L, Krohel G, Wolf B. The spectrum of neurologic disorder from vitamin E deficiency. *Neurology*. 1986;36:917–921.
65. Kaplan PW, Rawal K, Erwin CW, D'Souza BJ, Spock A. Visual and somatosensory evoked potentials in vitamin E deficiency with cystic fibrosis. *Electroencephalogr Clin Neurophysiol*. 1988;71:266–272.
66. Jeffrey GP, Muller DPR, Burroughs AK, et al. Vitamin E deficiency and its clinical significance in adults with primary biliary cirrhosis and other forms of chronic liver disease. *J Hepatol*. 1987;4:307–317.
67. Sung JH, Stadlan EM. Neuroaxonal dystrophy in congenital biliary atresia. *J Neuropathol Exp Neurol*. 1966;25:341–361.
68. Traber MG, Sokol RJ, Ringel SP, Neville HE, Thellman CA, Kayden HJ. Lack of tocopherol in peripheral nerves of vitamin E-deficient patients with peripheral neuropathy. *N Engl J Med*. 1987;317:262–265.
69. Yokota T, Wada Y, Furukawa T, Tsukagoshi H, Uchihara T, Watabiki S. Adult-onset spinocerebellar syndrome with idiopathic vitamin E deficiency. *Ann Neurol*. 1987;22:84–87.
70. Tappel AL. Vitamin E and free radical peroxiadation of lipids. *Ann NY Acad Sci*. 1972;203:12–28.
71. Sokol RJ. Vitamin E and neurologic deficits. *Adv Pediatr*. 1990;37:119–148.
72. Muller DP, Harries JT, Lloyd JK. The relative importance of the factors involved in the absorption of vitamin E in children. *Gut*. 1974;15:966–971.
73. Harding AE, Matthews S, Jones S, Ellis CJ, Booth IW, Muller DP. Spinocerebellar degeneration associated with a selective defect of vitamin E absorption. *N Engl J Med*. 1985;313:32–35.
74. Sokol RJ, Kayden HJ, Bettis DB, et al. Isolated vitamin E deficiency in the absence of fat malabsorption–familial and sporadic cases: characterization and investigation of causes. *J Lab Clin Med*. 1988;111:548–559.
75. Ouahchi K, Arita M, Kayden H, et al. Ataxia with isolated vitamin E deficiency is caused by mutations in the α-tocopherol transfer protein. *Nat Genet*. 1995;9:141–145.
76. Gotoda T, Arita M, Arai H, et al. Adult-onset spinocerebellar dysfunction caused by a mutation in the gene for α-tocopherol transfer protein. *N Engl J Med*. 1995;333:1313–1318.
77. Harding AE, Muller DP, Thomas PK, Willison HJ. Spinocerebellar degeneration secondary to chronic intestinal malabsorption: a vitamin E deficiency syndrome. *Ann Neurol*. 1982;12:419–424.
78. Howard L, Ovensen L, Satya-Murti S, Chu R. Reversible neurological symptoms caused by vitamin E deficiency in a patient with short bowel syndrome. *Am J Clin Nutr*. 1982;36:1243–1249.
79. Cirignotta F, Manconi M, Mondini S, Buzzi G, Ambrosetto P. Wernicke–Korsakoff encephalopathy and polyneuropathy after gastroplasty for morbid obesity. *Arch Neurol*. 2000;57:1356–1359.
80. Harwood SC, Chodoroff G, Ellenberg MR. Gastric partitioning complicated by peripheral neuropathy with lumbosacral plexopathy. *Arch Phys Med Rehab*. 1987;68:310–312.

81. Somer H, Bergstrom L, Mustajoki P, Rovamo L. Morbid obesity, gastric application and a severe neurological deficit. *Acta Med Scand.* 1985;217:575–576.
82. Koffman BM, Greenfield LJ, Ali II, Pirzada NA. Neurologic complications after surgery for obesity. *Muscle Nerve.* 2006;33(2):166–176.
83. Feit H, Glasberg M, Ireton C, Rosenberg RN, Thal E. Peripheral neuropathy and starvation after gastric partitioning for morbid obesity. *Ann Intern Med.* 1982;96:453–455.
84. Williams JA, Hall GS, Thompson AG, Cooke WT. Neurological disease after partial gastrectomy. *Br Med J.* 1969;3:210–212.
85. Abarbanel JM, Berginer VM, Osimani A, Solomon H, Charuzi I. Neurologic complications after gastric restriction surgery for morbid obesity. *Neurology.* 1987;37:196–200.
86. Thaisetthawatkul P, Collazo-Clavell ML, Sarr MG, Noreel JE, Dyck PJ. A controlled study of peripheral neuropathy after bariatric surgery. *Neurology.* 2004;63:1462–1470.
87. Hoffman PM, Brody JA. Neurological disorders in patients following surgery for peptic ulcer. *Neurology.* 1972;22:450.
88. Rudnicki SA. Prevention and treatment of peripheral neuropathy after bariatric surgery. *Curr Treat Options Neurol.* 2010; 12:29–36.
89. Thaisetthawatkul P, Collazo-Clavell ML, Sarr MG, Norell JE, Dyck PJ. Good nutritional control may prevent polyneuropathy after bariatric surgery. *Muscle Nerve.* 2010;42:709–714.
90. Schleper B, Stuerenburg HJ. Copper deficiency-associated myelopathy in a 46-year-old woman. *J Neurol.* 2001;248:705–706.
91. Hedera P, Fink JK, Bockenstedt PL, Brewer GJ. Myelopolyneuropathy and pancytopenia due to copper deficiency and high zinc levels of unknown origin: further support for existence of a new zinc overload syndrome. *Arch Neurol.* 2003;60:1303–1306.
92. Kumar N, Gross JB Jr, Ahlskog JE. Myelopathy due to copper deficiency. *Neurology.* 2003;61:273–274.
93. Kumar N, McEvoy KM, Ahlskog JE. Myelopathy due to copper deficiency following gastrointestinal surgery. *Arch Neurol.* 2003;60:1782–1785.
94. Greenberg SA, Briemberg HR. A neurological and hematological syndrome associated with zinc and excess and copper deficiency. *J Neurol.* 2004; 251:111–114.
95. Prodan CI, Holland NR, Wisdom PJ, Burstein SA, Bottomley SS. CNS demyelination associated with copper deficiency and hyperzincemia. *Neurology.* 2002;59:1453–1456.
96. Nations SP, Boyer PJ, Love LA, et al. Denture cream: An unusual source of excess zinc, leading to hypocupremia and neurologic disease. *Neurology.* 2008;71:639–643.
97. Kumar N, Gross JB Jr, Ahlskog JE. Copper deficiency myelopathy produces a clinical picture like subacute combined degeneration. *Neurology.* 2004;63:33–39.
98. Kumar N. Copper deficiency myelopathy (human sway-back). *Mayo Clin Proc.* 2006;81(10):1371–1384.
99. Rowin J, Lewis SL. Copper deficiency myeloneuropathy and pancytopenia secondary to overuse of zinc supplementation. *J Neurol Neurosurg Psychiatry.* 2005;76(5):750–751.
100. Prodan CI, Bottomley SS, Holland NR, Lind SE. Relapsing hypocupraemic myelopathy requiring high-dose oral copper replacement. *J Neurol Neurosurg Psychiatry.* 2006;77(9):1092–1093.
101. Bottomley SS. Sideroblastic anemias. In: Lee GR, Foerster J, Lukens J, et al., eds. *Wintrobe's Clinical Hematology.* 10th ed. Baltimore, MD: Lippincott Williams & Wilkins; 1999:1022–1045.
102. Gregg XT, Reddy V, Prchal JT. Copper deficiency masquerading as myelodysplastic syndrome. *Blood.* 2002;100:1493–1495.
103. Solomons NW. Biochemical, metabolic, and clinical role of copper in human nutrition. *J Am Coll Clin Nutr.* 1985;4:83–105.
104. Irving JA, Mattman A, Lockitch G, Farrell K, Wadsworth LD. Element of caution: a case of reversible cytopenias associated with excessive zinc supplementation. *CMAJ.* 2003;169: 129–131.
105. Fiske DN, McCoy HE III, Kitchens CS. Zinc-induced sideroblastic anemia: report of a case, review of the literature, and description of the hematologic syndrome. *Am J Hematol.* 1994; 46:147–150.
106. Weintraub MI. Hypophosphatemia mimicking acute Guillain–Barré–Strohl syndrome: a complication of hyperalimentation. *JAMA.* 1976;235:1040–1041.
107. Yagnik P, Singh N, Burns R. Peripheral neuropathy with hypophosphatemia in patient receiving intravenous hyperalimentation. *Muscle Nerve.* 1982;5:562.
108. Casey EB, Le Quesne PM. Electrophysiological evidence for a distal lesion in alcoholic neuropathy. *J Neurol Neurosurg Psychiatry.* 1972;35:624–630.
109. Mawdsley C, Mayer RF. Nerve conduction in alcoholic polyneuropathy. *Brain.* 1985;88:335–356.
110. Shankar K, Maloney FP, Thompson C. An electrodiagnostic study in chronic alcoholic subjects. *Arch Phys Med Rehab.* 1987;68:803–805.
111. Shields RW Jr. Alcoholic polyneuropathy. *Muscle Nerve.* 1985; 8:183–187.
112. Walsh JC, McLeod JG. Alcoholic neuropathy: an electrophysiological and histological study. *J Neurol Sci.* 1970;10:457–469.
113. Tabaraud F, Vallat JM, Hugon J, Ramiandrisoa H, Dumas M, Signoret JL. Acute or subacute alcoholic neuropathy mimicking Guillain–Barré syndrome. *J Neurol Sci.* 1990;97:195–205.
114. Wöhrle JC, Spengos K, Steinke W, Goebel HH, Hennerici M. Alcohol-related acute axonal polyneuropathy. A differential diagnosis of Guillain–Barré syndrome. *Arch Neurol.* 1998;55:1329–1334.

CHAPTER 19

Neuropathies Associated with Malignancy

Patients with malignancy can develop peripheral neuropathies as the result of (1) a direct effect of the cancer by invasion or compression of the nerves, (2) a remote or paraneoplastic effect including vasculitis, (3) a direct toxic effect of treatment, or (4) an alteration of immune status caused by immunosuppression (Table 19-1).[1,2] It is difficult to estimate the frequency of polyneuropathy in patients with cancer because it is dependent on a number of factors including the type, stage, and location of the malignancy, as well as confounding variables such as malnutrition, the toxic effects of therapy, and the background incidence of neuropathy in this frequently older population. Nevertheless, some series indicate that 1.7–5.5% of patients with cancer have clinical symptoms or signs of a peripheral neuropathy, while neurophysiologic testing (quantitative sensory testing and nerve conduction studies [NCS]) demonstrates evidence of peripheral neuropathy in as many as 30–40% of patients with cancer.[3] The most common associated malignancy is lung cancer, but neuropathies also complicate carcinoma of the breast, ovaries, stomach, colon, rectum, and other organs including the lymphoproliferative system.

▶ PARANEOPLASTIC NEUROPATHIES

Neuropathies related to remote effects of carcinoma or the so-called paraneoplastic syndromes are quite interesting but quite rare.[1,2,4]

PARANEOPLASTIC SENSORY NEURONOPATHY/GANGLIONOPATHY

In 1948, Denny-Brown reported two patients with small-cell lung cancer (SCLC) and sensory neuronopathy (SN).[5] Autopsies revealed dorsal root ganglionitis with degeneration of the posterior columns as well as peripheral sensory axons. Subsequently, there have been many reports of patients presenting with paraneoplastic encephalomyelitis (PEM) and/or SN.[3,5–31] SCLC is the most common malignancy associated with PEM/SN, but cases of carcinoma of the esophagus, breast, ovaries, kidney, and lymphoma have also been reported.[3,5,6] Approximately 13% of patients with SCLC have another type of concomitant malignancy.[3] Therefore, finding a malignancy other than SCLC in a patient with PEM/SN does not obviate the need to look for concurrent lung cancer.

Clinical Features

PEM/SN most commonly develops in the sixth or seventh decade.[3,5,6,32] The disease is more common in women than in men (up to a 2:1 ratio). The neurologic symptoms usually precede the diagnosis of cancer. Most malignancies are detected within 4–12 months, although there are reports of cancer being diagnosed 8 years or more following the onset of the neurologic symptoms.[3,5] Patients usually present with numbness, dysesthesia, and paresthesia, usually in the distal extremities. These symptoms begin in the hands in up to 60% and may be asymmetric in 27–40% of cases, a pattern that provides a helpful clue in distinguishing a SN from the more typical length-dependent axonal sensory polyneuropathy.[3,5] The onset can be quite acute or insidiously progressive. Diminished touch, pain, and temperature sensation and prominent loss of vibratory and position sense occur, resulting in sensory ataxia and pseudoathetosis. The causes of sensory ataxia are limited and should lead to a malignancy workup in any patient who exhibits such signs (Table 19-2). Muscle stretch reflexes are diminished or absent. While sensory symptoms predominate, mild weakness is evident in at least 20% of patients.[3] Weakness can be secondary to an associated myelitis, motor neuronopathy, or concurrent Lambert–Eaton myasthenic syndrome (LEMS).[3,5,32] Autonomic neuropathy may occur as an isolated disturbance or as part of the spectrum of a paraneoplastic syndrome in up to 28% of patients and can be the presenting feature in as many as 12%.[3,5,32]

Another clue suggesting a paraneoplastic etiology is the concomitant involvement of other anatomically unrelated neurologic systems. As many as 21% of affected individuals present with limbic encephalitis manifesting as confusion, memory loss, depression, hallucinations, or seizures.[3,5,32] Approximately 32% of patients develop brainstem dysfunction (e.g., diplopia, vertigo, nausea, and vomiting). Cranial neuropathies, especially of the eighth cranial nerve, occur in up to 15% of patients. Cerebellar ataxia, scanning dysarthria, tremor, and peduncular reflexes attributed to cerebellar dysfunction are evident in 25% of patients. Abnormal

TABLE 19-1. NEUROPATHIES ASSOCIATED WITH CANCER

Direct effect of the cancer by invasion or compression of the nerves
Paraneoplastic
Sensory ganglionopathy (anti-Hu syndrome)
Sensorimotor neuropathy
Autonomic neuropathy
Direct toxic effect of treatment
Neurotoxicity secondary to chemotherapy
Radiation toxicity
Alteration of immune status caused by immunosuppressive medications
Often occur in setting of bone marrow transplantation or treatment of GVHD

ocular movements such as nystagmus, opsoclonus, and internal and external ophthalmoplegia are seen in up to 32% of patients. Myoclonus develops in approximately 1% of patients. Myelitis with secondary degeneration of the anterior horn is the presenting feature in as many as 14% of those affected.

Laboratory Features

Polyclonal antineuronal antibodies (IgG) directed against a 35–40 kDa protein or complex of proteins, the so-called Hu antigen or antineuron nuclear antigen 1 (ANNA1), are found in the sera or cerebrospinal fluid (CSF) in the majority of patients with paraneoplastic PEM/SN.[3,5–13,32] The presence of anti-Hu antibodies in the serum correlates with SN,[11] while antibodies in the CSF are associated with the development of PEM.[12] In a study of 49 patients with paraneoplastic sensory neuropathy, anti-Hu antibodies were present in the serum of 40 out of 49 patients.[6] In 77 patients with idiopathic sensory neuropathy, anti-Hu antibodies were found in only 1 patient.[6] Thus, the sensitivity and specificity of the anti-Hu antibodies are high. However, 12% of patients with paraneoplastic SN did not have anti-Hu antibodies. Therefore, all patients suspected of having PEM/SN should undergo periodic screening for an underlying malignancy, regardless of their anti-Hu antibody status.

CSF may be normal or may demonstrate mild lymphocytic pleocytosis and elevated protein.[3,5,12,32] Oligoclonal bands and increased CSF IgG synthesis and index are evident in the majority of patients suggestive of intrathecal synthesis of the autoantibody. Magnetic resonance imaging (MRI) of the brain is usually unremarkable. However, some patients with encephalomyelitis have signal abnormalities on T2-weighted and FLAIR images in the temporal or frontal lobes.[3] Periventricular white matter hypodensities, and atrophy of the frontal and temporal lobes and cerebellum also have been reported.

NCS in pure SN reveal low-amplitude or absent sensory nerve action potentials (SNAPs).[33] Compound muscle action potentials (CMAPs) and needle electromyography (EMG) are normal unless the patient has a concurrent motor neuropathy or LEMS. The blink reflex study is usually abnormal, while the masseter reflex study can be normal.[14,15]

TABLE 19-2. CAUSES OF SENSORY NEUROPATHY/ GANGLIONOPATHY

Paraneoplastic (anti-Hu syndrome)
Sjögren's syndrome
Human immunodeficiency virus infection
Toxic agents (e.g., chemotherapy, pyridoxine, antinucleosides)

Reproduced with permission from Amato AA, Anderson MP. A 51 year old women with lung cancer and neuropsychiatric abnormalities (Case 38—2001). *N Engl J Med.* 2001;345(24):1758–1765.

Histopathology

Sural nerve biopsies may demonstrate perivascular inflammation comprised of plasma cells, macrophages, B cells, and T cells.[33] Autopsy studies reveal inflammation and degeneration of the dorsal root ganglia with secondary degeneration of sensory neurons and the posterior columns (Fig. 19-1).[2,3,13,16,31] In addition, inflammation and degeneration of neurons in the autonomic ganglia, including the myenteric plexus, may be evident.[16,17,19] Lennon et al. reported autoantibodies (presumably anti-Hu) directed against a nuclear antigen of myenteric neurons in patients with intestinal pseudo-obstruction due to autonomic involvement.[17] In patients with PEM, autopsies have revealed perivascular and perineuronal inflammation and degeneration of neurons in the brainstem and limbic system (medial temporal lobe, cingulate gyrus, piriform cortex, orbital surface of the frontal lobes, and the insular cortex) (Fig. 19-2).[3,8,13,32] The thalamus, hypothalamus, subthalamic nucleus, deep cerebellar nuclei, and Purkinje cells may also be involved. Inflammation and degeneration of the anterior horn cells and the ventral spinal roots are evident in patients with myelitis. In addition to deposition on tumor cells, deposits of anti-Hu antibody have been demonstrated in areas of the nervous system that correlate with the clinical symptoms.[13,16–19]

Pathogenesis

PEM/SN is probably the result of antigenic similarity between proteins expressed in the tumor cells and the neuron cells (e.g., Hu antigens), leading to an immune response directed against both tumor and neuronal cells.[3,5,20,21,32] The Hu antigen is a family of four similar RNA-binding proteins (HuD, HuC/ple21, Hel-N1, and Hel-N2). The Hu antigen is expressed in the nuclei and to a lesser extent in the cytoplasm of neurons and SCLC cells.[10] The function of this group of proteins is not known, but these are thought to be crucial in the development and maintenance of the nervous system.[21] The role of the anti-Hu antibodies in the development of PEM/NS is also unclear. The antibodies appear to bind

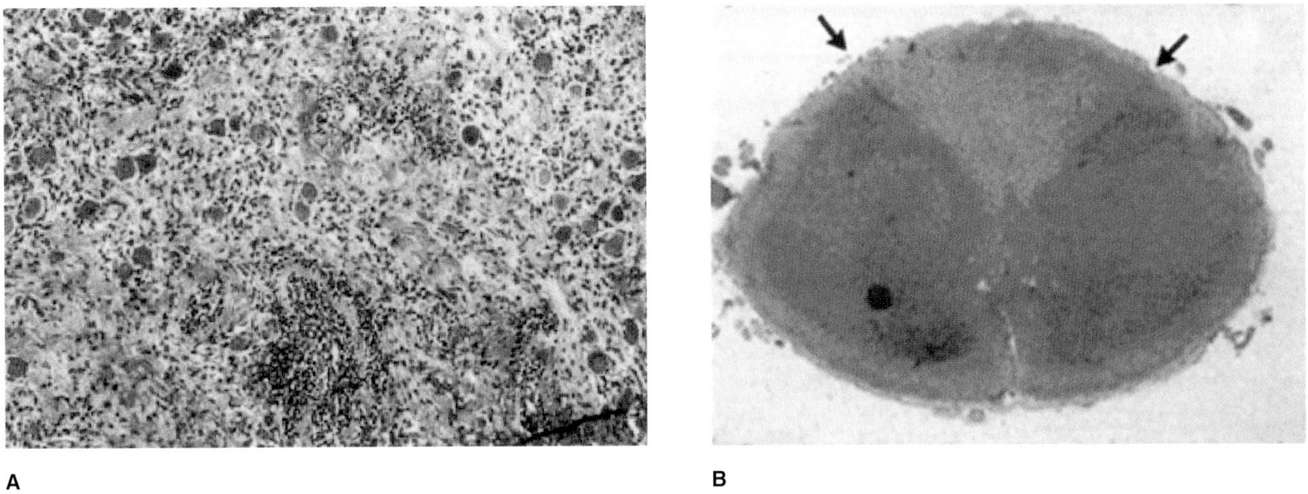

Figure 19-1. **(A)** Dorsal-root ganglia of the cervical cord, showing marked parenchymal and perivascular inflammation, loss of ganglion cells, and fibrosis (H&E, ×100). **(B)** Section of cervical spinal cord showing marked pallor of the dorsal columns (*arrows*) (Luxol Fast Blue—H&E, ×5). (Reproduced with permission from Amato AA, Anderson MP. A 51 year old woman with lung cancer and neuropsychiatric abnormalities (Case 38—2001). *N Engl J Med.* 2001;345(24):1758–1765.)

to CNS and PNS neurons affected in the syndrome.[13,16–19] There is a correlation of high anti-Hu titers in the CSF and the development of PEM,[12] and the serum titer with the occurrence of SN.[11] However, the anti-Hu antibodies have not been proved to be pathogenic. Passive transfer of autoantibodies from patients with PEM/SN and immunization with purified HuD protein have failed to reproduce the disease in animal studies.[24] Further, the anti-Hu antibodies exhibit only weak complement activation.[19,25]

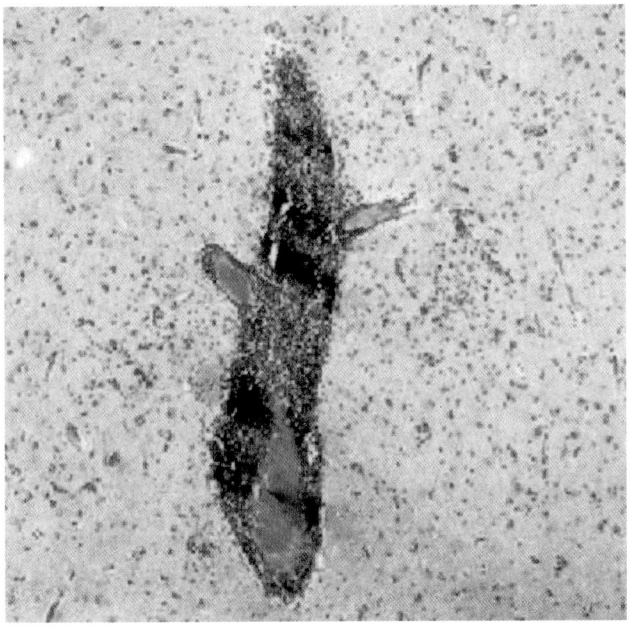

Figure 19-2. Amygdalar complex with a perivascular lymphocytic infiltrate and microglial nodules (H&E, ×100). (Reproduced with permission from Amato AA, Anderson MP. A 51 year old woman with lung cancer and neuropsychiatric abnormalities (Case 38—2001). *N Engl J Med.* 2001;345(24): 1758–1765.)

The cellular immune response also appears to be involved in the pathogenesis of PEM/SN.[26] The perivascular infiltrate in tumors and the nervous system consists mainly of CD4+ cells, B cells, and macrophages, while CD8+ cells, cytotoxic T cells, and microglia-like cells predominate in the tissue immediately surrounding neurons.[19,26] T-cell receptor studies on the inflammatory infiltrates in the nervous system and within the tumors of anti-Hu-positive PEM/SN patients reveal a limited Vβ repertoire and clonal expansion suggestive of an antigen-driven cytotoxic T-cell response.[27] Studies have demonstrated an increase of CD45RO+CD4+ memory helper T cells in the peripheral blood of patients with anti-PEM/SN.[26] Antigen-specific proliferation of these T cells occurs following in vitro stimulation of cultured lymphocytes with purified HuD antigen. In addition, the cells secreted interferon-γ, suggesting that these lymphocytes were primarily of the Th1 helper subtype. The authors speculated that neoplastic cells express the Hu antigen previously produced by fetal cells but lie sequestered in adult neurons. Autoreactive CD4+ T cells that escaped thymic deletion may become activated by the tumor expressing the Hu antigen. These cells, in turn, activate CD4+ Th1 T cells that migrate to the tumor and into the nervous system as well, inducing a direct cytotoxic effect on tumor cells and on neurons.

Treatment

Treatment of the underlying cancer generally does not affect the course of PEM/SN.[3,33] However, some patients may improve with treatment of the tumor. Unfortunately, plasmapheresis (PE), intravenous immunoglobulin (IVIg), rituximab, and immunosuppressive agents have been disappointing.[3,5,30,34]

PARANEOPLASTIC SENSORIMOTOR POLYNEUROPATHY

Clinical Features

Sensorimotor polyneuropathies occasionally can be paraneoplastic in nature. While sensory symptoms predominate in PEM/SN, mild weakness is evident in many patients as noted above.[6] It is unclear if there is truly a paraneoplastic sensorimotor polyneuropathy distinct from PEM/SN described previously. Besides generalized symmetric sensorimotor polyneuropathies, multiple mononeuropathies attributed to paraneoplastic vasculitis have been reported in patients with lymphoma, SCLC, adenocarcinoma of the lungs, endometrium, prostate, and kidneys.[35–40]

Laboratory Features

Sensory NCS show absent or low-amplitude SNAPs with normal or only borderline slowing of conduction velocities and slightly prolonged distal latencies, while motor studies demonstrated normal or only mild abnormalities reflective of axon loss.[4] A primarily demyelinating neuropathy may be seen as a complication of melanoma, lymphoma, and myeloma/plasmacytoma.[41,42] CV2/CRMP5-antibodies are associated mainly with SCLC and thymoma. Patients with CV2/CRMP5-Ab may present with a sensorimotor polyneuropathy but frequently also have cerebellar ataxia, chorea, uveo/retinal symptoms, and myasthenic syndrome (LEMS or myasthenia gravis).[43]

Histopathology

Nerve biopsies may reveal a generalized reduction in numbers of myelinated fibers, often with perivascular inflammation.[4] Necrotizing vasculitis is extremely rare.

Pathogenesis

The pathogenic basis of the neuropathy is not known. Perhaps, there is immune response directed at both the sensory and the motor components of peripheral nerves.

PARANEOPLASTIC AUTONOMIC NEUROPATHY

Autonomic dysfunction can occur as an isolated disturbance or as part of the spectrum of the anti-Hu–associated PEM/SN.[6,33] Autonomic neuropathy is most commonly described as a paraneoplastic effect of SCLC but has also occurred with adenocarcinoma and carcinoid tumor of the lungs, breast, testicular and ovarian cancer, pancreatic malignancy, and lymphoma.[6,44] Symptoms and signs of autonomic neuropathy include orthostatic hypotension, gastroparesis, intestinal pseudo-obstruction, urinary retention, dry eyes and mouth, and pupillary dysfunction. In a study of 71 patients with anti-Hu–associated PEM/SN, 10% presented with severe orthostatic hypotension and 28% had varying degrees of dysautonomia during the course of their illness.[6] Autopsies have demonstrated loss of neurons and inflammatory infiltrate in the dorsal root and autonomic ganglia (e.g., myenteric plexus). Autoantibodies directed against a nuclear antigen in myenteric neurons have been shown.[44]

COINCIDENTAL IDIOPATHIC SENSORY OR SENSORIMOTOR POLYNEUROPATHY ASSOCIATED WITH MALIGNANCY

Clinical Features

Idiopathic sensory or sensorimotor polyneuropathy complicating cancer is much more common than paraneoplastic neuropathies. The polyneuropathy is more frequent in individuals with SCLC but can be seen in most cancer. In the majority of cases, etiology of sensory or sensorimotor polyneuropathy complicating cancer remains unknown.

Most patients develop slowly progressive, distal, symmetric numbness beginning in the feet and later progressing to involve the hands. All sensory modalities can be affected, but the prominent sensory ataxia associated with PEM/SN does not occur. If weakness is appreciated it is usually mild and distal. Muscle stretch reflexes are diminished or absent distally.

Laboratory Features

There are no specific laboratory abnormalities. NCS demonstrate features of a length-dependent, axonal, sensory, or sensorimotor polyneuropathy with reduced or absent amplitudes and relatively preserved distal latencies and conduction velocities.[2] EMG may reveal mild denervation changes distally.

Histopathology

Nerve biopsies and autopsies reveal axonal degeneration and regeneration with secondary segmental demyelination and remyelination.

Pathogenesis

The pathogenic basis for this neuropathy is not known. Neuropathies can develop in untreated patients, so neurotoxicity from chemotherapies is not the cause in all. Patients with cancer may lose weight and appear cachectic; however, the neuropathy can manifest before they appear malnourished, and vitamin supplementation does not help. Perhaps, toxic or cytokine factors released by an inflammatory response to the tumor lead to neuronal damage. Alterations in protein and fat metabolism that are associated with cancers conceivably might cause neuropathy.

Treatment

There is no specific treatment for the neuropathy other than treating the underlying malignancy and maintaining adequate nutrition.

▶ NEUROPATHY SECONDARY TO TUMOR INFILTRATION

Malignant cells, in particularly leukemic and lymphomatous cells, can occasionally infiltrate peripheral nerves, leading to mononeuropathy, multifocal neuropathy/multiple mononeuropathies, polyradiculopathy, plexopathy, or even a generalized symmetric distal or proximal and distal polyneuropathy.[45–52] The neuropathy can begin acutely or have a more slow, insidious onset. Neuropathy related to tumor infiltration can be the presenting clinical manifestation of leukemia or lymphoma or the heralding of a relapse. The neuropathy may improve with treatment of the underlying leukemia or lymphoma or corticosteroids.

LEUKEMIA

Peripheral neuropathy occurs in up to 5.5% of patients with leukemia.[48,52–56] Mononeuropathy or multifocal neuropathy/multiple mononeuropathies can occur due to hemorrhage or leukemic infiltration into cranial or peripheral nerves, including the spinal roots. As one might expect, symmetric polyneuropathy due to leukemic infiltration of the nerves is unusual but has been described.

Electrophysiologic studies typically demonstrate features of a multifocal axonal sensorimotor neuropathy. Nerve biopsies can demonstrate leukemic infiltration of the nerve, axonal degeneration, and segmental demyelination. Vasculitic neuropathy may complicate hairy cell leukemia.[36,37]

ANGIOTROPHIC LARGE-CELL LYMPHOMA

This rare malignancy is characterized by intravascular proliferation of large, atypical, lymphoid B cells.[46,47,57–59] The CNS and skin are the most common sites of involvement. Nearly a quarter of patients develop a radiculopathy or polyradiculopathy, while 5% develop mononeuropathies. The diagnosis is made difficult by the absence of malignant cells in the peripheral blood or lymph nodes. Biopsy of affected nerves demonstrates intravascular and endoneurial lymphocytic infiltration (primarily B cells).

LYMPHOMATOID GRANULOMATOSIS

This angiocentric immunoproliferative disorder is associated with a pleomorphic lymphoid infiltrate of blood vessels. Infection of T cells by Epstein–Barr virus drives this inflammatory response of reactive T cells.[60] There is a predisposition for evolution into non-Hodgkin lymphoma. Distal symmetric polyneuropathy, multifocal neuropathy/multiple mononeuropathies, polyradiculoneuropathies, and cranial neuropathies develop in 10–15% of patients.[61–64] Electrophysiologic studies are suggestive of a multifocal axonal sensorimotor neuropathy. Nerve biopsies can demonstrate perivascular lymphoplasmatoid infiltrates in the epineurium, necrosis, thrombosis of the vessels, and asymmetric loss of axons between and within nerve fascicles due to ischemic injury.

▶ CRANIAL NEUROPATHIES AND RADICULOPATHIES

INFILTRATING TUMORS

The leptomeninges, cranial nerves, and nerve roots can also be invaded by tumor cells. Polyradiculopathies manifest as radicular pain and sensory loss, weakness, and hypo- or areflexia. Widespread involvement can mimic a generalized sensorimotor polyneuropathy. If the spinal cord is involved, superimposed upper motor neuron signs are seen. Multiple cranial neuropathies can occur due to local spread of a tumor (i.e., nasopharyngioma) or by metastasis. The sixth and fifth cranial nerves are most commonly affected in nasopharyngiomas, while the sixth cranial nerve followed by the third, fifth, and seventh are more commonly affected in metastatic processes. The so-called "numb chin syndrome," characterized by numbness of the lower lip and chin, is particularly worrisome for malignant invasion of the mental or alveolar branches of the mandibular nerve.

Imaging studies (e.g., MRI, CT, or PET) may demonstrate infiltration or compression of the nerve roots by the tumor (Figs. 19-3 and 19-4). CSF may be abnormal, revealing increased protein, an increased cell count, and malignant cytology. Electrodiagnostic studies can be useful to localize the site of the lesion(s).

Patients with leukemia and lymphoma may respond to irradiation and intrathecal chemotherapy. However, the response rate is much lower in other types of tumors with the possible exception of breast cancer.

BRACHIAL PLEXOPATHY

The brachial plexus can be involved due to regional spread of a local tumor (i.e., Pancoast tumor), metastases, or radiation-induced injury. Metastatic disease is responsible for most causes of brachial plexopathy in cancer patients, 78% in one large series.[65] Lung and breast cancers are the most common culprits. The tumors most often spread via the lymphatics to

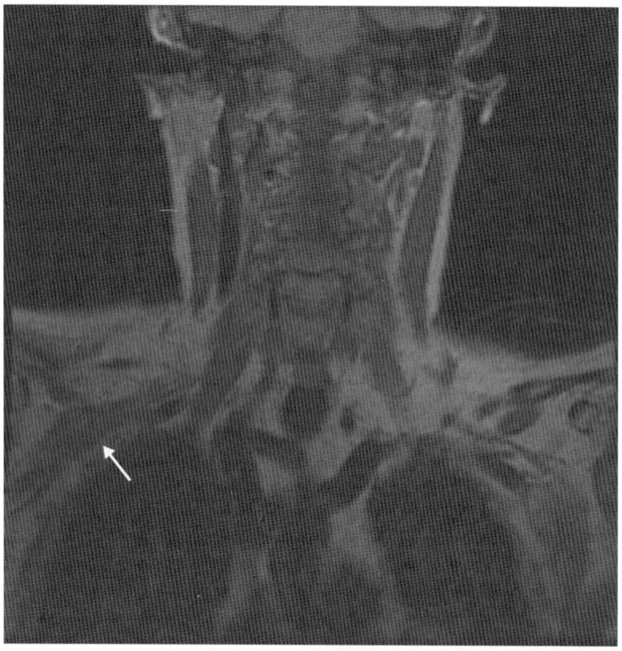

A

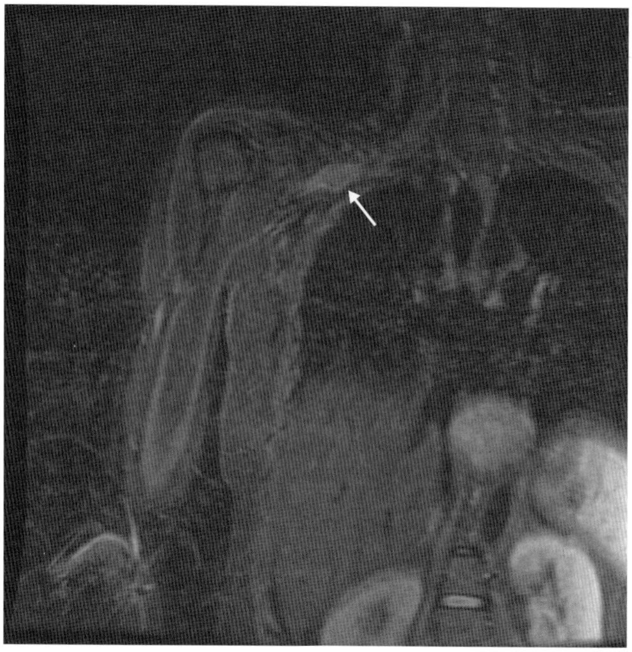

B

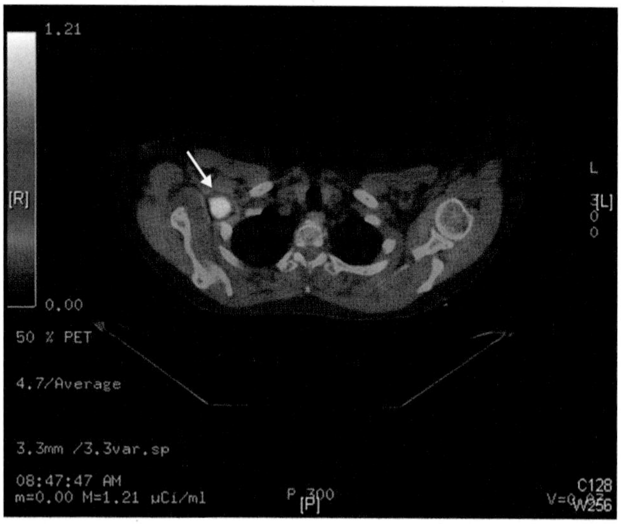

C

Figure 19-3. MRI T1 without contrast **(A)** and with contrast **(B)** demonstrates lymphoma compressing the right brachial plexus. PET/CT scan shows increased signal highlighting the tumor in the plexus **(C)**.

the lateral group of axillary lymph nodes, where divisions of the lower trunk of the brachial plexus are located. Lung cancers in the apices of the lungs may also invade the paravertebral space, the extraspinal C8–T3 mixed spinal nerves, the sympathetic chain, and the stellate ganglia.

Most patients complain of pain in the shoulder area radiating down the arm into the fingers, in particular the fourth and fifth digits. Sensory loss and weakness usually conform to the distribution of the lower trunk, and Horner's syndrome may be seen due to involvement of the superior cervical sympathetic ganglionitis often seen. The arm may appear swollen because of associated lymphedema. Signs and symptoms attributable to involvement of the upper and middle trunk of the brachial plexus are much less common and, when present, suggest epidural extension of the tumor or radiation-induced injury.

Radiation plexitis is usually associated with doses greater than 6,000 rads and can present 3 months to 26 years (mean 6 years) following radiation treatment to the region.[65] Paresthesias and lymphedema of the affected arm are common. Pain occurs in only 15% of patients and is usually not severe, which may help distinguish radiation-induced plexitis from tumor invasion. Further, the upper plexus is involved in 77% and diffuse plexus involvement occurs in 23% of patients with radiation plexitis. Some studies note that the entire plexus is more commonly involved than just the upper trunk.

Imaging studies may demonstrate malignant invasion of the plexus and perhaps extension to the epidural space

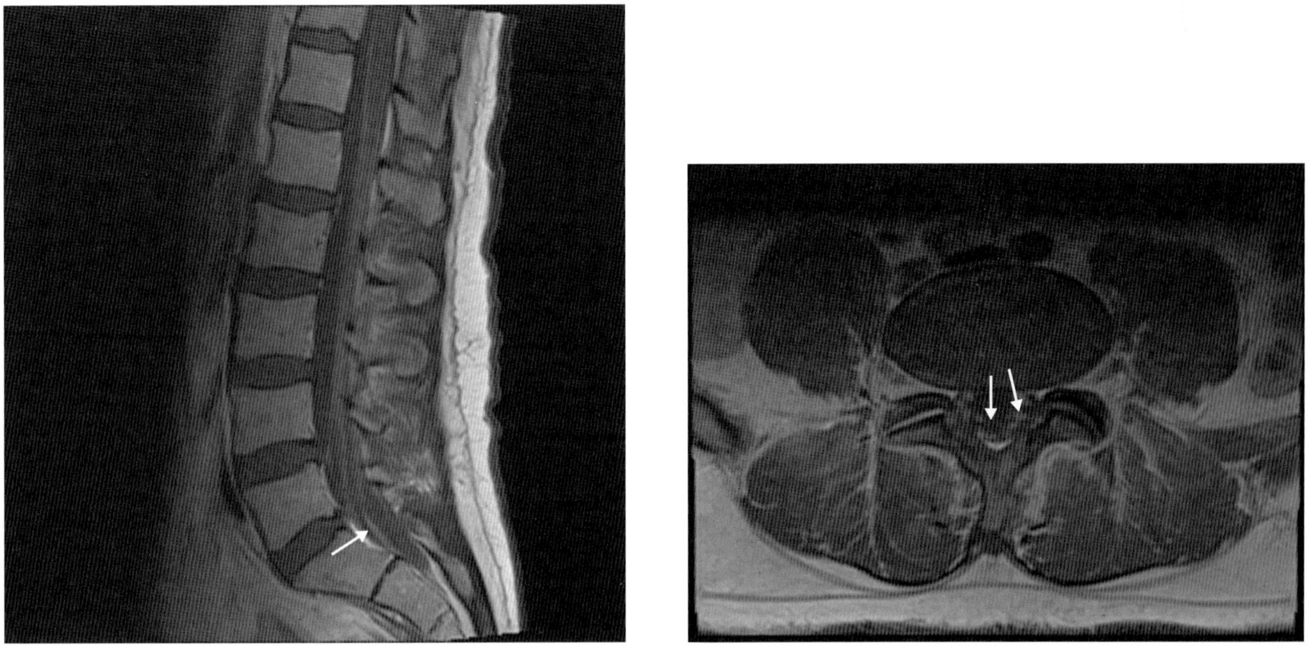

A B

Figure 19-4. Lumbosacral MRI (T1 with contrast) demonstrates enhancement of roots in sagittal **(A)** and axial sections **(B)** in a patient with lymphomatous polyradiculopathy.

(Fig. 19-3). Motor and sensory NCS reveal reduced amplitudes of involved nerves. Myokymic discharges may be appreciated on EMG and, when seen, are highly suggestive of radiation-induced damage. However, the absence of myokymia does not exclude radiation plexopathy. When noninvasive testing cannot differentiate between metastatic and radiation diseases, surgical exploration and biopsy may be required for definitive diagnosis.

Neoplastic invasion of the brachial plexus can be treated with radiation therapy. Pain may be improved but the prognosis for return of motor function is poor. Treatment of the pain with transcutaneous stimulation, sympathetic blockage, and dorsal rhizotomies has been disappointing.

LUMBOSACRAL PLEXOPATHY

The lumbosacral plexus may be invaded by local extension of intra-abdominal tumors (73%) or metastasis of distant neoplasms (27%).[66] Colorectal, cervical, and breast cancers, lymphoma, and sarcoma are the most common associated malignancies. The lumbar plexus is involved in 31%, lumbosacral trunk in 51%, and entire lumbosacral plexus in 18% of patients with malignant invasion of the plexus.[66,67] Patients usually complain of an insidious onset of pain, numbness, weakness, and edema of the lower limb. Approximately 25% of patients have involvement of both legs. Fewer than 10% of patients develop bowel or bladder incontinence or impotence.

Radiation-induced lumbosacral plexopathy can develop 1–31 years (mean 5 years) after completion of treatment. It usually manifests as slowly progressive weakness, and, unlike plexopathy secondary to tumor invasion, pain is present in only half the patients and typically is not as severe. Typically, there is symmetrical involvement of both legs, with the distal muscles being more affected than proximal muscles. Bowel and bladder incontinence may occur secondary to nerve injury or due to radiation-induced proctitis or cystitis.

MRI or CT of the lumbosacral spine and pelvis can demonstrate the tumor invading the lumbosacral plexus and perhaps extension into the epidural space. On EMG, fibrillation potentials and positive sharp waves are found in the paraspinal muscles in approximately 50% of patients with radiation-induced damage, suggesting that the disorder is more appropriately termed a radiation-induced radiculoplexopathy. Myokymic discharges are seen on EMG in over 50% of patients with radiation-induced lumbosacral radiculoplexopathy.

▶ NONINFILTRATIVE PERIPHERAL NEUROPATHIES ASSOCIATED WITH LYMPHOPROLIFERATIVE DISORDERS AND PLASMACYTOMAS

There is increased incidence of monoclonal gammopathies in patients with peripheral neuropathy, and neuropathies may be more frequent in patients with monoclonal gammopathies than in the general population.[68] Approximately 10% of patients with otherwise idiopathic peripheral neuropathies have monoclonal proteins compared to 2.5% of patients with peripheral neuropathies secondary to other diseases.[69,70] A causal relationship of demyelinating sensorimotor polyneuropathy and monoclonal IgM has been established (see Chapter 14, and discussion on DADS neuropathy).[70,71] Antibodies directed against myelin-associated glycoprotein (MAG) are present in at least 50% of these patients. However, what relationship, if any, IgA and IgG monoclonal gammopathies have to the pathogenesis of the peripheral neuropathies is not clear. Unlike IgM-associated demyelinating neuropathies, IgA and IgG immunoglobulin deposition is generally not seen on nerve sheaths in patients with neuropathies and concurrent IgA or IgG monoclonal gammopathy.

We test all patients with peripheral neuropathies for the presence of monoclonal gammopathies in the serum and urine. Serum and urine protein electrophoresis (SPEP and UPEP) are useful screening tests but are not as sensitive as immunoelectrophoresis, immunofixation, or assessment of serum free light chains. Therefore, our workup of neuropathies includes serum and urine immunoelectrophoresis or immunofixation and assessment for serum free light chains. In patients with suspected POEMS (see below) we also order vascular endothelial growth factor (VEGF) levels. A workup for amyloidosis, multiple myeloma, osteosclerotic myeloma, plasmacytoma, Waldenström macroglobulinemia, lymphoma, leukemia, and cryoglobulinemia should be performed in any patient in whom a monoclonal gammopathy is identified.[70,72–75] We order a radiologic skeletal survey to assess for osteolytic or sclerotic lesions and hematology consultation to consider a bone marrow biopsy. Although most patients with monoclonal gammopathies have no underlying malignancy (deemed monoclonal gammopathies of undetermined significance or MGUS), approximately 20% of MGUS patients subsequently develop lymphoma, leukemia, myeloma, or plasmacytoma.[70] In our experience, an acutely or subacutely developing neuropathy in a patient with a monoclonal protein may herald the conversion of MGUS to one of these malignant disorders.

LYMPHOMA

Clinical Features

Lymphoma may cause neuropathy by infiltration or direct compression of nerves,[50] but the neuropathies can also be paraneoplastic in nature.[76] Both Hodgkin disease and non-Hodgkin lymphoma are associated with polyneuropathies.[47,55,77–79] A prospective study reported clinical symptoms or signs of neuropathy in 8% and electrophysiologic evidence of neuropathy in 35% of patients with lymphoma.[76] The neuropathy can be purely sensory[76] or motor,[79] but most commonly is sensorimotor.[76] Autonomic neuropathy may also be seen. The pattern of involvement may be symmetric, asymmetric, or multifocal; the course may be acute,[55,77] subacute,[55,58] chronic progressive,[76,78] or relapsing and remitting.[77,78]

Laboratory Features

CSF may reveal lymphocytic pleocytosis and elevated protein.[50,76] Motor and sensory NCS reveal reduced amplitudes with preserved conduction velocities suggestive of a generalized axonal sensorimotor neuropathy[76] or demonstrate prolonged distal and F-wave latencies, slow conduction velocities, temporal dispersion, and conduction block,[55] similar to those observed in acute inflammatory demyelinating polyneuropathy (AIDP) and chronic inflammatory demyelinating polyneuropathy (CIDP). MRI scans may show enhancement of the nerves.[79]

Histopathology

Nerve biopsy may demonstrate endoneurial inflammatory cells in both the infiltrative and the presumed paraneoplastic neuropathies complicating lymphoma (Fig. 19-5). A monoclonal population of cells would favor lymphomatous invasion.[76,77]

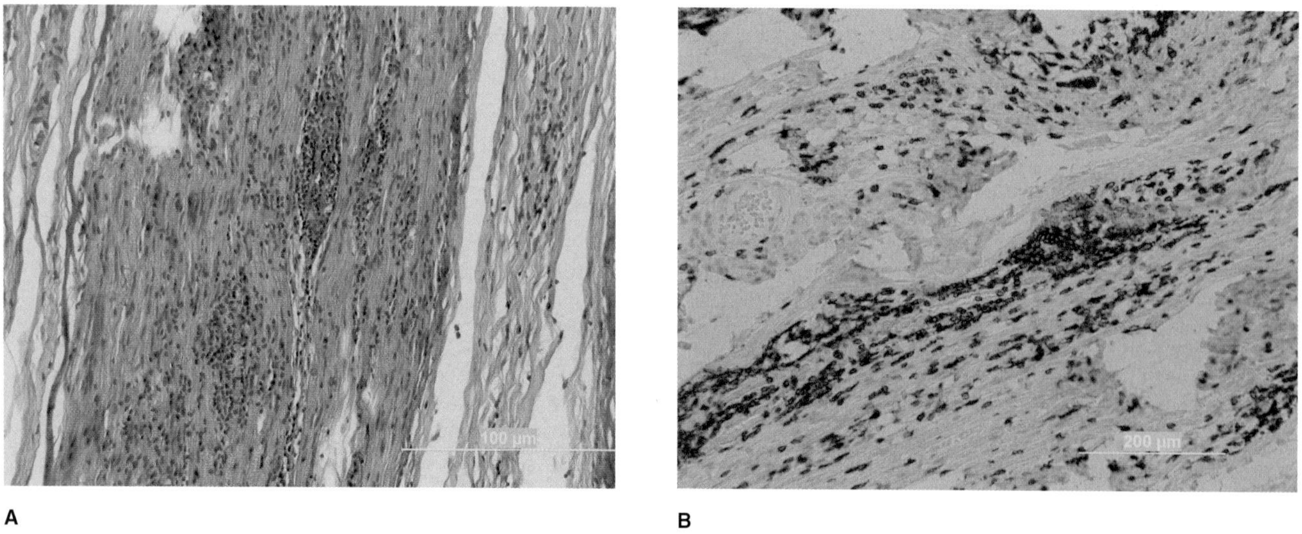

Figure 19-5. Lymphoma. Sural nerve biopsy demonstrates perivascular and endoneurial infiltration of lymphomatous cells on routine H&E **(A)** and immunoperoxidase stain using CD3 antibody **(B)**.

Pathogenesis

The paraneoplastic neuropathy associated with lymphomas is presumably autoimmune in nature, but the exact antigen(s) and trigger for the immune attack are not known.

Treatment

The neuropathy may respond to treatment of the underlying lymphoma or immunomodulating therapies.[50,55,80]

MULTIPLE MYELOMA

Multiple myeloma usually presents in the fifth to seventh decade of life with fatigue, bone pain, anemia, and sometimes hypercalcemia. Clinical signs and symptoms of peripheral neuropathies develop in 3–13% of patients,[69,74,81,82] while NCS demonstrate that as many as 40% of patients have a subclinical peripheral neuropathy.[82] The most common pattern is that of a distal, axonal, sensory, or sensorimotor polyneuropathy.[81,81] Less frequently, a chronic demyelinating polyneuropathy may develop.[81] Multiple myeloma can be complicated by amyloid polyneuropathy, which should be considered in patients with painful paresthesias, loss of pinprick and temperature discrimination, and autonomic dysfunction (suggestive of a small fiber neuropathy) and/or patients who develop atypically rapid and severe carpal tunnel syndrome (CTS). Expanding plasmacytomas can compress cranial nerves and spinal roots as well.

Laboratory Features

Multiple myeloma is the most common hematologic malignancy associated with a monoclonal gammopathy. The monoclonal protein is usually γ heavy chains or κ light chains and may be identified in the serum or urine. Anemia and hypercalcemia are common. Skeletal survey typically reveals osteolytic lesions. Diagnosis of multiple myeloma requires the demonstration of at least 10% plasma cells on a bone marrow biopsy. Motor and sensory NCS usually reveal reduced amplitudes with normal or only mildly abnormal distal latencies and conduction velocities.[81,82] Superimposed median neuropathy at the wrist is common.

Histopathology

Abdominal fat-pad, rectal, or sural nerve biopsy can be performed to look for amyloid deposition. Nerve biopsies usually reveal axonal degeneration along with mild segmental demyelination,[82] Amyloid deposition is seen in approximately two-thirds of nerve biopsies.[81] In CTS, amyloid may be deposited in the flexor retinaculum of the wrist, which is worthwhile biopsying if a patient with suspected amyloidosis undergoes carpal tunnel release surgery.

Pathogenesis

The mechanism of the neuropathy in multiple myeloma is multifactorial. The neuropathy may be related to primary amyloidosis with infiltration of the nerves. Other mechanisms of neuropathy may be due to the systemic consequences of multiple myeloma or (e.g., cytokines) or amyloidosis (e.g., renal failure). Chemotherapies employed to treat multiple myeloma (e.g., bortezomib and thalidomide) are commonly associated with neuropathy. A paraneoplastic effect is speculated in demyelinating neuropathies associated with polyneuropathy, organomegaly, endocrinopathy, monoclonal gammopathy, skin changes (POEMS) syndrome (discussed next).

Treatment

Unfortunately, the treatment of the underlying multiple myeloma does not usually affect the course of the neuropathy.

OSTEOSCLEROTIC MYELOMA (POEMS SYNDROME)

Clinical Features

Osteosclerotic myeloma is rare and is responsible for less than 3% of myelomas. Symptomatic polyneuropathy develops in near 50% of patients with osteosclerotic myeloma and often is the presenting feature.[83] Systemic manifestations include hepatosplenomegaly, cutaneous pigmentation, hypertrichosis, edema, pericardial and pleural effusions, leukonychia, finger clubbing, gynecomastia, testicular atrophy with impotence in men, amenorrhea in women, diabetes mellitus, arterial occlusive disease, and hypothyroidism. This complex constitutes the Crow–Fukase or POEMS syndrome.[74,83–91] Importantly, not every patient displays all the features of POEMS syndrome. Most individuals with POEMS syndrome have osteosclerotic myeloma, but the syndrome can also occur with Castleman disease (angiofollicular lymphoid hyperplasia), extramedullary plasmacytomas, Waldenström macroglobulinemia, and solitary lytic plasmacytoma. Some patients have no identifiable malignancy.

POEMS syndrome usually presents as symmetric tingling, numbness, and weakness that gradually progresses to involve proximal and distal arms and legs similar to CIDP. Rarely, the onset may be acute or subacute such that it resembles AIDP/Guillain–Barré syndrome (GBS).[90] The sensory modalities mediated by large fibers are affected most, with decreased but relative sparing of pain and temperature sensation. Muscle stretch reflexes are reduced or absent. The cranial nerves and respiratory muscles can be affected. Papilledema is evident in 29–55% of patients,[88] a finding that is uncommon in idiopathic CIDP. Patients can also develop a myopathy secondary to associated hypothyroidism or rarely an inflammatory myopathy.[91]

Laboratory Features

POEMS is usually associated with an IgG or IgA lambda chain monoclonal gammopathy, but in up to 20% of patients, the monoclonal protein is demonstrated in the urine but not in the serum.[74] Further, because the amount of monoclonal protein can be small, immunoelectrophoresis and immunofixation are much more sensitive than protein electrophoresis.[88,89] In addition, CSF protein levels are often markedly elevated, even more so than typical CIDP. POEMS syndrome is associated with high levels of serum VEGF and, conversely, low levels of serum erythropoietin.[92,93] Serum levels of VEGF and erythropoietin normalize with a response to therapy.[92]

Skeletal survey reveals characteristic sclerotic (two-thirds of cases) or mixed sclerotic and lytic bony lesions (one-third of cases) usually in the vertebral bodies, pelvis, or ribs (Fig. 19-6). In 50% of cases, these skeletal lesions are multiple and represent focal plasmacytomas. NCS can demonstrate features of a primary demyelinating or mixed axonal and demyelinating sensorimotor peripheral neuropathy.[81–83,86,94–97] NCS are usually indistinguishable from CIDP. However, conduction block is much less common in POEMS as compared to idiopathic CIDP.

Histopathology

Nerve biopsies usually reveal a combination of segmental demyelination and axonal degeneration.[86,98] A few endomysial or perivascular inflammatory cells may be seen. VEGF is highly expressed in blood vessels and some non-myelin-forming Schwann cells in nerve biopsies of patients with POEMS.[92] Light microscopy reveals an increased thickness of the basal lamina and a narrowing of the lumina of endoneurial vessels, while electron microscopy (EM) demonstrates proliferation of endothelial cells and opening of tight junctions.[92] EM may also reveal uncompacted myelin.[98]

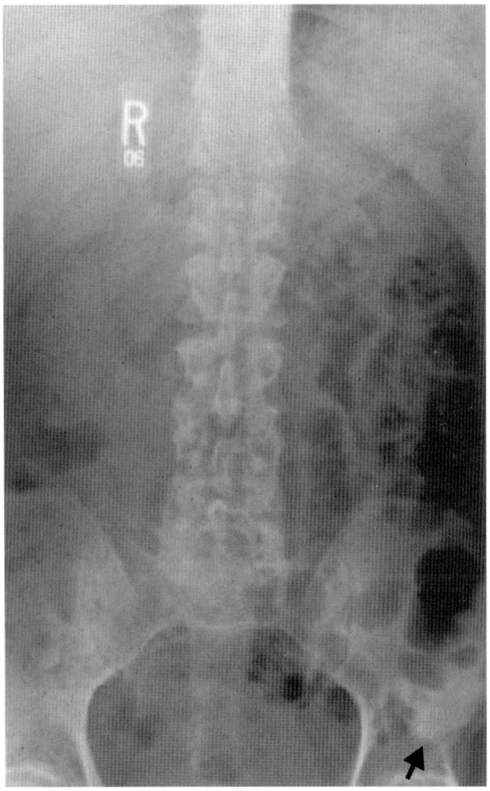

Figure 19-6. POEMS. Pelvic x-ray demonstrates a large osteosclerotic lesion (*arrow*) in the left iliac crest.

Pathogenesis

The pathogenesis of POEMS syndrome is not clear, but likely autoimmune in nature. Various cytokines including VEGF and matrix metalloproteinases are elevated in patients with POEMS syndrome and appear to correlate with the severity of the neuropathy.[92,93,99,100] Over expression of VEGF may increase nerve microvascular permeability, thereby inducing endoneurial edema and allowing neurotoxic cytokines and other chemicals access the nerve parenchyma, which lead to demyelination and secondary axonal degeneration.[90]

Treatment

The neuropathy is difficult to treat but may respond to radiation or surgical excision of the isolated plasmacytoma or to chemotherapy. The neuropathy can also improve with usual treatment given to patients with idiopathic CIDP (e.g., corticosteroids). However, the neuropathy is more refractory to treatment than typical CIDP, and POEMS needs to be suspected and re-evaluated for in all cases of refractory CIDP with repeated serum and urine immunofixation/immunoelectrophoresis and skeletal surveys. Refractory cases may respond to autologous peripheral blood stem cell transplantation.[93,100]

CASTLEMAN DISEASE (ANGIOFOLLICULAR LYMPH NODE HYPERPLASIA)

Castleman disease or angiofollicular lymph node hyperplasia is characterized by lymphoid hyperplasia associated with capillary proliferation and can be associated with POEMS syndrome (except for absence of the osteosclerotic lesions).[94] The angiofollicular lymph node hyperplasia and neuropathy may be related to increases in serum cytokine levels and VEGF, which are associated with the disorder.

WALDENSTRÖM MACROGLOBULINEMIA

Waldenström macroglobulinemia is associated with a malignant proliferation of lymphoplasmacytoid cells, which produce an IgM monoclonal protein, usually with a κ light chain.[74,101–105] It most commonly occurs in men between the ages of 50 and 70 years and usually presents with an insidious onset of progressive fatigue, weight loss, lymphadenopathy, hemorrhages (especially nose bleeds), anemia, and weakness. It commonly evolves from a patient with known IgM-MGUS. Hepatomegaly and splenomegaly may be appreciated on physical examination. Nearly 50% of patients have symptoms or signs of neuropathy on clinical examination and/or electrophysiologic testing.[105] Patients initially complain of numbness and paresthesias beginning in the feet, which then progresses proximally in the lower limbs and also affects the hands. Patients may develop difficulty in walking and loss of fine motor control of the fingers due to a sensory ataxia. Strength is normal or only slightly affected distally.

Laboratory Findings

Waldenström macroglobulinemia is responsible for about 2% of cases of monoclonal gammopathies with over 80% associated with a κ light chain. Diagnosis requires demonstration of an IgM monoclonal protein in a concentration greater than 3 g/L. The disorder is distinguished from IgM myeloma by the absence of lytic bone lesions and hypercalcemia and by the presence of hepatosplenomegaly and lymphadenopathy. Antibodies directed against MAG or sulfatide can be detected in the serum in as many as 38% of patients.[74] NCS may demonstrate features of a demyelinating sensorimotor polyneuropathy, of an axonal sensorimotor neuropathy, or may be normal suggesting a small fiber polyneuropathy.[74,101–105]

Histopathology

In cases of demyelinating neuropathy with MAG antibodies, nerve biopsies may show prominent demyelination and IgM deposition on the outer myelin membranes and occasionally in the periaxonal space but not on compact myelin.[105] Deposition of light chains in the endoneurium and epineurium resulting in massive fascicular hyalinosis and epineural arteries disruption has also been reported.[106]

Pathogenesis

The mechanism of the neuropathy is unknown. The demyelinating neuropathy may be related to MAG antibodies, although a causal relationship has not been established. Some neuropathies are associated with POEMS syndrome or caused by secondary amyloidosis or nerve fiber ischemia related to serum hyperviscosity.[87]

Treatment

Some patients benefit from corticosteroids, chlorambucil, or plasma exchange. However, prospective, blinded, controlled trials have not been performed. Rituximab, a monoclonal antibody directed against CD20 that is present on B lymphocytes, can be an effective treatment for Waldenström macroglobulinemia. However, there have been a few reports that rituximab may initially paradoxically worsen the associated neuropathy, rather than improve it.[107,108]

NEUROPATHIES ASSOCIATED WITH MGUS

Clinical Features

MGUS neuropathy is heterogeneous in regards to clinical, laboratory, and electrophysiologic features.[70,74,109–111] Neuropathies associated with an IgM monoclonal protein are typically demyelinating, while IgG and IgA monoclonal gammopathies can be axonal or demyelinating in nature. Patients with a demyelinating neuropathy can present with proximal and distal weakness and sensory symptoms typical of CIDP or just distal symptoms of distal acquired demyelinating sensory (DADS) neuropathy (see Chapter 14).[73,74,110–113] Individuals who are affected describe numbness and tingling in both the upper and the lower limbs beginning in the distal regions and progressing proximally. Weakness can also develop but is usually restricted to the distal limbs in the IgM-MGUS neuropathies, while patients with demyelinating neuropathies associated with IgG- and IgA-MGUS are more likely to have symmetrical proximal and distal weakness typical of idiopathic CIDP. Deep tendon reflexes are reduced or absent throughout.

Patients with an axonal neuropathy usually present with sensory symptoms in a length-dependent fashion. Their clinical, laboratory, histopathology, and electrophysiologic features are indistinguishable from idiopathic sensory or sensorimotor polyneuropathies.

Laboratory Features

At least 50% of the patients with IgM-MGUS neuropathy have antibodies directed against MAG.[70,112,113] Elevated CSF levels are common in patients with a demyelinating neuropathy. NCS in patients with IgG- and IgA-MGUS neuropathies can be either axonal or demyelinating in nature. The IgM-MGUS neuropathies are typically demyelinating with marked prolonged distal latencies, and moderately slow conduction velocities are variably reduced. Motor NCS reveal markedly prolonged distal latencies with moderate slowing of conduction velocities, but there is usually no evidence of temporal dispersion or conduction block.[72,111–114]

Histopathology

Nerve biopsy reveals a loss of large myelinated nerve fiber population, with relative sparing of the small myelinated and unmyelinated fibers. Segmental demyelination and remyelination are also appreciated in some patients. In some patients, there is a predominance of demyelination, while in others axonal loss may be somewhat more significant. In patients with IgM-MGUS, immunohistochemistry reveals immunoglobulin deposition on the outer myelin membranes and occasionally in the periaxonal space but not on compact myelin.[75] On EM the myelin sheaths appear to be separated, and IgM deposits are evident in these zones of myelin splitting.

Pathogenesis

IgM-MGUS is typically associated with a demyelinating neuropathy. Endoneurial injection or passive transfer of serum from patients with IgM-MAG antibodies to animals leads to conduction block and demyelination. However, response to PE and other immunotherapies is less satisfactory in this IgM-MGUS subgroup than in IgG/IgA demyelinating neuropathies where a causal link is even less well established.

Except for cases of amyloid neuropathy, there is no pathogenically proven causal relationship of monoclonal gammopathy and axonal sensorimotor polyneuropathy.

Treatment

Patients with MGUS neuropathy who fulfill clinical and electrophysiologic criteria for CIDP with proximal and distal weakness can improve with immunotherapy (discussed in Chapter 14).[112,113] However, those demyelinating neuropathies with mainly sensory symptoms and only mild distal weakness, particularly the IgM-MAG neuropathies, are usually refractory to treatment. Rare patients may respond to rituximab.[115,116] The demyelinating sensorimotor polyneuropathies associated with IgG-MGUS and IgA-MGUS are more amenable to treatment than the IgM-MGUS neuropathies.[117] There is no strong medical evidence that treating the MGUS in patients has any impact on axonal neuropathies.

▶ NEUROPATHY AS A COMPLICATION OF BONE MARROW TRANSPLANTATION/ GRAFT-VERSUS-HOST DISEASE

Neuropathies may develop in patients who undergo bone marrow transplantation because of toxic effects of chemotherapy, radiation, infection, or an autoimmune response directed against the peripheral nerves.[35,118,119] Carcinomatous or infectious meningitis with infiltration of nerves, malnutrition, and sepsis with multiorgan failure are other causes of polyneuropathy in critically ill patients. Many cranial neuropathies and radiculopathies are related to herpes zoster infection. Thrombocytopenia can lead to hemorrhage within the nerve or plexus.

Peripheral neuropathy in bone marrow transplantation patients is often associated with graft-versus-host disease (GVHD).[35] Chronic GVHD shares many features with a variety of autoimmune disorders, and it is possible that an immune-mediated response can be directed against peripheral nerves. Patients with chronic GVHD may develop cranial neuropathies including loss of olfactory and gustatory sensation,[120] sensorimotor polyneuropathy, multifocal neuropathy/multiple mononeuropathies, and severe generalized peripheral neuropathy resembling GBS[118,121,122] or CIDP.[35] Myositis, myasthenia gravis, and Lambert-Eaton myasthenic syndrome can also complicate GVHD. In patients with neuropathy, NCS may demonstrate primarily axonal, demyelinating, or mixed features. Some cases of GBS have been attributed to chemotherapy, cytomegalovirus, or *Campylobacter jejuni* infections and have improved with plasma exchange[121] or IVIg. The neuropathy may also improve with increased immunotherapy and resolution of the GVHD.[35]

▶ TOXIC NEUROPATHIES SECONDARY TO CHEMOTHERAPY

Many of the commonly used chemotherapy agents can cause a toxic neuropathy (Table 19-3).[1,2] The mechanisms by which these agents cause toxic neuropathies vary, as can the specific type of neuropathy. The risk of developing a toxic neuropathy or more severe neuropathy appears to be greater in patients with a pre-existing neuropathy (e.g., Charcot–Marie–Tooth disease and diabetes) and in those who concomitantly take more than one neurotoxic drugs (e.g., nitrofurantoin, isoniazid, disulfiram, pyridoxine, etc.). Chemotherapeutic agents usually cause a sensory greater than motor length-dependent axonal neuropathy or SN/ganglionopathy.

CISPLATIN

Clinical Features

Cisplatin is used for a variety of cancers and can cause a predominantly sensory neuropathy (ganglionopathy), usually at cumulative doses of 225–500 mg/m^2.[123–131] There is a predilection for involvement of large myelinated nerve fibers leading to paresthesia, hypesthesia, loss of vibratory perception and proprioception, often resulting in gait ataxia and pseudoathetoid movements. Muscle stretch reflexes are reduced or absent throughout. Interestingly, as many as 40% of patients can develop Lhermitte's sign, perhaps due to demyelination and edema of the posterior columns. Only a few patients (approximately 2%) develop weakness.[125] Onset of symptoms can appear as late as 8 weeks after the drug has been stopped and may progress up to 6 months following discontinuation of cisplatin, a phenomenon known as coasting.

Laboratory Features

NCS demonstrate low-amplitude or absent SNAPs with normal or only slightly prolonged distal latencies and slow sensory conduction velocities.[127–129] Vibratory perception is usually impaired on quantitative sensory testing. Motor NCS and needle EMG are usually normal.

Histopathology

Sural nerve biopsies reveal a predominant loss of large myelinated nerve fibers with axonal degeneration, segmental demyelination, and regenerating axonal sprouts.[124,126,127] Degeneration of neurons in the dorsal root ganglion and secondary axonal degeneration on both central and peripheral nerve processes are seen in rats given toxic doses of cisplatin.[128]

Pathogenesis

Cisplatin covalently binds DNA creating inter- and intrastrand cross-links. Pathologic and electrophysiologic studies suggest that neurons in the dorsal root ganglion are preferentially

TABLE 19-3. TOXIC NEUROPATHIES SECONDARY TO CHEMOTHERAPY

Drug	Mechanism of Neurotoxicity	Clinical Features	Nerve Histopathology	EMG/NCS
Vinca alkaloids (vincristine, vinblastine, vindesine, vinorelbine)	Interfere with axonal microtubule assembly; impairs axonal transport	Symmetric, S-M, large/small fiber PN; autonomic symptoms common; infrequent cranial neuropathies	Axonal degeneration of myelinated and unmyelinated fibers; regenerating clusters, minimal segmental demyelination	Axonal sensorimotor PN; distal denervation on EMG; abnormal QST, particularly vibratory perception
Cisplatin	Preferential damage to dorsal root ganglia: • binds to and cross-links DNA • inhibits protein synthesis • impairs axonal transport	Predominant large fiber sensory neuronopathy; sensory ataxia	Loss of large > small myelinated and unmyelinated fibers; axonal degeneration with small clusters of regenerating fibers; secondary segmental demyelination	Low-amplitude or unobtainable SNAPs with normal CMAPs and EMG; abnormal QST, particularly vibratory perception
Taxanes (paclitaxel, docetaxel)	Promotes axonal microtubule assembly; interferes with axonal transport	Symmetric, predominantly sensory, PN; large fiber modalities affected more than small fiber	Loss of large > small myelinated and unmyelinated fibers; axonal degeneration with small clusters of regenerating fibers; secondary segmental demyelination	Axonal sensorimotor PN; distal denervation on EMG; abnormal QST, particularly vibratory perception
Suramin				
Axonal PN	Unknown; • inhibition of neurotrophic growth factor binding; • neuronal lysosomal storage	Symmetric, length-dependent, sensory-predominant, PN	None described	Abnormalities consistent with an axonal S-M PN
Demyelinating PN	Unknown; • immunomodulating effects	Subacute, S-M PN with diffuse proximal and distal weakness; areflexia; increased CSF protein	Loss of large and small myelinated fibers with primary demyelination and secondary axonal degeneration; occasional epi- and endoneurial inflammatory cell infiltrates	Features suggestive of an acquired demyelinating sensorimotor PN (e.g., slow CVs, prolonged distal latencies and F-wave latencies, conduction block, and temporal dispersion)
ARA-C	Unknown; • selective Schwann cell toxicity; • immunomodulating effects	GBS-like syndrome; pure sensory neuropathy; brachial plexopathy	Loss of myelinated nerve fibers; axonal degeneration; segmental demyelination; no inflammation	Axonal, demyelinating, or mixed S-M PN; denervation on EMG
Etoposide (VP-16)	Unknown; • selective dorsal root ganglia toxicity	Length-dependent, sensory predominant PN; autonomic neuropathy	None described	Abnormalities consistent with an axonal S-M PN
Bortezomib (Velcade)	Unknown	Length-dependent, sensory, predominantly small fiber PN	Not described	Abnormalities consistent with an axonal sensory neuropathy with early small fiber involvement (abnormal autonomic studies)

S-M, sensorimotor; PN, polyneuropathy; EMG, electromyography; NCS, nerve conduction studies; QST, quantitative sensory testing; GBS, Guillain–Barré syndrome.
Modified with permission from Amato AA, Collins MP. Neuropathies associated with malignancy. *Semin Neurol.* 1998;18(1):125–144.

affected. Binding of the drug to neuronal DNA may inhibit transcription of important proteins and impair axonal transport.

OXALIPLATIN

Oxaliplatin is a third-generation platin derivative used mainly for treatment of colorectal cancer. Oxaliplatin has been associated with an acute sensory neuropathy that is often, but not always, reversible[132,133] The neuropathic symptoms are often aggravated by exposure to cold. NCS demonstrate features of a sensory greater than motor, axonal neuropathy. A reduction of intraepidermal nerve fiber density is evident with skin biopsy.[133]

VINCRISTINE

Clinical Features

Vincristine is commonly associated with a toxic sensorimotor and autonomic neuropathy.[134–136] Affected patients develop paresthesias and numbness, which can at times occur in the fingers before the toes. The loss of ankle jerks often precedes the subjective loss of sensation. Weakness of the hands and feet may occur in 25–35% of patients with increased dosage. Autonomic neuropathy characterized by constipation, urinary retention, impotence, and orthostatic hypotension may occur as well. Cranial neuropathies are uncommon, but optic neuropathy, oculomotor palsies, facial weakness, hearing loss, and laryngeal paralysis have been described. Neuropathic symptoms and signs are more prominent after a cumulative dose of 12 mg of vincristine.[113] However, neuropathy can develop as early as 2 weeks following a single 2 mg/m^2 dose. A coasting effect can be seen such that 24–30% of patients continue to worsen the first month after discontinuation of vincristine.[134] The median duration of symptoms after stopping the medication is around 3 months.[134]

Laboratory Features

Sensory and motor NCS reveal diminished amplitudes or absent responses with normal or only mildly prolonged distal latencies and slow conduction velocities.[134,137] The SNAP and CMAP amplitudes improve usually following discontinuation of cisplatin, but do not usually return to pretreatment levels. Active denervation in the form of fibrillation potentials and positive sharp waves may be seen on EMG in distal muscles.

Histopathology

Nerve biopsies demonstrate axonal degeneration and loss of myelinated and unmyelinated nerve fibers and clusters of regenerating axonal sprouts.

Pathogenesis

Vinca alkaloids inhibit microtubule formation by binding to tubulin. This, in turn, impairs axoplasmic transport and leads to cytoskeletal disarray and axonal degeneration.[138]

VINORELBINE

Clinical Features

Vinorelbine is a semisynthetic vinca alkaloid that causes a dose-related peripheral neuropathy in 20–50% of patients.[139–141] It is less neurotoxic than vincristine, and the associated neuropathy is severe in only 1% of cases. Patients present with distal sensory loss and paresthesia, and motor weakness can occur after 3–6 months of treatment. After 12 cycles of vinorelbine, most patients have reduced or absent muscle stretch reflexes at the ankles.[141] As with vincristine, symptoms and signs of autonomic neuropathy may develop but are less common.

Laboratory Features

Serial NCS reveal a dose-dependent reduction of SNAP and CMAP amplitudes, with preservation of distal latencies and conduction velocities.[141] The SNAP and CMAP amplitudes improve following discontinuation of the vinorelbine.

Histopathology

Nerve pathology has not been reported.

Pathogenesis

The pathogenesis is presumably similar to that of vincristine.

ETOPOSIDE

Clinical Features

Etoposide is a semisynthetic derivative of podophyllotoxin, which causes a moderate-to-severe predominantly sensory axonal neuropathy or ganglionopathy in 4–10% of patients.[142] Severe autonomic neuropathy can develop, leading to orthostatic hypotension and gastroparesis. The neuropathy gradually improves over several weeks or months following discontinuation.

Laboratory Features

NCS reveal low-amplitude SNAPs and CMAPs.

Histopathology

In mice, etoposide causes degeneration of the cell bodies within the dorsal root ganglion.[142] However, histopathology has not been well described in humans with the neuropathy.

Pathogenesis

Etoposide inhibits microtubule function, and the pathogenic basis of the neuropathy is probably similar to vincristine and vinorelbine.

PACLITAXEL (TAXOL)

Clinical Features

Taxol is used as adjuvant treatment of breast cancer and has been associated with a dose-dependent, predominantly sensory neuropathy.[143–152] A subclinical or mild neuropathy develops in up to 85% of patients after three to seven cycles of taxol at doses of 135–200 mg/m^2. A severe neuropathy occurs in 2% of patients at this lower dose range. However, at doses between 250 and 350 mg/m^2, neuropathic symptoms develop after first or second cycle, sometimes within 24 hours of the initial infusion. As many as 70% of patients have a severe neuropathy after high-dose paclitaxel with cumulative doses above 1,500 mg/m^2.[145,146] Pre-existing neuropathy and prior or concurrent exposure to neurotoxic agents are additional risk factors for developing a severe neuropathy.[146]

Laboratory Features

Sensory and motor NCS demonstrate reduced SNAP and CMAP amplitudes, which correlate with the cumulative dose of taxol.[143–159] Distal latencies and conduction velocities are usually normal, although demyelinating features have been described.[144,148] NCS abnormalities may predate occurrence of neuropathic symptoms.[152] Quantitative sensory testing reveals impairment of vibratory perception more often than abnormal thermal thresholds.[143,149] Needle EMG may reveal fibrillation potentials in distal limb muscles.[144,147]

Histopathology

Sural nerve biopsies reveal a preferential loss of large myelinated nerve fibers along with axonal degeneration with secondary demyelination and remyelination.[147,148] Regenerating axonal sprouts are uncommon. On EM, one may find accumulation of tubular and membranous structures within the axons.[147]

Pathogenesis

Taxol may have a toxic effect on the neuronal cell body, the axon, or both. In contrast to the vinca alkaloids, which disassemble microtubules, the taxanes (taxol and taxotere) promote microtubule assembly by increasing tubulin polymerization. The subsequent aggregation and accumulation of abnormal bundles of microtubules in dorsal root ganglia, axons, and Schwann cells impair axoplasmic transport.[153]

DOCETAXEL (TAXOTERE)

Clinical Features

Taxotere, a semisynthetic analogue of taxol, is also associated with a dose-dependent, predominantly sensory neuropathy. Neuropathies are less frequent and severe than that seen with taxol.[154–158] Patients describe pain in the hands and feet and also may have a Lhermitte's sign. On examination, large fiber sensory modalities are preferentially affected and most patients have reduced or absent muscle stretch reflexes at the ankles. Mild proximal and distal weakness is evident in 5–19% of patients. Most patients improve 1–2 months after cessation of the chemotherapy; however, neuropathic symptoms can continue to worsen for several months after discontinuation of the docetaxel.

Laboratory Features

Sensory and motor NCS reveal diminished amplitudes with only mild slowing of conduction velocities.[154,156]

Histopathology

Sensory nerve biopsy may reveal a loss of large myelinated fibers, with scattered fibers undergoing axonal degeneration.[156]

Pathogenesis

The pathogenic mechanism is presumably similar to taxol.

SURAMIN

Clinical Features

Suramin is a hexasulfonated naphthylurea that causes a peripheral neuropathy in 25–90% treated patients.[159–161] Neurotoxicity is the dose-limiting side effect, and there appears to be two distinct types of toxic neuropathy: (1) a dose-dependent, distal, axonal sensorimotor polyneuropathy and (2) a subacute demyelinating polyradiculoneuropathy.

The distal axonopathy is more common and manifests with distal numbness and paresthesias.[159,161] Examination reveals reduced light touch, pain, and vibratory perception; mild weakness of the distal limbs (e.g., toe extensors); and diminished ankle reflexes. This neuropathy is reversible upon suramin discontinuation.

A subacute sensorimotor demyelinating polyradiculoneuropathy is more severe and develops in 10–20% of patients after 1–5 months of treatment.[159–161] It is associated with peak plasma concentrations of over 300 μg/L, exposure to greater than 200 μg/L for more than 25 days per month, or cumulative dose of 40,000 mg/L. Patients present with numbness and paresthesias of the distal limbs or face, followed by symmetric, proximal greater than distal weakness. Muscle stretch reflexes are decreased or absent throughout. The weakness is insidiously progressive and can involve the respiratory muscles. Up to 25% of affected patients become bedridden and require mechanical ventilation. The neuropathy can continue to progress for 1 month following suramin discontinuation. It can take several months for patients to recover, and there frequently are residual numbness and weakness. Plasma exchange has been tried in an uncontrolled fashion with mixed results.

Laboratory Features

CSF protein may be elevated in patients with subacute demyelinating polyradiculoneuropathy.[159,161] NCS in the more common distal sensorimotor polyneuropathy reveal decreased amplitudes of SNAPs and CMAPs with relatively preserved distal latencies and conduction velocities.[159,161] Abnormal vibratory and cooling thresholds are seen with quantitative sensory testing.[159] Needle EMG may reveal fibrillation potentials and neurogenic MUAPs in distal muscles.

Electrodiagnostic studies in the subacute sensorimotor polyradiculoneuropathy reveal features of demyelination: prolonged distal latencies and F-waves, slow conduction velocities, temporal dispersion, and conduction block.[159–161] As in the distal axonopathy, quantitative sensory testing shows increased vibratory and cooling thresholds.[159] EMG demonstrates decreased recruitment of MUAPs in proximal and distal muscles and occasional fibrillation potentials.

Histopathology

Sural nerve biopsies in patients with the subacute demyelinating polyradiculoneuropathy demonstrate loss of large and small myelinated nerve fibers, demyelination and remyelination, and secondary axonal degeneration.[159–161] Epi- and endoneurial mononuclear inflammatory infiltrates may be seen. In animal models, suramin induces a length-, dose-, and time-dependent axonal sensorimotor polyneuropathy associated with axonal degeneration, atrophy, and accumulation of glycolipid lysosomal inclusions.[162]

Pathogenesis

The mechanism of neurotoxicity is unknown. Suramin may inhibit the interaction of neurotrophic factors with its peripheral nerve receptors[163] or induce a form of lysosomal storage disease. The demyelinating neuropathy may be immune mediated, related to the immunomodulating effects of suramin.[164]

CYTOSINE ARABINOSIDE

Clinical Features

Cytosine arabinoside (ARA-C) is an antimetabolite used in the treatment of leukemia and lymphoma. Sensory neuropathy and severe sensorimotor polyneuropathy resembling GBS[165–170] have been reported with cumulative doses ranging from 60 mg/m^2 to 36 g/m^2. These neuropathies can begin within hours or weeks following treatment.

Laboratory Features

Patients with a GBS-like neuropathy have increased CSF protein.[168] EMG and NCS can be compatible with a primary axonal[169] or an acquired demyelinating sensorimotor polyneuropathy.[166]

Histopathology

Sural nerve biopsies may reveal demyelination or axonal degeneration.[165,168,169]

Pathogenesis

The pathophysiologic mechanism(s) for the neuropathies are not known. The antimetabolite action of ARA-C may inhibit proteins necessary for myelin production, axonal structure, or axonal transport. Alternatively, the immunomodulating effects of ARA-C may predispose patients to an immune attack against the peripheral nerves.

IFOSFAMIDE

Ifosfamide, a cyclophosphamide analog, has been associated with polyneuropathy with total doses of 14 g/m^2 or more.[171] Patients manifest numbness, and painful paresthesias that begin in the hands and feet 10–14 days after treatment and gradually resolve but recur if they are rechallenged with the chemotherapy. Electrodiagnostic and histopathologic data are lacking, but the occasional onset beginning in the hands rather than the feet is suggestive of a ganglionopathy.

BORTEZOMIB (VELCADE)

Bortezomib, a selective, reversible inhibitor of the proteasome, is most commonly used for treatment of multiple myeloma.[172] Treatment-emergent neuropathy or symptomatic worsening of a pre-existent neuropathy developed in a third to two-thirds of myeloma patients in treatment trials.[172–176] Polyneuropathy also occurred in 9 out of 21 patients with renal cell carcinoma treated with bortezomib.[174] The risk of neuropathy correlates with the cumulative dose of bortezomib. Patients usually complain of paresthesia, burning dysesthesia, and numbness in a length-dependent distribution. The neuropathy usually improves when the dose is reduced or drug is discontinued. The electrophysiologic characteristics of the treatment-emergent neuropathy suggest a length-dependent, axonal, sensory polyneuropathy.[173,175] The absence of electrophysiologic changes in some patients with symptoms of burning and dysesthesias in their feet suggests involvement of small-diameter nerve fibers (i.e., a small fiber neuropathy) as well.

Laboratory Features

NCS may demonstrate a reduction or loss of amplitudes of SNAPs in a length-dependent pattern.[173,176] Motor studies are usually spared and EMG is typically normal. Autonomic studies, in particular, quantitative sweat testing may be abnormal.

Histopathology

Skin biopsies have shown a reduction in intraepidermal nerve fiber density.[176,177] Nerve biopsies of patients with the characteristic toxic neuropathy have not been reported. However, in Wistar rats, pathologic examination reported shows a dose-dependent axonopathy of the unmyelinated fibers in nerves of treated animals.[178] In mice, histopathologic findings have demonstrated a mild reduction of myelinated and unmyelinated fibers), mostly involving large and C fibers, with abnormal vesicular inclusion bodies in unmyelinated axons.[179] In addition, degeneration of dorsal root ganglia has been observed in mice treated with bortezomib.[180]

Pathogenesis

The pathophysiologic mechanism is not known. Bortezomib may block the ubiquitin–proteasome pathway, possibly causing a "toxic" buildup of proteins that should be degraded by the proteasome, resulting in impairment of neuronal function, initially in the dorsal root ganglia, and then leading to a retrograde (or "dying-back") axonopathy of small nerve fibers followed by larger nerve fibers.

CARFILZOMIB

Carfilzomib is a second-generation selective proteasome inhibitor that is also used to treat refractory multiple myeloma. Peripheral neuropathy can occur, but appears to be less common in patients receiving carfilzomib compared to bortezomib.[181]

▶SUMMARY

Neuropathy is not an uncommon complication in a cancer patient. Although a paraneoplastic etiology is often considered, most neuropathies in the setting of cancer are not the result of a remote, immune-mediated effect of cancer. The neuropathy is more commonly due to a direct, adverse side effect of chemotherapeutic agents (toxic neuropathy), or as a consequence of nutritional deficiency. In some cases, it may be due to compression or infiltration of the tumor. Treatment and prognosis are dependent on the etiology and mechanism of the neuropathy.

REFERENCES

1. Briemberg HR, Amato AA. Neuromuscular complications of cancer. *Neurol Clin*. 2003;21(1):141–165.
2. Amato AA, Dumitru D. Acquired neuropathies. In: Dumitru D, Amato AA, Swartz MJ, eds. *Electrodiagnostic Medicine*, 2nd edn. Philadelphia, PA: Hanley & Belfus; 2002:937–1041.
3. Amato AA, Collins MP. Neuropathies associated with malignancy. *Semin Neurol*. 1998;18:125–144.
4. Campbell MJ, Paty DW. Carcinomatous neuromyopathy: 1. Electrophysiological studies. *J Neurol Neurosurg Psychiatry*. 1974;37:131–141.
5. Denny-Brown D. Primary sensory neuropathy with muscular changes associated with carcinoma. *J Neurol Neurosurg Psychiatry*. 1948;11:73–87.
6. Dalmau J, Graus F, Rosenblum MK, Posner JB. Anti-Hu associated paraneoplastic encephalomyelitis/sensory neuronopathy. A clinical study of 71 patients. *Medicine*. 1992;71:59–72.
7. Lucchinetti CF, Kimmel DW, Lennon VA. Paraneoplastic and oncologic profiles of patients seropositive for type 1 antineuronal nuclear autoantibodies. *Neurology*. 1998;50:652–657.
8. Molinuevo JL, Graus F, Serrano C, Rene C, Guerrero C, Illa I. Utility of anti-Hu antibodies in the diagnosis of paraneoplastic sensory neuropathy. *Ann Neurol*. 1998;44:976–980.
9. Wilkinson PC, Zeromski J. Immunofluorescent detection of antibodies in sensory carcinomatous neuropathy. *Brain*. 1965;88:529–583.
10. Graus F, Elkon KB, Cordon-Cardo C, Posner JB. Sensory neuronopathy and small cell lung cancer. Antineuronal antibody that also reacts with the tumor. *Am J Med*. 1986;80:45–52.
11. Graus F, Elkon KB, Lloberes P, et al. Neuronal antinuclear antibody (anti-Hu) in paraneoplastic encephalomyelitis simulating acute polyneuritis. *Acta Neurol Scand*. 1987;75:249–252.
12. Dalmau J, Furneaux HM, Cordon-Cardo C, Posner JB. The expression of the Hu (encephalomyelitis/sensory neuronopathy) antigen in human normal and tumor tissues. *Am J Pathol*. 1992;141;881–886.
13. Dalmau J, Furneaux HM, Rosenblum MK, Kris MG, Posner JB. Detection of the anti-Hu antibody in the serum of patients with small cell lung cancer. A quantitative western blot analysis. *Ann Neurol*. 1990;27:544–552.
14. Vega F, Graus F, Chen QM, Poisson M, Schuller E, Delattre JY. Intrathecal synthesis of the anti-Hu antibody in patients with paraneoplastic encephalomyelitis or sensory neuronopathy: Clinical–immunological correlation. *Neurology*. 1994;44:2145–2147.
15. Dalmau J, Furneaux HM, Rosenblum MK, Graus F, Posner JB. Detection of the anti-Hu antibody in specific regions of the nervous system and tumor from patients with paraneoplastic encephalomyelitis/sensory neuronopathy. *Neurology*. 1991;41:1757–1764.
16. Auger RG. The role of the masseter reflex in the assessment of subacute sensory neuropathy. *Muscle Nerve*. 1998;21:800–801.
17. Auger RG, Windebank AJ, Lucchinetti CF, Chalk CH. Role of the blink reflex in the evaluation of sensory neuronopathy. *Neurology*. 1999;53:407–408.
18. Wanschitz J, Hainfellner JA, Kristoferitsch W, Drlicek M, Budka H. Ganglionitis in paraneoplastic subacute sensory neuronopathy: A morphologic study. *Neurology*. 1997;49:1156–1159.
19. Lennon VA, Sas DF, Busk MF, et al. Enteric neuronal autoantibodies in pseudo-obstruction with small-cell lung carcinoma. *Gastroenterology*. 1991;100:137–142.
20. Altermatt HJ, Rodriguez M, Scheithauer BW, Lennon VA. Paraneoplastic anti-Purkinje and type-1 anti-neuronal nuclear autoantibodies bind selectively to central, peripheral, and autonomic nervous system cells. *Lab Invest*. 1991;65:412–420.
21. Jean WC, Dalmau J, Ho A, Posner JB. Analysis of the IgG subclass distribution and inflammatory infiltrates in patients with anti-Hu-associated paraneoplastic encephalomyelitis. *Neurology*. 1994;44:140–147.

22. Rosenblum MK. Paraneoplastic and autoimmunologic injury of the nervous system: The anti-Hu syndrome. *Brain Pathol.* 1993;3:199–212.
23. Voltz RD, Graus F, Posner JB, Dalmau J. Paraneoplastic encephalomyelitis: An update on the effects of the anti-Hu immune response. *J Neurol Neurosurg Psychiatry.* 1997;63:133–136.
24. Sillevis-Smith PA, Manley GT, Posner JB. Immunization with the paraneoplastic encephalomyelitis antigen HuD does not cause disease in mice. *Neurology.* 1995;45:1873–1878.
25. Panegyres PK, Reading MC, Esiri MM. The inflammatory reaction of paraneoplastic ganglionitis and encephalitis: An immunohistochemical study. *J Neurol.* 1993;240:93–97.
26. Benyahia B, Liblau R, Merle-Béral H, Tourani JM, Dalmau J, Delattre JY. Cell-mediated autoimmunity in paraneoplastic neurological syndromes with anti-Hu antibodies. *Ann Neurol.* 1999;45:162–167.
27. Voltz R, Dalmau J, Posner JB, Rosenfeld MR. T-cell receptor analysis in anti-Hu associated paraneoplastic encephalomyelitis. *Neurology.* 1998;51:1146–1150.
28. Bastson OA, Fantle DM, Stewart JA. Paraneoplastic encephalomyelitis. Dramatic response to chemotherapy alone. *Cancer.* 1992;69:1291–1293.
29. Keime-Guibert F, Graus F, Broët P, et al. Clinical outcome of patients with the anti-Hu-associated encephalomyelitis after treatment of the cancer. *Neurology.* 1999;53:1719–1723.
30. Graus F, Vega F, Delattre JY, et al. Plasmapheresis and antineoplastic treatment in CNS paraneoplastic syndromes and antineuronal antibodies. *Neurology.* 1992;42:536–540.
31. Antoine JC, Mosneir JF, Honnorat J, et al. Paraneoplastic demyelinating neuropathy, subacute sensory neuropathy, and anti-Hu antibodies: Clinicopathological study of an autopsy case. *Muscle Nerve.* 1998;21:850–857.
32. Graus F, Keime-Guibert F, Rene R, et al. Anti-Hu-associated paraneoplastic encephalomyelitis: Analysis of 200 patients. *Brain.* 2001;124:1138–1148.
33. Amato AA, Anderson MP. A 51 year old woman with lung cancer and neuropsychiatric abnormalities (Case 38—2001). *N Engl J Med.* 2001;354:1758–1765.
34. Antoine JC, Camdessanché JP. Treatment options in paraneoplastic disorders of the peripheral nervous system. *Curr Treat Options Neurol.* 2013;15:210–223.
35. Amato AA, Barohn RJ, Sahenk Z, Tushka PJ, Mendell JR. Polyneuropathy complicating bone marrow and solid organ transplantation. *Neurology.* 1993;43:1513–1518.
36. Gabriel SE, Conn DL, Phyliky RL, Pittelkow MR, Scott RE. Vasculitis in hairy cell leukemia: Review of literature and consideration of possible pathogenic mechanisms. *J Rheumatol.* 1986;13:1167–1172.
37. Hasler P, Kistler H, Gerber H. Vasculitis in hairy cell leukemia. *Semin Arthritis Rheum.* 1995;25:134–142.
38. Johnson PC, Rolak LA, Hamilton RH, Laguna JF. Paraneoplastic vasculitis of the nerve: A remote effect of cancer. *Ann Neurol.* 1979;5:437–444.
39. Kurzrock R, Cohen PR, Markowitz A. Clinical manifestations of vasculitis in patients with solid tumors: A case report and review of the literature. *Arch Neurol.* 1994;154:334–340.
40. Oh SJ, Slaughter R, Harrell L. Paraneoplastic vasculitic neuropathy: A treatable neuropathy. *Muscle Nerve.* 1991;14:152–156.
41. Bird SJ, Brown MJ, Shy ME, Scherer SS. Chronic inflammatory demyelinating polyneuropathy associated with malignant melanoma. *Neurology.* 1996;46:822–824.
42. Weiss MD, Luciano CA, Semino-Mora C, Dalakas MC, Quarles RH. Molecular mimicry in chronic inflammatory demyelinating polyneuropathy and melanoma. *Neurology.* 1998;51:1738–1741.
43. Honnorat J, Cartalat-Carel S, Ricard D, et al. Onco-neural antibodies and tumour type determine survival and neurological symptoms in paraneoplastic neurological syndromes with Hu or CV2/CRMP5 antibodies. *J Neurol Neurosurg Psychiatry.* 2009;80:412–416
44. Levin KH, Lutz G. Angiotrophic large-cell lymphoma with peripheral nerve and skeletal muscle involvement: Early diagnosis and treatment. *Neurology.* 1996;47:1009–1011.
45. Grisold W, Piza-Katzer H, Jahn R, Herczeg E. Intraneural nerve metastasis with multiple mononeuropathies. *J Peripher Nerv Syst.* 2000;5(3):163–167.
46. Oei ME, Kraft GH, Sarnat HB. Intravascular lymphomatosis. *Muscle Nerve.* 2002;25(5):742–746.
47. Kelly JJ, Karcher DS. Lymphoma and peripheral neuropathy: A clinical review. *Muscle Nerve.* 2005;31:301–313.
48. Bobker DH, Deloughery TG. Natural killer cell leukemia presenting with a peripheral neuropathy. *Neurology.* 1993;43:1853–1854.
49. Borit A, Altrocchi PH. Recurrent polyneuropathy and neurolymphomatosis. *Arch Neurol.* 1971;24:40–49.
50. Krendel DA, Stahl RL, Chan WC. Lymphomatous polyneuropathy. Biopsy of clinically involved nerve and successful treatment. *Arch Neurol.* 1991;48:330–332.
51. Thomas FP, Vallejos U, Foitl DR, et al. B cell small lymphocytic lymphoma and chronic lymphocytic leukemia with peripheral neuropathy: Two cases with neuropathological findings and lymphocyte marker analysis. *Acta Neuropathol (Berl).* 1990;80:198–203.
52. Aregawi DG, Sherman JH, Douvas MG, Burns TM, Schiff D. Neuroleukemiosis: case report of leukemic nerve infiltration in acute lymphoblastic leukemia. *Muscle Nerve.* 2008;38:1196–1200.
53. Créange A, Theodorou I, Sabourin JC, Vital C, Farcet JP, Gherardi RK. Inflammatory neuromuscular disorders associated with chronic lymphoid leukemia: Evidence for clonal B cells within muscle and nerve. *J Neurol Sci.* 1996;137:35–41.
54. Krendel DA, Albright RE, Graham DG. Infiltrative polyneuropathy due to acute monoblastic leukemia in hematologic remission. *Neurology.* 1987;37:474–477.
55. Sumi SM, Farrell DF, Knauss TA. Lymphoma and leukemia manifested by steroid-responsive polyneuropathy. *Arch Neurol.* 1983;40:577–582.
56. Vital C, Bonnaud E, Arne L, Barrat M, Leblanc M. Polyneuritis in chronic lymphoid leukemia. Ultrastructural study of the peripheral nerve. *Acta Neuropathol.* 1975;32:169–172.
57. Vital C, Heraud A, Coquet M, Julien M, Maupetit J. Acute mononeuropathy with angiotropic lymphoma. *Acta Neuropathol (Berl).* 1989;78:105–107.
58. Dubas F, Saint-Andre JP, Poulard BA, Delestre F, Emile J. Intravascular malignant lymphomatosis (so-called malignant angioendotheliomatosis): A case confined to the lumbosacral spinal cord and nerve roots. *Clin Neuropathol.* 1990;9:115–120.
59. Glass J, Hochberg FH, Miller DC. Intravascular lymphomatosis: A systemic disease with neurologic manifestations. *Cancer.* 1993;71:3156–3164.
60. Wilson WH, Kingma DW, Raffeld M, Wittes RE, Jaffe ES. Association of lymphomatoid granulomatosis with Epstein–Barr viral infection of B lymphocytes and response to interferon-α2B. *Blood.* 1996;87:4531–4537.

61. Calatayud T, Vallejo AR, Dominguez L, Sotelo T, Peña P, Jimenez M. Lymphomatoid granulomatosis manifesting as a subacute polyradiculoneuropathy: A case report and review of the neurological manifestations. *Eur Neurol.* 1980;19:213–223.
62. Katzenstein AL, Carrington CB, Liebow AA. Lymphomatoid granulomatosis: A clinicopathologic study of 152 cases. *Cancer.* 1979;43:360–373.
63. Liebow AA, Carrington CR, Friedman PJ. Lymphomatoid granulomatosis. *Hum Pathol.* 1972;3:457–558.
64. Kasamon YL, Nguyen TN, Chan JA, Nascimento AF. EBV-associated lymphoma and chronic inflammatory demyelinating polyneuropathy in an adult without overt immunodeficiency. *Am J Hematol.* 2002;69(4):289–293.
65. Kori SH, Foley KM, Posner JB. Brachial plexus lesions in patients with cancer: 100 cases. *Neurology.* 1981;31:45–50.
66. Jaeckle KA, Young DF, Foley KM. The natural history of lumbosacral plexopathy in cancer. *Neurology.* 1985;35:8–15.
67. Evans RJ, Walton CPN. Lumbosacral plexopathy in cancer patients. *Neurology.* 1985;35:1392–1393.
68. Vrethem M, Cruz M, Wen-Xin H, Malm C, Holmgren H, Ernerudh J. Clinical, neurophysiological and immunological evidence of polyneuropathy in patients with monoclonal gammopathies. *J Neurol Sci.* 1993;114:193–199.
69. Kelly JJ Jr, Kyle RA, O'Brien PC, Dyck PJ. Prevalence of monoclonal protein in peripheral neuropathy. *Neurology.* 1981; 31:1480–1483.
70. Latov N. Prognosis of neuropathy with monoclonal gammopathy. *Muscle Nerve.* 2000;23:150–152.
71. Latov N, Sherman WH, Nemni R, Galassi G, Shyong JS, Penn AS. Plasma cell dyscrasia and peripheral neuropathy with a monoclonal antibody to peripheral nerve myelin. *N Engl J Med.* 1980;303:618–621.
72. Kelly JJ. The electrodiagnostic findings in peripheral neuropathy associated with monoclonal gammopathy. *Muscle Nerve.* 1983;6:504–509.
73. Kelly JJ. Peripheral neuropathies associated with monoclonal proteins: A clinical review. *Muscle Nerve.* 1985;8:138–150.
74. Kissel JT, Mendell JR. Neuropathies associated with monoclonal gammopathies. *Neuromuscul Disord.* 1996;6:3–18.
75. Vital A, Vital C, Julien J, Baquey A, Steck AJ. Polyneuropathy associated with IgM monoclonal gammopathy. *Acta Neuropathol (Berl).* 1989;79:160–167.
76. Walsh JC. Neuropathy associated with lymphoma. *J Neurol Neurosurg Psychiatry.* 1971;34:42–50.
77. Cameron DG, Howell DA, Hutchinson JL. Acute peripheral neuropathy in Hodgkin's disease. *Neurology.* 1958;8:575–577.
78. Lisak RP, Mitchell M, Zweiman B, Orrechio E, Asbury AK. Guillain–Barre syndrome and Hodgkin's disease: Three cases with immunological studies. *Ann Neurol.* 1977;1:72–78.
79. Flanagan EP, Sandroni P, Pittock SJ, Inwards DJ, Jones LK Jr. Paraneoplastic lower motor neuronopathy associated with Hodgkin lymphoma. *Muscle Nerve.* 2012;46:823–827.
80. Sagar HJ, Read DJ. Subacute sensory neuropathy with remission: An association with lymphoma. *J Neurol Neurosurg Psychiatry.* 1982;45:83–85.
81. Kelly JJ Jr, Kyle RA, Miles JM, O'Brien PC, Dyck PJ. The spectrum of peripheral neuropathy in myeloma. *Neurology.* 1981;31:24–31.
82. Walsh JC. The neuropathy of multiple myeloma. An electrophysiological and histological study. *Arch Neurol.* 1971;25: 404–414.
83. Kelly JJ Jr, Kyle RA, Miles JM, Dyck PJ. Osteosclerotic myeloma and peripheral neuropathy. *Neurology.* 1983;33:202–210.
84. Bardwick PA, Zvaifler NJ, Gill GN, Newman D, Greenway GD, Resnick DL. Plasma cell dyscrasia with polyneuropathy, organomegaly, endocrinopathy, M-protein and skin changes: The POEMS syndrome. *Medicine (Baltimore).* 1980;59:311–322.
85. Nakanishi T, Sobue I, Toyokura Y, et al. The Crow–Fukase syndrome: A study of 102 cases in Japan. *Neurology.* 1984;34: 712–720.
86. Ohi T, Kyle RA, Dyck PJ. Axonal attenuation and secondary segmental demyelination in myeloma neuropathies. *Ann Neurol.* 1985;17:255–261.
87. Kihara Y, Hori H, Murakami H, et al. A case of POEMS syndrome associated with reactive amyloidosis and Waldenström's macroglobulinaemia. *J Intern Med.* 2002;252(3):255–258.
88. Dispenzieri A, Kyle RA, Lacy MQ, et al. POEMS syndrome: Definitions and long-term outcome. *Blood.* 2003;101(7): 2496–2506.
89. Dispenzieri A. POEMS syndrome: 2011 update on diagnosis, risk-stratification, and management. *Am J Hematol.* 2011;86:591–601.
90. Isose S, Misawa S, Kanai K, et al. POEMS syndrome with Guillain-Barré syndrome-like acute onset: A case report and review of neurological progression in 30 cases. *J Neurol Neurosurg Psychiatry.* 2011;82:678–680.
91. Goebels N, Walther EU, Schaller M, Pongratz D, Mueller-Felber W. Inflammatory myopathy in POEMS syndrome. *Neurology.* 2000;55:1413–1414.
92. Scarlato M, Previtali SC, Carpo M, et al. Polyneuropathy in POEMS syndrome: Role of angiogenic factors in the pathogenesis. *Brain.* 2005;128:1911–1920.
93. Kuwabara S, Misawa S, Kanai K, et al. Autologous peripheral blood stem cell transplantation for POEMS syndrome. *Neurology.* 2006;66(1):105–107.
94. Donaghy M, Hall P, Gawler J, et al. Peripheral neuropathy associated with Castleman's disease. *J Neurol Sci.* 1989;89:253–267.
95. Donofrio PD, Albers JW, Greenberg HS, et al. Peripheral neuropathy in osteosclerotic myeloma: Clinical and electrodiagnostic improvement with chemotherapy. *Muscle Nerve.* 1984;7:137–141.
96. Ohi T, Nukada H, Kyle RA, et al. Detection of an axonal abnormality in myeloma neuropathy. *Ann Neurol.* 1983;14:120.
97. Sung JY, Kuwabara S, Ogawara K, Kanai K, Hattori T. Patterns of nerve conduction abnormalities in POEMS syndrome. *Muscle Nerve.* 2002;26(2):189–193.
98. Vital C, Vital A, Ferrer X, et al. Crow–Fukase (POEMS) syndrome: A study of peripheral nerve biopsy in five new cases. *J Peripher Nerv Syst.* 2003;8(3):136–144.
99. Michizono K, Umehara F, Hashiguchi T, et al. Circulating levels of MMP-1, -2, -3, -9, and TIMP-1 are increased in POEMS syndrome. *Neurology.* 2001;56(6):807–810.
100. Dyck PJ, Engelstad J, Dispenzieri A. Vascular endothelial growth factor and POEMS. *Neurology.* 2006;6(1):10–12.
101. Gotham JE, Wein H, Meyer JS. Clinical studies of neuropathy due to macroglobulinemia (Waldenström's syndrome). *Can Med Assoc J.* 1963;89:806–809.
102. Iwashita H, Argyrakis A, Lowitzsch K, et al. Polyneuropathy in Waldenström's macroglobulinemia. *J Neurol Sci.* 1974;21: 341–354.
103. Propp RP, Means E, Deibel R, Sherer G, Barron K. Waldenström's macroglobulinemia and neuropathy. *Neurology.* 1975; 25:980–988.

104. Vital C, Vallat JM, Deminiere C, Loubet A, Leboutet MJ. Peripheral nerve damage during multiple myeloma and Waldenström's macroglobulinemia. *Cancer*. 1982;50:1491–1497.
105. Levine T, Pestronk A, Florence J, et al. Peripheral neuropathies in Waldenström's macroglobulinaemia. *J Neurol Neurosurg Psychiatry*. 2006;77(2):224–228.
106. Luigetti M, Frisullo G, Laurenti L, et al. Light chain deposition in peripheral nerve as a cause of mononeuritis multiplex in Waldenström's macroglobulinaemia. *J Neurol Sci*. 2010;291:89–91.
107. Gironi M, Saresella M, Ceresa L, et al. Clinical and immunological worsening in a patient affected with Waldenström macroglobulinemia and anti-mag neuropathy after treatment with rituximab. *Haematologica*. 2006;91(6 suppl):ECR17.
108. Noronha V, Fynan TM, Duffy T. Flare in neuropathy following rituximab therapy for Waldenström's macroglobulinemia. *J Clin Oncol*. 2006;24(1):e3.
109. Gosselin S, Kyle RA, Dyck PJ. Neuropathy associated with monoclonal gammopathies of undetermined significance. *Ann Neurol*. 1991;30:54–61.
110. Kelly JJ, Adelman LS, Berkman E, Bhan I. Polyneuropathies associated with IgM monoclonal gammopathies. *Arch Neurol*. 1988;45:1355–1359.
111. Suarez GA, Kelly JJ. Polyneuropathy associated with monoclonal gammopathy of undetermined significance: Further evidence that IgM-MGUS neuropathies are different than IgG-MGUS. *Neurology*. 1993;43:1304–1308.
112. Katz JS, Saperstein DS, Gronseth G, Amato AA, Barohn RJ. Distal acquired demyelinating symmetric (DADS) neuropathy. *Neurology*. 2000;54:615–620.
113. Saperstein DS, Katz JS, Amato AA, Barohn RJ. The spectrum of the acquired chronic demyelinating polyneuropathies. *Muscle Nerve*. 2001;24:311–324.
114. Donofrio PD, Kelly JJ Jr. AEE case report #17: Peripheral neuropathy in monoclonal gammopathy of undetermined significance. *Muscle Nerve*. 1989;12:1–8.
115. Niermeijer JM, Eurelings M, Lokhorst HL, et al. Rituximab for polyneuropathy with IgM monoclonal gammopathy. *JNNP*. 2009;80:1036–1039.
116. Dalakas MC, Rakocevic G, Salajegheh M, et al. Placebo-controlled trial of rituximab in IgM anti-myelin-associated glycoprotein antibody demyelinating neuropathy. *Ann Neurol*. 2009;65:286–293.
117. Larue S, Bombelli F, Viala K, et al. Non-anti-MAG DADS neuropathy as a variant of CIDP: Clinical, electrophysiological, laboratory features and response to treatment in 10 cases. *Eur J Neurol*. 2011;18:899–905.
118. Eliashiv S, Brenner T, Abramsky O, et al. Acute inflammatory demyelinating polyneuropathy following bone marrow transplantation. *Bone Marrow Transplant*. 1991;8:315–317.
119. Openshaw H, Hinton DR, Slatkin NE, Bierman PJ, Hoffman FM, Snyder DS. Exacerbation of inflammatory demyelinating polyneuropathy after bone marrow transplantation. *Bone Marrow Transplant*. 1991;7:411–414.
120. Greenspan A, Deeg HG, Cottler-Fox M, Sirdofski M, Spitzer TR, Kattah J. Incapacitating peripheral neuropathy as a manifestation of chronic graft-versus-host disease. *Bone Marrow Transplant*. 1990;5:349–352.
121. Bashir RM, Bierman P, McComb R. Inflammatory peripheral neuropathy following high dose chemotherapy and autologous bone marrow transplantation. *Bone Marrow Transplant*. 1992;10:305–306.
122. Myers SE, Williams SF, Iveson T, Treleaven J, Powles R. Guillain–Barré syndrome after bone marrow transplantation. *Bone Marrow Transplant*. 1994;14:165–167.
123. Ashraf M, Scotchel PL, Krall JM, Flink EB. Cis-platinum induced hypomagnesemia and peripheral neuropathy. *Gynecol Oncol*. 1983;16:309–318.
124. Barajon I, Bersani M, Quartu M, et al. Neuropeptides and morphological changes in cis-platin-induced dorsal root ganglion neuronopathy. *Exp Neurol*. 1996;138:93–104.
125. Cerosimo RJ. Cisplatin neurotoxicity. *Cancer Treat Rev*. 1989; 16:195–211.
126. Gregg RW, Molepo JM, Monpetit VJ, et al. Cisplatin neurotoxicity: The relationship between dosage, time, and platinum concentration in neurologic tissues, and morphologic evidence of toxicity. *J Clin Oncol*. 1992;10:795–803.
127. Krarup-Hansen A, Fugleholm K, Helweg-Larsen S, et al. Examination of distal involvement in cisplatin-induced neuropathy in man. *Brain*. 1993;116:1017–1041.
128. LoMonaco M, Milone M, Batocchi AP, Padua L, Restuccia D, Tonali P. Cisplatin neuropathy: Clinical course and neurophysiological findings. *J Neurol*. 1992;239: 199–204.
129. Mollman JE, Hogan WM, Glover DJ, McCluskey LF. et al. Unusual presentation of cis-platinum neuropathy. *Neurology*. 1988;38:488–490.
130. Mollman JE, Glover DJ, Hogan WM, Furman RE. Cisplatin neuropathy: Risk factors, prognosis, and protection by WR-2721. *Cancer*. 1998;61:2192–2195.
131. Russell JW, Windebank AJ, McNiven MA, Brat DJ, Brimijoin WS. Effect of cisplatin and ACTH4-9 on neural transport in cisplatin induced neurotoxicity. *Brain Res*. 1975;676:258–267.
132. Grothey A. Oxaliplatin-safety profile: Neurotoxicity. *Semin Oncol*. 2003;30(4 suppl 15):5–13.
133. Burakgazi AZ, Messersmith W, Vaidya D, Hauer P, Hoke A, Polydefkis M. Longitudinal assessment of oxaliplatin-induced neuropathy. *Neurology*. 2011;77:980–986.
134. Verstappen CC, Koeppen S, Heimans JJ, et al. Dose-related vincristine-induced neuropathy with unexpected off-therapy worsening. *Neurology*. 2005;64:1076–1077.
135. Casey EB, Jellife AM, Le Quense M, Millett YL. Vincristine neuropathy: Clinical and electrophysiological observations. *Brain*. 1973;96:69–86.
136. Legha SS. Vincristine neurotoxicity: Pathophysiology and management. *Med Toxicol*. 1986;1:421–427.
137. Pal PK. Clinical and electrophysiological studies in vincristine induced neuropathy. *Electromyogr Clin Neurophysiol*. 1999; 39:323–330.
138. Sahenk Z, Brady ST, Mendell JR. Studies on the pathogenesis of vincristine-induced neuropathy. *Muscle Nerve*. 1987;10:80–84.
139. Goa KL, Faulds D. Vinorelbine: A review of its pharmacological properties and clinical use in cancer chemotherapy. *Drugs Aging*. 1994;5:200–234.
140. O'Reilly S, Kennedy MJ, Rowinsky EK, Donehower RC. Vinorelbine and the topoisomerase 1 inhibitors: Current and potential roles in breast cancer chemotherapy. *Breast Cancer Res Treat*. 1994;33:1–17.
141. Pace A, Bove L, Nistico C, et al. Vinorelbine neurotoxicity: Clinical and neurophysiological findings in 23 patients. *J Neurol Neurosurg Psychiatry*. 1996;61:409–411.
142. Bregman CL, Buroker RA, Hirth RS, Crosswell AR, Durham SK. Etoposide- and BMY-40481-induced sensory neuropathy in mice. *Toxicol Pathol*. 1994;22:528–535.

143. Forsyth PA, Balmaceda C, Peterson K, Seidman AD, Brasher P, DeAngelis LM. Prospective study of paclitaxel-induced peripheral neuropathy with quantitative sensory testing. *J Neurooncol.* 1997;35:47–53.
144. Lipton RB, Apfel SC, Dutcher JP, et al. Taxol produces a predominantly sensory neuropathy. *Neurology.* 1989;39:368–373.
145. Postma TJ, Vermorken JB, Liefting AJ, Pinedo HM, Heimans JJ. Paclitaxel-induced peripheral neuropathy. *Ann Oncol.* 1995;6:489–494.
146. Rowinsky EK, Chaudhry V, Forastiere AA, et al. Phase 1 pharmacologic study of paclitaxel and cisplatin with granulocyte colony-stimulation factor: Neuromuscular toxicity is dose-limiting. *J Clin Oncol.* 1993;11:2010–2020.
147. Sahenk Z, Barohn RJ, New P, Mendell JR. Taxol neuropathy: An electrodiagnostic and sural nerve biopsy finding. *Arch Neurol.* 1994;51:726–729.
148. van den Bent MJ, van Raaij-van den Aarssen VJ, Verweij J, et al. Progression of paclitaxel-induced neuropathy following discontinuation of treatment. *Muscle Nerve.* 1997;20:750–752.
149. van Gerven JM, Moll JW, van den Bent MJ, et al. Paclitaxel (Taxol) induces cumulative mild neurotoxicity. *Eur J Cancer.* 1994;30A:1074–1077.
150. Kuroi K, Shimozuma K. Neurotoxicity of taxanes: Symptoms and quality of life assessment. *Breast Cancer.* 2004;11(1):92–99.
151. Makino H. Treatment and care of neurotoxicity from taxane anticancer agents. *Breast Cancer.* 2004;11(1):100–104.
152. Park SB, Lin CS, Krishnan AV, Friedlander ML, Lewis CR, Kiernan MC. Early, progressive, and sustained dysfunction of sensory axons underlies paclitaxel-induced neuropathy. *Muscle Nerve.* 2011;43:367–374.
153. Roytta M, Raine CS. Taxol-induced neuropathy: Chronic effects of local injection. *J Neurocytol.* 1986;15:483–496.
154. Freilich RJ, Balmaceda C, Seidman AD, Rubin M, DeAngelis LM. Motor neuropathy due to docetaxel and paclitaxel. *Neurology.* 1996;47:115–118.
155. Hilkens PH, Verweij J, Stoter G, et al. Peripheral neurotoxicity induced by docetaxel. *Neurology.* 1996;46:104–108.
156. New PZ, Jackson CE, Rinaldi D, Burris H, Barohn RJ. Peripheral neuropathy secondary to docetaxel (Taxotere). *Neurology.* 1996;46:108–111.
157. Hsu Y, Sood AK, Sorosky JI. Docetaxel versus paclitaxel for adjuvant treatment of ovarian cancer: Case-control analysis of toxicity. *Am J Clin Oncol.* 2004;27(1):14–18.
158. Guastalla JP III, Dieras V. The taxanes: Toxicity and quality of life considerations in advanced ovarian cancer. *Br J Cancer.* 2003;89(suppl 3):S16–S22.
159. Chaudhry V, Eisenberber MA, Sinibaldi VJ, et al. A prospective study of suramin-induced peripheral neuropathy. *Brain.* 1996;119:2039–2052.
160. La Rocca RV, Meer J, Gilliat RW, et al. Suramin-induced polyneuropathy. *Neurology.* 1990;40:954–960.
161. Soliven B, Dhand UK, Kobayashi K, et al. Evaluation of neuropathy in patients on suramin treatment. *Muscle Nerve.* 1997;20:83–91.
162. Russell JW, Gill JS, Sorenson EJ, Schultz DA, Windebank AJ. Suramin-induced neuropathy in an animal model. *J Neurol Sci.* 2001;192(1–2):71–80.
163. Sullivan KA, Kim B, Buzdon M, Feldman EL. Suramin disrupts insulin-like growth factor-II (IGF-II) mediated autocrine growth in human SH-SY5Y neuroblastoma cells. *Brain Res.* 1997;744:199–206.
164. Czernin S, Gessl A, Wilfing A, et al. Suramin affects human peripheral blood mononuclear cells in vitro: Inhibition of Y cell growth and modulation of cytokine secretion. *Int Arch Allergy Immunol.* 1993;101:240–246.
165. Borgeat A, De Muralt B, Stalder M. Peripheral neuropathy associated with high-dose Ara-C therapy. *Cancer.* 1986; 58:852–853.
166. Johnson NT, Crawford SW, Sargar M. Acute acquired polyneuropathy with respiratory failure following high-dose systemic cytosine arabinoside and bone marrow transplantation. *Bone Marrow Transplant.* 1987;2:203–207.
167. Nevill TJ, Benstead TJ, McCormick CW, Hayne OA. Horner's syndrome and demyelinating peripheral neuropathy caused by high-dose cytosine arabinoside. *Am J Hematol.* 1989;32:314–315.
168. Openshaw H, Slatkin NE, Stein AS, Hinton DR, Forman SJ. Acute polyneuropathy after high-dose cytosine arabinoside in patients with leukemia. *Cancer.* 1996;78:1899–1905.
169. Paul M, Joshua D, Rehme N, et al. Fatal peripheral neuropathy associated with high-dose cytosine arabinoside in acute leukemia. *Br J Haematol.* 1991;79:521–523.
170. Russell JW, Powles RL. Neuropathy due to cytosine arabinoside. *Br Med J.* 1974;4:652–653.
171. Patel SR, Forman AD, Bejamin RS. High-dose ifosfamide-induced exacerbation of peripheral neuropathy. *J Natl Cancer Inst.* 1994;86:305–306.
172. Richardson PG, Barlogie B, Berenson J, et al. A phase 2 study of bortezomib in relapsed, refractory myeloma. *N Engl J Med.* 2003;348:2609–2617.
173. Richardson PG, Briemberg H, Jagganath S, et al. The frequency, severity, and reversibility of peripheral neuropathy during treatment of advanced multiple myeloma with bortezomib. *J Clin Oncol.* 2006;24:3113–3120.
174. Davis NB, Taber DA, Ansari RH, et al. Phase II trial of PS-341 in patients with renal cell cancer: A University of Chicago phase II consortium study. *J Clin Oncol.* 2004;22:115–119.
175. Stubblefield MD, Slovin S, MacGregor-Cortelli B, et al. An electrodiagnostic evaluation of the effect of pre-existing peripheral nervous system disorders in patients treated with the novel proteasome inhibitor bortezomib. *Clin Oncol (R Coll Radiol).* 2006;18:410–418.
176. Richardson PG, Xie W, Mitsiades C, et al. Single-agent bortezomib in previously untreated multiple myeloma: Efficacy, characterization of peripheral neuropathy, and molecular correlations with response and neuropathy. *J Clin Oncol.* 2009;27:3518–3525.
177. Giannoccaro MP, Donadio V, Gomis Pèrez C, Borsini W, Di Stasi V, Liguori R. Somatic and autonomic small fiber neuropathy induced by bortezomib therapy: An immunofluorescence study. *Neurol Sci.* 2011;32:361–363.
178. Meregalli C, Canta A, Carozzi VA, et al. Bortezomib-induced painful neuropathy in rats: A behavioral, neurophysiological and pathological study in rats. *Eur J Pain.* 2010;14:343–350.
179. Bruna J, Udina E, Alé A, et al. Neurophysiological, histological and immunohistochemical characterization of bortezomib-induced neuropathy in mice. *Exp Neurol.* 2010;223:599–608.
180. Carozzi VA, Canta A, Oggioni N, et al. Neurophysiological and neuropathological characterization of new murine models of chemotherapy-induced chronic peripheral neuropathies. *Exp Neurol.* 2010;226:301–309.
181. Lue J, Goel S, Mazumder A. Carfilzomib for the treatment of multiple myeloma. *Drugs Today (Barc).* 2013;49:171–179.

CHAPTER 20

Toxic Neuropathies

This chapter reviews neuropathies associated with various drugs and other environmental exposures (Table 20-1). Toxic neuropathies due to chemotherapeutic agents are discussed in Chapter 19. The associated neuropathy for most of these is an axonal, length-dependent predominantly sensory neuropathy. The history of exposure and sometimes the involvement of other organ systems help to suggest the correct diagnosis. Although we mention features that have been reported on nerve biopsy, this is not typically part of the workup as in most cases the abnormalities are nonspecific.

▶ TOXIC NEUROPATHIES ASSOCIATED WITH MEDICATIONS

METRONIDAZOLE

Clinical Features

Metronidazole is used to treat a variety of protozoan infections and Crohn disease.[1–8] Metronidazole is a member of the nitroimidazole group and has been associated with hyperalgesia and hypesthesia in a length-dependent pattern. Autonomic dysfunction may develop as well. Motor strength is typically normal. The cumulative dose at which neuropathy occurs is wide, ranging from 3.6 to 228 g. Although there is no clear dose effect, neuropathy appears to occur more frequently in patients receiving greater than 1.5 g daily of metronidazole for 30 or more days The neuropathic symptoms usually improve upon discontinuation of the drug, but there can be a coasting effect such that the symptoms may continue to worsen for several weeks. Some patients are left with residual sensory symptoms.

Laboratory Features

Nerve conduction studies (NCS) may be normal, as typical of a small fiber neuropathy, or reveal reduced amplitudes or absent sensory nerve action potentials (SNAPs) in the legs worse than in the arms. Motor conduction studies are usually normal.

Histopathology

Nerve biopsies are not routinely performed for this but have demonstrated loss of myelinated nerve fibers.

Pathogenesis

The pathogenic basis of the neuropathy is not known. Some have found that metronidazole binds to DNA and/or RNA, which could lead to breaks and impair transcription or translation to normal proteins.[7,8] Others have speculated that toxicity may arise from the production of nitro radical anions that bind and disrupt normal protein/enzyme function.[8] Furthermore, the histological abnormalities in metronidazole-treated rodents and abnormalities on brain MRI scans in patients with metronidazole-associated encephalopathy resemble thiamine (vitamin B1) deficiency. It has been postulated that there may be enzymatic conversion of metronidazole to an analog of thiamine, which may act as a B1 antagonist.[9]

MISONIDAZOLE

Clinical Features

Misonidazole is used as an adjuvant agent in the treatment of various malignancies.[10–13] As with metronidazole, misonidazole is a member of the nitroimidazole group. Some patients have developed painful paresthesias and sometimes distal weakness in a length-dependent pattern after approximately 3–5 weeks of therapeutic drug administration (total dose greater than 18 g). Vibratory and temperature perception are usually reduced, but muscle stretch reflexes are preserved. The neuropathy usually improves following discontinuation of the drug.

Laboratory Features

Sensory NCS reveal reduced amplitudes or unobtainable responses in the legs more than the arms. Motor conduction studies are typically normal.

Histopathology

A reduction in the large myelinated fibers with axonal degeneration and segmental demyelination and remyelination has been found on sural nerve biopsies. Accumulation of neurofilaments with axonal swellings can be found on electron microscopy (EM).

Pathogenesis

The pathogenic basis of the neuropathy is not known, but may be similar to metronidazole.

▶ TABLE 20-1. **TOXIC NEUROPATHIES**

Drug	Mechanism of Neurotoxicity	Clinical Features	Nerve Histopathology	EMG/NCS
Misonidazole	Unknown	Painful paresthesias, loss of large and small fiber sensory modalities, and sometimes distal weakness in length-dependent pattern	Axonal degeneration of large myelinated fibers; axonal swellings; segmental demyelination	Low-amplitude or unobtainable SNAPs with normal or only slightly reduced CMAP amplitudes
Metronidazole	Unknown	Painful paresthesias, loss of large and small fiber sensory modalities, and sometimes distal weakness in length-dependent pattern	Axonal degeneration	Low-amplitude or unobtainable SNAPs with normal CMAP
Chloroquine and hydroxychloroquine	Amphiphilic properties may lead to drug–lipid complexes that are indigestible and result in accumulation of autophagic vacuoles	Loss of large and small fiber sensory modalities and distal weakness in length-dependent pattern; superimposed myopathy may lead to proximal weakness	Axonal degeneration with autophagic vacuoles in nerves as well as muscle fibers	Low-amplitude or unobtainable SNAPs with normal or reduced CMAP amplitudes; distal denervation on EMG; irritability and myopathic-appearing MUAPs proximally in patients with superimposed toxic myopathy
Amiodarone	Amphiphilic properties may lead to drug–lipid complexes that are indigestible and result in accumulation of autophagic vacuoles	Paresthesia and pain with loss of large and small fiber sensory modalities and distal weakness in length-dependent pattern; superimposed myopathy may lead to proximal weakness	Axonal degeneration and segmental demyelination with myeloid inclusions in nerves and muscle fibers	Low-amplitude or unobtainable SNAPs with normal or reduced CMAP amplitudes; can also have prominent slowing of CVs; distal denervation on EMG; irritability and myopathic-appearing MUAPs proximally in patients with superimposed toxic myopathy
Colchicine	Inhibits polymerization of tubulin in microtubules and impairs axoplasmic flow	Numbness and paresthesia with loss of large fiber modalities in a length-dependent fashion; superimposed myopathy may lead to proximal in addition to distal weakness	Nerve biopsies demonstrate axonal degeneration; muscle biopsies reveal fibers with vacuoles	Low-amplitude or unobtainable SNAPs with normal or reduced CMAP amplitudes; irritability and myopathic-appearing MUAPs proximally in patients with superimposed toxic myopathy
Podophyllin	Binds to microtubules and impairs axoplasmic flow	Sensory loss, tingling, muscle weakness, and diminished muscle stretch reflexes in length-dependent pattern; autonomic neuropathy	Axonal degeneration	Low-amplitude or unobtainable SNAPs with normal or reduced CMAP amplitudes
Thalidomide	Unknown	Numbness, tingling, burning pain, and weakness in a length-dependent pattern	Axonal degeneration; Autopsy studies reveal degeneration of dorsal root ganglia	Low-amplitude or unobtainable SNAPs with normal or reduced CMAP amplitudes
Disulfiram	Accumulation of neurofilaments and impaired axoplasmic flow	Numbness, tingling, and burning pain in a length-dependent pattern	Axonal degeneration with accumulation of neurofilaments in the axons	Low-amplitude or unobtainable SNAPs with normal or reduced CMAP amplitudes
Dapsone	Unknown	Distal weakness that may progress to proximal muscles; sensory loss	Axonal degeneration and segmental demyelination	Low-amplitude or unobtainable CMAPs with normal or reduced SNAP amplitudes
Leflunomide	Unknown	Paresthesia and numbness in a length-dependent pattern	Unknown	Low-amplitude or unobtainable SNAPs with normal or reduced CMAP amplitudes

(continued)

▶ TABLE 20-1. (CONTINUED)

Drug	Mechanism of Neurotoxicity	Clinical Features	Nerve Histopathology	EMG/NCS
Nitrofurantoin	Unknown	Numbness, painful paresthesia, and severe weakness that may resemble GBS	Axonal degeneration; autopsy studies reveal degeneration of dorsal root ganglia and anterior horn cells	Low-amplitude or unobtainable SNAPs with normal or reduced CMAP amplitudes
Pyridoxine (vitamin B6)	Unknown	Dysesthesia and sensory ataxia; impaired large fiber sensory modalities on examination	Marked loss of sensory axons and cell bodies in dorsal root ganglia	Reduced amplitudes or absent SNAPs
Isoniazid	Inhibit pyridoxal phosphokinase leading to pyridoxine deficiency	Dysesthesia and sensory ataxia; impaired large fiber sensory modalities on examination	Marked loss of sensory axons and cell bodies in dorsal root ganglia and degeneration of the dorsal columns	Reduced amplitudes or absent SNAPs and to a lesser extent CMAPs
Ethambutol	Unknown	Numbness with loss of large fiber modalities on examination	Axonal degeneration	Reduced amplitudes or absent SNAPs
Antinucleosides	Unknown	Dysesthesia and sensory ataxia; impaired large fiber sensory modalities on examination	Axonal degeneration	Reduced amplitudes or absent SNAPs
Phenytoin	Unknown	Numbness with loss of large fiber modalities on examination	Axonal degeneration and segmental demyelination	Low-amplitude or unobtainable SNAPs with normal or reduced CMAP amplitudes
Lithium	Unknown	Numbness with loss of large fiber modalities on examination	Axonal degeneration	Low-amplitude or unobtainable SNAPs with normal or reduced CMAP amplitudes
Acrylamide	Unknown; may be caused by impaired axonal transport	Numbness with loss of large fiber modalities on examination; sensory ataxia; mild distal weakness	Degeneration of sensory axons in peripheral nerves and posterior columns, spinocerebellar tracts, mamillary bodies, optic tracts, and corticospinal tracts in the CNS	Low-amplitude or unobtainable SNAPs with normal or reduced CMAP amplitudes
Carbon disulfide	Unknown	Length-dependent numbness and tingling with mild distal weakness	Axonal swellings with accumulation of neurofilaments	Low-amplitude or unobtainable SNAPs with normal or reduced CMAP amplitudes
Ethylene oxide	Unknown; may act as alkylating agent and bind DNA	Length-dependent numbness and tingling; may have mild distal weakness	Axonal degeneration	Low-amplitude or unobtainable SNAPs with normal or reduced CMAP amplitudes
Organophosphates	Binds and inhibits neuropathy target esterase	Early features are those of neuromuscular blockade with generalized weakness; later axonal sensorimotor PN ensues	Axonal degeneration along with degeneration of gracile fasciculus and corticospinal tracts	Early: repetitive firing of CMAPs and decrement with repetitive nerve stimulation Late: axonal sensorimotor PN
Hexacarbons	Unknown; may lead to covalent cross-linking between neurofilaments	Acute, severe sensorimotor PN that may resemble GBS	Axonal degeneration and giant axons swollen with neurofilaments	Features of a mixed axonal and/or demyelinating sensorimotor axonal PN-reduced amplitudes, prolonged distal latencies, conduction block, and slowing of CVs
Lead	Unknown; may interfere with mitochondria	Encephalopathy; motor neuropathy (often resembles radial neuropathy with wrist and finger drop); autonomic neuropathy; bluish-black discoloration of gums	Axonal degeneration of motor axons	Reduction of CMAP amplitudes with active denervation on EMG

▶ TABLE 20-1. (CONTINUED)

Drug	Mechanism of Neurotoxicity	Clinical Features	Nerve Histopathology	EMG/NCS
Mercury	Unknown; may combine with sulfhydryl groups	Abdominal pain and nephrotic syndrome; encephalopathy; ataxia; paresthesia	Axonal degeneration; degeneration of dorsal root ganglia, calcarine, and cerebellar cortex	Low-amplitude or unobtainable SNAPs with normal or reduced CMAP amplitudes
Thallium	Unknown	Encephalopathy; painful sensory symptoms; mild loss of vibration; distal or generalized weakness may also develop; autonomic neuropathy; alopecia	Axonal degeneration	Low-amplitude or unobtainable SNAPs with normal or reduced CMAP amplitudes
Arsenic	Unknown; may combine with sulfhydryl groups	Abdominal discomfort, burning pain, and paresthesia; generalized weakness; autonomic insufficiency; can resemble GBS	Axonal degeneration	Low-amplitude or unobtainable SNAPs with normal or reduced CMAP amplitudes may have demyelinating features: prolonged distal latencies and slowing of CVs
Gold	Unknown	Distal paresthesia and reduction of all sensory modalities	Axonal degeneration	Low-amplitude or unobtainable SNAPs

PN, polyneuropathy; EMG, electromyography; MUAPs, motor unit action potentials; NCS, nerve conduction studies; GBS, Guillain–Barré syndrome; CMAP, compound muscle action potential; SNAP, sensory nerve action potential; CV, conduction velocity.

CHLOROQUINE

Clinical Features

Chloroquine is used in the treatment of malaria, sarcoidosis, systemic lupus erythematosus, scleroderma, and rheumatoid arthritis (RA). Chloroquine is associated with a toxic myopathy characterized by slowly progressive, painless, proximal weakness and atrophy, which is worse in the legs than in the arms (discussed in Chapter 35).[14–16] A neuropathy can also develop with or without the myopathy, leading to sensory loss, distal weakness, and reduced muscle stretch reflexes. The "neuromyopathy" usually appears in patients taking 500 mg/d for a year or more but has been reported with doses as low as 200 mg/d. The signs and symptoms of the neuropathy and myopathy are usually reversible following discontinuation of chloroquine.

Laboratory Features

Serum creatine kinase (CK) levels are usually elevated due to the superimposed myopathy. NCS reveal mild slowing of motor and sensory nerve conduction velocities (NCVs) with a mild to moderate reduction in the amplitudes. NCS may be normal in patients with only the myopathy. Electromyography (EMG) demonstrates myopathic motor unit action potentials (MUAPs), increased insertional activity in the form of positive sharp waves, fibrillation potentials, and occasionally myotonic potentials, particularly in the proximal muscles. Neurogenic MUAPs and reduced recruitment are found in more distal muscles.

Histopathology

Nerve biopsies demonstrate autophagic vacuoles and inclusions within Schwann cells (Fig. 20-1). Vacuoles may also be evident in muscle biopsies.

Pathogenesis

The pathogenic basis of the neuropathy is not known but may be related to the amphiphilic properties of the drug. Chloroquine contains both hydrophobic and hydrophilic regions that allow chloroquine to interact with the anionic phospholipids of cell membranes and organelles. This drug–lipid complex may be resistant to digestion by lysosomal enzymes, leading to the formation of autophagic vacuoles filled with myeloid debris that may, in turn, cause degeneration of nerves and muscle fibers.

HYDROXYCHLOROQUINE

Hydroxychloroquine is structurally similar to chloroquine and, not surprisingly, has also been associated with a toxic neuromyopathy.[17] Weakness and histological abnormalities are usually not as severe as seen in chloroquine myopathy. Vacuoles are typically absent on biopsy, but EM still may

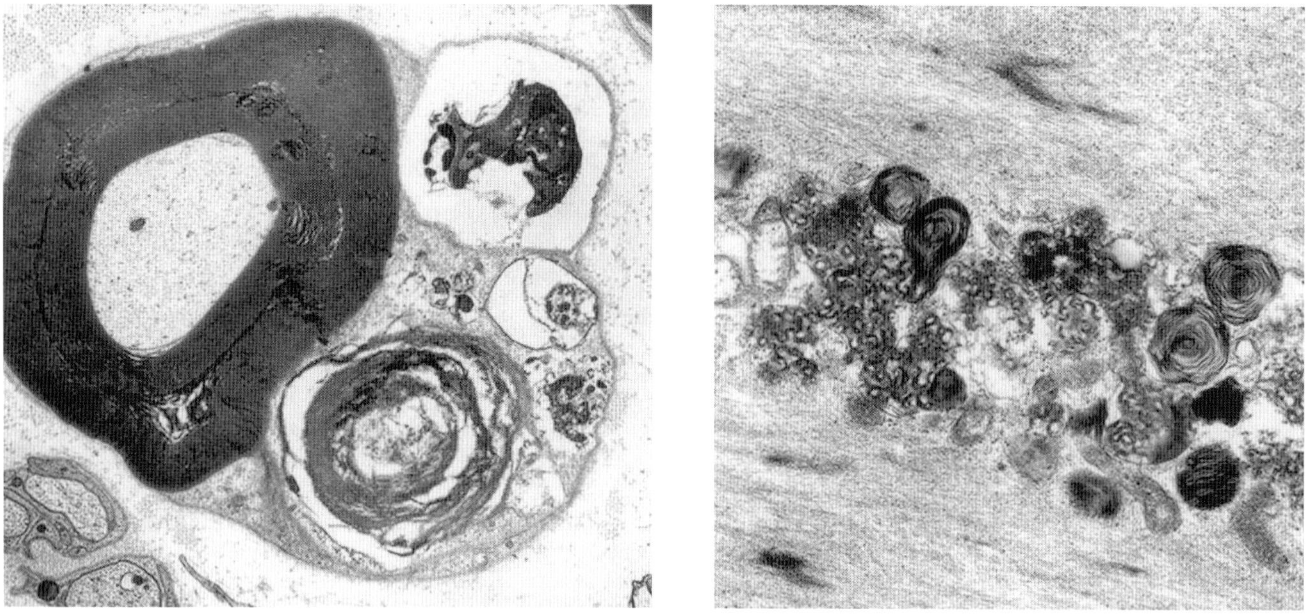

A B

Figure 20-1. Chloroquine neuropathy. Ultrastructural examination confirmed the presence of cytoplasmic lamellar inclusions in the Schwann cell cytoplasm **(A)**. Close examination shows the dimorphism of the inclusions made up of both curvilinear bodies and laminated (myeloid) osmophilic material in smooth muscle cell **(B)**. (Reproduced with permission from Bilbao JM: November 1998–70 year old woman with SLE, paraproteinemia and polyneuropathy. *Brain Pathol*. 1999;9(2):423–424.)

demonstrate abnormal accumulation of myeloid and curvilinear bodies.

AMIODARONE

Clinical Features

Amiodarone is an antiarrhythmic medication that is also associated with a neuromyopathy similar to chloroquine[18–23] Severe proximal and distal weakness can develop in the legs worse than in the arms, combined with distal sensory loss, tingling, and burning pain. In addition, amiodarone is also associated with tremor, thyroid dysfunction, keratitis, pigmentary skin changes, hepatitis, pulmonary fibrosis, and parotid gland hypertrophy. The neuromyopathy typically appears after patients have taken the medication for 2–3 years. Physical examination demonstrates arm and leg weakness, reduced sensation to all modalities, and diminished muscle stretch reflexes. The neuromyopathy usually improves following discontinuation of the drug.

Laboratory Features

Sensory NCS reveal markedly reduced amplitudes and, when obtainable, mild to moderately slow conduction velocities and prolonged distal latencies.[19,21,22] Motor NCS may also be abnormal, but usually not to the same degree as seen in sensory studies. EMG demonstrates fibrillation potentials, positive sharp waves, and occasionally myotonic discharges with a mixture of myopathic and neurogenic-appearing MUAPs.

Histopathology

Muscle biopsies demonstrate neurogenic atrophy, particularly in distal muscles, and autophagic vacuoles with myeloid and dense inclusions on EM. Sural nerve biopsies demonstrate a combination of segmental demyelination and axonal loss. EM reveals lamellar or dense inclusions in Schwann cells, pericytes, and endothelial cells. The inclusions in muscle and nerve biopsies have persisted as long as 2 years following discontinuation of the medication.

Pathogenesis

The pathogenesis is presumably similar to other amphiphilic medications (e.g., chloroquine).

COLCHICINE

Clinical Features

Colchicine is used primarily to treat patients with gout and is also associated with a toxic neuropathy and myopathy.[24–26] Affected individuals usually present with proximal weakness along with numbness and tingling in the distal extremities.

Reduced sensation to touch, vibration, position sense, and diminished muscle stretch reflexes are found on examination.

Laboratory Features

Motor and sensory NCS demonstrate reduced amplitudes.[24–26] The distal motor and sensory latencies can be normal or slightly prolonged and conduction velocities are normal or mildly slow. EMG demonstrates fibrillation potentials and positive sharp waves along with short-duration, low-amplitude MUAPs in the proximal limb muscles and long-duration, large-amplitude MUAPs distally.

Histopathology

Muscle biopsies reveal a vacuolar myopathy, while sensory nerve biopsies demonstrate axonal degeneration.

Pathogenesis

Colchicine inhibits the polymerization of tubulin into microtubules. The disruption of the microtubules probably leads to defective intracellular movement of important proteins, nutrients, and waste products in muscles and nerves.[25]

PODOPHYLLIN

Clinical Features

Podophyllin is a topical agent used to treat condylomata acuminata. Systemic side effects include pancytopenia and liver and renal dysfunction. Podophyllin is also potentially toxic to both the central and the peripheral nervous systems (PNS), leading to psychosis, altered consciousness, and polyneuropathy.[27,28] The neuropathy is characterized by slowly progressive sensory loss, paresthesias, muscle weakness, and diminished muscle stretch reflexes in a length-dependent pattern. Autonomic neuropathy with nausea, vomiting, gastrointestinal paresis, urinary retention, orthostatic hypotension, and tachycardia may also occur. The signs and symptoms of this toxic neuropathy can progress for a couple of months even after stopping the medication. The neuropathy gradually improves with discontinuation of the podophyllin, but it can take several months to over a year and residual deficits may remain.

Laboratory Features

Cerebrospinal fluid (CSF) protein levels can be elevated. Laboratory evaluation may also demonstrate pancytopenia, liver function abnormalities, and renal insufficiency. Sensory NCS reveal absent SNAPs or their reduced amplitudes. Motor NCS are less affected but can demonstrate reduced amplitudes.

Histopathology

Nerve biopsies demonstrate axonal degeneration.

Pathogenesis

Podophyllin binds to microtubules similar to colchicine and probably inhibits axoplasmic flow leading to axonal degeneration.[29]

THALIDOMIDE

Clinical Features

Thalidomide is an immunomodulating agent used to treat multiple myeloma, graft-versus-host disease, leprosy, and other autoimmune disorders.[30–36] Thalidomide is associated with severe teratogenic effects as well as peripheral neuropathy, which can be dose limiting. Most patients who develop the neuropathy have received a cumulative dose of at least 20 g of thalidomide.[34] Less than 10% of patients receiving less than 20 g of thalidomide develop polyneuropathy. Patients complain of numbness, painful tingling, burning discomfort in the feet and hands, and less commonly muscle weakness and atrophy. Even after stopping the drug for 4–6 years, as many as 50% of patients continue to have significant symptoms. Physical examination demonstrates a reduction in vibration and position sense, hypo- or areflexia, and occasionally proximal and distal weakness.

Laboratory Features

NCS demonstrate reduced amplitudes or complete absence of the SNAPs with preserved conduction velocities when obtainable.[30–36] Motor NCS are usually normal.

Histopathology

Nerve biopsies reveal a loss of large-diameter myelinated fibers and axonal degeneration.[35] Degeneration of dorsal root ganglion cells has been appreciated on autopsies.

Pathogenesis

The pathogenic basis of the neuropathy is not known.

DISULFIRAM

Clinical Features

Disulfiram (antabuse) is used to treat alcoholism. It is metabolized to carbon disulfide, which is a neurotoxin and can have adverse effects on both the PNS and the central nervous system (CNS).[37–44] A neuropathy with distal weakness (e.g., foot drop) and sensory loss may develop as early as 10 days to as long as 18 months after starting the drug.

Laboratory Features

NCS are suggestive of an axonal sensorimotor polyneuropathy with reduced amplitudes or absent SNAPs and CMAPs with normal or only moderately slow conduction velocities.[37,40,41] Needle EMG reveals fibrillation potentials and positive sharp waves in distal muscles along with decreased recruitment of neurogenic-appearing MUAPs.

Histopathology

Sural nerve biopsy has demonstrated axonal degeneration and segmental demyelination with a loss of predominately large-diameter fibers, although small-diameter fibers can be affected as well.[37–40] On EM, swollen axonal due to the accumulation of neurofilamentous debris within the myelinated and unmyelinated axons may be appreciated.

Pathogenesis

The neuropathy may be secondary to carbon disulfide, which is a metabolite of disulfiram. A similar axonal neuropathy characterized by accumulation of neurofilaments occurs with carbon disulfide toxicity.

DAPSONE

Clinical Features

Dapsone is used primarily for the treatment of leprosy and for various dermatologic conditions. A primarily motor neuropathy can develop as early as 5 days to as long as 5 years after starting the drug.[45–49] Weakness initially involves the hands and feet and over time progresses to affect more proximal muscles. Occasionally, patients complain of sensory symptoms without weakness.

Laboratory Features

Motor and sensory NCS usually demonstrate reduced amplitudes with normal or only slightly slow conduction velocities.[45–49] The NCS usually improve after the dapsone is discontinued.

Histopathology

Biopsy of the motor nerve terminal at the extensor brevis muscle has demonstrated axonal atrophy and Wallerian degeneration of the distal motor nerve terminals.[49] Sural nerve biopsy may reveal a loss of myelinated nerve fibers.

Pathogenesis

The pathogenic basis of the neuropathy is not known.

LEFLUNOMIDE

Clinical Features

Leflunomide is used for the treatment of RA. It is a prodrug for an active metabolite that reversibly inhibits dihydroorotate dehydrogenase. This enzyme catalyzes the rate-limiting step in the de novo synthesis of pyrimidines that are necessary for lymphocyte production. There have been several reports of patients treated with leflunomide who developed distal numbness and paresthesia.[50–55] The median duration of treatment at the onset of neuropathy was 7.5 months (range 3 weeks to 29 months) in one large study.[52]

Laboratory Features

NCS may demonstrate features of a primarily axonal, sensorimotor polyneuropathy.[50–55] More commonly, the NCS are normal and do not correlate with symptoms, which suggests that leflunomide may cause a small fiber neuropathy.[54] In this regard, a study of leflunomide treatment in patients with RA revealed abnormal cold detection on quantitative sensory testing compared to controls; vibratory thresholds were normal.[55]

Histopathology

There are no reports of nerve biopsies.

Pathogenesis

The pathogenic basis for the neuropathy is not known.

Treatment

The neuropathy usually improves after withdrawal of the medication.

NITROFURANTOIN

Clinical Features

Nitrofurantoin is an antibiotic most often used to treat urinary tract infections and may cause an acute and severe sensorimotor polyneuropathy [56–60] or a non–length-dependent small fiber neuropathy/ganglionopathy.[61] Patients may develop numbness, painful paresthesia, and sometimes quadriparesis. Elderly and those with baseline renal insufficiency are most at risk. Physical examination most often reveals decrease of all sensory modalities (except in cases of small fiber neuronopathy) in the distal regions of the upper and lower limbs. Muscle stretch reflexes are reduced or absent. Most patients slowly improve following discontinuation of the drug.

Laboratory Features

NCS may demonstrate reduced amplitudes or absent SNAPs and CMAPs suggestive of an axonopathy[58,59] or may be normal in cases of a small fiber neuropathy/ganglionopathy.[61]

Histopathology

Sural nerve biopsy may reveal loss of large myelinated fibers with signs of active Wallerian degeneration.[58] An autopsy study has shown degeneration of the spinal roots, dorsal more severely affected than ventral roots, and chromatolysis of the anterior horn cells.[57] Skin biopsies in patients with small fiber sensory neuropathy/ganglionopathy have shown distinctive morphologic changes with clustered terminal nerve swellings without a reduction in density.[61]

Pathogenesis

The pathogenic basis of the neuropathy is not known.

PYRIDOXINE (VITAMIN B6) TOXICITY

Clinical Features

Pyridoxine is an essential vitamin that serves as a coenzyme for transamination and decarboxylation. The recommended daily allowance in adults is 2–4 mg. However, at high doses (116 mg/d) patients can develop a severe sensory neuropathy with dysesthesia and sensory ataxia.[62–66] Some patients also complain of a Lhermitte's sign. There is one report of a patient taking 9.6 g pyridoxine per day who developed weakness as well.[67] Neurological examination reveals marked impaired vibratory perception and proprioception. Sensory loss can begin and be more severe in the upper than in the lower limbs. Muscle strength is usually normal, although there may be loss of fine motor control. Gait is wide based and unsteady secondary to the sensory ataxia. Muscle stretch reflexes are reduced or absent.

Laboratory Features

NCS usually reveal absent or markedly reduced SNAP amplitudes with relatively preserved CMAPs,[62–66] although one case with severe weakness reported reduced CMAP amplitudes and moderately slowing of CVs.[67]

Histopathology

Nerve biopsies have shown loss of axons of all fiber diameters.[65,66] Reduced numbers of dorsal root ganglion cells and subsequent degeneration of both the peripheral and the central sensory tracts have been appreciated in animal models.

Pathogenesis

The pathogenic basis for the neuropathy associated with pyridoxine toxicity is not known.

ISONIAZID

Clinical Features

Isoniazid (INH) is used for the treatment of tuberculosis. One of the most common side effects of INH is peripheral neuropathy.[68–70] Standard doses of INH (3–5 mg/kg/d) are associated with a 2% incidence of neuropathy, while neuropathy develops in at least 17% of patients taking in excess of 6 mg/kg/d of INH. The elderly, malnourished, and "slow acetylators" are at increased risk of developing the neuropathy. Patients present with numbness and tingling in their hands and feet. The neuropathy usually develops after 6 months in patients receiving smaller doses but can begin within a few weeks in patients on large doses. The neuropathic symptoms resolve after a few days or weeks upon stopping the INH, if done early. However, if the medication is continued, the neuropathy may evolve with more proximal numbness as well as distal weakness. Recovery at this stage can take months and may be incomplete. Examination reveals loss of all sensory modalities, distal muscle atrophy and weakness, reduced muscle stretch reflexes, and occasionally sensory ataxia. Prophylactic administration of pyridoxine 100 mg/d can prevent the neuropathy from developing.

Laboratory Features

NCS reveal decreased amplitudes of the SNAPs.

Histopathology

Sural nerve biopsies reveal axonal degeneration and loss of both myelinated and unmyelinated nerve fibers.[69] Autopsy studies have demonstrated degeneration of the dorsal columns.

Pathogenesis

INH inhibits pyridoxal phosphokinase resulting in pyridoxine deficiency. Because INH is metabolized by acetylation, individuals who are slow acetylators (an autosomal-recessive trait) maintain a higher serum concentration of INH and are more at risk of developing the neuropathy than people with rapid acetylation. Acetylation can also slow with age.

ETHAMBUTOL

Clinical Features

Ethambutol is also used to treat tuberculosis and has been associated with a sensory neuropathy and a severe optic neuropathy in patients receiving prolonged doses in excess of 20 mg/kg/d.[71,72] Patients develop numbness in the hands and feet without significant weakness. Examination reveals a loss of large fiber modalities and reduced muscle stretch reflexes distally. The peripheral neuropathy gradually improves after stopping of the medication; however, recovery of the optic neuropathy is more variable.

Laboratory Features

NCS reveal decreased amplitudes of the SNAPs with normal sensory distal latencies and conduction velocities. Motor conduction studies are usually normal.

Histopathology

A decreased number of myelinated nerve fibers due to axonal degeneration has been noted in human and animal studies.[73]

Pathogenesis

The pathogenic basis of the neuropathy is not known.

FLUOROQUINOLONES

The fluoroquinolones are wide-spectrum antibiotics that have been associated with a sensory polyneuropathy and optic neuropathy.[74,75] In a review, onset of adverse events was described as usually being rapid, with 33% of patients developing symptoms within 24 hours of initiating treatment, 58% within 72 hours, and 84% within one week.[74] There also has been a report that fluoroquinolones might unmask previously unrecognized hereditary neuropathy.[75]

NUCLEOSIDE NEUROPATHIES

Clinical Features

The nucleoside analogs zalcitabine (dideoxycytidine or ddC), didanosine (dideoxyinosine or ddI), stavudine (d4T), and lamivudine (3TC) are antiretroviral nucleoside reverse transcriptase inhibitor used to treat HIV infection. One of the major dose-limiting side effects of these medications is a predominantly sensory, length-dependent, symmetrically painful neuropathy.[76–79] ddC is the most extensively studied nucleoside analog and at doses greater than 0.18 mg/kg/d, is associated with a subacute onset of severe burning and lancinating pains in the feet and hands. One-third of patients on lower doses of ddC (0.03 mg/kg/d) develop a neuropathy within 1 week to a year (mean of 16 weeks) after starting the medication. On examination, hyperpathia, reduced pinprick, and temperature sensation, and to a lesser degree impaired touch and vibratory perception are found. Muscle stretch reflexes are diminished, particularly at the ankles. Occasionally, mild weakness of the ankles and of foot intrinsics is appreciated. Because of a "coasting effect," patients can continue to worsen even 2–3 weeks after stopping the medication. However, improvement in the neuropathy is seen in most patients following dose reduction after several months (mean time about 10 weeks).

Laboratory Features

Sensory NCS reveal decreased amplitudes or absent responses with normal distal latencies and CVs.[76–79] Motor NCS are usually normal. Impaired temperature and vibratory thresholds have been noted on QST.[76] The QST abnormalities, particularly vibratory perception precede clinical symptoms or standard nerve conduction abnormalities.

Pathogenesis

These nucleoside analogs inhibit mitochondrial DNA polymerase, which is the suspected pathogenic basis for the neuropathy. Acetyl-carnitine deficiency may contribute to the neurotoxicity of these nucleoside analogs.

PHENYTOIN

Clinical Features

Phenytoin is a commonly used antiepileptic medication. A rare side effect of phenytoin is a mild, primarily sensory neuropathy associated with reduced light touch, proprioception, and vibration as well as diminished or absent muscle stretch reflexes at the ankles.[80–84] Mild distal weakness may be seen. The neuropathy improves on discontinuation of the medication.

Laboratory Features

NCS reveal decreased amplitudes of the SNAPs with normal sensory distal latencies and conduction velocities. NCS demonstrate slightly reduced amplitudes and slow CVs in about 20% of patients taking only phenytoin. Motor NCS are usually normal.

Histopathology

Sural nerve biopsy has reportedly demonstrated a loss of the large myelinated axons along with segmental demyelination and remyelination.[84]

Pathogenesis

The pathogenic basis of the neuropathy is not known.

LITHIUM

Clinical Features

Lithium is more often associated with CNS toxicity (tremor, dysarthria, confusion, obtundation, sweating, and seizures), but some patients have developed sensorimotor peripheral neuropathies (distal motor and sensory loss and reduced muscle stretch reflexes).[85–87]

Laboratory Features

NCS reveal decreased amplitudes of the SNAPs with normal sensory distal latencies and conduction velocities. NCS demonstrate reduced amplitudes or absent SNAPs and CMAPs.

Histopathology

Nerve biopsies have demonstrated a loss of large myelinated fibers.

Pathogenesis

The pathogenic basis of the neuropathy is not known.

STATINS

Several case reports and epidemiologic series suggest that statin use may be associated with a small risk of peripheral neuropathy.[88–91] However, we must emphasize that these reports do not establish that statins cause peripheral neuropathy. Many patients on statins have other neuropathic comorbidities which confounds assignment of causal status. The neuropathy that has been associated with statin usage is predominantly sensory and typical of "idiopathic sensory polyneuropathy." Some, but not all patients, report improved symptoms following discontinuation of the statin. Because of the well-known benefits to statins, particularly in high-risk patients, and the unproven causal nature of statin use and neuropathies we do not typically advise our patients to discontinue statin use.

▶ TOXIC NEUROPATHIES ASSOCIATED WITH INDUSTRIAL AGENTS

ACRYLAMIDE

Clinical Features

Acrylamide, a vinyl monomer, is an important industrial agent used as a flocculating and grouting agent. It can be absorbed through the skin, ingested (following exposure to contaminated well water due to acrylamide grouting of the wells) or inhaled into the lungs. Following exposure, affected individuals may develop a distal sensorimotor polyneuropathy characterized by a loss of large fiber function.[92–96] Pain and paresthesia are uncommon. Some patients have ataxia and dysarthria; increasing irritability may also be seen. Chronic low-level exposure may cause mental confusion and hallucinations in addition to weakness, gait difficulties, and occasionally urinary incontinence. Exposure to the skin is associated with contact dermatitis.

On examination, there is a loss of vibration and proprioception with relatively good preservation of touch, pain, and temperature sensation. Patients may be ataxic and demonstrate a positive Romberg sign. Muscle stretch reflexes are reduced. Mild distal muscle atrophy and weakness may be appreciated. Patients with only low levels of exposure usually make a good recovery; however, those exposed to large amounts can take a year or more for significant improvement to occur and may not completely recover.

Laboratory Features

NCS reveal decreased amplitudes of the SNAPs with normal sensory distal latencies and conduction velocities. NCS reveal absent or markedly reduced amplitude in the SNAPs.[92–96] The CMAP amplitudes are normal or only slightly reduced, but temporal dispersion of the CMAPs may be observed in patients exposed to high levels of the substance.

Histopathology

Sural nerve biopsies reveal axonal degeneration with loss of the large myelinated fibers. The earliest histological abnormality in animals exposed to acrylamide is paranodal accumulation of 10-nm neurofilaments at the distal ends of the peripheral nerves. Subsequently, the distal axons enlarge and degenerate as can the posterior columns, spinocerebellar tracts, optic tracts, mammillary bodies, and the corticospinal tracts.

Pathogenesis

The exact pathogenic basis for the toxic neuropathy is unknown but is felt that acrylamide impairs fast bidirectional axonal transport as well as slow antegrade transport.

CARBON DISULFIDE

Clinical Features

Carbon disulfide is used to make rayon and cellophane and can be inhaled or absorbed through the skin. Acute exposure to high levels of carbon disulfide may lead to CNS abnormalities (e.g., psychosis), which resolve with elimination of exposure. Chronic low-level exposure to carbon disulfide has also been associated with a toxic peripheral neuropathy characterized by length-dependent numbness and tingling.[97] Examination reveals a loss of all sensory modalities and diminished muscle stretch reflexes. Mild muscle atrophy and weakness may be evident distally.

Laboratory Features

NCS reveal slowing of sensory and perhaps motor CVs.

Histopathology

Detailed descriptions of the histopathology in humans are lacking. However, experimental studies in animals have shown accumulation of 10-nm neurofilaments and axonal swellings similar to that seen in acrylamide and hexacarbon toxicity.

Pathogenesis

The pathogenic basis for the neuropathy is not known.

ETHYLENE OXIDE

Clinical Features

Ethylene oxide may be used to sterilize heat-sensitive materials, and exposure to ethylene oxide usually is associated with dermatologic lesions, mucosal membrane irritation, nausea, vomiting, and altered mentation. Exposure to high levels can lead to a severe sensorimotor peripheral neuropathy characterized by distal numbness and paresthesia.[98,99] Examination demonstrates a loss of all sensory modalities and occasionally distal weakness. Dysmetria due to a sensory ataxia, unsteady gait, and diminished muscle stretch reflexes are also seen.

Laboratory Features

NCS demonstrate reduced amplitudes or absent SNAPs and CMAPs.

Histopathology

Sensory nerve biopsies reveal the loss of primarily, but not exclusively, the large myelinated fibers.

Pathogenesis

The pathogenic basis of the neuropathy is not known. Ethylene oxide can act as an alkylating agent and can bind with many organic molecules, including DNA.

ORGANOPHOSPHATE POISONING

Clinical Features

The organophosphates are used in the production of insecticides, plastics, petroleum products, and as toxic nerve agents for biological warfare. Exposure to organophosphates can lead to severe neurological CNS and PNS side effects.[100–105] These compounds inhibit acetylcholinesterase and result in the accumulation of acetylcholine at cholinergic synapses. Thus, toxic exposure to organophosphate esters may produce acute clinical symptoms and signs referable to peripheral muscarinic and nicotinic receptors as well as in the CNS. The CNS side effects include anxiety, emotional lability, ataxia, altered mental status, unconsciousness, and seizures. The muscarinic effects can cause nausea, vomiting, abdominal cramping, diarrhea, pulmonary edema, and bradycardia. Side effects at nicotinic synapses at the neuromuscular junction result in generalized weakness and fasciculations.

Some patients with acute organophosphate toxicity later develop a distal sensorimotor peripheral neuropathy [organophosphate-induced delayed polyneuropathy (OPIDP)].[100–105] OPIDP evolves after several weeks following exposure and maximizes within several weeks. Cramping in the calf muscles, burning or tingling in the feet, and distal weakness are early symptoms. Symptoms and signs may then progress to involve the hands. Increased tone and hyperreflexia may be seen because of superimposed CNS dysfunction. The prognosis is good in patients with mild peripheral neuropathy. However, those individuals with severe peripheral and CNS insults generally do not fully recover and are left with significant residual deficits.

Laboratory Features

In the acute and subacute stages of toxic exposure, there is electrophysiological evidence of neuromuscular dysfunction secondary to compromise of acetylcholinesterase.[100–105] Motor NCS may demonstrate repetitive firing of the CMAPs following a single nerve stimulus. On low rates of repetitive stimulation, a decrementing response is seen, and this can persist for about 4–11 days. At both low (2–5 Hz) and high (20 Hz) rates of repetitive stimulation, the CMAP amplitudes initially decrement but then recover— approaching the baseline amplitudes. In OPIDP, NCS reveal decreased amplitudes of SNAPs and CMAPs consistent with an axonal sensorimotor polyneuropathy.

Histopathology

Autopsy studies have demonstrated a distal axonopathy and degeneration of the gracile fasciculus and the corticospinal tract. In addition, marked loss of both myelinated and unmyelinated nerve fibers in the sural nerve and a moderate loss of nerve fibers in the sciatic nerve were observed on autopsy of a patient who died from exposure to sarin gas.[100]

Pathogenesis

The pathogenic basis for OPIDP is not clear. Organophosphates bind to and inhibit an enzyme called neuropathy target esterase (NTE).[103] However, inhibition of NTE is not sufficient for the development of OPIDP. The organophosphate–NTE complex must age, whereby a lateral side chain of NTE is cleaved. Downstream this leads to the degeneration of nerves.

HEXACARBONS (*n*-HEXANE, METHYL *n*-BUTYL KETONE)/GLUE SNIFFER'S NEUROPATHY

Clinical Features

n-Hexane and methyl *n*-butyl ketone are water-insoluble industrial organic solvents, which are also present in some glues. Exposure through inhalation, accidentally or intentionally (glue sniffing), or through skin absorption can lead to a profound subacute sensorimotor polyneuropathy progressing over the course of 4–6 weeks.[106–111] The neuropathy presents with numbness and tingling in the feet and later involves the proximal legs and arms. Progressive weakness also develops. Ventilatory muscles are usually spared.

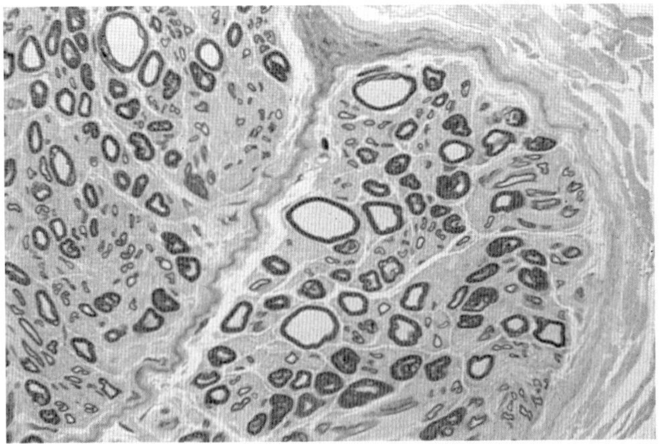

Figure 20-2. Hexacarbon toxicity. Giant axons are appreciated on this nerve biopsy in an individual who developed a severe neuropathy associated with chronic glue sniffing. (Reproduced with permission from Amato AA, Dumitru D. Acquired neuropathies. In: Dumitru D, Amato AA, Swartz MJ, eds. *Electrodiagnostic Medicine*, 2nd ed. Philadelphia, PA: Hanley & Belfus, 2002.)

Laboratory Features

NCS demonstrate decreased amplitudes of the SNAPs and CMAPs with slightly slow CVs.[106,109,110] Partial conduction block has also been appreciated in motor conduction studies in some patients.[111]

Histopathology

Nerve biopsy have revealed a loss of myelinated nerve fibers and the presence of giant axons (Fig. 20-2).[107] Segmental demyelination may be seen. EM reveals that the swollen axons are filled with 10-nm neurofilaments.

Pathogenesis

The exact mechanism by which hexacarbons cause a toxic neuropathy is not known. Hexacarbon exposure may lead to covalent cross-linking between axonal neurofilaments, which results in their aggregation, impaired axonal transport, swelling of the axons, and eventual axonal degeneration.

VINYL BENZENE (STYRENE)

Vinyl benzene or styrene is used to make some plastics and synthetic rubber. Toxic exposure leads to a primarily sensory neuropathy with burning pain and paresthesia in the legs.[112] Neurological examination demonstrates a reduction in pain and temperature, with relatively good preservation of proprioception, vibration sense, and muscle stretch reflexes. Strength is normal. NCS demonstrate a mild reduction in motor conduction velocities in the lower limbs.

► NEUROPATHIES ASSOCIATED WITH HEAVY METAL INTOXICATION

Heavy metal toxicity can be associated with axonal polyneuropathy. The severity of the neuropathy is usually related to the amount of metal that entered the patient's system either acutely or chronically. Clinical improvement is dependent on cessation of the exposure and supportive measures. Multiple organ systems can be involved besides the peripheral nervous system.

LEAD

Clinical Features

Lead neuropathy is uncommon, but it can be seen in children who accidentally ingest lead-based paints in older buildings and in industrial workers exposed to lead-containing products. The most common presentation of lead poisoning is an encephalopathy; however symptoms and signs of a primarily motor neuropathy can also occur.[113–119] The neuropathy is characterized by an insidious and progressive onset of weakness usually beginning in the arms, particularly involving the wrist/finger extensor muscles such that it resembles a radial neuropathy. Foot drop can be seen. Weakness can be asymmetric. Sensation is generally preserved; however, the autonomic nervous system can be affected, leading to constipation. Muscle stretch reflexes are diminished and plantar responses are flexor. Bluish black discoloration of gums near the teeth may be appreciated.

Laboratory Features

Laboratory investigation can reveal microcytic/hypochromic anemia with basophilic stippling of erythrocytes and an elevated serum coproporphyrin level. A 24-hour urine collection may demonstrate elevated levels of lead excretion. The NCS typical reveal reduced CMAP amplitudes, while the SNAPs are usually normal.

Histopathology

Nerve biopsy may show a loss of large myelinated axons.

Pathogenesis

The pathogenic mechanism of nerve injury is unclear but may be related to abnormal porphyrin metabolism (see Chapter 12). It is not known if the primary target of the toxic insult is the anterior horn cell or more distally in the peripheral nerve.

Treatment

The most important treatment is removing the source of the exposure. Chelation therapy with calcium disodium ethylenediaminetetraacetate, British anti-Lewisite, and penicillamine has been tried with variable success.

MERCURY

Clinical Features

Mercury toxicity may occur as a result of exposure to either organic or inorganic mercurials. The organic form of mercury is usually found in methyl or ethyl mercury. Organic mercury poisoning presents with paresthesias in hands and feet, which progress proximally and may involve the face and tongue.[120–125] Also, patients may have dysarthria, ataxia, reduced mentation, and visual and hearing loss.

The inorganic mercury compounds are primarily used for industrial purposes and consist of various mercury salts. Toxicity may arise from ingestion or inhalation of the compounds. Gastrointestinal symptoms and nephrotic syndrome are the primary clinical features associated with acute toxicity with inorganic mercury, but encephalopathy and sensorimotor polyneuropathy can also develop.

Laboratory Features

Organic mercury intoxication is difficult to diagnose because the metal is highly lipid soluble and thus remains in the body, so urinary excretion can be scant. Inorganic mercury is more readily excreted and a 24-hour urine collection can reveal an increased concentration of this metal. Sensory NCS may reveal low-amplitude SNAPs and borderline CVs.[120,122–125] Motor conductions are normal or show borderline CVs. Somatosensory-evoked potentials of the median nerve demonstrate absent cortical but present peripheral potentials.[125] Needle EMG is usually normal, but occasionally, there is abnormal spontaneous activity in the form of positive sharp waves and fibrillation potentials.

Histopathology

Autopsies of patients with organic mercury toxicity through eating contaminated fish in Minimata Bay demonstrated degeneration of the calcarine aspect of the cerebral cortex, cerebellum, and axons in the sural nerves and lumbar dorsal roots that likely account for the visual loss, ataxia, and polyneuropathy.

Pathogenesis

Mercury may bind to sulfhydryl groups of enzymatic or structural proteins, thereby impairing their proper function and leading to degeneration of the neurons. The primary site of neuromuscular pathology appears to be the dorsal root ganglia.

Treatment

The mainstay of treatment is removing the source of exposure. Too few patients have been treated with chelating agents such as penicillamine to adequately assess efficacy.

THALLIUM

Clinical Features

Thallium can exist in a monovalent or trivalent form and is primarily used as a rodenticide. Thallium poisoning usually manifests as burning paresthesias of the feet, abdominal pain, and vomiting.[126–129] Increased thirst, sleep disturbances, and psychotic behavior may be noted. Within the first week, patients develop pigmentation of the hair, an acne-like rash in the malar area of the face, and hyperreflexia. By the second and third weeks, autonomic instability with labile heart rate and blood pressure may be seen in addition. Hyporeflexia and alopecia also occur but may not be evident until the third or fourth week following exposure.

On examination, there is a reduction in pain and temperature sensation along with a mild decrease in vibratory perception and proprioception. Muscle stretch reflexes are reduced distally but generally preserved proximally. Distal muscle atrophy and weakness gradually ensue. With severe intoxication, proximal weakness and involvement of the cranial nerves can occur. Some patients require mechanical ventilation due to respiratory muscle involvement. The lethal dose of thallium is variable, ranging from 8 to 15 mg/kg of body weight. Death can result in less than 48 hours following a particularly large dose.

Laboratory Features

Serum and urine levels of thallium are increased. Routine laboratory testing can reveal anemia, renal insufficiency, and abnormal liver function tests. CSF protein levels are also elevated. NCS demonstrate features of a primarily axonal, sensorimotor polyneuropathy.[126–129] Within the first few days of intoxication NCS can be normal. After 1–2 weeks, the SNAPs and CMAPs in the legs have reduced amplitudes and H-reflexes are lost.

Histopathology

Autopsy studies and nerve biopsies demonstrate chromatolysis of cranial and spinal motor nuclei, dorsal spinal ganglia, and axonal degeneration of motor and sensory nerves.[126–129]

Pathogenesis

The pathogenic basis for the toxicity is not known.

Treatment

With acute intoxication, potassium ferric ferrocyanide II may be effective in preventing absorption of thallium from the gut. However, there may be no benefit once thallium has been absorbed. Unfortunately, chelating agents are not very efficacious. Adequate diuresis is essential to help eliminate thallium from the body without increasing tissue availability from the serum.

ARSENIC

Clinical Features

Arsenic is another heavy metal that is associated with a toxic sensorimotor polyneuropathy.[130–135] The neuropathy manifests 5–10 days after ingestion of arsenic and progresses for several weeks and can mimic Guillain–Barré syndrome clinically. The presenting symptoms are typically an abrupt onset of abdominal discomfort, nausea, vomiting, pain, and diarrhea, followed, within several days, by burning pain in the feet and hands. Subsequently, distal weakness ensues, and, with severe intoxication, proximal muscles and the cranial nerves are also affected. Muscle stretch reflexes are reduced. Some patients require mechanical ventilation because of ventilatory muscle involvement. Increased morbidity and mortality are associated with ventilatory muscle weakness and autonomic instability. Some patients appear confused due to a superimposed encephalopathy.

Examination of the skin can be helpful in diagnosing arsenic poisoning. The loss of the superficial epidermal layer results in patchy regions of increased or decreased pigmentation on the skin several weeks after an acute exposure or with chronic low levels of ingestion. Mee's lines, which are transverse lines at the base of fingernails and toenails, do not become evident until 1 or 2 months after exposure. Multiple Mee's lines may be appreciated in patients with long fingernails with more chronic exposure to arsenic. Mee's lines are not specific for arsenic toxicity, as these can also be seen following thallium poisoning. These arise from transient episodes of growth arrest.

Laboratory Features

Because arsenic is cleared from blood rapidly, assessing serum concentration of arsenic is not a reliable method to diagnose toxicity. However, arsenic levels are increased in the urine, hair, or fingernails of patients exposed to arsenic. Anemia with stippling of erythrocytes is common and occasionally pancytopenia and aplastic anemia can develop. Increased CSF protein levels without pleocytosis can be seen, which again can lead to a misdiagnosis of Guillain–Barré syndrome. NCS are usually more suggestive of an axonal sensorimotor polyneuropathy; however, demyelinating features can be present.[130–135] Sensory NCS reveal low-amplitude or absent SNAPs with relatively preserved distal latencies and CVs. Motor conduction studies may demonstrate possible conduction block and prolongation of F-wave latencies. Serial studies may show progressive deterioration of the CMAP amplitudes to distal stimulation associated with slowing of the conduction velocities. Needle EMG reveals positive sharp waves and fibrillation potentials with reduced numbers of motor units in the distal muscles progressing proximally in patients exposed to significant amounts of arsenic.

Histopathology

Nerve biopsies demonstrate axonal degeneration, reduced large- and small-diameter myelinated fibers, and occasional onion-bulb formations. Autopsy studies have revealed a loss of anterior horn cells.

Pathogenesis

The pathogenic basis of arsenic toxicity is not known. Arsenic may react with sulfhydryl groups of enzymatic (e.g., pyruvate dehydrogenase complex) and structural proteins in the neurons leading to their degeneration.

Treatment

Chelation therapy with British anti-Lewisite has yielded inconsistent results and its effect is not dramatic; therefore, it is not generally recommended.

GOLD

Clinical Features

Gold therapy (e.g., sodium aurothiomalate) was used in the past to treat RA. Some patients treated with gold salts develop a sensorimotor neuropathy several months following drug initiation manifesting as distal paresthesias in the hands and feet and occasionally mild weakness.[136,137] In addition, a systemic reaction (e.g., rash and pruritus) to the gold usually accompanies the neuropathic symptoms. Examination reveals reduced sensation to all modalities and diminished muscle stretch reflexes. Fasciculations or myokymia may be evident on examination. It may be impossible to distinguish the toxic neuropathy related to gold to the other more common neuropathies associated with RA (see Chapter 16).

Laboratory Features

NCS reveal reduced amplitudes of SNAPs with relative preservation of motor studies.

Histopathology

Nerve biopsies demonstrate axonal degeneration and segmental demyelination.

Pathogenesis

The pathogenic basis for the neuropathy is not known. It may be related to an immunological reaction triggered by the gold therapy.

Treatment

Treatment consists of stopping the gold therapy. British anti-Lewisite has been tried as well in a few patients, but it is unclear if this therapy is effective.

▶ NEUROPATHY ASSOCIATED WITH ALCOHOL ABUSE

Alcohol-related peripheral neuropathy has largely been assumed to be the result of nutritional deficiency based on observations made decades ago that the neuropathy seemed to be similar to that observed with thiamine deficiency (see Chapter 18).[138] Some studies suggest that alcohol may affect thiamine utilization rather than cause thiamine deficiency. Treatment with thiamine typically does not reverse the neuropathic symptoms and signs of patients with alcohol-related neuropathy. In addition, recent studies on animals and humans have supported a toxic etiology, likely affecting small unmyelinated and myelinated fibers early in the course, and progressing to more symptomatic clinical involvement as a large-fiber sensorimotor axonal neuropathy develops.[138]

▶ SUMMARY

Many drugs and environmental exposures have been associated with a toxic neuropathy, and thus the need for taking extensive medication and exposure history in any patient being evaluated for a neuromuscular disorder. The mechanisms by which these agents cause neuropathy are variable. These may have a primary effect on the neuronal cell body (ganglionopathy, the Schwann cells and myelin sheath, or axons). Most of the time, the neuropathies stabilize and improve after discontinuing the offending agent. However, there can be a coasting effect such that the neuropathy clinically worsens for a few months even after stopping the medication.

REFERENCES

1. Coxon A, Pallis CA. Metronizdazole neuropathy. *J Neuro Neurosurg Psychiatry*. 1976;39:403–405.
2. Takeuchi H, Yamada A, Touge T, Miki H, Nishioka M, Hashimoto S. Metronidazole neuropathy: A case report. *Jpn J Psychiatry Neurol*. 1988;42:291–295.
3. Zivkovic SA, Lacomis D, Giuliani MJ. Sensory neuropathy associated with metronidazole: Report of four cases and review of the literature. *J Clin Neuromuscul Dis*. 2001;3:8–12.
4. Gondim FAA, Brannagan TH 3rd, Sander HW, Chin RL, Latov N. Peripheral neuropathy in patients with inflammatory bowel disease. *Brain*. 2005;128:867–879.
5. Tan CH, Chen YF, Chen CC, Chao CC, Liou HH, Hsieh ST. Painful neuropathy due to skin denervation after metronidazole-induced neurotoxicity. *J Neurol Neurosurg Psychiatry*. 2011;82:462–466.
6. Hobson-Webb LD, Roach ES, Donofrio PD. Metronidazole: Newly recognized cause of autonomic neuropathy. *J Child Neurol*. 2006;21:429–431.
7. Bradley WG, Karlsson IJ, Rassol CG. Metronidazole neuropathy. *Br Med J*. 1977;2:610–611.
8. Leitsch D, Kolarich D, Binder M, Stadlmann J, Altmann F, Duchêne M. Trichomonas vaginalis: Metronidazole and other nitroimidazole drugs are reduced by the flavin enzyme thioredoxin reductase and disrupt the cellular redox system. Implications for nitroimidazole toxicity and resistance. *Mol Microbiol*. 2009;72:518–536.
9. Alston TA, Abeles RH. Enzymatic conversion of the antibiotic metronidazole to an analog of thiamine. *Arch Biochem Biophys*. 1987;257:357–362.
10. Melgaard B, Hansen HS, Kamieniecka Z, et al. Misonidazole neuropathy: A clinical, electrophysiological, and histological study. *Ann Neurol*. 1982;12:10–17.
11. Walker MD, Strike TA. Misonidazole peripheral neuropathy: Its relationship to plasma concentration and other drugs. *Cancer Clin Trials*. 1980;3:105–109.
12. Mamoli B, Wessely P, Kogelnik HD, Müller M, Rathkolb O. Electroneurographic investigations of misonidazole polyneuropathy. *Eur Neurol*. 1979;18:405–414.
13. Paulson OB, Melgaard B, Hansen HS, et al. Misonidazole neuropathy. *Acta Neurol Scand*. 1984;70(suppl 100):133–136.
14. Estes ML, Ewing-Wilson D, Chou SM, et al. Chloroquine neuromyotoxicity. Clinical and pathological perspective. *Am J Med*. 1987;82:447–455.
15. Mastaglia FL, Papadimitriou JM, Dawkins RL, Beveridge B. Vacuolar myopathy associated with chloroquine, lupus erythematosus and thymoma. *J Neurol Sci*. 1977;34:315–328.
16. Wasay M, Wolfe GI, Herrold JM, Burns DK, Barohn RJ. Chloroquine myopathy and neuropathy with elevated CSF protein. *Neurology*. 1998;51:1226–1227.
17. Stein M, Bell MJ, Ang LC. Hydroxychloroquine neuromyotoxicity. *J Rheumatol*. 2000;27:2927–2931.
18. Charness ME, Morady F, Scheinman MM. Frequent neurologic toxicity associated with amiodarone. *Neurology*. 1984;34:669–671.
19. Fraser AG, McQueen IN, Watt AH, Stephens MR. Peripheral neuropathy during longterm high-dose amiodarone therapy. *J Neurol Neurosurg Psychiatry*. 1985;48:576–578.
20. Jacobs JM, Costa-Jussa FR. The pathology of amiodarone neurotoxicity. *Brain*. 1985;108:753–769.
21. Meier C, Kauer B, Muller U, Ludin HP. Neuromyopathy during chronic amiodarone treatment. *J Neurol*. 1979;220:231–239.
22. Pellissier JF, Pouget J, Cros D, De Victor B, Serratrice G, Toga M. Peripheral neuropathy induced by amiodarone chlorohydrate. *J Neurol Sci*. 1984;63:251–266.
23. Orr CF, Ahlskog JE. Frequency, characteristics, and risk factors for amiodarone neurotoxicity. *Arch Neurol*. 2009;66:865–869.
24. Kuncl RW, Duncan G, Watson D, Alderson K, Rogawski MA, Peper M. Colchicine myopathy and neuromyopathy. *N Engl J Med*. 1987;316:1562–1568.
25. Kuncl RW, Cornblath DR, Avila O, Duncan G. Electrodiagnosis of human colchicine myoneuropathy. *Muscle Nerve*. 1989;12:360–364.
26. Riggs JE, Schochet SS Jr, Gutman L, Crosby TW, DiBartolomeo AG. Chronic human colchicine neuropathy and myopathy. *Arch Neurol*. 1986;43:521–523.
27. Filley CM, Graff-Radford NR, Lacy JR, Heitner MA, Earnest MP. Neurologic manifestations of podophyllin toxicity. *Neurology*. 1982;32:308–311.
28. Campbell AN. Accidental poisoning with podophyllin. *Lancet*. 1980;1:206–207.
29. Paulson JC, McClure WO. Microtubules and axoplasmic transport: Inhibition of transport by podophyllotoxin: An interaction with microtubule protein. *J Cell Biol*. 1975;67:461–467.
30. Fullerton PM, Kremer M. Neuropathy after intake of thalidomide (Distaval). *Br Med J*. 1961;2:855–858.

31. Fullerton PM, O'Sullivan DJ. Thalidomide neuropathy: A clinical, electrophysiological, and histological follow-up study. *J Neurol Neurosurg Psychiatry*. 1968;31:543–551.
32. Lagueny A, Rommel A, Vignolly B, et al. Thalidomide neuropathy: An electrophysiologic study. *Muscle Nerve*. 1986;9:837–844.
33. Powell RJ, Jenkins JS, Smith NJ, et al. Peripheral neuropathy in thalidomide treated patients. *Br J Rheumatol*. 1987;26:12.
34. Cavaletti G, Beronio A, Reni L, et al. Thalidomide sensory neurotoxity. A clinical and neurophysiologic study. *Neurology*. 2004;62:2291–2293.
35. Chaudhry V, Cornblath DR, Corse A, Freimer M, Simmons-O'Brien E, Vogelsang G. Thalidomide-induced neuropathy. *Neurology*. 2002;59(12):1872–1875.
36. Plasmati R, Pastorelli F, Cavo M, et al. Neuropathy in multiple myeloma treated with thalidomide: A prospective study. *Neurology*. 2007;69:573–581.
37. Ansbacher LE, Bosch EP, Cancilla PA. Disulfiram neuropathy: A neurofilamentous distal axonopathy. *Neurology*. 1982;32:424–428.
38. Bergouignan FX, Vital C, Henry P, Eschapasse P. Disulfiram neuropathy. *J Neurol*. 1988;235:382–383.
39. Borrett D, Ashby P, Bilbao J, Carlen P. Reversible late onset disulfiram induced neuropathy and encephalopathy. *Ann Neurol*. 1985;17:396–399.
40. Mokri B, Ohnishi A, Dyck PJ. Disulfiram neuropathy. *Neurology*. 1981;31:730–735.
41. Palliyath SK, Schwartz BD, Gant L. Peripheral nerve functions in chronic alcoholic patients on disulfiram: A six month follow-up. *J Neurol Neurosurg Psychiatry*. 1990;53:227–230.
42. Olney RK, Miller RG. Peripheral neuropathy associated with disulfiram administration. *Muscle Nerve*. 1980;3:172–175.
43. Palliyath SK, Schwartz BD, Gant L. Peripheral nerve functions in chronic alcoholic patients on disulfiram: A six month follow-up. *J Neurol Neurosurg Psychiatry*. 1990;53:227–230.
44. Filosto M, Tentorio M, Broglio L, et al. Disulfiram neuropathy: Two cases of distal axonopathy. *Clin Toxicol*. 2008;46:314–316.
45. Navarro JC, Rosales RL, Ordinario AT, Izumo S, Osame M. Acute dapsone induced peripheral neuropathy. *Muscle Nerve*. 1989;12:604–606.
46. Ahrens EM, Meckler RJ, Callen JP. Dapsone induced peripheral neuropathy. *Internat J Derm*. 1986;25:314–316.
47. Gutmann L, Martin JD, Welton W. Dapsone motor neuropathy-an axonal disease. *Neurology*. 1976;26:514–516.
48. Rapoport AM, Guss SB. Dapsone induced peripheral neuropathy. *Arch Neurol*. 1972;27:184–185.
49. Sirsat AM, Lalitha VS, Pandya SS. Dapsone neuropathy report of three cases and pathologic features of a motor nerve. *Int J Leprosy*. 1987;55:23–29.
50. Gabelle A, Antoine JC, Hillaire-Buys D, Coudeyre E, Camu W. Leflunomide-related severe axonal neuropathy. *Rev Neurol (Paris)*. 2005;161(11):1106–1109.
51. Kho LK, Kermode AG. Leflunomide-induced peripheral neuropathy. *J Clin Neurosci*. 2007;14:179–181.
52. Martin K, Bentaberry F, Dumoulin C, et al. Neuropathy associated with leflunomide: A case series. *Ann Rheum Dis*. 2005;64:649–650.
53. Metzler C, Arlt AC, Gross WL, Brandt J. Peripheral neuropathy in patients with systemic rheumatic diseases treated with leflunomide. *Ann Rheum Dis*. 2005;64:1798–1800.
54. Richards BL, Spies J, McGill N, et al. Effect of leflunomide on the peripheral nerves in rheumatoid arthritis. *Intern Med J*. 2007;37(2):101–107.
55. Kim HK, Park SB, Park JW, et al. The effect of leflunomide on cold and vibratory sensation in patients with rheumatoid arthritis. *Ann Rehabil Med*. 2012;36:207–212.
56. De Olivarius BF. Polyneuropathy due to nitrofurantoin therapy. *Ugeskr Laeger*. 1956;118:753.
57. Lhermitte F, Fardeau M, Chedru F. Polynevrites au cours de traitments par la nitrofuantoine. *Presse Med (Paris)*. 1963; 71:768.
58. Yiannikas C, Pollard JD, McLeod JG. Nitrofurantoin neuropathy. *Aust N Z J Med*. 1981;11:400–405.
59. Toole JF, Parrish ML. Nitrofurantoin polyneuropathy. *Neurology*. 1973;23:554–559.
60. Kammire LD, Donofrio PD. Nitrofurantoin neuropathy: A forgotten adverse effect. *Obstet Gynecol*. 2007;110(2, pt 2): 510–512.
61. Tan IL, Polydefkis MJ, Ebenezer GJ, Hauer P, McArthur JC. Peripheral nerve toxic effects of nitrofurantoin. *Arch Neurol*. 2012;69:265–268.
62. Dalton K, Dalton JT. Characteristics of pyridoxine overdose neuropathy syndrome. *Acta Neurol Scand*. 1987;76:8–11.
63. Albin RL, Albers JW, Greenberg HS, et al. Acute sensory neuropathy-neuronopathy from pyridoxine overdose. *Neurology*. 1987;37:1729–1732.
64. Albin RL, Albers JW. Long-term follow-up of pyridoxine induced acute sensory neuropathy/neuronopathy. *Neurology*. 1990;40:1319.
65. Schaumburg HH, Kaplan J, Windbank A, et al. Sensory neuropathy from pyridoxine abuse. *New Engl J Med*. 1983;309:445–448.
66. Parry GJ, Bredesen DE. Sensory neuropathy with low-dose pyridoxine. *Neurology*. 1985;35:1466–1468.
67. Gdynia HJ, Müller T, Sperfeld AD, et al. Severe sensorimotor neuropathy after intake of highest dosages of vitamin B6. *Neuromuscul Disord*. 2008;18:156–158.
68. Jones WA, Jones GP. Peripheral neuropathy due to isoniazid; report of two cases. *Lancet*. 1953;1:1073–1074.
69. Ochoa J. Isoniazid neuropathy in man: Quantitative electron microscope study. *Brain*. 1970;93:831–850.
70. Ohnishi A, Chua CL, Kuroiwa Y. Axonal degeneration distal to the site of accumulation of vesicular profiles in the myelinated fiber axon in experimental isoniazid neuropathy. *Acta Neuropathol*. 1985;67:195–200.
71. Tugwell P, James SL. Peripheral neuropathy with ethambutol. *Postgrad Med J*. 1972;48:667–670.
72. Nair VS, LeBrun M, Kass I. Peripheral neuropathy associated with ethambutol. *Chest*. 1980;77:98–100.
73. Matsuoka Y, Takayanagi T, Sobue I. Experimental ethambutol neuropathy in rats. Morphometric and teased-fiber studies. *J Neurol Sci*. 1981;51:89–99.
74. Cohen JS. Peripheral neuropathy associated with fluoroquinolones. *Ann Pharmacother*. 2001;35:1540–1547.
75. Panas M, Karadima G, Kalfakis N, Vassilopoulos D. Hereditary neuropathy unmasked by levofloxacin. *Ann Pharmacother*. 2011;45:1312–1313.
76. Berger AR, Arezzo JC, Schaumburg HH, et al. 2′,3′-Dideoxycytidine (ddC) toxic neuropathy: A study of 52 patients. *Neurology*. 1993;43:358–362.
77. Blum AS, Dal Pan GJ, Feiberg J, et al. Low-dose zalcitabine-related toxic neuropathy: Frequency, natural history, and risk factors. *Neurology*. 1996;46:999–1003.
78. Dubinsky RM, Yarchoan R, Dalakas M, Broder S. Reversible axonal neuropathy from treatment of AIDS and related

disorders with 2′,3′-dideoxycytidine (ddC). *Muscle Nerve.* 1989;12:856–860.
79. Verma A, Schein RM, Jayaweera DT, Kett DH. Fulminant neuropathy and lactic acidosis associated with nucleoside analog therapy. *Neurology.* 1999;53:1365–1367.
80. Dobkin BH. Reversible subacute peripheral neuropathy induced by phenytoin. *Arch Neurol.* 1977;34:189–190.
81. Chokroverty S, Sayeed ZA. Motor nerve conduction study in patients on diphenylhydantoin therapy. *J Neurol Neurosurg Psychiatry.* 1975;38:1235–1239.
82. Lovelace RE, Horwitz SJ. Peripheral neuropathy in long-term diphenylhydantoin therapy. *Arch Neurol.* 1968;18:69–77.
83. Shorvon SD, Reynolds EH. Anticonvulsant peripheral neuropathy: A clinical and electrophysiological study of patients on single drug treatment with phenytoin, carbamazepine or barbiturates. *J Neurol Neurosurg Psychiatry.* 1982;45:620–626.
84. Ramirez JA, Mendell JR, Warmolts JR, Griggs RC. Phenytoin neuropathy: Structural changes in the sural nerve. *Ann Neurol.* 1986;19:162–176.
85. Brust JC, Hammer JS, Challenor Y, Healton EB, Lesser RP. Acute generalized polyneuropathy accompanying lithium poisoning. *Ann Neurol.* 1979;6:360–362.
86. Pamphlett RS, Mackenzie RA. Severe peripheral neuropathy due to lithium intoxication. *J Neurol Neurosurg Psychiatry.* 1982; 45:656.
87. Johnston SR, Burn D, Brooks DJ. Peripheral neuropathy associated with lithium toxicity. *J Neurol Neurosurg Psychiatry.* 1991; 54:1019–1020.
88. Chong PH, Boskovich A, Stevkovic N, Bartt RE. Statin-associated peripheral neuropathy: Review of the literature. *Pharmacotherapy.* 2004;24:1194–1203.
89. Gaist D, Jeppesen U, Andersen M, García Rodríguez LA, Hallas J, Sindrup SH. Statins and risk of polyneuropathy: A case-control study. *Neurology.* 2002;58:1333–1337.
90. Corrao G, Zambon A, Bertù L, Botteri E, Leoni O, Contiero P. Lipid lowering drugs prescription and the risk of peripheral neuropathy: An exploratory case-control study using automated databases. *J Epidemiol Community Health.* 2004;58 (12):1047–1051.
91. Tierney EF, Thurman DJ, Beckles GL, Cadwell BL. Association of statin use with peripheral neuropathy in the US population 40 years of age or older. *J Diabetes.* 2013;5(2):207–215.
92. Leswing RJ, Ribelin WE. Physiologic and pathologic changes in acrylamide neuropathy. *Arch Environ Health.* 1969;18:23–29.
93. Davenport JG, Farrell DF, Sumi M. "Giant axonal neuropathy" caused by industrial chemicals: Neurofilamentous axonal masses in man. *Neurology.* 1976;26:919–923.
94. Sumner AJ, Asbury AK. Acrylamide neuropathy: Selective vulnerability of sensory fibers. *Trans Am Neurol Assoc.* 1974; 99: 79–83.
95. LoPachin RM, Balaban CD, Ross JF. Acrylamide axonopathy revisited. *Toxicol Appl Pharmacol.* 2003;188:135–153.
96. Kjuus H, Goffeng LO, Heier MS, et al. Effects on the peripheral nervous system of tunnel workers exposed to acrylamide and N-methylolacrylamide. *Scand J Work Environ Health.* 2004; 30:21–29.
97. Corsi G, Maestrelli P, Picotti G, Manzoni S, Negrin P. Chronic peripheral neuropathy in workers with previous exposure to carbon disulphide. *Br J Ind Med.* 1983;40:209–211.
98. Finelli PF, Morgan TF, Yaar I, Granger CV. Ethylene oxide induced polyneuropathy. *Arch Neurol.* 1983;40:419–421.
99. Kuzuhara S, Kanazawa I, Nakanishi T, Egashira T. Ethylene oxide polyneuropathy. *Neurology.* 1983;33:377–380.
100. Himuro K, Murayama S, Nishiyama K, et al. Distal sensory axonopathy after sarin intoxication. *Neurology.* 1998;51: 1195–1197.
101. Besser R, Gutmann L, Dillmann U, Weilemann LS, Hopf HC. End-plate dysfunction in acute organophosphate intoxication. *Neurology.* 1989;39:561–567.
102. de Jager AEJ, van Weerden TW, Houthoff HJ, de Monchy JG. Polyneuropathy after massive exposure to parathion. *Neurology.* 1981;31:603–605.
103. Lotti M, Becker CE, Aminoff MJ. Organophosphate polyneuropathy: Pathogenesis and prevention. *Neurology.* 1984;34:658–662.
104. Vasilescu C, Alexianu M, Dan A. Delayed neuropathy after organophosphorus insecticide (Dipterex) poisoning: A clinical, electrophysiological, and nerve biopsy study. *J Neurol Neurosurg Psychiatry.* 1984;47:543–548.
105. Wadia RS, Chitra S, Amin RB, Kiwalkar RS, Sardesai HV. Electrophysiological studies in acute organophosphate poisoning. *J Neurol Neurosurg Psychiatry.* 1987;50:1442–1448.
106. Korobkin R, Asbury AK, Sumner AJ, Nielsen SL. Glue-sniffing neuropathy. *Arch Neurol.* 1975;32:158–162.
107. Towfighi J, Gonatas NK, Pleasure D, Cooper HS, McCree L. Glue sniffer's neuropathy. *Neurology.* 1976;26:238–243.
108. Spencer PS, Schaumburg HH, Raleigh RL, Terhaar CJ. Nervous system degeneration produced by the industrial solvent methyl n-butyl ketone. *Arch Neurol.* 1975;32:219–222.
109. Allen N, Mendell JR, Billmaier DJ, Fontaine RE, O'Neill J. Toxic polyneuropathy due to methyl *n*-butyl ketone. *Arch Neurol.* 1975;32:209–218.
110. King PJL, Morris JG, Pollard JD. Glue Sniffing neuropathy. *Aust N Z J Med.* 1985;15:293–299.
111. Pastore C, Izura V, Marhuenda D, Prieto MJ, Roel J, Cardona A. Partial conduction blocks in *N*-hexane neuropathy. *Muscle Nerve.* 2002;26:132–135.
112. Behari M, Choudhary C, Roy S, Maheshwari MC. Styrene-induced peripheral neuropathy. *Eur Neurol.* 1986;25:424–427.
113. Feldman RG, Haddow J, Kopito L, Schwachman H. Altered peripheral nerve conduction velocity: Chronic lead intoxication in children. *Am J Dis Child.* 1973;125:39–41.
114. Feldman RG, Hayes MK, Younes R, Aldrich FD. Lead neuropathy in adults and children. *Arch Neurol.* 1977;34:481–488.
115. Jeyaratnam J, Devathasan G, Ong CN, Phoon WO, Wong PK. Neurophysiological studies on workers exposed to lead. *J Neurol Neurosurg Psychiatry.* 1985;42:173–177.
116. Seppalainen AM, Hernberg S. Sensitive technique for detecting subclinical lead neuropathy. *Br J Industr Med.* 1972;29:443–449.
117. Seppalainen AM, Tola S, Hernberg S, Kock B. Subclinical neuropathy at "safe" levels of lead exposure. *Arch Environ Health.* 1975;30:180–183.
118. Seto DS, Freeman JM. Lead neuropathy in childhood. *Am J Dis Child.* 1964;107:337–342.
119. Simpson JA, Seaton DA, Adams JF. Response to treatment with chelating agents of anaemia, chronic encephalopathy, and myelopathy due to lead poisoning. *J Neurol Neurosurg Psychiatry.* 1964;27:536–541.
120. Albers JW, Cavender GD, Levine SP, Langolf GD. Asymptomatic sensorimotor polyneuropathy in workers exposed to elemental mercury. *Neurology.* 1982;32:1168–1174.
121. Adams CR, Ziegler DK, Lin JT. Mercury intoxication simulating amyotrophic lateral sclerosis. *JAMA.* 1983;250:642–643.

122. Iyer K, Goodgold J, Eberstein A, Berg P. Mercury poisoning in a dentist. *Arch Neurol.* 1976;33:788–790.
123. Shapiro IM, Cornblath DR, Sumner AJ, et al. Neurophysiological and neuropsychological functions in mercury-exposed dentists. *Lancet.* 1982;1:1147–1150.
124. Le Quesne PM, Damluji SF, Rustam H. Electrophysiological studies of peripheral nerve in patients with inorganic mercury poisoning. *J Neurol Neurosurg Psychiatry.* 1974;37:333–339.
125. Tokuomi H, Uchino M, Imamura S, Yamanaga H, Nakanishi R, Ideta T. Minimata disease (organic mercury poisoning): Neuroradiologic and electrophysiologic studies. *Neurology.* 1982;32:1369–1375.
126. Dumitru D, Kalantri A. Electrophysiologic investigation of thallium poisoning. *Muscle Nerve.* 1990;13:433–437.
127. Bank WJ, Pleasure DE, Suzuki K, Nigro M, Katz R. Thallium Poisoning. *Arch Neurol.* 1972;26:456–464.
128. Limos LC, Ohnishi A, Suzuki N, et al. Axonal degeneration and focal muscle fiber necrosis in human thallotoxicosis: Histopathological studies of nerve and muscle. *Muscle Nerve.* 1982;5:698–706.
129. Davis LE, Standefer JC, Kornfel M, Abercrombie DM, Butler C. Acute thallium poisoning: Toxicological and morphological studies of the nervous system. *Ann Neurol.* 1981;10:38–44.
130. Difini JA, Santos JF, Barton B, Ayyar D. Misdiagnosis of acute arsenical neuropathy. *Muscle Nerve.* 1990;13:854.
131. Donofrio PD, Wilbourn AJ, Albers JW, Rogers L, Salanga V, Greenberg HS. Acute arsenic intoxication presenting as Guillain–Barré-like syndrome. *Muscle Nerve.* 1987;10:114–120.
132. Goddard MJ, Tanhehco JL, Dau PC. Chronic arsenic poisoning masquerading as Landry–Guillain–Barré syndrome. *Electromyogr Clin Neurophysiol.* 1992;32:419–423.
133. Murphy MJ, Lyon LW, Taylor JW. Subacute arsenic neuropathy: Clinical and electrophysiological observations. *J Neurol Neurosurg Psychiatry.* 1981;44:896–900.
134. Oh SJ. Electrophysiological profile in arsenic neuropathy. *J Neurol Neurosurg Psychiatry.* 1991;54:1103–1105.
135. Greenberg SA. Acute demyelinating polyneuropathy with arsenic ingestion. *Muscle Nerve.* 1996;19:1611–1613.
136. Katrak SM, Pollock M, O'Brien CP, et al. Clinical and morphological features of gold neuropathy. *Brain.* 1980;103:671–693.
137. Mitsumoto H, Wilbourn AJ, Subramony SH. Generalized myokymia and gold therapy. *Arch Neurol.* 1982;39:449–450.
138. Mellion M, Gilchrist JM, de la Monte S. Alcohol-related peripheral neuropathy: Nutritional, toxic, or both? *Muscle Nerve.* 2011;43:309–316.

CHAPTER 21

Neuropathies Associated with Endocrinopathies

Various peripheral neuropathies are associated with the different endocrinopathies (Table 21-1). In particular, peripheral neuropathy associated with diabetes mellitus (DM) is one of the most common causes worldwide.

▶ DIABETIC NEUROPATHY

DM is the most common endocrinopathy and can be separated into two major subtypes: (1) insulin-dependent DM (IDDM or type 1 DM) and (2) non–insulin-dependent DM (NIDDM or type 2 DM). DM is the most common cause of peripheral neuropathy in developed countries. DM is associated with several types of polyneuropathies: distal symmetric sensory or sensorimotor polyneuropathy, autonomic neuropathy, diabetic neuropathic cachexia (DNC), polyradiculoneuropathies, cranial neuropathies, and other mononeuropathies (Table 21-1).[1,2] The exact prevalence of each subtype of neuropathy among diabetic patients is not accurately known, but it has been estimated that between 5 and 66% of patients with diabetes develop a neuropathy.[3] Diabetic neuropathy can occur in children and adults.[4]

Long-standing, poorly controlled DM, and the presence of retinopathy and nephropathy are risk factors for the development of peripheral neuropathy in diabetic patients.[5] In a large community-based study, 1.3% of the population had DM (27% type 1 DM and 73% type 2 DM).[5] Of these, approximately 66% of individuals with type 1 DM had some form of neuropathy: generalized polyneuropathy, 54%; asymptomatic median neuropathy at the wrist, 22%; symptomatic carpal tunnel syndrome, 11%; autonomic neuropathy, 7%; and various other mononeuropathies alone or in combination (3%) such as ulnar neuropathy, peroneal neuropathy, lateral femoral cutaneous neuropathy, and diabetic polyradiculoneuropathy. In the type 2 DM group, 45% had generalized polyneuropathy, 29% had asymptomatic median neuropathy at the wrist, 6% had symptomatic carpal tunnel syndrome, 5% had autonomic neuropathy, and 3% had other mononeuropathies/multiple mononeuropathies. Considering all forms of DM, 66% of patients had some objective signs of neuropathy, but only 20% of patients with DM were symptomatic from neuropathy.

DIABETIC DISTAL SYMMETRIC SENSORY AND SENSORIMOTOR POLYNEUROPATHY

Clinical Features

Distal symmetric sensory polyneuropathy (DSPN) is the most common form of diabetic neuropathy.[1,2] It is a length-dependent neuropathy in which affected individuals develop sensory loss beginning in the toes, which gradually progresses over time up the legs and into the fingers and arms.[6,7] When severe, a patient may also develop sensory loss in the trunk (chest and abdomen) in the midline that spreads out laterally toward the spine. Sensory loss is often accompanied by paresthesia, lancinating pains, burning, or a deep aching discomfort in 40–60% of patients with DSPN.[1,8] A severe loss of sensation can lead to increased risk of infection, ulceration, and Charcot joints. Patients with small fiber neuropathy can also develop symptoms and signs of an autonomic dysfunction, as the autonomic nervous system is mediated by small myelinated and unmyelinated nerve fibers. Poor control of DM and the presence of nephropathy correlate with an increased risk of developing or worsening of DSPN.[3,5]

Neurological examination reveals loss of small fiber function (pain and temperature sensation) only or panmodality sensory loss. Those individuals with large fiber sensory loss have reduced muscle stretch reflexes, particularly at the ankles, but reflexes can be normal in patients with only small fiber involvement or in patients whose neuropathy has not ascended far enough proximally to affect the reflex arc of the Achilles deep tendon reflex. Muscle strength and function are typically normal, although mild atrophy and weakness of foot intrinsics and ankle dorsiflexors may be detected. Because patients without motor symptoms or signs on clinical examination often still have electrophysiological evidence of subclinical motor involvement, the term "distal symmetric or length-dependent sensorimotor peripheral neuropathy" is also appropriate.[9]

Laboratory Features

DSPN can be the presenting manifestation of DM as many patients may be unaware of their abnormal glucose metabolism. There may be an increased risk of impaired glucose tolerance (IGT) on oral glucose tolerance test even in those individuals with normal fasting blood sugars (FBS) and

▶ **TABLE 21-1. NEUROPATHIES ASSOCIATED WITH ENDOCRINOPATHIES**

Diabetes Mellitus
Distal symmetric sensory and sensorimotor polyneuropathy
Autonomic neuropathy
Diabetic neuropathic cachexia
Polyradiculoplexus neuropathy
Mononeuropathy/multiple mononeuropathies
Acute treatment–induced painful neuropathy
Hypoglycemia/Hyperinsulinemia
Generalized sensory or sensorimotor polyneuropathy
Acromegaly
Generalized sensory or sensorimotor polyneuropathy
Carpal tunnel syndrome
Hypothyroidism
Carpal tunnel syndrome
Generalized sensory or sensorimotor polyneuropathy

hemoglobin A1 C levels. Some studies report IGT (defined as 2-hour glucose of >140 and <200 mg/dL) in as many as 36% and DM (defined as 2-hour glucose of >200 mg/dL or FBS of >126 mg/dL) in up to 31% of patients with sensory neuropathy.[10–12] In patients with painful sensory neuropathy, the incidence of IGT or DM may be even higher. Although we have been impressed with the prevalence of IGT in our patients with burning feet, the linkage of IGT with DSPN remains controversial as other authorities have not found an association.[13,14]

Up to 50% of patients with DM have reduced sensory nerve action potential (SNAP) amplitudes and slow conduction velocities of the sural or plantar nerves, while up to 80% of symptomatic individuals have abnormal sensory nerve conduction studies (NCS).[1,15,16] Quantitative sensory testing may reveal reduced vibratory and thermal perception. Autonomic testing may also be abnormal, in particular quantitative sweat testing.[17]

Motor NCS are less severely affected than the sensory studies but still are frequently abnormal with low amplitudes and normal or only slightly prolonged distal latencies and slow nerve conduction velocities (NCVs).[1,15] Rarely, the NCV slowing can be within the "demyelinating range" (e.g., less than 30% below the lower limit of normal); however, conduction block and temporal dispersion are not usually appreciated.[15,18] Needle electromyography (EMG) examination may demonstrate fibrillation potentials, positive sharp waves, and large motor unit action potentials (MUAPs) in the distal muscles.

Histopathology

Nerve biopsies are not routinely done in patients with DSPN. In part, this is because of the nonspecific nature of the nerve pathology and the potential for poor wound healing in diabetics. If performed, nerve biopsy can reveal axonal degeneration, clusters of small regenerated axons, and segmental demyelination that is more pronounced distally, as expected in a length-dependent process (Fig. 21-1).[17] An asymmetric loss of axons between and within nerve fascicles may be appreciated. There is often endothelial hyperplasia of epi- and endoneurial arterioles and capillaries along with redundant basement membranes around these small blood vessels and thickening of the basement membrane of the perineurial cells (Fig. 21-2).[20] In addition, perivascular infiltrate consisting predominantly of CD8+ T cells can sometimes be seen.

Nerve biopsies may appear normal in patients with pure small fiber neuropathy. However, skin biopsies can demonstrate a reduction of small myelinated intraepidermal nerve fibers in such cases.[21–23] Reduced intraepidermal nerve fiber

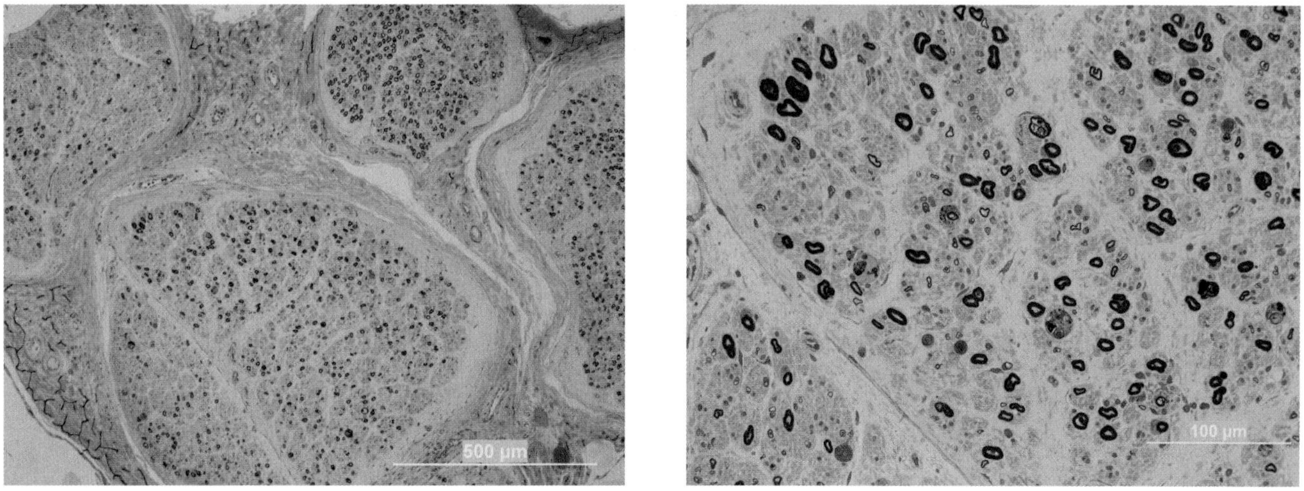

A **B**

Figure 21-1. Diabetic neuropathy. Sural nerve biopsy demonstrates asymmetric loss of myelinated nerve fibers between and within nerve fascicles **(A)**. Higher power reveals loss of large and small fibers and active axonal degeneration **(B)**. Plastic sections stained with toluidine blue.

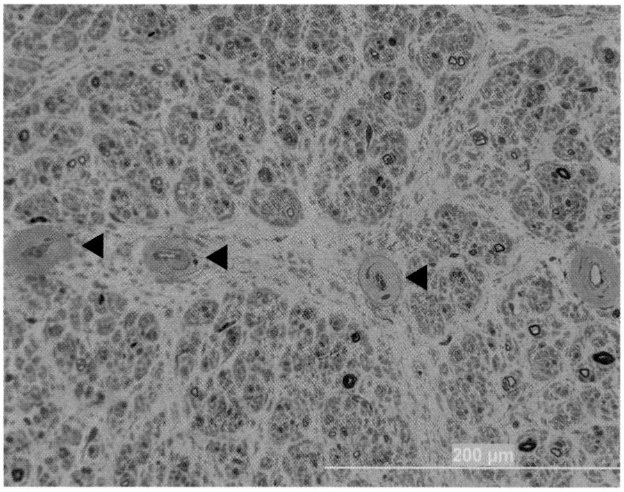

Figure 21-2. Diabetic neuropathy. Sural nerve biopsy demonstrates marked loss of myelinated nerve fibers and blood vessels with markedly thickened basement membrane (*arrowheads*). Plastic sections stained with toluidine blue.

densities correlate with impaired temperature thresholds on quantitative sensory testing (QST) and the duration of the DM.[23] Patients with IGT are more likely to have a predominantly small fiber neuropathy, compared to patients with DM, who have more involvement of large nerve fibers.[12]

Pathogenesis

The pathogenic basis for DSPN is unknown. Suspected pathogenic mechanisms include abnormalities in various metabolic processes, microangiopathic ischemia, and inflammation (Fig. 21-3).[1,19,24–27] In regard to aberrant metabolism, diabetes is associated with hyperglycemia, dyslipidemia, and impaired insulin signaling. Increased intracellular glucose may damage neurons by causing excessive glycolysis that overloads mitochondria, resulting in the production of reactive oxygen species (ROS).[1] Furthermore, polyol pathway activity may be increased leading to hyperosmolarity and oxidative stress. Hyperglycemia is also associated with glycosylation of reactive carbohydrate groups to various proteins, lipids, nucleic acids, and so-called glycation end products (AGEs), which impair their normal function.[1] Also, these AGEs may bind to a receptor (RAGE), which in turn, leads to activation of inflammatory cascades and oxidative stress. Increased free fatty acids and triglycerides bind to receptors on neurons and Schwann cells leading to increased oxidative stress and inflammation. Diminished insulin production (as seen in type 1 DM) and insulin resistance (seen in type 2 DM) may be associated with abnormal neurotrophic effects.[1]

Treatment

The mainstay of treatment is tight control of glucose, as studies have shown that this can reduce the risk of developing neuropathy or improve the underlying neuropathy.[28–31] Pancreatic transplantation may stabilize or slightly improve sensory, motor, and autonomic function but is not a pragmatic solution for most patients.[17,30] More than 20 trials of aldose reductase inhibitors have been performed and most have been negative or associated with unacceptable side effect profiles.[2,32] However, a double-blind, placebo-controlled study of Fidarestat was associated with improvement of subjective symptoms and five of eight electrophysiological parameters.[33] Trials of neurotrophic growth factors have also been disappointing.[34,35] A double-blind study of alpha-lipoic acid, an antioxidant, found significant improvement in neuropathic sensory symptoms such as pain and several other neuropathic end points.[36]

A variety of medications have been used to treat painful symptoms associated with DSPN, including antiepileptic medications, antidepressants, sodium channel blockers, and other analgesics with variable success (Table 21-2).[37–45] Our first step in patients with just distal leg pain is a trial of lidoderm patches on the feet, as this is associated with fewer systemic side effects. If this is insufficient or patients have more generalized pain, we often start gabapentin at a dose of 300 mg TID or pregabalin (50 mg TID). We typically go with gabapentin initially because it is less expensive. We gradually increase the dosage as tolerated and necessary. If this is still ineffective, we usually add an antidepressant medication: duloxetine (30–120 mg daily), venlafaxine (37.5–225 mg daily), or a tricyclic antidepressant medication (amitriptyline). For breakthrough pain, we prescribe tramadol 50 mg every 6 hours.[41] If this does not control the pain, oxycodone, morphine, or dextromethorphan may be tried. In general, we prefer to limit opioid use to the nighttime, both in an attempt to improve sleep, and to limit opioid exposure and minimize tachyphylaxis. There is little evidence that oxcarbazepine, lamotrigine, topiramate, lacosamide, mexiletine. magnets, or Reiki therapy are of any significant benefit.[1,37,38]

DIABETIC AUTONOMIC NEUROPATHY

Clinical Features

Autonomic neuropathy typically is seen in combination with DSPN and only rarely in isolation.[1,46,47] The autonomic neuropathy can manifest as abnormal sweating, dry feet, dysfunctional thermoregulation, dry eyes and mouth, pupillary abnormalities, cardiac arrhythmias, postural hypotension, gastrointestinal abnormalities (e.g., gastroparesis, postprandial bloating, chronic diarrhea, or constipation), and genitourinary dysfunction (e.g., impotence, retrograde ejaculation, and incontinence). Importantly, the presence of autonomic neuropathy doubles the risk of mortality.[48]

Laboratory Features

Tests of autonomic function are generally abnormal, including sympathetic skin responses and quantitative sudomotor

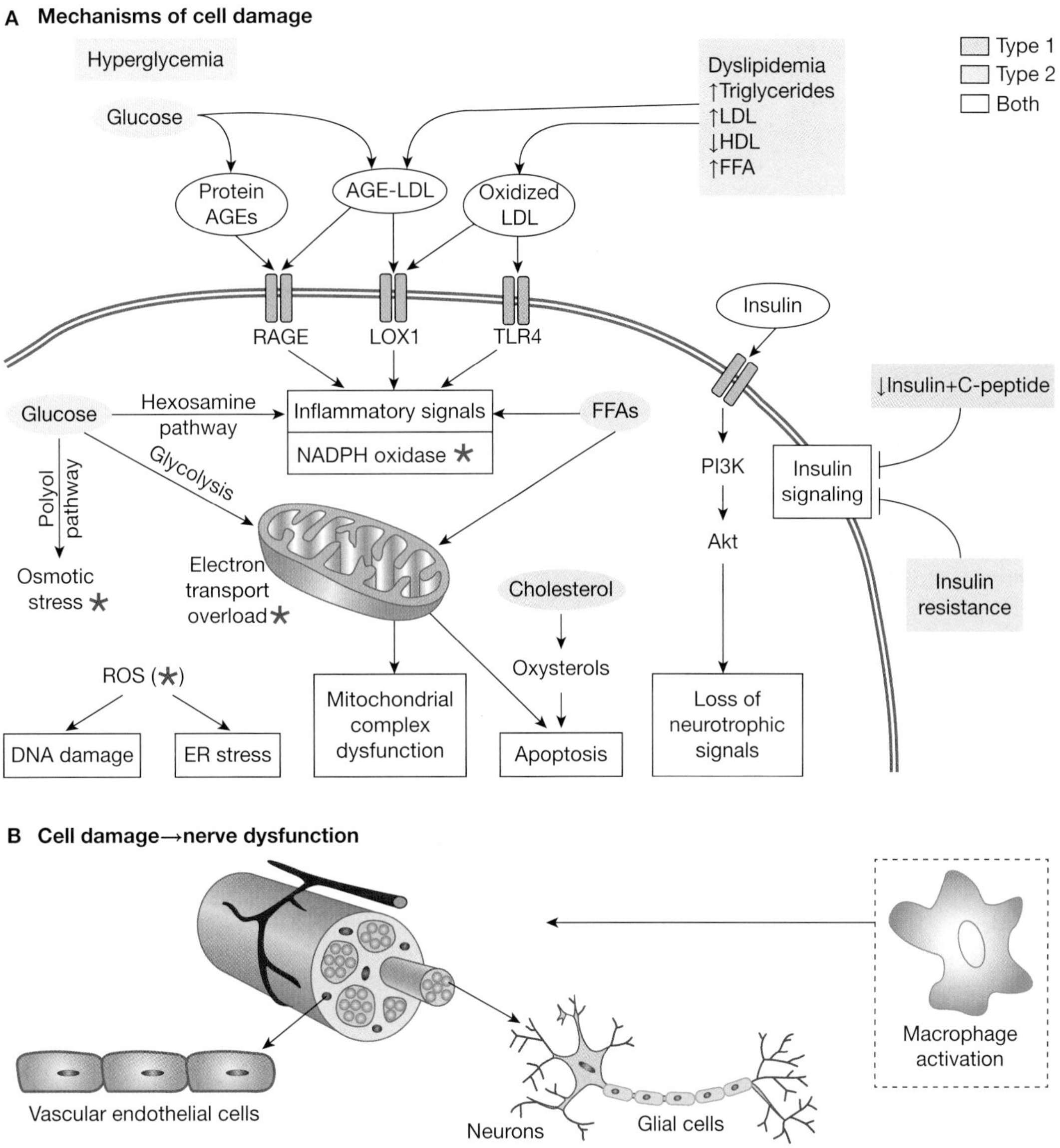

Figure 21-3. Mechanisms of diabetic neuropathy. Factors linked to type 1 diabetes (*orange*), type 2 diabetes (*blue*), and both (*green*) cause DNA damage, endoplasmic reticulum stress, mitochondrial complex dysfunction, apoptosis, and loss of neurotrophic signaling **(A)**. This cell damage can occur in neurons, glial cells, and vascular endothelial cells, as well as trigger macrophage activation, all of which can lead to nerve dysfunction and neuropathy **(B)**. The relative importance of the pathways in this network will vary with cell type, disease profile, and time. AGE, advanced glycation end products; LDL, low-density lipoprotein; HDL, high-density lipoprotein; FFA, free fatty acids; ROS, reactive oxygen species (*red star*); ER, endoplasmic reticulum; PI3 K, phosphatidylinositol-3-kinase; LOX1, oxidized LDL receptor 1; RAGE, receptor for advanced glycation end products; TLR4, toll-like receptor 4. (Reproduced with permission from Callaghan BC, Cheng HT, Stables CL, et al: Diabetic neuropathy: Clinical manifestations and current treatments. *Lancet Neurol.* 2012;11(6):521–534).

axon reflex testing.[46,47] Sensory and motor NCS generally demonstrate the same features described above with DSPN.

Histopathology

Degeneration of sympathetic and parasympathetic neurons along with inflammatory infiltrates within the ganglia have been appreciated.[49]

Pathogenesis

The pathogenic basis for autonomic neuropathy is unknown but may be similar to DSPN.

Treatment

Pancreatic transplantation may stabilize or slightly improve autonomic function.[17] In patients with symptomatic

▶ TABLE 21-2. TREATMENT OF PAINFUL SENSORY NEUROPATHIES

Therapy	Route	Dose	Side Effects
First Line			
Pregabalin	PO	50–200 mg TID	Cognitive changes, sedation
Gabapentin	PO	300–1,200 mg TID	Cognitive changes, sedation
Serotonin-norepinephrine reuptake inhibitors (e.g., duloxetine, venlafaxine)	PO	Duloxetine, 30–120 mg daily Venlafaxine, 37.5–225 mg daily	Cognitive changes, sedation
Tricyclic antidepressants (e.g., amitriptyline)	PO	10–100 mg qhs	Cognitive changes, sedation, dry eyes and mouth, urinary retention, constipation
Second line			
Tramadol	PO	50–100 mg QID	Cognitive changes, sedation, GI upset, addiction
Opioids (oxycodone, morphine)	PO	10–120 mg daily	Cognitive changes, sedation, GI upset, addiction
Dextromethorphan	PO	400 mg daily	Drowsiness, dizziness, nausea, vomiting
Other agents			
Lidocaine, 2.5%/pylocaine, 2.5% cream	Apply cutaneously	QID	Local irritation
Lidoderm, 5% patch	Apply to painful area	Up to three patches daily for 12 h at a time	Local irritation
Capsaicin, 0.025–0.075% cream	Apply cutaneously	QID	Painful burning skin

orthostatic hypotension, we try as many nonpharmacologic treatments as possible, including pressure stockings, small frequent meals, raising the head of the bed at night, and avoidance of alcohol. When drug treatment is required, we initiate treatment with fludrocortisone (starting at 0.1 mg BID) or midodrine (10 mg TID).[47] Pyridostigmine may also be helpful. It is important to note that asymptomatic standing time, rather than improvement in standing blood pressure, is the most important parameter to monitor. Nonsteroidal anti-inflammatory agents may also be of benefit. Metoclopramide is used to treat diabetic gastroparesis, while clonidine may help with persistent diarrhea. Sildenafil and other similar medications are used to treat erectile dysfunction.

DIABETIC NEUROPATHIC CACHEXIA

Clinical Features

DNC is very rare but can be the presenting manifestation of DM.[51–53] This form of diabetic neuropathy is more common in men (usually associated with type 2 DM) than in women (most cases associated with type 1 DM) and generally occurs in their sixth or seventh decade of life. Patients with DNC develop an abrupt onset of severe generalized painful paresthesias involving the trunk and all four limbs, usually setting off significant precipitous weight loss. Mild sensory loss may be detected on examination along with reduced muscle stretch reflexes. Weakness and atrophy are evident in some patients. DNC tends to gradually improve spontaneously, usually preceded by recovery of the weight loss. Rarely, DNC can recur.

Laboratory Features

Cerebrospinal fluid (CSF) protein may be increased. SNAPs may be absent or have very low amplitudes.[51,52] Normal or slightly diminished compound muscle action potential (CMAP) amplitudes with mild slowing of conduction velocities can also be observed. Needle EMG typically demonstrates evidence of active denervation in the form of fibrillation potentials and positive waves in affected muscles.

Histopathology

Nerve biopsies demonstrate severe loss of large myelinated axons with relative sparing of small myelinated and unmyelinated fibers.[52]

Pathogenesis

The pathogenic basis for the disorder is not known.

Treatment

Most patients improve spontaneously, with control over the DM within 1–3 years. Symptomatic treatment of the painful paresthesias is the same as that described for DSPN.

DIABETIC POLYRADICULOPATHY OR RADICULOPLEXUS NEUROPATHY

Two categories of diabetic radiculoplexus neuropathy can be made on the basis of clinical differences: (1) the more common asymmetric, painful, radiculoplexus neuropathy (i.e., diabetic amyotrophy) and (2) the rare symmetric, relatively painless, radiculoplexus neuropathy.[54] The latter form is controversial. It may represent chronic inflammatory demyelinating polyneuropathy (CIDP) in a patient with diabetes, a distinct form of diabetic neuropathy, or may just fall within the spectrum of diabetic amyotrophy.

ASYMMETRIC, PAINFUL DIABETIC POLYRADICULOPATHY OR RADICULOPLEXUS NEUROPATHY (DIABETIC AMYOTROPHY)

Clinical Features

This is the most common form of polyradiculopathy or radiculoplexus neuropathy associated with DM (also known as diabetic amyotrophy, Bruns–Garland syndrome, diabetic lumbosacral radiculoplexopathy, and proximal diabetic neuropathy).[54–62] It more commonly affects older patients with DM type 2, but it can affect type 1 diabetic patients. It can be the presenting manifestation of DM in approximately one-third of patients. Typically, patients present with severe pain in the low back, hip, and thigh in one leg. Rarely, the diabetic polyradiculoneuropathy begins in both legs at the same time. Nevertheless, in such cases nerve involvement is generally asymmetric. About 50% of patients also complain of numbness and paresthesia. Atrophy and weakness of proximal and distal muscles in the affected leg become apparent within a few days or weeks. The term "proximal diabetic neuropathy" stems from the observation that muscles innervated by the L2–L4 myotomes are the most commonly affected, producing weakness of hip flexion, hip adduction, and knee extension. The knee jerk on the affected side is virtually always diminished or lost in many cases. However, any leg muscle may be affected.[55] In fact, we have seen cases with L5 or S1 monoradiculopathy patterns of pain and weakness in newly diagnosed diabetics without compressive lesions. Conversely and unfortunately, we have seen many patients undergo unnecessary laminectomies because of incidental magnetic resonance imaging (MRI) findings in the presence of severe radicular pain and weakness suggesting structural impingement. Although the onset is typically unilateral, it is not uncommon for the contralateral leg to become affected several weeks or months later. As with DNC, the polyradiculoneuropathy is often accompanied or heralded by severe weight loss. Weakness progresses gradually or in a stepwise fashion, usually over several weeks or months, but can continue to progress for 18 months or more.[55] Most patients usually have underlying DSPN. Eventually, the disorder stabilizes, and slow recovery ensues over 1–3 years. However, in many cases there is significant residual weakness, sensory loss, and pain.

Rather than the more typical lumbosacral radiculoplexus neuropathy, some patients develop thoracic radiculopathy.[50,60] Patients describe pain radiating from the posterolateral chest wall anteriorly to the abdominal region, with associated loss of sensation anterolaterally. Weakness of the abdominal wall may lead to herniations of the viscera. A cervical variant of diabetic radicular plexus neuropathy manifesting as acute pain, weakness, and sensory loss in one or both upper limbs can rarely occur as well.[57,58]

Laboratory Features

Lumbar puncture usually reveals an elevated CSF protein with a normal cell count. Erythrocyte sedimentation rate is often increased. MRI scans of the nerve roots and plexus can reveal enhancement.[55,59] NCS reveal features suggestive of multifocal axonal damage to the roots and plexus with reduced or low amplitudes of SNAPs and CMAPs.[55–57,60,62] Conduction velocities in the affected limbs are normal or mildly slow. Autonomic studies may be abnormal as well.[57,60] Needle EMG reveals positive sharp waves and fibrillation potentials and reduced recruitment of affected proximal and distal muscles in the affected limbs and paraspinal muscles in keeping with the radiculoplexus localization. Large-amplitude, long-duration, polyphasic MUAPs are seen after 3–6 months as reinnervation occurs.

Histopathology

Sural, superficial peroneal, and lateral femoral cutaneous nerve biopsies, if performed, reveal loss of myelinated nerve fibers, which is often asymmetric between and within nerve fascicles.[55,57,61,63–67] Active axonal degeneration and clusters of small, thinly myelinated regenerating fibers are appreciated. Mild perivascular inflammation and, less commonly, vasculitis with fibrinoid necrosis involving epineurial and perineurial blood vessels have been noted on some nerve biopsies (Fig. 21-4).[57,61,62] Again, nerve biopsy is not recommended in the vast majority of cases.

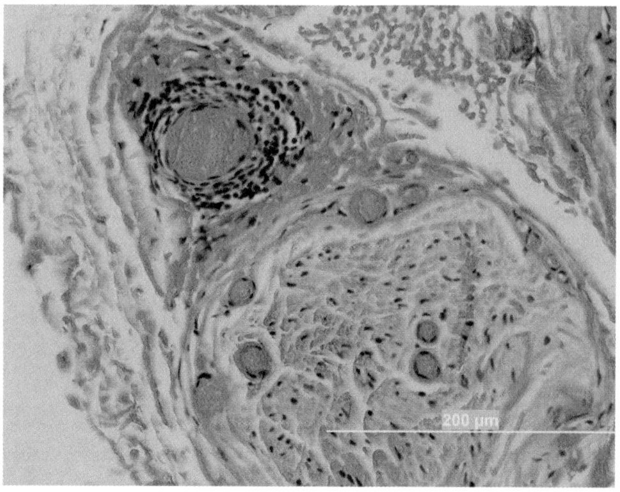

Figure 21-4. Lumbosacral radiculoplexus neuropathy. Superficial peroneal nerve biopsy reveals perivascular inflammation of a small epineurial vessel. H&E stain.

Pathogenesis

Some authorities have speculated that diabetic radiculoplexus neuropathy is an immune-mediated microangiopathy; however, the pathogenic mechanism is unclear.[61–63]

Treatment

Small retrospective studies have reported that intravenous immunoglobulin (IVIG), prednisone, and other forms of immunosuppressive therapy appear to be helpful in some patients with diabetic amyotrophy.[54,60–63] We have been impressed by that short courses of corticosteroids ease the pain associated with the severe radiculoplexus neuropathy; this can allow the patients to undergo physical therapy. However, the natural history of this neuropathy is gradual improvement, so the actual effect, if any, of these immunotherapies on the radiculoplexus neuropathy is not known. Prospective, double-blind, placebo-controlled trials are necessary to define the role of various immunotherapies in this disorder.

SYMMETRIC, PAINLESS, DIABETIC POLYRADICULOPATHY OR RADICULOPLEXUS NEUROPATHY

Clinical Features

The second major group of diabetic polyradiculopathy or radiculoplexus neuropathy manifests as progressive, relatively painless, symmetrical proximal and distal weakness that typically evolves over weeks to months, such that it clinically resembles CIDP.[57,60,63,66–73] Whether this neuropathy represents the coincidental occurrence of CIDP in a patient with DM, or this is a distinct form of diabetic neuropathy, is unclear and controversial.[73] This type of neuropathy occurs in both type 1 and type 2 DM.

The pattern of weakness resembles CIDP in that there is symmetric distal and proximal weakness affecting the legs more than the arms. Distal muscles are more affected than proximal muscles. In our experience there is usually distal arm weakness, but proximal arm involvement is often less noticeable than that seen in patients with idiopathic CIDP. Unlike the more common "diabetic amyotrophy" discussed in the previous section, the onset of weakness is not heralded or accompanied by such severe back and proximal leg pain, and the motor weakness is relatively symmetric. However, distal dysesthesias, perhaps secondary to a superimposed DSPN, are occasionally present.

Laboratory Features

CSF protein concentration is often increased. NCS demonstrate mixed axonal and demyelinating features, with absent or reduced SNAP and CMAP amplitudes combined with slowing of NCVs, prolongation of distal latencies, and absent or prolonged latencies of F waves.[57,63,66,68,69,73] Rarely, conduction block and temporal dispersion are found.[57,66,69] Occasionally, the electrophysiological features can fulfill research criteria for demyelination, but these patients generally have patterns that are more axonal in nature than seen in idiopathic CIDP.[66,67,69] EMG reveals fibrillation potentials and positive sharp waves diffusely, including multiple levels of the paraspinal musculature. Autonomic studies may demonstrate abnormalities in sudomotor, cardiovagal, and adrenergic functions.[57,60]

Histopathology

Sural nerve biopsies, if performed, demonstrate a loss of large and small myelinated nerve fibers with axonal degeneration and clusters of small regenerating fibers as well as perivascular inflammation or the so-called "microvasculitis."[57,60,63,66,68,73] Nerve biopsies may show immunoreactivity for matrix metalloproteinase-9 as seen in idiopathic CIDP.[72] A study out of the Mayo Clinic compared pathological features of nerve biopsies of this painless, symmetric, diabetic radiculoplexus neuropathy to the more typical painful, asymmetric, diabetic radiculoplexus neuropathy and to 25 CIDP biopsies.[73] Nerve biopsies of two types of diabetic radiculoplexus neuropathies were similar, showing features of ischemic injury (multifocal fiber loss), perineurial thickening, injury neuroma, neovascularization, and microvasculitis (epineurial perivascular inflammation, prior bleeding, vessel wall inflammation). In contrast, CIDP biopsies did not show ischemic injury or microvasculitis but revealed demyelination and onion bulbs. However, the study did not include any biopsies of patients who may have had diabetes and coincidental CIDP that was responsive to immunotherapy.

Pathogenesis

The pathogenic basis for this form of polyradiculoneuropathy is unknown and perhaps is multifactorial. This neuropathy may represent part of the spectrum of diabetic amyotrophy, believed by some to result from microvasculitis.[73] We suspect that rare cases represent CIDP occurring coincidentally in patients with DM, as some appear to improve with various immunotherapies. However, this apparent response does not imply that the patients have CIDP, because these patients can improve spontaneously without treatment and because microvasculitis may be responsive to immunotherapies as well.[57,60] Alternatively, the disorder in some patients may represent a distinct form of diabetic neuropathy caused by associated metabolic disturbances, such as uremia.

Treatment

As noted, some patients improve with immunotherapy [i.e., IVIG, plasma exchange (PE), and corticosteroids], suggesting that this type of diabetic neuropathy may be immune mediated.[57,60,63,66,68,70] We often perform lumbar puncture on these patients. If the CSF protein is normal, then we would not proceed with immunotherapy, as it is highly unlikely that the patient has CIDP. If the CSF protein is elevated, one does not know if the patient has CIDP or the protein is elevated because of the diabetes. In these cases, we give a trial of plasmapheresis, because it generally works quickly in patients with CIDP, and we can avoid the potential side effects of corticosteroids and IVIG in these patients. If PE is effective, then we would continue with courses of PE or consider IVIG or prednisone, suspecting that they have an immune-mediated neuropathy and concluding that the benefit of these agents may offset the risks.

DIABETIC MONONEUROPATHIES OR MULTIPLE MONONEUROPATHIES

Diabetic patients are vulnerable to developing mononeuropathies and multiple mononeuropathies, including cranial neuropathies.[1,74] Most of the time patients have underlying DSPN. The mononeuropathies are usually insidious in onset and presumably mechanical in nature due to entrapment or compressive mechanisms. Mononeuropathies that have an abrupt onset and a presumed ischemic mechanism (e.g., a diabetic third nerve palsy), are more likely to occur in individuals not yet identified as being diabetic. The most common neuropathies are median neuropathy at the wrist and ulnar neuropathy at the elbow, but peroneal neuropathy at the fibular head and sciatic, lateral femoral cutaneous, and cranial neuropathies also occur. In regard to cranial mononeuropathies, a seventh nerve palsy is most common, followed by third, sixth, and, less frequently, fourth nerve palsies. The multiple mononeuropathies, perhaps in combination with a radiculoplexus neuropathy, may give the appearance of a mononeuropathy multiplex pattern.

ACUTE TREATMENT-INDUCED PAINFUL NEUROPATHY

Clinical Features

As mentioned previously, chronic painful neuropathies are common in diabetic patients. However, some patients suffer from severe acute neuropathic pain. This may occur in the setting of DNC or anorexia associated with severe weight loss. Rarely, severe pain develops soon after starting intensive glycemic treatment with rapid control of the glycemia, so-called treatment-induced neuropathy or insulin neuritis.[75–79] This can occur in patients with type 1 or type 2 diabetes following treatment with insulin or oral hypoglycemic agents. The pain is usually in a length-dependent distribution but can be diffuse. Many patients, particularly those with type 1 DM, suffer from autonomic symptoms (orthostatic lightheadedness, nausea, vomiting, diarrhea, early satiety, and erectile dysfunction in men). Worsening retinopathy also parallels the course of the neuropathic pain. On examination, pain and temperature sensation are reduced, while most patients have hyperalgesia and allodynia. Muscle strength is not impaired.

Laboratory Features

NCS may be normal or abnormal, similar to DSPN. Autonomic testing usually reveals abnormal heart rate response to deep breathing and abnormal Valsalva ratio with diminished variability in the heart rate as well as orthostatic hypotension.[75]

Histopathology

When performed, sural nerve biopsies have revealed variable loss of myelinated fibers, acute axonal degeneration, and some clusters of regenerating myelinated fibers which is indistinguishable from other forms of diabetic neuropathy.[75] Skin biopsies usually demonstrate a reduction in intraepidermal nerve fiber density.[75]

Pathogenesis

The pathogenic basis of acute treatment-induced neuropathy is not known, but the phenotype suggests diffuse damage to the unmyelinated and lightly myelinated nerve fibers.[75]

Treatment

The pain associated with this neuropathy is very difficult to control. Fortunately, it is a spontaneously reversible disorder, and typically patients report pain improvement after many months of continued glucose control.

▶ NEUROPATHIES ASSOCIATED WITH OTHER ENDOCRINOPATHIES

HYPOGLYCEMIA/HYPERINSULINEMIA

Clinical Features

Polyneuropathy has been associated with persistent hypoglycemia secondary to an islet cell tumor of the pancreas, hyperinsulinemia, or in early stages of treatment of DM.[80–83] The neuropathy is characterized by progressive numbness and paresthesias in the hands and feet. Over time, distal motor weakness and atrophy may develop. Muscle stretch reflexes are generally reduced in a length-dependent fashion. With correction of the hypoglycemia, the sensory symptoms usually improve; however, muscle atrophy and weakness often remain to some extent.

Laboratory Features

NCS reveal SNAPs that are reduced in amplitude or absent.[81,83] The CMAP amplitudes are slightly decreased, while the conduction velocities are normal or only mildly reduced. Needle EMG may demonstrate fibrillation potentials, positive sharp waves, and reduced recruitment of large polyphasic MUAPs in the distal limb muscles.[80–83]

Histopathology

Very few nerve biopsies have been performed on individuals with this disorder, but axonal loss primarily affecting the large myelinated fibers has been reported.[81]

Pathogenesis

The basis for the polyneuropathy is not known but is felt to be directly attributable to reduced glucose levels in peripheral nerves. A rat model of recurrent episodes of severe hypoglycemia was associated with early vascular anomalies in endoneurial microvessels in rat sciatic nerves without any observable changes in nerve fibers.[84] Other studies demonstrated that acute lowering of glucose levels under hypoxic conditions in rats leads to apoptosis of dorsal root ganglia neurons.[85] Hypoxia-induced cell death was decreased when dorsal root ganglia neurons were maintained in high-glucose medium, suggesting that high levels of substrate protected against hypoxia. Apoptosis was completely prevented by increasing the concentration of nerve growth factor.

Treatment

Patients should be treated for the underlying cause of the hyperinsulinemia.

ACROMEGALY

Clinical Features

Acromegaly can be associated with several types of neuropathy, in addition to myopathy.[86–90] Carpal tunnel syndrome is the most common neuropathy complicating acromegaly.[86,88] A generalized sensorimotor peripheral neuropathy, characterized by numbness, paresthesias, and mild distal weakness beginning in the feet and progressing to the hands, is less frequent. Clinical or electrophysiological evidence of carpal tunnel syndrome has been demonstrated in 82% of patients and a generalized sensorimotor peripheral neuropathy in 73% of patients with acromegaly.[86] In addition, the bony overgrowth in or about the spinal canal and neural foramina can result in spinal cord compression or polyradiculopathies.

Laboratory Features

NCS in patients with generalized polyneuropathy demonstrate reduced amplitudes of SNAPs with prolonged distal latencies and slow CVs.[86] The CMAPs are usually normal, but there may be slightly reduced amplitudes, prolonged distal latencies, and slow motor conduction velocities.

Histopathology

Nerve biopsies in patients with acromegaly and generalized polyneuropathy may reveal an increase in endoneurial and subperineurial connective tissue and an overall increase in the fascicular area, combined with a loss of myelinated and unmyelinated nerve fibers.[86,90]

Pathogenesis

The pathogenic basis of the polyneuropathy associated with acromegaly is unknown. The neuropathy may be related to superimposed DM in some cases. Increased growth hormone and upregulation of insulin-like growth factor receptors may result in proliferation of endoneurial and subperineurial connective tissue, which could make the nerve fibers more vulnerable to pressure and trauma.

Treatment

It is unclear at this time if the polyneuropathy improves with treatment of this endocrinopathy.

HYPOTHYROIDISM

Clinical Features

Hypothyroidism is more commonly associated with a proximal myopathy, but patients are predisposed to develop carpal tunnel syndrome.[91–96] Rarely, a generalized sensory polyneuropathy, characterized by painful paresthesias and numbness in both the hands and the legs, also complicates hypothyroidism.[92,93,97]

Laboratory Features

NCS features suggestive of carpal tunnel syndrome are most common, but a generalized sensorimotor polyneuropathy may be demonstrated.[91–93] In patients with a generalized neuropathy, the SNAP amplitudes are reduced and distal latencies may be slightly prolonged.[94,95] CMAPs reveal normal or slightly reduced amplitudes, mild-to-moderate slowing of CVs, and slight prolongation of motor distal latencies.

Histopathology

Nerve biopsies, when performed, have revealed a loss of myelinated nerve fibers, mild degrees of active axonal degeneration, and segmental demyelination with small onion-bulb formations.[91,94] Skin biopsies have shown reduced intraepidermal nerve fiber density in patients with hypothyroid neuropathy, but also in patients with asymptomatic hypothyroidism.[97,98]

Pathogenesis

Carpal tunnel syndrome is most likely the result of reduced space within the flexor retinaculum as a result of associated edematous changes. The etiology of the generalized neuropathy associated with hypothyroidism is not known.

Treatment

Correction of the hypothyroidism usually at least halts further progression of the polyneuropathy, and in some cases leads to improvement.

▶ SUMMARY

DM is the most common etiology of neuropathy (at least in industrialized nations) when the cause of the neuropathy is found. There are several types of neuropathy associated with DM as discussed. Treatment is aimed at control of the blood sugar and symptomatic management of pain. Aside from diabetic neuropathies, the endocrine-related neuropathies are relatively uncommon, although hyperinsulinemia, hypothyroidism, and acromegaly have also been associated with neuropathy.

REFERENCES

1. Callaghan BC, Cheng HT, Stables CL, Smith AL, Feldman EL. Diabetic neuropathy: Clinical manifestations and current treatments. *Lancet Neurol.* 2012;11:521–534.
2. Podwall D, Gooch C. Diabetic neuropathy: Clinical features, etiology, and therapy. *Curr Neurol Neurosci Rep.* 2004;4(1):55–61.
3. Partanen J, Niskanen L, Lehtinen J, Mervaala E, Siitonen O, Uusitupa M. Natural history of peripheral neuropathy in patients with non-insulin-dependent diabetes mellitus. *N Engl J Med.* 1995;333:89–94.
4. Bao XH, Wong V, Wang Q, Low LC. Prevalence of peripheral neuropathy with insulin-dependent diabetes mellitus. *Pediatr Neurol.* 1999;20:204–209.
5. Dyck PJ, Kratz KM, Litchy WJ, et al. The prevalence by staged severity of various types of diabetic neuropathy, retinopathy, and nephropathy in a population-based cohort: The Rochester diabetic neuropathy study. *Neurology.* 1993;43:817–824.
6. Brown MJ, Martin JR, Asbury AK. Painful diabetic neuropathy: A morphometric study. *Arch Neurol.* 1976;33:164–171.
7. Dyck PJ, Davies JL, Litchy WJ, O'Brien PC. Longitudinal assessment of diabetic polyneuropathy using composite score in the Rochester Diabetic Neuropathy Study cohort. *Neurology.* 1997;49:229–239.
8. Boulton AJ, Knight G, Drury J, Ward JD. The prevalence of symptomatic diabetic neuropathy in an insulin-treated population. *Diabetes Care.* 1985;8:125–128.
9. Dyck PJ, Karnes JL, O'Brien PC, et al. The Rochester diabetes neuropathy study: Reassessment of tests and criteria for diagnosis and stages severity. *Neurology.* 1992;42:1164–1170.
10. Singleton JR, Smith AG, Bromberg MB. Painful sensory polyneuropathy associated with impaired glucose tolerance test. *Muscle Nerve.* 2001;24:1225–1228.
11. Novella SP, Inzucchi SE, Goldstein JM. The frequency of undiagnosed diabetes and impaired glucose tolerance in patients with idiopathic sensory neuropathy. *Muscle Nerve.* 2001;24:1229–1231.
12. Sumner CJ, Seth S, Griffin JW, Cornblath DR, Polyswdkia M. The spectrum of neuropathy in diabetes and impaired glucose tolerance. *Neurology.* 2003;60:108–111.
13. Hughes RA, Umapathi T, Gray IA, et al. A controlled investigation of the cause of chronic idiopathic axonal polyneuropathy. *Brain.* 2004;127:1723–1730.
14. Dyck PJ, Overland CJ, Davies JL, et al. Does impaired glycemia cause polyneuropathy and other diabetic complications? *J Peripheral Nervous Soc.* 2011;16(suppl 3):30–31.
15. Wilson JR, Stittsworth JD Jr, Kadir A, Fisher MA. Conduction velocity versus amplitude analysis: Evidence for demyelination in diabetic neuropathy. *Muscle Nerve.* 1998;21:1228–1230.
16. Krarup C. An update on electrophysiological studies in neuropathy. *Curr Opin Neurol.* 2003;16:603–612.
17. Navarro X, Sutherland DE, Kennedy WR. Long-term effects of pancreatic transplantation on diabetic neuropathy. *Ann Neurol.* 1997;42:727–736.
18. Abu-Shukra SR, Cornblath DR, Avila OL, et al. Conduction block in diabetic neuropathy. *Muscle Nerve.* 1991;14:858–862.
19. Dyck PJ, Sherman WR, Halcher LM, et al. Human diabetic endoneurial sorbitol, fructose, and myo-inositol related to sural nerve morphometry. *Ann Neurol.* 1980;8:590–596.
20. Hill RE, Williams PE. Perineurial cell basement membrane thickening and myelinated nerve fibre loss in diabetic and nondiabetic peripheral nerve. *J Neurol Sci.* 2004;217(2):157–163.
21. Herrman DN, Griffin JW, Hauer P, Cornblath DR, McArthur JC. Intraepidermal nerve fiber density, sural nerve morphometry and electrodiagnosis in peripheral neuropathies. *Neurology.* 1999;53:1634–1640.
22. Polydefkis M, Griffin JW, McArthur J. New insights into diabetic polyneuropathy. *JAMA.* 2003;290:1371–1376.
23. Shun CT, Chang YC, Wu HP, et al. Skin denervation in type 2 diabetes: Correlations with diabetic duration and functional impairments. *Brain.* 2004;127:1593–1605.
24. Gillon KR, Hawthorne JN, Tomlinson DR. Myo-inositol and sorbitol metabolism in relation to peripheral nerve function in experimental diabetes in the rat: Effect of aldose reductase inhibition. *Diabetologia.* 1983;25:365–371.
25. Vlassara H. Recent progress in advanced glycosylation end products and diabetic complications. *Diabetes.* 1997;46:S19–S25.
26. Dyck PJ, Zimmerman BR, Vilen TH, et al. Nerve glucose, fructose, sorbitol, myo-inositol, and fiber degeneration and regeneration in diabetic neuropathy. *N Engl J Med.* 1998;319:542–548.
27. Sima AA. New insights into the metabolic and molecular basis for diabetic neuropathy. *Cell Mol Life Sci.* 2003;60:2445–2464.
28. Diabetes Control and Complications Trial Research Group. The effect of diabetes on the development and progression of long-term complications in insulin-dependent diabetes mellitus. *N Engl J Med.* 1993;329:977–986.
29. Diabetes Control and Complications Trial. Effect of intensive diabetes treatment on nerve conduction in the diabetes control and complications trial. *Ann Neurol.* 1995;38:869–880.
30. Kennedy WR, Navarro X, Goetz FC. Sutherland DE, Najarian JS. Effects of pancreatic transplantation on diabetic neuropathy. *N Engl J Med.* 1990;322:1031–1037.
31. Writing Team for the Diabetes Control and Complications Trial/Epidemiology of Diabetes Interventions and Complications Research Group. Effect of intensive therapy on the microvascular complications of type 1 diabetes mellitus. *JAMA.* 2002; 287(19):2563–2569.
32. Greene DA, Arezzo JC, Brown MB, The Zenarestat Study Group. Effect of aldose reductase inhibition on nerve conduction and morphometry in diabetic neuropathy. *Neurology.* 1999;53:580–591.
33. Hotta N, Toyota T, Matsuoka K, et al; SNK-860 Diabetic Neuropathy Study Group. Clinical efficacy of fidarestat, a novel aldose reductase inhibitor, for diabetic peripheral neuropathy:

A 52-week multicenter placebo-controlled double-blind parallel group study. *Diabetes Care*. 2001;24:1776–1782.
34. Apfel SC, Schwartz S, Ardonato BT, et al; The RHNGF Clinical Investigator Group. Efficacy and safety of recombinant human nerve growth factor in patients with diabetic polyneuropathy. A randomized controlled trial. *JAMA*. 2000;284:2215–2221.
35. Wellmer A, Misra VP, Sharief MK, Kopelman PG, Anand P. A double-blind placebo-controlled clinical trial of recombinant human brain-derived neurotrophic factor (RHBDNF) in diabetic polyneuropathy. *J Peripher Nerv Syst*. 2001;6:204–210.
36. Ametov AS, Barinov A, Dyck PJ, et al; SYDNEY Trial Study Group. The sensory symptoms of diabetic polyneuropathy are improved with alpha-lipoic acid: The SYDNEY trial. *Diabetes Care*. 2003;26:770–776.
37. Attal N, Cruccu G, Baron R, et al. EFNS guidelines on the pharmacological treatment of neuropathic pain: 2010 revision. *Eur J Neurol*. 2010;17:1113-e88.
38. Bril V, England J, Franklin GM, et al. American Academy of Neurology; American Association of Neuromuscular and Electrodiagnostic Medicine; American Academy of Physical Medicine and Rehabilitation. Evidence-based guideline: Treatment of painful diabetic neuropathy: Report of the American academy of neurology, the American association of neuromuscular and electrodiagnostic medicine, and the American academy of physical medicine and rehabilitation. *Neurology*. 2011;76:1758–1765.
39. Backonja M, Beydoun A, Edwards KR, et al. Gabapentin for the symptomatic treatment of painful neuropathy in patients with diabetes mellitus: A randomized control trial. *JAMA*. 1998;280:1831–1836.
40. The Capsaicin Study Group. Treatment of painful diabetic peripheral neuropathy with topical capsaicin: A multi-center, double-blind, vehicle-controlled study. *Arch Intern Med*. 1991; 151:2225–2229.
41. Harati Y, Gooch C, Swenson M, et al. Double-blind randomized trial of tramadol for the treatment of the pain of diabetic neuropathy. *Neurology*. 1998;50:1842–1846.
42. Max MB, Lynch SA, Muir J, et al. Effects of desipramine, amitriptyline, and fluoxetine on pain in diabetic neuropathy. *N Engl J Med*. 1992;326:1250–1256.
43. Morello CM, Leckband SG, Stoner CP, Morhouse DF, Sahagian GA. Randomized double-blind study comparing the efficacy of gabapentin with amitriptyline on diabetic neuropathy pain. *Arch Intern Med*. 1999;159:1931–1937.
44. Wolfe GI, Trivedi JR. Painful peripheral neuropathy and its nonsurgical treatment. *Muscle Nerve*. 2004;30:3–19.
45. Kochar DK, Rawat N, Agrawal RP, et al. Sodium valproate for painful diabetic neuropathy: A randomized double-blind placebo-controlled study. *QJM*. 2004;97:33–38.
46. Cohen JA, Jeffers BW, Faldut D, Marcoux M, Schrier RW. Risks for sensorimotor peripheral neuropathy and autonomic neuropathy in non-insulin-dependent diabetes mellitus (NIDDM). *Muscle Nerve*. 1998;21:72–80.
47. Vinik AI, Freeman R, Erbas T. Diabetic autonomic neuropathy. *Semin Neurol*. 2003;23(4):365–372.
48. Soedamah-Muthu SS, Chaturvedi N, Witte DR, et al. Relationship between risk factors and mortality in type 1 diabetic patients in Europe: The EURODIAB Prospective Complications Study (PCS). *Diabetes Care*. 2008;31:1360–1366.
49. Duchen LW, Anjorin A, Watkins PJ, Mackay JD. Pathology of autonomic neuropathy in diabetes mellitus. *Ann Intern Med*. 1980;92:301–303.
50. Ellenberg M. Diabetic truncal mononeuropathy—A new clinical syndrome. *Diabetes Care*. 1978;1:10–13.
51. Godil A, Berriman D, Knapik S, Normal M, Godil F, Firek AF. Diabetic neuropathic cachexia. *West J Med*. 1996;165:882–885.
52. Jackson CE, Barohn RJ. Diabetic neuropathic cachexia: Report of a recurrent case. *J Neurol Neurosurg Psychiatry*. 1998;64: 785–787.
53. Neal JM. Diabetic neuropathic cachexia: A rare manifestation of diabetic neuropathy. *South Med J*. 2009;102:327–329.
54. Amato AA, Barohn RJ. Diabetic lumbosacral radiculoneuropathies. *Curr Treat Options Neurol*. 2001;3:139–146.
55. Barohn RJ, Sahenk Z, Warmolts JR, Mendell JR. The Bruns-Garland syndrome (diabetic amyotrophy): Revisited 100 years later. *Arch Neurol*. 1991;48:1130–1135.
56. Stewart JD. Diabetic truncal neuropathy: Topography of the sensory deficit. *Ann Neurol*. 1989;25:233–238.
57. Pascoe MK, Low PA, Windebank AJ, Litchy WJ. Subacute diabetic proximal neuropathy. *Mayo Clin Proc*. 1997;72: 1123–1132.
58. Katz JS, Saperstein DS, Wolfe G, et al. Cervicobrachial involvement in diabetic radiculoplexopathy. *Muscle Nerve*. 2001;24:794–798.
59. O'Neil BJ, Flanders AE, Escandon S, Tahmoush AJ. Treatable lumbosacral polyradiculitis masquerading as diabetic amyotrophy. *J Neurol Sci*. 1997;151:223–225.
60. Jaradeh SS, Prieto TE, Lobeck LJ. Progressive polyradiculoneuropathy in diabetes: Correlation with variables and clinical outcome after immunotherapy. *J Neurol Neurosurg Psychiatry*. 1999;67:607–612.
61. Dyck PJ, Norell JE, Dyck PJ. Microvasculitis and ischemia in diabetic lumbosacral radiculoplexus neuropathy. *Neurology*. 1999;53:2113–2121.
62. Dyck PJ, Windebank AJ. Diabetic and nondiabetic lumbosacral radiculoplexus neuropathies: New insights into pathophysiology and treatment. *Muscle Nerve*. 2002;25:477–491.
63. Krendel DA, Costigan DA, Hopkins LC. Successful treatment of neuropathies in patients with diabetes mellitus. *Arch Neurol*. 1995;52:1053–1061.
64. Said G, Goulon-Goeau C, Lacroix C, Moulonguet A. Nerve biopsy findings in different patterns of proximal diabetic neuropathy. *Ann Neurol*. 1994;35:559–569.
65. Said G, Elgrably F, Lacroix C, et al. Painful proximal diabetic neuropathy: Inflammatory nerve lesions and spontaneous favorable outcome. *Ann Neurol*. 1997;41:762–770.
66. Gorson KC, Ropper AH, Adelman LS, Weinberg DH. Influence of diabetes mellitus on chronic inflammatory demyelinating polyneuropathy. *Muscle Nerve*. 2000;23:37–43.
67. Riley DE, Shields RE. Diabetic amyotrophy with upper limb involvement. *Neurology*. 1984;34(suppl 1):173.
68. Stewart JD, Mckelvey R, Durcan L, Carpenter S, Karpati G. Chronic inflammatory demyelinating polyneuropathy (CIDP) in diabetics. *J Neurol Sci*. 1996;142:59–64.
69. Sharma KR, Cross J, Farronay O, Ayyar DR, Shebert RT, Bradley WG. Demyelinating neuropathy in diabetes mellitus. *Arch Neurol*. 2002;59:758–765.
70. Sharma KR, Cross J, Ayyar DR, Martinez-Arizala A, Bradley WG. Diabetic demyelinating polyneuropathy responsive to intravenous immunoglobulin therapy. *Arch Neurol*. 2002;59:751–757.
71. Haq RU, Pendlebury WW, Fries TJ, Tandan R. Chronic inflammatory demyelinating polyradiculoneuropathy in diabetic patients. *Muscle Nerve*. 2003;27:465–470.

72. Jann S, Bramerio MA, Beretta S, et al. Diagnostic value of sural nerve matrix metalloproteinase-9 in diabetic patients with CIDP. *Neurology*. 2003;61:1607–1610.
73. Garces-Sanchez M, Laughlin RS, Dyck PJ, Engelstad JK, Norell JE, Dyck PJ. Painless diabetic motor neuropathy: A variant of diabetic lumbosacral radiculoplexus neuropathy? *Ann Neurol*. 2011;69:1043–1054.
74. Albers JW, Brown MB, Sima AA, Greene DA. Frequency of median mononeuropathy in patients with mild diabetic neuropathy in the early diabetes intervention trial (EDIT). *Muscle Nerve*. 1996;19:140–146.
75. Gibbons CH, Freeman R. Treatment-induced diabetic neuropathy: A reversible painful autonomic neuropathy. *Ann Neurol*. 2010;67:534–541.
76. Caravati CM. Insulin neuritis: A case report. *VA Med Monthly*. 1933;59:745–746.
77. Tesfaye S, Malik R, Harris N, et al. Arterio-venous shunting and proliferating new vessels in acute painful neuropathy of rapid glycaemic control (insulin neuritis). *Diabetologia*. 1996;39:329–335.
78. Dabby R, Sadeh M, Lampl Y, Gilad R, Watemberg N. Acute painful neuropathy induced by rapid correction of serum glucose levels in diabetic patients. *Biomed Pharmacother*. 2009;63:707–709.
79. Vital C, Vital A, Dupon M, Gin H, Rouanet-Larriviere M, Lacut JY. Acute painful diabetic neuropathy: Two patients with recent insulin-dependent diabetes mellitus. *J Peripher Nerv Syst*. 1997;2:151–154.
80. Danta G. Hypoglycemic peripheral neuropathy. *Arch Neurol*. 1969;21:121–132.
81. Jaspan JB, Wollman RL, Berstein L, Rubenstein AH. Hypoglycemic peripheral neuropathy in association with insulinoma: Implication of glucopenia rather than hyperinsulinism. *Medicine (Baltimore)*. 1982;61:33–44.
82. Mulder DW, Bastron JA, Lambert EH. Hyperinsulin neuronopathy. *Neurology*. 1956;6:627–635.
83. Wilson JL, Sokol DK, Smith LH, Snook RJ, Waguespack SG, Kincaid JC. Acute painful neuropathy (insulin neuritis) in a boy following rapid glycemic control for type 1 diabetes mellitus. *J Child Neurol*. 2003;18:365–367.
84. Ohshima J, Nukada H. Hypoglycaemic neuropathy: Microvascular changes due to recurrent hypoglycaemic episodes in rat sciatic nerve. *Brain Res*. 2002;947:84–89.
85. Honma H, Podratz JL, Windebank AJ. Acute glucose deprivation leads to apoptosis in a cell model of acute diabetic neuropathy. *J Peripher Nerv Syst*. 2003;8(2):65–74.
86. Low PA, McLeod JG, Turtle JR, et al. Peripheral neuropathy in acromegaly. *Brain*. 1974;97;139–152.
87. Khaleeli AA, Levy RD, Edwards RH. The neuromuscular features of acromegaly: A clinical and pathological study. *J Neurol Neurosurg Psychiatry*. 1984;47:1009–1015.
88. Pickett JBE, Layzer RB, Levin SR, Scheider V, Campbell MJ, Sumner AJ. Neuromuscular complications of acromegaly. *Neurology*. 1975;25:638–645.
89. Dinn JJ, Dinn EI. Natural history of acromegalic peripheral neuropathy. *Q J Med*. 1985;57:833–842.
90. Dinn JJ. Schwann cell dysfunction in acromegaly. *J Clin Endocrinol*. 1970;31:140–143.
91. Martin J, Tomkin GH, Hutchinson M. Peripheral neuropathy in hypothyroidism–an association with spurious polycythemia (Gaisbock's syndrome). *J R Soc Med*. 1983;76:187–189.
92. Meier C, Bischoff A. Polyneuropathy in hypothyroidism. *J Neurol*. 1977;215:103–114.
93. Nemni R, Bottacchi E, Fazio R, et al. Polyneuropathy in hypothyroidism: Clinical, electrophysiologic and morphologic findings in four cases. *J Neurol Neurosurg Psychiatry*. 1987; 50:1454–1460.
94. Dyck PJ, Lambert EH. Polyneuropathy associated with hypothyroidism. *J Neuropathol Exp Neurol*. 1970;29:631–658.
95. Fincham RW, Cape CA. Neuropathy in myxedema. *Arch Neurol*. 1968;19:464–466.
96. Eslamian F, Bahrami A, Aghamohammadzadeh N, Niafar M, Salekzamani Y, Behkamrad K. Electrophysiologic changes in patients with untreated primary hypothyroidism. *J Clin Neurophysiol*. 2011;28:323–328.
97. Penza P, Lombardi R, Camozzi F, Ciano C, Lauria G. Painful neuropathy in subclinical hypothyroidism: Clinical and neuropathological recovery after hormone replacement therapy. *Neurol Sci*. 2009;30:149–151.
98. Magri F, Buonocore M, Oliviero A, et al. Intraepidermal nerve fiber density reduction as a marker of preclinical asymptomatic small-fiber sensory neuropathy in hypothyroid patients. *Eur J Endocrinol*. 2010;163:279–284.

CHAPTER 22

Idiopathic Polyneuropathy

In our experience and others, a cause for neuropathy will not be found in as many as 50% of cases despite an extensive work-up.[1–11] The chronic idiopathic polyneuropathies are likely a heterogeneous group of neuropathies. Most individuals have only sensory symptoms, but some may have mild weakness (e.g., toe extension) or slight abnormalities on motor conduction studies. The neuropathy may affect large- and/or small-diameter nerve fibers. As the etiology is unknown, only symptomatic management of the neuropathic pain is available.

► CHRONIC, IDIOPATHIC, LENGTH-DEPENDENT SENSORY OR SENSORIMOTOR POLYNEUROPATHY

CLINICAL FEATURES

Most individuals present with numbness, tingling, or pain (e.g., sharp stabbing paresthesias, burning, or deep aching sensation) in the feet between the ages of 45 and 70 years.[1–11] This is a common problem occurring in approximately 3% of adults as they age. In a large series of 93 patients with idiopathic sensory polyneuropathy, 63% presented with numbness and paresthesia along with pain, 24% with numbness or paresthesia without pain, and 10% with pain alone.[9] Eventually, 65–80% of affected individuals develop neuropathic pain.[6,9–11] Sensory symptoms are first noted in the toes and slowly progress up the legs and later into the arms. The average time to involvement of the hands is approximately 5 years.[6,9]

Neurological examination reveals the typical length-dependent pattern of sensory loss.[6,7,9,11] Vibratory perception is reduced in 80–100%, proprioception is impaired in 20–30%, pinprick sensation is diminished in 75–85%, and light touch is decreased in 54–92% of those with the neuropathy. Strength is usually normal, although mild distal weakness and atrophy involving toe muscles may be appreciated in 40–75% of cases, and rarely of ankle dorsiflexors and plantar flexors.[6,9,11] However, upper limb strength, including the hand intrinsics, should be normal. Muscle stretch reflexes are usually absent at the ankle and diminished at the knees and arms. Generalized areflexia though is less common and would point to a hereditary or acquired demyelinating neuropathy.

Within the category of idiopathic sensory or sensorimotor polyneuropathies are people who have only a small fiber sensory neuropathy.[2,3,7,9] By definition, these individuals should have normal nerve conduction studies (NCS), and nerve biopsies, if performed, demonstrate a relatively normal density of large myelinated nerve fibers. Most people with small fiber neuropathy (approximately 80%) complain of burning pain in the feet, while 40–60% describe sharp, lancinating pain; paresthesias; or just numbness. Symptoms may involve the distal upper extremities. Rarely, the neuropathy is restricted to the arms and face or involves the autonomic nervous system.[2,3] Examination reveals reduced pinprick or temperature sensation in almost all patients, while vibratory perception is impaired in half. Muscle strength is preserved. Likewise, muscle stretch reflexes are also usually normal, but a few patients have reduced reflexes at the ankles.

LABORATORY FEATURES

The diagnosis of chronic idiopathic polyneuropathy is one of exclusion. Laboratory testing should include fasting blood glucose (FBS), hemoglobin A1 C (HgbA1 C), antinuclear antibody, anti-Ro and anti-La antibodies (SSA and SSB), erythrocyte sedimentation rate, B12, serum and urine immunoelectrophoresis/immunofixation, and thyroid, liver, and renal function tests.[12,13] If the FBS and HgbA1 C are normal, we typically order an oral glucose tolerance test (GTT). The most common abnormality, when one is found, in patients with sensory neuropathy is diabetes or impaired glucose tolerance (IGT). IGT (defined as glucose of >140 and <200 mg/dL on 2-hour GGT) is seen in 17–61% and frank diabetes mellitus (DM) (defined as 2-hour glucose of >200 mg/dL on GGT or FBS of >126 mg/dL) in 20–31% of patients with sensory neuropathy (Table 22-1).[14–18] In patients with painful sensory symptoms (not just numbness), the likelihood of IGT or DM is even higher. However, some authorities have not found increased risk of IGT in their patients with idiopathic neuropathy compared to age-matched controls.[19] Thus, although the risk of both previously undetected DM and IGT may be increased in patients with sensory neuropathy, this is still controversial and a causal relationship has not been firmly established.[20,21]

About 5% of patients with chronic idiopathic sensory or sensorimotor polyneuropathy have a monoclonal protein detected in the serum or urine, but this is not much

▶ TABLE 22-1. RESULTS OF GLUCOSE TOLERANCE TESTING IN OTHERWISE IDIOPATHIC POLYNEUROPATHY[14–17]

Authors (References)	No. of Patients	Mean Age (Range)	Total with Abnormal Glucose Metabolism	Impaired Glucose Tolerance	Diabetes Mellitus
Singleton et al.	89 (total) 33 (painful sensory neuropathy)	64 years (44–92 years)	43/89 (56%) 20/33 (60%)	15/89 (25%) 7/33 (21%)	28/89 (31%) 13/33 (39%)
Novella et al.	48 (total) 24 (painful sensory neuropathy)	64 years (41–82 years)	24/48 (50%) 18/28 (65%)	13/48 (27%) 10/28 (36%)	11/48 (23%) 8/28 (29%)
Sumner et al.	73 (total)	61 years (44–91 years)	41/73 (56%)	26/73 (36%)	15/73 (20%)
Harris et al.	2,884 (normal age-matched population)		18.5% in patients aged 40–74 years	15.8% in patients aged 40–74 years 20.7% in patients 60–74 years	2.7% in patients 40–74 years

higher than the age-matched normal controls. Furthermore, the relationship of these monoclonal proteins to the pathogenesis of most neuropathies is unclear. There is a strong pathogenic relationship established in people with demyelinating sensorimotor polyneuropathies with IgM monoclonal proteins, half of whom have myelin-associated glycoprotein (MAG) antibodies (discussed in Chapters 14 and 19). However, most individuals with chronic idiopathic sensory or sensorimotor polyneuropathy have axonal neuropathies both histologically and electrophysiologically. Amyloidosis is the other condition in which a pathogenic relationship between the neuropathy and the monoclonal protein is clear. Thus, amyloid neuropathy needs to be excluded in patients with a monoclonal gammopathy before concluding that the neuropathy is idiopathic in nature (see Chapter 16). This may require a fat pad, rectal, bone marrow, or nerve biopsy.

Although some studies have suggested that antisulfatide antibodies are common with painful small fiber neuropathy,[22,23] subsequent reports suggest that these antibodies have a very low sensitivity and poor specificity.[6,10] We never order them as we have found them to be of little use clinically, and a pathogenic relationship has never been demonstrated. That is, the presence of these antibodies does not imply that the patients have an immune-mediated neuropathy and that they may respond to treatment with immunotherapy. We also feel that there is no role for screening various antiganglioside and other antinerve antibodies (e.g., GM1 and Hu antibodies) in the workup of patients with chronic, indolent, sensory predominant, length-dependent polyneuropathies. CSF examination is usually normal and is also unwarranted.

In people with a large fiber neuropathy, the sensory NCS reveal either absent or reduced amplitudes that are worse in the legs.[1,3,4,6–12] Sensory NCV are normal or only mildly slow. Quantitative sensory testing (QST) demonstrates abnormal thermal and vibratory perception in as many as 85% of patients.[7,9] In addition, autonomic testing (e.g., quantitative sudomotor axon reflex and heart rate testing with deep breathing or Valsalva) is abnormal in some patients. Despite the fact that sensory symptoms predominate, motor NCS are often abnormal. Wolfe et al.[9] reported that 60% of their patients with idiopathic polyneuropathy had abnormal motor NCS. The most common motor abnormalities are reduced peroneal and posterior tibialis compound muscle action potentials (CMAP) amplitudes, while distal latencies and conduction velocities of the peroneal and posterior tibial CMAPs are normal or only slightly impaired. Abnormalities of median and ulnar CMAPs are much less common. Fibrillation potentials and positive waves on needle EMG are also commonly found in intrinsic foot muscles as a further indicator of frequently subclinical motor involvement. In the authors' experience, they may be the only indicator of motor involvement in what may otherwise appear to be a pure sensory neuropathy.

In patients with pure small fiber neuropathies, motor and sensory NCS are, by definition, normal. The peripheral autonomic nervous system is often affected in small fiber neuropathies; thus, autonomic testing can be useful.[13,24–27] The quantitative sudomotor axon reflex test (QSART) can be performed in the distal and proximal aspects of the legs and arms (Fig. 22-1). Sweat glands are innervated by small nerve fibers, and impaired QSART is highly specific and sensitive for small fiber damage, with 59–80% of patients having an abnormal study (Table 22-2).[24–27] Other autonomic tests [e.g., heart rate (HR) variability with deep breathing (DB) or Valsalva maneuver] may also be abnormal in affected individuals.[7] In this regard, assessments include variability of HR to DB (Fig. 22-2) and response of the HR and blood pressure to Valsalva maneuvers and positional changes (e.g., response to tilt table or supine to standing position).

Abnormal thermal and vibratory perception thresholds may be demonstrated using QST.[28] Unlike NCS that

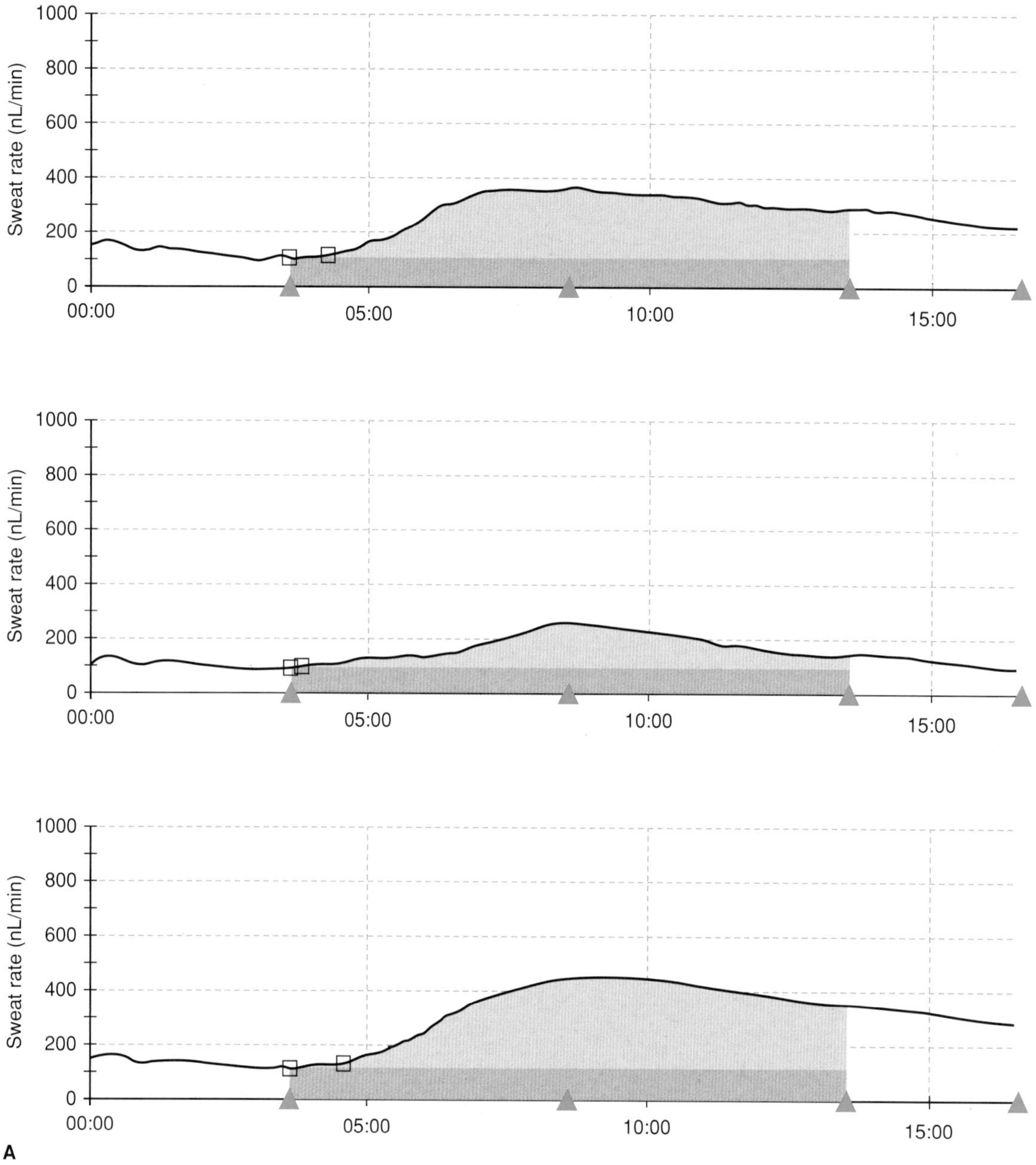

Figure 22-1. Quantitative sudomotor axon reflex test (QSART). Sudomotor function can be quantitated by measuring the amount of sweat produced in the distal and proximal aspects of the legs and arms. In **(A)**, a normal response is seen (lower panel recorded from foot, middle panel for shin, and upper panel from thigh). Individuals with small fiber neuropathy may have reduced cumulative sweat. In length-dependent process, the QSART is worse distally (e.g., at the foot compared to more proximally **(B)**, lower panel recorded from foot, middle panel for shin, and upper panel from thigh).

only assess the physiology of large-diameter sensory fibers, QST of heat and cold perception can evaluate small fiber function. Abnormal QST has been reported in 60–85% of patients with predominantly painful sensory neuropathy (Table 22-2).[9,25,29,30] However, QST depends on patient attention and cooperation; it cannot differentiate between simulated sensory loss and sensory neuropathy. Furthermore, the sensitivity and specificity of QST are lower than QSART and skin biopsies.[31,32]

HISTOPATHOLOGY

Nerve biopsies in patients with chronic, sensory predominant, length-dependent neuropathies may reveal axonal degeneration, regenerating axonal sprouts, or axonal atrophy with or without secondary demyelination.[5–7,9,33] Quantitative morphometry may reveal loss of large- and small-diameter myelinated fibers and small unmyelinated fibers. Occasionally, scattered perivascular and endoneurial lymphocytes

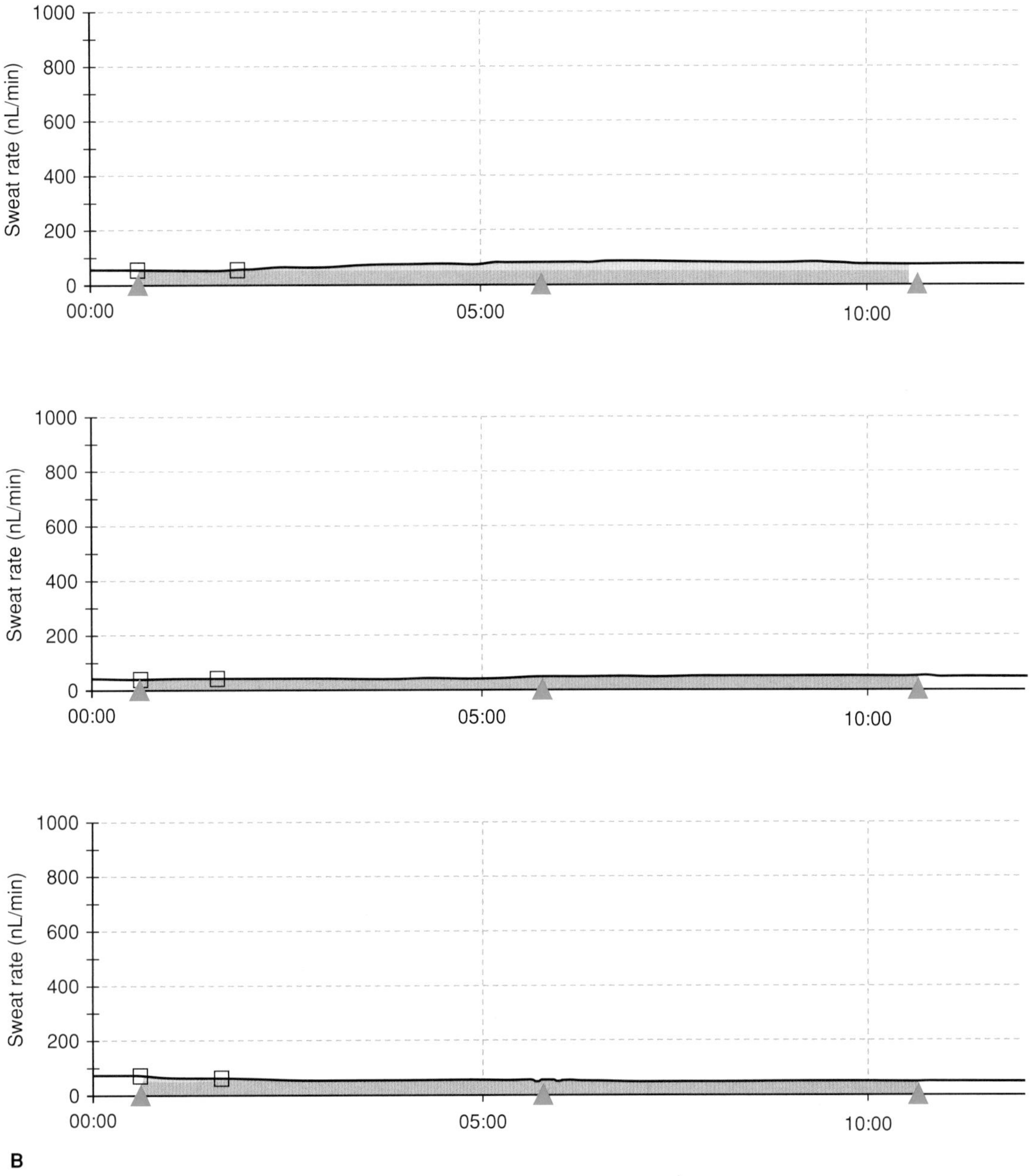

Figure 22-1. *(Continued)*

may be seen on nerve biopsy,[33,34] although necrotizing vasculitis is not a feature. A clonal restriction of the variable T-cell receptor γ-chain gene has been demonstrated by one group of researchers.[35] Basal lamina area thickness, endoneurial cell area, and number of endothelial cell nuclei may be increased. However, the abnormalities on nerve biopsy are nonspecific and are generally not helpful in finding an etiology for the neuropathy. There, we do not routinely perform nerve biopsies on all patients with unexplained polyneuropathies. We consider doing a biopsy in people with autonomic sign or monoclonal gammopathies to assess for amyloidosis, those with multiple mononeuropathies, and in patients with underlying diseases associated with vasculitis (e.g., connective tissue disorders, cryoglobulinemia, and hepatitis B or C).

Nerve biopsies in individuals with small fiber neuropathies may show selective loss of small myelinated nerves and unmyelinated nerve fibers, but this requires quantitative analysis by electron microscopy (Fig. 22-3).[13] A more sensitive and less invasive means of assessing these small fiber neuropathies histopathologically is by measuring intraepidermal nerve fiber (IENF) density on skin biopsies (Fig. 22-4).[3,7,29,36,37,38–42] Assessment of IENF density also appears to be more sensitive in identifying patients with small fiber neuropathies than sural nerve biopsies, NCS, or QST

▶ TABLE 22-2. COMPARISON OF DIAGNOSTIC TESTS IN PATIENTS WITH PREDOMINANTLY PAINFUL, SENSORY NEUROPATHY[3,7,9,24–26,29–30,37]

Authors (References)	No. of Patients	Antinerve Antibodies No. of Patients (%)	Abnormal QST Cold or Heat Pain No. of Patients (%)	Abnormal Cardiovagal (HR to DB or Valsalva) No. of Patients (%)	Abnormal QSART No. of Patients (%)	Reduced Epidermal Nerve Fiber Density No. of Patients (%)	Abnormal Sural Nerve Biopsy No. of Patients (%)	Abnormal NCS No. of Patients (%)
Stewart et al.	**40**			11 (28%)	32 (80%)			0 (0%)
Holland et al.	20 (total)		14/17 (82%)			10/20 (50%)		8/12 (67%)
	10 (idiopathic)		7/9 (78%)			7/10 (70%)		6/9 (67%)
Holland et al.	**32**	N.D.	17/27 (63%)			26/31 (81%)	4/6 (67%)	0 (0%)
Tobkin et al.			67%	75%	80%			
Periquet et al.	117 (total)	1 (<1%)	23/32 (72%)[a]		19/32 (59%)[a]	28/32 (87.5%)[a]		51%
	Group 1, 60 (51%)	1 (2%)				(0%) (by definition)		100%
	Patients with abnormal NCS	0 (0%)						0% (by definition)
	Group 2, 44 (38%)							0% (by definition)
	Patients with normal NCS but abnormal IENF density							
	Group 3, 13 (11%)							
	Patients with normal NCS and IENF density							
Novak et al.	92 (total)		66/75 (88%)	58 (63%)	67 (73%)	51/60 (85%)		45 (49%)
	47 with "small fiber neuropathy and normal NCS"		34/40 (85%)[a]	27 (57%)	32 (68%)	29/37 (74%)		
Smith et al.[b]	14		4/7 (57%)			11/14 (76%)		8/14 (57%)
Wolfe et al.	92 (<5% pure small fiber neuropathy)	0/41	32/39 (82%)				13/14 (93%)	58/81(72) with abnormal sural SNAPs
Herrmann et al.	26 (total)					12/26 (46%)		10/22 (45%)
	Four (small fiber neuropathy)					4/4 (100%)		(0 by definition)

[a]Included abnormal QST to cold or vibratory perception. Table includes only those 32 patients who each had QST, QSART, and IENF density.
[b]Patients with diabetes or impaired glucose tolerance.
Bold, idiopathic, predominantly small fiber neuropathy; QST, quantitative sensory testing; QSART, quantitative sudomotor axon reflex test; N.D., not done or not reported; NCS, nerve conduction studies.

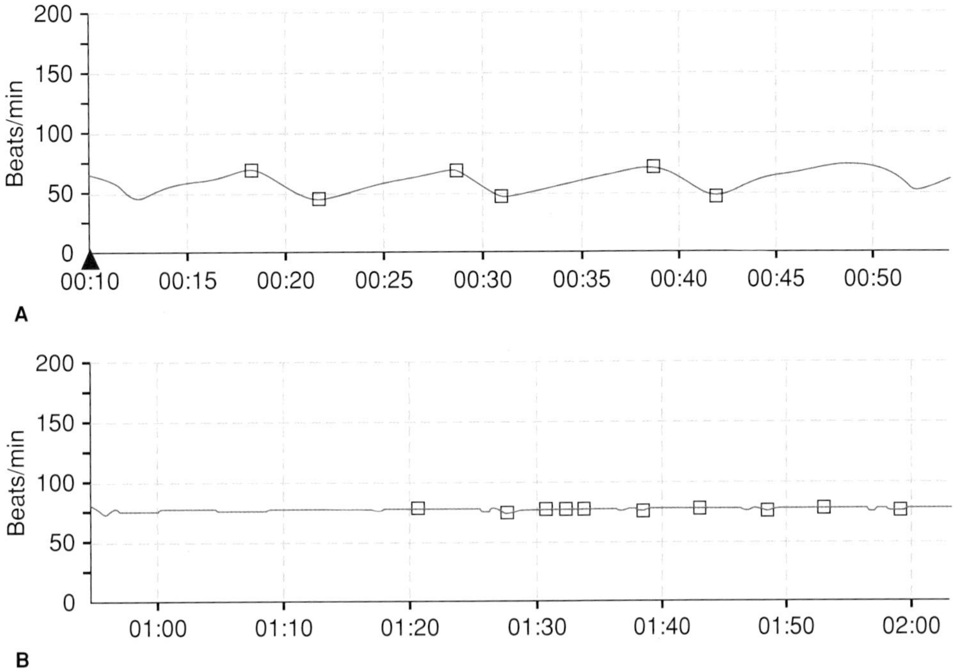

Figure 22-2. Heart rate variability. Normally, the heart rate varies with respiration **(A)**. Some individuals with small fiber involvement have an autonomic neuropathy with cardiovagal abnormalities, as demonstrated by reduced heart rate variability with deep breathing **(B)**.

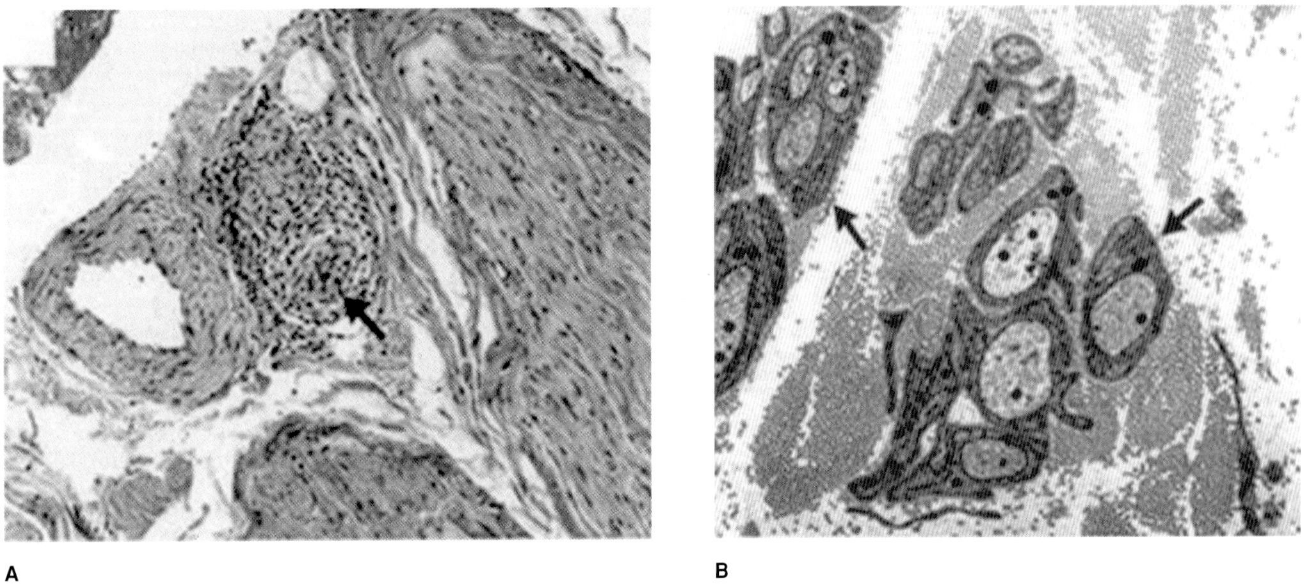

Figure 22-3. Specimen from a sural nerve biopsy. The nerve is morphologically normal on light microscopy **(A)**. There is a focal perivascular lymphocytic infiltrate, and in one small perineurial vessel (*arrow*) the infiltrate extends through the wall (hematoxylin and eosin, ×125). There is no necrosis or other evidence of vasculitis or intraneural inflammation. An electron micrograph **(B)** shows empty Schwann-cell processes (*arrows*) that are consistent with the loss of small, unmyelinated fibers (×8,000). (Used with permission of Doctors Lawrence Hayward and Thomas Smith, University of Massachusetts Medical School, Worcester, MA.)

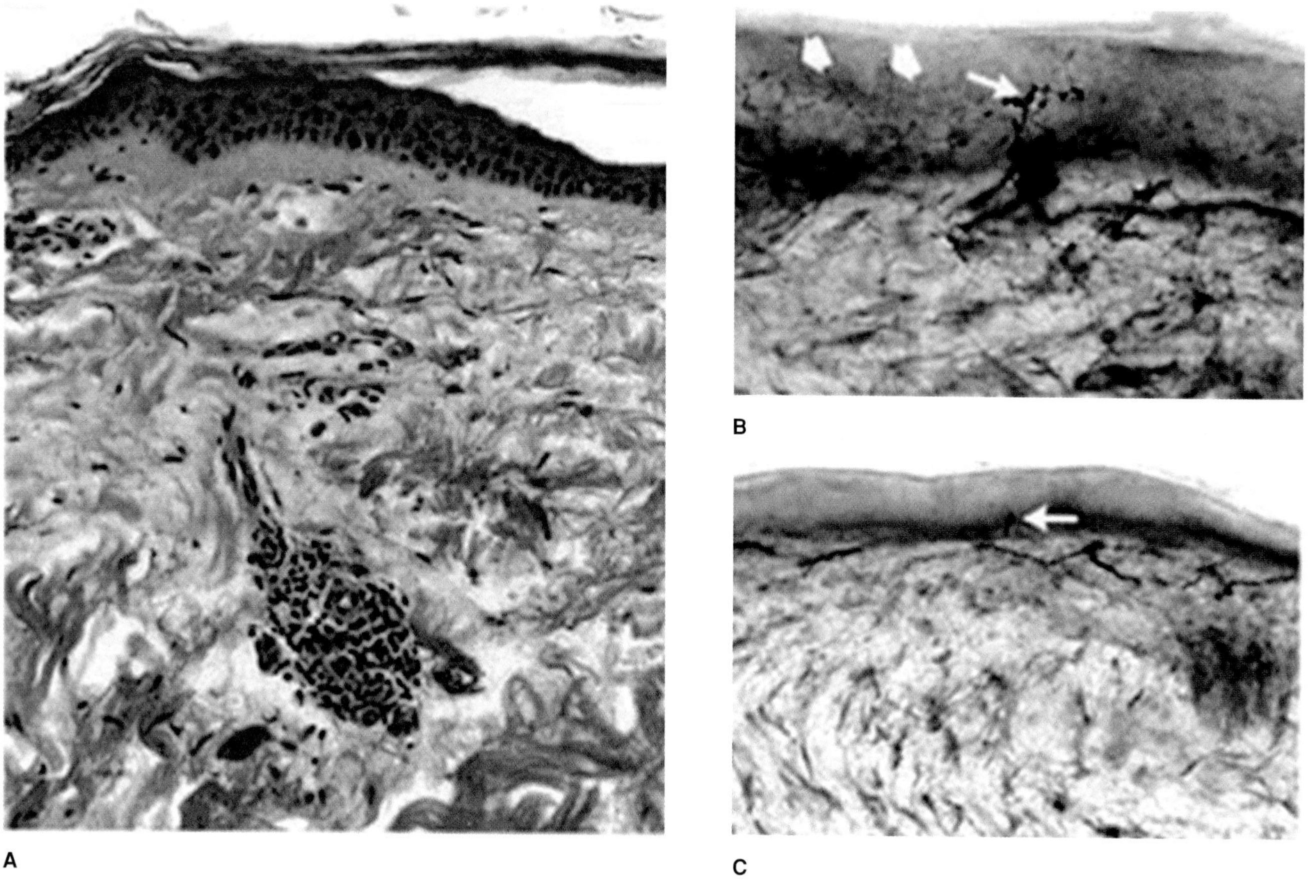

Figure 22-4. Specimens from skin-punch biopsies. A specimen obtained at the time of the patient's first evaluation at this hospital **(A)** shows a focal perivascular lymphocytic infiltrate (hematoxylin and eosin, ×125). A section immunolabeled against protein gene product 9.5 to reveal neural processes or axons (*thick arrows*) **(B)** shows an epidermal neurite with axonal swellings, which are abnormal (*thin arrow*). The density of nerve fibers is greater than normal (immunoperoxidase, ×500). A specimen obtained 11 months later **(C)** shows marked reduction in neurite density and axonal swelling (*arrow*) in a remaining neurite (×300). (Reproduced with permission from Amato AA, Oaklander AL. Case 16–2004: A 76-year-old woman with numbness and pain in the feet and legs. *N Engl J Med*. 2004;350:2181–2189.)

(Table 22-2). Punch biopsy of the skin can be obtained at the foot, calf, or thigh, and immunohistochemistry using antibodies directed against protein gene product 9.5 (PGP 9.5) is used to stain small intraepidermal fibers. Intraepidermal nerve fibers arising entirely from the dorsal root ganglia represent the terminals of C and Aδ nociceptors. The density of these nerve fibers is reduced in patients with small fiber neuropathies, in which NCS, QST, and routine nerve biopsies are often normal. In at least a third of people with painful sensory neuropathies, IENF density on skin biopsies represents the only objective abnormality present following extensive evaluation.[7]

PATHOGENESIS

As the name implies, the pathogenic basis of chronic, idiopathic, length-dependent sensory or sensorimotor polyneuropathy is unknown, but is likely multifactorial in etiology.[19] Some may have genetic causes, while others may have a primary degenerative or immunological basis. Prediabetes is part of the metabolic syndrome, which also includes hypertension, hyperlipidemia, and obesity. Individual aspects of the metabolic syndrome influence risk and progression of diabetic neuropathy and may play a causative role in neuropathy for those with both prediabetes and otherwise idiopathic neuropathy.[54]

TREATMENT

Unfortunately, there is no treatment for slowing the progression or reversing the "numbness" or lack of sensation. Therapies are aimed at symptomatic management of neuropathic pain and reducing the risk of falling through the use of durable medical equipment.[8,9,44–48] Most of the randomized controlled trials addressed patients with postherpetic neuralgia or painful neuropathy mainly caused by diabetes. A large number of such class I trials provide level A evidence for the efficacy of tricyclic antidepressants, gabapentin, pregabalin,

▶ TABLE 22-3. **TREATMENT OF PAINFUL SENSORY NEUROPATHIES**

Therapy	Route	Dose	Side Effects
Lidoderm 5% patch	Apply cutaneously	Up to three patches daily for 12 h at a time	Local irritation
Gabapentin	p.o.	300–1,200 mg TID	Cognitive changes and sedation
Pregabalin	p.o.	50–100 mg TID	Cognitive changes and sedation
Tricyclic antidepressants (e.g., amitriptyline and nortriptyline)	p.o.	10–100 mg qhs	Cognitive changes, sedation, dry eyes and mouth, urinary retention, and constipation
Duloxetine	p.o.	60 mg daily	Cognitive changes, dizziness, sedation, insomnia, nausea, and constipation
Venlafaxine	p.o.	75–150 mg daily	Asthenia, sweating, nausea, constipation, anorexia, vomiting, somnolence, dry mouth, dizziness, nervousness, anxiety, tremor, and blurred vision as well as abnormal ejaculation/orgasm and impotence
Carbamazepine	p.o.	200–400 mg q 6–8 h	Cognitive changes, dizziness, leukopenia, and liver dysfunction
Phenytoin	p.o.	200–400 mg qhs	Cognitive changes, dizziness, and liver dysfunction
Tramadol	p.o.	50 mg QID	Cognitive changes and GI upset
Other agents			
Mexiletine	p.o.	200–300 mg TID	Arrhythmias
Capsaicin 0.025–0.075% cream	Apply cutaneously	QID	Painful burning skin

GI, gastrointestinal.
Modified with permission from Amato AA, Dumitru D. Acquired neuropathies. In: Dumitru D, Amato AA, Swartz MJ, eds. *Electrodiagnostic Medicine*, 2nd ed. Philadelphia, PA: Hanley & Belfus; 2002.

and opioids followed by topical lidocaine (in postherpetic neuralgia) and the newer antidepressants venlafaxine and duloxetine (in painful neuropathy).[48]

Our approach to treating the painful paresthesias and burning sensation associated with chronic idiopathic sensory neuropathy is uniform regardless of etiology (e.g., painful sensory neuropathies related to DM, HIV infection, and herpes zoster infection) (Table 22-3). We start off with Lidoderm 5% patches to the feet, as this treatment is associated with less systemic side effects.[49] If this does not suffice (and it usually does not), our next step is to add an antiepileptic (e.g., gabapentin, pregabalin) or antidepressant (e.g., nortriptyline, duloxetine). We usually start at a low dose and gradually increase as necessary and as tolerated. A combination of an antiepileptic and antidepressant medication should be tried if monotherapy with either medication class fails. Tramadol is used to treat breakthrough pain.

▶ IDIOPATHIC SENSORY NEURONOPATHY/ GANGLIONOPATHY

This disorder is believed to be caused by an autoimmune attack directed against the dorsal root ganglia. The differential diagnosis of sensory neuronopathy includes a paraneoplastic syndrome, which is typically associated with anti-Hu antibodies, and a sensory ganglionitis related to Sjögren syndrome. Certain medications or toxins (e.g., various chemotherapies, vitamin B6), infectious agents (e.g., HIV), and other systemic disorders are also associated with a sensory neuronopathy. Despite extensive evaluation, many cases of sensory neuronopathy have no clear etiology, the so-called idiopathic sensory neuronopathy. The acute cases may represent a variant of GBS, although the onset can be insidiously in nature and slowly progressive.

CLINICAL FEATURES

Idiopathic sensory neuronopathy is a rare disorder that usually presents in adulthood (mean age of onset 49 years, with range 18–81 years) and has a slight female predominance.[50–55] Symptoms can develop over a few hours or evolve more insidiously over several months or years, and the course can be monophasic with a stable or remitting deficit, chronic progressive, or chronic relapsing. Unlike typical GBS, only rare patients report a recent antecedent infection. The presenting complaint is numbness and tingling face, trunk, or limbs, which can be painful. Symptoms begin asymmetrically and in the upper limbs in nearly half of the patients, suggesting a ganglionopathy as opposed to a length-dependent process. Usually, the sensory symptoms become generalized, but they can remain asymmetric. Patients also describe clumsiness of the hands and gait instability. Severe autonomic symptoms develop in some.[55]

On examination, marked reduction in vibration and proprioception are found, while pain and temperature sensations are less affected. Manual muscle testing is usually normal. Some muscle groups may appear weak, but this is usually secondary to impaired modulation of motor activity due to the proprioceptive defect. Most patients have sensory ataxia, which can be readily demonstrated by having the patient perform the finger–nose–finger test with their eyes open and then closed. Patients may have only mild dysmetria with their eyes open, but when their eyes are closed, they consistently miss their nose and the examiner's stationed finger. Pseudoathetoid movements of the extremities may also be appreciated. Patients exhibit a positive Romberg sign and, not surprisingly, describe more gait instability in the dark or with their eyes closed while in the shower. Muscle stretch reflexes are decreased or absent, while plantar reflexes are flexor.

A detailed history and examination are essential to exclude a toxic neuronopathy, paraneoplastic syndrome, or disorder related to a connective tissue disease (i.e., Sjögren syndrome). Importantly, the sensory neuronopathy can precede the onset of malignancy or SICCA symptoms (i.e., dry eyes and mouth); therefore, these disorders should always be kept in mind. Pertinent laboratory and malignancy workup should be ordered. A rose bengal stain or Schirmer's test may be abnormal in patients with sicca symptoms. A lip or parotid gland biopsy likewise can be abnormal revealing inflammatory cell infiltration and destruction of the glands. Subacute sensory neuronopathy has also been associated with recent Epstein–Barr virus infection.[56]

LABORATORY FEATURES

The CSF protein is normal or only slightly elevated in most patients. However, the CSF protein can be markedly elevated (reportedly as high as 300 mg/dL) when examined within a few days in cases with a hyperacute onset. Only rare patients exhibit CSF pleocytosis. MRI scan can reveal gadolinium enhancement of the posterior spinal roots or increased signal abnormalities on T2-weighted images in the posterior columns of the spinal cord.[55,57] Some patients have a monoclonal gammopathy (IgM, IgG, or IgA). Ganglioside antibodies, particularly GD1b antibodies, have been demonstrated in some cases of idiopathic sensory neuronopathy associated with IgM monoclonal gammopathy.[58]

Antineuronal nuclear antibodies (e.g., anti-Hu antibodies) should be assayed in all individuals with sensory neuronopathy to evaluate for a paraneoplastic syndrome. Likewise, antinuclear, SS-A, and SS-B antibodies should be ordered to look for evidence of Sjögren syndrome, which can also present with a sensory neuronopathy.

The characteristic NCS finding is low-amplitude or absent SNAPs in the arms, while the SNAPs in the legs may be normal,[51,52,54,57] a pattern that can also be seen in sensory nerve conductions in acquired inflammatory demyelinating neuropathy. In the either case, this pattern indicates the non-length-dependent nature of these disorders. When SNAPs are obtainable, the distal sensory latencies and nerve conduction velocities are normal or only mildly abnormal. In contrast, motor NCS either are normal or reveal only mild abnormalities. In addition, H reflexes and blink reflexes are typically be unobtainable.[59] An abnormal blink reflex favors a nonparaneoplastic etiology for a sensory neuronopathy but does not exclude an underlying malignancy.[60] The masseter reflex or jaw jerk is abnormal in patients with sensory neuropathy but is usually preserved in patients with sensory neuronopathy.[59] The masseter reflex is unique among the stretch reflexes in that the cell bodies of the afferent limb lie in the mesencephalic nucleus within the CNS. This differs from the sensory cell bodies innervating the limbs, which reside in the dorsal root ganglia of the PNS. The blink reflex can be impaired in sensory ganglionopathies, because the afferent cell bodies lie in the gasserian ganglia that are outside the CNS.

HISTOPATHOLOGY

Sensory nerve biopsies may reveal a preferential loss of large myelinated or small unmyelinated fibers. Mild perivascular inflammation may be seen, but prominent endoneurial infiltrate is not appreciated. There is no evidence of segmental demyelination.

Autopsies performed in a couple of patients with acute idiopathic sensory neuronopathy have revealed widespread inflammation involving sensory and autonomic ganglia, with loss of associated neurons and wallerian degeneration of the posterior nerve roots and dorsal columns being evident in one.[50] The motor neurons and roots were normal. Immunohistochemistry suggested a CD8+ T-cell mediated attach directed against sensory ganglia. In another autopsy, there was severe neuronal cell loss in the thoracic sympathetic and dorsal root ganglia, and Auerbach's plexus with well-preserved anterior horn cells.[55] Myelinated fibers in the anterior spinal root were preserved, while those in the posterior spinal root and the posterior column of the spinal cord were depleted.

PATHOGENESIS

In some cases, the sensory neuronopathies may be caused by an autoimmune attack directed against the dorsal root ganglia. Serum from affected patients immunostain dorsal root ganglia cells in culture and inhibits neurite formation.[61] The neuronal epitope is unknown, but the ganglioside GD1b has been hypothesized to be the target antigen.[58] GD1b localizes to neurons in the dorsal root ganglia, and antibodies directed against this ganglioside have been detected in some patients with idiopathic sensory neuronopathy.[50] Furthermore, rabbits immunized with purified GD1b develop ataxic sensory neuropathy associated with loss of the cell bodies in the dorsal root ganglia and axonal degeneration of the dorsal column of the spinal cord but without demyelination or an inflammatory infiltrate.

TREATMENT

Various modes of immunotherapy have been tried, including corticosteroids, PE, and IVIG.[55,57] However, there have been no prospective, double-blind, placebo-controlled trials. Occasionally, patients appear to improve with therapy; however, some improve spontaneously and many stabilize without treatment. In our experience, most patients have not experienced a dramatic improvement following treatment. Perhaps, this is because once the cell body of the sensory neuron is destroyed, it will not regenerate. However, in patients seen in the acute setting or those who have a chronic progressive deficit, a trial of immunotherapy may be warranted.

▶ IDIOPATHIC SMALL FIBER SENSORY NEURONOPATHY

This may represent a subtype of sensory neuropathy/ganglionopathy discussed in the preceding section but clinically only involved small fiber neurons.

CLINICAL FEATURES

Most patients with small fiber neuropathies typically present insidious with slowly progressive burning pain and paresthesia in a length-dependent fashion beginning in the feet. Most are idiopathic in nature, but DM, amyloidosis, Sjögren syndrome, and hereditary sensory and autonomic neuropathy need to be excluded. However, some individuals present with symptoms suggestive of a small fiber neuropathy that are not be length-dependent.[62–64] Often the neuropathy begins acutely and an antecedent infection is common. Affected individuals often describe numbness, tingling, or burning pain in the face, trunk, or arms before or more severe than in the distal lower extremities. Patients with non–length-dependent small fiber neuronopathy may more often report an "itchy" quality and allodynia to light touch.[64] Neurological examination discloses normal muscle strength and a non–length-dependent sensory loss for pain or temperature. Proprioception, vibratory perception, and reflexes are normal. The burning dysesthesia usually disappears within 4 months; however, the numbness and objective sensory loss tended to persist longer.

LABORATORY FEATURES

CSF examination may reveal albuminocytological dissociation. Motor and sensory conduction studies that primarily assess large fiber function are normal. Autonomic testing may be abnormal.

HISTOPATHOLOGY

In an autopsy case, there was severe neuronal cell loss in the thoracic sympathetic and dorsal root ganglia, and Auerbach's plexus with well-preserved anterior horn cells.[55] Myelinated fibers in the anterior spinal root were preserved, while those in the posterior spinal root and the posterior column of the spinal cord were depleted. Skin biopsies in some patients have shown reduced nerve fiber density, which in most cases was worse in the thigh compared to calf.[63]

PATHOGENESIS

The acute clinical presentation often following an infection and CSF findings suggests that this is a rare variant of GBS.

TREATMENT

A trial of IVIG would seem warranted in patients who present in the acute phase of the illness.

▶ FACIAL ONSET SENSORY AND MOTOR NEURONOPATHY

This is a non–length-dependent neuronopathy/ganglionopathy that starts with loss of facial sensation and overtime also involves motor neurons.

CLINICAL FEATURES

Patients usually developed paraesthesia and numbness initially in a trigeminal nerve distribution that slowly progresses to involve sensory neurons innervating the scalp, neck, upper trunk, and upper limbs in a descending pattern.[66–69] Over 5 to 10 years, dysphagia and dysarthria occur along with cramps, fasciculations and weakness, and atrophy in the arms due to slowly progressive lower motor neuron involvement. Ventilatory failure may also develop. Upper motor neuron signs do not typically appear.

LABORATORY FEATURES

NCS typically reveal reduced amplitudes or absent SNAPs in arms, while SNAPs are normal in the legs. Blink reflexes are abnormal. Subsequently, CMAP amplitudes may diminish and active denervation is apparent on EMG. MRI scans may demonstrate mild atrophy of the brainstem and spinal cord. Some patients have been reported with antisulfatide or GD1b antibodies.[66]

HISTOPATHOLOGY

Autopsy in one patient disclosed loss of motor neurons in the hypoglossal nucleus and cervical anterior horns, along with loss of sensory neurons in the main trigeminal sensory nucleus and dorsal root ganglia.[66]

PATHOGENESIS

The pathogenic basis of facial onset sensory and motor neuronopathy (FOSMN) is unknown. The presence in some patients of autoantibodies has suggested a possible autoimmune basis. However, treatment with a variety of immunotherapies has not resulted in improvement or halt of progression, a finding which supports FOSMN being a primary neurodegenerative disorder.

TREATMENT

Although a few patients have been reported with transient clinical benefit or subclinical improvement with immunotherapies, most continue to progress.

▶ SUMMARY

Chronic idiopathic polyneuropathies are quite common in clinical practice despite extensive laboratory evaluation. A standard laboratory workup, including NCS, is important to perform before concluding that the neuropathy is idiopathic in nature. Many of the patients may have IGT, particularly those with a small fiber phenotype, if an oral GTT is performed, even if they have normal FBS and HgbA1C levels. Nerve biopsies are generally not indicated. Although skin biopsy may be informative by showing reduced epidermal nerve fibers when other studies (e.g., NCS, QST, and autonomic studies) are normal, they do not define etiology and often tell you nothing that you don't already know based on the history and clinical examination. That is, persons with burning and tingling pain in their feet with normal reflexes and NCS probably have a small fiber neuropathy, regardless of what the skin biopsy shows. Patients need reassurance that it is not all that unusual for an etiology of neuropathy to be undetermined despite workup. Primary treatment is directed and symptomatic management of their pain.

REFERENCES

1. Amato AA, Oaklander AL. Case records of the Massachusetts general hospital. Weekly clinicopathological exercises. Case16-2004. A 76-year-old woman with numbness and pain in the feet and legs. *N Engl J Med.* 2004;350(21):2181–2189.
2. Gorson KC, Ropper AH. Idiopathic distal sensory small fiber neuropathy. *Acta Neurol Scand.* 1995;92(5):376–382.
3. Holland NR, Crawford TO, Hauer P, Cornblath DR, Griffin JW, McArthur JC. Small-fiber sensory neuropathies: clinical course and neuropathology of idiopathic cases. *Ann Neurol.* 1998;44(1):47–59.
4. Lacomis D. Small-fiber neuropathy. *Muscle Nerve.* 2002; 26(2): 173–188.
5. McLeod JG, Tuck RR, Pollard JD, Cameron J, Walsh JC. Chronic polyneuropathy of undetermined cause. *J Neurol Neurosurg Psychiatry.* 1984;47(5):530–535.
6. Notermans NC, Wokke JH, Franssen H, et al. Chronic idiopathic polyneuropathy presenting in middle or old age: a clinical and electrophysiological study of 75 patients. *J Neurol Neurosurg Psychiatry.* 1993;56(10):1066–1071.
7. Periquet MI, Novak V, Collins MP, et al. Painful sensory neuropathy: prospective evaluation of painful feet using electrodiagnosis and skin biopsy. *Neurology.* 1999;53(8): 1641–1647.
8. Wolfe GI, Barohn RJ. Cryptogenic sensory and sensorimotor polyneuropathies. *Semin Neurol.* 1998;18(1):105–111.
9. Wolfe GI, Baker NS, Amato AA, et al. Chronic cryptogenic sensory polyneuropathy: clinical and laboratory characteristics. *Arch Neurol.* 1999;56(5):540–547.
10. Grahmann F, Winterholler M, Neundörfer B. Cryptogenic polyneuropathies: an out-patient follow-up study. *Acta Neurol Scand.* 1991;84(3):221–225.
11. Notermans NC, Wokke JH, van den Berg LH, et al. Chronic idiopathic axonal polyneuropathy. Comparison of patients with and without monoclonal gammopathy. *Brain.* 1996;119 (pt 2):421–427.
12. England JD, Gronseth GS, Franklin G, et al. Evaluation of distal symmetric polyneuropathy: the role of laboratory and genetic testing (an evidence-based review). *Muscle Nerve.* 2009;39(1):116–125.
13. England JD, Gronseth GS, Franklin G, et al. Evaluation of distal symmetric polyneuropathy: the role of autonomic testing, nerve biopsy, and skin biopsy (an evidence-based review). *Muscle Nerve.* 2009;39:106–115.
14. Singleton JR, Smith AG, Bromberg MB. Painful sensory polyneuropathy associated with impaired glucose tolerance test. *Muscle Nerve.* 2001;24(9):1225–1228.
15. Novella SP, Inzucchi SE, Goldstein JM. The frequency of undiagnosed diabetes and impaired glucose tolerance in patients with idiopathic sensory neuropathy. *Muscle Nerve.* 2001;24(9):1229–1231.
16. Sumner CJ, Seth S, Griffin JW, Cornblath DR, Polyswdkia M. The spectrum of neuropathy in diabetes and impaired glucose tolerance. *Neurology.* 2003;60(1):108–111.
17. Harris MI, Flegal KM, Cowie CC, et al. Prevalence of diabetes, impaired fasting glucose, and impaired glucose tolerance in U.S. adults. The third national health and nutrition examination survey,1988–1994. *Diabetes Care.* 1998;21(4):518–524.
18. Smith AG, Singleton JR. The diagnostic yield of a standardized approach to idiopathic sensory-predominant neuropathy. *Arch Intern Med.* 2004;164(9):1021–1025.
19. Hughes RA, Umapathi T, Gray IA, et al. A controlled investigation of the cause of chronic idiopathic axonal polyneuropathy. *Brain.* 2004;127(Pt 8):1723–1730.
20. Russell JW, Feldman EL. Impaired glucose tolerance–does it cause neuropathy? *Muscle Nerve.* 2001;24(9):1109–1112.
21. Dyck PJ, Dyck PJ, Klein CJ, Weigand SD. Does impaired glucose metabolism cause polyneuropathy? Review of previous studies and design of a prospective controlled population-based study. *Muscle Nerve.* 2007;36(4):536–541.
22. Nemni R, Fazio R, Quattrini A, Lorenztti I, Mamoli D, Canal N. Antibodies to sulfatide and to chondroitin sulfate C in patients with chronic sensory neuropathy. *J Neuroimmunol.* 1993;43(1–2):79–86.
23. Pestronk A, Li F, Griffin J, et al. Polyneuropathy syndromes associated with serum antibodies to sulfatide and myelin-associated glycoprotein. *Neurology.* 1991;41(3):357–362.

24. Stewart JD, Low PA, Fealy RD. Distal small fiber neuropathy: results of tests of sweating and autonomic cardiovascular reflexes. *Muscle Nerve*. 1992;15(6):661–665.
25. Novak V, Freimer ML, Kissel JT, et al. Autonomic impairment in painful neuropathy. *Neurology*. 2001;56(7):861–868.
26. Tobkin K, Guiliani MJ, Lacomis D. Comparison of different modalities for detection of small fiber neuropathy. *Clin Neurophysiol*. 1999;110(11):1909–1912.
27. Low VA, Sandroni P, Fealey RD, Low PA. Detection of small-fiber neuropathy by sudomotor testing. *Muscle Nerve*. 2006;34(1):57–61.
28. Dyck PJ, O'Brien PC. Quantitative sensory testing in epidemiological and therapeutic studies of peripheral neuropathy. *Muscle Nerve*. 1999;22(6):659–662.
29. Holland NR, Stocks NR, Hauer P, Cornblath DR, Griffin JW, McArthur JC. Intraepidermal nerve fiber density in patients with painful sensory neuropathy. *Neurology*. 1997;48(3):708–711.
30. Smith AG, Raachandran P, Tripp S, Singleton JR. Epidermal nerve innervation in impaired glucose tolerance and diabetes-associated neuropathy. *Neurology*. 2001;57(9):1701–1704.
31. Mendell JR, Sahenk Z. Painful sensory neuropathy. *N Engl J Med*. 2003;348(13):1243–1255.
32. Freeman R, Chase KP, Risk MR. Quantitative sensory testing cannot differentiate simulated sensory loss from sensory neuropathy. *Neurology*. 2003;60(3):465–470.
33. Kelkar P, McDermott WR, Parry GJ. Sensory-predominant, painful, idiopathic neuropathy: Inflammatory changes in sural nerves. *Muscle Nerve*. 2002;26:413–416.
34. Bosboom WM, Van den Berg LH, De Boer L, et al. The diagnostic value of sural nerve T cells in chronic inflammatory demyelinating polyneuropathy. *Neurology*. 1999;53(4):837–845.
35. Gherardi RK, Farcet J-P, Créange A, et al. Dominant T-cell clones of unknown significance in patients with idiopathic sensory neuropathies. *Neurology*. 1998;51(2):384–389.
36. Vlcková-Moravcová E, Bednarík J, Dusek L, Toyka KV, Sommer C. Diagnostic validity of epidermal nerve fiber densities in painful sensory neuropathies. *Muscle Nerve*. 2008;37(1):50–60.
37. Herrmann DN, Griffin JW, Hauer P, Cornblath DR, McArthur JC. et al. Epidermal nerve fiber density, sural nerve morphometry and electro-diagnosis in peripheral neuropathies. *Neurology*. 1999;53(8):1634–1640.
38. McCarthy BG, Hseih ST, Stocks A, et al. Cutaneous innervation in sensory neuropathies: evaluation by skin biopsy. *Neurology*. 1995;45(10):1845–1855.
39. Wendelschafer-Crabb G, Kennedy WR, Walk D. Morphological features of nerves in skin biopsies. *J Neurol Sci*. 2006;242 (1–2):15–21.
40. Hays AP. Utility of skin biopsy to evaluate peripheral neuropathy. *Curr Neurol Neurosci Rep*. 2010;10(2):101–107.
41. Devigili G, Tugnoli V, Penza P, et al. The diagnostic criteria for small fibre neuropathy: From symptoms to neuropathology. *Brain*. 2008;131(pt 7):1912–1925.
42. Walk D, Wendelschafer-Crabb G, Davey C, Kennedy WR. Concordance between epidermal nerve fiber density and sensory examination in patients with symptoms of idiopathic small fiber neuropathy. *J Neurol Sci*. 2007;255(1–2):23–26.
43. Gordon Smith A, Robinson Singleton J. Idiopathic neuropathy, prediabetes and the metabolic syndrome. *J Neurol Sci*. 2006;242(1–2):9–14.
44. Galer BS. Painful polyneuropathy. *Neurol Clin*. 1998;16(4): 791–812.
45. Wolfe GI, Trivedi JR. Painful peripheral neuropathy and its non-surgical treatment. *Muscle Nerve*. 2004;30(1):3–19.
46. Gilron I, Bailey JM, Dongsheng T, Holderen RR, Weaver DF, Houlden RL. Morphine, gabapentin, or other combination for neuropathic pain. *N Engl J Med*. 2005;352(13):1324–1334.
47. Singleton JR. Evaluation and treatment of painful peripheral polyneuropathy. *Semin Neurol*. 2005;25(2):185–195.
48. Attal N, Cruccu G, Haanpaa M, et al. EFNS guidelines on pharmacological treatment of neuropathic pain. *Eur J Neurol*. 2006;13(11):1153–1169.
49. Herrmann DN, Barbano RL, Hart-Gouleau S, Pennella-Vaughan J, Dworkin RH. An open-label study of the lidocaine patch 5% in painful idiopathic sensory polyneuropathy. *Pain Med*. 2005;6(5):379–384.
50. Hainfellner JA, Kristferitsch W, Lassmannn H, et al. T cell-mediated ganglionitis associated with acute sensory neuronopathy. *Ann Neurol*. 1996;39(4):543–547.
51. Knazan M, Bohlega S, Berry K, et al. Acute sensory neuronopathy with preserved SEPs and long-latency reflexes. *Muscle Nerve*. 1990;13(5):381–384.
52. Sterman AB, Schaumburg HH, Asbury AK. The acute sensory neuronopathy syndrome: A distinct clinical entity. *Ann Neurol*. 1980;7(4):354–358.
53. Kuntzer T, Atoine JC, Steck AJ. Clinical features and pathophysiological basis of sensory neuronopathies (ganglionopathies). *Muscle Nerve*. 2004;30(3):255–268.
54. Camdessanché JP, Jousserand G, Ferraud K, et al. The pattern and diagnostic criteria of sensory neuronopathy: a case-control study. *Brain*. 2009;132(pt 7):1723–1733.
55. Koike H, Atsuta N, Adachi H, et al. Clinicopathological features of acute autonomic and sensory neuropathy. *Brain*. 2010;133(10):2881–2896.
56. Rubin D, Daube JR. Subacute sensory neuropathy associated with Epstein–Barr virus. *Muscle Nerve*. 1999;22(11):1607–1610.
57. Wada M, Kato T, Yuki N, et al. Gadolinium-enhancement of the spinal posterior roots in acute sensory ataxic neuropathy. *Neurology*. 1997;49(5):1470–1471.
58. Dalakas MC. Autoimmune ataxic neuropathies (sensory ganglionopathies): are glycolipids the responsible autoantigens? *Ann Neurol*. 1996;39(4):419–422.
59. Auger RG. The role of the masseter reflex in the assessment of subacute sensory neuropathy. *Muscle Nerve*. 1998;21(6): 800–801.
60. Auger RG, Windebank AJ, Lucchinetti CF, Chalk CH. Role of the blink reflex in the evaluation of sensory neuronopathy. *Neurology*. 1999;53(2):407–408.
61. Van Dijk GW, Wokke JH, Notermans NC, van den Berg LH, Bär PR. Indications for an immune-mediated etiology of idiopathic sensory neuronopathy. *J Neuroimmunol*. 1997;74 (1–2):165–172.
62. Seneviratne U, Gunasekera S. Acute small fibre sensory neuropathy: another variant of Guillain–Barre syndrome? *J Neurol Neurosurg Psychiatry*. 2002;72(4):540–542.
63. Gorson KC, Herrmann DN, Thiagarajan R, et al. Non-length dependent small fibre neuropathy/ganglionopathy. *J Neurol Neurosurg Psychiatry*. 2008;79(2):163–169.
64. Gemignani F, Giovanelli M, Vitetta F, et al. Non-length dependent small fiber neuropathy. a prospective case series. *J Peripher Nerv Syst*. 2010;15(1):57–62.
65. Koike H, Sobue G. Small neurons may be preferentially affected in ganglionopathy. *J Neurol Neurosurg Psychiatry*. 2008;79 (2):113.

66. Vucic S, Tian D, Chong PS, Cudkowicz ME, Hedley-Whyte ET, Cros D. Facial onset sensory and motor neuronopathy (FOSMN syndrome): a novel syndrome in neurology. *Brain.* 2006;129(pt 2):3384–3390.
67. Isoardo G, Troni W. Sporadic bulopsinal muscle atrophy with facial-onset sensory neuropathy. *Muscle Nerve.* 2008;37(5): 659–662.
68. Hokonohara T, Shigeto H, Kawano Y, Ohyagi Y, Uehara M, Kira J. Facial onset sensory and motor neuronopathy (FOSMN) syndrome responding to immunotherapies. *J Neurol Sci.* 2008;275(1–2):157–158.
69. Fluchere F, Verschueren A, Cintas P, et al. Clinical features and follow-up of four new cases of facial-onset sensory and motor neuronopathy. *Muscle Nerve.* 2011;43(1):136–140.

CHAPTER 23

Focal Neuropathies of the Upper Extremities and Trunk: Radiculopathies, Brachial Plexopathies, and Mononeuropathies

Numbness, pain, and/or weakness involving one or both arms are common reasons for referral to the neuromuscular clinician. These symptoms may be due to radiculopathy, brachial plexopathy, or one or more mononeuropathies. Some systemic etiologies for these focal neuropathic disorders have been discussed in preceding chapters (e.g., Lyme disease, vasculitis, and diabetes mellitus). This chapter will focus mainly on radiculopathies secondary to compression (e.g., degenerative joint disease and herniated discs), brachial plexitis, traumatic plexopathies, and focal mononeuropathies related to compression or entrapment. Before discussing the evaluation and management of these disorders, a review of the normal anatomy would be helpful.

▶ ANATOMY

SPINAL NERVES

Recall that there are seven cervical vertebrae, the first of which, the atlas, articulates with the skull's occipital condyles. The orientation of this joint allows primarily for flexion/extension movements. The second cervical vertebra, the axis, has a superiorly directed bony prominence, the dens, which articulates with the atlas and allows for rotational movements of the head and neck. The third through seventh cervical vertebrae are composed of the vertebral bodies themselves as well as short pedicles giving rise to laminae, which end in comparatively short and often bifid spinous processes. The transverse processes arise near the junctional zone of the pedicle and lamina. Between the transverse processes at each vertebral level lies a sulcus for the spinal nerves.

The spinal nerves are composed of a dorsal root and a ventral root (Fig. 23-1). The dorsal root consists of sensory fibers emanating from the dorsal root ganglia that lie outside the spinal cord. These dorsal root fibers enter the posterolateral aspect of the spinal cord and into the dorsal horn. Along the anterior aspect of the spinal cord, two or as many as 12 individual rootlets arising from anterior horn cells, fila radicularia, fuse to form the ventral root. Just distal to the dorsal root ganglion, the ventral and dorsal roots merge to form the spinal nerve. In the cervical region, there are eight cervical spinal roots on each side but only seven cervical vertebrae (Fig. 23-2). The first cervical spine nerve arises between the skull and atlas. As a result, each numbered cervical nerve root is related to the bony level immediately inferior to it down to the T1 vertebra. For example, the fifth cervical nerve root exits the spinal column just superior to the fifth cervical vertebrae. The eighth cervical nerve root exits the spinal column superior to the first thoracic vertebra.

At the intervertebral foramina, the spinal nerves are joined by the gray rami from the cervical sympathetic chain ganglia (Fig. 23-1). The superior cervical ganglion communicates with C1–4 spinal roots, the middle cervical ganglion with the C5 and C6 spinal nerves, and the inferior cervical ganglion with C8 and T1 spinal roots. Importantly, the sympathetic nerves to head and neck arise from the first thoracic segment. Thus, injuries to the T1 nerve root may result in ipsilateral Horner syndrome (miosis, ptosis, and anhidrosis). Just distal to the entry point of the gray rami, the cervical spinal nerves branch to form an anterior and posterior primary ramus. The nerve fibers in the posterior primary ramus innervate the paraspinal muscles, while the anterior primary rami of C5–T1 cervical spinal nerves form the brachial plexus (Fig. 23-3).

A dermatome refers to the cutaneous region supplied by a specific spinal nerve root segment (Fig. 23-4). Notably, there is some overlap of the cutaneous innervation by individual spinal nerves. The motor fibers emanating from the anterior horn cells, which course through the ventral root, spinal root, brachial plexus, and finally individual nerves, innervate specific muscle groups. Most muscles are supplied by motor nerves arising from at least two spinal cord segments (e.g., the deltoid muscle is innervated by motor fibers within the C5 and C6 spinal roots).

BRACHIAL PLEXUS

The brachial plexus is composed of three trunks (upper, middle, and lower), with two divisions (anterior and posterior)

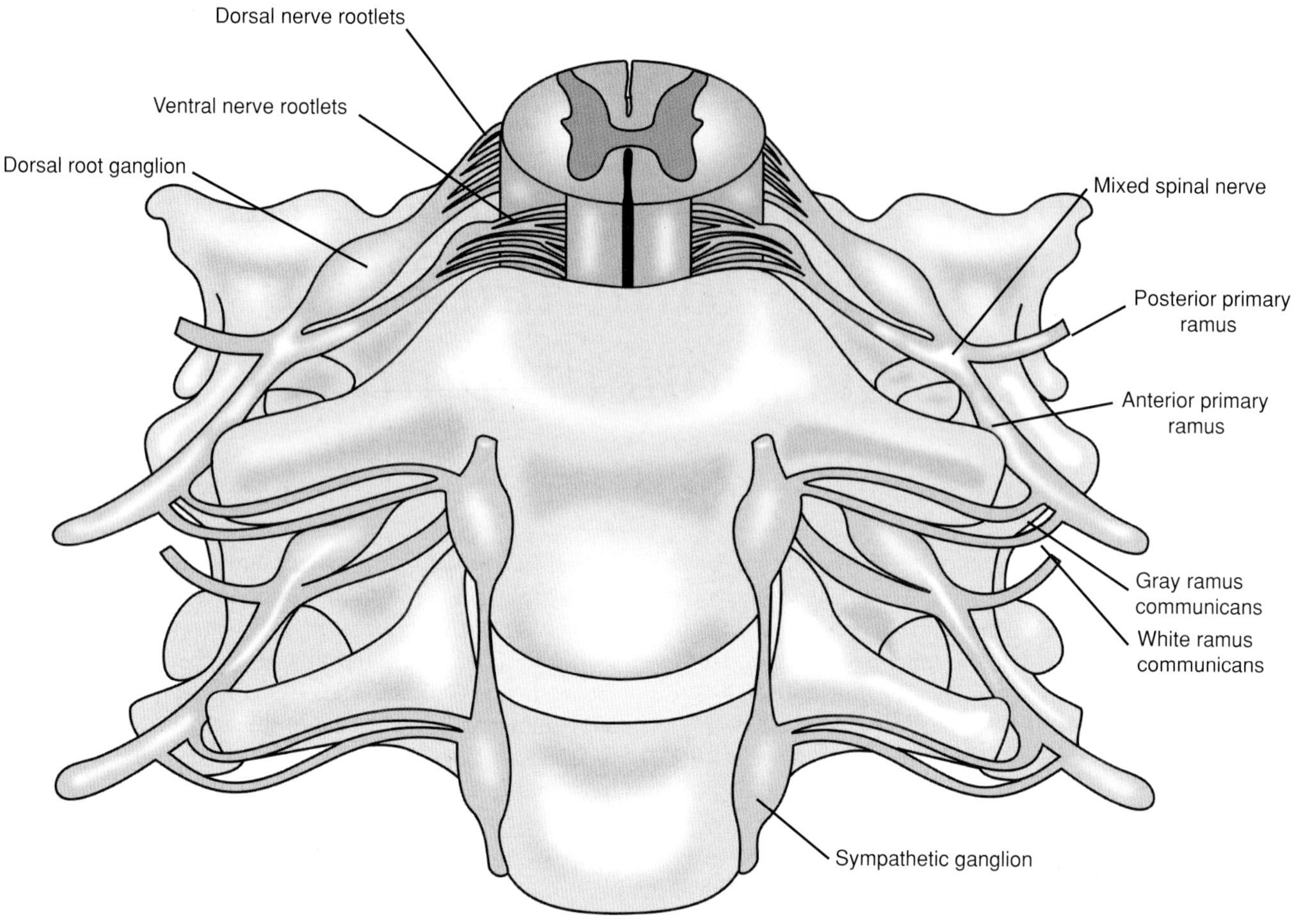

Figure 23-1. The spinal cord is depicted with multiple ventral and dorsal rootlets joining to form the mixed spinal nerve root. Communications between the sympathetic ganglia and the spinal nerves are appreciated, and the gray and white rami are seen as well. (Reproduced with permission from Ferrante MA. Brachial plexopathies: classification, causes, and consequences. *Muscle Nerve*. 2004;30(5):547–568.)

per trunk. Subsequently, the trunks divide into three cords (medial, lateral, and posterior), and from these arise the multiple terminal nerves innervating the arm (Table 23-1, Fig. 23-4).[1-3] More specifically, the anterior primary rami of C5 and C6 fuse to form the upper trunk; the anterior primary ramus of C7 continues as the middle trunk, while the anterior rami of C8 and T1 join to form the lower trunk. Of note, in approximately 62% of anatomic dissections of the brachial plexus, the C4 spinal nerve contributes to the upper trunk.[1,4] In this situation, the brachial plexus is said to be a "prefixed plexus," in which all of the spinal nerve contributions usually are shifted up one level. As a result, the contribution from the T1 spinal segment to the lower trunk of the brachial plexus may be minimal. In contrast, in approximately 7% of anatomic dissections of the brachial plexus, C5 contributes minimally to the brachial plexus, a so-called "postfixed plexus."[1] In such cases, the spinal nerve contributions may be shifted down by one level; therefore, C7 contributes to the upper trunk while the lower trunk might receive nerves from the T2 spinal segment. However, the frequency of contributions of C4 and T2 to the brachial plexus is controversial, based on surgical explorations in patients following trauma.[1,5]

The anterior divisions of the upper and middle trunks fuse to form the lateral cord, while the anterior division of the lower trunk continues as the medial cord. The three posterior divisions of the upper, middle, and lower trunks join forming the posterior cord. The designations medial, lateral, and posterior cords refer to their respective anatomic positions relative to the axillary artery. The cords constitute the longest subsections of the brachial plexus.[6] There is some anatomic variation and communication between nerve fibers running between the different cords.[1,4]For example, some nerve fibers may exit the lateral cord and join the medial cord. Thus, the ulnar nerve may have contributions from the C7 spinal nerve.

TERMINAL NERVES

The terminal nerves arise from the brachial plexus and may be purely sensory, motor, or mixed sensorimotor

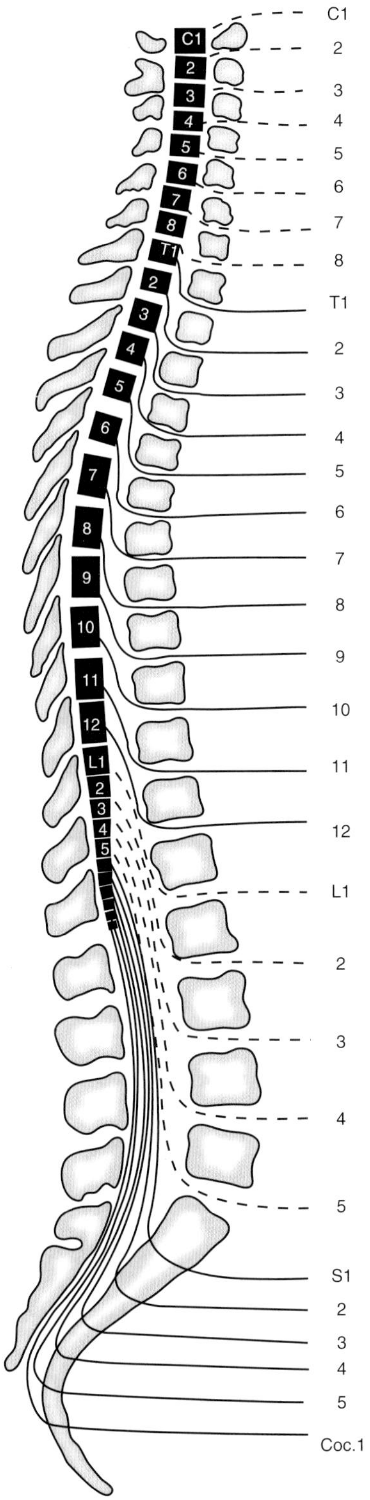

Figure 23-2. A sagittal section of the adult spinal column is depicted with the spinal cord demarcated by individual neural segments. Note the anatomic discrepancy between the termination of the spinal cord and vertebral column. The disparity between the spinal cord's neural segment and associated bony level with respect to spinal nerve exit is also shown. (Modified with permission from Haymaker W, Woodhall B. Peripheral Nerve Injuries: *Principles of Diagnosis*. Philadelphia, PA: WB Saunders; 1953.)

(Fig. 23-3). The dorsal scapular nerve, long thoracic nerve, and a branch to the phrenic nerve arise directly from the spinal roots. The only two terminal nerves arising from the trunks are the subclavian and suprascapular nerves, and these both leave from the upper trunk. No terminal nerves come directly from the middle and lower trunk. The upper and lower subscapular and thoracodorsal nerves depart from the posterior cord, while the posterior cord terminates as the axillary and radial nerves. From the proximal aspect of the medial cord arises a single motor branch innervating the pectoral muscle, the medial pectoral nerve. The purely sensory medial brachial and medial antebrachial cutaneous nerves originate from the distal aspect of the medial cord. The medial cord terminates by sending a medial branch to the median nerve with the remnant continuing as the ulnar nerve. The lateral pectoral nerve comes off the proximal portion of the lateral cord. The lateral cord terminates as the musculocutaneous nerve and a lateral branch that joins a branch from the medial cord to form the median nerve. Individual terminal nerves are discussed in more detail below.

Spinal Accessory Nerve

Although not a nerve arising from the brachial plexus, the spinal accessory nerve or cranial nerve XI courses through the neck and shoulder region and is often affected in brachial plexus injuries. The nerve consists of a bulbar or accessory component that arises from the medulla and a spinal portion that arises from the anterior horn cells in the cervical cord down to C6. The nerves from the bulbar origin supply the soft palate and contribute to the recurrent laryngeal and possibly parasympathetic fibers, which then merge into the vagal nerve to the heart. The spinal component ascends between the ligamentum denticulatum and posterior spinal nerve roots, enters the cranium through the foramen magnum, and then exits the skull via the jugular foramen. The nerve descends posterior to the digastric and stylohyoid muscles to the sternocleidomastoid muscle, which it innervates, and terminates in the trapezius muscle, which it also supplies.

Terminal Nerves Arising from Cervical Roots

Phrenic Nerve

The phrenic nerve is derived primarily from the C4 spinal nerve, but C3 and C5 roots may also contribute (Fig. 23-3). The phrenic nerve crosses the anterior scalene and enters the thorax, where it innervates the diaphragm.

Dorsal Scapular Nerve

The dorsal scapular nerve usually arises directly from the C5 spinal nerve shortly after it exits the intervertebral foramen (Fig. 23-5). The nerve courses between the middle and posterior scalene musculature and innervates the major and minor rhomboid muscles and the levator scapulae.

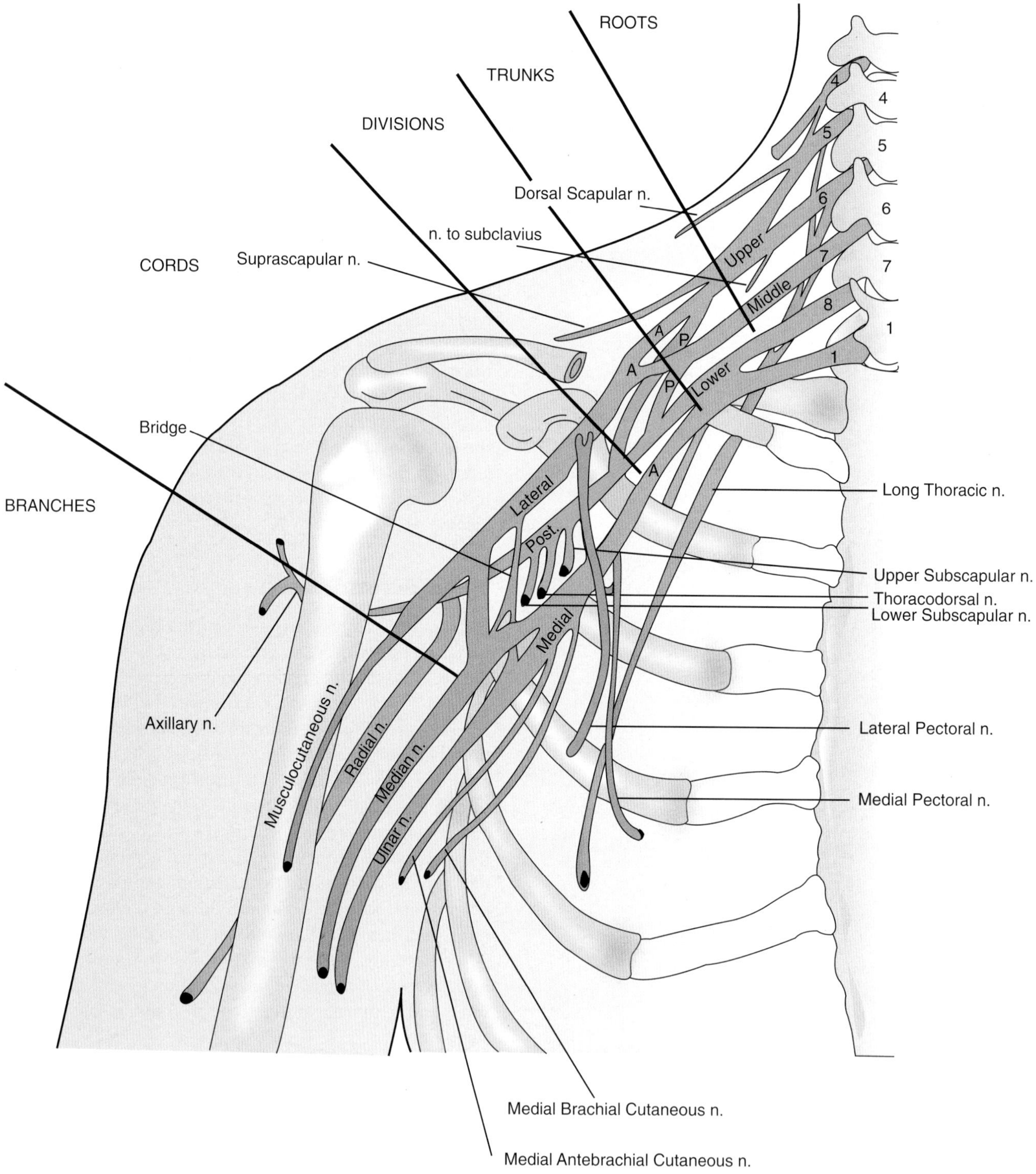

Figure 23-3. Diagrammatic representation of the brachial plexus (trunks, cords, and divisions) as well as its terminal nerves are depicted. A, anterior division; P, posterior division; n, nerve. (Modified with permission from Dumitru D, Zwarts MJ. Brachial plexopathies and proximal mononeuropathies. A, anterior division; P, posterior division; n, nerve. In: Dumitru D, Amato AA, Zwarts MJ, eds. *Electrodiagnostic Medicine*. 2nd ed. Philadelphia: Hanley & Belfus; 2002.)

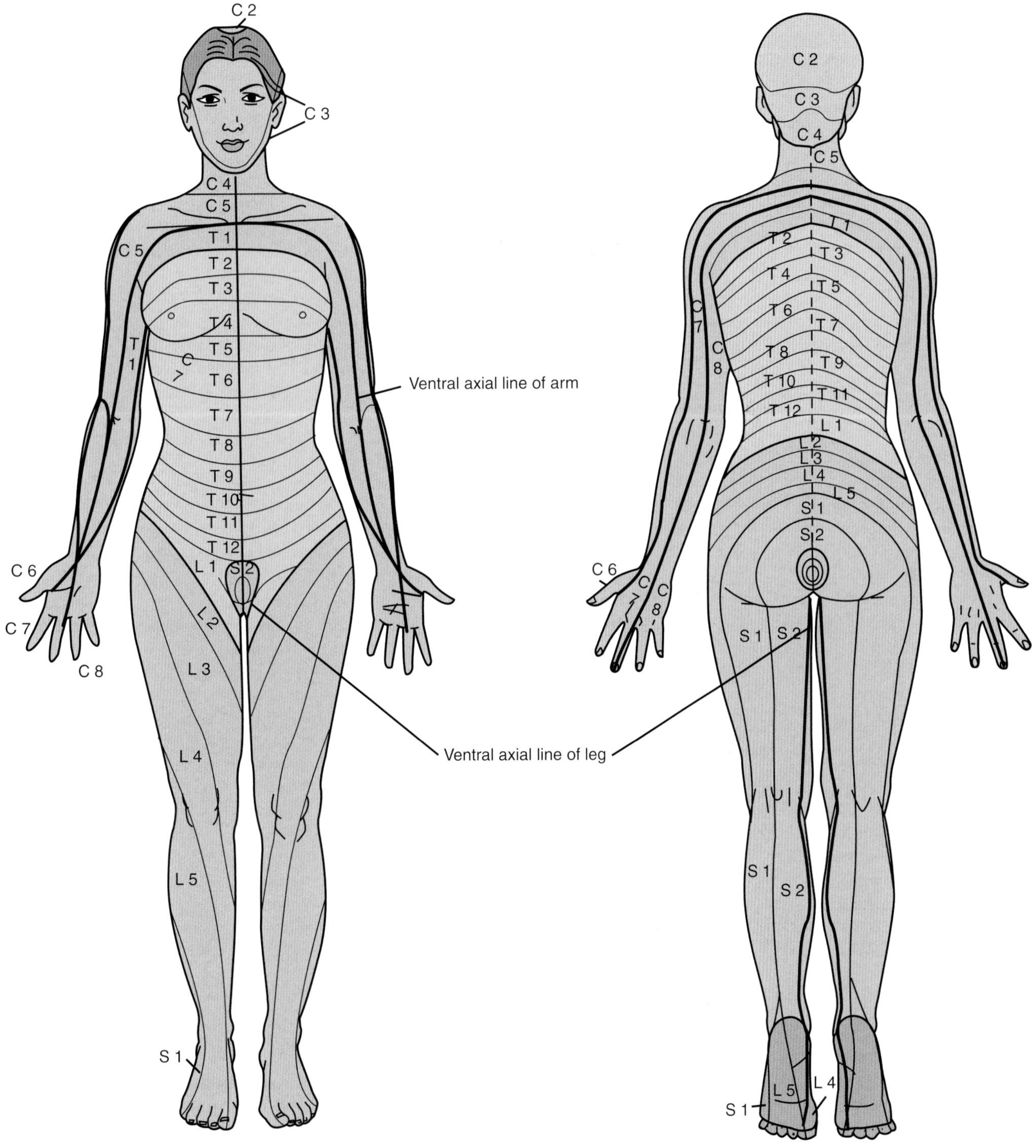

Figure 23-4. Dermatomal representation. (Modified with permission from Keegan JJ, Garret FD. Segmental distribution of the cutaneous nerves in the limbs of man. *Anat Rec*. 1948;102(4):409–437.)

Long Thoracic Nerve

Branches arising from the C5, C6, and C7 spinal nerves join forming the long thoracic nerve. The nerve descends to the lateral chest wall, where it innervates the serratus anterior muscle.

Terminal Nerves Arising from Trunks

Suprascapular Nerve

The suprascapular nerve arises from the upper trunk shortly after it is formed (Fig. 23-3). The nerve descends posteriorly between the omohyoid and the trapezius muscles. In

▶ TABLE 23-1. **INNERVATION OF THE MUSCLES IN THE UPPER LIMB**

Muscle	Root(s)	Trunk	Cord	Nerve
Trapezius				Spinal accessory (cranial nerve XI)
Rhomboid major and minor	(C4), C5			Dorsal scapular
Serratus anterior	C5, C6, C7			Long thoracic
Supraspinatus/infraspinatus	C5, C6	Upper		Suprascapular
Pectoralis major	C5, C6	Upper/middle	Lateral	Lateral pectoral
Pectoralis major and minor	C7, C8, T1	Lower	Medial	Medial pectoral
Latissimus dorsi	C6, C7, C8	Upper/middle/lower	Posterior	Thoracodorsal
Teres major	C5, C6, C7	Upper/middle	Posterior	Lower subscapular
Teres minor	C5, C6	Upper	Posterior	Axillary
Deltoid	C5, C6	Upper	Posterior	Axillary
Brachioradialis	C5, C6	Upper	Posterior	Radial
Biceps brachii	C5, C6	Upper	Lateral	Musculocutaneous
Brachialis	C5, C6	Upper	Lateral/(posterior)	Musculocutaneous/(radial)
Triceps	C6, C7, C8	Upper/middle/lower	Posterior	Radial
Anconeus	C7, C8	Middle/lower	Posterior	Radial
Supinator	C7, C8	Middle/lower	Posterior	Posterior interosseous
Extensor carpi radialis	C6, C7	Middle/lower	Posterior	Radial
Extensor carpi ulnaris	C6, C7, C8	Upper/middle/lower	Posterior	Posterior interosseous
Extensor digitorum communis	C7, C8	Middle/lower	Posterior	Posterior interosseous
Extensor indicis proprius	C7, C8	Middle/lower	Posterior	Posterior interosseous
Extensor pollicis	C7, C8	Middle/lower	Posterior	Posterior interosseous
Pronator teres	C6, C7	Middle/lower	Lateral/medial	Median
Flexor digitorum superficialis	C7, C8, T1	Middle/lower	Lateral/medial	Median
Flexor digitorum profundus I and II	C7, C8, T1	Middle/lower	Lateral/medial	Anterior interosseous (median)
Flexor digitorum profundus III and IV	C7, C8, T1	Middle/lower	Lateral/medial	Ulnar
Flexor carpi radialis	C6, C7, (C8)	Middle/lower	Lateral/medial	Median
Flexor carpi ulnaris	C7, C8, T1	(Middle)/lower	(Lateral)/medial	Ulnar
Flexor policis longus	(C7), C8, T1	(Middle)/lower	(Lateral)/medial	Anterior interosseous (median)
Pronator quadratus	C8, T1	Lower	Medial	Anterior interosseous (median)
Abductor pollicis brevis	C8, T1	Lower	Medial	Median
Adductor pollicis	C8, T1	Lower	Medial	Ulnar
Opponens pollicis	C8, T1	Lower	Medial	Median
Abductor digiti minimi	C8, T1	Lower	Medial	Ulnar
Dorsal and volar interossei	C8, T1	Lower	Medial	Ulnar
First and 2nd lumbrical	C8, T1	Lower	Medial	Median
Third and 4th lumbrical	C8, T1	Lower	Medial	Ulnar

In parentheses are roots, trunks, cords, or nerves that may have mild contribution to innervation of the muscle group in some patients.

the posterior shoulder, it courses through the suprascapular notch under the scapula's superior transverse ligament to innervate the supraspinatus muscle, then through the spinoglenoid notch to innervate the infraspinatus muscle (Fig. 23-5).

Nerve to the Subclavius

This is a small nerve that arises from the C5 root or upper trunk, which innervates the small subclavius muscle that runs between the clavicle and first rib.

Terminal Nerves Arising from Cords

Medial Pectoral Nerves

The medial pectoral nerve arises from the medial trunk (Fig. 23-3). This nerve innervates both the pectoralis major and the pectoralis minor muscles. The major spinal contributions to this nerve are C8 and T1.

Lateral Pectoral Nerves

The lateral pectoral nerve innervates the pectoralis major. It usually comes from the lateral cord, but occasionally arises from the anterior division of the upper and middle trunks just prior to the formation of the lateral cord. This anatomic variation may explain the observation that in plexus injuries affecting the medial and lateral cords resulting in a flail arm, the strength of the pectoralis major muscle may be relatively preserved. The major spinal contributions of this nerve are C5–7.

Subscapular Nerves

The upper and lower subscapular nerves originate from the posterior cord in the axilla. The upper subscapular nerve

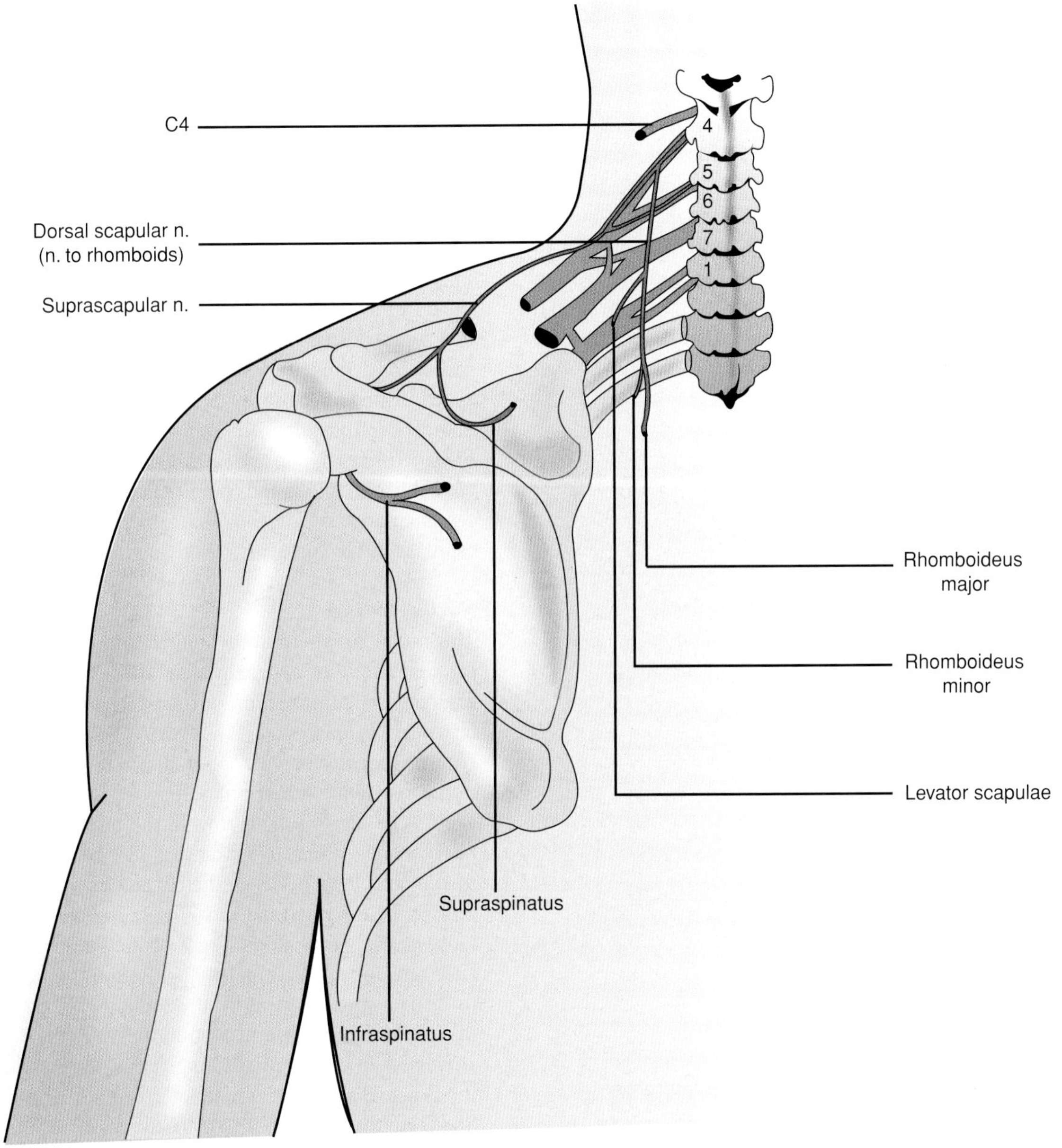

Figure 23-5. The posterior aspect of the thorax is shown, with the dorsal scapular and suprascapular nerves coursing to their respective muscles. The suprascapular nerve passes beneath the suprascapular notch (not depicted) as well as around the spinoglenoid notch, which are two potential areas of compromise. (Modified with permission from Haymaker W, Woodhall B. *Peripheral Nerve Injuries: Principles of Diagnosis*. Philadelphia, PA: WB Saunders; 1953.)

innervates the subscapularis muscle, while the lower subscapular nerve supplies subscapularis and the teres major muscle. The major spinal contributions to this nerve are from C5 and C6.

Thoracodorsal Nerve

The thoracodorsal nerve, also known as the middle subscapular nerve, comes off the posterior cord and innervates the latissimus dorsi muscle. This nerve can also arise in some cases from the radial and axillary nerves.[4] The major spinal nerves contributing to the thoracodorsal nerve are C5–7, particularly C7.

Medial Cutaneous Nerve of the Arm

The medial cutaneous nerve of the arm (medial brachial cutaneous nerve) originates from the medial cord and supplies sensation to the medial aspect of the arm. Its primary contribution comes from the C8 and T1 spinal nerves.

Medial Cutaneous Nerve of the Forearm

The medial cutaneous nerve of the forearm (medial antebrachial cutaneous nerve) usually projects from the medial cord, but it may arise from the medial cutaneous nerve of the arm.[4] The nerve supplies sensation from the medial forearm and also originates from the C8 and T1 spinal nerves.

Musculocutaneous Nerve

The lateral cord terminates as a bifurcation resulting in the musculocutaneous nerve and a lateral branch that combines with a branch from the medial cord to form the median nerve (Fig. 23-6). In about 5% of individuals, the musculocutaneous nerve originates from the anterior division of the upper trunk, in which case the lateral root to the median nerve arises from the middle trunk only.[4] The major spinal nerves contributing to the musculocutaneous nerve are C5 and C6. In addition, C7 contributes to this nerve in at least half but less than two-thirds of cadavers examined.[4] The musculocutaneous nerve innervates the coracobrachialis, biceps brachii, and brachialis muscles. It terminates as the lateral cutaneous nerve of the forearm, supplying sensation to the lateral aspect of the volar surface of the forearm.

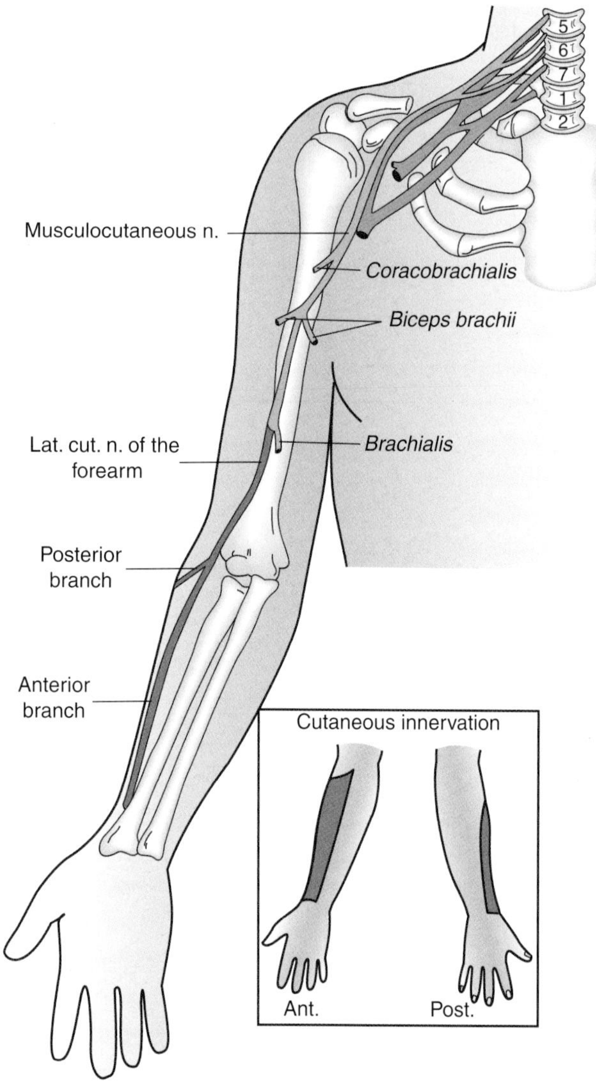

Figure 23-6. The musculocutaneous nerve is the termination of the lateral cord and supplies the coracobrachialis, biceps brachii, and brachialis muscles. It terminates as the lateral antebrachial cutaneous nerve, which splits into two cutaneous branches to supply the radial aspect of the forearm. (Modified with permission from Haymaker W, Woodhall B. *Peripheral Nerve Injuries: Principles of Diagnosis*. Philadelphia, PA: WB Saunders; 1953.)

Axillary Nerve

The axillary nerve contains portions of the spinal nerves arising from C5 and C6 and is one of the two terminal branches of the posterior cord (Fig. 23-7). The nerve usually originates near the subscapularis muscle posterior to the pectoralis minor muscle and then traverses the quadrangular or quadrilateral space formed inferiorly by teres major, laterally by the long head of the triceps brachii, medially by the humerus, and superiorly by the teres minor. Upon exiting this space, the axillary nerve innervates the teres minor and deltoid muscles. The axillary nerve also sends cutaneous branches that supply sensation to the lateral aspect of the proximal arm overlying the deltoid muscle.

Radial Nerve

The radial nerve contains contributions from mainly C5–8 (as well as T1 in approximately 10% of individuals) and, in essence, is a continuation of the posterior cord after the axillary nerve branches off (Fig. 23-8).[1,7] While still in the axillary region, a posterior cutaneous nerve branches off the radial nerve to provide sensation to the posterior aspect of the upper arm to the level of the elbow. In the proximal arm, the radial nerve travels medial to the humerus and descends between the medial and long heads of the triceps muscle along the spiral groove. In the proximal arm, the radial nerve innervates the long, medial, and lateral heads of the triceps brachii and the anconeus muscles. Upon leaving the spiral groove in the mid- to distal aspect of the arm, the radial nerve courses down to the lateral aspect of the arm and innervates the brachioradialis and extensor carpi radialis longus as well as a small branch to the brachialis muscle, the latter receiving its main contribution from the musculocutaneous nerve. An additional branch, the posterior antebrachial cutaneous nerve, separates from the radial nerve in the mid-arm region and descends to supply sensation to the posterior aspect of the forearm.

In the elbow region, the radial nerve splits to form the purely sensory superficial radial nerve and the purely motor posterior interosseous nerve. In this area is the so-called radial tunnel bound by the radius, the capsule of the radiocapitellar joint, the brachialis and biceps brachii tendons (forming the medial walls), and the brachioradialis, extensor carpi radialis, and extensor carpi ulnaris muscles (forming the lateral and anterior walls). The radial tunnel ends at the fibrous band around the superficial head of the supinator muscle, which is known as the arcade of Fröhse. The superficial radial nerve travels on the undersurface of the brachioradialis, outside the radial tunnel, into the forearm. Around the mid-forearm, the nerve moves more superficially and travels along the extensor aspect of the distal forearm. After the superficial radial nerve passes the wrist, it supplies sensation to the lateral, extensor

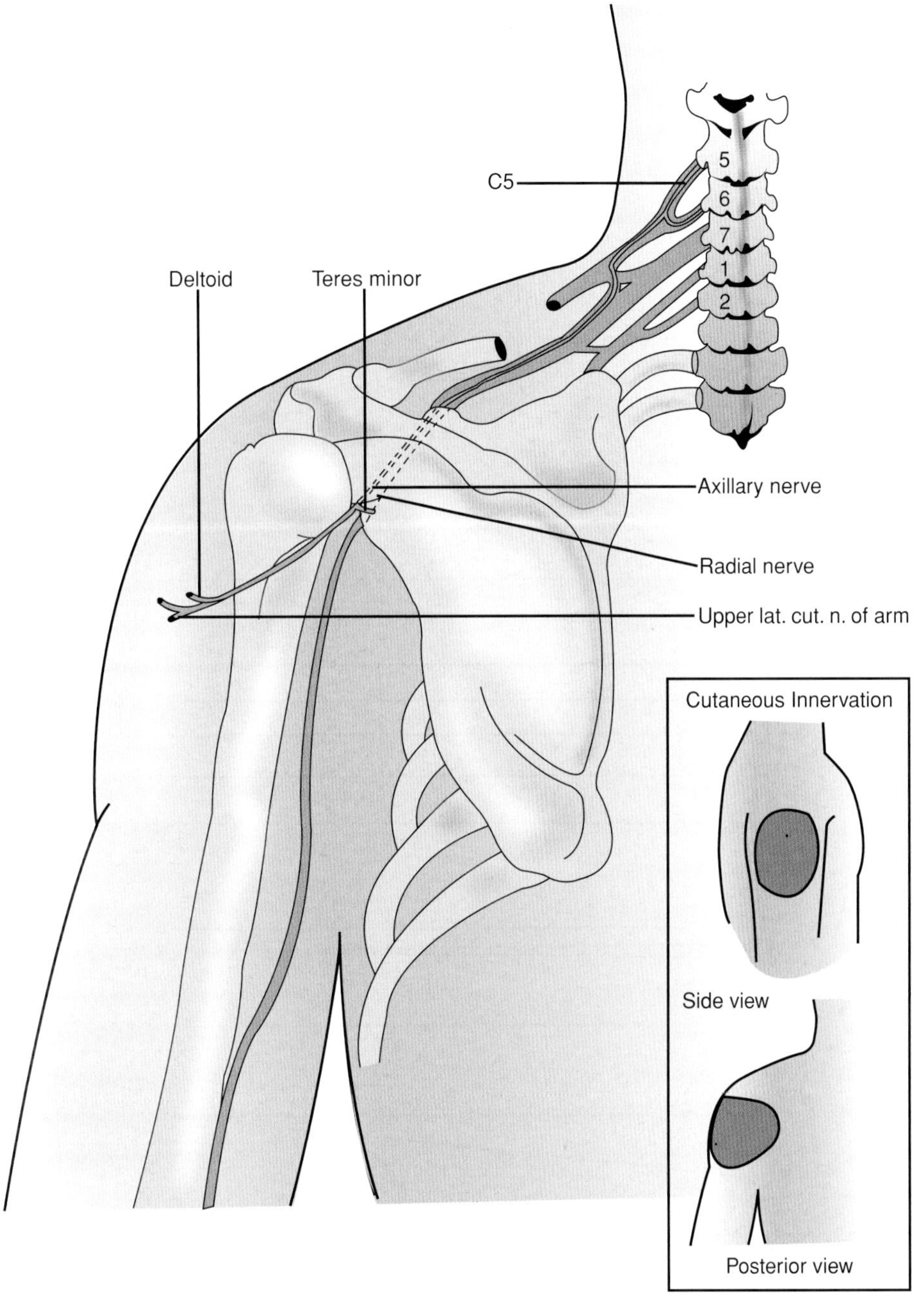

Figure 23-7. One of the terminal branches of the posterior cord is the axillary nerve. It supplies both the teres minor and the deltoid muscles as well as providing cutaneous sensation to the skin overlying the deltoid muscle (upper lateral cutaneous nerve of the arm). (Modified with permission from Haymaker W, Woodhall B. *Peripheral Nerve Injuries: Principles of Diagnosis*. Philadelphia, PA: WB Saunders; 1953.)

surface of the hand and fingers, analogous to the median distribution on the palmar surface (except the distal aspects of the fingertips on the dorsal surface which are supplied by the median nerve). The posterior interosseous nerve traverses the radial tunnel and then descends under the arcade of Fröhse. The posterior interosseous nerve continues down the extensor aspect of the forearm. Along the way it innervates the supinator, extensor digitorum communis, extensor carpi radialis brevis, extensor digiti minimi, extensor carpi ulnaris, abductor pollicis longus, extensor pollicis longus and brevis, and the extensor indicis proprius.

Median Nerve

The median nerve is formed by the fusion of branches from the lateral and medial cords (Fig. 23-9). The main spinal nerve contributions to the median nerve are C6–T1. Motor fibers arise from C6–T1 spinal segments, while sensory fibers are derived primarily from the C6 and C7 segments. Occasionally,

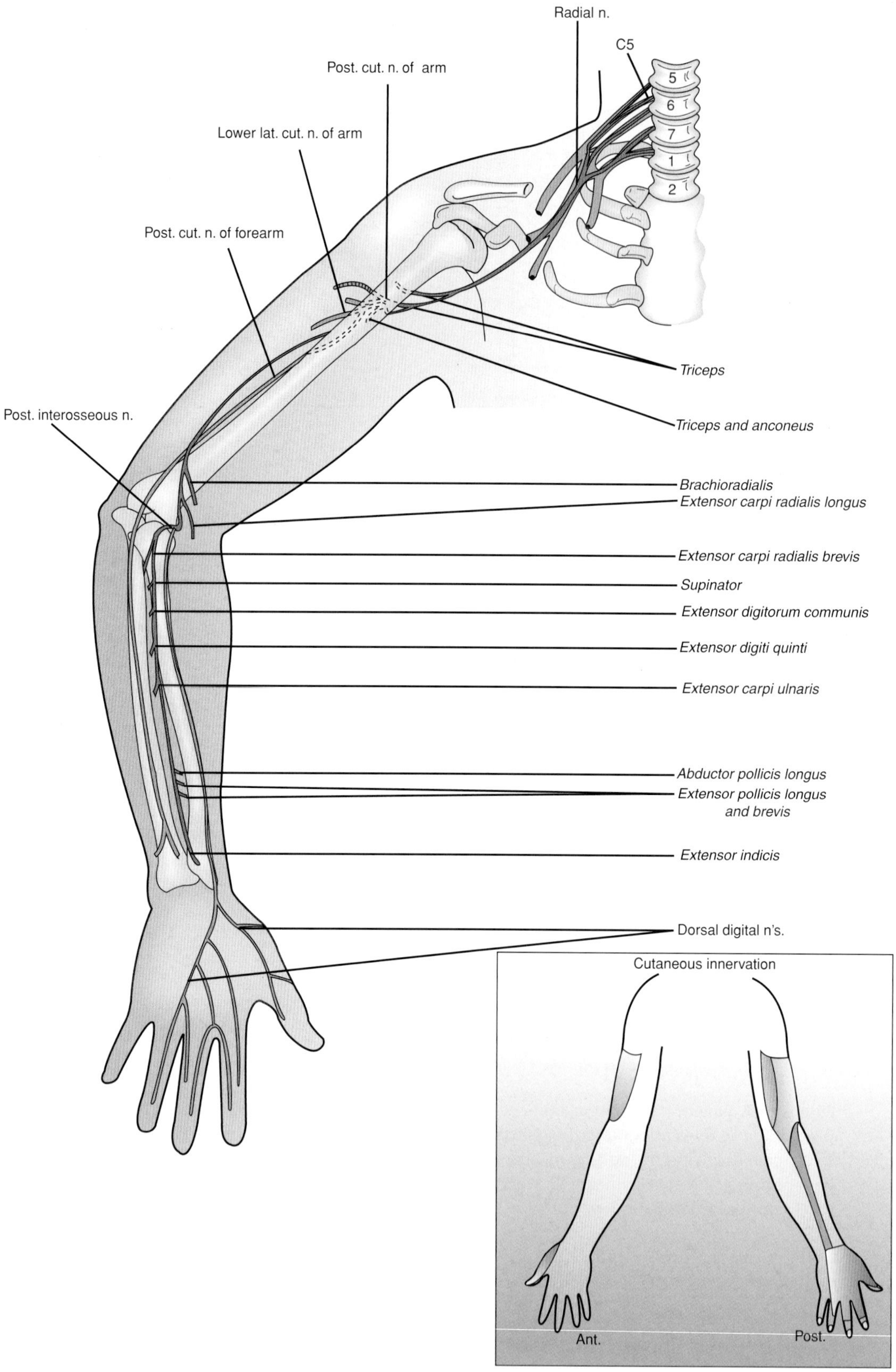

Figure 23-8. The course and muscular innervation of the radial nerve is depicted. In the axilla and proximal arm, the triceps muscle is innervated, and the three sensory branches originate. Sensory disturbances can help localize a lesion at or proximal to the spiral groove. (Modified with permission from Haymaker W, Woodhall B. *Peripheral Nerve Injuries: Principles of Diagnosis*. Philadelphia, PA: WB Saunders; 1953.)

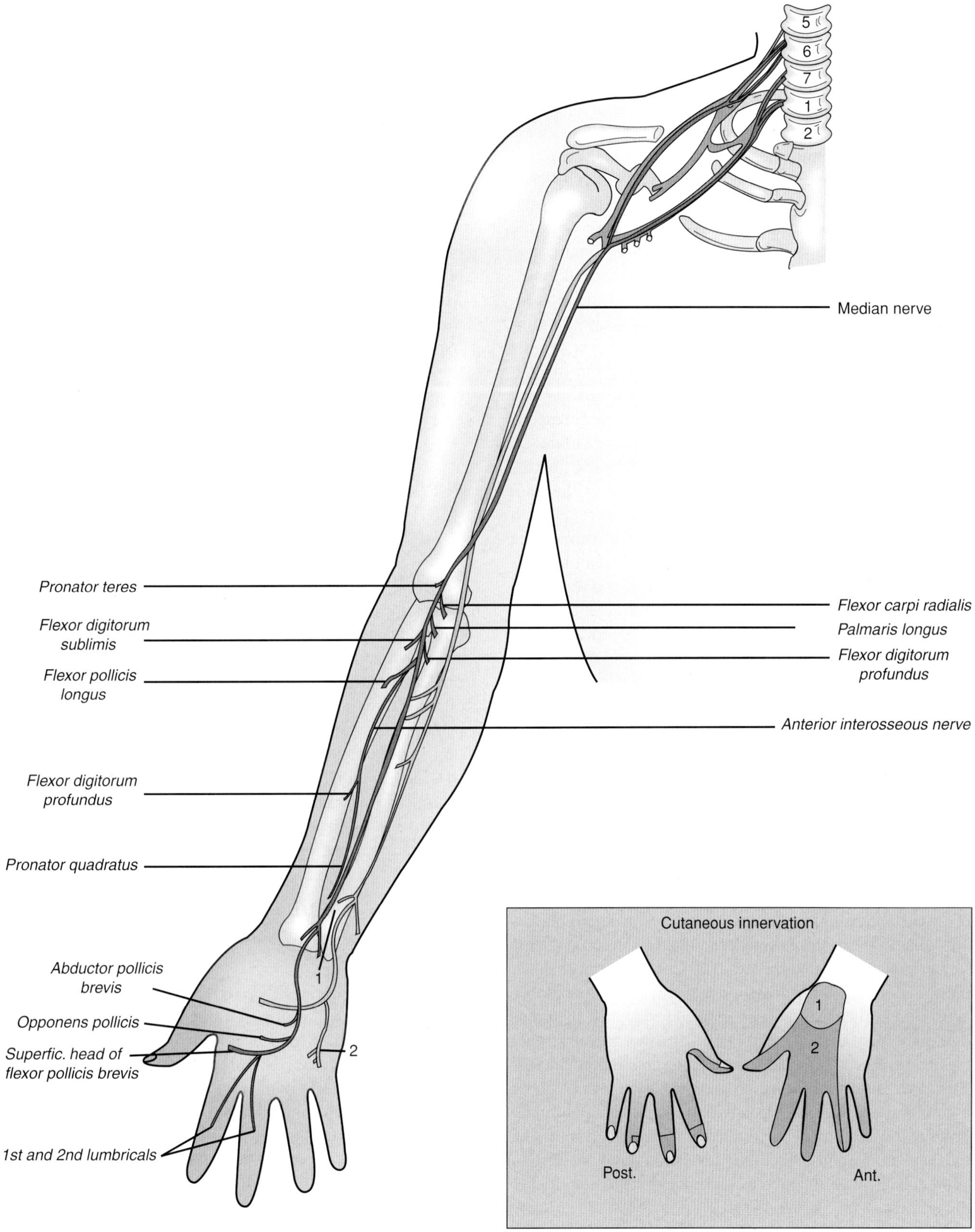

Figure 23-9. There are no muscular or cutaneous branches arising from the median nerve in the axillary region or arm. The first branch originating from the median nerve is to the pronator teres in the proximal forearm. (Modified with permission from Haymaker W, Woodhall B. *Peripheral Nerve Injuries: Principles of Diagnosis*. Philadelphia, PA: WB Saunders; 1953.)

C5 can also contribute to the median nerve.[1] The sensory fibers travel through the upper and middle trunks to the lateral cord into the median nerve, while the motor fibers pass through all the trunks as well as the medial and lateral cords.

The median nerve descends in the anterior compartment of the arm on the medial side to the antecubital fossa region. Past the elbow, the median nerve courses through the two heads of the pronator teres muscle and then between the flexor digitorum superficialis and profundus muscles to the wrist. In the forearm, the median nerve innervates the pronator teres, flexor carpi radialis, palmaris longus, and flexor digitorum superficialis muscles. In the upper to mid-forearm level, the anterior interosseous nerve branches from the main median nerve. This is a pure motor nerve that supplies the flexor digitorum profundus 1 and 2, flexor pollicis longus, and pronator quadratus muscle. The main median nerve trunk continues distally down the forearm to the wrist. Just before entering the carpal tunnel, the palmar cutaneous branch arises to supply sensation over the thenar eminence. The nerve then enters the carpal tunnel bounded by the carpal bones with the transverse ligament serving as the roof. Also within the carpal tunnel lie the nine flexor tendons to the fingers. Within or just distal to the carpal tunnel, the recurrent branch of the median nerve arises and innervates the abductor pollicis brevis, opponens pollicis, and the superficial head of the flexor pollicis brevis. The terminal branches of the median nerve supply the first and second lumbrical muscles, while the digital branches provide sensation to the volar aspects (and the tips of the dorsal aspects) of the thumb, index, and middle fingers, and the lateral half the ring finger.

Ulnar Nerve

The ulnar nerve arises at the termination of the medial cord distal to the medial cutaneous nerves of the arm and forearm and the medial branch of the median nerve (Fig. 23-10). The spinal nerve contributions are mainly C8 and T1, but C7 fibers may also be present in 43–92% of cases, as suggested by brachial plexus dissections.[1,4] The C7 contribution derives from a branch of the lateral cord and innervates the flexor carpi ulnaris muscle. The ulnar nerve descends anterior to the teres major and latissimus dorsi muscles into the arm. Then the nerve travels down the posterior compartment of the upper arm to the ulnar groove at the elbow. The ulnar groove is formed by the medial epicondyle of the humerus and the olecranon process of the ulna, with the ulnar collateral ligament serving as the floor. Approximately 1.0–2.5 cm distal to the ulnar groove, the nerve traverses under a fibrous aponeurotic arch connecting the humeral and ulnar heads of the flexor carpi ulnaris muscle. The area encompassing the ulnar groove and aponeurotic arch is commonly referred to as the cubital tunnel. Of note, the ulnar nerve yields no branches in the arm proximal to the elbow.

Distal to the elbow, the ulnar nerve travels between the flexor carpi ulnaris and flexor digitorum profundus muscles descending to the wrist. In the forearm, it innervates the flexor carpi ulnaris and the flexor digitorum profundus III and IV muscles. The dorsal ulnar cutaneous nerve originates in the mid or distal forearm to provide sensation to the dorsum of the medial aspect of the hand and fourth and fifth digits. Just before entering Guyon's canal at the wrist, the palmar branch arises to provide sensation to the hypothenar eminence and motor innervation to the palmaris brevis muscle. The remaining components of the ulnar nerve travel into Guyon's canal, formed by the hook of the hamate bone (on the radial aspect), the pisiform bone (on the ulnar aspect), the pisohamate ligament (serves as the floor), and the transverse carpal ligament (serves as the roof). Within or just distal to Guyon's canal, the ulnar nerve splits into its terminal branches. A superficial terminal branch supplies sensation to the palmar aspect of the little finger and half of the ring finger, plus some of the distal aspects of these digits dorsally. A deep motor branch innervates the hypothenar muscles and then turns and continues across the hand to innervate the third and fourth lumbricals, interossei, adductor pollicis, and deep head of the flexor pollicis brevis muscle.

▶ PATHOPHYSIOLOGY OF RADICULOPATHIES, PLEXOPATHIES, AND MONONEUROPATHIES

Before discussing the approach to patients with focal nerve lesions in the arm, it is important to understand the pathophysiologic basis of these neuropathies. Clinicians need to be aware of the mechanisms of nerve injury so that they can plan, time, and interpret the electrodiagnostic evaluation in order to offer the most accurate prognoses and treatment options. The pathophysiologic bases of nerve injury are limited: demyelination, conduction block, or axonal degeneration. The method by which an individual nerve is injured (e.g., gun shot wound to upper arm, prolonged hyperextension of the arm during surgery, and falling asleep on arm) often provides insight into the underlying pathophysiology.

TYPES OF NERVE FIBER DAMAGE

Neuropraxia

The term "neuropraxia," also known as first-degree injury, refers to neuronal dysfunction due to transient conduction block.[1,8–10] In regard to focal peripheral nerve lesions, neuropraxia may arise from ischemia or demyelination. Compression of a nerve can result in segmental ischemia, which if of only short duration, results in a rapidly reversible physiologic conduction block lasting minutes or perhaps a few hours. However, experimental studies suggest that pressure related to compression on the nerve can result in distortion of the underlying nerve segment with paranodal and then segmental demyelination.[11] Neuropraxia due to demyelination may resolve after several weeks following remyelination of the nerve segment. Thus, prognosis in lesions associated with only conduction block resulting from mechanical (as opposed to immune-mediated or radiation) mechanisms without secondary axonal loss is excellent.

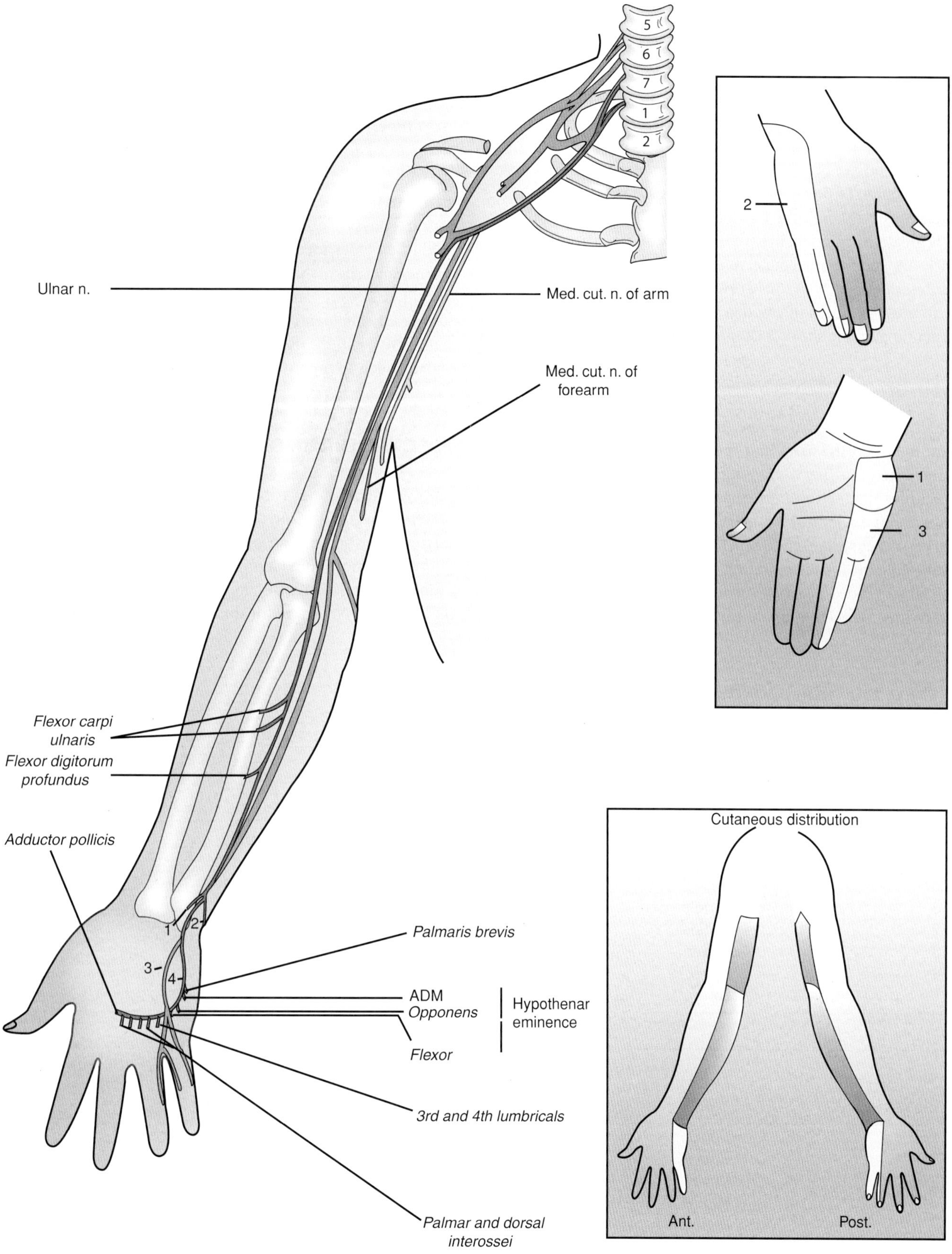

Figure 23-10. The ulnar nerve does not have any motor or cutaneous branches in the arm. ADM, abductor digiti minimi. The cutaneous branches of the medial cutaneous nerves of the arm and forearm are depicted. (Modified with permission from Haymaker W, Woodhall B. *Peripheral Nerve Injuries: Principles of Diagnosis*. Philadelphia, PA: WB Saunders; 1953.)

Axonotmesis

Axonotmesis or second-degree injury refers to nerve injuries in which the axon is interrupted but the epineurium is intact.[1,8–10] Following this type of nerve injury, the axon distal to the lesion, now separated from its cell body, will degenerate over the next 7–10 days. Subsequently, regenerating nerve sprouts emerge from the proximal stump of the sectioned nerve to attempt reinnervation of previously denervated tissues (e.g., muscle or cutaneous skin). Because the endoneurium is preserved, there is a greater likelihood that the regenerating axons can grow back and reinnervate denervated tissues than in neurotmesis described below. Axons grow back at a rate of 1 mm/d, so restoration of function can take many months to over a year, depending on the site of the lesion and length of the nerve.

Neurotmesis

Neurotmesis refers to severe, often penetrating nerve injuries, in which the axon and the supporting epineurium are interrupted (i.e., nerve transaction).[1,8–10] Present technology precludes distinction between axonotmesis and neurotmesis without exploratory surgery and direct inspection of the nerve. Because the endoneurium is also interrupted, it is more difficult for regenerating nerve sprouts to reinnervate the target tissues. Scarring secondary to the disruption of the overlying connective tissue can also impede reinnervation. Regenerating nerves may become entwined with the scar tissue creating a neuroma. Thus, the prognosis for spontaneous recovery following this type of lesion is poor.

▶ APPROACH TO PATIENTS

As with other neuromuscular disorders, the most important step is trying to localize the site of the lesion based on the history and physical examination. Following this, electrodiagnostic studies are performed to confirm the localization or try to localize the exact site of the lesion more accurately, if not apparent by the clinical examination. Often radiologic studies are done to further assist in identifying the site of the lesion and the possible cause. We begin the discussion of the approach of such patients with a review of electrodiagnostic studies that can be helpful.

ELECTRODIAGNOSTIC STUDIES

The evaluation of the arm for possible cervical radiculopathy, brachial plexopathy, or mononeuropathy(ies) requires performing sensory, motor, and mixed sensorimotor nerve conduction studies (NCS) along with electromyography (EMG) (Table 23-2). This text is not meant to be a "how-to book" on EMG and NCS, and for this we refer the reader to several

▶ TABLE 23-2. **NERVE CONDUCTION STUDIES**

Sensory Studies				
	Brachial Plexus			
Spinal Root	Trunk	Cord	Peripheral Nerve	
C6	Upper	Lateral	Lateral antebrachial cut.	
C6	Upper	Lateral	Median to first/second digit	
C6	Upper	Posterior	Radial to base of first digit	
C6	Middle	Lateral	Median to second digit	
C7	Middle	Lateral	Median to third digit	
C8	Lower	Medial	Ulnar to fifth digit	
C8	Lower	Medial	Dorsal ulnar cutaneous	
T1	Lower	Medial	Medial antebrachial cut.	
Motor Studies				
	Brachial Plexus			
Spinal Root	Trunk	Cord	Peripheral Nerve	Muscle
C5,C6	Upper	Lateral	Musculocutaneous	Biceps
C5,C6	Upper	Posterior	Axillary	Deltoid
C5,C6	Upper		Suprascapular	SS, IS
C7,C8	Middle	Posterior	Radial	EIP
C8,T1	Lower	Medial	Median	APB
C8,T1	Lower	Medial	Ulnar	ADM, FDI

Cut, cutaneous; SS, supraspinatus; IS, infraspinatus; FIP, extensor indicis proprius; ABP, abductor pollicis brevis; FDI, first dorsal interosseous; ADM, abductor digiti minimi.
Modified with permission from Wilbourn AJ. Electrodiagnosis of plexopathies. *Neurol Clin*. 1985;3:511–529.

excellent reference books regarding electrodiagnostic medicine (more details can also be obtained in Chapter 2 of this book).[6,12–15] However, clinicians taking care of patients with neuromuscular disorders need to be aware of the utility and limitations of these studies. The electrodiagnostic studies also need to be tailored to the individual patients depending on their symptoms and signs and as the results of the ongoing EMG and NCS are being analyzed.

Sensory NCS

Evaluating the sensory nerve action potentials (SNAPs) is important in distinguishing a radiculopathy from a more distal process. The lesion in most radiculopathies is proximal to the dorsal root ganglia (DRG). Because the cell bodies and distal axons are intact in cervical radiculopathies, the SNAPs should be normal. In contrast, in brachial plexopathies and mononeuropathies (in nerves with sensory fibers), in which the lesion is distal to the dorsal root ganglion, one would expect to see reduced amplitudes of SNAPs in the distribution of the affected nerve, provided there is significant axonal injury. In cases of a demyelinating lesion or conduction block (as the case in neuropraxic injuries), the SNAP distal to the site of the lesion is usually normal. When the injury to the plexus or peripheral nerve is axonal in nature, one also needs to remember that it takes several days from the time of the injury for Wallerian degeneration of the axons to occur distally. Thus, it takes approximately 7–10 days for the SNAPs to disappear, even if the nerve is completely severed. After this period of time there is sufficient degeneration of axons to begin to distinguish postganglionic axonal loss from conduction block/demyelination or a preganglionic lesion. However, an abnormal SNAP does not imply that the spinal root is normal. For example, in traumatic brachial plexopathies, avulsion of nerve root may occur concurrently with injury to nerve distal to the DRG.

It is very important to compare the SNAPs in the affected arm to the analogous nerves in the contralateral arm. It is possible that the SNAP amplitude(s) in an affected arm may still fall "within normal limits" for that electrodiagnostic laboratory even if injured. An asymptomatic limb provides better normative data for that individual than does normative data derived from populations. We, like most electrodiagnosticians, consider SNAP amplitude(s) less than half of that obtained from the analogous nerve in an asymptomatic limb to be abnormal. This of course is not helpful if the symptoms are bilateral.

The specific sensory studies performed are again dependent on the possibilities for the site of the lesion (Table 23-3).[16] If one is evaluating a patient with sensory symptoms affecting the thumb, the possibilities include a C6 radiculopathy, upper trunk, lateral cord, median or radial mononeuropathies, or injury to the digital branches of these nerves. The sensory studies most helpful would be a median SNAP from the thumb or index finger and the superficial radial SNAP, and perhaps the lateral antebrachial cutaneous SNAP. In addition, the median and ulnar mixed nerve palmar studies are helpful to look for carpal tunnel syndrome. As with all electrodiagnostic evaluations, it is important to define the boundaries of abnormality by identifying a normal response in a nerve that is not felt to be clinically affected (e.g., an ulnar SNAP in this situation). If the patient has symptoms involving little finger, then the investigator needs to conduct studies to differentiate a C8/T1 radiculopathy, lower trunk, medial cord, and ulnar neuropathy from one another.

Motor NCS

Evaluation of a motor nerve is performed by stimulating the nerves at several locations and recording the compound muscle action potential (CMAP) from accessible muscle bellies, as discussed in Chapter 2 (Table 23-3).[16] As with sensory studies, the majority of accessible motor stimulation sites are remote from the proximally located lesions associated with a radiculopathy or plexopathy. Thus, it is technically very difficult to assess for a demyelinating/conduction block lesion in these proximal sites. Further, most electrodiagnostic laboratories routinely perform median, ulnar, and radial motor conductions recording from muscles that innervated primarily by the C8–T1 segments. These motor studies are most useful in lower trunk and medial cord injuries as well as median, ulnar, or radial neuropathies. They are of limited value in pathology affecting the C5–7 segments or the elements of the brachial plexus through which these fibers descend. Motor conduction studies can assist in localizing the site and nature of the lesion (e.g., axonal or demyelinating/conduction block) involving testable nerves. Again, following an axonal lesion, one needs to wait about 7–10 days until Wallerian degeneration has occurred and CMAP amplitudes become reliably reduced. Furthermore, in demyelination/conduction block, one could identify this type of lesion

TABLE 23-3. CAUSES OF RADICULOPATHY

Herniated nucleus proposus
Degenerative joint disease
Rheumatoid arthritis
Trauma
Vertebral body compression fracture
Pott's disease
Compression by extradural mass (e.g., meningioma, metastatic tumor, hematoma, abscess)
Primary nerve tumor (e.g., neurofibroma, Schwanomma, neurioma)
Carcinomatous meningitis
Perineural spread of tumor (e.g., prostate cancer)
Acute inflammatory demyelinating polyradiculopathy
Chronic inflammatory demyelinating polyradiculopathy
Sarcoidosis
Amyloidoma
Diabetic radiculopathy
Infection (Lyme disease, Herpes Zoster, Cytomegalovirus, Syphilis, Strongyloides)

only by stimulating the nerve proximal and distal to the site of the lesion. Axillary CMAPs recorded from the deltoid or musculocutaneous CMAPs recorded from the biceps brachii are technically more difficult to perform and interpret and are limited by patient tolerance of the intensity of stimulus often required to achieve a supramaximal CMAP in deeply positioned nerves. In such cases, it would be important to study the contralateral asymptomatic side as a comparison. Radiculopathies are not usually associated with an abnormal CMAP, unless there has been severe end-stage neurogenic atrophy of the muscle. This is a product of most muscles being innervated by more than one nerve root, and by the difficulty of identifying conduction block at the root level. Thus, detecting reduced CMAP amplitudes in cervical radiculopathies is uncommon unless it is severe or there are multiple roots affected.

F-Waves

F-wave studies have limited value in the evaluation of most radiculopathies and entrapment neuropathies. The reason for this is clear if one understands the pathogenesis of most of these focal neuropathies and the limitations inherent in F-wave assessment. The length of a possible compressive/demyelinating lesion is small in most radiculopathies and even mononeuropathies due to entrapment/compression (e.g., ulnar neuropathy at the elbow or median neuropathy at the wrist). Remember, the F-wave latency takes into account the time for the stimulus to travel antegrade through the motor nerve, stimulate a pool of anterior horn cells, and then travel back down the motor axon to stimulate the muscle. Thus, even if there were focal slowing across a small site of demyelination, this may be obscured by the normal conduction to and from the spine across the majority of the nerve. Further, most criteria regarding F-waves use the shortest latencies of multiple responses to define if the study is abnormal. Thus, one only needs to have one normal axon for the F-wave study to be deemed normal. Finally, amplitude measurement, the most important parameter obtained in NCS, cannot be reliably assessed in F-wave studies. However, if one is looking for a large proximal demyelinating lesion, as can be seen in some focal forms of chronic inflammatory demyelinating neuropathy, then F-waves are of some value.

H-Reflex

The only reliable H-reflex in the arm is from the flexor carpi radialis muscle following median nerve stimulation at the antecubital fossa.[17] This study is not routinely performed, as it usually does not assist in localizing the lesion apart from what is gained from the clinical examination, routine motor and sensory NCS, and the EMG. Nevertheless, the H-reflex for the flexor carpi radialis muscle may be abnormal in C6 or C7 radiculopathies, upper or middle trunk plexopathies, lateral cord lesions, or proximal median neuropathies. The major value of the H-reflex in the upper extremities occurs when H-reflexes are recognized during routine NCS. This implicates the presence of pyramidal tract pathology affecting that limb and may shift the investigation of the patient's complaints from the peripheral to central nervous system.

Somatosensory-Evoked Potentials

Somatosensory-evoked potentials have limited utility in radiculopathies and most neuropathies for much the same reason as discussed with F-waves. However, somatosensory-evoked potentials may be of value in assessment of brachial plexopathies because routine sensory NCS will not pick up a demyelination or conduction in the plexus.[18–21]

Needle EMG

The EMG examination is essential in the evaluation of patients for radiculopathy, plexopathy, and mononeuropathy. In combination with the clinical examination and carefully performed motor and sensory NCS, EMG of muscles supplied by different spinal roots, trunks, divisions, and cords of the brachial plexus, and different terminal nerves solidifies the localization of the site of the lesion. As discussed in Chapter 2, with EMG we assess the presence of abnormal insertional and spontaneous activity, the morphology of motor unit action potentials (MUAPs), and the recruitment properties of these units. Abnormal insertional or spontaneous activity in the form of positive sharp waves or fibrillation potentials implies membrane instability, which in neurogenic processes is typically due to axonal degeneration. Irritation of the nerve with or without axonal degeneration may result in fasciculation potentials, complex repetitive discharges, or myokymic discharges. The detection of myokymic discharges in a patient with history of cancer and radiation, who is now presenting with focal deficits in an arm, would strongly suggest radiation-induced injury to the roots or plexus as opposed to tumor infiltration. The demonstration of abnormal spontaneous activity in the paraspinal muscles suggests that there is at least some injury to the anterior horn cells or spinal nerves but also does not exclude an injury more distally (e.g., double crush).

Importantly, fibrillation potentials and positive sharp waves may not be present for up to 1 week in a paraspinal muscle and 3 weeks in limb muscles following axonal injury to a nerve root. However, voluntary recruitment of MUAPs is affected immediately. Thus, any injury to the nerve that results in a significant loss of muscle strength should be accompanied by reduced recruitment (e.g., fast-firing) of MUAPs. In neuropraxic injuries in which there is demyelination or conduction block without axonal degeneration, fibrillation potentials and positive sharp waves are not seen and the only abnormality apparent on the EMG is reduced recruitment of MUAPs. Reduced recruitment in the absence of abnormal spontaneous activity, NCS abnormalities, and morphological change in MUAPs more than 3 weeks subsequent to symptom onset implicates conduction block.

Following an axonal injury and muscle fiber reinnervation, fibrillation potentials and positive sharp waves are no longer evident. Reinnervation is more complete in muscles closer to the site of axonal injury (e.g., paraspinal muscles in a radiculopathy). If reinnervation occurs by successful axonal regrowth, then reestablishment of a near-normal number of motor units and innervation ratio, motor unit number and morphology may appear normal. In contrast, if reinnervation takes place via collateral sprouting, the motor units of an effected muscle will remain chronically reduced in number and increased in size, even if strength is reestablished. Muscle groups more distal to the site of the lesion (e.g., hand intrinsic muscles in a cervical radiculopathy) may be less likely to be completely reinnervated, and thus fibrillation potentials and positive sharp waves may persist indefinitely.

Another important point is that because of fascicular arrangement of axons running through various segments of the nerve trunk from the spine to the target muscle, an incomplete nerve injury may not necessarily demonstrate an abnormality in every muscle innervated by an affected spinal nerve root, trunk, cord, or terminal nerve.

RADIOLOGICAL STUDIES

Imaging studies such as a myelogram or magnetic resonance imaging (MRI) of the cervical spinal and brachial plexus are extremely valuable and complement the clinical examination and electrodiagnostic medicine study. MRI has, for the most part, replaced myelogram and computerized axial tomographic (CT) scans except in individuals in whom MRI is contraindicated (e.g., those with magnetic implants) for evaluation of radiculopathies. CT scans, particularly with contrast within the subarachnoid space can be useful[22] but high-resolution MRI is much more sensitive for radiculopathies, plexopathies, and focal neuropathies (Figs. 23-11 to 23-13).[23–29] Several studies have investigated the utility of ultrasound in focal neuropathies.[30–36]

▶ SPECIFIC DISORDERS

CERVICAL RADICULOPATHIES

Recall the disparity between the number of cervical vertebrae (seven) and nerve roots (eight) (Fig. 23-2). As a result, each numbered cervical nerve root is related to the bony level immediately inferior to it. For example, the C5 spinal root exits the spinal column between the fourth and fifth cervical vertebra, and it is vulnerable to compression from a herniated disc (herniated nucleus pulposus or HNP) between C4 and C5. The C6 spinal root exits the spinal column between the fifth and the sixth cervical vertebrae and may be injured from an HNP between C5 and C6. In the same manner, an HNP between C6 and C7 levels may damage the C7 root, while an HNP at the C7 and C8 vertebrae may impinge the C8 nerve root. The T1 spinal nerve exists between the eighth cervical and first thoracic vertebrae and may be damaged by an HNP at this level.

Most cervical radiculopathies involve the C5–8 spinal nerve roots (C7 occurring in 31–81%, C6 in 19–25%, C8 in 4–10%, and C5 in 2–10%).[13,37–41] Causes of cervical radiculopathy are multiple (Table 23-3), and most commonly involve compression of nerve root by an HNP or osteophytes in the case of degenerative spine disease. Individuals with a cervical radiculopathy typically present with neck or posterior shoulder pain in the scapular region that radiates down the affected arm. Turning the head toward the painful arm, particularly with neck extension, can narrow the neural foramen further compressing the nerve root and thus exacerbating the pain, as can downward pressure on the affected individual's head. The patient may have weakness in the distribution of the affected myotome and sensory loss in the dermatome that is involved. The deep tendon reflexes of affected segment may also be reduced. Because there is much overlap in the territories supplied by individual spinal roots, symptoms and signs can be similar to a plexopathy or focal neuropathy. Therefore, as previously discussed, EMG and NCS combined with imaging studies are extremely valuable in localization. Imaging studies are also important to assess structural etiology (e.g., HNP, osteophyte impinging on root, tumor of the nerve or extrinsic tumor/mass compression of the nerve, or inflammatory process). Further, nerve root avulsion may accompany nearly 80% of severe brachial plexopathies due to trauma.

C5 Radiculopathy

People with a C5 radiculopathy may have weakness of shoulder abduction, external rotation, elbow flexion, and supination of the wrist along with sensory loss in the shoulder region although sensory signs and symptoms may be absent in many cases. The biceps brachii and brachioradialis deep tendon reflexes may be asymmetrically reduced compared to the unaffected limb. Routine median and ulnar motor and sensory NCS are normal, as these do not carry any fibers emanating from the C5 spinal root. Electrodiagnostic localization is dependent on the EMG examination (Table 23-1). Abnormalities in the mid-cervical paraspinal, supraspinatus, infraspinatus, deltoid, biceps brachii, supinator, and brachioradialis muscles are seen in C5 radiculopathies. However, these muscles are also innervated by C6. The rhomboids are primarily innervated by C5, so abnormalities in this group strongly support a C5 radiculopathy. Further, if one sees membrane instability in the triceps brachii, pronator teres, extensor carpi radialis, or flexor carpi radialis that are innervated by C6, but not by C5, the above findings are

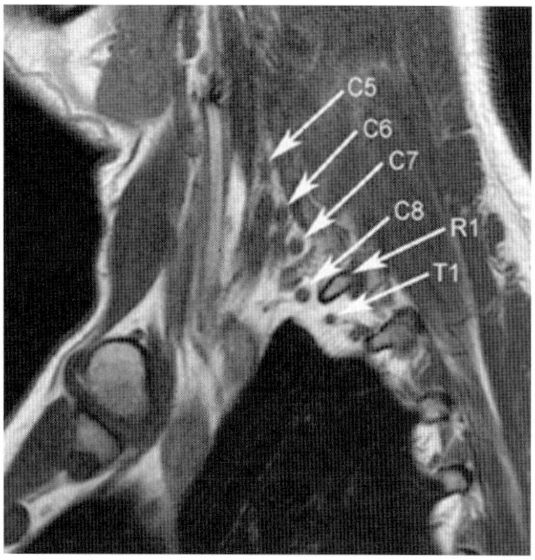

A

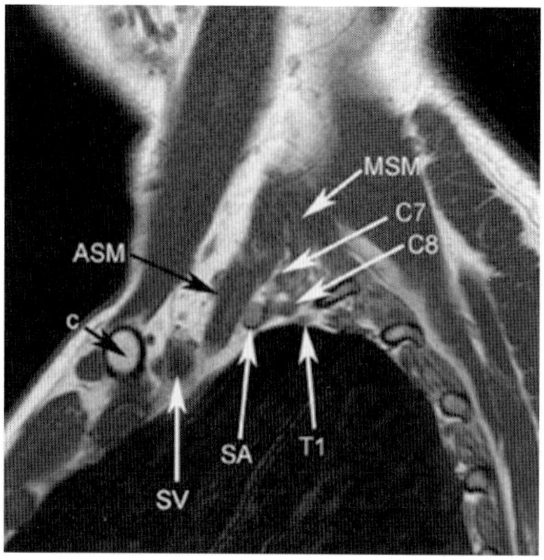

B

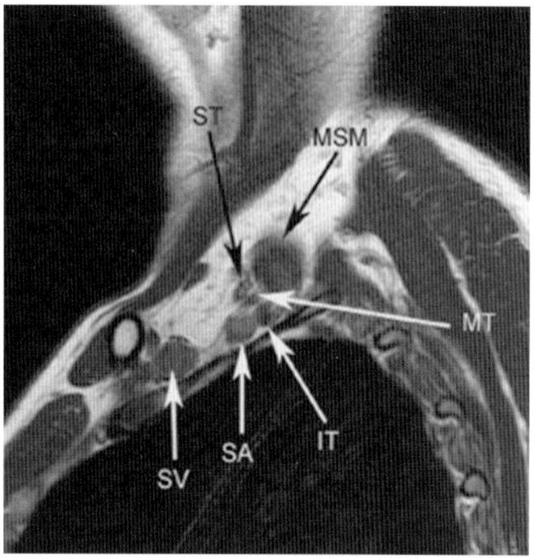

C

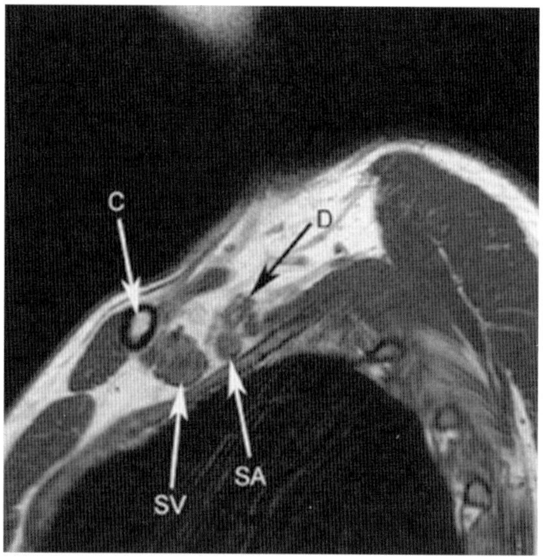

D

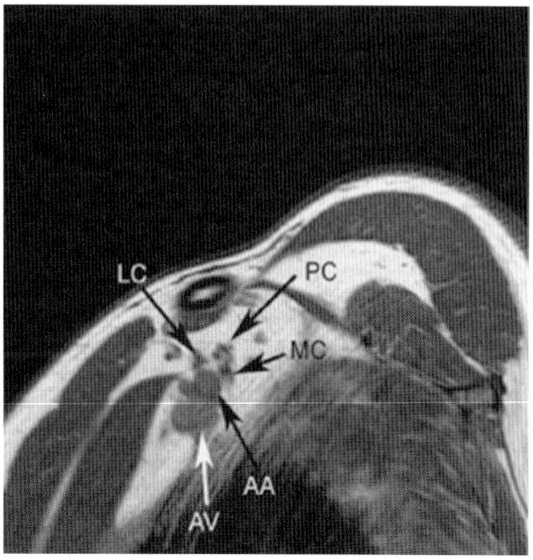

E

Figure 23-11. MRI of brachial plexus. Normal sagittal anatomy. **(A)** Roots C5–T1 just lateral to the intervertebral foramina, T1 is located below and C8 above the first rib (R1). **(B)** Subclavian artery (SA) and the roots C7, C8, and T1 are seen within the interscalene triangle between the anterior scalene muscle (ASM) and middle scalene muscle (MSM). The subclavian vein (SV) is positioned between the ASM and the clavicle (c). **(C)** Just lateral to the interscalene triangle the three trunks are formed, the superior (ST), the middle (MT), and inferior trunk (IT). **(D)** The divisions (D) are formed at the level where the brachial plexus crosses the clavicle. **(E)** Around the axillary artery (AA) the three cords are located, the lateral (LC) most anterior, the posterior (PC) most superior, and the medial (MC) most posterior. AV, axillary vein. (Reproduced with permission from van Es HW, Bollen TL, van Heesewijk HP. MRI of the brachial plexus: a pictorial review. *Eur J Radiol*. 2010;74(2):391–402.)

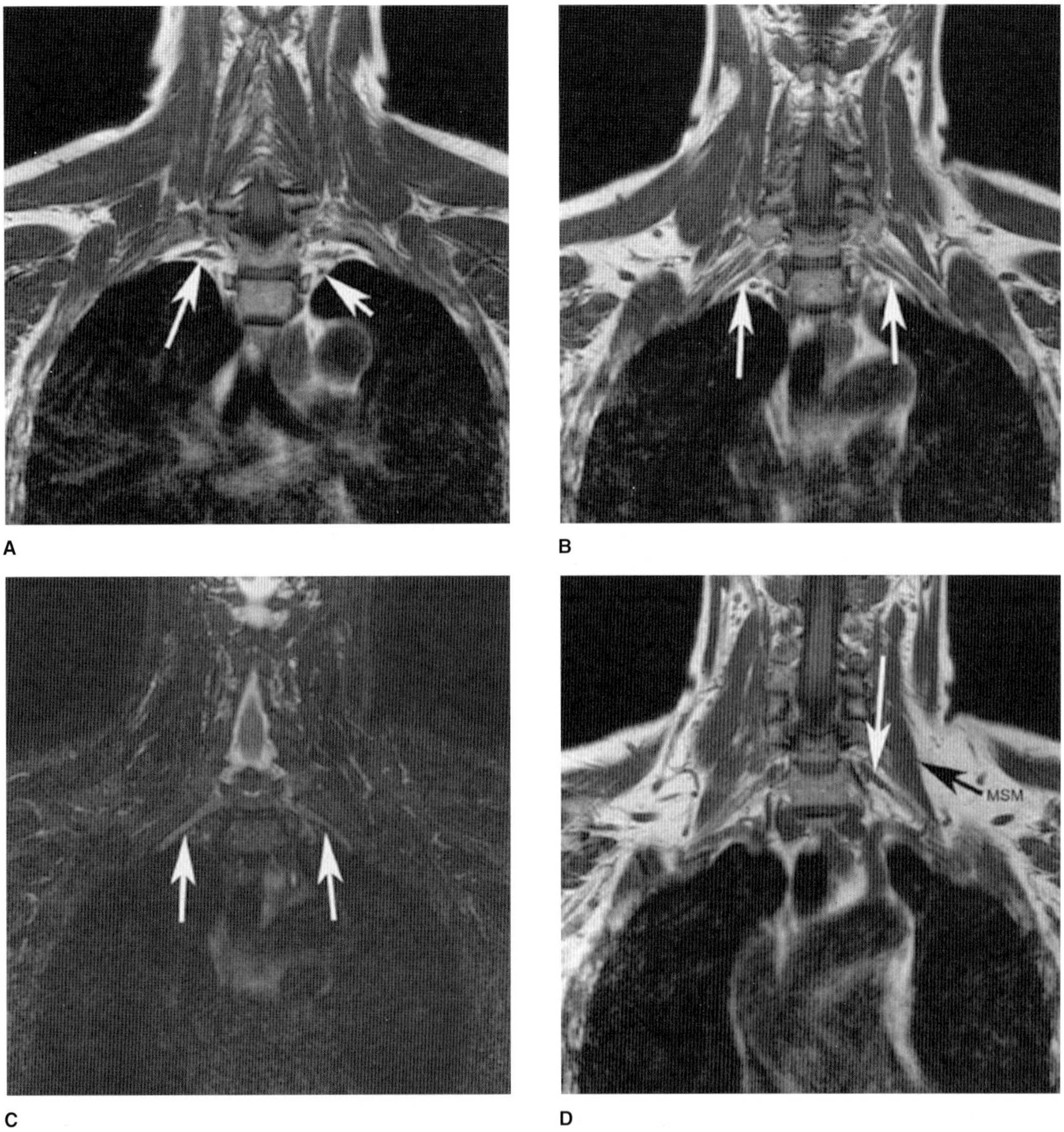

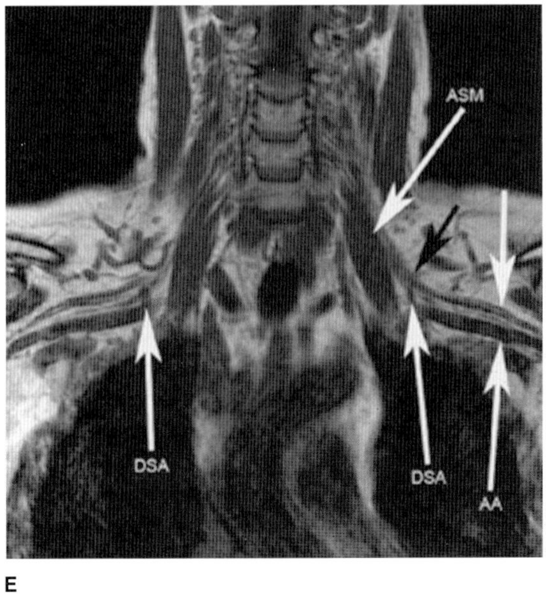

Figure 23-12. MRI of brachial plexus. Normal coronal anatomy. **(A)** Most posterior image with the horizontal course of the T1 nerve root (*long arrow*), very close to the lung apex. Short arrow points to the stellate ganglion. **(B)** Image just anterior to **(A)** with the C8 nerve roots (*arrows*). **(C)** T2-STIR image at the same level as **(B)** shows the slightly increased signal intensity of the normal C8 nerve roots (*arrows*). **(D)** *Arrow* points to the C7 nerve root. MSM, middle scalene muscle. **(E)** The cords (*white arrow*) are seen as linear structures above the axillary artery (AA). The dorsal scapular artery (DSA) courses between the trunks of the brachial plexus, black *arrow* points to the superior trunk. ASM, anterior scalene muscle. (Reproduced with permission from van Es HW, Bollen TL, van Heesewijk HP. MRI of the brachial plexus: a pictorial review. *Eur J Radiol*. 2010;74(2):391–402.)

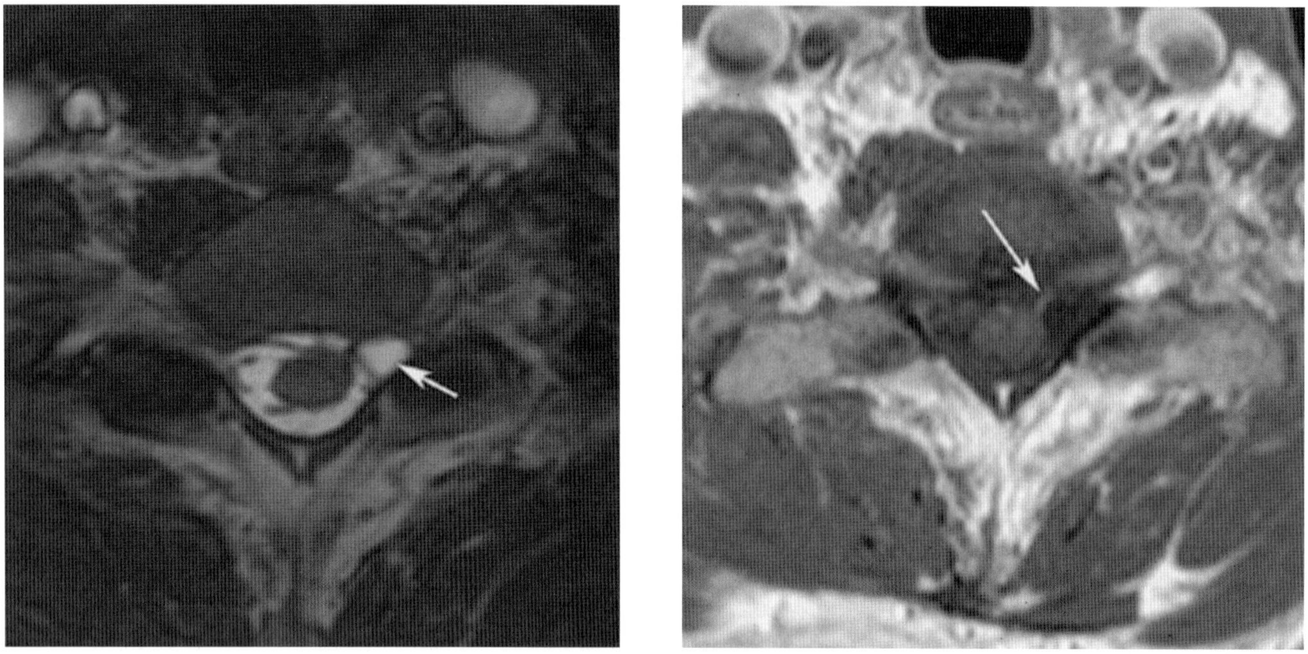

A B

Figure 23-13. MRI of cervical spine. Traumatic nerve root avulsion. **(A)** Axial balanced fast field echo (FFE) image demonstrates a traumatic pseudomeningocele (*arrow*). **(B)** Axial T1-weighted image with intravenous gadolinium shows the enhancement of an avulsed nerve root (*arrow*). (Reproduced with permission from van Es HW, Bollen TL, van Heesewijk HP. MRI of the brachial plexus: a pictorial review. *Eur J Radiol*. 2010;74(2):391–402.)

more consistent with a C6 nerve root lesion or multiple root involvement.

A common differential diagnostic consideration in a patient with C5 radiculopathy is rotator cuff injury, which may also produce shoulder pain and weakness in arm abduction and external rotation. Clinical distinction can be made be reproduction of discomfort by passive movement of the shoulder, rather than at the neck, and by the preservation of biceps strength and reflex in most rotator cuff injuries. Other differential diagnostic considerations not related to trauma or degenerative spine disease include brachial plexopathy, diseases that may present as multifocal neuropathies, and in the absence of pain or paresthesia, motor neuron disease.

▶ TABLE 23-4. **BRACHIAL PLEXUS CLASSIFICATION: NATURE OF INJURY**

Closed	Open
Idiopathic brachial plexus neuropathy	Trauma
Traction injuries (obstetric, postsurgical)	(e.g., Gunshot
Closed trauma	wound,
Radiation related	shrapnel,
Tumor (primary/secondary)	lacerations)
Neurogenic thoracic outlet syndrome	
Rucksack palsy	
Genetic (HNA, HNPP)	

HNA, hereditary neuralgia amyotrophy; HNPP, hereditary neuropathy with liability to pressure palsy.
Modified with permission from Wilbourn AJ. Brachial plexus disorders. In: Dyck PJ, Thomas PK, Griffin JU, et al eds. *Peripheral Neuropathy*. 3rd ed. Philadelphia, PA: W.B. Saunders; 1992.

C6 Radiculopathy

Individuals with a C6 radiculopathy can present in a similar manner to that described above with a C5 radiculopathy. However, weakness may also involve extension of the elbow (triceps), pronation, and extension of the wrist (extensor carpi radialis). Patients often complain of paresthesia localized to the thumb. In a patient with suspected C6 radiculopathy, one needs to consider an upper trunk or lateral cord lesion, median neuropathy, or radial neuropathy. Therefore, at the very least, we usually perform median and radial SNAPs and a median CMAP. In addition, we obtain lateral antebrachial cutaneous SNAPs, if we are suspicious of a brachial plexopathy affecting the upper trunk. As discussed, these NCS should be normal in a C6 radiculopathy, but the flexor carpi radialis H-reflex may be abnormal. However, localization hinges on the EMG study (Table 23-1). There is significant overlapping of findings in C6 and C5 as well as C7 radiculopathies. Needle EMG may demonstrate abnormalities in the mid to low cervical paraspinals, supraspinatus, infraspinatus, deltoid, biceps brachii, triceps brachii, pronator teres, brachioradialis, supinator, extensor carpi radialis, and flexor carpi radialis muscles. Rotator cuff injury, multifocal neuropathies, and brachial plexus neuritis are likely to be the most common differential diagnostic considerations unrelated to trauma or degenerative joint disease of the cervical spine.

C7 Radiculopathy

People with a C7 radiculopathy often have pain or sensory symptoms radiating down the arm into the middle digit. Weakness of elbow extension and wrist flexion or finger extension may be evident along with a diminished triceps reflex. In patients with suspected C7 radiculopathy, a median CMAP, median SNAP to the third digit, and radial SNAP can be done to assess for a more distal lesion. But again, one should expect routine NCS to be normal in a C7 radiculopathy except for perhaps the flexor carpi radialis H-reflex. On EMG, abnormalities may be detected particularly in the triceps brachii, anconeus, pronator teres, flexor carpi radialis, extensor digitorum communis, and less commonly the extensor digitorum indicis, extensor pollicis longus and brevis, and flexor pollicis longus muscles (Table 23-1). The differential diagnosis of C7 radiculopathy is limited and is probably mimicked most closely by radial mononeuropathies. Most radial neuropathies occur at or distal to the spiral groove, thus resulting in sparing of triceps and prominent weakness of wrist extension. C7 root lesions, on the other hand, typically affect the triceps but rarely produce severe weakness of wrist extension.

C8/T1 Radiculopathy

It is often very difficult to distinguish a C8 from a T1 radiculopathy, so these are discussed together. Individuals who are affected have sensory disturbance affecting the medial aspect of the hand and forearm along with hand weakness. The differential diagnosis included a lower trunk plexopathy such as neurogenic thoracic outlet syndrome, a medial cord lesion, an ulnar neuropathy, and in the absence of pain and sensory symptoms, motor neuron disease. In cases of ulnar neuropathy, the site of the lesion may be at the wrist, elbow, or elsewhere. The NCS are very helpful in terms of localization. It is important to perform ulnar and median CMAPs and SNAPs as well as a medial antebrachial cutaneous SNAP to exclude a plexus or root lesion unless unequivocal focal abnormalities of the ulnar motor conduction studies can be demonstrated (Table 23-3). The SNAPs should be normal in a radiculopathy, but in a lower trunk or medial cord injury the ulnar and medial antebrachial cutaneous SNAP amplitude may be reduced. A reduction in the median CMAP amplitude with a normal median SNAP would further support a lower trunk or medial cord injury (Table 23-2). On EMG, one may see abnormalities in any of the median- or ulnar-innervated muscles innervated by C8 and T1 spinal roots (Table 23-1). The thenar eminence may be predominantly innervated by T1, so the median CMAP amplitude may be disproportionately reduced compared to the ulnar CMAP in a T1 radiculopathy. Most of the radial-innervated muscles supplying the fingers originate from the C7 and C8 spinal segments but not T1. Therefore, EMG of these muscle groups can help distinguish a C8 from a T1 radiculopathy. In the case of a lower trunk lesion, muscles innervating radial muscles via the C8 nerve root will be affected as well as intrinsic hand muscles, whereas this will not be the case in medial cord lesions.

Multiple Cervical Radiculopathies

Most cervical radiculopathies involve only one root, but approximately 12–30% may involve multiple levels.[38,40] If this is the case, CMAP amplitudes are more likely to be reduced although SNAPS will remain spared. The presence of EMG abnormalities suggesting a polyradiculopathy must raise the suspicion of other diseases, particularly motor neuron disease. In such cases, it is important to study the lower extremity, thoracic paraspinals, and even selected cranial nerves (e.g., the tongue and sternocleidomastoid).

THORACIC RADICULOPATHIES

For the sake of completeness, we will briefly discuss thoracic radiculopathies although these are relatively uncommon. HNPs in the thoracic region account for only 0.22–5.3% of all disc protrusions.[42–45] Approximately 75% of symptomatic thoracic radiculopathies occur between T8 and T12, with most occurring between T11 and T12. Central and centrolateral HNPs can compress the spinal cord, leading to symptoms and signs of a myelopathy. Patients may present circumferential chest or abdominal pain and/or paresthesias, leg pain or weakness, or bowel or bladder difficulties (e.g., constipation, urinary retention, and incontinence). At the T11–12 region, the conus medullaris or cauda equina may be affected with ensuing bowel/bladder and lower extremity deficits.

Trauma is the most common cause of a herniated thoracic disc accounting for 14–63% of cases.[46,47] Degenerative changes of the spine account for a minority of cases. Other structural causes for thoracic radiculopathies that need to be considered include compression due to metastatic disease, vertebral collapse, Pott's disease, and primary nerve tumors. Perhaps, the most common etiology of thoracic radiculopathy is diabetes mellitus (e.g., diabetic radiculoneuropathy). Additional nonstructural causes of thoracic radiculopathies include Lyme disease, herpes zoster, cytomegalovirus, sarcoidosis, and carcinomatous meningitis. Of note, thoracic disc herniations on imaging are far more common than causally related clinical syndromes, and clinicians need to be cautious before attributing nonspecific clinical symptoms to an imaging abnormality.

The electrodiagnostic evaluation of thoracic radiculopathies is limited. NCS are not helpful. EMG may demonstrate abnormal insertional and spontaneous activity in the thoracic paraspinal muscles. Care must be taken not to insert the needle too far so as to avoid a pneumothorax. EMG of abdominal muscles may be of value, as one can also assess for MUAP morphology and recruitment abnormalities.

TREATMENT OF RADICULOPATHIES

Treatment is dependent on the etiology of the radiculopathy. For the sake of discussion, we will focus here on treatment of radiculopathies related to HNPs or spondylotic disease, as radiculoneuropathies related to other entities (e.g., Lyme disease, diabetes) are discussed in other chapters in this book. It is difficult to make evidence-based medical decisions regarding the best therapeutic approach to patients with cervical radiculopathies due to the lack of well-designed, prospective, controlled, and blinded trials. That said, it is important to realize that the natural history of radiculopathies related to compression from HNPs is favorable. In a large series of patients with cervical radiculopathy followed for up to 5 years, 90% were asymptomatic or had only slight pain at last follow-up; however, 26% of all patients underwent surgery.[48]

Treatment of acute radiculopathy is focused on relief of pain. Injections of corticosteroids or local anesthetic agents have been employed, but again there is no strong medical evidence that these are beneficial. Likewise, there is no proven efficacy for bed rest, cervical traction, corticosteroids, nonsteroidal anti-inflammatory drugs, or muscle relaxants. Commonly used medications for neuropathic pain such as antiepileptic agents or tricyclic antidepressants can be tried, as can short courses of narcotics. In patients with intractable pain or those with significant weakness, decompressive surgery may be warranted. Small trials assessing the effects of surgery versus conservative management for cervical spondylotic radiculopathy or myelopathy have shown little or no difference in the long-term, though there was quicker pain relief in the surgical group.[49,50]

BRACHIAL PLEXOPATHY

Brachial plexopathies can be classified on the basis of the nature of the injury (i.e., an open or closed brachial plexopathy), the anatomic location of the lesion, or the mechanism of injury (Table 23-2).[1–3] MRI can be helpful in identifying both the site and cause of the lesion because anatomical resolution of the roots, trunks, divisions, and cords is very well depicted due to the inherent contrast differences between the nerves and surrounding fat (Figs. 23-11 and 23-4).[23] However, MRI is expensive, and usually we can make an accurate diagnosis on the basis of clinical examination, supplemented when necessary by electrodiagnostic studies. Therefore, we will begin by reviewing clinical and electrodiagnostic features that one may expect to see with lesions affecting various trunks and cords of the brachial plexus.

Upper Trunk

Individuals with upper trunk lesions have weakness in the deltoid and biceps brachii muscles (Fig. 23-3). Therefore, they commonly complain of difficulty lifting their arms. Sensory loss involves the lateral arm and forearm down to the lateral aspect of the hand and fingers. The biceps brachii and brachioradialis reflexes are typically reduced. Injuries in isolation are relatively common when compared to isolated middle or lower trunk lesions.

EMG and NCS are useful in differentiating an upper trunk lesion from a C5 or C6 radiculopathy. Remember that upper trunk lesions are distinguished from C5–6 injuries in that the posterior primary rami are spared, as are the nerve branches to the rhomboid and serratus anterior muscles. Also, trunk lesions are distal to the dorsal root ganglion. Therefore, if the nature of upper trunk injury is axonal damage and not just neuropraxia (i.e., conduction block and/or demyelination), the radial, median recording from the thumb and possibly the index finger, and lateral antibrachial cutaneous SNAPs may have reduced amplitudes, particularly when compared to the asymptomatic contralateral arm (Table 23-2). These SNAPs would be normal in a cervical radiculopathy or in a neuropraxic or demyelinating process affecting the trunk. Routine median and ulnar CMAPs are not particularly helpful other than excluding involvement of other trunks or nerves. A musculocutaneous CMAP can be done by recording from the biceps brachii, but this is usually not useful in distinguishing a C5 or C6 radiculopathy from an upper trunk lesion. However, the EMG can be localizing in combination with the sensory studies. Recall that the posterior primary rami to the paraspinal muscles, the dorsal scapular nerve to the rhomboid, and long thoracic nerve to the serratus anterior come off the cervical roots before the formation of the upper trunk. EMG of these muscles may show evidence of denervation in a C5 or C6 radiculopathy, but would be spared if the lesion only involved the upper trunk. One should do an extensive EMG to ensure that abnormalities are restricted to muscles innervated by the upper trunk, with sparing of muscles innervated by the middle and lower trunk (Table 23-1).

Middle Trunk

Isolated middle trunk lesions are extremely rare and middle trunk lesions most often occur in combination with other plexus lesions (Fig. 23-3). Symptoms and signs would resemble a C7 radiculopathy. Affected people may experience weakness of elbow, wrist, and finger extension and sensory loss or pain in the posterior forearm and the dorsal and palmar aspect of the middle finger. The triceps reflex may be reduced.

Provided the injury is axonal in nature, a diminished amplitude of the median SNAP to the third digit may be evident as the cutaneous fibers that supply this finger usually traverse the middle trunk (Table 23-2). Also, the radial CMAP recorded from the extensor indicis proprius may have reduced amplitude, if there is sufficient axon loss. However, the EMG is most important in delineating the extent of motor involvement. Remember that the middle trunk contains the C7 spinal nerves and after passing through the middle trunk these diverge and traverse the posterior and lateral cords (Table 23-1, Fig. 23-3). Thus, most muscles innervated by the radial nerve with the exception of the brachioradialis would be affected in addition to some median-innervated forearm muscles (e.g., those muscles with C6 and C7 and lateral cord innervation). Additionally, EMG abnormalities may be appreciated in the pectoralis major, latissimus dorsi, and teres major muscles, as these muscles are, in part, innervated by the C7 spinal nerves and middle trunk via the medial and posterior cords. However, the serratus anterior muscle, which has C7 innervation in common but not the middle trunk, would be spared with a middle trunk lesion (recall the long thoracic nerve branches directly off the roots). There are no nerve branches arising directly from the middle trunk, and so it can be difficult to distinguish a lesion involving the middle trunk from those affecting portions of the lateral and posterior cords.

Lower Trunk

Lesions affecting the lower trunk have symptoms similar to a C8/T1 radiculopathies, medial cord plexopathies, and ulnar neuropathies (Fig. 23-3). Affected individuals have sensory loss of the medial aspect of the forearm and hand along with weakness of ulnar-, median-, and radial-nerve–innervated wrist/hand muscles. Involvement of radial-nerve and posterior cord–innervated C8/T1 muscles puts the lesion more proximal than the medial cord.

NCS are valuable in localizing the lesion (Table 23-2). With axonal lesions, one would expect to see reduced amplitudes of ulnar and medial antebrachial cutaneous SNAPs in both lower trunk and medial cord lesions, but not in a C8 or T1 radiculopathy. A reduction in the amplitude of the median and ulnar CMAPs may be seen in a severe radiculopathy, lower trunk, or medial cord axonopathies. EMG should show signs of denervation in radial-, median-, and ulnar-innervated distal arm muscles, as the nerves supplying these muscles all course through the lower trunk (Table 23-1). However, the lower cervical paraspinal muscles should be spared in brachial plexus lesions. Compared to other plexus injuries, the prognosis for recovery is comparatively poor because of the long distance a regenerating nerve must cover to reinnervate the muscles in the distal arm.[1]

Posterior Cord

The nerves originating from the posterior cord include the thoracodorsal, the upper and lower subscapular, axillary, and radial nerves (Fig. 23-3). Depending on where the lesion is in the cord, individuals who are affected may have weakness of shoulder abduction, shoulder extension, supination of the wrist, and elbow/wrist/finger extension along with sensory disturbance in shoulder area, posterior arm and forearm, and the dorsum of the hand.

Provided the lesion is axonal in nature, both the superficial radial and posterior cutaneous nerve of the forearm SNAP amplitudes may be reduced in a posterior cord lesion (Table 23-2). However, the sensory studies of the lateral antebrachial cutaneous nerves, which also courses through the upper trunk but the lateral cord as opposed to the posterior cord, would be normal. A radial CMAP recording from the extensor indicis proprius would be expected to show reduced amplitude, when there has been significant axonal loss involving the C7 and C8 spinal nerve fibers coursing through the posterior cord. EMG would be expected to demonstrate abnormalities of the latissimus dorsi, teres major (though difficult to study), deltoid, and the radial-innervated muscles (Table 23-1).

Lateral Cord

The lateral cord is the continuation of the anterior division of the upper trunk (Fig. 23-3). Individuals with a lateral cord lesion may experience weakness of shoulder flexion and abduction, elbow flexion and pronation, and wrist flexion. In addition, sensory disturbance would involve the lateral, volar aspect of the upper arm and forearm along with the lateral and palmar aspect of the hand and fingers. The biceps brachii reflex should be reduced with sparing of the brachioradialis reflex.

Median SNAPs to the first three digits, superficial radial nerve to the thumb, and the lateral antebrachial cutaneous nerve should be studied to help localize pathology to the lateral cord (Table 23-3). With axonal lesions to the lateral cord, the median and lateral antebrachial SNAPs are expected to have decreased amplitude, but the radial SNAP should be normal as this arises from the posterior cord. A musculocutaneous CMAP recording from the biceps brachii muscles may have reduced amplitude. EMG can demonstrate evidence of denervation in the biceps brachii, pronator teres, flexor carpi radialis muscles, and perhaps the infraclavicular and midsternal fibers of the pectoralis major (Table 23-1). These findings coupled with normal EMG of the cervical paraspinal, supraspinatus, infraspinatus, deltoid, and triceps muscles localize the lesion distal to the upper trunk and out of the territory of the posterior cord.

Medial Cord

The medial cord is a continuation of the anterior division of the lower trunk (Fig. 23-3). A medial cord injury clinically resembles a lower trunk lesion except that radial-nerve–innervated C8/T1wrist/hand muscles would be spared. Remember that nerves to radial-innervated muscles in the forearm course through the lower trunk and then enter the posterior cord rather than the medial cord. Therefore, the ulnar-, median-, and radial-innervated muscles to the digits are affected in a lower trunk lesion; only the ulnar- and median-innervated muscles will be abnormal with medial cord damage.

The medial antebrachial cutaneous and ulnar SNAPs may be reduced in amplitude provided that there is axonal injury, but this does not help distinguish a medial cord from a lower trunk lesion (Table 23-2). The medial antebrachial cutaneous response is disproportionately reduced in comparison to the ulnar SNAP in neurogenic thoracic outlet syndrome, however, presumably due to a larger component from the T1 spinal nerve. Conversely, the ulnar SNAP is typically more affected from poststernotomy plexopathies as the C8 spinal nerve appears to be the primary structure injured. Decreased amplitudes of median and ulnar CMAPs recording from thenar and hypothenar muscles do not discriminate between injury to the lower trunk and medial cord. One way to try to differentiate a medial cord from a lower trunk lesion would be by assessing the radial CMAP recorded from the extensor indicis proprius muscles. EMG is more helpful in distinguishing between a lower trunk and a medial cord injury. Again, if EMG demonstrates signs of denervation in C8/T1 radial- as well as median- and ulnar-innervated musculature, then a lower trunk as opposed to medial cord injury should be considered (Table 23-1).

SPECIFIC BRACHIAL PLEXUS DISORDERS

In the following section, we will go into more detail about the common types of brachial plexopathy.

Immune-Mediated Brachial Plexus Neuropathy

Immune-mediated brachial plexus neuropathy (IBPN) goes by various terminologies, including acute brachial plexitis or neuritis, neuralgic amyotrophy, and Parsonage–Turner syndrome.[2,3,51–55] IBPN usually presents with an acute, often nocturnal, onset of severe pain in the shoulder region. The pain is frequently described like a hot poker jammed into the upper arm. Sometimes the pain involves the forearm or may be restricted to this segment of the arm (as seen in individuals with anterior interosseous syndrome as a forme fruste of IBPN). The pain is often exacerbated by movement of the arm. The intense pain usually lasts several days to a few weeks, but a dull ache can persist for 3 years or more.[55] Individuals who are affected may not appreciate weakness of the arm early in the course because the pain limits movement. However, as the pain dissipates, weakness and often, a lesser degree sensory loss are appreciated. Attacks can occasionally recur.[55] This disorder is usually clinically unilateral, but the opposite arm may be affected occasionally to a lesser degree.

Clinical findings are dependent on the distribution of involvement (e.g., specific trunks, divisions, cords, or terminal nerves). Occasional mild abnormalities of the cerebrospinal fluid (increased protein or pleocytosis) are found indicative of presumed inflammatory process also extending to the roots.[53] One large study suggested that 36% of patients recovered most functions within the first year, 75% by the second year's end, and 89% by the end of the third year.[53] However, another large study of 246 cases found that approximately two-thirds of patients still had persistent pain and weakness after 3 years and <8% had a full recovery according to the patients.[55] Mild paresis was still evident in 69%, with severe weakness in 3%. Proximally located muscles are more likely to regain strength than the more distal hand muscles.

The most common pattern of IBPN involves the upper trunk or a single or multiple mononeuropathies primarily involving the suprascapular, long thoracic, or axillary nerves.[1,54–58] Additionally, the phrenic[59,60] and anterior interosseous[55,61–63]nerves may be concomitantly affected. Any of these nerves may also be affected in isolation as a forme fruste of IBPN. In most IBPNs, the paraspinal muscles are normal on EMG, suggesting that the lesion is distal to the root/spinal nerve level, but occasionally signs of active denervation are apparent, suggesting root involvement. Rarely, multiple cranial nerves (IX, X, XI, and XII) may be involved.[64] In this regard, an isolated spinal accessory neuropathy presenting as acute unilateral suboccipital and neck pain and weakness of the trapezius muscle may also represent a forme fruste of IBPN.[65]

The pathogenic basis of IBPN is unknown but presumed to be immunologic. Circumstantial evidence of an inflammatory basis is that IBPN may develop following immune system provocation by infection, vaccination, bone transplantation, or following treatment with immune-modulating agents (e.g., interferons, interleukin-2, and tumor necrosis-alpha blockers).[53,66–70] In addition, some series have reported antibodies directed against peripheral nerve myelin and soluble terminal complement complexes.[71] Biopsies of the brachial plexus are not typically performed for IBPN, but there are few descriptions of such biopsies revealing perivascular epineurial and endoneurial inflammatory cell infiltrates. The antigen(s) of which the autoimmune attack is directed is not known, but the electrodiagnostic abnormalities suggest a primary insult against the axons of the nerves as opposed to the myelin.

The electrodiagnostic findings are dependent on the site(s) of involvement and can be rather multifocal.[1–3,51,56] The upper trunk is primarily involved in most patients. Thus, it is not surprising that median and ulnar motors studies are abnormal in only about 15% of patients with IBPN.[56] Median, lateral antebrachial cutaneous, and radial SNAPs are more likely to be abnormal. Also, CMAPs recorded from the deltoid and biceps muscles can demonstrate abnormalities. Other laboratory abnormalities include slightly increased cerebrospinal fluid protein with or without mild pleocytosis in a little over 10% of patients.[53,55] MRI scan of the plexus may demonstrate increased T2 signal suggestive of inflammation or edema.[28,29,55]

We often treat patients presenting acutely who continue to have severe pain with a short course of corticosteroids (e.g., prednisone 50 mg daily tapering by 10 mg every 4–5 days), although there are very few evidence-based studies that have demonstrated any efficacy. However, in our anecdotal experience, corticosteroids seem to help alleviate the pain, which can be useful in allowing the patient to proceed with physical therapy. They do not appear to expedite return of strength. If the pain has already resolved by the time we see them, we do not treat with corticosteroids. The mainstay of treatment is physical and occupational therapy to prevent contractures in an immobilized arm, improve function, and maintain strength in unaffected muscles.

Other Immune-Mediated Neuropathies

Rarely, a painful or painless brachial plexopathy may be the sole manifestation of an asymmetric form of chronic inflammatory demyelinating neuropathy, multifocal acquired motor and sensory demyelinating neuropathy, or multifocal motor neuropathy.[72] Diagnosis of these entities requires demonstration of conduction block or focal slowing localized to the brachial plexus, which is often technically difficult. The importance of identifying multifocal acquired motor and sensory demyelinating neuropathy or multifocal motor neuropathy is their potential responsiveness to immunotherapy. See Chapter 14 on "Chronic Inflammatory Demyelinating Polyneuropathy and Related Disorders" for more details.

Obstetrically Related Plexopathies

The annual incidence of obstetrically related plexus injuries ranges between 0.38 and 2.0 per 1,000 live births.[1–3,73–79] Three types of brachial plexus injury complicate childbirth: (1) diffuse plexopathy, (2) upper trunk plexopathy (Erb palsy), or (3) lower trunk plexopathy (Klumpke paralysis). The plexus can be damaged during childbirth due to traction on the arm and thereby the nerves. Increased risk is associated with heavy birth weight of the infant, mothers with short stature, breech presentation, long and difficult labor, and heavily sedated mothers (resulting in diminished muscle tone during delivery).[1,74,75,80–82] In addition, forceful downward traction applied to the head after the fetal third rotation is a risk factor of obstetric brachial plexus palsy in vaginal deliveries in cephalic presentation.[83]

Erb palsy, the most common type of obstetric paralysis, results from stretch of the nerves of the upper trunk of the brachial plexus.[18,74,76] Severe traction injury may also lead to avulsion of the C5 or C6 spinal nerves. Traction of the upper trunk can occur with shoulder dystocia in a vertex presentation or difficulty delivering the aftercoming head in a breech presentation. Upper trunk lesion leads to weakness of the supraspinatus, infraspinatus, deltoid, biceps brachii, teres minor, brachioradialis, extensor carpi radialis longus/brevis, and supinator muscles. An infant who is affected typically lies with their arm adducted and internally rotated (unopposed pull of the sternal portion of the pectoralis major and latissimus dorsi muscles), elbow extended and forearm pronated (unopposed triceps and pronator teres/quadratus muscles), and wrist/fingers flexed (weak wrist extensors—the so-called "waiter's tip position").[1] Diaphragmatic or serratus anterior weakness suggests the possibility of root avulsion, as the nerves to these muscles arise proximal to the upper trunk.

Rarely, the lower trunk or C8 or T1 roots are injured during childbirth (Klumpke paralysis).[78] These usually occur in the setting of face presentation and hyperextension of the neck but can also complicate breech deliveries with hyperabduction of the arm. Infants will have good proximal arm strength, but weakness of hand muscles is evident. Finally, the entire plexus can also be affected to varying degrees.[84,85]

Radiological imaging is essential to assess for the possibility of associated humeral or clavicular fractures as well as diaphragmatic paralysis. In addition, MRI should be done to assess for nerve root avulsion.[2,86,87]

Electrodiagnostic studies are useful to determine the site and severity of injury and prognosis and to decide about the appropriateness and timing of any operative intervention.[1,2,74,75,80] Abnormalities in SNAPs and CMAPs may be evident in 7–10 days. Electrodiagnostic studies are typically performed 4–6 weeks following delivery, as it can take this long for active signs of denervation to be evident on EMG. However, detection of voluntary MUAPs at any time, even before the 4–6-week period, demonstrates that there is at least partial continuity between the anterior horn cells and the target muscle SNAPs are typically more vulnerable to injury than CMAPs. A pattern of where SNAP amplitude(s) are low, but CMAP amplitude(s) are disproportionately reduced suggests pathology both proximal and distal to the level of the dorsal root ganglia and raises the possibility of avulsion. Prognosis is better, if the nerve is not completely severed. If SNAPs or CMAPs are low or absent and there is initially no MUAP on EMG, serial studies can be performed every 6–8 weeks to assess for evidence of reinnervation.

The natural history is not well defined, but patients with upper trunk lesions often have significant improvement within 3 months. Those with lower trunk lesions are more likely to have a more prolonged course and incomplete recovery. Unfortunately, there is no chance for regeneration of the nerves following a root avulsion. Reconstructive surgical procedures may be employed in order to help restore elbow flexion and shoulder abduction in patients with severe axonal injury.[60,88–90]

Neurogenic Thoracic Outlet Syndrome

The term "thoracic outlet syndrome" has been ascribed to disorders, including those attributed to compromise of blood vessels between the base of the neck and the axilla.[1–3] Our discussion is limited to the rare neurogenic form of thoracic outlet syndrome, which, in essence, is a lower trunk plexopathy. Most cases of alleged thoracic outlet syndrome are unassociated with any objective clinical, electrophysiological, or imaging evidence of vascular or nerve compromise. Most individuals with true neurogenic thoracic outlet syndrome are women with a prominent C7 transverse process or true cervical rib that can be appreciated on plain films of the cervical spine (Fig. 23-14). These cases are often associated with a sharp fibrous band extending from the tip of the elongated C7 transverse process or cervical rib to the first thoracic rib. This band usually cannot be visualized on imaging studies, including MRI scans. Its presence is however suggested by demonstration of the bony anomalies described above. The proximal aspect of the lower trunk becomes angulated or stretched as it passes over this fibrous band. Because the T1 fibers lie below the C8 fibers, these are usually distorted and thus are more likely to be damaged. Thus, affected individuals have muscle atrophy and weakness that is often greater in the thenar muscles, which have more T1 innervation than the hypothenar muscles, which have more C8 innervation. In addition, patients complain of numbness, paresthesia, and pain along the medial aspects of the arm, forearm, and hand. Electrodiagnostic studies demonstrate that the median CMAP and medial antebrachial cutaneous SNAP amplitudes are reduced to a greater extent than the ulnar SNAP and CMAP, because the former studies primarily assess T1 fibers, while ulnar studies primarily assess C8 fibers.[2,58,91–94] Neurogenic thoracic outlet syndrome is typically treated by surgical resection of the taut band. In our experience, surgery may arrest progression and relieve pain but would uncommonly restore bulk or strength of hand muscles.

Plexopathies Associated with Neoplasms

Neoplasms involving the brachial plexus may be primary nerve tumors, local cancers expanding into the plexus (e.g., Pancoast lung tumor or lymphoma), and metastatic tumors.[95,96] Primary brachial plexus tumors are less common than the secondary tumors and include schwannomas, neurinomas, and neurofibromas.[25,42,97–99] These primary tumors may present as mass lesions in the supraclavicular fossa region or axilla. Pain and paresthesias are early symptoms, while motor and sensory losses occur later as the tumor may initially distort the nerve fibers but do not result in conduction block, demyelination, or axon loss right away.

Schwannomas are commonly benign and well encapsulated, affect the proximal segments of the plexus, and may be surgically removed with minimal damage to the nearby nerve fibers (Fig. 23-15).[97,99,100] However, malignant schwannomas do rarely occur.[101] Neurofibromas are the most common form of peripheral nerve tumor and are typically benign. However, when seen in the context of neurofibromatosis, these are often multiple and affect a larger portion of the brachial plexus.[97] Additionally, neurofibromas interdigitate more with nerve fibers within the nerve fascicle and are more commonly associated with neurological deficits than schwannomas. Further, it is difficult to remove these surgically without damaging the affected nerve. These tumors can also convert to a more malignant form, particularly in neurofibromatosis.

Secondary tumors affecting the brachial plexus are more common and are always malignant. These may arise from local tumors expanding into the plexus. For example, a Pancoast tumor of the upper lobe of the lung may invade or compress the lower trunk, while a primary lymphoma arising from the cervical or axillary lymph nodes may also infiltrate the plexus.[95,96] Pancoast tumors typically present as an insidious onset of pain in the upper arm, sensory disturbance in the medial aspect of the forearm and hand, and weakness and atrophy of the intrinsic hand muscles along with an ipsilateral Horner syndrome. Chest CT scans or MRI can demonstrate extension of the tumor into the plexus. Metastatic involvement of the brachial plexus may occur with spread of breast cancer into the axillary lymph nodes and the nearby nerves (Fig. 23-16). Pain is usually the presenting manifestation due to spread of the cancer into the plexus and is accompanied by widespread paresthesias. Weakness and sensory loss conform to the distribution of the affected nerves. Likewise, electrodiagnostic abnormalities are dependent on the nerves that are involved as previously discussed.[14,21]

Recurrent Neoplastic Disease or Radiation

The treatment for various malignancies (e.g., lung, breast, and lymphoma) often involves radiation therapy, the field of which may include parts of the brachial plexus. It can be difficult in such situations to determine if a new brachial plexopathy is related to tumor within the plexus or from radiation-induced nerve damage. Radiation can be associated with microvascular abnormalities and fibrosis of surrounding tissues, which can damage the axons and the Schwann cells.[1,102] Radiation-induced plexopathy can develop months or years following therapy and is dose dependent.[7,96,103]

Tumor invasion is usually painful and more commonly affects the lower trunk, while radiation injury is often painless and affects the upper trunk.[96] Imaging studies such as MRI and CT scans are useful but can be insensitive in detecting microscopic invasion of the plexus. EMG can be informative, if myokymic discharges are appreciated, as this finding strongly suggests radiation-induced damage. However, absence of myokymic discharges does not rule out radiation as the cause of the plexopathy.

Backpack or Rucksack Palsy

This condition refers to paresis of the arms occurring in soldiers or civilians wearing heavy backpacks or rucksacks strapped around the shoulders.[1–3,104,105] Motor and sensory losses most typically are in the distribution of the upper trunk but can be more widespread. The injury is usually neuropraxic in nature, although secondary axonal degeneration may occur. If one sees electrophysiological features of multifocal demyelination at common compression sites (e.g., at the carpal tunnel, across the elbow, and across the fibular

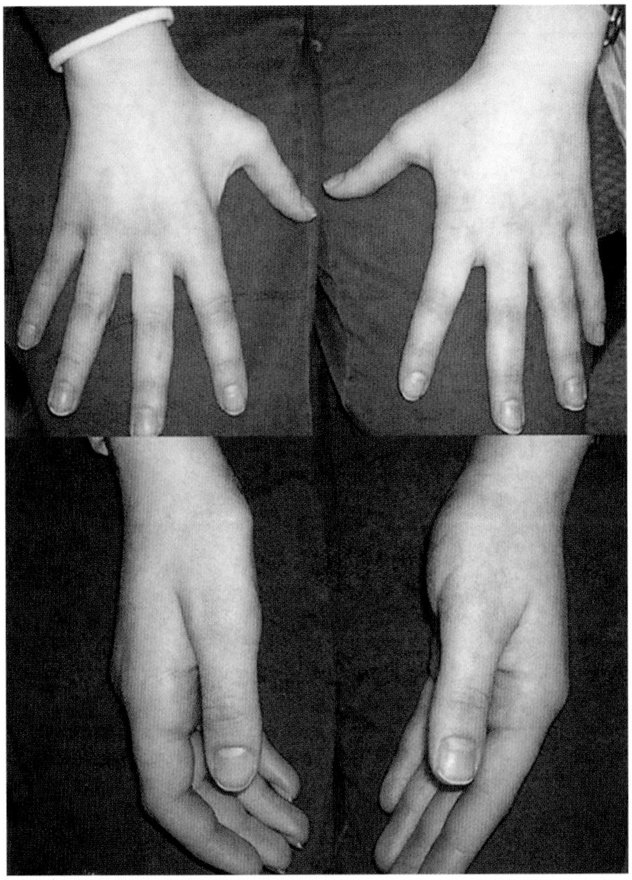

A

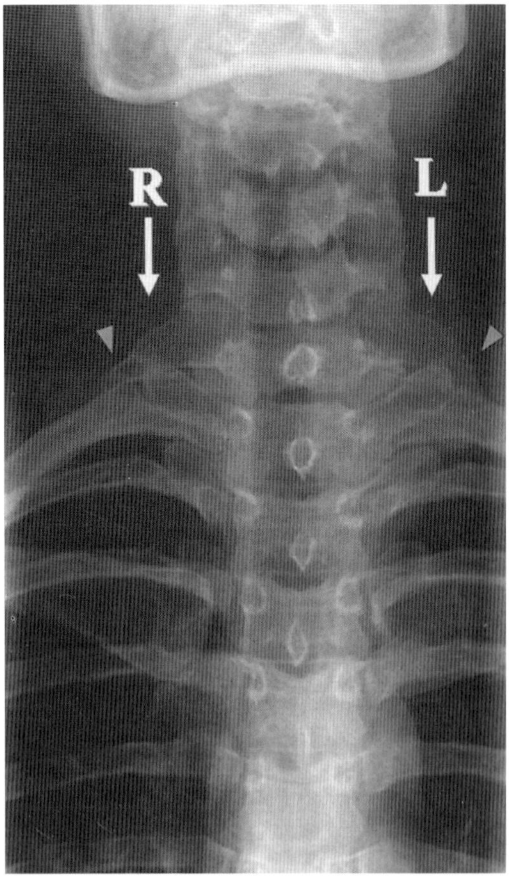

B

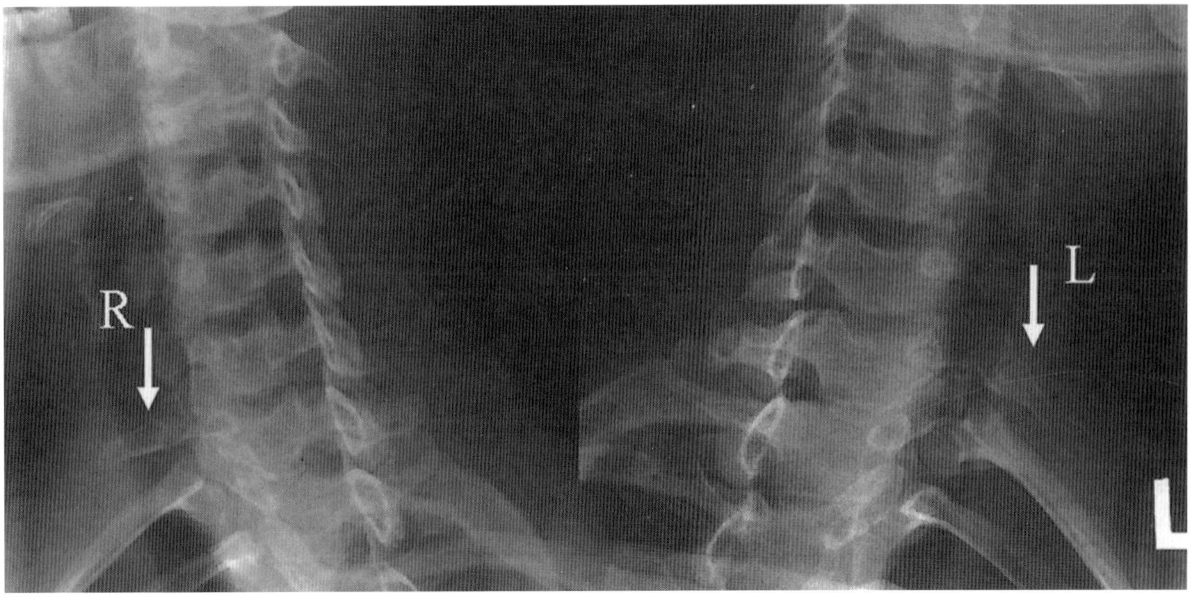

C

Figure 23-14. Neurogenic thoracic outlet syndrome. Atrophy of the right thenar eminence and first dorsal interosseous muscles are evident **(A)**. Plain cervical spine films demonstrate small cervical ribs (*arrows*) bilaterally on AP view **(B)** and oblique view **(C)**. (Reproduced with permission from of Steven A. Greenberg, MD. Reproduced with permission from Greenberg SA, Amato AA. *EMG Pearls*. Philadelphia, PA: Hanley & Belfus; 2004.)

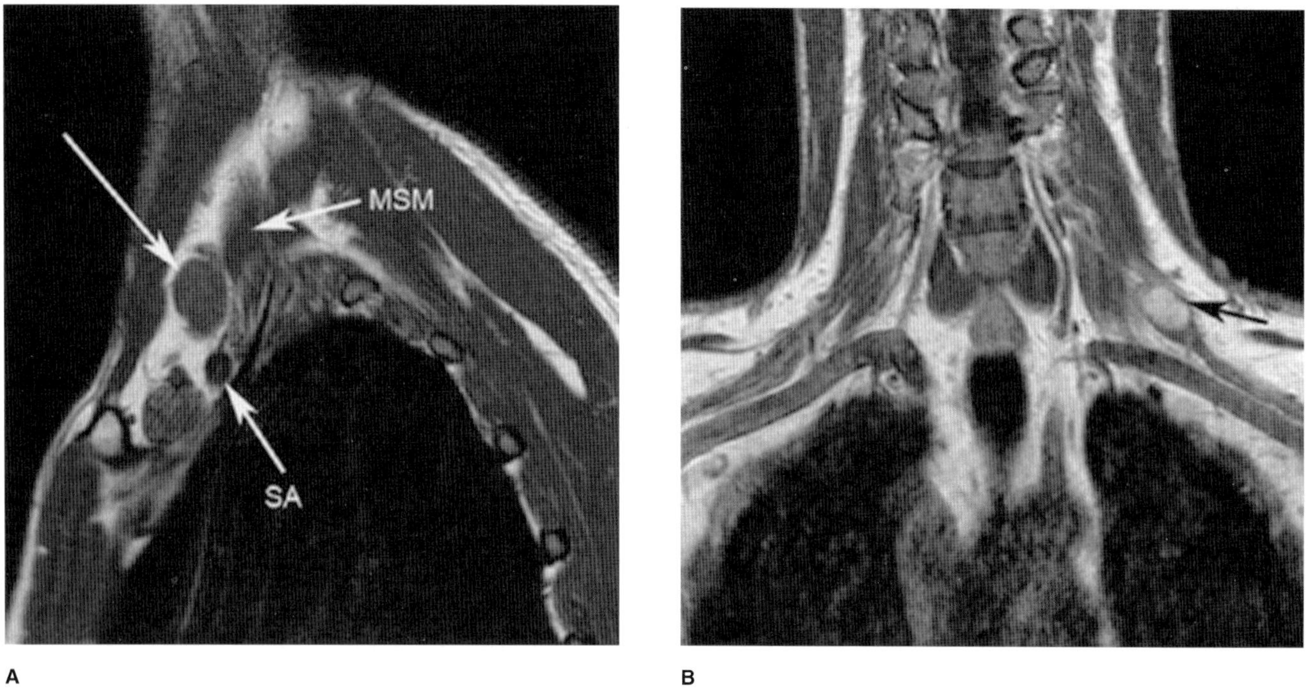

Figure 23-15. MRI of brachial plexus. Schwannoma of the superior trunk. **(A)** Sagittal T1-weighted image, *arrows* point to the tumor which is located in the superior trunk just lateral to the interscalene triangle and above the subclavian artery (SA). MSM, middle scalene muscle. **(B)** Coronal T1-weighted image with intravenous gadolinium shows the enhancing tumor (*arrow*). (Reproduced with permission from van Es HW, Bollen TL, van Heesewijk HP. MRI of the brachial plexus: a pictorial review. *Eur J Radiol*. 2010;74(2): 391–402.)

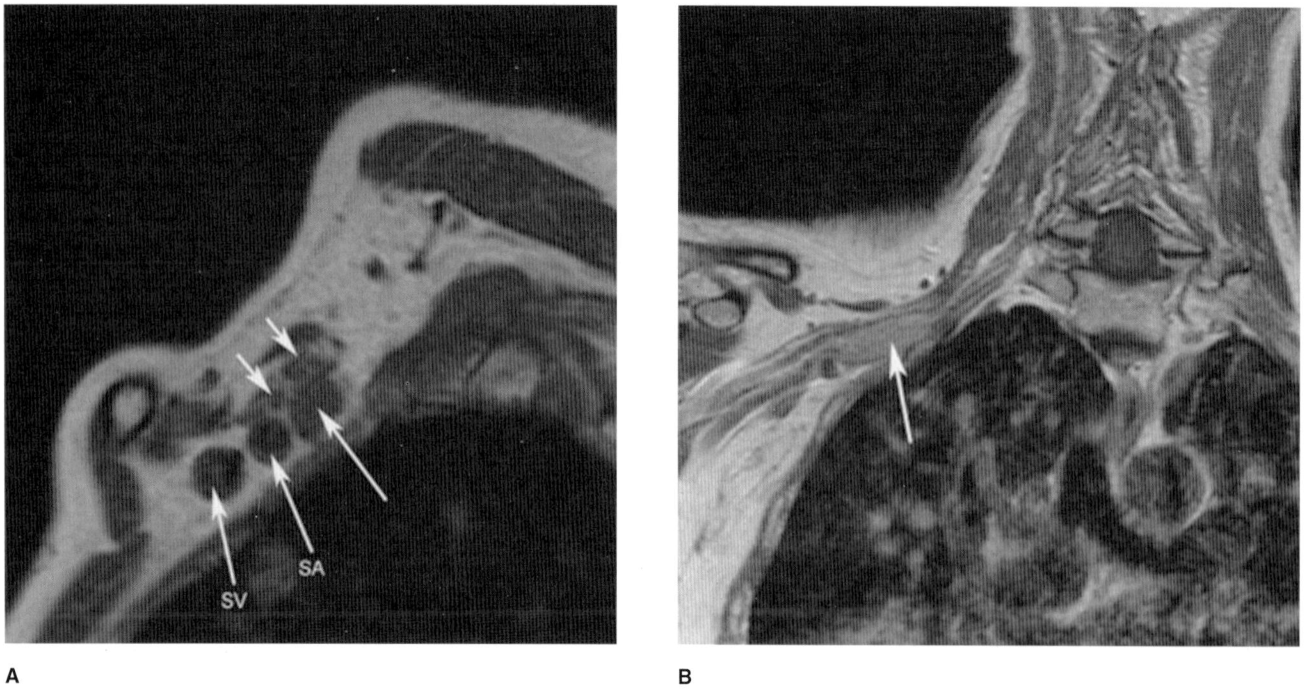

Figure 23-16. MRI of brachial plexus. Metastatic plexopathy of breast carcinoma. **(A)** Sagittal T1-weighted image shows a mass at the level of the divisions of the brachial plexus (long *arrows*). Note the normal neighboring nerves of the brachial plexus (short *arrows*). SA, subclavian artery; SV, subclavian vein. **(B)** Coronal T1-weighted image with intravenous gadolinium demonstrates the enhancement of the metastasis (*arrow*). (Reproduced with permission from van Es HW, Bollen TL, van Heesewijk HP. MRI of the brachial plexus: a pictorial review. *Eur J Radiol*. 2010;74(2):391–402.)

head) then hereditary neuropathy with liability to pressure palsy (HNPP) needs to be considered.

Perioperative Plexopathies (Median Sternotomy)

The most common surgical procedures associated with brachial plexopathy as a complication are those that involve median sternotomies (e.g., open heart surgeries and thoracotomies). Brachial plexopathies occur in as many as 5.0% of patients following a median sternotomy and typically affects the spinal nerve of the C8 root.[1–3,106–108] Thus, individuals manifest with sensory disturbance affecting the medial aspect of forearm and hand along with weakness of the intrinsic hand muscles, as discussed previously. Because of the location of the sensory symptoms, these lesions are often incorrectly blamed on ulnar neuropathies resulting from poor intraoperative elbow positioning or padding. The mechanism of this plexopathy is felt to be related to the stretch of the spinal nerve of the C8 root. These injuries are usually neuropraxic in nature, so most individuals who are affected recover in a few months.[107,109] However, some patients with significant axon loss may have a longer and incomplete recovery. Neurophysiological features are those previously discussed for lower trunk lesions.

Burners/Stingers

Burners and stingers refer to brachial plexus injuries caused by impact to shoulder region usually in the course of contact sports (e.g., football).[1,2] Usually, the affected athlete notes severe pain and sensory disturbance in the arms without any motor loss. The symptoms typically resolve after a few minutes. The mechanism is unclear, but the rapid recovery in most cases suggests a neuropraxic injury to the cervical roots or plexus, particularly the upper trunk.

Hereditary Neuropathies Manifesting as Brachial Plexopathy

Hereditary neuralgic amyotrophy (HNA) is an autosomal-dominant disorder characterized by recurrent attacks of pain, weakness, and sensory loss in the distribution of the brachial plexus, often beginning in childhood.[55,110] The clinical and electrophysiological features of HNA resemble those of IBPN. HNA should be considered in patients with recurrent attacks of brachial plexitis, even though the nonhereditary, idiopathic cases can recur.[55] In addition, HNPPs can present as painless brachial plexopathy. This may be one etiology of backpack palsy that was discussed in a previous section. In contrast to HNA, HNPP is a generalized or multifocal process, which is demyelinating in nature. HNA can be caused by mutations in the gene encoding septin 9, (*SEPT9*), while HNPP is usually caused by deletions in chromosome 17p11.2, resulting in a loss of function of peripheral myelin protein 22 (PMP-22). See Chapter 11 regarding "Charcot–Marie–Tooth Disease and Related Disorders" for more details.

SURGICAL TREATMENT OF BRACHIAL PLEXOPATHIES

The treatment of traumatic brachial plexopathies and timing of any surgical intervention are dependent on the type and severity of the injury, the location, and the time frame.[90] Most closed injuries result in neuropraxis or axonotmesis that may recover spontaneously. As a result, they are initially treated conservatively with physical and occupational therapy. Patients are followed closely with serial clinical and electrodiagnostic assessments to assess for recovery. If patients show no signs of recovery after 2–3 months in upper trunk lesions or 4–5 months for middle or lower trunk lesions, then surgical intervention should be considered.[90] Injuries associated with high-energy trauma or those associated with near-total paralysis may be observed for a shorter period of time (3 weeks to 3 months) prior to surgery.[111] Injuries associated with sharp penetrating trauma are more likely associated with severing of nerves and should be repaired within 72 hours, if possible.[17,89,97,112] Worsening neurological function, hematoma formation, concomitant bone or vascular injuries, and compartment syndrome are other indications for more acute surgical intervention.[90] Various surgical techniques including neurolysis, nerve grafting, neurotization, and free muscle transfer are performed in order to assist in regaining shoulder abduction and elbow flexion and some use of the hand function.[111,113–115]

► TERMINAL NERVE LESIONS

In this section, we discuss mononeuropathies of the upper limb mainly due to trauma, compression, or entrapment, or those that are idiopathic in nature. Any of these nerves may be affected alone or in combination with other nerve lesions in other settings such as vasculitis (isolated or systemic), infection (e.g., Lyme disease, leprosy, HIV, cytomegalovirus, and hepatitis), immune-mediated demyelination (e.g., multifocal motor neuropathy and multifocal acquired demyelinating motor and sensory neuropathy), and other inflammatory neuropathies (e.g., perineuritis and sarcoidosis), as discussed in other chapters in this book.

SPINAL ACCESSORY

As discussed previously, the spinal accessory nerve does not arise from the brachial plexus. Since it is often damaged with trauma to the neck and shoulder region with or without brachial plexus involvement, we discuss spinal accessory neuropathy in this chapter. Lymph node biopsy and other surgical procedures in the posterior triangle are very common etiologies for spinal accessory neuropathies. The nerve can also be involved in IBPN. Injury of the nerve is often painful, presumably due to the mechanical effects from the dropped shoulder it produces. The shoulder drop is best observed

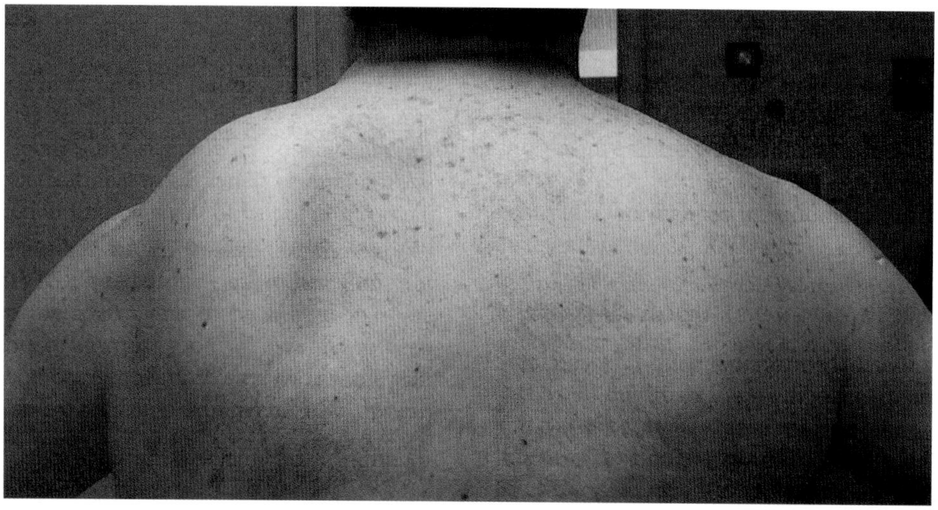

Figure 23-17. Spinal accessory neuropathy. Winging of the left scapula is appreciated and is brought out by abduction of the shoulder. (Reproduced with permission from Steven A. Greenberg, MD. Reproduced with permission from Greenberg SA, Amato AA. *EMG Pearls*. Philadelphia, PA: Hanley & Belfus; 2004.)

from behind the patient. An accessory nerve palsy often results in scapular winging as well and a reduced capability of flexing the arm fully at the shoulder in the sagittal plane. (Fig. 23-17). Winging from a spinal accessory nerve lesion is distinguished from winging from rhomboid and serratus anterior weakness by a number of observations and provocative maneuvers. Winging from trapezius weakness is accentuated by resisted external rotation of the arm at the shoulder. This occurs as the trapezius normally acts to hold the entire medial border of the scapula against the chest wall to provide the resistance necessary for effective external rotation. The winging typically affects the entire medial border of the scapula equally so the inferior angle and posterior angle tend to be at near-equivalent distances from both the spine and chest wall, maintaining the medial scapular border in a vertical orientation. Trapezius weakness can also be detected and distinguished from serratus anterior weakness by the patient's inability to flex the arm at the shoulder in the prone position. This maneuver results in compensatory lumbar hyperlordosis and producing the triangle sign (the three sides of the triangle being the table, anterior chest wall, and undersurface of the arm with the axilla being the apex. [116,117] Most lesions are distal to the innervation of the sternocleidomastoid muscles; however, proximal damage may result in weakness of turning the head to the contralateral side. CMAPs recorded from the trapezius muscle may demonstrate reduced amplitude compared to the contralateral side, but electrodiagnosis usually relies on demonstrating denervation changes in this muscle.

DORSAL SCAPULAR NERVE

The dorsal scapular arises mainly from C5 spinal root but may have contributions from the C4 segment. The nerve innervates the rhomboid major and minor along with the levator scapula, which assist in retraction (draw medial border closer to rib cage and midline), elevation, and medial inferior angle rotation of the scapula. Therefore, damage to the dorsal scapular nerve leads to scapular winging, with the inferior angle rotated laterally. Elevation of the arm overhead will accentuate the scapular winging. It is very unusual to have an isolated dorsal scapular nerve injury. NCS are not particularly helpful. Electrodiagnostic confirmation requires demonstration of EMG abnormalities isolated to the rhomboid and levator scapula muscles.

LONG THORACIC NERVE

The long thoracic nerve originates from the fusion of branches from the C5, C6, and often C7 spinal roots, and it innervates the serratus anterior muscle (Fig. 23-3). This muscle stabilizes the scapula and helps hold it tight against the chest wall during movement of the shoulder girdle. In addition, it assists in rotating the scapula laterally to allow for full elevation of the arm as the glenohumeral joint provides for only 90 degrees of arm flexion and abduction at the shoulder. A long thoracic neuropathy manifests as scapular winging, a reduction in the ability to elevate the arm in a sagittal and coronal plane, and with reduced strength in pushing activities. The whole scapula is winged. As the muscle originates from the bottom half of the scapula, the inferior angle of the scapula tends to be more affected than the superior angle resulting in the inferior angle to be rotated toward the spine and to be farther off the chest wall than the superior angle. (Fig. 23-18). This winging is accentuated by having the patient flex the arm forward at the shoulder against resistance.

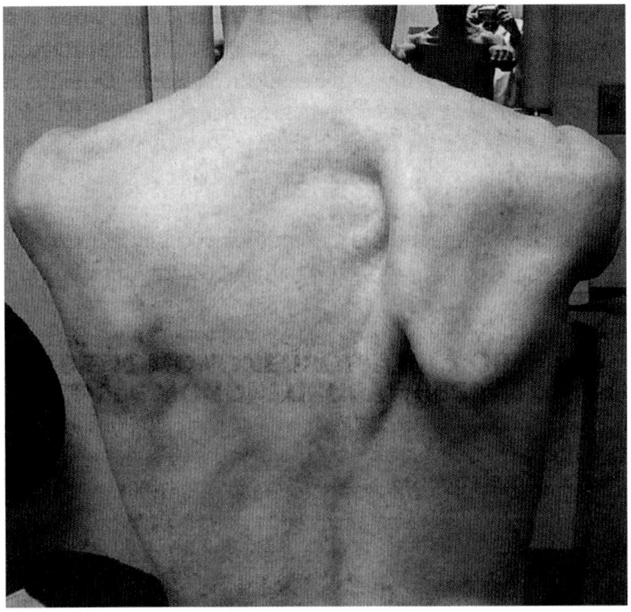

Figure 23-18. Long thoracic neuropathy. Winging of the right scapula is appreciated and is enhanced by having the patient flex the arm forward at the shoulder. There is also atrophy of the infraspinatus secondary to a superimposed suprascapular nerve injury. (Reproduced with permission from Steven A. Greenberg, MD. Reproduced with permission from Greenberg SA, Amato AA. *EMG Pearls*. Philadelphia, PA: Hanley & Belfus; 2004.)

The long thoracic nerve may be damaged from trauma[118–120] or during surgical procedures, particularly mastectomies and thoracotomies (Table 23-5).[121,122] Most often, we see long thoracic neuropathies either isolated or in combination with other neuropathies in the setting of IBPN.[53] Motor NCS of the long thoracic nerve is not typically performed, and electrodiagnostic confirmation of a long thoracic neuropathy requires demonstration of EMG abnormalities isolated to the serratus anterior muscle. Needle EMG of this muscle should be done cautiously due to risk of pneumothorax.

Long thoracic neuropathies are usually managed conservatively depending on etiology. Open injuries due to trauma may require surgery. Otherwise, in most instances we start with physical and occupational therapy along with bracing. Scapulothoracic stabilization braces can be used to help keep the shoulder abutted against the thorax. If the shoulder function does not improve over time, surgery can be considered to stabilize the scapula.[123,124]

TABLE 23-5. CONDITIONS ASSOCIATED WITH PROXIMAL LONG THORACIC NEUROPATHY

Trauma
Surgical injury (postthoracotomy, radical mastectomy, axillary surgery, rib resection)
Immune-mediated brachial plexus neuropathy

SUPRASCAPULAR NERVE

The suprascapular nerve arises from the upper trunk and innervates the supraspinatus and infraspinatus muscles (Fig. 23-5). The supraspinatus muscle assists in the initial aspects of shoulder abduction, while the infraspinatus muscle is used to externally rotate the arm at the shoulder. Thus, these movements are limited, depending on the location of the suprascapular nerve injury.

The nerve may be damaged with trauma to the shoulder region, particularly if there is a dislocation or fracture of the shoulder.[125–129] The nerve may be injured at the suprascapular notch affecting both muscles, or rarely in the spinoglenoid notch with weakness confined to the infraspinatus.[130,131] More commonly, this suprascapular nerve is affected in the setting of IBPN and involvement may be isolated to this nerve.[53,54]

Motor conduction studies to this nerve are technically limiting, so electrodiagnosis relies on EMG demonstration of denervation changes in the supraspinatus and infraspinatus muscle, if the lesion is proximal to the suprascapular notch or limited to the infraspinatus muscle, if the lesion occurs in the region of the spinoglenoid.

Management is dependent on the etiology of the neuropathy. Surgery is warranted for open lesions related to trauma, otherwise conservative therapy with pain control is recommended. Local injections of corticosteroids can be tried if the cause is felt to be related to compression of the nerve in the suprascapular or supraglenoid notch, and some even advocate surgery; however, entrapment of the nerves at this site remains a controversial etiology.[132,133]

MEDIAL/LATERAL PECTORAL NERVES

The medial and lateral pectoral nerves are discussed together as both innervate the pectoralis minor and major muscles (Fig. 23-3). The large pectoralis major muscle assists in internal rotation, anterior flexion, and adduction of the arm at the shoulder, while the pectoralis minor assists in scapula stabilization during arm extension at the shoulder. These nerves may be damaged rarely, usually during surgical procedures in the anterior chest and axillary region. Again, motor conduction studies of these nerves are not routinely performed and electrodiagnostic confirmation requires demonstration of EMG abnormalities in the pectoralis minor and major muscles.

SUBSCAPULAR NERVE

Injury to the subscapular nerve has not been described in detail and rarely occur in isolation but may be involved in more generalized plexopathy. As the lower subscapular nerve innervates the teres major muscle, damage to this nerve may result in weakness of internal rotation and adduction of the arm at the shoulder. There are no motor NCS for this nerve, and needle EMG of the muscle is difficult given its deep location.

THORACODORSAL NERVE

The thoracodorsal nerve arises form the posterior cord and innervates the latissimus dorsi muscle (Fig. 23-3). Weakness of this muscle results in impaired ability to adduct, internally rotate, and extend the arm at the shoulder. Slight winging of the inferior margin of the scapula may be observed when the patient is asked to place the dorsum of the hand of the affected arm on the buttock.[10,121]

The nerve is usually affected in association with posterior cord or more proximal brachial plexus injuries. NCS are not routinely done on this nerve, but EMG of the latissimus dorsi muscle is easy to perform and helps in localizing the lesion to C5–7 nerve fibers at or proximal to the posterior cord.

MUSCULOCUTANEOUS NERVE

The musculocutaneous nerve represents a continuation of the lateral cord and innervates the coracobrachialis, biceps brachii, and to some extent the brachialis (Fig. 23-6). After innervating these muscles, it terminates as the lateral antebrachial cutaneous nerve to supply sensation to the lateral aspect of the forearm from the elbow to the wrist. Damage to the musculocutaneous nerve may therefore result in sensory loss in this distribution and weakness of elbow flexion accompanied by a reduced deep tendon reflex of the biceps brachii. The musculocutaneous nerve may be damaged by anterior dislocations of the shoulder and prolonged hyperextension of the arm, secondary to weight lifting (perhaps compressed within hypertrophic muscle) (Table 23-6).[8,121,134–136] It is also often affected in IBPN.[53]

The lateral antebrachial cutaneous SNAP is easy to obtain and would be expected to be reduced in axonal lesions affecting the musculocutaneous nerve (Table 23-2). This is nonlocalizing in and of itself as the SNAP could also be reduced with lateral cord or upper trunk lesions; however, it would be normal in C6 radiculopathy. A musculocutaneous CMAP can be obtained by stimulating the brachial plexus in the supraclavicular fossa and recording from the biceps brachii. It can provide valuable prognostic information. A normal CMAP recording from biceps and stimulating in the axilla occurring 10 days after injury in a patient who cannot activate the biceps strongly implicates conduction block and suggests a rapid and excellent return of function. Comparing the CMAP amplitude to the opposite side can provide an estimate of the degree of axon loss. EMG may show denervation abnormalities in the coracobrachialis, biceps brachii, and brachialis muscles (Table 23-1). Again abnormalities in the supraspinatus, deltoid, biceps brachii, and pronator teres muscles, but not in serratus anterior, rhomboids, or paraspinal regions, would imply an upper trunk injury, while denervation changes in the latter three regions would suggest a radiculopathy or anterior horn cell disease. On the other hand, only finding abnormalities in the biceps brachii and pronator teres, sparing deltoid, is more consistent with a lateral cord injury.

Initial management depends on the etiology of the neuropathy. Those caused by severe trauma may require surgical treatment. However, in most cases a conservative approach is warranted.

▶ TABLE 23-6. CONDITIONS ASSOCIATED WITH MUSCULOCUTANEOUS NEUROPATHY

Trauma (fracture or dislocation of shoulder, fracture of humerus, missile injuries, stab wounds, blunt force injuries)
Injection injury
Immune-mediated brachial plexus neuropathy
Soft tissue or peripheral nerve tumor
Ischemia (e.g., vasculitis)
Multifocal motor neuropathy or multifocal acquired demyelinating motor and sensory neuropathy
Compression within hypertrophied biceps brachii muscle after vigorous exercise
Compression by sharp free margin of biceps aponeurosis

AXILLARY NERVE

The axillary nerve originates from the posterior cord and innervates the teres minor and deltoid muscle (Fig. 23-7). In addition, the lateral cutaneous nerve of the arm arises from the axillary nerve. Thus, axillary neuropathies may manifest with weakness of abduction of the arm and sensory loss in the region of skin overlying the deltoid muscle.

Axillary neuropathies may occur in the setting of IBPN, trauma to the shoulder, fractures of the upper humerus, or stretch injury (Table 23-7).[8,9,121,137–139] Axillary CMAPs may be recorded from the deltoid muscle following supraclavicular stimulation of the brachial plexus to see if there is asymmetrical loss of amplitude on the affected site or a disconnect between the amount of movement and the size of the CMAP. A superficial radial SNAP would be expected to be normal in an axillary neuropathy and can help distinguish an axillary neuropathy from a posterior cord lesion or upper trunk lesion (Table 23-2).

▶ TABLE 23-7. CONDITIONS ASSOCIATED WITH AXILLARY NEUROPATHY

Trauma (e.g., fracture or dislocation of shoulder, fracture of humerus, missile injuries, stab wounds, blunt force injuries)
Stretch injury (e.g., hyperabduction during sleep, surgery)
Injection injury
Immune-mediated brachial plexus neuropathy
Soft tissue or peripheral nerve tumor
Ischemia (e.g., vasculitis)
Multifocal motor neuropathy or multifocal acquired demyelinating motor and sensory neuropathy

Furthermore, EMG should show evidence of denervation in the deltoid and teres minor muscles with sparing of radial-innervated muscles in an isolated axillary neuropathy (Table 23-1). In addition, a normal EMG of the supraspinatus, infraspinatus, rhomboids, biceps brachii, pronator teres, and brachioradialis suggests that the lesion is distal to the C5/C6 roots or upper trunk when combined with denervation of the deltoid.

Axillary neuropathies related to penetrating injuries should be surgically explored. Otherwise, these are managed conservatively with pain management and PT/OT. If there is no improvement within 6 months, surgical treatment and grafting can be considered.[140]

RADIAL NERVE

The radial nerve is one of the major terminations of the posterior cord and is composed of fibers from spinal segments C5–8 and occasionally contains T1 fibers (Fig. 23-8). The radial nerve is quite long and provides innervation to upper arm and forearm muscles as well as for cutaneous sensation of large aspects of the arm. The clinical and electrodiagnostic features of radial neuropathies depend on the site of the lesion. The superficial radial SNAP should be abnormal, if there is significant axonal nerve injury, except with posterior interosseous nerve damage, as this is a purely motor nerve. Radial CMAP to the radial-innervated muscles such as the extensor indicis proprius should be performed with short incremental stimulation of the radial nerve through the spinal groove to assess for focal conduction block or slowing across this site. With significant axonal injury, the CMAP amplitude should be reduced regardless of stimulation site. EMG is more helpful in localizing the site of the lesion with axonal injury. Evidence of active denervation in the form of fibrillation potentials and positive sharp waves would be expected in an axonal nerve injury, provided there has been substantial time for Wallerian degeneration to occur. In a pure neuropraxic injury, only reduced recruitment of MUAPs would be appreciated on EMG, although many predominantly demyelinating injuries may have some element of axon loss. A few fibrillation potentials do not preclude a good recovery as they may originate from a very small number of injured axons.

▶ TABLE 23-8. CONDITIONS ASSOCIATED WITH PROXIMAL RADIAL NEUROPATHY

Trauma
Fracture of humerus
Improper use of crutches (e.g., compression in axilla)
Stretch injury (e.g., hyperabduction of arm during surgery, sleep)
Saturday night palsy (external compression by arm being compressed against firm edge at the spiral groove—usually in intoxicated individuals)
Other external compression (partner falling asleep on arm)
Immune-mediated brachial plexus neuropathy
Soft tissue or peripheral nerve tumor
Ischemia (e.g., A-V fistulas, vasculitis)
Multifocal motor neuropathy or multifocal acquired demyelinating motor and sensory neuropathy

Proximal Radial Neuropathy

Damage to the nerve in the axilla or proximal arm is uncommon but can result from compression (e.g., crutches, intoxicated patients who fall asleep with outstretched arm pressed against a hard surface, missile injuries, and other trauma to the axilla) (Table 23-8).[8,9,121] Of course, a radial neuropathy can also occur in the setting of a more widespread multifocal process (e.g., vasculitis, IBPN). Proximal radial nerve injuries can result in weakness of elbow, wrist, and finger extension as well as supination of the forearm. In addition, sensory disturbance may be evident in the posterior aspect of the forearm and back of the hand and fingers. Provided there is sufficient axon loss, the superficial radial SNAP and radial CMAP recorded from the extensor indicis proprius may have reduced amplitudes (Table 23-2). EMG should demonstrate signs of denervation in the triceps as well as more distal radial-innervated forearm muscles (Table 23-1).

Radial neuropathy in the arm distal to the branches innervating the triceps arises from various mechanisms. One of the most common radial neuropathies is the so-called "Saturday night palsy" and is usually the result of prolonged compression of the radial nerve in the spiral groove in an individual who is intoxicated. Proximal radial nerve lesions have also been speculated to be the result of anomalous muscle compression or damage secondary to triceps muscle contraction.[141,142] On clinical examination, one would expect to find weakness of the radial-innervated muscles distal to the triceps in addition to sensory loss in the posterior aspect of the forearm and back of the hand and fingers. Again, a superficial radial SNAP and a radial CMAP may have reduced amplitudes, if the injury is axonal. EMG should demonstrate signs of denervation of radial-innervated forearm muscles, unless it is caused by a pure conduction block, with sparing of the more proximal triceps muscles.

Proximal radial neuropathies caused by penetrating trauma should be surgically explored and treated with end-to-end anastomosis or grafting. Closed traumas, including humeral fractures, are often due to neuropraxia and recover gradually on their own. A trial of conservative therapy is employed prior to any surgery. Proximal radial neuropathies related to pressure or stretch injuries (e.g., Saturday night palsy) or IBPN are also treated conservatively. Finger and wrist splints, pain control, and physical and occupational therapy are employed.

Posterior Interosseous Neuropathy

Damage to the posterior interosseous nerve will result in weakness of wrist and finger extensors with sparing of sensation. The posterior interosseous nerve can be damaged from multiple mechanisms (Table 23-9). Although some have speculated that the nerve can be entrapped within the

▶ **TABLE 23-9. CONDITIONS ASSOCIATED WITH POSTERIOR INTEROSSEOUS NEUROPATHY**

Immune-mediated brachial plexus neuropathy
Trauma
Compression by tumors, ganglion cysts, lipoma, bursitis
Compression by the arcade of Fröhse
Compression by facial bands connecting the brachialis to the brachioradialis muscle at the radial head
Compression by edge or fibrous bands within the supinator muscle
Compression by a bifid extensor carpi radialis brevis muscle
Rheumatoid arthritis
Soft tissue or peripheral nerve tumor
Ischemia (e.g., A-V fistulas, vasculitis)
Multifocal motor neuropathy or multifocal acquired demyelinating motor and sensory neuropathy

supinator muscle (arcade of Fröhse), this is quite rare in our opinion. Many such cases probably represent a forme fruste of an IBPN or another immune-mediated neuropathy (e.g., multifocal motor neuropathy) (Fig. 23-19). On NCS, the superficial radial SNAP should be normal, but the radial CMAP recorded from the extensor indicis proprius may reveal a reduction in amplitude, provided there is significant axon loss (Table 23-2). EMG should demonstrate signs of denervation in muscles innervated by the posterior interosseous nerve.

Unless the posterior interosseous neuropathy is related to open trauma, it is managed conservatively as discussed with proximal radial neuropathies. Rare cases of the so-called radial tunnel syndrome with compression of the posterior interosseous nerve may improve with surgery.[143] Again, we feel that such entrapment is quite rare and the existence is controversial.

▶ **TABLE 23-10. CONDITIONS ASSOCIATED WITH SUPERFICIAL RADIAL NEUROPATHY**

External compression (handcuffs, tight wrist bands, casts)
De Quervain tenosynovitis
Trauma
Soft tissue or peripheral nerve tumor

Superficial Radial Neuropathy

The superficial radial nerve is a pure sensory branch of the radial nerve that provides sensation to the dorsum of the hand. It can be damaged by various means (Table 23-10). In particular, compression by tight bands, watches, and handcuffs can lead to a superficial radial neuropathy. The superficial radial SNAP is usually decreased in amplitude, while motor studies and EMG would be normal. This type of neuropathy is usually due to neuropraxia and improves spontaneously. Cases related to laceration or other trauma may require surgery.

MEDIAN NERVE

As previously discussed, the median nerve contains fibers originating from spinal segments C6–T1, which then course

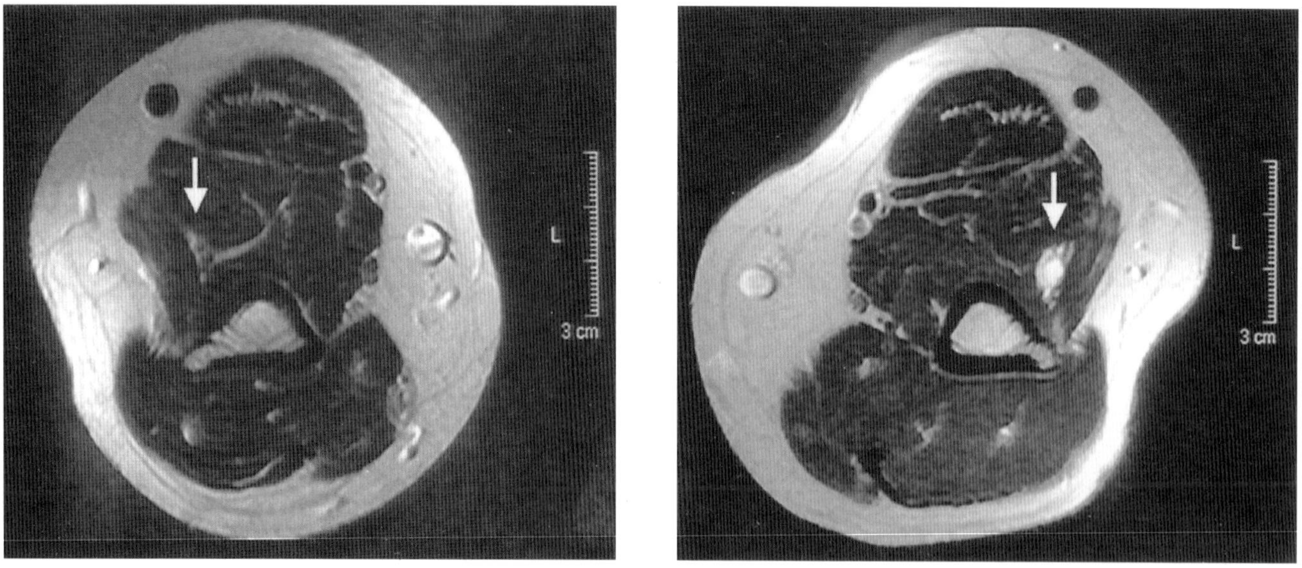

Right radial nerve Left radial nerve

Figure 23-19. MRI of (T2) forearms in a patient with multifocal motor neuropathy affecting the left radial nerve demonstrates focal enlargement and enhancement of the radial nerve (*arrows*) in the forearm on the left side. (Reproduced with permission from Steven A. Greenberg, MD. Reproduced with permission from Greenberg SA, Amato AA. *EMG Pearls*. Philadelphia, PA: Hanley & Belfus; 2004.)

through all three trunks and the medial and lateral cords. The median nerve is formed by the merging of branches from the medial and lateral cords (Fig. 23-9). Axons from spinal segments C5–7 that course through the upper and middle trunks and lateral cords are responsible for providing cutaneous sensation to the palmar aspect of the hand and digits 1–3 and usually the lateral half of digit 4. In addition, these segments also innervate several forearm muscles, primarily the pronator teres and flexor carpi radialis. On the other hand, C8 and T1 nerve fibers course through the lower trunk and medial cord and innervate muscles controlling finger movements and provide no sensory input.

Proximal Median Neuropathy

Proximal median neuropathies in the axilla, upper arm, and forearm may result from misuse of crutches, missile injuries, and laceration of the nerve by trauma (Table 23-11) (Fig. 23-20).[8,9,144,145] Compression of the nerve can also occur due to an awkward sleeping position—often in individuals who are intoxicated. Ischemic damage to the median nerve can occur as a complication of nerve ischemia due to arterial diversion resulting from creation of shunts of fistulas for renal dialysis.[146] The median nerve can be affected as well in the setting of IBPN. Proximal median neuropathies have been reported to be caused by compression by the ligament of Struthers, but this is controversial.[147–150] Compression by the lacertus fibrosus or bicipital aponeurosis at the elbow have also been implicated as possible etiologies.[151]

TABLE 23-11. CONDITIONS ASSOCIATED WITH PROXIMAL MEDIAN NEUROPATHY

Improper use of crutches (e.g., compression in axilla)
Trauma (e.g., dislocation of shoulder, fracture of humerus, missile injuries, stab wounds, tourniquets)
Compression by ligament of Struthers
Pronator teres syndrome
Thickened lacertus fibrosus
Fibrous arch of the flexor digitorum superficialis
Tendinous band or hypertrophied pronator teres muscle
Sleep palsies
Compartment syndrome
Ischemia (e.g., A-V fistulas, vasculitis)
Immune-mediated brachial plexus neuropathy
Soft tissue or peripheral nerve tumor
Multifocal motor neuropathy or multifocal acquired demyelinating motor and sensory neuropathy

Individuals with proximal median neuropathies present with weakness of the median-innervated forearm and hand muscles and reduced sensation in the palmar aspect of the hand, digits 1–3, and the lateral aspect of digit 4. In our experience, it is not uncommon for proximal median neuropathies to clinically manifest as predominantly anterior interosseous syndromes, even though electrodiagnosis suggests that the entire nerve is affected. In these cases, median SNAPs to any of these digits would be expected to show reduced amplitudes again, provided there is sufficient axonal injury. The

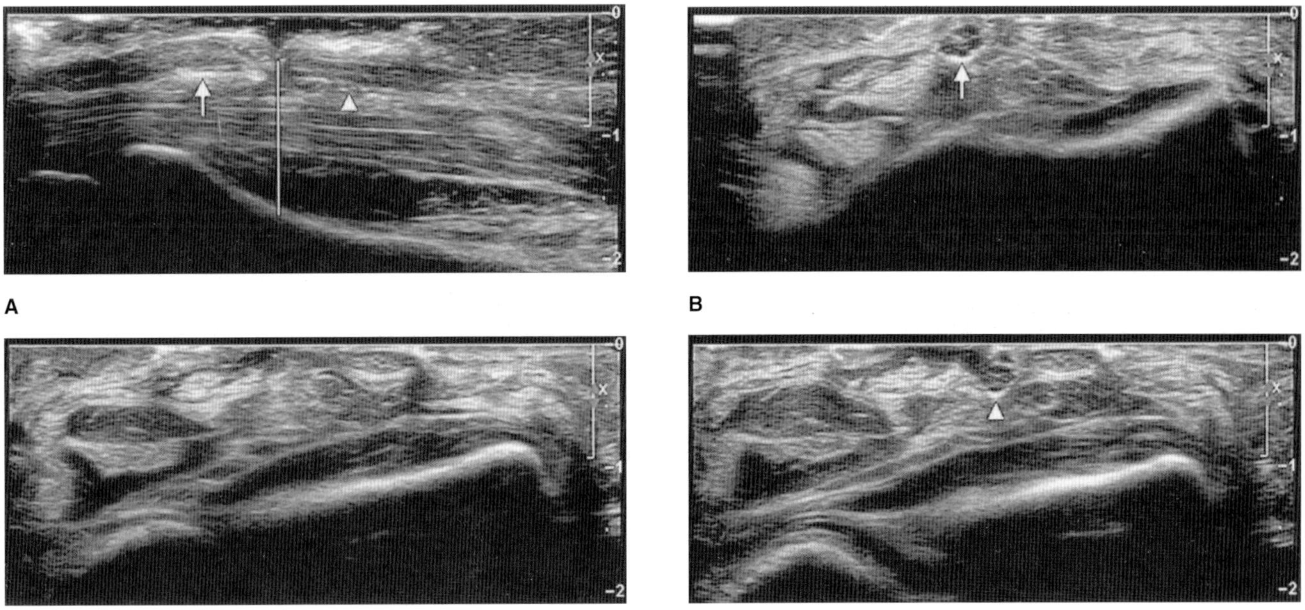

A B C D

Figure 23-20. Ultrasound images depicting transection of the median nerve in the forearm. **(A)** Sagittal view showing the distal nerve stump (*arrow*), proximal stump (*arrowhead*), and the transection (*line*). Cross-sectional views at the level of the distal nerve **(B)**, site of transection **(C)**, and proximal nerve **(D)**. The median nerve is seen in images **(B)** and **(D)**, but it is not present in image **(C)** at the site of transection. (Reproduced with permission from Cartwright MS, Chloros GD, Walker FO, Wiesler ER, William W, Campbell WW. Diagnostic ultrasound for nerve transaction. *Muscle Nerve*. 2007;796–799.)

distal latency or conduction velocity of the median SNAP would be expected to be normal or only slightly impaired compared to the loss of amplitude. Similarly, the median CMAP amplitude recorded from the abductor pollicis studies may be reduced. It is important in these proximal median neuropathies to look for evidence of slowing of CV, temporal dispersion, or focal conduction block (discussed in Chapters 2 and 12). EMG would be expected to demonstrate abnormalities in median-innervated muscles in the forearm and hand (Table 23-1).

A controversial entity is the so-called pronator teres syndrome. In this disorder, the median nerve is thought to be compressed where it passes under the fibrous arch connecting the two heads of the pronator teres muscle. The major clinical manifestation is pain and tenderness in the volar aspect of the forearm and paresthesias in the distribution of the median nerve. These symptoms are exacerbated by having the patient actively trying to pronate the forearm against resistance. We remain rather skeptical of this diagnosis, as there is usually no objective clinical or electrodiagnostical evidence of median nerve injury.

Proximal median neuropathies carry a poor prognosis if there is significant axonal degeneration. The reason is the long distance the nerve must grow in order for complete reinnervation to occur. As long as there are some voluntary MUAPs in the forearm and hand muscles, there is potential for recovery.

The proximal median neuropathies are usually treated conservatively unless trauma is involved. Decompression surgeries have not been adequately studied in a scientific fashion, owing in part to the rarity of proximal median compressive neuropathies.

Anterior Interosseous Syndrome

The anterior interosseous nerve can be damaged from multiple mechanisms (Table 23-12). Most commonly, in our experience, an anterior interosseous neuropathy arises either in conjunction with or as a forme fruste of an IBPN. As mentioned, proximal median neuropathies may masquerade as anterior interosseous syndrome. As the anterior interosseous nerve is a pure motor nerve, patients do not have sensory loss. However, severe pain in the forearm for several days or weeks is typical in cases related to IBPN. Individuals have weakness in the flexor digitorum profundus I and II, flexor hallucis longus, and pronator quadratus muscles. This leads to difficulty with pinching maneuvers or forming the letter "O" with their thumb and index or middle fingers, as they have weakness of flexion of the distal aspects of these digits. Most cases should be managed conservatively. However, if there is no improvement in function after 4–6 months, surgical exploration to assess for compression can be considered.[139,152]

TABLE 23-12. CAUSES OF ANTERIOR INTEROSSEOUS NEUROPATHY

Immune-mediated brachial plexus neuropathy
Trauma
Fibrous band within the pronator teres
Compartment syndrome
Soft tissue or peripheral nerve tumor
Ischemia (e.g., A-V fistulas, vasculitis)
Multifocal motor neuropathy

Median Neuropathy at the Wrist or Carpal Tunnel Syndrome

Median neuropathy at the wrist or carpal tunnel syndrome (CTS) is the most common mononeuropathy. There are multiple causes of median neuropathy at the wrist, although the vast majority are thought to be related to tenosynovitis of the flexor tendons which also occupy the carpal tunnel along with the median nerve (Table 23-13).[8,9] Some clinicians restrict the term "CTS" only to those median neuropathies at the wrist caused by tenosynovitis. People with median neuropathy at the wrist usually complain of intermittent numbness and tingling of their fingers particularly at night or in other situations where the carpal tunnel is narrowed by wrist extension or extension, for example, holding a steering wheel, telephone, or hairdryer. Sometimes the numbness and tingling as well as the pain patients describe extend beyond the territory of the median nerve (e.g., these may describe sensory symptoms in the little finger and aching in the forearm as well). The symptoms may be exacerbated by repetitive activity. However, the discomfort often occurs at rest. The painful paresthesias may be briefly alleviated by shaking the hands, the so-called 'flick sign."[153]

Clinical examination is frequently normal when the nerve is predominantly irritated, not injured. When axon loss occurs, patients may develop constant numbness and the examination may reveal loss of sensation in the median

TABLE 23-13. CONDITIONS ASSOCIATED WITH MEDIAN NEUROPATHY AT THE WRIST

Idiopathic
Flexor tenosynovitis
Degenerative joint disease
Rheumatoid arthritis
Sarcoidosis
Space occupying lesions (e.g., ganglion cysts, lipomas, hemangiomas, giant cell tumors, osteomas)
Trauma (e.g., Colles' fracture, dislocation/fracture of carpal bones)
Pregnancy
Endocrine (e.g., hypothyroid, acromegaly, diabetes mellitus[a])
Amyloidosis (familial and primary)
Hereditary neuropathy with liability to pressure palsies
Soft tissue or peripheral nerve tumor

[a]It is unclear if individuals with typical generalized diabetic polyneuropathy may be predisposed to focal mononeuropathies related to compression.

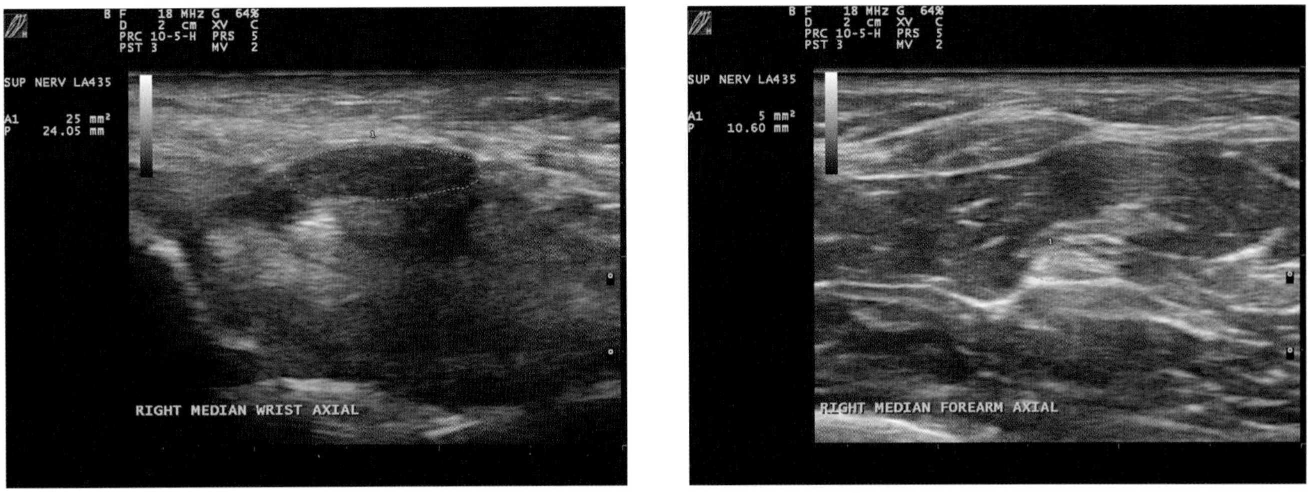

A B

Figure 23-21. Sonograms of a patient with symptomatic right carpal tunnel syndrome. The right median nerve had a markedly increased cross-sectional area (CSA) of 25 mm^2 at the distal wrist crease (normal <12 mm^2) **(A)**, and 5 mm^2 in the forearm **(B)**, as outlined by the green dashes resulting in an increased wrist/forearm CSA ratio of 5 (normal <1.5).

nerve distribution to the fingers. Motor function is generally spared, unless the injury is severe at which point weakness of atrophy of the thenar muscles is appreciated. Tapping over the wrist may elicit increased paresthesias in the fingers (Tinel sign), but this is not very specific. Having the persons maintain their wrists in the flexed posture may also exacerbate the discomfort in the fingers (Phalen sign), and this is more specific for CTS.

Sonography of the median nerve at the wrist may demonstrate flattening of the median nerve at the wrist (Fig. 23-21).[30,31,36,154] A recent meta-analysis reported that the sensitivity and specificity of ultrasound in the diagnosis of CTS are 77.6% and 86.8%, respectively.[154] MRI of the wrist may show reduction of the cross-sectional diameter of the carpal tunnel.[25,26] Swelling of the tendons, boney and cystic lesions, as well as compression of the nerve may be visualized by MRI. The major drawback of MRI is that it is very expensive. Despite the potential benefits, imaging of the carpal tunnel is not routinely applied by most clinicians.

There are various NCS that can be performed to confirm the clinical impression of a median neuropathy at the wrist. It should be recognized that NCS like all tests are imperfect, in part because it tests for nerve injury, not irritation. It is estimated that approximately 10% of patients with histories highly suggestive of CTS will have normal NCS. In addition to performing median sensory and motor studies, it is essential to also include motor and sensory studies of other nerves (e.g., ulnar or radial) to ensure that the neuropathy is not more generalized. The studies should also be tailored according to the individual's symptoms. If a patient complains of sensory disturbance mainly in the third digit, then a median SNAP to the third digit should be performed as opposed to doing the median SNAP to the thumb or second digit. Median SNAPs are more sensitive than CMAPs in detecting abnormalities associated with CTS. Mixed compound nerve action potentials (CNAPs), which are obtained by stimulating the median and ulnar mixed nerves in the palm and recording over the respective nerves at the wrist, are often even more sensitive as they are usually performed across a shorter distance. Significantly prolonged distal latencies of the median palmar mixed CNAP compared to the ulnar study would support the clinical impression of CTS. In addition to stimulating at the wrist and recording at the digit, it is sometimes useful to do a mid-palm stimulation (half-way between site of wrist stimulation and the recording electrodes) when performing the median SNAPs. If one sees a prolonged distal latency/slow CV and reduced amplitude following wrist stimulation, this should be compared to latency/CV and amplitude after stimulation in the palm to see if there was more focal slowing or conduction block across the wrist. This is particularly valuable in people who have a coexisting generalized polyneuropathy, in order to see if there is a superimposed median neuropathy at the wrist.

The earliest electrodiagnostic abnormalities on NCS in CTS are prolonged distal latencies or slowing of the median SNAP or palmar mixed CNAP across the palm. Subsequently, there may be a reduction in SNAP or mixed CNAP amplitude due to either axon loss or conduction block. Subsequently, distal latencies of the median CMAP become prolonged. Amplitudes of the median CMAP are usually affected much later in the course. In severe cases of CTS, median SNAPs and median CMAPs recorded from the abductor pollicis brevis may be unobtainable. Thus, from an NCS standpoint, one cannot localize the site of the median neuropathy, as a lesion may be anywhere from the hand to the origin of the median nerve in the plexus. In such cases, it is useful to perform median CMAP to the second lumbrical and ulnar CMAP to the second interosseous muscles while stimulating the median and ulnar nerves, respectively, at the wrist. The reason is that the median CMAP from the second lumbrical is often less affected in CTS than the CMAP from the APB. Therefore, a CMAP from this muscle may be obtained when one from the APB cannot. Thus, a prolonged distal latency and reduced amplitude of the median CMAP (second lumbrical) compared to the ulnar CMAP (second interosseous) may be appreciated and confirm the localization of the lesion to the wrist. EMG is often done to further assess the degree of axonal damage and assess the localization of the lesion. Often the EMG is normal in mild CTS. Reduced recruitment of normal appearing MUAPs suggests conduction block. Given its chronic nature, enlarged MUAPs in the APB commonly occur. Signs of active denervation (e.g., fibrillation potentials) are less common but may become evident in rapidly progressive or severe cases.

The treatment of CTS has been the subject of several recent reviews.[155–158] Treatments of CTS include modification of activities, splinting of the wrist, corticosteroid injections, nonsteroidal anti-inflammatory drugs, diuretics, and surgery. To complicate matters, there are various surgical techniques that can be employed as well (standard open surgery with exploration and release versus minimally invasive endoscopic approach). Unfortunately, most studies of CTS have lacked scientific rigor, and thus recommendations for the best therapeutic approach are debatable.

Twenty to seventy percent of patients with CTS treated nonsurgically improve to some extent.[155,159–161] Corticosteroid injections into the carpal tunnel have become an increasingly used alternative to surgery. Risks include cutaneous atrophy, depigmentation, and inadvertent puncture of the median nerve, blood vessels, or tendons within the carpal tunnel.[155] Median nerve injury and tendon rupture are the most severe complications, but each occurs in <0.1% of injections. Approximately 30% of patients have no or only mild improvement following local corticosteroid injection, while 70% have a very good response (complete relief or only minor residual symptoms).[155,162] A study comparing corticosteroid injection versus surgery demonstrated similar short-term efficacy of both treatments, but the relapse rate was common in the injection group and rare in the surgical group after 1 year.[101] In this regard, there are no good studies assessing the safety and efficacy of repeated corticosteroid injections. A recent randomized trial comparing surgery to conservative management with wrist splints and nonsteroidal medications demonstrated a modest benefit of unclear clinical significance with surgery.[161]

The average success rate from surgery is approximately 75% (range 27–100%), but 8% of patients actually worsen.[155] Failure rates may relate to patients being operated on who do not actually have CTS. In this regard, improvement following surgery is noted in only half of patients who had normal electrodiagnostic testing prior surgery, while success rates are much higher in those with NCS that were abnormal. Another common cause of failed surgery is incomplete division of the transverse carpal ligament, perhaps owing to poor choice of incision and inadequate exposure.[155] Another reason for failed surgery is such end-stage denervation resulting from delayed treatment. There may be a <50% success rate for surgery in patients with marked thenar atrophy and weakness, no recordable median CMAPs and SNAPS, and active denervation on EMG.[155,162] In our opinion, CTS surgery in this population should only be considered for reasons of pain relief, not with the expectation that strength or sensation will return in any meaningful way.

Complications of surgery occur in 1–2% of cases and include injury to the recurrent motor and cutaneous branches of the median nerve, lesions of the main trunk of the median nerve, the main trunk and deep motor branch of the ulnar nerve, postoperative hematoma, wound infection, scarring, and complex regional pain syndrome type II.[155]

With the above caveats, we initially try conservative management having patients wear neutral angle wrist splints, particularly those individuals with only sensory abnormalities on NCS. In patients with objective motor deficits, we still try a short trial of wrist splints along with corticosteroid injections. However, we refer them for surgery if there is no benefit after a couple of months. We usually do not recommend surgery when NCS are normal.

ULNAR NERVE

The ulnar nerve is the anatomic continuation of the medial cord and contains nerve fibers originating from the C8 and T1 spinal roots, which course through the lower trunk and then median cord (Fig. 23-10). As previously discussed, there may also be a contribution from C7 in some individuals. This is a long nerve and lesions may occur anywhere along its course. Therefore, the clinical and electrophysiological findings are dependent on the site and nature of the lesion.

Proximal Ulnar Neuropathy (Axilla to Upper Elbow Region)

Similar mechanisms that cause proximal median and radial neuropathies can cause a proximal ulnar neuropathy (Table 23-14).[8,9] There are no ulnar-innervated muscles in the upper arm; therefore, any proximal lesion will clinically resemble those caused by more common ulnar neuropathy at the elbow (discussed in next section). Ulnar neuropathies in the upper arm related to open trauma usually require surgical repair.

TABLE 23-14. CONDITIONS ASSOCIATED WITH PROXIMAL ULNAR NEUROPATHY

Trauma
Compression during sleep
Soft tissue or peripheral nerve tumor
Ischemia (e.g., A-V fistulas, vasculitis)
Multifocal motor neuropathy or multifocal acquired demyelinating motor and sensory neuropathy

Provided there is significant axonal loss, the ulnar and dorsal ulnar SNAPs would be expected to have reduced amplitudes, while the medial antebrachial cutaneous SNAP should be normal. The ulnar CMAP may demonstrate reduced amplitude without focal slowing or conduction block across the elbow. EMG should show abnormalities confined to ulnar-innervated muscles in the hand and forearm (Table 23-1). However, these SNAPs and EMG alterations do not distinguish between a proximal ulnar neuropathy in the upper arm and one across the elbow. Electrophysiologically, the only way one can localize an ulnar neuropathy to the proximal upper arm is by demonstrating focal conduction block or slowing of ulnar CV between axillary and above the elbow stimulation sites.

Ulnar Neuropathy at the Elbow

This is the second most common mononeuropathy aside from CTS, and it is usually the result of compression of the nerve at this level. As the nerve is superficial around the ulnar groove, it is more susceptible to extrinsic compression (e.g., from leaning on the elbow). There are numerous intrinsic mechanisms by which the ulnar nerve may be injured in this region (Table 23-15).[8,9] The term "tardy ulnar palsy" is applied to ulnar neuropathies that occur on a delayed basis following bone injuries at the elbow. It is speculated that the nerve may become stretched or compressed by exuberant callus formation or altered angle of the elbow joint. The nerve may also become entrapped or compressed by the humeroulnar aponeurotic retinaculum or by other anatomic structural variants in and around the ulnar groove and cubital tunnel. Also, the nerve can occasionally prolapse out of the ulnar groove although this happens in many normal individuals and should not be assumed to be pathological.

Regardless of the etiology, the clinical signs and symptoms of an ulnar neuropathy at the elbow are similar. Individuals who are affected often complain of discomfort and perhaps tenderness in the medial elbow. They will typically describe numbness and tingling in the medial aspect of the hand and the fifth digit along with the medial half of the fourth digit (both palmar and dorsal aspects of these fingers). It is important to realize that the vast majority of ulnar neuropathies present with sensory symptoms. Compressive or entrapment ulnar neuropathies presenting with purely motor signs and symptoms are extremely rare in our experience.

Tapping the nerve in the elbow often exacerbates these symptoms (e.g., positive Tinel sign). Weakness may involve any or all of the ulnar-innervated muscles in the hand and forearm. This can lead to decreased muscle grip and spreading out or bringing fingers closer together. It is not uncommon for an ulnar neuropathy at the elbow to produce detectable hand but not forearm muscle weakness. We have found assessing for weakness of the flexion of little finger at the distal interphalangeal joint to be the most reliable means by which to detect ulnar forearm muscle weakness when it is present. With axonal degeneration, atrophy of the hypothenar and interossei muscles may be seen (most notably appreciated in the first dorsal interosseous).

Imaging studies such as MRI and, in particular, ultrasound have been used to assist in diagnosis (Fig. 23-22).[32,33] Ulnar and dorsal ulnar cutaneous SNAP amplitudes should be reduced if there is significant axonal damage at or near the elbow. However, if there is only a neuropraxic or demyelinating lesion in the elbow these SNAPs are typically normal, as these do not assess slowing of conduction across the elbow. Localization is dependent on the ulnar motor conductions and EMG.[6,163–165] We usually perform ulnar motor conductions recording from both the first dorsal interosseous and the abductor digiti minimi muscles with stimulation sites at the wrist, below the elbow, and above the elbow. Because of the fascicular arrangement of nerves destined to innervate these muscles, one may find abnormalities in one but not the other muscle. Most of the lesions in the elbow initially lead to demyelination in this segment. One would expect to see normal distal latencies, amplitudes, and CV between the wrist and below-elbow stimulation sites. However, slowing of CV may be appreciated between the below- and above-elbow sites.[164] As the size of the demyelinating lesion may be small, the shorter the distance between the below- and above-elbow sites, the more likely one will be able to demonstrate focal slowing (we try to keep the distance at most 8–10 cm). In addition, conduction block may be appreciated between these sites of stimulation. To further localize where in the elbow the nerve is damaged and to increase the sensitivity if routine ulnar CMAPs across the elbow are normal, one can do inching studies. Perhaps, a more appropriate term is "centimetering" as the nerve is stimulated every 1–2 cm, beginning 5 cm below to 5 cm above the elbow.[6,163,165] In most patients with focal demyelinating lesions in this location detected with this technique, both an abrupt latency shift and change in CMAP morphology can be reproducibly

TABLE 23-15. CONDITIONS ASSOCIATED WITH ULNAR NEUROPATHY AT THE ELBOW

Tardy ulnar palsy (due to deformities of elbow related to previous fractures of humerus or other trauma to the joint)
Subluxation of the ulnar nerve
Compression by arcade of Struthers (medial intramuscular septum)
Compression by aponeurotic band between heads of flexor carpi ulnaris
Compression by ligament/band (retrocondylar)
Trauma
Soft tissue tumor or masses
Leprosy
Diabetes mellitus[a]

[a]It is unclear if individuals with typical generalized diabetic polyneuropathy may be predisposed to focal mononeuropathies related to compression.

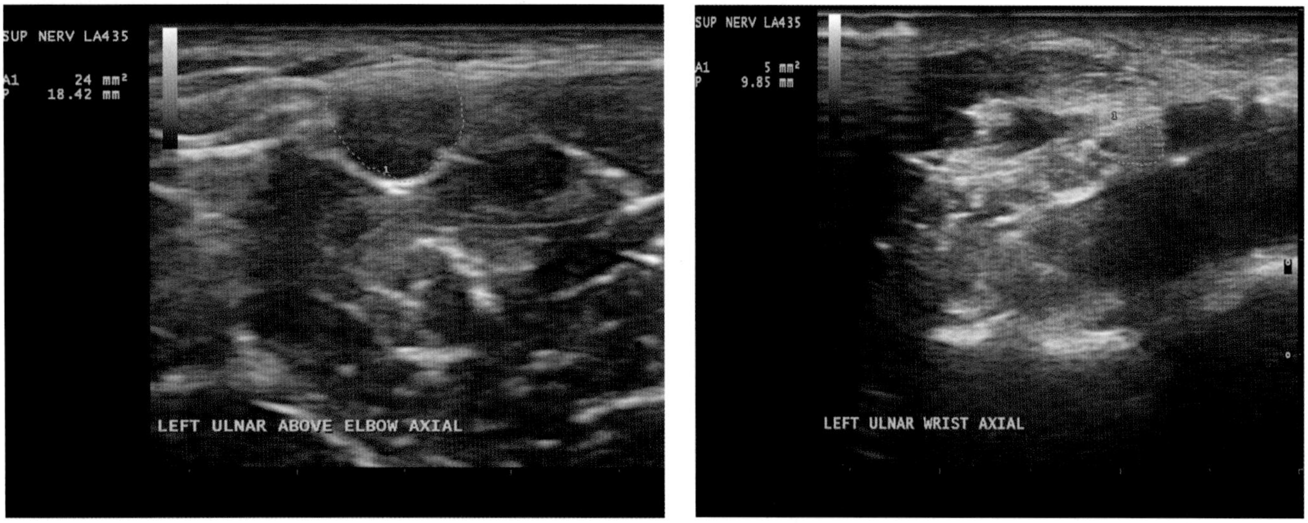

A B

Figure 23-22. Ultrasound of ulnar nerve reveals marked increase in area above the elbow of 24 mm^2 (normal ≤10 mm^2) and normal area at the wrist of 5 mm^2 (normal ≤6 mm^2) resulting in an increased elbow/wrist ratio of 4.8 (normal <2).

demonstrated. Assessing for slowing of the ulnar CNAPs across the elbow may be informative in some patients.[166] If secondary axonal degeneration occurs then focal slowing of conduction velocity or conduction block may no longer be apparent. In such cases, the ulnar CMAP does not help in differentiating an ulnar neuropathy at the wrist from a more proximal lesion. The dorsal ulnar cutaneous SNAP is thus important, because an abnormality in this study implies a lesion proximal to the wrist as do EMG abnormalities in ulnar-innervated forearm muscles (e.g., flexor carpi ulnar and flexor digitorum III and IV). Unfortunately, in a significant number of cases of ulnar mononeuropathy, predominantly those without a demyelinating component, the site of the lesion cannot be precisely localized. Again, in neuropraxic or demyelinating lesions, the EMG may just demonstrate reduced recruitment of MUAPs. One particular pitfall in assessment of potential ulnar neuropathies is the demonstration of a greater than 20% drop in ulnar CMAP amplitude comparing below elbow to wrist stimulation. Although this could implicate a demyelinating ulnar neuropathy in the forearm, a Martin-Gruber anastomosis provides a far more common possibility and needs to be excluded.

There is a lack of randomized, prospective studies aimed at assessing the efficacy of various treatments of the more common ulnar neuropathy at the elbow.[167] Most studies have been retrospective and subject to bias. Individuals with intermittent sensory symptoms may respond to conservative measures.[168] Nonsurgical measures include elbow pads, avoidance of leaning on the elbow, splinting the elbow in extension at night, and nonsteroidal anti-inflammatory drugs. Surgical procedures may be more beneficial in patients who have motor signs and symptoms, but not everyone improves. There are various surgical approaches (e.g., simple decompression, medial epicondylectomy, and nerve transposition), and there does not seem to be any significant differences in clinical outcomes,[169] but none has been rigorously studied in a scientific fashion. There may be increased risks with nerve transposition including infarction due to devascularization of the nerve and increased scarring. We are particularly reluctant to recommend this procedure to diabetics with their increased risk of microvasculopathy.

Ulnar Neuropathy in the Hand

The ulnar nerve can be damaged at various locations within the wrist or hand and by different mechanisms (Table 23-16). One of the most common etiologies is a compression by a ganglion cyst, which can easily be seen on MRI (Fig. 23-23) or ultrasound of the hand.[35] The ulnar nerve can be damaged

▶ **TABLE 23-16. CONDITIONS ASSOCIATED WITH ULNAR NEUROPATHY AT THE WRIST**

External compression (e.g., bicyclist)
Space occupying lesions (e.g., ganglion cysts, lipoma, nerve sheet tumors)
Trauma (fracture to metacarpals, pisiform, hamate, dislocation of distal ulna, laceration
Degenerative arthritis
Rheumatoid arthritis
Diabetes mellitus[a]

[a]It is unclear if individuals with typical generalized diabetic polyneuropathy may be predisposed to focal mononeuropathies related to compression.

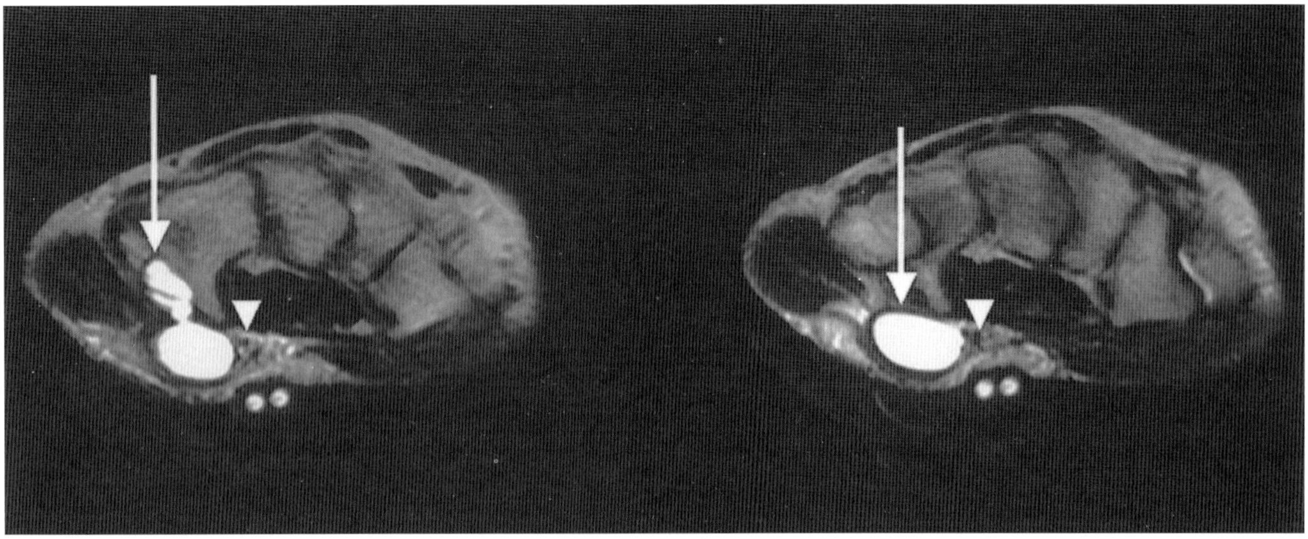

Figure 23-23. MRI of the wrist in a patient with ulnar neuropathy. MRI reveals a ganglionic cyst (*arrow*) adjacent to the hamate in Guyon's canal that is displacing the ulnar nerve and artery (*arrowhead*). (Reproduced with permission from of Steven A. Greenberg, MD. Reproduced with permission from: Greenberg SA, Amato AA. *EMG Pearls*. Philadelphia, PA: Hanley & Belfus, Inc; 2004.)

in one of four sites within the hand, and the clinical and electrophysiological findings are dependent on the site and nature of the lesion (Fig. 23-24).

1. The entire nerve may be damaged just proximal to or within Guyon's canal. This type of lesion affects the superficial sensory and deep motor branches of the distal ulnar nerve, resulting in sensory loss of the volar aspect of the fifth digit and usually the medial half of the fifth digit and weakness of all ulnar-innervated hand muscles. In contrast to more proximal ulnar lesions (e.g., ulnar neuropathy at the elbow), the dorsal ulnar cutaneous nerve is spared; thus, individuals have normal sensation of the dorsum of the ulnar aspect of the hand. In addition, there is normal strength of the flexor carpi ulnaris and flexor digitorum profundus III and IV. The ulnar SNAP may demonstrate prolonged distal latency or reduced amplitude depending on the degree of axon loss, while the dorsal ulnar cutaneous SNAP should be normal. The ulnar CMAP recorded from both the abductor digiti minimi and the first dorsal interosseous may show prolonged distal latencies or reduced amplitudes, again dependent on the nature and severity of the lesion. EMG may demonstrate evidence of denervation in the first dorsal interosseous and abductor digiti minimi but the flexor carpi ulnaris and flexor digitorum profundus III and IV should be normal.
2. The nerve may be compressed just outside Guyon's canal such that only the superficial sensory branch is affected. In this case, sensation is decreased but all motor functions are spared. Electrodiagnostic studies would only show abnormalities of the ulnar SNAP.
3. The nerve may be damaged distal to the take off of the superficial sensory branch and affect only the deep motor branch. In such cases, sensation is spared, but motor function affecting any or all of the ulnar hand intrinsic muscles in the hand may be affected. The ulnar SNAPs would be normal, but ulnar CMAPs to both the first dorsal interosseous and the abductor digiti minimi should be abnormal, as would EMG of these muscles.
4. Finally, the nerve may be compressed distal to the branch innervating the hypothenar eminence. Thus, only the interossei and adductor pollicis muscles are affected. A lesion may be even more distal such that only the adductor pollicis or perhaps the first dorsal interosseous are abnormal. Ulnar SNAPs and ulnar CMAPs to the abductor digiti minimi would be normal. Only the ulnar CMAP from the dorsal interosseous would show abnormalities. Likewise, on EMG the abductor digiti minimi would be spared and denervation may be appreciated only in the dorsal interossei and adductor pollicis muscles.

Ulnar neuropathy in the hand due to external compression (e.g., bicyclist) may be treated conservatively. If caused by a fracture of the hamate or pisiform bones, exploratory surgery with decompression and neurolysis are often required. Also, ulnar neuropathies in the hand related to open trauma or internal compression (e.g., ganglion cyst) are usually managed with surgery.

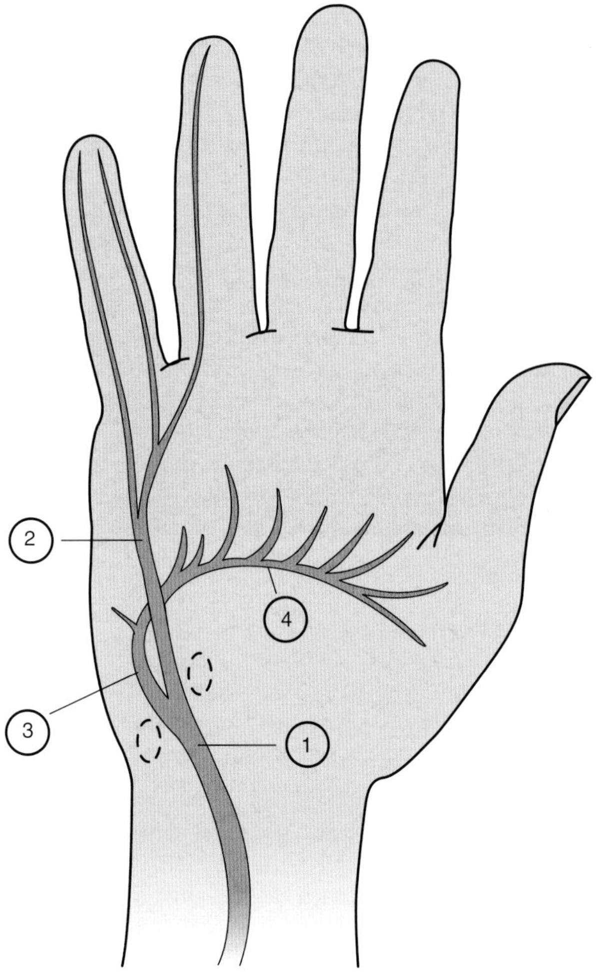

Figure 23-24. There are four main areas in which the ulnar nerve can be damaged at the wrist, and each leads to different clinical and electrophysiological abnormalities as discussed in the text. (Modified with permission from Stewart JD. *Focal Peripheral Neuropathies*. New York, NY: Elsevier; 1987.)

▶ CONCLUSION

The multiple etiologies of focal neuropathies affecting the upper extremity (including radiculopathies, plexopathies, and mononeuropathies) can be quite daunting even to the experienced clinician. The key to the evaluation of patients with these types of focal neuropathies begins with localization. This is accomplished by a good physical examination and electrodiagnostic study. Other studies such as various modes of radiological imaging can assist in localizing and identifying an etiology. Prognosis is dependent on the cause and nature of the neuropathy. Neuropraxic lesions secondary to minor compression or stretch usually of the nerve tend to recover well; however, those associated with severe axonal degeneration take much longer to regenerate and recover. Treatment likewise is dependent on the nature of the nerve injury. Most focal neuropathies are initially managed conservatively, but severe nerve injuries may require surgical intervention.

REFERENCES

1. Dumitru D, Zwarts MJ. Brachial plexopathies and proximal mononeuropathies. In: Dumitru D, Amato AA, Zwarts MJ, eds. *Electrodiagnostic Medicine*. 2nd ed. Philadelphia, PA: Hanley & Belfus; 2002:777–836.
2. Ferrante MA. Brachial plexopathies: Classification, causes, and consequences. *Muscle Nerve*. 2004;30(5):547–568.
3. Wilbourn AJ. Plexopathies. *Neurol Clin*. 2007;25(1):139–171.
4. Kerr AT. The brachial plexus of nerves in man, the variations in its formation and branches. *Am J Anat*. 1918;23:285–395.
5. Millesi H. Brachial plexus injuries—management and results. *Clin Plast Surg*. 1984;11:115–120.
6. Greenberg SA, Amato AA. *EMG Pearls*. Philadelphia, PA: Hanley & Belfus; 2004.
7. Haymaker W, Lindgreen M. Nerve disturbances following exposure to ionizing radiation. In: Vinken PJ, Bruyn GW, eds. *Handbook of Clinical Neurology*. Vol 7. Amsterdam: North Holland; 1970:338.
8. Dawson DM, Hallett M, Wilbourn AJ, Campbell WW. *Entrapment Neuropathies*. 3rd ed. Boston, MA: Little, Brown and Company; 1999.
9. Stewart JD. *Focal Peripheral Neuropathies*. New York, NY: Elsevier; 1987.
10. Sunderland S. *Nerve and Nerve Injuries*. Edinburgh: Churchill-Livingstone; 1978.
11. Ochoa J. Nerve fiber pathology in acute and chronic compression. In: Omer GE, Spinner M, eds. *Management of Peripheral Nerve Problems*. Philadelphia, PA: Saunders; 1980.
12. Aminoff MJ. Clinical electromyography. In: Aminoff MJ, ed. *Electrodiagnosis in Clinical Neurology*. 2nd ed. New York, NY: Churchill Livingstone; 1986:231–263.
13. Dumitru D, Amato AA, Swartz MJ. *Electrodiagnostic Medicine*, 2nd ed. Philadelphia, PA: Hanley & Belfus; 2002.
14. Kimura J. *Electrodiagnosis of Diseases of Nerve and Muscle: Principles and Practice*. 3rd ed. Philadelphia, PA: FA Davis; 2001.
15. Oh SJ. *Clinical Electromyography. Nerve Conduction Studies*. 3rd ed. Baltimore, MD: William & Wilkins; 2004.
16. Dumitru D, Amato AA, Swartz MJ. Nerve conduction studies. In: Dumitru D, Amato AA, Swartz MJ, eds. *Electrodiagnostic Medicine*. 2nd ed. Philadelphia, PA: Hanley & Belfus; 2002: 159–223.
17. Schimseider RJ, de Visser BW, Kemp B. The flexor carpi radialis H reflex in lesions of the sixth and seventh cervical roots. *J Neurol Neurosurg Psychiatry*. 1985;48:445–449.
18. Eisen A, Hoirch M. Electrodiagnostic evaluation of radiculopathies and plexopathies using somatosensory evoked potentials. *Electroencephalogr Clin Neurophysiol*. 1982;36(suppl): 349–357.
19. Jones SJ, Parry W, Landi A. Diagnosis of brachial plexus traction lesions by sensory nerve action potentials and somatosensory evoked potentials. *Injury*. 1981;12:376–382.
20. Jones SJ. Diagnostic value of peripheral and spinal somatosensory evoked potentials in traction lesions of the brachial plexus. *Clin Plast Surg*. 1984;11:167–172.

21. Lederman RJ, Wilbourn AJ. Brachial plexopathy: Recurrent cancer or radiation? *Neurology*. 1984;34:1331–1335.
22. Rapoport S, Blair DN, McCarthy SM, Desser TS, Hammers LW, Sostman HD. Brachial plexus: Correlation of MR imaging with CT and pathologic findings. *Radiology*. 1988;167:161–165.
23. van Es HW, Bollen TL, van Heesewijk HP. MRI of the brachial plexus: A pictorial review. *Eur J Radiol*. 2010;74:391–402.
24. Daily AT, Tsuruda JS, Filler AG, Maravilla KR, Goodkin R, Kliot M. Magnetic resonance neurography of peripheral nerve regeneration. *Lancet*. 1997;350:1221–1222.
25. Filler AG, Maravilla KR, Tsuruda JS. MR neurography and muscle MR for image diagnosis of disorders affecting the peripheral nerves and musculature. *Neurol Clin*. 2004;22:643–682.
26. Grant GA, Britz GW, Gookdkin R, Jarvik JG, Maravilla K, Kliot M. The utility of magnetic resonance imaging in evaluating peripheral nerve disorders. *Muscle Nerve*. 2002;25:314–331.
27. Gupta RK, Mehta VS, Banerji AK, Jain RK. MR evaluation of brachial plexus lesions. *Neuroradiology*. 1989;31:377–381.
28. Sherrier RH, Sostman JD. Magnetic resonance imaging of the brachial plexus. *J Thoracic Imaging*. 1993;8:27–33.
29. Wittenberg KH, Adkins MC. MR imaging of non-traumatic brachial plexopathies: Frequency and spectrum of findings. *Radiographics*. 2000;20:1023–1032.
30. Altinok T, Baysal O, Karakas HM, et al. Ultrasonographic assessment of mild and moderate idiopathic carpal tunnel syndrome. *Clin Radiol*. 2004;59(10):916–925.
31. Bayrak IK, Bayrak AO, Tilki HE, Nural MS, Sunter T. Ultrasonography in carpal tunnel syndrome: Comparison with electrophysiological stage and motor unit number estimate. *Muscle Nerve*. 2007;35:344–348.
32. Beekman R, Wokke JH, Schoemaker MC, Lee ML, Visser LH. Ulnar neuropathy at the elbow: Follow-up and prognostic factors determining outcome. *Neurology*. 2004;63(9):1675–1680.
33. Beekman R, Schoemaker MC, van der Plas JP, et al. The diagnostic value of high-resolution sonography in ulnar neuropathy at the elbow. *Neurology*. 2004;62:767–773.
34. Cartwright MS, Chloros GD, Walker FO, Wiesler ER, William W, Campbell WW. Diagnostic ultrasound for nerve transaction. *Muscle Nerve*. 2007;35(6):796–799.
35. Jacob A, Moorthy TK, Thomas SV, Sarada C. Compression of the deep motor branch of the ulnar nerve: An unusual cause of pure motor neuropathy and hand wasting. *Arch Neurol*. 2005;62(5):826–827.
36. Ziswiler HR, Reichenbach S, Vogelin E, Bachmann LM, Villiger PM, Juni P. Diagnostic value of sonography in patients with suspected carpal tunnel syndrome: A prospective study. *Arthritis Rheum*. 2005;52(1):304–311.
37. Kelsey JL, Githens PB, Walter SD, et al. An epidemiological study of acute prolapsed cervical intervertebral disc. *J Bone Joint Surg*. 1984;66A:907–914.
38. Lunsford LD, Bissonette DJ, Janetta PJ, Sheptak PE, Zorub DS. Anterior surgery for cervical disc disease. *J Neurosurg*. 1980;53:1–11.
39. Martins AN. Anterior cervical discectomy with and without interbody bone graft. *J Neurosurg*. 1976;44:290–295.
40. Negrin P, Lelli S, Fardin P. Contribution of electromyography to the diagnosis, treatment, and prognosis of cervical disc disease: A study of 114 patients. *Electromyogr Clin Neurophysiol*. 1991;31:173–179.
41. Scoville WB, Dohrmann GJ, Corkill G. Late results of cervical disc surgery. *J Neurosurg*. 1976;45:203–210.
42. Abbott KH, Retter RH. Protrusions of thoracic intervertebral disks. *Neurology*. 1956;6:1–10.
43. Arce CA, Dohrmann GJ. Herniated thoracic discs. *Neurol Clin*. 1985;3:383–392.
44. Arseni C, Nash F. Thoracic intervertebral disc protrusion: A clinical study. *J Neurosurg*. 1960;17:418–430.
45. Otani K, Yoshida M, Fujii E, Nakai S, Shibasaki K. Thoracic disc herniation: Surgical treatment. *Spine*. 1988;13:1262–1267.
46. Benson MK, Byrnes DP. The clinical syndromes and surgical treatment of thoracic intervertebral disc prolapse. *J Bone Joint Surg*. 1975;57B:471–477.
47. Bohlman HH, Zdeblick TA. Anterior excision of herniated thoracic discs. *J Bone Joint Surg*. 1988;70A:1038–1047.
48. Radhakrishnan K, Litchy WJ, O'Fallon WM, Kurland LT. Epidemiology of cervical radiculopathy: A population-based study from Rochester, Minnesota, 1976 through 1990. *Brain*. 1994;117:325–335.
49. Persson LC, Carlson CA, Carlson JY. Long-lasting cervical radiculopathy pain managed with surgery, physiotherapy, or a cervical collar. *Spine*. 1997;22:751–758.
50. Nikolaidis I, Fouyas IP, Sandercock PA, Statham PF. Surgery for cervical radiculopathy or myelopathy. *Cochrane Database Syst Rev*. 2010;1:CD001466.
51. England JD, Sumner AJ. Neuralgic amyotrophy: An increasingly diverse entity. *Muscle Nerve*. 1987;10:60–68.
52. Parsonage MJ, Turner AJ. Neuralgic amyotrophy. The shoulder-girdle syndrome. *Lancet*. 1948;1:973–978.
53. Tsairis P, Dyck PJ, Mulder DW. Natural history of brachial plexus neuropathy: Report on 99 cases. *Arch Neurol*. 1972;27:109–117.
54. Turner AJ, Parsonage MJ. Neuralgic amyotrophy (paralytic brachial neuritis): With special reference to prognosis. *Lancet*. 1957;1:209–212.
55. van Alfen N, van Engelen BG. The clinical spectrum of neuralgic amyotrophy in 246 cases. *Brain*. 2006;129:438–450.
56. Cwik VA, Wilbourn AJ, Rorick M. Acute brachial neuropathy: Detailed EMG findings in a large series. *Muscle Nerve*. 1990;13:859.
57. Flaggman PD, Kelly JJ. Brachial plexus neuropathy: An electrophysiologic evaluation. *Arch Neurol*. 1980;37:160–164.
58. Weikers NJ, Mattson RH. Acute paralytic brachial neuritis: A clinical and electrodiagnostic study. *Neurology*. 1969;19:1153–1158.
59. Cape CA, Fincham RW. Paralytic brachial neuritis with diaphragmatic paralysis. *Neurology*. 1965;15:191–193.
60. Walsh NE, Dumitru D, Kalantri A, Roman A. Brachial neuritis involving the bilateral phrenic nerves. *Arch Phys Med Rehabil*. 1987;68:46–48.
61. Kiloh L, Nevin S. Isolated neuritis of the anterior interosseous nerve. *Br Med J*. 1952;1:850–851.
62. Renneis GD, Ochoa J. Neuralgic amyotrophy manifesting as anterior interosseous nerve palsy. *Muscle Nerve*. 1980;3:160–164.
63. Smith BE, Herbst B. Anterior interosseous nerve palsy. *Arch Neurol*. 1974;30:330–331.

64. Pierre PA, Laterre CE, van den Bergh PY. Neuralgic amyotrophy with involvement of cranial nerves IX, X, XI and XII. *Muscle Nerve.* 1990;13:704–707.
65. Eisen A, Bertrand G. Isolated accessory nerve palsy of spontaneous origin. A clinical and electromyographic study. *Arch Neurol.* 1972;27:496–502.
66. Bernsen PL, Wong Chung RE, Vinergoets HM, Janssen JT. Bilateral neuralgic amyotrophy induced by interferon treatment. *Arch Neurol.* 1988;45(4):449–451.
67. Cruz-Martinez A, Barrio JM, Arpa J. Neuralgic amyotrophy: Variable expression in 40 patients. *J Peripher Nerv Sys.* 2002;7:198–204.
68. Kiwit JC. Neuralgic amyotrophy after administration of tetanus toxoid. *J Neurol Neurosurg Psychiatry.* 1984;47:320.
69. Loh FL, Herskovitz S, Berger AR, Swerdlow ML. Brachial plexopathy associated with interleukin-2 therapy. *Neurology.* 1992;42:462–463.
70. Weintraub MI, Chia DT. Paralytic brachial neuritis after swine flu vaccination. *Arch Neurol.* 1977;34:518.
71. Vriesendorp FJ, Dmytrnko GS, Dietrich T, Koski CL. Anti-peripheral nerve myelin antibodies and terminal activation products of complement in serum of patients with acute brachial plexus neuropathy. *Arch Neurol.* 1993;50:1993.
72. Amato AA, Jackson CE, Kim JY, Worley KL. Chronic relapsing brachial plexus neuropathy with persistent conduction block. *Muscle Nerve.* 1997;20:1303–1307.
73. Adler JB, Patterson RL. Erb's palsy: Long term results of treatment in eighty-eight cases. *J Bone Joint Surg.* 1967;49A: 1052–1064.
74. Eng GD. Brachial plexus palsy in newborn infants. *Pediatrics.* 1971;48:18–28.
75. Eng GB, Koch B, Smokvina MD. Brachial plexus palsy in neonates and children. *Arch Phys Med Rehabil.* 1978;59:458–464.
76. Erb W. Ueber eine eigenthumliche localisation von lahmengen im plexus brachialis. *Verhandl d Naturhist-Med Heidelberg.* 1874;2:130–137.
77. Greenwald AG, Shute PC, Shiveley JL. Brachial plexus birth palsy: A 10 years report on the incidence and prognosis. *J Pediatr Orthop.* 1984;4:689–692.
78. Klumpke A. Contribution a l'etude des paralysies radiculaires du plexus brachial. Paralysies radiculaires totales. Paralysies radiculaires inferieures. De la participation des filest sympathiques oculo-pupillaires dans ces paralysies. *Rev Med.* 1885; 5:591.
79. Specht EE. Brachial plexus palsy in newborn: Incidence and prognosis. *Clin Orthop.* 1975;110:32–34.
80. Johnson EW, Alexander MA, Koenig WC. Infantile Erb's palsy (Smellie's palsy). *Arch Phys Med Rehabil.* 1977;58:175–178.
81. McFarland LV, Raskin M, Daling JR, Benedetti TJ. Erb/Duchenne's palsy: A consequence of fetal macrosomia and method of delivery. *Obstet Gynecol.* 1986;68:784–788.
82. Meyer RD. Treatment of adult and obstetrical brachial plexus injuries. *Orthopedics.* 1986;9:899–903.
83. Mollberg M, Wennergren M, Bager B, Ladfors L, Hagberg H. Obstetric brachial plexus palsy: A prospective study on risk factors related to manual assistance during the second stage of labor. *Acta Obstet Gynecol Scand.* 2007;86(2):198–204.
84. Boome RS, Kaye JC. Obstetric traction injuries of the brachial plexus. *J Bone Joint Surg.* 1988;70B:571–576.
85. Rossi LN, Vassella F, Mumenthaler M. Obstetrical lesions of the brachial plexus: Natural history in 34 personal cases. *Eur Neurol.* 1982;21:1–7.
86. Kneeland JB, Kellman GM, Middleton WD, et al. Diagnosis of disease of the supraclavicular region by use of MR imaging. *Am J Roentgenol.* 1987;148:1149–1151.
87. Popovich MJ, Taylor FC, Helmer E. MR imaging of birth-related brachial plexus avulsion. *AJNR AM J Neuroradiol.* 1989;10(suppl 5):S98.
88. Kline DG. Surgical repair of peripheral nerve injury. *Muscle Nerve.* 1990;13:843–852.
89. Kline DG, Hudson AR. *Nerve Injuries.* Philadelphia, PA: WB Saunders; 1995:611.
90. Spinner RJ, Kline DG. Surgery for peripheral nerve and brachial plexus injuries or other nerve lesions. *Muscle Nerve.* 2000;23:680–695.
91. Aminoff MJ, Olney RK, Parry GJ, Raskin NH. Relative utility of different electrophysiologic techniques in the evaluation of brachial plexopathies. *Neurology.* 1988;38:546–550.
92. Cuetter AC, Bartoszek DM. The thoracic outlet syndrome: Controversies, over diagnosis, over treatment, and recommendations for management. *Muscle Nerve.* 1989;12:410–419.
93. Gilliat RW, Le Quesne PM, Logue V, Sumner AJ. Wasting of the hand associated with a cervical rib or band. *J Neurol Neurosurg Psychiatry.* 1970;33:615–624.
94. Gilliatt RW, Willison RG, Dietz V, Williams IR. Peripheral nerve conduction in patients with a cervical rib and band. *Ann Neurol.* 1978;4:124–129.
95. Jaeckle KA. Nerve plexus metastases. *Neurol Clin.* 1991;9: 857–866.
96. Kori SH, Foley KM, Posner JB. Brachial plexus lesions in patients with cancer: 100 cases. *Neurology.* 1981;31:45–50.
97. Lusk MD, Kline DG, Garcia CA. Tumors of the brachial plexus. *Neurosurgery.* 1987;21:439–453.
98. Richardson RR, Siqueira EB, Oi S, Nunez C. Neurogenic tumors of the brachial plexus: Report of two cases. *Neurosurgery.* 1979;4:66–70.
99. Sell PJ, Semple JC. Primary nerve tumours of the brachial plexus. *Br J Surg.* 1987;74:73–74.
100. Godwin JT. Encapsulated neurilemoma (schwannoma) of the brachial plexus: Report of 11 cases. *Cancer.* 1952;5:708–720.
101. Ly-Pen D, Andreu JL, de Blas G, Sanchez-Olaso A, Millan I. Surgical decompression versus local steroid injection in carpal tunnel syndrome: A one-year, prospective, randomized, open, controlled clinical trial. *Arthritis Rheum.* 2005;52: 612–619.
102. Harper CM, Thomas JE, Cascino TL, Litchy WJ. Distinction between neoplastic and radiation-induced brachial plexopathy, with emphasis on the role of EMG. *Neurology.* 1989;39:502–506.
103. Thomas JE, Cascino TL, Earle JD. Differential diagnosis between radiation and tumor plexopathy of the pelvis. *Neurology.* 1985;35:1–7.
104. Corkill G, Lieberman JS, Taylor RG. Pack-palsy in backpackers. *West J Med.* 1980;132:569–572.
105. Daube JR. Rucksack paralysis. *J Am Med Assoc.* 1969;208: 2447–2452.
106. Graham JF, Pye IF, McQueen IN. Brachial plexus injury after median sternotomy. *J Neurol Neurosurg Psychiatry.* 1981; 44:621–625.

107. Hanson MR, Breuer AC, Furland AJ, et al. Mechanism and frequency of brachial plexus injury in open-heart surgery: A prospective study. *Ann Thorac Surg*. 1983;36:675–679.
108. Morin JE, Long R, Elleker MG, Eisen AA, Wynands E, Ralphs-Thibodeau S. Upper extremity neuropathies following median sternotomy. *Ann Thorac Surg*. 1982;34:181–185.
109. Seyfer AE, Grammer NY, Bogumill GP, Provost JM, Chandry U. Upper extremity neuropathies after cardiac surgery. *J Hand Surg*. 1985;10:16–19.
110. Chance PF, Lensch MW, Lipe H, Brown RH Sr, Brown RH Jr, Bird TD. Hereditary neuralgic amyotrophy and hereditary neuropathy with liability to pressure palsies: Two distinct genetic disorders. *Neurology*. 1994;44:2253–2257.
111. Hentz VR. Is microsurgical treatment of brachial plexus palsy better than conventional treatment? *Hand Clin*. 2007;23(1): 83–89.
112. Hentz VR. Brachial plexus injuries. In: Omer GE Jr, Spinner M, Van Beek AL, eds. *Management of Peripheral Nerve Problems*. 2nd ed. Philadelphia, PA: WB Saunders; 1998: 445–453.
113. Shin AY, Spinner RJ, Steinmann SP, Bishop AT. Adult traumatic brachial plexus injuries. *J Am Acad Orthop Surg*. 2005;13(6): 382–396.
114. Terzis JK, Kostas I, Soucacos PN. Restoration of shoulder function with nerve transfers in traumatic brachial plexus palsy patients. *Microsurgery*. 2006;26(4):316–324.
115. Terzis JK, Kostopoulos VK. The surgical treatment of brachial plexus injuries in adults. *Plast Reconstr Surg*. 2007;119(4):73e–92e.
116. Levy O, Relwani JG, Mullett H, Haddo O, Even T. The active elevation lag sign and the triangle sign: New clinical signs of trapezius palsy. *J Shoulder Elbow Surg*. 2009;18:573–576.
117. Chan PK, Hems TE. Clinical signs of accessory nerve palsy. *J Trauma*. 2005;60:1142–1144.
118. Goodman CE, Kenrick MM, Blum MV. Long thoracic nerve palsy: A follow-up study. *Arch Phys Med Rehabil*. 1976;56: 352–355.
119. Johnson JT, Kendall HO. Isolated paralysis of the serratus anterior muscle. *J Bone Joint Surg*. 1955;37A:567–574.
120. Kaplan PE. Electrodiagnostic confirmation of long thoracic nerve palsy. *J Neurol Neurosurg Psychiatry*. 1980;43:50–52.
121. Haymaker W, Woodhall B. *Peripheral Nerve Injuries: Principles of Diagnosis*. Philadelphia, PA: WB Saunders; 1953.
122. Petrera JE, Trojaborg W. Conduction studies of the long thoracic nerve in serratus anterior palsy of different etiology. *Neurology*. 1984;34:1033–1037.
123. Warner JJ, Navarro RA. Serratus anterior dysfunction: Recognition and treatment. *Clin Orthop*. 1998;349:139.
124. Wiater JM, Flatow EL. Long thoracic nerve injury. *Clin Orthop*. 1999;368:17.
125. Clein LJ. Suprascapular entrapment neuropathy. *J Neurosurg*. 1975;43:337–342.
126. Edeland HG, Zachrisson BE. Fracture of the scapular notch associated with lesion of the suprascapular nerve. *Acta Orthop Scand*. 1975;46:758–763.
127. Swafford AR, Lichtman DH. Suprascapular nerve entrapment: A case report. *J Hand Surg*. 1982;7:57–60.
128. Toon TN, Bravois M, Guillen M. Suprascapular nerve injury following trauma to the shoulder. *J Trauma*. 1981;21:652–655.
129. Zoltan JD. Injury to the suprascapular nerve associated with anterior dislocation of the shoulder: Case report and review of the literature. *J Trauma*. 1979;19:203–206.
130. Aiello I, Serra G, Traina GC, Tugnoli V. Entrapment of the suprascapular nerve of the spinoglenoid notch. *Ann Neurol*. 1982;12:314–316.
131. Carlson JA, Baruah JK. Suprascapular nerve entrapment at spinoglenoid notch. *Neurology*. 1985;35:78.
132. Antoniadis G, Richeter HP, Rath S. Suprascapular nerve entrapment: Experience with 28 cases. *J Neurosurg*. 1996;85:1020.
133. Antoniou J, Tae SK, Williams GR, Bird S, Ramsey ML, Iannotti JP. Suprascapular neuropathy: Variability in the diagnosis, treatment, and outcome. *Clin Orthop Relat Res*. 2001;386:131–138.
134. Braddom RL, Wolfe C. Musculocutaneous nerve injury after heavy exercise. *Arch Phys Med Rehabil*. 1978;59:290–293.
135. Kim SM, Goodrich JA. Isolated proximal musculocutaneous nerve palsy: Case report. *Arch Phys Med Rehabil*. 1984;65: 735–736.
136. Liveson JA. Nerve lesions associated with shoulder dislocation: An electrodiagnostic study of 11 cases. *J Neurol Neurosurg Psychiatry*. 1984;47:742–744.
137. Aita JF. An unusual compressive neuropathy. *Arch Neurol*. 1984;41:341.
138. Berry H, Bril V. Axillary nerve palsy following blunt trauma to the shoulder region: A clinical and electrophysiological review. *J Neurol Neurosurg Psychiatry*. 1982;45:1027–1032.
139. Kirby JF, Kraft GH. Entrapment neuropathy of anterior branch of axillary nerve: Report of case. *Arch Phys Med Rehabil*. 1972;53:338–340.
140. Steinnman SP, Moran EA. Axillary nerve injury: Diagnosis and treatment. *J Am Acad Orthop Surg*. 2003;9:328.
141. Kameda Y. An anomalous muscle (accessory scapularis-teres-latissimus muscle) in the axilla penetrating the brachial plexus in man. *Acta Anat*. 1976;96:513–533.
142. Lotem N, Fried A, Levy M, Solzi P, Najenson T, Nathan H. Radial palsy following muscular effort. A nerve compression syndrome possibly related to a fibrous arch of the lateral head of the triceps. *J Bone Joint Surg*. 1971;53B:500–506.
143. Kim DH, Murovic JA, Kim YY, Kline DG. Surgical treatment and outcomes in 45 cases of posterior interosseous nerve entrapments and injuries. *J Neurosurg*. 2006;104(5): 766–777.
144. Boswick JA, Stromberg WB. Isolated injury to the median nerve above the elbow. *J Bone Joint Surg*. 1967;49A:653–658.
145. Staal A, Van voorthuisen AE, Van Dijk LM. Neurological complications following arterial catheterization by the axillary approach. *Br J Radiol*. 1966;39:115–116.
146. Bolton CF, Driedger AA, Lindsay RM. Ischaemic neuropathy in uraemic patients caused by bovine arteriovenous shunt. *J Neurol Neurosurg Psychiatry*. 1979;42:810–814.
147. Al-Naib I. Humeral supracondylar spur and Struther's ligament: A rare cause of neurovascular entrapment in the upper limb. *Int Orthop*. 1994;18:393.
148. Aydinlioglu A, Cirik B, Akpina F, Tosun N, Dogan A. Bilateral median nerve compression at the level of Struthers ligament. *J Neurosurg*. 2000;92:693.
149. Bilbe T, Yalaman O, Bilge S, Cokneşeli B, Barut S. Entrapment of the median nerve at the level of the ligament of Struthers. *Neurosurgery*. 1990;27:787–789.
150. Schrader PA, Reina CR. Struther's ligament neuropathy in a juvenile. *Orthopedics*. 1994;17:723.
151. Spinner RJ, Carmichael SW, Spinner M. Partial median nerve entrapment in the distal arm because of an accessory bicipital aponeurosis. *J Hand Surg Am*. 1991;16:236.

152. Schantz K, Riegels-Nielsen P. The anterior interosseous nerve syndrome. *J Hand Surg Br*. 1992;17:510.
153. Pyrse-Phillips WE. Validation of a diagnostic sign in carpal tunnel syndrome. *N Engl J Med*. 1993;329:2013–2018.
154. Fowler JR, Gaughan JP, Ilyas AM. The sensitivity and specificity of ultrasound for the diagnosis of carpal tunnel syndrome: A meta-analysis. *Clin Orthop Relat Res*. 2011;469(4):1089–1094.
155. Bland JDP. Treatment of carpal tunnel syndrome. *Muscle Nerve*. 2007;36:167–171.
156. Marshall S, Tardif G, Ashworth N. Local corticosteroid injection for carpal tunnel syndrome. *Cochrane Database Syst Rev*. 2007;18(2):CD001554.
157. O'Connor D, Marshall S, Massy-Westropp N. Non-surgical treatment (other than steroid injection) for carpal tunnel syndrome. *Cochrane Database Syst Rev*. 2003;(1):CD003219.
158. Scholten RJ, Gerritsen AA, Uitdehaag BM, van Geldere D, de Vet HC, Bouter LM. Surgical treatment options for carpal tunnel syndrome. *Cochrane Database Syst Rev*. 2004;(4):CD003905.
159. Padua L, Padua R, Aprile I, Pasqualetti P, Tonali P. Multiperspective follow-up of untreated carpal tunnel syndrome: A multicenter study. *Neurology*. 2001;56:1459–1466.
160. Verdugo RJ, Salinas RS, Castilo J, Cea JG. Surgical versus non-surgical treatment for carpal tunnel syndrome. *Cochrane Database Syst Rev*. 2003;3:CD0011552.
161. Jarvik JG, Comstock BA, Kliot M, et al. Surgery versus non-surgical therapy for carpal tunnel syndrome: A randomised parallel-group trial. *Lancet*. 2009;374:1074–1081.
162. Bland JD. Do nerve conductions predict the outcome of carpal tunnel decompression. *Muscle Nerve*. 2001;24:935–940.
163. American Association of Electrodiagnostic Medicine, American Academy of Physical Medicine and Rehabilitation, American Academy of Neurology. Practice parameter for electrodiagnostic studies in ulnar neuropathy at the elbow: Summary statement. *Arch Phys Med Rehabil*. 1999;80:357–359.
164. Kincaid JC, Phillips LH, Daube JR. The evaluation of suspected ulnar neuropathy at the elbow. *Arch Neurol*. 1986;43:44–47.
165. Visser LH, Beekman R, Franssen H. Short-segment nerve conduction studies in ulnar neuropathy at the elbow. *Muscle Nerve*. 2005;31(3):331–338.
166. Raynor EM, Shefner JM, Preston DC, Logigian EL. Sensory and mixed nerve conduction studies in the evaluation of ulnar neuropathy at the elbow. *Muscle Nerve*. 1994;17:785–792.
167. Mowlawi A, Andrews K, Lille S, Verhulst S, Zook EG, Milner S. The management of cubital tunnel syndrome: A meta-analysis of clinical studies. *Plast Reconstr Surg*. 2000;106:327–334.
168. Dellon AL, Hament W, Gittelshorn A. Nonoperative management of cubital tunnel syndrome: An 8-year prospective study. *Neurology*. 1993;43:1673–1677.
169. Macadam SA, Gandhi R, Bezuhly M, Lefaivre KA. Simple decompression versus anterior subcutaneous and submuscular transposition of the ulnar nerve for cubital tunnel syndrome: A meta-analysis. *J Hand Surg Am*. 2008;33:1314.e1–e12.

CHAPTER 24

Focal Neuropathies of the Lower Extremities: Radiculopathies, Plexopathies, and Mononeuropathies

Limb pain, diminished sensation (numbness), altered sensory perception (paresthesias and dysesthesias) and impaired function due to weakness are exceedingly common complaints in the practice of medicine. Many individuals with one or more of these symptoms, particularly pain in isolation, have musculoskeletal problems. Some of these individuals may have sensory symptoms as well. Although this suggests nerve involvement, it is not uncommon to be unable to find objective evidence of nerve pathology particularly if the sensory symptoms are intermittent and vague in their anatomic distribution. By the same token, many of these patients have the perception of weakness that may result from limitations imposed by pain. Not uncommonly, however, patients with complaints of limb pain, sensory symptoms, and altered function will have focal nerve injuries affecting the nerve roots, lumbosacral plexus, or individual peripheral nerves, the subject matter of this chapter.

The purpose of this chapter is to provide a conceptual framework by which to evaluate and manage patients with focal lower limb complaints. The specific goals are to provide strategies to accurately diagnose and then manage focal nerve injuries. This begins by distinguishing them from the musculoskeletal causes of monomelic symptoms described in Chapter 36. Subsequently, as with all neurologic problem-solving exercises, localization is attempted to nerve roots, plexus or one or more individual nerves. As etiologies of nerve injury vary with anatomic locus, the benefit of localization is to limit differential diagnostic considerations, facilitate etiologic diagnosis and provide optimal management. Consideration of chronologic course and risk factors will aid in differential diagnosis.

The format of this chapter will parallel that of the preceding chapter on analogous disorders of the upper extremities to which the reader is referred regarding relevant anatomy, pathophysiology, and electrodiagnostic (EDX) evaluation. To avoid redundancy, these subjects will only be addressed when there are relevant differences between the upper and lower extremities. A detailed review of the clinical features, etiologies, evaluation, and management of individual focal neuropathies of the lower extremities will be provided. As in other chapters in this book, descriptions will rest on a foundation of published data but will be expanded upon by the personal experiences of the authors.

▶ ANATOMY

LUMBOSACRAL NERVE ROOTS

There are a few, clinically relevant differences in anatomy and nomenclature between the upper and lower limbs that require repetition. The organization of nerve roots is in many ways identical to that in cervical spine. One notable exception is that dorsal root ganglia may reside in an intraspinal location within the lumbosacral spine. In some cases, this results in mechanical nerve root compression distal rather than proximal to the dorsal root ganglion, producing a potentially confusing pattern of EDX findings to those unfamiliar with this anatomical variant.[1]

In the lumbosacral cord the nerve roots have a more oblique, descending trajectory than their cervical counterparts, due to the differing length of the spinal cord and vertebral column (Fig. 24-1). The nerve roots need to descend for a considerable distance from the conus medullaris through the spinal canal before they exit the spinal canal from their designated foramen. Understandably, the root will exit the foramen from the most rostral position within the foramen possible, immediately beneath the pedicle of the vertebral body with the same numerical designation. As this is typically above the plane in which disc material extrudes, or spondylotic bars are most likely to develop, the tendency is to compress the next nerve root which has not yet exited the spinal column and the one corresponding to the lower of the two vertebrae constituting that particular foramen.

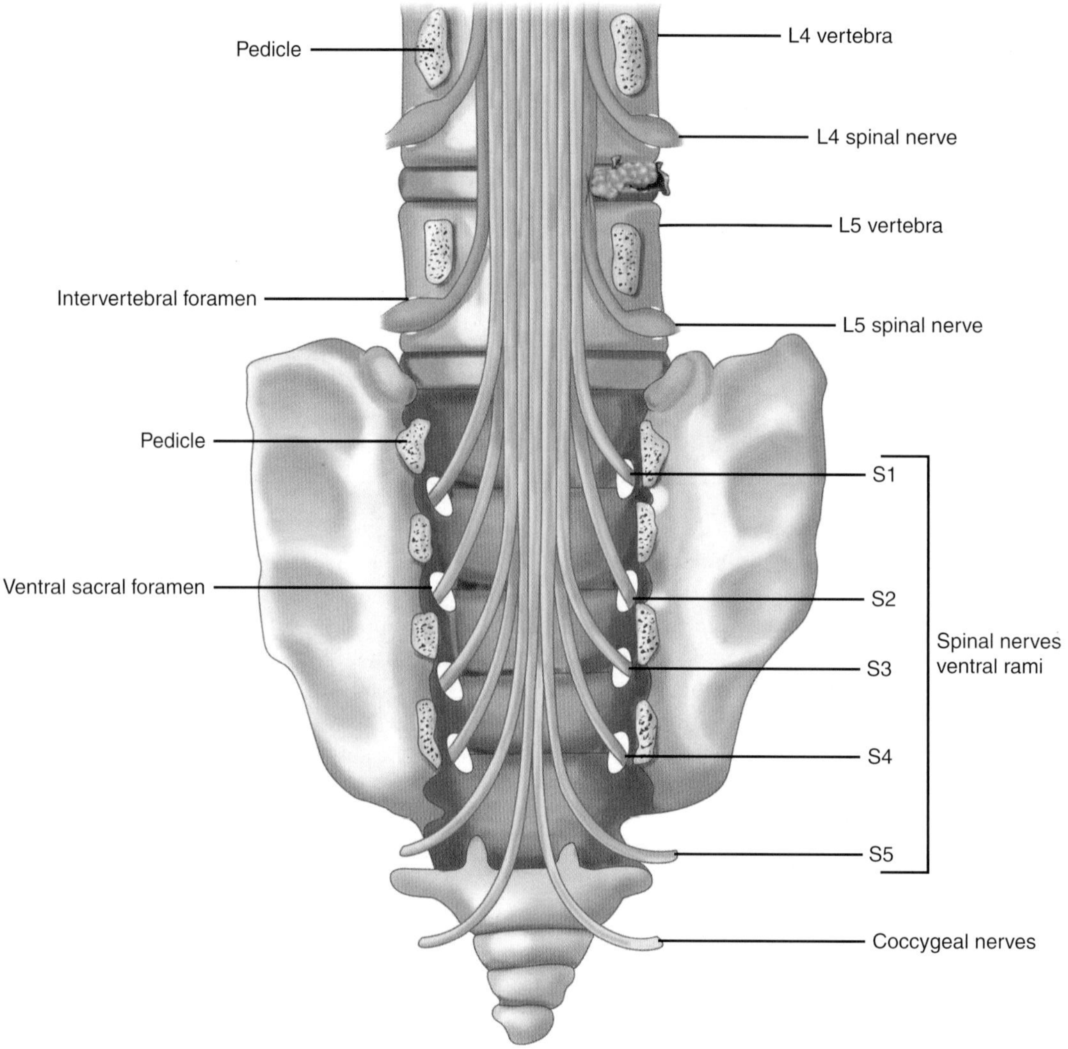

Figure 24-1. Anatomic correlations between disc herniation and affected nerve root in the lumbosacral spine.

In consideration of these influences, disc material extruding from the C5–6 intervertebral disc would preferentially come in contact with a nerve root lying directly above it (C6) in the absence of a pre- or postfixed plexus as mentioned in Chapter 23.[2] Similarly, in the lumbosacral spine, pathology of the L4–5 disc is most likely to impinge upon the L5 root, not where it exits the foramen but as it traverses the L4–5 disc on its way to the more caudal foramen formed by the L5 and S1 vertebral bodies (Fig. 24-1). There is one additional consideration. In the cervical spine the C5–6 disc pathology preferentially affects the C6 root as their courses parallel each other. With a lumbosacral disc herniation however, as the descending nerve roots traverse the disc perpendicularly, the nerve root that is preferentially compressed is related to how far medial or lateral the disc material protrudes from the rent in the annulus fibrosis. For example, disc herniation at L4–5 near the midline preferentially compresses a more medially positioned S1 or other sacral nerve roots. Alternatively, the more typical posterior-lateral disc herniation that occurs lateral to the posterior longitudinal ligament may preferentially affect the L5 root. A far lateral herniation may compress the laterally placed L4 root against its pedicle or overlying lamina (Fig. 24-1).

It is important to recognize two other potential variations from typical compressive radiculopathy. Segmental patterns of injury do not necessarily originate from pathology of nerve roots but can originate from injury to analogous segments of the spinal cord, particularly if the pathology is affecting the anterior horn but sparing the centrifugally placed descending motor and ascending sensory tracts. These segmental deficits may also result from compressive cord injury that may be at a level more rostral than the clinical deficits. Hypothetically, this results from an ischemic mechanism similar to what has been proposed in neoplastic spinal cord compression. Lower motor neuron deficits resulting from presumed ischemic anterior horn cell injury has been described in both cervical spondylotic myelopathy and from dural arteriovenous injury.[3,4]

It is also true that radiculopathy can be obscured by myelopathy, particularly in the cervical and thoracic regions.

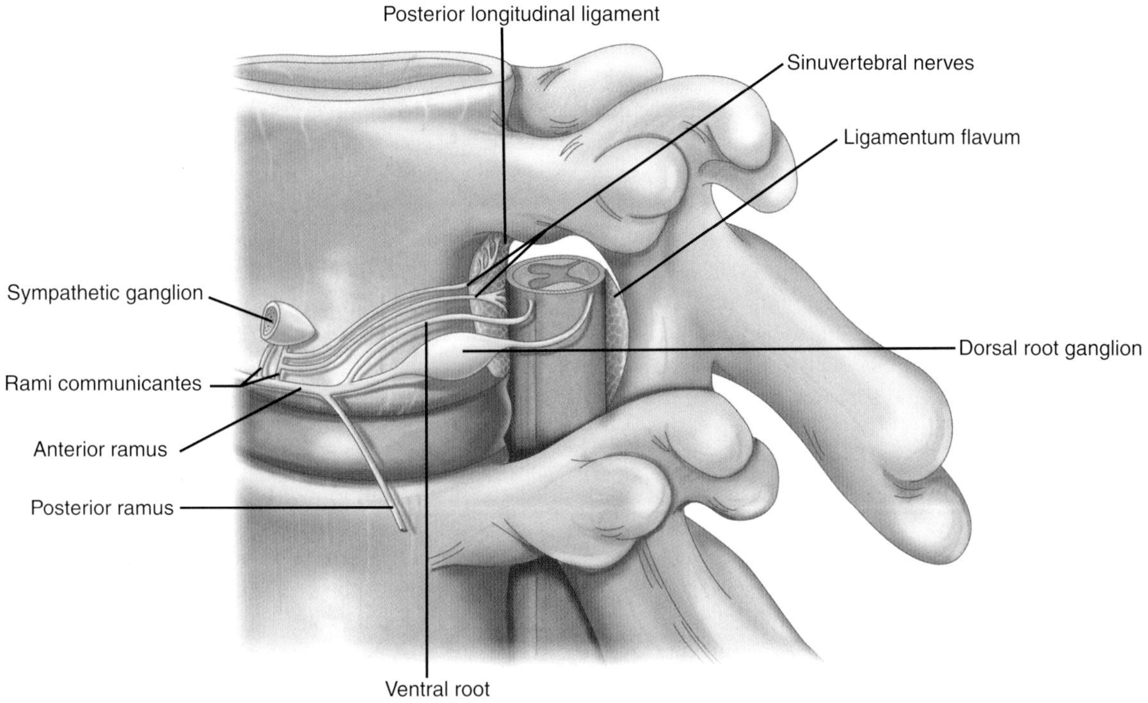

Figure 24-2. Anatomy of the spine.

A spondylotic bar encroaching on the spinal canal in the neck is more likely to be manifest with tract rather than segmental signs and symptom whereas this same bar in the lumbosacral spine can have radiculopathic but not myelopathic manifestations.

Musculoskeletal conditions are estimated to underlie 70% or more of back pain cases.[5] Understanding back and radicular pain requires a basic understanding of the lumbosacral spine anatomy (Fig. 24-2).[6] The articular surfaces that contribute to both the mobility and stability of the spine include the intervertebral discs and two pairs of synovial joints that together form the articular connections between contiguous vertebrae. These synovial joints include the zygapophyseal or facet joints that are formed by extensions of two contiguous vertebral laminae and constitute the roof of the neural foramina. These latter joints are innervated by branches of the posterior ramus of the spinal nerve. Diseases affecting these structures are one of many potential sources of nonradiating back pain. The second synovial joint system, the uncovertebral joints of Luschka, arises from the posterior-lateral surfaces of the vertebral bodies. These joints along with the disc itself constitute the floor or ventral boundary of the neural foramina through which nerve roots exit. The rostral and caudal boundaries of the neural foramen are formed by the pedicles of the vertebrae immediately above and below the foramen in question.

There are two major ligamentous structures within the spinal canal: the posterior longitudinal ligament and the ligamentum flavum. Both are longitudinally oriented, the former running along the anterior aspect of the central canal just posterior to the vertebral bodies and disc spaces. The latter runs along the posterior aspect of the spinal canal just underneath the spinous processes. The posterior longitudinal ligament is half the width of its cervical counterpart in the lumbar spinal canal. This may add to an increased risk of paramedian disc herniation with potential consequence related to bowel and bladder control. The posterior longitudinal ligament is innervated by the sinuvertebral (recurrent meningeal or recurrent nerves of Luschka) nerves that arise from the rami communicantes outside the neural foramina. These travel posteriorly to innervate the dura, annulus fibrosis, the walls of intraspinal blood vessels as well as the posterior longitudinal ligaments (Fig. 24-2). The ligamentum flavum contains few nociceptive fibers. Its major clinical significance may be to contribute to canal stenosis by its tendency to hypertrophy as part of the spondylotic process. The diameter of the central canal averages 18 mm in most normal adults with a range of between 15 and 23 mm. As in the cervical canal, it widens by a few millimeters when the patient bends forward.

Although this is a text of neuromuscular disorders, it is appropriate to mention potential sources of back, buttock, thigh, and leg pain. It is safe to say that isolated back pain without radicular pain or neurologic signs or symptoms may occur as the initial symptom of disorders which may eventually have neurologic consequences. It is equally safe to say that it may be difficult to initially distinguish common non-neurologic and often musculoskeletal causes of back pain from less common ones that have or may develop neurologic consequences. In the former category, potential anatomic sources of back pain include many spinal structures, such as the posterior longitudinal and other ligaments, capsules of the facet and sacroiliac joints, vertebral periosteum, dura, the paravertebral musculature and fascia, blood vessels, annulus fibrosus, spinal nerve roots, epidural veins and arterioles, and epidural fibroadipose tissue.[5] Although it has long been suggested that paraspinal muscle pain originates from muscular spasm promoting constriction of intramuscular blood vessels, the lack of continuous EMG activity in hardened, tender muscles suggests that myoedema rather than continuous muscle activity promotes back stiffness and discomfort. In any event, identifying the anatomic source of back pain in an individual patient is an extremely difficult undertaking. Due to their lack or relative lack of nociceptive nerve endings, neither the nucleus pulposus nor the ligamentum flavum appear to be likely culprits.

Degenerative spine disease, i.e., spondylosis, affects a number of different structures, which may individually or collectively narrow the diameter of the neural foramen or the central canal of the spinal column. As a consequence, nerve root integrity may be compromised in either location by enlargement of normal anatomic structures. Degeneration of the zygapophyseal and uncovertebral joints promotes osteophyte formation and space occupying joint enlargement. Intraspinal ligaments hypertrophy. Degeneration of the intervertebral disc results in bulging of the annular ring and loss of its vertical height reducing intrapedicular distances and contributing to foraminal narrowing. If spondylolysis and resulting spondylolisthesis occurs, that is the shifting of one vertebral body on another in an anterior–posterior direction, both central canal and foraminal cross-sectional area is compromised.

The intervertebral disc consists of a gelatinous center, the nucleus pulposus, and a cartilaginous margin, the annulus fibrosis. As mentioned, the concept of discogenic pain is somewhat nebulous in that there are a paucity of nociceptive pain fibers innervating the outer annulus and none within the nucleus pulposus itself. Although the pain and pathophysiology of nerve root disease are typically attributed to direct compression of the nerve root and the inflammation that accompanies it, it is important to remember that other potentially pain-sensitive structures such as the sinuvertebral nerves traverse the neural foramina as well.[7–9] Although there is a rich anastomotic blood supply to the spinal cord and nerve roots, ischemic injury resulting from radicular vascular compression may represent an alternative mechanism of nerve root injury.

LUMBOSACRAL PLEXUS

There is considerable variation in the anatomy of the lumbosacral plexus (Figs. 24-3 and 24-4). It may have contributions from as many as 11 spinal nerves but is typically composed of 8 (L1–S3). The lumbar plexus is predominantly composed of branches from L1 to L4, with variable contributions from T11, T12, and L5. Typically, the majority of L4 fibers travel with the lumbar plexus, with a much smaller contribution from L4 joining with L5 to form the lumbosacral trunk. In a "prefixed" plexus, the plexus shifts downward so that there is more of an L1 contribution to the lumbar plexus, the femoral and obturator nerves become comprised of L2–3-rather than L3–4 segmental contributions and the majority of L4 fibers end up in the sacral plexus. In the so-called "postfixed" plexus, the plexus is shifted upward so that virtually all of L4 and some of L5 are now confined within the lumbar rather than sacral plexuses.

The lumbar plexus is formed in the retroperitoneum, just inferior to the kidney and just behind the psoas muscle. Its blood supply originates from the internal iliac artery. Ischemic injury may occur from distal aortic or internal iliac arterial occlusion. The major branches of the upper lumbar plexus are the ilioinguinal, genitofemoral, and lateral femoral cutaneous nerve (LFCN) or lateral cutaneous nerve of the thigh. The femoral, obturator, and lumbosacral trunks are the major components of the lower aspect of the lumbar plexus.

The sacral plexus is formed within the concavity of the ventral surface of the sacrum, behind and lateral to the rectum. The L4 and L5 contributions to the sacral plexus and to the sciatic nerve are provided by the lumbosacral trunk, the conduit between the lumbar and the sacral plexuses. The lumbosacral trunk traverses the pelvic brim at the posterior aspect of the pelvis, over the sacral alae, and just lateral to the sacroiliac joints (Fig. 24-3). In this location, it is vulnerable to compressive injury during parturition. The major branches of the sacral plexus are the superior and inferior gluteal nerves, the posterior cutaneous nerve of the thigh, the fibular (formerly peroneal) and tibial divisions of the sciatic nerve, and the pudendal nerve.

As mentioned, the embryologic rotation of the limb results not only in the spiral orientation of the dermatomes and hip ligaments but in relocation of muscles from their original anatomic positions. Muscles that were originally located on the posterior surface of the lower limb are innervated by the posterior branches of the lumbosacral plexus, for example, femoral, fibular (formerly peroneal), superior and inferior gluteal nerves as well as the lateral cutaneous nerve of the thigh. Muscles that were originally in an anterior location are innervated by anterior branches, for example, genitofemoral, obturator, and tibial nerves.

INDIVIDUAL PERIPHERAL NERVES OF THE LOWER EXTREMITIES

Identification of lower extremity mononeuropathies is dependent on knowledge of patterns of muscle weakness, sensory symptoms and reflex loss if relevant. As the pattern of muscle weakness arguably provides the most objective localizing information, knowledge of the muscles that promote the major movements of the thigh, leg, foot, and toes and the nerves that innervate them is invaluable (Tables 24-1 and 24-2). Determination of potential etiology however is enhanced by a detailed understanding of the relationship between the nerves and contiguous anatomic structures. The

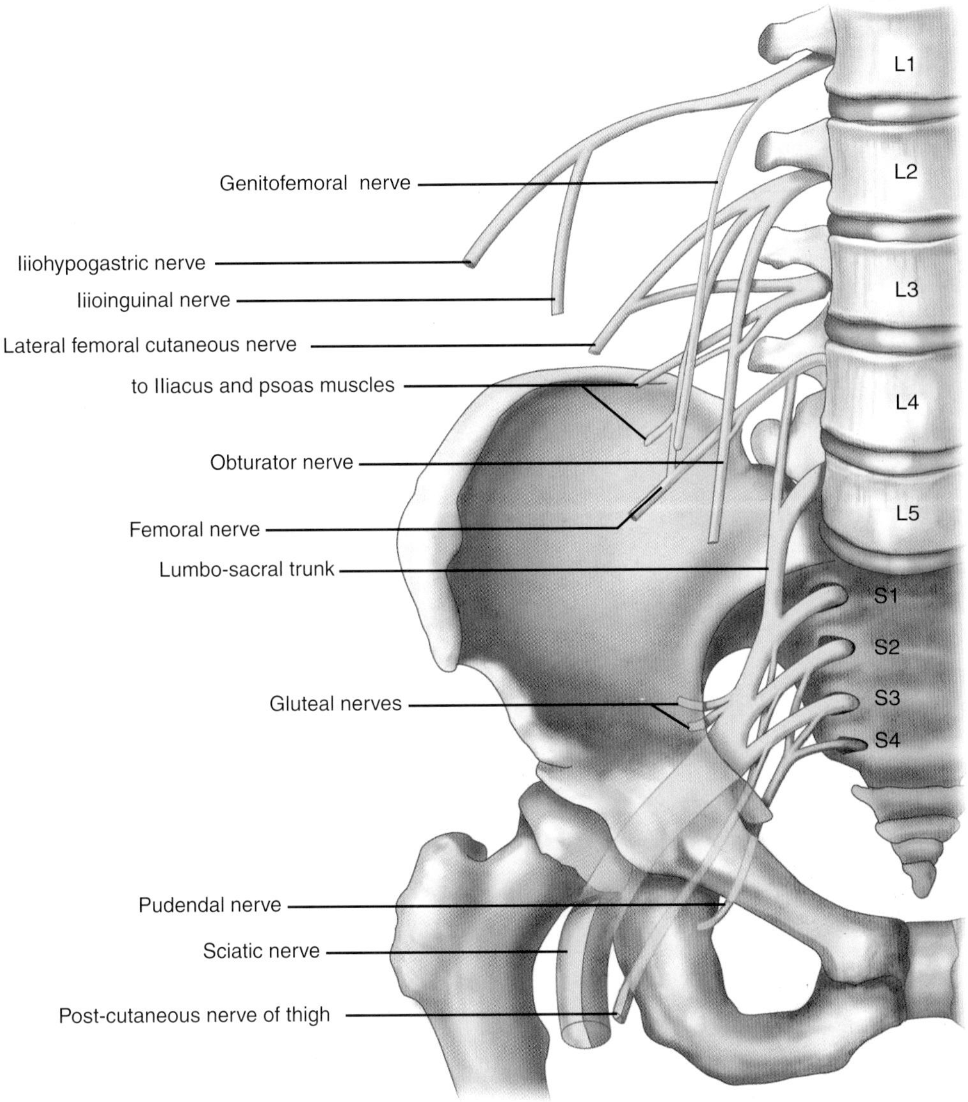

Figure 24-3. Lumbosacral plexus.

following paragraphs summarize the relevant lower extremity peripheral nerve anatomy.

The iliohypogastric nerve is primarily an extension of the L1 nerve root with some contribution from T12. It exits on the lateral border of the psoas muscle in proximity to the lower pole of the kidney and traverses the ventral surface of the quadratus lumborum muscle. It exits the abdominal wall superior to the iliac crest. It provides partial innervation to the transverse abdominus and internal oblique muscles of the abdominal wall. There are two cutaneous branches, one overlying the iliac crest in the posterior axillary line and a second innervating a small transverse patch above the pubic symphysis (Fig. 24-5).

The ilioinguinal nerve has a similar L1 segmental origin and anatomic course. Its course is parallel but caudal to the iliohypogastric nerve along the upper border of the iliac crest. Its course is retrocolic along the posterior abdominal wall. The nerve passes through the superficial inguinal ring to supply the skin overlying the inguinal ligament, extending to the regions just above and lateral to the base of the penis and scrotum (or labia). In other words, the area just above the genitals and just below the pubic symphysis (Fig. 24-5). Like the iliohypogastric nerve, the ilioinguinal nerve innervates the transverse abdominus and internal oblique muscles.

The genitofemoral nerve has near equal contributions from the L1 and L2 segments. It penetrates the psoas muscle in the retroperitoneum and descends vertically along its ventral surface. It lies in close proximity to the external iliac artery, ureters, terminal ileum on the right, and sigmoid colon on the left. Like the iliohypogastric nerve, it has two separate sensory branches. The larger of the two, the femoral branch, innervates the anterior, proximal thigh in the midline, just distal to the inguinal ligament. The second, smaller genital branch, supplies a small cutaneous zone on the lateral aspect of the root of the penis and scrotum or corresponding area of the labia. Its cutaneous distribution overlaps with

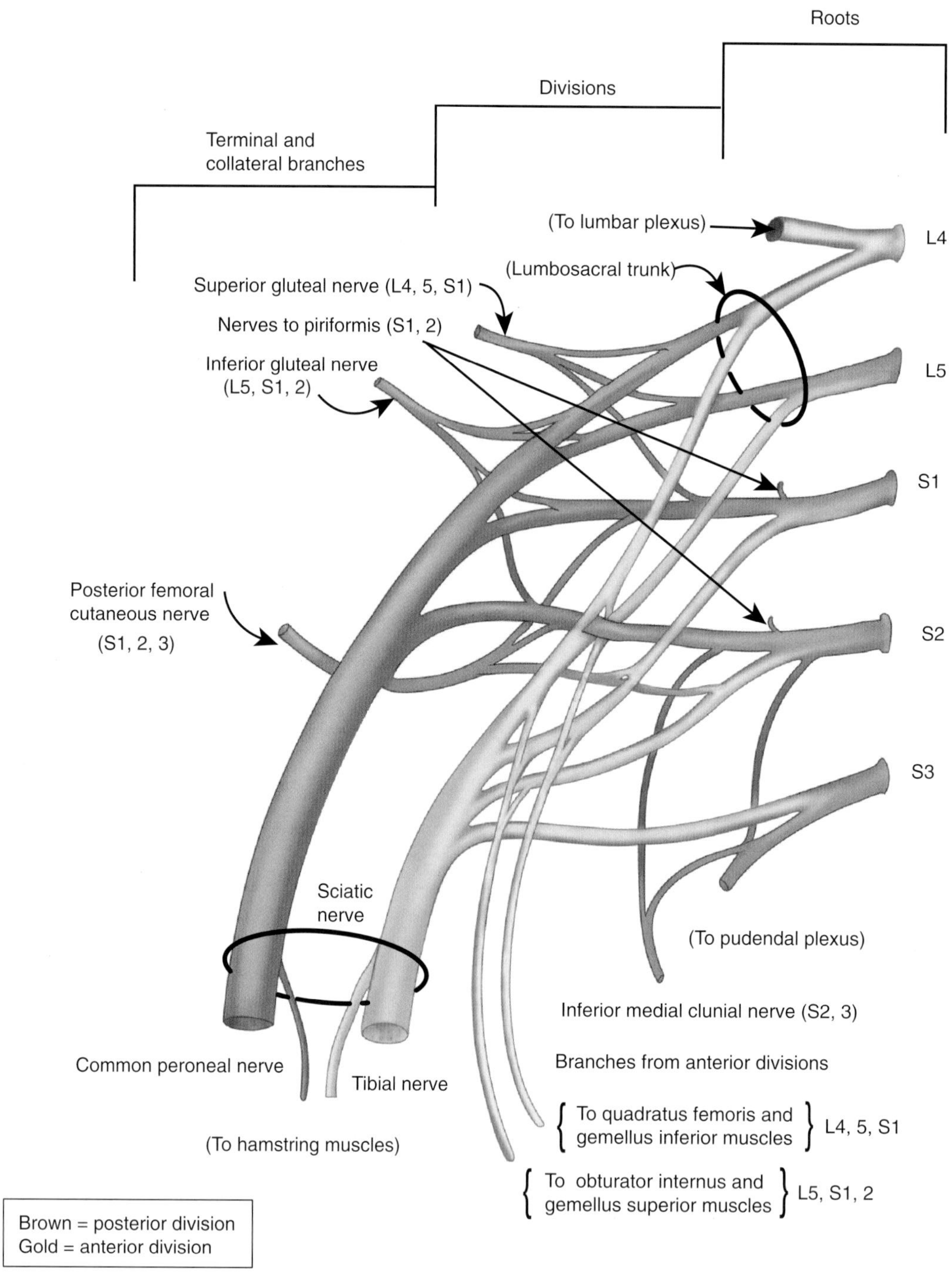

Figure 24-4. Lumbosacral trunk, sacral plexus, and sciatic nerve.

portions of the ilioinguinal and iliohypogastric territories (Figs. 24-3 and 24-5). The only muscular branch is the cremaster muscle which controls the ascent/descent of the testes in order to maintain spermatic temperature homeostasis.

The obturator nerve receives contributions from the second through fourth lumbar segments (Figs. 24-3, 24-5 to 24-7). It emerges from the medial border of the psoas muscle just rostral to the pelvic brim and descends through the pelvis vertically, medial to the course of the femoral nerve, to exit the pelvis through the obturator foramen. It innervates the adductor longus, brevis, and a portion of the adductor magnus muscle, as well as the gracilis, and obturator externus muscles. The major function of these muscles is to adduct the thigh with contributions to thigh flexion and external rotation. Cutaneous sensation is supplied to a small patch on the inner thigh.

The femoral nerve is also an extension of the L2–4 segments (Figs. 24-3 and 24-7). It arises in a retroperitoneal location and passes between the psoas and the iliacus muscles before traveling under the iliacus fascia in the lateral

▶ TABLE 24-1. **LUMBOSACRAL PLEXUS ANATOMY**

Muscles Innervated	Cutaneous Distribution	Segmental Contribution	Plexus	Nerve
Transverse abdominus and internal oblique	Superior iliac crest at the posterior axillary line and small patch above the symphysis pubis	T12, L1	Lumbar	Iliohypogastric
Transverse abdominus and internal oblique	Skin overlying the inguinal ligament extending to the base of penis	L1	Lumbar	Ilioinguinal
Cremaster	Anterior proximal thigh in midline just caudal to the inguinal ligament and the serotum, labia majora, and adjacent thigh	L1, L2	Lumbar—anterior	Genitofemoral
None	Anterolateral thigh	L2–3	Lumbar—posterior	Lateral cutaneous nerve of the thigh
Psoas minor	None	L1–2–3	Lumbar	Branches of lumbar plexus and femoral
Iliacus and psoas major	None	L2–3–4	Lumbar	Branches of lumbar plexus and femoral
Sartorius	Anterior thigh	L2–3–4	Lumbar—posterior	Femoral
Rectus femoris, vastus lateralis–medialis–intermedius, and pectineus	Anterior thigh	L2–3–4	Lumbar	Femoral
None	Medial leg	L4	Lumbar	Saphenous
Gracilis, adductor magnus–longus–brevis, and obturator internus	Small patch of medial thigh	L2–3–4	Lumbar—anterior	Obturator
None	Posterior thigh, inferior buttock, lateral perineum, proximal medial thigh	S1–2–3	Sacral	Posterior cutaneous nerve of the thigh
Gluteus medius–minimus and tensor fascia lata	None	L4–5, S1	Lumbosacral trunk Sacral—posterior	Superior gluteal
Gluteus maximus	None	L5, S1–2	Lumbosacral trunk Sacral—posterior	Inferior gluteal
External anal sphincter	Distal anal canal and perianal skin	S2–3–4	Sacral	Pudendal—inferior rectal
Muscles of the pelvic floor, external urethral sphincter, and the erectile tissue of the penis	Perineum ventral to the rectum as well as the scrotum and labia	S2–3–4	Sacral	Pudendal—perineal
None	Penis or labia	S2–3–4	Sacral	Pudendal—dorsal nerve of the penis/labia
Semimembranosis/semitendinosis	NA	L5, S1–2	Lumbosacral trunk Sacral—anterior	Sciatic—tibial
Long head of biceps	NA	L5, S1–2	Lumbosacral trunk Sacral—anterior	Sciatic—tibial
Short head of biceps	NA	L5, S1–2	Lumbosacral trunk Sacral—posterior	Sciatic—common peroneal
Tibialis anterior, extensor digitorum longus and brevis, and extensor hallucis longus	Interspace between first and second digits	L4–5, S1	Lumbosacral trunk Sacral—posterior	Common peroneal—deep peroneal

(*continued*)

▶ TABLE 24-1. (CONTINUED)

Muscles Innervated	Cutaneous Distribution	Segmental Contribution	Plexus	Nerve
Peroneus longus and brevis	Distal-lateral leg and dorsum of foot	L4–5, S1	Lumbosacral trunk Sacral—posterior	Common Peroneal—superficial peroneal
Flexor hallucis longus, flexor digitorum longus, and tibialis posterior	NA	L5, S1	Lumbosacral trunk Sacral—anterior	Tibial
Medial and lateral gastrocnemius, soleus, plantaris, and popliteus	NA	S1–2	Sacral—anterior	Tibial
None	Lateral surface of foot	S1	Sacral	Sural
Intrinsic foot muscles (toe flexors–adductors–abductors)	Sole of the foot	S1–2	Sacral—anterior	Tibial—medial and lateral plantar nerves, calcaneal nerve

pelvis, where it is potentially vulnerable to an iliacus compartment syndrome. It exits the pelvis below the inguinal ligament and lateral to the femoral artery. From a motor perspective, the femoral nerve innervates the psoas and the iliacus muscles in the pelvis and six muscles in the thigh, including the four components of the quadriceps, the sartorius, and the pectineus muscles. The primary function of the majority of these muscles is to extend the leg at the knee joint. In addition, the iliopsoas, sartorius, pectineus, and the rectus femoris all contribute to hip flexion. The rectus femoris is the only quadriceps muscle that originates from the pelvis and is therefore the only one of the quadriceps capable of contributing to hip flexion. The sartorius is an unusual muscle as it contributes to external rotation at the hip joint, flexion at the knee joint, and hip flexion. The pectineus muscle contributes both to external rotation and adduction of the thigh. From a sensory perspective, the femoral nerve supplies sensation to the anterior surface of the thigh and the medial aspect of the leg through its terminal sensory branch, the saphenous nerve.

The LFCN is an extension of the second and third lumbar nerve roots (Figs. 24-3 and 24-6). It also emerges from the lateral border of the psoas and traverses the lateral pelvis deep to the iliacus fascia. It exits the pelvis at the anterior superior iliac spine, often penetrating the lateral margin of the inguinal ligament. It has no motor function and provides cutaneous innervation to the anterolateral thigh as well as the underlying fascia.

Prior to the actual formation of the sciatic nerve, there are four nerves originating from the upper sacral segments. The pudendal nerve is the more proximate of these, originating from the S2–4 segments. In a slightly more caudal location, the posterior cutaneous nerve of the thigh is formed by two or more S1–3 segments before these segments merge with the lumbosacral trunk to form the sciatic nerve which occurs just lateral and anterior to the sacrum. The last branches departing the sacral plexus prior to the formation of the sciatic nerve are the superior and inferior gluteal nerves. They are comprised of the L4–S1 and L5–S2 segments, respectively. The superior gluteal nerve is typically the only nerve to exit the sciatic notch above the piriformis muscle, the sciatic, inferior gluteal, pudendal and posterior cutaneous nerves of the thigh all typically exiting the sciatic notch caudal to this horizontally oriented muscle. Intramuscular injections are avoided in the inferior, medial quadrant of the buttocks, in order to avoid injury to these nerves which travel deep to this topographical location. The superior gluteal nerve innervates the gluteus medius, gluteus minimus, and tensor fascia lata muscles. Thigh abduction at the hip joint is their major action. All contribute to internal rotation of the thigh as well. The gluteus minimus provides a minor contribution to hip flexion, and the posterior aspect of the gluteus medius contributes partially to external rotation of the thigh. The inferior gluteal nerve innervates the gluteus maximus, which is the primary hip extensor, but provides a minor contribution to external rotation as well. Neither nerve has cutaneous representation.

The sciatic nerve receives contributions from the last two lumbar roots via the lumbosacral trunk and the first three sacral segments (Figs. 24-3 and 24-4). In reality, it is really two nerves that are conjoined, the tibial and the fibular (formerly peroneal) nerves. As many sciatic neuropathies preferentially affect the fibular nerve and may mimic a fibular neuropathy at a more distal location, it may be helpful to conceptualize the sciatic nerve as two separate nerves. The segmental contribution to these two nerves is somewhat different. The peroneal nerve contains few, if any, S3 fibers, whereas there is no meaningful L4 contribution to the tibial nerve in the majority of individuals. The sciatic nerve exits the pelvis through the sciatic notch, typically beneath the piriformis muscle, but at times traversing through or above it. The former provides the anatomic basis for the controversial piriformis syndrome. The sciatic nerve descends lateral to the ischial tuberosity of the pelvis and medial to the greater

▶ TABLE 24-2. **MUSCLES CONTRIBUTING TO SPECIFIC LOWER EXTREMITY MOVEMENTS**

Thigh						Leg		Foot			
Flexion	Extension	Abduction	Adduction	External Rotation	Internal Rotation	Extension	Flexion	Dorsiflexion	Plantar Flexion	Inversion	Eversion
Iliopsoas	Gluteus maximus	Gluteus medius	Adductor magnus	Sartorius	Tensor fascia lata	Vastus medialis	Semimembranosis	Tibialis anterior	Medial gastrocnemius	Tibialis posterior	Peroneus longus
Rectus femoris	Adductor magnus	Gluteus minimus	Adductor longus	Iliopsoas	Gluteus medius	Vastus lateralis	Semitendinosis	Extensor digitorum longus	Lateral gastrocnemius	Tibialis anterior	Peroneus brevis
Sartorius	Long head of biceps femoris	Tensor fascia lata	Adductor brevis	Pectineus	Gluteus minimus	Vastus intermedius	Short head of biceps femoris		Soleus	Flexor digitorum longus	Extensor digitorum longus
Pectineus	Semitendinosis	Piriformis	Gracilis	Adductor longus		Rectus femoris	Long head of biceps femoris		Peroneus longus	Flexor hallucis longus	Extensor hallicus longus
Adductor longus	Semimembranosis	Obturator internus	Iliopsoas	Adductor magnus		Tensor fascia lata	Sartorius		Peroneus brevis		
Adductor brevis		Gemelli	Pectineus	Gluteus maximus			Gracilis		Plantaris		
Adductor magnus				Gluteus medius			Popliteus		Flexor hallucis longus		
Gluteus minimus				Piriformis			Gastrocnemius		Flexor digitorum longus		
Tensor fascia lata				Obturator internus			Plantaris		Tibialis posterior		
				Gemelli							
				Obturator externus							
				Quadratus femoris							

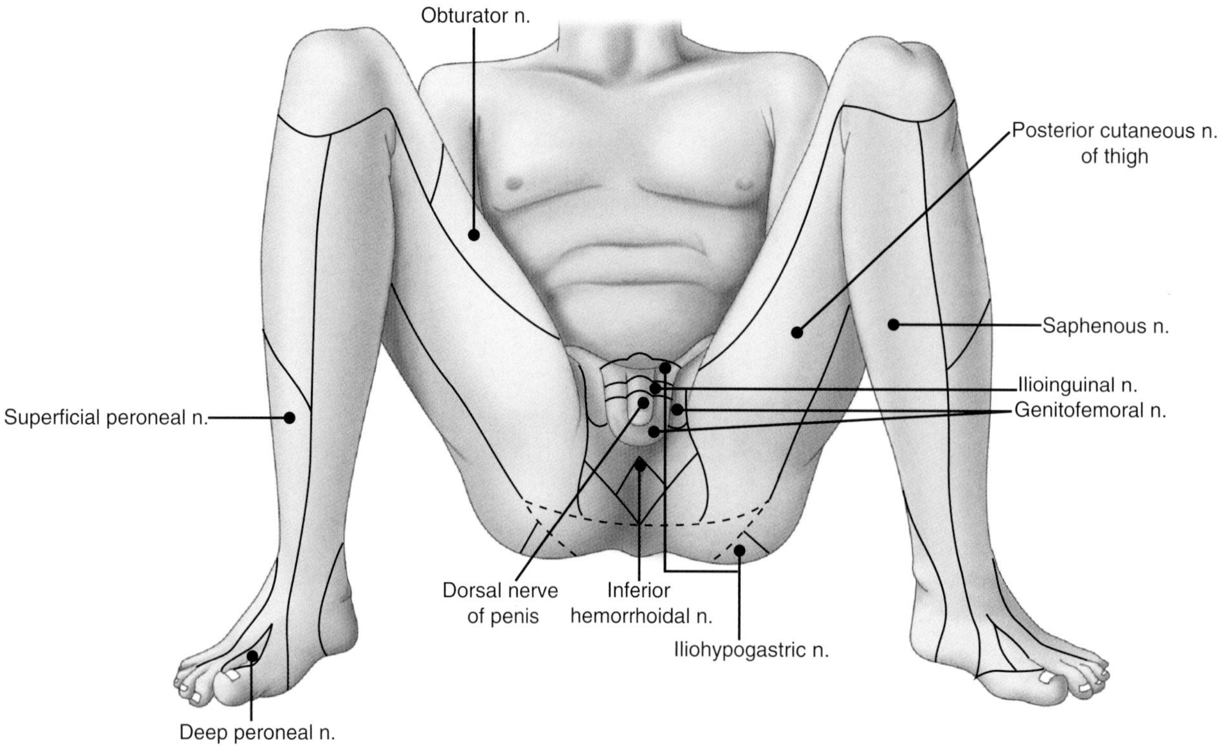

Figure 24-5. Cutaneous innervation of the groin, perineum, and genitals.

trochanter of the proximal femur, where it is potentially vulnerable not only to misplaced injections but also to displaced hip fractures or inadvertent injury during arthroplasty.

In the thigh, the sciatic nerve innervates the hamstrings, the short head of the biceps innervated by the lateral trunk or fibular (peroneal) portion of the nerve. The remaining three muscles; the semitendinosus, semimembranosus, and long head of the biceps; are innervated by the medial trunk or tibial division. The lateral two muscles are largely S1 innervated whereas the medial two muscles are predominantly L5. In addition, the adductor magnus may receive partial innervation by the sciatic nerve, providing a potential source of electrodiagnostic confusion for the unwary. A lesion of the sciatic nerve proximal to the knee will produce a pattern of sensory symptoms or sensory loss that includes the entire foot and the distal half of the lateral surface of the leg, sparing the L4/saphenous innervated medial leg. The blood supply to the sciatic nerve originates predominantly from branches of the inferior gluteal artery and popliteal arteries. This creates a watershed at mid-thigh level, which has been proposed as an explanation for both the location and prevalence of sciatic neuropathies in vasculitis.

The posterior cutaneous nerve of the thigh exits the pelvis through the lower sciatic notch, medial to the sciatic nerve and lateral to the pudendal nerve. Like the sciatic nerve, it may travel through the piriformis muscle in some individuals. It travels deep to the gluteus maximus which protects it. At the level of the gluteal crease, cluneal branches exit and ascend to supply the skin of the inferior buttock. There are perineal branches as well, which supply the skin and fascia of the lateral perineum, the proximal medial thigh, and the posterolateral aspect of the scrotum/labia as well as root of penis/clitoris. The terminal branch descends vertically to provide sensory capability to the posterior thigh and often proximal aspect of the posterior calf. The posterior cutaneous nerve of the thigh has no motor function.

In the leg, the common fibular nerve bifurcates below the level of the fibular head into its deep fibular (peroneal) and superficial fibular divisions (Figs. 24-4 and 24-8). The deep fibular nerve innervates the muscles of the anterior compartment: the tibialis anterior (TA), the extensor hallucis, the extensor digitorum longus, and the peroneus tertius, a muscle of electrodiagnostic interest. In the foot, it innervates a solitary muscle: the extensor digitorum brevis (EDB). Collectively, the major function of these muscles is to dorsiflex the foot at the ankle and the toes at the metatarsal–phalangeal joints although the peroneus tertius contributes to ankle eversion as well. The superficial fibular (peroneal) nerve innervates the lateral compartment of the leg, including the peroneus longus and brevis muscles. The major function of these muscles is to evert the foot at the ankle. The deep fibular nerve has a predominantly motor function with a very small cutaneous contribution to the interdigital space between the first and second digits. The superficial fibular nerve innervates the skin of the dorsal surface of the foot and the distal-lateral surface of the leg.

The tibial nerve receives contributions from the L5–S3 nerve roots and is the continuation of the medial cord of the

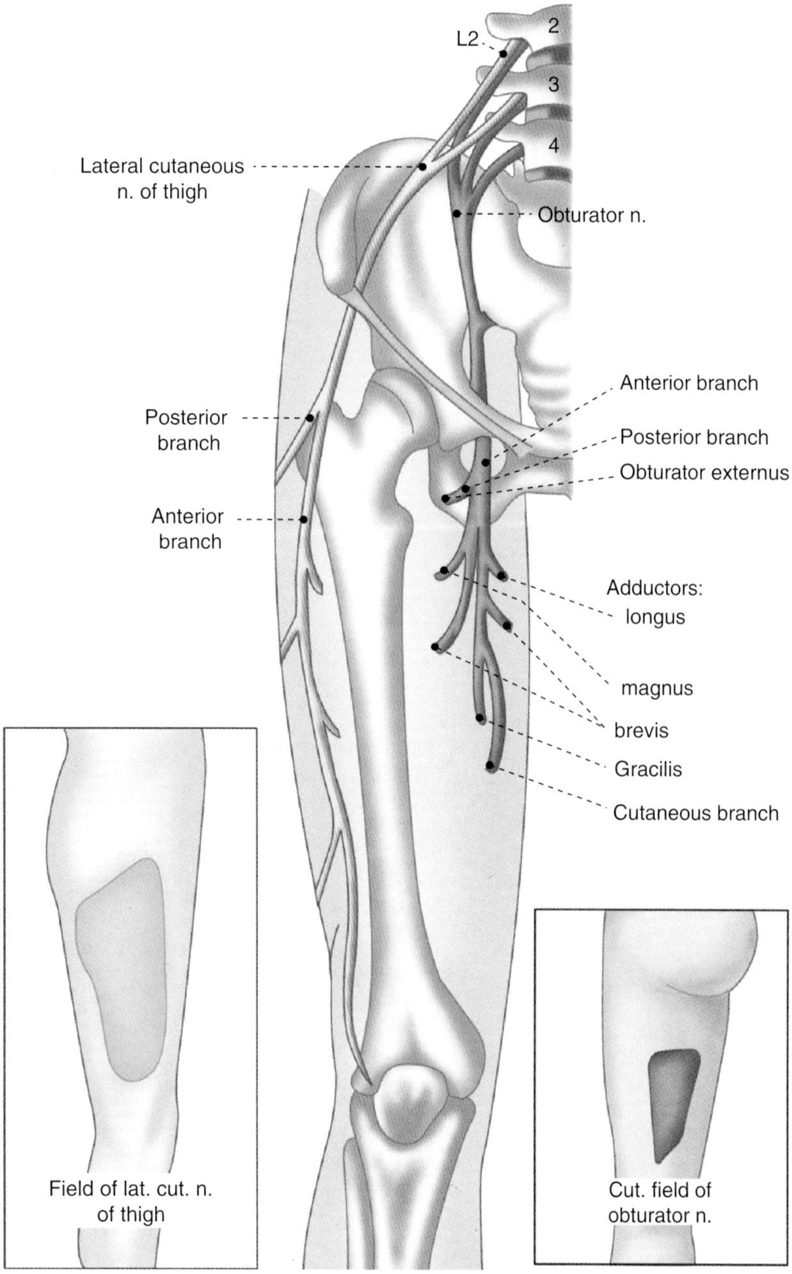

Figure 24-6. Obturator and lateral femoral cutaneous nerves. Cut, cutaneous.

sciatic nerve (Figs. 24-4 and 24-9). It physically separates itself from its fibular (peroneal) counterpart in the distal thigh, passes through the popliteal fossa before passing between the two heads of the gastrocnemius muscle. As previously mentioned, it innervates three of the four hamstring muscles in the thigh. In the leg, it supplies the posterior compartment including the two heads of the gastrocnemius, soleus, tibialis posterior, flexor digitorum longus, and flexor hallucis longus muscles. In the foot, it supplies all intrinsic foot muscles except the EDB. Its primary functions are to flex the leg at the knee, to plantar flex and invert the foot at the ankle, and to flex, abduct, and adduct the toes. The three cutaneous branches of the tibial nerve all branch at the level of the medial malleolus and include the medial and lateral plantar and calcaneal nerves. These provide the cutaneous innervation for the medial sole, lateral sole, and heel surface, respectively.

The sural nerve is formed in the popliteal fossa by anastomotic contributions from the common fibular and tibial nerves. It is derived primarily from the S1 nerve root. It descends in a fairly superficial, posterior position in the calf, moving somewhat laterally as it passes behind the lateral malleolus. It provides cutaneous innervation to the lateral foot.

The pudendal nerve has a convoluted course. It first exits the pelvis through the greater gluteal foramen only to reenter through a narrow aperture and potential site of entrapment between the sacrotuberous and sacrospinous ligaments. It then

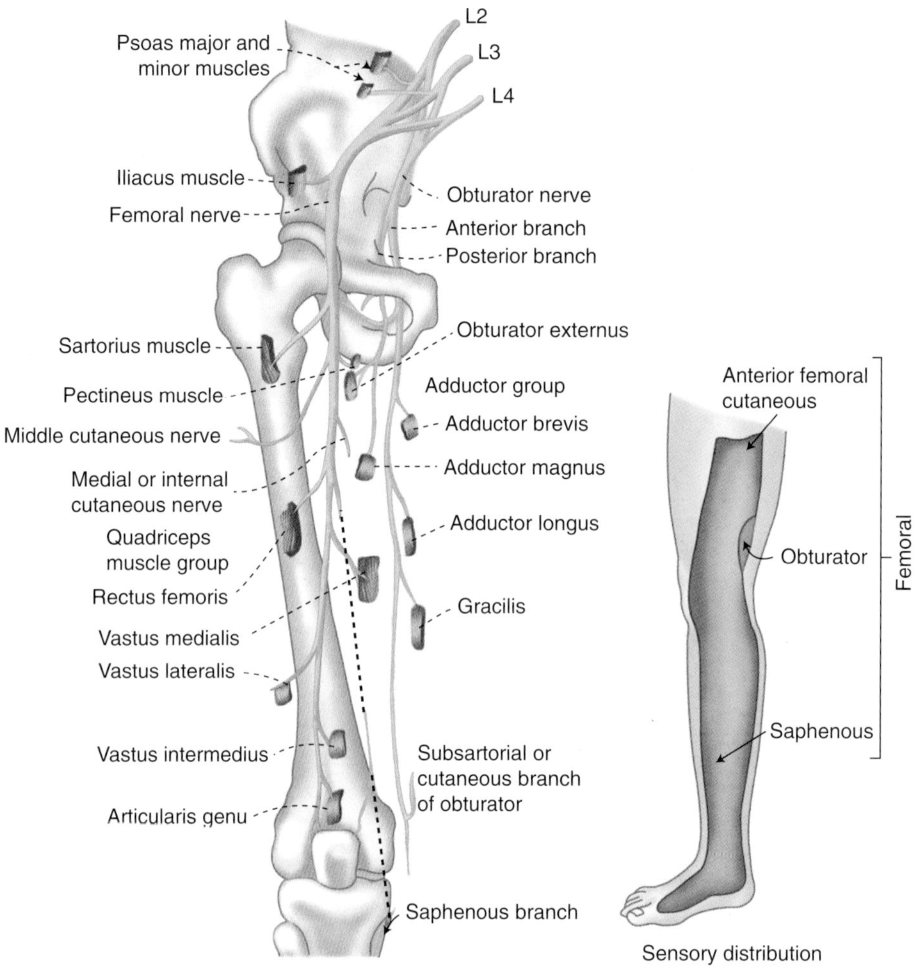

Figure 24-7. Femoral and obturator nerves.

passes through Alcock's canal created by the obturator muscle posteriorly and the ischial tuberosity anteriorly before exiting the pelvis for good just below the symphysis pubis.[10] It has three major branches: the inferior rectal or hemorrhoidal, the perineal, and the dorsal nerve of the penis/clitoris (Figs. 24-3 to 24-5). The inferior rectal nerve innervates the external anal sphincter and supplies sensation to the distal anal canal and perianal skin. The perineal nerve innervates the muscles of the pelvic floor, the external urethral sphincter, and the erectile tissue of the penis. Its cutaneous innervation includes the perineum anterior to the rectum as well as the scrotum and labia. The dorsal nerve of the penis is a purely sensory branch whose cutaneous representation is the skin of the penis and labia.

PATHOPHYSIOLOGY

The pathophysiology of peripheral nerve injury has been described in detail in Chapters 2 and 22. Axon loss with Wallerian degeneration typically results from disorders that infiltrate or infarct nerves and may result when nerves are sufficiently inflamed or mechanically injured by compression or stretch of adequate intensity or duration. Axon loss is often accompanied by pain, often deep, aching and burning in character. It is common, particularly with acute or subacute pathological processes. Muscle weakness and atrophy, sensory loss that affects all modalities, loss of deep tendon reflexes if relevant to the nerve injured, and even dysautonomic manifestations including sweating and vasomotor abnormalities are anticipated. Electrodiagnostically, amplitudes of involved sensory and motor nerves diminish on nerve conductions and fibrillation potentials and eventually a reduced number of enlarged, reconfigured motor unit action potentials (MUAPs) develop.

Many experimental models of nerve compression support the belief that myelin is preferentially damaged in the early stages of external compression or internal entrapment. Electrodiagnostically, this may express itself by any combination of focal and uniform slowing of affected fibers, nonuniform slowing (i.e., temporal dispersion), or conduction block. Demyelinating nerve injuries are, in general, less painful than their axonal counterparts but this is etiologically dependent. Clinically, focal slowing may produce paresthesias but no objective deficits. Differential slowing may impair modalities

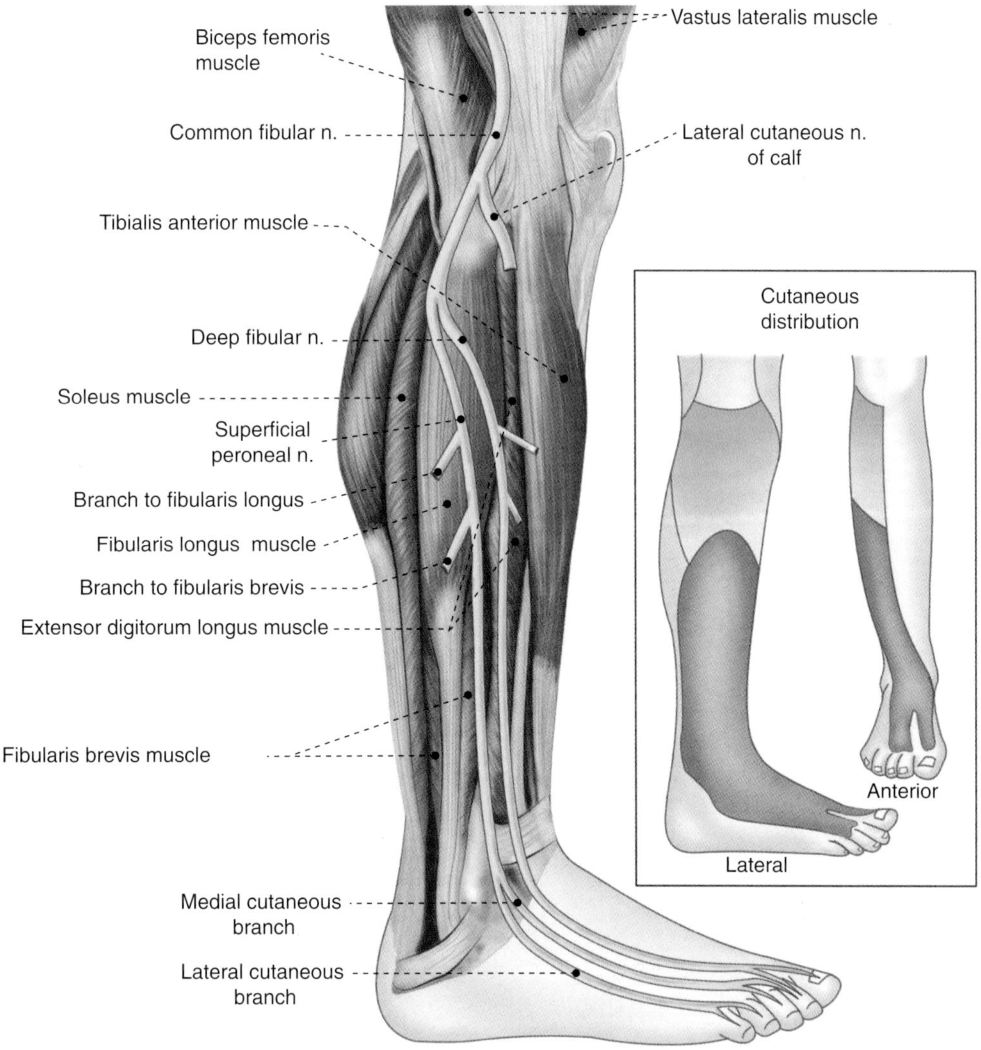

Figure 24-8. Fibular (peroneal) nerve.

that are dependent on the synchrony of impulse transmission such as deep tendon reflexes and the perception of vibration. Conduction block causes weakness without atrophy (other than that attributable to disuse) and loss of sensory modalities dependent on large myelinated fibers including vibration and position sense. Needle examination of muscles innervated by nerves affected by conduction block demonstrates reduced recruitment of MUAPs but neither fibrillation potentials nor abnormal motor unit action potential morphology as there is no axon loss or reinnervation. As implied above, individual fibers may be affected by focal slowing, demyelinating conduction block, or axon loss, leading to an mixed axonal demyelinating EDX pattern.

ELECTRODIAGNOSTIC STUDIES

Electrodiagnosis (EDX) has a significant role in determination of the existence, location, pathophysiology, severity, and prognosis of focal lower extremity neuropathies. Detailed description of EDX as a diagnostic tool can be found in Chapter 2 and many of the principles of EDX relevant to focal neuropathies of the upper extremities found in Chapter 23 and in the previous section apply here as well.

In general, monoradiculopathies are characterized by normal sensory nerve action potentials (SNAPs) in relevant dermatomes, normal or reduced compound muscle action potential amplitudes (CMAP) in relevant myotomes depending on the degree and type of injury, and evidence of acute and/or chronic denervation in muscles innervated by a single segment but by more than one peripheral nerve. Denervation is frequently, but not universally, found in analogous paraspinal segments. Presumably, failure to demonstrate paraspinal denervation in radiculopathy reflects sampling error, and demyelinating pathophysiology or in more longstanding cases, successful reinnervation. Practically speaking, monoradiculopathies that can be confirmed electrodiagnostically have at least some component of axon loss as the ability to identify demyelinating lesions in proximal locations is limited by anatomic and other considerations.

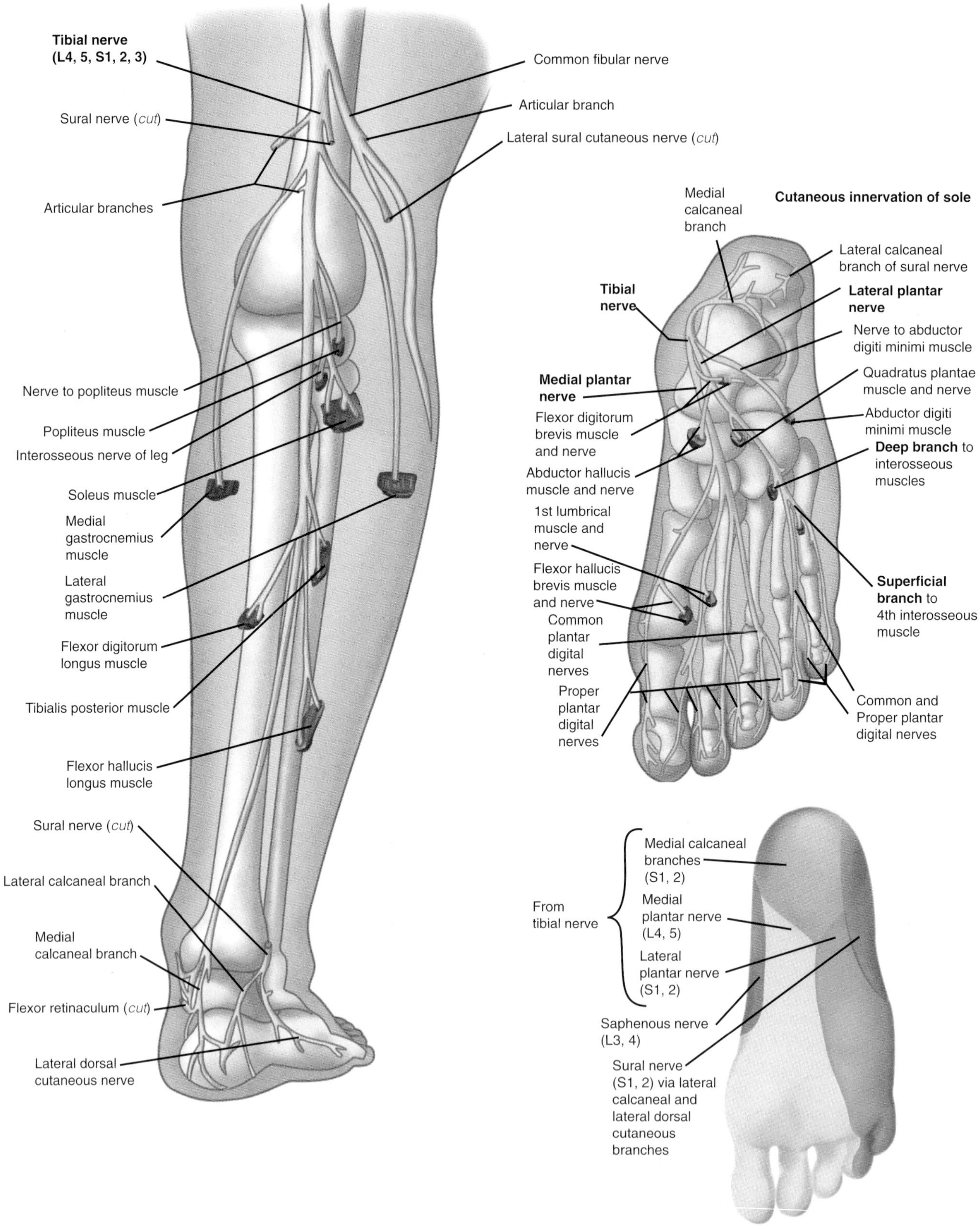
Tibial nerve
(L4, 5, S1, 2, 3)
Sural nerve (cut)
Articular branches
Common fibular nerve
Articular branch
Lateral sural cutaneous nerve (cut)
Nerve to popliteus muscle
Popliteus muscle
Interosseous nerve of leg
Soleus muscle
Medial gastrocnemius muscle
Lateral gastrocnemius muscle
Flexor digitorum longus muscle
Tibialis posterior muscle
Flexor hallucis longus muscle
Sural nerve (cut)
Lateral calcaneal branch
Medial calcaneal branch
Flexor retinaculum (cut)
Lateral dorsal cutaneous nerve
Medial calcaneal branch
Cutaneous innervation of sole
Lateral calcaneal branch of sural nerve
Tibial nerve
Lateral plantar nerve
Nerve to abductor digiti minimi muscle
Quadratus plantae muscle and nerve
Medial plantar nerve
Flexor digitorum brevis muscle and nerve
Abductor digiti minimi muscle
Deep branch to interosseous muscles
Abductor hallucis muscle and nerve
1st lumbrical muscle and nerve
Flexor hallucis brevis muscle and nerve
Superficial branch to 4th interosseous muscle
Common plantar digital nerves
Proper plantar digital nerves
Common and Proper plantar digital nerves
From tibial nerve
Medial calcaneal branches (S1, 2)
Medial plantar nerve (L4, 5)
Lateral plantar nerve (S1, 2)
Saphenous nerve (L3, 4)
Sural nerve (S1, 2) via lateral calcaneal and lateral dorsal cutaneous branches

Figure 24-9. Tibial nerve. Cut, cutaneous.

For example, the EDX pattern of an L5 radiculopathy would include a normal superficial peroneal SNAP and normal or reduced CMAP amplitude recording from the EDB or TA muscles and evidence of denervation in muscles such as the TA, the flexor digitorum longus, the tensor fascia lata as well as lumbosacral paraspinal muscles. These share L5 segmental innervation but are innervated by four different peripheral nerves. Like the clinical examination however, not all muscles innervated by the L5 segment will be denervated in all cases or denervated to the same degree.[11]

Polyradiculopathy has a near identical EDX pattern. The major exception is the pattern of denervation on needle EMG, which is commonly bilateral and by definition found in multiple segmental distributions. The major distinction between polyradiculopathy and multifocal neuropathy or plexopathy is the sparing of SNAPs in polyradiculopathy. There may be variables such as age, intraspinal positioning of the dorsal root ganglia, lower extremity edema, or concomitant but unrelated polyneuropathy which may be confounding. In addition, particularly in chronic polyradiculopathies such as spinal stenosis, denervation may take on a pseudo-length–dependent pattern suggesting a polyneuropathy.[12] CMAP amplitudes are more likely to be reduced as the protection offered to individual muscles by multisegmental innervation is less prevalent.

Polyradiculoneuropathy or radiculoplexus neuropathy is a pattern that is arguably more relevant to the lower extremities in view of the predilection for diabetes to affect lumbar nerve roots and contiguous plexus and nerve elements. It is a pattern that may occur with acquired, inflammatory demyelinating neuropathies as well but these are usually easily distinguished both by phenotype and by the characteristic demyelinating features found on nerve conduction studies. In general, polyradiculoneuropathies are electrodiagnostically defined by concomitant paraspinal denervation and abnormal SNAPs.

Plexopathies are typically monomelic but may affect the contralateral limb concomitantly or on a delayed basis, depending on etiology. Both clinically and electrodiagnostically, the pattern is typically one of both motor and sensory involvement involving multiple nerve and nerve root distributions. Relevant SNAP and CMAP amplitudes are reduced. Denervation will be found in proximal as well as distal limb muscles innervated by the same elements of the plexus, for example, both the tensor fascia lata and the TA in a lumbosacral trunk lesion, but should not occur in the representative areas of the lumbosacral paraspinal muscles. Demyelinating features may occur in plexopathies but are again often obscured by the proximal location of the pathology inaccessible to routine nerve conduction studies. Uncommonly focal, acquired demyelinating neuropathies such as multifocal acquired demyelinating sensory and motor neuropathy (MADSAM or Lewis-Sumner syndrome) may initially occur in a pattern that is both clinically and electrodiagnostically suggestive of plexopathy although this is usually more of an issue in the upper extremities.[13]

With axon loss mononeuropathies, reduced SNAP and CMAP amplitudes are expected assuming they are performed late enough to allow completion of Wallerian degeneration. By definition, these abnormalities will be confined to the affected nerve. Mild degrees of axon loss may be more readily detected by comparing the amplitude of the affected to the unaffected side rather than to population norms. This is particularly true for SNAPs. Most electrodiagnosticians consider an amplitude of less than 50% of the unaffected side to be abnormal. Denervation on needle examination would be confined to muscles innervated by the peripheral nerve in question but may be limited by site of injury along the length of the nerve as well as by selective fascicular involvement. As an example, denervation would understandably occur in the TA but not the peroneus longus muscle in an axon-loss deep peroneal neuropathy. The same pattern of denervation however, could be conceivably found in more proximal neuropathy affecting the common peroneal or even sciatic nerve due to selective fascicular involvement. Nerve fibers destined to innervate specific muscles may be sequested to specific fasicles in proximal nerve locations. As a result, partial nerve injury in a proximal location may result in selective fascicular injury resulting in an incomplete pattern of denervation.[14,15]

The EDX pattern in predominantly demyelinating mononeuropathies differs considerably from their axonal predominant counterparts. Again, by definition, the pattern of abnormalities would be confined to a singular nerve distribution. Sensory nerve conductions should be normal unless there is an axonal component to the injury or there is conduction block that exists between the stimulation and recording sites. Demyelination will have no effect on the conductive properties of a nerve if the lesion is either proximal or distal (as opposed to within) the tested segment of nerve. For example, with a demyelinating common fibular neuropathy at the fibular head, the superficial fibular SNAP amplitude obtained from a location distal to the site of pathology will be normal. Similarly, the CMAP amplitude will be normal if the stimulation site is below the demyelinated segment. For that reason, in any suspected demyelinating mononeuropathy, an attempt should be made if technically possible to stimulate the nerve in question above and if at all possible across (inching) the affected site. This has the benefit of not only identifying the existence of the abnormality, but also precisely localize it, while at the same time providing valuable prognostic information. Needle examination findings in a demyelinating mononeuropathy consist only of reduced recruitment of normal appearing MUAPs and then only if the pathophysiology is that of conduction block. Focal slowing and temporal dispersion are not associated with abnormalities on needle examination. As many nerve injuries include demyelinating and axonal components, it is not uncommon to identify EDX features associated with both types of injuries.

IMAGING

Historically, x-rays of the lumbosacral spine were performed routinely in patients with back or radicular pain. In consideration of radiation exposure and their very limited yield in this clinical context, we agree with those who would utilize routine back x-rays for those with significant trauma, those with symptoms or at high risk for systemic disease, or those with histories suggesting recent compression fracture.[5] When indicated and when feasible, magnetic resonance imaging (MRI) imaging is the imaging procedure of choice for suspected mono- or polyradiculopathy. Although we have a low threshold for ordering MRIs in individuals with radiculopathy and neurologic deficits, we do not consider it mandatory. We are comfortable following someone clinically when all information points to a routine compressive radiculopathy due to disc herniation, as long as improvement with subsequent evaluations can be demonstrated. Information gleaned from imaging studies requires careful clinical correlation as incidental findings are exceedingly frequent. Depending on age, herniated discs are identifiable in 20–40% of asymptomatic individuals.[5] Bulging discs are even more prevalent, identifiable in up to 80% of asymptomatic volunteers.[5] The decision to utilize gadolinium is individualized. It provides limited benefit in typical discogenic or spondylotic disease and poses some risk, particularly in those with reduced glomerular filtration. Gadolinium is most likely to be helpful in those with prior back surgery or when there is suspicion of systemic disease as a cause of radiculopathy. When MRI is precluded for any reason, post-myelographic CT scans provide an excellent imaging surrogate for nerve root disease. Although ultrasound appears to have an increasing role in neuromuscular disease, it is felt to be of limited or no utility in the evaluation of radiculopathy.[16]

MRI has become the modality of choice for evaluation of lumbosacral plexopathy or radiculoplexopathy as well, particularly utilizing 3 T or higher neurography techniques.[17] It is of value not only with structural pathology of nerve like neurofibromatosis but is of benefit in presumed inflammatory, ischemic injury in disorders such as non-diabetic lumbosacral radiculoplexus neuropathy (non-DLRPN).[17,18] Its resolution is in general superior to CT, and it provides the added benefit of readily providing axial, sagittal, and coronal viewing planes. Gadolinium is often of value, as neoplastic and inflammatory conditions are both relatively common causes of plexopathy whose visualization and characterization will be enhanced with the addition of gadolinium.[19]

Imaging of mononeuropathies in the lower extremities, particularly in proximal locations, is rendered difficult by the small diameter and circuitous course of the nerves in conjunction with the complex anatomy of the region. MRI and ultrasound imaging of at least seven nerves (femoral, lateral femoral cutaneous, obturator, sciatic, superior and inferior gluteal, and pudendal) are feasible and warranted in the case of unexplained or progressive neuropathies identified by clinical and/or EDX means.[10] The imaging may allow for identification of focal T2 signal abnormalities at sites of compression, nerve enlargement and enhancement from neural tumors, enhancement from focal inflammatory lesions, or external compression from any contiguous mass.[17] Imaging may also have a therapeutic application, allowing for more precise application of steroid injections, for example, in obese individuals with meralgia paresthetica in whom normal anatomic landmarks may be difficult to identify.[10] Recently, diffusion tensor imaging has been utilized axonal changes in patients with peripheral neuropathy. Conceivably, this or similar technologies may provide the ability to image and monitor axonal regrowth subsequent to injury and potential therapeutic intervention.[20]

▶ SPECIFIC DISORDERS

MONORADICULOPATHIES

Lumbosacral radiculopathies are more prevalent than their cervical or thoracic counterparts. For the most part, they occur as a consequence of mechanical compression from some aspect of spondyloarthropathy that is narrowing of the central canal or lateral recesses, and/or neural foramina by disc material, osteophyte, hypertrophied ligament or some combination thereof. Less commonly, they may result from compression from benign or malignant neoplasm, hematoma or abscess. They may result as well from neoplastic, infectious and inflammatory disorders with a predilection to attack or invade nerve roots or meninges (Table 24-3 and Fig. 24-10).

▶ **TABLE 24-3. MONORADICULOPATHIES: PATTERNS OF CLINICAL INVOLVEMENT**

Nerve Root	Muscle Action Most Commonly Weak	Other Muscle Actions That May Be Weak	Characteristic Areas of Sensory Symptoms/Sensory Loss	Reflex Loss
L2	Thigh flexion	NA	Anterior thigh	Cremasteric
L3	Leg extension (one leg partial squat)	Hip flexion and adduction	Medial knee	Quadriceps reflex
L4	Leg extension (one leg partial squat)	Hip flexion and adduction	Medial leg	Quadriceps reflex
L5	Great toe dorsiflexion	Dorsiflexion of digits II–V and foot, ankle inversion and eversion, knee flexion, and hip abduction	Great toe, dorsum of foot, and distal-lateral leg	+/− Internal hamstring
S1	Foot plantar flexion (single leg heel lift)	Toe and knee flexion and hip extension	Digits IV and V, lateral foot, and heel and plantar surface	Achilles reflex

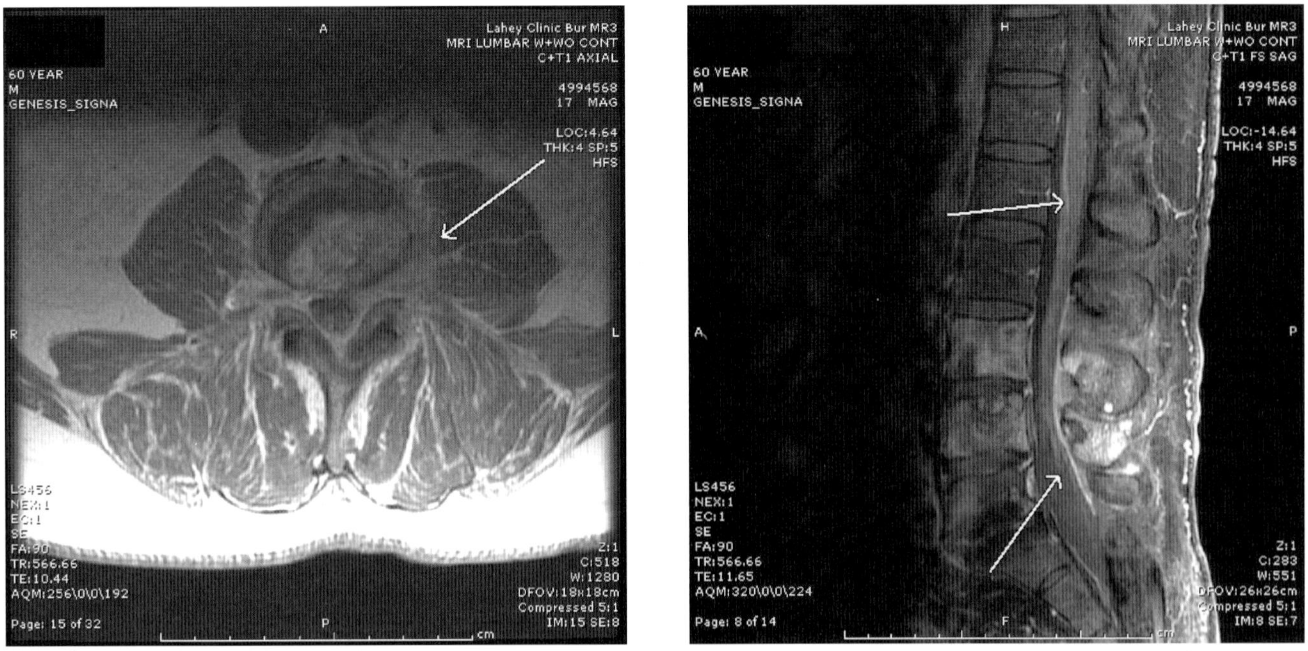

A B

Figure 24-10. Gadolinium-enhanced T1 **(A)** axial and **(B)** sagittal MR images of the lumbar spine in a 60-year-old male with atypical, progressive left L3–L4 radiculopathy demonstrating abnormal enhancement of multiple vertebral bodies, epidural space, cauda equina, and left L2–3, 3–4, and 4–5 neural foramina resulting from previously asymptomatic B-cell lymphoma.

A heightened index of suspicion is required for these less common causes. The primary symptom of monoradiculopathy is pain, commonly described as radicular or sciatic due to its linear trajectory following the course of the sciatic nerve in most cases. It has been estimated that disc herniations associated with objective neurologic deficits occur in the complete absence of pain in only 1/1,000 patients.[5]

Radicular pain in the lower extremity often occurs in the absence of significant back pain and often begins in the sacroiliac or gluteal regions. Although commonly continuous, it may be interrupted, for example, affecting the buttock and anterior leg but skipping the thigh. The pain is often positional depending on the exact site and vector of compression, often related to specific back postures which may increase or decrease the cross-sectional area of the central canal or neural foramina. Limb pain that is aggravated by side-bending toward the affected side or by straight leg raising of the ipsilateral or contralateral leg is likely to be due to nerve root compression. Radicular pain induced by straight leg raising of less than 60 degrees is a sensitive but nonspecific sign estimated to occur in 90% of patients with radiculopathy secondary to disc herniation.[21] Conversely, reproduction of ipsilateral radicular pain by raising the opposite limb, that is, reverse straight leg raising, is a highly specific but fairly insensitive provocative test.[5] In upper lumbar disc disease, pain may be reproduced by reverse straight raising, that is, by passively extending rather than flexing the thigh at the hip joint.[22]

Pain may also be increased by increased pressure within the intraspinal canal. The latter is frequently provoked by maneuvers that increase intrathoracic pressure resulting in increased volume of the epidural venous plexus. Pain radiating down the leg provoked by straining or coughing is therefore a helpful although inconsistent clinical clue.

Regarding the examination of a patient with neurologic complaints of the lower extremity, there are a number of notable differences in comparison to the upper limb. The lower extremity has fewer testable muscles and actions than the upper extremity. For example, there is no pronation or supination at the knee, and the testable options of the toes is limited in comparison to the fingers. In the lower extremities, there may be greater difficulty in distinguishing a nerve from a nerve root lesion as there is greater overlap in both the motor and sensory functions of specific nerves and nerve roots. For example, there are more similarities than differences in the motor, sensory, and reflex findings in an L3–4 radiculopathy and femoral neuropathy. One advantage that the lower extremity holds over the upper extremity however, both clinically and electrodiagnostically, is that that muscles belonging to the same myotome can be found in both proximal and distal locations. For example, the L5 segment contributes significantly to both toe extension and hip abduction, whereas the C5 segment has no meaningful contribution to distal upper extremity functions such as wrist or finger movement.

It is also important for a clinician to recognize that clinically evident motor deficits in monoradiculopathy may be subtle if evident at all due to the typical multisegmental innervation of virtually all muscles. As a corollary of this,

▶ **TABLE 24-4. MONORADICULOPATHY: ETIOLOGIES**

Herniated nucleus pulposus
Spondylosis, that is, osteophyte formation and ligamentous hypertrophy
Nerve sheath tumors
Diabetes (rare)
Herpes zoster
Initial manifestation of eventual polyradiculopathy (see Table 24-5)

weakness from monoradiculopathy when present should not produce complete paralysis of any muscle. It is also important to recognize that the pattern of weakness in monoradiculopathy although segmental, typically does not affect all muscles innervated by a single myotome to the same extent (Table 24-4). This is particularly true for muscles that are more proximally located in a given segment. For example, the weakness in an L5 radiculopathy may be confined to great toe extension and is infrequently detected in hip abduction. Relevant deep tendon reflexes in monoradiculopathies are typically reduced or are absent in the affected segment.

As previously emphasized, sensory symptoms in monoradiculopathy, like many neurologic diseases, are a more sensitive indicator of sensory involvement than sensory signs. Again, with suspected L5 radiculopathy, a complaint of a numb big toe should be considered as a valid complaint even in the absence of convincing sensory deficits on examination. In addition, it is not uncommon for paresthesias and sensory loss to persist long after radicular pain and demonstrable weakness have resolved. Another potential source of error in the interpretation of radicular sensory involvement is the failure to recognize that the topographical area of sensory involvement described by the patient or demonstrable on examination is typically far smaller than predicted on the basis of the commonly published dermatomal maps (Fig. 24-11).

Although the vast majority of compressive monoradiculopathies have pain as their cardinal symptom at some point in their natural history as described above, it is important to recognize that there appear to be exceptions. Patients may have either dermatomal sensory symptoms or myotomal motor signs in the absence or relative absence of pain. On occasion, patients will have radicular pain with paresthesia that will abruptly resolve, only to be replaced by weakness in

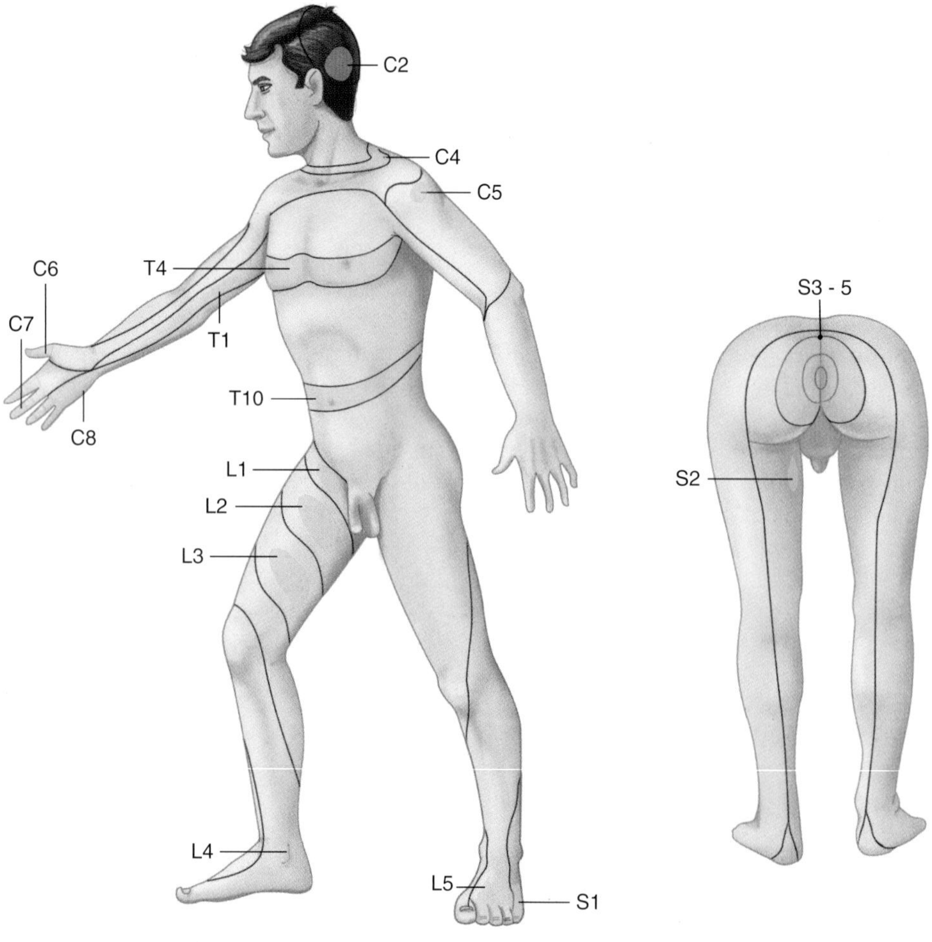

Figure 24-11. Clinical dermatome map.

a segmental pattern. It has been hypothesized that this may occur as a result of disc sequestration and migration.[23,24] The authors' personal observations of this syndrome occurring in the immediate aftermath of spinal manipulation would support this contention.

L1–2

Monoradiculopathies affecting these roots are uncommon and typically present with pain referred into the inguinal region and perhaps the proximal, anterior thigh. Pain in this region is however, uncommonly neurogenic in nature. Other than L1–2 radiculopathies, neurogenic pain with this topographic distribution may result from mononeuropathies of the ilioinguinal or genitofemoral nerves. Although discogenic L1/L2 radiculopathy may occur, suspected L1/L2 radiculopathy should generate an increased level of suspicion for an unusual etiology of root disease (Fig. 24-12). Paresthesias occur in the trochanteric and/or upper groin regions in L1 lesions and the anterior thigh in L2. Weakness is uncommon but may be detectable in hip flexion with L2 root disease. The ipsilateral cremasteric reflex may be lost.

L3–4

L3–4 monoradiculopathies have the potential for substantial morbidity if quadriceps weakness occurs. Pain and sensory symptoms of the thigh and medial knee imply L3 involvement, whereas involvement of the medial leg implicates the L4 root. Either lesion may lead to a diminished or absent knee jerk and weakness of hip flexion and adduction in addition to the critical function of knee extension. As the quadriceps is a particularly strong muscle, mild weakness may only be detectable in a younger, nonobese patient by asking the patient to get up from a chair on one leg at a time without using the arms. Alternatively, mild weakness may be detected by asking the patient to do a partial squat while weight bearing on one leg alone. Both tests should be applied cautiously. In either case, the examiner must position themselves in such a manner and be confident that they can support the patient and prevent a fall should one occur with either maneuver. Many texts suggest that the TA receives partial innervation through the L4 segment. In the authors' experience and in the published experience of others, weakness of foot dorsiflexion and denervation of the TA rarely occur in documented L4 monoradiculopathies.[15] The differential diagnosis of L3–4 radiculopathy includes femoral mononeuropathies, lumbar plexopathies, and radiculoplexus neuropathies. Clinical and electrodiagnostic sparing of hip abductors distinguishes a femoral mononeuropathy from any of the other disorders. The more difficult distinction is from lumbar radiculoplexus neuropathies or plexopathies which may share a similar pattern of pain, sensory involvement, weakness, and denervation. A combination of imaging of the back and retroperitoneum, EDX, and the clinical contextual features may be required to resolve this differential diagnostic dilemma.

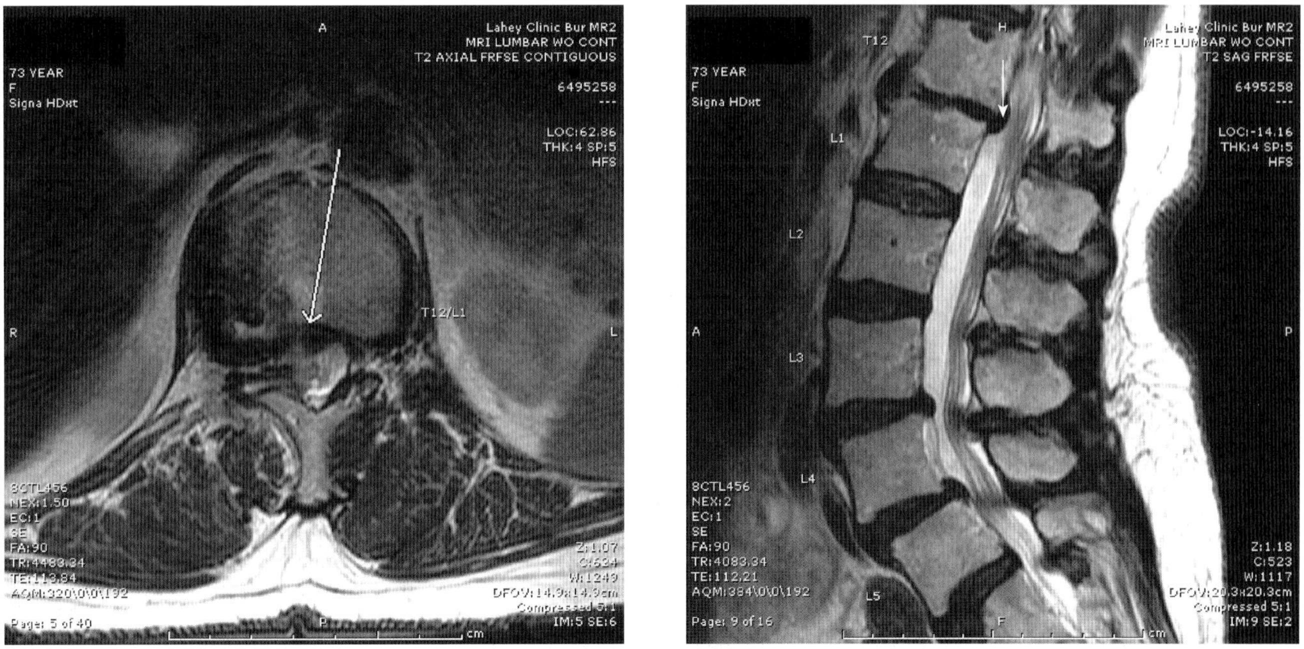

A B

Figure 24-12. T2 **(A)** axial and **(B)** sagittal MR images of the lumbar spine demonstrating right T12–L1 disc herniation in a patient with ipsilateral neuropathic groin pain.

L5

L5 is the most common lower extremity monoradiculopathy. The pain typically extends from buttock to posterolateral thigh to anterolateral leg. Sensory symptoms are felt in the lateral leg, instep, dorsum of the foot, and particularly in the big toe. In most people, weakness will be most commonly and readily detected in great toe extension. Weakness of foot dorsiflexion and typically inversion > eversion may occur as well. Weakness of knee flexion and hip abduction are less frequent and/or are more difficult to detect. The differential diagnosis of L5 radiculopathies is essentially the differential diagnosis of foot drop. As many causes of polyneuropathy, motor neuron disease, and even myopathy have a predilection to affect foot dorsiflexion, this differential diagnosis is expansive. As the most commonly occurring of these is a common fibular neuropathy, it is extremely important to assess the strength of ankle inversion which should not be affected in a common fibular (peroneal) neuropathy.

As suggested, a diagnosis of L5 monoradiculopathy should be made cautiously in the absence of pain and/or sensory symptoms, when foot dorsiflexion weakness exceeds toe extension weakness or when the ipsilateral ankle jerk is depressed. The former raises the possibility of motor neuron disease, rarely myasthenia or distal myopathy particularly if bilateral and symmetric. Foot drop greater than or without toe drop suggests distal myopathy or upper motor neuron disease. An absent ankle jerk should not occur in an L5 monoradiculopathy and suggests more proximal pathology of the sciatic nerve in which the fibular nerve is more severely affected, or concomitant involvement of the S1 nerve root.

S1

This is the second most common lower extremity monoradiculopathy. The radicular or "sciatic" pain of S1 root disease typically extends from buttock down the posterior surface of thigh and leg into the heel and at times into the lateral toes. Sensory symptoms are most pronounced in the posterior lateral leg and particularly in the lateral and plantar surfaces of the foot and little toe. Muscle weakness, if present, most commonly occurs in foot plantar flexion. Detection of S1 weakness may be hampered by the considerable baseline strength of foot plantar flexion, knee flexion, and hip extension. Functional testing, for example, the ability to elevate the heel fully off the floor while standing on one leg alone while keeping the knee fully extended is helpful in this regard. As this is a test of strength, not balance, the patients should be supported by either their examiner or a nearby wall. Detectable weakness in S1-innervated hip extension is uncommon and is most rigorously tested by having the patient extend the thigh at the hip while in the prone position. A suppressed or absent ankle jerk is expected.

The differential diagnosis of an S1 radiculopathy is not as extensive as its L5 counterpart. Tibial, sural, and plantar neuropathies are uncommon. Sciatic neuropathies are more common. Most cases are dominated however by deficits arising from its fibular division. Sacral plexopathies are usually readily distinguished from S1 root disease by the more widespread pattern of weakness and sensory loss.

▶ ETIOLOGIES OF MONORADICULOPATHIES

Table 24-4 lists the more common causes of monoradiculopathies. Herniation of intervertebral discs causes the vast majority of monoradiculopathies in those younger than 50 years. Spondylosis is a far more common cause of root disease in older adults. Typically, the clinical deficits are more evident in a monoradiculopathy caused by disc herniation than in spondylosis, presumably due to its relative acuity. Spondylotic disease is typically more insidious in its development and commonly affects multiple levels bilaterally in an older population, a pattern that may be evident only through electrodiagnostic evaluation. Contrary to common belief, disc herniations are rarely the result of significant traumas such as motor vehicle accidents. Nonspondylotic causes of monoradiculopathy deserve a higher index of suspicion in individuals at risk (e.g., individuals who are immunosuppressed or with prior history of malignancy); those with fever, weight loss, or other symptoms of systemic disease; or those whose neurologic deficits progress.

The differential diagnosis of monoradiculopathy is limited. Neoplasms, either nerve sheath tumors or malignancies affecting vertebrae or meninges are one cause of nondiscogenic/spondylytic monoradiculopathy (Fig. 24-10). Any slowly progressive monoradiculopathy should prompt a careful discussion of family history and search for neurocutaneous stigmata, including subcutaneous and Lisch nodules, café-au-lait spots, and axillary freckles. Diabetes is not commonly considered as a cause of monoradiculopathy, but self-limited monoradiculopathies will occasionally occur in diabetics in the absence of other apparent causes. Herpes zoster (shingles), is a fairly common cause of radicular pain and sensory loss but on occasion can produce "zoster motor paresis" in approximately 5% of affected individuals, presumably due to retrograde viral movement from the dorsal root ganglia into the anterior horn.[25–30] Other disorders with an affinity for nerve roots may occasionally present as a monoradiculopathy as an initial manifestation of an evolving polyradiculopathy (Table 24-5).

▶ EVALUATION OF SUSPECTED MONORADICULOPATHIES

Imaging and EDX play complementary roles in the evaluation of monoradiculopathies of the lower extremity. There is no universal diagnostic algorithm. Clinical judgment should be blended with individual patient characteristics and goals. The major benefit of imaging is the potential for identifying

▶ TABLE 24-5. POLYRADICULOPATHY: ETIOLOGIES

Arachnoiditis
Degenerative
Spondylosis (spinal stenosis)
Central disc herniation
Epidural lipomatosis
Diabetes (polyradiculoplexus neuropathy)
Iatrogenic (epidural and caudal anesthesia)
Ischemic
Dural vascular malformations
Spinal cord infarction
Nonsystemic vasculitic neuropathy
Infectious
CMV
HIV (CMV, herpes simplex, syphilis, *Cryptococcus*, and atypical mycobacteria)
Lyme disease
Schistosomiasis
Spinal epidural abscess
Inflammatory
Sarcoidosis
Neoplastic
Meningitis
Primary spinal cord tumors—ependymomas, lipomas, dermoid, epidermoid, hemangioblastoma, paraganglioma, and ganglioneuroma
Primary nerve sheath tumors—neurofibromas and schwannomas
Primary vertebral tumors—cordomas, multiple myeloma, and osteoma
Primary paravertebral tumors—lymphomas
Metastatic vertebral tumors—breast, lung, and prostate
Intravascular tumor—lymphoma
Osseous
Paget disease
Inflammatory spondyloarthropathies, e.g., ankylosing spondylitis
Radiation

CMV, cytomegalovirus.

disease etiology, something that EDX may imply but rarely accomplishes. As previously mentioned, the significance of imaging abnormalities is hampered by the frequent occurrence of clinically irrelevant anatomic abnormalities.[31–33] Imaging is also limited in its ability to identify causes of radiculopathy unassociated with structural pathology.

EDX, on the other hand, is a physiologic test, capable of detecting disordered nerve function in the absence of imaging abnormalities. Like imaging, it frequently detects abnormalities irrelevant to the problem at hand, which may result from pre-existing nerve pathology or again be a consequence of the vagaries of aging. As a general rule, we use EDX primarily when there is a lack of concordance between clinical and imaging data. As alluded to, we are comfortable following a patient with a typical presentation of a discogenic monoradiculopathy clinically, without initial ancillary testing. If patients fail to improve or worsen or develop symptoms of systemic disease, imaging should be obtained. We also consider imaging to be a mandatory predecessor to any surgical procedure. Other diagnostic modalities have been described in the evaluation of lumbosacral radiculopathy such as somatosensory-evoked potentials and lumbar puncture. In general, they add little to the evaluation for the majority of patients.

▶ MANAGEMENT OF MONORADICULOPATHY

The rational management of lumbosacral monoradiculopathies requires an understanding of the natural history of the disease. It is estimated that 90% of patients with symptomatic radiculopathy associated with imaging confirmed disc herniations will respond favorably to time or conservative measures.[5,34] Clinical improvement seems to correlate with MR evidence disc involution that occurs in two-thirds of cases within 6 months. Despite these favorable statistics, there is a paucity of evidence to support individual treatment modalities. For example, the efficacy of the time-honored treatment of bed rest for acute monoradiculopathies has been called into question.[35] If used, prolonged bed rest may actually have a deleterious effect on functional recovery in comparison to short periods of immobilization.[36] Currently, most physicians favor maintenance of activity over immobilization with the exception of activities that involve heavy lifting, repetitive torsion, or prolonged axial loading of the trunk such as prolonged sitting. Despite their popularity, physical measures including traction, physical therapy, and manipulative therapy by osteopathic and chiropractic technique may provide short-term relief but appear to have no protracted benefit.[37,38] We are more comfortable with manipulative therapy in the musculoskeletal back pain population than we are in individuals with acute disc herniations. In the latter group, we have observed the abrupt onset of neurologic deficit such as foot drop chronologically linked to back manipulation.

As inflammation is believed to be at least partly responsible for pain production in nerve root compression, short courses of corticosteroids may be used in patients in whom their use is not contraindicated. Although there is evidence suggesting lack of benefit, it provides both a rational and an anecdotally efficacious means of promoting rapid pain relief.[39] We have prescribed a 10-day regimen of 55 dexamethasone tablets (1 mg) beginning with 10 mg on day one and reducing the dose by 1 mg every day. Alternatively, a methylprednisolone dose pack may be prescribed. As always, would be reluctant to do this if there were any suspicion of indolent infection with an opportunistic infection such as tuberculosis or strongyloidiasis that might be exacerbated by the addition of steroids.

Nonsteroidal anti-inflammatory agents are frequently prescribed for this purpose as well. The short-term use of narcotic analgesia is reasonable when required. If this need persists for more than 2–4 weeks, then alternative etiologies, consideration of confounding psychosocial factors, or when relevant, surgical intervention should be considered. Muscle relaxants are of value in musculoskeletal causes of back pain but have a limited role in the treatment of nerve root compression. Epidural and facet joint steroid injections have enjoyed recent popularity as treatment options.[40–43] Evidence would suggest that short-term pain amelioration may occur as a result of their use although their use is not without risk.[44] There is no evidence that would indicate a reduction in the duration of functional impairment, the need for surgery, or the incidence of pain beyond 3 months.[40,41] Other techniques such as traction, fluoroscopically guided blockade of selective nerve roots or facet joints or transcutaneous nerve stimulation appear to have limited if any benefit.[42,43,45,46] Although predominantly of historical interest, chymopapain injections and lumbar traction are mentioned here for sake of completeness as treatments whose time has come and gone.

The decision to proceed to surgical intervention is dependent on the demonstration of surgically amenable pathology that is anatomically concordant with the patient's phenotype. The typical indication is a patient with refractory pain despite a reasonable trial (2–4 weeks) of conservative therapy. The primary goal of surgery in these situations is to provide accelerated pain relief which appears to be supported by current evidence.[47] Patients with surgical intervention however, do not return to work faster than those treated conservatively.[5] Surgical outcomes appear comparable between microdiscectomy and the more traditional open discectomy technique.[47] Decision making may be confounded however by the recognition that some patients will experience the paradoxical dissipation of pain at the same time their neurologic deficits are worsening.[31] Most clinicians would also consider it prudent to move rapidly to surgical decompression in the less common situations where acute–subacute involvement of multiple nerve roots with genitourinary dysfunction occurs (cauda equina syndrome) or with particularly severe (MRC 3 or less) weakness. Although there is no evidence basis to support early surgical intervention in these less common situations, it remains the recommended approach by most neurologists and neurosurgeons.[31] Although it is hoped that early surgical intervention will favorably alter the natural history and outcome in these situations, available studies, although not specifically addressing the more severe phenotypes of acute cauda equina syndrome or severe limb weakness, suggest that the eventual outcome relevant to both pain and neurologic deficit are independent of whether surgical or conservative treatment is applied.[48–50]

POLYRADICULOPATHIES

Clinically apparent polyradiculopathy occurs more commonly in the lumbosacral than cervical region. The most common cause is spinal stenosis resulting from degenerative spondylotic disease and/or congenital narrowing of the central spinal canal and/or neural foramina. As a result compression of the cauda equina occurs, the symptoms of which are often positional in nature.[51–53] The signs and symptoms of spinal stenosis are limited to the back and lower extremities and occasionally to bowel, bladder, and sexual function. Onset is typically insidious and protean in nature with nonspecific low back discomfort and morning stiffness, relieved by activity. The most recognizable symptomatic expression of spinal stenosis is neurogenic claudication (i.e., pain), numbness and the perception of weakness in the back, buttocks, or legs that is often bilateral and typically exacerbated by back extension, standing, or walking.[52] Symptoms are typically diminished by sitting, lying down, or assuming a flexed lumbar posture. The patient may not benefit from walking behind a shopping cart or walker which promotes this positioning. This same effect may be noted by the relative ease of ascending rather than descending stairs and by activities that encourage lumbar spine flexion (e.g., riding an exercise bicycle) in comparison to those that do not (e.g., walking).

The clinical examination of a patient with symptomatic spinal stenosis is normal in the majority of cases.[52] Straight leg raising does not reproduce symptoms. Although it may be possible to elicit abnormal findings on the neurologic examination after the patient is rendered symptomatic by walking, the yield of this strategy is low in our experience. Although less well recognized and somewhat controversial, it has been suggested that sensory symptoms or even weakness occurring without significant pain may be the dominant initial symptoms of this disorder.[12,54] The former may mimic a length-dependent polyneuropathy, presumably due to the more successful reinnervation process in proximal limb locations. Paradoxically, unilateral calf hypertrophy has also been reported to occur in lumbosacral spinal stenosis.[55,56] Our personal experience would support the validity of these uncommon presentations (Fig. 24-13).

Alternatively, polyradiculopathy may result from harm to nerve roots as a consequence of meningeal-based pathology. In these cases, cervical and thoracic roots and cranial nerves may be affected as well as their lumbosacral counterparts. The majority of these disorders are painful and are commonly associated with systemic disorders that produce constitutional or other symptoms indicative of non-neurologic end-organ involvement. These are most readily recognized by the sequential development of motor, sensory, and reflex deficits, which are segmental in their pattern and often asymmetric and haphazard in their distribution. Eventually, these deficits may become confluent and with their localization becoming less recognizable unless the history can be recalled in a detailed and chronologic fashion.

The differential diagnosis of lumbosacral polyradiculopathy includes disorders of the conus medullaris, multifocal neuropathy, plexopathy, and radiculoplexopathy. Multifocal neuropathies are potentially distinguished by their nerve rather than segmental distribution of symptoms, with a tendency to spare the trunk and cranial nerves. Lumbosacral plexopathies commonly affect either the lumbar or sacral

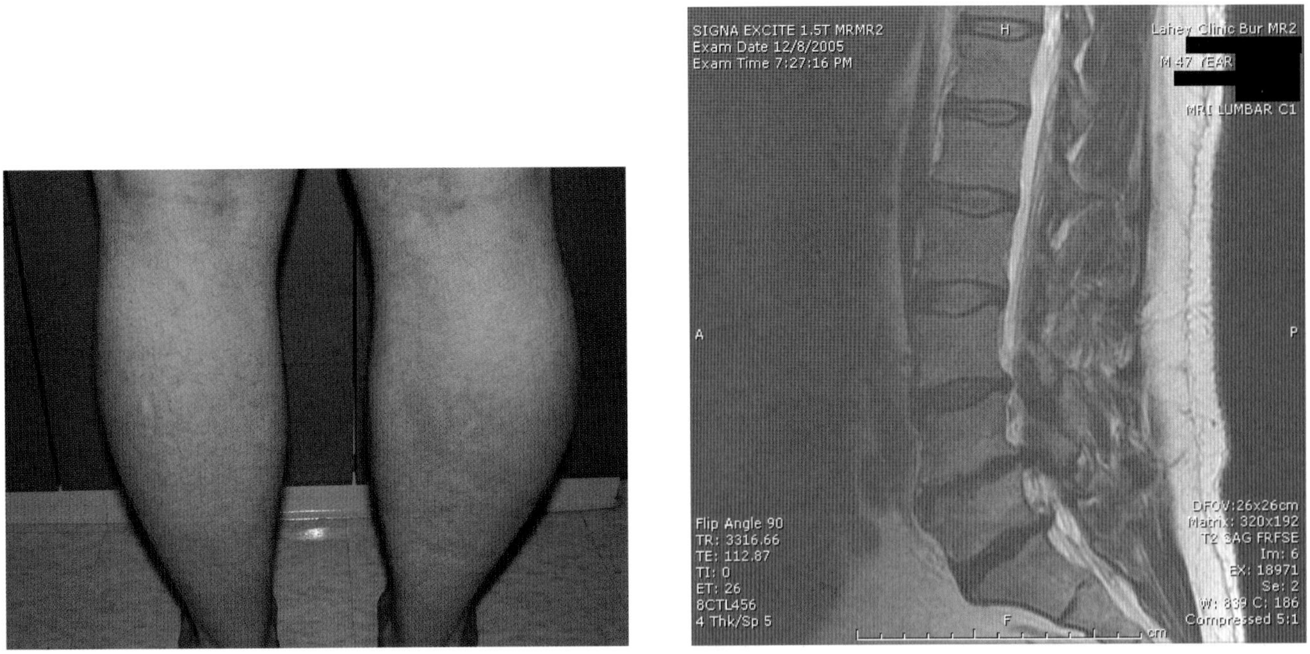

A

B

Figure 24-13. **(A)** Calf hypertrophy in a 47-year-old male with neurogenic claudication with **(B)** T2 MR sagittal imaging demonstrating spinal stenosis (gastrocnemius muscle biopsy not shown demonstrating neurogenic atrophy).

portions of the plexus individually and are often unilateral in presentation. Disorders of the lower spinal cord parenchyma (i.e., the conus medullaris syndrome) may produce motor and sensory deficits typically confined to the lower extremities, which appear segmental in nature, in addition to the common and often initial symptoms of bowel, bladder, and sexual dysfunction. Because of their intraparenchymal location, pain is typically less of an issue than in cauda equina syndromes which it may otherwise closely mimic. For the most part, unlike polyradiculopathy from systemic disease and multifocal neuropathy, signs and symptoms would be expected to remain confined to the lower extremities and genitourinary function.

ETIOLOGIES OF POLYRADICULOPATHY

The potential etiologies of lumbosacral polyradiculopathy are more extensive than monoradiculopathy (Table 24-5).[57] The more notable etiologies will be elaborated on here. Spondylosis producing the syndrome of spinal stenosis is far and away the most common cause of lumbosacral polyradiculopathy, estimated to occur with a prevalence of 5 in every 1,000 Americans older than 50 years.[57–59] Spinal stenosis may be congenital in nature as well which may synergistically predispose to symptomatic disease with acquired spondylosis later in life. Conversely, the syndrome may be created by a normal canal size with hypertrophic nerve roots in chronic inflammatory demyelinating polyneuropathy and Charcot–Marie–Tooth disease (Fig. 24-14).[60–64] Large, midline disc herniations may produce an acute or subacute cauda equina syndrome but are relatively uncommon, presumably due to the protective nature of the posterior longitudinal ligament.

There are numerous, less common causes of polyradiculopathy or conus medullaris lesions that may mimic

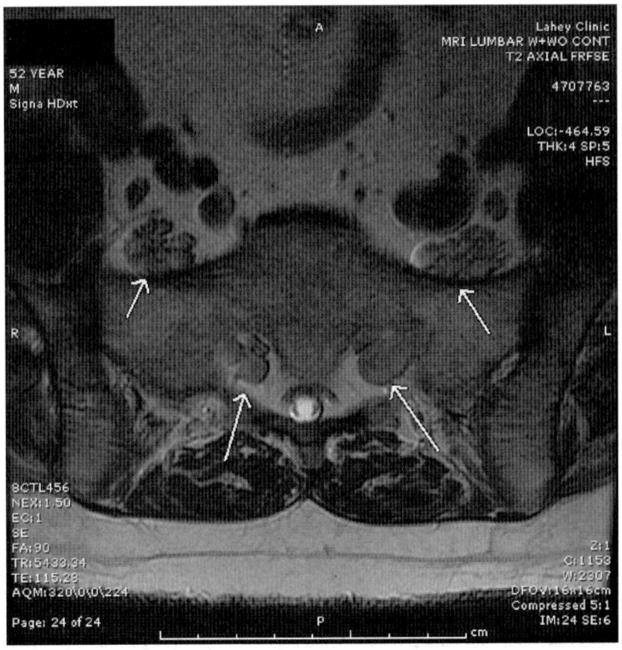

Figure 24-14. T2 MRI axial images of hypertrophied sacral nerve roots extending into the sacral plexus in a patient with Charcot–Marie–Tooth disease.

polyradiculopathy by anterior horn cell loss produced by intramedullary ischemic change. Some of these disorders may present as monoradiculopathies that subsequently evolve. Increased suspicion for these secondary causes should occur with acute to subacute symptom onset or disease progression, concurrence of constitutional symptoms or other clues of potential systemic disease, or unusual pain patterns such as worsening at night suggesting neoplastic, infectious, or inflammatory disease.[5]

Considerations for secondary causes of polyradiculopathy (or conus medullaris syndrome) include primary neoplasms of the spine or spinal cord,[65] metastatic disease to the spine with secondary cauda equina compression, or meningeal-based disease-causing neoplastic meningitis.[66–69] Primary tumors with an affinity for lower spine or spinal cord include glioma, ependymoma, chordoma, schwannomas, neurofibromas, meningiomas, hemangioblastomas, or dermoid tumors. Prostate, myeloma, breast, and lung cancers are the more common causes of tumors with an affinity to metastasize to bone. Back pain as a presenting feature of malignancy is rare. Less than 1% of individuals presenting with back pain in one large series were found to have cancer. Older age, an elevated sedimentation rate and anemia were helpful diagnostic clues in this series.[65] Leukemia, non-Hodgkin lymphoma, breast, lung, melanoma, and gastroesophageal malignancies are the most common causes of neoplastic meningitis.

Ischemic disorders of the lower spinal cord and nerve roots may cause or mimic polyradiculopathy. Causes include spinal dural vascular malformations[3,70–73] and occlusive diseases of the aorta and its different branches.[74–76] Dural vascular malformations commonly present with the stepwise progression of lower extremity sensory and motor signs and symptoms, with or without signs and symptoms of genitourinary tract involvement. Technically, it should be classified as a myeloradiculopathy, as both spinal cord parenchyma and nerve roots are vulnerable to the ischemic change. Symptoms may initiate with some traumatic event and may be noted to intensify with either the upright position or the Valsalva maneuver. Approximately half of patients who are afflicted will experience pain. Although both upper and lower motor neuron features typically occur, approximately 30% of patients with dural malformations will have motor features that are predominantly or exclusively lower motor neuron in character. If imaging is focused on the lower lumbar spine, the enlarged, edematous conus characteristic of this disorder may be overlooked (Fig. 24-15). At times, the sensory signs and symptoms created by dural malformations are minor and may be overlooked. In this situation, both the clinical and the electrodiagnostic patterns may suggest motor neuron disease. Abnormalities in the H reflex, which may occur in dural malformations, are a potentially helpful means to distinguish these disorders.[70]

There are numerous infectious disorders with a predilection for lumbosacral nerve roots. Spinal epidural abscess may present as a monoradiculopathy evolving into polyradiculopathy.[77–82] Suspicion should be heightened in context of fever or other constitutional symptoms, intravenous drug abuse or indwelling catheters, percussion tenderness of the spine, or recent bacteremia. Polyradiculopathy is one

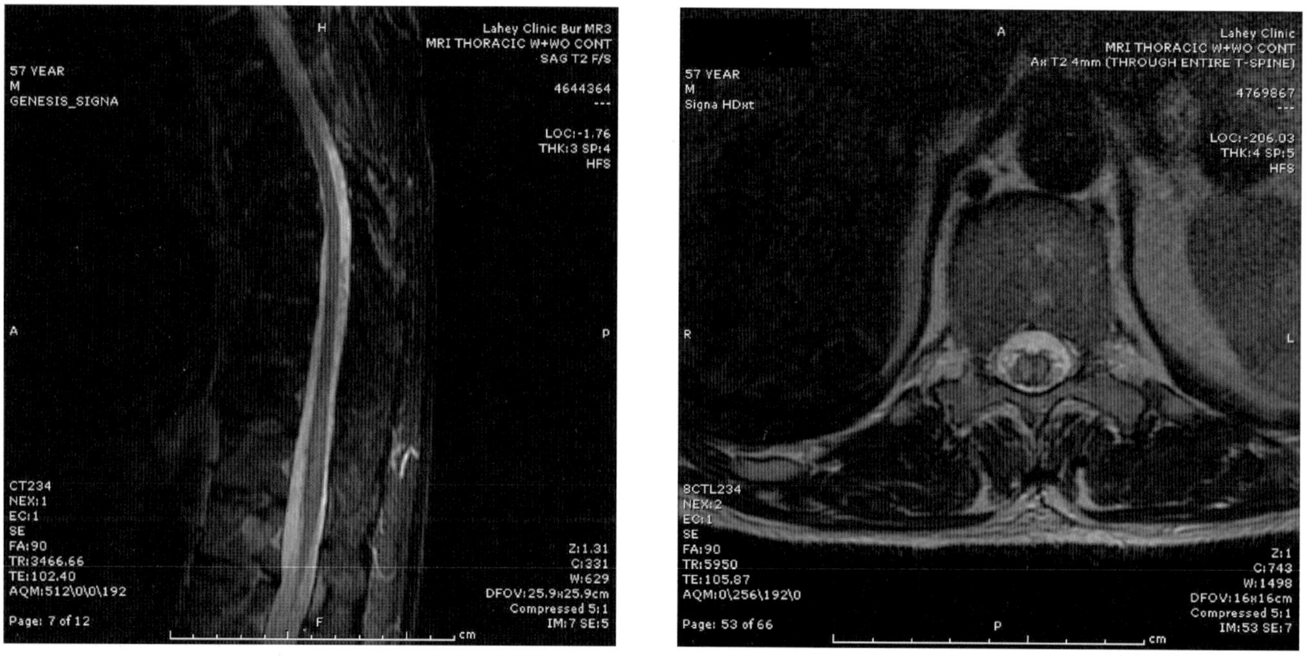

A B

Figure 24-15. MRI **(A)** sagittal and **(B)** axial T2 MR images demonstrating enlargement and hazy T2 signal increase in the conus medullaris concentrated in the intramedullary gray matter images secondary to more rostrally located dural venous malformation.

of the numerous HIV-related neurologic syndromes.[83] It is estimated to affect approximately 2% of patients who are infected, typically patients with established acquired immunodeficiency syndrome (AIDS) and CD4 counts <100 cell/μL. It may present as a pure motor syndrome.[84] Polyradiculopathy may also result from infections with cytomegalovirus, herpes simplex, atypical mycobacteria, cryptococcus, and treponemal agents in this patient population as well as with lymphoma.[85–87]

Polyradiculopathy is one of the more common neurologic manifestations of Lyme disease, affecting approximately half of the patients with peripheral nerve involvement.[88] Dermatomal sensory loss and pain are the most common symptoms. Segmental weakness occurs but is less prevalent. Lyme polyradiculopathy typically occurs within days to weeks of the characteristic rash, seemingly linked to the hematogenous dissemination of the organism. In addition to the meninges and nerve roots, joints, peripheral nerves, and the cardiac conduction system seem to be the end organs at particular risk. Potential or known exposure risk to the transmitting Ixodes tick species, seasonal predilection, prior rash, arthralgias, truncal pain secondary to thoracic and upper abdominal root involvement, and facial palsy are helpful diagnostic clues.[89,90] Schistosomiasis may present as a lumbosacral polyradiculopathy as well.[91]

The most notable inflammatory disorder with an affinity for the lumbosacral nerve roots is sarcoidosis.[92–94] Sarcoidosis has diverse phenotypic manifestations that may affect peripheral and central nervous system manifestations in addition to other potential end-organ involvement. It is estimated that 5% of individuals will have symptomatic nervous system involvement. Although many publications addressing neurosarcoidosis emphasize that neurologic manifestations typically occur in patients with established disease, this perspective is not always accurate from the viewpoint of a neurologist. In one series of sarcoidosis associated with a focal neuropathy, polyradiculopathy was the most common pattern affecting 22 of 57 reported patients.[92] The cauda equina, in particular, is at risk.[93,94] Other neuropathic patterns that may result from sarcoidosis include radiculoplexus neuropathy, multifocal neuropathy, or length-dependent polyneuropathy. Sarcoidosis can also cause a distal myopathy that can be confused with a radiculopathy in a patient with ankle dorsiflexion weakness. Pain and sensory symptoms occur more frequently than motor signs in most cases, being typically multifocal and nonlength dependent in distribution and monophasic in their chronologic course. Constitutional symptoms as well as symptoms referable to other end organs frequently affected by this disease are commonplace. Although more commonly associated with a multifocal or length-dependent neuropathy pattern, a polyradiculopathy phenotype has been reported with vasculitis.[95] We have also seen multiple sclerosis present with conus medullaris involvement initially mimicking a polyradiculopathy.

Structural disorders may cause or mimic polyradiculopathy. These include occult myelodysplasia with or without syringomyelia [96] and has been to occur in epidural lipomatosis as well.[97] Lumbosacral polyradiculopathy may result from iatrogenic disorders. Arachnoiditis is a syndrome in which the arachnoid becomes thickened, scarred, and adherent with presumed secondary ischemic consequences to nerve elements. Historically, the syndrome was most closely linked to the use of myelographic contrast agents. Arachnoiditis may also be caused as an unintended consequence of intended intrathecal injection of therapeutic agents, for example, chemotherapy, or the unintended intrathecal injection of agents that are potentially toxic. Radiation-induced nerve injury, also discussed in Chapter 9, may result in a neuropathy affecting the lower extremities.[98–109] Symptom onset is typically delayed by an average of 6 years after exposure. The range, however, is exceedingly broad, with onset latency varying between 4 months and 25 years. It most commonly occurs in the context of treatment of testicular cancer or lymphoma. Radiation doses typically exceed 4,000 cGY. As postirradiation neuropathy is frequently a pure motor syndrome, the actual localization of nerve injury has been in dispute. Less than a third of patients have notable sensory symptoms or signs. Whether the pathology preferentially occurs in the anterior horn cells of the conus medullaris, the ventral roots, the lumbosacral plexus, or a combination of any of the aforementioned elements is uncertain.[99] Current evidence, including reports of root enhancement on MRI in some patients, favors a polyradiculopathic localization.[98,99,107,108] Typically the deficits are bilateral and asymmetric, although monomelic presentations do occur.[102] Any segment may be affected, with L5 and S1 deficits being the most frequent. Pain may occur but typically follows the development of weakness and is usually not a major issue. Nodular enhancement of nerve roots and the conus medullaris with MR imaging resulting from radiation effect have been reported.[109] Understandable confusion with polyradiculopathy secondary to neoplastic meningitis will occur under this circumstance. Polyradiculopathy has also been reported as an iatrogenic complication of epidural injections for both analgesic and anesthetic purposes.[44] Patients with pre-existing spinal stenosis would appear to be at greater risk of this apparently rare and unintended consequence of a common procedure.

▶ EVALUATION OF SUSPECTED POLYRADICULOPATHY

In patients with suspected polyradiculopathy, the evaluation, as always is dictated by clinical context and likely differential diagnostic considerations. Imaging, preferably with MRI is the first step. It is imperative however that imaging be correlated with clinical findings. We do not believe that decisions regarding spinal stenosis surgery be dominated by imaging appearance in consideration of the significant incidence of asymptomatic stenosis.[110] Asymptomatic spinal stenosis is estimated to occur in 65% of asymptomatic volunteers, particularly in an older population.[5,111] As neurologic examinations in patients with spondylotic spinal stenosis are commonly normal, EMG can be very useful in identifying subclinical denervation in a characteristic pattern with signs of chronic denervation and reinnervation, and in some cases ongoing denervation. Studies have suggested that there is a strong correlation between abnormal EDX studies, imaging findings, and characteristic symptoms of spinal stenosis, a correlation that does not exist with severity of imaging findings alone without symptoms. Electrodiagnostic confirmation of symptomatic spinal stenosis has been identified to occur in 50–93% of individuals.[110–112] The EDX pattern of polyradiculopathy is not specific for spinal stenosis however as it can be seen with any condition affecting multiple nerve roots or with anterior horn cell disease. For this reason, EDX studies should be interpreted cautiously in patients with a polyradiculopathy pattern in the absence of pain or sensory symptoms.

The threshold for lumbar puncture performance is much lower in polyradiculopathy as opposed to monoradiculopathy and is typically performed in anyone with concern for systemic disease, particularly in patients who have clinically evident polyradiculopathy without proportionate structural pathology on imaging. In these cases, routine CSF analysis for white cells, protein, and glucose should be obtained in addition to cytologic analysis and appropriate additional testing for disorders such as sarcoid, Lyme, CMV, and HIV among others. If cord enlargement with T2 signal changes over multiple segments on MR images within the conus is identified, consideration of imaging of the proximal spinal cord in consideration of spinal dural malformation should be considered. The diagnosis of spinal dural arteriovenous fistulas requires a high index of suspicion. A more specific, although less commonly seen, feature is the presence of serpiginous flow voids representing engorged venous structures typically located dorsal to the spinal cord.

MANAGEMENT OF POLYRADICULOPATHY

Optimal management of spinal stenosis in a given patient is hampered by the variable natural history of the disorder. It is an indolent disorder for the most part. It is estimated that over 4 years, 15% will improve, an equal number will worsen, and 70% will remain the same.[5] Conservative measures are largely supported by anecdotal evidence.[110] Abdominal and back strengthening exercises benefit some patients. Durable medical equipment including rolling walkers which encourage favorable postures often improve the duration and distance of comfortable ambulation. Epidural injections may provide short-term although rarely durable relief.[40] The current weight of evidence favors but does not mandate an operative approach. In the majority of cases, there is no urgency to intervene and an initial conservative course is reasonable, particularly in patients with minimal clinical deficits.[51] It is estimated that 75–85% of well-selected individuals will experience significant improvement of lower extremity symptoms that may last for years with 10–15% of patients experiencing complications.[31,52] Considerable controversy persists relating to the nature of the surgical procedure, a discussion of which is beyond the scope of this chapter. Many patients require intervention at multiple levels. There is no consensus regarding the relative benefits of fusion versus decompression alone, and whether fusion should include the introduction of costly hardware. One less invasive surgical procedure potentially performed under local anesthesia involves the placement of an intralaminar spacing device in individuals who experience positional relief of symptoms. The device mechanically limits extension and promotes a posture of relative lumbar flexion. Reports suggest a beneficial effect on symptom relief in a significant proportion of selected individuals.[113]

Spinal dural arteriovenous fistulas are typically managed by a combination of selective catheterization and embolization of feeding arterial structures and surgical decompression, assuming that the diagnosis is made prior to complete and permanent ischemic injury to the spinal cord. As it is associated with abnormal CSF findings, implying CNS involvement, current recommendations for the treatment of Lyme polyradiculopathy are to treat with parenteral antibiotics, typically a cephalosporin.[89,90] Symptomatic sarcoidosis is typically treated with corticosteroids or other immunomodulating agents. Neoplastic meningitis may be treated with local radiation or intrathecal chemotherapy. Aggressive treatment is most likely undertaken with the hope of preserving rather than reclaiming a good quality of life. An extensive disease burden and significant morbidity typically warrant a more palliative approach in consideration of the poor natural history of the disease even with aggressive treatment regimens.

► PLEXOPATHIES AND RADICULOPLEXUS NEUROPATHIES

Plexopathies are typically recognized when motor, sensory, and, if applicable, reflex deficits occur in multiple nerve and segmental distributions confined to one extremity. Although lumbar plexopathies may be bilateral, they rarely occur concurrently, involvement of the second limb typically occurring in a chronologically dissociated manner. Sacral plexopathies however are more likely to manifest bilaterally due to the more proximate anatomic relationship between the left- and right-sided nerve elements. Radiculoplexus neuropathies have a near identical phenotype to plexopathies. As the name implies, the distinction is based upon pathology that involves nerve roots as well as plexus elements. This may be demonstrable by imaging but is much more likely to be identified electrodiagnostically where concomitant denervation in lumbosacral paraspinal muscles and abnormalities of anatomically analogous SNAPs implicates both root and spinal nerve/plexus involvement. In the author's opinion, the concept of radiculoplexus neuropathy has value as it is very disease specific. The pattern was likely coined in response to the almost unique tendency of diabetes to affect the peripheral nervous system in this way.[114]

The differential diagnosis of plexopathy includes disorders of the conus medullaris and cauda equina (polyradiculopathy). If there is a paucity of pain and sensory involvement, motor neuron disease needs to be considered as well. In general, intraspinal causes of lower extremity neuropathy affecting the conus medullaris or cauda equina are more likely to be bilateral than causes of lumbosacral plexopathy. Exceptions are frequent enough, however, to diminish the value of this rule in the evaluation of the individual patient. Otherwise the patterns of pain, sensory symptoms, weakness, and reflex loss may overlap considerably. At times, the clinical context may be helpful but imaging and EDX evaluation are often necessary to sort out anatomic localization in individual cases.

ETIOLOGIES OF LUMBOSACRAL PLEXOPATHY OR RADICULOPLEXUS NEUROPATHY

The numerous causes of lumbosacral plexopathies and radiculoplexus neuropathies are listed in Table 24-6. Diabetic lumbosacral radiculoplexus neuropathy (DLRPN) is a fairly common cause of painful leg weakness. It has been historically referred to by many names, including diabetic amyotrophy, diabetic femoral neuropathy, and the Bruns–Garland syndrome among others.[114–118] Current thinking implicates that DLRPN is a spectrum disorder.[118] The classical form is characterized by the acute to subacute onset of severe unilateral hip and/or thigh pain as the initial symptom, followed within days by awareness of ipsilateral leg weakness. Adjectives such as aching, stabbing, lancinating, and burning have all been used. The exact onset of weakness may be obscured by pain. The syndrome evolves over weeks to months in most cases. DLRPN may become bilateral in a substantial proportion of individuals who are affected, usually with an interval of weeks–months.

The weakness of DLRPN is typically restricted to muscles innervated by the lumbar plexus, affecting hip flexion, adduction, and particularly knee extension. The latter is a considerable source of morbidity. There is a frequent need for durable equipment in order to minimize fall risk, particularly walkers or crutches, and in some cases knee–ankle–foot orthoses or even wheelchairs. Two-thirds of individuals will have weakness in the L5 myotome and half in the S1 dermatome in addition to the muscles innervated by the L2–4 roots.[119] L5 and S1 myotomal weakness may occur without concomitant involvement of proximal myotomes. The reference to diabetic monoradiculopathies earlier in this chapter probably represents a limited expression of this disorder. Paresthesias and sensory loss may occur but are typically overshadowed by the pain and weakness. A small percentage will have a concurrent or chronologically proximate truncal neuropathy, which is a helpful clue in support of a diabetic etiology. Weight loss, the so-called diabetic cachexia, is a common comorbidity. Approximately a half of individuals who are afflicted will have signs and symptoms attributable to dysautonomia if sought after, including orthostatic intolerance, urinary dysfunction, constipation and diarrhea, tachycardia, and impotence.[116] Concurrent, sensory predominant, length-dependent, and symmetric polyneuropathy occurs frequently based on clinical and EDX assessments but may be absent in approximately a quarter of patients.[119]

Less frequently, a radiculoplexus neuropathy occurs in diabetics that differs from the classic form in that it is symmetric in distribution, more insidious in onset, and predominantly motor in its manifestations with limited pain and sensory symptomatology.[118] Like DLPRN, lower extremity muscles bear the brunt of the disease. Unlike the classic syndrome, the weakness typically begins distally rather than proximally and can affect the arms in some cases. In consideration of these clinical features, it has been suggested that this syndrome may represent chronic inflammatory demyelinating polyradiculoneuropathy (CIDP) rather than DLPRN. Data provided through electrodiagnosis, biopsy of peripheral nerve and the natural history of the disease however, suggests that this phenotype is part of the DLRPN spectrum and distinctive from CIDP.[118] In addition, there appears to be no increased incidence of classic CIDP in the diabetic population.[120]

DLRPN, like other focal diabetic neuropathies, but in contrast to the more common length-dependent symmetric diabetic polyneuropathy, is not clearly related to disease duration or control and appears to have a more favorable natural history.[117,121] It is not rare for the onset DLPRN to lead to the discovery of impaired glucose tolerance or diabetes.[118,122] It has been reported that impaired glucose tolerance

TABLE 24-6. LUMBOSACRAL PLEXOPATHIES AND RADICULOPLEXUS NEUROPATHIES

Retroperitoneal hematoma
Psoas abscess
Malignant neoplasm
Benign neoplasm
Radiation
Amyloid
Diabetic radiculoplexus neuropathy
Idiopathic radiculoplexus neuropathy
Sarcoidosis
Aortic occlusion/surgery
Lithotomy positioning
Hip arthroplasty
Pelvic fracture
Obstetric injury

may be identified in approximately two-thirds of individuals with apparent idiopathic lumbosacral plexopathy.[121] The typical natural history is for pain to relent within weeks to months. Eventual improvement in strength and significant functional recovery occurs in the majority patients over the course of months to a year or two although many will have some residual weakness if carefully sought for. As in most neuropathies in which proximal and distal muscle weakness occurs, return of function occurs most successfully in proximal muscles.

The preponderance of evidence suggests that DLPRN occurs as a result of an inflammatory disorder, directed at the microvasculature resulting in ischemic nerve injury.[116,118,123] Peripheral nerve biopsies demonstrate in about 80% of classic asymmetric DLPRN and 50% of the motor predominant symmetric phenotype evidence of multifocal nerve fiber degeneration within or between fascicles, strongly implicating an ischemic mechanism.[118] Other common pathologic findings include infiltrates of lymphocytes (CD45) and macrophages (CD68) most commonly surrounding epineurial arterioles, venules, and capillaries but at times infiltrating vessel walls (microvasculitis) with occasional evidence of prior hemorrhage.[118]

A similar, perhaps identical, phenotype has been described as an idiopathic condition.[117,124–130] Again, the lumbar plexus appears to be predominantly affected in most cases, although both sacral plexopathies and pan-plexopathies may occur as well. As in its diabetic counterpart, delayed involvement of the opposite side may occur. The disorder is also monophasic in most individuals but can be relapsing or progressive in some.[127,130] As in its brachial plexus analog, an antecedent immunization or symptoms of infection may occur. This phenomenon appears to be more common in children than in adults.[129] Nerve pathology in apparent idiopathic lumbosacral radiculoplexus neuropathy appears to be similar if not identical to DLRPN.[118,126,177]

Acute lower extremity monoplegia has been reported as a rare presenting manifestation of acute aortic occlusion.[131] The localization of nerve injury in this condition is uncertain but is classified here as a plexopathy due to its phenotype.[74] Lumbar plexopathies are a well-recognized complication of retroperitoneal hemorrhage.[132,133] Various primary and metastatic malignancies can affect the lumbosacral plexus as well as treatment with radiation and interarterial chemotherapy.[104] Primary tumors known to infiltrate the plexus include those originating from the cervix, endometrium, ovary, testes, prostate, bone, and colon as well as hematologic malignancies such as myeloma, lymphoma, and acute myelogenous leukemia.[105,134–136] Radiation of cervical and endometrial cancer is a recognized cause of lumbar plexopathy.[100,105,134,137] Other reported etiologies include psoas abscess, intraneural spread of amyloid, pelvic fracture, benign tumors such uterine leiomyoma, sarcoidosis, lithotomy positioning, and hip arthroplasty.[138–141] Obstetrical injury often associates with a phenotype that approximates a lumbosacral trunk injury, both clinically and electrodiagnostically.[142,143] Woman of short stature seem to be at particular risk.

EVALUATION OF SUSPECTED LUMBOSACRAL PLEXOPATHIES OR RADICULOPLEXUS NEUROPATHIES

Most patients with plexopathies will undergo both imaging and EDX evaluations. It is logical to begin with EDX in an attempt to localize pathology and focus imaging. Again, the absence of paraspinal denervation and abnormalities of anatomically relevant SNAPs serve to distinguish plexopathies from radiculopathies.[117,128,129,144] Distinction of plexopathies from mononeuropathies is more dependent on the pattern of abnormalities on needle examination and less on the pattern of nerve conductions. For example, sacral plexopathies are distinguished from sciatic neuropathies by denervation of muscles innervated by the superior and inferior gluteal nerves which would not occur with sciatic neuropathies. Although the yield of imaging in DLRPN is extremely low, we feel obligated to image them nonetheless.[17,18] Although the clinical syndrome is fairly distinctive, particularly in patients with concomitant paraspinal denervation, the tendency for the weakness to progress over weeks to months makes both patient and physician uncomfortable with a watch-and-wait approach without the reassurance provided by imaging that is either normal or consistent with idiopathic or diabetic LRPN.[18] As with all suspected diabetic neuropathies, we do not advocate for the routine use of nerve biopsy in plexopathy or radiculoplexus neuropathy unless there are clinical, imaging, or laboratory features that would suggest a disorder capable of infiltrating nerve in which a nerve biopsy would be diagnostic, for example, amyloid, sarcoid, or lymphoma. We also do not advocate for the routine use of CSF evaluation in cases where plexus localization can be confidently made through clinical, EDX or imaging means.

▶ MANAGEMENT OF LUMBOSACRAL PLEXOPATHY OR RADICULOPLEXUS NEUROPATHY

There are no known effective treatments for either the idiopathic or the diabetic forms of lumbosacral radiculoplexus neuropathy. Various immunomodulating agents such as corticosteroids, intravenous immunoglobulin (IVIG), plasma exchange, and cyclophosphamide have been used both in diabetic and in idiopathic forms of radiculoplexus neuropathy.[117,118,129,145–148] A suggested benefit has been suggested, in some, but not all reports.[144–147] Case reports suggest a benefit of IVIG in idiopathic lumbosacral radiculoplexus neuropathy.[144,149] This suggested benefit is described more as a tendency to arrest progression rather than to result in immediate improvement. In a recent poll of a popular blog attended by many in the neuromuscular community [Rick's Real Neuromuscular Friends (RRNMF)], there was considerable ambivalence concerning immunomodulating treatment for this population. If any treatment is to be used prior to proof of efficacy, it is suggested that it be used early in the clinical course.

With retroperitoneal hemorrhage, it is not known whether surgical decompression alters the natural history of the condition. If surgery is to be done, it is rational to do it expeditiously rather than on a delayed basis after axon loss is more likely to have occurred. Similarly, there are no known effective treatments for radiation-induced nerve injury. Many patients with plexopathy or radiculoplexus neuropathies will benefit from evaluation by a physiatrist or physical therapist, particularly if there is significant quadriceps weakness. Consideration should be given to relevant orthotic devices such as knee–ankle–foot orthoses and/or durable medical equipment such as canes, crutches, or walkers as discussed in Chapter 5. Neuropathic pain should be treated with medications that may have an acceptable benefit to side effect ratio such as tricyclic antidepressants, anticonvulsants such as carbamazepine, gabapentin or pregabalin, or serotonin norepinephrine reuptake inhibitors such as duloxetine or venlafaxine.

MONONEUROPATHIES AND MONOMELIC POLYNEUROPATHIES

Mononeuropathies are usually the result of compression or entrapment. For purposes of this discussion, we will consider compression as a force that originates outside of the body that irritates or injures a nerve structure. In contrast, we will consider entrapment to represent an internal force created by altered anatomy of a normal structure. The mechanism of compressive injury may result from direct stretch and distortion of nerve elements, indirect injury from concussive effects from, for example, a bomb blast, or ischemic injury resulting from the concomitant compression of blood supply to nerve. It is suspected that there are a number of conditions make nerve more susceptible to pressure injury. Hereditary neuropathy with liability to pressure palsy (HNPP) is perhaps the best established example of this. Both diabetes and prior radiation are also suspected to render peripheral nerves more susceptible to mechanical injury, presumably as both are thought to compromise the vaso nevorum and the blood supply of peripheral nerves.[150] Although the vast majority of mononeuropathies occur from mechanical injury, mononeuropathy may uncommonly occur due to alternative mechanisms. Specifically, mononeuropathy may be the first manifestation of a systemic disorder with a predilection to infarct, inflame, or infiltrate peripheral nerve which then commonly evolves into a multifocal neuropathy pattern.

Mononeuropathies may be painful or painless, depending on multiple factors such as the etiology, acuity, and pathophysiology of the injury. The presence of motor or sensory symptoms, typically the reason why nerve injury is suspected, is largely dependent on the makeup of the nerve. For example, meralgia paresthetica, one of the more common lower extremity mononeuropathies may produce pain, paresthesias, and sensory loss but would not cause motor weakness. Like all nerve injuries, the pattern of weakness, usually the most objective means to determine the existence and localization of nerve injury either clinically or electrodiagnostically, may not always precisely localize the nerve injury site. As previously mentioned, certain fascicles and therefore certain muscles may be spared with a given injury, falsely localizing the problem to a more distal location than is actually the case.[14,15] Reflex loss is dependent on the nerve affected, being the norm in femoral and sciatic neuropathies but unexpected in any other lower extremity mononeuropathy. Table 24-7 provides a list of many of the reported causes of the common lower extremity mononeuropathies.

▶ EVALUATION OF SUSPECTED MONONEUROPATHIES

EDX of suspected mononeuropathies has numerous potential benefits. Needle electromyography may demonstrate abnormalities in muscles that are not clinically weak, aiding both in localization process to a single nerve and within that nerve. This is particularly true with axon loss injury. For example, in patient with an apparent fibular (peroneal neuropathy) denervation of the short head of the biceps implicates a sciatic neuropathy rather than the more common fibular (peroneal) neuropathy at the fibular head. Nerve conductions may not only help to confirm localization to a single nerve, but will even more precisely localize a nerve injury if focal demyelination in any of its three forms can be demonstrated. For example, 45% of common peroneal neuropathies can be localized to the fibular head region as a result of demyelinating features identified by sequential, segmental stimulation in this region.[151] Identifying a predominantly demyelinating injury is also beneficial for prognostic reasons, a predominantly demyelinating injury typically having a much quicker and complete recovery than its predominantly axonal counterpart. Finally nerve conduction studies may provide additional insights. The demonstration of a focal demyelinating lesion at a location where compression or entrapment does not typically occur may suggest that an apparent mononeuropathy may be the first manifestation of an imminent multifocal neuropathy, for example, MADSAM. Also, nerve conductions may reveal evidence of a more widespread polyneuropathy in a patient with a demyelinating mononeuropathy at a typical compression site, suggesting the possibility of a hereditary disorder like HNPP.

The use of imaging in the evaluation of mononeuropathies has expanded considerably.[10,17,152–156] It provides a far greater probability for an etiologic diagnosis than EDX. As a general rule, we consider imaging in patients with apparent mononeuropathies occurring in the absence of a clear compression/entrapment mechanism, in a clinical context that would suggest a noncompressive/entrapment cause, or in the setting of unexplained progression.

With MRI, increased T2 signal within nerve is thought to correlate with the lesion site in acute axonal injury.[156] MRI with the addition of gadolinium is the test of choice to identify a suspected nerve sheath tumor (Fig. 22-16). MRI may also be used to identify an abnormal structure that is

TABLE 24-7. MONONEUROPATHIES: ETIOLOGIES

Iliohypogastric
- Lower quadrant surgery—appendectomy and nephrectomy
- Retroperitoneal tumor

Ilioinguinal
- Surgery—herniorrhaphies, suprapubic (Pfannenstiel), nephrectomy, and appendectomy incisions
- Parturition
- Bone harvesting from the iliac crest
- Abdominal wall entrapment syndrome

Genitofemoral
- Surgery—herniorrhaphy and appendectomy
- Psoas abscess

Obturator
- Tumor—transitional cell carcinoma of the bladder, cervical carcinoma, lymphoma, prostatic carcinoma and sarcoma, histologically undefinable
- Parturition
- Prolonged lithotomy position
- Hip arthroplasty
- Surgical tourniquets
- Myositis ossifications
- Obturator hernias
- Pelvic surgery including those done laparoscopically
- Pelvic fracture

Femoral
- Retroperitoneal or iliacus hematoma
- Lithotomy positioning
- Hip arthroplasty or dislocation
- Iliac artery occlusion
- Femoral arterial procedures—diagnostic or therapeutic
- Femoral artery aneurysms or pseudoaneurysms
- Infiltration by hematogenous malignancies
- Penetrating groin trauma
- Pelvic surgery
- Idiopathic
- Mechanical pressure clamp on the femoral artery

Lateral cutaneous nerve of the thigh
- Meralgia paresthetica
- Bone graft harvesting
- Retrocecal appendectomy
- Hip arthroplasty
- Cesarean section
- Pelvic fracture
- Aortobifemoral bypass surgery

Sciatic
- Gluteal compartment syndrome from hematoma and "toilet seat" neuropathy
- Hip arthroplasty and fracture—dislocation
- Femoral fracture
- Groin injury including gunshot wound
- Infarction due to vasculitis or vascular surgical procedures of the lower extremity
- Lithotomy positioning
- Gluteal injection injury
- Immobilization with impaired consciousness
- Intraoperative thigh tourniquet
- Infiltration by lymphoma
- Endometriosis
- Gluteal artery aneurysms
- Gluteal varicosities
- Compression from lipoma or nerve sheath tumor
- Umbilical artery injections in neonates
- Persistent sciatic artery
- Cardiac surgery
- Compression from prominent lesser trochanter
- Piriformis syndrome

Peroneal
- External compression—stockings, casts, and leg crossing Weight loss
- Stretch—bungee jumping, acute plantar flexion/inversion, and prolonged knee flexion during childbirth
- Prolonged squatting
- Cysts and tumors of the tibiofibular joint
- Postoperative
- Closed or open trauma
- Fibular fractures
- Dislocated knees
- Surgery in the popliteal fossa
- Vasculitis
- Baker cyst
- Acute occlusion of femoral or popliteal arteries

Tibial
- Trauma—compression from casts or tourniquets, hip arthroplasty, gunshot and other penetrating wounds, tibial plateau fracture/dislocations, and gluteal injections
- Ischemia—acute large artery occlusive disease or posterior
- Compartment syndrome
- Tumor—neurofibroma, neurosarcoma, osteochondroma, and lymphoma
- Miscellaneous—ruptured Baker cyst, popliteal hemorrhage, sclerosing treatment of varicose veins, and repetitive foot plantar flexion occupations
- Tarsal tunnel syndrome

Sural
- Ankle injury
- Vein stripping procedures
- Schwannomas
- Ganglionic cysts
- Baker's cyst or surgery
- Fracture of the base of the fifth metatarsal
- Compression from the hard upper edges of ski boots
- Vasculitis
- Calf muscle biopsy
- Arthroscopic surgery
- Idiopathic

compressing and injuring a peripheral nerve such as an osteochondroma of the fibular head or a Baker cyst within the popliteal fossa. MRI can also provide indirect evidence of nerve injury by demonstrating abnormal signal change in muscles.[152] For example, the presence of increased T2 signal (suggesting edema) or increased T1 signal (suggesting fatty infiltration) confined to the gluteus medius, minimus, and tensor fascia lata would strongly implicate a superior gluteal

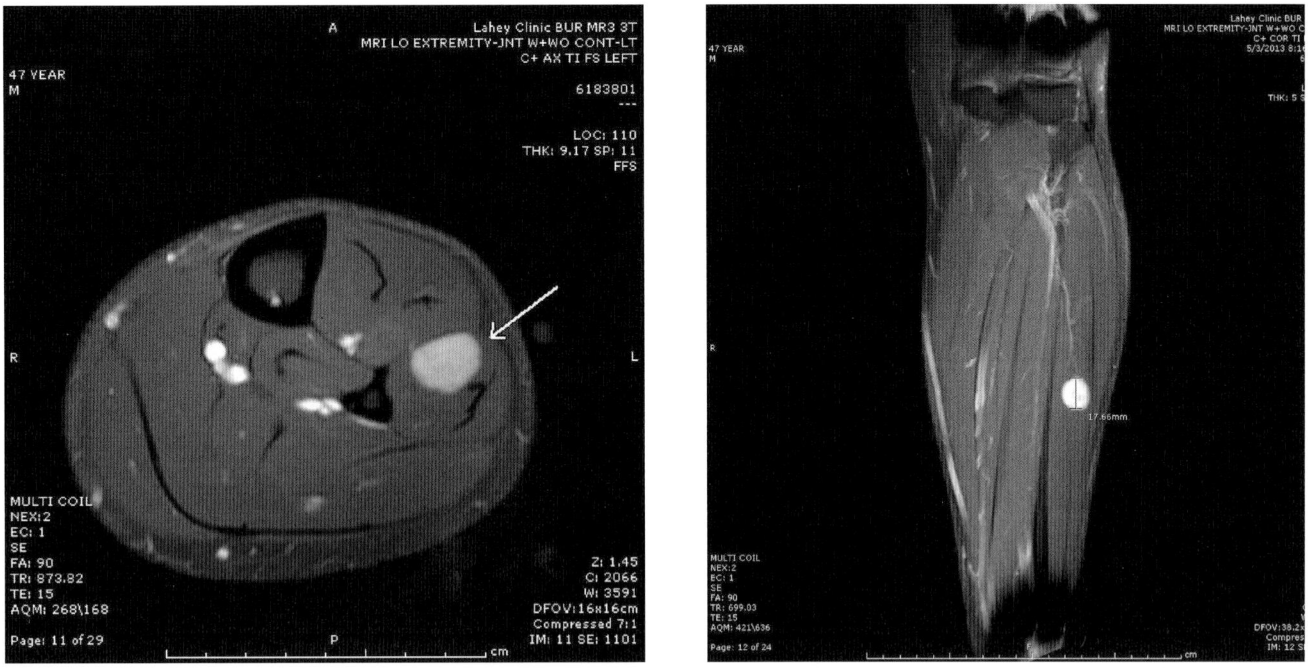

A B

Figure 24-16. **(A)** Axial and **(B)** coronal Gadolinium-enhanced T1 MR images demonstrating a Schwannoma in a 47-year-old male who would experience a Tinel sign every time his lateral left leg was struck by a crawling child in his wife's day care facility.

mononeuropathy. MRI can demonstrate muscle enlargement and signal change in a given anatomic compartment that help to define a compartment syndrome. Finally, MR imaging may demonstrate focal nerve swelling and increased T2 signal in nerve, particularly within the brachial plexus, that may be helpful in the diagnosis of multifocal neuropathy syndromes such as multifocal motor neuropathy that may present as mononeuropathies and be initially diagnostically elusive.[157]

Ultrasonography of nerve and muscle disease is also an expanding field. The information that it provides overlaps considerably with that provided by MRI although it has both benefits and limitations (Fig. 24-17).[153–155] It can be difficult

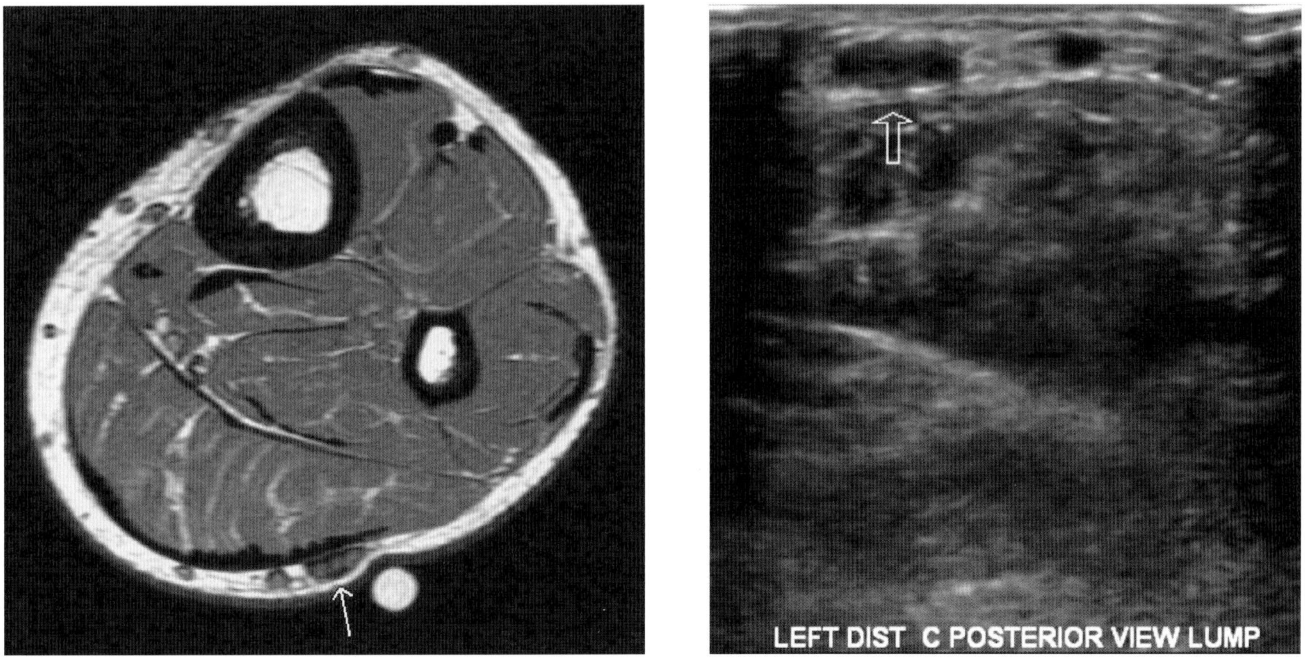

Figure 24-17. T1 MR (**left**) and ultrasonic (**right**) images of nodular enlargement of cutaneous nerves in Hansen disease.

to utilize when nerves are deeply situated in regions with complex anatomy.[10] Conversely, it may be easier to follow a nerve along its longitudinal course with ultrasound in comparison to MRI. Ultrasound is obviously more portable than MRI and does not have the limitations imposed by pacemakers and other devices. We do not routinely obtain blood work in mononeuropathy patients unless the clinical context directs us to do so.

▶ MANAGEMENT OF MONONEUROPATHIES

Management is dependent on the etiology, location, severity, and duration of nerve injury. With rare exception, monophasic compressive nerve injuries are treated conservatively. If it can be determined that a nerve injury is progressive and due to a definable cause of external compression, the source of compression should be surgically altered or removed. Surgical intervention in diabetics with mononeuropathies should be undertaken cautiously, as the already potentially compromised microvasculature may be further injured with nerve manipulation or transposition.

In case of trauma from "clean" penetrating injuries such as knife or glass wounds in which complete loss of function implicates potential nerve transaction, immediate exploration with attempted primary reanastomosis is considered. If potential nerve transaction occurs from trauma associated with considerably surrounding tissue damage such as a gunshot wound, exploration is typically delayed for a month or more, assuming that there is no suggestion of recovery from either a clinical or an EDX perspective. If the nerve is transected, nerve grafting will be required if anastomosis is attempted, as the retraction of the severed ends will prevent primary reanastomosis on a delayed basis. If the nature of the injury makes nerve transaction unlikely, even in the setting of complete or near-complete nerve injury, surgical exploration is usually not attempted for at least 6 months. If there is partial but convincing improvement measured either clinically or electrically, it is unlikely that surgical intervention will improve outcome. If there is no evidence of improvement, exploration may be considered. The goals in this case would be to perform nerve grafting if the nerve is transected, to identify and remove any external source of nerve compression (external neurolysis), and to potentially perform internal neurolysis. The latter is considered if the epineurium is intact, but intraoperative nerve conductions indicate that there is no impulse transmission through the injured segment. The intent is to dissect out individual fascicles and to potentially free them from any scarring that has taken place within the confines of the epineurial sheath. Alternatively if upon dissection, all fascicles are anatomically discontinuous despite preservation of epineurial continuity, a predictably rare event, nerve grafting may be attempted.[158]

The outcome of surgical intervention for peripheral nerve injury is often disappointing. The age of the patient, comorbid illnesses, and the distance between injury and reinnervating target are key variables. In general, muscles in proximity to axon loss lesions are more likely to recover meaningful function than those at a distance, regardless of whether surgical intervention takes place or not.

As discussed in the plexopathy section, bracing and other forms of durable equipment may improve both mobility and safety. With common peroneal or sciatic neuropathies, custom-fitted ankle–foot orthoses (AFO) are recommended if the patients "catch their toes" and trip. Some patients benefit from AFOs by improving their gait as well as by diminishing their risk of falling. Selected patients with femoral neuropathies may benefit from a knee–ankle–foot orthoses. In addition, a cane, walker, or even wheelchair may be necessary, depending on the severity of quadriceps weakness and the strength of unaffected muscles. Patients with quadriceps weakness may also benefit from lift chairs, which will aid them in getting to their feet, and stair lifts if access to second floors or basements in their homes or places of work is required and cannot be accomplished by some other means.

▶ INDIVIDUAL MONONEUROPATHIES OF THE LOWER EXTREMITIES

- Ilioinguinal neuropathy

  Clinical recognition of an ilioinguinal mononeuropathy is based on sensory complaints in the appropriate topographic area, typically occurring in a postoperative context.[159] The ilioinguinal nerve provides cutaneous innervation most reliably to the base of penis (mons pubis, labia majora) as well as along the inguinal ligament or in the most proximal aspect of the anteromedial thigh. Either reduced or heightened sensibility may be found on tactile stimulation of these areas. The most problematic symptom is "neuralgic" pain along the inguinal ligament, medial groin, scrotum, or labia that often has burning or lancinating characteristics. This pain is typically reproducible by groin pressure or by extending the thigh at the hip. As a result, patients often maintain a flexed posture while walking. The ilioinguinal nerve also provides motor branches to the transverse abdominus and internal oblique muscles of the lower abdominal wall. Paresis in the ipsilateral lower abdominal musculature may be demonstrable either by having the patient contract the abdominal wall by attempting a sit up. Involvement of the abdominal musculature may be more readily detected by needle electromyography, particularly in those with an endomorphic body habitus. The differential diagnosis is largely that of L1 radiculopathies, iliohypogastric or genitofemoral mononeuropathies, and non-neurologic causes of groin pain.

  The prevalence of ilioinguinal neuropathy probably relates to the frequency of potentially causative surgical procedures. Herniorrhaphies are the most notorious, either open or laparoscopic, with an incidence reported as high as 10%.[160–162] When explored, the mechanism of neuropathy appears to be nerve transaction, entrapment, or traumatic neuroma.[162] Other pelvic procedures including suprapubic (Pfannenstiel) incision, nephrectomy, femoral catheter placement, hysterectomy, orchiectomy, and appendectomy have been associated with this injury as well. Ilioinguinal neuropathy has been rarely described as a complication of parturition, bone harvesting from the iliac crest, and presumed tearing of the external oblique aponeurosis in hockey players. Spontaneously and idiopathically occurring ilioinguinal neuropathies have also been described, attributed to anatomic variation in anatomy and presumed entrapment from surrounding musculoaponeurotic structures.[159]

Diagnosis may be aided by reproduction of the typical pain pattern by palpation (Tinel sign) or hip extension, EDX demonstration of denervation confined to abdominal wall muscles, and/or by pain relief achieved by nerve block with local anesthetic. With nerve percussion, the pain typically radiates into the medial thigh and/or genitalia. Treatment may involve pharmacologic attempts at neuropathic pain relief with drugs such as gabapentin, nerve blocks with steroids and local anesthetics, or unproven noninvasive measures such as transcutaneous nerve stimulation or pulsed radiofrequency therapy to the upper lumbar roots. Surgical interventions for intractable cases including neurectomy have been favorably reported.[163–165]

- Iliohypogastric neuropathy

Iliohypogastric neuropathies are far less common than their ilioinguinal counterparts.[159,162] The nerve has anterior and lateral branches. The lateral branch provides sensation to a vertically oriented patch that descends from the superior margin of the iliac crest in the posterior axillary line to a position just posterior to the head of the trochanter. The anterior branch supplies a small area just rostral to the symphysis pubis. Like the ilioinguinal nerve, it provides motor branches to the transverse abdominus and internal oblique muscles of the lower abdominal wall. There is considerable overlap in the signs and symptoms of ilioinguinal and iliohypogastric nerve injury and they may be indistinguishable from one another.

Iliohypogastric neuropathies typically result from surgery in the lower quadrants including appendectomy, hysterectomy, inguinal herniorrhaphy, and nephrectomy or from pathology in the retroperitoneum. They may occur in the third trimester or as a result of sports injury. Diagnostic strategies and treatment options are identical to ilioinguinal nerve injury.[165]

- Genitofemoral neuropathy

The phenotype of genitofemoral neuropathy is similar to ilioinguinal and iliohypogastric neuropathies.[159] If distinction is to be made, it is most likely to occur as a result of the topographic area that is affected. Sensory loss or hyperesthesia in genitofemoral neuropathies occurs in a small zone in the anterior thigh just inferior to the mid-inguinal ligament (femoral branch) and immediately lateral to part of the cutaneous distribution of the ilioinguinal nerve. The sensory distribution of the genital branch includes the labia majorus and scrotum and is probably indistinguishable in this location from ilioinguinal and iliohypogastric nerve injury. The phenotype usually consists of sensory complaints in medial groin, exacerbated by walking, rotation of the hip joint, or by tactile stimulation of the nerve. The loss of the cremasteric reflex on the symptomatic side provides diagnostic support but inexplicably is not invariably lost with injuries to this nerve.

Once again, the most likely cause is a complication of a preceding lower abdominal surgery including herniorrhaphy, appendectomy, biopsy, cesarean section, or as a complication of retroperitoneal hematoma or pregnancy. Fortunately, these injuries are rare. Anesthetic block of the L1–L2 roots is reported to reliably predict a good response to surgical intervention if required. When required, neurectomy is the procedure of choice and has been reported to be very effective in well-chosen patients.[165,166]

- Superior and inferior gluteal neuropathies

The superior and inferior gluteal nerves are virtually never affected in isolation. They have been reported subsequent to hip arthroplasty either due to direct injury from instrumentation or indirectly from stretch. It has been suggested that these nerves may be compressed by pelvic osteophytes and post-traumatic bone spurs as well.[10] There have been reports of superior gluteal nerve injuries in response to injection injuries and inferior gluteal nerve injuries with pelvic malignancy. The latter usually occurs with concurrent injury to the sciatic, pudendal, and/or posterior cutaneous nerve of the thigh. Posterior cutaneous nerve of the thigh injuries has been reported to occur with injection injuries, lacerations, and prolonged bike riding. Recognition is based on sensory complaints/loss of the posterior thigh and inferior buttock. An intermittent neuralgia of this nerve has been reported.[167]

- LFCN/ "meralgia paresthetica"

One of the first documented and certainly more eloquent descriptions of meralgia paresthetica was by Sigmund Freud regarding his personal experience. He described a "furry sensation, a feeling of alien skin almost imperceptible at rest but exacerbated by walking, frequently accompanied by painful short, pricking at right angles to the skin as well as a disagreeable sensitivity to the rubbing of underclothes."[168] Like Freud, the majority of patients experience pain, often burning in character. Typically, there is either a diminished or increased response to tactile stimulus in the anterior lateral thigh, typically in an area analogous to the positioning of a hand in a pants' pocket.[169] In the majority of individuals, symptoms are unilateral. In the 10% whose symptoms are bilateral, there is still unilateral dominance.[170] Weakness and reflex loss are notable for their absence.

The diagnosis of meralgia paresthetica is largely clinical.[171] It has been suggested that placing a patient in the lateral recumbent position with the asymptomatic side downward and placing pressure on the symptomatic iliac crest for 45 seconds will relieve the symptoms of meralgia paresthetica in 95% of cases with similar specificity.[159] EDX may be helpful if the LFCN SNAP is reduced in amplitude or absent on the symptomatic side. Unfortunately, it is not uncommon for the response to be absent bilaterally, which may be related to technical factors such as patient body habitus. In some cases the LFCN SNAP may be normal bilaterally in the setting of a credible clinical diagnosis.[170] Presumably, this is a consequence of a predominantly demyelinating lesion at the inguinal ligament, proximal to both the stimulation and recording site. The differential diagnosis of meralgia paresthetica includes L2–L3 radiculopathy, lumbar plexopathy, or a non-neuropathic cause of thigh pain, for example, hip joint disease.

Meralgia paresthetica, literally thigh pain, is most commonly attributed to entrapment or injury to the nerve as it passes through the lateral portion of the inguinal ligament, just medial to the anterior superior iliac spine. This belief is supported by observations made during therapeutic neurectomy in patients with chronic, intractable meralgia.[170] This is a common disorder with an estimated overall incidence of $32/10^5$.[169] The incidence appears to climb with increasing age although seems to peak between ages 55 and 65 at approximately double that rate.[169] Risk factors include obesity and diabetes, the latter thought to be independent from body mass index.[170] The disorder seems to be most commonly idiopathic. Identifiable causes that have been reported include retrocecal appendectomy, hip surgery, cesarean section, pelvic fracture, seat belt injury, iliac crest bone marrow harvesting, prone positioning during spinal surgery, and aortobifemoral bypass grafting.[172,173]

The natural history of the disorder is variable.[171] The disorder can be self-limited or persist chronically. There are no controlled trials that we are aware of that identify the effect of weight loss on the natural history. Treatment paradigms, if necessary include the use of medications to treat neuropathic pain, injection in proximity of the presumed site of entrapment at the lateral aspect of inguinal ligament at the anterior superior iliac spine, or neurolysis or neurectomy in chronic, intractable cases. Surgical intervention has been demonstrated to have a favorable outcome in small case series.[170,173,174] At the time of neurectomy, four of seven resected nerves demonstrated focal indentation of the nerve at the inguinal ligament, a finding not demonstrable in control individuals. Nonetheless, a Cochrane review concludes that no intervention has proven benefit over the natural history of the disease.[175] Pathologic examination of the nerve demonstrated findings described in animal models of chronic nerve compression with multifocal fiber loss. In addition, there was evidence of inflammation in the majority of cases.[170]

- Femoral neuropathy

The phenotype of a femoral mononeuropathy phenotype is typically dominated by weakness of knee extension, and depending on the location, weakness of hip flexion as well. Sensory symptoms occurring on either the anterior thigh and/or the medial leg occur in only half of reported cases. A prominent painful component is the exception rather than the rule. It may be delayed and is often self-limited in nature. Preservation of the quadriceps (patellar) reflex would be unusual and call the diagnosis into question.[176]

The diagnosis is typically made by clinical examination supported by electrodiagnostic findings. Imaging of the pelvis is recommended if a readily available cause is not apparent. This is particularly true if the deficits are progressive or if the clinical context suggests an increased risk of hematoma or abscess. The EDX evaluation may include motor conduction studies of the femoral nerve although we do not find them particularly helpful in most cases. The diagnosis is supported by an abnormal saphenous SNAP with preservation of the other ipsilateral sensory responses. As the saphenous SNAP may be technically difficult to obtain, we do not place a great deal of weight on a low amplitude or absent response unless it is readily acquired on the opposite side. Depending on how proximal or distal the lesion, needle EMG findings should be confined to some or all the eight femoral innervated muscles if tested. The differential diagnosis of femoral neuropathies consists of lumbar plexopathies and radiculoplexus neuropathies, L3/L4 radiculopathies and non-neurogenic causes of pelvic, hip or thigh pain in which there may be perceived weakness resulting from pain.

The reported causes of femoral mononeuropathies are varied and include retroperitoneal or iliacus hematoma, lithotomy positioning, hip arthroplasty or dislocation, iliac artery occlusion, and femoral arterial procedures that are either diagnostic or therapeutic, mechanical clamping following those procedures, infiltration by hematogenous malignancy, penetrating groin trauma, and pelvic surgery including hysterectomy and renal transplantation, or idiopathic.[177–186] Femoral neuropathies have been reported to occur with compression from giant iliopsoas bursa or acetabular ganglia as the nerve passes under the inguinal ligament.[10] We, and others, have seen femoral neuropathy with apparent infarction of femoral innervated muscles in the setting of IV drug abuse.[187]

Management is largely determined by etiology but is conservative in most cases. Pain management and physical therapy are the primary therapeutic modalities. As described in Chapter 5, bracing such as knee–ankle–foot orthoses and durable medical equipment such as canes, crutches, walkers, or even wheelchairs may allow for independent mobility associated with a diminished risk of falling that these patients are at particular risk for.

- Saphenous neuropathy

The saphenous is the terminal sensory branch of the femoral nerve, passing through Hunter's canal on the medial surface of the knee after innervating the anteromedial surface of the leg, the medial malleolar region, and the medial surface of the foot. This is the only region of the lower extremity below the knee innervated by nonsciatic nerve branches. Affected patients have pain and paresthesia in the aforementioned zone. There may be a Tinel sign at the most common entrapment point at the medial knee.[159,188,189] Saphenous neuropathy has been reported to occur as a result of a ganglion cyst or following surgery in the popliteal fossa.[190,191] Many patients respond to conservative treatment or to nerve block although success with neurectomy may occur as well.[188,189] As expected, the latter procedure results in residual sensory loss in the medial leg and ankle.

- Obturator neuropathy

Obturator mononeuropathy typically presents with pain in the groin, anterior, and/or medial thigh which is the initial symptom in the majority of patients. Paresthesias in the medial thigh occur, but are often obscured by pain. Weakness may not be evident clinically, and EDX evidence of denervation confined to obturator-innervated muscles may be required. Weakness occurs predominantly in hip adduction, although weakness in hip flexion may coexist.[192] Ipsilateral leg edema may occur. The differential diagnosis is largely that of lumbar plexopathy or radiculoplexus neuropathy in addition to non-neurologic causes of pelvic and thigh pain. In the author's as well as others' experience, diabetic radiculoplexus neuropathy may occasionally mimic an obturator mononeuropathy with apparent clinical and electrodiagnostic sparing of the quadriceps.[193] The clinical diagnosis of obturator neuropathy is confirmed electrodiagnostically.[193] Imaging of the pelvis is recommended if the etiology is not apparent.[10]

These mononeuropathies occur infrequently. Etiologies include pelvic instrumentation, occult or previously recognized malignancy.[192,193] Reported malignancies include transitional cell carcinoma of the bladder, cervical carcinoma, lymphoma, prostatic carcinoma and sarcoma, or tumors that are histologically undefinable. The majority of cases are related to mechanical injury. Reported causes are similar to femoral mononeuropathies and include childbirth, osteitis pubis, acetabular labral cysts, the prolonged lithotomy position, total hip arthroplasty, surgical tourniquets, myositis ossifications, obturator hernias, pelvic surgery including those done laparoscopically, and pelvic fracture.[10,193] Prognosis is in large part determined by etiology and is favorable with neuropathies that occur acutely.[193]

- Sciatic Neuropathies

Sciatic neuropathies are often painful and may lead to a causalgic syndrome. Sensory complaints and sensory loss occur in the entire foot and the distal-lateral leg. The ankle jerk and, on occasion, the internal hamstring reflex are diminished or absent on the affected side. Ambulation is significantly impaired. A severe sciatic neuropathy results in weakness involving all motions of the ankle and toes as well as flexion of the leg at the knee. Abduction and extension of the thigh at the hip should be spared. As previously mentioned, the peroneal functions of the sciatic nerve are typically involved disproportionately to their tibial counterparts.[194,195] Misdiagnosis of a common peroneal neuropathy may occur with incomplete sciatic neuropathies which may be the most common differential diagnostic consideration. Other considerations include length-dependent monomelic polyneuropathies from lower extremity arterial occlusion, sacral plexopathy, or lumbosacral polyradiculopathy. Distinction between sciatic mononeuropathy and these entities can usually be easily made by careful EDX evaluation. If the cause of sciatic neuropathy is inapparent, MRI with gadolinium from sciatic notch to popliteal fossa is suggested.

Sciatic neuropathies are most commonly traumatic, most notably related to hip arthroplasty or fracture/dislocations.[185,194–197] There are numerous other diverse causes including penetrating trauma, intramuscular injections, hemorrhage into the piriformis region, aneurysm of the inferior gluteal artery, prolonged lithotomy positioning, vasculitis, endometrial implants leading to catamenial sciatica, prolonged immobility leading to a gluteal compartment syndrome sometimes resulting from sitting on a hard surface, also known as "toilet seat" neuropathy, infiltration by lymphoma, intraoperative thigh tourniquet, persistent sciatic arteries, gluteal varicosities, and nerve sheath tumors.[198–204] Sciatic neuropathy has been reported to occur in association with cardiac surgery, presumably due to an ischemic mechanism related to intra-arterial balloon placement or concomitant peripheral vascular disease.[205] Sciatic neuropathies in the pediatric population have different causes including inadvertent injection into the umbilical artery in a newborn.[206]

A potential and controversial cause of sciatic nerve entrapment is the piriformis syndrome.[207,208,209] Symptoms consist of buttock and posterior thigh pain reproduced by maneuvers that stretch the sciatic nerve. Provocative diagnostic maneuvers such as tenderness to palpation in the inferior medial quadrant of the buttock, or exacerbation of pain by passively internally rotating, adducting and flexing the thigh while the patient is in supine position, actively abducting the thigh against resistance in the seated position, or abducting the thigh of the symptomatic side while in the left lateral recumbent positions have been reported.[209] Objective clinical and EDX evidence of nerve injury are notable for their absence. Demonstrating a prolonged H reflex latency in the symptomatic leg when the thigh is maintained in a flexed, internally rotated, and adducted position is a reported but unvalidated means by which to support the diagnosis.[209] It has been reported that ipsilateral evidence of piriformis enlargement coupled with MR evidence of nerve edema has a 93% specificity and 64% sensitivity in identifying this syndrome as determined by surgical outcome.[210] Conversely, the piriformis has been reported to be atrophied ipsilaterally in chronic cases. The proposed mechanism for the piriformis syndrome is sciatic nerve compression by an abnormal piriformis muscle or an abnormal relationship between nerve and muscle as the nerve exits the pelvis at the sciatic notch. The nerve typically exits below the muscle, but on occasion exits above or traverses through it.

We favor conservative therapy with stretching or targeted injections with local anesthetics and steroids.[209] Recently, injection with botulinum toxin utilized in an attempt to relax the piriformis muscle and relieve pressure on the sciatic nerve has been reported to have beneficial result.[209] We avoid any consideration of exploration in the absence of objective, clinical, EDX, or convincing imaging abnormalities.

- Common fibular neuropathy

Common fibular mononeuropathies along with meralgia paresthetica are the most commonly occurring lower extremity mononeuropathies. Fibular neuropathies often occur with a paucity of pain, present in only a fifth of patients, and typically with minimal sensory symptoms.[151] As a result, recognition is commonly prompted by the development of foot drop. The pattern of weakness is distinctive, affecting foot and toe dorsiflexion and foot eversion alone, thus distinguishing it from other causes of foot drop. Like all partial nerve injuries, there may be either diminished sensation or hypersensitivity. This tends to be subtle and found on the distal-lateral leg and/or the dorsum of the foot. Deep tendon reflexes are spared in the absence of a second confounding problem. The differential diagnosis includes an L5 radiculopathy, a partial sciatic neuropathy, a lumbosacral trunk lesion, motor neuron disease, or a distal myopathy if foot drop is bilateral.

Causes of common fibular neuropathy include structural pathology of the fibular head including cysts of the tibiofibular joint, external compression particularly following weight loss or habitual leg crossing, casts or compression stockings, surgery, closed or open trauma, prolonged squatting, fibular fractures, dislocated knees, surgery in the popliteal fossa, vasculitis, fibular tumors, Baker cysts, stretch injuries from acute plantar flexion/inversion or prolonged knee flexion during childbirth, and acute occlusion of femoral or popliteal arteries.[151,211–215] Thirteen of 103 patients in one series were diabetic, representing a possible predisposition to compressive injury.[151] Peroneal neuropathies occur in childhood as well.[216]

- Tibial neuropathy

Tibial neuropathies proximal to the ankle are uncommon. The pattern of weakness of a tibial mononeuropathy in isolation varies by location. Knee flexion is weak with a lesion near or proximal to the hip joint but is spared with lesions located distal to the proximal thigh. Lesions in the distal thigh or proximal leg are typically associated with weakness of foot plantar flexion and inversion, toe flexion, and, if detectable, toe abduction. Sensory symptoms and sensory loss are confined to the sole of the foot and the very distal aspect of the dorsal surface of the toes. Depression or loss of the ankle jerk is invariable. Tibial mononeuropathies are most commonly confused with S1 monoradiculopathies.

Tibial neuropathies typically result from trauma, tumor, or ischemia. Traumatic causes account for approximately half of all cases. The nature of the trauma is variable and may include compression from casts or tourniquets, hip arthroplasty, gunshot and other penetrating wounds, tibial fractures, and gluteal injections. Acute limb ischemia was the most common nontraumatic cause in one series affecting approximately 20% of patients (see length-dependent monomelic neuropathy below).[217] Coexistent fibular neuropathies may occur in both traumatic and ischemic etiologies. Rare causes include idiopathic hypertrophic nerve lesions, ruptured Baker cysts, and hematoma formation in the popliteal fossa.

Tarsal tunnel syndrome is a controversial entity most closely associated with external compression from tight-fitting foot wear or prior ankle injury.[218–221] Arguably, it is associated with symptoms more than signs. In a manner analogous to carpal tunnel syndrome, patients may be typically plagued by pain in the ankle and foot and dysesthesias often burning in of the sole that are intermittent and worse nocturnally. As weakness of tibial innervated intrinsic foot muscles may be difficult to clinically detect, objective motor deficits are uncommon. Due to the frequent calloused condition of the sole of the foot, detection of credible sensory loss may be challenging. The validity of Tinel sign at the flexor retinaculum is uncertain. It is estimated that only 10% of patients referred to neurologists with suspected tarsal tunnel syndrome will receive that diagnosis when subjected to careful clinical and EDX scrutiny.[218] The majority of these individuals will be found to have plantar fasciitis or sensory neuropathy.

- Sural neuropathy

  Sural mononeuropathies are uncommon other than as a consequence of nerve biopsy. Sural neuropathies present with some combination of numbness, pain, or paresthesias on the lateral foot in the cutaneous distribution of the nerve. Sural neuropathies are most commonly traumatic in etiology associated with ankle injury, surgery, or vein stripping procedures. Schwannomas, ganglionic cysts, Baker cysts or their surgery, fracture of the base of the fifth metatarsal, arthroscopic knee surgery, muscle biopsy of the calf, compression from the hard upper edges of ski boots, vasculitis, and idiopathic are other recognized causes.[222–224] Electrodiagnostic confirmation is readily obtained unless confounded by comorbidity such as polyneuropathy.

- Pudendal neuropathy

  Pudendal neuropathy typically presents with chronic perineal pain. It is typically aggravated by sitting, relieved by standing, and resolves when supine or sitting without pressure placed on the perineum, for example, a toilet seat.[10] Distinguishing pudendal neuropathy from the more common indeterminate causes of perineal pain may be aided by the concomitant description of numbness or other sensory symptoms of the penis, scrotum, labia majora, and perineum. If bilateral, disturbances in micturition, defecation, erection, and ejaculation may occur.[225]

  Pudendal neuropathy may result from pelvic and hip fractures, injection injuries, hemorrhage into piriformis, neoplastic invasion, surgical procedures, childbirth, or prolonged or inordinate pressure on perineum from ill-fitting bicycle seats or pressure devices that may be used to reduce hip dislocations.[225,226] Predisposition to entrapment or compression is thought to be facilitated by the relationship of the pudendal nerve with the sacrotuberous and sacrospinous ligaments or the ischial tuberosity as the nerve exits the pelvis through Alcock's canal where fibrosis of the obturator internus muscle has been described.[10,227]

  The diagnosis of pudendal neuropathy is challenging as there are limited objective findings to distinguish true neuropathy from the seemingly far more prevalent cases of undefined perineal and genital pain and sensory symptoms such as vulvodynia and proctalgia fugax that may defy objective diagnosis. Some of these have been attributed to pudendal neuralgia presumed but unproven to represent an entrapment syndrome.[228] A number of EDX techniques have been applied to the evaluation of the pudendal nerves including nerve conduction studies but we have limited confidence in either their sensitivity or specificity in the identification of pudendal nerve injury.[229] Identifying evidence of denervation confined to the external anal sphincter would provide strong supportive evidence of axon loss injury to the pudendal nerve. MRI is of value in selective cases.[10] Relief of symptoms with pudendal nerve block would serve both a diagnostic and therapeutic purpose.[230] Surgical intervention should be undertaken judiciously and is recommended only in those cases with significant morbidity and definable pathology.[231]

▶ MONOMELIC POLYNEUROPATHY

The monomelic polyneuropathies are relatively uncommon disorders that typically directly or indirectly result from acute limb ischemia. Occlusion of major limb vessels such as the aortic bifurcation, external iliac, or superficial femoral artery resulting from embolus or instrumentation such as intra-aortic balloon pumping or arterial cannulation associated with coronary bypass grafting are the typical causes in the lower extremities.[75,232,233,234] Implicit in the description of this syndrome is the belief that nerve is either more readily injured or less readily recoverable with acute limb ischemia than are other limb tissues. Chronic limb ischemia has been reported to associate with electrodiagnostic findings, suggesting length-dependent axon loss.[234–238] Whether this ever translates into a clinically evident neuropathy in the absence of other tissue damage is a matter of controversy.

Most disorders that affect multiple nerves or multiple nerve roots are systemic disorders that typically affect more than one extremity. Monomelic polyneuropathies bear resemblance to plexopathies in that both motor and sensory deficits occur, affecting more than one nerve distribution but confined to a single extremity. The dominant feature is deep, persistent, burning pain in the foot associated with cutaneous hypersensitivity. The distribution of motor and sensory deficits is typically length dependent, affecting all nerves below the knee and typically below mid calf. Muscle innervated by those same nerves and segments more proximally located are spared.[232] Although motor deficits occur, like length-dependent axonal polyneuropathies, these are typically less evident from a clinical perspective. Part of this stems from the clinical difficultly in clinically assessing the most severely affected intrinsic foot muscles. From an EDX standpoint, this syndrome may resemble a sciatic neuropathy. Notable differences are that the hamstring muscles tend to be spared and the saphenous sensory response will be abnormal in monomelic polyneuropathy if it can be reliably contrasted to the uninvolved opposite limb. The EDX pattern of monomelic polyneuropathy is unique in that it is a multifocal neuropathy, but one that is both length dependent and confined to one limb as the name implies in the majority of cases.

Compartment syndromes refer to ischemic tissue damage within confined anatomic spaces typically bordered by taut fascial membranes. Peripheral nerves are at risk from the cycle of ischemia that is created by increased compartmental pressure. Typically, an initial injury promotes edema and increased compartment pressure. This impairs compartment perfusion and promotes further ischemic injury and, as a result, further swelling. A vicious positive feedback cycle is thus created. Pressure blisters, a swollen limb, and/or myoglobinuria are potentially associated clinical features that may warn of impending nerve injury or aid to clarify the mechanism of nerve injury.[239,240] Many of the mononeuropathies previously mentioned in this chapter are at risk of injury from immobilization, either due to a direct pressure or in association with nerve injury occurring from more diffuse compartmental pressure. Recognized compartment syndromes in the lower extremity include sciatic neuropathy from the gluteal compartment or posterior compartment of the thigh syndromes, femoral neuropathy from the iliacus compartment or within the anterior thigh, and a peroneal palsy resulting from an anterior compartment syndrome in the leg.[240,241]

Imaging of the involved area will typically identify swelling and signal changes within the muscle of that compartment. Manometric measurements may confirm elevated pressure within that compartment, pressures as low as 30 mm Hg being potentially injurious to nerve.[239] A compartment syndrome is a surgical emergency that requires decompression and potentially debulking of the involved anatomic compartment(s).

▶SUMMARY

Focal neuropathies of the lower extremities are common neurologic problems that are frequently caused by compressive mechanisms. Clinically directed localization supplemented by electrodiagnostic testing (when required) provides the foundation for the evaluation of these disorders. When the neuropathy cannot be readily attributed to a common compressive mechanism, imaging rationally directed by the localization process facilitates identification of less commonly occurring secondary causes of individual nerve injury.

Focal neuropathies are potentially more amenable to surgical intervention than are the majority of disorders described elsewhere in this text. Many of these disorders will have natural histories that are self-limited and a decision to surgically intervene should not be based solely on EDX or imaging data. Once again, the skilled and judicious neuromuscular clinician is in a unique position to provide both accurate disease identification and optimal management.

REFERENCES

1. Levin KH. L5 radiculopathy with reduced superficial peroneal sensory responses: intraspinal and extraspinal causes. *Muscle Nerve*. 1998;2:3–7.
2. Pellerin M, Kimball Z, Tubbs RS, et al. The prefixed and postfixed brachial plexus: a review with surgical implications. *Surg Radiol Anat*. 2010;32:251–260.
3. Jellema K, Tijssen CC, van Jin JC. Spinal dural arteriovenous fistulas: a congestive myelopathy that initially mimics a peripheral nerve disorder. *Brain*. 2006;129:3150–3164.
4. Mathews JA. Wasting of small hand muscles in upper and mid-cervical cord lesions. *Q J Med*. 1998;91:691–700.
5. Deyo RA, Weinstein JN. Low back pain. *N Engl J Med*. 2001; 344(5):363–370.
6. Devereaux MW. Anatomy and examination of the spine. *Neurol Clin*. 2007;25:331–351.
7. Furusawa N, Baba H, Miyoshi N, et al. Herniation of cervical intervertebral disc: immunohistochemical examination and measurement of nitric oxide production. *Spine*. 2001;26: 1110–1116.
8. Kang JD, Georgescu HI, McIntyre-Larkin L, Stefanovic-Racic M, Evans CH. Herniated cervical intervertebral discs spontaneously produce matrix metalloproteinases, nitric oxide, interleukin-6 and prostaglandin E2. *Spine*. 1995;20: 2373–2378.
9. Kang JD, Stefanovic-Racic M, McIntyre LA, Georgescu HI, Evans CH. Toward a biochemical understanding of human intervertebral disc degeneration and herniation: contributions of nitric oxide, interleukins, prostaglandin E2 and matrix metalloproteinases. *Spine*. 1997;22:1065–1073.
10. Martinoli C, Miguel-Perez M, Padua L, Gandolfo N, Zicca A, Tagliafico A. Imaging of neuropathies about the hip. *Eur J Radiol*. 2013;82(1):17–26.
11. Burakgazi AZ, Kelly JJ, Richardson P. The electrodiagnostic sensitivity of proximal lower extremity muscles in the diagnosis of L5 radiculopathy. *Muscle Nerve*. 2012;45:891–893.
12. Rutkove SB, Nardin RA, Raynor EM, Levy ML, Landrio MA. Lumbosacral radiculopathy mimicking distal polyneuropathy. *J Clin Neuromuscul Dis*. 2000;2:65–69.
13. Tramontozzi LA III, Russell JA. Orthostatic intolerance in multifocal acquired demyelinating sensory and motor neuropathy. *J Clin Neuromusc Dis*. 2012;14(1):34–39.
14. Stewart JD. Magnificent MRI and fascinating selective nerve fascicle damage. *Neurology*. 2014;82:554–555.
15. Pham M, Bäumer P, Meinck HM, et al. Anterior interosseous nerve syndrome: fascicular motor lesions of median nerve trunk. *Neurology*. 2014;82:598–606.
16. Therapeutics and Technology Assessment Subcommittee of the American Academy of Neurology. Review of the literature on spinal ultrasound for the evaluation of back pain and radicular disorders. *Neurology*. 1996;51:343–344.

17. Delaney H, Bencardino J, Rosenberg ZS. Magnetic resonance neurography of the pelvis and lumbosacral plexus. *Neuroimaging Clin N Am*. 2014;24(1):127–150.
18. Filosto M, Pari E, Cotelli M, et al. MR neurography in diagnosing nondiabetic lumbosacral radiculoplexus neuropathy. *J Neuroimaging*. 2013;23(4):543–544.
19. Ishii K, Tamaoka A, Shoji S. MRI of idiopathic lumbosacral plexopathy. *Neurology*. 2004;63:E6.
20. Mathys C, Aissa J, Hörste GM, et al. Peripheral neuropathy: assessment of proximal nerve integrity by tensor imaging. *Muscle Nerve*. 2013;48:889–896.
21. Spangfort E. LaSègue's sign in patients with lumbar disc herniation. *Acta Orthop Scand*. 1971;42:459–460.
22. Dyck P. The femoral nerve traction test with lumbar disc protrusions. *Surg Neurol*. 1976;6:166–166.
23. Bozzao A, Gallucci M, Masciocchi C, Aprile I, Barile A, Passariello R. Lumbar disc herniation: MR imaging assessment of natural history in patients treated without surgery. *Radiology*. 1992;185:135–141.
24. Delauche-Cavallier MC, Budet C, Laredo JD, et al. Lumbar disc herniation: computed tomography scan changes after conservative treatment of nerve root compression. *Spine*. 1992; 17:927–933.
25. Tilki HE, Mutluer N, Selcuki D, Stalberg E. Zoster paresis. *Electromyogr Clin Neurophysiol*. 2003;43(4):231–234.
26. Akiyama N. Herpes zoster infection complicated by motor paralysis. *J Dermatol*. 2000;27(4):252–257.
27. Cockerell OC, Ormerod IE. Focal weakness following herpes zoster. *J Neurol Neurosurg Psychiatry*. 1993;56(9):1001–1003.
28. Kawajiri S, Tani M, Noda K, Fujishima K, Hattori N, Okuma Y. Segmental zoster paresis of limbs: report of three cases and review of literature. *Neurologist*. 2007;13(5):313–317.
29. Thomas JE, Howard F. Segmental zoster paresis—a disease profile. *Neurology*. 1972;22:459–466.
30. Bahadir C, Kalpakcioglu EB, Kurtulus D. Unilateral diaphragmatic paralysis and segmental motor paresis following herpes zoster. *Muscle Nerve*. 2008;38:1070–1073.
31. Bartleson JD. *Update in Spine Disorders. Annual Meeting of the American Academy of Neurology*. Course 72 – Neurology Update 1. Philadelphia, PA: American Academy of Neurology; 2014.
32. Boden SD, Davis DO, Dina TS, Patronas NJ, Wiesel SW. Abnormal magnetic resonance scans of the lumbar spine in asymptomatic subjects: a prospective investigation. *J Bone Joint Surg Am*. 1990;72:403–408.
33. Jensen M, Brant-Zawadzki M, Obuchowski N, Modic MT, Malkasian D, Ross JS. Magnetic resonance imaging of the lumbar spine in people without back pain. *N Engl J Med*. 1994;331: 69–73.
34. Malmivarra A, Hakkinen U, Aro T, et al. The treatment of acute low back pain—bed rest, exercise or ordinary activity? *N Engl J Med*. 1995;332:331–335.
35. Deyo RA, Diehl AK, Rosenthal M. How many days of bed rest for acute low back pain? *N Engl J Med*. 1986;315:1064–1070.
36. Weber H. Lumbar disc herniation: a prospective study of prognostic factors including a controlled trial. *J Oslo City Hosp*. 1978;28:33–64, 89–120.
37. Cherkin DC, Deyo RA, Battié M, Street J, Barlow W. A comparison of physical therapy, chiropractic manipulation, and provision of an educational booklet for the treatment of patients with low back pain. *N Engl J Med*. 1998;339:1021–1029.
38. Andersson GB, Lucente T, Davis AM, Kappler RE, Lipton JA, Leurgans S. A comparison of osteopathic spinal manipulation with standard care for patients with low back pain. *N Engl J Med*. 1999;341:1426–1431.
39. Haimovic IC, Beresford HR. Dexamethasone is not superior to placebo for treating lumbosacral radicular pain. *Neurology*. 1986;36:1593–1594.
40. Armon C, Argoff C, Samuels J, Backonja MM. Assessment: use of epidural steroid injections to treat radicular lumbosacral pain: report of the Therapeutics and Technology Assessment Subcommittee of the American Academy of Neurology. *Neurology*. 2007;68:723–729.
41. Carette S, Leclaire R, Marcous S, et al. Epidural corticosteroid injections for sciatica due to herniated nucleus pulposus. *N Engl J Med*. 1997;336:1634–1640.
42. Carette S, Marcoux S, Truchon R, et al. A controlled trial of corticosteroid injections into facet joints for chronic low back pain. *N Engl J Med*. 1991;325:1002–1007.
43. MacVicar J, King W, Landers MH, Bogduk N. The effectiveness of lumbar transforaminal injection of steroids: a comprehensive review with systematic analysis of the published data. *Pain Med*. 2013;14:14–28.
44. Yuen EC, Layzer RB, Weitz SR, Olney RK. Neurologic complications of lumbar epidural anesthesia and analgesia. *Neurology*. 1995;45:1795–1801.
45. Deyo RA, Walsh NE, Martin DC, Schoenfeld LS, Ramamurthy S. A controlled trial of transcutaneous electrical nerve stimulation (TENS) and exercise for chronic low back pain. *N Engl J Med*. 1990;322:1627–1634.
46. Beurskens AJ, de Vet HC, Koke AJ, et al. Efficacy of traction for nonspecific low back pain: 12-week and 6-month results of a randomized clinical trial. *Spine*. 1997;22:2756–2762.
47. Gibson AJ, Waddell G. Surgical interventions for lumbar disc prolapse. *Cochrane Database Syst Rev*. 2008.
48. Hakelius A. Prognosis in sciatica: a clinical follow-up of surgical and non-surgical treatment. *Acta Orthop Scand (Suppl)*. 1970;129:1–76.
49. Nashold BS, Hrubec A. *Lumbar Disc Disease: A 20-Year Clinical Follow-Up Study*. St Louis, MO: Mosby; 1971.
50. Weber H. Lumbar disc herniation: a controlled, prospective study with 10 years of observation. *Spine*. 1983;8:131–140.
51. Chad DA. Lumbar spinal stenosis. *Neurol Clin*. 2007;25: 407–418.
52. Hall S, Bartleson JD, Onofrio BM, Baker HL Jr, Okazaki H, O'Duffy JD. Lumbar spinal stenosis: clinical features, diagnostic procedures, and results of surgical treatment in 68 patients. *Ann Intern Med*. 1985;103:271–275.
53. Katz JN, Harris MB. Lumbar spinal stenosis. *N Engl J Med*. 2008;358:818–825.
54. Guigui P, Benoist M, Delecourt C, Delhoume J, Deburge A. Motor deficit in lumbar spinal stenosis: a retrospective study of a series of 50 patients. *J Spinal Disord*. 1998; 11(4):238–288.
55. Montagna OM, Nartubekku OM, Rasi F, Girignotta F, Govoni E, Lugaresi E. Muscular hypertrophy after chronic radiculopathy. *Arch Neurol*. 1984;41:397–398.
56. Swartz KR, Fee DB, Trost GR, Waclawik AJ. Unilateral calf hypertrophy seen in lumbosacral stenosis. *Spine*. 2002;27:E406–E409.
57. Levin KH, Covington EC, Devereaux MW, et al. *Neck and Back Pain*. Vol 7. Philadelphia, PA: Continuum, American

Academy of Neurology, Williams, Wilkins and Lippincott; 2001:60

58. Moreland L, Lopez-Mendez A, Alarcon G. Spinal stenosis: a comprehensive review of the literature. *Semin Arthritis Rheum.* 1989;19:127–149.
59. Porter R. Spinal stenosis and neurogenic claudication. *Spine.* 1996;21:2046–2052.
60. Choi SK, Bowers RP, Buckthal PE. MR Imaging in hypertrophic neuropathy: a case of hereditary motor and sensory neuropathy, type I (Charcot-Marie-Tooth). *Clin Imaging.* 1990;14:204–207.
61. Diederichs G, Hoffmann J, Klingebiel R. CIDP-induced spinal canal obliteration presenting as lumbar spinal stenosis. *Neurology.* 2007;68(9):701.
62. De Silva RN, Willison HJ, Doyle D, Weir AI, Hadley DM, Thomas AM. Nerve root hypertrophy in chronic inflammatory demyelinating polyneuropathy. *Muscle Nerve.* 1994;17:168–170.
63. Ginsberg L, Platts AD, Thomas PK. Chronic inflammatory demyelinating polyneuropathy mimicking a lumbar spinal stenosis syndrome. *J Neurol Neurosurg Psychiatry.* 1995;59: 189–191.
64. Goldstein JM, Parks BJ, Mayer PL, Kim JH, Sze G, Miller RG. Nerve root hypertrophy as the cause of lumbar stenosis in chronic inflammatory demyelinating polyradiculoneuropathy. *Muscle Nerve.* 1996;19(7):892–896.
65. Deyo RA, Diehl A. Cancer as a cause of back pain: frequency, clinical presentation, and diagnostic strategies. *J Gen Intern Med.* 1988;3(3):230–238.
66. Kaplan JG, DeSouza TG, Farkash A, et al. Leptomeningeal metastases: comparison of clinical features and laboratory data of solid tumors, lymphomas and leukemias. *J Neurooncol.* 1990;9(3):225–229.
67. Little JR, Dale AJ, Okazaki H. Meningeal carcinomatosis. *Arch Neurol.* 1974;30(2):138–143.
68. Viali S, Hutchinson DO, Hawkins TE, et al. Presentation of intravascular lymphomatosis as lumbosacral polyradiculopathy. *Muscle Nerve.* 2000;23:1295–1300.
69. Wasserstrom W, Glass J, Posner J. Diagnosis and treatment of leptomeningeal metastases from solid tumors: experience with 90 patients. *Cancer.* 1982;49:759–772.
70. Armon C, Daube JR. Electrophysiological signs of arteriovenous malformations of the spinal cord. *J Neurosurg Neurol Psychiatry.* 1989;52:1176–1181.
71. Atkinson JL, Miller GM, Krauss WF, et al. Clinical and radiographic features of dural arteriovenous fistula, a treatable cause of myelopathy. *Mayo Clin Proc.* 2001;76:1120–1130.
72. Linden D, Berlit P. Spinal arteriovenous malformations: clinical and neurophysiologic findings. *J Neurol.* 1996;243:9–12.
73. Schrader V, Koenig E, Thron A, Dichgans J. Neurophysiologic characteristics of spinal arteriovenous malformations. *Electro Clin Neurophys.* 1989;29:169–177.
74. Lee SB, Hall CW, Wijdicks EF. Monoplegia due to acute aortic occlusion. *Muscle Nerve.* 2005;32(5):686–687.
75. Larson Wl, Wald JJ. Foot drop as a harbinger of aortic occlusion. *Muscle Nerve.* 1995;18:899–903.
76. Levin KH, Daube JR. Spinal cord infarction: another cause of "lumbosacral polyradiculopathy." *Neurology.* 1984;34:389–390.
77. Baker AS, Ojemann RG, Swartz MN, Richardson EP Jr. Spinal epidural abscess. *N Engl J Med.* 1975;293:463–468.
78. Davis DP, Wold RM, Patel RJ, et al. The clinical presentation and impact of diagnostic delays on emergency department patients with spinal epidural abscess. *J Emerg Med.* 2004;26(3):285–291.
79. Del Burling O, Gower DJ, McWhorter JM. Changing concepts in spinal epidural abscess: a report of 29 cases. *Neurosurgery.* 1990;27(2):185–192.
80. Heusner AP. Nontuberculous spinal epidural infections. *N Engl J Med.* 1948;239(23):845–854.
81. Mackenzie AR, Laing RB, Smith CC, Kaar GF, Smith FW. Spinal epidural abscess: the importance of early diagnosis and treatment. *J Neurol Neurosurg Psychiatry.* 1998;65(2):209–212.
82. Nussbaum ES, Rigamonti D, Standiford H, Numaguchi Y, Wolf AL, Robinson WL. Spinal epidural abscesses: a report of 40 cases and review. *Surg Neurol.* 1992;38(3):225–231.
83. Corral I, Querada C, Casado JL, et al. Acute polyradiculopathies in HIV-infected patients. *J Neurol.* 1997;244(8):499–504.
84. Benatar MG, Eastman RW. Human immunodeficiency virus-associated pure motor lumbosacral polyradiculopathy. *Arch Neurol.* 2000;57(7):1034–1039.
85. de Gans J, Portegies P, Tiessens G, Troost D, Danner SA, Lange JM. Therapy for cytomegalovirus polyradiculomyelitis in patients with AIDS: treatment with ganciclovir. *AIDS.* 1990;4(5):421–425.
86. So YT, Olney RK. Acute lumbosacral polyradiculopathy in acquired immunodeficiency syndrome: experience in 23 patients. *Ann Neurol.* 1994;35(1):53–58.
87. Whitely RJ, Jacobson MA, Friedberg DN, et al. Guidelines for the treatment of cytomegalovirus diseases in patients with AIDS in the era of potent antiretroviral therapy: recommendations of an international panel. *Arch Intern Med.* 1998;158(9):957–969.
88. Logigian EL, Steere AC. Clinical and electrophysiologic findings in chronic neuropathy of Lyme disease. *Neurology.* 1992;42:303–311.
89. Halperin JJ. Lyme disease and the peripheral nervous system. *Muscle Nerve.* 2003;28(2):133–143.
90. Halperin JJ, Shapiro ED, Logigian E, et al. Practice parameter: Treatment of nervous system Lyme disease (an evidence-based review). Report of the quality standards subcommittee of the American Academy of Neurology. *Neurology.* 2007;69(1):91–102.
91. Carod Artal FJ, Vargas AP, Horan TA, Marinho PB, Coelho Costa PH. Schistosoma mansoni myelopathy: clinical and pathologic findings. *Neurology.* 2004;63(2):388–391.
92. Burns TM, Dyck PJ, Aksamit AJ, Dyck PJ. The natural history and long-term outcome of 57 limb sarcoidosis neuropathy cases. *J Neurol Sci.* 2006;244(1–2):77–87.
93. Koffman B, Junck L, Elias ST, Feit HW, Levine SR. Polyradiculopathy in sarcoidosis. *Muscle Nerve.* 1999;22(5):608–613.
94. Verma KK, Forman AD, Fuller GN, Dimachkie MM, Vriesendorp FJ. Cauda equina syndrome as the isolated presentation of sarcoidosis. *J Neurol.* 2000;247:573–574.
95. Molyneux PD, Barker R, Thomas PK, King RH, Miller DH. Non-systemic vasculitic neuropathy presenting with a painful polyradiculopathy. *J Neurol.* 2000;247(8):645–646.
96. Muhn N, Baker SK, Hollenberg RD, Meaney BF, Tarnopolsky MA. Syringomyelia presenting as rapidly progressive foot drop. *J Clin Neuromuscul Dis.* 2002;2(3):133–134.
97. Miller DW, Katirji F, Preston DC. Idiopathic epidural lipomatosis. *J Clin Neuromuscul Dis.* 2005;6:144–146.
98. Berlit P, Schwechheimer K. Neuropathological findings in radiation myelopathy of the lumbosacral cord. *Eur Neurol.* 1987;27:29–34.

99. Bowen J, Gregory R, Squier M, Donaghy M. The post-irradiation lower motor neuron syndrome: neuronopathy or radiculopathy. *Brain*. 1996;119:1429–1439.
100. Greenfield MM, Stark FM. Post-irradiation neuropathy. *AJR Am J Roentgenol*. 1948;60:617–622.
101. Kristensen O, Melgard B, Schiodt AV. Radiation myelopathy of the lumbo-sacral spinal cord. *Acta Neurol Scand*. 1977;56:217–222.
102. Lamy C, Mas JL, Varet B, Ziegler M, de Rocondo J. Post-radiation lower motor neuron syndrome presenting as monomelic amyotrophy. *J Neurol Neurosurg Psychiatry*. 1991; 54:648–649.
103. Maier JG, Perry RH, Saylor W, Sulak MH. Radiation myelitis of the dorsolumbar spinal cord. *Radiology*. 1969;93:153–160.
104. Pettigrew LC, Glass JP, Maor M, Zornoza J. Diagnosis and treatment of lumbosacral plexopathies in patients with cancer. *Arch Neurol*. 1984;41:1282–1285.
105. Thomas JE, Cascino TL, Earle JD. Differential diagnosis between radiation and tumor plexopathy of the pelvis. *Neurology*. 1985;35:1–7.
106. van der Sluis RW, Wolfe GI, Nations SP, et al. Post-radiation lower motor neuron syndrome. *J Clin Neuromuscul Dis*. 2000;2:10–17.
107. Feistner H, Weissenborn K, Munte FT, Heinze HJ, Malin JP. Post-irradiation lesions of the caudal roots. *Acta Neurol Scand*. 1989;80:277–281.
108. Mitsunaga Y, Yoshimura T, Hara H, Yamada T, Kira J, Kobayashi T. A case of cervical radiation radiculopathy resembling motor neuron disease. *Rinsho Shinkeigaku*. 1998;38:450–452.
109. Hsia AW, Katz JS, Hancock SL, Peterson K. Post-irradiation polyradiculopathy mimics leptomeningeal tumor on MRI. *Neurology*. 2003;60:1694–1696.
110. Haig AJ, Tomkins CC. Diagnosis and management of lumbar spinal stenosis. *JAMA*. 2010;303(1):71–72.
111. Haig AJ, Tong HC, Yamakawa KS et al. Spinal stenosis, back pain, or no symptoms at all? A masked study comparing radiologic and electrodiagnostic diagnosis to the clinical impression. *Arch Phys Med Rehabil*. 2006;87(7):897–903.
112. Wilbourn AJ, Aminoff MJ. AAEM minimonograph 32: the electrodiagnostic examination in patients with radiculopathies. *Muscle Nerve*. 1998;21:1612–1631.
113. Kuchta J, Sobottke R, Eysel P, Simons P. Two year results of interspinous spacer (X-Stop) implantation in 175 patients with neurologic intermittent claudication due to lumbar spinal stenosis. *Eur Spine J*. 2009;18:1823–1829.
114. Bastron JA, Thomas JE. Diabetic polyradiculopathy, clinical and electromyographic findings in 105 patients. *Mayo Clin Proc*. 1981;56:725–732.
115. Barohn R, Sahenk Z, Warmolts JR, Mendell JR. The Bruns-Garland syndrome (diabetic amyotrophy) revisited 100 years later. *Arch Neurol*. 1991;48:1130–1135.
116. Dyck PJ, Norell JE, Dyck PJ. Microvasculitis and ischemia in diabetic lumbosacral radiculoplexus neuropathy. *Neurology*. 1999;53(9):2113–2121.
117. Dyck PJ, Windebank AJ. Diabetic and non-diabetic lumbosacral radiculoplexus neuropathies: new insights into pathophysiology and treatment. *Muscle Nerve*. 2002;25(4):477–491.
118. Garces-Sanchez M, Laughlin RS, Dyck PJ, Engelstad JK, Dyck PJ. Painless diabetic motor neuropathy: a variant of diabetic lumbosacral radiculoplexus neuropathy. *Ann Neurol*. 2011;69:1043–1054.
119. Levin KH, Wilbourn AJ. Diabetic radiculopathy without peripheral neuropathy. *Muscle Nerve*. 1991;14:889.
120. Laughlin RS, Dyck PJ, Melton LJ, Leibson C, Ransom J, Dyck PJ. Incidence and prevalence of CIDP and the association of diabetes mellitus. *Neurology*. 2009;73:39–45.
121. Kelkar P, Hammer-White S. Impaired glucose tolerance in nondiabetic lumbosacral radiculoplexus neuropathy. *Muscle Nerve*. 2005;31(2):273–274.
122. Sumner CJ, Sheth S, Griffin JW, Cornblath DR, Polydefkis M. The spectrum of neuropathy in diabetes and impaired glucose tolerance. *Neurology*. 2003;60(1):108–111.
123. Said G, Elgrably F, Lacroix C, et al. Painful proximal diabetic neuropathy: Inflammatory nerve lesions and spontaneous favorable outcome. *Ann Neurol*. 1997;41(6):762–770.
124. Sander JE, Sharp FR. Lumbosacral plexus neuritis. *Neurology*. 1981;31:470–473.
125. Bradley WG, Chad D, Verghese JP. Painful lumbosacral plexopathy with elevated erythrocyte sedimentation rate: a treatable inflammatory syndrome. *Ann Neurol*. 1984;15:457–464.
126. Dyck PJ, Engelstad J, Norell J, Dyck PJ. Microvasculitis in nondiabetic lumbosacral radiculoplexus neuropathy (LSRPN): similarity to the diabetic variety (DLSRPN). *J Neuropathol Exp Neurol*. 2000;59(6):525–538.
127. Dyck PJ, Norell JE, Dyck PJ. Non-diabetic lumbosacral radiculoplexus neuropathy: natural history, outcome and comparison with the diabetic variety. *Brain*. 2001;124:1197–1207.
128. Evans BA, Stevens JC, Dyck PJ. Lumbosacral plexus neuropathy. *Neurology*. 1981;31:1327–1330.
129. Tarulli A, Rutkove SB. Lumbosacral plexitis. *J Clin Neuromuscul Dis*. 2005;7:72–78.
130. Yee T. Recurrent idiopathic lumbosacral plexopathy. *Muscle Nerve*. 2000;23:1439–1442.
131. Gloviczki P, Cross SA, Stanson AW, et al. Ischemic injury to the spinal cord or lumbosacral plexus after aorto-iliac reconstruction. *Am J Surg*. 1991;162:131–136.
132. Chiu WS. The syndrome of retroperitoneal hemorrhage and lumbar plexus neuropathy during anticoagulant therapy. *South Med J*. 1976;69(5):595–599.
133. Emery S, Ochoa J. Lumbar plexus neuropathy resulting from retroperitoneal hemorrhage. *Muscle Nerve*. 1978;1:330–334.
134. Aho K, Sainio K. Late irradiation-induced lesions of the lumbosacral plexus. *Neurology*. 1983;33:953–955.
135. Jaeckle KA, Young DF, Foley KM. The natural history of lumbosacral plexopathy in cancer. *Neurology*. 1985;35:8–15.
136. Ladha SS, Spinner RJ, Suarez GA, Amrami KK, Dyck PJ. Neoplastic lumbosacral radiculoplexopathy in prostate cancer by direct perineural spread: an unusual entity. *Muscle Nerve*. 2006;34(5):659–665.
137. Georgiu A, Grigsvy PW, Perez DA. Radiation induced lumbosacral plexopathy in gynecologic tumors: clinical findings and dosimetric analysis. *Int J Oncol Biol Phys*. 1993;26:479–482.
138. Ladha SS, Dyck PJ, Spinner RJ, et al. Isolated amyloidosis presenting with lumbosacral radiculoplexopathy: description of two cases and pathogenic review. *J Peripher Nerv Syst*. 2006;11(4):346–352.
139. Kutsy RL, Robinson LR, Routt ML. Lumbosacral plexopathy in pelvic trauma. *Muscle Nerve*. 2000;23:1757–1760.
140. Felice KJ, Donaldson JO. Lumbosacral plexopathy due to benign uterine leiomyoma. *Neurology*. 1995;45:1943–1944.
141. Zuninga G, Ropper A, Frank J. Sarcoid peripheral neuropathy. *Neurology*. 1991;41:1558–1561.

142. Hudcova J, Schumann R, Russell JA. Epidural analgesia and postpartum lumbosacral neurologic deficit: a dilemma. *Anesthesiology*. 2004;100(suppl 1):69, A123.
143. Katirji MB, Wilbourn A, Scarberry S, Preston DC. Intrapartum maternal lumbosacral plexopathy. *Muscle Nerve*. 2002;26 (3):340–347.
144. Kawagashira Y, Watanabe H, Oki Y, et al. Intravenous immunoglobulin therapy markedly ameliorates muscle weakness and severe pain in proximal diabetic neuropathy. *J Neurol Neurosurg Psychiatry*. 2007;78(8):899–901.
145. Dyck PJ, Norell JE, Dyck PJ. Methylprednisolone may improve lumbosacral radiculplexus neuropathy. *Can J Neurol Sci*. 2001;28:224–227.
146. Krendel DA, Costigan DA, Hopkins LC. Successful treatment of neuropathies in patients with diabetes mellitus. *Arch Neurol*. 1995;52:1053–1061.
147. Zochodne DW, Isaac D, Jones C. Failure of immunotherapy to prevent, arrest or reverse diabetic lumbosacroal plexopathy. *Acta Neurol Scand*. 2003;107:299–301.
148. Dyck JB, O'Brien PC, Bosch EP, et al. Results of a controlled trial of IV methylprednisolone in diabetic lumbosacral radiculoplexus neuropathy (DLPRN): a preliminary indication of efficacy. *J Peripher Nerve Syst* 2005;10(suppl 1):21.
149. Verma A, Bradley WG. High-dose intravenous immunoglobulin therapy in chronic progressive lumbosacral plexopathy. *Neurology*. 1994;44(2):248–250.
150. Pradat P-F, Bouche P, Delanian S. Sciatic nerve mononeuropathy: an unusual late effect of radiotherapy. *Muscle Nerve*. 2009;40:872–874.
151. Katirji MB, Wilbourn AJ. Common peroneal mononeuropathy: a clinical and electrophysiologic study of 116 lesions. *Neurology*. 1988;38:1723–1728.
152. Grant GA, Britz GW, Goodkin R, Jarvik JG, Maravilla K, Kliot M. The utility of magnetic resonance imaging in evaluating peripheral nerve lesions. *Muscle Nerve*. 2002;25:314–331.
153. Halford H, Graves A, Bertorinie T. Muscle and nerve imaging techniques in neuromuscular diseases. *J Clin Neuromusc Dis*. 2000;2:41–51.
154. Walker FO, Cartwright MS, Wiesler ER, Caress J. Ultrasound of nerve and muscle. *Clin Neurophysiol*. 2004;115:495–507.
155. Cartwright MS, Chloros GD, Walker FO, Wiesler ER, Campbell WW. Diagnostic ultrasound for nerve transaction. *Muscle Nerve*. 2007;35:796–799.
156. Koltzenburg M, Bendszus M. Imaging of peripheral nerve lesions. *Curr Opin Neurol*. 2004;17:621–626.
157. Briani C, Cacciavillani M, Lucchetta M, Cecchin D, Gasparotti R. MR neurography findings in axonal multifocal motor neuropathy. *J Neurol*. 2013;260(9):2420–2422.
158. Robinson LR. Traumatic injury to peripheral nerves. *Muscle Nerve*. 2000;23:863–873.
159. Toussaint CP, Perry EC II, Pisansky MT, Anderson DE. What's new in the diagnosis and treatment of peripheral nerve entrapment neuropathies. *Neurol Clin*. 2010;28:979–1004.
160. Miller JP, Acar F, Kaimaktchiev VB, Gultekin SH, Burchiel KJ. Pathology of ilioinguinal neuropathy produced by mesh entrapment: case report and literature review. *Hernia*. 2008;12(2): 213–216.
161. Ndiaye A, Diop M, Ndoye JM, et al. Anatomical basis of neuropathies and damage to the ilioinguinal nerve during repairs of groin hernias (about 100 dissections). *Surg Radiol Anat*. 2007;29(8):675–681.
162. Vuillemier H, Hubner M, Demartines N. Neuropathy after herniorraphy: indication for surgical treatment and outcome. *World J Surg*. 2009;33(4):841–845.
163. Hahn L. Clinical findings and results of operative treatment in ilioinguinal nerve entrapment syndrome. *Br J Obstet Gynaecol*. 1989;96(9):1080–1083.
164. Nahabedian MY, Dellon AL. Outcome of the operative management of nerve injuries in the ilioinguinal region. *J Am Coll Surg*. 1997;184(3):265–268.
165. Lee CH, Dellon AL. Surgical management of groin pain of neural origin. *J Am Coll Surg*. 2000;191(2):137–142.
166. Murovic JA, Kim DH, Tiel RL, Kline DG. Surgical management of 10 genitoremoral neuralgias at the Louisiana State University Health Sciences Center. *Neurosurgery*. 2005;56(2):298–303.
167. Chutkow JG. Posterior femoral cutaneous neuralgia. *Muscle Nerve*. 1988;11:1146–1148.
168. Schiller F. Sigmund Freud's meralgia paresthetica. *Neurology*. 1985;35:557–558.
169. Parisi TJ, Mandrekar J, Dyck PJ, Klein C. Meralgia paresthetica: relation to obesity, advanced age and diabetes mellitus. *Neurology*. 2011;77:1538–1542.
170. Berini SE, Spinner RJ, Jentoft ME, et al. Chronic meralgia paresthetica and neurectomy: a clinical pathologic study. *Neurology*. 2014;82:1551–1555.
171. Seror P, Seror R. Meralgia paresthetica: clinical and electrophysiological diagnosis in 120 cases. *Muscle Nerve*. 2006;33: 650–654.
172. Grossman MG, Ducey SA, Nadler SS, Levy AS. Meralgia paresthetica: diagnosis and treatment. *J Am Acad Orthop Surg*. 2001;9(5):336–344.
173. Nahabedian MY, Dellon AL. Meralgia paresthetica: etiology, diagnosis, and outcome of surgical decompression. *Ann Plast Surg*. 1995;35(6):590–594.
174. Ducic I, Dellon AL, Taylor NS. Decompression of the lateral femoral cutaneous nerve in the treatment of meralgia paresthetica. *J Reconstruct Microsurg*. 2006;22(2):113–118.
175. Khalil N, Nicotra A, Rakowicz W. Treatment for meralgia paraesthetica. *Cochrane Database Syst Rev*. 2008;(3): CD004159.
176. Kuntzer T, van Melle G, Regli F. Clinical and prognostic features in unilateral femoral neuropathies. *Muscle Nerve*. 1997;20:205–211.
177. Van Veer H, Coosemans W, Pirenne J, Monbaliu D. Acute femoral neuropathy: a rare complication after renal transplantation. *Transplant Proc*. 2010;42(10):4384–4388.
178. Peirce C, O'Brien C, O'Herlihy C. Postpartum femoral neuropathy following spontaneous vaginal delivery. *J Obstet Gynaecol*. 2010;30(2):203–204.
179. Al-Ajmi A, Rousseff RT, Khuraibet AJ. Iatrogenic femoral neuropathy: two cases and literature update. *J Clin Neuromusc Dis*. 2010;12(2):66–75.
180. Moore AE, Stringer MD. Iatrogenic femoral nerve injury: a systematic review. *Surg Radiol Anat*. 2011;33(8):649–658.
181. Young MR, Norris JW. Femoral neuropathy during anticoagulant therapy. *Neurology*. 1976;26:1173–1175.
182. Massey EW, Tim RW. Femoral compression neuropathy from a mechanical pressure clamp. *Neurology*. 1989;39:1263.
183. Frew N, Foster P, Maury A. Femoral nerve palsy following traumatic posterior dislocation of the hip. *Injury, Int J Care Injured*. 2013;44:261–262.

184. Clarke-Pearson DL, Geller EJ. Complications of hysterectomy. *Obstet Gynecol.* 2013;121:654–673.
185. Schmalzried TP, Amstutz HC, Dorey FJ. Nerve palsy associated with total hip replacement. *J Bone Joint Surg.* 1991;73A(7):1074–1080.
186. Mastroiannia PP, Roberts MP. Femoral neuropathy and retroperitoneal hemorrhage. *Neurosurgery.* 1983;13(1):44–47.
187. Kaku DA, So YT. Acute femoral neuropathy and iliopsoas infarction in intravenous drug users. *Neurology.* 1990;40:1317–1318.
188. Romanoff ME, Cory PC Jr, Kalenak A, Keyser GC, Marshall WK. Saphenous nerve entrapment at the adductor canal. *Am J Sports Med.* 1997;17(4 a):478–481.
189. Worth RM, Kettelkamp DB, Defalque RJ, Duane KU. Saphenous nerve entrapment. A cause of medial knee pain. *Am J Sports Med.* 1984;12(1):80–81.
190. Sole JS, Pingree MJ, Spinner RJ, Murthy NS, Sellon JL. Saphenous neuropathy secondary to extraneural ganglion cyst 15 years after reconstruction of the anterior cruciate ligament. *PM R.* 2014;6(5):451–455.
191. Shenoy AM, Wiesman J. Saphenous mononeuropathy after popliteal vein aneurysm repair. *Neurologist.* 2010;16(1):47–49.
192. Rogers LR, Borkowski GP, Albers JW, Levin KH, Barohn RJ, Mitsumoto H. Obturator mononeuropathy caused by pelvic cancer: six cases. *Neurology.* 1993;43:1489–1492.
193. Sorenson EJ, Chen JJ, Daube JR. Obturator neuropathy: causes and outcome. *Muscle Nerve.* 2002;25(4):605–607.
194. Yuen EC, Olney RK, So YT. Sciatic neuropathy: clinical and prognostic features in 73 patients. *Neurology.* 1994;44:1669–1674.
195. Yuen EC, So YT, Olney RK. The electrophysiologic features of sciatic neuropathy in 100 patients. *Muscle Nerve.* 1995;18:414–420.
196. Goldberg G, Goldstein H. AAEM case report 32: nerve injury associated with hip arthroplasty. *Muscle Nerve.* 1998;21:519–527.
197. Nercessian OA, Macaulay W, Stinchfield FE. Peripheral neuropathies following total hip arthroplasty. *J Arthroplasty.* 1994; 9:645–651.
198. Salazar-Grueso E, Roos R. Sciatic endometriosis: a treatable sensorimotor mononeuropathy. *Neurology.* 1986;36:1360–1363.
199. Holland NR, Schwarz-Williams L, Blotzer JW. Toilet seat" sciatic neuropathy. *Arch Neurol.* 1999;56:116.
200. Kornetzky L, Linden D, Berlit P. Bilateral sciatic nerve "Saturday night palsy". *J Neurol.* 2001;248(5):425.
201. Preston DC, Shapiro BE. Lymphoma of the sciatic nerve. *J Clin Neuromuscul Dis.* 2001;2:227–228.
202. Gasecki AP, Ebers GC, Vellet AD, Buchan A. Sciatic neuropathy associated with persistent sciatic artery. *Arch Neurol.* 1992;49:967–968.
203. Bendszus M, Rieckmann P, Perez J, Koltzenburg M, Reiners K, Solymosi L. Painful vascular compression syndrome of the sciatic nerve caused by gluteal varicosities. *Neurology.* 2003;61:985–987.
204. Flanagan W, Webster GD, Brown MW, Massey EW. Lumbosacral plexus stretch injury following the use of the modified lithotomy position. *J Urol.* 1985;134:567–568.
205. McManis PG. Sciatic nerve lesions during cardiac surgery. *Neurology.* 1994;44:684–687.
206. Srinivasan J, Ryan MM, Escolar DM, Darras B, Jones HR. Pediatric sciatic neuropathies: a 30-year prospective study. *Neurology.* 2011;76(11):976–980.
207. Stewart JD. The piriformis syndrome is overdiagnosed. *Muscle Nerve.* 2003;28(5):644–646.
208. Fishman LM, Schaefer MP. The piriformis syndrome is underdiagnosed. *Muscle Nerve.* 2003;28(5):646–649.
209. Kirschner JS, Foye PM, Cole JL. Piriformis syndrome, diagnosis and treatment. *Muscle Nerve.* 2009;40:10–18.
210. Filler AG, Haynes J, Jordan SE, et al. Sciatica of non-disc origin and piriformis syndrome: diagnosis by magnetic resonance neurography and interventional magnetic resonange imaging with outcome study of resulting treatment. *J Neurosurg Spine.* 2005;2:99–115.
211. Iverson DJ. MRI detection of cysts of the knee causing common peroneal neuropathy. *Neurology.* 2005;65:1829–1831.
212. Sotaniemi KA. Slimmer's paralysis—peroneal neuropathy during weight reduction. *J Neurol Neurosurg Psychiatry.* 1984;47:564–566.
213. Campellone JV. Peroneal neuropathy from antithrombotic stockings. *J Clin Neuromuscul Dis.* 1999;1:14–16.
214. Uncini A, Di Muzio A, Awad J, Gambi D. Compressive bilateral peroneal neuropathy: serial electrophysiologic studies and pathophysiological remarks. *Acta Neurol Scand.* 1992;85: 66–70.
215. Adornato B, Carlini WG. Pushing palsy: a case of self-induced bilateral peroneal palsy during natural childbirth. *Neurology.* 1992;42(4):936–937.
216. Jones HR, Felice KJ, Gross PT. Pediatric peroneal mononeuropathy: a clinical and electromyographic study. *Muscle Nerve.* 1993;16:1167–1173.
217. Drees C, Wilbourn AJ, Stevens GH. Main trunk tibial neuropathies. *Neurology.* 2002;59:1082–1084.
218. Alsharabati M, Oh SJ. How common is tarsal tunnel syndrome? *Muscle Nerve.* 2009;40:689–690.
219. Delisa JA, Saeed MA. The tarsal tunnel syndrome. *Muscle Nerve.* 1983;6:664–670.
220. Goodgold J, Kopell HP, Spielholz NI. The tarsal-tunnel syndrome: objective diagnostic criteria. *N Engl J Med.* 1965; 273(14):742–745.
221. Oh SJ, Sarala PK, Kuba T, Elmore RS. Tarsal tunnel syndrome: electrophysiological study. *Ann Neurol.* 1979;5:327–330.
222. Li Y, LedermanRJ. Sural mononeuropathy: a report of 36 cases. *Muscle Nerve.* 2014;49:443–445.
223. Smith HB, Litchy WJ. Sural mononeuropathy: a clinical and electrophysiological study. *Neurology.* 1989;39(suppl 1):296.
224. Stickler DE, Morley KN, Massey EW. Sural neuropathy: etiologies and predisposing factors. *Muscle Nerve.* 2006;34: 482–484.
225. Silbert PL, Dunne JW, Edis RH, Stewart-Wynne EG. Bicycling induced pudendal nerve pressure neuropathy. *Clin Exp Neurol.* 1991;28:191–196.
226. Andersen KV, Bovim G. Impotence and nerve entrapment in long distance amateur cyclists. *Acta Neurol Scand.* 1997;95:233–240.
227. Insola A, Granata G, Padua L. Alcock canal syndrome due to obturator internus. *Muscle Nerve.* 2010;42:431–432.
228. Stav K, Dwyer PL, Roberts L. Pudendal neuralgia. Fact or fiction? *Obstet Gynecol Surg.* 2009;64(3):190–199.
229. O'Brien C, O'Herlihy C, O'Connell PR. Pudendal neuropathy is best determined by full neurophysiologic assessment. *Am J Obstret Gynecol.* 2004;191(5):1836.
230. Hough DM, Wittenberg KH, Pawlina W, et al. Chronic perineal pain caused by pudendal nerve entrapment: anatomy and CT-

guided perineural injection technique. *AJR Am J Roentgenol.* 2003;181:561–567.
231. Hruby S, Dellon L, Ebmer J, Höltl W, Aszmann OC. Sensory recovery after decompression of the distal pudendal nerve: anatomical review and quantitative neurosensory data of a prospective clinical study. *Microsurgery.* 2009;29(4): 270–274.
232. Wilbourn AJ, Furlan AJ, Hulley W, Ruschhaupt W. Ischemic monomelic neuropathy. *Neurology.* 1983;33:447–451.
233. Lachance DH, Daube JR. Acute peripheral arterial occlusion: electrophysiologic study of 32 cases. *Muscle Nerve.* 1991;14(7):633–639.
234. Levin KH. AAEE case report #19: ischemic monomelic neuropathy. *Muscle Nerve.* 1989;12:791–795.
235. England JD, Ferguson MA, Hiatt WR, Regensteiner JG. Progression of neuropathy in peripheral arterial disease. *Muscle Nerve.* 1995;18:380–387.
236. Nukada H, van Rij AM, Packer SG, McMorran PD. Pathology of acute and chronic ischaemic neuropathy in atherosclerotic peripheral vascular disease. *Brain.* 1996;119:1449–1460.
237. Weber F, Ziegler A. Axonal neuropathy in chronic peripheral arterial occlusive disease. *Muscle Nerve.* 2002;26:471–476.
238. Weinberg DH, Simovic D, Isner J, Ropper AH. Chronic ischemic monomelic neuropathy from critical limb ischemia. *Neurology.* 2001;57:1008–1012.
239. Shields RW, Root KE, Wilbourn AJ. Compartment syndromes and compression neuropathies in coma. *Neurology.* 1986;36:1370–1374.
240. Farrell CM, Rubin DI, Haidukewych GJ. Acute compartment syndrome of the leg following diagnostic electromyography. *Muscle Nerve.* 2003;27:374–377.
241. Poppi M, Giuliani G, Gambari PI, Acciarri N, Gaist G, Calbucci F. A hazard of craniotomy in the sitting position: the posterior compartment syndrome of the thigh. *J Neurosurg.* 1989;71:618–619.

CHAPTER 25

Autoimmune Myasthenia Gravis

Acquired, autoimmune myasthenia gravis (MG), the most common noniatrogenic disorder of neuromuscular transmission (DNMT), remains the favorite child of many neuromuscular clinicians. Arguably, it provides more professional satisfaction than any other neuromuscular disease. This fulfillment is derived in part from the intellectual satisfaction that comes from understanding disease pathogenesis. At the same time, satisfaction is gained by the ability to make meaningful improvements in patient function and quality of life through the application of rational and effective treatment. MG represents one of medicine's most notable translational successes in bringing basic science to the bedside.

Although descriptions of individuals likely to have been affected by MG can be traced to antiquity, our current understanding of disease mechanism(s) originates from a series of seminal observations and discoveries. Thomas Willis, a seventeenth-century physiologist, is frequently credited for initially describing the clinical syndrome of MG. The concept of MG as a DNMT and the first therapeutic triumph are often credited to British clinician Mary Walker. She described the benefits of cholinesterase inhibitors in the 1930s; her discovery extrapolated from her observations related to the similarities between MG and curare toxicity. In 1960, Simpson first promoted the hypothesis of an autoimmune basis for MG on the basis of his observations of an increased prevalence in young women and in individuals with other autoimmune diseases.[1] In that same decade, support for MG as a DNMT was provided by the in vitro electrophysiological demonstration that miniature end plate potential (EPP) amplitudes in MG were greatly reduced.[2] In 1973 Daniel Drachman et al. solidified the concept of MG as a postsynaptic DNMT by demonstrating loss of acetylcholine receptors (AChR) in MG patients through α-bungarotoxin labeling techniques.[3] In the same year, Patrick and Lindstrom confirmed the autoimmune nature of MG with the development of an experimental MG model in rabbits who became weak when immunized with AChR.[4] In 1976, the seminal article describing the value of AChR autoantibody testing in the diagnosis of myasthenia was published.[5] In 2001, Hoch et al. first reported the association between MG and autoantibodies directed against muscle-specific kinase (MuSK).[6] In 2008, unnamed autoantibodies directed at clustered AChRs were found in low titer in the serum of approximately two-thirds of AChR and MuSK seronegative patients.[7,8] In 2011, patient's with autoantibodies directed at the lipoprotein receptor protein 4 (LPR4) were identified as a third MG serotype.[9]

Historically, seronegative MG referred to patients lacking AChR autoantibodies. With the discovery of MuSK autoantibodies, the concept of double seronegative MG patients was coined. As our knowledge of LPR4 MG is somewhat limited, and as LPR4 autoantibody tests are not commercially available at the time of writing this, seropositive will be used in this chapter to refer only to AChR and MuSK MG.

The incidence of MG and its serodistribution may vary with geography and/or ethnicity.[10] MG has been estimated to occur in 2–10/10^6 individuals/year in the Eastern United States and the Netherlands but up to 20/10^6 people/year in Eastern Spain.[11–13] The prevalence is estimated to be as infrequent as 2 and as frequent as 200/10^6 individuals.[13–24] The age of onset may also be influenced by geographical and/or ethnic differences. Juvenile onset MG is uncommon in occidental populations but may represent more than half of cases in Asian populations.[25] Heritable MG is rare, estimated to occur in approximately 2% of cases although the concordance rate in monozygotic twins is estimated at 40%.[23,26–28] Under the age of 40, AChR MG is almost three times more common in women. Men and women in their 40s however, are affected with equal frequency whereas in older individuals, the prevalence is greater in men at a ratio of 1.5:1.[29,30]

Understanding normal and abnormal neuromuscular transmission (NMT) is relevant not only to MG but to other DNMT that may be either acquired or heritable, resulting from genetic, infectious/toxic, or paraneoplastic/autoimmune mechanisms. These mechanisms typically act individually, but be synergistic. For example, a family has been recently reported in which there appears to be synergy between genetic and autoimmune influences. Multiple family members with seropositive MG were found to have mutations in the ecto-NADH oxidase 1 gene (ENOX1), a gene expressed in both thymus and skeletal muscles.[31] The mechanism by which this mutation, posited to predispose to autoimmunity, might cause MG remains unknown. It is thought to relate to sequence homologies between ENOX1 and the main immunogenic region (MIR) of the alpha-1 subunit of the AChR. This provides a theoretical explanation for a heritable and anatomically targeted autoimmune disorder.[32]

This chapter will focus on acquired, autoimmune MG, a postsynaptic disorder representing the prototype of DNMT. Chapter 26 will discuss the less frequently occurring infectious/toxic and genetic (i.e., CMS or congenital myasthenic syndromes) DNMT, both categories which can be conceptualized and categorized as adversely affecting NMT at the presynaptic, synaptic, or postsynaptic levels.

▶ CLINICAL FEATURES

Acquired MG typically evolves subacutely over days to months and reaches its clinical nadir within 2 years.[33] The majority of patients are seropositive and usually have similar phenotypes regardless of the existence or type of autoantibody. Individual cases may have differing clinical features and natural histories, that may allow prediction of an individual serotype and different responsiveness to treatment.[10] Each section of this chapter will describe the general features of the disease in its classical form associated with binding autoantibodies directed toward the AChR, and will then distinguish the differing features of other serotypes when applicable.

The natural history of myasthenia is difficult to predict in an individual patient. Information is, in a large part, derived from historical data accumulated prior to the availability of current therapeutic options.[13] It is recognized that approximately 15–20% of Caucasian patients with initial signs and symptoms restricted to the oculomotor system will retain this restricted phenotype.[33] Ninety percent of those destined to develop generalized disease will do so within 2 years of symptom onset and a similar number will reach the nadir of their disease within a 7-year period.[13,34,35] It has been suggested, but by no means universally accepted, that immunomodulating treatment may diminish the risk of evolving into generalized disease.[36,37] Spontaneous, remissions unrelated to treatment are estimated to occur in between 10-22% of MG patients.[13,30] These remissions may occur at any time in the course of the disease. Half of the patient's who achieve spontaneous remission, relapse within 6 months and 90% within a year.[13,30] Regarding therapeutic decisions, however, there is no apparent correlation between the existence and length of remission and maximal disease severity.[13] Mortality statistics in MG has been undoubtedly altered by therapeutic intervention. At the turn of the twentieth century it was approximated at 70%, reduced to 23–30% by the 1950s, with contemporary estimates in the 1.2–2.2% range.[13,23,38]

The diagnosis of myasthenia is clinically established by two phenotypic features, the pattern of weakness and its tendency to fluctuate. There are theories underlying the selected vulnerability of certain muscles in MG that will be addressed in the pathophysiology section. The basis for the characteristic patterns of weakness in MG remains, however, largely speculative.[39] It may be related to the distribution of different types of neuromuscular junctions (NMJs) in different muscles.

The fluctuating nature of myasthenic symptoms is related to the dynamic biology of the NMJ.[40] It is a quality of the disease that may be a dominant feature of the patient's history or may be overlooked. MG patients may recognize that their symptoms may vary on a minute-to-minute, diurnal, or week-to-week basis.[41–44] For example, a patient may describe normal articulation at the onset of a telephone conversation and may have unintelligible speech 5 minutes later. Patients may observe normal eyelid position upon awakening and then develop ptosis as the day wears on. Fluctuation may not be simply diurnal and patients may have functional hardships one month that seem to improve on their own the next month without apparent explanation. Fluctuations may also occur in response to identifiable variables such as temperature, systemic infection, menses, anxiety, emotional stress, and pregnancy.[18,45–50] Myasthenic visits to emergency rooms are known to increase in frequency in early morning hours in equatorial countries where electricity and therefore air conditioning may not be available at night, making this potentially the warmest period of the day. Variability may also occur not only in the timing but in the pattern of weakness. Alternating ptosis represents the most notable example of this phenomenon. It should be emphasized that diurnal worsening of strength and stamina is not pathognomonic of MG as the weakness of any neuromuscular disease may worsen as the day goes on.

MG may also be suspected by the pattern of weakness. MG should be considered in any patient with painless weakness, particularly when the weakness is multifocal or diffuse in distribution or when weakness of ocular and bulbar muscles predominates. Asymmetry is not uncommon, particularly with ptosis. Most myasthenics will experience ptosis, diplopia, dysphagia, dysphonia, difficulty chewing, or symptoms referable to facial or neck weakness, either in isolation or in combination. Identification of weakness in muscles innervated by anatomically unrelated cranial nerves, for example, concomitant weakness of eyelid opening and eyelid closure represents a common and diagnostically useful example.

Initial symptoms restricted to ptosis or diplopia will be the presenting symptoms of MG patients in 65–85% of cases and 95% will experience oculomotor involvement at some point in their illness.[33,37,43,51,52] Overt diplopia may be preceded by nonspecific visual blurring when ocular malalignment is minimal and insufficient to produce two distinct images. The presence of other signs and symptoms of myasthenia or the resolution of blurring the covering of either eye aids in the identification of blurring due to ocular malalignment. Other than the levator palpebrae, the medial rectus appears to be most susceptible of the extraocular muscles. Any pattern of ophthalmoparesis may occur, however, potentially mimicking an individual cranial nerve palsy or intranuclear ophthalmoplegia, or at times even producing nystagmus.[53,54,55]

Bulbar symptoms typically refer to disordered speech and swallowing but will be extended here to include weakness of jaw, facial, and neck muscles. Bulbar onset of MG is quite common particularly in our experience in older men, and is estimated to occur in approximately 15% of cases.[55] Weakness of bulbar muscles is estimated to occur in >40% of MG patients sometime in their illness. As bulbar weakness may be associated with considerable morbidity, we consider bulbar symptoms to be indicative of generalized MG; ocular MG being restricted to ptosis and diplopia. Speech may be adversely affected in a number of ways. The voice may be hypophonic due to vocal cord paresis or expiratory muscle weakness.[56–58] It may have a nasal quality due to palatal insufficiency and nasal air leak. The patient may be dysarthric as a result of weakness of the lips, tongue, or cheeks. Nasal regurgitation of food and liquid, difficulty manipulating food due to tongue weakness, as well as ineffective sniffing, coughing, nose blowing, or throat clearing may be noted.

Facial weakness is common. Lower facial weakness may result in dysarthria or sialorrhea, or in difficulty whistling, inflating balloons, or drinking from a straw. It may also interfere with the accuracy of pulmonary function testing due to poor oral seal. Weakness of upper facial muscles is equally prevalent but less likely to be symptomatic. Occasionally, patients may complain of visual blurring due to lower lid weakness resulting in pooling of tears. Facial weakness can be easily missed if not sought for, particularly if bilateral. Patients who are affected may be unable to bury their eyelashes or maintain eye closure against resistance. They may be unable to whistle, make a kissing noise, or hold air in their distended cheeks against resistance. A "myasthenic snarl," may occur in which the mid-portion of the upper lip elevates without elevation of the corners of the mouth during an attempted smile.

Symptoms and signs referable to jaw weakness, particularly jaw closing, occur fairly commonly in MG. Although jaw weakness may occur in other neuromuscular diseases, many of the other causes, for example, Guillain–Barré syndrome, are unlikely to have a phenotype readily confused with MG.[59] Like most neuromuscular diseases, neck flexor weakness is more common and more pronounced than neck extensors weakness in the majority but not in all MG patients. Head drop is not rare however, and may be the presenting symptom. Like other causes of head drop, posterior neck pain relieved by head support may be the most prominent symptom associated with this sign, presumably related to the stretch placed on posterior cervical muscles and ligaments by the weight of the head. Ventilatory insufficiency is a rare presenting symptom of MG but may develop in a significant percentage of patients with untreated or refractory generalized disease.[58,60] Along with dysphagia, it is undoubtedly the predominant basis for mortality in MG unrelated to complications of treatment or immobility.

Limb weakness occurs in 20–30% of affected individuals. Limb weakness preferentially affects proximal muscles.[61,62] One potential but undoubtedly partial explanation is the warmer temperature of the proximal limbs.[63] Typically, limb weakness occurs in concert with the signs and symptoms of oculobulbar disease. In approximately 10% of patients with limb involvement, MG may be initially restricted to distal limb muscles, with foot or finger drop being notable presentations that have been reported and that we have seen.[64–69] Again, the pattern may be focal, multifocal, or diffuse.[43]

MUSK MG

Approximately 7–15% of all MG patients or 40% of seronegative patients with generalized MG are estimated to have MuSK autoantibodies.[6,10,55,70–76] On average, MuSK MG patients are younger and more severely affected than their AChR MG counterparts although MuSK MG rarely if ever develops in an individual in the first decade of life.[10,77,78] Disease prevalence in MuSK MG is highest in the third and fourth decades of life in non-Asian populations. In some series, males and females are affected equally whereas in other series, females have predominated.[73,77,79–81]

Most MuSK MG patients will have a phenotypic pattern indistinguishable from AChR MG patients. Nonetheless, there are certain clinical features that suggest an increased or decreased probability of MuSK MG.[70–88] For example, purely ocular disease is a rare MuSK MG phenotype.[71–73,77,86,87] Patterns that suggest an increase probability of MuSK MG include persistent bulbar symptoms refractory to treatment, prominent neck, facial, and ventilatory muscle weakness and the presence of muscle atrophy in an otherwise typical MG patient, notably in the tongue.[10,72] The latter finding may render the clinical distinction from bulbar amyotrophic lateral sclerosis (ALS) more difficult.[55,77,79,88] As MuSK is known to facilitate reinnervation, it is plausible that the atrophy noted in this serotype may be related to a "denervating" effect of MuSK autoantibodies.[89] MuSK MG patients in general have more severe disease both at onset and disease nadir, are less likely to achieve complete remission with treatment, and are more likely to experience myasthenic crises than either their AChR or seronegative counterparts.[10,77–79]

SERONEGATIVE MG INCLUDING PATIENTS WITH LPR4 AUTOANTIBODIES

Seronegative MG may represent up to 34% of MG patients depending on the study and the ethnic background of the cohort studied.[10] In 2008, a high sensitivity assay discovered IgG1 autoantibodies in two-thirds of these seronegative MG patients.[7] In 2011, an epitope on the LPR4 protein was found to be the target of IgG1 autoantibodies, presumably the same autoantibodies described 3 years previously.[9] These patients, historically included in the seronegative group, represent a very small percentage of MG patients.[89] Studies to date have estimated that LPR4 autoantibodies are found in 3%, 9%, and 50% of seronegative MG patients.[9,25,90] These significant differences may represent differences between ethnicities, differences in methodology, or accuracies relevant to small sample size; the 50% figure originating from a study of only 13 patients.[90]

The weight of current evidence suggests seronegative MG, with or without LPR4 autoantibodies, manifests phenotypic, natural history and response to treatment features similar, if not identical, to AChR MG.[7,10,91] Otherwise seronegative patients possessing low titers of IgG1 autoantibodies

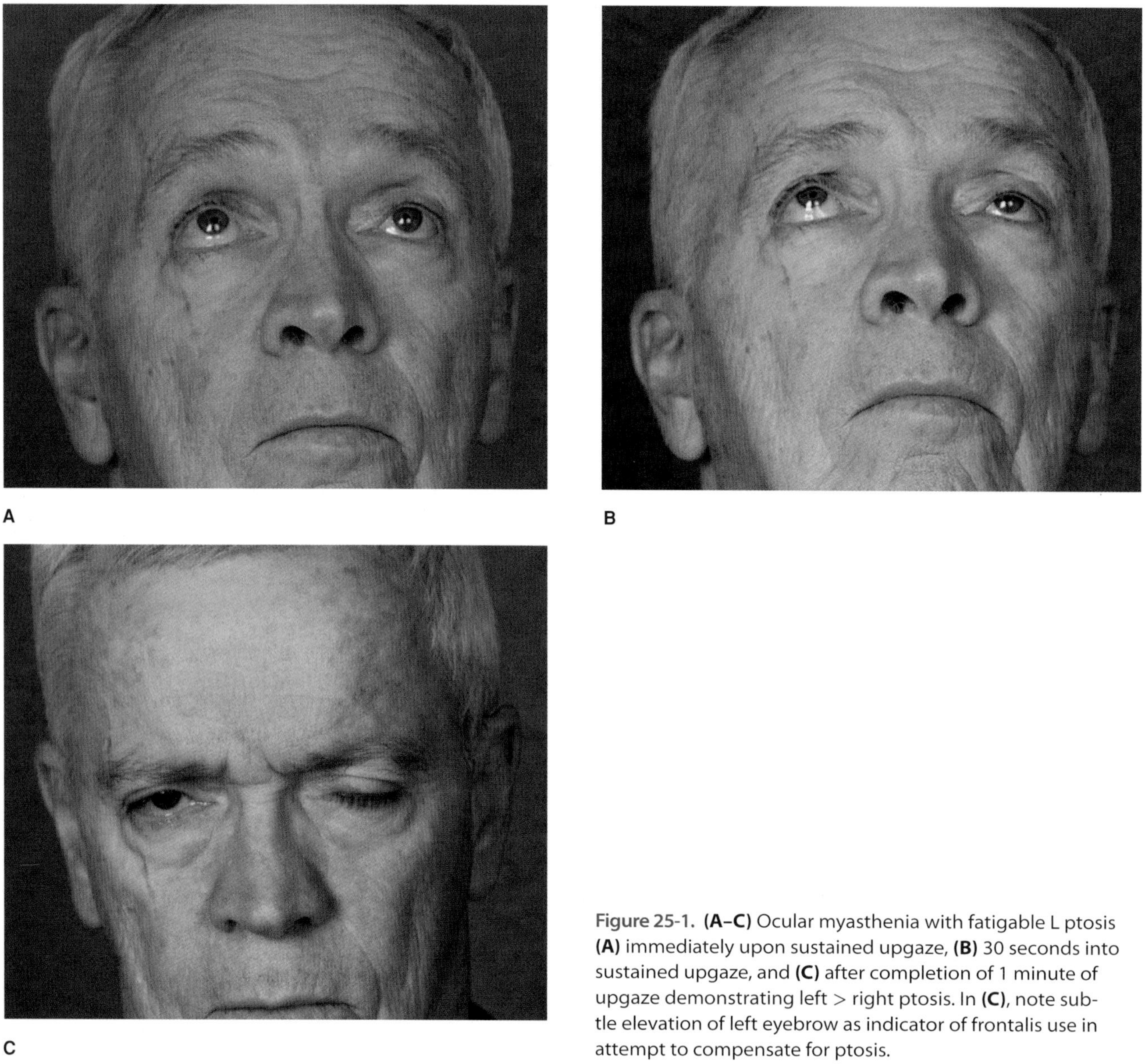

Figure 25-1. **(A–C)** Ocular myasthenia with fatigable L ptosis **(A)** immediately upon sustained upgaze, **(B)** 30 seconds into sustained upgaze, and **(C)** after completion of 1 minute of upgaze demonstrating left > right ptosis. In **(C)**, note subtle elevation of left eyebrow as indicator of frontalis use in attempt to compensate for ptosis.

directed toward clustered AChRs have been reported to exist in approximately two-thirds of all seronegative AChR/MuSK MG and half of ocular seronegative MG patients, potentially explaining at least in part the high prevalence of conventional seronegativity in this latter population.[7,8,91]

The examination of the suspected or established MG patient includes a number of unique or relatively unique features. As ptosis is such a common manifestation of MG, documentation of the baseline upper and lid positions in relationship to the pupil is recommended prior to provocative testing and to distinguish ptosis from squinting, both of which narrow the palpebral fissure.

In MG, pupil function is spared although physiological anisocoria is common enough to provide a potentially confounding feature. In order to unmask or exacerbate ptosis or extraocular muscle weakness, the suspected MG patient is asked to sustain either up or lateral gaze for a minute while limiting blinking as much as possible (Fig. 25-1A–C). Drifting of lid or eyeball position is watched for. Cogan's lid twitch is another sign thought to be a relatively specific, although not necessarily sensitive, sign in MG assessment. With this maneuver, the patient is first asked to look down and then rapidly saccade to reassume the primary position. Normally the eyelid moves synchronously with the eyeball. A positive sign is defined by the eyelid overshooting the eyeball position leading to a transient scleral exposure and upper lid oscillation.

Another maneuver with potential diagnostic benefit has been referred to as enhanced ptosis.[92] This maneuver has been described in patients with bilateral asymmetric ptosis but is conceptually of value in apparent unilateral ptosis as well. In this maneuver, the clinician manually elevates the most affected eyelid which may result in the revelation or exacerbation of ptosis on the opposite side in an MG patient. The proposed explanation for this phenomenon is Hering's law of equal innervation. Theoretically, with manual lid elevation, there is less need for supranuclear stimulation of the levator subnucleus of the oculomotor nerve. As this is a single midline nucleus which innervates both levator palpebrae muscles, lifting the more severely affected lid leads to the need for less supranuclear stimulation of this subnucleus affecting the contralateral as well as ipsilateral levator palpebrae.

The last bedside maneuver relative to the evaluation of ptosis is the icepack test which relies on the recognized physiological enhancement of NMT by cooling. In this maneuver, an ice pack applied to a closed eyelid may result in notable improvement of existing ptosis. As the icepack is potentially noxious, exposure should be limited to a minute or less.

As motor neuron disease is often the major differential diagnostic consideration in patients with painless weakness who do not have ptosis or diplopia, the clinical assessment of the suspected MG patient includes careful observation of muscles for atrophy and fasciculations. Although muscle atrophy may occur in MG patients, particularly in those with MuSK autoantibodies, it is typically notable for its absence. Demonstrating weakness at the bedside that worsens with sustained or repetitive use in limb and trunk muscles is of theoretical, but in our experience, limited value in suspected MG patients. Any cause of neuromuscular weakness may produce reduced strength on repeated effort and normal patients may be reluctant to sustain effort resulting in a false perception of fatigable weakness. A careful assessment of cranial muscle strength is, however, very important in the assessment of suspected or known MG patients. We typically assess the strength of eyelid and lip closure, jaw opening and closing, tongue protrusion, and neck flexion and extension. In our experience, residual evidence of eye closure weakness in patients who otherwise seem to be in remission is a fairly common finding and should not by itself represent a justification to alter treatment. Again, demonstrating weakness in two or more muscles innervated by anatomically unrelated nerves, in the absence of atrophy and fasciculations, pain, sensory, or autonomic symptoms is likely to represent MG. As symptoms suggesting inadequate breathing warrant serious attention, we find bedside or telephone-based estimates of ventilatory muscle strength helpful. We do this by having the patients count out loud as far as one's vital capacity will allow after full inspiration. The vital capacity in cubic centimeters can be estimated with reasonable accuracy by multiplying this number by one hundred.

MG IN SPECIFIC POPULATIONS

There are special considerations in pregnant women with myasthenia, their newborn children, and children with myasthenia.[93–97] In an extensive review of the literature involving 322 pregnancies in 225 myasthenic mothers, 31% of mothers had no change in their myasthenic symptoms, 28% improved, and 41% deteriorated during the pregnancy.[98] During the postpartum period, 30% had a disease exacerbation. There is a theoretical risk of transmitting IgG AChR antibodies in breast milk, although most infants have no problem with breastfeeding.

Transient neonatal autoimmune MG develops in approximately 10% of infants born to mothers with MG.[100–112] It has been reported to occur in MuSK MG.[113] Maternal treatment seems to significantly lower the risk of infantile disease.[114] Onset is usually within the first 3 days of life. The most notable features include a weak cry, difficulty feeding due to a poor suck, hypotonia, respiratory difficulty, ptosis, and diminished facial expression resulting from facial muscle weakness. The disorder is temporary in most cases, with a mean duration of about 18–20 days. In rare cases, in utero paralysis may lead to a child born with multiple joint contractures.[114] Other than recognition and symptomatic treatment, the most important aspect of this disorder is that there appears to be no increased risk of the child developing MG in later life.

Juvenile MG represents a "subclassification" of autoimmune MG.[96–98,115–118] It is estimated that approximately 10% of acquired (non-neonatal) autoimmune MG cases will occur before 18 years of age in occidental populations, the majority subsequent to puberty.[114,115,117] This statistic may be inflated, as some reported juvenile, seronegative cases could easily represent congenital myasthenic syndromes (CMS). The clinical features are similar to adult-onset MG, with the majority of patients initially presenting with primarily ocular symptoms.[117] Serum AChR antibodies are present in the majority of affected children. The electrophysiologic findings are also identical to the adult form of the disease.[118]

ASSOCIATED DISORDERS

Effective management of MG requires knowledge of disorders that occur with an increased incidence in patients with MG, particularly thymic abnormalities and other autoimmune diseases which may occur separately or overlap. Thymus gland pathology is the most notorious disease association.[23,71,119] As many as 80% of patients with seropositive MG have thymic hyperplasia while approximately 12% have thymoma.[23,120–122] Hyperplasia is more common in younger patients. Thymomas occur equally in men and women and occur with the greatest frequency in middle-aged and older individuals.[23] Patients with thymoma, on average, have more severe clinical presentations and higher AChR antibody titers than their nonthymomatous counterparts. Thymic abnormalities have been documented to occur in MuSK MG but are thought to occur far less frequently.[10,23,71,74,78,81,123] Thymic pathology, either hyperplasia or thymoma, occurs in seronegative and presumably in LPR4 MG.[23] In patients with thymoma, slightly more than half will be found to have or will develop MG.[23]

Thymomas are not uniquely associated with MG and may coexist with other autoimmune disorders, other autoantibodies, and a host of other neurological and neuromuscular disorders (Fig. 25-2A,B).[124] Reported associations include granulomatous myositis, myocarditis, Isaacs'

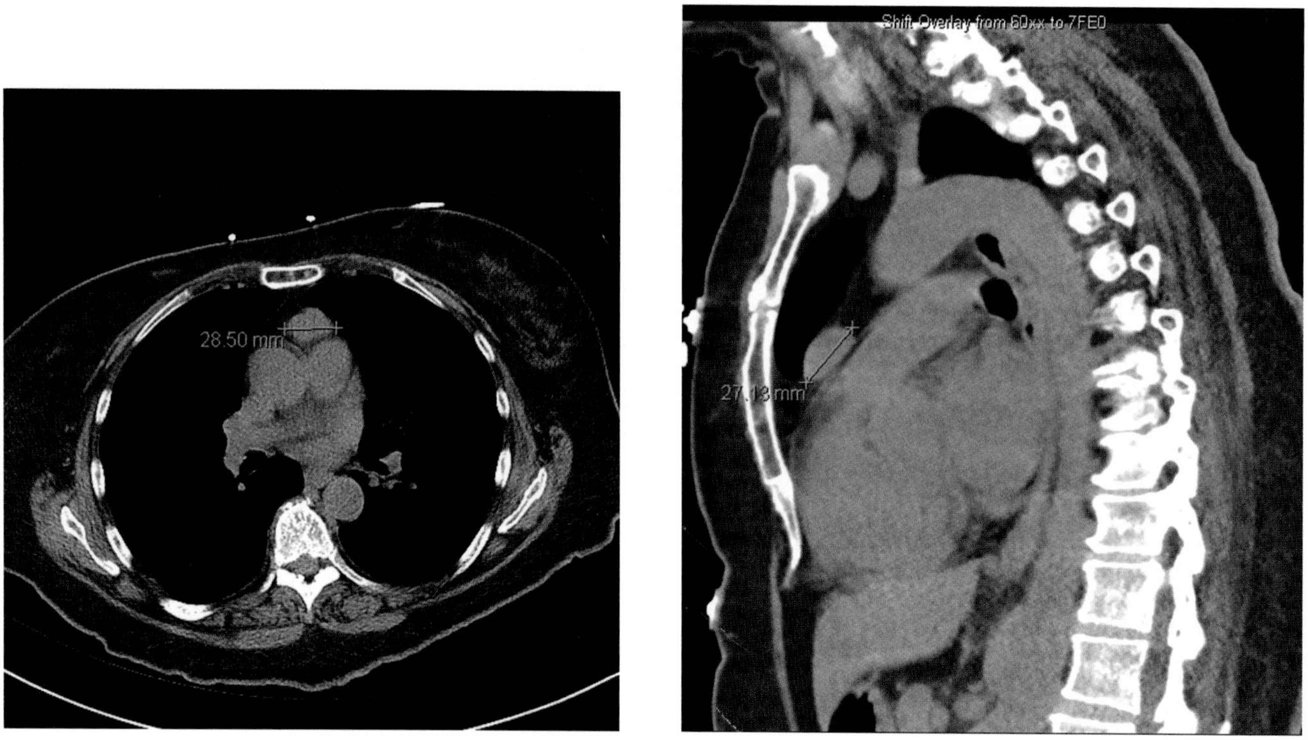

A B

Figure 25-2. CT scan of the chest in axial **(A)** and sagittal **(B)** orientation revealing thymoma in an MG patient.

syndrome, rippling muscle disease, limbic and cerebellar encephalitis, and autonomic neuropathy including the syndrome of intestinal pseudoobstruction.[125–130] Eleven patients with a particularly severe phenotype characterized by bulbar involvement, myasthenic crises, thymoma, myocarditis, and prolonged QT electrocardiographic interval have been described associated with Kv1.4 voltage-gated potassium channel in addition to AChR-binding autoantibodies.[129]

Other autoimmune diseases, most notably Hashimoto's disease, occur with increased frequency in MG in addition to rheumatoid arthritis, systemic lupus erythematosus, Sjögren's syndrome, red blood cell aplasia, ulcerative colitis, sarcoidosis, Addison's disease, and hyperparathyroidism.[131–135] Predictably, these disorders may occur with or without thymic abnormalities. Other neurological or neuromuscular disorders reported to coexist with MG include acute and chronic inflammatory demyelinating polyneuropathies, autonomic neuropathy (e.g., intestinal pseudoobstruction) with or without encephalopathy, Lambert–Eaton myasthenic syndrome (LEMS), acquired neuromyotonia or Isaacs' syndrome, acquired rippling muscle disease and stiff person syndrome,[125,128,136–153] In addition, approximately 5% of patients with MG also have an inflammatory myopathy.[137,154–157] Most of these patients also have a thymoma with or without myocarditis. The histopathology often reveals a giant cell or granulomatous myositis. Serum CK levels are usually elevated with concomitant inflammatory myopathy, which would not be expected in MG alone. It is estimated that the coexistence of other autoimmune diseases approximates 30% in AChR or in seronegative MG as opposed to MuSK MG where the prevalence of other autoimmune disease is estimated to approximate 20%.[71]

▶ DIAGNOSIS AND DIFFERENTIAL DIAGNOSIS

The diagnosis of myasthenia is usually established clinically and supported by a positive response to one or more of the following tests:

- serological—autoantibodies against the AChR or MuSK
- pharmacological—response to edrophonium
- electrophysiological—repetitive nerve stimulation (RNS) or single-fiber electromyography (SFEMG)

As has been repeatedly emphasized, MG should be considered in any patient with painless weakness, occurring in a regional, multifocal, diffuse, or even a seemingly focal pattern. The likelihood of MG increases substantially with the objective demonstration of fatigable weakness, particularly in an oculobulbar distribution. Weakness may be asymmetric and occurs in the absence of fasciculations and in most cases, muscle atrophy.

The differential diagnosis of MG includes other disorders in which signs and symptoms reside predominantly if not exclusively within the voluntary motor system (Table 25-1).

▶ **TABLE 25-1. DIFFERENTIAL DIAGNOSIS OF MG**

Brain
Wernicke encephalopathy[a]
Rabies[a]
Brainstem neoplasm[a]
Anterior horn cell
ALS
Kennedy syndrome[a]
Spinal muscular atrophy[a]
Enterovirus infection[a]
Root/nerve
Chronic meningitis[a]
Miller Fisher syndrome[a]
Diphtheria[a]
Immune-mediated motor neuropathies[a]
NMJ
Congenital myasthenic syndromes
Lambert Eaton myasthenic syndrome
Botulism
Tick paralysis
Muscle
Oculopharyngeal MD
Myotonic MD[a]
Mitochondrial myopathy
Congenital myopathy[a]
Inflammatory myopathy[a]
Miscellaneous
Depression[a]
Chronic fatigue[a]
Dysthyroid ophthalmopathy[a]
Orbital pseudotumor[a]

[a]Unlikely source of confusion.

Considerations include other DNMT such as the CMS, other acquired DNMT such as LEMS or botulism, motor neuron diseases such as spinal muscular atrophy (SMA), ALS, or X-linked spinal bulbar muscular atrophy (SBMA), numerous myopathies, particularly those with a predilection for cranial musculature, or motor neuropathies when the weakness is largely confined to the limbs.

Due to frequently overlapping phenotypes, and potentially similar electrophysiological features and pharmacological response, the most vexing of these considerations are the CMS. CMS should be seriously considered in any child, adolescent, or young adult with apparent seronegative MG. A history suggesting other involved relatives and/or consanguinity increases the probability of CMS. The CMS will be considered in more detail in the subsequent chapter.

In adults with bulbar weakness, considerations other than MG include but are not limited to the progressive bulbar palsy form of ALS, Kennedy disease, LEMS, botulism, and both acquired and hereditary myopathies. Congenital myasthenia cannot be entirely excluded from consideration as the DOK-7 and rapsyn mutations in particular may be associated with a late-onset phenotype and be readily misidentified as seronegative MG.[158] Most causes of multiple cranial neuropathies typically produce sensory in addition to motor symptoms but occasionally these syndromes may be motor predominant. As the presence of ptosis or ophthalmoparesis essentially excludes motor neuron disease or inflammatory myopathy from consideration, careful surveillance for these abnormalities provides valuable differential diagnostic insight. LEMS is usually dominated by symptoms referable to proximal limb muscles with prominent fatigue and symptoms of cholinergic dysautonomia, but ptosis and bulbar symptoms do occur and can make its distinction from MG challenging in some cases.[159,160] Botulism can affect children and adults and as a presynaptic disorder, can produce cholinergic dysautonomia with constipation and enlarged, unreactive pupils. Its acuity and the clinical context in which it occurs are helpful features to help distinguish it from MG. A number of inherited muscle diseases such as oculopharyngeal muscular dystrophy, mitochondrial myopathy, myotonic muscular dystrophy, and rare adult-onset cases of congenital myopathy such as centronuclear myopathy may produce oculobulbar syndromes.

As mentioned above, MG may rarely present with weakness restricted itself to limb or trunk muscles. The pattern of weakness may be predominantly proximal and symmetric or distal and asymmetric. Accordingly, the differential diagnostic considerations are broad and include anterior horn cell diseases, myopathies, neuropathies with motor predominance including some cases of inflammatory demyelinating polyneuropathy, multifocal motor neuropathy in more chronic and focal cases, as well as other forms of DNMT such as LEMS, botulism and acute organophosphate poisoning. Many of these diseases commonly have cranial nerve involvement as well. In children, SMA, congenital myasthenia, botulism, tick paralysis, and various myopathies would be the primary considerations. Poliomyelitis or other enteroviral infections would readily distinguish themselves in most cases but require consideration along with botulism and tick paralysis in any acute–subacute-onset case due to their pure motor characteristics.

PATHOPHYSIOLOGY

Successful NMT is dependent on the anatomical and physiological capabilities of the NMJ to translate and amplify a peripheral nerve action potential (NAP) into a transsynaptic chemical signal mediated by the neurotransmitter acetylcholine (ACh). Subsequently, the NMJ promotes the generation of a postsynaptic EPP, which unlike an action potential, varies in amplitude. If this EPP achieves the necessary magnitude, an action potential will be generated in the corresponding muscle fiber. This single muscle fiber action potential (SMFAP) tranduces the electrical event into a chemical and eventually mechanical event. The SFMAP promotes calcium release into the sarcoplasmic reticulum which is responsible for myofiber contraction and the generation of force.[161] The amount of force generated is dependent on the number of motor units activated, and ultimately, the number of muscle fibers in which this sequence of events takes place.

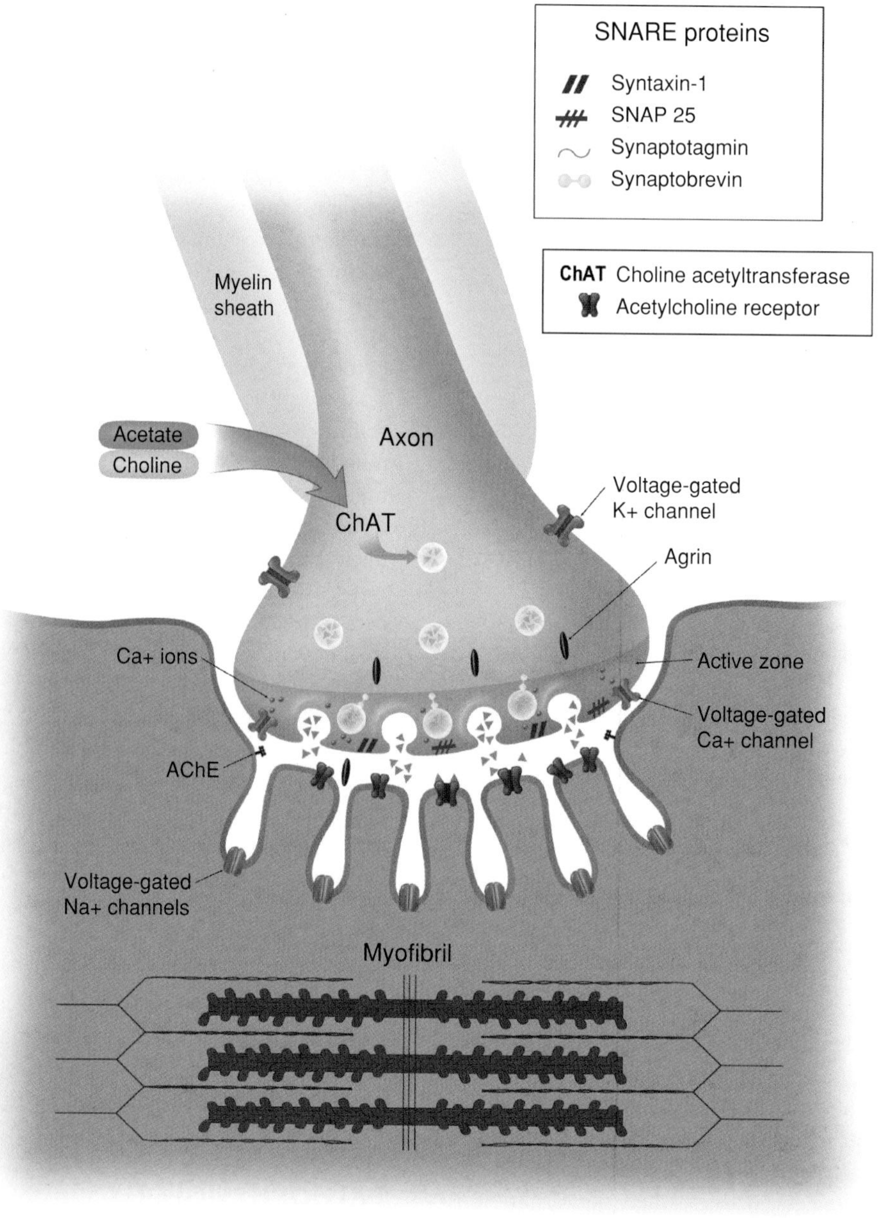

Figure 25-3. Normal neuromuscular junction—presynapse.

NMT is a process that is highly conserved between species. It has evolved into an extremely efficient system empowered with a substantial safety factor allowing for fail-safe repetitive and sustained muscle contraction in normal individuals. We have obtained considerable knowledge about the complexities of both normal and abnormal NMT. This section will address NMT and DNMT from a very superficial, clinically relevant perspective.

In view of the sophisticated evolution of NMT into a highly efficient system, external influences are more likely to compromise rather than enhance this efficiency. When NMT is compromised, it typically results in a phenotype typically dominated by fatigue and skeletal muscle weakness. As the neuromuscular junction lies beyond the protection of the blood–nerve barrier and is composed of a large number of proteins essential to its optimal function, it is vulnerable to a large number of immune-mediated, toxic, and genetic influences that can adversely affect both its function and structure. DMNT may result from anatomical and/or physiological disruption of one or more of the three components of the NMJ: (1) the presynaptic nerve terminal in which the synthesis, packaging, storage, presynaptic membrane binding, and/or release of ACh and the vesicles (quanta) that contain it take place, (2) the synaptic cleft through which ACh migrates and is eventually metabolized, and/or (3) the postsynaptic muscle membrane where specialized ACh receptors/channels are optimally positioned and organized (Figs. 23-3 and 23-4). Postsynaptic DNMT

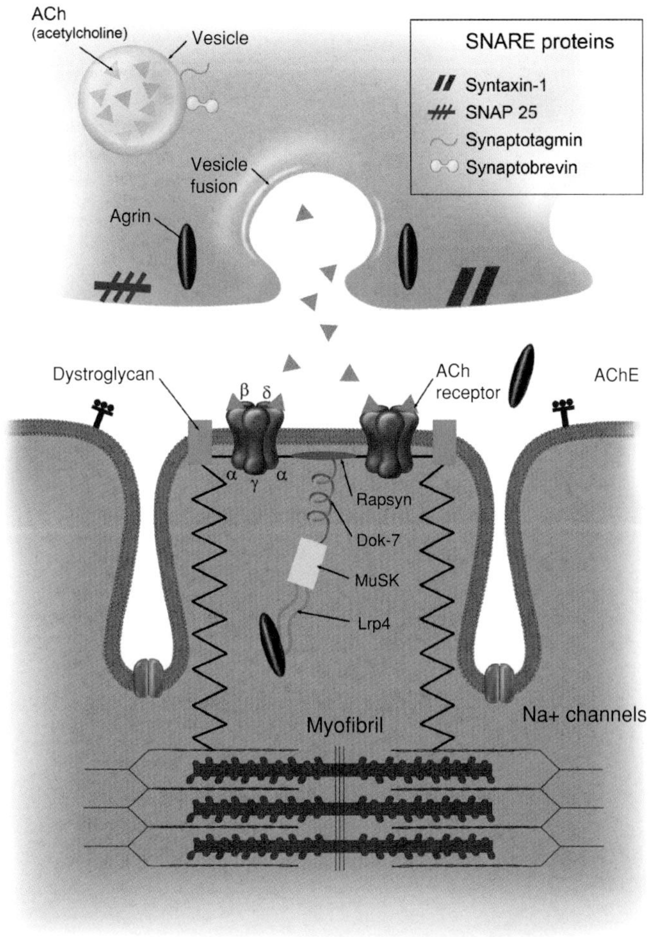

Figure 25-4. Normal neuromuscular junction—postsynapse.

may result from multiple potential mechanisms including interference with ACh binding, AChR organization, increased AChR turnover, or overt anatomic disruption (Fig. 23-5).[38,55] This section will review the anatomical, biochemical, and physiological aspects of normal and abnormal NMT.

Although DNMT are usually categorized as belonging to one of the three aforementioned anatomical domains, it would be overly simplistic to assume that all NMJs are the same, that each of the three anatomic NMJ domains develops embryologically in isolation, that any domain functions independently of the other two, or that any DNMT results solely from dysfunction of an individual domain. For example, the presynaptic configurations may differ between different NMJs in different muscles with terminal twigs having either an "en plaque" or "en grappe configuration." The former refers to large, single contacts on each muscle fiber. It is the predominant form in most mammalian muscles. The latter array refers to multiple, smaller contact points on individual fibers. This configuration seems to correlate with the need for tonic muscle contraction and is most prevalent in nonmammalian systems, but exists in humans in extraocular muscles in particular and in the tensor tympani, stapedius, laryngeal muscles, and tongue as well.[39] The greater concentration of fetal-type AChR in extraocular muscles represents one hypothesis as to why these muscles appear to be disproportionately susceptible to AChBR autoantibodies and why they are relatively spared in MuSK MG.[162]

In addition, AChR structure may differ between muscles as well. Muscles innervated by terminal twigs with en grappe morphologies are more likely to have fetal-type AChRs (described below) whose physiological properties may differ from their en plaque counterparts.[1] NMT also differs between different fiber types. Type 2 muscle fibers (fast twitch) have greater sensitivity to ACh than their type 1 counterparts translating to a larger safety factor in NMT. This results from larger nerve terminals, a greater average quantal content, an increased number of postsynaptic folds, and a greater density of sodium channels.[39,162] This is teleologically logical, as firing frequencies in fast twitch fibers are much higher than their slow twitch counterparts, translating to greater ACh depletion in the active zone of the presynaptic

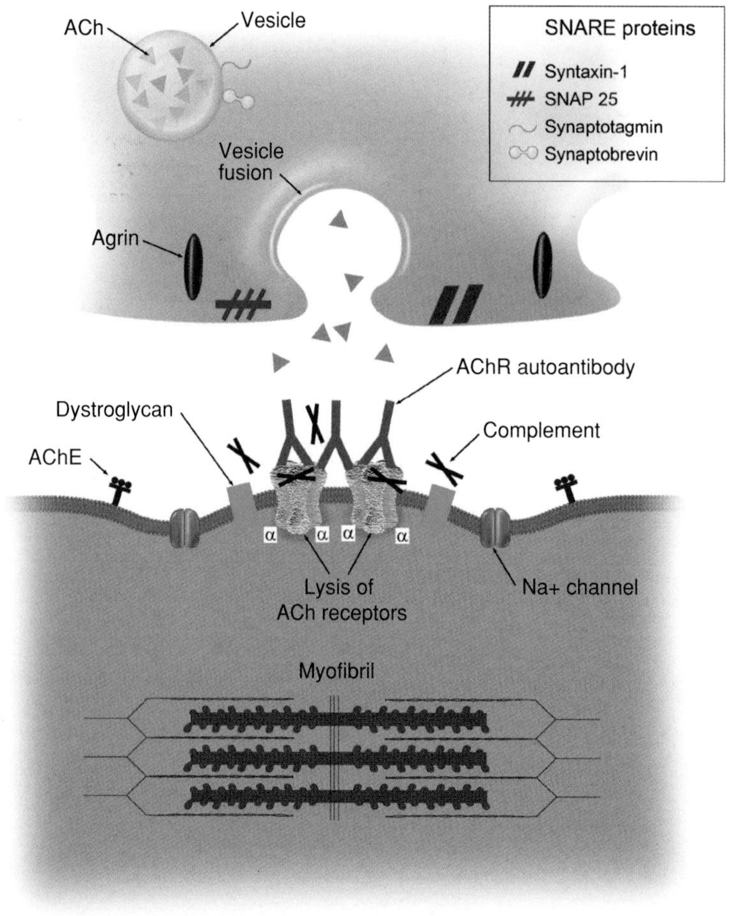

Figure 25-5. Neuromuscular junction in AChBR MG.

region, thereby requiring a greater safety factor in type 2 fibers to ensure uniformly successful NMT.[162]

Lastly, there is a significant interdependence on the three anatomical domains of the NMJ that is evident not only during synaptogenesis but in disease. Optimal postsynaptic architecture and function is very dependent on presynaptic influence.[90] As an example, acquired postsynaptic MuSK MG and the inherited synaptic form (end plate acetylcholinesterase (AChE) deficiency of CMG both have adverse effects on more than one domain of the NMJ anatomy.[90] AChE deficiency will have presynaptic effects such as reduction in quantal content and in the size of the presynaptic nerve terminal as well as a postsynaptic effect in the generation of an end plate myopathy.[163]

The sequence of events in normal, successful NMT can be conceptualized as beginning with the synthesis and resynthesis of ACh in the presynaptic terminal and can be schematically followed in (Figs. 25-3 and 25-4). This is accomplished primarily by the enzyme choline acetyltransferase (ChaT) that combines acetate and choline after their reuptake into the presynaptic terminal. Synthesized ACh molecules are packaged into vesicles or quanta that exist in three separate zones; a large storage pool, a mobilization pool, and in clusters close to the presynaptic membrane referred to as the active (immediate release) zone.[164] Although there are non–calcium-dependent mechanisms of ACh release, the efficient function of these active zones is dependent on calcium entry into the distal motor nerve terminal. The P/Q type voltage-gated calcium channels (VGCC) integral to this process are distributed along the active zones at vesicle fusion sites on the presynaptic membrane. In response to a NAP, the presynaptic calcium concentration increases to the 100–1000 μM range.[162,165] Vesicle release occurs after a delay of approximately 100 μs following the NAP with the presynaptic calcium concentration dissipating after approximately 200 μs. As calcium channels are not fully activated by a normal NAP, the capacity to increase quantal content exists by other mechanisms not involved in normal NMT.

In mammalian systems, the contents of 50–300 vesicles are typically released in response to a single NAP, referred to in the aggregate as the quantal content.[39] There are approximately 200–400 $\times 10^3$ individual synaptic vesicles contained in the average nerve terminal. In mammalian NMJs, approximately 20% of these are positioned for immediate release in the active zones.[166,167] Within each vesicle, there are between 5–10 × 10^3 molecules of ACh, the number varying somewhat between individual vesicles.[168,169] In at least one form of congenital MG associated with the impaired synthesis of ACh due to a mutation of the ChaT gene, reduction of the number of ACh molecules within a single synaptic vesicle is reduced sufficiently to interfere with NMT.[39]

The mobilization pool is estimated to contain 300 × 10^3 vesicles that can be moved readily to the active zone region.[168] Following vesicle fusion with the presynaptic membrane and exocytosis, ACh resynthesis and repackaging (endocytosis) take place. Experimental data suggest that the rate of resynthesis parallels the rate of ACh release under normal physiological conditions and is capable of increasing to keep pace with neuromuscular activation.[170]

The process of ACh synthesis and resynthesis, vesicle packaging, migration, docking, and exocytotic release into the synaptic cleft is dependent on greater than 1000 functional presynaptic proteins (Fig. 25-3). Detailed description of this obviously complex system is incompletely understood and beyond the scope of this chapter. The key proteins underlying vesicular fusion with the presynaptic membrane are referred to as the SNARE protein complex (**s**oluble **N**SF **a**ttachment protein **r**eceptor). Key components of the SNARE complex are synaptotagmin and synaptobrevin (bound to the vesicular membrane), and syntaxin-1 and SNAP 25 (bound to the presynaptic plasmalemma). Interaction between synaptobrevin and syntaxin-1 and SNAP 25 prime the binding and fusion process that culminates by the subsequent binding of calcium to synaptotagmin that triggers quantal release into the synaptic space.[39] Subsequent to its role in this process, calcium may freely diffuse away from the active sites, be removed from the nerve terminal by a coupled sodium/calcium exchange mechanism, or be sequestered in the smooth endoplasmic reticulum or mitochondria.[171] To the best of our knowledge, there are no recognized acquired or heritable disorders related to the proteins discussed in this paragraph.

The quantal content varies in response to each NAP. Under normal circumstances, the quantal content produces an EPP that far exceeds that necessary to produce a postsynaptic muscle fiber action potential ensuring the fail-safe generation of muscle fiber action potentials with repetitive or sustained attempts at voluntary muscle activation. Although largely irrelevant to normal physiology, presynaptic release of ACh can be augmented as mentioned previously. This effect may be either pathological or therapeutic, depending on the context in which it occurs. In disorders of NMT, the EPP may be augmented by pharmacological intervention at the presynaptic terminal that either prolongs depolarization by blocking potassium channels or the duration and effect of calcium. 3,4 diaminopyridine is an example of the former and guanidine is an example of the latter.[39,162,165] In addition, autoantibodies directed at components of the presynaptic potassium channels may produce a pathological condition of muscular hyperactivity (Isaacs' syndrome) as reviewed in Chapter 10.

Another presynaptic contribution to NMJ development in particular, and to its maintenance and function as well, is the protein agrin. Agrin, synthesized in and released from the presynapse, contributes significantly to postsynaptic differentiation and to the stabilization of end plate receptors[172] This process of end plate differentiation requires interaction with a number of crucial postsynaptic proteins including LPR4, MuSK, downstream of kinase-7 (Dok7), and receptor-aggregating protein at the synapse (rapsyn).[90] As will be described in this and the subsequent chapter, impaired NMT may result as a consequence of either heritable defects in many of these proteins (agrin, MuSK, rapsyn, Dok7) or in some cases autoantibodies directed against them (MuSK, LPR4).[90]

The morphology of the synaptic space may be subdivided into the major or primary gap (cleft) between the nerve terminal and muscle and multiple secondary clefts formed by the postjunctional folds extending into the postsynaptic region.[39] This folding increases the surface area of the postjunctional membrane by 10-fold in comparison to the presynaptic membrane.[173,174] This allows for an increase in the density of AChRs/channels as described below, thereby improving the efficiency of NMT. The synaptic cleft is narrow with an average distance of 50 nm between the presynaptic membrane and the summits of the postsynaptic folds.[39] This narrow gap facilitates rapid NMT. Once released into the synapse, the quanta will briefly bind to and interact with ACh receptors or channels that control the ingress of cations into the muscle fibers on which the receptors are located.

ACh binding to the end plate is short-lived, due in part to diffusion away from the receptor and in large part due to catabolism by the enzyme AChE that is anchored to the basal lamina by its collagen tail, the outer layer of the postsynaptic muscle membrane.[39] It is encoded by the triple-stranded collagen Q gene (COLQ) which is relevant to one form of CMS that will be described in Chapter 26. Drugs that reversibly inhibit AChE are used both diagnostically (edrophonium) and therapeutically (pyridostigmine) in MG whereas irreversible anticholinesterases (organophosphates) are utilized for their toxic properties as insecticides or in warfare. There are multiple isoforms of AChE.[175] The primary form is AChE-S (synaptic) which is bound to the basal lamina. Other forms, AChE-E (erythropoietic) and AChE-R (read-through) do not play significant roles in ACh catalysis under normal circumstances but compensatory increases in AChR-R in response to chronic treatment with cholinesterase inhibitors may have detrimental clinical effects as described below.[175]

ACh catalysis by AChE is one of the fastest enzymatic processes known and occurs at a rate of five ACh molecules per millisecond.[176] Despite this, ACh enjoys a competitive advantage as the density of AChR (15–30 K × m^2) is 5–10 times greater than the molecular density of AChE (2–3 × $10^3/m^2$).[177] This allows 50–75% of the quantal content to achieve successful interaction with AChR under normal circumstances.[178]

Temperature changes affect NMT in a variety of ways that may have both electrodiagnostic (EDX) and clinical significance.[44,45,48,49,179,180] These effects will be addressed here as the most notable physiological effect of temperature change on NMT is on AChE. Reduced temperature slows the rate of AChE hydrolysis of ACh, prolonging the duration of EPPs by allowing ion channels to remain open for longer periods of time and enhancing end-plate responsiveness to ACh.[181,182] The net effect of cooling is to enhance NMT. Electrodiagnostically, this may diminish the probability of demonstrating a decremental response to slow repetitive stimulation. Clinically, cooling may improve function, for example, patient recognition that cold liquids are easier to swallow than warm ones.

Cooling has other non-AChE effects on the physiology of NMT. Both the duration and amplitude of the NAP at the presynaptic terminal are increased by cooling.[163–185] This may be a consequence of prolonged calcium channel open time and augmented quantal content.[186] Reducing the affected muscle's temperature is known to increase the AChR's open time as well.[182] Finally, a reduction in muscle temperature leads to a lowering of the resting membrane potential, bringing it closer to threshold, allowing a myofiber action potential to be triggered with a smaller EPP. These four factors, and perhaps others as well, serve to improve NMT in response to cooling.

The organization of the postsynaptic membrane provides for efficiency in NMT (Fig. 25-4). The development and maintenance of end plate complexity is related to the proximity of nerve terminals both embryologically and during adult life and to the influence of ACh and agrin produced and released by these nerve terminals. The key anatomic structure on the end plate is the AChR receptor or channel. Each AChR channel is a glycoprotein composed of five subunits that are arranged in a manner similar to barrel staves turned inside out, resulting in a transmembrane structure with a sagittal appearance similar to the cooling tower of a nuclear power plant. In an adult, the channel consists of two α subunits with singular copies of β, δ, and ε subunits.[39,162,187] Embryologically, the AChR has a γ subunit instead of an ε subunit. The transition to an adult configuration occurs at least in part due to the trophic influence of the presynaptic nerve terminal during the innervation process. Fetal AChRs are typically downregulated during adult life but their presence may have two notable clinical influences. As mentioned above, they may persist to some degree in certain adult muscles, particularly those with en grappe nerve presynaptic morphology, and may contribute to the selected vulnerability of ocular and bulbar muscles in acquired MG. Their persistence in some forms of congenital myasthenia may allow for survival in what would otherwise be a lethal condition.

At the NMJ, AChRs preferentially reside in at the apices of the junctional folds of the muscle end plate and span the postsynaptic membrane. These channels are topographically clustered with their density estimated to approach 10,000 molecules per μm^2.[188] The density of these channels falls to approximately 10 molecules per μm^2 within a few microns of the end plate.[39,162] The topography of AChR channel distribution both on and within the muscle end plate is essential for optimal NMT. The placement of these channels is established embryologically and maintained during adult life through the contributions of a number of numerous proteins that are essential for the development and maintenance of channel distribution and their optimal function.[114] The initiation of this process is through the effects of the presynaptically synthesized and released protein agrin and ACh, both of which are essential to this process. Agrin knockout mice have normal numbers of AChRs but no evidence of clustering. Agrin appears to bind postsynaptically to LRP4 which in turn results in MuSK activation.[189] MuSK is required not only for proper synaptogenesis, but for the stabilization and maintenance of end plates in postnatal life. Knockout MuSK mice embryos fail both to develop AChR clusters or to survive.[39] Deletion of MuSK in adult muscle leads to the degradation and complete loss of NMJs. MuSK reacts in turn with Dok-7 to activate certain downstream signaling pathways and with rapsyn. ACh clustering is maintained by rapsyn which directly binds with the cytoskeleton and dystrophin-glycoprotein complex, specifically through α- and β- dystroglycan.[39,162,190,191] Despite the apparent importance of Dok-7 in this process, defects in this protein do not appear to adversely affect AChR clustering on junctional folds.[162] An additional protein, neuregulin (NRG-1) also appears to play a role in the clustering of AChRs at the NMJ.[39,162]

As mentioned, the AChR is a ligand-gated channel that spans the postsynaptic muscle membrane with its long axis oriented perpendicular to this membrane. It has a hydrophilic central pore with the ACh-binding site located on the extracellular surface of each subunit.[192] In the resting state, the central narrow region or waist created by the apex of the convexity of all five subunits meet in opposition, effecting channel closure. Channel opening is dependent on the simultaneous binding of two molecules of ACh with each channel, which then leads to a conformational change, allowing transient opening of the channel pore and, as a result, ion movement. The agonist binding sites for ACh straddle the α/δ or α/ε (α/γ when relevant), identical to the binding site for α bungarotoxin.[114,162] They appear to be distinct from, but close to the MIR which resides on the α subunit and is the locus for AChR autoantibody binding.[114,162] The α/γ binding site appears to have the highest affinity for ACh which could in turn have relevance in regard to the selective vulnerability of certain muscles which have a greater prevalence of this channel type. Although potassium, calcium, and sodium ions are all capable of traversing the channel, sodium conductance is most dynamic due to favorable size, concentration, and electrical gradient considerations.

In response to the random spontaneous release of singular quanta, unrelated to NAPs, individual channels will open and a miniature end plate potential (MEPP) will be created in that muscle fiber. This is presumed to have a trophic influence on muscle but produces no myofiber contraction. MEPPs occur at a frequency of about 0.2–0.03 times per second, resulting in the activation of $1–2 \times 10^3$ AChR channels and the generation of a nonpropagated waveform with a magnitude of 0.5–1 mV.[193,194]

The nonpropagating EPP generated by the normal quantal content release typically exceeds 50 mV in amplitude, and in normal individuals, produces a propagating SMFAP in each muscle fiber stimulated.[195] In health there is a "safety factor", that being an EPP whose magnitude far exceeds that which is required to depolarize the muscle fiber. A typical mammalian resting membrane potential is approximately −80 mV. The threshold for depolarization may be achieved by a change in voltage of only 10–15 mV, thus providing the three- to fourfold safety margin that normally exists in NMT transmission. The magnitude of the EPP is decreased with repetitive stimuli occurring at a frequency of 5 Hz or less, which, at least initially, deplete ACh-containing vesicles in the active zone. Because of the aforementioned safety margin however, this effect has no significance in the normal individual.

The decline in the EPP in response to "slow" repetitive stimulation will not persist indefinitely as the EPP amplitudes begin to increase after the fourth or fifth stimulus attributed to ACh arrival from the mobilization pool. Conversely, and perhaps counterintuitively, the EPP may be augmented substantially by repetitive stimuli at frequencies of 5 Hz or more. This phenomenon of post-tetanic facilitation is attributed, in large part, to enhanced quantal release related to lingering calcium effects within the presynaptic terminal. Again, this phenomenon bears no consequence in the normal individual, as MFAP occurs in each muscle fiber in response to each and every stimulus. This post-tetanic facilitation does not last indefinitely, and the EPP will begin to decline after approximately 1 minute in normal people due to declining ACh availability. This latter phenomenon is referred to as post-tetanic or postexercise exhaustion and can also be utilized as a diagnostic tool with repetitive stimulation studies in patients with suspected DNMT.[196,197] Although post-tetanic exhaustion will not result in NMT failure in normal individuals, it may do so in patients with DNMT whose safety margin for the generation of muscle fiber action potentials is compromised at baseline by disease. In all DNMT, reduction and eventual loss of the EPP safety margin by whatever means is the universal mechanism by which NMT failure and weakness are created.

In addition to the AChR channel, Nav 1.4 sodium channels are also integral to the generation of the muscle fiber action potential.[166] Unlike the AChR, they are clustered at the base rather than the peak of the synaptic folds.[39,175] Their density is 5–10-fold higher in the end plate than in other regions of the sarcolemma and have a greater density in type 2 than in type 1 muscle fibers.[162] Sodium ingress at the NMJ facilitates the EPP generated by ACh channel opening and adds to the safety margin of NMT. Mutation of Nav 1.4 channel gene is a rare form of CMS.

The half-life of an AChR in the junctional membrane is about 8–10 days.[198] Under normal circumstances, there is a normal turnover of AChR which are internalized and degraded. The senescent receptors are internalized by the process of endocytosis and transported to lysosomes for degradation through an intricate network of intracellular tubules. This process is accelerated in disease as described in more detail below, being expedited by cross-linking of channels with AChR autoantibodies.[162] The AChR are not recycled but are replaced by newly synthesized receptors, one reason why DNMT are more treatment responsive than other neuromuscular disorders in which damaged components are not as readily restored, even if the disease process is arrested.

Integral to the pathogenesis of ACHR MG is the reduction of AChR at the end plate as initially demonstrated by Fambrough and Drachman in 1973 through radiolabeled α-bungarotoxin techniques.[3] The pathogenic AChBR autoantibodies of MG are of the IgG1 and IgG3 types and bind predominantly to the MIRs of the AChR which exist on the two alpha subunits of the channel.[32,73,114,199–201] Once bound to the AChR, these antibodies initiate a number of irreversible processes, all of which are directed at the AChR and postsynaptic membrane. The most potent of these appears to be complement-mediated, membrane-attack complex lysis of AChR.[202,203] Resultant end plate changes not only reduce receptor number but have other anatomic consequence of physiological significance that include simplification of the normal corrugated structure of the end plate (Fig. 25-5). This not only reduces the cross-sectional area but widens the synaptic cleft, thus further reducing the probability of ACh/AChR interaction.[173,204,205] Other potential pathophysiological mechanisms include steric hindrance, with autoantibodies physically blocking ACh binding sites on adjacent channels or preventing the conformational change resulting in opening of the ion pore.[206]

The autoantibodies not only bind to the AChR but also cross-link with other antibodies.[207,208] When the AChRs are cross-linked in this manner, these are reabsorbed by the postsynaptic membrane by a process known as endocytosis. This process takes place under normal circumstances but accelerates up to three times faster in the presence of AChBR autoantibodies. As a result, the normal NMJ AChR half-life of 5–10 days is dramatically reduced and the AChR population diminished.[209–211] As synthesis of new AChRs remains unchanged, there is a significant net reduction of 70–90% AChRs per NMJ.[3] Although AChR MG is conceptually a disorder mediated by autoantibodies, there is a significant T-cell-mediated, CD4 lymphocyte component as well.[55,212] T lymphocytes specific to AChRs are found in patients with myasthenia.[213,214] T cell-targeted therapies hold therapeutic promise for MG.[212,215]

MG also reduces the number of sodium channels that are clustered at the depths of the end plate folds.[166] This appears to increase the threshold for muscle fiber action potentials.[162] In any event, reduction in the number or function of sodium channels at the muscle end plate will further erode the safety margin of NMT.

MuSK MG

The pathogenesis of MuSK myasthenia is not as well understood as AChR MG but is clearly different. The association between MuSK and MG is based on a number of lines of evidence. There appears to be a strong association between the presence of MuSK autoantibodies and patients with seronegative myasthenic phenotypes. MuSK autoantibodies produce weakness and reduction in MEPP amplitudes in mice and a weakness associated with impaired AChR clustering in rabbits when passively transferred. Children born of MuSK MG mothers may develop transient neonatal MG and respond to plasma exchange (PLEX) treatment.[74,83,216,217] Lastly, MEPP amplitude reduction has been demonstrated in vitro in an intercostal muscle biopsy specimen acquired from a MuSK MG patient.[218]

Current knowledge suggests that MuSK MG is a disease of disordered AChR distribution as opposed to one of AChR destruction. There appears to be a good clinical pathological correlation between those muscles where clustering is impacted the most and selectively vulnerable muscles such as sternocleidomastoid, diaphragm, and masseter.[79] Histological studies of MuSK MG patients suggest that unlike AChBR MG, substantial loss of AChR content and IgG/complement does not occur.[79] Unlike AChBR autoantibodies, MuSK autoantibodies are of the IgG4 subtype and do not activate complement.[72,219] Their primary action in hampering NMT in MuSK MG appears to be fragmentation of the normal AChR clustering at the junctional peaks of the postsynaptic membrane. In addition, MuSK autoantibodies may have synaptic and presynaptic effects including impaired binding of the collagen tail of the AChE molecule and presynaptic reduction in quantal content instead of the usual compensatory increase that occurs in other forms of MG.[178,219] In fact, recent studies suggest that the primary binding site for MuSK autoantibodies is the site of interaction between MuSK and the collagen tail of AChE (ColQ) responsible for the anchoring of AChE on the basal lamina.[220] This may provide an explanation for why MuSK MG patients, as will be subsequently described, uncommonly respond favorably to cholinesterase inhibitors.[79] Accordingly, MuSK MG may be eventually classified as a synaptic rather than postsynaptic disorder. Like most other postsynaptic proteins, mutation of the MuSK gene may result in rare reported cases of CMG.[221]

LPR4 MG

The pathogenesis of LPR4 MG is incompletely understood. In support of a pathogenetic role of LPR4 autoantibodies, serum from LPR4 MG patients reduces MEPP amplitudes in mice.[8] The preponderance of evidence suggests that LPR4 MG is an IgG1-complement–mediated disease similar to AChBR MG.[8,9,25,222] Accordingly, patients with LPR4 MG respond to immunomodulating agents in a manner similar to AChR MG patients although these two autoantibodies rarely, if ever, coexist.[25] In contrast, as the normal function of LPR4 involves interaction with MuSK in AChR clustering during synaptogenesis, one would predict a disease mechanism similar to MuSK MG in which complement-mediated end plate destruction does not appear to have a role. Unlike AChR MG, a small percentage of LPR4 MG patients will also harbor MuSK autoantibodies.[9,25]

Transient Neonatal MG

The pathophysiology of transient neonatal myasthenia results from the passive transplacental transfer of the mother's IgG AChR antibodies which bind to the interface of alpha and gamma subunits.[114] The reason why this disorder does not happen with greater frequency is unknown.

No discussion of MG pathophysiology would be complete without attempting to provide a cogent explanation for the selective vulnerability of certain muscle groups and the notable asymmetries that may occur in a disease occurring as a consequence of equitable distribution of circulating autoantibodies. Two potential explanations have already been discussed: (1) differing pathophysiological mechanisms with differing autoantibodies and (2) differences in the AChR channel types in different muscles. It has also been hypothesized that the preferential involvement of the external ocular muscles may be related to the elevated temperature of the head compared to limbs. This of course, would provide an inadequate explanation for asymmetry. In the end, adequate pathophysiological explanations for the myasthenic phenotype remain elusive.[223,224]

Lastly, the major gap that remains in our understanding of acquired, autoimmune MG pathogenesis is the knowledge of what initiates the disease process.[32] As mentioned, Mendelian genetics appears to have a minimal causative role in acquired, autoimmune MG. We agree with those who believe that the future will identify a significant genetic role in disease susceptibility to adverse environmental influence.[23,26,31,32] The role of infectious agents such as the Epstein–Barr virus as one of these potential environmental precipitants remains uncertain.[225] The thymus gland continues to occupy center stage in any MG etiology discussion.[23,226–228] One potential explanation involves the recognition that the thymus contains myoid cells and other types of stem cells that may serve as autoantigens by the expression of AChRs or AChR antigens on their surface.[23] In this same vein, AChR-specific B lymphocytes are found within the thymus gland of MG patients that are capable of generating antibodies to AChR in culture.

▶ LABORATORY FEATURES

The reader is referred to Chapter 2 where the testing modalities used in support of an MG diagnosis are reviewed. In this

▶ TABLE 25-2. **DIAGNOSTIC YIELD OF TESTS USED IN THE DIAGNOSIS OF AUTOIMMUNE MG**[6,9,10,25,37,55,71–74,76,91,230,232,275,296,417]

		AChR							
Type	Tensilon	Binding	Blocking	Modulating	MuSK	LPR4[a]	Distal Rep Stim	Prox Rep Stim	SFEMG
Remission		81%	19%	75%					
Ocular	86%	36–79%	30%	72%	Rare	? 50%	0–35%	45–50%	59–63%
Mild generalized		75–94%	52–66%	89%			55%	76%	91%
Moderate–severe generalized	95%			91%			86–99%	96–99%	99%
All		66–94%	52%	86%	7–15%		37–62%	62–77%	86–92%
Seronegative				5%	40%	3–50%			

[a]LPR4, lipoprotein-related protein 4 (not commercially available).
MuSK, muscle-specific kinase; AChR, antiacetylcholine receptor; SFEMG, single-fiber electromyography.

section, we will briefly review the serological, EDX, pharmacological, and imaging methods available to aid in the diagnosis and management of myasthenic patients. We will focus on their strengths and weaknesses, and the strategies that we employ in their use. The relative sensitivities of different tests used to support the clinical diagnosis of MG have been estimated and are summarized in Table 25-2.[6,9,10,25,37,55,72–74,77,91,160,229–232]

Diagnostic strategies in MG undoubtedly vary between clinicians and institutions due to individual bias and preference, test availability, and relevant differential diagnostic considerations in individual cases. Even in the most clinically straightforward cases, we believe that diagnostic confirmation should be obtained whenever possible, particularly if immunomodulating treatment or thymectomy is contemplated. The most sensitive test for MG is SFEMG (92–100%) followed by RNS of distal and proximal nerves (0–99%) depending on the muscle tested and whether the disease is limited or generalized in its manifestations.[229] Neither modality is, however, specific for MG. AChR antibody testing is slightly less sensitive (36–94%) depending also on whether the patient has ocular or generalized disease as well as the nature of the assay utilized, but is highly specific.

SEROLOGICAL TESTING

Identification of AChR autoantibodies is the most expeditious means to confirm MG. Although there are different types of AChR autoantibodies as will be subsequently described, the AChR binding antibody is the principal pathogenic antibody tested for. It will be considered synonymous with AChR autoantibodies throughout this chapter unless otherwise specified. Typically, this is the only diagnostic test that we initially order unless there are phenotypic features that would suggest MuSK MG. As mentioned, the sensitivity is estimated at approximately 36–79% in ocular MG, 75–94% in generalized MG, and 66–93% in all MG patients.[5,37,114,231,233] They are however, highly specific for the MG, being rarely reported as false positives in patients with other autoimmune diseases such as systemic lupus, rheumatoid arthritis, hepatitis, thymoma without MG, inflammatory neuropathy, motor neuron disease, 13% of patients with LEMS, 3% of patients with lung cancer without an apparent neurological disorder and in some asymptomatic relatives of MG patients.[160] We consider the diagnosis to be confirmed if these autoantibodies are present in the appropriate clinical context.

The value of these autoantibodies is for all intents and purposes in establishing the diagnosis initially. Although titers may decline with treatment, in particular following thymectomy, it is generally held that this test cannot reliably determine disease severity, response to treatment, or to predict either remission or relapse.[55,234] Unlike many other tests used in everyday practice, mild elevations in the AChR autoantibody titer are often significant. Conversely, patients without AChR autoantibodies may have a different disease, harbor a different MG autoantibody, have seronegative MG, or on occasion have a false negative result. This latter situation may arise with testing that has been done too early, or in an individual in whom autoantibody formation has been suppressed by immunomodulating treatment or thymectomy.[233,234] For these reasons, testing prior to the initiation of immunomodulating treatment or thymectomy is ideal. As initially seronegative patients may develop autoantibodies over time, repeat testing in a recommended interval of 6 months in the appropriate clinical context may be considered.[231]

AChR-modulating and AChR-blocking autoantibodies are also commercially available but play a less significant clinical role.[160,235] AChR modulating autoantibodies measure degradation of the AChR in cultured human myotubes.[232] Both of these autoantibodies are most likely to coexist in individuals who are AChR binding autoantibody seropositive and are unlikely to occur in isolation.[126,160,235] In one report, AChR modulating autoantibodies were found in 75% of patients with AChR binding autoantibodies but in only 5% of seronegative patients.[232] It is our practice to order these autoantibodies only in this latter population. High titers of AChR modulating autoantibodies also play a potential role in the detection of thymoma. Seventy three percent of patients afflicted with both thymoma and MG harbor AChR modulating autoantibodies producing a >90% receptor loss.[125,126,142] Although this potentially justifies their use as a screening tool for thymoma detection, we preferentially rely on imaging for this purpose.

AChR-blocking autoantibodies bind to the same site as ACh or α-bungarotoxin, close to but distinct from the MIR on the extracellular domain of the ACh channel.[232] They are found in approximately half of patients with generalized MG, but in only 30% of patients with ocular disease.[160,235] In one study, these autoantibodies were found in 30% of MG patients seropositive for AChR-binding autoantibodies but in no seronegative MG patient. As a result of this insensitivity, we find AChR-blocking autoantibody testing to have limited clinical value.

It is estimated that approximately 40–70% of AChR seronegative patients will have MuSK autoantibodies.[6,73,236] Our practice is to screen for MuSK autoantibodies as a first step along with AChR-binding autoantibodies if the phenotype is suggestive of MuSK MG. We also order MuSK autoantibodies in any MG suspect who is AChR seronegative. MuSK and AChR antibodies rarely coexist.[6,73,89,237] Although somewhat controversial, there appears, unlike AChR seropositive patients, to be a correlation between anti-MuSK titers, disease severity, and treatment responsiveness, thymectomy being the notable exception.[73,79,89]

Striated muscle antibodies refer to a class of antibodies directed against components of skeletal muscle including titin, the ryanodine receptor, myosin, and α-actinin.[238] These are found in approximately 30% of adult patients with MG without thymoma, 24% of patients with thymoma without MG, and 70–80% of patients who have both.[126,160,239] We have had numerous experiences where the occurrence of these autoantibodies even in high titer appears to have no detectable clinical correlation. Again, we largely rely on imaging to detect thymoma, and in view of the questionable sensitivity of the test, we find their utility limited. It is reasonable however, to measure these antibodies before and after thymectomy as a failure to reduce the titer suggests incomplete resection and as an increasing striational autoantibody titer postthymectomy has been reported to herald thymoma recurrence.

We routinely obtain a thyroid stimulating hormone level as the incidence of hypo- or hyperthyroidism is fairly high in MG patients and as a failure to recognize dysthyroidism may affect treatment efficacy. It is not uncommon for other autoantibodies to coexist with MG and/or thymoma such as ganglionic (as opposed to the nicotinic found on muscle) AChR antibodies, voltage-gated potassium channel antibodies, and CRMP-5-IgG autoantibodies.[125,126,130] We do not routinely test for autoantibodies more closely related to other autoimmune diseases in MG patients unless there is clinical suspicion to do so. Antibodies directed against the Kv1.4 subunit of voltage-gated potassium channels have been described to occur in a percentage of patients with MG but not in patients with thymoma, inflammatory myopathy, or in healthy controls.[129] These were found exclusively in patients who were also AChR-binding antibody positive and are not commercially available. Their role in the diagnosis of MG, if any, has yet to be defined.

ELECTROPHYSIOLOGICAL TESTING

The role of EDX testing in MG has undoubtedly diminished in an era of readily available, affordable, and accurate serological testing. EDX provides the greatest utility in the seronegative patient where its purpose is to identify a pattern of abnormalities that support a diagnosis of a postsynaptic DNMT, in turn consistent with MG.[240] At the same time, it attempts to identify or exclude a pattern of abnormalities suggestive of an alternative cause of painless weakness. Electrodiagnosis is used by some in MG to monitor the response to treatment but we do not find this necessary in the vast majority of patients. One uncommon use of EDX in the MG patient is to identify afterdischarges on routine motor conduction studies that would support overdosing with cholinesterase inhibitors.[241] The actual mechanics involved in the performance of repetitive stimulation of motor nerves and SFEMG are provided in Chapter 2.[218,242] In this section, we will focus on the strategies and pitfalls involved in MG EDX and its interpretation, including a summary of characteristic pattern of abnormalities.[243]

The EDX evaluation of a patient with suspected MG begins with routine nerve conductions. Typically we obtain, one motor and one sensory conduction from an upper and lower limb, four conductions in total. We would expect these to be normal in a postsynaptic DNMT in the absence of an alternative or additional confounding diagnosis. If the compound muscle action potential (CMAP) amplitudes are reduced in a patient with a phenotype resembling MG, a motor neuron disease or a presynaptic DNMT such as LEMS or botulism should be considered. If this occurs, we would attempt facilitation with 10 seconds of exercise followed by a second, supramaximal stimulus immediately thereafter, attempting to identify a presynaptic DNMT. We then proceed to repetitive stimulation testing at 2–3 Hz. In general, we typically study the ulnar, accessory, and facial nerves although readily adapt this menu if warranted by clinical circumstance. If possible, we start with a weak muscle, particularly if it is in the hand where the study is technically easier to perform. If there is no weakness, or the weakness is proximal, we would go straight to the accessory nerve as the best compromise between diagnostic yield and technical ease. If a patient has only ocular or bulbar weakness, we usually start with a facial muscle such as the orbicularis oculi or the nasalis.

If repetitive stimulation reveals a decrement at baseline, we reproduce it to ensure its validity and then exercise the muscle studied. We then attempt to repair the decrement by exercising the muscle for 10 seconds and then repeating the

RNS. However, if no convincing decrement is seen, we then exercise the muscle for a full minute and then repeat repetitive stimulation trains of 10 at 2–3 Hz every 30 seconds for up to 5 minutes, looking for postexercise exhaustion.

If RNS is normal, we proceed to EMG to look for motor unit instability as evidence of DNMT, or features of other possible neuromuscular disorders that may mimic MG (e.g., myopathy, motor neuron disease). If both repetitive stimulation and concentric needle EMG are nondiagnostic, we proceed to SFEMG. This testing order is based on the knowledge that SFEMG is a very sensitive but not specific test. The choice of muscle(s) for SFEMG depends on the patient phenotype. The majority of patients in whom SFEMG is performed in our laboratories have either isolated ocular complaints or on occasion generalized fatigue for which the referring physician wishes to exclude MG. In the former circumstance, we typically study the frontalis or orbicularis oculi muscle whereas in the latter, the extensor digitorum communis is our typical site. Each case should be individually assessed however, with the choice of nerves and muscles tested based on clinical evaluation. In a myasthenic, diagnostic yield will always be greatest in a clinically weak muscle. Again, failure to demonstrate a decremental response, increased jitter, and neuromuscular blockade in a clinically weak muscle implicates a diagnosis other than MG.

There are a number of important caveats to consider in the EDX testing of an MG suspect. Temperature change has a number of significant and at times conflicting physiological effects on NMT.[45,244] In the aggregate, however, the maintenance of surface temperature to an optimal temperature of 35°C or above is required to minimize the risk of either a false negative repetitive stimulation or single-fiber study. A false negative study may also occur as a result of anticholinesterase medication exposure. Ideally, potential MG patients should be tested prior to exposure to any medication that might significantly affect the disease, particularly through interference with NMT (Table 25-3). In particular, pyridostigmine should be discontinued if possible at least 12–24 hours before the study.

False positives are an even larger potential pitfall in the EDX testing of an MG suspect. The most common cause of a false positive examination is undoubtedly technical, particularly with repetitive stimulation testing. Unwanted movement by either the patient or technician can result in movement of the stimulator resulting in submaximal stimulation and the appearance of a "pseudodecrement." Unwanted movement resulting in baseline deviation is a particular problem both in large proximal muscles and in the face. The latter often occurs from grimacing in response to facial nerve stimulation and the undesired coactivation of other facial innervated muscles. Any technique that will reduce unwanted muscle contraction and movement and unwanted artifact is desirable.

To minimize the risk of a false positive interpretation, we require that all characteristics of a typical postsynaptic decremental response be fulfilled. These include: (1) a normal baseline CMAP amplitude, (2) a nadir that occurs at the fourth or fifth response of a 10-stimulus train, (3) the greatest decrease in CMAP amplitude between consecutive responses occurring between the first and second responses and (4) a steady rise in the CMAP amplitude after the fifth response that allows the CMAP amplitude to approach but not achieve that of the first response, producing a "tilted saucer," "ski jump," or "inverted banana" configuration (Fig. 25-6).

The other false positive scenario is assigning EDX abnormalities to MG, when the abnormal NMT is due to a different disease. As discussed below, there is potential overlap between the needle EMG findings in MG and other neuromuscular diseases. In addition, an abnormal repetitive stimulation or SFEMG study is not specific for MG and can be seen in any neuromuscular disease that may cause a secondary effect on NMT. Of these disorders, ALS may be the most common typically resulting in a decremental response of <10%.[245–249] The EDX features

TABLE 25-3. DRUGS THAT MAY ADVERSELY AFFECT NEUROMUSCULAR TRANSMISSION[303,418]

1. Drugs that may unmask or exacerbate myasthenia gravis
   a. Antiarrhythmic agents—lidocaine, quinidine, quinine, procainamide, and trimethaphan camsylate
   b. Antimicrobial agents including aminoglycosides, polymyxin B, colistin, clindamycin, ciprofloxacin, netilmicin, azithromycin, pefloxacin, norfloxacin, and erythromycin
   c. Corticosteroids
   d. Magnesium (parenteral)
   e. Neuromuscular blocking agents—depolarizing and nondepolarizing including botulinum toxin, d-tubocurarine, succinylcholine, vecuronium, pancuronium, atracurium, and gallamine
2. Drugs potentially implicated in unmasking or exacerbating myasthenia gravis
   a. Anesthetics—diazepam, ketamine
   b. Anticonvulsants—phenytoin, mephenytoin, ethosuximide, barbiturates, carbamazepine, and gabapentin
   c. Antimicrobial agents—tetracyclines and ampicillin
   d. Antirheumatics—chloroquine
   e. Beta blockers—propranolol, oxprenolol, timolol, practolol, and betaxolol
   f. Drugs of abuse—cocaine
   g. Gastrointestinal—cimetidine
   h. Miscellaneous—D-L-carnitine, tropicamide, iodinated radiographic contrast, and trihexyphenidyl
   i. Ophthalmics—echothiophate
   j. Psychotropic drugs—phenothiazines and lithium
3. Drugs that cause myasthenia gravis or mimic myasthenia gravis
   a. D-Penicillamine
   b. Alpha-interferon
   c. Case reports: trimethadione, riluzole, ritonavir, chloroquine, statins, and beta-interferon
   d. Tandutinib

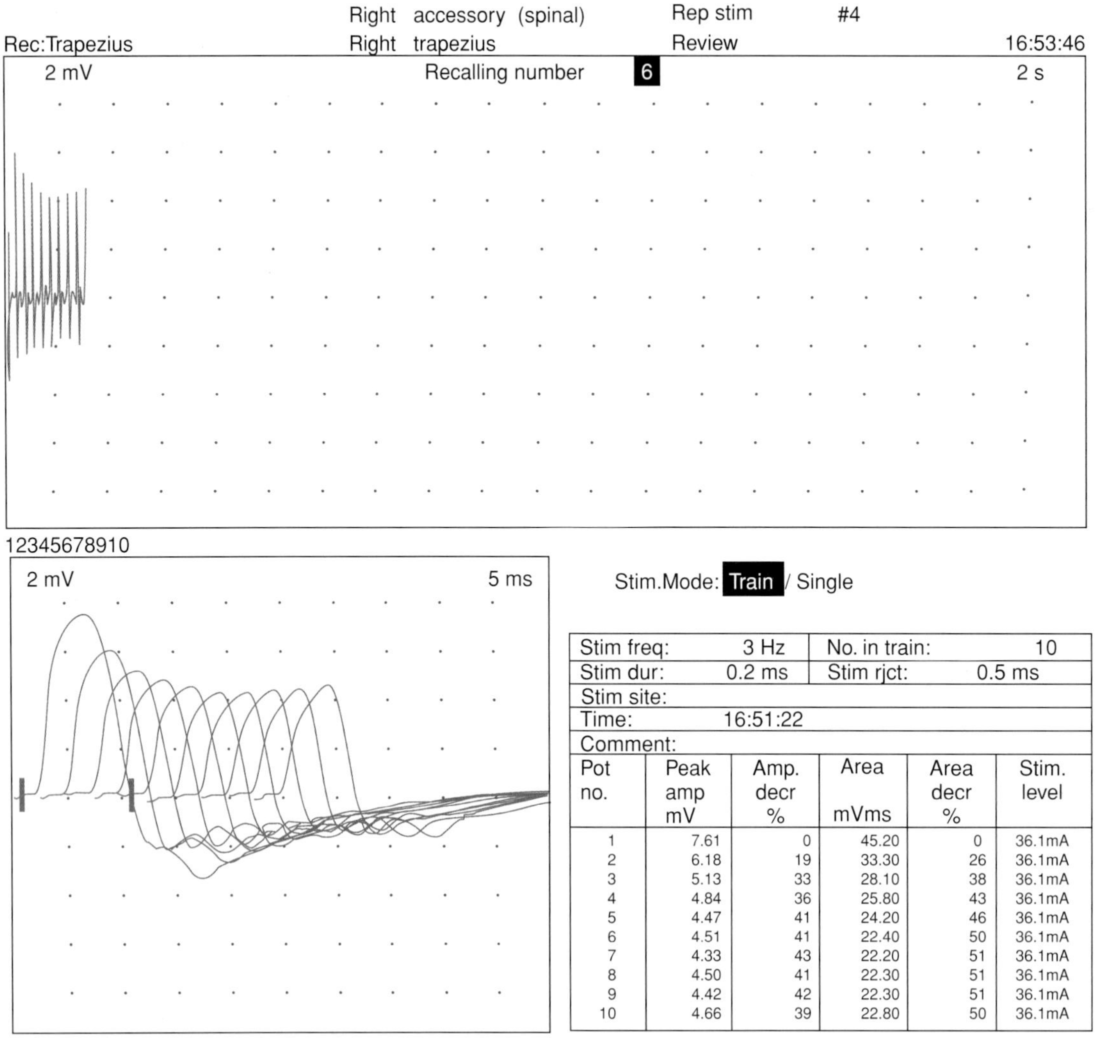

Stim freq:	3 Hz	No. in train:	10
Stim dur:	0.2 ms	Stim rjct:	0.5 ms
Stim site:			
Time:	16:51:22		
Comment:			

Pot no.	Peak amp mV	Amp. decr %	Area mVms	Area decr %	Stim. level
1	7.61	0	45.20	0	36.1mA
2	6.18	19	33.30	26	36.1mA
3	5.13	33	28.10	38	36.1mA
4	4.84	36	25.80	43	36.1mA
5	4.47	41	24.20	46	36.1mA
6	4.51	41	22.40	50	36.1mA
7	4.33	43	22.20	51	36.1mA
8	4.50	41	22.30	51	36.1mA
9	4.42	42	22.30	51	36.1mA
10	4.66	39	22.80	50	36.1mA

Figure 25-6. Typical pattern of a pathological decremental response to "slow" (2–5 Hz) repetitive stimulation.

characteristic of a postsynaptic DNMT that occur in other neuromuscular disease may have multiple mechanisms. In ALS and other denervating disorders, they are hypothesized to result from immature NMJ occurring as a consequence of attempted reinnervation.

Neither increased insertional activity nor abnormal spontaneous activity is typically identified in an MG patient. Fibrillation potentials and positive waves may occur however, particularly in paraspinal, bulbar, and proximal muscles.[250] Presumably, they result from severe end plate destruction and effective denervation. In support of this, their prevalence appears to correlate with patients who are significantly affected by generalized disease.

Two different types of abnormal motor unit action potential (MUAP) change may occur in MG. Both may be easily overlooked. Short-duration, low-amplitude MUAPs associated with early recruitment may occur. This pattern results from neuromuscular blockade and an effective reduction in the number of functional myofibers within a given motor unit, analogous to what may occur with myopathies.[251,252] Small MUAPs have been reported in MuSK MG as well, also consistent with a reduced number of normally functioning muscle fibers per motor unit resulting from either NM blockade, muscle fiber loss, or muscle fiber atrophy.

A more sensitive and valuable needle EMG tool is the demonstration of MUAP variability (instability) (Fig. 25-7). MUAP variability is the analog of clinical weakness and fatigue, a decremental response with repetitive stimulation, and blocking on SFEMG. It represents NMT failure of one or more single-fiber components to the MUAP that is typically intermittent, resulting in constant variation in the size, shape, and sound produced by an isolated MUAP. Unstable MUAPs are readily identified by the trained ear, and visualized with the use of a trigger and delay line. Their value is to provide evidence of abnormal NMT in muscles not easily studied by repetitive stimulation without necessarily undergoing the rigor of the SFEMG examination.

The EDX yield in MG varies depending on the serotype, severity, the EDX technique chosen, and the nerve/muscle

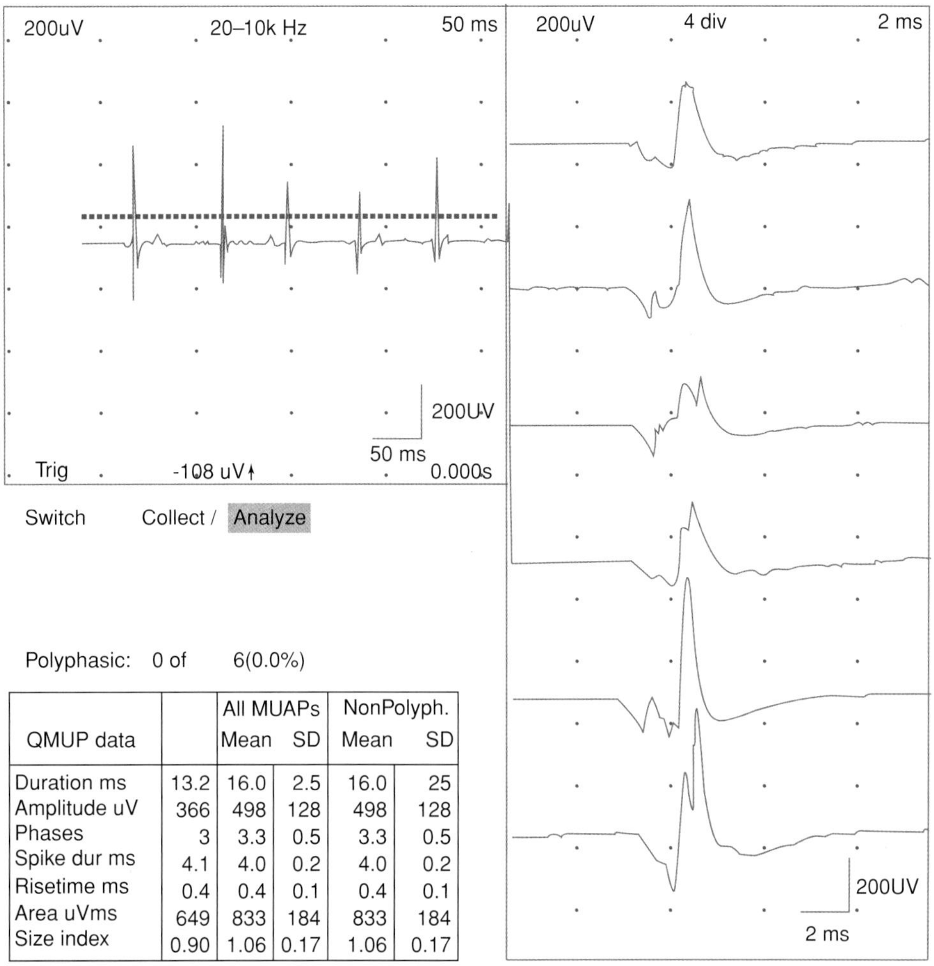

QMUP data		All MUAPs Mean	SD	NonPolyph. Mean	SD
Duration ms	13.2	16.0	2.5	16.0	25
Amplitude uV	366	498	128	498	128
Phases	3	3.3	0.5	3.3	0.5
Spike dur ms	4.1	4.0	0.2	4.0	0.2
Risetime ms	0.4	0.4	0.1	0.4	0.1
Area uVms	649	833	184	833	184
Size index	0.90	1.06	0.17	1.06	0.17

Figure 25-7. Motor unit instability—that is, variable MUAP size and shape with consecutive firings.

studied. To reinforce a previous point, absent technical difficulties, the diagnostic yield in a muscle rendered weak by myasthenia should be 100%. Conversely, the value of EDX relies on its ability to demonstrate disordered NMT in muscles that do not appear to be clinically affected.

To be considered abnormal, most laboratories require demonstration of a decrement of ≥10% in two muscles. These criteria are met in response to "slow" repetitive stimulation (2–5 Hz) in 37–62% of all individuals with MG.[252–256] The yield is lowest with intrinsic hand muscles which lack a decremental response in 50–70% of patients with moderately severe MG.[257] Proximal muscles, for example, the biceps, deltoid, and the trapezius, have higher yields. Erb's point stimulation with deltoid recording may be 80–90% sensitive in patients with myasthenia, but brachial plexus stimulation is both uncomfortable and technically difficult in view of the movement it creates. Accessory nerve stimulation has similar sensitivity and is usually better tolerated with an easier-to-establish stable baseline.[258] Facial nerve activation with recordings from the orbicularis oculi or nasalis muscles has a higher yield than limb muscles.

In patients with ocular MG, repetitive stimulation of a distal upper extremity nerve yields positive results in up to 35% of patients. Adding a proximal nerve increases the yield slightly to 45%. Patients who are MuSK antibody positive tend to have both a lesser incidence estimated at 60% and a lesser degree of decrement in limb muscles compared to other MG populations.[73,78,81] A higher yield of abnormal decrement will be found in facial muscles in the anti-MuSK patient population.[259] Estimates of incidence of abnormal decrement in these patients range from 25% to 50% in limb muscles as opposed to 50–85% in facial muscles.[77,82]

The EDX assessment of children with suspected MG is analogous to adults. In normal infants, the limited data available suggest that with stimulation rates between 1 and 2 Hz, there is no alteration in the CMAP.[260–262] Repetitive stimulation at rates between 2 and 5 Hz yields variable results, with some normal infants demonstrating a decrement and others revealing no change. In summary, premature infants and some term infants will have a reduced NMJ reserve capacity, especially at the higher rates of stimulation. Repetitive stimulation can be performed and interpreted confidently in term infants as long as this caveat is kept in mind.

The electrical findings in transient neonatal MG are analogous to those found in adults.[101,263] A decremental CMAP response is typically demonstrable at low rates of stimulation, which can be minimized with postactivation excitation (20–50 Hz repetitive stimulation) and augmented with postactivation exhaustion (repetitive trains of 2–5 Hz stimulation performed at 30 seconds to 1 minute intervals over a protracted period). Frequently, a decrement occurring at high rates of stimulation occurs as well, depending on the severity of the disease.

SFEMG is the most sensitive and least specific of EDX testing procedures for MG.[264] It can be performed either voluntary activation of a tested muscle or by electrical stimulation of a motor nerve branch innervating that muscle. Either method has its benefits and drawbacks. One strength of stimulated SFEMG is that it is less reliant on patient cooperation than voluntary SFEMG, making it the technique of choice in infants, an elderly person who may not be able to steadily sustain a minimal level of muscle activation, or any potentially uncooperative individual.[265–269] Stimulated SFEMG is typically faster to perform than voluntary SFEMG, providing an additional advantage. Its major disadvantage occurs when a muscle rather than nerve fiber is stimulated leading to a falsely reduced jitter value. Both voluntary and stimulated SFEMG are specialized techniques that many electromyographers do not receive training in. One benefit of SFEMG, stimulated or voluntary, is that it allows access to muscles frequently affected in MG not accessible to repetitive stimulation. The major benefit of SFEMG, however, and the one that translates to its high diagnostic sensitivity is its ability to detect abnormalities in NMT prior to development of overt NMT failure.

As described in Chapter 2, SFEMG assesses NMT by comparing the discharge intervals of two or more SMFAPs belonging to the same MUAP. This is technically accomplished by limiting the recording radius of the EMG needle. Historically, this was accomplished both by increasing the low frequency filter settings of the EMG machine and by using a special needle with a very limited recording radius. These needles are, however, expensive and reusable, necessitating sterilization after each use as well as periodic sharpening. For practical reasons, many institutions now use disposable, concentric needles which are adequate surrogates providing acceptable accuracy if attention is paid to detail during performance and interpretation.[270–273]

Two parameters are typically measured in the SFEMG assessment of a suspected MG patient. Jitter refers to the variation in the interval between the two single-muscle fiber action potentials mentioned above. Because of the normal variation in EPP amplitude, jitter is a property of normal muscle, typically lying in the 15–45 μs range depending on age and the muscle studied.[274,275] It becomes abnormal only when it is either smaller or in the case of MG, larger than normal (Fig. 25-8A,B). Increased jitter reflects abnormal or delayed, not failed NMT. As a result, abnormal jitter does not translate to weakness. With an increase in jitter values to 80 μs or above, however, NMT becomes tenuous and begins to intermittently fail. As a result, blocking, the equivalent of a decremental response to repetitive stimulation, motor unit instability, and clinical weakness, becomes manifest (Fig. 25-8B).

SFEMG is abnormal in 77–100% of patients, depending on disease severity and the number and distribution of muscles tested.[252,276–280] Specifically, the sensitivity of SFEMG is estimated at 97% if both a limb and a facial muscle are studied.[263] SFEMG abnormalities are found in the frontalis or orbicularis oculi in 87–99% of patients with oculobulbar weakness.[264] Studying the frontalis as opposed to a limb muscle will increase diagnostic yield from the 22–66% to the 54–100% range in all MG patients.[276,278] SFEMG abnormalities, like every other aspect of MG, can be patchy. We have observed instances while recording three SMFAPs belonging to the same motor unit where jitter is markedly increased in one pair while normal in the other. As a quantitative reflection of this, one study of 433 potential pairs from 32 patients with MG revealed normal jitter in 9%, increased jitter in 38%, and abnormal jitter with blocking in 53% of the potentials.[252,277] Although jitter measurements improve following successful treatment,[276,281–283] jitter abnormalities may persist even in those in clinical remission.[276,284] As in "slow" repetitive stimulation, SFEMG abnormalities in patients with MuSK MG are more likely to be found in facial or proximal muscles rather than in distal limb muscles such as the extensor digitorum communis, with a lower yield in limb muscles in general than expected in other MG populations.[75,86]

Historically, regional applications of both ischemia and d-tubocurarine curare were used in addition to "slow" repetitive stimulation, in an effort to increase diagnostic yield in MG. As these are cumbersome and potentially risky maneuvers, SFEMG represents the preferred EDX alternative in most EMG laboratories where "slow" repetitive stimulation is nondiagnostic.

PHARMACOLOGICAL TESTING

The edrophonium (i.e., Tensilon) test is a useful diagnostic adjunct in MG.[285–287] Edrophonium is a short-acting anticholinesterase, the administration of which will result in a transient increase in ACh availability at the NMJ and amplify the EPP. To perform the edrophonium test, a butterfly needle is placed in an accessible vein. A 2 mg (0.2 mL) test dose of edrophonium is administered initially. A small initial dose is necessary as some patients are extremely sensitive to the medication and may respond favorably to a small dose but not respond to a full 10 mg dose, leading to a potential false-negative conclusion in these individuals. If there is no

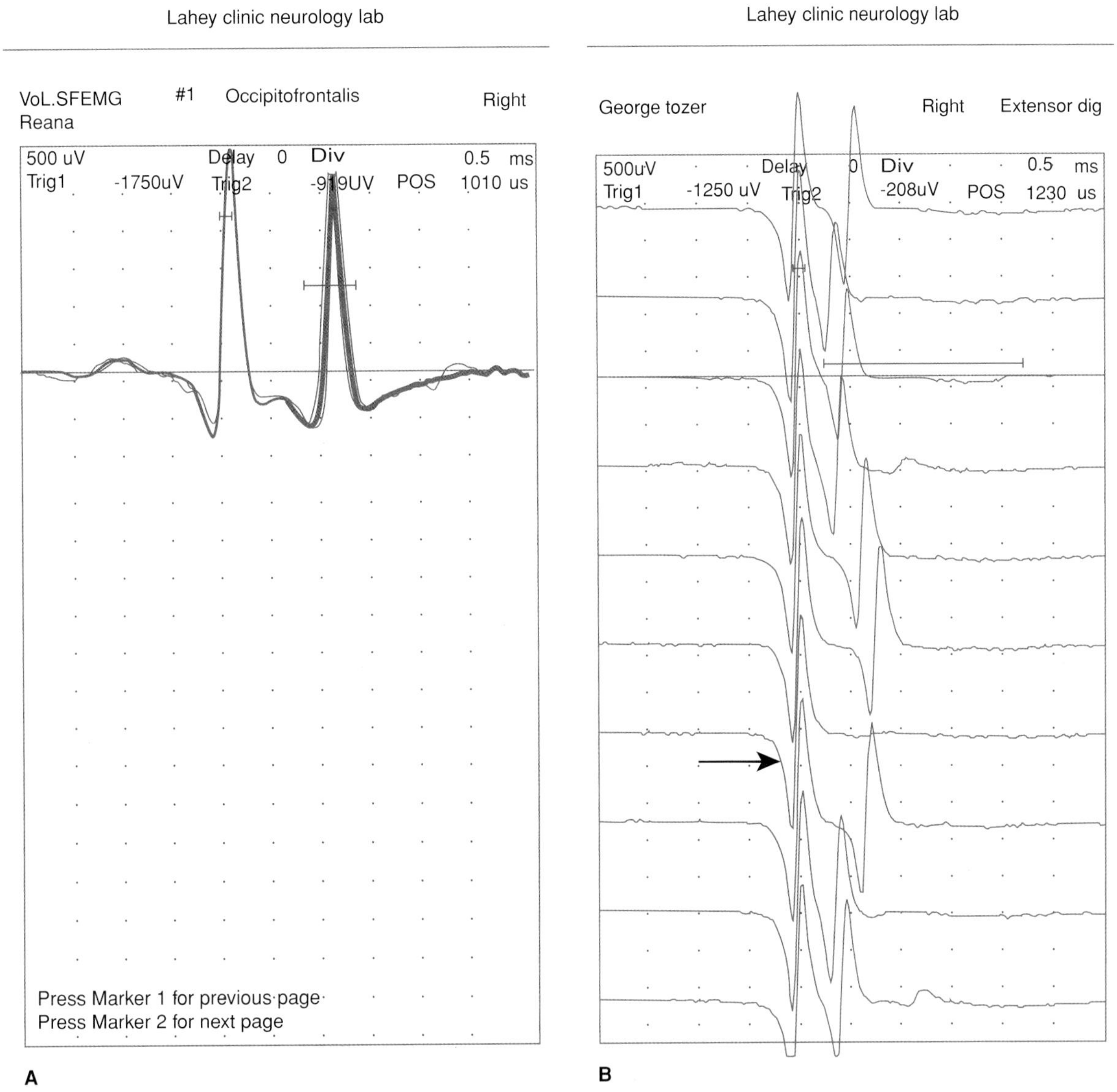

Figure 25-8. Single-fiber electromyography demonstrating a normal recording (**A**) and increased jitter and blocking (**B**—seventh pair from top—*arrow*) from an MG patient.

response to the initial 2 mg after 60 seconds, the remaining 8 mg are administered in 2 mg increments every 10–15 seconds. If the patient has an objective improvement or a severe side effect, the rest of the injection is aborted.

Performance of edrophonium testing should only be done in patients in whom objective weakness is present. In this regard, evaluating improvement of ptosis, ophthalmoparesis, or dysarthria is more useful than a complaint of dysphagia or fatigue. We have attempted tensilon testing in conjunction with modified barium swallow or pulmonary function testing as a means of identifying an objective response but have not had great success.

The sensitivity of edrophonium testing in MG is reported to be 86% for ocular and 95% for generalized MG.[288] Like repetitive stimulation, an abnormal test signifies abnormal NMT but does not define a singular disease. False positive responses have been reported in LEMS, ALS, CMS, botulism, Guillain–Barré syndrome, dysthyroid ophthalmopathy, and brainstem tumors.[37,289–292] Edrophonium testing is reported to have less utility in MuSK MG with a reported sensitivity of 50–70%.[78,82]

Edrophonium testing is not without risk. Historically, these were office-based procedures, performed without incident in most cases. Some patients would experience transient, disquieting but ultimately harmless symptoms such as nausea, vomiting, increased tearing, lacrimation, fasciculations, borborygmi, and eructation. Rarely however, serious reactions including bradycardia or heart block may occur. For consideration of patient safety, these tests are now routinely performed in monitored settings with individuals who are trained in resuscitation with adequate resources including parenteral atropine available.

Edrophonium has also been used in an attempt to distinguish weakness resulting from MG as opposed to that created by cholinergic excess. The availability of other effective MG treatments has limited the need for high dose anticholinesterase treatments in recent years. In addition, myasthenic crises and cholinergic crisis can be clinically distinguished in most individuals based on both the amount of anticholinesterase received and the presence of muscarinic symptoms that frequently occur in association with cholinergic crisis. For these reasons, this application of edrophonium is largely of historical interest.

IMAGING

Pathological changes in the thymus are found in >80% of patients with MG, detectable by imaging in many cases. In approximately 50% of those with MG, the histology will be that of lymphoreticular hyperplasia.[293] In the minority estimated at between 10–30%, either a benign low-grade thymoma of the thymic epithelium may be encountered, or on occasion an invasive thymoma.[23] Although chest x-ray may detect thymic enlargement from either hyperplasia or thymoma, either computerized tomography or magnetic resonance provide better resolution and are preferable studies. Although the thymus is typically located in the anterior mediastinum, it may be found ectopically in the neck or other regions of the chest.[293,294] In normal individuals, the CT appearance of normal thymus is homogeneous with attenuation characteristics similar to muscle, decreasing in size with age as fatty replacement takes place. The gland loses its appearance as a discreet structure somewhere between ages 25 and 40.[293] With MR, the normal childhood thymic appearance is also homogeneous with signal characteristics somewhere between muscle and fat. In addition to these features, a normal thymus gland is also characterized by its size and shape. A focal abnormality of the contour of the gland suggests an underlying neoplasm.

With thymic hyperplasia, the CT attenuation properties are normal. In slightly more than half of cases, the gland will appear abnormal because of its enlargement or in some cases, a focal mass.[293] MR characteristics are similar with gland enlargement but with normal signal characteristics. With thymoma, CT typically identifies sharply demarcated round or lobulated masses, commonly associated with low attenuation components that represent cysts, hemorrhage or necrosis (Fig. 25-2A,B). Calcifications occur and do not distinguish between invasive and noninvasive tumors.[293] Thymomas may enhance with iodinated contrast but the benefit is likely outweighed by the risk of an allergic response or a myasthenic exacerbation.[295]

The MR appearance of thymoma is also that of a gland incorporating a round, oval, or lobulated mass.[293] Signal intensity is low on T1-weighted images similar to that of muscle and relatively high signal intensity with T2-weighting. T2-weighted images may also define a lobulated structure characteristic of thymoma. One potential advantage of MR over CT in the evaluation of thymoma is the identification of characteristics suggestive of invasive thymoma such as obliteration of the adjacent fat planes.[293] Thymic abnormalities in patients with anti-MuSK antibodies are uncommon and typically minimal when they occur.[77] This point is emphasized in a study of 167 patients with thymoma.[126] Of the 92 who had MG, only one was seropositive for MuSK antibodies.

Recently, the bright tongue sign has been reported in ALS patients, representing fatty replacement of the genioglossus muscle demonstrable with MR imaging. This finding is not unique to ALS and has been reported in MuSK MG patients, in keeping with the muscle atrophy that can be seen in some of these patients, and providing another potentially confounding feature in the distinction of MG from bulbar ALS.[89]

▶ HISTOPATHOLOGY

Presumably, the majority of muscle biopsies performed in MG patients is done inadvertently in seronegative individuals with phenotypes that mimic myopathy. Muscle biopsy has no role in the majority of MG patients and much of what we know about myasthenic muscle histology comes from postmortem specimens.[296] These reports need to be interpreted with caution. Although MG is a systemic disease, described abnormalities often existed in limb muscles whereas the majority of these patients had oculobulbar phenotypes. Consequently, the abnormalities described are not necessarily disease-related.[296] Conversely, if muscle biopsy were to be performed, consideration of a false negative result should be given in view of sampling error and the patchy nature of the disease. Interpretation of historical publications of muscle histology in MG should be made with the knowledge that many preceded the availability of contemporary histochemical analysis. Lastly, interpretation of muscle histology in MG should be made with consideration of the effects from potential coexistence of other disorders that occur with increased frequency in MG such as dysthyroidism or autoimmune muscle disease.

The findings on light microscopic analysis of MG muscle are nonspecific. The muscle may be normal in appearance.[296] When abnormal, the most common findings are type 1 fiber predominance, mild fiber type grouping, or type 2 fiber atrophy.[296,297] Focal interstitial inflammatory infiltrates, historically referred to as lymphorrhages, are not uncommon, and have been described predominantly within proximity of necrotic fibers, blood vessels, and muscle end plates (Fig. 25-9).[296–299] Histological features of myopathy are not a characteristic feature of myasthenic muscle.[296]

Muscle biopsies in MuSK MG patients have been reported to demonstrate myofiber atrophy and minor simplification of some end plates.[73] Despite the known function of MuSK in synaptogenesis, the density and distribution of AChR in patients with MuSK appear normal in the

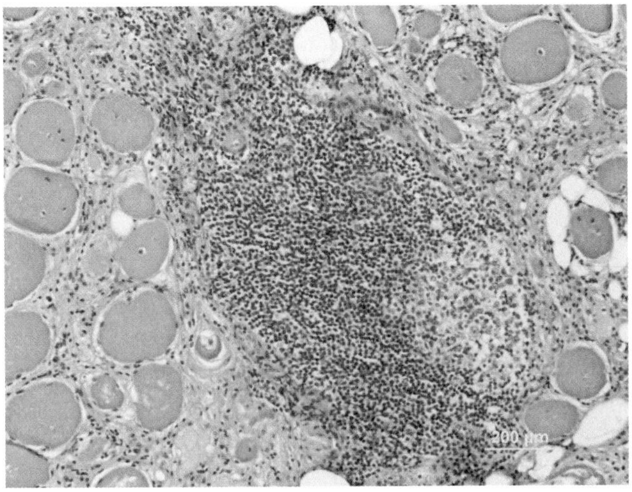

Figure 25-9. Cross section of muscle biopsy in a myasthenic patient demonstrating a focal inflammatory response "lymphorrhage."

studies reported to date. Complement deposition or other markers of an immune-mediated disease have not been identified.[212,300]

Ultrastructural abnormalities are more evident in MG. Immunoelectron microscopy of the postsynaptic membrane region in patients with myasthenia demonstrates IgG and complement precipitation on the membrane, a widened synaptic space, reduced postsynaptic membrane complexity with fewer postjunctional folds, and decreased numbers of AChRs. Many of the remaining AChRs are bound with IgG.[173,203–205,301] In contrast, the presynaptic portion of the NMJ appears completely normal.

There has been some historical concern pertaining to potential adverse structural effects on muscle in response to chronic or excessive anticholinesterase exposure.[176] In animals, degeneration of postsynaptic folds has been described. SFEMG studies have suggested increased fiber density in patients treated with anticholinesterase medications, suggested of denervation and reinnervation and consistent with some of the histological findings described above. In addition, prolonged exposure to anticholinesterases leads to an overexpression of the AChE-R isoform. Overexpressed AChE-R in transgenic mice leads to myopathic muscle changes including atrophic and vacuolated muscle fibers as well as neurogenic muscle changes.[302] The clinical relevance of these observations is uncertain, given the relatively minor histological findings reported in patients largely studied in an era when anticholinesterase medications were the primary therapy for MG, commonly used in large doses for prolonged periods of time.

Although relevant to myasthenia, the histological abnormalities of the thymus gland are beyond the scope of this chapter. The reader is referred to an excellent review of the thymus gland in myasthenia for more detailed information on this subject.[23]

▶ TREATMENT

Managing a myasthenic patient requires consideration of numerous variables. Patient age, gender, comorbidities, concurrent medication, patient functional expectations, serotype, clinician experience and preference, treatment availability and cost, and whenever available, an evidence-based perspective all require consideration in treatment decisions. Many excellent reviews are available that address these options and strategies.[38,55,303] The ideal of a fully evidence-based therapeutic approach is hampered by the lack of adequate studies. This impediment is multifactorial. MG is a relatively uncommon disease with multiple treatment options, many of which are considered effective, if imperfectly so. In support of this perception of therapeutic efficacy is the previously mentioned mortality statistics which unequivocally demonstrate an improvement in MG care over the course of the last century.[13,23,38] The strategies suggested in this chapter represent our approach, based in part on the teaching of our mentors and in part our personal experience, heavily blended with guidance from the literature. Our approach is intended to provide guidance and is not intended to be dogmatic or inflexible in its application.

One management consideration is disease serotype. AChR and seronegative MG are largely considered to have overlapping but non-identical phenotypes and treatment responsiveness. Reports suggest that seronegative MG patients respond better to most treatment modalities than either MuSK or AChR MG but less well to thymectomy than AChBr disease.[71,80,304] In general, the weight of existing evidence suggests that MuSK MG is a more severe disease, less treatment responsive, and requires in part a different therapeutic strategy.[10,71] Cholinesterase inhibitors are thought to be ineffective and may worsen the disease. Current thinking suggests that thymectomy has a limited role in MuSK MG unless thymoma is identified, an extremely rare occurrence.[71,73,77,83,123] Steroids may or may not be effective.[78] Expert opinion indicates that MuSK MG responds to other immunomodulating therapies.[73,74,80,81,82,305,306–308] Intravenous immunoglobulin (IVIG) may work in some cases of MuSK MG patients refractory to other modalities.[308,311] We and others have been impressed with rituximab in refractory MG, both AChR-MG and MuSK-MG.[310–313] With LPR4 MG, a distinct therapeutic strategy has not been developed. Current strategy is to treat it identically to traditional AChR MG.

Therapeutic strategies in MG include attempts to treat the disease symptomatically (cholinesterase inhibitors, noninvasive positive pressure ventilation, percutaneous gastrostomy), remove a potential contributor to disease pathogenesis (thymectomy), suppress components of disease immunopathogenesis (immunomodulation through the use of drugs, IVIG, or PLEX), prevent when possible and address when necessary potential exacerbating factors (e.g., avoidance of drugs with neuromuscular blocking properties, treating intercurrent infections and comorbidities such as dysthyroidism), and potentially prevent the escalation from mild to more severe disease. In that regard, it has been suggested that corticosteroids may reduce the conversion frequency of purely ocular to generalized disease.[36,37] Although we frequently treat disabling ocular symptoms refractory to pyridostigmine with immunomodulating agents, we do not do so routinely with the goal of reducing the probability of disease generalization.

In general, our philosophy is to treat the patient, not the disease. We attempt to achieve an optimal sense of patient well-being and function, while at the same time considering what an acceptable level of risk might be. This would include consideration of both probability and magnitude of potential side effects. Along those lines, we do not dogmatically adhere to historical therapeutic recommendations such as avoidance of thymectomy in patients >65 years of age or in patients with ocular myasthenia. The reluctance to thymectomize older individuals (without thymoma) is based largely on the atrophic nature of the gland in older individuals. We are unaware of any evidence that supports either decreased efficacy or increased procedural risk based on chronological age alone. Similarly we would consider thymectomy or immunosuppression in a pyridostigmine-resistant individual with limited ocular disease if their visual morbidity significantly interfered with their vocation or quality of life.[314–316] Our management strategies are summarized at the end of this section.

SYMPTOMATIC TREATMENT

Although most patients will not adequately respond to peripheral cholinesterase inhibitors alone, they are frequently used as the initial treatment. This practice evolves from the consideration of their cost and favorable side effect profile. In patients with minor morbidity, they may suffice as the sole treatment. Pyridostigmine is the drug of choice as it has a more favorable duration of action and side effect profile than other drugs of its class. The initial oral dose is typically 15–60 mg three times a day. In a patient with dysphagia, it is typically prescribed 30–60 minutes before meals. We rarely use more than 240 mg a day as higher doses are commonly associated with adverse rather than beneficial effect. If the patient does not achieve the desired therapeutic effect by 360 mg per day, it is our experience that they are unlikely to benefit by further dose escalation. It is also important to recognize that the beneficial effects of pyridostigmine may wane with time if autoimmunity remains unchecked, with unabated destruction of motor end plates resulting in depletion of ACh binding sites. For these reasons, we typically initiate immunomodulating therapy if 240 mg of daily pyridostigmine (60 mg every 6 hours) does not achieve or maintain the desired effect. As we tend to avoid large anticholinesterase doses, cholinergic crisis is a disorder of largely historical interest in our experience.

There are different peripheral cholinesterase inhibitors with different delivery models. Neostigmine can be given parenterally at a dose of 7.5–15 every 4–6 hours and may be the drug of choice for intramuscular delivery.[303] Pyridostigmine is also available in a 180 timespan capsule, utilized primarily for treatment of nocturnal symptoms. The timespan formulation is rarely used diurnally due to its variable absorption.[38] It is also available in a liquid form (12 mg/ml) and in a parenteral form that can be used in patients who cannot or should not swallow. It is important to be aware that the parenteral dose pyridostigmine is 1/30th to 1/60th of its oral counterpart. The most common side effects are related to the gastrointestinal tract such as abdominal discomfort, nausea and diarrhea. As these symptoms are related to muscarinic, not nicotinic side effects, they may be treated with anticholinergic drugs without adversely affecting the beneficial effects on nicotinic NMT.

The role of parenteral pyridostigmine is primarily in the treatment of MG patients undergoing elective surgery during the period where their oral intake is prohibited. We are less likely to use it during myasthenic crisis in an intubated patient as its potential beneficial effect may be outweighed by increased secretion production as an unwanted side effect.[38] Pyridostigmine by itself will rarely, if ever, prevent myasthenic crises or rescue patients from it once it occurs.

Noninvasive positive pressure ventilation has a limited but important role in the management of MG patients. It is used to delay or avoid intubation in a patient with imminent crisis, to help wean a patient from invasive ventilation recovering from crisis, or to treat sleep-disordered breathing when present, which MG patients, like all neuromuscular patients, are susceptible to.[317] Percutaneous gastrostomy is virtually never required in MG due to the typical efficacy and relative rapid onset of available MG treatments in restoring functional swallowing and minimizing aspiration risk. We have encountered rare MG patients who have received percutaneous gastrostomy as a result of diagnostic delay, for example, for an anterior cervical osteophyte misidentified as the cause of dysphagia, the gastrostomy tube subsequently removed once effective swallowing was restored.

Symptomatic treatments may be used locally as well. Lid crutches for the treatment of ptosis may be tried but is in our experience rarely tolerated. Topical naphazoline, a sympathomimetic drug with preferential $\alpha 2$ activity, has been reported to provide a marked response in 30% and a worthwhile benefit in an additional 40% of MG patients with ptosis.[318] Presumably, the drug acts on the sympathetically innervated lid elevator, Müller's muscle.

Thymectomy

The association with thymic hyperplasia and an apparent therapeutic benefit of thymectomy were first described by Blalock in MG patients in the World War II era[319–321] Thymectomy for nonthymomatous patients remains an accepted, but unproven therapeutic option for MG treatment.[71,294,322] Estimates suggest the 50–60% of MG patients undergoing thymectomy, particularly those with thymic hyperplasia, will achieve symptomatic remission. This data, however does not account for potential contamination by the known spontaneous remission that may occur as part of the natural history of the disease.[71,303] Regarding thymectomy and serotype, complete symptomatic remission is estimated to occur in 54% in AChBR MG, in 40% of patients with seronegative disease, and in 20% of MuSK MG patients with or without thymic hyperplasia.[323] Current consensus recommends avoidance of thymectomy in nonthymomatous MuSK MG patients.[71,73,77,83,123]

The American Academy of Neurology Practice Parameter that reviewed 21 published level II studies of nonthymomatous thymectomy in MG patients found that patients undergoing thymectomy were 1.7 times as likely to improve, 1.6 times as likely to become asymptomatic, and twice as likely to attain medication-free remission.[322] The apparent benefits of thymectomy are often delayed with a median time to achieve complete stable remission judged to be in the 17–20 month range.[322] Current beliefs are that the benefits of thymectomy are greatest if performed within 3 years of initial symptoms.[38] The neuromuscular community awaits the results of an international prospective trial intended to identify the frequency and magnitude of thymectomy benefit in MG patients.[323–325]

Response appears to vary by thymectomy technique and disease serotype. Historically, remission rate is thought to increase proportionately to the extent of thymic removal, and a transcervical, transsternal "complete" thymectomy is thought to provide the greatest chance of achieving this goal.[294] We acknowledge however, that more recent data suggest similar efficacy with less invasive techniques such as video-assisted thoracoscopic surgery.[326,327]

There is a consensus that all patients with thymoma should have thymectomy to minimize the risk of the morbidity and potential mortality of local invasion, or the smaller risk of disseminated metastasis. It is generally held that MG in patients with thymoma are less responsive to thymectomy in comparison to MG patients with thymic hyperplasia.[38]

Immunomodulating Treatment

Details pertaining to specific immunomodulating treatments have been provided in Chapter 4. This chapter will focus on specific principles and practices related to the management of the MG patient.

Prior to the initiation of any immunomodulating agent, we attempt to exclude any indolent infectious disease such as tuberculosis or strongyloidiasis that may become symptomatic with treatment. We attempt to identify patients at increased risk because of potential prior exposure to these diseases (e.g., someone who has emigrated from a country where strongyloidiasis is endemic) and liberally obtain skin and serological testing, quantiferon gold assessments and chest x-rays. With corticosteroid use, we obtain baseline bone density determinations and vitamin D levels. All patients on corticosteroids are advised to take calcium carbonate (approximately 1000 mg/day) and vitamin D (approximately 2000 IU/day) supplements. There is an increased risk of symptomatic osteoporosis and pneumocystis in patients treated with corticosteroids or other immunomodulating drugs. Bisphosphonate prophylaxis of glucocorticoid-induced osteopenia has been shown to reduce adverse effects on bone density but has equivocal results regarding reducing the rate of bone fracture.[328] Studies provide varying results depending on patient gender, prophylactic drug utilized and dose chosen. We do not routinely provide pneumocystis prophylaxis as we are unaware of any literature that provides adequate guidance regarding risk and risk reduction relevant to the number and type of immunomodulating agents that are used.

Corticosteroids are estimated to benefit 80–90% of myasthenic patients, typically within 2 weeks with maximum benefit occurring on average within 3 months and within 6 months in all patients destined to respond.[38,329–332]

There are two approaches commonly used in treating patients with corticosteroids. Regardless of the dosage used, the prednisone is typically prescribed as a single morning dose, attempting to mimic the normal physiological diurnal variation of endogenous glucocorticoids as much as possible. Unfortunately, again there is no literature to support any one approach being more effective than the others.

The first approach is the start low, go slow approach advocated by the Johns Hopkins group.[44] We typically use this in patients with ocular myasthenia or mild generalized MG. In such cases, we usually initiate prednisone at 20 mg daily with instructions for the patient to increase the dose by 5 mg every 5–7 days as needed to control their symptoms up to a total daily dose of 1.0 mg/kg. We have patients stay on whatever the effective dosage is for one month before slowly tapering down by 5 mg a month to 20 mg daily and then by 2.5 mg every month until we find the lowest possible dose that controls their disease. The downside of this start low, go slow approach is that it takes longer from initiation of steroids to see an effect and does not guarantee avoidance of corticosteroid exacerbation.[305]

The second approach is to start patients on high dose daily prednisone (e.g., 0.75–1.0 mg/kg) at onset. The benefit of this approach is that patients usually improve faster. The downside is that approximately 10–15% of myasthenics who are started on high-dose prednisone may experience an initial decline in strength during the first week or so.[330,332–334] For this reason, we usually reserve this approach to patients with moderate-to-severe MG who are or who will be hospitalized. The mechanism of the exacerbation is not clear. It would appear to be related to NMT as opposed to adverse nerve or muscle effect as it is associated with worsening of the decremental response to repetitive stimulation if employed.[334] This weakness tends to dissipate even with continued use of high steroid dosage. It is also possible that the apparent worsening represents situational bias. That is, the patients who are started on high dose prednisone most often have newly diagnosed or progressive MG. The worsening of the MG may be because of the progression of the disease itself and not the addition of the steroids.

There are different approaches even with high dose prednisone treatment. Some authorities advocate for maintaining patients on daily steroids, while others would taper to an alternate day schedule. We typically start patients on daily prednisone for at least 2 weeks and then try the alternate day approach unless the patient has diabetes as this approach renders it more difficult to control glucose levels. As soon as the patient demonstrates clinical benefit, we begin to wean on an every other day basis. Again, there are multiple approaches. One is to double the dose on the odd day and provide no steroids on the even day. The odd day dosage is then gradually reduced. Alternatively, and perhaps preferable due to its less abrupt pattern, we will wean by maintaining the initial dose on the odd day, for example, 60 mg, and with the dose reduction occurring initially on even days, for example, 50 mg. The subsequent wean occurs by continuing the reduction on the lower dose day until it reaches zero. At that point, the wean is continued by sequential reduction of the odd day amount. The rate of weaning depends on how the patient responds. Typically, if the patient is responding, we reduce the dose by 10 mg at a time. If the patient is deemed unresponsive to steroids, or develops unacceptablel side effects, the wean occurs much more rapidly. Once the total dose reaches a semi-arbitrary dose of 20 mg every other day, we typically reduce to the dose by no more than 5 mg or less at each interval. We consider 20 mg every other day, again based on arbitrary data, as the highest acceptable steroid dose that we feel comfortable using on a chronic basis. If another immunomodulating agent is started simultaneously as is commonly the case (see below), we space the dose reduction intervals so as to ideally discontinue the steroids within a 6–12-month time frame. In our experience on average, more problems are created by weaning too fast, than weaning too slow. If the patient demonstrates no benefit within 2 months of institution of corticosteroids, they are rapidly weaned and discontinued.

If immunomodulating treatment is indicated, we commonly initiate a second-line drug along with corticosteroids. The benefit of steroids is their relatively rapid onset of action whereas many of the second- and third-line agents require at least 3 months and typically more time in order to demonstrate efficacy. As we prefer to avoid the long-term effects of corticosteroids that seem inevitable at higher doses, we attempt to provide long-term therapeutic remission with other immunomodulating drugs that are often better tolerated in the long term. Our goal is to achieve a satisfactory response with a second-line, or if necessary a third-line, agent as a monotherapy over the course of the first year. We recognize that the evidence basis by which to justify the use of or to choose a specific nonsteroidal immunomodulating drug for MG treatment is limited. We consider azathioprine[333,335–339] as the second-line treatment of choice. Some prefer mycophenolate[341–351] as a second-line choice though two randomized clinical trials (discussed below) failed to demonstrate efficacy. Improvement is noted in 70–90% of patients with myasthenia treated with azathioprine, including some patients who are steroid- resistant.[333] Although some patients will display early intolerance to azathioprine, we have numerous patients in clinical and side-effect-free remission for over 20 years while on azathioprine monotherapy. Deficiency of enzyme thiopurine methyltransferase predisposes to bone marrow toxicity in patients exposed to azathioprine. We remain uncertain as to whether routine screening for levels of this enzyme is beneficial prior to the initiation of this drug.

Mycophenolate is attractive both for its ease of use and relatively benign side effect profile for an immunomodulating drug. Although the two randomized, blinded, clinical trials reported in 2008 failed to demonstrate a benefit, this may have been a consequence of trial design (studies too short in duration for a response to occur).[340,341] A retrospective study demonstrating a therapeutic benefit after 6 months would support this contention.[351] Alternatively, the concurrent small prednisone dose, 20 mg daily, that patients received in both the treatment and placebo arm in the MSG study suggests efficacy from this drug that might have masked a potential benefit from mycophenolate. We, as well as others, believe it to be an effective, well-tolerated drug in some patients.

We have had positive experiences with other immunomodulating agents, typically prescribed in those patients who have had inadequate or adverse responses to pyridostigmine, corticosteroids, azathioprine, and/or mycophenolate. In view of their side effect profiles, uncertainty of benefit, monitoring requirements or cost considerations, we tend to use cyclosporine,[352–356] tacrolimus,[357–367] cyclophosphamide,[368–371] and rituximab[305–307,310–313,372–374] as third-line treatment agents. We also use methotrexate as third-line agent while awaiting the results of a large randomized, double-blind trial. As mentioned above, rituximab, cyclophosphamide, and cyclosporine have been specifically, albeit anecdotally, reported to benefit MuSK MG patients.[305,307,356,369] We have used rituxan in either two or four infusions over the course of 1 month and found it to be quite effective in refractory MuSK and AChR patients (Chapter 4). In our experience, the response to rituximab is durable and often exceeds a year of more before tretreatment is required. We have had a limited experience with sirolimus and remain uncertain regarding its efficacy. We reserve cyclophosphamide for patients' refractory to other aforementioned treatments.

As the specter of opportunistic infection and neoplasm exists in all patients treated with long-term immunomodulating agents, we give consideration to gradual withdrawal of these agents in any patient who has been in a stable, apparent remission for 2 years or more. It is our impression that many MG patients will have mild, asymptomatic, residual weakness of eye closure despite otherwise excellent disease control. We do not consider this finding to represent a contraindication to attempted weaning from immunomodulating therapy. Given the statistical uncertainty of risk versus benefit, this decision is heavily influenced by patient perspective. We have been successful in this approach in a number of individuals, with or without thymectomy, although are uncertain whether this represents the effect of treatment or the natural history of the disease.

IVIG[98,116,375–385] and PLEX[381,384,386–398] are considered to be effective treatments for MG.[381,384,393,399–402] Their therapeutic support however, has not been without controversy. Historically, many neurologists have considered PLEX superior to IVIG.[393] IVIG, however, has been demonstrated to benefit MG patients in a prospective randomized trial whereas no analogous PLEX study has been conducted.[377] In addition, IVIG has been suggested to be particularly effective in the treatment of MuSK MG.[73,77,308,309,403] As a result, American Academy of Neurology guidelines have identified IVIG as "probably effective and should be considered" in contrast to PLEX where "there is insufficient evidence to support or refute the use of plasma exchange" in MG.[385,390] The latter position generated a considerable editorial response from the journal's readership including many individuals recognized for their expertise in MG management.[397] These critics aptly pointed out that PLEX was penalized due to its competitive disadvantage, that is, the unlikelihood of a class 1 study of PLEX in MG ever being conducted. A subsequently published head-to-head class 1 study reinforced the opinion that PLEX performed slightly better than IVIG, although both treatments were found to be statistically equivalent relative to both the degree of efficacy and the number of MG patients that benefitted from their use.[399,402]

We primarily use IVIG and PLEX in two situations, to avert or treat myasthenic crisis or to "tune up" an MG patient with residual weakness prior to thymectomy.[404] This is done hoping to minimize the risk of postoperative complications such as aspiration or prolonged ventilator dependency.[400] Typical algorithms involving five infusions or exchanges are used for each. Due to the cost, lifestyle inconvenience and in some cases risk (e.g., need for central venous access in PLEX), we tend to avoid chronic treatment with these two modalities unless other therapeutic options are precluded.

Their greatest benefit of IVIG and PLEX is their relatively rapid onset of action, often within days.[381,401] Both are costly although IVIG may enjoy a cost advantage, particularly in the hospitalized patient as it can characteristically be completed in a shorter period of time resulting in a potentially shorter length of stay. PLEX has been reported to have a 90% efficacy in one retrospective study and 65% in a prospective one.[396,399] IVIG has been reported to achieve a significant benefit in 69% of patients.[399] Exchange can be successfully accomplished in an outpatient setting through peripheral access in the majority of patients. Peripheral versus central venous access minimizes risk, particularly that of a serious risk.[396] One additional potential drawback of PLEX is the need to coordinate its timing in relation to immunomodulatory drug administration.

Other novel treatments for MG have been suggested, all intended to address adverse effects while sparing beneficial aspects of immune surveillance.[215] One such attempt that appears to have been successful in an in vitro rat model of autoimmune myasthenia is vaccination with cytoplasmic epitopes of the ACh subunits. The intended strategy is to deflect the potentially destructive aspects of autoimmunity away from the extracellular domains of these ACh subunits that the disease targets.[405] A second strategy is the development of synthesized anti-sense RNA molecules that target the gene expression of the AChE-R isoform. By doing so, NMT is augmented and potential adverse effects of increased AChE-R levels on muscle that may result from chronic anticholinesterase use are avoided.[215] Another apparent successful in vitro strategy is to utilize genetically engineered dendritic cells to present AChR epitopes. The intent here is to specifically kill the T cells responsible for the initiation of the autoimmune response.[212] The engineering of monoclonal antibodies that target specific components of disease-specific autoimmunity represents an additional strategy. Blocking of complement activation by eculizumab that is currently being studied in clinical trial is one such strategy. The C5 complement inhibitor rEV576 has also been utilized.[406] The tumor necrosis factor alpha blocker etanercept was reported in a small trial to have modest efficacy.[407] Allogenic hematopoietic stem cell transplantation has been utilized successfully in one case.[408]

Special Circumstances

The treatment of MG in children and adolescents provides a number of additional challenges.[96–98,115–117] In adolescents with MG, we attempt to avoid corticosteroids and other immunomodulating drugs if possible in view of the adverse effects on growth and the concern for the suspected increased risk of neoplasm over a patient's lifetime. Avoidance in adolescent females is of particular concern due to the potential teratogenicity in future pregnancies. We are uncertain of the potential for teratogenicity resulting from immunomodulating drug exposure in males. We have been very supportive of thymectomy in the adolescent female population in the hope of achieving drug-free remission during the patient's reproductive years. Removal of the thymus in children does not appear to have any deleterious effect on immune system development.[333] In a large retrospective series of 149 patients with juvenile MG, 85 patients had a thymectomy while 64 patients were managed medically.[97] In the thymectomy group, 82% of patients improved, while 48% went into remission compared to a 63% improvement rate and a 34% remission rate in the patients who are nonthymectomized.[97] In another retrospective series of 79 patients with juvenile MG, 65 patients (82%) underwent thymectomy. Of the patients who were thymectomized, remission occurred in 60% compared to 29% in the nonthymectomized group.[96] Neither of these studies controlled for baseline severity or concomitant medical treatment, thus the role of thymectomy in juvenile MG like adults remaining unproven.[322]

Management of MG is challenging both in anticipation of and during pregnancy. Evidence-based guidance is limited. Myasthenics should be treated as high-risk pregnancies both for the mother's and the child's welfare. In general, the pregnant myasthenic may be managed with a philosophy similar to the pregnant epileptic. Concerns regarding potential teratogenic effects of drugs need to be balanced with the recognition of harm that could befall both mother and child with inadequate treatment. In both diseases, the smallest effective doses of the safest potential therapies are sought.

MG is not recognized to have any adverse effects on pregnancy, for example, increasing the risk of eclampsia. Pregnancy may influence MG, however, particularly regarding management decisions. Existing information suggests that 1/3 of MG patients will improve, worsen or remain the same during pregnancy.[99,409] The first trimester and the postpartum periods are the periods where exacerbation is estimated to most commonly occur.[409] Myasthenic morbidity may stem not only from the disease itself but may result from the mechanical effects of the enlarging fetus on diaphragmatic movement.

Regarding management, cholinesterase inhibitors have been used anecdotally without apparent harm. There appears to be little, if any, risk of unwanted stimulation of the myometrium. Magnesium, potentially used for the treatment of pregnancy-related hypertension, is optimally avoided in a pregnant MG patient. There are theoretical concerns that PLEX may adversely affect pregnancy by unwanted effects on hormonal levels, potentially increasing the risk of premature delivery.[409] The risks of IVIG during pregnancy are largely unknown. Of the immunomodulating treatment options, corticosteroids are probably the safest although they do pose a slightly increased risk of fetal cleft lip and of premature rupture of the membranes.[409] As a general rule, although successful pregnancies have been accomplished under their influence, other immunomodulating drugs are avoided prior to conception and during pregnancy if at all possible.

Prevention and Treatment of Potential Exacerbating Factors

The effects of pregnancy on MG have already been described. Intercurrent infections and other coexisting autoimmune diseases if uncontrolled are both believed to aggravate MG. Drugs remain the most noteworthy category of influences that aggravates, and in some cases even causes, MG (Table 25-3).

Monitoring

We monitor our patient's treatment response primarily through clinical assessment. We feel that in most cases, it is at least as effective and undoubtedly more efficient and cost-effective than other testing modalities. As mentioned in Chapter 1, hand-held dynamometry can be a very effective tool for this purpose. As mentioned, monitoring autoantibody titers has little or no role other than potentially assessing the efficacy of thymectomy or monitoring for thymoma reoccurrence. Although electrophysiological parameters can be utilized as an indicator of treatment responsiveness, we find them to be unnecessary in the vast majority of cases. We tend to use them only in confounding situations, that is, attempting to separate myasthenic weakness from that of another potential cause. Cost, time expenditure, and patient comfort are factors that dissuade us from their routine use in patient monitoring. Again, in the spirit of treating the patient, not the disease, electrophysiological monitoring may be too sensitive and potentially lead to excessive treatment. As an example, increased jitter in an asymptomatic muscle is not an indication for treatment initiation or modification.

Assessment scales designed specifically for MG have been used both to stage disease severity, to accurately monitor response to treatment, and to assess quality of life in MG patients.[410,411] They are, to the best of our knowledge, utilized more as clinical research tools rather than assessment tools routinely used in the clinic. The Osserman scale is primarily a staging tool.[18] Adult MG is subdivided into Group 1 (ocular: 15–20%), Group 2A (mild generalized: 30%), Group 2B (moderately severe generalized: 20%), Group 3 (acute fulminating: 11%), and Group 4 (late severe: 9%). In Europe, the myasthenic muscle score (MMS) developed in 1983 is the preferred metric for determining efficacy in MG clinical trials.[412] It is a 100-point scale that assesses trunk as well as oculobulbar, limb and muscle strength. In the United States, the quantified MG score (QMS), also initially proposed in 1983 and later modified, is the preferred instrument. It is a 39-point scale that has considerable overlap with the MMS although it incorporates ventilatory muscle strength and does not address trunk strength beyond neck flexors.[412–414]

In summary, our typical management strategy for MG is not dogmatic and often varies in consideration of patient and physician preference and individual patient context and comorbidities. We attempt to document a patient's clinical deficits as quantitatively as possible at baseline in order to improve our ability to make future rational treatment decisions. We obtain baseline thyroid function studies and chest imaging (typically CT) in all patients including those with MuSK autoantibodies in whom demonstration of thymic abnormalities would be extremely unlikely. We would be vigilant for any clinical clues suggesting a synergistic cause of weakness (e.g., hypokalemia) or coexistent autoimmune disease and test accordingly. In patients with minor morbidity, we initiate pyridostigmine, typically at a dose of 60 mg tid. In patients with generalized myasthenia who do not appear to be at the imminent risk of aspiration or ventilatory failure, we typically initiate both corticosteroids at a 1 mg/kg dose (prednisone or methylprednisolone if parenteral therapy is required) along with a second immunomodulating drug, potentially as an outpatient if adequate monitoring can be assured. Hospital admission is suggested to any generalized MG patient placed on high dose corticosteroids; (1) who cannot be reliably monitored as an outpatient, (2) who is symptomatic from a breathing or swallowing perspective, or

(3) who appears to be at increased risk of falling if their limb weakness transiently worsens . We have a very low threshold to admitting anyone with symptoms of swallowing or ventilatory muscle weakness to the ICU and would recommend prophylactic intubation when the forced vital capacity declines to <15 mL/kg or the negative inspiratory pressure is <30 cm H_2O. Myasthenic crisis is typically treated with intravenous corticosteroids and either IVIG or PLEX with a second-line immunomodulating agent typically added prior to discharge.[415,416]

Thymectomy is offered to virtually every patient with thymoma, unless comorbidities negate any reasonable chance of benefit. We also offer thymectomy to the majority of adolescents and adults with generalized myasthenia without MuSK autoantibodies assuming that they are strong enough and otherwise healthy enough to safely undergo this treatment. We do so based upon the anecdotal belief that it will increase the probability of future drug-free remission. As a general rule, we do not offer this treatment initially, allowing the patient the opportunity to accept and adapt to their diagnosis. By the same token, based again on the anecdotal suggestion that the efficacy of thymectomy wanes in patients with longstanding MG, we typically offer this option within the first two years of disease if possible.

REFERENCES

1. Simpson JA. Myasthenia gravis: A new hypothesis. *Scott Med J.* 1960;5:419–436.
2. Vincent A. Unravelling the pathogenesis of myasthenia gravis. *Nat Rev Immunol.* 2002;2(10):797–804.
3. Fambrough DM, Drachman DB, Satyamurti S. Neuromuscular junction in myasthenia gravis: Decreased acetylcholine receptors. *Science.* 1973; 182:293–295.
4. Patrick J, Lindstrom J. Autoimmune response to acetylcholine receptor. *Science.* 1973;180(4088):871–872.
5. Lindstrom JM, Seybold ME, Lennon VA, Whittingham S, Duane DD. Antibody to acetylcholine receptor in myasthenia gravis: Prevalence, clinical correlates and diagnostic value. *Neurology.* 1976;26(11):1054–1059.
6. Hoch W, McConville J, Hels S, Newsom-Davis J, Melms A, Vincent A. Autoantibodies to the receptor tyrosine kinase MuSK in patients with myasthenia gravis without acetylcholine receptor antibodies. *Nat Med.* 2001;7:365–368.
7. Leite MI, Jacob S, Viegas S, et al. IgG1 antibodies to acetylcholine receptors in seronegative myasthenia gravis. *Brain.* 2008;131:1940–1952.
8. Jacob S, Viegas S, Leite MI, et al. Presence and pathogenic relevance of antibodies to clustered acetylcholine receptor in ocular and generalized myasthenia gravis. *Arch Neurol.* 2012; 69(8):994–1001.
9. Higuchi O, Hamuro J, Motomura M, Yamanashi Y. Autoantibodies to low-density lipoprotein receptor-related protein 4 in myasthenia gravis. *Ann Neurol.* 2011;69:418–422.
10. Baggi F, Andreetta F, Maggi L, et al. Complete stable remission and autoantibody specificity in myasthenia gravis. *Neurology.* 2013;80:188–195.
11. Phillips LH 2nd, Torner JC. Epidemiologic evidence for a changing natural history of myasthenia gravis. *Neurology.* 1996;47(5):1233–1238.
12. Aragones JM, Bolibar I, Bonfill X, et al. Myasthenia gravis. A higher than expected incidence in the elderly. *Neurology.* 2003;60(6):1024–1026.
13. Oosterhuis HJ. The natural course of myasthenia gravis: A long term follow up study. *J Neurol Neurosurg Psychiatry.* 1989;52:1121–1127.
14. Alter M, Talbert OR, Kurland LT. Myasthenia gravis in a southern community. *Arch Neurol.* 1960;3:65–69.
15. Cohen MS. Epidemiology of myasthenia gravis. *Mongr Allergy.* 1987;21:246–251.
16. Garland H, Clark AN. Myasthenia gravis: A personal study of 60 cases. *Br Med J.* 1956;1:1259–1262.
17. Hokkanen E. Epidemiology of myasthenia gravis in Finland. *J Neurol Sci.* 1969;9:463–478.
18. Osserman KE, Genkins G. Studies in myasthenia gravis: A review of a 20-year experience in over 1200 patients. *Mt Sinai J Med.* 1971;38:497–537.
19. Phillips LH, Torner JC, Anderson MS, Cox GM. The epidemiology of myasthenia gravis in central and western Virginia. *Neurology.* 1992;42:1888–1893.
20. Somnier FE, Keidling N, Paulson OB. Epidemiology of myasthenia gravis in Denmark: A longitudinal and comprehensive population survey. *Arch Neurol.* 1991;48:733–739.
21. Storm-Mathisen A. Epidemiological and prognostical aspects of myasthenia gravis in Norway. *Acta Neurol Scand.* 1976; 54:120.
22. Storm-Mathisen A. Epidemiology of myasthenia gravis in Norway. *Acta Neurol Scand.* 1984;70:274–284.
23. Cavalcante P, Le Panse R, Berrih-Aknin S, et al. The thymus in myasthenia gravis: Site of "innate autoimmunity". *Muscle Nerve.* 2011;44:467–484.
24. Phillips LH 2nd. The epidemiology of myasthenia gravis. *Ann N Y Acad Sci.* 2003;998:407–412.
25. Zhang B,Tzartos JS, Belimezi M, et al. Autoantibodies to lipoprotein-related protein 4 in patients with double-seronegative myasthenia gravis. *Arch Neurol.* 2012;69(4):445–451.
26. Lisak RP. The clinical limits of myasthenia gravis and differential diagnosis do it. *Neurology.* 1997;48(Suppl 5):S36–S39.
27. Herrmann C. The familial occurrence of myasthenia gravis. *Ann N Y Acad Sci.* 1971;183:334–350.
28. Hokkanen E, Emeryk-Szajewska B, Rowinska-Marcinska K. Evaluation of the jitter phenomena in myasthenic patients and their relatives. *J Neurol.* 1978;219:73–82.
29. Grob D. Course and management of myasthenia gravis. *JAMA.* 1953;153:529–532.
30. Grob D, Brunner NG, Namba T. The natural course of myasthenia gravis and effects of therapeutic measures. *Ann N Y Acad Sci.* 1981;377:652–669.
31. Landouré G, Knight MA, Stanescu H, et al. A candidate gene for autoimmune myasthenia gravis. *Neurology.* 2012;79:342–347.
32. Lindstrom J. What initiates the autoimmune response to muscle AChRs in myasthenia gravis? *Neurology.* 2012;79: 304–305.
33. Grob D, Brunner N, Namba T, Pagala M. Lifetime course of myasthenia gravis. *Muscle Nerve.* 2008;37:141–149.
34. Bever CT, Aquino AV, Penn AS, Lovelace RE, Rowland LP. Prognosis of ocular myasthenia. *Ann Neurol.* 1983;14:516–519.

35. Grob D, Arsura EL, Brunner NG, Namba T. The course of myasthenia gravis and therapies affecting outcome. *Ann N Y Acad Sci.* 1987;505:472–499.
36. Mee J, Paine M, Byrne E, King J, Reardon K, O'Day J. Immunotherapy of ocular myasthenia gravis reduces conversion to generalized myasthenia gravis. *J Neuroophthalmol.* 2003;23:251–255.
37. Kupersmith MJ. Ocular myasthenia gravis: Long-term treatment successes and failures with long-term follow up. *J Neurol.* 2008;256:1314–1320.
38. Kumar V, Kaminski HJ. Treatment of myasthenia gravis. *Curr Neurol Neurosci Rep.* 2011;11:89–86.
39. Hughes BW, Kusner LL, Kaminski HJ. Molecular architecture of the neuromuscular junction. *Muscle Nerve.* 2006;33: 445–461.
40. Keesey JC. Clinical evaluation and management of myasthenia gravis. *Muscle Nerve.* 2004;29:484–505.
41. Grob D, Brunner NG, Namba T. The natural course of myasthenia gravis and effect of therapeutic measures. *Ann New York Acad Sci.* 1971;38:497.
42. Lopate G, Pestronk A. Autoimmune myasthenia gravis. *Hosp Pract (Office Ed).* 1993;28:109–112.
43. Beekman R, Kuks JB, Oosterhuis HJ. Myasthenia gravis: Diagnosis and follow-up of 100 consecutive patients. *J Neurol.* 1997;244:112–118.
44. Drachman DB. Myasthenia gravis. *N Engl J Med.* 1994;330: 1797–1810.
45. Borenstein S, Desmedt JE. Temperature and weather correlates of myasthenic fatigue. *Lancet.* 1974;2:63–66.
46. Borenstein S, Desmedt JE. Local cooling in myasthenia: Improvement on neuromuscular failure. *Arch Neurol.* 1975;32:152–157.
47. Fennell DF, Ringle SP. Myasthenia gravis and pregnancy. *Obstet Gynecol Surv.* 1987;41:414–421.
48. Gutmann L. Heat exacerbation of myasthenia gravis. *Neurology.* 1978;28:398.
49. Gutmann L. Heat-induced myasthenic crisis. *Arch Neurol.* 1980;37:671–672.
50. Mitchell P, Bebbington M. Myasthenia gravis in pregnancy. *Obstet Gynecol.* 1992;80:178–181.
51. Evoli A, Batocchi AP, Minisci C, Di Schino C, Tonali P. Therapeutic options in ocular myasthenia gravis. *Neuromuscul Disord.* 2001;11:208–216.
52. Simpson JF, Westerberg MR, Magee KR. Myasthenia gravis: An analysis of 295 cases. *Acta Neurol Scand.* 1966;42(Suppl 23): 1–27.
53. Acers TE. Ocular myasthenia gravis mimicking pseudonuclear ophthalmoplegia and variable esotropia. *Am J Ophthalmol.* 1979;88:319–321.
54. Spooner JW, Baloh RW. Eye movement fatigue in myasthenia gravis. *Neurology.* 1979;29:29–33.
55. Meriggioli MN, Sanders DB. Autoimmune myasthenia gravis: Emerging clinical and biological heterogeneity. *Lancet Neurol.* 2009;8(5):475–490.
56. Maher J, Grand'maison F, Nicolle MW, Strong MJ, Bolton CF. Diagnostic difficulties in myasthenia gravis. *Muscle Nerve.* 1998;21:577–583.
57. Mao VH, Abaza M, Speigel JR, et al. Laryngeal myasthenia gravis: Report of 40 cases. *J Voice.* 2001;15(1):122–130.
58. Mier A, Laroche C, Green M. Unsuspected myasthenia gravis presenting as respiratory failure. *Thorax.* 1990;45:422–423.
59. Pal S, Sanyal D. Jaw muscle weakness: A differential indicator of neuromuscular weakness-preliminary observations. *Muscle Nerve.* 2011;43:807–811.
60. Gracey DR, Divertie MB, Howard FM. Mechanical ventilation for respiratory failure in myasthenia gravis: 2-year experience with 22 patients. *Mayo Clin Proc.* 1983;58:597–602.
61. Oh SJ, Kuruoglu R. Chronic limb-girdle myasthenia gravis. *Neurology.* 1992;42:1153–1156.
62. Rodolico C, Toscano M, Autunno S, et al. Limb-girdle myasthenia: Clinical, electrophysiological and morphological features in familial and autoimmune cases. *Neuromuscul Disord.* 2002;12: 964–969.
63. Jablecki C, Benton A. The frequency of muscle involvement in myasthenia gravis correlates with mean muscle temperature. *Muscle Nerve.* 1982;5:491–492.
64. Gilad R, Sadeh M. Bilateral foot drop as a manifestation of myasthenia gravis. *J Clin Neuromuscul Dis.* 2000;2:22–23.
65. Musser WS, Barbano RL, Thornton CA, Moxley RT, Hermann DN, Logigian EL. Distal myasthenia gravis with a decrement, and increment, and denervation. *J Clin Neuromuscul Dis.* 2001;3:16–19.
66. Nations SP, Wolfe GI, Amato AA, Jackson CE, Bryan WW, Barohn RJ. Distal myasthenia gravis. *Neurology.* 1999;52: 632–632.
67. Nicolle MW. Wrist and finger drop in myasthenia gravis. *J Clin Neuromuscul Dis.* 2006;8:65–69.
68. Ozturk A, Deymeer F, Serdarogly P, et al. Distribution of muscle weakness in myasthenia gravis [abstract]. *Neuromuscul Disord.* 1999;9:6–7.
69. Janssen JC, Larner AJ, Harris J, Sheean GL, Rossor MN. Myasthenic hand. *Neurology.* 1998;51:913–914.
70. Ponseti JM, Caritg M, Gamez J, López-Cano M, Vilallonga R, Armengol M. A comparison of long-term post-thymectomy outcome of anti-AChR positive, anti-AChR negative, and anti-MuSK-positive patients with non-thymomatous myasthenia gravis. *Expert Opin Bio Ther.* 2009;9(1):1–8.
71. McConville J, Farugia ME, Beeson D, et al. Detection and characterization of MuSK antibodies in seronegative myasthenia gravis. *Ann Neurol.* 2004;55:580–584.
72. Sanders DB, El-Salem K, Massey JM, McConville J, Vincent A. Clinical aspects of MuSK antibody positive seronegative MG. *Neurology.* 2003;60:1978–1980.
73. Zhou L, McConville J, Chaudhry V, et al. Clinical comparison of muscle-specific tyrosine kinase (MuSK) antibody-positive and -negative myasthenic patients. *Muscle Nerve.* 2004;30: 55–60.
74. Stickler DE, Massey JM, Sanders DB. MuSK-antibody positive myasthenia gravis: Clinical and electrodiagnostic patterns. *Clin Neurophysiol.* 2005;116:2065–2068.
75. Yeh J-H, Chen W-H, Chiu H-C, Vincent A. Low frequency of MuSk antibody in generalized seronegative myasthenia gravis among Chinese. *Neurology.* 2004;62:2131–2132.
76. Wolfe GI, Trivedi JR, Oh SJ. Clinical review of muscle-specific tyrosine kinase-antibody positive myasthenia gravis. *J Clin Neuromuscul Dis.* 2007;8:217–224.
77. Evoli A, Tonali PA, Padua L, et al. Clinical correlates with anti-MuSK antibodies in generalized seronegative myasthenia. *Brain.* 2003;126:2304–2311.
78. Bartoccioni E, Scuderi F, Minicuci GM, Marino M, Ciaraffa F, Evoli A. Anti-MuSK antibodies: Correlation with myasthenia gravis severity. *Neurology.* 2006;67(3):505–507.

79. Deymeer F, Gungor-Tuncer O, Yiolmaz V, et al. Clinical comparison of anti-MuSK- vs. anti-AChR-positive and seronegative myasthenia gravis. *Neurology*. 2007;60:609–611.
80. Guptill JG, Sanders DB, Evoli A. Anti-MuSK antibody myasthenia gravis: Clinical findings in response to treatment into large cohorts. *Muscle Nerve*. 2011;44:36–40.
81. Pasnoor M, Wolfe GI, Nations S, et al. Clinical findings in MuSK-antibody positive myasthenia gravis: A US experience. *Muscle Nerve*. 2010;41:370–374.
82. Lavrnic D, Losen M, Vujic A, et al. The features of myasthenia gravis with autoantibodies to MuSK. *J Neurol Neurosurg Psychiatry*. 2005;76:1099–1102.
83. Lee JY, Sung JJ, Cho JY, et al. MuSK antibody-positive, seronegative myasthenia gravis in Korea. *J Clin Neurosci*. 2006;13:353–255.
84. Niks EH, Kuks JB, Vershuuren JJ. Epidemiology of myasthenia gravis with anti-muscle specific kinase antibodies in the Netherlands. *J Neurol Neurosurg Psychiatry*. 2007;78:417–418.
85. Padua L, Tonali P, Aprile I, Caliandro P, Bartoccioni E, Evoli A. Seronegative myasthenia gravis: Comparison of neurophysiological picture in MuSK+ and MUSK– patients. *Eur J Neurol*. 2006;13:273–276.
86. Caress JB, Hunt CH, Batish SD. Anti-MuSK myasthenia gravis presenting with purely ocular findings. *Arch Neurol*. 2005;62:1002–1003.
87. Hanisch F, Eger K, Zierz S. MuSK-antibody positive pure ocular myasthenia gravis. *J Neurol*. 2006;253:659–660.
88. Farrugia ME, Robson MD, Clover L, et al. MRI and clinical studies of facial and bulbar muscle involvement in MuSK antibody-associated myasthenia gravis. *Brain*. 2006;129:1481–1492.
89. Punga AR, Ruegg MA. Signaling and aging at the neuromuscular synapse: Lessons learnt from neuromuscular diseases. *Clin Opin Pharmacol*. 2012;12:340–346.
90. Pevzner A, Schoser B, Peters K, et al. Anti-LRP4 autoantibodies in AchR- and MuSK-antibody-negative myasthenia gravis. *J Neurol*. 2012;259:427–435.
91. Vincent A, McConville J, Farrugia ME, Newsom-Davis J. Seronegative myasthenia gravis. *Semin Neurol*. 2004;24:125–133.
92. Gorelick PB, Rosenberg M, Pagano RJ. Enhanced ptosis in myasthenia gravis. *Arch Neurol*. 1981;38:531.
93. Batocchi AP, Majolini L, Evoli A, Lino MM, Minisci C, Tonali P. Course and treatment of myasthenia gravis during pregnancy. *Neurology*. 1999;52:447–452.
94. Hoff JM, Dalveit AK, Gilhus NE. Myasthenia gravis: Consequences for pregnancy, delivery, and the newborn. *Neurology*. 2003;61:1362–1366.
95. Lindner A, Schalke B, Toyka KV. Outcome in juvenile-onset myasthenia gravis: A retrospective study with long-term follow-up of 79 patients. *J Neurol*. 1997;244:515–520.
96. Rodriguez M, Gomez MR, Howard FM, Taylor WF. Myasthenia gravis in children: Long-term follow-up. *Ann Neurol*. 1983;13:504–510.
97. Selcen D, Dabrowski ER, Michon AM, Nigro MA. High-dose immunoglobulin therapy in juvenile myasthenia gravis. *Pediatr Neurol*. 2000;22:40–43.
98. Plauche WC. Myasthenia gravis in mothers and their newborns. *Clin Obstet Gynecol*. 1991;34:82–99.
99. Bartoccioni E, Evoli A, Casali C, Scoppetta C, Tonali P, Provenzano C. Neonatal myasthenia gravis: Clinical and immunological study of seven mothers and their newborn infants. *J Neuroimmunol*. 1986;12:155–161.
100. Branch CE, Swift TR, Dyken PR. Prolonged neonatal myasthenia gravis: Electrophysiological studies. *Ann Neurol*. 1978;3:416–418.
101. Eymard B, Vernet-der Garabedian B, Berrih-Aknin S, Pannier C, Bach JF, Morel E. Anti-acetylcholine receptor antibodies in neonatal myasthenia gravis: Heterogeneity and pathogenic significance. *J Autoimmun*. 1991;4:185–195.
102. Geddes AK, Kidd HM. Myasthenia gravis of newborn. *Can Med Assoc J*. 1951;64:152–156.
103. Keesey J, Lindstrom J, Cokeley H. Anti-acetylcholine receptor antibody in neonatal myasthenia gravis. *N Engl J Med*. 1977; 296:55.
104. Lefvert AK, Osterman PO. Newborn infants to myasthenic mothers: A clinical study and an investigation of acetylcholine receptor antibodies in 17 children. *Neurology*. 1983;33:133–138.
105. Morel E, Eymard B, Vernet-der Garabedian B, Pannier C, Dulac O, Bach JF. Neonatal myasthenia gravis: A new clinical and immunologic appraisal on 30 cases. *Neurology*. 1988;38:138–142.
106. Namba T, Brown SB, Grob D. Neonatal myasthenia gravis: Report of two cases and review of the literature. *Pediatrics*. 1970;45:488–504.
107. Ohta M, Matsubara F, Hayashi K, Nakao K, Nishitani H. Acetylcholine receptor antibodies in infants of mothers with myasthenia gravis. *Neurology*. 1981;31:1019–1022.
108. Papazian O. Transient neonatal myasthenia gravis. *J Child Neurol*. 1992;7:135–141.
109. Seybold ME, Lindstrom JM. Myasthenia gravis in infancy. *Neurology*. 1981;31:476–480.
110. Strickroot FL, Schaeffer BL, Bergo HL. Myasthenia gravis occurring in an infant born of a myasthenic mother. *J Am Med Assoc*. 1942;120:1207–1209.
111. Tzartos SJ, Efthimiadis A, Morel E, Eymard B, Bach JF. Neonatal myasthenia gravis: Antigenic specificities of antibodies in sera from mothers and their infants. *Clin Exp Immunol*. 1990;80:376–380.
112. Elias ST, Butler I, Appel SH. Neonatal myasthenia gravis in the infant of a myasthenic mother in remission. *Ann Neurol*. 1979;6:72–75.
113. Murray EL, Kedar S, Vedanarayanan VV. Transmission of maternal muscle-specific tyrosine kinase (MuSK) to offspring: Report of two cases. *J Clin Neuromuscul Dis*. 2010;12(2):76–79.
114. Vincent A. *Neuromuscular Junction and Other Inherited Disorders*. Amsterdam, Netherlands: Elsevier; 2009:575–583.
115. Evoli A, Batocchi AP, Bartoccioni E, Lino MM, Minisci C, Tonali P. Juvenile myasthenia gravis with prepubertal onset. *Neuromuscul Disord*. 1998;8:561–567.
116. Herrmann DN, Carney PR, Wald JJ. Juvenile myasthenia gravis: Treatment with immune globulin and thymectomy. *Pediatr Neurol*. 1998;18:63–66.
117. Snead OC, Benton JW, Dwyer D, et al. Juvenile myasthenia gravis. *Neurology*. 1980;30:732–739.
118. Vial C, Charles N, Chauplannaz G, Bady B. Myasthenia gravis in childhood and infancy: Usefulness of electrophysiologic studies. *Arch Neurol*. 1991;48:847–849.
119. Evoli A, Minisci C, Di Schino C, et al. Thymoma in patients with MG: Characteristics and long-term outcome. *Neurology*. 2002;59:1844–1850.
120. Hohlfeld R, Wekerle H. The thymus in myasthenia gravis. *Neurol Clin*. 1994;12:331–342.
121. Lovelace RE, Younger DS. Myasthenia gravis with thymoma. *Neurology*. 1997;48(Suppl 5):S76–S81.

122. Drachman DB. Myasthenia gravis. *N Engl J Med.* 1997; 330(25):1797–1809.
123. Leite MI, Ströbel P, Jones M, et al. Fewer thymic changes in MuSK antibody-negative than in MuSK positive MG. *Ann Neurol.* 2005;57:444–448.
124. Witt NJ, Bolton CF. Neuromuscular disorders and thymoma. *Muscle Nerve.* 1988;2:398–405.
125. Vernino S, Lennon VA. Ion channel and striational antibodies define a continuum of autoimmune neuromuscular excitability. *Muscle Nerve.* 2002;26:702–707.
126. Vernino S, Lennon VA. Muscle and neuronal autoantibody markers of thymoma: Neurological correlations. *Ann N Y Acad Sci.* 2003;998:359–361.
127. Khella SL, Souyah N, Dalmau J. Thymoma, myasthenia gravis, encephalitis, and a novel anticytoplasmic neuronal antibody. *Neurology.* 2007;69:1302–1303.
128. Martinelli P, Patuelli A, Minardi C, Cau A, Riviera AM, Dal Posso F. Neuromyotonia, peripheral neuropathy and myasthenia gravis. *Muscle Nerve.* 1996;19:505–510.
129. Suzuki S, Satoh T, Yasouka H, et al. Novel antibodies to a voltage-gated potassium channel K,1.4 in a severe form of myasthenia gravis. *J Neuroimmunol.* 2005;170:141–149.
130. Vernino S, Lennon VA. Autoantibody profiles and neurological correlations of thymoma. *Clin Cancer Res.* 2004;10:7270–7275.
131. Osserman KE, Tsairis P, Weiner LB. Myasthenia gravis and thyroid disease: Clinical and immunological correlation. *J Mt Sinai Hosp.* 1967;34:469–483.
132. Becker KL, Titus JH, McConahey WM, Woolner LB. Morphologic evidence of thyroiditis in myasthenia gravis. *J Am Med Assoc.* 1964;187:994–996.
133. Downes JM, Greenwood BM, Wray SH. Autoimmune aspects of myasthenia gravis. *Q J Med.* 1966;35:85–105.
134. Penn AS, Schotland DL, Rowland LP. Immunology of muscle disease. *Res Publ Assoc Res Nerv Ment Dis.* 1971;49:215–240.
135. Wolf SM, Rowland LP, Schotland DL, McKinney AS, Hoefer PF, Aranow H Jr. Myasthenia as an autoimmune disease: Clinical aspects. *Ann N Y Acad Sci.* 1966;135:517–535.
136. Lee EK, Maselli RA, Ellis WG, Agius MA. Morvan's fibrillary chorea: A paraneoplastic manifestation of thymoma. *J Neurol Neurosurg Psychiatry.* 1998;65:857–862.
137. Mygland A, Vincent A, Newsom-Davis J, et al. Autoantibodies in thymoma-associated myasthenia gravis with myositis or neuromyotonia. *Arch Neurol.* 2000;57:527–531.
138. Aarli JA. Neuromyotonia and rippling muscles. Two infrequent concomitants to myasthenia gravis with thymoma. *Acta Neurol Scand.* 1997;96:342.
139. Heidenreich F, Vincent A. Antibodies to ion-channel proteins in thymoma with myasthenia, neuromyotonia, and peripheral neuropathy. *Neurology.* 1998;50:1483–1485.
140. Newsom-Davis J, Mills KR. Immunological associations of acquired neuromyotonia (Isaacs' syndrome): Report of 5 cases and literature review. *Brain.* 1993;116:453–469.
141. Perini M, Ghezzi A, Basso PF, Montanini R. Association of neuromyotonia with peripheral neuropathy, myasthenia and thymoma: A case report. *Ital J Neurol Sci.* 1994;15:307–310.
142. Vernino S, Auger R, Emslie-Smith A, Harper CM, Lennon VA. Myasthenia, thymoma, presynaptic antibodies, and a continuum of neuromuscular hyperexcitability. *Neurology.* 1999;53:1233–1239.
143. Ansevin CF, Agamanolis DP. Rippling muscles and myasthenia gravis with rippling muscles. *Arch Neurol.* 1996;53:197–199.
144. Muller-Felber W, Ansevin CF, Ricker K, et al. Immunosuppressive treatment of rippling muscles in patients with myasthenia gravis. *Neuromuscul Disord.* 1999;9:604–607.
145. Nicholas AP, Chatterjee A, Arnold MM, Claussen GC, Zorn GL, Oh SJ. Stiff-persons' syndrome associated with thymoma and subsequent myasthenia gravis. *Muscle Nerve.* 1997;20: 493–498.
146. Piccolo G, Martino G, Moglia A, Arrigo A, Cosi CV. Autoimmune myasthenia gravis with thymoma following spontaneous remission of stiff-man syndrome. *Ital J Neurol Sci.* 1990;11:177–180.
147. Anderson NE, Hutchinson DO, Nicholson GI, Aitcheson F, Nixon JM. Intestinal pseudo-obstruction, myasthenia gravis, and thymoma. *Neurology.* 1996;47:985–987.
148. Pande R, Leis AA. Myasthenia gravis, thymoma, intestinal pseudo-obstruction, and neuronal nicotinic acetylcholine receptor antibody. *Muscle Nerve.* 1999;1600–1602.
149. Katz JS, Wolfe GI, Bryan WW, Tintner R, Barohn FU. Acetylcholine receptor antibodies in the Lambert–Eaton myasthenic syndrome. *Neurology.* 1998;50:470–475.
150. Newsom-Davis J, Leys K, Ferguson I, Modi G, Mills K. Immunological evidence for the co-existence of the Lambert–Eaton myasthenic syndrome and myasthenia gravis in two patients. *J Neurol Neurosurg Psychiatry.* 1991;54:452–453.
151. Oh SJ. Overlap myasthenic syndrome. *Neurology.* 1987;37: 1411–1414.
152. Tabbaa MA, Leschner RT, Campbell WW. Malignant thymoma with dysautonomia and disordered neuromuscular transmission. *Arch Neurol.* 1986;43:955–957.
153. Taphoorn MJB, Van Duijn H, Wolters ECH. A neuromuscular transmission disorder: Combined myasthenia gravis and Lambert–Eaton syndrome in one patient. *J Neurol Neurosurg Psychiatry.* 1988;51:880–882.
154. Namba T, Brunner NG, Grob D. Idiopathic giant cell polymyositis. Report of a case and review of the literature. *Arch Neurol.* 1974;31:27–30.
155. Johns TR, Crowley WJ, Miller JQ, Campa JF. The syndrome of myasthenia and polymyositis with comments on therapy. *Ann N Y Acad Sci.* 1971;183:64–71.
156. Burke JS, Medline NM, Katz A. Giant cell myocarditis and myositis associated with thymoma and myasthenia gravis. *Arch Pathol Lab Med.* 1969;88:359–366.
157. Pascuzzi RM, Roos KL, Phillips LH. Granulomatous inflammatory myopathy associated with myasthenia gravis. A case report and review of the literature. *Arch Neurol.* 1986;43:621–623.
158. Alseth EH, Maniaol AH, Elsais A, et al. Investigation for RAPSN and DOK-7 mutations in a cohort of seronegative myasthenia gravis patients. *Muscle Nerve.* 2011;43:574–577.
159. Burns TM, Russell JA, LaChance D, Jones HR. Oculobulbar involvement is typical with Lambert–Eaton myasthenic syndrome. *Ann Neurol.* 2003;53:270–273.
160. Lennon VA. Serologic profile of myasthenia gravis and distinction from the Lambert-Eaton myasthenic syndrome. *Neurology.* 1997;48(Suppl 5):S23–S27.
161. Ruff RL, Rutecki P. Faster, slower, but never better: Mutations of the skeletal muscle acetylcholine receptor. *Neurology.* 2012;79:404–405.
162. Kaminski HJ, Suarez J, Ruff RL. Neuromuscular junction physiology in myasthenia gravis: Isoforms of the acetylcholine receptor in extraocular muscle and the contribution of sodium channels to the safety factor. *Neurology.* 1997;48:S8–S17.

163. Engel AG, Shen X-M, Selcen D. What we learned from the congenital myasthenic syndromes. *J Mol Neurosci.* 2010;40: 143–153.
164. Birks RI, Huxley HE, Katz B. The fine structure of the neuromuscular junction in the frog. *J Physiol.* 1960;150:134–144.
165. Ruff RL, Lennon V. End-plate voltage-gated sodium channels are lost in clinical and experimental myasthenia gravis. *Ann Neurol.* 1998;43:370–379.
166. Barrett EF, Magleby KL. Physiology of cholinergic transmission. In: Goldberg AM, Hahn P, eds. *Biology of Cholinergic Function.* New York, NY: Raven Press; 1976:29–100.
167. Steinbach JH, Stevens CF. Neuromuscular transmission. In: Llinas R, Precht W, eds. *Progress Neurobiology.* Berlin: Springer-Verlag; 1976:35–92.
168. Kuffler SW, Yoshikami D. The number of transmitter molecules in a quantum: An estimate from iontophoretic application of acetylcholine at the neuromuscular synapse. *J Physiol.* 1975;251:465–482.
169. Martin AR. Quantal nature of synaptic transmission. *Physiol Rev.* 1986;46:51–66.
170. Potter LT. Synthesis, storage and release of 14 C acetylcholine in isolated rat diaphragm muscles. *J Physiol.* 1970;206:145–166.
171. Rahamimoff R, Erulkar SD, Lev-Tov A, Meiri H. Intracellular and extracellular calcium ions in transmitter release at the neuromuscular synapse. *Ann N Y Acad Sci.* 1978;307:583–598.
172. Gautam M, Noakes PG, Moscoso L, et al. Defective neuromuscular synaptogenesis in agrin-deficient mutant mice. *Cell.* 1996;85(4):525–535.
173. Engel AG, Santa T. Histometric analysis of the ultra-structure of the neuromuscular junction in myasthenia gravis and the myasthenic syndrome. *Ann N Y Acad Sci.* 1971;183:46–63.
174. Engel AG, Tsujihata M, Lindstrom JM, Lennon VA. The motor end-plate in myasthenia gravis and in experimental autoimmune myasthenia gravis. A quantitative ultrastructural study. *Ann N Y Acad Sci.* 1976;274:60–79.
175. Punga AR.Stalberg E. Acetylcholinesterase inhibitors in MG: To be or not to be? *Muscle & Nerve.* 2009;39(6):724–728.
176. Vigny M, Bon S, Massoulie J, Leterrier F. Active-site catalytic efficiency of acetylcholinesterase molecular forms in Electrophorus, torpedo, rat, and chicken. *Eur J Biochem.* 1978;85:317–323.
177. Hubbard JI. Microphysiology of vertebrate neuromuscular junction transmission. *Physiol Rev.* 1973;53:674–723.
178. Pennefather P, Quasterl DM. Relation between subsynaptic receptor blockade and response to quantal transmitter at the mouse neuromuscular junction. *J Gen Physiol.* 1981;78: 313–344.
179. Ricker K, Hertel G, Stodieck S. Influence of temperature on neuromuscular transmission in myasthenia gravis. *J Neurol.* 1977;216:273–282.
180. Stamboulis E, Lygidakis C. Local warming in myasthenia gravis. *Electromyogr Clin Neurophysiol.* 1984;24:429–435.
181. Foldes FF, Kuze S, Vizi ES, Deery A. The influence of temperature on neuromuscular performance. *J Neural Transm.* 1978;43:27–45.
182. Lass Y, Fischback GD. A discontinuous relationship between the acetylcholine-activated channel conductance and temperature. *Nature.* 1976;263:150–151.
183. Lang H, Trontelj J. Effect of temperature on NCV and NAP of human nerve. *Muscle Nerve.* 1986;9:573.
184. Bolton CF, Sawa GM, Carter K. The effects of temperature on human compound action potentials. *J Neurol Neurosurg Psychiatry.* 1981;44:407–413.
185. Louis AA, Hotson JR. Regional cooling of human nerve and slowed NA+ inactivation. *Electroenceph Clin Neurophysiol.* 1986;63:371–375.
186. Hubbard JI, Jones SF, Landau EM. The effect of temperature change upon transmitter release, facilitation and post-tetanic potentiation. *J Physiol.* 1971;216:591–609.
187. Kistler J, Stroud RM, Klymkowsky MW, Lalancette RA, Fairclough RH. Structure and function of an acetylcholine receptor. *Biophys J.* 1982;37:371–383.
188. Gillespie SK, Balasubramanian S, Fung ET, Huganir RL. Rapsyn clusters and activates the synapse-specific receptor tyrosine kinase MuSK. *Neuron.* 1996;16:953–962.
189. Evoli A, Lindstrom J. Myasthenia gravis with antibodies to MuSK. *Neurology.* 2011;77:1783–1784.
190. Frail DE. McLaughlin LL. Mudd J. Merlie JP. Identification of the mouse muscle 43,000-dalton acetylcholine receptor-associated protein (RAPsyn) by cDNA cloning. *J Biol Chem.* 1988;263(30):15602–15607.
191. Lonenzoni PJ, Scola RH, Kay CS, Werneck LC. Congenital myasthenic syndrome: A brief review. *Pediatr Neurol.* 2012; 46:141–148.
192. Conti-Tronconi B, Raferty M. The nicotinic cholinergic receptor: Correlation of molecular structure with functional properties. *Annu Rev Biochem.* 1982;51:491–530.
193. Anderson CR, Stevens CF. Voltage clamp analysis of acetylcholine produced end-plate current fluctuations at frog neuromuscular junction. *J Physiol.* 1973;235:655–691.
194. Katz B, Miledi R. The statistical nature of the acetylcholine potential and its molecular components. *J Physiol.* 1972; 224:665–699.
195. Boyd IA, Martin AR. Spontaneous subthreshold activity at mammalian neuromuscular junctions. *J Physiol.* 1956;132: 61–73.
196. Desmedt JE. Nature of the defect of neuromuscular transmission in myasthenic patients: Post-tetanic exhaustion. *Nature.* 1957;179:156–157.
197. Desmedt JE. Myasthenic-like features of neuromuscular transmission after administration of an inhibitor of acetylcholine synthesis. *Nature.* 1958;182:1673–1674.
198. Salpeter MM, Harris R. Distribution and turnover rate of acetylcholine receptors throughout the function folds at a vertebrate neuromuscular junction. *J Cell Biol.* 1983;96:1781–1785.
199. Tzartos S, Seybold M, Lindstrom J. Specificities of antibodies to acetylcholine receptors in sera from myasthenia gravis patient measured by monoclonal antibodies. *Proc Natl Acad Sci USA.* 1982;79:188–192.
200. Bray J, Drachman D. Binding affinities of anti-acetylcholine receptor autoantibodies in myasthenia gravis. *J Immunol.* 1982;128:105–110.
201. Masuda T, Motomura M, Utsugisawa K, et al. Antibodies against the main immunogenic region of the acetylcholine receptor correlate with disease severity of myasthenia gravis. *J Neurol Neurosurg Psychiatry.* 2012;83:935–940.
202. Engel AG, Sahashi K, Fumagalli G. The immunopathology of acquired myasthenia gravis. *Ann N Y Acad Sci.* 1981;377: 158–174.
203. Engel AG, Lambert EH, Howard FM. Immune complexes (IgG and C3) at the motor end-plate in myasthenia gravis. Ultrastructural and light microscopic localization and electrophysiological correlations. *Mayo Clin Proc.* 1977;52: 267–280.

204. Engel AG, Lindstrom JM, Lambert EH, Lennon VA. Ultrastructural localization of the acetylcholine receptor in myasthenia gravis and in its experimental autoimmune model. *Neurology*. 1977;27:307–315.
205. Santa T, Engel AG, Lambert EH. Histometric study of neuromuscular junction ultrastructure. *Neurology*. 1972;22:71–82.
206. Schonbeck S, Chrestel S, Hohlfeld R. Myasthenia gravis: Prototype of the antireceptor autoimmune diseases. *Int Rev Neurobiol*. 1990;32:175–200.
207. Fumagalli G, Engel AG, Linstrom J. Ultrastructural aspects of acetylcholine receptor turnover at the normal end-plate and in autoimmune myasthenia gravis. *J Neuropathol Exp Neurol*. 1982;41:567–579.
208. Stanley EF, Drachman DB. Effect of myasthenic immunoglobulin on acetylcholine receptors of intact mammalian neuromuscular junctions. *Science*. 1978;200:1285–1289.
209. Drachman DB. The biology of myasthenia gravis. *Annu Rev Neurosci*. 1981;4:195–225.
210. Drachman DB, Adams RN, Josifek LF, Pestronk A, Stanley EF. Antibody-mediated mechanisms of ACh receptor loss in myasthenia gravis: Clinical relevance. *Ann N Y Acad Sci*. 1981;377:175–188.
211. Kao I, Drachman DB. Myasthenic immunoglobulin accelerates acetylcholine receptor degradation. *Science*. 1977;196:527–529.
212. Sun W, Adams RN, Miagkov A, Lu Y, Juon HS, Drachman DB. Specific immunotherapy of experimental myasthenia gravis in vitro and in vivo: The guided missile strategy. *J Neuroimmunol*. 2012;251:25–32.
213. Newsom-Davis J, Willcox N, Scadding G, Calder L, Vincent A. Antiacetylcholine receptor antibody synthesis by cultured lymphocytes in myasthenia gravis: Thymic and peripheral blood cell interactions. *Ann N Y Acad Sci*. 1981;377:393–402.
214. Scadding GK, Vincent A, Newsom-Davis J, Henry K. Acetylcholine receptor antibody synthesis by thymic lymphocytes: Correlation with thymic histology. *Neurology*. 1981;31:935–943.
215. Kim JY, Park KD, Richman DP. Treatment of myasthenia gravis based on its immunopathogenesis. *J Clin Neurol*. 2011;7:173–183.
216. Shigemoto K, Kubo S, Maruyama N, et al. Induction of myasthenia by immunization against muscle-specific kinase. *J Clin Invest*. 2006;116(4):1016–1024.
217. Klooster R, Plomp JJ, Huijbers MG, et al. Muscle-specific kinase myasthenia gravis IgG4 autoantibodies cause severe neuromuscular junction dysfunction in mice. *Brain*. 2012; 135:1081–1101.
218. Shiraishi H, Motomura M, Yoshimura T, et al. Acetylcholine receptors loss and postsynaptic damage in MuSK antibody-positive myasthenia gravis. *Ann Neurol*. 2005;57:289–293.
219. Slater C. Diverse aspects of vulnerability at the neuromuscular junction. *Brain*. 2012;135:997–1001.
220. Kawakami Y, Ito M, Hirayama M, et al. Anti-MuSK autoantibodies block binding of collagen Q to MuSK. *Neurology*. 2011;77:1819–1826.
221. Mihaylova V, Salih MA, Mukhtar MM, et al. Refinement of the clinical phenotype in MuSK-related congenital myasthenic syndromes. *Neurology*. 2009;73:1926–1928.
222. Richman DP. Antibodies to low density lipoprotein receptor-related protein 4 in seronegative myasthenia gravis. *Arch Neurol*. 2012;69(4):434–435.
223. Verschuuren JJ, Palace J, Gilhus NE. Clinical aspects of myasthenia explained. *Autoimmunity*. 2010;43(5–6):344–352.
224. MacLennan C, Beeson D, Buijs A-M, Vincent A, Newsom-Davis J. Acetylcholine receptor expression in human extraocular muscles and their susceptibility to myasthenia gravis. *Ann Neurol*. 1997;41:423–431.
225. Serafini B, Cavalcante P, Bernasconi P, Aloisi F, Mantegazza R. Epstein-Barr virus in myasthenia gravis thymus: A matter of debate. *Ann Neurol*. 2011;70(3):519.
226. Genkins G, Papatestas AE, Horowitz SH, Kornfield P. Studies in myasthenia gravis: Early thymectomy. Electrophysiologic and pathologic correlations. *Am J Med*. 1975;58:517–524.
227. Papatestas AE, Genkins G, Horowitz SH, Kornfeld P. Thymectomy in myasthenia gravis: Pathologic, clinical, and electrophysiologic correlations. *Ann N Y Acad Sci*. 1976;274:555–573.
228. Rivner MH, Swift TR. Thymoma: Diagnosis and management. *Semin Neurol*. 1990;10:83–88.
229. Oh SJ, Kim DE, Kuruoglu R, Bradley RJ, Dwyer D. Diagnostic sensitivity of the laboratory tests in myasthenia gravis. *Muscle Nerve*. 1992;15:720–724.
230. Vincent A, Newsom-Davis J. Acetylcholine receptor antibody as a diagnostic test for myasthenia gravis: Results in 153 validated cases and 2967 diagnostic assays. *J Neurol Neurosurg Psychiatry*. 1985;48:1246–1252.
231. Vincent A. Acetylcholine receptor antibody as a diagnostic test for myasthenia gravis: Results in 153 validated cases and 2967 diagnostic assays. *J Neurol Neurosurg Psychiatry*. 2012;83(3): 237–238.
232. Sanders DB, Andrews I, Howard JF, Massey JM. Seronegative myasthenia gravis. *Neurology*. 1997;48(Suppl 5):S40–S45.
233. Vincent A, Newsom-Davis J, Newton P, Beck N. Acetylcholine receptor antibody and clinical response to thymectomy in myasthenia gravis. *Neurology*. 1983;33:1276–1282.
234. Chan KH, Lachance DH, Harper CM, Lennon VA. Frequency of seronegativity in adult-acquired generalized myasthenia gravis. *Muscle Nerve*. 2007;36:651–658.
235. Howard FM, Lennon VA, Finley J, Matsummoto J, Elvebach LR. Clinical correlations of antibodies that bind, block, or modulate human acetylcholine receptors in myasthenia gravis. *Ann N Y Acad Sci*. 1987;505:526–538.
236. Ohta K, Shigemoto K, Kubo S, et al. MuSK antibodies in AChR Ab-seropositive MG vs AChR Ab-seronegative MG. *Neurology*. 2004;62:2132–2133.
237. Zouvelou V, Kyriazi S, Rentzos M, et al. Double-seropositive myasthenia gravis. *Muscle Nerve*. 2013;47(3):465–466.
238. Yamamoto AM, Gajdos P, Eymard B, et al. Anti-titin antibodies in myasthenia gravis: Tight association with thymoma and heterogeneity of nonthymoma patients. *Arch Neurol*. 2001;58: 885–890.
239. Lanska DJ. Diagnosis of thymoma in myasthenics using anti-striated muscle antibodies: Predictive value and gain in diagnostic certainty. *Neurology*. 1991;41:520–524.
240. Lange DJ. Electrophysiological testing of neuromuscular transmission. *Neurology*. 1995;48(suppl 5):S18–S22.
241. Punga AR, Sawada M, Stalberg EV. Electrophysiological signs and the prevalence of adverse effects of acetylcholinesterase inhibitors in patients with myasthenia gravis. *Muscle Nerve*. 2008;37(3):300–307.
242. Howard JF Jr, Sanders DB, Massey JM. The electrodiagnosis of myasthenia gravis and the Lambert-Eaton myasthenic syndrome. *Neurol Clin*. 1994;12(2):305–330.
243. Keesey JC. Electrodiagnostic approach to defects of neuromuscular transmission. *Muscle Nerve*. 1989;12:613–626.

244. Stalberg E, Sanders DB. Effect of temperature on neuromuscular transmission. *Muscle Nerve.* 1986;9:573.
245. Daube JR. Electrodiagnostic studies in ALS and other motor neuron disorders. *Muscle Nerve.* 2000;23:1488–1502.
246. Yamashita S, Sakaguchi H, Mori A, et al. Significant CMAP decrement by repetitive nerve stimulation is more frequent in median than ulnar nerves of patients with amyotrophic lateral sclerosis. *Muscle Nerve.* 2012;45(3):426–428.
247. Henderson RD, Daube JR. Decrement in surface-recorded motor unit potentials in amyotrophic lateral sclerosis. *Neurology.* 2004;63:1670–1674.
248. Maselli RA, Wollman RL, Leung C, et al. Neuromuscular transmission in amyotrophic lateral sclerosis. *Muscle Nerve.* 1993;16:1193–1203.
249. Wang FC, DePasqua V, Gérard P, Delwaide PJ. Prognostic value of decremental responses to repetitive nerve stimulation in ALS patients. *Neurology.* 2001;57:897–899.
250. Barbieri S, Weiss GM, Daube JR. Fibrillation potentials in myasthenia gravis. *Muscle Nerve.* 1982;5:S50.
251. Oosterhuis HJ, Hootsmans WJ, Veenhuyzen HB, van Zadelhoff I. The mean duration of motor unit action potential in patients with myasthenia gravis. *Electroencephalogr Clin Neurophysiol.* 1972;32:697–700.
252. Stalberg E. Clinical electrophysiology in myasthenia gravis. *J Neurol Neurosurg Psychiatry.* 1980;43:622–633.
253. Gilchrist JM, Sanders DB. Double-step repetitive stimulation in myasthenia gravis. *Muscle Nerve.* 1987;10:233–237.
254. Kelly JJ, Daube JR, Lennon VA, Howard FM Jr, Younge BR. The laboratory diagnosis of mild myasthenia gravis. *Ann Neurol.* 1982;12:238–342.
255. Liam Oey P, Wieneke GH, Hoogenraad TU, van Huffelen AC. Ocular myasthenia gravis: The diagnostic yield of repetitive stimulation and stimulated single fiber EMG of orbicularis oculi muscle and infrared reflection oculography. *Muscle Nerve.* 1993;16:142–149.
256. Oh SJ, Eslami N, Nishihira T, et al. Electrophysiological and clinical correlation in myasthenia gravis. *Ann Neurol.* 1982;12:348–354.
257. Ozdemir C, Young RR. The results to be expected from electrical testing in the diagnosis of myasthenia gravis. *Ann N Y Acad Sci.* 1976;274:203–222.
258. Schumm F, Stohr M. Accessory nerve stimulation in the assessment of myasthenia gravis. *Muscle Nerve.* 1984;7:147–151.
259. Oh SJ, Hatanaka Y, Hemmi S, et al. Repetitive nerve stimulation of facial muscles in MuSK antibody-positive myasthenia gravis. *Muscle Nerve.* 2006;33:500–504.
260. Churchill-Davidson HC, Wise RP. Neuromuscular transmission in the newborn infant. *Anesthesiology.* 1963;24:271–278.
261. Gatev V, Stamatova B, Angelova B, Ivanov I. Effects of repetitive stimulation on the electrical and mechanical activities of muscles in normal children. *Electromyogr Clin Neurophysiol.* 1975;15:339–355.
262. Koenigsberger MR, Patten B, Lovelace RE. Studies of neuromuscular function in the newborn: 1. A comparison of myoneural function in the full term and premature infant. *Neuropaediatrie.* 1973;4:350–361.
263. Hays RM, Michaud LJ. Neonatal myasthenia gravis: Specific advantages of repetitive stimulation over edrophonium testing. *Pediatr Neurol.* 1988;4:245–247.
264. Sanders DB. Clinical impact of single-fiber electromyography. *Muscle Nerve.* 2002;11(Suppl):15–20.
265. Jabre JF, Chirico-Post J, Weiner M. Stimulation SFEMG in myasthenia gravis. *Muscle Nerve.* 1989;12:38–42.
266. Trontelj JV, Mihelin M, Fernandez JM, Stalberg E. Axonal stimulation for end-plate jitter studies. *J Neurol Neurosurg Psychiatry.* 1986;49:677–685.
267. Trontelj JV, Khuraibet A, Mihelin M. The jitter in stimulated orbicularis oculi muscle: Technique and normal values. *J Neurol Neurosurg Psychiatry.* 1988;51:814–819.
268. Trontelj JV, Stalberg E, Mihelin M. Jitter in the muscle fiber. *J Neurol Neurosurg Psychiatry.* 1990;53:49–54.
269. Trontelj JV, Stalberg E, Mihelin M. Jitter of the stimulated motor axon. *Muscle Nerve.* 1992;15:449–454.
270. Stålberg EV, Sanders DB. Jitter recordings with concentric needle electrodes. *Muscle Nerve.* 2009;40:331–339.
271. Farrugia ME, Weir AI, Cleary M, Cooper S, Metcalfe R, Mallik A. Concentric and single fiber needle electrodes yield comparable jitter results in myasthenia gravis. *Muscle Nerve.* 2009;39(5):579–585.
272. Benatar M, Hammad M, Doss-Riney H. Concentric-needle single-fiber electromyography for the diagnosis of myasthenia gravis. *Muscle Nerve.* 2006;34(2):163–168.
273. Sanders DB. Measuring jitter with concentric needle electrodes. *Muscle Nerve.* 2013;47:317–318.
274. Gilchrist JM. Single fiber EMG reference values: A collaborative effort. *Muscle Nerve.* 1992;15:151–161.
275. Kouyoumdjian JA, Stålberg EV. Reference jitter values for concentric needle electrodes in voluntarily activated extensor digitorum communis and orbicularis oculi muscles. *Muscle Nerve.* 2008;37(6):694–699.
276. Cruz Martinez A, Ferrer MT, Diez Tejedor E, Perez Conde MC, Anciones B, Frank A. Diagnostic yield of single fiber electromyography and other electrophysiological technique in myasthenia gravis I. Electromyography, automatic analysis of the voluntary pattern, and repetitive nerve stimulation. *Electromyogr Clin Neurophysiol.* 1982;22:377–393.
277. Stalberg E, Ekstedt J, Broman A. Neuromuscular transmission in myasthenia gravis studied with single fiber electromyography. *J Neurol Neurosurg Psychiatry.* 1974;37:540–547.
278. Sanders DB, Howard JF, Johns TR. Single fiber electromyography in myasthenia gravis. *Neurology.* 1979;29:68–76.
279. Massey JM, Sanders DB. Single fiber electromyography in myasthenia gravis during pregnancy. *Muscle Nerve.* 1993;16: 458–460.
280. Murga L, Sanchez F, Menedez C, Castilla JM. Diagnostic yield of stimulated and voluntary single-fiber electromyography in myasthenia gravis. *Muscle Nerve.* 1998;21:1081–1083.
281. Sanders DB, Massey JM. Does change in neuromuscular jitter predict or correlate with clinical change in myasthenia gravis? *Neurology.* 2013;80:P02.204.
282. Konishi T, Nishitani H, Matsubara F, Ohta M. Myasthenia gravis: Relation between jitter in single-fiber EMG and antibody to acetylcholine receptor. *Neurology.* 1981;31:386–392.
283. Sitzer G, Brune GG. Effect of cholinesterase inhibitors and thymectomy on single fiber EMG in myasthenia gravis. *Ann N Y Acad Sci.* 1981;377:884–886.
284. Emeryk B, Rowinska K, Nowad-Michalska T. Do true remissions in myasthenia gravis really exist? An electrophysiological study. *J Neurol.* 1985;231:331–335.
285. Osserman KE, Kaplan LI. Rapid diagnostic test for myasthenia gravis: Increased muscle strength, without fasciculations, after intravenous administration of edrophonium (Tensilon) chloride. *J Am Med Assoc.* 1952;150:265–268.

286. Osserman KE, Genkins G. Clinical reappraisal of the use of edrophonium (Tensilon) chloride tests in myasthenia gravis and significance of clinical classification. *Ann N Y Acad Sci.* 1965;135:312–326.
287. Seybold ME, Daroff RB, Hachinski V. The office tensilon test for ocular myasthenia gravis. *Arch Neurol.* 1986;43:842–844.
288. Phillips LH 2nd, Melnick PA. Diagnosis of myasthenia gravis in the 1990s. *Semin Neurol.* 1990;10:62–69.
289. Moorthy G, Behrens MM, Drachman DB, et al. Ocular pseudomyasthenia or ocular myasthenia "plus": A warning to clinicians. *Neurology.* 1989;39:1150–1154.
290. Mulder DW, Lambert EH, Eaton LM. Myasthenic syndrome in patients with ALS. *Neurology.* 1959;9:627–631.
291. Ragge NK, Hoyt WF. Midbrain myasthenia: Fatigable ptosis, lid twitch sign, and ophthalmoparesis from a dorsal midbrain glioma. *Neurology.* 1992;42:917–919.
292. Dirr LY, Donofrio PD, Patton JF, Troost BT. A false-positive edrophonium test in a patient with a brainstem glioma. *Neurology.* 1989;39:865–867.
293. Takahashi K, Al-Janabi NJ. Computed tomography and magnetic resonance imaging of mediastinal tumors. *J Magn Reson Imaging.* 2010;32(6):1325–1339.
294. Jaretzki A III. Thymectomy for myasthenia gravis: Analysis of the controversies regarding technique and results. *Neurology.* 1997;48:52S–63S.
295. Chagnac Y, Hadani M, Goldhammer Y. Myasthenic crisis after intravenous administration of iodinated contrast agent. *Neurology.* 1985;35(8):1219–1220.
296. Fenichel GM, Shy GM. Muscle biopsy experience in myasthenia gravis. *Arch Neurol.* 1963;9(3):237–243.
297. Engel WK, McFarlin DE. Muscle lesions in myasthenia gravis. Discussion. *Ann N Y Acad Sci.* 1966;135(1):68–78.
298. Maselli RA, Richman DP, Willmann RI. Inflammation at the neuromuscular junction in myasthenia gravis. *Neurology.* 1991;41:1497–1504.
299. Pascuzzi RM, Campa JF. Lymphorrhage localized to the muscle end-plate on myasthenia gravis. *Arch Pathol Lab Med.* 1988;112:934–937.
300. Selcen D, Fukuda T, Shen X-M, Engel AG. Are MuSK antibodies the primary cause of myasthenic symptoms? *Neurology.* 2004;62:1945–1950.
301. Lindstrom J, Lambert EH. Content of acetylcholine receptor and antibodies bound to receptor in myasthenia gravis, experimental autoimmune myasthenia gravis, and Eaton–Lambert syndrome. *Neurology.* 1978;28:130–138.
302. Lev-Lehmann E, Evron T, Broide RS, et al. Synaptogeneis and myopathy under acetylcholinesterase overexpression. *J Mol Neurosci.* 2000;14:93–105.
303. Massey JM. Treatment of acquired myasthenia gravis. *Neurology.* 1997;48(Suppl 5):S46–S51.
304. Soliven BC, Lange DJ, Penn AS, et al. Seronegative myasthenia gravis. *Neurology.* 1988;38:514–517.
305. Baek WS, Bashey A, Sheean GL. Complete remission induced by rituximab in refractory, seronegative, muscle-specific kinase positive myasthenia gravis. *J Neurol Neurosurg Psychiatry.* 2007;78:771.
306. Díaz-Manera J, Martínez-Hernandez E, Querol L, et al. Long-lasting treatment effect of rituximab in MuSK myasthenia. *Neurology.* 2012;78:189–193.
307. Hain B, Jordan K, Deschauer M, Zierz S. Successful treatment of MuSK antibody-positive myasthenia gravis with rituximab. *Muscle Nerve.* 2006;33(4):575–580.
308. Shibata-Hamaguchi, A, Samuraki M, Furui E, et al. Long-term effect of intravenous immunoglobulin on anti-MuSK antibody-positive myasthenia gravis. *Acta Neurol Scand.* 2007;116:406–408.
309. Takahashi H, Kawaguchi N, Nemoto Y, Hattori T. High-dose intravenous immunoglobulin for the treatment of MuSK antibody-positive seronegative myasthenia gravis. *J Neurol Sci.* 2006;247:239–241.
310. Nowak RJ, Dicapua DB, Zebardast N, Goldstein JM. Response of patients with refractory myasthenia gravis to rituximab: A retrospective study. *Ther Adv Neurol Disord.* 2011;4:259–266.
311. Collongues N, Casez O, Lacour A, et al. Rituximab in refractory and non-refractory myasthenia: A retrospective multicenter study. *Muscle Nerve.* 2012;46:687–691.
312. Steiglbauer K, Topakian R, Schäffer G, Aichner FT. Rituximab for myasthenia gravis: Three case reports and review of the literature. *J Neurol Sci.* 2009;280:120–122.
313. Blum S, Gillis D, Brown H, et al. Use and monitoring of low-dose rituximab in myasthenia gravis. *J Neurol Neurosurg Psychiatry.* 2011;82:659–663.
314. Agius MA. Treatment of ocular myasthenia gravis with corticosteroids: Yes. *Arch Neurol.* 2000;57:750–751.
315. Kaminski HJ, Daroff RB. Treatment of ocular myasthenia. Steroids only when compelled. *Arch Neurol.* 2000;57:752–753.
316. Benatar M, Kaminski HJ. Evidence report: The medical treatment of ocular myasthenia (an evidence-based review). *Neurology.* 2007;68:2144–2149.
317. Nicolle MW, Rask S, Koopman WJ, George CF, Adams J, Wiebe S. Sleep apnea in patients with myasthenia gravis. *Neurology.* 2006;67(1):140–142.
318. Nagane Y, Utsugisawa K, Suzuki S, et al. Topical naphazoline in the treatment of myasthenic blepharoptosis. *Muscle Nerve.* 2011;44:41–44.
319. Blalock A, Mason MF, Morgan HJ, Riven SS. Myasthenia gravis and tumors of the thymic region. Report of a case in which the tumor was removed. *Ann Surg.* 1939;110:544–561
320. Blalock A. Thymectomy in the treatment of myasthenia gravis. Report of twenty cases. *J Thorac Surg.* 1944;13:316–339.
321. Blalock A, Harvey AM, Ford FR, Lilientha JL Jr. The treatment of myasthenia gravis by removal of the thymus gland. Preliminary report. *JAMA.* 1945;127:1089–1096.
322. Gronseth GA, Barohn RB. Practice parameter: Thymectomy for autoimmune myasthenia gravis (an evidence-based review): Report of the Quality Standards Subcommittee of the American Academy of Neurology. *Neurology.* 2000;55:1–7.
323. Wolfe GI, Kaminski HJ, Jaretzki A III, Swan A, Newsom-Davis J. Development of a thymectomy trial in nonthymomatous myasthenia gravis patients receiving immunosuppressive therapy. *Ann NY Acad Sci.* 2003;998:473–480.
324. Aban IB, Wolfe GI, Cutter GR, et al. The MGTX experience: Challenges in planning and executing an international, multicenter clinical trial. *J Neuroimmunol.* 2008;201–202:80–84.
325. Newsome-Davis J, Cutter G, Wolfe GI, et al. Status of thymectomy trial for nonthymomatous myasthenia gravis patients receiving prednisone. *Ann NY Acad Sci.* 2008;1132:344–347.
326. Matee MJ, Mack MJ. Surgical approaches to the thymus in patients with myasthenia gravis. *Thorac Surg Clin.* 2009;19:83–89.
327. Manlulu A, Lee TW, Wan I, et al. Video-assisted thoracic surgery thymectomy for nonthymomatous myasthenia gravis. *Chest.* 2005;128:3454–3460.

328. Pereira RM, Carvalho JF, Paula AP, et al. Guidelines for the prevention and treatment of glucocorticoid-induced osteoporosis. *Rev Bras Rheumatol.* 2012;52(4):580–593.
329. Pascuzzi RM, Coslett HB, Johns TR. Long-term corticosteroid treatment of myasthenia gravis: Report of 116 patients. *Ann Neurol.* 1984;15:291–298.
330. Johns TR. Long-term corticosteroid treatment of myasthenia gravis. *Ann NY Acad Sci.* 1987;505:568–583.
331. Schneider-Gold C, Gajdos P, Toyka KV, Hohlfeld RR. Corticosteroids for myasthenia gravis. *Cochrane Database Syst Rev.* 2005;2:CD002828.
332. Bae JS, Go SM, Kin BJ. Clinical predictors of steroid-induced exacerbation in myasthenia gravis. *J Clin Neurosci.* 2006;13:1006–2010.
333. Sanders DB, Scoppetta C. The treatment of patients with myasthenia gravis. *Neurol Clin.* 1994;12:343–368.
334. Miller RG, Milner-Brown HS, Mirka A. Prednisone-induced worsening of neuromuscular function in myasthenia gravis. *Neurology.* 1986;36:729–732.
335. Palace J, Newsom-Davis J, Lecky B. A randomized double-blind trial of prednisolone alone or with azathioprine in myasthenia gravis. Myasthenia Gravis Study Group. *Neurology.* 1998;50:1778–1783.
336. Herrllinger U, Weller M, Dichgans J, Melms A. Association of primary central nervous system lymphoma with long-term azathioprine therapy for myasthenia gravis. *Ann Neurol.* 2000;47:682–683.
337. Hohlfeld R, Michels M, Heininger K, Besinger U, Toyka KV. Azathioprine toxicity during long-term immunosuppression of generalized myasthenia gravis. *Neurology.* 1988;38: 258–261.
338. Kissel JT, Levy RJ, Mendell JR, Griggs RC. Azathioprine toxicity in neuromuscular disease. *Neurology.* 1986;36:35–39.
339. Gajdos P, Elkharrat D, Chevret S, Chastang C. A randomized clinical trial comparing prednisone and azathioprine in myasthenia gravis. Results of the second interim analysis. *J Neurol Neurosurg Psychiatry.* 1993;56:1157–1163.
340. The Muscle Study Group. A trial of mycophenolate mofetil with prednisone as initial immunotherapy in myasthenia gravis. *Neurology.* 2008;71:394–399.
341. Sanders DB, Hart IK, Mantegazza R, et al. An international, phase III, randomized trial of mycophenolate mofetil in myasthenia gravis. *Neurology.* 2008;71:400–406.
342. Bromberg MB, Wald JJ, Forshew DA, Feldman EL, Albers JW. Randomized trial of azathioprine or prednisone for initial immunosuppressive treatment of myasthenia. *J Neurol Sci.* 1997;150:59–62.
343. Meriggioli MN, Rowin J, Richman JG, Leurgans S. Mycophenolate mofetil for myasthenia gravis: A double-blind, placebo-controlled pilot study. *Ann N Y Acad Sci.* 2003;998:494–499.
344. Meriggioli MN, Ciafaloni E, Al-Hayk KA, et al. Mycophenolate mofetil for myasthenia gravis: An analysis of efficacy, safety, and tolerability. *Neurology.* 2003;61:1438–1440.
345. Sanders D, McDermott M, Thornton C, Tawil A, Barohn R; the Muscle Study Group. A trial of mycophenolate mofetil (MMF) with prednisone as initial immunotherapy in myasthenia gravis (MG) [abstract]. *Neurology.* 2007;68: A107.
346. Ciafaloni E, Massey JM, Tucker-Lipscomb B, Sanders DB. Mycophenolate mofetil for myasthenia gravis: An open-label pilot study. *Neurology.* 2001;56:97–99.
347. Vernino S, Salomao DR, Habermann TM, O'Neill BP. Primary CNS lymphoma complicating treatment of myasthenia gravis with mycophenolate mofetil. *Neurology.* 2005;65:639–641.
348. Hauser RA, Malek AR, Rosen R. Successful treatment of a patient with severe refractory myasthenia gravis using mycophenolate mofetil. *Neurology.* 1998;51:912–913.
349. Sollinger HW; Renal Transplant Mycophenolate Mofetil Study Group. Mycophenolate mofetil for the prevention of acute rejection in primary cadaveric renal allograft recipients. U.S. Renal Transplant Mycophenolate Mofetil Study Group. *Transplantation.* 1995;60:225–232.
350. Chaudhry V, Cornblath DR, Griffin JW, O'Brien R, Drachman DB. Mycophenolate mofetil: A safe and promising immunosuppressant in neuromuscular diseases. *Neurology.* 2001;56:94–96.
351. Hehir MK, Burns TM, Alpers J, Conaway MR, Sawa M, Sanders DB. Mycophenolate mofetil in AChR-antibody-positive myasthenia gravis: Outcomes in 102 patients. *Muscle Nerve.* 2010;41(5):593–598.
352. Ciafaloni E, Nikhar NK, Massey JM, Sanders DB. Retrospective analysis of the use of cyclosporine in myasthenia gravis. *Neurology.* 2000;55:448–450.
353. Sanders DB, Ciafaloni E, Nikhar NK, Massey JM. Retrospective analysis of the use of cyclosporine in myasthenia [abstract]. *Neurology.* 2000;54(Suppl 3):A394.
354. Tindall RS, Rollins JA, Phillips JT, Greenlee RG, Wells L, Belendiuk G. Preliminary results of a double-blind, randomized, placebo-controlled trial of cyclosporine in myasthenia gravis. *N Engl J Med.* 1987;316:719–724.
355. Tindall RS, Phillips JT, Rollins JA, Wells L, Hall K. A clinical therapeutic trial of cyclosporine in myasthenia gravis. *Ann N Y Acad Sci.* 1993;681:539–551.
356. Kurokawa T, Nishiyama T, Yamamoto R, Kishida H, Hakii Y, Kuroiwa Y. Anti-MuSK antibody positive myasthenia gravis with HIV infection successfully treated with cyclosporin: A case report. *Rinsho Shinkeigaku.* 2008;48(9):666–669.
357. Yoshikawa H, Kiuchi T, Saida T, Takamori M. Randomised double blind, placebo controlled study of tacrolimus in myasthenia gravis. *J Neurol Neurosurg Psychiatry.* 2011;82:970–977.
358. Ponseti JM, Gamez J, Azem J, et al. Post-thymectomy combined treatment of prednisone and tacrolimus versus prednisone alone for the consolidation of complete stable remission in patients with myasthenia gravis: A non-randomized, non-controlled study. *Curr Med Res Opin.* 2007;23:1269–1278.
359. Ponseti JM, Azem J, Fort JM, et al. Long-term results of tacrolimus in cyclosporine- and prednisone-dependent myasthenia gravis. *Neurology.* 2005;64:1641–1643.
360. Nagane Y, Utsugisawa K, Obara D, Kondoh R, Terayama Y. Efficacy of low-dose FK506 in the treatment of myasthenia gravis-a randomized pilot study. *Eur Neurol.* 2005;53: 146–150.
361. Benatar M, Sanders D. the importance of studying history: Lessons learnt from a trial of tacrolimus in myasthenia gravis. *J Neurol Neurosurg Psychiatry.* 2011;82:945.
362. Evoli A, Di Schino C, Marsili F, Punzi C. Successful treatment of myasthenia gravis with tacrolimus. *Muscle Nerve.* 2002;25(1):111–114.
363. Konishi T, Yoshiyama Y, Takamori M, Yagi K, Mukai E, Saida T; Japanese FK506 MG Study Group. Clinical study of FK506 in patients with myasthenia gravis. *Muscle Nerve.* 2003;28(5):570–574.

364. Sanders DB, Aarli JA, Cutter GR, Jaretzki A III, Kaminski HJ, Phillips LH II. Long-term results of tacrolimus in cyclosporine- and prednisone-dependent myasthenia gravis [comment]. *Neurology*. 2006;66(6):954–955.
365. Schneider-Gold C, Hartung HP, Gold R. Mycophenolate mofetil and tacrolimus: New therapeutic options in neuroimmunological diseases. *Muscle Nerve*. 2006;34(3):284–291.
366. Tada M, Shimohata T, Tada M, et al. Long-term therapeutic efficacy and safety of low-dose tacrolimus (FK506) for myasthenia gravis. *J Neurol Sci*. 2006;247(1):17–20.
367. Wakata N, Saito T, Tanaka S, Hirano T, Oka K. Tacrolimus hydrate (FK506): Therapeutic effects and selection of responders in the treatment of myasthenia gravis. *Clin Neurol Neurosurg*. 2003;106(1):5–8.
368. Lewis RA, Lisak RP. "Rebooting" the immune system with cyclophosphamide: Taking risks for a "cure"? *Ann Neurol*. 2003;53:7–9
369. Lin PT, Martin BA, Winacker AB, So YT. High-dose cyclophosphamide in refractory myasthenia with MuSK antibodies. *Muscle Nerve*. 2006;33:433–435.
370. DeFeo LG, Schottlender J, Martelli NA, Molfino NA. Use of intravenous pulsed cyclophosphamide in severe, generalized myasthenia gravis. *Muscle Nerve*. 2002;26:32–36.
371. Drachman DB, Jones RJ, Brodsky RA. Treatment of refractory myasthenia: "Rebooting" with high-dose cyclophosphamide. *Ann Neurol*. 2003;53:29–34.
372. Kuntzer T, Carota A, Novy J, Cavassini M, Du Pasquier RA. Rituximab is successful in an HIV positive patient with MuSK myasthenia. *Neurology*. 2011;76:757–758.
373. Maddison P, McConville J, Farrugia ME, et al. The use of rituximab in myasthenia gravis and Lambert-Eaton myasthenic syndrome. *J Neurol Neurosurg Psychiatry*. 2011;82:671–673.
374. Gajra A, Vajpayee N, Grethlein SJ. Response of myasthenia gravis to rituximab in a patient with non-Hodgkin lymphoma. *Am J Hematol*. 2004;77(2):196–197.
375. Gajdos P, Chevret S, Toyka K. Intravenous immunoglobulin for myasthenia gravis. *Cochrane Database Syst Rev*. 2006;19: CD002277.
376. Gajdos P, Tranchant C, Clair B, et al. Myasthenia Gravis Clinical Study Group Treatment of myasthenia gravis exacerbation with intravenous immunoglobulin 1 g/kg versus 2 g/kg: A randomized double blind clinical trial. *Ann Neurol*. 2005;62: 1689–1693.
377. Zinman L, Ng E, Bril V. IV immunoglobulin in patients with myasthenia gravis: A randomized controlled trial. *Neurology*. 2007;68:837–841.
378. Achiron A, Barak Y, Miron S, Sarova-Pinhas I. Immunoglobulin treatment in refractory myasthenia gravis. *Muscle Nerve*. 2000;23:551–555.
379. Cosi V, Lombardi M, Piccolo G, Erbetta A. Treatment of myasthenia gravis with high-dose intravenous immunoglobulin. *Acta Neurol Scand*. 1991;84:81–84.
380. Dwyer JM. Manipulating the immune system with immune globulin. *N Engl J Med*. 1992;326:107–116.
381. Gajdos P, Chevret S, Clair B, Tranchant C, Chastang C. Clinical trial of plasma exchange and high-dose intravenous immunoglobulin in myasthenia gravis. *Ann Neurol*. 1997;41:789–796.
382. Howard JF Jr. Intravenous immunoglobulin for the treatment of acquired myasthenia gravis. *Neurology*. 1998;51(Suppl 5): S30–S36.
383. Jongen JL, van Doorn PA, van der Meche FG. High-dose intravenous immunoglobulin therapy for myasthenia gravis. *J Neurol*. 1998;245:26–31.
384. Qureshi AI, Choudhry MA, Akbar MS, et al. Plasma exchange versus intravenous immunoglobulin treatment in myasthenic crisis. *Neurology*. 1999;52:629–632.
385. Li HF, Gao X, Hong Y, et al. Evidence-based guideline: Intravenous immunoglobulin in the treatment of neuromuscular disorders: Report of the Therapeutics and Technology Assessment Subcommittee of the American Academy of Neurology. *Neurology*. 2012;78:1009–1015.
386. NIH Consensus Conference. The utility of therapeutic plasmapheresis for neurological disorders. *JAMA*. 1986;256:1333–1337.
387. Pinching AF, Peters DK, Newsom-Davis J. Remission of myasthenia gravis following plasma exchange. *Lancet*. 1976;2:1373–1376.
388. Antozzi C, Gemma M, Regi B, et al. A short plasma exchange protocol is effective in severe myasthenia gravis. *J Neurol*. 1991;238:103–107.
389. Mandawat A, Mandawat A, Kaminski H, Shaker Z, Alawi AA, Alshekhlee A. Outcome of plasmapheresis in myasthenia gravis: Delayed therapy is not favorable. *Muscle Nerve*. 2011;43:578–584.
390. Cortese I, Chaudhry V, So YT, Cantor F, Cornblath DR, Rei-Grant A. Evidence-based guideline update: Plasmapheresis in neurologic disorders: Report of the Therapeutics and Technology Assessment Subcommittee of the American Academy of Neurology. *Neurology*. 2011;76:294–300.
391. Gajdos P, Chevret S, Toyka K. Plasma exchange for myasthenia gravis. *Cochrane Database of Syst Rev*. 2002;(4):CD002275.
392. Yeh JH, Chiu HC. Plasmapheresis in myasthenia gravis. A comparative study of daily versus alternately daily schedule. *Acta Neurol Scand*. 1999;99:147–151.
393. Stricker RB, Kwiatkowski BJ, Habis JA, Kiprov DD. Myasthenic crisis: Response to plasmapheresis following failure of intravenous gamma-globulin. *Arch Neurol*. 1993;50:837–840.
394. Howard JF. The treatment of myasthenia gravis with plasma exchange. *Semin Neurol*. 1982;2:273–279.
395. Mahalati K, Dawson RB, Collins JO, Mayer RF. Predictable recovery for myasthenia gravis crisis with plasma exchange: 36 cases and review of current management. *J Clin Apher*. 1999;14:1–8.
396. Guptill JT, Oakley D, Kuchibhatla M, et al. A retrospective study of complications of therapeutic plasma exchange in myasthenia. *Muscle Nerve*. 2013;47:170–176.
397. Kaminski H, Cutter G, Ruff RL, Wolfe G. Evidence-based guideline update: Plasmapheresis in neurologic disorders. *Neurology*. 2011;77:e101–e102.
398. Dau PC, Lindstrom JM, Cassel CK, Denys EH, Shev EE, Spitler LE. Plasmapheresis and immunosuppressive drug therapy in myasthenia gravis. *N Engl J Med*. 1977;297:1134–1140.
399. Barth D, Nabavi Noure M, Ng E, Nwe P, Bril V. Comparison of IVIg and PLEX in patients with myasthenia gravis. *Neurology*. 2011;76:2017–2023.
400. Mandawat A, Kaminski HJ, Carter G, Katirji B, Alshekhlee A. Comparative analysis of therapeutic options used for myasthenia gravis. *Ann Neurol*. 2010;68(6):797–805.
401. Ronager J, Ravnborg M, Hermansen I, Vorstrup S. Immunoglobulin treatment versus plasma exchange in patients with chronic moderate to severe myasthenia gravis. *Artif Organs*. 2001;25:967–973.
402. Bril V, Barnett-Tapia C, Barth D, Katzberg HD. IVIG and PLEX in the treatment of myasthenia gravis. *Ann N Y Acad Sci*. 2012;1275(1):1–6.
403. Sanders DB, Massey J, Juel V. MuSK antibody positive myasthenia gravis: Response to treatment in 31 patients [abstract]. *Neurology*. 2007;68:A299.

404. Huang C-S, Hsu H-S, Kao K-P, Huang M-H, Huang B-S. Intravenous immunoglobulin in the preparation of thymectomy for myasthenia gravis. *Acta Neurol Scand.* 2003;108: 136–138.
405. Luo J, Kuryatov A, Lindstrom JM. Specific immunotherapy of experimental myasthenia gravis by a novel mechanism. *Ann Neurol.* 2010;67:441–451.
406. Soltys J, Kusner LL, Young A, et al. A novel complement inhibitor limits severity of experimental myasthenia gravis. *Ann Neurol.* 2009;65:67–75.
407. Rowin J, Meriggioli MN, Tüzün E, Leurgans S, Christadoss P. Etanercept treatment in in corticosteroid-dependent myasthenia gravis. *Neurology.* 2004;63:2390–2392.
408. Strober J, Cowan MJ, Horn BN. Allogeneic hematopoietic cell transplantation for refractory myasthenia gravis. *Arch Neurol.* 2009;66:659–661.
409. Berlit S, Tuschy B, Spaich S, Sütterlin M, Schaffelder R. Myasthenia gravis in pregnancy: A case report. *Case Rep Obstet Gynecol.* 2012;2012:736024.
410. Burns TM. More than meets the eye: The benefits of listening closely to what our patients with myasthenia gravis are telling us. *Muscle Nerve.* 2012;46:153–154.
411. Farrugia ME, Vincent A. Autoimmune mediated neuromuscular junction defects. *Curr Opin Neurol.* 2010;23:489–495.
412. Gajdos P, Sharshar T, Chevret S. Standards of measurements in myasthenia gravis. *Ann N Y Acad Sci.* 2003;998:445–452.
413. Barohn RJ, McIntire D, Herbelin L, Wolfe GI, Nations S, Bryan WW. Reliability testing of the quantitative myasthenia gravis score. *Ann N Y Acad Sci.* 1998;841:769–772.
414. Bedlack RS, Simel DL, Bosworth H, Samsa G, Tucker-Lipscomb B, Sanders DB. Quantitative myasthenia gravis score: Assessment of responsiveness and longitudinal validity. *Neurology.* 2005;64(11):1968–1970.
415. Berrouschot J, Baumann I, Kalischewski P, Sterker M, Schneider D. Therapy of myasthenic crisis. *Crit Care Med.* 1997;25:1228–1235.
416. Thomas CE, Mayer SA, Gunger Y, et al. Myasthenic crisis: Clinical features, mortality, complications, and risk factors for prolonged intubation. *Neurology.* 1997:48–1253–1260.
417. Vincent A, Leite MI. Neuromuscular junction autoimmune disease: Muscle specific kinase antibodies and treatments for myasthenia gravis.. *Curr Opin Neurol.* 2005;18(5):519–525.
418. Lehky TJ, Iwamoto FM, Kreisel TN, Floeter MK, Fine HA. Neuromuscular junction toxicity with tandutanib induces and myasthenic-like syndrome. *Neurology.* 2011;76:236–241.

CHAPTER 26

Other Disorders of Neuromuscular Transmission

This chapter describes the disorders of neuromuscular transmission (DNMT) other than myasthenia gravis (MG) (Table 26-1). The neuromuscular junction (NMJ) is a physiologically complex structure. Its ability to function optimally requires the integration of a large number of proteins including ion channels that are correctly configured and distributed. As a result of numerous potential sites of vulnerability, DNMTs may occur as a consequence of multiple, albeit infrequent disorders. Autoimmune, genetic, or toxic mechanisms may disrupt the ultrastructure or physiology of the NMJ, thus interfering with effective NMT.

► LAMBERT–EATON MYASTHENIC SYNDROME

CLINICAL FEATURES

The Lambert–Eaton myasthenic syndrome (LEMS) can be conceptualized as an acquired presynaptic DNMT typically presenting with symptoms of proximal lower extremity weakness and fatigue. The first single case description of LEMS was provided by Anderson in 1953. Its eponym however is credited to Edward Lambert and Lee Eaton who along with Edward Rooke described in 1956 the electrophysiological as well as clinical characteristics of the disorder in six cases.[1,2] LEMS is a rare disorder with an estimated incidence of 1 and prevalence of 3.5 per million people.[1–10] LEMS is largely a disease of adults although rare pediatric cases have been described [both acquired autoimmune condition and as a congenital myasthenic syndrome (CMS)].[11] LEMS is paraneoplastic disorder in many cases, but can be seen as a primary autoimmune disorder without an underlying cancer. The epidemiology between those cases of LEMS associated with a malignancy differs from those cases without an underlying neoplasm. Nonneoplastic LEMS appears to have two peaks, 35 and 60 years of age, occurring far frequently in women in the younger group. Paraneoplastic LEMS peaks in incidence at age 60 with two-thirds of this group being men.[2]

In adult LEMS, there is a strong support for a causative relationship for autoantibodies directed against voltage-gated calcium channels (VGCC) which are detectable in the majority of afflicted individuals, regardless of the presence of an underlying malignancy.[12] Paraneoplastic LEMS comprises approximately two-thirds of cases. Small-cell carcinoma of the lung (SCLC) is the underlying malignancy in approximately 90% of these cases and 50–60% of all cases.[13–15] Thymic tumors, non-SCLC lung cancers, lymphoproliferative disorders, and prostate cancer are the next most common associations.[2,16–19] Pancreatic, breast and ovarian carcinomas, and Wilms' tumor may represent chance associations.[12,20,21] Conversely, it is estimated that between 0.5 and 4% of all SCLC patients will develop the clinical features of LEMS and approximately 8% will develop VGCC autoantibodies.[22,23] The LEMS symptoms usually precede tumor recognition. Historically, this latency has been typically estimated to be less than 1 year, but may extend beyond 5 years in rare cases. These figures may however, represent a bias generated by surveillance techniques less sensitive than those currently available. In a more recent study of 100 LEMS patients followed for a minimum of 3 and a median of 8 years, 91% of those with malignancy were identified by 3 months of symptom onset and 96% by the end of the first year.[15]

The phenotypic and electrophysiological characteristics of paraneoplastic and nonparaneoplastic LEMS for all intents and purposes are indistinguishable in individual cases.[24] Suspicion for an underlying malignancy should increase however, if the patient is over 50 years, has a history of tobacco use, progresses rapidly, or develops weight loss, erectile dysfunction, or bulbar symptoms within 3 months of symptom onset.[2] A person with all six of these characteristics has a greater than 90% chance of harboring an underlying malignancy.[2] Presumably, symptoms suggestive of other paraneoplastic disorders would increase the probability of an underlying malignancy as well. In general, paraneoplastic LEMS progresses more rapidly than its nonparaneoplastic counterpart.[25] Other autoimmune diseases such as rheumatoid arthritis, thyroiditis, systemic lupus erythematosus, inflammatory bowel disease, primary biliary cirrhosis, vitiligo, celiac disease, or even MG occur in approximately 25% of cases and their presence favors a nonneoplastic form of the disease.[14,26,27] Although the phenotype of LEMS appears homogeneous, independent of underlying cause or serology, the natural history of LEMS however, may be influenced by serotype. On average, seronegative LEMS patients appear to have a shorter life expectancy. An explanatory hypothesis for this observation is a potential therapeutic role for autoantibodies (see below).

▶ **TABLE 26-1. DISORDERS OF NEUROMUSCULAR TRANSMISSION OTHER THAN AUTOIMMUNE MYASTHENIA GRAVIS**

Presynaptic
Lambert–Eaton myasthenic syndrome (LEMS)
Botulism and botulinum toxin
Tick paralysis (Australian)
Congenital myasthenia gravis
Choline acetyltransferase deficiency (ChAT)
Paucity of synaptic vesicles
Congenital LEMS
Toxins
Envenomation
Elapid snake species (kraits, mambas, coral snakes)
Arthropods (black and brown widow spiders, scorpions)
Marine species (cone snails, sea snakes)
Drugs
Aminoglycosides and other antibiotics
Calcium channel blocking agents (minor)
Aminopyridines
Corticosteroids
Hemicholinium-3
Synaptic/basal lamina
Congenital myasthenic syndromes
Acetylcholine esterase deficiency (COLQ)
Laminin β2 (LAMB2)
Drugs and toxins
Reversible cholinesterase inhibitors—edrophonium, pyridostigmine, and neostigmine
Irreversible—organophosphates and carbamates
Postsynaptic
Drug-induced myasthenia gravis
Penicillamine
Alpha-interferon
Congenital myasthenic syndromes
Agrin deficiency (AGRN)
AChR (subunit) deficiency with or without kinetic defect [slow (opening) or fast (opening) channel syndromes]
εAChR subunit (CHRNE)
αAChR subunit (CHRNA1)
βAChR subunit (CHRNB1)
δAChR subunit (CHRND)
γAChR subunit (Escobar syndrome)
AChR—structural or organizational defects
Dok-7 deficiency (DOK7)
MuSK deficiency (MuSK)
Rapsyn deficiency (RAPSN)
Sodium channel myasthenia (SCN4A)
Plectin deficiency (PLEC)
Glutamine-fructose-6-phosphate transaminase 1 MG (GFPT1)
Dolichyl-phosphate N-acetylglucosamine-phosphotransferase 1 MG (DPAGT1)
Drugs and toxins
d-Tubocurarine, vecuronium, and other nondepolarizing blocking agents
Succinylcholine, decamethonium, and other depolarizing blocking agents
Tetracyclines, lincomycin, and other antibiotics

Lack of stamina and fatigue are the most common presenting symptoms of LEMS.[1,3,5,7–10,28,29] In our experience, the described morbidity often seems disproportionate to the degree of objective weakness. It has been our perspective as well that this discordance may contribute to the suspicion of a psychogenic disorder, particularly in young women. Symptomatic weakness in LEMS typically relates to functions requiring proximal, particularly lower extremity muscles and is noted in approximately 80% of patients during the course of the illness. A third of patients complain of muscle aching and stiffness during or following physical exertion. Approximately 20% of patients note that their weakness and fatigue are exacerbated by hot weather or baths. Ocular and bulbar symptoms are not as common or as severe as seen in MG but do occur.[15,30,31] They typically develop later in the disease and are rarely the sole or initial manifestation.[2,31,32] Symptomatic diplopia without overt ophthalmoparesis is typically transient and mild when it occurs. Ptosis is more common in our experience and is estimated to occur in a third to a half of cases. In those with cranial muscle involvement, neck flexor, extensor, and facial muscles are among the most commonly affected. Head drop has been reported as a presenting manifestation.[33] Some patients develop dysarthria or dysphagia. Ventilatory muscle involvement is rare although breathing issues related to smoking, chronic lung disease, and lung cancer are not. Ventilatory failure as a rare presenting manifestation of LEMS has been described.[34–36]

As a presynaptic DNMT, in contrast to MG, LEMS frequently affects both nicotinic and muscarinic function with resultant cholinergic dysautonomia. This may manifest as blurred vision (impaired accommodation), xerostomia, xerophthalmia, constipation, hypohydrosis, and/or impotence.[12] Xerostomia may contribute to dysphagia and dysarthria. Complaints of numbness and paresthesias in the distal extremities occur less frequently. They are not related to disordered NMT but more likely result from any of the mechanisms relevant to cancer patients. Patients with LEMS may have coexistent paraneoplastic syndromes such as sensory neuronopathy, cerebellar ataxia, and/or limbic encephalitis with frequently coexistent Hu autoantibodies.[37]

One potential explanation for the apparent discordance between the severity of patient symptoms and their actual strength logically extrapolates from disease pathophysiology. As brief exercise can transiently enhance neuromuscular transmission in presynaptic disorders, the patient's strength should be ideally assessed at the initiation of contraction, not several seconds later. This transient improvement in strength usually dissipates with sustained muscle contraction. It is most readily identified in hip and shoulder girdle muscles. Repetitive squatting may be one means to demonstrate this phenomenon. Exercise may also be used to evaluate ptosis, which may be temporarily improved with sustained voluntary lid elevation in a manner opposite to MG.[38]

There are other potential, noteworthy observations to be made in an LEMS patient. Typical of DNMTs, muscle bulk in LEMS tends to be preserved. In advanced stages of the disease however, muscle atrophy can be observed. Sluggish pupillary reaction in response to a light stimulus or diminished sweating in response to a provocative challenge are means by which to identify cholinergic dysautonomia. Deep tendon reflexes are typically diminished or absent in LEMS. Like assessments of strength, this phenomenon may be obscured if manual muscle testing is done prior to deep tendon reflex assessment.

A small number of patients will present with what seems to be an MG/LEMS overlap syndrome.[39–41] Most MG cases overlapping with LEMS are based on the presence of acetylcholine receptor (AChR) antibodies in patients who otherwise appear to have LEMS on a clinical and electrophysiological basis. As many as 13% of patients with LEMS have AChR-binding autoantibodies.[42] The AChR autoantibodies may be epiphenomenal rather than pathogenic in at least some LEMS patients.[42,43] Nonetheless, rare patients may exhibit clinical features of both LEMS and MG.[39,42,44,46]

DIAGNOSIS AND DIFFERENTIAL DIAGNOSIS

As a disorder characterized by a subacute limb-girdle weakness and fatigue, the primary differential diagnostic considerations for LEMS are limb-girdle myopathies and MG. MG may readily be confused with LEMS, particularly if signs and symptoms of oculobulbar weakness are readily evident with LEMS or if they are inapparent in MG. As a general rule, oculobulbar signs occur early and are prominent in MG and tend to be less frequent, less severe, and occur later in the disease course in LEMS.[2,31] Exceptions do exist.[15,30] Botulism has similar clinical features to LEMS including the pattern of weakness and the presence of cholinergic dysautonomia. Both its typically acute onset and the clinical context in which it occurs are the usual discriminating factors. LEMS can present in childhood and CMS may first manifest itself in adulthood. Consequently, CMS deserve consideration in any LEMS suspect as well. Motor neuron diseases that produce a limb-girdle pattern of weakness such as Kennedy disease are distinguished by their chronicity, and the presence of atrophy and fasciculations. The pattern and evolution of the weakness produced by multifocal motor neuropathy are, as the name implies, usually distinctive from LEMS. Motor predominant forms of CIDP may represent a very relevant diagnostic consideration in an LEMS suspect, particularly as both abolish deep tendon reflexes and affect the autonomic nervous system. The majority of these disorders can be readily distinguished from LEMS by electrodiagnostic (EDX) testing.

Electrodiagnostic Testing (EDX)

Diagnostic confirmation of LEMS is obtained by electrophysiological and/or autoantibody testing. As with all DNMTs, sensory conductions are normal unless paraneoplastic sensory neuropathy, chemotherapy-induced neuropathy, or other confounding disorders coexist. H reflexes may be absent upon initial attempts at elicitation but may appear following muscle contraction, an observation more likely to be of academic interest rather than pragmatic benefit.[46]

In LEMS and other presynaptic DNMTs, the baseline compound muscle action potential (CMAP) amplitudes are significantly reduced in contrast to typical MG. Reduced CMAP amplitudes are in many cases widespread in the distribution. In a large study of 73 patients with LEMS (42% with lung cancer), the CMAP amplitude was reduced in the abductor digiti quinti (ADQ) in 95%, abductor pollicis in 85%, extensor digitorum brevis in 80%, and in the trapezius in only 55% of cases.[47] This diffuse pattern of reduced CMAP amplitudes in the presence of normal sensory nerve action potentials (SNAPs) may provide the initial suspicion for LEMS. The CMAP response to exercise and/or repetitive stimulation along with serological testing provide confirmation.[5,6,8,48–55]

On occasion, the EDX pattern in LEMS may be confused with MG. LEMS patients will typically demonstrate both an incremental pattern to fast repetitive stimulation (10–50 Hz) or brief exercise as well as a decremental response to slow (2–5 Hz) repetitive stimulation (Fig. 26-1A and B).[47,53–57] If a patient with LEMS is seen early enough in

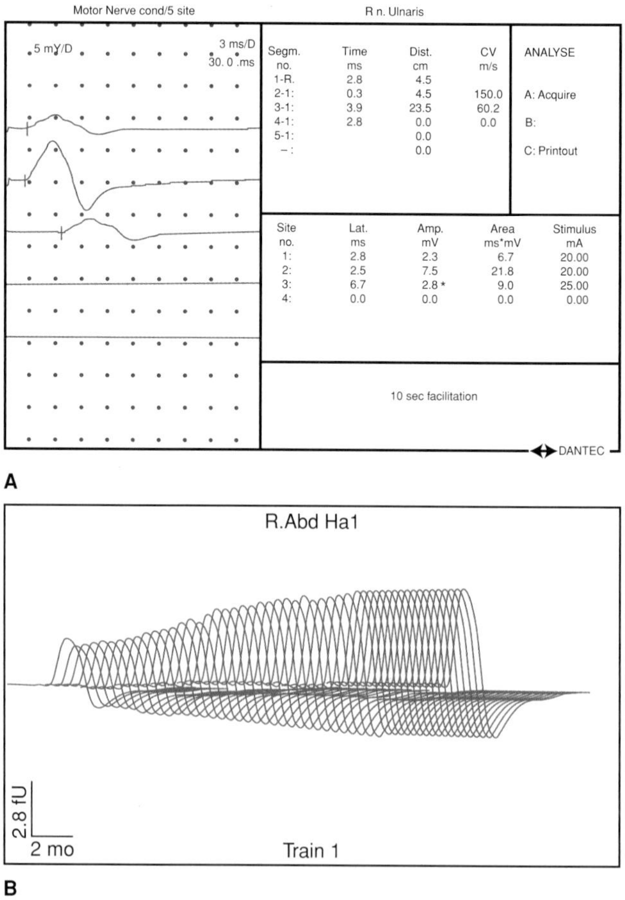

Figure 26-1. Incremental response to brief (10 seconds) exercise in a patient with LEMS **(A)** (trace 1 ulnar CMAP at baseline, trace 2 ulnar CMAP immediately after 10 seconds of isometrically resisted finger abduction, trace 3 ulnar CMAP 1 minute later). Incremental response to 20-Hz fast repetitive stimulation **(B)**.

their illness however, their baseline CMAP amplitudes may fall within population norms. In this situation, the incremental response characteristic of a presynaptic deficit may not be either evident or sought for. The demonstration of a decrement in response to slow (2–5 Hz) repetitive stimulation, characteristic of both LEMS and MG, without demonstration of an increment may lead to misdiagnosis. If LEMS is suspected but cannot be confirmed either electrodiagnostically or serologically, the evolution into the typical presynaptic DNMT pattern may be disclosed with repeated nerve conduction studies.[58,59]

This decremental pattern in LEMS is similar although not necessarily identical to that described in MG. In MG, following the initial decrement between the first and fifth stimuli, there is an increase in CMAP amplitude between the fifth and tenth stimuli. The CMAP amplitudes in LEMS plateau continue to decline between the fifth and tenth responses in LEMS.[60,61] In LEMS, decrement in response to 3-Hz stimulation has been demonstrated in the ADQ in 98%, APB in 98%, EDB in 84%, and trapezius in 89% of cases.[47]

In a cooperative patient, incremental testing can be rapidly and easily performed. A supramaximal baseline CMAP is obtained after suitable hand warming. The muscle tested is then subjected to 10–15 seconds of isometric resistance. Immediately thereafter, a second, supramaximal electrical stimulus is applied. In normal individuals, there may be a mild increase in CMAP amplitude (<40%) associated with a shorter duration and similar area under the curve (pseudofacilitation). The actual basis of this phenomenon is poorly understood. It has been postulated to represent improved motor unit synchronization due to a disproportionate increase in the conduction velocity of the slowest conducting muscle fibers.[62,63] In the majority of patients with LEMS, brief exercise will produce a 100–400% increase in CMAP amplitude. It is important to recognize that patients with end-stage LEMS may fail to mount this dramatic of an incremental response.[64] In individuals who cannot cooperate with isometric exercise for whatever reason, "fast" repetitive stimulation of 20 Hz or higher represents a more uncomfortable means by which to demonstrate the characteristic increment.

Abnormal insertional and spontaneous activity on needle examination such as fibrillation potentials are typically absent in LEMS.[5,6,28,50,51,58,65] Abnormalities of motor unit action potential (MUAP) morphology are apparent in weak muscles if carefully assessed. Neuromuscular blockade at individual myoneural junctions effectively reduces the number of single fiber action potentials contributing to the MUAP, resulting in shorter duration and lower amplitude waveforms. Consequently, the twitch tension of motor units decline and compensatory early (increased) recruitment results. In addition, the random blockade of single myofiber action potentials desynchronizes the MUAP leading to an increased percentage of polyphasic MUAPs. Motor unit variability (instability) is readily evident in LEMS if sought for but will be less apparent with the facilitation promoted by increased MUAP firing frequencies.

Predictably, both volitional and stimulated single fiber electromyography (SFEMG) evaluations of patients with LEMS yield abnormal results.[8,48,50,51,53,56,66–77] Jitter values in patients with LEMS are significantly elevated and statistically exceed that observed in MG. In essentially all NMJs examined, irrespective of muscle chosen, markedly abnormal jitter values are evident. This is disparate from MG where a spectrum of jitter values from normal to highly abnormal exists within and between individual muscles. Unlike MG, the jitter in patients with LEMS is not dependent on the degree of weakness in a particular muscle. Blocking is often more prevalent and severe in LEMS in comparison to MG. Some of the highest percentages of blocked potentials occur in LEMS.

Frequency-dependent alterations in jitter and blocking are also observed in LEMS if sought for as implied in the previous statements regarding frequency-dependent MUAP variability (instability). Specifically, at low rates of voluntary firing, jitter and blocking can be quite impressive. Further increase in the duration of muscle activation or rate of individual MUAP firing will result in reduced jitter and blocking. These observations can be quantitated by using stimulated SFEMG.[72,73,76,78,79] Stimulating an intramuscular neural branch and recording a single muscle fiber potential allow jitter measurement with quantifiable stimulus rates. One study of patients with LEMS demonstrated that the jitter decreased from a mean of 150 μs at a stimulation rate of 2 Hz to about 90 μs at a firing rate of 15 Hz.[70,72] Similarly, when changing the stimulus frequency from 2 to 15 Hz, the percent of blockings decreased from 70% to fewer than 10%. Distinguishing MG from LEMS by contrasting stimulated SFEMG responses is theoretically possible but impractical in most circumstances. Muscle temperature affects EDX responses in LEMS as well.[79–82] Decreasing muscle temperature results in an improvement in the CMAP amplitude at rest, reduces the magnitude of decrement at low rates of stimulation, and prolongs the duration of postactivation facilitation. Like MG, the yield of EDX testing will be increased not only by ensuring that limbs are adequately warm but also by discontinuing cholinesterase inhibitors 24 hours before testing.[83]

As dysautonomia in LEMS is commonplace, abnormal autonomic nervous system testing is anticipated. In a series of 30 patients with LEMS, autonomic testing revealed abnormalities of sudomotor function in 83% of patients, abnormal cardiovagal reflexes in 75%, decreased salivation in 44%, and abnormal adrenergic function in 37% of tested individuals in keeping with the predominantly cholinergic dysautonomia of the disease.[10,12]

Serological Testing

Antibodies directed against the P/Q-type VGCC of the motor nerve terminals are believed to be pathogenic and are highly sensitive and specific for LEMS. They are detected by immunoprecipitation of VGCC from human brain, labeled with ω-conotoxin derived from the fish-eating Conus species of snails, incubated with serum from LEMS patients.[2,84] These antibodies are detectable in the serum in 98% or more of paraneoplastic and >80% of nonparaneoplastic LEMS patients.[12,24,42] Conversely, as previously mentioned, it is estimated that 4% of patients with SCLC will develop VGCC autoantibodies.[25] In addition, antibodies directed against the N-type VGCCs, which are located on autonomic and peripheral nerves as well as cerebellar, cortical, and spinal neurons, are present in 74% of patients with paraneoplastic LEMS and 40% of nonparaneoplastic LEMS patients.[12,42]

LEMS patients may harbor other autoantibodies. The SOX1 antigen was originally found as a result of antiglial nuclear antibodies cross reacting with Bergmann glia of the Purkinje cell layer of rat cerebellum. The SOX1 antigen also plays a role in the development of airway epithelia and is found in SCLC. SOX autoantibodies are of potential clinical value as they are highly specific for LEMS and SCLC. They are found in two-thirds of LEMS patients with SCLC, 12% of SCLC without LEMS, and <5% of LEMS without cancer.[85,86] Despite the cerebellar location of the antigen, there is no consistent association with paraneoplastic cerebellar degeneration or other paraneoplastic disorders. These antibodies are commercially available as antiglial nuclear antibodies as part of the Mayo Clinic paraneoplastic antibody panel. As previously mentioned, some patients with paraneoplastic LEMS will also harbor Hu autoantibodies associated with a sensory ganglionopathy, cerebellar degeneration, and/or limbic encephalopathy.[12,37,42] Autoantibodies against the presynaptic protein synaptotagmin have also been described in LEMS patients but have no current clinical application.[2]

Serological testing for VGCC and AChR autoantibodies usually accurately discriminate between LEMS and MG when there is phenotypic overlap. Nonetheless, as previously mentioned, AChR-binding antibodies are found in as many as 13% of patients with LEMS.[42] Conversely, as previously mentioned, autoantibodies against the P/Q VGCCs are found in <5% of patients who have the phenotypic and electrophysiological characteristics of MG.[42,43] The concurrence of both antibodies is thought to be epiphenomenal in most cases.[42]

Pharmacological Testing

Edrophonium testing in LEMS produces variable results and is not normally employed.

Imaging

Surveillance for a potential underlying neoplasm should be undertaken to some extent in any patient with LEMS. There is published guidance as to how extensive the initial evaluation should be, and how frequently it should be repeated if the initial evaluation is negative.[15] Although paraneoplastic LEMS is largely a disorder of older people who have smoked, we are of the opinion that every LEMS patient should have a careful physical examination, and some form of imaging. Chest x-ray is considered an insufficiently sensitive imaging procedure in this context.[15] In a younger individual without a smoking history, we lobby for a total body positron emission tomographic scan (FDG-PET) while remaining aware that problems with both availability and reimbursement may be encountered. FDG-PET is likely the most sensitive means by which to detect an underlying malignancy.[15] In an older patient with a smoking history, CT of the thorax will detect the majority of tumors that are initially detectable.[15] If CT of the thorax is normal, FDG-PET is also suggested.[15] Regarding subsequent surveillance in individuals in whom no tumor is initially detected, evaluation has been suggested at 6-month intervals for 2 years.[15] Our personal preference is to apply this strategy only to those individuals with a smoking history. As contemporary data indicates that a very high percentage of individuals with initially occult neoplasms will be detected within the first year of LEMS onset, we would limit rescreening to 1 year. Once again, we prefer FDG-PET rather than CT in consideration with radiation exposure as well as the probable greater sensitivity of the former for malignancy detection outside of the central nervous system (CNS).

HISTOPATHOLOGY

One reason to perform EDX in patients with limb-girdle patterns of weakness is to distinguish LEMS from myopathy and avoid muscle biopsy in these patients. If performed, muscle biopsy reveals only nonspecific type II fiber atrophy.[8] On quantitative electron microscopic analysis, nerve terminals appear normal in both their size and the number of synaptic vesicles they contain.[87] Similarly, the postsynaptic membrane is intact but with an increase in the postsynaptic fold area and number of secondary synaptic clefts, presumably as a compensatory mechanism in response to reduced quantal release. The total number and activation properties of individual AChRs appear normal. Freeze-fracture analysis of the presynaptic membrane demonstrates a marked decrease in the number of intramembranous proteinaceous particles, which are assumed to be P/Q VGCC. These presumptive channels are disorganized and aggregated in clumps.[88–90]

PATHOGENESIS

In summary, the preponderance of evidence suggests that LEMS is a disorder of impaired presynaptic ACh release resulting from autoantibody mediated–VGCC dysfunction. The mechanism appears to be downregulation of channels and endocytosis rather than mechanical blockade.[27] As a consequence of this autoimmune assault, reduced presynaptic calcium ion concentrations occur in response to a motor nerve action potential.[12,42] Quantal ACh content, that is, the number of active vesicles released in response to a nerve action potential is reduced and neuromuscular transmission compromised.[12,14,27,90,92]

Presynaptic function includes concentrating and storing ACh within vesicles, facilitating their movement to active release zones where they dock and fuse, thus setting the stage for ACh release into the synaptic cleft in response to a motor nerve action potential. The migration, docking, and fusion with the presynaptic plasma membrane and subsequent exocytosis into the synaptic cleft are all dependent on the complex interaction of an extensive number of proteins. Some of the more notable constituents of this complex neuromuscular transmission process include synaptobrevin and synaptotagmin (associated with the synaptic vesicles), NSF (N-ethylamide sensitive ATPase) and α-SNAP (both found in the cytosol), syntaxin and SNAP-25 (synaptic vesicle–associated 25-kDa protein), and membrane-bound VGCCs.[93] Synaptobrevin, syntaxin, and SNAP-25 are collectively known as SNARE (SNAP receptor) proteins. The known specificity of tetanus and botulism toxins for SNARE proteins and the impaired ACh release that results from their exposure to the NMJ illustrate the essential function of SNARE proteins in presynaptic vesicular exocytosis.

In normal individuals, a motor nerve action potential transiently opens presynaptic VGCCs resulting in an increased motor nerve terminal intracellular calcium concentration. The effect does not achieve the magnitude that it potentially could as the duration of the nerve action potential of <1.0 ms undershoots the activation time constant of the VGCC of 1.3 ms.[91] The intracellular calcium concentration peaks by 200 μs and persists for approximately 800 μs following the nerve action potential, numbers critical to the understanding of repetitive stimulation responses in DNMT.

An intracellular calcium concentration of 200–300 μM is achieved under normal circumstances. It is estimated that 60 VGCCs need to open to allow the ingress of the approximately 13,000 calcium ions to promote required for exocytosis of a solitary vesicle. In mammalian systems, the response to a motor nerve action potential is a quantal content of 50–300 whereas in LEMS, the mean is roughly 8 (3.3–15).[91] Similar effects on quantal content are achieved by reducing the calcium concentration or increasing the magnesium concentration in the extracellular fluid bathing the nerve terminal.[93]

The facilitatory effect of intracellular calcium on ACh release initiates with its binding to synaptotagmin, subsequently with syntaxin and SNAP-25, and eventually with synaptobrevin to complete the vesicular, exocytotic cascade. Calcium is believed to be essential in cleaving the bonds holding ACh vesicles to the intraneural cytoskeletal framework which is largely composed of actin and microtubules, thus hindering the vesicle's ability to fuse or dock with recognition proteins at the active zones.[93,94]

There are six types of VGCCs in mammalian systems (L, N, P, Q, R, T) distinguished by their pharmacological and biophysical properties. The predominant channel in mammalian NMJs is the P/Q channel. The P/Q channel is composed of a pore-forming α_{1a} subunit as well as $\alpha 2\delta$, γ, and β_{4a} subunits. The VGCCs are normally closed by neural repolarization promoted by the opening of presynaptic voltage-gated potassium channels. Failure of these channels to close promptly results in prolonged depolarization, and certain disorders of neuromuscular hyperactivity described in Chapter 10.

In normal individuals, these P/Q-type VGCCs are present on both the granule and Purkinje cells of the cerebellum and in presynaptic motor nerve terminals. They exist as well on small-cell carcinoma cells, providing a logical substrate for an autoimmune, paraneoplastic mechanism. In support of this, autoantibodies reacting with the P/Q-type VGCCs are found in 90% of patients with LEMS.

Autoantibody binding appears to specify the α_{1a} subunit. As a consequence, there appears to be a downregulation in the number of calcium channels, resulting in a decrease in total current flow without a reduction of current flow in individual channels.[96] Complement does not appear to be involved in this process. The nerve terminal maintains a grossly normal appearance without evidence of lytic destruction.[88] A causative role for these autoantibodies is supported by the induction of all of the electrophysiological, morphological, and clinical manifestation of LEMS by passive transfer of IgG from patients with paraneoplastic and nonparaneoplastic LEMS to animals, or from mother to fetus.[24,96,97] In addition, similar results utilizing the serum of seronegative patients supports an autoimmune mechanism in this group as well. The trigger for this autoimmune response is unknown. In patients with cancer, it is speculated that molecular mimicry results in the presynaptic motor nerve terminal becoming the innocent bystander in an immune response initially directed at the neoplasm.[90,91,98] As LEMS occurs in only a small proportion of patients harboring SCLC, a genetic predisposition is hypothesized.[99] Sixty-five percent of LEMS patients have the HLA haplotype HLA-B8-DR3, lending some support for this hypothesis although its prevalence appears greatest in the younger, non-neoplastic cohort.[2]

TREATMENT

Identification and treatment of an underlying neoplasm, if present, is the foundation of LEMS treatment. If the tumor can be successfully treated, the morbidity of LEMS can be substantially reduced in a number of patients with concomitant improvement in their electrophysiological studies.[48,98–102] If the patient remains symptomatic, with or without successful tumor treatment, adjuvant treatment with drugs that either enhance neuromuscular transmission or address autoimmunity can be utilized.[2,9,29,103–105] Like myasthenia, the treatment regimen should be individually tailored in consideration with disease severity and the degree to which it affects a patient's lifestyle, as well as numerous other contextual features including cost, availability, and relevant comorbidities. Like MG, avoidance of drugs with known neuromuscular blocking properties is recommended.

Pharmacological treatment for LEMS is largely based on clinical experience.[103] As of this writing, only 3,4 diaminopyridine (3,4 DAP) and intravenous immunoglobulin (IVIG) have been systematically studied.[107]

Anticholinesterase medications can be used in a manner identical to patients with MG.[6,48,49,57,106] Analogous to MG, pyridostigmine provides symptomatic treatment without addressing the root cause of the disease. Electrophysiologically, its application may result in a 50–100% increase in the baseline CMAP amplitude. In our experience, the drug is effective although the response is often modest, and probably insufficient by itself in controlling the morbidity of the disease.

Guanidine, a drug that is believed to prolong the motor nerve action potential and augment quantal content, was used historically in LEMS treatment.[48,52,59,107,108] A small open-label trial demonstrated that both strength and CMAP amplitude are improved in all patients tested. Unfortunately, gastrointestinal side effects and the serious risk of renal failure and bone marrow suppression have made it largely a drug of historical interest.

The aminopyridines are a class of drugs that block voltage-dependent potassium channel conductance. 3,4 DAP is the drug of choice, when available, for the symptomatic treatment of LEMS.[2,48,103,106,109–112] It may be used in addition to pyridostigmine. Four prospective, randomized placebo-controlled trial of 3,4 DAP in LEMS patients (paraneoplastic and nonparaneoplastic) have identified improvements in multiple outcome measures including strength, quantitative myasthenic scales, and CMAP amplitudes.[106,110,113] Our practice is to start cautiously with a dose of 10 mg t.i.d. The medication is generally well tolerated, with a few patients experiencing perioral and acral paresthesias. It is recommended that doses should not exceed 100 mg/day, as higher doses may result in seizures although its blood–brain barrier penetration is less than other aminopyridines.[2,110] Cardiac conduction defects, particularly prolonged QT intervals are an additional concern and warrant EKG screening both before and during treatment. Like others, we have had no adverse cardiac experiences.[2] In our experience, although beneficial, 3,4 DAP rarely restores either strength or stamina fully. It is not FDA approved and its availability is limited in the United States. It is available on a compassionate use basis through Jacobus Pharmaceuticals. Clinical trials for LEMS patients with both 3,4 DAP and an alternative formulation amifampridine are available (www.clinicaltrials.gov). The drug may also be acquired through compounding pharmacists.

An alternative pharmacological approach is attempted immunomodulation with drug treatment, plasma exchange, or intravenous immunoglobulin.[2,29,48,103,109,114–119] A single crossover trial of IVIg demonstrated a benefit in strength and a decline in VGCC autoantibody titres but failed to demonstrate a statistically significant improvement in CMAP amplitudes.[116] Plasma exchange has been reported to have a clinical and electrical benefit in LEMS but has never been subjected to a prospective clinical trial.[117–119] Improvements in CMAP amplitudes at rest, following exercise, or in response to high rates of repetitive stimulation following plasmapheresis may be seen.[117–119] The peak response is observed by about 2 weeks after the treatment, with a diminution in effectiveness by the end of 3–4 weeks. There are no controlled trials in LEMS of any of the commonly used immunomodulating agents. The most common regimen used in LEMS is probably a combination of prednisone and azathioprine which has been shown to induce clinical remission in some patients.[104,116] It may improve CMAP amplitudes as well as patient strength and stamina. Case reports have suggested a benefit from rituximab.[120,121]

One theoretical concern with LEMS or any other paraneoplastic neuromuscular disorder is the potential risk that suppressing the patient's immune system will have adverse effects on tumor control. One hypothesis as to why LEMS often precedes tumor detection is that the same immune response that produces LEMS simultaneously limits tumor growth. Limited data suggests that immunomodulation can be utilized in LEMS without an adverse effect on tumor control.[98]

► CONGENITAL MYASTHENIC SYNDROMES

CLINICAL FEATURES

The CMS may be conceptualized as inherited DNMT that typically, but not universally, become evident at birth, in infancy, or in childhood. Juvenile and adult-onset cases do occur and are characteristic of specific genotypes (Tables 26-2 and 26-3).[122–128] It is not uncommon for early-onset cases to go undiagnosed until later life, often misdiagnosed as seronegative myasthenia, myopathy, or spinal muscular atrophy. CMS are rare or at least uncommonly recognized conditions that are caused by specific protein deficiencies whose normal functions are requisite to successful neuromuscular transmission at presynaptic, synaptic, and/or postsynaptic locations. The majority of CMS are related to proteins unique to the NMJ resulting in a purely neuromuscular syndrome. A few of the CMS are related to proteins affecting other organ systems including cardiac and smooth muscle, skin, and kidney.[128,129] Rarely, there may be CNS involvement with microcephaly, seizures ocular, and auditory abnormalities.[128] Connective tissue involvement with skeletal deformities or contractures occur in some cases most notably in rapsyn deficiency, AChR γ deficiency (Escobar syndrome) and some of the more recently described, later-onset, limb-girdle syndromes associated with abnormal glycosylation.[125,130–138]

The prevalence of genetically identifiable CMS is estimated at 3.8×10^6.[131] Currently there are at least 18 recognized CMS and 17 recognized genotypes that are characteristically categorized by the primary anatomic region of the NMJ that is adversely affected and the identity of the mutated protein (Table 26-1).[139] Of these genotypes, the most commonly occurring are postsynaptic with deficiencies of the ε subunit of the AChR, downstream of tyrosine kinase (Dok-7), and rapsyn deficiency constituting up to 75% of identifiable cases.[126]

▶ TABLE 26-2. **CONGENITAL MYASTHENIC SYNDROMES**

CMS Subtype	Gene/Protein Deficiency	Clinical Features	Electrophysiological Features	Response to AChE Inhibitors	Treatment
Presynaptic disorder					
CMS with paucity of ACh release	ChAT	AR; early onset; respiratory failure at birth; episodic apnea; improvement with age	Decremental response with RNS	Improve	AChE inhibitors; 3,4 DAP
Synaptic disorder					
AChE deficiency	COLQ	AR; early onset; variable severity; axial weakness with scoliosis; apnea; ±EOM involvement, slow or absent pupillary responses	Afterdischarges on nerve stimulation and decrement with RNS	Worsen	Albuterol; ephedrine; 3,4 DAP; avoid AChE inhibitors
Postsynaptic disorders involving AChR deficiency or kinetics					
Primary AChR deficiency	AChR subunit genes	AR; early onset; variable severity; fatigue; typical MG features	Decremental response with RNS	Improve	AChE inhibitors; 3,4 DAP
AChR kinetic disorder: slow channel syndrome	AchR subunit genes	AD; onset childhood to early adult; weak forearm extensors and neck; respiratory weakness; variable severity	Afterdischarges on nerve stimulation and decrement with RNS	Worsen	Fluoxetine and Quinidine; avoid AChE inhibitors
AChR kinetic disorder: fast channel syndrome	AchR subunit genes	AR; onset early; mild to severe; ptosis, EOM involvement; weakness and fatigue	Decremental response with RNS	Improve	AChE inhibitors; caution with 3,4 DAP
Postsynaptic disorders involving abnormal clustering/function of AChR					
	Dok-7	AR; limb-girdle weakness with ptosis but no EOM involvement	Decremental response with RNS	Variable	Albuterol; ephedrine; may worsen with AChE inhibitors
	Rapsyn	AR; early onset with hypotonia, respiratory failure, and arthrogryposis at birth to early adult onset resembling MG	Decremental response with RNS	Variable	Albuterol
	Agrin	AR; limb-girdle or distal weakness; apnea	Decremental response with RNS	Variable	Albuterol; may worsen with AChE inhibitors
	MuSK	AR; congenital or childhood onset of ptosis, EOM land progressive limb-girdle weakness	Decremental response with RNS	Variable	Variable response to AChE inhibitors and 3,4, DAP; positive response to albuterol
	LPR4	AR; congenital onset with hypotonia; ventilatory failure; mild ptosis and EOM weakness, proximal weakness	Decremental response with RNS	Worsen	Worsen with AChE inhibitors
Other postsynaptic disorders					
Limb-girdle CMS with tubular aggregates	GFPT1; DPAGT1; ALG2; ALG14	AR; limb-girdle weakness usually without ptosis or EOM weakness; onset in infancy or early adult	Decremental response with RNS	Variable	Albuterol; ephedrine; variable response to AChE inhibitors and 3,4, DAP; albuterol
Congenital muscular dystrophy with myasthenia	Plectin	AR; infantile or childhood onset of generalized weakness including ptosis and EOM; epidermolysis bullosa simplex; elevated CK	Decremental response with RNS	Variable	No response to AChE and 3,4 DAP

AD, autosomal dominant; AR, autosomal recessive; CHAT, choline acetyl transferase; CMS, congenital myasthenic syndrome; COLQ, collaganic tail of endplate acetylcholinesterase; Dok7, downstream of tyrosine kinase 7; DPAGT1, UDP-N-acetylglucosamine-dolichyl-phosphate N-acetylglucosamine phosphotransferase; GFPT1, glutamine-fructose-6-phosphate amidotransferase 1; LRP4, lipoprotein receptor-related protein 4; MuSK, muscle-specific kinase; RNS, repetitive nerve stimulation; 3,4 DAP, 3,4-diaminopyridine.

TABLE 26-3. DIAGNOSTIC CLUES USED TO IDENTIFY AND CLASSIFY CONGENITAL MYASTHENIC SYNDROMES

General clues (relative, not absolute)

- Early onset (inutero, neonatal, or infantile)
- Consanguinity, affected relatives suggesting an AR pedigree
- Seronegativity for autoimmune MG
- Refractoriness to cholinesterase inhibitors
- Failure to respond to immunomodulating agents
- Nonspecific light microscopic changes in muscle (if performed)

Epidemiology

- **Ethnicity**
  - German, Western/Central Europe
    - Dok-7, Rapsyn deficiencies
  - Brazil, Portugal, Spain, Tunisia, Algeria
    - AChR ε deficiency—CHRNE
  - Near-Eastern Jewish
    - Rapsyn deficiency
- **Age of onset**
  - Severe, lethal, akinetic syndrome
    - AChR γ deficiency
    - AChR α, β, δ subunit deficiencies
    - Rapsyn deficiency
    - Dok-7 deficiency
  - Typical onset—birth or infancy
    - ChAT deficiency
    - AChE deficiency
    - AChR subunit deficiencies
    - AChR deficiency with kinetic defect—fast channel syndrome
    - Rapsyn deficiency
    - LRP4
  - Variable including potential late-onset
    - Rapsyn deficiency (some cases)
    - Dok-7 deficiency
    - GFPT1 myasthenia (some cases)
    - DPAGT1 myasthenia
    - AChR (subunit) deficiency with kinetic defect—slow channel syndrome
    - MuSK deficiency
    - ALG2 and ALG14
- **Symptoms worsened by cold**
  - AChE deficiency
- **Periodic exacerbations**
  - Intercurrent infection
    - Rapsyn deficiency
    - ChAT deficiency
    - AChR (subunit) deficiency and fast channel syndrome
  - Pregnancy and menstruation
    - Dok-7
    - MuSK deficiency
  - Indeterminate reasons
    - DPAGT1 MG
- **Dominant inheritance**
  - AChR deficiency—kinetic disorder—slow channel

Electrophysiology

- **Afterdischarges**
  - AChE deficiency (not universal)
  - AChR deficiency—kinetic disorder—slow channel
  - Agrin deficiency
- **CMAP incremental response**
  - Congenital LEMS
- **Decremental response to repetitive stimulation at 2–5 Hz**
  - AChR (subunit) deficiency
  - Dok-7
  - ChAT deficiency (some cases)
  - AChE deficiency
  - Congenital LEMS
  - DPAGT1 CMS
  - GFPT1 CMS
  - ALG2/ALG14 CMS
  - LRP4 CMS
- **CMAP decremental response to variable rates**
  - ChAT deficiency (10 Hz RS for 5 min)

Muscle histology

- **End plate myopathy**
  - AChR deficiency—kinetic disorder—slow channel
  - AChE deficiency
- **Tubular aggregates**
  - GFPT1 CMS
  - DPAGT1 CMS
  - ALG2/ALG14 CMS

Response to treatment

- **Refractory to or exacerbated by cholinesterase inhibitors**
  - AChE deficiency (COLQ) (relative contraindication)
  - Laminin β2 myasthenia (relative contraindication)
  - AChR (subunit)—kinetic disorder—slow channel syndrome
  - Dok-7 deficiency
  - Agrin deficiency
  - Rapsyn deficiency
  - Plectin
  - LRP4 CMS
- **Responsive to cholinesterase inhibitors**
  - Laminin β2 myasthenia
  - GFPT1 myasthenia
  - DPAGT1 myasthenia
  - ChAT deficiency (variable)
  - AChR (subunit) deficiency or fast channel syndrome (partial)
  - CMS with a paucity of synaptic vesicles
  - MuSK deficiency (partial)
  - Congenital LEMS
- **Refractory to 3,4 DAP**
  - AChE deficiency
  - Congenital LEMS
  - Agrin defect
  - AChR deficiency—kinetic disorder—slow channel
  - AChR deficiency—kinetic disorder—fast channel syndrome (relatively contraindicated)
  - Dok-7 deficiency
- **Responsive to 3,4 DAP**
  - ChAT deficiency (variable)
  - AChR (subunit) deficiency
  - Rapsyn deficiency
  - Agrin deficiency
  - MuSK deficiency (limited)
  - Congenital LEMS
  - GFPT1 myasthenia

TABLE 26-3. (CONTINUED)

- **Responsive to sympathomimetic amines (albuterol, ephedrine, salbutamol)**
  - AChR deficiency—kinetic disorder—slow channel
  - AChE deficiency (some cases)
  - Agrin deficiency
  - MuSK deficiency
  - Dok-7 deficiency (some cases)
  - Laminin β2 myasthenia
  - DPAGT1 MG
- **Responsive to open channel blockers (quinidine, quinine, fluoxetine)**
  - Slow channel syndrome
- **Responsive to guanidine**
  - Congenital LEMS

Phenotype

- **Pattern of weakness**
  - Typical oculobulbar pattern
    - CMS with a paucity of synaptic vesicles
    - ACh receptor deficiency
    - MuSK deficiency
  - Ophthalmoparesis limited or absent
    - AChR deficiency with kinetic defect—slow channel syndrome
    - Dok-7 myasthenia
    - GFPT1 deficiency
    - Rapsyn deficiency
    - ChAT deficiency
    - Congenital LEMS
    - Agrin deficiency
    - ALG2/ALG14 CMS
  - Significant involvement of limb and axial muscles
    - ACh receptor deficiency
    - Dok-7 deficiency
    - GFPT1 MG
    - DPAGT1 MG
    - Rapsyn (some cases)
    - Agrin deficiency (some cases)
    - MuSK deficiency
    - ALG2/ALG14
  - Preferential involvement of distal muscles or distinctive muscle groups
    - Rapsyn (late-onset) (foot drop)
    - AChR deficiency—kinetic disorder—slow channel (cervical muscles, wrist/finger drop)
    - Agrin deficiency
    - GFPT1 myasthenia (scapular winging, foot drop, wrist/finger drop)
    - DPAGT1 MG (foot drop, wrist/finger drop)
  - Stridor/vocal cord paralysis
    - Dok-7 deficiency
  - Infantile hypotonia
    - ChAT deficiency
    - AChR deficiency
    - LRP4
  - Episodic apnea
    - ChAT deficiency
    - Na—channel myasthenia
    - Rapsyn deficiency
    - AChE deficiency
    - Dok-7 deficiency
    - MuSK deficiency
    - GFPT1
- **Contractures or dysmorphic features**
  - Rapsyn deficiency (facial deformities)
  - ACh receptor deficiency (particularly the gamma and fetal γ subunit)
  - GFPT1 myasthenia
  - ALG2/ALG14 CMS
- **Delayed pupillary light reflex**
  - Acetylcholinesterase deficiency
  - Laminin β2 myasthenia
- **Systemic features**
  - Nephrotic syndrome, ocular abnormalities
    - Laminin β2 myasthenia
  - Epidermolysis bullosa simplex
    - Plectin deficiency

CMS are phenotypically heterogeneous, even within the limited manifestations of the neonate and child. This heterogeneity exists both within and between different CMS genotypes.[122,128,130,140] It is attractive to suggest that the more consistent phenotype of autoimmune MG and LEMS is a consequence of what is essentially a singular target in both conditions, the AChR and VGCC, respectively. Conversely, the CMS result from the disordered structure of nerve terminals, individual AChRs, abnormal AChR distribution, or abnormal NMT physiology at either the presynaptic, synaptic, or postsynaptic level.

There are phenotypic manifestations of CMS that serve both to suggest not only a CMS, but also in some cases implicating one or more specific CMS genotypes. These features are outlined in Tables 26-2 and 26-3. As is the case in all DNMT, the CMS phenotype is typically dominated by symptoms attributable to skeletal muscle weakness. Like autoimmune MG, oculobulbar muscles are commonly involved but sparing or limited involvement of oculobulbar musculature may occur. This pattern has been most commonly associated with choline acetyltransferase (ChAT), acetylcholinesterase (AChE, COLQ) rapsyn, agrin, Dok-7, glutamine-fructose-6-phosphate transaminase 1 (GFPT1), dolichyl-phosphate N-acetylglucosamine-phosphotransferase 1 (DPAGT1), ALG2, and ALG deficiencies.[125,128–130,132,133,135–138,140,141]

CMS may become evident in utero with maternal recognition of reduced fetal movement. This phenotype is most commonly associated with AChR γ subunit gene mutations and to a lesser extent with mutations of the α, β, and δ subunits, Dok-7, and rapsyn genes.[125] More commonly, CMS present at birth or at infancy as a "floppy infant" with neonatal hypotonia in combination with a poor suck and weak cry, or with apneic episodes. Stridor, choking spells, and/or ventilatory difficulties are less-specific manifestations that

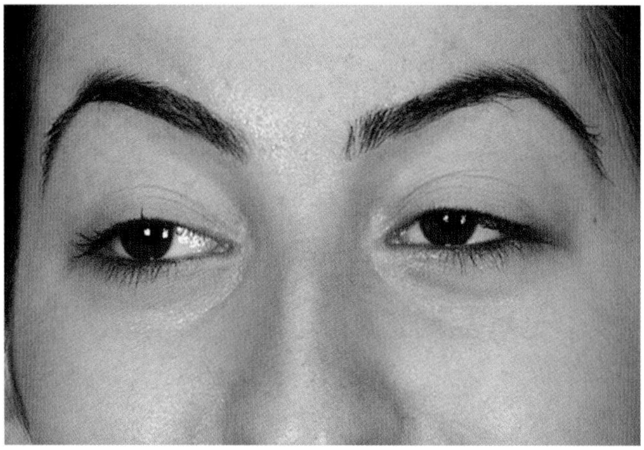

Figure 26-2. Ptosis, compensatory frontalis contraction, and partial ophthalmoparesis in a 15-year-old female with epsilon subunit deficiency. (Used with permission from Prof. Feza Deymeer, University of Istanbul, Istanbul, Turkey.)

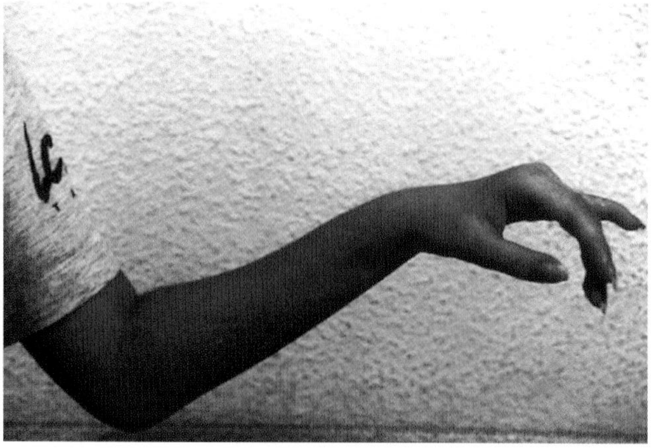

Figure 26-3. Weakness of wrist and finger extension in slow channel syndrome. (Used with permission from Prof. Feza Deymeer, University of Istanbul, Istanbul, Turkey.)

are not uncommon particularly in this period. Contractures are another potential neonatal manifestation and have been reported in rapsyn deficiency (associated with facial deformities), ACh receptor deficiency (particularly the γ and fetal γ subunit), GFPT1, ALG2, and ALG14 deficiencies.[130–133]

When present, ptosis, is typically but not universally symmetric and diurnally variable. Ptosis and opthalmoparesis when present, are helpful clues in distinguishing CMS from other causes of weakness in all age groups (Fig. 26-2).[123] In some patients, particularly in later onset cases, limb-girdle weakness may predominate with relative sparing of oculobulbar musculature. Historically, this was referred to as limb-girdle MG.[142–145] This nomenclature has been supplanted by classification based on genotype as mutations correlating with this phenotype continue to be uncovered. Currently Dok-7, GFPT1, DPAGT1, ALG2, and ALG14 deficiencies are the most frequent causes of this syndrome.[131–138,146]

Prominent scapular winging may be seen in some subtypes. CMS may affect not only proximal upper and lower extremity muscles but also can be associated with foot and finger drop. The latter may affect some digits more than others and suggest an increased likelihood of specific CMS genotypes in the appropriate context (Tables 26-2 and 26-3; Figs. 26-3 and 26-4). Despite NMJ localization, muscle atrophy is not rare in older individuals. In older individuals, limited stamina and prominent fatigue may be the predominant morbidity.

Both diurnal variation and periodic exacerbation of CMS may occur, the latter commonly resulting from fever or intercurrent illness, pregnancy, menstruation, or even stress.[125,126,128] Involvement of other end organs with certain CMS genotypes may produce recognizable syndromes providing an additional source of diagnostic information. Cardiac and smooth muscles are however, uncommonly involved in the majority of syndromes (Tables 26-2 and 26-3).[147] We are unaware of significant dysautonomia occurring in these disorders.

The natural history of CMS is quite variable. Delayed motor milestones are the norm in those affected in infancy. Some individuals have a seemingly static course whereas insidious disease progression is anticipated in two of the syndromes. Only one of the currently recognized syndromes (slow channel syndrome) is typically inherited in a dominant fashion, the remaining disorders being autosomal recessive.[148,149] Recognition of recessive inheritance pattern or parenteral consanguinity are supportive diagnostic clues for CMS although in small or fragmented families, cases may appear to be sporadic.

Because of its infrequency, CMS may not be considered in the differential diagnosis of a weak patient. Predictably this pitfall is more likely to be encountered in older individuals,

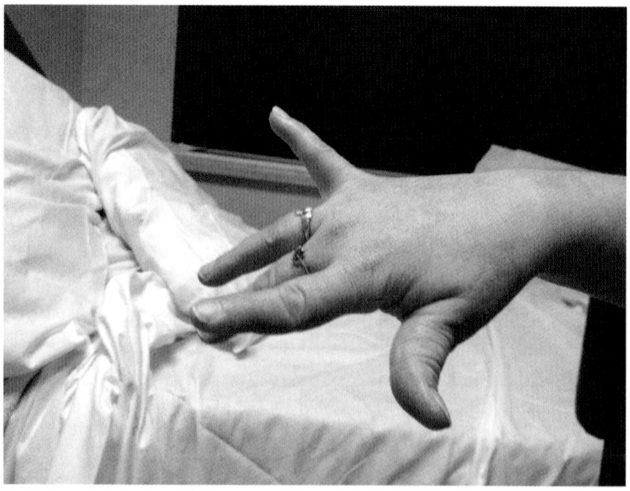

Figure 26-4. Weakness of finger extension in adult female with neonatal dysphagia and apneic episodes attributed to nonspecific myopathy. Became ventilator dependent following scoliosis surgery at age 11, and walked unassisted until age 15. Developed unilateral ptosis in adulthood. Diagnosed with CMS secondary to agrin deficiency at age 43.

particularly in those with a predominantly limb-girdle patterns of weakness. Even in an older individual with a typical MG phenotype, CMS should be given at least brief consideration in any patient with suspected seronegative myasthenia, myopathy of indeterminate cause, or spinal muscular atrophy.[150]

The following summarizes the notable clinical features of specific CMS . Associated genes are listed in parentheses after each disorder heading (Tables 26-2 and 26-3).

Presynaptic (Estimated as 5% of All CMS Cases)

ChAT Deficiency[127,128,151,152,154]

This disorder characteristically manifests as a distinctive phenotype of episodic bulbar weakness with a weak cry and poor sucking capability, and ventilatory distress with potential apnea. Ptosis is common, ophthalmoparesis is rare. The natural history is variable. Apneic episodes may begin in the neonatal period, infancy, or childhood and may be lethal. They may resolve or recur episodically even into adult life. Exacerbations may be triggered by intercurrent infection or other stress.

Paucity of Synaptic Vesicles[125,154,155]

The single reported case of this phenotype described ptosis, ophthalmoparesis, facial weakness, and generalized fatigable weakness of the extremities that began in infancy. The molecular basis of this disorder is unknown.

Congenital Lambert–Eaton Like Myasthenic Syndrome[125,156]

Rare cases of this disorder have been described, predominantly recognized by the characteristic presynaptic EDX pattern described in the diagnostic section. The two described cases involved a severely affected neonate with hypotonia, bulbar weakness, and ventilator dependency and a young child with less-severe manifestations including delayed motor milestones without eye movement or other distinctive abnormalities.

Synaptic CMS (Estimated as 15% of All CMS Cases)

Acetylcholine Esterase Deficiency (COLQ)[127–129,152,157–160]

This the most common cause of synaptic CMS, inherited in a recessive fashion. The natural history is again variable ranging from a typical neonatal disorder with severe morbidity to later-onset, more indolent cases. Early-onset cases tend to be dominated by hypotonia and delayed motor milestones, ventilatory and bulbar difficulties, associated with ptosis and ophthalmoparesis in some but not all cases. Slow pupillary responses to light are reported as a distinctive although not necessarily unique feature of this genotype. In later life, limb weakness, muscle atrophy, and skeletal deformities particularly involving the spine may become apparent. Survival into adulthood is the norm.

Laminin β2 Deficiency (LAMB2)[128,129,151,161]

This is a rare, severe form of CMS. As the β2 chain of laminin is found in other tissues, mutations of the LAMB2 gene may result in Pierson syndrome as well as CMS with associated congenital nephrotic syndrome and ocular defects. The described phenotype includes delayed motor milestones with facial and limb-girdle weakness, with or without ptosis and ophthalmoparesis, pupillary and macular abnormalities, and the potential for ventilatory muscle weakness.

Postsynaptic (Estimated as 80% of CMS Cases)

Agrin Deficiency[128,129,161,162]

Despite the presynaptic site of its synthesis, the major role of agrin is to initiate AChR clustering by binding to lipoprotein receptor-related protein 4 (LRP4) resulting in phosphorylation of muscle-specific kinase (MuSK). Activated MuSK interacts in turn with Dok-7 and rapsyn to promote AChR aggregation. Agrin CMS is a rarely reported, with a mild phenotype characterized by ptosis, delayed motor milestones and mild proximal weakness. We have seen prominent wrist and finger drop when the diagnosis was delayed until adulthood (Fig. 26-5). Ophthalmoparesis is an inconsistent feature. Facial and ventilatory muscle weakness occur in some cases.

Acetylcholine Receptor (AChR) (Subunit Deficiency), with or Without Kinetic Defect [i.e., Slow (Closing) Channel Syndrome or Fast (Closing) Channel Syndrome] (CHRNA1, CHRNB1, CHRND0, and CHRNE)[127,128,148,149,151,152,164]

Subunit mutations are the most common forms of the postsynaptic CMS. The ACh channel typically consists of two α subunits, one β, one δ, and one ε, the latter which normally supplants the fetal γ subunit late in gestation. Adult subunits are encoded by the individual genes listed above. The ε subunit gene (CHRNE) is the most common subunit deficiency and the most common CMS in most series.[126] This mutation

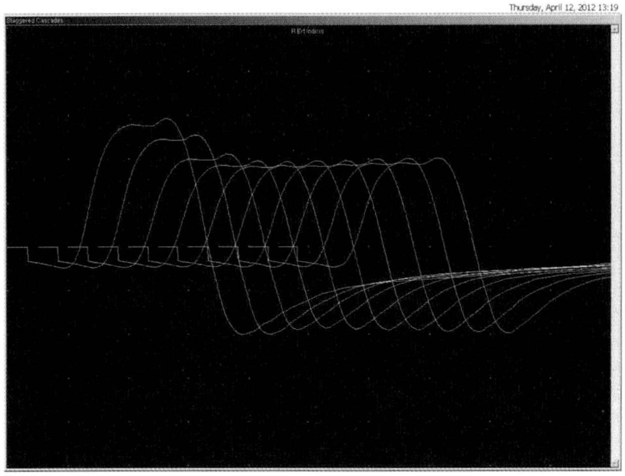

Figure 26-5. Decremental response to repetitive stimulation from extensor indicis proprius leading to diagnosis of CMS.

tends to be more benign than other CMS as the ε subunit deficiency may be buffered to some extent by persistent fetal γ subunit function. This compensatory mechanism is not an option for other subunit mutations. Subunit mutations may adversely affect neuromuscular transmission by at least two mechanisms which may occur individually or concurrently. They may either reduce subunit expression and consequently receptor function and/or alter ACh channel kinetic properties. Kinetic alterations may produce either a slow channel (i.e., slow to close resulting in increased ionic passage) or fast channel (i.e., fast to close resulting in truncation of normal ionic passage from extracellular to intracellular compartments) syndrome. As previously implied, impaired NMT may result from either subunit deficiency and/or abnormal kinetic function and are not mutually exclusive.

The phenotype of AChR subunit mutations is again variable although more likely static than progressive. As described, mutations in the AChR ε subunit gene with reduced subunit expression typically correlates with a mild phenotype. Affected patients tend to have a nonprogressive phenotype typically manifesting as feeding problems and ptosis at birth or in infancy. Ophthalmoparesis is common although may not be present at birth (Fig. 26-2). Limb weakness occurs but ventilatory muscle involvement is rare. In contrast, non-ε AChR subunit gene mutations typically correlate with a more severe phenotype with ventilatory crises precipitated by choking and consequential shortening of life expectancy.

With a kinetic defect producing a slow channel syndrome, the clinical course is typically indolent, often sparing cranial musculature, and frequently affecting cervical muscles as well as wrist/finger extensors (Figs. 26-3 and 26-4). Spinal deformities may develop later in life. The fast channel syndrome tends to arise from the mutations in the α, δ, and ε subunit genes.[166] Neonatal onset is the norm with a severe phenotype incorporating ptosis and ophthalmoparesis, bulbar and ventilatory weakness.

The Escobar syndrome results from mutations in the fetal γ subunit. As the contributions of the fetal subunit are largely dissipated by 33 weeks of gestation, neonates born with γ subunit mutations are typically born with arthrogryposis and ventilatory difficulties and do not develop a typical CMS phenotype.

Acetylcholine Receptor Deficiency—Structural or Organizational

Dok-7 Deficiency[124,128,141,167–171]

This disorder most frequently presents with delayed onset in childhood but may present as late as the third decade. Although infantile onset may occur, normal motor milestones are commonly achieved before deterioration begins. Disease severity is variable, ranging from the mildly to severely symptomatic individuals. A progressive course is the most common. The typical phenotype is a limb-girdle pattern of weakness with the development of ambulatory difficulties during childhood. Ptosis may occur in later life. Ophthalmoparesis is infrequent and typically mild. Facial weakness is common. Significant bulbar symptoms including vocal cord paralysis, stridor, and poor feeding may occur in infancy. Severe disability including ventilatory failure may occur by the third decade in some cases. Worsening during pregnancy has been described.

MuSK Deficiency[128,171–173]

The few reported cases of this disorder describe onset variability ranging from the neonatal period to later life. There is variability in disease severity as well. Ptosis, partial ophthalmoparesis, and mild facial weakness are commonplace. Weakness affecting proximal limbs, particularly shoulder abductors and ventilatory muscles occur in some but not all individuals.

Rapsyn Deficiency[122,123,125,128,130,152]

This is one of the more common CMS, constituting approximately 15–20% of cases. The phenotype including age of onset is variable. Most cases present at birth or at infancy although cases presenting as late as the 20s occur. Neonatal arthrogryposis is common and prognathism and high-arched palate may occur. Crises may be precipitated by intercurrent infection. Ptosis, facial, jaw, and neck weakness are common whereas ophthalmoparesis is rare. Limb weakness is more common in later-onset cases. Although often proximal and symmetric, foot drop in late-onset cases is well recognized. If children survive the neonatal period, improvement with aging is not uncommon.

LPR4 Deficiency[139]

Predictably, a CMS patient with an LPR4 gene mutation has been recently described. The phenotype included hypotonia at birth with ventilatory and feeding difficulties. Motor milestones were delayed. As the child aged, prominent fatigue with proximal greater than distal extremity weakness became evident along with mild ptosis and ophthalmoparesis. A decremental response to repetitive stimulation was identified that responded favorably to edrophonium. Treatment with pyridostigmine however, aggravated weakness.

Sodium Channel CMS[174]

This disorder has been described in a single individual with recurrent apneic episodes and learning difficulties, perhaps related to hypoxic-ischemic injury.

Plectin Deficiency[140]

Plectin is a protein that links different cytoskeletal elements to target organelles in different body tissues. It provides crucial support for the junctional folds of the NMJ. As a result, the phenotype includes the potential for multiorgan involvement including skin [epidermolysis bullosa simplex (EBS)], skeletal muscle (muscular dystrophy), smooth muscle (esophageal atresia), and cardiac muscle (cardiomyopathy). The phenotype typically begins in infancy as EBS and evolves into a disorder producing ptosis and ophthalmoparesis, dysphagia, facial and limb weakness associated with a decremental response to slow repetitive stimulation. Modest CK elevations may occur.

Glutamine-Fructose-6-Phosphate Transaminase 1 Deficiency (GFPT1)[131,135,146]

Like many of the CMS, this genotype has phenotypic heterogeneity. Onset of reported cases range from in utero recognition to 19 years of age. The course is typically slowly progressive. Neonatal cases may be arthrogrypotic, with poor bulbar function and apneic episodes. The most common phenotype is a later-onset syndrome dominated by a proximal > distal pattern of weakness. The distal muscles most commonly involved include forearm extensors, intrinsic hand muscles, and the anterior compartment of the leg. Serum CK values are elevated in 50% of cases.

Dolichyl-Phosphate N-Acetylglucosamine-Phosphotransferase 1 Deficiency (DPAGT1)[132,136,137]

Like GFPT1, DPAGT1 is an enzyme thought to be necessary for the glycosylation of the nicotinic AChR and integral to the assembly and insertion of the channel into the postsynaptic membrane. It shares other features with GFPT1 CMS including a propensity to begin beyond the neonatal period and to produce a limb-girdle pattern of weakness. It does not seem to significantly affect life expectancy and individuals in their sixth decade have been reported. Other features common to GFPT1 and DPAGT1 CMS are tubular aggregates on muscle biopsy, decremental responses to slow repetitive stimulation and responsiveness to cholinesterase inhibitors, and 3,4 DAP. Unlike GFPT1 CMS, CK values are reported to be normal. Consistent with DPAGT1's role in glycosylation in locations other than the NMJ, mutations of this gene may also produce a severe, neonatal multisystem disorder referred to as type 2 that may include seizures, microcephaly, ventilatory distress, hypotonia, and behavioral abnormalities. The determination of phenotype appears to be based on mutation location.

ALG2 and ALG14 CMS[133,138]

Asparagine-related glycosylation plays a critical role in protein folding, transport, localization, and folding. Recessively inherited mutations in these two genes that contribute to this process have been recently reported to result in CMS that bear many similarities to DPAGT1 and GFPT1 CMS. Most affected individuals reported to date have had a limb-girdle phenotype affecting limb muscles preferentially, typically symmetrically with proximal predominance. Scapular winging may occur, contractures are commonplace and a high-arched palate has been described. Facial weakness may occur but extraocular muscle involvement is not a typical feature of the disease. Learning disability may occur. Onset age may range from infancy with hypotonia to adulthood although initial symptoms in the late first decade would seem to be the norm. Wheelchair dependency may or may not occur. A decremental response to slow repetitive stimulation and responsiveness to cholinesterase inhibitors are the norm. Tubular aggregates may be found on muscle biopsy. CK is usually normal but may be minimally elevated.

DIAGNOSIS AND DIFFERENTIAL DIAGNOSIS

The differential diagnosis of CMS in the neonatal period is largely that of the floppy infant (Table 1-1). In the presence of ptosis and ophthalmoparesis, particular consideration should be given to transient neonatal autoimmune MG, certain congenital myopathies, mitochondrial myopathy, and myotonic muscular dystrophy (Table 1-8). Later in infancy, infantile botulism should be considered, particularly with an acute to subacute onset, and symptoms of cholinergic dysautonomia such as sluggish pupils and constipation. In childhood, autoimmune MG and rarely autoimmune LEMS require consideration. When the phenotype is dominated by a limb-girdle pattern of weakness, numerous myopathies and spinal muscular atrophy are the primary considerations. The latter may be suspected by the presence of fasciculations, tremor, or a neurogenic pattern with EDX, or if necessary, muscle biopsy.

Routine laboratory testing is of limited value in CMS. Serum CK levels are of little value in that they are characteristically normal or modestly elevated similar to other neuromuscular disorders with which CMS might be confused.[124] CK testing may be helpful in distinguishing two similar phenotypes DPAGT1 and GFPT1 CMS as it is elevated in approximately half of the latter patients but is normal in all reported cases of the former to date.[134] These two disorders as well as deficiencies in ALG2 and ALG14 may also be distinguished from all other CMS as they are the only CMS reported to demonstrate tubular aggregates with light microscopy and oxidative staining of a muscle biopsy specimen.[132,133,138]

The diagnosis of CMS, if clinically suspected, is further supported by the combination of abnormal EDX testing results and edrophonium testing when present, coupled with the absence of serological markers of autoimmune MG and LEMS. Edrophonium testing is positive in most CMS including the presynaptic disorders, AChR deficiency, and the fast-channel syndromes. End plate AChE deficiency, occasional cases of the slow-channel syndrome, and Dok-7 syndromes are notable exceptions.

At times, identification of motor unit variability, after discharges with routine motor conductions, or a decremental response to slow repetitive stimulation may lead to an unanticipated discovery of a CMS. None of these EDX findings are however, adequately sensitive or specific to allow for a definitive CMS diagnosis in many cases. Afterdischarges are typically identified in only three forms of CMS: AChE, agrin, and AChR receptor (associated with the slow-channel syndrome) deficiency. In all three, the afterdischarges represent prolonged postsynaptic depolarization. Afterdischarges may also occur with neuromyotonia, envenomation with K^+ channel poisons, intoxication with organophosphate or other anticholinesterase agents, and certain muscle channelopathies.

As described below and summarized in Tables 26-2 and 26-3, not all CMS may be identified by abnormal EDX testing. Repetitive stimulation at various frequencies and stimulated SFEMG are the most frequently used techniques in the pediatric age group. Caution in interpretation is required however, as there is limited normative data in infancy.[175] It would appear that in a full-term normal newborn, no decremental response to slow repetitive stimulation is demonstrable in spite of what may be an immature NMJ. A decrement in response to frequencies of 5 Hz or more has been reported in normal newborns so that techniques that utilize higher stimulation frequencies including stimulated SFEMG must be interpreted with caution.[175]

Decremental responses to repetitive stimulation have been described in all forms of CMS although certain forms (ChAT deficiency) require prolonged stimulation at higher rates (10 Hz) in order to provoke the decrement (Fig. 26-5).[126,128,131,133,138,139] As with autoimmune MG, a decremental response in these syndromes is expected in any clinically weak muscle and in some but not necessarily all clinically unaffected muscles. Standard repetitive nerve stimulation (RNS) protocols may have to be modified in order to identify abnormal NMT in some syndromes. The decrement in AChE deficiency and the slow-channel syndrome typically becomes greater with faster rates of stimulation.[126] In ChAT deficiency, 10-Hz RNS for 5 minutes may be required to identify a decremental response.[125,127,152] A small increment in response to fast repetitive stimulation has been reported in ChAT deficiency as well.[127] Like acquired, autoimmune LEMS, the Lambert–Eaton form of CMS is characterized by a low baseline CMAP and an incremental response of up to 2000% with 20–50-Hz repetitive stimulation.[156]

MUAPs that are polyphasic and smaller in both amplitude and duration may occur in CMS as a result of at least two mechanisms. Neuromuscular blockade at individual NMJs may reduce the number of single fiber action potentials that contribute to the normal MUAP size and configuration. In addition, in AChE deficiency and the slow-channel syndrome, an end plate myopathy may develop as a result of excessive end plate stimulation resulting in smaller MUAPs as well.[127]

A definitive diagnosis of CMS remains challenging in most cases. Historically, a CMS diagnosis was arrived at with the confluence of a characteristic phenotype in a young person with negative serological testing for autoimmune MG, EDX evidence of a DNMT, with or without a positive response to cholinesterase inhibitors and when present, a compatible family history. Confirmation was achievable only by a selected group of laboratories capable of ultrastructural analysis of NMJs and in vitro physiological testing of NMT.

Genetic testing now provides at least in principle, a more direct and efficient manner in which to not only confirm a CMS diagnosis but also to identify the genotype as well. To date, 18 CMS genotypes have been identified.[139] Genetic testing in CMS however, is fraught with a number of limitations including availability and cost considerations.[125] Identification of pathogenic mutations from benign polymorphisms is not always easy. Mutational analysis is also incapable of defining a kinetic defect in association with an identified subunit mutation. Kinetic defects, important in therapeutic decision making, are identified only with the use of in vitro microelectrode or single-channel patch clamp recordings.[166] It is estimated that successful genotyping can occur in half to as many as 90% of CMS cases.[126,127,176] If genotyping is an available option, test selection should be judicious. Considerations should be directed by the phenotypic and epidemiological clues provided in Tables 26-2 and 26-3 as well as by genotype frequency.

HISTOPATHOLOGY

Light microscopic examination of muscle biopsy is of limited value in CMS but is often performed in consideration of the more likely possibility of myopathy, particularly in older individuals. Perhaps the most specific potential finding would be the presence of tubular aggregates. Although neither sensitive nor specific for CMS, they are a potential finding in limb-girdle phenotypes of CMS including GFPT1, DPAGT1, and ALG2/ALG14.[124,131–133,135–138] Otherwise, light microscopic findings are of limited benefit. In the majority of cases, they neither distinguish CMS from other neuromuscular diseases nor do they aid in the definition of a specific CMS genotype.

A number of nonspecific, largely myopathic findings have been described in muscle biopsy specimens from CMS patients. Type 1 fiber predominance is perhaps the most common of these and has been described in rapsyn, Dok-7, GFPT1, and MuSK CMS.[124,130,141,146,171] Other features described in other CMS including Dok-7, GFPT1, plectin, and MuSK include type 2 fiber atrophy/hypotrophy, isolated myofiber necrosis and regeneration, diminished oxidative stain uptake, ragged red fibers, increased frequency of internal nuclei, fiber splitting, and subsarcolemmal nuclear chains.[124,140,141,146,171] Autophagic vacuoles that may stain with acid phosphatase and may contain glycogen have been described in DPAGT1 and GFPT1 CMS.[131,132] Neurogenic features of small grouped atrophy and target formations have been described.[131,132,146,156]

Ultrastructural abnormalities of the NMJ occur in most CMS.[125] They are not syndrome specific. Simplified junctional folds appear to be the most common abnormality in some but not all end plates in many of the disorders and are frequently associated with reduction in the number of AChRs.[131,140] This finding has been reported in a number of syndromes including the slow-channel AChR kinetic disorder, and the AChE, LAMB2, rapsyn, plectin, MuSK, LRP4, GFPT1, and Dok-7 forms of CMS.[125,130,131,139,140,171] The pattern of simplification of the junctional folds varies however, being focal in synaptic disorders and diffuse in many postsynaptic disorders such as AChR ε subunit or rapsyn deficiency.[129] In the synaptic CMS, that is, LAMB2, agrin, and AChE deficiency, as well as in MuSK CMS, the ultrastructural findings may include reduction of the axon terminal size, partial encasement of the nerve endings by Schwann cells, widening of the primary synaptic cleft, and invasion of the synaptic cleft by the processes of Schwann cells in addition to focal simplification of postsynaptic folds.[129] This observation of abnormal presynaptic morphology in a synaptic disorder reflects that the pathophysiology of individual CMS may extend beyond the primary site of involvement. In Dok-7 myasthenia, myeloid structures may populate the junctional cytoplasm. Nerve terminals ending as growth cones without AChR contact has been described in MuSK CMS.[173]

In AChE deficiency and the slow-channel syndrome, prolonged end plate current produces postsynaptic cationic overloading resulting in an end plate myopathy.[129] The histological features of this are characterized by subsynaptic degenerative abnormalities, autophagic vacuoles, dilated sarcotubular elements, increased lipid droplets, and apoptosis of junctional nuclei occurring as a consequence of postsynaptic cationic overloading. In the presynaptic disorder, CMS with a paucity of synaptic vesicles, electron microscopy demonstrates the feature that defines the condition.[127] Ultrastructural abnormalities do not occur routinely however, in all CMS. In agrin deficiency, congenital LEMS, and the fast-channel kinetic syndrome of AChR deficiency, the postsynaptic regions are reported to be ultrastructurally normal.[152]

PATHOGENESIS

The efficiency of NMT is dependent on numerous interrelated components. Optimal NMT requires adequate synthesis of ACh and its packaging and positioning of the resultant synaptic vesicles at the active zones of the presynaptic terminal. Equally important is adequate quantal content or the number of vesicles released as a result of a nerve action potential and the resultant amplitude and duration of the end plate current that the vesicular–end plate interaction produces. This is in turn dependent on synaptic metabolism of ACh that is neither inadequate nor excessive, as well as the normal positioning, clustering, positioning and kinetics of both the ACh and Na+ channels on the peaks and troughs of the end plate folds, respectively.

CMS result from single-gene mutations resulting in abnormal structure or function in one or more of these components of NMT. In each instance, there is a resulting alteration in end plate current, impaired generation of myofiber action potentials, and as a consequence, reduced strength and stamina of voluntary muscles. With the majority of genotypes, a reduction in end plate current occurs. In two of these disorders however, AChE deficiency and the slow-channel kinetic disorder of the AChR, the current is excessively prolonged.[165] Although adverse pathophysiological events are typically characterized as occurring at a singular presynaptic, synaptic, or postsynaptic region, many of the CMS will have secondary consequences that affect additional NMJ loci.

In ChAT deficiency, impaired resynthesis of ACh compromises NMT by progressively depleting quantal content. This along with miniature end-plate potential (MEPP) and EPP amplitude are normal at rest but decline with repetitive stimulation at 10 Hz for 5 minutes with subsequent gradual recovery.[152] CMS with a paucity of synaptic vesicles is associated with a reduced density of synaptic vesicles at the active zones. The probability of quantal release, that is, proportion of vesicles released/nerve action potential, is normal.[125] Conversely, the LEMS variant of CMS is associated with reduced quantal content with a reduced probability of quantal release.[125] Like its autoimmune counterpart, it is defined by the characteristic EDX pattern of a reduced CMAP amplitude at rest, a decremental response to 2–5 Hz repetitive stimulation and an incremental response to faster rates of repetitive stimulation or exercise. The exact mechanism by which this occurs is not fully understood.[125] No mutations of VGCC-related proteins have been identified to date.[127] A failure to respond to 3,4 DAP suggests that congenital LEMS is not a consequence of disordered calcium channels.[152]

With AChE deficiency, the most common of the synaptic disorders, the absence of AChE prolongs the lifetime of ACh in the synaptic space and as a consequence, the duration of the MEPP and EPP. The duration of the synaptic current outlasts the refractory period of the muscle fiber which overstimulates the postsynaptic region. Neuromuscular transmission is impaired by multiple mechanisms including loss of AChR from the degenerating junctional folds and desensitization from ACh overexposure. In addition, there are presynaptic effects with the small and often Schwann cell–encased nerve terminals associated with reduced quantal release. In addition, the excessive stimulation promotes cationic overloading resulting in an end plate myopathy.

In view of the integral role of laminin as a component of the basal lamina, and the critical role of the basal lamina in the creation and configuration of the motor end plates, LAMB2 deficiency is hypothesized to adversely affect the development of the complex end plate anatomy.[127] LAMB2 deficiency also associates with abnormal nerve terminals that are both small and encased by Schwann cells. Widening of the synaptic space and junctional fold are additional consequences as is the demonstration of decreased MEPP amplitude.[125,152] Agrin is bound to laminin on the synaptic basement membrane with the possibility that agrin deficiency (described below) has a synaptic as well as postsynaptic pathogenesis.[151]

The most common postsynaptic disorders involve mutations of AChR subunits, most commonly ε. Again, mutations may produce a deficiency and/or a kinetic disorder. With receptor deficiency, as the name implies, the AChRs at the NMJ are patchy in distribution and reduced in number with a proportionate reduction in end plate current.[125,165]

The pathophysiology of the AChR mutations resulting in kinetic disorders differs dependent on whether the problem is one of delayed (slow channel) or premature (fast channel) AChR closure subsequent to the generation of an initial muscle fiber action potential. The pathophysiology of the slow-channel syndrome is similar to AChE deficiency including depolarization block and the development of an end plate myopathy from excessive stimulation.[125] The pathophysiology of the fast-channel syndrome includes reduced ACh affinity for the AChR, shortened duration of the EPP and as a consequence, diminished Na^+ activation.[165] AChR density on the postsynaptic fold is normal.[177]

Many of the CMS relate to mutations of genes that produce proteins integral to the proper placement and aggregation of AChRs on which optimal NMT is dependent. Agrin is secreted by the distal motor nerve terminal and binds to LRP4. The LRP4-agrin complex activates MuSK which in turn with Dok-7 stimulates rapsyn to concentrate and anchor AChR at the NMJ.[93,151]

CMS due to LPR4, MuSK, rapsyn, and Dok-7 can all be conceptualized as impairing NMT through impaired AChR clustering. In CMS due to rapsyn deficiency, AChR clustering is impaired, the number of AChRs per end plate reduced, and as a consequence, the amplitude of the MEPPs.[125,130,178] The presumed mechanism of impaired NMT in MuSK CMS is the failure of normal MuSK to bind LPR4 and promote agrin-induced AChR clustering.[125] In CMS related to Dok-7 mutations, there is loss of AChR from degenerating postsynaptic folds.[141] Na+ channels are also reduced in number. Consequently, MEPP and predictably EPP amplitudes are reduced in most but not all patients.[169] There are presynaptic effects as well including encasement of nerve terminals with Schwann cell processes resulting in reduced quantal content in some cases.[125,169] DPAGT1, GFPT1, and ALG2/ALG14 play roles in AChR subunit glycosylation.[131–133,138,179] All have been hypothesized to adversely affect NMT by impeding the normal assembly and transport of AChRs into the postsynaptic membrane resulting in simplified postsynaptic membranes with decreased end plate AChR density.[127,138,180]

Plectin is a versatile protein that links cytoskeletal proteins in different locations explaining its potential multisystem phenotype. One area which is concentrated is the NMJ providing at least an anatomical correlation with the CMS that may associate with plectin gene mutations. The mechanism of impaired NMT is uncertain but is associated with reduced MEPP amplitudes. Morphological changes in muscle may correlate with the limb-girdle dystrophic pattern that occurs in some patients.[125] Na+ channel CMS is a rare disorder that understandably diminishes the end plate current as a result of SCN4 A mutations affecting Nav 1.4 channel function.[125]

TREATMENT

Many of the CMS will respond to pharmacological treatment (Table 26-2). Unfortunately, few if any respond as dramatically as can often be achieved in patients with autoimmune MG. One benefit of accurate CMS genotyping is the ability to choose the appropriate treatment. Specific syndromes are predictably responsive or unresponsive to particular agents. In certain syndromes, for example AChE deficiency and the slow-channel syndrome associated with excessive end plate current, anticholinesterases have adverse effects and are contraindicated.

Cholinesterase inhibitors typically benefit most of the presynaptic CMS , and some of the postsynaptic disorders. Conversely, cholinesterase inhibitors are ineffective or contraindicated in others particularly those in which the end plate is overstimulated, for example, AChE deficiency and the slow-channel syndrome. The reader is referred to Tables 26-2 and 26-3 for the effect of AChE in different CMS. In children, the typical dose for pyridostigmine, which is available in syrup form, is 1 mg/kg given four to six times per day orally with the maximum dose being 7 mg/kg/day.[127]

Similarly, 3,4 DAP may be effective or ineffective. It has been reported to be helpful in ChAT, AChR subunit, rapsyn, agrin, and MuSK deficiencies as well as GFPT1 and DPAGT1 deficiency. Patients with AChE deficiency, both the slow- and fast-channel syndrome, congenital LEMS, and agrin deficiency do not typically respond. Patients with Dok-7 deficiency may benefit in some but not all cases. The recommended dose of 3,4 DAP is up to 1 mg/kg/day in divided doses.

Sympathomimetic amines may be effective in certain CMS, particularly those who are refractory to 3,4 DAP and cholinesterase inhibitors.[180,181] Albuterol employed in divided doses of 4–18 mg/day is commonly utilized.[180] These include the slow-channel syndrome, some cases of AChE, agrin, MuSK, and Dok-7 deficiency and DPAGT1 and LAMB2 CMS. The slow-channel syndrome may respond to open-channel blockers including quinidine, quinine, or fluoxetine.[182]

Like the majority of NM diseases, supportive treatments may be required. Parents with children with CMS associated with episodic ventilatory crises may be instructed how to deliver intramuscular neostigmine at a dose of 0.01–0.04 mg/kg.[127] These households are ideally equipped with apnea and oxygen saturation monitors, and breathing aids such as Ambu bags along with the training necessary for their proper use.[125] In addition, patient counseling to avoid drugs that might further impair neuromuscular transmission is advised (Table 25-3). If anesthesia is required for any purpose, neuromuscular blocking agents should be avoided. Gastrostomy tubes may be required in individual patients.

▶ BOTULISM

The disease we know as botulism was named following an 18th-century outbreak caused by improper preparation of sausage (botolus—Latin). Botulism is a relatively unique disease in consideration with the multiple mechanisms by which it can be acquired and the clinical contexts in which these mechanisms operate. The disease may occur as either an infection or an intoxication. Either the spores (infancy) or preformed toxin (adults) may be inadvertently ingested. The latter often results as a consequence of improperly prepared foods or beverages. The organisms may incubate in wounds that facilitate growth under anaerobic conditions, particularly in the setting of parenteral drug abuse. In view of its potency, botulism represents a feared weapon in the arsenal of bioterrorists.[183,184] Inadvertent toxic effects may also occur as the unintended, iatrogenic consequence of the toxin use as a therapeutic agent.

CLINICAL FEATURES

In an adult, botulism is most commonly acquired as a foodborne illness or through wounds. Foodborne botulism is a rare disease, with fewer than 35 cases reported annually in the United States. Infantile botulism is more prevalent, with 80–100 cases estimated to occur annually in the United States.[185] In Canada, there were 205 foodborne cases reported in a 10-year span for an annual incidence of 0.03×10^5.[186] The commercial preparation of food and the typically adverse conditions for spore formation within the adult GI tract are the primary reasons for this low incidence. Reported cases are often related to unusual regional or cultural food preparation or storage practices. Even in foodborne botulism, most reported cases are sporadic with outbreaks of more than 2–3 people being unusual.[185]

The morbidity of botulism is considerable, 30–67% of patients requiring intubation in different series.[186,187] Mortality rates have dropped considerably from historical estimates and are estimated to be between 3 and 5% in this era of intensive care units and the availability of the heptavalent antitoxin.[185,186] Although uncontrolled, one report described a statistically significant reduction in the length of hospital stay for patients receiving antitoxin.[186] The mortality for infantile botulism is less. With appropriate intensive care and use of the human source antitoxin, the survival rate is estimated at nearly 100%.[185] Although the effects of botulinum toxin are permanent once bound to peripheral nerve terminals, recovery occurs with adequate support, presumably on the basis of growth of new nerve terminals. Typically this recovery is measured in months and may take longer for autonomic than somatic functions. It may be dependent on serotype, type A botulinum toxin having the most protracted effect.[188] Full recovery is estimated to occur in 95% of individuals if adequately supported.[185] Of interest, three children born to women who developed botulism during pregnancy were unaffected by the disease.[186] In addition, children born to women receiving therapeutic botulinum toxin injections have not been reported to develop adverse effects.

Botulism is commonly categorized by one of five different mechanisms of intoxication or infection. The clinical presentation of botulism is similar, regardless of the mechanism of inoculation.[189–192] Foodborne botulism in adults is the classic form, first recognized in 1897, with symptoms typically occurring within 2–72 hours of ingestion of food contaminated with the preformed toxin. The initial symptoms are typically related to impaired GI motility including constipation, emesis, abdominal cramping, and/or diarrhea. Neurological impairment follows in short order. The severity of the illness is thought to be related largely to the amount of toxin ingestion. Signs and symptoms referable to motor functions of cranial nerves are virtually always the initial neurological manifestation. Signs and symptoms of dysautonomia, particularly of cholinergic function soon follow. For purposes of easy recall, the clinical manifestations have been referred to as the "dozen Ds." They include dry mouth, diplopia, dilated pupils, droopy eyelids, droopy face, diminished gag reflex, dysphagia, dysarthria, dysphonia, difficulty lifting the head, descending paralysis, and dyspnea related to diaphragmatic paralysis.

Dysautonomic manifestations may include blurred vision from impaired accommodation, urinary retention, ileus, and postural hypotension. The latter is presumably related to impaired cholinergic release at vasomotor, preganglionic sympathetic neurons. Of potential symptoms, xerostomia, diplopia, and dysphagia are the most frequent and occur in over 90% of reported cases. Dyspnea and ventilatory muscle weakness occur in a large proportion of patients. The need for ventilator support has been reported to occur in 32–81% of patients.[191,192] The duration of required mechanical ventilation is dependent on the severity of the illness and serotype of the infecting organism, with a mean of 58 days for type A and 26 days for type B botulism.[191,192] Careful observation suggests that ventilatory muscle weakness precedes the recognition of limb and trunk weakness. The latter is common, typically occurring in a descending pattern affecting arms before legs, and typically although not always symmetric in distribution.[190] Deep tendon reflexes may be normal or diminished initially, with progression to complete loss in severely affected individuals. The sensorium and sensory system are unaffected unless CO_2 retention from ventilatory muscle weakness ensues.

Infantile botulism was first described in 1976. It is the most common form of botulism in the United States with an incidence that is approximately twice that of foodborne disease. Unlike foodborne disease, it can be conceptualized as infection, not an intoxication as the organisms colonize the vulnerable intestine of the infant. It typically affects children in the first 6 months of life and is strongly related to the use of honey which has been shown to harbor clostridial spores (particularly type B) in up to 25% of products.[190] Only 20% of infantile cases are attributable to honey ingestion however.[185] The clinical manifestations, in consideration of the child's maturational age are understandably more protean than in adults. The severity of the phenotype is variable. Constipation is the usually the first and in some cases the only manifestation. Children typically develop a weak cry, a poor suck and swallowing capabilities. Excessive drooling accompanied by a weak cry is particularly worrisome. Ptosis and "smoothing" of facial expression may be noted. Hypotonia, particularly of the neck, occurs in the more severe cases. Tachycardia and urinary retention are additional dysautonomic manifestations.

Like infantile botulism, wound botulism represents an infection rather than an intoxication. It was first described in 1943 as a consequence of trauma or surgery presumably related to the anaerobic environment created by necrotic tissue. Ironically, in some cases it may have been related to the use of honey which has been applied to wounds to facilitate healing through its bactericidal and hygroscopic properties.[190] Wound botulism is now however most commonly associated with recreational drug use, most commonly subcutaneous injection of black tar heroin but has been reported with subcutaneous injection of cocaine as well.[185,193] This may occur as a result of abscess formation at injection sites which can be quite subtle and appear as no more than a furuncle or small area of cellulitis. As the toxin can penetrate mucous membranes as well disrupted skin, it has been associated with the inhalation of cocaine as well.[190] The clinical manifestations of wound botulism are similar to foodborne botulism with the exception that gastrointestinal complaints are less common. Wound botulism is more likely to affect an individual as opposed to a group as might be anticipated in foodborne disease. The incubation period is longer in wound botulism, typically 4–14 days in comparison to hours for toxin or spore ingestion.

Hidden botulism was first described in 1977 and can be conceptualized as the adult variant of infantile botulism. The acidic milieu of the normal adult gastrointestinal tract is not normally conducive to proliferation of the *Clostridium botulinum* organism once introduced. Adults with abnormal gastrointestinal tracts however, due to surgery, inflammatory bowel disease, antimicrobial use, or achlorhydria may be at risk for bacterial colonization. The diagnosis in these cases is often rendered more challenging as there is no history of the more common forms of contact with either the spores or the toxin, that is, suspicious food ingestion or drug use.[190]

Inadvertent botulism, first described in 1997, refers largely to the unintentional consequences of therapeutic botulinum toxin use. This practice may, in some cases, result in inadvertent weakness of nearby muscles. Systemic effects of local intramuscular injections have been reported as well. These are typically occult and measurable only through SFEMG. Rarely, however, actual botulism has resulted from injection of doses well within therapeutic ranges. An additional inadvertent mechanism of botulism is through aerosolization and inhalation of the toxin, as has been reported in laboratory workers where the organism is stored and studied.[190]

Botulinum toxin as an instrument of terrorists would be most likely delivered as a contaminant of food preparations or in an aerosolized form. As the toxin rapidly denatures with exposure to sunlight or chlorine, contamination of public water supplies would be an unlikely strategy.[183,184]

DIAGNOSIS AND DIFFERENTIAL DIAGNOSIS

Practically speaking, botulism remains a clinical diagnosis. The diagnosis should be strongly suspected with the acute onset of multiple cranial nerve abnormalities confined to the motor domain, particularly when preceded by gastrointestinal symptoms and accompanied by signs and symptoms of dysautonomia, impaired ventilation, and a descending pattern of limb weakness. The Centers for Disease Control (CDC) criteria for foodborne botulism require this phenotype occurring with identification of the toxin or the cultured organism. As identification of the organism or the toxin takes time and is imperfect, a heightened clinical index of suspicion is key. When suspected, it is important to obtain a detailed history of potential exposures early in the course as the opportunity to do so may be quickly lost if intubation is required. Even when the diagnosis is strongly supported or confirmed by ancillary testing, treatment decisions are required prior to the identification of toxin or organism.

Confirmation of foodborne botulism can be achieved by detection of the neurotoxin and identification of its subtype in serum, stool, gastric aspirate, or samples of ingested food. This opportunity dissipates rapidly however as the yield declines to <30% after 2 days. Samples need to be obtained before the administration of antitoxin which nullifies the result of the mouse bioassay.[184] In all other forms of botulism except inadvertent botulism, the focus is on isolating the organism, not the toxin. In infantile or hidden botulism, the intent is to culture *C. botulinum* from fecal material or gastric aspirate/vomitus.[186] The sensitivity of stool cultures is estimated at 60% but declines to 36% after 3 days.[190] The presence of the bacillus is considered de facto evidence of botulism, as they are virtually never found in healthy individuals. In cases of suspected wound botulism, the integument should be carefully searched, not only for gross disruption and wound contamination, but also for minor bruising with or without signs of infection. Culture of these areas should be performed for anaerobic organisms. The nasal mucosa should be visualized and nasal swabs with anaerobic culture media utilized. Diagnostic criteria allow for a definite diagnosis to be made in someone with a characteristic phenotype who is epidemiologically linked to one or more other individuals who have had laboratory confirmation. This may occur in foodborne disease but is essentially nonexistent in wound botulism and other forms of the disease.

The primary differential diagnostic considerations for botulism are acute–subacute disorders that result in multiple cranial nerve deficits.[184] If more than one case were to occur simultaneously, the likelihood of botulism would be significantly increased as most differential diagnostic considerations would be less apt to cluster. An outbreak of carbamate (insecticide) toxicity used on watermelons, although a somewhat different phenotype, represents a notable potential exception.[194] Based on its prevalence alone, stroke is probably the primary emergency room suspicion.[195] To a neurologist, Guillain–Barré syndrome (GBS) variants, tick paralysis, neuropathy related to marine intoxications, and MG are the most likely considerations. This is particularly true in consideration of the motor predominance, the cranial nerve predilection, and the associated dysautonomia that Miller Fisher syndrome and the GBS pharyngeal-cervical-brachial variants may produce.[196] Any acute to subacute cause of cranial and limb weakness including disorders with an affinity for the meninges such as viral infections like polio and West Nile virus, neoplastic meningitis, sarcoidosis, marine intoxications, and Lyme disease should be considered. Many will have sensory rather than motor symptoms and are more likely to affect the limb rather than cranial nerve function. Although characterized by pharyngitis and a swollen neck, the local penetration of the diphtheria exotoxin can produce palatal paralysis, dysphonia, and dysphagia as well as a demyelinating polyneuropathy. The red, painful throat that may accompany the xerostomia of botulism may serve to confound the distinction between the two conditions. CMS would have to be considered in children although the time course should be distinctive from botulism in most cases. LEMS is also a potential consideration given that it produces muscle weakness in concert with a cholinergic dysautonomia. Cranial nerve findings are less prevalent in LEMS and the clinical context is usually different, thus allowing confident distinction from botulism in most cases.

LABORATORY FEATURES

EDX evaluation typically provides strong diagnostic support in the appropriate context.[190,197–201] The pattern is typical of a presynaptic DNMT in many but not all cases. Sensory nerve conduction studies are normal. CMAP amplitudes are frequently reduced in 85% of tested nerves. A decremental response to slow repetitive stimulation (2-5 Hz) and an incremental response to fast repetitive stimulation (10-50 Hz) are frequent but not invariable findings.[190,202] It is generally accepted that rates of 20 Hz or higher have greater diagnostic yields. At times however, either the decremental or incremental response may be elusive. There is a belief that EDX abnormalities in limb muscles including reduced CMAP amplitudes may be less commonly encountered in individuals whose phenotype is restricted to cranial nerve signs and symptoms. Conversely, the inability to convincingly demonstrate an incremental response also appears to correlate with very low amplitude or even absent CMAPs at baseline.[201] In keeping with this, the incremental response when present tends to be of lesser magnitude than identified in LEMS. To distinguish this increment from a physiological increment, it should achieve a maximal amplitude of greater than 40% of baseline. In botulism, the increment is commonly less than 100% as opposed to LEMS in which the diagnostic threshold exceeds 100% of baseline CMAP amplitude in any given muscle.[190] The duration of the increment is brief, often in the 30–60 second range when subsequent, single stimuli are delivered. It is estimated that incremental responses are demonstrable in only 60% of patients.[190] Needle examination findings are often abnormal but not specific. With needle electromyography, low amplitude, short duration, polyphasic MUAPs with increased recruitment, and fibrillation potentials may be demonstrable. Increased jitter values with blocking on SFEMG are to be expected but again indicate only the existence of a neuromuscular transmission abnormality, not the cause.

The diagnosis of botulism is confirmed by the demonstration of toxin or organism in appropriately symptomatic individuals. Currently, the gold standard for the detection of botulinum toxin in foodborne botulism is the mouse bioassay, which is performed by designated BSL-3 containment facilities. It is traditionally used to confirm the presence of toxin in serum, gastric content, stool or the food that the inoculum is thought to originate from. Unfortunately, its sensitivity is insufficient to detect low toxin levels. No more than 45% of patients will test positive, depending on factors such as how rapidly the specimen is obtained and the specific serotype.[185,203] The duration of toxin detection is limited and declines rapidly following exposure. The detection of botulinum toxin type B in the system may be possible for up to 12 days in contrast to type A which is estimated to persist for 4 days or less.[187] In general, specimens obtained more than 7 days postexposure are unlikely to be positive.[185] In addition, availability of assay result requires a minimum of 24 hours and up to 4 days. Newer methodologies utilizing functional dual coating (FDC) and polymerase chain reaction (PCR) technologies promise higher diagnostic yield.[204,205] Specimens obtained for purposes of toxin identification should be refrigerated, not frozen, until they can be shipped to the CDC or limited number of state laboratories equipped to perform the assays.

Stool culture is considered the diagnostic test of choice in infantile and hidden botulism and anaerobic culture of the abscess site in wound botulism. As many patients will be constipated, acquisition of stool with the administration of a sterile water enema may be required. Cultures of nasal swabs may be helpful in rare inhalational cases related to vocational exposures or cocaine use.

Other testing is of limited diagnostic value in suspected botulism. Cerebrospinal fluid (CSF) protein if checked, is universally normal as a potentially distinguishing feature from GBS.[185] Tensilon testing is generally considered to have a limited value in botulism. A positive response is rarely dramatic and occurs in only a quarter of affected individuals.[184,185,206–208] Although of limited diagnostic value, assessment of forced vital capacity or negative inspiratory force are important tools for disease management purposes.

HISTOPATHOLOGY

There is no role for either nerve or muscle biopsy in botulism in most if not all cases. In one autopsied case, the findings in muscle were degenerating muscle fibers and scattered angular atrophic fibers. Sural and peroneal nerves displayed no significant histopathology in this individual.[209]

PATHOGENESIS

Botulinum toxin is an exotoxin produced by the anaerobic, spore-forming bacillus *C. botulinum* in most cases with *C. butyricum* and *C. baratii* reported as being neurotoxigenic in India and China.[185] The toxin exists in seven currently recognized serotypes, designated A to G, that have similar but not identical biological properties. In North America, disease is associated with toxin types A, B, E, and to a lesser extent type F. Type E is the most common strain causing foodborne disease in North America.[185] Botulinum toxicity is substantial, rivaled by few other substances. Parenteral exposure requires a far smaller inoculum than inhalational exposure which is more potent in turn than ingestion.[185]

Foodborne disease has been linked to a long list (often exotic) of food types or food preparation practices that may be both geographically and culturally based.[186,200] One of the more interesting and contemporary forms of foodborne botulism are outbreaks that have occurred in prison populations attributed to the production and ingestion of an illicit fermented beverage known as "pruno."[210] Despite the name, it is likely that the botulinum spores in reported outbreaks of pruno ingestion originated from potato. The *C. botulinum* bacillus reverts to a spore form under stress. Ideal conditions for spore germination include an anaerobic milieu, nonacidic pH, and low salt and sugar content.[185] These conditions are most commonly achieved with inadequate home canning procedures without achievement of adequate duration or degree of temperatures. Outbreaks of foodborne botulism are also reported in cultures that prepare particular foods by allowing them to ferment while avoiding cooking altogether.[185,186] Although spores are susceptible to heat, their elimination requires temperatures (85°C) that may be difficult to attain and maintain at higher altitudes. Outbreaks of foodborne disease appear to be more common with home canning in these regions.[190] Poorly prepared or stored root vegetables such as potatoes or mushrooms appear to be frequent culprits due to their significant soil exposure where the clostridial organisms are ubiquitous.[210] In view of that, it is not surprising that ingestion of botulism spores may occur commonly without causing disease. In adults, either a large inoculum (poorly prepared or stored food) or gut conditions conducive to spore germination (achlorhydria) are required for foodborne botulism to occur. Unlike the spores, the botulinum toxin itself is readily denatured by heat.

Botulinum toxin can be absorbed as an active process by the inhalational route. The toxin does not traverse unbroken skin but is bound to and can be transported across the membranes of epithelial cells including through the nasal mucosa with cocaine inhalation or aerosolization in laboratories or potentially during terrorist acts.[190,211] It can also be introduced through broken skin via inadvertent wounds, or through recreational (heroin) or therapeutic (botox) injections. Once absorbed the toxin migrates to the perineuronal microcompartment in the vicinity of vulnerable cholinergic nerve endings. Only these cells have the ability to selectively accumulate the molecule and do so by receptor-mediated endocytosis and translocator mechanisms.[211] The toxins then interfere with the release of ACh through slightly different mechanisms affecting the SNARE protein complex. They all gain entrance to the presynaptic terminal through endocytosis via synaptic vesicles, a "Trojan horse" effect. There botulinum toxin serotypes A, C, and E target SNAP-25 whereas botulinum toxin B, D, F, and G cleave VAMP/synaptobrevin, the net effect in each case being disruption of quantal release.[188] In vitro electrophysiological studies indicate that there is a significant reduction in the EPP amplitude far below the 7–20 mV necessary to bring the myofiber from its resting membrane potential to action potential threshold. Intuitively, the frequency of MEPPs is reduced, but not MEPP amplitude.[212,213]

TREATMENT

Botulism treatment involves early acquisition of diagnostic specimens and the earliest possible administration of botulinum antitoxin. It is important to have a high diagnostic suspicion of botulism in any case of acute polycranial neuropathy particularly if preceded by gastrointestinal symptoms. Botulism may represent the most important reason to obtain emergent EDX testing. Other than antitoxin administration, intensive care support, when necessary, is the other critical component of successful botulism treatment. Because of potential public health implications, it is recommended that every case of botulism be reported to the state public health department who may also aid the physician in the necessary epidemiological investigation.

Consensus opinion is that heptavalent botulinum antitoxin (HBAT), which only binds to circulating toxin, should be administered expeditiously, prior to availability of any supportive or confirmatory testing results.[195] As of March 2010, HBAT is the only botulinum antitoxin available in the United States for naturally occurring noninfant botulism.[214] It is available only through the CDC. Unlike prior monovalent or bivalent products, it addresses all seven serotypes. Baby botulism immune globulin (BIG) remains available for infant botulism through the California Infant Botulism Treatment and Prevention Program.[214] One observational study reported that the mean length of hospitalization was 5 days shorter in adults for those who received the antitoxin.[185] In infants, it has been reported to reduce the average length of hospitalization from 6 to 3 weeks.[185]

Botulinum toxoid was previously available as an investigational pentavalent (ABCDE) botulinum toxoid vaccine for workers at risk for occupational exposure to botulinum toxins. The CDC discontinued this product as of 2011.[215]

Local measures may be employed with specific botulism mechanisms. In suspected foodborne botulism, gastric lavage, or enemas may be employed if ingestion is recent in an attempt to remove as much unabsorbed toxin from the gastrointestinal tract as possible. With wound botulism, it is recommended that any potential abscess be debrided and cultured with antimicrobials being administered as required to address other potential, concomitant infections.

Pharmacologically, both pyridostigmine, guanidine, and 3,4 DAP have been used in the treatment of botulism.[216] They appear to have limited benefit and have not been recommended for routine use. Avoidance of any drugs with significant NMJ blocking properties is strongly recommended (Table 25-3).

▶ TOXINS/ENVENOMATIONS

There are many environmental intoxications or envenomations whose morbidity results largely from disordered neuromuscular transmission. Many are rare and exotic. This section will review some of the more notable examples. Table 26-1 provides a list of the more well-known NM toxins and attempts to categorize them by their presumed site of action as pre-, post-, or synaptic disorders.

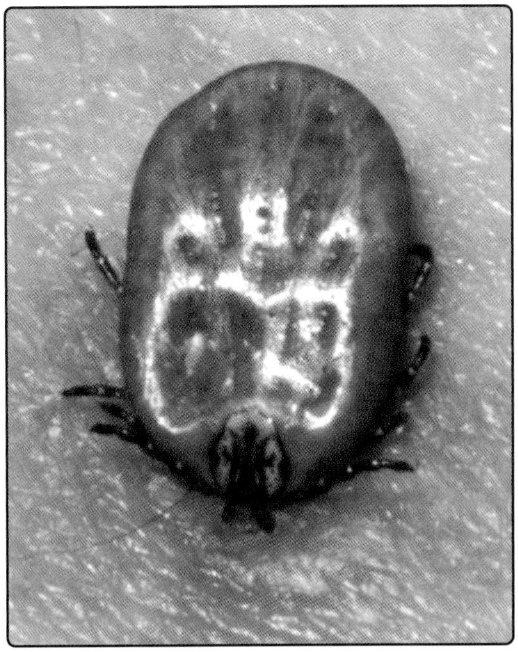

Figure 26-6. *Dermacentor variabilis* feeding. The tick has been attached for 24 hours. (Reproduced from Goldsmith LA, Katz SI, Gilchrest BA, Paller AS, Leffell DJ, Wolff K. *Fitzpatrick's Dermatology in General Medicine*. 8th ed. New York, NY: McGraw-Hill; 2012.)

TICK PARALYSIS

Tick paralysis is a caused by exposure to the saliva of the Ixodid (hard shelled) tick family. Its history is colorful and entertaining.[217] The first presumed cases were reported in southeastern Australia in 1824.[217,218] It is a disease that affects multiple animal species including dogs, cats, and cattle in addition to humans.[217] In Australia, its prevalence in domestic animals makes it a disease of considerable economic consequence.[217] Of the two major endemic regions in North America, Dermacentor andersoni (Rocky Mountain wood tick) is the most common vector in the Pacific Northwest and Canada. Dermacentor variabilis (dog tick) is the predominant vector in the Southeastern United States where the disease is less frequently identified (Fig. 26-6). Other less common vectors include Amblyomma americanum and maculatum, and Ixodes scapularis and pacificus in the United States, and *Ixodes holocyclus*, the major vector in Australia.[219] Like botulism, tick paralysis usually presents as isolated cases but may present with clusters as well.[219] Tick paralysis is believed to be a DNMT in which the predominant effect of the toxin is to impair the presynaptic release of ACh.[220,221]

Clinical Features

The phenotype of tick paralysis is strikingly similar to GBS. As the time of the tick attachment is often uncertain, the time between tick attachment and symptom onset is usually imprecise but is estimated at a mean of 5 days although experiments in sheep suggest that feeding for a week by a gravid female tick is typical.[217,219] Once the patient becomes symptomatic, the disorder moves rapidly with the nadir occurring on an average of 1.5 days after initial symptom.[218,219,222–234]

Once the tick is identified and removed, full neurological recovery takes place at an average of 1.5 days in North America but is more protracted in Australia where tick paralysis is a more severe disease.[218,219]

Affected individuals, particularly children, characteristically experience a prodrome of irritability, somnolence, myalgias, asthenia, and ataxia.[217] The ataxia may be so prominent in some cases as to be categorized as a cerebellar syndrome. Despite the "flu-like" prodrome, fever is not a part of the illness. Diarrhea may occur but unlike botulism, gastrointestinal symptoms are otherwise limited. Paresthesias or dysesthesia may precede the development of weakness, affecting the hands and feet in keeping with a non–length-dependent neuropathy. They may have a pruritic or burning characteristic although significant pain is uncharacteristic.[217] Despite these complaints, objective sensory loss is mild if evident at all.

Like typical GBS, sensory symptoms are rapidly overshadowed by the evolution of flaccid weakness which ascends, affecting legs before arms, unlike the descending pattern of botulism. This evolution typically occurs over hours to days.[217] Cranial nerve and autonomic function are typically impaired subsequent to the development of limb weakness. Bulbar involvement including hoarseness, dysphagia, and sialorrhea occur as does bifacial weakness.[218] Both internal (mid-position, unreactive pupils) and external ophthalmoparesis including ptosis occur, particularly in the more severe Australian form of the disease.[218] Ventilatory muscle weakness with the need for assisted mechanical ventilation is estimated to occur in 10% of patients.[219] Patients are typically areflexic, but like GBS, this may not be the case initially.[217,218,235] The mortality of tick paralysis has been reported at between 6 and 11% but the majority of these cases seem to have occurred in the pre-ICU era.[219]

As previously mentioned, tick paralysis in Australia appears to be a more severe disease.[217,218,236] An atypical pattern of focal weakness, mimicking Bell palsy or a brachial plexopathy has been reported in Australian but not North American cases.[217,237] Pupillary involvement occurs commonly in Australian cases but is rare in North Americans and should prompt consideration of botulism or Miller Fisher syndrome.[217] Hypertension is a common manifestation of tick paralysis in Australia but not in North America. Worsening paralysis may continue following removal of the *I. holocyclus* tick for up to 48 hours whereas continued progression following tick removal is unusual in the United States where dramatic improvement within hours may occur.[235] Prolonged need for mechanical ventilation for a week or more is not uncommon in Australia but uncharacteristic in the United States.[218]

Diagnosis and Differential Diagnosis

Tick paralysis may be unique in that the mechanisms for the diagnosis and treatment are for all intents and purposes identical, that is, identification and removal of the tick. The definitive diagnosis involves simply clinical improvement of the characteristic syndrome temporally related to tick removal. In that spirit, the key to diagnosis is a heightened index of suspicion for tick paralysis in patients with apparent GBS, particularly in the spring and summer months, particularly with young girls with a history of outdoor exposure in the endemic areas mentioned above.[219] Unfortunately, the diagnosis may be impeded in some cases as the tick may have completed feeding and detached itself prior to its identification.[217] Like botulism, tick paralysis cases are usually sporadic but may occur in clusters. None of these epidemiological features are absolute however as tick paralysis has been reported in adults in 20% of cases, in nonendemic regions including urban areas, and at attachment sites other than the scalp (particularly behind the ear), the neck, and the groin.[217,219,238]

The major differential diagnostic consideration for tick paralysis is GBS for which tick paralysis is often misdiagnosed.[219] There are relative, but no absolute differences between the two disorders. Tick paralysis tends to evolve more rapidly, has few if any demyelinating features on motor nerve conduction studies, spares sensory nerve action potentials, is less likely to be painful, and is accompanied by a normal CSF profile. Again, in consideration with this sizeable overlap, is imperative that any GBS suspect undergoes a thorough body search particularly of the scalp before the initiation of plasma exchange or IVIg. Other causes of acute motor weakness require consideration as well. These include acute myelopathies such as transverse myelitis, poliomyelitis, and other enteroviral infections, botulism, myasthenia, diphtheria, porphyria, metabolic disturbances such as severe hypokalemia or hypophosphatemia and potentially other intoxications or envenomations discussed in this chapter and other chapters affecting nerve, NMJ, or muscle.

Laboratory Features

Spinal fluid analysis is of potential value in tick paralysis as it is characteristically normal, unlike GBS or many of the other differential diagnostic considerations.[217,218] As CSF protein may be normal in early GBS as well, it is not an absolute discriminator for these two diseases. Although atypical for DNMT, elevated CK has been reported in some cases.[218] Edrophonium is felt to have no effect on the weakness produced by tick paralysis.[217,218,235] Ironically, the greatest value of an EEG in tick paralysis is the possibility that the tick may be identified by EEG technicians during scalp electrode placement.[235]

The major EDX finding in tick paralysis is a reduction in CMAP amplitudes with normal SNAPs.[218,223,235,239–243] This nerve conduction pattern is not pathognomonic and is consistent with any presynaptic DNMT, or a disorder of anterior horn cells, ventral roots, or motor nerves. Although minor slowing of motor conduction velocities have been reported in North American cases, they are not of any apparent diagnostic significance.[217] It may become evident however with sequential testing before and after tick removal that distal latencies may be mildly affected by the disease.[235,239] Theoretically, this may reflect disordered neuromuscular transmission time or potentially slowed conduction in terminal nerve twigs. Features suggesting acquired demyelination such as CMAP temporal dispersion or conduction block as occurs commonly in GBS are not generally described.[235,239] We are aware of one report of proximal nerve inexcitability with normal motor conduction parameters on distal stimulation.[237] This has been attributed to sodium channel dysfunction within nerve in a manner similar to certain marine toxins or the acute motor axonal neuropathy form of GBS. Neither repetitive stimulation at either low and high frequency nor exercise either brief or prolonged seem to affect CMAP amplitudes in tick paralysis in contrast to other DNMT.[235,239] Needle electromyographic results are normal other than for one extreme case of a child with more than 50 attached ticks in which fibrillation potentials were identified.[241]

Histopathology

There is no apparent role for muscle or peripheral nerve biopsy.

Pathogenesis

Children, particularly girls, are three times as likely to be afflicted with tick paralysis as are adults.[218,222–224,244] One hypothesis for this discrepancy is that a child's short stature makes their head more accessible to ticks. In addition, long hair in girls is hypothesized to provide a covert location for the protracted feeding necessary to cause disease. The fact that other illnesses transmitted by the same species of tick occur more commonly in males supports this hypothesis.[217] Other considerations potentially relevant to the increased incidence in children is that the toxin load is diluted in a larger adult and that the adult is more likely to find and remove the tick at an earlier stage.[217] On the other hand, adult men are more likely to be affected than women presumptively because of increased exposure to wooded areas.

Tick paralysis, at least that produced by *I. holocyclus*, results from holocyclotoxin that is secreted into the salivary glands of the offending vector.[217] The concentration of toxin has been demonstrated to increase as the tick feeds, explaining in part the latency between tick attachment and symptom onset. North American ticks are presumed to have a slightly different toxin with a similar mechanism of action. In both Northern and Southern hemisphere disease however, the toxin is believed to interfere with the presynaptic release of ACh from presynaptic terminals of NMJs and presumably autonomic neurons as well although pupillary abnormalities are the only common dysautonomic manifestation of the disease.[217,220,221] In addition, there is experimental evidence implicating an additional effect on nerve conduction, hypothetically via sodium channel dysfunction providing a potential explanation for the sensory symptoms or prolonged distal latencies that may accompany the disease.[217,237] Regardless of mechanism, it is unlikely to be associated with any structural injury as electrophysiological recovery can begin within hours of tick removal.[237]

Treatment

Treatment strategies include prevention, supportive care, and tick removal. When outdoors in endemic areas, limiting exposed skin surfaces, utilizing light clothing to improve tick detection, and spraying or impregnating clothing with insect repellants such as those containing pyrethrin/pyrethroid are deterrent strategies.[237] Supportive care is similar to any paralyzing neuromuscular illness including prophylaxis against deep vein thrombosis, skin breakdown, nerve compression, and surveillance for and when necessary treatment of dysautonomia and ventilatory failure.

The most important aspect of care is the identification and removal of the offending tick. The fact that there are historical cases in which the tick was found postmortem emphasizes this point.[230] It is strongly recommended that ticks be removed with slow and steady pressure applied with tweezers placed as close to the skin as possible, to ensure removal of mouth parts.[219] In addition, as individual ticks can harbor multiple different pathogenic organisms, it is important to avoid the expression of further material into the wound by fingertip pressure.[218] Heating or covering the tick with vasoline or similar substances impervious to air is not generally recommended.[217]

A polyclonal antitoxin is available for the treatment of *I. holocyclus*. It is a canine derivative and is associated with a high incidence of adverse allergic responses including serum sickness and anaphylaxis.[217,218] It is only used in severe cases. No antitoxin exists for North American disease not would it be recommended due to the rapid response to tick removal.[217] It also has to be utilized rapidly to provide any benefit. Attempts have been made to develop a vaccine for tick paralysis with some reported success in the laboratory.[236,245] We are unaware however of either the availability or effectiveness of a vaccine for humans.

ACUTE ORGANOPHOSPHATE AND CARBAMATE POISONING

Organophosphates and carbamates are chemicals that respectively irreversibly or reversibly inactivate AChE. They are used as insecticides or as instruments of homicide, suicide, or chemical warfare.[246] Inadvertent exposure occurs, most prevalently in the developing world. The World Health Organization estimates that globally, the majority of the more than 200,000 deaths that occur each year are self-inflicted, a problem particularly prevalent in Sri Lanka.[247–249] Mortality is estimated at 15–30% or more, particularly where intensive care is not readily available.[248]

CLINICAL FEATURES

Organophosphate toxicity produces both an acute and a delayed neurological syndrome with different mechanisms of action and different phenotypes. The neuropathy, referred to as organophosphate-induced delayed polyneuropathy or OPIDP, develops as a delayed response to toxic exposure through a different mechanism unrelated to AChE inhibition. It is discussed in Chapter 20. This section will focus exclusively on the manifestations of acute exposure. Unlike the majority of the disorders in this and the preceding chapter, the effects of acute organophosphate or carbamate exposure enhance rather than impair the effects of ACh at the NMJs and autonomic synapses through irreversible inhibition of AChE although the clinical features often evolve into manifestations of synaptic exhaustion. The phenotype of acute organophosphate toxicity is distinctive from other DNMT for two reasons. One is the initial manifestations of cholinergic excess. The other relates to the ability of organophosphates to cross the blood–brain barrier producing CNS as well as PNS cholinergic disruption.

Acute organophosphate toxicity manifests within 24 hours of exposure, typically less. Some of the more notable symptoms pertain largely to the autonomic manifestations of the disease are referred to by the acronym SLUDGE, standing for salivation, lacrimation, urination, defecation, increased gastrointestinal motility, and emesis.[248,250] One report identified that 75% of affected patients have miotic pupils and CNS symptoms.[251] CNS side effects more commonly occur in organophosphates than in carbamates which have less-effective CNS penetration. CNS manifestations may include agitated delirium and potentially coma, with or without seizures. Two-thirds of patients in the aforementioned series of 47 patients were noted to have hypersalivation and roughly half-experienced agitation and muscle fasciculations.[251] Other muscarinic symptoms include bronchospasm, bronchorrhea, and bradycardia. Both hypotension and hypertension may occur, attributed to overstimulation of muscarinic parasympathetic and nicotinic sympathetic neurons, respectively.[248] Diaphoresis may occur as well. Muscarinic symptoms may dissipate with the development of large pupils in some cases presumably due to cholinergic bombardment and postsynaptic exhaustion in a manner similar to succinylcholine effect. Muscle weakness is presumably related to the same mechanism.

In addition to paresis of limbs, ophthalmoparesis and ventilatory muscles that may require mechanical ventilation and intensive care may occur.[252] In one study, approximately 20% of intoxicants required mechanical ventilation.[251] Death most commonly results from respiratory or ventilatory failure that may stem from a combination of excessive pulmonary secretions, diaphragmatic or intercostal muscle weakness, or most commonly from impaired CNS ventilatory drive.[248,250] The term "intermediate syndrome" has been coined to describe ventilatory failure that may suddenly occur from diaphragmatic and intercostal muscle weakness after the patient has been treated and stabilized relating to the initial symptoms of muscarinic excess.[248] Assessing the patient's ability to lift their head off the bed has been suggested as a means of indirectly monitoring the development of ventilatory muscle weakness.[248]

DIAGNOSIS AND DIFFERENTIAL DIAGNOSIS

The diagnosis of organophosphate toxicity is typically based on clinical suspicion, generated by the recognition of characteristic clinical signs, smell of pesticides or solvents, and supported by characteristic EDX features and reduced butyrylcholinesterase or AChE activity in the blood.[248] The initial clinical picture commonly includes miotic pupils, excessive sweating, and altered level of consciousness and hypoventilation.[248]

The major differential diagnosis of organophosphate toxicity is carbamate toxicity.[248,253] Any acute disorder producing signs and symptoms of both muscle weakness and dysautonomia such as GBS, botulism, tick paralysis, and other phenotypically similar intoxications/envenomations should be considered.

LABORATORY FEATURES

Unlike presynaptic disorders of NMT, CMAP amplitudes at rest are typically normal in acute organophosphate poisoning.[252] Repetitive stimulation at both low and high frequencies result in a decremental response.[252] Like two forms of CMS, the slow-channel syndrome and AChE deficiency, nerve conduction studies in organophosphate toxicity are distinctive from most DNMT in that afterdischarges of CMAPs occur in response to a single supramaximal stimulus (Fig. 2-4) and are estimated to occur in 60% of intoxicated individuals.[252] The afterdischarge, like the parent CMAP will decrement with repetitive stimulation.[252]

Inhibition of plasma butyrylcholinesterase, also known as pseudocholinesterase or plasma cholinesterase, aids in determining the existence but not severity of organophosphate effect. A decline in the degree of butyrylcholinesterase inhibition may signify the elimination of organophosphate from the body.[250] As mentioned, AChE exists on red cells as well as at cholinergic synapses. Red cell cholinesterase levels measured in whole blood provide an additional means by which to determine not only organophosphate exposure but the severity of AChE inhibition.[248] The accuracy of both assays is highly dependent on technical considerations, specifically the need to cool the patient's blood immediately after acquisition. Methodology also exists for the detection of organophosphates in air and water samples as well as on the clothing of exposed individuals.

HISTOLOGY

There is no role for nerve or muscle biopsy in acute organophosphate toxicity.

PATHOGENESIS

Organophosphates gain access to the human body through ingestion (usually intentional) or through inhalation or dermal exposure either of which could be accidental or intentional.[246] They adversely affect AChE at synapses and on red cell membranes and additionally inhibit butyrylcholinesterase in plasma. The latter effect appears to have little or no associated morbidity.[248] Organophosphates work by irreversibly preventing the ability of an AChE molecule from metabolizing ACh, by depositing a phosphoryl group at the active serine hydroxyl site of AChE at both nicotinic and muscarinic synapses.[249,250] OPIDP is due to inhibition of a different enzyme, neurotoxic esterase.

TREATMENT

Like all acutely paralyzing diseases capable of resulting in ventilatory failure, ICU care is integral to the care of many acutely intoxicated patients.[248] Once stabilized, in cases where the toxin has been ingested, gastric lavage with or without activated charcoal is routinely utilized in an attempt to reduce the toxin burden.[247,248] Intravenous fluids, usually normal saline, is delivered with a goal of maintaining systolic blood pressure above 80 mm Hg and urine output above 0.5 mL/kg/hour.[248] Nasal oxygen is commonly administered. Positioning the patient on their left side may aid in secretion clearance, reduce risk of aspiration, and decrease pyloric emptying and toxin absorption in patients who have injected the toxin.[248]

The recommended pharmacological treatment of proven benefit is intravenous atropine used to lessen adverse muscarinic and CNS morbidity, atropine being capable of crossing the blood–brain barrier. Various regimens have been recommended. An initial IV bolus of 1–3 mg is suggested.[248] A second bolus, double the original, is recommended if the pupil size, blood pressure, pulse, breath sounds, or sweat production do not improve in 5 minutes. Alternative regimens include either continuous IV infusion of atropine at an initial rate of 0.02–0.08 mg/kg or intermittent intravenous injections of 4 mg every 15 minutes until secretions control has been achieved have been recommended as well.[251] Use of intravenous β- or calcium channel blockers have been suggested for cardioprotection if heart rates exceed 130 bpm.[251] Benzodiazepines are used as a matter of routine in intubated patients and in those who have seized, and are indicated as well along with atropine for the treatment of agitation. Magnesium sulfate, α2 adrenergic agonists such as clonidine, sodium bicarbonate, butyrylcholinesterase, hemodialysis/hemofiltration and bacterially derived phospho triesterases, or hydrolases that break down organophosphates enzymatically represent suggested treatments of unproven benefit.[248.]

Pralidoxime is the most commonly used agent of the oxime class whose utility is relevant only in organophosphate toxicity. It has no effect on the toxicity of other carbamylated cholinesterases such as physostigmine or neostigmine. Its mechanism of action is to reactivate AChE. It does so by binding the cholinesterase molecule and by doing so, inducing a conformational change in the organophosphate molecule attached to the other end of AChE. This allows for dissociation of the otherwise irreversible bond between AChE and organophosphate.[249] Unlike atropine, pralidoxime does not cross the blood–brain barrier and does not benefit CNS morbidity. The World Health Organization recommended regimen is a 30 mg/kg pralidoxime chloride bolus followed by 8 mg/kg/hour infusion.[247] An alternative regimen employed in Asia is 1 g of pralidoxime every 4–6 hours for 1–3 days.[254] Despite repeated evidence of a benefit in animals however, benefit in humans remains unproven with some reports suggesting a deleterious effect.[247,251,254] There are numerous proposed hypotheses as to why a disparity exists in vitro and in vivo effects.[251]

There are numerous species of venomous arthropods, snakes, and marine species whose bite or at times ingestion may produce weakness or other symptoms referable to the neuromuscular system.[255–259] Although uncommon in North America, it is estimated that there are more than 150,000 envenomation deaths that occur in the world annually as a result of venomous bites.[257] The land and surrounding waters of Australia and Southeast Asia are the home for many of these species. Although many of these toxins have systemic effects as well as direct effects on peripheral nerve and muscle, the morbidity of a number of these toxins relate to adverse effects on neuromuscular transmission. As many of these disorders indirectly affect neuromuscular transmission by affecting sodium or potassium channels on presynaptic nerve terminals, separating envenomations considered as neuropathic from those whose mechanisms of action appear to be focused on NMT alone is somewhat arbitrary and artificial. As neuropathies caused by envenomations often produce sensory as well as motor consequences, this separation has some clinical validity and will be maintained throughout this text. This section, although not intended to be comprehensive, will highlight some of the more noteworthy toxins that produce neuromuscular disorders largely attributable to disordered NMT.

SNAKES

Serpents belonging to some but not all of the Elapid (cobras, kraits, mambas, coral snakes, sea snakes, and a number of terrestrial Australian) species produce venom that adversely affects NMT at either the presynaptic or postsynaptic level.[256] Kraits (Bungarus sp.) secrete both presynaptic toxins referred to as β-neurotoxins and the postsynaptic α- or γ-neurotoxins that have curare-like effects.[256,258] These actions are not mutually exclusive although it is the β-neurotoxin that is felt to be the predominant source of morbidity.[258] The β-neurotoxin is a phospholipase that results in a loss of synaptophysin and a reduction in synaptic vesicles presynaptically.

The Eastern Green Mamba (Dendroaspis sp.) release two toxins, dendrotoxin and fasciculin. The former specifically binds neuronal potassium channels and prolongs depolarization in nerve terminals, thus facilitating ACh release. The latter is a cholinesterase inhibitor.[260] Cobra species (Naja sp.) secrete cobrotoxin that inhibits binding of ACh at nicotinic receptors (κ-neurotoxin).[258,260] Coral snakes (Micrurus sp.), the only Elapids indigenous to the United States secrete an α neurotoxin (postsynaptic).[261] Vipers and rattlesnake (Crotalid sp.) envenomation may have neurological consequences, for example, generalized myokymia as a consequence of rattlesnake envenomation, but do not typically affect neuromuscular transmission.

Snake envenomation regardless of species may, and often do affect other organ systems as a result of other toxic components, particularly those that incite inflammation with a prominent local wound reaction or that have either procoagulant or anticoagulant effects. Snake venom does not cross the blood–brain barrier but can adversely affect the CNS through thrombotic or hemorrhagic complications.[256] Optic neuritis, a cerebellar syndrome and a diffuse encephalomyelitis have been rarely described as a delayed complication of venomous snake bites.[256] The mechanism is unknown but may represent a hypersensitivity reaction to antivenin.

The presence or absence of local reaction depends on the species and the constituency of the venom. With krait and coral snake envenomation, it tends to be negligible. Systemic symptoms typically begin within 1–4 hours but may be delayed for up to 12 hours. Initial systemic symptoms may be nonspecific including chest and abdominal discomfort and tightness, myalgias, and nausea among others. CNS symptoms are thought to result from hypoxia or hypotension as these toxins do not cross the blood–brain barrier. Although DNMT is in the exclusive domain of the Elapid species, it is not a universal consequence of envenomation.[256] Symptoms referable to cholinergic excess such as fasciculations and hypersalivation may or may not occur. The following description is prototypical when weakness occurs. The pattern, like botulism, is descending. Ptosis and ophthalmoparesis typically precede facial weakness. Neck flexor weakness is a harbinger of ventilatory muscle involvement. Arms weakness may be observed to precede leg weakness if affected individuals are observed carefully.[256,259] A direct myotoxic effect of neurotoxins resulting in rhabdomyolysis may occur, typically associated with β-neurotoxicity but reported with α-neurotoxicity as well.[258,261] Mortality rates vary but are high without adequate medical care and death may occur within 48 hours of envenomation.[258] During the Vietnam War, American soldiers referred to the multibanded krait as the two-step snake due to the exaggerated claim that death occurred within two steps of being bit. With Mamba envenomation, local swelling and nausea precede descending paralysis which includes cranial nerve palsies, ventilatory muscle and limb weakness.[260]

EDX evaluations have been rarely reported in Elapid envenomation.[259] The pattern is one of reduced CMAP amplitudes at baseline with a mild decremental response with slow repetitive stimulation.

Treatment considerations are individualized.[256] As a general rule, the involved limb should be immobilized and kept in a dependent position to limit toxin dissemination. Intubation and mechanical ventilation should be instituted early with any indication of breathing difficulties. Volume repletion should be provided and antihistamines, corticosteroids, and epinephrine considered with any indication of shock or allergic reaction to antivenin. Monitoring for and treatment of adverse procoagulant or anticoagulant effects is important. In the case of bleeding, the use of fresh frozen plasma, cryoprecipitates, and human fibrinogen concentrates is indicated. Monitoring for compartment syndrome in the vicinity of the wound is important. Fasciotomy should be undertaken cautiously however, due to considerations of hemostatic difficulties that these patients may experience. Monitoring CK levels in anticipation of possible rhabdomyolyis and myoglobinuric renal failure is recommended.[258] Wound debridement may be required if local tissue necrosis ensues. If there is any doubt of the patient's vaccination status, tetanus toxoid should be provided. Cholinesterase inhibitors may be considered if the species of snake is known and the venom recognized to be an α-neurotoxin with reversible postsynaptic blocking properties. Antivenin, delivered as soon as possible, is recommended and is felt to reduce the mortality rates of envenomation significantly. Antivenins exist in the preferable monovalent (species specific) or polyvalent forms.[260] Elapid envenomation is rare in North America but does rarely occur in natural habits in the southern US and Latin America from Coral snakes or with exotic species in pet owners and zoo employees.[261,262] Antivenoms for Elapids may be difficult to obtain, particularly in the United States. Valuable resources include the poison center hotline (800–222–1222) and the Association of Zoological Parks and Aquariums (301–562–0777).[260] As antivenins are developed in nonhuman species, there is a significant risk of allergic response that should be monitored for and treated as necessary.

ARTHROPODS

α-Latrotoxin is the active constituent of black widow and brown widow spider venom.[263–266] The venom stimulates the release of a number of neurotransmitters including norepinephrine, dopamine, and acetylcholine resulting in vesicle depletion.[260,267] The mechanism of depleted ACh at presynaptic terminals of the NMJ appears to be independent of the normal calcium dependent ACh-release mechanisms. Both the PNS and CNS are affected. The syndrome differs from most DNMT described in this chapter as the disordered NMT results in symptoms of neuromuscular hyperactivity. Paralysis does not occur. Local pain is a characteristic symptom of the spider bite. Initial symptoms are those of overstimulation with autonomic overactivity including vasoconstriction, and hypertension, diaphoresis and neuromuscular overactivity including painful muscle rigidity and cramping which typically begin at the bite site and spreads centrifugally. Spasms of the abdominal wall may mimic a surgical abdomen. Understandably, serum CK values may be elevated. Headache, dyspnea secondary to bronchoconstriction, emesis, priapism, lethargy, irritability, tremor, fasciculation, and/or ataxia are other common manifestations.[256,260] Myocarditis is a reported, a potentially fatal manifestation.[268] Treatment includes antivenom which should be used judiciously and with prophylactic antihistamine and epinephrine in view of the high rates of allergic reaction including anaphylaxis. Airway management is as always, a priority. Symptomatic use of benzodiazepines, infusions of calcium gluconate to address cramping and atropine may be considered as well as tetanus immunization.

Scorpion intoxication is also thought to manifest through an increase in presynaptic ACh release as well as a direct effect on muscle, both believed to occur as a result of impaired deactivation of sodium channels.[267] The clinical picture of scorpion envenomation is dominated by muscle weakness associated with arterial hypertension, cardiac arrhythmias, myocarditis, or pulmonary edema. These latter manifestations result from the catecholamine release or direct cardiac toxicity.[256] Treatment with vasodilators are commonly required to counteract the hyperadrenergic aspects of scorpion stings.

MARINE ENVENOMATIONS

There are numerous marine species that transmit toxins to humans. The transmission may occur through bites, stings, or ingestion. Only a few of these toxins impair NMT as their primary mechanism of action.[269,270]

Sea snakes, formerly considered as members of the Hydrophiidae family, are now classified as Elapids and share many of the toxic properties described above. They reside almost exclusively in the warm waters of the South Pacific and Indian oceans. Symptom onset is usually 1–6 hours after the bite has occurred. The local reaction is limited. Morbidity stems from both direct myotoxic effects as well as disordered NMT. The former include myalgia aggravated with movement, trismus, and rhabdomyolysis with the risk of myoglobinuric renal failure. The latter include dysphagia, ptosis, and ophthalmoplegia, and ascending paralysis. Seizures, coma, and potentially death from ventilatory failure may occur. Identification of a specific sea snake species (52) is less likely to occur than with bites of their terrestrial cousins. Sea snake antivenom appears equally effective regardless of species. The availability is limited in the Western hemisphere but may be obtained at the Long Beach (CA) aquarium. Again, the risk of allergic reaction needs to be taken into consideration. Management is otherwise similar to that recommended for terrestrial Elapid envenomations.

The cone snail resides in habits similar to sea snakes.[269] A dart-like barb coated in toxin can be fired from between the edges of its shell if handled. Envenomation with conotoxin, intended to paralyze its prey, has resulted in numerous human deaths. The conotoxins have affinity for nicotinic AChRs, neuronal calcium channels, muscle sodium channels, vasopressin receptors, and N-methyl-D-aspartate receptors. Presumably, its affinity for presynaptic calcium channels provides the basis for the paralysis it can cause.[271–273] A local reaction to snail envenomation produces variable degrees of discomfort followed or accompanied by local swelling and numbness, blanching, cyanosis, and necrosis. Systemically patients may experience nausea and pruritus in addition to dysphagia, blurred vision, paralysis, and in the most severe cases ventilatory failure. Cardiovascular collapse can occur as well. Without support, death may occur as rapidly as 2 hours after envenomation. No antivenin has been developed for the cone snail.

DRUGS AND METABOLIC DISTURBANCES

There are multiple drugs and notable metabolic disturbances that can affect neuromuscular transmission, and multiple mechanisms by which they can do so that can occur at either a presynaptic, synaptic, or postsynaptic location.[267,274–281] Those that are capable of augmenting neuromuscular transmission may be therapeutically useful in DNMT. Guanidine, rarely used now because of side effects but used historically in the treatment of LEMS, enhances NMT by inhibiting calcium egress from the presynaptic terminal and thereby increasing the probability of vesicle fusion and quantal release. Pyridostigmine, edrophonium, neostigmine, and physostigmine are used both diagnostically and therapeutically to enhance NMT by their reversible cholinesterase inhibition. They can be used to both diagnose MG, treat MG as well as other DNMT, or in case of physostigmine that crosses the blood–brain barrier, be used as a treatment for the CNS toxicity of drugs with anticholinergic properties.

When drugs that augment cholinergic function are used in normal individuals where NMT is already optimal, they may achieve either desired or undesired symptoms of cholinergic excess at muscarinic, nicotinic, and depending on blood–brain barrier penetration, CNS synapses. Conversely, with certain drugs such as succinylcholine, this effect can be of sufficient magnitude to exhaust the NMJ resulting in potentially therapeutic paralysis. This effect can be used to ensure immobility during surgery or to reduce resistance to mechanical ventilation. This same therapeutic paralytic effect can be obtained by nondepolarizing neuromuscular blockers whose mechanism of action is post- rather than presynaptic. The most notorious of these nondepolarizing neuromuscular blocking agents is curare which is a naturally occurring derivative of the plant *Strychnos toxifera*.[276] Although first utilized as a toxin in hunting or in war, like botulinum toxin it can be used therapeutically as well as a paralyzing agent (d-tubocurarine) and was once used to augment the diagnostic yield of repetitive stimulation testing in patients with suspected MG.

There are many other drugs whose primary therapeutic target is not the NMJ but which have neuromuscular blocking properties that vary in degree. These drugs may have little or no effect on normal people with a full neuromuscular reserve but may uncover or increase morbidity in an individual with a pre-existing DNMT such as myasthenia. Finally, there are drugs, most notably penicillamine and αinterferon, that are believed to induce autoimmune myasthenia.[282–300] The reader is referred to Table 25-3 for list of agents known to adversely affect neuromuscular transmission.

Although the release of ACh at presynaptic terminals is calcium dependent, an effect theoretically compromised by increased concentrations of its competing cation, magnesium, there is a paucity of information that either hypocalcemia or hypermagnesemia have significant impacts on neuromuscular transmission on most individuals. Autoantibodies (VGCC autoantibodies in LEMS) and environmental toxins (conotoxin in Cone snails) that specifically react with presynaptic VGCCs impair NMT and produce weakness. Despite that, tetany, not weakness is the typical effect of hypocalcemia and appears to result from an effect on the sarcoplasmic reticulum in muscle, not the NMJ. In addition, drugs with calcium channel blocking properties seem to have little if any significant adverse clinical or electrophysiological effects on NMT.[301] Conversely, hypermagnesemia has rarely been reported as a cause of significant neuromuscular weakness by competitively inhibiting calcium entry into the nerve terminal.[302–306] Serum levels of >5 mEq/L may abolish deep tendon reflexes, with generalized weakness typically present with levels >9–10 mEq/L.[307] The reported EDX pattern when reported is consistent with a presynaptic DNMT, that is, reduced CMAP amplitude at rest, a decremental response to slow (2–5 Hz) repetitive stimulation and an incremental response to brief exercise or more rapid stimulation frequencies (10–50 Hz).[304,306]

▶SUMMARY

Neuromuscular transmission is a complex physiological event that can be readily disrupted by numerous acquired or heritable conditions affecting one or more of its presynaptic, synaptic, or postsynaptic components. Acquired MG is the most common of these disorders. This chapter describes other, less common disorders that require an increased index of suspicion in an individual(s) presenting with painless weakness. This is particularly true when the history reveals a clinical context predisposing to one of these disorders, or when weakness is accompanied by symptoms referable to autonomic or CNS cholinergic dysfunction.

REFERENCES

1. Lambert EH, Eaton LM, Rooke ED. Defect of neuromuscular conduction associated with malignant neoplasms. *Am J Physiol.* 1956;187:612–613.
2. Titulaer MJ, Lang B, Verschuuren JJ. Lambert–Eaton myasthenic syndrome: From clinical characteristics to therapeutic strategies. *Lancet Neurol.* 2011;10:1098–1107.
3. Eaton LM, Lambert EH. Electromyography and electric stimulation of nerves in diseases of motor unit: Observations on myasthenic syndrome associated with malignant tumors. *JAMA.* 1957;163(13):1117–1124.
4. Elmqvist D, Quastel DM. Presynaptic action of hemicholinium at the neuromuscular junction. *J Physiol.* 1965;177:463–482.
5. Elmqvist D, Lambert EH. Detailed analysis of neuromuscular transmission in a patient with the myasthenic syndrome sometimes associated with bronchogenic carcinoma. *Mayo Clin Proc.* 1968;43:689–713.
6. Lambert EH, Rooke ED. Myasthenic state and lung cancer. In: Brain L, Norris F, eds. *The Remote Effects of Cancer on the Nervous System.* New York: Grune & Stratton;. 1965:362–410.
7. Lambert EH, Lennon VA. Neuromuscular transmission in nude mice bearing oat cell tumors from Lambert–Eaton myasthenic syndrome. *Muscle Nerve.* 1982;5(Suppl):S39–S45.
8. O'Neill JH, Murray NM, Newsom Davis J. The Lambert–Eaton myasthenic syndrome: A review of 50 cases. *Brain.* 1988;111:577–596.
9. Pascuzzi RM, Kim YI. Lambert–Eaton syndrome. *Semin Neurol.* 1990;10:35–41.
10. Rubenstein AE, Horowitz SH, Bender AN. Cholinergic dysautonomia and Eaton–Lambert syndrome. *Neurology.* 1979; 29:720–723.
11. Morgan-Followell B, de Los Reyes E. Child neurology: Diagnosis of Lambert-Eaton myasthenic syndrome in children. *Neurology.* 2013;80(21):e220–e222.
12. Lennon VA, Kryzer TJ, Griesmann GE, et al. Calcium-channel antibodies in Lambert–Eaton myasthenic syndrome and other paraneoplastic syndromes. *N Engl J Med.* 1995;332:1467–1474.
13. Farrugia ME, Vincent A. Autoimmune mediated neuromuscular junction defects. *Curr Opin Neurol.* 2010;23:489–495.
14. Lang B, Newsom-Davis J, Wray D, Vincent A, Murray N. Autoimmune aetiology for myasthenic (Eaton-Lambert) syndrome. *Lancet.* 1981;2(8240):224–226.
15. Titulaer MJ, Wirtz PW, Willems LN, van Kralingen KW, Smitt PA, Verschuuren JJ. Screening for small-cell lung cancer: A follow-up study of patients with Lambert-Eaton myasthenic syndrome. *J Clin Oncol.* 2008;26:4276–4281.
16. Fernandez-Torron R, Arocha J, Lopez-Picazo JM, et al. Isolated dysphagia due to paraneoplastic myasthenic syndrome with anti-P/Q voltage-gated calcium-channel and anti-acetylcholine receptor antibodies. *Neuromuscul Disord.* 2011;21:126–128.
17. Lauritzen M, Smith T, Fischer-Hansen B, Sparup J, Olesen J. Eaton-Lambert syndrome and malignant thymoma. *Neurology.* 1980;30:634–638.
18. Murimoto M, Osaki T, HNagara Y, Kodate M, Motomura M, Murai H. Thymoma with Lambert-Eaton myasthenic syndrome. *Ann Thorac Surg.* 2010;89:2001–2003.
19. Pasquoloni E, Aubart F, Brihaye B, et al. Lambert-Eaton myasthenic syndrome and follicular thymic hyperplasia in systemic lupus erythematosus. *Lupus.* 2011;20:745–748.
20. Argov Z, Shapira Y, Averbuch-Heller L, Wirguin I. Lambert-Eaton myasthenic syndrome (LEMS) in association with lymphoproliferative disorders. *Muscle Nerve.* 1995;18:715–719.
21. Petersen CL, Hemker BG, Jacobson RD, Warwick AB, Jaradeh SS, Kelly ME. Wilms tumor presenting with Lambert-Eaton myasthenic syndrome. *J Pediatr Hematol Oncol.* 2013;35(4):267–270.
22. Maddison P, Newsom-Davis J, Mills KR, Souhami RL. Favourable prognosis in Lambert-Eaton myasthenic syndrome and small-cell lung carcinoma. *Lancet.* 1999;353:117–118
23. Wirtz PW, Lang B, Graus F, et al. P/Q-type calcium channel antibodies, Lambert-Eaton myasthenic syndrome and survival in small cell lung cancer. *J Neuroimmunol.* 2005;164:161–165.
24. Nakao YK, Motomura M, Fukudome T, et al. Seronegative Lambert–Eaton myasthenic syndrome: Study of 110 Japanese patients. *Neurology.* 2002;59:1773–1775.

25. Titulaer MJ, Klooster R, Potman M, et al. SOX antibodies in small-cell lung cancer and Lambert-Eaton myasthenic syndrome: Frequency and relation with survival. *J Clin Oncol.* 2009;27:4260–4267.
26. Wirtz PW, Bradshaw J, Wintzen AR, Verschuuren JJ. Associated autoimmune disease in patients with the Lambert-Eaton myasthenic syndrome. *J Neuroimmunol.* 2005;159:230–237.
27. Gutmann L, Crosby TW, Takamori M, Martin JD. The Eaton–Lambert syndrome and autoimmune disorders. *Am J Med.* 1972;53:354–356.
28. Lambert EH, Rooke ED, Eaton LM, et al. Myasthenic syndrome occasionally associated with bronchial neoplasm: Neurophysiologic studies. In: Viets HR, ed. *Myasthenia Gravis.* Springfield, IL: C C Thomas Publishers; 1961:362–410.
29. McEvoy KM. Diagnosis and treatment of Lambert–Eaton myasthenic syndrome. *Neurol Clin.* 1994;12:387–399.
30. Rudnicki SA. Lambert-Eaton myasthenic syndrome with pure ocular weakness. *Neurology.* 2007;68:1863–1864.
31. Wirtz PW, Sotodeh M, Nijnuis M, et al. Different distribution of muscle weakness between myasthenia gravis and the Lambert-Eaton myasthenic syndrome. *J Neurol Neurosurg Psychiatry.* 2002;73:766–768.
32. Burns TM, Russell JA, LaChance D, Jones HR. Oculobulbar involvement is typical with Lambert–Eaton myasthenic syndrome. *Ann Neurol.* 2003;53:270–273.
33. Rácz A, Giede-Jeppe A, Schramm A, Schwab S, Maihöfner C. Lambert-Eaton myasthenic syndrome presenting with a "dropped head syndrome" and associated with antibodies against N-type calcium channels. *Neurol Sci.* 2012;34(7):1253–1254.
34. Nicolle MW, Stewart DJ, Remtulla H, Chen R, Bolton CF. Lambert–Eaton myasthenic syndrome presenting with severe respiratory failure. *Muscle Nerve.* 1996;19:1328–1333.
35. Smith AG, Wald J. Acute ventilatory failure in Lambert–Eaton myasthenic syndrome and its response to 3,4-diaminopyridine. *Neurology.* 1996;46:1143–1145.
36. Barr CW, Claussen G, Thomas D, Fesenmeier JT, Peralman RL, Oh SJ. Primary respiratory failure as the presenting symptom in Lambert–Eaton myasthenic syndrome. *Muscle Nerve.* 1993;16:712–715.
37. Mason WP, Graus F, Lang B, et al. Small cell lung cancer, paraneoplastic cerebellar degeneration, and Lambert–Eaton myasthenic syndrome. *Brain.* 1997;120:1279–1300.
38. Breen LA, Gutmann L, Brick JF, Riggs JR. Paradoxical lid elevation with sustained upward gaze: A sign of Lambert–Eaton syndrome. *Muscle Nerve.* 1991;14:863–866.
39. Oh SJ, Dwyer DS, Bradley RJ. Overlap myasthenic syndrome: Combined myasthenia gravis and Eaton-Lambert syndrome. *Neurology.* 1987;37:1411–1414.
40. Boiardi A, Bussone G, Negri S. Alternating myasthenia and myastheniform syndromes in the same patient. *J Neurol.* 1979; 220:57–64.
41. Dahl DS, Sato S. Unusual myasthenic state in a teenage boy. *Neurology.* 1974;24:897–901.
42. Lennon VA. Serologic profile of myasthenia gravis and distinction from the Lambert–Eaton myasthenic syndrome. *Neurology.* 1997;48(Suppl 5):S23–S27.
43. Katz JS, Wolfe GI, Bryan WW, Tintner R, Barohn RJ. Acetylcholine receptor antibodies in the Lambert–Eaton myasthenic syndrome. *Neurology.* 1998;50:470–475.
44. Newsom-Davis J, Leys K, Vincent A, Ferguson I, Modi G, Mills K. Immunological evidence for the co-existence of the Lambert–Eaton myasthenic syndrome and myasthenia gravis in two patients. *J Neurol Neurosurg Psychiatry.* 1991;54:452–453.
45. Kim JA, Lim YM, Jang EH, Kim KK. A patient with coexisting myasthenia gravis and Lambert-Eaton myasthenic syndrome. *J Clin Neurol.* 2012;8(3):235–237.
46. Joy JL, Baysal AI, Oh SJ. Reflex improvement after exercise in the Eaton–Lambert syndrome. *Muscle Nerve.* 1987;10:671–672.
47. Tim RW, Massey JM, Sanders DB. Lambert–Eaton syndrome: Electrodiagnostic findings and response to treatment. *Neurology.* 2000;54:2176–2178.
48. Jablecki C. Lambert–Eaton myasthenic syndrome. *Muscle Nerve.* 1984;7:250–257.
49. McQuillen MP, Johns RJ. The nature of the defect in the Eaton–Lambert syndrome. *Neurology.* 1967;17:527–536.
50. Cruz Martinez A, Ferrer MT, Morales C, et al. Electromyography, single fiber electromyography, and necropsy findings in myasthenic syndrome associated with bronchogenic carcinoma. *Electromyogr Clin Neurophysiol.* 1982;22:531–548.
51. Henriksson KG, Nilsson O, Rosen I, Schiller HH. Clinical, neurophysiological and morphological findings in Eaton–Lambert syndrome. *Acta Neurol Scand.* 1977;56:117–140.
52. Lambert EH. Defects of neuromuscular transmission in syndromes other than myasthenia gravis. *Ann N Y Acad Sci.* 1966;135:367–384.
53. Oh SJ, Kim DE, Kuruoglu R, Brooks J, Claussen GW. Electrophysiological and clinical correlations in the Lambert–Eaton myasthenic syndrome. *Muscle Nerve.* 1996;19:903–906.
54. Oh SJ, Kurokawa K, Glaussen GC, Ryan HR Jr. Electrophysiological diagnostic criteria of Lambert–Eaton, myasthenic syndrome. *Muscle Nerve.* 2005;32:515–520.
55. Tim RW, Sanders DB. Repetitive nerve stimulation studies in the Lambert–Eaton myasthenic syndrome. *Muscle Nerve.* 1994;17:995–1001.
56. Oh SJ. The Eaton–Lambert syndrome in ocular myasthenia gravis. *Arch Neurol.* 1974;31:183–186.
57. Ingram DA, Davis GR, Schwartz MS, Traub M, Newland AC, Swash M. Cancer associated myasthenic (Eaton–Lambert) syndrome: Distribution of abnormality and effect of treatment. *J Neurol Neurosurg Psychiatry.* 1984;47:806–812.
58. Brown JC, Johns RJ. Diagnostic difficulties encountered in the myasthenic syndrome sometimes associated with carcinoma. *J Neurol Neurosurg Psychiatry.* 1974;37:1214–1224.
59. Scopetta C, Csali C, Vaccario ML, Provenzano C. Difficult diagnosis of Eaton–Lambert syndrome. *Muscle Nerve.* 1984;7:680–681.
60. Baslo MB, Deymeer F, Serdaroglu P, Parman Y, Ozdemir C, Cuttini M. Decrement pattern in Lambert-Eaton myasthenic syndrome is different from myasthenia gravis. *Neuromuscul Disord.* 2006;16:454–458.
61. Sanders DB, Cao L, Massey JM, Juel VC, Hobson-Webb L, Guptill JT. Is the decremental pattern in Lambert-Eaton syndrome different from that in myasthenia gravis? *Clin Neurophysiol.* 2014;125(6):1274–1277.
62. Desmedt JE. The neuromuscular disorder in myasthenia gravis: I. Electrical and mechanical responses to nerve stimulation in hand muscles. In: Desmedt JE, ed. *New Developments in Electromyography and Clinical Neurophysiology.* Basel: Karger; 1973:241–304.
63. Stalberg E, Trontelj JV. *Single Fiber Electromyography.* Old Woking: Mirvalle Press; 1979.

64. Oh SJ. *Electromyography: Neuromuscular Transmission*. Baltimore, MD: Williams & Wilkins; 1988.
65. Rooke DE, Eaton LM, Lambert EH, Hodgson CH. Myasthenia and malignant intrathoracic tumor. *Med Clin North Am*. 1960;44:977–988.
66. Schwartz MS, Stalberg E. Myasthenic syndrome studied with single fiber electromyography. *Arch Neurol*. 1975;32:815–817.
67. Schwartz MS, Stalberg E. Myasthenia gravis with features of the myasthenic syndrome. *Neurology*. 1975;25:80–84.
68. Cruz Martinez A, Ferrer MT, Diez Tejedor E, Perez Conde MC, Anciones B, Frank A. Diagnostic yield of single fiber electromyography and other electrophysiological technique in myasthenia gravis I. Electromyography, automatic analysis of the voluntary pattern, and repetitive nerve stimulation. *Electromyogr Clin Neurophysiol*. 1982;22:377–393.
69. Cruz Martinez A, Ferrer MT, Perez Conde MC, Diez Tejedor E, Barreiros P, Ribacoba R. Diagnostic yield of single fiber electromyography and other electrophysiologic techniques in myasthenia gravis II. Jitter and motor unit fiber density studies. Clinical remission and thymectomy. *Electromyogr Clin Neurophysiol*. 1982;22:395–417.
70. Trontelj JV, Stalberg E, Mihelin M. Jitter in the muscle fiber. *J Neurol Neurosurg Psychiatry*. 1990;53:49–54.
71. Trontelj JV, Stalberg E. Single motor end-plates in myasthenia gravis and LEMS at different firing rates. *Muscle Nerve*. 1991;14:226–232.
72. Trontelj JV, Stalberg E, Khuraibet AJ. Tetanic potentiation and depression at single motor end-plates in myasthenia and LEMS. *J Neurol Sci*. 1990;98(Suppl):289–290.
73. Kim DE, Claussen GC, Oh SJ. Single-fiber electromyography improvement with 3,4 diaminopyridine in Lambert–Eaton myasthenic syndrome. *Muscle Nerve*. 1998;21:1107–1108.
74. Oh SJ. SFEMG improvement with remission in the cancer-associated Lambert–Eaton myasthenic syndrome. *Muscle Nerve*. 1989;12:844–848.
75. Oh SJ, Hurwitz EL, Lee KW, Change CW, Cho HK. The single fiber EMG in the Lambert–Eaton myasthenic syndrome. *Muscle Nerve*. 1989;12:159–161.
76. Sadeh M, River Y, Argov Z. Stimulated single-fiber electromyography in Lambert–Eaton myasthenic syndrome before and after 3,4-diaminopyridine. *Muscle Nerve*. 1997;20:735–739.
77. Torbergsen T, Stalberg E, Bless JK. Subclinical neuromuscular involvement in patients with lung cancer. *Acta Neurol Scand*. 1984;69(Suppl 98):190–191.
78. Trontelj JV, Mihelin M, Fernandez JM, Stalberg E. Axonal stimulation for end-plate jitter studies. *J Neurol Neurosurg Psychiatry*. 1986;49:677–685.
79 Chaudhry V, Watson DF, Bird SJ, Cornblath DR. Stimulated single fiber electromyography in Lambert–Eaton syndrome. *Muscle Nerve*. 1991;14:1227–1230.
80. Ricker K, Hertel G, Stodieck S. The influence of local cooling on neuromuscular transmission in the myasthenic syndrome of Eaton and Lambert. *J Neurol*. 1977;217:95–102.
81. Ricker K, Hertel G, Stodieck S. Influence of temperature on neuromuscular transmission in myasthenia gravis. *J Neurol*. 1977;216:273–282.
82. Ward CD, Murray NM. Effect of temperature on neuromuscular transmission in the Eaton–Lambert syndrome. *J Neurol Neurosurg Psychiatry*. 1979;42:247–249.
83. AAEM Quality Assurance Committee. American Association of Electrodiagnostic Medicine. Practice parameter for repetitive nerve stimulation and single fiber EMG evaluation of adults with suspected myasthenia gravis of Lambert-Eaton myasthenic syndrome: Summary statement. *Muscle Nerve*. 2001;24:1236–1238.
84. Leys K, Lang B, Johnston I, Newsom-Davis J. Calcium channel autoantibodies in the Lambert-Eaton myasthenic syndrome. *Ann Neurol*. 1991;29(3):307–314.
85. Lipka AF, Verschuuren JJ, Titulaer MJ. SOX1 antibodies in Lambert-Eaton myasthenic syndrome and screening for small cell lung carcinoma. *Ann N Y Acad Sci*. 2012;1275:70–77.
86. Sabater L, Titulaer M, Saiz A, Verschuuren J, Güre AO, Graus F. SOX1 antibodies are markers of paraneoplastic Lambert–Eaton myasthenic syndrome. *Neurology*. 2008;70:924–928.
87. Engel AG, Santa T. Histometric analysis of the ultra-structure of the neuromuscular junction in myasthenia gravis and the myasthenic syndrome. *Ann N Y Acad Sci*. 1971;183:46–63.
88. Engel AG. Review of evidence for loss of motor nerve terminal calcium channels in Lambert–Eaton myasthenic syndrome. *Ann N Y Acad Sci*. 1991;635:246–258.
89. Fukunaga H, Engel AG, Osame M, et al. Paucity and disorganization of presynaptic membrane active zones in the Lambert–Eaton syndrome. *Muscle Nerve*. 1982;5:686–697.
90. Fukunaga H, Engel AG, Lang B, Newsom-Davis J, Vincent A. Passive transfer of Lambert–Eaton myasthenic syndrome with IgG from man to mouse depletes the presynaptic membrane active zones. *Proc Natl Acad Sci USA*. 1983;80:7636–7640.
91. Hughes BW, Kusner LL, Kaminski HJ. Molecular architecture of the neuromuscular junction. *Muscle Nerve*. 2006;33: 445–461.
92. Kim YI. Passively transferred Lambert–Eaton syndrome in mice receiving purified IgG. *Muscle Nerve*. 1986;9:523–530.
93. Engel AG. The neuromuscular junction. In: Aminoff M, Boller F, Swaab D, eds. *Handbook of Clinical Neurology*. Chapter 3, Vol. 91. Amsterdam, Netherlands: Elsevier; 2008:103–148.
94. Leveque C, Hoshino T, David P, et al. The synaptic vesicle protein synaptotagmin associates with calcium channels and is a putative Lambert–Eaton myasthenic syndrome antigen. *Proc Natl Acad Sci USA*. 1992;89:3625–3629.
95. Pinto A, Kazuo I, Newland C, Newson-Davis J, Lang B. The action of Lambert-Eaton myasthenic syndrome immunoglobulin B on cloned human voltage-gated calcium channels. *Muscle Nerve*. 2002;25:715–724.
96. Lecky BR. Transient neonatal Lambert-Eaton syndrome. *J Neurol*. 2006;77:1094.
97. Reuner U, Kamin G, Ramantani G, Reichmann H, Dinger J. Transient neonatal Lambert-Eaton syndrome. *J Neurol*. 2008;255:1827–1828.
98. Chalk CH, Murray NM, Newsom-Davis J, O'Neill JH, Spiro SG. Response of the Lambert–Eaton myasthenic syndrome of associated small-cell lung carcinoma. *Neurology*. 1990;40:1552–1556.
99. De Aizpurua HJ, Lambert EH, Griesmann GE, et al. Antagonism of voltage-gated calcium channels in small cell carcinomas of patients with and without Lambert–Eaton myasthenic syndrome by autoantibodies w-conotoxin and adenosine. *Cancer Res*. 1988;48:4719–4724.
100. Hawley RJ, Cohen MH, Saini N, Armbrustmacher VW. The carcinomatous neuromyopathy of oat cell lung cancer. *Ann Neurol*. 1980;7:65–72.
101. Jenkyn LR, Brooks PL, Forcier RJ, Maurer LH, Ochoa J. Remission of the Lambert–Eaton syndrome and small cell anaplastic

carcinoma of the lung induced by chemotherapy and radiotherapy. *Cancer*. 1980;46:1123–1127.

102. Maddison P, Newsom-Davis J. Treatment for Lambert-Eaton myasthenic syndrome. *Cochrane Database Syst Rev*. 2005;18(2):CD003279.
103. Skeie GO, Apostolski S, Evoli A, et al. Guidelines for treatment of autoimmune neuromuscular transmission disorders. *Eur J Neurol*. 2010;17:893–902.
104. Maddison P. Treatment in Lambert-Eaton myasthenic syndrome. *Ann N Y Acad Sci*. 2012;1275:78–84.
105. Tim RW, Massey JM, Sanders DB. Lambert-Eaton myasthenic syndrome (LEMS) clinical and electrodiagnostic features and response to therapy in 59 patients. *Ann N Y Acad Sci*. 1988; 841:823–826.
106. Lundh H, Nilsson O, Rosen I. Treatment of Lambert–Eaton syndrome: 3,4-diaminopyridine and pyridostigmine. *Neurology*. 1984;34:1324–1330.
107. Oh SJ, Lee YW, Rutsky E. Eaton–Lambert syndrome: Reflex improvement with guanidine. *Arch Phys Med Rehabil*. 1977;58: 457–459.
108. Oh SJ, Kim KW. Guanidine hydrochloride in the Eaton–Lambert syndrome: Electrophysiological improvement. *Neurology*. 1973;23:1084–1090.
109. Keogh M, Sedehizadeh S, Maddison P. Treatment for Lambert-Eaton myasthenic syndrome. *Cochrane Database Syst Rev*. 2011;(2):CD003279.
110. Sanders DB, Massey JM, Sanders LL, Edwards LJ. A randomized trial of 3,4-diaminopyridine in Lambert–Eaton myasthenic syndrome. *Neurology*. 2000;54:603–607.
111. Oh SJ, Claussen GG, Hatanaka Y, Morgan MB. 3,4-Diaminopyridine is more effective than placebo in a randomized, double-blind, cross-over drug study in LEMS. *Muscle Nerve*. 2009;40(5):795–800.
112. McEvoy KE, Windebank AJ, Daube JR. Low PA. 3,4- diaminopyridine in Lambert-Eaton myasthenic syndrome. *N Engl J Med*. 1989;321(23):1567–1571.
113. Wirtz PW, Verschuuren JJ, van Dijk JG, Efficacy of 3,4- diaminopyridine and pyridostigmine in the treatment of Lambert-Eaton myasthenic syndrome: A randomized, double-blind, placebo-controlled, crossover study. *Clin Pharmacol Ther*. 2009;86(1):44–48.
114. Streib EW, Rothner AD. Eaton–Lambert myasthenic syndrome. Long term treatment of three patients with prednisone. *Ann Neurol*. 1981;10:448–453.
115. Kimura I, Ayyar DR. The Eaton–Lambert myasthenic syndrome and long-term treatment with prednisone. *Tohoku J Exp Med*. 1984;143:405–408.
116. Newsom-Davis J, Murray NM. Plasma exchange and immunosuppressive drug treatment in the Lambert–Eaton myasthenic syndrome. *Neurology*. 1984;34:480–485.
117. Bain PG, Motomura M, Newsom-Davis J, et al. Effects of intravenous immunoglobulin on muscle weakness and calcium-channel autoantibodies in the Lambert-Eaton myasthenic syndrome. *Neurology*. 1996;47(3):678–683.
118. Dau PC, Deny EH. Plasmapheresis and immunosuppressive drug therapy in the Eaton–Lambert syndrome. *Ann Neurol*. 1982;11:570–575.
119. Denys EH, Dau PC, Lindstrom JM. Neuromuscular transmission before and after plasmapheresis in myasthenia gravis and myasthenic syndrome. In: Dau PC, ed. *Plasmapheresis and Immunobiology of Myasthenia Gravis*. Boston, MA: Houghton Mifflin; 1979:248–257.
120. Maddison P, McConville J, Farrugia ME, et al. The use of rituximab in myasthenia gravis and Lambert-Eaton myasthenic syndrome. *J Neurol Neurosurg Psychiatry*. 2011;82:671–673.
121. Pellkofer HL, Voltz R, Kuempfel T. Favorable response to rituximab in a patient with anti-VGCC positive Lambert-Eaton myasthenic syndrome and cerebellar dysfunction. *Muscle Nerve*. 2009;40:305–308.
122. Burke G, Cossins J, Maxwell S, et al. Rapsyn mutations in hereditary myasthenia: Distinct early- and late-onset phenotypes. *Neurology*. 2003;61(6):826–828.
123. Beeson D, Hantai D, Lochmuller H, Engel AG. 126th International Workshop: Congenital myasthenic syndromes, 24–26 September. 2004, Naarden, the Netherlands. *Neuromuscul Disord*. 2005;15:498–512.
124. Müller JS, Herczegfalvi A, Vilchez JJ, et al. Phenotypical spectrum of DOK7 mutations in congenital myasthenic syndromes. *Brain*. 2007;130:1497–1506.
125. Engel AG. Current status of the congenital myasthenic syndromes. *Neuromuscular Disorders*. 2012;22:99–111.
126. Finlayson S, Beeson D, Palace J. Congenital myasthenic syndromes: An update. *Pract Neurol*. 2013;13:80–91.
127. Lorenzoni PJ, Scola RH, Kay CS, Werneck LC. Congenital myasthenic syndrome: A brief review. *Pediatr Neurology*. 2012;46:141–148.
128. Barašić N, Chaouch A, Müller JS, Lochmüller S. Genetic heterogeneity and pathophysiological mechanisms in congenital myasthenia syndromes. *Eur J Pediatr Neurol*. 2011;15:189–196.
129. Maselli RA, Arredondo J, Ferns MJ, Wollmann RL. Synaptic basal lamina-associated congenital myasthenic syndromes. *Ann N Y Acad Sci*. 2012;1275:36–48.
130. Milone M, Shen XM, Selcen D, et al. Myasthenic syndrome due to defects in rapsyn: Clinical and molecular findings in 39 patients. *Neurology*. 2009;73:228–235.
131. Selcen D, Shen XM, Milone M, et al. GFPT1 myasthenia. *Neurology*. 2013;81:370–378.
132. Finlayson S, Pallace J, Belaya K, et al. Clinical features of congenital syndrome due to mutations in DPAGT1. *J Neurol Neurosurg Psychiatry*. 2013;84:1119–1125.
133. Cossins J, Belaya K, Hicks D, et al. Congenital myasthenic syndromes due to mutations in ALG2 and ALG14. *Brain*. 2013;136:944–956.
134. Ohno K. Glycosylation defects as an emerging novel cause leading to a limb-girdle type of congenital myasthenic syndromes. *J Neurol Neurosurg Psychiatry*. 2013;84:1064.
135. Senderek J, Muller JS, Dusl M, et al. Hexosamine biosynthetic pathway mutations cause neuromuscular transmission defect. *Am J Hum Genet*. 2011;88:162–172.
136. Belaya, K, Finlayson S, Cossins J, et al. Identification of DPAGT1 as a new gene in which mutations cause a congenital myasthenic syndrome. *Ann N Y Acad Sci*. 2012;1275:29–35.
137. Belaya K, Finlayson S, Slater CR, et al. Mutations in DPAGT1 cause a limb-girdle myasthenic syndrome with tubular aggregates. *Am J Hum Genet*. 2012;91:193–201.
138. Monies DM, Al-Hindi HN, Al-Muhaizea MA, et al. Clinical and pathological heterogeneity of a congenital disorder of glycosylation manifesting as a myasthenic/myopathic syndrome. *Neuromuscul Disord*. 2014;24(4):353–359.
139. Ohkawara B, Cabrera-Serrano M, Nakata T, et al. LRP4 third β-propeller domain mutations cause novel congenital myasthenia by compromising agrin-mediated MuSK signaling in a

position- specific manner. *Hum Mol Genet*. 2014;23(7):1856–1868.
140. Selcen D, Juel VC, Hobson-Webb LD, et al. Myasthenic syndrome caused by plectinopathy. *Neurology*. 2011;76:327–336.
141. Selcen D, Milone M, Shen XM, et al. Dok-7 myasthenia: Phenotypic and molecular genetic studies in 16 patients. *Ann Neurol*. 2008;64:71–87.
142. Dobkin BH, Verity MA. Familial neuromuscular disease with type 1 fiber hypoplasia, tubular aggregates, cardiomyopathy, and myasthenic features. *Neurology*. 1978;28:1135–1140.
143. Furui E, Fukushima K, Sakashita T, Sakato S, Matsubara S, Takamori M. Familial limb-girdle myasthenia with tubular aggregates. *Muscle Nerve*. 1997;20:599–603.
144. Johns TR, Campa JF, Crowley WJ, et al. Familial myasthenia with tubular aggregates. *Neurology*. 1971;21:449.
145. McQuillen MP. Familial limb-girdle myasthenia. *Brain*. 1966; 89:121–132.
146. Guergueltcheva V, Müller JS, Dusl M, et al. Congenital myasthenic syndrome with tubular aggregates caused by GFPT1 mutations. *J Neurol*. 2012;259:838–850.
147. Abicht A, Müller J, Lochmüller H. Congenital myasthenic syndromes. In: Pagon RA, Adam MP, Bird TD, Dolan CR, Fong CT, Stephens K, eds. *GeneReviews™ [Internet]*. Seattle, WA: University of Washington; http://www.ncbi.nlm.nih.gov/gtr/. 2012:1993–2013.
148. Engel AG, Ohno K, Milone M, et al. New mutations in acetylcholine receptor subunit genes reveal heterogeneity in the slow channel congenital myasthenic syndrome. *Hum Mol Genet*. 1996;5:1217–1227.
149. Engel AG, Lambert EH, Mulder DM, et al. A newly recognized congenital myasthenic syndrome attributed to a prolonged open time of the acetylcholine induced ion channel. *Ann Neurol*. 1982;11:553–569.
150. Alseth EH, Maniaol AH, Elsais A, et al. Investigation for rapsyn and Dok-7 mutations in a cohort of seronegative myasthenia gravis. *Muscle Nerve*. 2011;43:574–577.
151. Punga AR, Ruegg MA. Signaling and aging at the neuromuscular synapse: Lessons learnt from neuromuscular disease. *Curr Opin Pharmacol*. 2012;12:340–346
152. Engel AG, Shen XM, Selcen D, Sine SM. What have we learned from the congenital myasthenic syndromes. *J Mol Neurosci*. 2010;40:143–153.
153. Ohno K, Tsujino A, Brengman JM, et al. Choline acetyltransferase mutations cause myasthenic syndrome associated with episodic apnea in humans. *Proc Natl Acad Sci USA*. 2001;98:2017–2022.
154. Walls TJ, Engel AG, Nagel AS, Harper CM, Trastek VF. Congenital myasthenic syndrome associated with paucity of synaptic vesicles and reduced quantal release. *Ann N Y Acad Sci*. 1993;681:461–468.
155. Engel AG, Walls TJ, Nagel A, Uchitel O. Newly recognized congenital myasthenic syndromes: I. Congenital paucity of synaptic vesicles and reduced quantal release, II. High-conductance fast-channel syndrome, III. Abnormal acetylcholine receptor (AChR) interaction with acetylcholine, IV. AChR deficiency and short channel-open time. *Prog Brain Res*. 1990;84:125–137.
156. Bady B, Chauplannaz G, Carrier H. Congenital Lambert-Eaton myasthenic syndrome. *J Neurol Neurosurg Psychiatry*. 1987;50(4):476–478.
157. Engel AG, Lambert EH, Mulder DM, et al. Recently recognized congenital myasthenic syndromes: (a) end-plate acetylcholine (ACh) esterase deficiency (b) putative abnormality of the ACh induced ion channel (c) putative defect of ACh resynthesis or mobilization—clinical features, ultrastructure and cytochemistry. *Ann N Y Acad Sci*. 1981;377:614–616.
158. Engel AG, Lambert EH, Gomez MR. A new myasthenic syndrome with end-plate acetylcholinesterase deficiency, small nerve terminals and reduced acetylcholine release. *Ann Neurol*. 1977;1:315–330.
159. Hutchinson DO, Walls TJ, Nakano S, et al. Congenital acetylcholinesterase deficiency. *Brain*. 1993;116:633–653.
160. Jennekens FG, Hesselmans LF, Veldman H, Jansen EN, Spaans F, Molenaar PC. Deficiency of acetylcholine receptors in a case of end-plate acetylcholinesterase deficiency: A histochemical investigation. *Muscle Nerve*. 1992;15:63–72.
161. Maselli RA, Ng JJ, Anderson JA, et al. Mutations in LAMB2 causing a severe form of synaptic congenital myasthenic syndrome. *J Med Genet*. 2009;46:203–208.
162. Maselli RA. Fernandez JM, Arredondo J. et al. LG2 agrin mutation causing severe congenital myasthenic syndrome mimics functional characteristics of non-neural (z-) agrin. *Hum Genet*. 2012;131:1123–1135.
163. Huz´e C, Bauché S, Richard P. et al. Identification of an agrin mutation that causes congenital myasthenia and affects synapse function. *Am J Hum Genet*. 2009;85:155–167.
164. Burke G, Cossins J, Maxwell S, et al. Distinct phenotypes of congenital acetylcholine receptor deficiency. *Neuromuscul Disord*. 2004;14:356–364.
165. Ruff RL, Putecki P. Faster, slower, but never better. Mutations of the skeletal muscle acetylcholine receptor. *Neurology*. 2012;79:404–405.
166. Shen X-M, Ohno K, Fukudome T, et al. Congenital myasthenic syndrome caused by low-expressor fast-channel AChR δ subunit mutation. *Neurology*. 2002;59:1881–1889.
167. Palace J, Lashley D, Newsom-Davis J, et al. Clinical features of the DOK7 neuromuscular junction synaptopathy. *Brain*. 2007;130:1507–1515.
168. Selcen D, Milone M, Shen XM, et al. Dok-7 myasthenia: Clinical spectrum, endplate (EP) electrophysiology and morphology, 12 novel DNA rearrangements, and genotype–phenotype relations in a Mayo cohort of 13 patients. *Neurology*. 2007;68(Suppl 1):A106–A107.
169. Anderson JA, Ng JJ, Bowe C, et al. Variable phenotypes associated with mutations in Dok-7. *Muscle Nerve*. 2008;37:448–456.
170. Beeson D, Higuchi O, Palace J, et al. Dok-7 mutations underlie a neuromuscular junction synaptopathy. *Science*. 2006;313:1975–1978.
171. Maselli RA, Arredondo J, Cagney O, et al. Mutations in MUSK causing congenital myasthenic syndrome impair MuSK-Dok-7 interaction. *Hum Mol Genet*. 2010;19:2370–2379.
172. Mihaylova V, Salih MA, Mukhtar MM, et al. Refinement of the clinical phenotype in musk-related congenital myasthenic syndromes. *Neurology*. 2009;73:1926–1928.
173. Chevessier F, Faraut B, Ravel-Chapuis A, et al. MUSK, a new target for mutations causing congenital myasthenic syndrome. *Hum Mol Genet*. 2004;13:3229–3240.
174. Tsujino A, Maertens C, Ohno K, et al. Myasthenic syndrome caused by mutation of the SCN4 A sodium channel. *Proc Natl Acad Sci USA*. 2003;100:7377–7382.
175. Kosac A, Gavillet E, Whittaker RG. Neurophysiological testing in congenital myasthenic syndromes: A systematic review of published normal data. *Muscle Nerve*. 2013;48:711–715.

176. Scara U, Della Marina A, Abicht A. Congenital myasthenic syndromes: Current diagnostic and therapeutic approaches. *Neuropediatrics*. 2012;43:184–193.
177. Engel AG, Brengman J, Edvardson S, Shen X-M. Highly fatal lowaffinity fast-channel congenital myasthenic syndrome caused by a novel AChR e subunit mutation at the agonist binding site. *Neurology*. 2011;76(Suppl 4):A644.
178. Cheung J, Cossins J, Liu W, Belaya K, Palace J, Beeson D. Pathogenic mechanisms of RAPSN mutations in congenital myasthenic syndromes. *Muscle Ne*rve. 2013;S11.
179. Zoltowska K, Webster R, Finlayson S, Maxwell S, Cossins J, Beeson D. GFPT1 mutations that underlie congenital myasthenic syndrome reduce AChR expression. *Muscle Nerve*. 2013:S10.
180. Liewluck T, Selcen D, Engel AG. Beneficial effects of albuterol in congenital endplate acetylcholinesterase deficiency and Dok-7 myasthenia. *Muscle Nerve*. 2011;44(5):789–794.
181. Lashley D, Palace J, Jayawant S, Robb S, Beeson D. Ephedrine treatment in congenital myasthenic syndrome due to mutations in Dok-7. *Neurology*. 2010;74:1517–1523.
182. Harper CM, Fukodome T, Engel AG. Treatment of slow-channel congenital myasthenic syndrome with fluoxetine. *Neurology*. 2003;60:1710–1713.
183. Balali-Mood M, Moshiri M, Etemad L. Medical aspects of bioterrorism. *Toxicon*. 2013;69:131–142.
184. Arnon SS, Schechter R, Inglesby TV, et al. Botulinum toxin as a biological weapon. *JAMA*. 2001;285(8):1059–1070.
185. Sobel J. Botulism. *Clin Infect Dis*. 2005;41(8):1167–1173.
186. Leclair D, Fung J, Isaac-Renton JL, et al. Foodborne botulism in Canada. 1985–2005. *Emerg Infect Dis*. 2013;19(6):961–968.
187. Woodruff BA, Griffin PM, McCroskey LM, et al. Clinical and laboratory comparison of botulism from toxin types A, B, and E in the United States. 1975–1988. *J Infect Dis*. 1992;166:1281–1286.
188. Rossetto O, Megighian A, Scorzeto M, Montecucco C. Botulinum neurotoxins. *Toxicon*. 2013;67(1):31–36.
189. Maselli R, Bakshi N. Botulism. *Muscle Nerve*. 2000;23:1137–1144.
190. Cherington M. Clinical spectrum of botulism. *Muscle Nerve*. 1998;21:701–710.
191. Donadia JA, Gangarosa EJ, Faich GA. Diagnosis and treatment of botulism. *J Infect Dis*. 1971;124:108–112.
192. Schmidt-Nowara WW, Samet JM, Rosario PA. Early and late pulmonary complications of botulism. *Arch Intern Med*. 1983;143:451–456.
193. Rapoport S, Watkins PB. Descending paralysis resulting from occult wound botulism. *Ann Neurol*. 1984;16:359–361.
194. Green MA, Heumann MA, Wehr HM, An outbreak of watermelon-borne pesticide toxicity. *Am J Public Health*. 1987; 77: 1431–1434.
195. Forss N, Ramstead R, Bäcklund T, Lindström M, Kolho E. Difficulties in diagnosing food-borne botulism. *Case Rep Neurol*. 2012;4:113–115.
196. Wakerley BR, Yuki N. Pharyngeal-cervical-brachial variant of Guillain-Barré syndrome. *J Neurol Neurosurg Psychiatry*. 2014;85(3):339–344.
197. Cherington M, Electrophysiologic methods as an aid in diagnosis of botulism: A review. *Muscle Nerve*. 1982;5:S28–S29.
198. Cornblath DR, Sladky JT, Sumner AJ: Clinical electrophysiology of infantile botulism. *Muscle Nerve*. 1983;6:448–452.
199. Gutmann L, Bodensteiner J, Gutierrez A. Electrodiagnosis of botulism (letter). *J Pediatr*. 1992;121:835.
200. Kongsaengdao S, Samintarapanya K, Rusmeechan S, Sithinamsuwan P, Tanprawate S. Electrophysiological diagnosis and patterns of response to treatment of botulism with neuromuscular respiratory failure. *Muscle Nerve*. 2009;40(2):2 71–278.
201. Oh SJ. Botulism: Electrophysiological studies. *Ann Neurol*. 1977;1:481–485.
202. Cherington M. Botulism: Ten year experience. *Arch Neurol*. 1974;30:432–437.
203. Vasa M, Baudendistel TE, Ohikhuare CE, et al. Clinical problem-solving. The eyes have it. *N Engl J Med*. 2012:367(10): 938–943.
204. Jones RG, Marks JD. Use of a new functional dual coating (FDC) assay to measure low toxin levels in serum and food samples following an outbreak of human botulism. *J Med Microbiol*. 2013;62:828–835.
205. Mazuet C, Ezan E, Volland H, Popoff MR, Becher F. Toxin detection in patients' sera by mass spectrometry during two outbreaks of type A botulism in France. *J Clin Microbiol*. 2012; 50(12):4091–4094.
206. Kuruoglu R, Cengiz B, Tokcaer A. Botulism with sensory symptoms diagnosed by neuromuscular transmission studies associated with edrophonium responsiveness. *Electromyogr Clin Neurophysiol*. 1996;36:477–480.
207. Athwal BS, Gale AN, Brett MM, Youl BD. Wound botulism in the UK. *Lancet*. 2001;357:234.
208. Hughes JM, Blumenthal JR, Merson MH, Lombard GL, Dowell VR Jr, Gangarosa EJ. Clinical features of types A and B foodborne botulism. *Ann Intern Med*. 1981;95:442–445.
209. Devers KG, Nine JS. Autopsy findings in botulinum toxin poisoning. *J Forensic Sci*. 2010;55(6):1649–1651.
210. Thurston D, Risk I, Hill MB, et al. Botulism from drinking prison-made alcohol - Utah. 2011. *MMWR Morb Mortal Wkly Rep*. 2012;61(39):782–784.
211. Simpson L. The life history of a botulinum toxin molecule. *Toxicon*. 2013;68:40–59.
212. Maselli RA, Burnett ME, Tonsgard JH. In vitro microelectrode study of neuromuscular transmission in a case of botulism. *Muscle Nerve*. 1992;15:273–276.
213. Maselli RA, Ellis W, Mandler RN, et al. Cluster of wound botulism in California: Clinical, electrophysiologic, and pathologic study. *Muscle Nerve*. 1997;20:1284–1295.
214. Centers for Disease Control and Prevention (CDC). Investigational heptavalent botulinum antitoxin (HBAT) to replace licensed botulinum antitoxin AB and investigational botulinum antitoxin E. *MMWR Morb Mortal Wkly Rep*. 2010;59(10):299.
215. Centers for Disease Control and Prevention (CDC). Notice of CDC's discontinuation of investigational pentavalent (ABCDE) botulinum toxoid vaccine for workers at risk for occupational exposure to botulinum toxins. *MMWR Morb Mortal Wkly Rep*. 2011;60(42):1454–1455.
216. Friggeri A, Marçon F, Marciniak S, et al. 3,4-Diaminopyridine may improve neuromuscular block during botulism. *Crit Care*. 2013;17(5):449.
217. Edlow JA, McGillicuddy DC. Tick paralysis. *Infect Dis Clin North Am*. 2008;22:397–413.
218. Grattan-Smith PJ. Morris JG, Johnston HM, et al. Clinical and neurophysiological features of tick paralysis. *Brain*. 1997; 120:1975–1987.

219. Diaz JH. A 60 year meta-analysis of tick paralysis in the United States: A predictable, preventable, and often misdiagnosed poisoning. *J Med Toxicol.* 2010;6:15–21.
220. Cooper BJ, Spence I. Temperature-dependent inhibition of evoked acetylcholine release in tick paralysis. *Nature.* 1976; 263(5579):693–695.
221. Emmons P, McLennan H. Failure of acetylcholine release in tick paralysis. *Nature.* 1959;183(4659):474–475.
222. Dworkin MS, Shoemaker PC, Anderson DE. Tick paralysis: 33 human cases in Washington state, 1946–1996. *Clin Infect Dis.* 1999;29:1435–1439.
223. Felz MW, Smith CD, Swift TR. Brief report: A 6-year-old girl with tick paralysis. *N Engl J Med.* 2000;342:90–94.
224. Schaumburg HH, Herskowitz S. The weak child–a cautionary tale. *N Engl J Med.* 2000;342:127–129.
225. Abbott KH. Tick paralysis: A review. *Proc Staff Meet Mayo Clin.* 1943;18:39–64.
226. Adler K. Tick paralysis. *Can Med Assoc J.* 1966;94:550–551.
227. Gorman RJ, Snead OC. Tick paralysis in three children: The diversity of neurologic presentations. *Clin Pediatr (Phila).* 1978;17:249–251.
228. Mongan PF. Tick toxicosis in North America. *J Fam Pract.* 1979;5:939–944.
229. Pearn J. Neuromuscular paralysis caused by tick envenomation. *J Neurol Sci.* 1977;34:37–42.
230. Rose I. A review of tick paralysis. *Can Med Assoc J.* 1954; 70:175–176.
231. Rose I, Gregson JD. Evidence of neuromuscular block in tick paralysis. *Nature.* 1956;178:95–96.
232. Stanbury JB, Huyck JH. Tick paralysis: A critical review. *Medicine.* 1945;24:219–242.
233. Wright SW, Trott AT. North American tickborne diseases. *Ann Emerg Med.* 1988;17:964–972.
234. Kincaid JC. Tick bite paralysis. *Semin Neurol.* 1990;10:32–34.
235. Swift TR, Ignacio OJ. Tick paralysis: Electrophysiologic studies. *Neurology.* 1975;25(12):1130–1133.
236. Masina S, Broady KW. Tick paralysis: Development of a vaccine. *Int J Parasitol.* 1999;29:535–541.
237. Krishnan AV, Lin CS, Reddel SW, McGRath R, Kiernan MC. Conduction block and impaired axonal function in tick paralysis. *Muscle Nerve.* 2009;40:358–362.
238. Pecina CA. Tick paralysis. *Semin Neurol.* 2012;32:531–532.
239. Cherington M, Snyder RD. Tick paralysis: Neurophysiologic studies. *N Engl J Med.* 1968;278:95–97.
240. DeBusk FL, O'Connor S. Tick toxicosis. *Pediatrics.* 1972;50: 328–329.
241. Donat JR, Donat JF. Tick paralysis with persistent weakness and electromyographic abnormalities. *Arch Neurol.* 1981;38:59–61.
242. Morris HH 3rd. Tick paralysis: Electrophysiologic measurements. *South Med J.* 1977;70:121–123.
243. Vedanarayanan VV, Evans OB, Subramony SH. Tick paralysis in children: Electrophysiology and possibility of misdiagnosis. *Neurology.* 2002;59:1088–1090.
244. Schmitt N, Bowmer EJ, Gregson JD. Tick paralysis in British Columbia. *Can Med Assoc J.* 1969;100:417–421.
245. Stone BF, Neish AL. Tick-paralysis toxoid: An effective immunizing agent against the toxin of Ixodes holocyclus. *Aust J Exp Biol Med Sci.* 1984;62:189–191.
246. Nakajima T, Ohta S, Morita H, Midorikawa Y, Mimura S, Yanagisawa N. Epidemiological study of sarin poisoning in Matsumoto City, Japan. *J Epidemiol.* 1998;8:33–41.
247. Buckley NA, Eddleston M, Li Y, Bevan M, Robertson J. Oximes for acute organophosphate pesticide poisoning (Review). *Cochrane Database Syst Rev.* 2011;(2):CD005085.
248. Eddleston M, Buckley NA, Eyer P, Dawson AH. Management of acute organophosphorus pesticide poisoning. *Lancet.* 2008; 371:597–607.
249. Jokanović M, Prostran M. Pyridinium oximes as cholinesterase reactivators. Structure-activity relationship and efficacy in the treatment of poisoning with organophosphorus compounds. *Curr Med Chem.* 2009;16(17):2177–2188.
250. Janković M. Medical treatment of acute poisoning with organophosphorus and carbamate pesticides. *Toxicol Lett.* 2009;190(2):107–115.
251. Sungur M, Güven M. Intensive care management of organophosphate insecticide poisoning. *Crit Care.* 2001;5:211–215.
252. Besser R, Gutmann L, Dillman U, Weilemann LS, Hoff HC. End-plate dysfunction in acute organophosphate intoxication. *Neurology.* 1989;39:561–567.
253. Green MA, Heumann MA, Wehr HM, et al. An outbreak of watermelon-borne pesticide toxicity. *Am J Public Health.* 1987;77:1431–1434.
254. Eddleston M, Eyer P, Worek F, et al. Pralidoxime in acute organophosphate poisoning – a randomised controlled trial. *PLoS Med.* 2009;6(6):e10000104.
255. Kularatne SA, Senanayake N. Venomous snake bites, scorpions, and spiders. *Handb Clin Neurol.* 2014;120:987–1001.
256. Del Brutto OH. Neurological effects of venomous bites and stings: Snakes, spiders, and scorpions. *Handb Clin Neurol.* 2013;114:349–368.
257. White J. Bites and stings from venomous animals: A global overview. *Ther Drug Monit.* 2000;22(1):65–68.
258. Faiz A, Ghose A, Ahsan F, et al. The greater black krait (Bungarus niger), a newly recognized cause of neuro-myotoxic snake bite envenoming in Bangladesh. *Brain.* 2010;133:3183–3193.
259. Singh G, Pannu HS, Chawla PS, Malhotra S. Neuromuscular transmission failure due to common krait (Bungarus Caeruleus) envenomation. *Muscle Nerve.* 1999;22:1637–1643.
260. Tormoehlen L. Toxins and disorders of neuromuscular transmission. Annual Meeting of the American Academy of Neurology. 2013
261. Norris RL, Pfalzgraf RR, Gavin Laing G. Death following coral snake bite in the United States – First documented case (with ELISA confirmation of envenomation) in over 40 years. *Toxicon.* 2009;53(6):693–697.
262. Pettigrew LC, Glass JP. Neurologic complication of a coral snake bite. *Neurology.* 1985;35:589–592.
263. Allen C. Arachnid envenomations. *Emerg Med Clin North Am.* 1992;10(2):269–298.
264. Clark RF, Wethern-Kestner S, Vance MV, Gerkin R. Clinical presentation of black widow spider envenomation: A review of 163 cases. *Ann Emerg Med.* 1992;21:782–787.
265. Howard BD, Gundersen CB Jr. Effects and mechanisms of polypeptide neurotoxins that act presynaptically. *Annu Rev Pharmacol Toxicol.* 1980;20:307–336.
266. Russel FE. Venomous arthropods. *Vet Hum Toxicol.* 1991; 33:505–508.
267. Swift TR. Disorders of neuromuscular transmission other than myasthenia gravis. *Muscle Nerve.* 1981;4:334–353.
268. Golcuk Y, Velibey Y, Gonullu H, Sahin M, Kocabas E. Acute toxic fulminant myocarditis after a black widow spider

envenomation: Case report and literature review. *Clin Toxicol (Phila)*. 2013;51(3):191–192.
269. Auerbach PS. Marine envenomations. *N Engl J Med*. 1991;325 (7):486–493.
270. Balhara KS, Stolbach A. Marine envenomations. *Emerg Med Clin North Am*. 2014;32(1):223–243.
271. Kerr LM, Yoshikami D. A venom peptide with a novel presynaptic blocking action. *Nature*. 1984;308:282–284.
272. Olivera BM, Gray WR, Zeikus R, et al. Peptide neurotoxins from fish-hunting cone snails. *Science*. 1985;230:1338–1343.
273. Sano K, Enomoto K, Maeno T. Effects of synthetic ω-conotoxin, a new type of $Ca2^+$ antagonist, on frog and mouse neuromuscular transmission. *Eur J Pharmacol*. 1987;141:235–241.
274. Hunter JM. New neuromuscular blocking drugs. *N Engl J Med*. 1995;332(95):1691–1699.
275. Gooch JL, Moore MH, Ryser DK. Prolonged paralysis after neuromuscular junction blockade: Case report and electrodiagnostic findings. *Arch Phys Med Rehabil*. 1993;74:1007–1011.
276. Riddings LW, Jackson CE, Rogers S, et al. Electrophysiologic evidence for neuromuscular blockade following prolonged paralysis with curare-like agents. *Muscle Nerve*. 1992;15:1205–1206.
277. Yee WC, Lopate G, Peeples D, et al. Postparalysis paralysis syndrome: Sequential electrodiagnostic studies. *Muscle Nerve*. 1992;15:1206.
278. Howard JF Jr. Adverse drug effects on neuromuscular transmission. *Semin Neurol*. 1990;10:89–102.
279. Atchison WD, Adgate L, Beaman CM. Effects of antibiotics on uptake of calcium into isolated nerve terminals. *J Pharmacol Exp Ther*. 1988;245:394–401.
280. Argov Z, Mastaglia FL. Disorders of neuromuscular transmission caused by drugs. *N Engl J Med*. 1979;301:409–413.
281. Klopstock T. Drug-induced myasthenic syndromes. www.medlink.com. 2009.
282. Bever CT Jr, Chang HW, Penn AS, Jaffe IA, Bock E. Penicillamine-induced myasthenia gravis: Effects of penicillamine on acetylcholine receptor. *Neurology*. 1982;32:1077.
283. Albers JW, Hodach RJ, Kimmel DW, Treacy WL. Penicillamine-associated myasthenia gravis. *Neurology*. 1980;30:1246–1249.
284. Albers JW, Beals CA, Levine SP. Neuromuscular transmission in rheumatoid arthritis, with and without penicillamine treatment. *Neurology*. 1981;31:1562–1564.
285. Russell AS, Lindstrom JM. Penicillamine-induced myasthenia gravis associated with antibodies to acetylcholine receptor. *Neurology*. 1978;28:847–849.
286. Batocchi AP, Evoli A, Servidei S, Palmisani MT, Apollo F, Tonali P. Myasthenia gravis during interferon-alpha therapy. *Neurology*. 1995;45:382–383.
287. Andonopoulos AP, Terzis E, Tsibri E, Papasteriades CA, Pappetropoulos T. D-Penicillamine induced myasthenia gravis in rheumatoid arthritis: An unpredictable common occurrence? *Clin Rheumatol*. 1994;13:568–588.
288. Bruggeman W, Herath H, Ferbert A. Follow-up and immunologic findings in drug-induced myasthenia. *Med Klin*. 1996;91:268–271.
289. Buchnall RC, Dixon A, St J, Glick EN, Woodland J, Zutshi DW. Myasthenia gravis associated with penicillamine treatment for rheumatoid arthritis. *Br Med J*. 1975;1:600–602.
290. Drosos AA, Christou L, Galanopoulou V, Tzioufas AG, Tsiakou EK. D-Penicillamine induced myasthenia gravis: Clinical, serological and genetic findings. *Clin Exp Rheumatol*. 1993;11:387–391.
291. Fawcett PR, McLachlan SM, Nicholson LV, Argov Z, Mastaglia FL. D-Penicillamine-associated myasthenia gravis: Immunological and electrophysiological studies. *Muscle Nerve*. 1982;5:328–334.
292. Liu GT, Bienfang DC. Penicillamine-induced ocular myasthenia gravis in rheumatoid arthritis. *J Clin Neurol Ophthalmol*. 1990;10:201–205.
293. Masters CL, Dawkikns RL, Zilko PJ, Simpson JA, Leedman RJ. Penicillamine-associated myasthenia gravis, antiacetylcholine receptor and antistriational antibodies. *Am J Med*. 1977;63:689–694.
294. Raynauld JP, Lee YS, Kornfeld P, Fries JF. Unilateral ptosis as an initial manifestation of D-penicillamine induced myasthenia gravis. *J Rheumatol*. 1993;20:1592–1593.
295. Vincent A, Newsom-Davis J, Martin V. Anti-acetylcholine receptor antibodies in D-penicillamine-associated myasthenia gravis [letter]. *Lancet*. 1978;1:1254.
296. Vincent A, Newsom-Davis J. Acetylcholine receptor antibody characteristics in myasthenia gravis. II. Patients with penicillamine-induced myasthenia or idiopathic myasthenia of recent onset. *Clin Exp Immunol*. 1982;49:266–272.
297. Lensch E, Faust J, Nix WA, Wandel E. Myasthenia gravis after interferon-alpha treatment. *Muscle Nerve*. 1996;19:927–928.
298. Mase G, Zorzon M, Biasutti E, et al. Development of myasthenia gravis during interferon-alpha treatment for anti-HCV positive chronic hepatitis. *J Neurol Neurosurg Psychiatry*. 1996;60:348–349.
299. Perez A, Perella M, Pastor E, Cano M, Secudero J. Myasthenia gravis induced by alpha-interferon therapy. *Am J Hematol*. 1995;49:365–366.
300. Piccolo G, Franciotta D, Versino M, Alfonsi E, Lombardi M. Poma G. Myasthenia gravis in a patient with chronic active hepatitis C during interferon-alpha treatment. *J Neurol Neurosurg Psychiatry*. 1996;60:348.
301. Adams RJ, Rivner MH, Salazar J, Swift TR. Effects of oral calcium antagonists on neuromuscular transmission. *Neurology*. 1984;34 (Suppl 1) 132–133.
302. Streib EW. Adverse effects of magnesium salt cathartics in a patient with the myasthenic syndrome (Lambert–Eaton syndrome). *Ann Neurol*. 1977;2:175–176.
303. Bashuk RG, Krendel DA. Myasthenia gravis presenting as weakness after magnesium administration. *Muscle Nerve*. 1990;13:708–712.
304. Castlebaum AR, Donofrio PD, Walker FO, Troost BT. Laxative abuse causing hypermagnesemia, quadriparesis, and neuromuscular junction defect. *Neurology*. 1989;39:746–747.
305. Krendel DA. Hypermagnesemia and neuromuscular transmission. *Semin Neurol*. 1990;10:42–45.
306. Swift TR. Weakness from magnesium containing cathartics. *Muscle Nerve*. 1979;2:295–298.
307. Flowers CJ Jr. Magnesium in obstetrics. *Am J Obstet Gynecol*. 1965;91:763–776.
308. Kaire GH. Isolation of tick paralysis toxin from Ixodes holocyclus. *Toxicon*. 1966;4:91–97.

CHAPTER 27

Muscular Dystrophies

Muscular dystrophies are hereditary, progressive muscle diseases in which there is necrosis of muscle tissue and replacement by connective and fatty tissues, which helps to distinguish them from other hereditary myopathies. Before discussing specific types of muscular dystrophies, it is important to have an understanding of the relevant muscle proteins that are affected in the various dystrophies. The different forms of muscular dystrophies result from mutations affecting proteins localizable to the sarcolemma, myonuclei, basement membrane and extracellular matrix surrounding muscle fibers, sarcomere and nonstructural enzymatic proteins.[1,2]

▶ DYSTROPHIN–GLYCOPROTEIN COMPLEX AND RELATED PROTEINS

DYSTROPHIN

The identification and characterization of dystrophin as the abnormal gene product in Duchenne and Becker muscular dystrophies (DMD and BMD) were the major discoveries underlying our current understanding of muscular dystrophies (Fig. 27-1).[1–3] Dystrophin is located on the cytoplasmic face of skeletal and cardiac muscle membrane and constitutes approximately 5% of the sarcolemmal cytoskeletal proteins. Dystrophin is a rod-shaped molecule composed of four domains.[3] The amino-terminal domain binds to the cytoskeletal filamentous actin. The second domain bears similarity to spectrin and provides structural integrity to red blood cells. The third domain is a cysteine-rich region, and the fourth domain is the carboxy terminal. The cysteine-rich domain and the first half of the carboxy-terminal domain of dystrophin are important in linking dystrophin to β-dystroglycan and the glycoproteins that span the sarcolemma.

Dystrophin is also present in the brain where it localizes subcellularly to the postsynaptic density, a disc-shaped structure beneath the postsynaptic membrane in chemical synapses. The postsynaptic density may play an important role in synaptic function by stabilizing the synaptic structure, anchoring postsynaptic receptors, and transducing extracellular matrix–cell signals.

DYSTROPHIN-ASSOCIATED PROTEINS/GLYCOPROTEINS

Dystrophin is tightly associated with a large oligomeric complex of sarcolemmal proteins referred to as the dystrophin–glycoprotein complex (Fig. 27-1).[3–6] Mutations in the various genes, which encode for the different proteins of the dystrophin–glycoprotein complex, are now known to be responsible for many forms of muscular dystrophy (Table 27-1). In addition to dystrophin, the dystrophin–glycoprotein complex is composed of an entirely cytoplasmic group of proteins referred to as the syntrophin complex, the dystroglycan complex, and the sarcoglycan complex (Fig. 27-1).

The syntrophin complex binds to the carboxy terminus of dystrophin and is composed of three distinct 59-kD dystrophin-associated proteins (DAPs), which are encoded by separate genes. α-syntrophin is expressed only in muscle and the gene has been localized to chromosome 20q11.2. β1- and β2-syntrophin are more widely expressed, and their genes have been localized to chromosomes 8q23–24 and 16q22–23, respectively. Dystrobrevin is encoded on chromosome 2p22–23 and is a cytoplasmic protein, which binds to the syntrophin complex and to the C terminus of dystrophin.

The dystroglycan complex is composed of α- and β-dystroglycan. β-dystroglycan spans the sarcolemmal membrane and has a cytoplasmic tail that binds to dystrophin, while the extracellular tail binds α-dystroglycan. α-dystroglycan, which is entirely extracellular, also binds to α-laminin (merosin), a basal lamina protein. Of note, a gene located on chromosome 3p21 encodes for both the α- and β-dystroglycan. Importantly, α-dystroglycan undergoes N-linked and extensive O-linked glycosylation, which appears to be important for normal binding to merosin and perhaps other extracellular matrix proteins.[7]

The sarcoglycan complex includes four membrane-spanning proteins: (1) α-sarcoglycan (previously known as adhalin), (2) β-sarcoglycan, (3) γ-sarcoglycan, and (4) δ-sarcoglycan. In addition, there is a 25-kD transmembrane protein, sarcospan, which colocalizes with the sarcoglycan complex. The sarcoglycan complex associates with the cysteine-rich domain and/or the first half of the carboxy terminal of dystrophin directly or indirectly via the dystroglycan complex. The exact relationship between the sarcoglycan complex and the dystrophin–dystroglycan complex is still unclear. Mutations in the various sarcoglycan genes are responsible for limb-girdle muscular dystrophies (LGMDs) 2C, 2D, 2D, and 2F.

MEROSIN/LAMININ

The basal lamina surrounding each muscle fiber closely adheres to the sarcolemma and is composed of type I and IV collagen, heparan sulfate, proteoglycan, entactin, fibronectin,

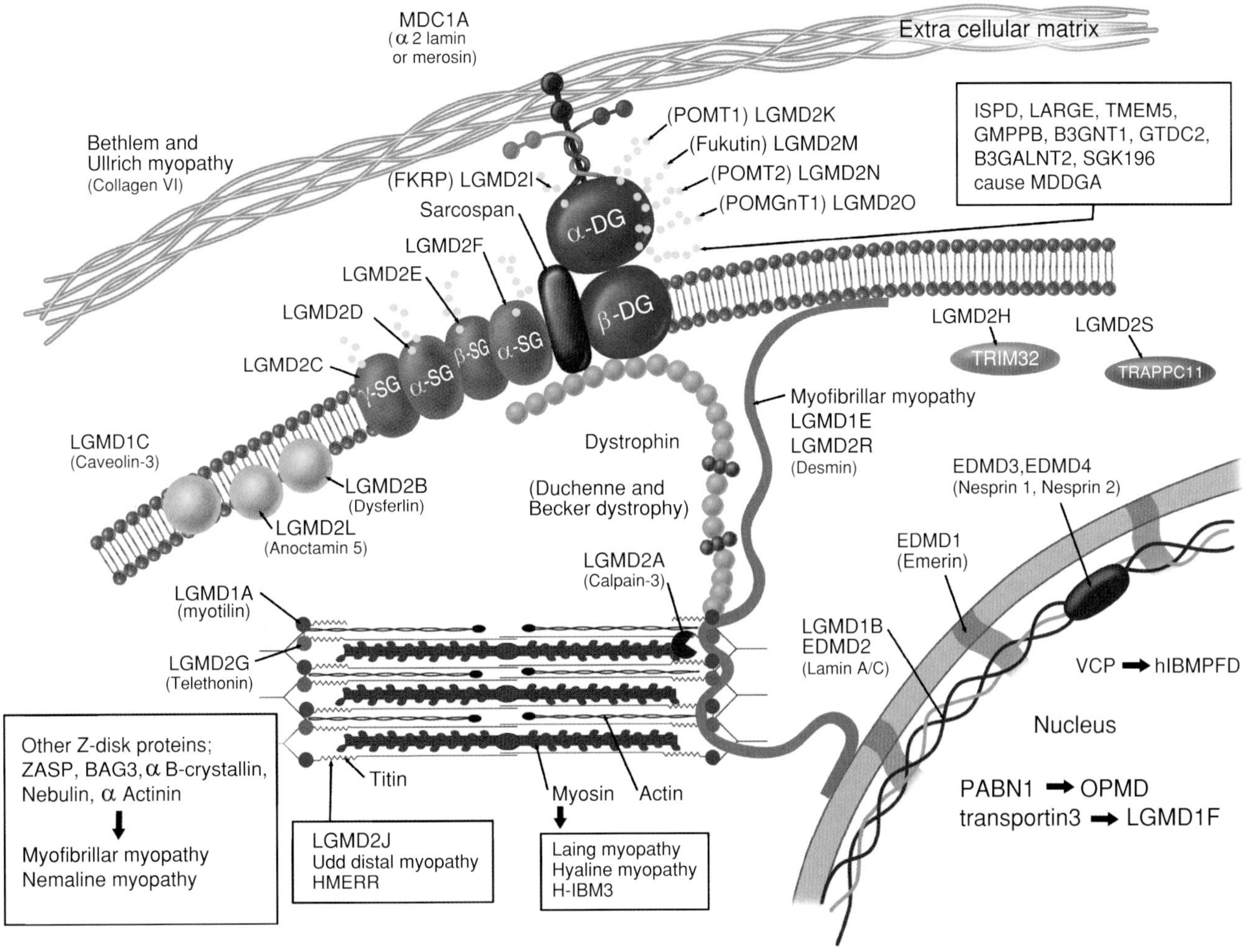

Figure 27-1. Proteins involved in muscular dystrophies. This schematic shows the location of various sarcolemmal, sarcomeric, nuclear, and enzymatic proteins associated with muscular dystrophies. The diseases associated with mutations in the genes responsible for encoding these proteins are shown in boxes. Dystrophin, via its interaction with the dystroglycan complex, connects the actin cytoskeleton to the extracellular matrix. Extracellularly, the sarcoglycan complex interacts with biglycan, which connects this complex to the dystroglycan complex and the extracellular matrix collagen. Various enzymes are important in the glycosylation of the α-dystroglycan and mediate its binding to the extracellular matrix and usually cause a congenital muscular dystrophy with severe brain and eye abnormalities, but may cause milder LGMD phenotype. Mutations in genes that encode for sarcomeric and Z-disc proteins cause forms of LGMD and distal myopathies (including myofibrillar myopathy, forms of hereditary inclusion body myopathy) as well as nemaline rod myopathy and other "congenital" myopathies. Mutations affecting nuclear membrane proteins are responsible for most forms of EDMD. Mutations in other nuclear genes cause other forms of dystrophy.

and laminin. Laminin is a large flexible heterotrimer composed of three different but homologous α, β, and γ chains, held together by disulfide bonds. There are five different α chains, three β chains, and two γ chains that have been characterized. The major isoform of laminin heavy chains in muscle is laminin-2, which is composed of α2, β1, and γ1 chains. Muscle also contains laminin-4, composed of α2, β2, and γ1 subunits. Merosin is the collective name for laminins that share a common α2 chain. α-dystroglycan binds specifically to laminin-2, but not to the other extracellular components (Fig. 27-1). Ligands for the sarcoglycan complex are unknown, but it has been postulated that the complex is directly or indirectly linked to laminin-4.[8]

Merosin is also expressed in the endoneurial basement membrane surrounding the myelin sheath of peripheral nerves.[9] Likewise, α- and β-dystroglycan are found in peripheral nerves. Expression of α- and β-dystroglycan is restricted to the outer membrane of Schwann cells and is not present in the inner membrane or on compact myelin. Transmembrane β-dystroglycan anchors extracellular α-dystroglycan to the outer membrane of Schwann cells and myelin. As in muscle, merosin serves as a ligand in the Schwann cell dystroglycan complex by binding to α-dystroglycan. This complex appears to have a role in peripheral myelinogenesis. Mutations involving the merosin gene not only result in a form of congenital muscular dystrophy (MDC), but they also

► TABLE 27-1. **MOLECULAR DEFECTS OF MUSCULAR DYSTROPHIES**

Disease	Inheritance	Chromosome	Affected Protein
X-LINKED DYSTROPHIES			
Duchenne/Becker	XR	Xp21	Dystrophin
Emery–Dreifuss	XR	Xq28	Emerin
Scapuloperoneal/reducing body myopathy	XR	Xq26.3	Four-and-a-half LIM domain 1 (FHL1)
LIMB-GIRDLE DYSTROPHIES (LGMD)			
LGMD1A	AD	5q22.3-31.3	Myotilin
LGMD1B	AD	1q11-21	Lamin A and C
LGMD1C	AD	3p25	Caveolin-3
LGMD1D	AD	6q23	DNAJB6
LGMD1E	AD	2q35	Desmin
LGMD1F	AD	7q32	Transportin 3
LGMD2A	AR	15q15.1–21.1	Calpain 3
LGMD2B	AR	2p13	Dysferlin
LGMD2C	AR	13q12	γ-sarcoglycan
LGMD2D	AR	17q12–21.3	α-sarcoglycan
LGMD2E	AR	4q12	β-sarcoglycan
LGMD2F	AR	5q33–34	δ-sarcoglycan
LGMD2G	AR	17q11–12	Telethonin
LGMD2H	AR	9q31–33	E3-ubiquitin-ligase (TRIM 32)
LGMD2I	AR	19q13	Fukutin-related protein (FKRP)
LGMD2J	AR	2q31	Titin
LGMD2K	AR	9q31	POMT1
LGMD2L	AR	11p14.3	Anoctamin 5
LGMD2M	AR	9q31–33	Fukutin
LGMD2N	AR	14q24	POMT2
LGMD2O	AR	1p32	POMGnT1
LGMD2P	AR	3p21	α-Dystroglycan
LGMD2Q	AR	8q24	Plectin 1
LGMD2R	AR	2q35	Desmin
LGMD2S	AR	4q35.1	TRAPPC11
CONGENITAL MUSCULAR DYSTROPHIES (MDC)			
MDC1 A	AR	6q22–23	Laminin-α_2 chain
α_7-Integrin-related MDC	AR	12q13	α_7-Integrin
MDC1 C	AR	19q13	FKRP
MDDGA1	AR	9q31	POMT1
MDDGA2	AR	14q24	POMT2
MDDGA3	AR	1p32	POMGnT1
MDDGA4	AR	9q31–33	Fukutin
MDDGA5	AR	19q13	FKRP
MDDGA6	AR	22q12.3	LARGE
MDDGA7	AR	7p21.2	ISPD
MDDGA8	AR	3p22.1	GTDC2
MDDGA10	AR	12q14.2	TMEM5
MDDGA11	AR	3p22.1	B3GALNT2
MDDGA12	AR	8p11.21	SGK196
MDDGA13	AR	11q13	B3GNT1
MDDGA13	AR	3p21.31	GMPPB
Rigid spine syndrome	AR	1p35–36	Selenoprotein N1
Ullrich/Bethlem	AR/AD	21q22.3 and 2q37	Collagens 6A1, 6A2, and 6A3

▶ TABLE 27-1. (CONTINUED)

Disease	Inheritance	Chromosome	Affected Protein
DISTAL DYSTROPHIES/MYOPATHIES			
Welander	AD	2p13	TIA1
Udd	AD	2q31	Titin
Markesbery-Griggs	AD	10q22.3–23.2	ZASP
Nonaka	AR	9p1-q1	GNE
Miyoshi 1	AR	2p13	Dysferlin
Miyoshi 3	AR	11p14.3	Anoctamin 5
Laing (MPD1)	AD	14q11	MyHC 7
Williams	AD	7q32	Filamin C
Distal myopathy with vocal cord and pharyngeal weakness (VCPDM or MPD2)	AD	5q31	Matrin 3
OTHER DYSTROPHIES			
Facioscapulohumeral type 1	AD	4q35	Deletion in D4Z4 region with secondary increase in DUX4
Facioscapulohumeral type 2	AD	18p11.32	SMCHD1 with secondary increase in DUX4
Scapuloperoneal dystrophy	AD	2q35	Desmin
	AD	14q11	MyHC 7
	XR	Xq26.3	Four-and-a-half LIM domain 1 (FHL1) protein
Emery–Dreifuss type 3	AD	6q24	Nesprin-1
Emery–Dreifuss type 4	AD	14q23	Nesprin-2
Emery–Dreifuss type 5	AD	3p25.1	TMEM43
Oculopharyngeal	AD	14q11.2–13	PABP2
Myotonic dystrophy 1	AD	19q13.3	DMPK
Myotonic dystrophy 2	AD	3q21	ZNF9
Myofibrillar myopathy	AD	5q22.3–31.3	Myotilin
	AD	10q22.3–23.2	ZASP
	AD	7q32.1	Filamin-c
	AD	11q21–23	αB-crystallin
	AD/AR	2q35	Desmin
	AR	1p36	Selenoprotein N1
	AD	10q25–26	BAG-3
HEREDITARY INCLUSION BODY MYOPATHIES			
AR h-IBM	AR		GNE
h-IBMPFD	AD		VCP
h-IBM 3	AD		MyHC IIa

AD, autosomal dominant; *AR,* autosomal recessive; *B3GALNT2*, Beta-1,4-N-acetlyglucosaminyltransferase; *B3GNT1*, beta-1,3-N-acetylglucosaminyltransferase 1; *FRG1*, FSHD region gene 1; *FTD,* frontotemporal dementia; *GMPPB*, GDP-mannose pyrophosphorylase B; *GNE*, UDP-*N*-acetylglucosamine 2-epimerase/*N*-acetylmannosamine kinase; *GTDC2*,O-linked mannose beta-1,4-N-acetylglucosaminyltransferase; *h-IBM*, hereditary inclusion body myopathy; *h-IBMPFD*, hereditary inclusion body myopathy, Paget disease and frontotemporal dementia; *ISPD*, isoprenoid synthase domain-containing protein; *MDDGA1*, Muscular dystrophy–dystroglycanopathy with brain and eye anomalies (type A); *MyHC,* myosin heavy chain; *POMGnT1*, *O*-mannose-â-1,2-*N*-acetylglucosaminyl transferase; *POMT1*, *O*-mannosyltransferase; *SGK196*, protein-O-mannose kinase; *TIA1*, T-cell restricted intracellular antigen; *TMEM5*, transmembrane protein 5; *VCP,* valosin containing protein; *ZASP,* Z-band alternatively spliced PDZ motif-containing protein.

are associated with mild dysmyelination in the central and peripheral nervous systems.

INTEGRINS

Integrins are transmembrane, heterodimeric (α/β) receptors, which play key roles in establishing linkages between the extracellular matrix and the cytoskeleton, as well as in transducing extracellular matrix–cell signals.[10] Integrins are important in cell adhesion, migration, differentiation, proliferation, and cytoskeletal organization. The major integrin expressed throughout the sarcolemma in mature muscle fibers is α7β 1D. Studies have demonstrated that α7β 1D integrin binds to merosin in skeletal muscle, which appears to be as important as the linkage of α-dystroglycan to merosin in providing structural stability (Fig. 27-1). Mutations of the α7 subunit lead to abnormal binding of merosin to integrin and cause some forms of MDC.

UTROPHIN (DYSTROPHIN-RELATED PROTEIN)

Utrophin is an autosomal homolog of dystrophin. It is ubiquitously expressed but is localized exclusively at the neuromuscular junction in normal skeletal muscle. Utrophin associates with DAPs, suggesting that the utrophin–glycoprotein complex plays a role in the formation and integrity of the neuromuscular junction. Upregulation of utrophin is evident in the dystrophinopathies, perhaps as a compensatory mechanism.

▶ OTHER SARCOLEMMAL PROTEINS

DYSFERLIN

Dysferlin is another cytoskeletal protein present in skeletal and cardiac muscles. It is located predominantly on the subsarcolemmal surface of the muscle membrane, but it has a small transmembrane spanning tail (Fig. 27-1). The protein does not appear to be directly connected to the dystrophin–glycoprotein complex. The function of dysferlin is not entirely known. Dysferlin may have a role in membrane fusion and repair by regulating vesicle fusion with the membrane.[11,12] In addition, dysferlin may assist in stabilizing the sarcolemmal membrane or in signal transduction.[13,14] Mutations affecting the dysferlin gene result in LGMD2B and a form of Miyoshi type distal myopathy.

CAVEOLAE

Caveolae are 10–100-nm invaginations in the sarcolemma, derived by the oligomerization of approximately 14–16 caveolin-3 monomers that form a scaffolding complex of proteins and lipids (Fig. 27-1).[15,16] Caveolin-3 co-fractionates with the dystrophin–glycoprotein complex but is thought to be part of a discrete complex. It does not directly bind to dystrophin or the sarcoglycans but does apparently interact with dysferlin. Caveolin-3 is necessary for the proper formation of T tubules and may assist in organization of signaling complexes, calcium channels (i.e., dihydropyridine and ryanodine receptors), and sodium channels. Mutations in the *CAV3* gene encoding for caveolin-3 are responsible for causing LGMD 1C, rippling muscle disease, a form of distal myopathy, and some cases of idiopathic hyper-CK-emia.[17,18] Cavin is another protein that localizes to caveolae that when abnormally expressed leads to a myopathy.

▶ SARCOMERIC PROTEINS

In addition to the above sarcolemmal and related proteins, there are a number of important proteins that compose and support the sarcomere (Fig. 27-1). The major contractile myofibrillar proteins are the thick and thin filaments. The main component of the thick filaments is a polymer of myosin. A single thick filament is composed of nearly 300 myosin molecules. Each individual myosin molecule, in turn, consists of a single long "tail" attached to two "head" portions that project out from the tail. The head and its projecting part are referred to as a cross-bridge, which has two flexible hinges: one at the head/arm interface and the other at the arm/filament interface. The entire myosin filament is twisted about a central axis, allowing the cross-bridges to extend longitudinally and circumferentially 360°. The head or the myosin heavy chain (MyHC) includes ATP-binding sites that acts as an ATPase and also an actin-binding region. The energy liberated by this process is used to maintain the cross-bridge in the extended or "cocked" position. There are three major MyHC isoforms that are expressed in human skeletal muscle (type I, MyH7, expressed in type 1 fibers; IIa, MyH2, expressed in 2A fibers; and IIx, MyH1, expressed in 2B fibers).[19] Mutations in genes that encode for various MyHC isoforms cause various myopathies and cardiomyopathies.

The thin filament is composed of three subcomponents: actin, tropomyosin, and troponin. Polymerized globular or G-actin molecules form two helical strands of filamentous or F-actin. Each G-actin molecule binds one molecule of ADP. Two chains of tropomyosin molecules wind loosely within the helical structure of the F-actin. The tropomyosin molecules overlie "active sites" on the actin molecules that link with the myosin heads forming the cross-bridges. The third major subcomponent of the thin filament, troponin, consists of three globular proteins: troponin I, T, and C. Troponin I binds strongly to actin, troponin T is attached to tropomyosin, while troponin C has a large affinity for calcium. The troponin complex attaches the tropomyosin molecules to the actin molecules, thereby forming the complete thin filament. The interaction between the myosin cross-bridges and actin filaments causes the muscle fiber to shorten or contract because the above-noted filaments slide past each other.

One end of the actin filaments is firmly anchored to the Z-disc and the other end projects out between myosin filaments. These Z-discs extend from myofibril to myofibril across the diameter of a muscle fiber. The region of muscle or myofibril between two Z-discs is called a sarcomere. The major protein of the Z-disc is α-actinin. Nebulin is a giant protein, which is attached to α-actinin at the Z-disc and spans the entire length of the thin filament. There are two nebulin molecules for every thin filament. Desmin is an intermediate-size filament that encircles the Z-disc and helps to link the Z-disc to the sarcolemma, myonuclei, and adjacent myofibers. The cytoplasmic heat-shock protein, α B-crystallin, interacts with desmin in the assembly and stabilization of the Z-disc. Syncoilin, together with plectin, may also link desmin filaments to the Z-disc.[20] Furthermore, ZASP (Z-band alternatively spliced PDZ motif-containing protein) binds to α-actinin and assists in cross-linking thin filaments of adjacent sarcomeres.[21]

Other filamentous proteins are also important in providing stability to the sarcomere (Fig. 27-1). The giant protein titin (also known as connectin) is attached to the Z-disc and spans from the M-line to the Z-line of the sarcomere. Titin serves to connect the myosin filaments to the Z-disc. Telethonin is another sarcomeric protein present in skeletal and cardiac muscles. It colocalizes with titin to the Z-discs and along the thick filaments. Telethonin is also linked with myotilin, which in turn interacts with α-actinin and actin. In addition, filamin-c binds actin and is also involved in the formation of the Z-disc. Filamin-c also binds γ- and δ-sarcoglycan at the sarcolemma and may also play a role involved in signaling pathways from the sarcolemma to the myofibril.[22]

The interaction of all these sarcomeric proteins and Z-disc is important in myofibrillogenesis. As will be discussed, mutations affecting the genes encoding for these various sarcomeric proteins are responsible for causing different dystrophies, congenital myopathies, and inherited cardiomyopathies.

The myofibrils are surrounded by intracellular fluid called sarcoplasm. Within the sarcoplasm lies large numbers of mitochondria required for energy and other organelles. Within the sarcoplasma and surrounding the myofibrils there is an intricate series of channels called the sarcoplasmic reticulum. Longitudinal sarcoplasmic reticulum channels terminate along large terminal cisternae at either end of the sarcomere. T tubules closely associate with terminal cisternae. Two terminal cisternae are in close association with one T tubule forming a so-called triad. The T tubule conducts action potentials into the terminal cisternae and the depths of the muscle. The action potentials open voltage-gated L-type calcium channels, called the dihydropyridine receptor, located on the sarcolemmal membrane. The dihydropyridine receptor also serves as a voltage sensor for the calcium release channel, the ryanodine receptor, located on the sarcoplasmic reticulum. Mutations in these genes are responsible for hypokalemic periodic paralysis, malignant hyperthermia, and central core disease. In addition, there is a separate calcium reuptake channel located on the sarcoplasmic reticulum called sarcoplasmic reticulum calcium-ATPase. Mutations in the gene encoding for this protein (*SERCA1*) lead to Brody disease which is characterized by impaired relaxation of muscles.

▶ NUCLEAR PROTEINS

Emerin is a member of the nuclear lamina-associated protein (LAP) family and is located on the inner nuclear membranes of skeletal, cardiac, and smooth muscle fibers (Fig. 27-1).[23–26] The nuclear lamina is a multimeric matrix composed of a complex of intermediate-sized filaments (lamins A, B, and C), which associates with the nucleoplasmic surface of the inner nuclear membrane. Of note, lamins A and C are produced by alternative splicing of a single gene. Emerin is attached to the inner nuclear membrane through its carboxy-terminal tail, while the remainder of the protein projects into the nucleoplasm. The lamins bind to emerin, specific lamin receptors, and perhaps other LAPs located on the inner nuclear membrane. This complex of proteins is important in the organization and structural integrity of the nuclear membrane. In addition, LAPs, lamin receptors, and the lamins bind to chromatin and promote its attachment to the nuclear membrane. Nesprin 1 and 2 are located in the outer and inner nuclear membrane and bind to actin and interact with emerin and the lamins to provide support to the nuclear membrane. Abnormalities in these nuclear envelop proteins apparently disrupt the structure of the nuclear membrane, the organization of interphase chromatin, and perhaps also signal transduction between the nucleus and the sarcoplasm.[27,28] Mutations in the gene that code for emerin are responsible for X-linked Emery–Dreifuss muscular dystrophy (EDMD), while mutations involving the gene that encodes lamin A/C cause autosomal-dominant EDMD/limb-girdle dystrophy 1B. In addition, mutations in the genes that encode for nesprin 1 and 2 as well as transmembrane protein 43 also cause an autosomal dominant form of EDMD.

Valosin-containing protein (VCP) localizes to nuclei around nucleoli and is associated with a variety of cellular activities, including cell-cycle control, membrane fusion, and the ubiquitin–proteasome degradation pathway. It may also have a role in RNA processing. Mutations in the VCP gene cause hereditary inclusion body myopathy (h-IBM) with Paget disease and frontotemporal dementia (h-IBMPFD), in addition to a form of familial amyotrophic lateral sclerosis. The gene that encodes for another nuclear protein, poly(A) binding protein nuclear 1 (PABN1) is mutated in oculopharyngeal muscular dystrophy (OPMD).

▶ ENZYMATIC PROTEINS

Calpain-3 is a muscle-specific, calcium-dependent, nonlysosomal, proteolytic enzyme present in muscle. The pathophysiologic mechanism of how mutations involving this enzyme result in a dystrophic process is not completely understood. Calpain-3 exists in both the cytosol and the nuclei of skeletal muscle fibers (Fig. 27-1), where it may be directly involved or may participate in the activation of other enzymes involved in muscle metabolism. Mutations in the calpain-3 gene are responsible for LGMD 2A.

Tripartite motif-containing protein 32, also known as E3-ubiquitine ligase, is encoded by *TRIM32*. This enzyme may function by tagging proteins (e.g., ubiquitination) for degradation by proteasomes (Fig. 27-1). Mutations in *TRIM32* cause LGMD 2H.[29]

Fukutin is a glycosyltransferase, and its deficiency is associated with abnormal glycosylation of α-dystroglycan and results in Fukuyama congenital muscular dystrophy and LGMD2M (Fig. 27-1). Mutations in the fukutin-related protein gene (*FKRP*), are found in some patients with MDC with normal merosin (MDC 1C) and in LGMD 2I.[30–32] Interestingly, impaired glycosylation of α-dystroglycan is felt to be responsible for other forms of MDC (muscle–eye–brain disease [MEB] and Walker–Warburg syndrome [WWS]).[33] MEB is most commonly caused by mutations in the *O*-mannose-β-1,2-*N*-acetylglucosaminyl transferase gene

(*POMGnT1*), which also causes LGMD 2N. WWS is most commonly caused by mutations in the *O*-mannosyltransferase gene (*POMT1*) that also causes LGMD 2K. Mutations in numerous other genes that encode for enzymes that are important in glycosylation of α-dystroglycan can cause congenital muscular dystrophy or a milder LGMD syndrome (i.e., *POMT2, LARGE, ISPD, GTDC2, B3GALNT2, B3GNT1, TMEM5, GMPPB, SGK196, DPM1, DPM2, DPM3*).

Thus, it appears that normal glycosylation of α-dystroglycan is important for muscle function but also for normal development of the central nervous system, which is affected in these forms of MDC. A number of other genes that are important in the glycosylation of α-dystroglycan have recently been reported and will be discussed in the section regarding congenital muscular dystrophies. Interestingly, mutations in the gene encoding for α-dystroglycan itself have been found to cause LGMD2P. In addition, UDP-*N*-acetylglucosamine 2-epimerase/*n*-acetylmannosamine kinase, encoded by *GNE*, is involved in the post-translational glycosylation of proteins, is abnormal in some forms of autosomal-recessive inclusion body myopathy (also known as the Nonaka type of distal myopathy).

▶ OTHER PROTEINS

Anoctamin 5 is another sarcolemmal protein whose precise function is still unknown. It seems to have putative calcium-activated chloride channel function. Interestingly, mutations in *ANO-5* that encode the protein results in either LGMD phenotype (LGMD2L) or a Miyoshi myopathy-like distal myopathy (MM3), as will be discussed.

▶ MUSCULAR DYSTROPHIES

Muscular dystrophies traditionally have been classified according to their pattern of weakness (e.g., limb girdle, facioscapulohumeral, and scapuloperoneal) and mode of inheritance (Table 27-1). Advances in genetics have led to the classification of muscular dystrophies based on the responsible gene defect. As you will see, there are disparate phenotypes associated with similar genotypes and near identical phenotypes associated with many different genotypes.

▶ THE DYSTROPHINOPATHIES: DUCHENNE AND BMD

DUCHENNE MUSCULAR DYSTROPHY

Clinical Features

The best known of the muscular dystrophies is DMD.[36–38] DMD is an X-linked recessive disorder, but approximately one-third of patients with DMD are a result of spontaneous mutations. The incidence is roughly 1 per 3,500 male births, with a prevalence approaching 1 per 18,000 males.[39]

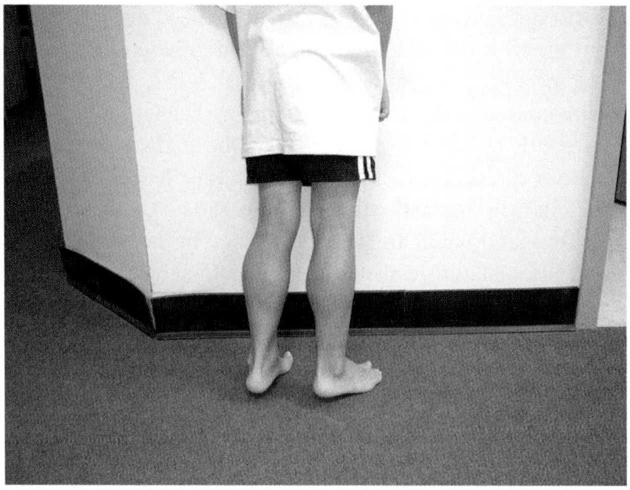

Figure 27-2. Duchenne muscular dystrophy. Enlarged calf muscles (pseudohypertrophy) and tight head cords resulting in toe walk are seen in this affected boy.

The natural history of children with DMD (not treated with corticosteroids) is well known.[38,40,41] Most boys appear quite normal at birth and achieve the anticipated milestones of sitting and standing with little or only slight delay. However, some affected boys are hypotonic and weak at birth. Careful inspection of neck flexors in infants and toddlers suspected of having the disease usually reveal some degree of weakness. A wide-base, waddling gait is noted by about 2–6 years of age, the waddling representing a compensatory action for hip abductor weakness. The affected child has difficulty running and jumping. There is a tendency for the child to walk on the toes, related to the center of balance being displaced anteriorly because of axial and hip girdle weakness and also from heel cord tightness. Calf hypertrophy may also be appreciated (Fig. 27-2). The progressive leg weakness leads to increasing falls between the ages of 2 and 6 years. Children also have difficulty arising from the floor and employ the characteristic Gower sign to enable them to rise to a standing position. Weakness is characteristically worse proximally and more so in the lower compared to upper limbs. Usually by 8 years of age, affected children have difficulty climbing stairs and need to pull themselves up the stairs using the handrails. Hyperlordosis of the lumbar spine is often noted during standing, a compensatory maneuver for hip extensor weakness. Between 6 and 12 years of age, weakness progresses to the point that the upper limb and torso muscles are profoundly affected. Ambulation becomes progressively more difficult, and affected children are confined to a wheelchair by 12 years of age. This in turn leads to the development of kyphoscoliosis and worsening of contractures. Nowadays as boys with DMD are usually treated with corticosteroids, they can ambulate past the age of 12 years. The biceps brachii, triceps, and quadriceps reflexes diminish and are absent in 50% of children by the age of 10 years. An interesting finding is the persistent ability to obtain an ankle jerk in at least a third of patients, even in end stages of the disease. Contractures about the hip and ankles also significantly impair posture.

Ventilatory function gradually declines and leads to death in most patients by the early twenties. This may be a consequence not only of ventilatory muscle weakness, but also due to the altered thoracic anatomy related to the aforementioned kyphoscoliosis. In addition to skeletal muscle, cardiac muscle is also involved. Most patients are asymptomatic early in the course; however, dysrhythmias and congestive heart failure (CHF) can occur late in the disease. Approximately 90% of patients have electrocardiogram (EKG) abnormalities, most commonly sinus tachycardia, tall right precordial R waves, and deep narrow Q waves in the left precordial leads.[42–44] Echocardiogram reveals dilation and/or hypokinesis of ventricular walls. Unfortunately, most patients with DMD die in their late teens or early twenties from ventilatory or cardiac failure. Smooth muscle is also affected, and patients can develop gastroparesis and intestinal pseudo-obstruction.

The central nervous system is also involved in DMD. The average IQ of the affected children is approximately one standard deviation below the normal mean.[45] The mechanism by which the central nervous system is affected is unclear, but, as noted above, dystrophin is expressed at some synapses in the brain.

Laboratory Features

The serum creatine kinase (CK) levels are markedly elevated (50–100 times normal or greater) at birth and peak at around 3 years of age. Subsequently, serum CK levels decline approximately 20% per year as a result of decreasing muscle bulk, although the CK levels never normalize.

Electrodiagnostic testing in dystrophinopathies is of limited value, particularly when there is a family history of the disorder. Diagnosis requires genetic testing for identifiable mutations in the dystrophin gene and, if that is unrewarding, a muscle biopsy utilizing immunostaining and/or immunoblotting techniques. Electrodiagnostic testing may be helpful in sporadic cases and in BMD in which CK levels can be only mildly elevated and the differential diagnosis is much broader. Needle electromyography (EMG) demonstrates increased insertional and spontaneous activity in the form of fibrillation potentials and positive sharp waves. However, as muscle tissue is progressively replaced with both adipose cells and connective tissue, insertional activity diminishes. The mean amplitudes of nonpolyphasic motor unit action potentials (MUAPs) are reduced, but large-amplitude polyphasic potentials can also be seen. Both short- and long-duration MUAPs can be demonstrated in individual muscles, the latter reflecting the chronicity of the myopathic process. An early recruitment pattern of MUAPs is evident at low force thresholds in weak muscles.

Histopathology

Muscle biopsies reveal scattered necrotic and regenerating muscle fibers, variability in muscle fiber size, increased endomysial and perimysial connective tissue, scattered hypertrophic and hypercontracted fibers in addition to small, rounded, regenerating fibers (Fig. 27-3). Fiber splitting and central nuclei can also be seen but occur less often than in other muscular dystrophies. The process of degeneration and regeneration continues until the limited regenerative capacity of the satellite cells is exceeded, at which time the necrotic muscle tissue is replaced with fat and connective tissue.

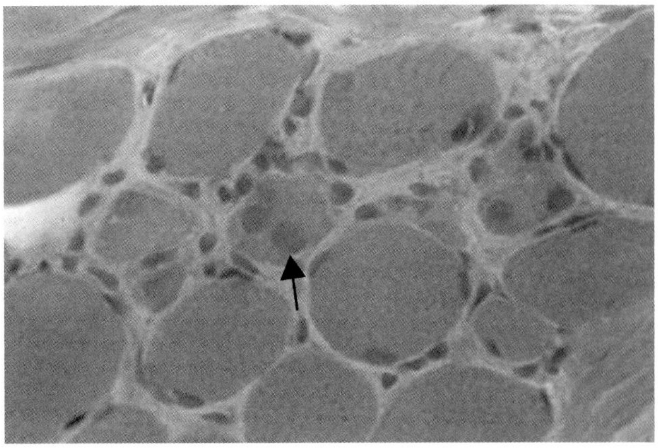

Figure 27-3. Duchenne muscular dystrophy. Muscle biopsy in a patient with DMD demonstrates mild variability in fiber size with small regenerating fibers that have enlarged nuclei (*arrow*). Hematoxylin and eosin (H&E).

Endomysial inflammatory cells consisting of cytotoxic T lymphocytes (two-thirds) and macrophages (one-third) are present to a variable degree and phagocytize necrotic fibers.[46] Rarely, non-necrotic fibers expressing major histocompatibility antigen are invaded by CD8+ cytotoxic T cells in a manner similar to inclusion body myositis (IBM) and polymyositis.

Immunohistochemistry demonstrates reduced or absent dystrophin on the sarcolemma (Fig. 27-4).[36,38] About 60% of patients with DMD will have some faint staining of the muscle membrane using antibodies directed against the amino terminal or rod domain of dystrophin. However, less than 1% of muscle fibers have sarcolemmal staining with antibodies directed against the carboxy terminal of dystrophin. The few dystrophin-positive muscle fibers are known as revertants. They arise secondary to spontaneous subsequent mutations that restore the "reading frame" and allows transcription of dystrophin, albeit abnormal size and shape. On the other hand, utrophin, which is normally restricted to the neuromuscular junction, is overexpressed in DMD and is present throughout the sarcolemma.

Immunoblot or western blot of muscle tissue assesses both the quantity and the size of the dystrophin present. With use of carboxy-terminal antibodies, the western blot reveals 0–3% of the normal amount of dystrophin present in muscle tissue, and the size of the remaining dystrophin is usually diminished.[4] With amino-terminal or rod-domain antibodies, approximately 50% of patients with DMD have some detectable truncated dystrophin. Immunohistochemical analysis in dystrophinopathies may also demonstrate a reduction of dystroglycan, dystrobrevin, and all the sarcoglycan proteins, including sarcospan.

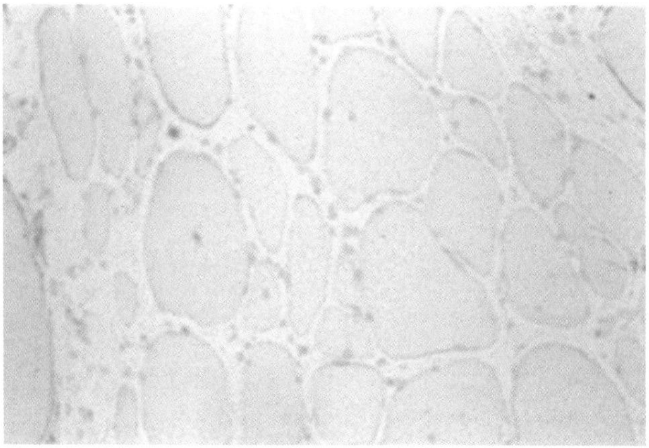

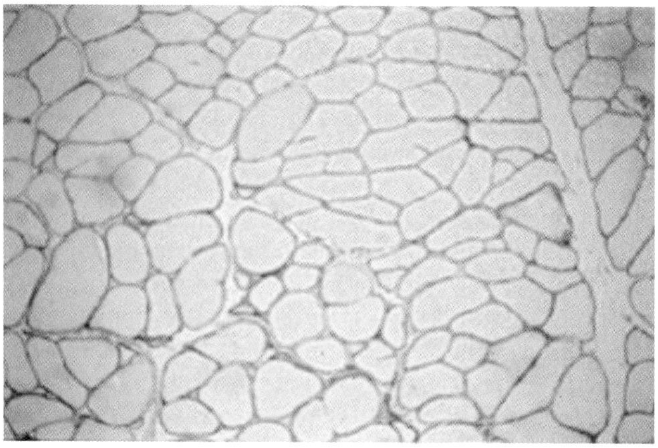

Figure 27-4. Immunoperoxidase staining using dystrophin (Dys 2) antibodies demonstrates absence of sarcolemmal staining on muscle fibers in DMD **(A)** and normal staining in a control biopsy **(B)**.

BECKER MUSCULAR DYSTROPHY

Clinical Features

BMD represents a milder form of dystrophinopathy. BMD can be distinguished from DMD clinically by its slower rate of progression and by dystrophin analysis.[2,38] The incidence of BMD is approximately 5 per 100,000.[39,47] Approximately 10% of cases are the result of spontaneous mutations. Clinical features that help with the diagnosis of possible BMD include (1) a family history compatible with X-linked recessive inheritance, (2) ambulation maintained past the age of 15 years (in absence of steroid treatment), (3) a limb-girdle pattern of muscle weakness, and (4) calf hypertrophy (pseudohypertrophy).[48] Some patients exhibit preferential involvement of the quadriceps muscle (quadriceps myopathy).[49] BMD patients, unlike DMD, typically have relative sparing of neck flexor strength as a distinctive clinical feature.

A wide spectrum of clinical phenotypes and variability can be seen even within families.[2,50] Most patients develop difficulty in walking; however, by definition, they remain ambulatory past the age of 15 years. Approximately 50% of affected individuals lose the ability to ambulate independently by the fourth decade. Some patients manifesting with isolated myalgias,[51] myoglobinuria,[52] cardiomyopathy,[53,54] and asymptomatic hyper-CK-emia have been demonstrated to have mild forms of dystrophinopathy. Cardiac abnormalities are similar to those described for DMD.[55] Mental abilities have not been investigated as thoroughly as in DMD, but some series have demonstrated a borderline or mildly impaired IQ in patients with BMD.[48,50] The life expectancy is reduced, although many patients live well into adulthood.[48]

Laboratory Features

Serum CK levels are elevated, often 20–200 times normal.[2] Patients with only exertional myalgias may have only slightly elevated serum CK levels. EMG is abnormal in weak muscles as discussed in DMD section. Skeletal muscle magnetic resonance imaging (MRI) scans can demonstrate fatty replacement of affected muscle groups (Fig. 27-5).

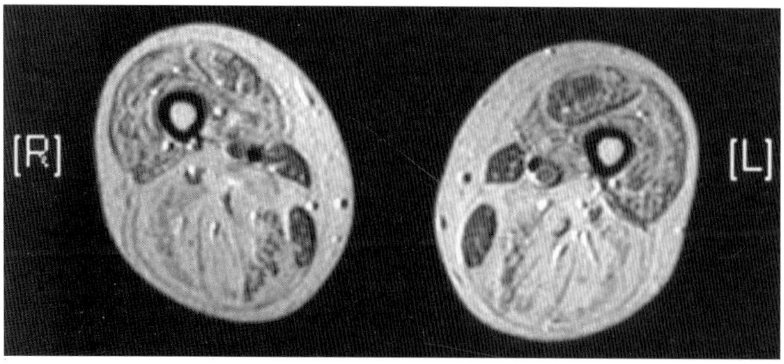

Figure 27-5. Becker muscular dystrophy. Skeletal muscle MRI (T1 weighted) of the thigh in a patient with BMD demonstrates the bright and feathery appearance of fat and connective tissue replacing muscle in the thighs.

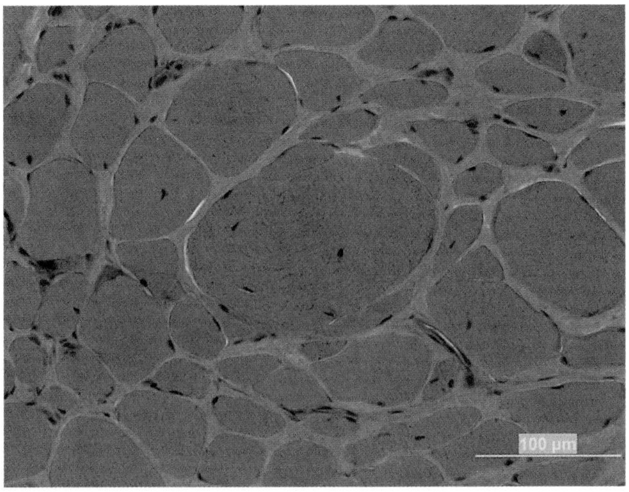

Figure 27-6. Becker muscular dystrophy. Muscle biopsy demonstrates increased endomysial connective tissue, marked variability in muscle fiber size, slightly increased internalized nuclei, and splitting of muscle fibers. H&E.

Histopathology

The histological features are similar to those observed for DMD, but are less severe (Fig. 27-6).[2,56] BMD may be distinguished histologically from DMD with immune staining, which demonstrates the presence of dystrophin using carboxy-terminal antibodies on muscle membranes in most cases of BMD. In contrast, immunostaining with antibodies directed against the carboxy terminal of dystrophin is usually negative in DMD. However, the degree and intensity of the dystrophin staining are usually not normal in BMD. The staining pattern may be uniformly reduced or can vary between and within fibers. Western blot analysis of muscle tissue typically reveals an abnormal quantity and/or size of the dystrophin protein.[2,4,36,38,57]

OUTLIERS

This older term was used for children who have a clinical phenotype in between that of DMD and BMD. In the pre-steroid era, these children were defined by the ability to ambulate after the age of 12 years, but required a wheelchair by the age of 15 years. In early childhood, outliers may be distinguished from children with more severe DMD clinical phenotype by the presence of antigravity neck flexion strength. Children with DMD cannot lift their heads fully against gravity when lying supine (Medical Research Council grade less than 3), unlike outliers and BMD children who typically can. Immunologic studies on muscle tissue usually reveal the presence of some dystrophin, although often reduced in amount and/or size.

WOMEN CARRIERS

The daughters of men with BMD (males with DMD are usually infertile) and the mothers of affected children, who also have a family history of DMD or BMD are obligate carriers of the mutated dystrophin gene. Mothers and sisters of isolated patients with DMD or BMD are at risk of being carriers. One of the most important aspects of caring for patients and families with dystrophinopathies is to determine the carrier status of "at-risk" females for the purpose of genetic counseling. There is a 50% chance that males born to women carriers will inherit the disease, and 50% of the daughters born will become carriers themselves. Women carriers are usually asymptomatic, but a few develop muscle weakness.[2,58] These cases are usually explained by the Lyon hypothesis: skewed inactivation of the normal X-chromosome and dystrophin gene results in increased transcription of the mutated dystrophin gene. Females with translocations at the chromosomal Xp21 site or Turner syndrome (XO genotype) may also develop dystrophinopathies.

Manifesting carriers typically have a mild limb-girdle phenotype similar to BMD.[2] Prior to the advances in molecular genetics, these women were often diagnosed with LGMD, particularly when there was no family history of DMD or BMD. Rarely, females can develop severe weakness as seen in DMD.

Laboratory and histologic features of manifesting carriers are similar to those discussed for DMD and BMD. Immunostaining for dystrophin demonstrates an absent, decreased, or mosaic pattern of staining in many women carriers (Fig. 27-7); however, staining can be normal.[58-61] Thus, immunostaining and western blot analysis are not very sensitive in identifying carrier status of asymptomatic females.

Serum CK levels are an insensitive measure of carrier status.[62,63] CK levels can be elevated early in life; however, a normal serum CK does not exclude a carrier status. Elevated serum CK levels are identified in less than 50% of obligate carriers. The most reliable method of detecting carrier status is with genetic testing. This is accomplished first by

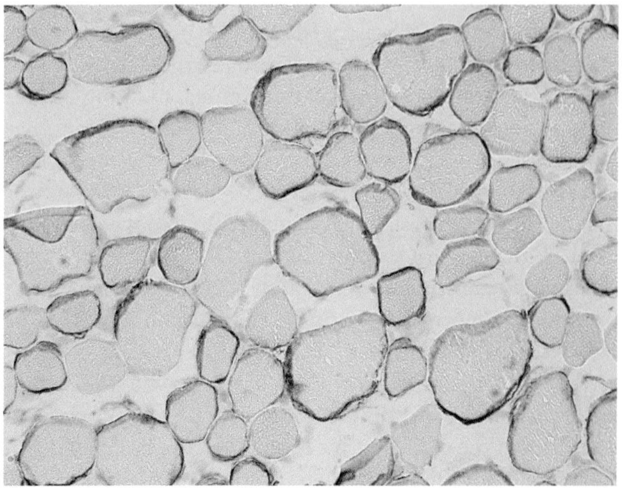

Figure 27-7. Muscle biopsy of a manifesting woman carrier of a dystrophin mutation demonstrates a mosaic pattern of dystrophin expression on the sarcolemma. Immunoperoxidase staining using dystrophin (Dys 2) antibodies.

identifying the specific mutation in an affected male relative. The detection of such a mutation makes carrier detection of at-risk female relatives much easier and also allows for subsequent prenatal detection in at-risk fetuses. If a mutation is demonstrated in an affected male relative, at-risk females can be screened for the same mutation. However, it should be noted that the carrier status of a mother of a sporadic DMD case must be interpreted cautiously because of the potential for germline mosaicism.[64] In a germline mosaic, the mutation involves only a percentage of the germ cells (i.e., oocytes) but are not present in the leukocytes in which DNA analysis is performed. In these rare cases, an affected child may have an identifiable mutation on DNA analysis, but the mother could have no demonstrable mutation in the leukocytes but is still capable of having other affected children. The recurrence rate in germline carriers is unknown and dependent on the number of mutated oocytes, but has been estimated to be as high as 14%.[64] Prenatal diagnosis can be made with DNA analysis of chorionic villi or amniotic fluid cells when there is an identifiable mutation in the family.

MOLECULAR GENETICS AND PATHOGENESIS OF THE DYSTROPHINOPATHIES

Dystrophin is a structural protein, which is intimately bound to the sarcolemma and provides structural integrity to the muscle membrane (Fig. 27-1).[6] Abnormal dystrophin quantity or quality results in the muscle losing its ability to maintain its integrity during contraction, leading to membrane tears and subsequent muscle fiber necrosis.

The dystrophin gene, located on chromosome Xp21, is composed of approximately 2.4 megabases of genomic DNA and includes 79 exons, which code for a 14-kb transcript.[3,5] The large size of the gene probably accounts for the high spontaneous mutation rate responsible for one-third of new cases. Large deletions, several kilobases to over 1 million base pairs, can be demonstrated in approximately two-thirds of patients with dystrophinopathy. Approximately 5–10% of DMD cases are caused by point mutations, resulting in premature stop codons.[65] Duplications are evident in another 5% of cases. Mutations occur primarily in the center (80%) and near the amino terminal (20%) of the gene.[65] Mutations that disrupt the translational reading frame of the gene lead to near total loss of dystrophin and DMD, while in-frame mutations result in the translation of semifunctional dystrophin of abnormal size and/or amount and in outlier or BMD clinical phenotypes.[4] Although there are exceptions to the "reading-frame rule," 92% of phenotypic differences are explained by in-frame and out-of-frame mutations.[65] It appears that the quality or remaining functional capability of the mutated dystrophin protein is more important than the actual quantity. The reduction in the various sarcoglycans, which is also evident in immunohistochemical studies of DMD and BMD, suggests that normal dystrophin is important for the integrity of the sarcoglycan complex.

TREATMENT OF THE DYSTROPHINOPATHIES

Corticosteroids

Prednisone (0.75 mg/kg/day) has been shown to increase strength and function (peaking at 3 months) and slow the rate of deterioration in children with DMD.[36,38,66–71] Steroids also appear to reduce the risk of scoliosis and stabilize pulmonary function. The beneficial effects are noted as early as 10 days and are sustained for at least 3 years. These apparent clinical benefits are accompanied by an increase in muscle mass and decline in the rate of muscle catabolism.[69] The mechanism is not felt to be related to the immunosuppressive action of prednisone on inflammatory infiltrates in the muscle but rather by altering muscle metabolism, particularly protein synthesis and/or breakdown. Lower doses of prednisone (<0.75 mg/kg/day) are not as effective in DMD. There have been no large, double-blinded, placebo-controlled studies assessing the efficacy of steroids in BMD, although small series suggest a possible benefit.[72]

Unfortunately, high-dose prednisone is associated with significant side effects including weight gain, stunted growth, cushingoid appearance, excessive hair growth, irritability, and hyperactivity. In addition, prednisone is also associated with an increased risk of infections, cataract formation, hypertension, glucose intolerance, osteoporosis, and osteonecrosis. Twice-weekly oral prednisone given on a weekend (5 mg/kg/day) appeared to be beneficial compared to historical controls in a small open-label study of 20 boys with DMD.[73]

An analog of prednisone, deflazacort (not FDA approved) has been studied in several clinical trials of DMD.[36,38,71,74,75] These studies suggest that deflazacort at doses of 0.9 and 1.2 mg/kg/day may be as effective as prednisone 0.75 mg/kg/day and associated with fewer side effects.

A randomized, double-blind, placebo-controlled trial of oxandrolone, a synthetic anabolic dihydrotestosterone derivative, at a dose of 0.1 mg/kg/d for 6 months in 51 boys with DMD demonstrated no statistically significant improvement in manual muscle strength.[76] Modest improvement in strength has been reported in a small number of patients with DMD and BMD treated with short courses of creatine monohydrate (5–10 g/day).[77,78] Creatine supplementation may increase the muscle supply of phosphocreatine and increase the ATP resynthesis.

Gene Therapy

Potential strategies for replacing the defective dystrophin protein are somatic gene therapy via myoblast or stem cell transplantation and direct gene replacement using modified viral vectors. Controlled trials of human myoblast transfer in DMD have not resulted in any significant clinical improvement.[79] Stem cell therapies are being evaluated in animal models and may proceed to human trials in the near future.

Antisense oligonucleotides designed to induce exon skipping of specific mutations and drugs that allow read-through of nonsense mutations have potential benefit.[38,80]

Such drugs can be designed to skip over specific exon such that the reading frame might be restored. This could lead to increased expression of dystrophin, albeit at a reduced size. Antisense oligonucleotides would theoretically be able to correct multiple DMD mutations. For example, skipping of exon 45 might theoretically correct both deletions of exons 46–47 and exons 46–48. It has been estimated that as many as 35% of DMD might theoretically improve by targeting a limited number of exons (44, 45, 51, and 53) and the yield may increase to over 80% with skipping of two exons.[38] A small study of intravenously administered AVI-4658, a phosphorodiamidate morpholino oligomer (PMO) designed to induce exon 51 skipping in DMD, was demonstrated to be associated with increased dystrophin expression.[81] A double-blind placebo-controlled trial of Eteplirsen, a PMO designed to skip exon 51, demonstrated increased dystrophin production and, perhaps, slightly improved or stabilized the 6-minute walk test (6MWT); however, two patients who lost the ability to ambulate early in the course of this study were excluded from the analysis of the 6MWT.[82] Drisapersen, another PMO designed to skip exon 51, also improved dystrophin expression in a small study.[80,83] Ataluren (PTC124), a drug that enables ribosomal read-through of premature stop codons, was studied in a large clinical trial of DMD and showed a possible effect (improved 6MWT) in the low dose cohort but not in a higher dose cohort.[84]

Supportive Therapy

Patients are best managed using a multidisciplinary approach.[2,36–38] Ideally, neuromuscular clinics should involve neurologists, physiatrists, physical therapists, occupational therapists, speech therapists, respiratory therapists, dietitians, cardiologists, pulmonologists, psychologists, and genetic counselors, in order to assess all the needs of individual patients. Physical therapy is a key component in the treatment of patients with muscular dystrophy. Because contractures develop early in the disease, particularly of the heel cords, iliotibial bands, and the hips, appropriate stretching exercises must be started early in the disease: Long leg braces may aid ambulation. Rehabilitation issues are discussed in greater detail in Chapter 5.

Cardiac function, including EKG and echocardiogram should be assessed at diagnosis of DMD or at least by the 6 years of age and then at least once every 2 years until the age of 10 years.[36–38] Afterwards, there should be annual cardiac assessments, sooner if cardiac symptoms and signs begin earlier. Holter monitoring should also be considered as arrhythmia may develop before signs of systolic dysfunction. Afterload reduction with angiotensin-converting enzyme inhibitors or angiotensin receptor blockers are considered standard treatments of cardiomyopathy.[36–38] β blockers and diuretics are also used to treat heart failure. Likewise, cardiac assessments and treatment are important in management of patients with BMD.[2]

Scoliosis is a universal complication of DMD, particularly once the child is nonambulatory.[36–38] We perform yearly spinal radiographs to assess progression once scoliosis is apparent on clinical examination. Scoliosis results in pain, aesthetic damage, and perhaps ventilatory compromise. Orthopedic consultation should be considered for curves past 20 degrees.[38] We consider spinal fusion in children with 35 degrees scoliosis or more and for those who are in significant discomfort. Ideally, forced vital capacity should be greater than 35% to minimize the risk of surgery. Quality of life seems to be improved following spinal stabilization; however, scoliosis surgery does not appear to increase ventilatory function.

DMD, GLYCEROL KINASE DEFICIENCY, AND ADRENAL HYPOPLASIA CONGENITA

DMD and glycerol kinase deficiency (GKD) can occur together as part of a contiguous gene syndrome at chromosome Xp21.[85–87] The gene order for the contiguous loci is Xpter—AHC–GKD–DYS—centromere, and thus patients may also have adrenal hypoplasia congenita (AHC) depending on the extent of the mutation. Microdeletions can span these contiguous genes, producing a clinical phenotype that is different from that seen in patients who have mutations only within the individual DMD, GK, or AHC genes. Most children with combined DMD and GKD exhibit severe psychomotor delay. In addition to muscular weakness due to DMD, children who are affected often experience episodic nausea, vomiting, and stupor from GKD. Further, mutations involving the DAX1 gene responsible for AHC can result in life-threatening adrenal insufficiency manifested by addisonian hyperpigmentation of the skin, hypogonadotropic hypogonadism/cryptorchidism, hyperkalemia, hyponatremia, and hypoglycemia. Glycerol kinase is responsible for the first step in glycerol metabolism and is important in glycolysis, gluconeogenesis, and triglyceride metabolism:

$$\text{glycerol} + \text{ATP} \Leftrightarrow \text{glycerol 3-phosphate} + \text{ADP}.$$

GKD results in glyceroluria and hyperglycerolemia. GKD should be considered in a young child with elevated serum triglyceride levels because the standard serum triglyceride test actually measures free glycerol. The neurological side effects of GKD are responsive to a fat-restricted diet and avoidance of prolonged fasting.

AHC is caused by mutations in the dosage-sensitive sex reversal AHC, X-chromosome, gene 1, or *DAX1*. The DAX1 protein is a member of the nuclear hormone receptor superfamily and functions to regulate the transcription of genes involved in the normal development of the adrenal glands. Decreased serum levels of gonadotropins and a subnormal increase in serum cortisol in response to exogenous administration of adrenocorticotropic hormone are found. Treatment of adrenal insufficiency is by replacement of glucocorticoids, mineralocorticoids, and testosterone.

Mutations involving the 3′ (carboxy-terminal) portion of the dystrophin gene usually span into the GK locus. Thus, patients with dystrophinopathies who have three mutations should be evaluated for the contiguous gene syndrome. Most patients have DMD; BMD can also occur. Diagnosis of X-chromosomal microdeletions can be made with Southern blotting, DNA amplification through PCR, or fluorescent in situ hybridization analysis. Further, fluorescent in situ hybridization provides a rapid and accurate evaluation for these microdeletions and can also be used for carrier detection and prenatal diagnosis.

LIMB-GIRDLE MUSCULAR DYSTROPHY

The LGMDs are a heterogeneous group of disorders that clinically resemble the dystrophinopathies, except for the equal occurrence in men and women (Table 27-1).[1,2,6] The prevalence rate of LGMD ranges from 80 to 700 per 100,000 while estimated prevalence of individual specific subtypes LGMDs is quite variable as well.[2] The LGMDs are inherited in an autosomal-recessive or autosomal-dominant fashion. Autosomal-dominant LGMDs are classified as type 1 (e.g., LGMD 1), while recessive forms are termed type 2 (e.g., LGMD 2). Further alphabetical subclassification has been applied to these disorders in the order they were discovered in consideration of their distinct genotypes. (e.g., LGMD 2A, LGMD 2B, etc.; see Table 27-1). For the most part, the clinical, laboratory, and histopathological features of the LGMDs are nonspecific, with the few exceptions to be discussed.

► AUTOSOMAL-DOMINANT LGMD

LGMD 1A (MYOTILIN)

Clinical Features

Gilchrist and colleagues described the original family (144 patients over seven generations) with this autosomal-dominant inherited LGMD (Table 27-1, Fig. 27-8).[88] Subsequently there have been many other reports, some under

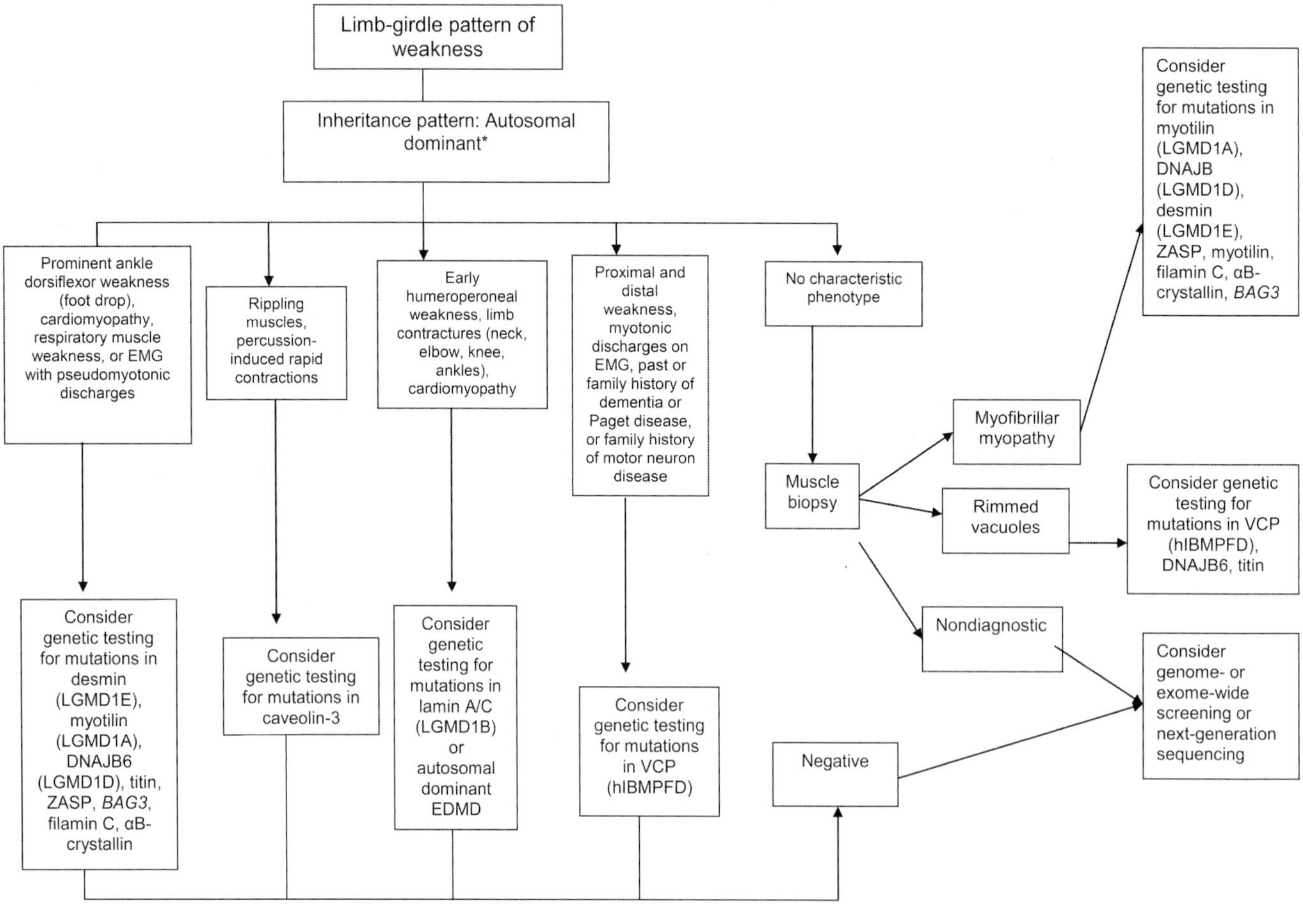

Figure 27-8. Diagnostic approach to patients with a limb-girdle pattern of weakness and suspected muscular dystrophy with an autosomal dominant inheritance pattern. Autosomal dominant, autosomal recessive, or X-linked inheritance may be responsible in sporadic cases. EDMD, Emery–Dreifuss muscular dystrophy; h-IBMPFD, hereditary inclusion body myopathy with Paget disease and frontotemporal dementia; LGMD, limb-girdle muscular dystrophy; VCP, valosin-containing protein. (Reproduced with permission from Narayanaswami P, Weiss M, Selcen D, et al: Evidence-based guideline summary: diagnosis and treatment of limb-girdle and distal dystrophies: report of the guideline development subcommittee of the American Academy of Neurology and the practice issues review panel of the American Association of Neuromuscular & Electrodiagnostic Medicine, *Neurology*. 2014;83(16):1453–1463.)

the category of myofibrillar myopathy (MFM).[2,89–99] The onset of weakness ranges from the teens to the eighth decade of life. There is often an early predilection for the scapular–humeral–pelvic muscles. However, distal leg and occasionally arm weakness can be weaker than proximal muscles in some patients.[2,20,98] Patients can also develop an associated cardiomyopathy. Unlike the dystrophinopathies and other LGMDs (e.g., the sarcoglycanopathies), calf hypertrophy is rare. Dysarthria[93,94] or hypernasal speech[95] occurs in some individuals.

Laboratory Features

Serum CK levels are normal or elevated up to nine times normal. Muscle imaging studies have revealed fibrofatty replacement and edema in the medial gastrocnemius, soleus, hip adductors, and biceps femoris with relative sparing of the semitendinosus muscles.[91,92,95]

Histopathology

Muscle biopsies are notable for the frequent occurrence of rimmed vacuoles and occasional nemaline rod-like inclusions.[2,89,90] Muscle biopsies can demonstrate features of MFM (see later section regarding MFM) on routine light microscopy, immunohistochemistry, and electron microscopy (EM).[2,20]

Molecular Genetics and Pathogenesis

LGMD 1A is caused by autosomal dominant mutations in the *MYOT* gene that encodes for myotilin located on chromosome 5q22.3–31.3.[2,20,90] Spontaneous mutations are common, so the lack of a family history should not exclude the diagnosis. Rare cases of MFM have been reported with autosomal recessive inheritance.[99] Myotilin is a sarcomeric protein that colocalizes with α-actinin at the Z-disc. Some of the clinical, laboratory, and histologic features are similar to those described in autosomal-dominant h-IBM and MFM, which is discussed in more detail in the section on MFM.[2,20]

LGMD 1B (LAMIN A/C)

Clinical Features

LGMD 1B can present with weakness in the hip and shoulder girdle or have a predilection for the humeral and peroneal muscles and is often associated with cardiac conduction defects; some affected individuals manifest only with a cardiomyopathy.[2,100–108] The cardiomyopathy and associated arrhythmias can result in sudden death and often require pacemaker or intracardiac defibrillator implantation.[2] Some patients require cardiac transplantation because of CHF from dilated cardiomyopathy. This clinical phenotype can resemble that seen in the more common X-linked EDMD. In this regard LGMD 1B and autosomal-dominant EDMD are allelic being caused by mutations in the lamin A/C gene, *LMNA*.[2,27,102]

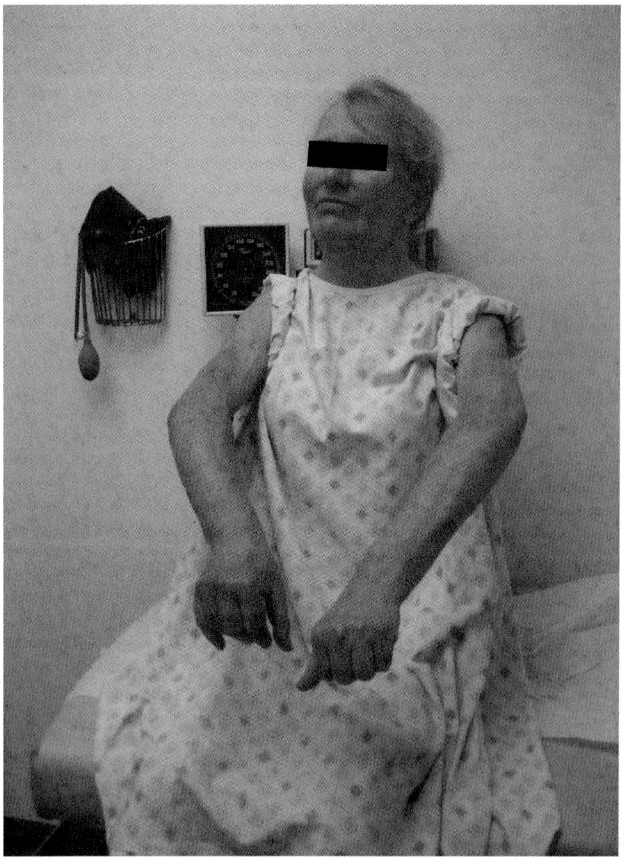

Figure 27-9. A patient with LGMD1B/EDMD2 caused by *LMNA* mutation demonstrated severe early elbow contractures.

The AD-EDMD phenotype is characterized by proximal arm weakness with preferential involvement of humeral muscles, both proximal and distal weakness in the lower extremities, ankle and elbow contractures (Fig. 27-9), and spinal rigidity (particularly in the neck). However, contractures may not be apparent until late in the disease course or not at all, which is a feature that may help distinguish it from X-linked EDMD caused by mutations in the emerin gene, in which contractures are invariably present early in the disease course.[103–108] The LGMD phenotype is associated with proximal leg more than arm weakness, but again often with preferential involvement of humeral muscles. Again, flexion contractures of elbows and Achilles tendons may be seen but can be subtle or not apparent until late in the course.

Laboratory Features

Serum CK levels may be normal or elevated up to 25 times normal. Skeletal muscle imaging with MRI or CT can show fatty infiltration in the posterior compartment of the thigh and calves.[2,109–112] One imaging study comparing AD-EDMD to Bethlem/Ullrich myopathies (collagen VI disorders), which clinically can resemble EDMD, except for the absence of cardiac involvement, found that the quadriceps were relatively spared and the hamstrings were more severely involved in AD-EDMD.[110]

Histopathology

Muscle biopsies demonstrate variation in fiber size, increased endomysial connective tissue, normal dystrophin, sarcoglycan, and emerin staining. Occasionally, rimmed vacuoles are evident on muscles biopsy.[100,101] Emerin and lamin A/C expressions on the nuclear membrane are typically normal with immunohistochemistry. On EM, myonuclei exhibit the loss of peripheral heterochromatin or its detachment from the nuclear envelop, altered interchromatic texture, and fewer nuclear pores compared to normal.[26]

Molecular Genetics and Pathogenesis

LGMD 1B is caused by mutations in *LMNA* that encodes for lamin A/C.[27,28,102] Of note, Dunnigan type familial partial lipodystrophy, mandibuloacral dysplasia, Hutchinson–Gilford progeria syndrome, restrictive dermopathy, and a form of dominant-intermediate Charcot–Marie–Tooth (CMT) neuropathy are also allelic disorders associated with *LMNA* mutations.[2] Interestingly, phenotypic variability occurs even within family members carrying the same mutation.[2,105] The pathogenic role of lamin A/C is discussed in more detail in the EDMD section.

LGMD 1C (CAVEOLIN-3)

Clinical Features

This autosomal-dominant LGMD is caused by mutations in the caveolin-3 gene and is associated with a heterogeneous phenotype.[2,15–18,113–125] Affected individuals may present in childhood or adult life with proximal weakness or exertional myalgias.[16] Calf hypertrophy may be evident.[2] The rate of progression is variable. Other patients manifest with muscle stiffness, rippling muscle disease, distal weakness (anterior or posterior compartment), asymptomatic hyper-CK-emia, and rarely myoglobinuria.[2,15–18,114,121] Generalized percussion-induced rapid contractions (PIRCs) were apparent in the face, neck, and extremities in all affected patients in one series, while actual rippling muscles were evident in approximately two-thirds.[124] Spontaneous mutations are not uncommon, so a lack of a family history does not exclude the diagnosis.[15]

Laboratory Features

Serum CK is usually elevated three to 30-fold.[2]

Histopathology

Muscle biopsies demonstrate nonspecific myopathic features with normal dystrophin, sarcoglycan, and merosin staining.[2] Reduced caveolin-3 staining may be appreciated along the sarcolemma. EM reveals a decreased density of caveolae on the muscle membrane as well.

Molecular Genetics and Pathogenesis

LGMD 1C is caused by mutations in the caveolin-3 gene (*CAV3*) located on chromosome 3p25.[2,15,16] Caveolin-3 is located on the sarcolemma (Fig. 27-1). It cofractionates with the dystrophin–glycoprotein complex but is thought to be part of a discrete complex. Caveolins play a role in the formation of caveolae membranes, where they act as scaffolding proteins to organize and concentrate caveolin-interacting lipids and proteins.[16] Caveolin-3 might also function to facilitate organization of signaling complexes, and the sodium channels that later function might contribute to the pathogenesis of rippling muscle disease.

LGMD 1D (DNAJB6)

Clinical Features

LGMD 1D is a rare dystrophy associated with slowly progressive weakness with onset usually in the third to sixth decade.[2,126–128] However, it can manifest in the teens. Affected individuals may develop proximal muscle weakness in the lower extremities (hamstrings worse than quadriceps) with normal or only mild proximal upper extremity strength.[128] However, the phenotype can be variable and some develop more distal lower extremity weakness with preferential involvement of the posterior compartment more than the anterior compartment.[127] Cardiac and ventilatory muscles are usually spared.

Laboratory Features

Serum CK levels range from normal to 10-fold elevated, but are usually 2–3 times the upper limit of normal.

Histopathology

Muscle biopsy reveal muscle fibers with rimmed vacuoles and other features suggestive of a MFM.[127]

Molecular Genetics and Pathogenesis

The disorder is caused by mutations in the DNAJ (Hsp40) homolog, subfamily B, member gene (*DNAJB6*) located on chromosome 7q36.[128]

LGMD 1E (DESMIN)

Clinical Features

LGMD 1E is an autosomal dominant disorder caused by mutations in the gene that encodes for desmin (*DES*). It is allelic with LGMD 2R, which is a desminopathy inherited in an autosomal recessive fashion. Mutations in *DES* are also one of the most common causes of MFM. The age of onset ranges from the first to sixth decade of life.[2] Although patients may have a limb-girdle pattern of weakness,[132–138] most have more distal involvement with the earliest manifestation being progressive foot drop.[2,135–138] In addition, some have proximal equal to distal weakness,[132–134,138] or a scapuloperoneal distribution.[133,137] Dysphagia or dysarthria can also occur.[132,136,138] Ventilatory muscle weakness[2,135,137,138] and cardiac involvement are common and may precede skeletal muscle weakness.[2,130,132–137] Cardiac manifestations include arrhythmia (e.g., atrioventricular conduction block, atrial fibrillation, other tachyarrhythmias, sudden cardiac death) and some patients require pacemaker or cardioverter defibrillator implantation. Dilated cardiomyopathy appears to be more frequent than hypertrophic or restrictive cardiomyopathy.[2] Some patients have had cardiac transplantation.[130]

Laboratory Features

Serum CK levels are normal or only moderately elevated (up to five times normal).[2,133–137] EMG is myopathic and often demonstrated increased insertional and spontaneous activity (fibrillation potentials, positive sharp waves). In addition, myotonic, or more appropriately, pseudomyotonic discharges (decrescendo as opposed to crescendo/decrescendo frequency and amplitude of discharges) is seen. Skeletal muscle imaging of the distal leg usually shows involvement of the tibialis anterior and peroneus group more than the posterior compartment (medial gastrocnemius and soleus).[2] In the thighs the earliest abnormalities may be in the semitendinosus and sartorius.[2]

Histopathology

Muscle biopsy reveals muscle fibers with rimmed vacuoles and other features suggestive of a MFM.

Molecular Genetics and Pathogenesis

The disorder is caused by mutations in the *DES* gene that encodes for desmin, an intermediate filament. In muscle, desmin forms a three-dimensional scaffold extending across the diameter of the myofibril surrounding the Z discs and linking the entire sarcomere (contractile proteins) to the sarcolemmal membrane, cytoplasmic organelles, and myonuclei.

LGMD 1F (TRANSPORTIN-3)

Clinical Features

This recently described dystrophy can present in infancy to late adult life with proximal greater than distal weakness, legs more than arms.[139,140]

Laboratory Features

CK level is normal to moderately elevated.

Histopathology

Muscle biopsy can show rimmed vacuoles and features of MFM.

Molecular Genetics and Pathogenesis

LGMD 1F is caused by mutation in *TNP03* which encodes for transportin-3, a nuclear import receptor for precursor-mRNA splicing factors.[139,140]

▶ AUTOSOMAL-RECESSIVE LGMD

LGMD 2A (CALPAIN-3)

Clinical Features

This LGMD was first described in inhabitants of Reunion Island in the Indian Ocean, but subsequently, the dystrophy has been reported throughout the world (Table 27-1, Fig. 27-10).[1,2,141–148] Most epidemiological series report that 18.5–35% of LGMD are calpainopathies (LGMD2A). It is the most common form of LGMD in people from eastern Europe, Spain, Italy, the Netherlands, northern England, and Brazil.[2] In this regard, LGMD2A is responsible for approximately 28% of LGMD cases in Italy,[146] 26.5% in northern England,[147] and 21% in the Netherlands.[148]

The onset of weakness ranges from early childhood to mid-adult life.[1,2,141–148] There is an early predilection for the pelvic-girdle muscles and posterior thigh (gluteus maximus, thigh adductors, hamstrings, and, to a lesser degree, the gluteus medius and psoas), followed 2–5 years later by periscapular and humeral muscle weakness and atrophy (latissimus dorsi, serratus anterior, rhomboids, pectoralis major, and the biceps brachii). The deltoid and brachioradialis are less severely affected, while the distal leg, supra- and infraspinati, triceps, brachialis, and forearm muscles are relatively spared. Only mild weakness of neck muscles can be detected. Scapular winging is present in the majority of patients. Facial muscles are usually unaffected. Ocular and velopharyngeal muscles are not involved. There is often slight scoliosis from truncal weakness. Abdominal muscles are more affected than paraspinal spinal muscles. Early contractures at the elbows and calves are typically present, such that patients may mimic EDMD. Calf hypertrophy may be seen, but is less common than in dystrophinopathies, sarcoglycanopathies, and LGMD 2I. Muscle stretch reflexes are absent or diminished. Progression is steady but variable between different affected kinships. However, there can be variability of phenotypic expression within families.[2,144] For the most part, the earlier onset of symptoms and signs correlates with a faster evolution of the disease process. Approximately 50% of patients are nonambulatory by the age of 20 years, but some are able to walk late in life. Ventilatory function is only moderately affected. Cardiac function is normal, and there is no intellectual impairment. Life expectancy is close to normal.

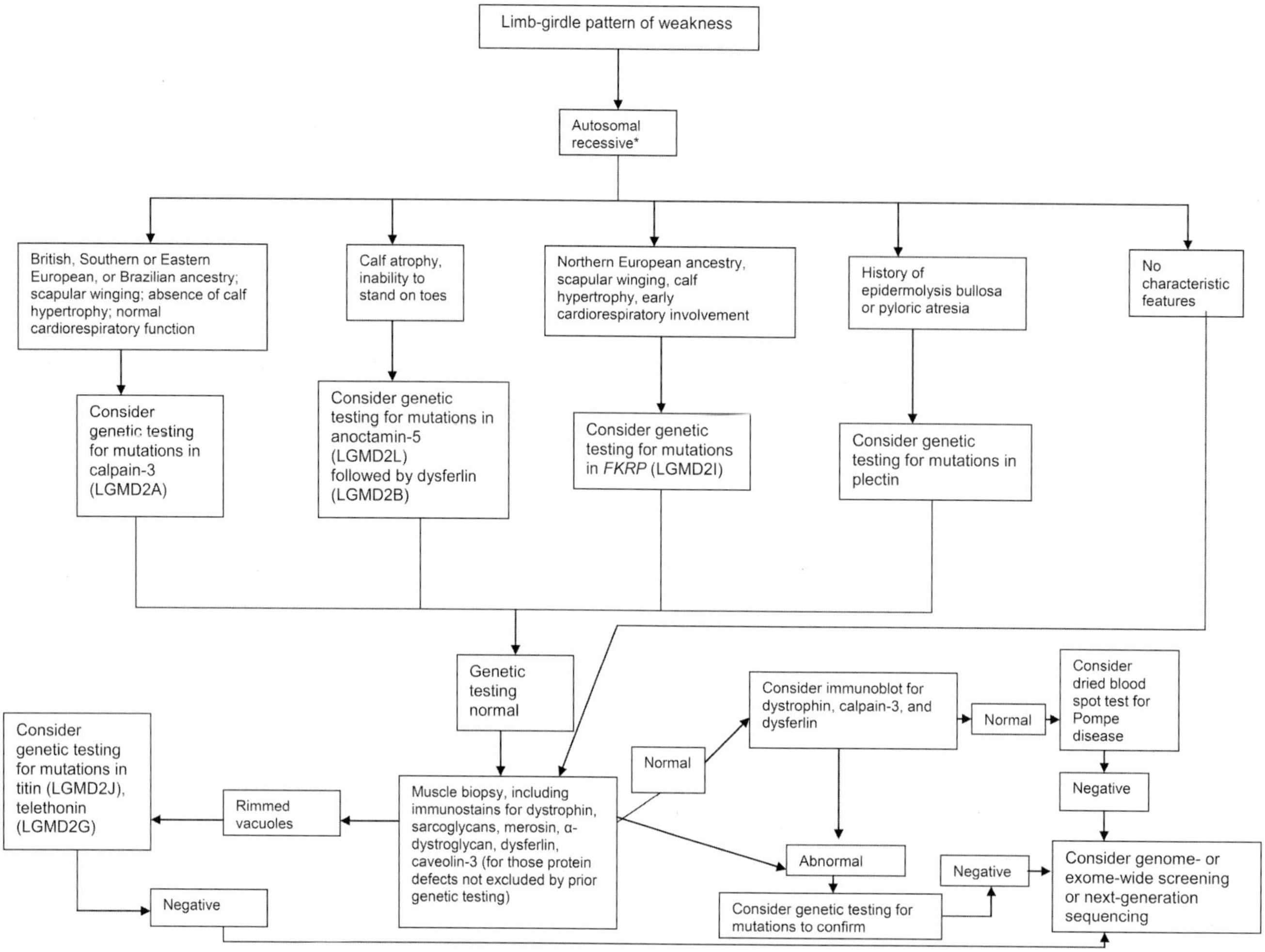

Figure 27-10. Diagnostic approach to patients with a limb-girdle pattern of weakness and suspected muscular dystrophy with an autosomal recessive inheritance pattern. Autosomal dominant, autosomal recessive, or X-linked inheritance may be responsible in sporadic cases. LGMD, limb-girdle muscular dystrophy. (Reproduced with permission from Narayanaswami P, Weiss M, Selcen D, et al: Evidence-based guideline summary: diagnosis and treatment of limb-girdle and distal dystrophies: report of the guideline development subcommittee of the American Academy of Neurology and the practice issues review panel of the American Association of Neuromuscular & Electrodiagnostic Medicine, *Neurology.* 2014;83(16):1453–1463.)

Laboratory Features

Serum CK levels are usually increased up to 20 times normal early in the disease, but decrease close to the normal range later when patients are wheelchair bound. Rare affected children have had peripheral eosinophilia. Skeletal muscle MRI scans demonstrate fat and connective tissue replacing normal muscle fibers. There is a predilection for the posterior thigh and adductors in the upper leg, as well as the soleus and medial gastrocnemius muscles in the lower leg (Fig. 27-11).[2,151–153]

Histopathology

Muscle biopsies demonstrate variation in fiber size associated with increased endomysial connective tissue. A lobulated appearance of muscle fibers on NADH staining is a frequent observation; however, this finding is not specific for calpainopathies. Interestingly, there was a report of six unrelated calpainopathy patients presenting as eosinophilic myositis in childhood.[149] We have also found mutations in the calpain-3 gene in adults who were originally misdiagnosed as having eosinophilic myositis that was refractory to immunosuppressive treatment (Fig. 27-12).[150]

As calpain-3 is a cytosolic enzyme immunostaining cannot be performed for diagnosis. Western blot analysis demonstrates reduced calpain-3 in most biopsies, but in 20% of cases the western blot is normal. The mutation in the gene may not alter the size or amount of calpain-3, but may affect the enzyme activity. Unfortunately, there are no readily available tests to assess enzyme activity at this time. In addition, definite diagnosis requires demonstration of a mutation in calpain-3 gene because secondary deficiency in calpain-3 can be seen in other dystrophies, most notably the dysferlinopathies and titinopathies.

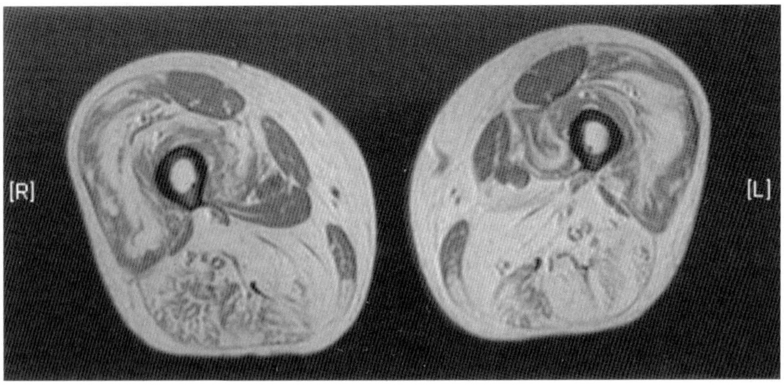

Figure 27-11. LGMD 2 A. Skeletal muscle MRI scan (T1 weighted) of the thigh reveals fat and connective tissue (bright signal) replacing normal muscle fibers with a predilection for the posterior thigh muscles.

Molecular Genetics and Pathogenesis

LGMD 2A is caused by mutations in the calpain-3 gene (*CPN3*)[1,2,145,154–159] Approximately 21–23% of patients in large series had only one identifiable mutation. Over two-thirds of patients with calpainopathy manifest with a BMD-like phenotype, approximately 10% present with severe childhood-onset weakness similar to DMD, while even fewer manifest with a distal myopathy, or have asymptomatic hyper-CKemia.[2] Prenatal diagnosis of LGMD 2A is possible through DNA analysis of fetal cells obtained by amniocentesis or chorionic villus sampling.

Calpain-3 is a muscle-specific, calcium-dependent, nonlysosomal, proteolytic enzyme. The mutation leads to an absence or a reduction in this enzyme, but how this results in the dystrophic process is not fully understood. Calpain-3 activates other enzymes involved in muscle metabolism.[156] Lack of calpain-3 might lead to the accumulation of toxic substances in muscle cells. Perhaps, calpain-3 plays a role in gene expression by regulating turnover or activity of transcription factors or their inhibitors.[156]

The reason for the peripheral eosinophilia and the eosinophilic infiltrate noted in biopsies of some affected individuals with LGMD 2A is not clear. Calpain-3 is highly expressed in T lymphocytes. These cells secrete interleukin-5 and interleukin-3, which are cytokines that are required for the growth and differentiation of eosinophils. Perhaps, the mutation in the gene causes not only LGMD, but also a perturbation of T-cell function leading to eosinophilia.[160]

LGMD 2B (DYSFERLIN)

Clinical Features

LGMD 2B usually presents in the late teens or early twenties, although onset as late as the age of 48 years has been reported.[1,2,161–171] The clinical phenotype is quite variable, with some patients having a "limb-girdle" pattern of weakness, others having early involvement of the posterior calf muscles (i.e., Miyoshi myopathy), and still others with anterior tibial weakness or combination of any of the above. Most patients manifest at least initially with a Miyoshi phenotype, with atrophy and weakness of the gastrocnemius and soleus muscles (Fig. 27-13). This is in contrast to many other forms of LGMD, which more typically have calf muscle hypertrophy or pseudohypertrophy. Not uncommonly, involvement of the calf muscles is asymmetric. A very uncommon presentation is early involvement of the paraspinal muscles leading to rigid spine syndrome or, on the opposite end of the spectrum, a lax spine with hyperlordosis or kyphosis. LGMD2B accounts for approximately 6% of the LGMDs.[2]

On examination, patients will have difficulty standing on their tip toes. Over time, the hamstrings and gluteal muscles are affected and then the distal arms. Less commonly, affected individuals manifest with proximal hip-girdle weakness followed by shoulder-girdle weakness. Mild scapular

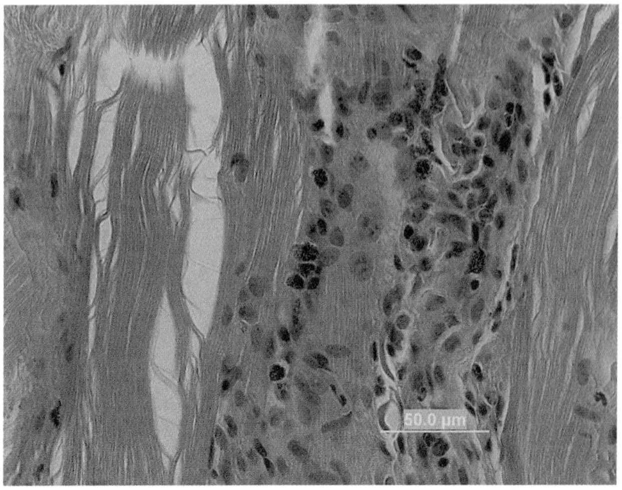

Figure 27-12. LGMD 2 A. Muscle biopsy demonstrates eosinophilic infiltrate that can be mistaken for eosinophilic myositis. Paraffin section, H&E.

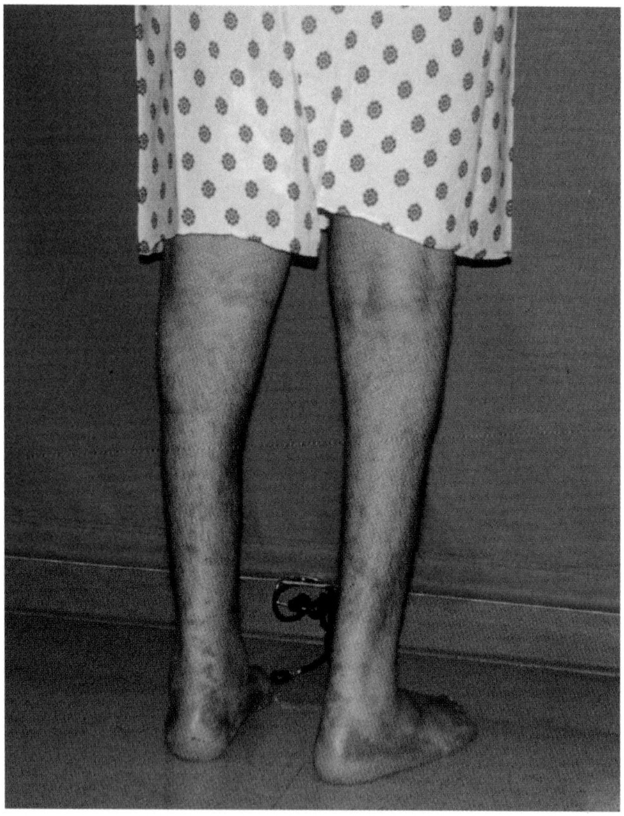

Figure 27-13. LGMD 2B/Miyoshi myopathy. Note the marked atrophy of the calves in a patient with Miyoshi myopathy.

winging may be evident at any stage of the disease. Still other patients have early, prominent involvement of the anterior tibial muscles. In our experience, a good examination will often detect atrophy and weakness of the calf muscles in patients with the "limb-girdle" and the "anterior tibial" phenotypes. A helpful sign in dysferlinopathies is the early loss of the Achilles' tendon reflexes. Usually, this is the most preserved reflex in other forms of LGMD but is the first to disappear in the dysferlinopathies. Of note, there is intra- and interfamilial variability in disease progression and pattern of muscle involvement.

Progression is usually slow, although we have seen several patients with a rather abrupt onset and rapid progression to a nonambulatory state. The subacute rapid progression and the prominent inflammatory cell infiltrate seen on muscle biopsy (see histopathology) can lead to the misdiagnosis of polymyositis.

Laboratory Features

Serum CK levels are usually markedly elevated (usually 35–200 times normal). Because dysferlin is present on white blood cells, western blot analysis on these cells for dysferlin represents a noninvasive method of making the diagnosis.[111] Skeletal muscle imaging with CT and MRI[2,169–171] has not shown preferential involvement of the posterior compartments of the distal and proximal legs. Interestingly, the pattern of muscle involvement is similar regardless of whether patients manifest with Miyoshi or limb-girdle phenotype in that there is early involvement of the gastrocnemius and thigh adductors with both presentations.[169]

Histopathology

Muscle biopsies demonstrate variation in fiber size, scattered necrotic and regenerating fibers, and increased endomysial connective tissue. Immunostaining reveals absent or diminished sarcolemmal staining with dysferlin antibodies. In contrast, there may be increased cytoplasmic staining. The reduced sarcolemmal immunostaining can be secondary and seen in other types of LGMD[172]; therefore, western blot needs to be performed on the muscle or white blood cells to confirm a primary deficiency. Not uncommonly, a prominent mononuclear inflammatory cell infiltrate is evident in the endomysium and surrounding blood vessels, which likely accounts for many cases of dysferlinopathy being misdiagnosed as polymyositis.[173] In contrast to polymyositis, the inflammatory cells do not typically appear to invade non-necrotic fibers. Another immunohistological feature that is helpful is the deposition of membrane attack complex on the sarcolemma of non-necrotic muscle fibers (Fig. 24-14).[174] This is an early finding in dysferlinopathies and other dystrophies with inflammation that is not seen in primary inflammatory myopathies such as polymyositis, dermatomyositis, and IBM. Interestingly, amyloid deposition in blood vessel walls, around the sarcolemma, and in the endomysial or perimysial connective tissue may be apparent with Congo red staining.[175] On EM, duplication of the basal lamina, disruption in the sarcolemma, invaginations or papillary exophytic defects of the muscle membrane, and subsarcolemma vesicles may be appreciated.[175]

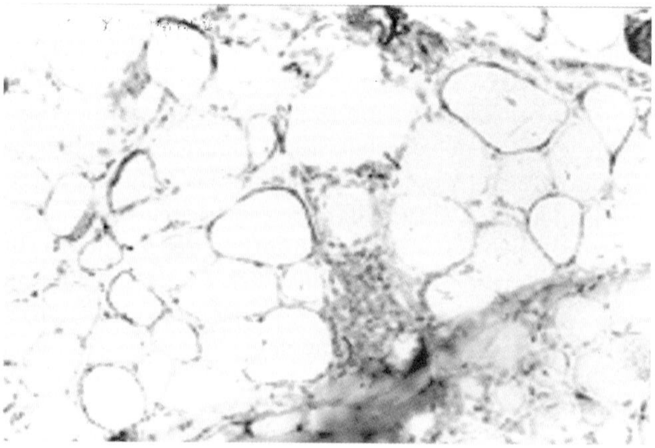

Figure 27-14. LGMD 2B/Miyoshi myopathy. Muscle biopsies often demonstrate endomysial inflammatory cell infiltrate that can lead to misdiagnosis as polymyositis (PM). An early observation is the demonstration of membrane attack complex (MAC) on the sarcolemma of non-necrotic muscle fibers in dysferlinopathies (also seen in FSHD) that is not appreciated in PM. Immunoperoxidase with anti-MAC antibodies.

Molecular Genetics and Pathogenesis

Mutations within the dysferlin gene are the cause of Miyoshi myopathy type 1, LGMD 2B, and some distal myopathies with anterior tibial weakness.[1,2,13,161,176] A study of 407 muscle biopsies from patients with unclassified myopathies (nondystrophinopathy and nonsarcoglycanopathy) demonstrated that 6.5% had abnormal dysferlin by western blot and immunostaining.[159] Dysferlinopathy accounted for 1% of patients with an unknown LGMD and 60% of patients with a distal myopathy. The clinical phenotype of patients with dysferlinopathy broke down as follows: 80% manifested with distal weakness, 8% had LGMD phenotype, and 6% presented with asymptomatic hyper-CK-emia. Dysferlin shares amino acid sequence homology with *Caenorhabditis elegans* spermatogenesis factor FER-1, thus the origin of its name. Dysferlin is located predominantly on the subsarcolemmal surface of the muscle membrane, but it has a small transmembrane spanning tail (Fig. 24-1). It does not appear to have a significant interaction with the dystrophin–glycoprotein complex, and immunostaining for dystrophin, dystroglycans, merosin, and the sarcoglycans is normal. Recent studies have suggested that at least one role of dysferlin is patching defects in skeletal membrane such that mutations in the gene result in defective membrane repair.[12]

SARCOGLYCANOPATHIES (LGMD 2C, LGMD 2D, LGMD 2E, AND LGMD 2F)

Clinical Features

The sarcoglycanopathies account for approximately 10% of LGMD in the following frequencies: α-sarcoglycan 6.6%, β-sarcoglycan 3.1%, γ-sarcoglycan 1.5%, and δ-sarcoglycan <1%.[1,2,6,177–187] The clinical, laboratory, and histologic features of the sarcoglycanopathies are quite similar to the dystrophinopathies, with some children developing severe weakness resembling DMD, and other patients having a later onset and slower progression similar to BMD.[2] Proximal leg and arm muscles are affected early, and calf pseudohypertrophy can often be appreciated. Cardiomyopathy can also occur similar to the dystrophinopathies.[2,179] In contrast to the dystrophinopathies, there are no significant intellectual impairments.

Laboratory Features

Serum CK levels are markedly elevated.[2] Echocardiogram may reveal evidence of cardiomyopathy.

Histopathology

Muscle biopsies demonstrate normal dystrophin; however, all of the sarcoglycans are usually absent or diminished on the sarcolemma, regardless of the primary sarcoglycan mutation.[2]

Molecular Genetics and Pathogenesis

LGMDs 2C, 2D, 2E, and 2F are caused by mutations in the γ-, α-, β-, and δ-sarcoglycan genes, respectively.[1,2,6,177–186] The clinical phenotypes appear to correlate with the expression of the sarcoglycans. The proteins of the sarcoglycan complex appear to function as a unit. Mutations involving any of the sarcoglycans result in destabilization of the entire complex and reduced expression of the other proteins. As apparent with the dystrophinopathies, the clinical severity of the sarcoglycanopathies may correlate with the type of mutation (i.e., whether the reading frame is preserved) and subsequent level of functional protein expression.

LGMD 2G (TELETHONIN)

Clinical Features

This myopathy is associated with prominent early weakness of the quadriceps and anterior tibial muscle groups with an onset between 2 and 15 years.[1,2,188,189] Some affected individuals manifest similar to Miyoshi myopathy with calf weakness. However, some have calf hypertrophy. Weakness affects the proximal more than distal muscles in the arms. Progression of weakness varies even within families. Cardiac involvement was noted in 3/6 affected members of one family; the type of involvement was not specified.

Laboratory Features

Serum CKs are elevated three to 30-fold.

Histopathology

Besides the usual dystrophic features, many muscle fibers had one or more rimmed vacuoles.[2] Immunohistochemistry and western blot analysis demonstrate a deficiency of telethonin.[189]

Molecular Genetics and Pathogenesis

LGMD 2G is caused by mutations in the telethonin gene, *TCAP*, located on chromosome 17q11-12.[189] Telethonin, also known as titin-cap, is a 19-kD sarcomeric protein that is expressed in skeletal and cardiac muscles, where it localizes to the central parts of the Z-disc.[190] It is a ligand for the giant sarcomeric protein, titin, which helps phosphorylate the C-terminal domain of telethonin in early differentiating myocytes. Telethonin may also overlap with myosin as well. It is amongst the most abundant proteins in muscle. The interaction of telethonin with titin appears to be important in myofibrillogenesis.[190,191]

LGMD 2H (E3-UBIQUITINE LIGASE OR TRIM 32)

Clinical Features

This genetically distinct LGMD was initially reported in families of Manitoba Hutterite origin.[1,2,29,192–195] Most affected individuals have exercise-induced myalgias and an examination revealing a limb-girdle pattern of weakness with scapular winging, facial weakness, calf hypertrophy, and heel cord contractures. The age at onset ranged from birth to the seventh decade of life. The myopathy is slowly progressive, and most affected individuals are still ambulatory without assistance in the fourth decade of life.

Laboratory Features

Serum CKs are elevated 5 to 50-fold. There may be nonspecific EKG changes.

Histopathology

Muscle biopsies demonstrate typical dystrophic features. In addition, many fibers (mostly type 2) contain small vacuoles that immunostain for sarcoplasmic reticulum-associated ATPase.[193,194] These vacuoles abut T-tubules and appear to be membrane bound on EM.

Molecular Genetics and Pathogenesis

LGMD 2H and sarcotubular myopathy (discussed in Chapter 28 with Congenital Myopathies) are allelic disorders caused by mutations in the gene, *TRIM32*, that encodes for E3-ubiquitine ligase (also known as tripartite motif-containing 32).[29] This enzyme may function by ubiquinating proteins that need proteasomal degradation.[195] The mechanism by which this leads to muscle destruction is unclear, but one might speculate on the possible toxic accumulation of "aged" or otherwise abnormal proteins not cleared by proteasomes.

LGMD 2I (FKRP)

Clinical Features

LGMD 2I was initially described in a large consanguineous Tunisian family with 13 affected members.[196] However, it subsequently has been demonstrated worldwide and is the most common form of LGMD in northern Europe. LGMD2I has constituted 4–30% of all LGMDs.[2,197–205] One class 1 study found this to be the cause of 19% of LGMDs.[147] The onset can range from infancy (MDC type 1C) to the fourth decade of life.[30,31] The pattern of weakness and course is variable. Some individuals have more hip-girdle involvement, while others are weaker in the proximal arms and neck flexors. Calves are often hypertrophic. Importantly, approximately one-half of patients develop a dilated cardiomyopathy and ventilatory muscle weakness.[2,197–198] Rare patients present with episodes of myoglobinuria.[203,204]

Laboratory Features

Serum CKs are elevated 10–30 times normal in some younger patients who are affected but may be normal in older individuals. PFTs often reveal reduced FVC while echocardiograms demonstrate a dilated cardiomyopathy.[2,200,202,205] MRI studies of the legs revealed abnormal signal and fatty infiltration, but the findings are not specific.[2,206]

Histopathology

Nonspecific dystrophic features are evident on muscle biopsy. Of note, immunohistochemistry demonstrates normal dystrophin and sarcoglycan staining. However, α-dystroglycan and occasionally merosin are reduced or absent with immunostaining (Fig. 27-15).

Molecular Genetics and Pathogenesis

LGMD 2I is caused by mutations in the gene that encodes for FKRP located on chromosome 19q13.3.[1,2] Mutations in this gene are also responsible for MDC type 1C; FKRP is a glycosyltransferase and its deficiency is associated with abnormal glycosylation of α-dystroglycan, which apparently disrupts the dystrophin–glycoprotein complex. Abnormalities in glycosylation of α-dystroglycan is a recurring theme in the MDCs, as this is also causative mechanism in Fukuyama disease, MEB, WWS, and LARGE-related CMD (MDC 1D). There is a correlation between a reduction in α-dystroglycan, the causal mutation, and the clinical phenotype in MDC 1C and LGMD 2I.[32]

FKRP localizes in rough endoplasmic reticulum, while fukutin localizes in the *cis*-Golgi compartment (ER).[207] Fukutin and FKRP appear to be involved at different steps in *O*-mannosylglycan synthesis of α-dystroglycan, and FKRP is most likely involved in the initial step in this synthesis. ER retention of mutant FKRP may play a role in the pathogenesis of these dystrophies and potentially explain why the allelic disorder LGMD 2I is milder, because the mutated protein is able to reach the Golgi apparatus.[208]

TITINOPATHY

Mutations in the titin gene (*TTN*) are associated with at least three different clinical phenotypes: autosomal recessive LGMD2J, autosomal dominant distal myopathy (Udd type distal myopathy), and autosomal dominant hereditary myopathy with early respiratory failure (HMERF).[1,2,209–220] The Udd type distal myopathy is the most common phenotype associated with TTN mutations is discussed in the Distal Myopathy section under Udd type distal myopathy. We will discuss the LGMD2J and HMERF phenotypes next.

LGMD 2J (TITIN)

Clinical Features

LGMD2J usually presents in the first three decades of life with proximal leg and arm with milder distal (anterior tibial, gastrocnemius, forearm, and hand) weakness.[2,210,211,216]

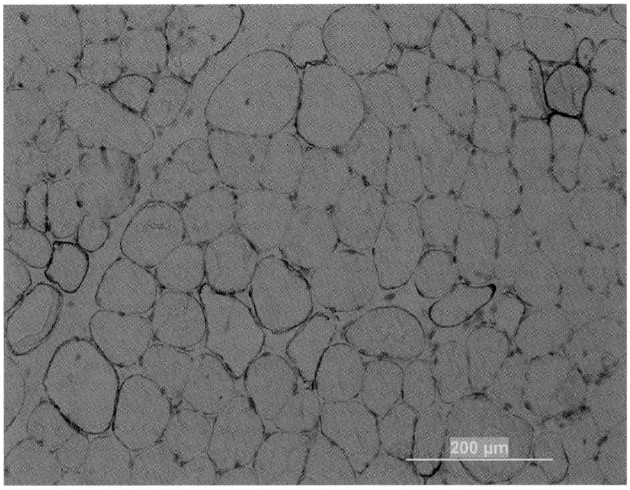

A

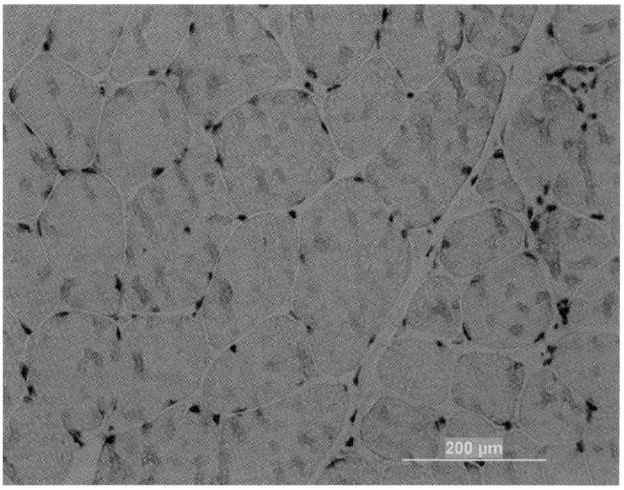

B

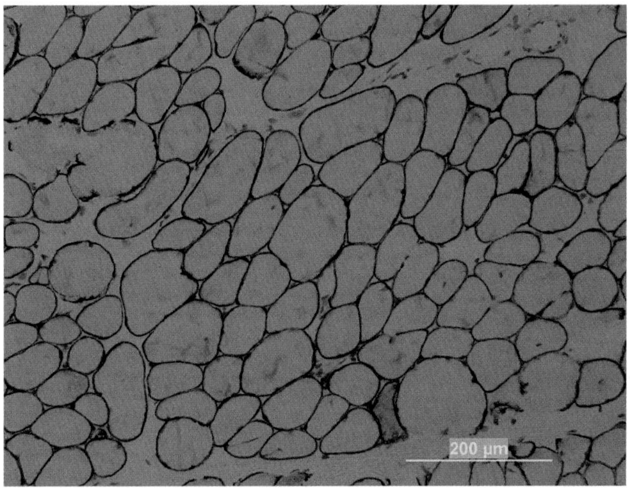

C

Figure 27-15. LGMD 2I. Muscle biopsies demonstrate reduced or patchy merosin staining **(A)**, absent α-dystroglycan staining **(B)**, but normal dystrophin staining **(C)** around the sarcolemma. Immunoperoxidase.

Many affected individuals are wheelchair dependent within 20 years of onset. Scapular winging is uncommon but may be evident.

A somewhat different presentation is that of an early-onset, proximal, and distal weakness leading to delayed motor milestones that is associated with a severe dilated cardiomyopathy.[219] Notably, some of these affected children exhibit hypertrophy of the thighs and calves along with atrophy of the arms. Spinal rigidity and moderate joint contractures appeared in the first decade. Affected individuals develop CHF and may suffer sudden death from fatal arrhythmias.[219]

Laboratory Features

CK elevation is usually 3–5 times normal. As mentioned, echocardiography may reveal features of a cardiomyopathy and PFTs can reveal signs of ventilatory muscle weakness. Skeletal muscle MRI has demonstrated fatty replacement of thigh (hamstrings more than quadriceps) and lower leg muscles (anterior more than posterior compartment).[215]

Histopathology

Muscle biopsies revealed dystrophic features and, unlike the allelic Udd type distal myopathy, rimmed vacuoles are absent or rare.[210,216,220]

Molecular Genetics and Pathogenesis

As mention previously, LGMD2J is caused by mutations in *TTN* that encodes the sarcolemmal protein, titin.

HEREDITARY MYOPATHY WITH EARLY RESPIRATORY FAILURE (TITIN)

Clinical Features

HMERF has been reported in Sweden and England.[217,218] The clinical phenotype overlaps with that seen in LGMD2J and Udd type distal myopathy.[2] Like Udd type distal myopathy, HMERF is associated with early progressive foot drop and an autosomal dominant inheritance. However, it tends to affect patients in early adulthood (but can develop in late teens to the eighth decade of life) and may affect the proximal muscles (legs greater than arms), as seen in LGMD2J. The majority of patients have prominent calf hypertrophy. As the name of the syndrome implies, HMERF is also associated with severe ventilatory muscle weakness. However, cardiomyopathy is not a common feature.

Laboratory Features

Serum CKs are usually mildly elevated. One study reported that skeletal muscle MRI identified the most commonly affected muscles to be the semitendinosus (20/21 subjects), the peroneus longus (16/21), and the obturator externus (15/21).[218]

Histopathology

Muscle biopsies reveal dystrophic features along with muscle fibers containing rimmed vacuoles and eosinophilic inclusions. Further, light microscopy and EM may reveal extensive myofibrillar degeneration with Z-disc as seen in MFM.

Molecular Genetics and Pathogenesis

HMERF is caused by mutations in *TTN.*

LGMD 2K (POMT1)

LGMD 2K is caused by mutations in the *POMT1* gene which is more commonly associated with WWS (discussed in section Congenital Muscular Dystrophy). However, rare patients have a milder LGMD phenotype.[2,221]

LGMD 2L/MIYOSHI MYOPATHY TYPE 3 (ANOCTAMIN-5)

Clinical Features

Patients with mutations in *ANO5* that encode for anoctamin 5 can manifested with a limb-girdle pattern of weakness (LGMD2L) or with distal weakness resembling Miyoshi myopathy (referred to as Miyoshi myopathy type III or MM3).[1,2,222–227] Similar to what is seen in the dysferlinopathies (i.e., LGMD2B and MM1), the clinical phenotypes often overlap in the anoctaminopathies. In addition, some patients have asymptomatic hyper-CK-emia, at least on presentation.[223–226] Epidemiological studies have suggested that anoctaminopathy may be one of the most common adult muscular dystrophies in Northern Europe, with a prevalence of about 20–25% in unselected undiagnosed cases.[227]

Onset of weakness usually ranges from 20–55 years with a mean in the mid 30s in both LGMD2L and MM3 presentations. As alluded, atrophy and weakness of the calf muscles (gastrocnemius or tibialis anterior) can be seen in combination with proximal muscle involvement. Asymmetric atrophy of the biceps brachii in the arms and quadriceps in the legs appears to be common.

Patients with MM3 manifest with early calf weakness and atrophy that is also often asymmetric.[2] However, some patients initially have calf hypertrophy before the atrophy occurs. The phenotype can merge with LGMD2L as some affected individuals develop atrophy or weakness of the quadriceps, biceps brachii, and pectoral muscles.[224–226]

Laboratory Features

CK levels are usually moderately elevated some 8 to over 20-fold.[2] Echocardiography, ECG, and PFTs are usually normal.[2,223–226] Skeletal muscle MRI has demonstrated atrophy and fat replacement of the long head of the biceps brachii in the arms and the medial gastrocnemius, soleus, adductor magnus, hamstrings, tensor fasciae latae, and to a lesser extent the quadriceps in the legs that is often asymmetric.[223,225]

Histopathology

Muscle biopsies reveal nonspecific dystrophic features.[223,225]

Molecular Genetics and Pathogenesis

LGMD2L is caused by mutations in *ANO5* that encode anoctamin 5.[222–227] This protein is located within the endoplasmic reticulum. The exact function of anoctamin 5 is unclear, but it belongs to a family of proteins found in calcium active chloride channels.

LGMD 2M (FUKUTIN)

LGMD 2M is caused by mutations in the fukutin gene that usually causes Fukuyama muscular dystrophy (discussed in more detail in the section on Congenital Muscular Dystrophy). However, mutations may rarely be associated with a more benign LGMD phenotype.[1,2,221,228,229]

LGMD 2N (POMT2)

LGMD 2N is caused by mutations in the *POMT2* gene that encodes for protein-O-mannosyltransferase. Mutations in *POMT2* usually cause MEB disease (discussed in more detail in section Congenital Muscular Dystrophies), but rarely can cause a more benign form of limb-girdle dystrophy.[1,2,221,230]

LGMD 2O (POMGnT1)

Mutations in *POMGnT1* also usually cause MEB disease (discussed in more detail in the section regarding Congenital Muscular Dystrophies), but have been associated with more benign LGMD 2O that has later onset of weakness and spared cognition.[1,2,228,221,231]

LGMD 2P (α-DYSTROGLYCAN)

Clinical Features

LGMD2P was recently reported in a child with unsteady gait and difficulty climbing stairs starting at 3 years of age.[232] Microcephaly and intellectual developmental delay was noted, and IQ at age 16 was 50.

Laboratory Features

CK levels were elevated at >4,000 U/L. Brain MRI was normal in the reported case.

Histopathology

Muscle biopsy revealed dystrophic features with a reduction of α-dystroglycan on immunohistochemistry.

Molecular Genetics and Pathogenesis

This dystrophy is caused by mutations in the *DAG1* gene that encode for α-dystroglycan. This disorder is in essence a primary α-dystroglycanopathy in which mutations lead to impaired binding to merosin and destabilization of the dystrophin–dystroglycan complex.

LGMD 2Q (PLECTIN-1)

Clinical Features

LGMD 2Q, also referred to as muscular dystrophy associated with epidermolysis bullosa, is caused my mutations in the gene that encodes for plectin 1.[2,233–246] Interestingly, in this regard, it is also allelic to a form of congenital myasthenia.[2,233,236,241,242,244] The characteristic clinical feature is the development in infancy or early childhood of epidermolysis bullosa, which manifests as blisters of the skin and mucous membranes, and nail bed abnormalities. Later in life, progressive weakness may ensue. Others manifest in early childhood or up to the fourth decade of life with limb girdle weakness without any skin abnormalities,[2,240] while some affected individuals may have ptosis, ophthalmoplegia, and facial weakness.[2,237,240] Other reported features include dental caries, scarring alopecia, urethral strictures, pyloric atresia, esophageal strictures, respiratory distress, and, rarely, cardiomyopathy.

Laboratory Features

CK levels may be slightly to markedly elevated. EMG demonstrates myopathic features with muscle membrane irritability and repetitive nerve stimulation, at least in cases of congenital myasthenia, have shown decrement. In vitro electrophysiologic studies showed normal quantal release by nerve impulse and small miniature EP potentials.[233]

Histopathology

Muscle biopsy may demonstrate type I fiber predominance and irregular oxidative staining. One study reported immunohistochemical loss of sarcolemmal staining using the antibody to the rod domain of plectin-1 in type I fibers, whereas type II fibers retained activity.[241] Plectin-1 deficiency may also be demonstrated on skin biopsy. EM has shown nonspecific myofibrillar disarray and Z-disc streaming. In those with features of congenital myasthenia, the endplates had focal degeneration of the junctional folds, but AChR content was normal.[233]

Molecular Genetics and Pathogenesis

LGMD 2Q is caused by mutations in the *PLEC1* that encodes for plectin-1. Plectin may serve as a scaffolding protein important for the formation of muscle fibers and neuromuscular transmission and also for the structural integrity of skin.[247,233]

LGMD 2R (DESMIN)

LGMD 2R manifests with progressive proximal muscle weakness and ventilatory failure in early childhood or adulthood. CK levels are mildly elevated. In contrast to most cases of primary desminopathy, it is associated with autosomal recessive inheritance as opposed to autosomal dominant.[247,248] It is allelic with LGMD1E and is discussed in more detail in the section regarding LGMD1E and myofibrillar myopathies.[2]

LGMD 2S (TRAPPC11)

This is recently reported LGMD in Syrians and Hutterites[249] is characterized by an infantile onset of choreiform, athetoid or dystonic movements, seizures, truncal ataxia, and mental intellectual disability. Proximal weakness developed in childhood along with scoliosis and hip dysplasia. CK is mild to moderately elevated. LGMD 2S is caused by mutations in the gene encoding transport (trafficking) protein particle complex, subunit 11 (*TRAPPC11*), which is important in trafficking proteins between endoplasmic reticulum and Golgi complex.

DIAGNOSIS AND TREATMENT OF LGMD

Diagnosis can be aided by the use of algorithms developed recently by a practice guideline committee of the American Academy of Neurology (AAN) and American Association of Neuromuscular and Electrodiagnostic Medicine (AANEM) (Figs. 27-8, 27-10, 27-16).[2] Treatment is largely supportive.[2] Physical and occupational therapy are important to prevent contractures and improve function. Large therapeutic trials

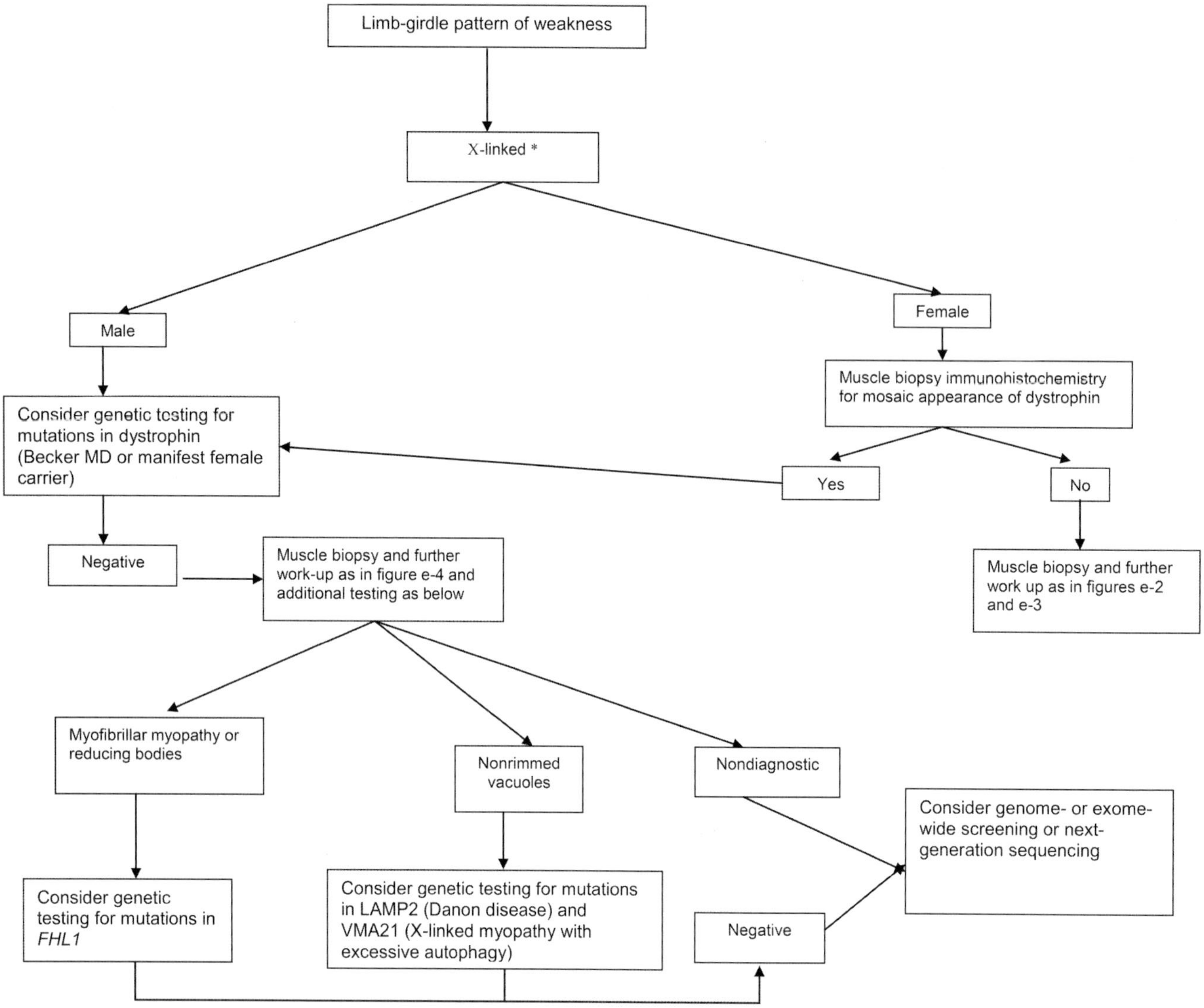

Figure 27-16. Diagnostic approach to patients with a limb-girdle pattern of weakness and suspected muscular dystrophy with an X-linked recessive inheritance pattern. In women, an X-linked disorder may be considered, if there is a familial presentation with men more affected than women. *Autosomal dominant, autosomal recessive, or X-linked inheritance may be responsible in sporadic cases. MD, muscular dystrophy. (Reproduced with permission from Narayanaswami P, Weiss M, Selcen D, et al: Evidence-based guideline summary: diagnosis and treatment of limb-girdle and distal dystrophies: report of the guideline development subcommittee of the American Academy of Neurology and the practice issues review panel of the American Association of Neuromuscular & Electrodiagnostic Medicine, *Neurology*. 2014;83(16):1453–1463.

of corticosteroids (similar to those conducted for DMD) have not been performed in patients with LGMD. Modest improvement in strength has been reported in a small number of patients with LGMD treated with short courses of creatine monohydrate (5–10 g/day). Advances in molecular genetics may lead to better forms of treatment in the future.

▶ CONGENITAL MUSCULAR DYSTROPHY

The congenital muscular dystrophies or MDCs are a heterogeneous group of autosomal-recessive disorders, characterized by the perinatal onset of hypotonia and weakness, dystrophic appearing muscle biopsies, and the exclusion of other recognizable causes of myopathy of the newborn (Table 27-1).[250] The abbreviation assigned by the Human Genome Organization is "MDC" for muscular dystrophy, congenital. The MDCs have been classified in the past according to clinical, ophthalmological, radiological, and pathological features. A more recent classification was proposed based on the location of the defective proteins and purported pathogeneses of the individual dystrophies.[250–252] The major categories of MDCs include (1) those associated with mutations in genes encoding structural proteins of the basal lamina, extracellular matrix, or sarcolemmal proteins that bind to the basal lamina; (2) those associated with impaired glycosylation of α-dystroglycan; and (3) those associated with selenoprotein 1 mutations.

▶ MDC ASSOCIATED WITH GENETIC DEFECTS OF STRUCTURAL PROTEINS OF THE BASAL LAMINA OR EXTRACELLULAR MATRIX

MDC 1A (ALSO KNOWN AS MDC WITH LAMININ α2 OR MEROSIN DEFICIENCY OR THE CLASSIC/OCCIDENTAL TYPE)

Approximately 30–40% of patients with MDC have absent or severely decreased merosin.[250–256] In addition, there are patients with partial merosin deficiency, analogous to the dystrophinopathies and sarcoglycanopathies.[254–262] However, some of these partial merosinopathies are now known to be secondary deficiencies related to glycosylation defects in α-dystroglycan.

Clinical Features

Children with MDC 1A usually present at birth with generalized weakness and hypotonia. There is a predilection for neck, shoulder, and hip-girdle muscles.[262] Calf hypertrophy may be appreciated early in the course. Contractures develop, but severe arthrogryposis is rare. Breathing and feeding problems can be present but usually not severe enough to require ventilator support at birth.[251] Some children develop a cardiomyopathy. Limited extraocular movements can be observed in the later stages.

Merosin-negative MDC typically has more severe weakness and is associated with a poorer prognosis compared with merosin-positive cases.[254] Most children with MDC 1A never ambulate independently, although rarely children are able to stand and occasionally walk with assistance. Individuals with only partial merosin deficiency have a milder course and can present in childhood with a DMD phenotype or in early adulthood with a phenotype similar to BMD or LGMD.[252–256,263]

Most children with MDC 1A have normal intelligence despite abnormal white matter changes apparent on MRI. However, there is a high incidence of epilepsy (12–30%) as well as a few reported cases of occipital dysplasia in merosin-deficient MDC.[213,257] Epilepsy can also occur in patients with partial merosin deficiency. Rare patients with MDC 1A with epilepsy and occipital agyria also have mental retardation.

Laboratory Features

Serum CK levels are markedly elevated, usually over 2,000 IU/L in the merosin-negative infants, while partial merosinopathies are associated with normal or mildly elevated serum CKs. Brain MRI often demonstrates diffuse white matter abnormalities in T2-weighted images suggestive of dysmyelination in most children after the age of 6 months (Fig. 27-17). In addition, occipital polymicrogyria/agyria and hypoplasia of pons and/or cerebellum are evident in rare cases.[250,251] Patients with partial merosin deficiency may or may not have cerebral hypomyelination on MRI. Visual- and somatosensory-evoked potential may reveal delayed latencies in MDC 1A.[264] Slowing of nerve conduction velocities is also commonly appreciated.[256]

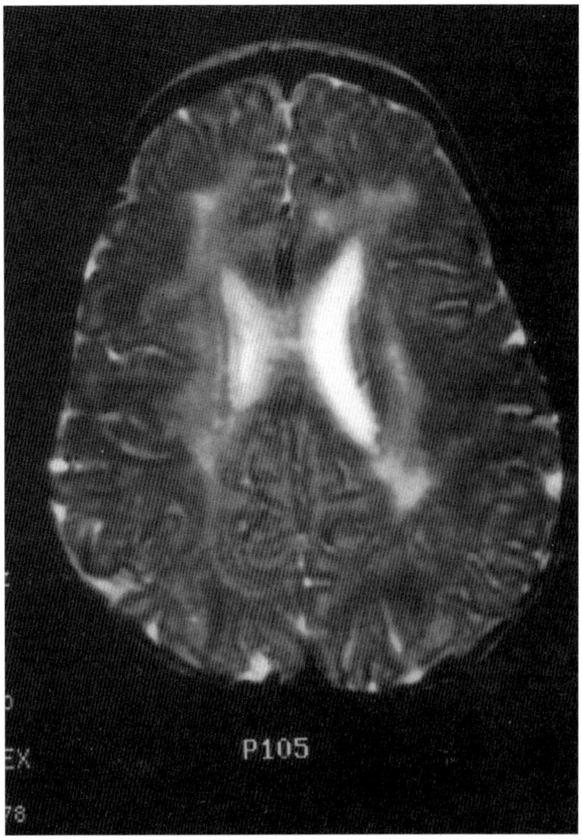

Figure 27-17. Congenital muscular dystrophy. T2-weighted MRI of the brain of an infant with merosin-negative congenital muscular dystrophy reveals increased signal of the subcortical white matter consistent with hypomyelination.

Histopathology

Muscle biopsies demonstrate variation in fiber size, increased endomysial connective tissue, and notably decreased or absent merosin (Fig. 27-18).

Molecular Genetics and Pathogenesis

MDC 1A is associated with mutations in the gene encoding α-2 subchain of merosin or alpha-laminin, *LAMA2*, on chromosome 6q21–22. The gene codes for a 390-kD protein, which is synthesized as one chain but processed into two fragments. On immunoblot, these two fragments have molecular masses of approximately 80 kD (C terminal) and 300 kD (N terminal).[255]

Merosin is also present in the basal lamina of myelinated nerves. Abnormal expression of merosin may interfere with myelinogenesis and may account for the hypomyelination evident in the central and peripheral nervous system. Importantly, merosin is expressed in the skin, and thus

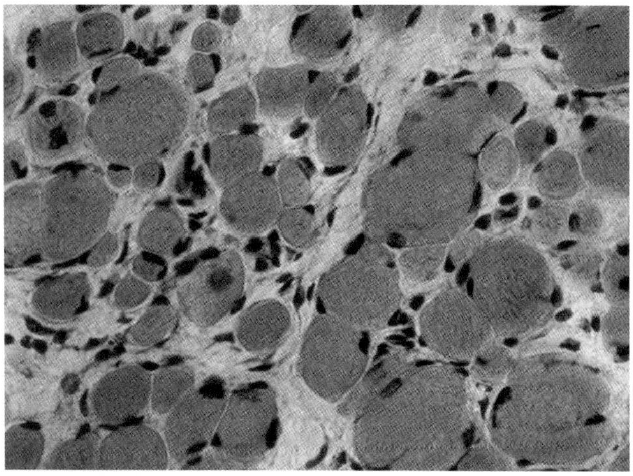

Figure 27-18. Congenital muscular dystrophy. Muscle biopsy demonstrates fiber size variability and increased endomysial and perimysial connective tissue consistent with a dystrophic process. H&E.

merosin-negative MDC can be diagnosed on skin biopsies.[259,265] Further, prenatal diagnosis of merosin-negative MDC can be made on chorionic villous sampling.[260,266]

Merosin binds to α-dystroglycan and α7β 1D integrin (Fig. 27-1). As with primary dystrophinopathies and adhalinopathies, merosinopathies may result in a disruption and loss of integrity of the dystrophin–glycoprotein complex. Mutations in the α-2 subchain of merosin result in a markedly diminished expression of α7β 1D integrin, but a normal or only mildly decreased expression of components of the dystroglycan or sarcoglycan complexes on the sarcolemma. Of note, mutations involving the α7 subunit of integrin that binds to merosin also results in a form of MDC.[267]

MEROSIN-POSITIVE CLASSIC MDC

As noted in the previous discussion, merosin-positive forms of classic MDC are clinically more benign than merosin-negative MDC. These merosin-positive MDC cases are genetically heterogeneous. Some partial merosin deficiency cases (the so-called MDC 1B) map to genetic loci on chromosome 1q42. The exact gene for MDC 1B has not as yet been identified. Some cases of partial merosin deficiency or MDCs with normal merosin are due to mutations in glycosyltransferases, which cause secondary α-dystroglycanopathy (these are discussed in a separate section).

Mutations of the α7 subunit of integrin gene, *ITGA7*, located on chromosome 12q13 have been demonstrated in three patients to date with merosin-positive MDC.[269] Children who are affected present with congenital onset of generalized weakness and hypotonia and had delayed motor milestones. Mental retardation was evident in one child who had a normal MRI of the brain and EEG. Serum CK was only mildly elevated (less than five times normal). Muscle biopsies only showed mild variation of fiber size with normal merosin expression on immunohistochemistry.

► ULLRICH DISEASE

Clinical Features

Ullrich congenital muscular dystrophy (UCMD) is associated with weakness at birth or early infancy, contractures of the proximal joints, hyperextensibility of the distal joints, high-arched palate, and protuberant calcanei.[250,268,269] UCMD is allelic with the more benign Bethlem myopathy. UCMD was initially felt to be autosomal recessive, while Bethlem myopathy was autosomal dominant, but UCMD can be autosomal dominant in inheritance.[270] UCMD is associated with congenital muscle weakness, delayed motor milestones, proximal joint contractures, scoliosis, and marked distal joint hyperextensibility. Intelligence is normal.

Laboratory Features

Serum CK is normal or mildly elevated.

Histopathology

Muscle biopsies reveal variation in muscle fiber size, scattered regenerating and degenerating fibers, and increased endomysial connective tissue. Immunohistochemistry reveals that collagen VI is present in the interstitium but absent from the sarcolemma.[269] EM demonstrates that collagen VI in the interstitium fails to anchor normally to the basal lamina surrounding muscle fibers.

Molecular Genetics and Pathogenesis

Collagen VI is composed of three chains, α1, α2, and α3, and is a ubiquitously expressed extracellular matrix protein. The three chains are encoded by the genes *COL6A1* and *COL6A2* on chromosome 21q22.3 and *COL6A3* on chromosome 2q37. UCMD and the less severe Bethlem myopathy are caused by mutations in these genes.[250,270] UCMD had been considered a recessive condition caused by homozygous or compound heterozygous mutations in COL6A2 and COL6A3. In contrast, the milder disorder Bethlem myopathy has dominant inheritance and is caused by single mutations in COL6A1, COL6A2, and COL6A3.[270] However, some studies have demonstrated that UCMD can be inherited in a dominant fashion as well.[270] Collagen VI deficiency in muscle or cultured fibroblasts was complete in severe cases and partial in the milder forms, which suggests a correlation between the degree of collagen VI deficiency and the clinical severity in UCMD.[271] Not all patients with Ullrich disease have mutations in collagen VI. However, the absence of collagen VI is seen even in these cases, suggesting a mutation involving other proteins that interact with collagen VI.

▶ MDC ASSOCIATED WITH IMPARIED GLYCOSLYLATION OF α-DYSTROGLYCAN

The primary sequence of α-dystroglycan predicts a molecular mass of 72 kD; however, the mass of α-dystroglycan in the skeletal muscle is 156 kDa.[251] The increase in size is due to posttranslational modification of α-dystroglycan. O-mannosyl and LARGE-dependent glycosylation of α-dystroglycan is apparently important for stable binding of this sarcolemmal to merosin in the basement membrane. The α-dystroglycanopathies are the result of mutation in the α-dystroglycan (*DAG1*) gene, but also in at least 13 other genes to date that are involved in the glycosylation pathway (*POMT1, POMT2, POMGnT1, FKRP, Fukutin, LARGE, ISPD, GTDC2, B3GALNT2, B3GNT1, TMEM5, GMPPB, SGK196*, and dolichyl-phosphate mannosyltransferase subunit genes-*DPM1, DPM2, DPM3*).[2,251,252,272–293]

The glycosyltransferase *O*-mannosyltransferase 1 (*POMT1*) forms a complex with a second putative *O*-mannosyltransferase (POMT2) to catalyze the first step in *O*-mannosyl glycosylation.[251,252] Subsequently, the transfer of *N*-acetylglucosamine to *O*-mannose of glycoproteins is catalyzed by *O*-mannose β-1,2-*N*-acetylglucosaminyltransferase (POMGnT1). Fukutin, FKRP, LARGE, and other enzymes mentioned above are other secretory enzymes involved in post-translational glycosylation of α-dystroglycan, although the exact reactions they catalyze are not known. Not only is glycosylation of α-dystroglycan important for proper muscle function, but impaired glycosylation of α-dystroglycan leads to defects in neuronal migration and the abnormalities in the central nervous system.

The nomenclature of these disorders has changed in recent years.[250] Muscular dystrophy–dystroglycanopathy with brain and eye anomalies (type A), MDDGA1, previously referred to as the WWS or MEB disease, is genetically heterogeneous and can be caused by mutation in other genes involved in DAG1 glycosylation. MDDGA1 is caused by mutation in the gene encoding protein O-mannosyltransferase-1 (*POMT1*); MDDGA2 is caused by mutations in the *POMT2* gene; MDDGA3 is caused by mutation in the *POMGNT1* gene; MDDGA4 is caused by mutations in the *FKTN* gene; MDDGA5 is caused by mutations in the *FKRP* gene; MDDGA6 is caused by mutations in the *LARGE* gene; MDDGA7 is caused by mutations in the *ISPD* gene; MDDGA8 is caused by mutations in the *GTDC2* gene; MDDGA10 is caused by mutations in the *TMEM5* gene; MDDGA11, caused by mutations in the *B3GALNT2* gene; MDDGA12 is caused by mutations in the *SGK196* gene; MDDGA13 is caused by mutations in the *B3GNT1* gene; and MDDGA14 is caused by mutations in the *GMPPB* gene.[250,272–293]

Muscle biopsy findings are indistinguishable from other forms of MDC using routine stains. A striking inflammatory infiltrate is occasionally present, which has led to the erroneous diagnosis of a congenital inflammatory myopathy or polymyositis. Importantly, abnormal glycosylation of α-dystroglycan can be appreciated by reduced immunostaining of the sarcolemmal membrane with antibodies directed against α-dystroglycan and merosin.[250,280–283]

▶ FUKUYAMA CONGENITAL MUSCULAR DYSTROPHY

Clinical Features

FCMD was originally described in Japan, where it is the most common form of MDC.[250–252,284] The myopathy presents with generalized proximal greater than distal weakness and hypotonia in infants. Mothers of affected children retrospectively recall decreased fetal movements. There is an increased frequency of spontaneous abortions of affected fetuses. Pseudohypertrophy of the calves is recognized in approximately half the children. Muscle stretch reflexes are reduced. Some children are born with arthrogryposis and contractures that are progressive.

In addition to the myopathy, FCMD is associated with severe structural abnormalities of the brain, including microcephaly, cortical dysplasia, lissencephaly, pachygyria, polymicrogyria, and hydrocephalus.[284,285] Intellectual function is markedly compromised. Approximately 50% of children who are affected have seizures. Both physical and mental developments are delayed, with the majority never being able to stand or ambulate independently. Most children die by the age of 10–12 years of age from ventilatory failure.

Laboratory Features

The serum CK level is usually elevated 10–50 times normal values. Electroencephalography is often abnormal, demonstrating epileptiform activity and generalized slowing. MRI and CT scans of the brain reveal structural abnormalities and evidence of hypomyelination.

Molecular Genetics and Pathogenesis

FCMD is caused by mutations in the fukutin gene, *FKTN*, which is located on chromosome 9q31.[284–287] Fukutin is a secretory enzyme that localizes to the *cis*-Golgi compartment and is thought to have a role in post-translational glycosylation of α-dystroglycan.[207] In addition to the skeletal muscle involvement, the disruption of normal glycosylation of α-dystroglycan or other proteins leads to defects in neuronal migration and differentiation, which accounts for the many abnormalities seen within the central nervous system.

▶ WALKER–WARBURG SYNDROME

Clinical Features

WWS, or cerebro-ocular dysplasia, is the most severe α-dystroglycanopathy and is associated with a life expectancy of less than 3 years. WWS presents as severe generalized weakness and hypotonia in infancy.[280–282] In addition, the infants are usually born blind secondary to ocular malformations, which include fixed pupils, hypoplasia of the optic nerves, microphthalmia, corneal opacities, cataracts, shallow anterior chambers, ciliary body abnormalities, iridolental synechiae, and retinal dysplasia and detachment. As with FCMD and MEB, WWS is associated with migrational and developmental disturbances of neurons in the brain, which include lissencephaly, polymicrogyria, hydrocephalus, hypomyelination of the subcortical white matter, and hypoplasia of the brainstem and vermis. Seizures are common.

Laboratory Features

Serum CK levels are elevated. Brain MRI scans reveal structural abnormalities, which are alluded to in the above section. Electroencephalography is often abnormal, revealing slowing of the background and epileptiform activity.

Molecular Genetics and Pathogenesis

WWS is caused by mutations in several genes (*POMT1 POMT2, FKRP, FKTN, ISPD, CTDC2, TMEM5, POMGNT1, B3GALNT2, GMPPB, B3GNT1, SGK196*).[250,251,280–282,288] Mutations in the *POMT1* gene are the most common and account for the 20% of WWS.[250,251] The clinical phenotype of patients with mutations in the POMT1 gene is also variable, with rare cases being reported with LGMD and mild mental retardation (LGMD 2K).[289]

▶ MUSCLE-EYE-BRAIN DISEASE

Clinical Features

MEB disease was initially described in Finnish patients, but has been subsequently reported in other populations.[250,281,282,290–292] As in WWS, brain and eye abnormalities accompany the muscle weakness; however, MEB is less severe. Although infants are weak and motor development is slow, most affected children eventually can sit and stand and some ambulate. There are severe cognitive impairments associated with structural abnormalities in the brain, which include pachygyria, polymicrogyria, abnormal midline structures, and hypoplasia of the vermis and pons. MEB is also associated with progressive myopia, glaucoma, and late cataracts.

Laboratory Features

Serum CK levels are elevated. MRI of the brain may demonstrate polymicrogyria, abnormal midline structures, hypoplastic vermis, and pons.[281,290–292]

Molecular Genetics and Pathogenesis

MEB is most commonly caused by mutations in the gene that encodes for *O*-mannose-β-1,2-*N*-acetylglucosaminyl transferase (*POMGnT1*) on chromosome 1p32-p34.[281,282,287] POMGnT1 catalyzes the transfer of *N*-acetylglucosamine to *O*-mannose of glycoproteins. Mutations in this gene has also been associated with a milder myopathy, LGMD 2M. Mutations in the *FKRP, FKTN, ISPD*, and *TMEM5* genes can also cause MEB.[250]

MDC 1C

Clinical Features

MDC 1C (also known as MDDGA5) is allelic to LGMD 2I and is caused by mutations in the gene that encodes for FKRP. The FKRP-related myopathies are very common, especially among patients of Northern European, including English, ancestry, and give rise to the largest phenotypical spectrum of muscular dystrophies so far connected to mutations of a single gene.[250–252] The age of onset can range from infancy (e.g., congenital) to the fourth decade of life, with a pattern of weakness similar to MDC 1A. A phenotype reminiscent of WWS can also be seen in patients with FKRP mutations. Early involvement of cardiac and respiratory muscles is common.[197–199]

Laboratory Features

CK levels are always very elevated (10–75× normal). Echocardiogram may reveal features of a dilated cardiomyopathy. Pulmonary function tests may reveal reduced forced vital capacity and inspiratory pressures. MRI of the brain may reveal microcephaly, cerebellar cysts, and hypoplasia of the vermis, and also white matter abnormalities on MRI as in other α-dystroglycanopathies.[250,293]

Molecular Genetics and Pathogenesis

MDC 1C is caused by mutations in *FKRP* that encodes for FKRP. FKRP localizes in rough endoplasmic reticulum and appears to be involved in one of the initial steps in *O*-mannosyl glycan synthesis of α-dystroglycan.[207] ER retention of mutant FKRP may play a role in the pathogenesis and potentially explain why the allelic disorder LGMD 2I is milder, because the mutated protein is able to reach the Golgi apparatus.[208] There is a correlation between a reduction in α-dystroglycan, the mutation, and the clinical phenotype in MDC 1C and LGMD 2I.[32] Patients with MDC 1C have a profound depletion of α-dystroglycan, those with a Duchenne-like phenotype have a moderate reduction in α-dystroglycan, and individuals with the milder form of LGMD 2I demonstrate a variable but subtle alteration in α-dystroglycan immunolabeling.

MDC 1D

Clinical Features

This is a very rare dystrophy, which as in other secondary α-dystroglycanopathies, is associated with generalized weakness, mental retardation, and global developmental delay.[34,35,250,272] Motor milestones are delayed, but individuals who are affected may be able to ambulate. Nystagmus may be evident on examination but no other ocular abnormalities are typically identified.

Laboratory Features

Serum CK is mild to moderately elevated. Mild structural abnormalities have been appreciated on brain MRI.

Molecular Genetics and Pathogenesis

Mutations in the human LARGE gene (also is required for glycosylation of α-dystroglycan) is responsible for this rare form of MDC.[34,35,272] This gene encodes for another putative glycosyltransferase.

► MDC ASSOCIATED WITH SELENOPROTEIN N1 MUTATIONS

RIGID SPINE SYNDROME

Clinical Features

The rigid spine syndrome or rigid spine muscular dystrophy (RSMD) is heterogeneous disorder. One subtype, RSMD1, manifests in infancy with hypotonia, proximal weakness, and delayed motor milestones.[250,294–301] Affected individuals develop progressive limitation of spine mobility often associated with scoliosis and contractures at the knees and elbows. Thus, these patients share many clinical features with EDMD and UCMD/Bethlem myopathy. Of note, some patients previously diagnosed with multi/minicore congenital myopathy have a rigid spine. Respiratory weakness can develop due to stiffness of the rib cage and involvement of the diaphragm. Many patients require noninvasive ventilator support.

Laboratory Features

Serum CK levels are normal to slightly elevated. Conduction defects may be evident on EKG. Pulmonary function tests reveal a reduced vital capacity in patients old enough to cooperate. EMG demonstrates myopathic appearing MUAPs, while insertional activity is typically normal and abnormal spontaneous activity is sparse.

Histopathology

Muscle biopsies reveal nonspecific myopathic features including variability in fiber size, increased internal nuclei, type 1 fiber predominance, and moth-eaten fibers and lobulated fibers on NADH-TR stains. Some cases are associated with multiple minicores. Cytoplasmic bodies, Mallory bodies, increased desmin expression, and sarcoplasmic and intranuclear tubulofilamentous inclusions may also be present similar to MFM.[181] Endomysial fibrosis is apparent, particularly in axial muscles (i.e., rectus abdominis and paraspinal muscles). Immunostains for dystrophin, sarcoglycans, and the dystroglycans are normal.

Molecular Genetics and Pathogenesis

Some cases of autosomal-recessive RSMD have been linked to mutations in the gene that encodes for selenoprotein N1, *SEPN1*, located on chromosome 1p35–36.[250,297,300] Mutations in this gene have also been shown in some patients with multi/minicore myopathy and MFM. Selenoprotein N1 is an endoplasmic reticulum glycoprotein. The function of this protein is not known.

► DIAGNOSIS AND TREATMENT OF MDC

With the various genes that can cause congenital muscular dystrophy, diagnosis can be daunting, particularly with those more familiar with taking care of adults. Assessment of ocular and brain abnormalities and other features can help point to the right direction of genetic testing (Fig. 27-19). Treatment of the MDCs is supportive. Corticosteroids have not been studied in a prospective, placebo-controlled, double-blind fashion as in DMD, but it is clear that corticosteroids have not been associated with any significant benefit even in those cases with associated significant inflammation on muscle biopsy. Antiepileptic medications are necessary for control of seizures. Physical therapy and range of motion exercise are important to reduce contractures. Ventilator support, invasive or noninvasive, may be beneficial in patients with ventilatory muscle involvement.

► OTHER REGIONAL FORMS OF MUSCULAR DYSTROPHY

FACIOSCAPULOHUMERAL MUSCULAR DYSTROPHY

Clinical Features

Facioscapulohumeral muscular dystrophy (FSHD) is an autosomal-dominant disorder, with an incidence of approximately 4 per million and a prevalence of roughly 50 per million.[302] There is a variable degree of penetrance of clinical findings within families, while around 30% of affected family members are unaware of their deficits. Thus, it is very important to examine family members of patients suspected of having FSHD.

Onset of weakness is usually appreciated between 3 and 44 years, although onset as late as 75 years has been reported.[303–306] As the name suggests, FSHD is characterized

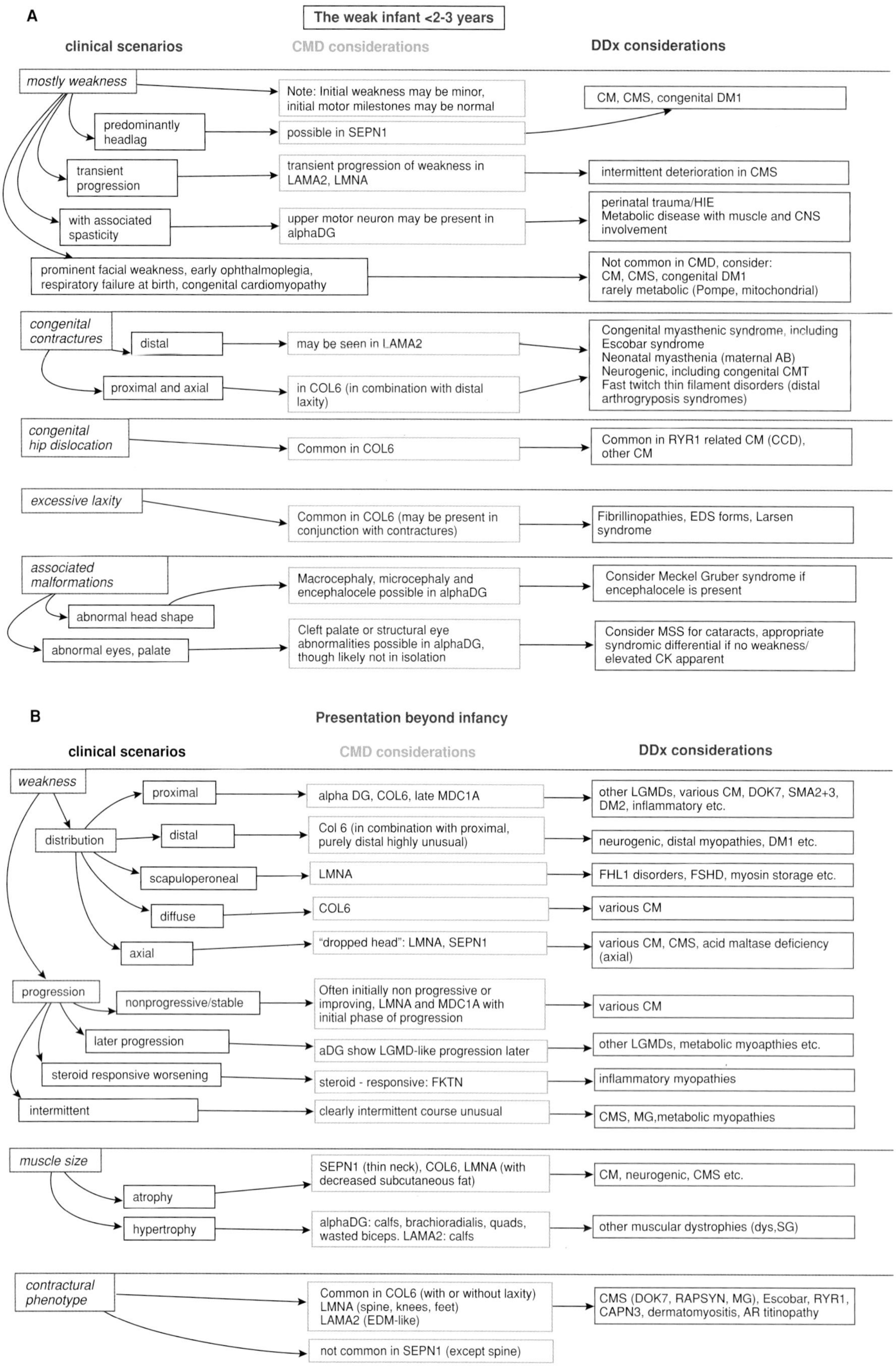

Figure 27-19. Differential diagnostic considerations for various clinical findings in infancy **(A)** and beyond infancy **(B, C)**, as well as for various laboratory findings that may be available at the outset of the diagnostic encounter **(D)**.

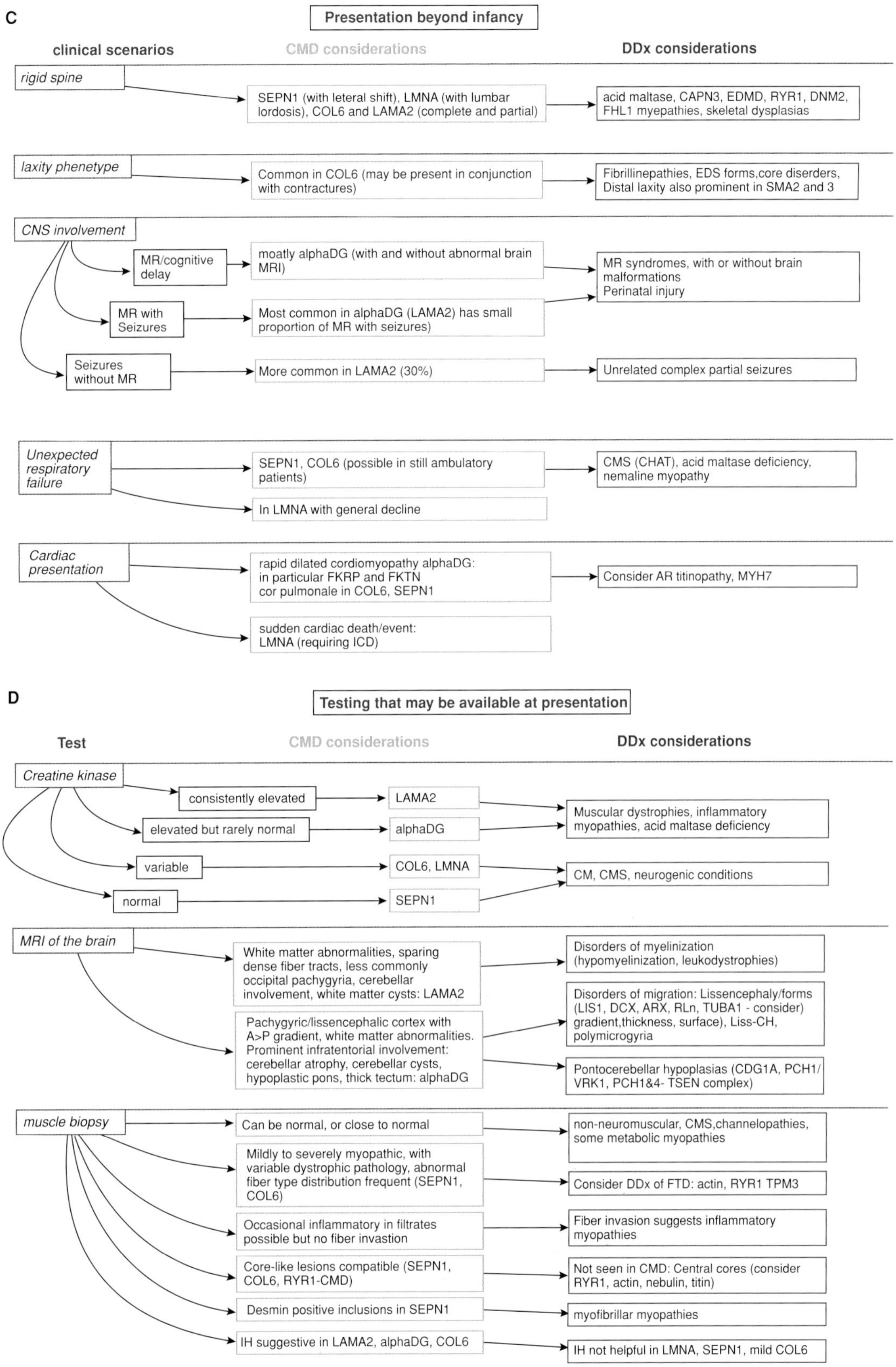

Figure 27-19. (*Continued*) *Note*: The most important tools in the clinical differential diagnosis are: EMG/NCV to diagnose neurogenic involvement, muscle biopsy, and selective biochemical and genetic testing. The differential diagnostic considerations are not exhaustive but highlight a few of the more relevant conditions to consider with a given clinical picture. To save space we are only using the gene/protein symbols to indicate specific diagnosis. (Reproduced with permission from Bönnemann CG, Wang CH, Quijano-Roy S, et al. Diagnostic approach to the congenital muscular dystrophies. *Neuromuscul Disord*. 2014;24(4):289–311.)

by muscle weakness and wasting in a rather specific distribution. The muscles of facial expression, particularly the orbicularis oculi, zygomaticus, and orbicularis oris muscles, are affected early. Patients may be unable to fully close their eyes against resistance and may sleep with incomplete eyelid closure. Affected persons can have a horizontal smile and weak puckering of the lips. Facial weakness may be strikingly asymmetric, mimicking a seventh nerve palsy. The muscles of mastication and the external ocular muscles are typically spared.

The scapula-stabilizer muscles (serratus anterior, rhomboid, middle trapezius, and, to some degree, latissimus dorsi muscles) are also weak and atrophic early in the course. Weakness of these muscles lead to upward and lateral rotation of the shoulder blades with scapular winging and the appearance of a "trapezius hump," which often is mistaken for muscle hypertrophy (Fig. 27-20). Although the deltoids are relatively spared during the early course of the disease, the sternocostal head of the pectoralis major is often atrophic and weak. The clavicles are displaced more horizontally and may angle downward from the sternum to the upper arm. Combined with the internal rotation of the upper arms, the anterior axillary folds, which are normally vertical, become horizontally displaced. There are also significant weakness and atrophy of the biceps brachii and triceps, with relatively normal bulk of the forearm muscles producing the so-called "Popeye arms." Wrist extensors are weaker than wrist flexors. The characteristic facial and upper torso appearance led to the designation of "facioscapulohumeral" muscular dystrophy. Some patients with FSHD manifest only with scapular winging or a limb-girdle pattern of weakness, thus mimicking an LGMD.[307] Further, there can be striking asymmetric and sometimes unilateral involvement of the facial, scapular stabilizers, or humeral muscles.

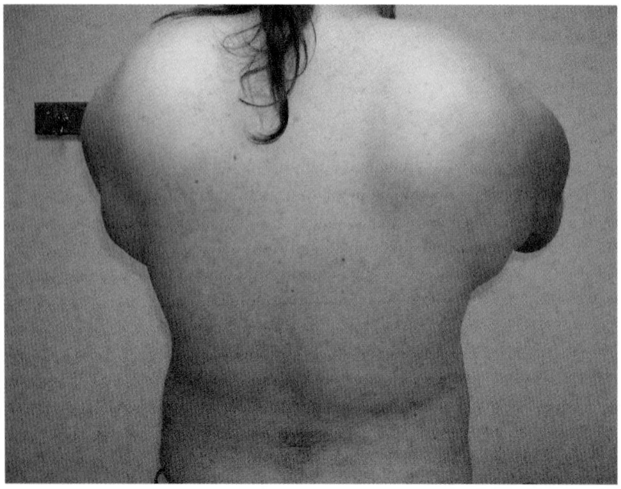

Figure 27-20. Facioscapulohumeral muscular dystrophy (FSHD). Characteristic appearance of a patient diagnosed with FSHD. On attempted forward flexion of the arms at the shoulders the scapulae elevates and laterally deviates off the posterior rib cage under the trapezius musculature, giving the false impression of very muscular individual. Palpation reveals the bone underlying the muscle tissue.

The tibialis anterior is usually the earliest lower limb muscle to manifest weakness, and occasionally patients present with foot drop.[306] The gastrocnemius muscles are usually normal, although rarely patients manifest with difficulty walking on their toes.[306] The muscle involvement may progress to the pelvic musculature, producing a hyperlordotic posture and a waddling gait. As in the face and arms, weakness in the legs is often asymmetric. Approximately 20% of patients with FSHD eventually will require wheelchairs.

Abdominal muscles may also be involved, producing a positive Beevor sign (the umbilicus may move up or down a few centimeters, when the patient is supine and attempts to flex the head because of upper or lower abdominal muscle weakness). Although seldom volunteered, asking a patient if they have to roll on their side or arise from a supine position, may provide insight into possible abdominal wall weakness. Sensation is intact to all modalities, and the reflexes are usually absent or diminished commensurate with the degree of muscle wasting.

Some patients with FSHD appear to experience a late exacerbation of muscle weakness. They may only have mild weakness for years and then suddenly have a marked increase of weakness in the typical distribution over the course of several years. Affected individuals usually have a normal life span; however, severe progressive ventilatory muscle weakness has been reported in approximately 1% of large series of patients with FSHD.[308] Severe extremity weakness, wheelchair dependency, and kyphoscoliosis appear to be risk factors for ventilatory failure. Further, rare patents develop cardiac involvement manifesting as conduction defects, supraventricular, or ventricular arrhythmias that may require pacemaker implantation.[309]

Infantile-onset FSHD is associated with severe weakness presenting in the first 2 years of life. A wheelchair is required to maintain mobility by the time the patient is 9 or 10 years of age. FSHD can also be associated with profound sensorineural hearing loss and retinal telangiectasias (Coats' disease). Some infants present with profound facial diplegia mimicking Mobius syndrome.[310]

Laboratory Features

Serum CK levels normal or moderately elevated.

Histopathology

The muscle biopsy demonstrates variation in muscle fiber size with atrophic and hypertrophic fibers, scattered necrotic and regenerating fibers, increased internalized nuclei, and increased endomysial connective tissue. Prominent mononuclear inflammatory infiltrate may be appreciated in the endomysium, which can lead to confusion with polymyositis (Fig. 27-21).[311] Immunostaining with antibodies directed against membrane attack complex may demonstrate deposition on the sarcolemma of non-necrotic muscle fibers.[312]

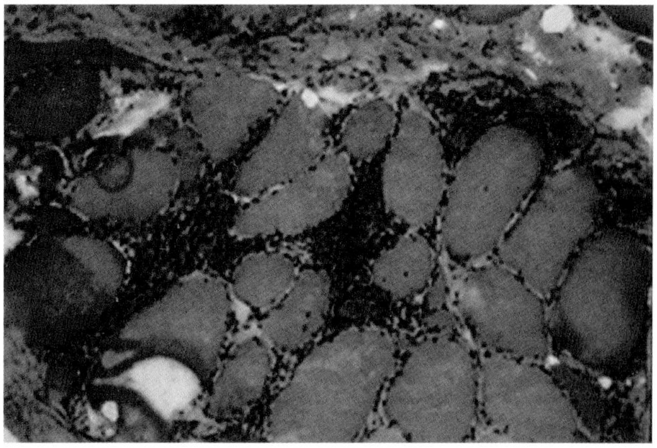

Figure 27-21. Facioscapulohumeral muscular dystrophy. Muscle biopsy demonstrates prominent inflammation (H&E). Physicians need to be aware that such prominent inflammation can be present in muscular dystrophies and can occasionally be misdiagnosed as an inflammatory myopathy (e.g., polymyositis). The inflammatory cells present in the dystrophic muscle usually do not invade non-necrotic muscle fibers, in contrast to the invasion of non-necrotic muscle fibers seen in polymyositis and inclusion body myositis.

Molecular Genetics and Pathogenesis

There are two genetic distinct causes of FSHD: FSHD type 1 (FSHD1) and FSHD type 2 (FSHD2), but the pathogenic mechanisms appear related. Both forms are inherited in an autosomal dominant fashion, but spontaneous mutations are common and penetrance is variable in both.

FSHD1 is responsible for 95% of cases and is linked to mutations in the telomeric region of chromosome 4q35 (Fig. 27-22).[302,303,313] An *Eco*RI polymorphism occurs and is variable in size; normally it is it normal 50–300 kB, but is reduced in FSHD1 to 10–30 kB).[304] Within this *Eco*RI polymorphism lies a tandem array of 11–100 *Kpn* I units, each 3.3 Kb in size, which is termed D4Z4.[302] Most patients with autosomal-dominant FSHD1 carry one array of 1–10 units. It is this decrease in the number of these KpnI units or 3.3 kB repeats that result in the decreased size of

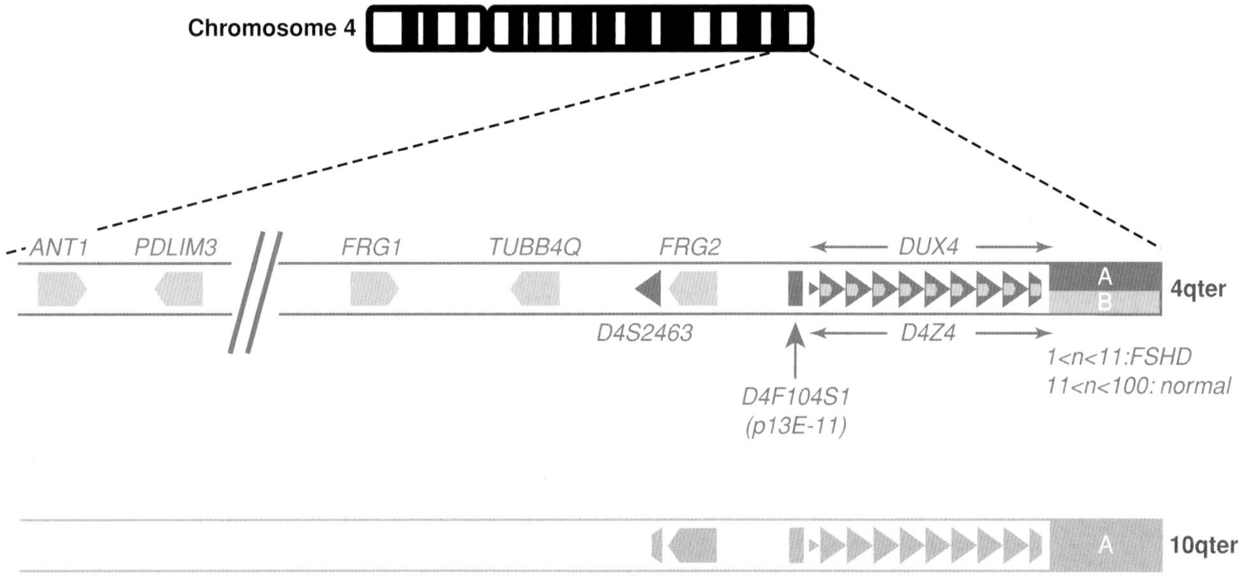

Figure 27-22. Schematic representation of the facioscapulohumeral muscular dystrophy (FSHD) locus. The polymorphic D4Z4 repeat array (*arrowheads*) in the subtelomere of chromosome 4 (blue) can vary between 11 and 100 units in the healthy population. One inversed copy of D4Z4 (D4S2463) is located 37 Kb proximally. Just preceding the D4Z4 repeat unit, probe p13E-11 (D4F104S1), used in the DNA diagnosis of FSHD, is situated. Within each unit, a putative open reading frame designated DUX4 (*block arrow*) is located, but expression of this gene has never been established. In a proximal direction, several additional genes have been identified (*block arrows*) including *FRG2, TUBB4Q* (a pseudogene), and *FRG1*. At a much larger distance, several other genes have been evaluated for their involvement in FSHD. Most notably, these include *ANT1* and *PDLIM3*. Distal to D4Z4, two allelic variants of 4qter have been identified: 4 qA (dark blue) and 4qB (light blue). Both variants are almost equally common in the population and vary by a few insertion and deletion events. FSHD alleles are exclusively linked with the 4 qA variant. The subtelomere of chromosome 10q is similarly organized as 4q due to an ancient duplication of the 4q subtelomere. The homology between 4qter and 10qter extends from the telomere to 40 kb proximally to D4Z4 within an incomplete inverted copy of D4Z4. In contrast to 4qter, there is no B variant of the 10q subtelomere. (Reproduced with permission from Tawil R, Van Der Maarel SM. Facioscapulohumeral muscular dystrophy. *Muscle Nerve.* 2006;34(1):1–15.)

the FSHD-associated polymorphism. In addition, there is normally an allelic variation of chromosome 4qter, designated 4qA and 4qB, which differs by a few insertion/deletion events in the region distal to D4Z4.[302] The 4qA allele contains a block of beta-satellite DNA directly distal to D4Z4 on 4qA, which is not present on the 4qB allele. Although occurring in similar frequency in the normal population, FSHD1 and FSHD2 causing mutations are associated exclusively in the 4qA type of allele. Similar reductions in D4Z4 in 4qB alleles are nonpathogenic.

There is an inverse correlation between the size of the D4Z4 repeat unit and the severity of the disease. Patients carrying one to three units are usually severely affected and often represent isolated (de novo mutations) cases, whereas patients carrying 4 to 10 units typically have an affected parent.[302] Anticipation phenomena may occur in some families, although the size of the mutation appears stable and there can be extreme variability in phenotype even within families.[314] The mutation in FSHD1 is unlike other described genetic disorders, in which anticipation is associated with an increased size of a polymorphic trinucleotide repeat mutation.

Approximately 5% of FSHD patients do not have a deletion affecting D4Z4 repeats. Rather, these FSHD2 patients have mutations in the *SMCHD1* gene on chromosome 18p11.32 that encodes the structural maintenance of chromosomes flexible hinge domain containing 1 protein.[315,316] Notably, the D4Z4 region in hypomethylated in FSHD1 and FSHD2. Methylation is an epigenic means of reducing transcription. Within the D4Z4 repeat lies the *DUX4* gene that is normally not expressed. Hypomethylation of the D4Z4 region seen in FSHD1 and FSHD2 leads to a toxic overexpression of this *DUX4* gene. *DUX4* encodes for double homeobox 4, which itself is a transcription factor controlling the expression of other genes. This in-turn likely leads to the under or overexpression of other genes.

Diagnosis

The diagnosis of FSHD is usually apparent on clinical grounds. Genetic testing is particularly useful for confirmation in patients without family history or unusual clinical phenotypes as well as for genetic counseling. We start off by testing for FSHD1 as it is much more common, and if this is unrevealing, test for FSHD2.

Treatment

A small open-label pilot study of prednisone 1.5 mg/kg/day for 12 weeks resulted in no significant improvement in strength or muscle mass.[305] An open-label trial of albuterol in 15 patients with FSHD for 3 months demonstrated increased lean body mass and muscle strength.[317] However, a subsequent larger, longer, double-blinded, placebo-controlled study of albuterol revealed no clear benefit.[318] Modest improvement in strength has been reported in a small number of patients with FSHD treated with short courses of creatine monohydrate (5–10 g/day).

Surgery to fix the scapula to the thorax, thereby increasing range of motion, is beneficial in some patients.[319,320] However, they need to have sufficient strength of the deltoid muscles in order to benefit from the procedure. Ankle–foot orthotics are useful in patients with foot drop secondary to tibialis anterior weakness.

SCAPULOPERONEAL MUSCULAR DYSTROPHY

Clinical Features

Patients with scapuloperoneal muscular dystrophy manifest with foot drop followed by scapular weakness within the first two decades of life.[2,321,327] Weakness is often asymmetric, and patients sometimes are misdiagnosed as having a peroneal neuropathy. Furthermore, some with a scapuloperoneal pattern of weakness do indeed suffer from a form of neuropathy or motor neuronopathy.[328] A few patients with myopathic scapuloperoneal syndromes may demonstrate compensatory hypertrophy of the extensor digitorum brevis with the ability to dorsiflex the foot more effectively than the big toe, an unlikely observation in a neurogenic foot drop. The hypertrophy may result from attempting to dorsiflex the foot with this muscle. Ankle contractures are prominent features of the disease secondary to the weak anterior compartment muscles. The weak scapular muscles result in an appearance of the shoulder-girdle similar to that seen in FSHD. However, unlike FSHD, the humeral musculature is usually relatively spared. On the other hand, the peroneal muscles are typically more severely affected in scapuloperoneal muscular dystrophy compared to FSHD. Rarely, some patients may manifest mild weakness of the facial muscles, creating a diagnostic confusion with FSHD. However, facial muscle weakness is usually much less prominent than that seen in FSHD. Muscle weakness is slowly progressive.

Laboratory Features

The serum CK levels can be normal or moderately abnormal. The motor and sensory nerve conductions are normal aside from reduced CMAPs in the more severely affected muscles.[2,322–327] Needle EMG may demonstrate sparse fibrillation potentials and myopathic units.

Histopathology

Muscle biopsies reveal nonspecific myopathic features, including fiber size variation with atrophic and hypertrophic fibers, split fibers, necrotic and regenerating fibers, and increased endomysial connective tissue.[325,327] Some biopsies demonstrate inclusions typical of MFM.[326]

Molecular Genetics and Pathogenesis

Mutations in the *DES* gene on chromosome 2q35 encoding for desmin[133] and in the *FHL1* on Xq26.3 encoding for four and a half LIM protein,[329] are the causes of some cases of scapuloperoneal dystrophy.[2] Mutations in these genes are also associated with MFM as will be discussed in a later section.

Treatment

There are no reported studies regarding medical therapy in scapuloperoneal muscular dystrophy. Ankle–foot orthoses are beneficial in patients with ankle dorsiflexor weakness. Surgery to stabilize the scapula may improve arm function in some patients.

X-LINKED EDMD (Fig. 27-23)

Clinical Features

EDMD is characterized by (1) early contractures of the Achilles' tendons, elbows, and posterior cervical muscles; (2) slowly progressive muscle atrophy and weakness, with a predominantly humeroperoneal distribution in early stages; and (3) cardiomyopathy with conduction defects.[2,330–335] Prominent contractures are evident in early childhood or in the teenage years, with an inability to fully extend the elbows secondary to elbow flexion contractures (Fig. 27-24). Patients may toe walk due to early heal cord contractures. There is reduced mobility of the spine such that EDMD is in the differential diagnosis of the so-called "rigid spine syndrome."[331] Patients have difficulty flexing their neck and trunk. Importantly, the contractures of the Achilles' tendons, elbows, and paraspinal muscles are evident before there is any significant weakness, which helps distinguish EDMD from other types of dystrophies associated with contractures.

Patients with EDMD usually appear normal at birth. Some children develop mild weakness. The characteristic pattern of muscle involvement helps distinguish EDMD from most other forms of dystrophy. There is an early predilection for weakness and atrophy affecting the humeroperoneal muscles (i.e., biceps brachii, triceps, anterior tibial, and peroneal muscles). Pes cavus deformities of the feet are common. Weakness is slowly progressive, and eventually the shoulder- and pelvic-girdle muscles can become involved. Most affected individuals are able to ambulate into the third decade. Unlike many of the LGMDs, which it may be confused with, there is no calf hypertrophy. Muscle stretch reflexes are diminished or absent early in the disease.

Importantly, EDMD is associated with potentially lethal cardiac arrhythmias by the end of the second or beginning of the third decade. Conduction defects range from first-degree A-V block to complete heart block. Syncope and sudden cardiac death can occur. Although women carriers do not manifest muscle weakness or contractures, they may develop a cardiopathy. Affected individuals with *FHL1* mutations (see below) are more apt to develop ventilatory muscle failure.[2,129,336,337–339]

Laboratory Features

The serum CK levels may be normal or moderately elevated. EKG frequently reveals sinus bradycardia, prolongation of the PR interval, or more severe degrees of conduction block. Motor and sensory nerve conduction studies are typically normal in these patients. EMG reveals myopathic MUAPs.

Histopathology

The muscle biopsy findings can be quite varied, depending on the degree of weakness of the biopsied muscle.[2,335] There is usually muscle fiber size variation with type 1 fiber atrophy. There can be a predominance of either type 1 or type 2 muscle fibers. Muscle fiber splitting, increased central nuclei, and endomysial fibrosis may be seen. Immunohistochemistry reveals the absence of emerin as well as abnormal lamin A/C and lamin B2 on the nuclear membrane.[24,25] Ultrastructural studies demonstrate the focal absence of peripheral heterochromatin in areas between the nuclear pores, irregular and uniform thickening of the nuclear lamina, and compaction of heterochromatin in areas of irregular thickening of the nuclear lamina and areas where the peripheral heterochromatin does not adhere to the nuclear lamina.[25] Diagnosis can be confirmed by immunostaining muscle or skin tissue for emerin or by immunoblot analysis of leukocytes.

Muscle biopsies in patients with *FHL1* mutations (EDMD-X2, see below) can be distinguished from those with more common emerin mutations, (EDMD-X1) as the former reveals reducing bodies, cytoplasmic bodies, and sometimes features of MFM.[2,129,336,340,341]

Molecular Genetics and Pathogenesis

Most cases of EDMD (EDMD-X1) are caused by mutations in *STA* located on chromosome Xq28, which encodes for emerin (Table 27-1).[2,342] Emerin is located on the inner nuclear membranes of skeletal, cardiac, and smooth muscle fibers as well as skin cells.[23,24] Its carboxy-terminal tail anchors the protein to the inner nuclear membrane, while the remainder of the protein projects into the nucleoplasm. Emerin is a member of the nuclear LAP family.[23–25] The nuclear lamina is composed of intermediate-sized filaments (e.g., lamins A, B, and C) associated with the nucleoplasmic surface of the inner nuclear membrane. These lamins bind to various LAPs, including LAP1, LAP2, and lamin B receptor, which are located on the inner

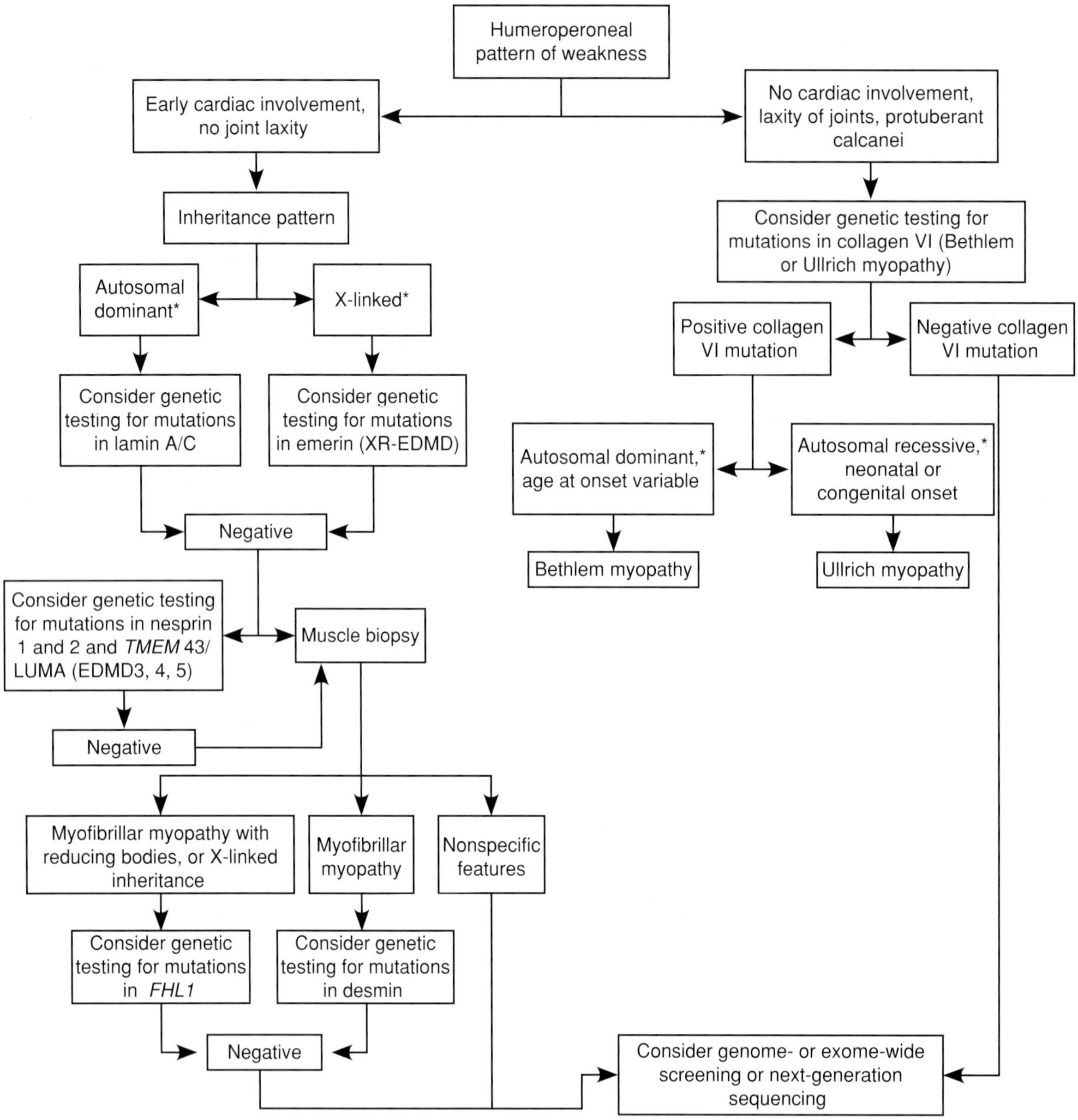

Figure 27-23. Diagnostic approach to patients with a humeroperoneal pattern of weakness and suspected muscular dystrophy (Emery–Dreifuss muscular dystrophy). *Autosomal dominant, autosomal recessive, or X-linked inheritance may be responsible in sporadic cases. EDMD, Emery–Dreifuss muscular dystrophy. (Reproduced with permission from Narayanaswami P, Weiss M, Selcen D, et al: Evidence-based guideline summary: diagnosis and treatment of limb-girdle and distal dystrophies: report of the guideline development subcommittee of the American Academy of Neurology and the practice issues review panel of the American Association of Neuromuscular & Electrodiagnostic Medicine, *Neurology*. 2014;83(16):1453–1463.)

nuclear membrane. LAP2, lamin B receptor, and the lamins also bind to chromatin and thereby promote its attachment to the nuclear membrane. Mutations in emerin conceivably lead to disorganization of the nuclear lamina and heterochromatin that is apparent on EM and immunohistochemistry.[25] In addition, mutations in *FHL1* gene that encodes the four-and-one-half LIM1 protein can present with an EDMD phenotype (EDMD-X2) or as a scapuloperoneal myopathy, LGMD, or even as rigid spine syndrome.[2,336–341]

Treatment

We obtain yearly EKGs on all our patients (as well as on possible female carriers) and 24-hour Holters and cardiology consultations on those with abnormalities (e.g., atrioventricular block) or cardiac symptoms. Affected individuals may require pacemakers or intracardiac defibrillators, and some authorities even recommend these prophylactically.[2] Physical therapy is aimed at minimizing contractures.

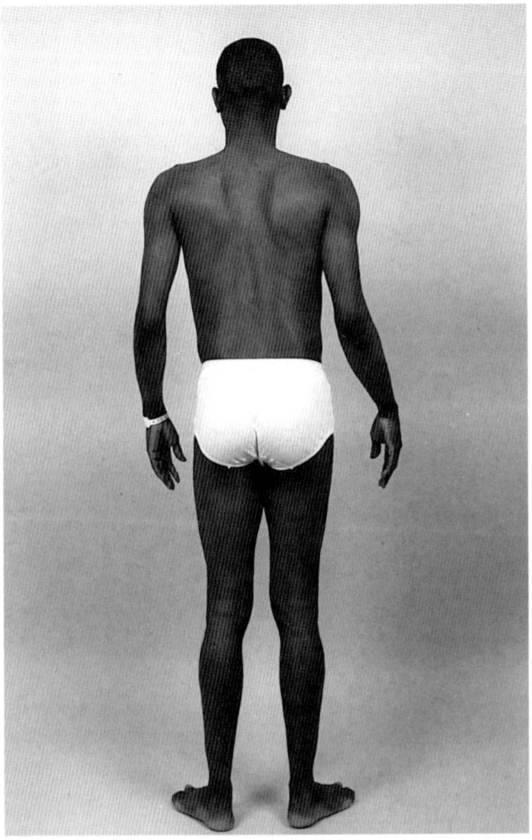

Figure 27-24. Emery–Dreifuss muscular dystrophy (EDMD). Posterior view of a patient with EDMD demonstrates atrophy of the triceps musculature, left more than right, and early contractures of the elbows (patient is unable to straighten the arms down at the side). There is also mild scapular winging.

AUTOSOMAL-DOMINANT EDMD2/LGMD 1B

The clinical, laboratory, and histopathological features of this LGMD 1B are identical to those described above for typical X-linked EDMD1, except for autosomal-dominant inheritance and equal frequency of affected females (Figs. 27-8 and 27-23).[27,27,28,102] They are also less likely to manifest with significant contractures, particularly early on. As noted previously, autosomal-dominant EDMD2 and LGMD 1B are allelic disorders caused by mutations in the lamin A/C gene (*LMNA*) located on chromosome 1q11–23.[2,27,102,343,344] Mutations in the rod domain of *LMNA* cause hereditary dilated cardiopathy and conduction defects with or without an underlying skeletal muscle involvement.[2,27,29,102] De novo mutations are responsible for 76% of cases; therefore, mutations in *LMNA* should be considered in all autosomal dominant and sporadic cases of EDMD and familial dilated cardiopathy.[27] Marked variability in the clinical phenotype can be seen within and between families with specific mutations in the *LMNA* gene.

Lamins A and C are produced by alternative splicing of the lamin A/C RNA transcript. As discussed in the pathogenesis discussion regarding X-linked EDMD, these lamins are important in the organization and integrity of the nuclear membrane. Muscle biopsies demonstrate variation in fiber size, increased endomysial connective tissue, normal emerin expression, and usually normal lamin A/C expression. EM reveals nuclear alterations similar to X-linked EDMD in 10% of muscle fibers.[23,26] There is loss of peripheral heterochromatin or detachment from the nuclear envelop, alterations in interchromatin texture, and fewer nuclear pores compared to normal.

AUTOSOMAL-RECESSIVE EDMD3

Clinical Features

This is a rare autosomal-recessive muscular dystrophy, with contractures and severe rigidity of the spine reported in five unrelated children (three boys and two girls).[345] Onset was in the first 2 years of life, and the children were unable to walk by the age of 8 years. However, they had no cardiac abnormalities.

Laboratory Features

Serum CK was moderately elevated.[345]

Histopathology

Muscle biopsies revealed nonspecific dystrophic changes with normal expression of emerin, dystrophin, the sarcoglycans, and laminins $\alpha 2$, $\alpha 5$, $\beta 1$, $\gamma 1$ chains.[345]

Molecular Genetics and Pathogenesis

Autosomal recessive EDMD is also caused by mutations in *LMNA*.[345]

OTHER EDMD

Over 60% patients with EDMD do not have mutations in the genes encoding emerin or lamin A/C.[346] Mutations in the genes that encode for nesprin-1 and -2 have been reported in several sporadic cases and autosomal dominant families with EDMD-like phenotypes.[346] Nesprin-1 and -2 (*n*uclear *e*nvelope *sp*ectrin *r*epeat proteins) are spectrin-repeat containing proteins that are anchored in the outer and inner nuclear membranes. Nesprin-1 and Nesprin-2 are transcribed from two genes, *SYNE1* on chromosome 6q24 and *SYNE2* on chromosome 14q23. Nesprin-1 and -2 bind actin and both emerin and lamins A/C, thereby linking the nuclear lamina with the actin cytoskeleton. In addition, rare causes of autosomal dominant EDMD are caused by mutations in *TMEM43* that encodes for transmembrane protein 43 or LUMA.[347] The clinical phenotype is essentially identical to that seen with emerin and lamin A/C mutations. LUMA is also a nuclear envelope protein that binds emerin and lamin A/C.

BETHLEM MYOPATHY

Clinical Features

Bethlem myopathy is an autosomal dominant disorder that is allelic to and a mild variant of UCMD discussed previously. The clinical features are very similar to EDMD.[348–356] Onset is usually at birth or early childhood. Decreased fetal movements may be noted in utero, and neonates may demonstrate generalized hypotonia. Motor milestones are often delayed, but are reached. However, weakness may not be evident until early adulthood. Variability in the age of onset and in clinical severity may even be seen within affected family members. There is proximal greater than distal muscle weakness, with the legs being more severely affected than the arms. Extensor muscles are weaker than flexor muscles. There can be mild neck and trunk involvement, but cranial muscles are spared. Muscle strength can be asymmetric. Calf hypertrophy may be seen. As in EDMD, contractures at the elbows and ankles are evident early in the course before any significant weakness manifests. Eventually, contractures develop in the wrists and fingers. Some patients manifest with only proximal hip- and shoulder-girdle weakness without evidence of contractures, thus resembling an LGMD. Muscle stretch reflexes may be normal or reduced.

Until recently, it was thought that the heart was spared in Bethlem myopathy—a feature that might help to distinguish it from EDMD. However, a recent study of patients with Bethlem myopathy revealed that eight of 74 had abnormal EKGs, four of 24 had abnormal Holters, and six of 51 had abnormal echocardiograms.[355] Abnormalities include atrial fibrillation, accelerated atrial rhythm, intraventricular conduction delay, right bundle branch, and pathological Q waves, and atrial dilatation. Thus, it appears that detailed cardiac investigations in Bethlem myopathy do reveal abnormalities in 10% of cases. However, the relationship of these cardiac abnormalities to Bethlem myopathy still remains to be established.

Ventilatory muscles appear to be involved in Bethlem myopathy and seems to be related to more severe weakness.[255] Pulmonary investigations performed in 56 patients revealed reduced vital capacity below 50% in five patients and 11 patients had vital capacities between 50% and 70%.[355] Two patients were on ventilatory support. Others have also reported progressive ventilatory insufficiency due to diaphragmatic muscle involvement.[352]

Laboratory Features

Serum CK is normal or mildly elevated. Cardiac studies (e.g., EKG, Holter monitor, and echocardiogram) may be abnormal as discussed in the previous section. Motor and sensory nerve conduction studies are normal. Insertional and spontaneous activity is usually normal on EMG, although a mixture of small-amplitude, short-duration polyphasic MUAPs with large-amplitude, long-duration MUAPs can be seen.[351,352]

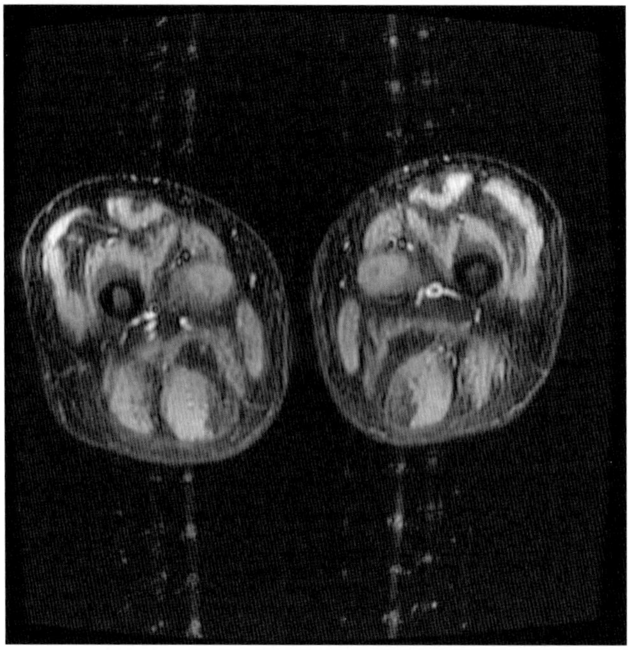

Figure 27-25. Skeletal muscle MRI of the thigh in patient with Bethlem myopathy reveals moderate involvement of thigh muscles with the "central shadow" within the rectus femoris, atrophy and increased abnormal signal at the periphery of the vastus lateralis, and fatty replacement between the vastus lateralis and the vastus intermedius.

Skeletal muscle MRI scans may reveal early involvement of the thigh muscles with a fairly specific pattern (Fig. 27-25) in which the preferential involvement of the rectus femoris with focus of fatty replacement in the anterior aspect of the muscle.[357,358] Other muscle fibers have fatty replacement in their periphery with relatively sparing the central regions.

Histopathology

Muscle biopsies demonstrate nonspecific myopathic features. There is variability in fiber size, increased splitting, central nuclei, and mild endomysial fibrosis. Lobulated type 1 fibers and moth-eaten fibers may be apparent on NADH-TR stains.

Molecular Genetics and Pathogenesis

Bethlem myopathy has been linked to dominant heterozygous mutations of the genes (COL6A1, COL6A2, and COL6A3) encoding for the α1 and α2 subunits of collagen VI located on chromosome 21q and α3 subunit of collagen VI located on 2q37.[270,353,358] Collagen VI bridges the extracellular matrix with the sarcolemma. Interestingly, compound heterozygous mutations have been defined in the COL6A2 and COL6A3 genes in the more severe UCMD (see the section Congenital Muscular Dystrophies).[270] Collagen VI deficiency in muscle or cultured fibroblasts was complete in severe cases and partial in the milder ones, which suggests a correlation between the degree of collagen VI deficiency and the clinical severity in UCMD.[271]

Treatment

Physical therapy is indicated to prevent progressive contractures that can impair mobility and function.

BENT SPINE/DROPPED HEAD SYNDROME

Clinical Features

Neck extensor weakness can be an early and prominent manifestation of several disorders, in particular myasthenia gravis and amyotrophic lateral sclerosis.[359] However, there are a number of patients with weakness that remains restricted to the cervical and, sometimes, also to the thoracic and paraspinal muscles leading to bent spine syndrome or camptocormia.[359–362] Onset of neck extensor weakness usually begins after 60 years of age leading to progressive head drop. Involvement of the thoracic paraspinal muscles leads to severe kyphosis or the bent spine posture upon standing (see Chapter 2, Figure 2–30). When patients are supine, their posture is normal, in contrast to patients with fixed contractures of the spine. Weakness may remain clinically isolated to the neck extensors even for several years, although there may be subclinical (radiographic or electromyographic) evidence of disease in the upper thoracic paraspinal muscles. In addition, mild shoulder girdle weakness may also develop. A family history of bent spine syndrome has been described.[361]

Laboratory Features

Serum CK is usually normal or only mildly elevated. Monoclonal gammopathy may be seen in cases of sporadic late-onset nemaline myopathy, which can occasionally present with a neck extensor myopathy.[363] CT and MRI of the low cervical and upper thoracic spine reveal atrophy and fatty or edematous changes in the paraspinal muscles (see Chapter 2, Figure 2–30A). Motor and sensory nerve conduction studies are normal. EMG reveals fibrillation potentials and positive sharp waves in cervical and thoracic paraspinals.[359,361] Short-duration, small-amplitude MUAPs with early recruitment are seen in the cervical and thoracic paraspinal muscles. EMG of the arms and legs is typically normal.

Histopathology

Muscle biopsies of the cervical paraspinal muscles demonstrate nonspecific myopathic features, including variability in fiber size with atrophic and hypertrophic muscle fibers, increased internalized nuclei, fiber splitting, moth-eaten fibers, fibers with rimmed vacuoles, and increased endomysial connective tissue. Rare cases with endomysial inflammation have been reported.[364,365] Biopsies of proximal limb muscles may be normal or may demonstrate similar, but less prominent, abnormalities. Ragged red fibers and cytochrome C oxidase (COX)-negative fibers suggestive of mitochondrial dysfunction are not uncommon but may be age related. Cores and minicores may also be appreciated in some cases (Fig. 27-26).[366,367] Late-onset nemaline myopathy also can occasionally present initially as an axial myopathy.[363]

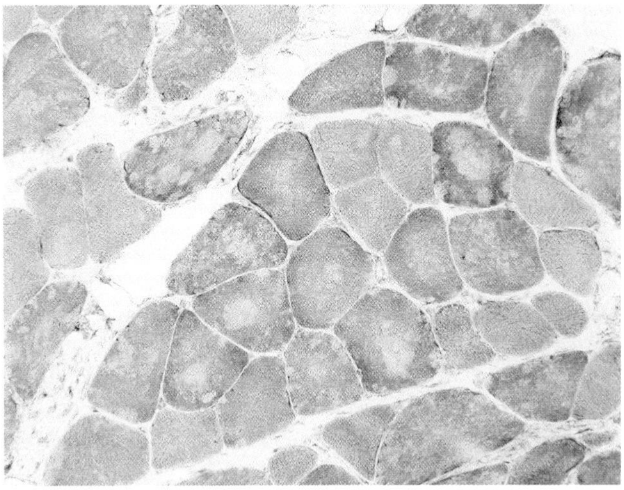

Figure 27-26. Muscle biopsy in patient with bent spine syndrome and ryanodine receptor gene (*RYR1*) mutation demonstrates central cores, multiminicores, and moth eaten fibers, NADH x 20x.

Pathogenesis

Isolated neck extensor myopathy may just represent a "forme fruste" of the bent spine syndrome. The cause of axial myopathy is heterogeneous. In some cases, the myopathy may be the result of a monophasic inflammatory process restricted to the paraspinal muscles.[360,364,365] We suspect that in most cases this disorder represents a regional form of muscular dystrophy or other hereditary myopathy that predominantly affects the paraspinal muscles. Rarely, dysferlinopathies and FSHD can present with a paraspinal myopathy that can lead to camptocormia. Myotonic dystrophies and late-onset Pompe disease have also been described to manifest initially with head drop or bent spine syndrome. Several series have reported mutations in *RYR1* (ryanodine receptor) in a number of patients, and we have seen this as well.[366,367] *RYR1* mutations are more commonly associated with other phenotypes such as malignant hyperthermia or congenital myopathy with central cores.

Treatment

Immunosuppressive therapy and pyridostigmine are not typically beneficial. However, improvement with corticosteroid and azathioprine[360,364] or intravenous immunoglobulin[365] has been reported in rare patients. Cervical collars may help stabilize the head drop.

OCULOPHARYNGEAL MUSCULAR DYSTROPHY

Clinical Features

OPMD is an autosomal-dominant disorder, which usually presents in the fourth to sixth decade of life with increasing ptosis.[368,369] The ptosis is almost always bilateral but can be asymmetric. The extraocular muscles are involved in approximately 50% of patients but is often subtle and double vision is uncommon. The pupils are spared. Approximately one-fourth of patients manifest initially with dysphagia, which is slowly progressive and leads to severe weight loss and aspiration.[369] Facial and masticatory muscles may be slightly weak in some patients. The gag reflex is impaired. Laryngeal involvement can also develop, resulting in dysphonia.

Some patients develop slight weakness of the neck and proximal limbs. Distal muscles weakness may also occur, particularly in the distal oculopharyngeal dystrophy variant (see below). Sensation is normal, but muscle stretch reflexes can be reduced or absent. Life span is not altered.

Laboratory Features

Serum CK levels are normal or only mildly elevated. Swallowing studies demonstrate impaired pharyngeal and esophageal motility.

Histopathology

The muscles most severely affected are the extraocular and pharyngeal muscles, although minor abnormalities may be detectable in the limb muscles in advanced cases. Muscle biopsies reveal variation in fiber size, degenerating and regenerating fibers, increased internal nuclei, and an increase in adipose and endomysial connective tissue.[368,369] Rimmed vacuoles similar to those found in inclusion body myositis/myopathy and some of the distal myopathies are often, although not universally, observed. On EM, intranuclear inclusions are evident in up to 9% of muscle nuclei.[370] These tubulofilamentous inclusions have an outer diameter of approximately 8.5 nm and an inner diameter of 3 nm, are up to 0.25 μm in length, and are often arranged in tangles or palisades.[370] In addition, 15–18-nm tubulofilaments may be evident in the cytoplasm, as seen in IBM, h-IBM, and some of the distal myopathies. OPMD can be distinguished from various mitochondrial myopathies, which can also cause ptosis and ophthalmoparesis, by the lack of ragged red fibers. However, there have been a few cases of OPMD with abnormal mitochondrial structure and quantity on EM, although these findings, for the most part, are suspected to be age related. Further, muscle biopsies of pharyngeal muscles (taken at the time of cricopharyngeal myotomy-anecdotal observations) reveal more severe abnormalities along with frequent rimmed vacuoles, ragged red fibers, and nemaline rods. Sural nerve biopsy in a few patients revealed a mild reduction in myelinated and unmyelinated nerve fibers; however, this could be a confounding variable related to the patients' advanced ages.

Molecular Genetics and Pathogenesis

OPMD is caused by expansions of a short GCG repeat within the *PABN1* gene located on chromosome 14q11.1 (Table 27-1).[368–371] Normally, there are six GCG repeats encoding for a polyalanine tract at the N terminus of the protein, but approximately 2% of the population has polymorphism with seven GCG repeats (GCG^{7}). In OPMD, there is an expansion to 8 to 13 repeats (GCG^{8-13}). These expansions are meitotically stable, explaining the lack of anticipation phenomena form one generation to the next. Patients who are homozygous for (GCG) expansions may manifest at an earlier age and have more severe weakness. Also, patients who are heterozygous for (GCG^{8-13}) and the (GCG^{7}) polymorphism are also more severely affected. Interestingly, a late-onset, autosomal-recessive form of OPMD can develop in patients who are homozygous for the (GCG^{7}) polymorphism. The (GCG^{7}) allele within *PABPN1* was the first example of a polymorphism that could act as a modifier of a dominant phenotype or as a recessive mutation.

The PABPN1 protein is found mostly in dimeric and oligomeric forms with the nuclei (Fig. 27-1).[372,373] PABPN1 is involved in polyadenylation of mRNA and is adjoined to the polyadenylated mRNA complex for transport through the nuclei pores into the cytoplasm. In the cytoplasm, the PABPN1 detaches from the mRNA. The mRNA is translated into protein and the PABPN1 is actively transported back into the nuclei. The expansion of the GCG repeats probably results in abnormal folding of the polyalanine domains of PABPN1. The misfolded proteins are ubiquitinated but are resistant to nuclear proteasomal degradation. The mutated PABPN1 oligomers then accumulate as the 8.5 nm intranuclear tubulofilamentous inclusions apparent on EM.[371–373] The more severe clinical phenotypes are associated with a large number of myonuclei containing intranuclear inclusions.[373] The aggregation of mutated PAPBN1 may lead to disruption of various nuclear or cytoplasmic processes leading to cell death.

Treatment

Noninvasive therapies include the use of eyelid crutches on glasses or even taping the eyelids, neither of which are commonly popular with patients due to the mechanical irritation of the eyelids they create. Ptosis surgery can also be performed, if patients have sufficient orbicularis oculi strength to allow complete closure of the eyelids postoperatively. There is the risk of corneal abrasions and keratitis, if the eyelids cannot close completely. Cricopharyngeal myotomy may be beneficial in patients with dysphagia. Patients with severe dysphagia resulting in aspiration or significant weight loss require percutaneous endogastric tube placement.

VARIANTS OF OPMD

There are a few genetically distinct variants of OPMD. Infantile or early childhood onset of ptosis, ophthalmoparesis, and severe generalized weakness with respiratory failure has been reported.[369] Another variant of OPMD is oculopharyngodistal myopathy. Most of the reports of oculopharyngodistal myopathy have come from Japan,[374,375] although the myopathy occurs in other ethnic groups.[376,377] Weakness develops earlier than classic OPMD, with onset in the first decade of life in some cases. We have seen a patient with distal OPMD and chronic intestinal pseudo-obstruction.[376]

The laboratory, histologic, and electrodiagnostic features of these variants are, for the most part, indistinguishable from OPMD. Intranuclear inclusions similar to OPMD may be found. Whether or not these variants have mutations in the *PABPN1* gene remains to be determined. Mutations in the *PABPN1* gene were not identified in one family with atypical OPMD (early onset in second–third decade, elevated serum CK, and profound ophthalmoplegia).[369]

DISTAL MYOPATHY/MUSCULAR DYSTROPHY

Although distal weakness is often presumed to be neuropathic in etiology, a variety of neuromuscular disorders, including myopathies, are associated with distal extremity weakness (Table 27-1, Fig. 27-27).[2,378,379] The distal myopathies are characterized clinically by progressive atrophy and weakness of distal arm or leg muscles and histologically by nonspecific myopathic features on muscle biopsy. We consider the distal myopathies to be forms of muscular dystrophy. Advances in the molecular genetics of these disorders support this notion, as some types of distal myopathy have been found to be allelic with specific types of LGMD (tibial myopathy and LGMD 2 J caused by titin mutations and Miyoshi myopathy and LGMD 2B caused by dysferlin mutations). Furthermore, there is a clear overlap of some distal myopathies with some forms of h-IBM and MFM. The distal myopathies can be subdivided, based on the clinical features, age of onset, CK levels, muscle histology, and mode of inheritance.

WELANDER DISTAL MYOPATHY

Clinical Features

Welander originally described the features of this autosomal dominant myopathy in a report of 249 cases from 72 Scandinavian families.[380] Onset of weakness usually begins in the fifth decade of life, with rare cases beginning before the age of 30 years (mean age of onset 47 years, range 20–77 years). Weakness is usually first noted in the wrist and finger extensors and slowly progresses to involve the distal lower limbs—ankle dorsiflexors more than the plantar flexors.[2,380–382] However, in approximately 10% of cases, weakness is initially appreciated in the legs or there is simultaneous involvement of the distal arms and legs. Although the extensor muscle groups are more severely affected, the flexor groups are involved in over 40% of cases. Rarely, proximal muscles become weak. Sensation is usually normal. Muscle stretch reflexes are initially preserved, but the brachioradialis and Achilles' reflexes diminish or disappear over time.

Laboratory Features

Serum CK levels are usually normal or only minimally abnormal.[2] Motor and sensory nerve conduction studies are usually normal for age. Diminished temperature and vibratory perception quantitative sensory testing has been demonstrated in some patients.[381–383] Needle EMG demonstrates early recruitment of small-amplitude, short-duration MUAPs.[2,381–383] Quantitative EMG further suggests a myopathic process.[381]

Histopathology

Muscle biopsies demonstrate variability in fiber size, increased central nuclei, split fibers, and increased endomysial connective tissue and adipose cells in longstanding disease.[2,381–386] Furthermore, rimmed vacuoles typical of IBM, h-IBM, and OPMD are seen in scattered muscle fibers. EM also reveals 15–18-nm cytoplasmic and nuclear filaments similar to those observed in IBM, h-IBM, and OPMD. In addition, disruption of myofibrils and accumulation of Z-disc-derived material similar to that found in MFM can also be demonstrated. Nerve biopsies may reveal a moderate reduction of mainly small-diameter, myelinated fibers.[383]

Molecular Genetics and Pathogenesis

Welander myopathy is caused by mutations in the *TIA1* gene that encodes for T-cell restricted intracellular antigen, which is a RNA-binding protein.[387] The TIA1 protein appears to aggregate in granules in muscle biopsy in patients with Welander myopathy. The mutations in *TIA1* may make the transcribed protein more prone to self-aggregation and aggregate with other proteins.[387,388]

UDD DISTAL MYOPATHY

Clinical Features

As previously discussed, this autosomal dominant distal myopathy is associated with mutations in the *TTN*. Udd distal myopathy usually presents after the age of 35 years (usually in the fifth to seventh decade), with weakness of

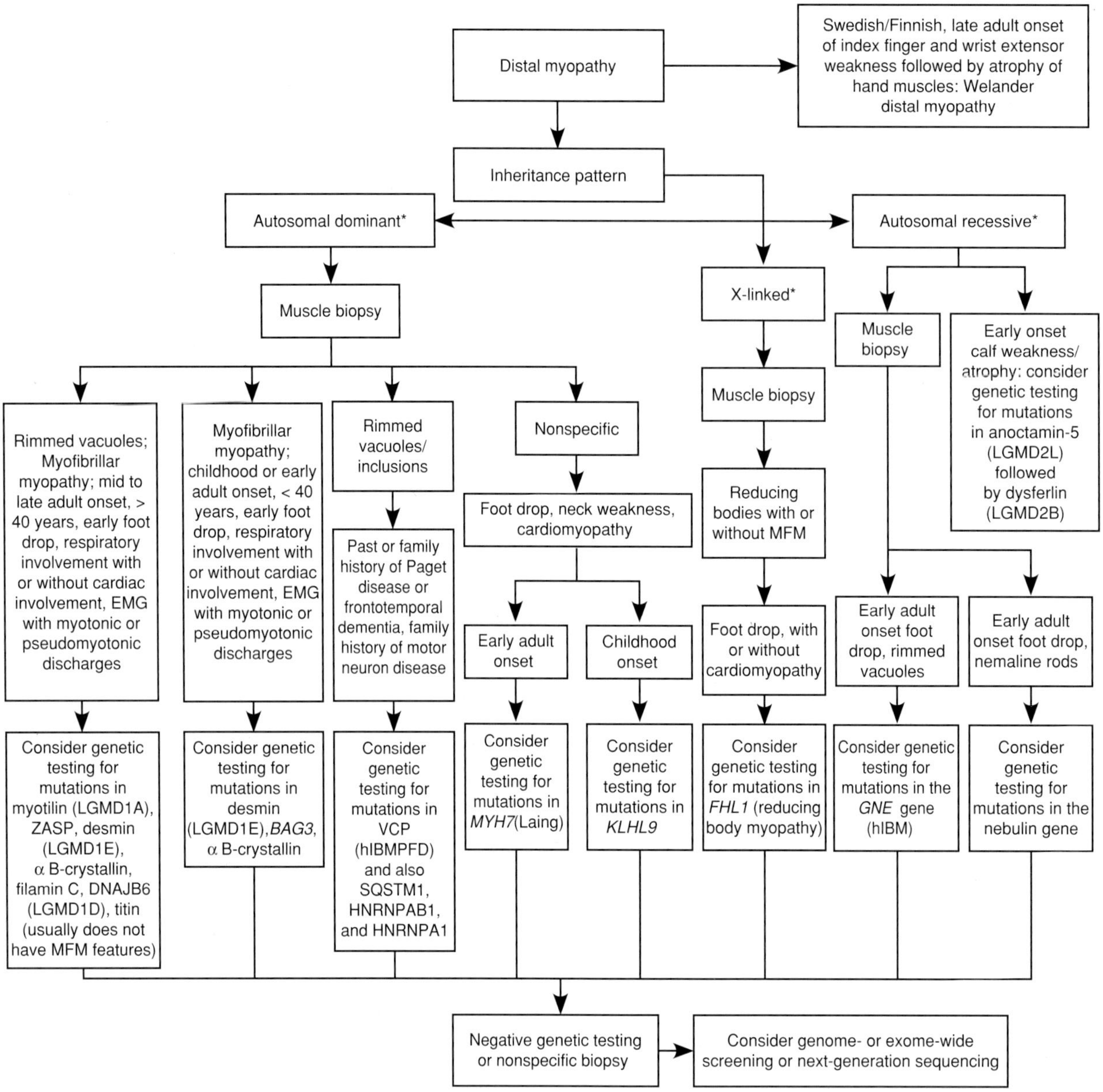

Figure 27-27. Diagnostic approach to patients with a distal pattern of weakness and suspected muscular dystrophy. *Autosomal dominant, autosomal recessive, or X-linked inheritance may be responsible in sporadic cases. h-IBM, hereditary inclusion body myopathy; h-IBMPFD, hereditary inclusion body myopathy with Paget Disease and Frontotemporal Dementia. (Reproduced with permission from Narayanaswami P, Weiss M, Selcen D, et al: Evidence-based guideline summary: diagnosis and treatment of limb-girdle and distal dystrophies: report of the guideline development subcommittee of the American Academy of Neurology and the practice issues review panel of the American Association of Neuromuscular & Electrodiagnostic Medicine, *Neurology*. 2014;83(16):1453–1463.)

the anterior compartment of the lower legs resulting in unilateral or bilateral foot drop.[2,209,210,211–220,389,390] The disorder is slowly progressive, beginning in the toe extensors and gradually involving anterior tibial muscles. Occasionally, the proximal legs and distal upper limbs (predominately the hand intrinsics and wrist extensors) are affected. Rarely, the arms are affected more than the legs, posterior calves are involved with sparing of the anterior tibial muscles, or patients have a limb-girdle distribution of weakness.[209] Facial muscles are usually spared, although bulbar weakness has been reported. Sensation is normal. Achilles' tendon reflexes are usually reduced. Unlike other forms of titinopathy, cardiac and ventilatory muscles are usually spared in Udd distal myopathy.

Laboratory Features

Serum CK is normal or only slightly elevated.[2,209,210–213,215–220,389,390] Motor and sensory NCS are normal. EMG of affected muscles reveals fibrillation potentials and positive sharp waves as well as small-amplitude, brief-duration MUAPs that recruit early.[2,212,390] Imaging scans of muscle revealed fatty infiltration in the anterior tibial and extensor digitorum longus more than the gastrocnemius muscles; the proximal pelvic muscles, gluteus medius and minimus may be affected later.[210,215]

Histopathology

Muscle biopsies reveal dystrophic features fibers with rimmed vacuoles.[2,212,388,390] Other features of MFM are usually not seen in titinopathy manifesting with the Udd distal myopathy, but may be seen in those with the HMERF presentation as discussed in LGMD2J section.

Molecular Genetics and Pathogenesis

Udd distal myopathy is caused by mutations in the *TTN* gene on chromosome 2q31–33 encoding for titin.[2,209,391] As previously discussed, the disorder is allelic to autosomal recessive LGMDJ and autosomal dominant HMERF. Why dominant mutations in the *TTN* typically lead to such different phenotypes and inheritance pattern is not entirely clear. A confounding factor is the variability of clinical phenotype sometimes seen even within families. The giant protein titin (also known as connectin) is attached to the Z-disc and spans from the M- to the Z-line of the sarcomere. Titin serves to connect the myosin filaments to the Z-disc and probably plays an important role in myofibrillogenesis.

MARKESBERY–GRIGGS DISTAL MYOPATHY

Clinical Features

This is another late-onset, autosomal dominant distal myopathy, typically beginning in the anterior compartment of the legs with onset in third to eighth decade of life.[2,392,393] Some patients develop proximal leg and distal arm weakness (wrist and finger extensors) as well. A dilated cardiomyopathy is common.

Laboratory Features

Serum CK is normal or only mildly elevated. Motor and sensory nerve conduction studies are usually normal. Serum CK is usually mildly elevated, and EMG reveals features of a myopathy with muscle membrane irritability.

Histopathology

Muscle biopsies demonstrate rimmed vacuoles and features of MFM.

Molecular Genetics and Pathogenesis

Markesbery–Griggs distal myopathy is caused by mutations in LIM domain binding 3 gene (*LDB3*) that encodes for Z-band alternatively spliced PDZ-motif containing protein or ZASP.[2,393]

NONAKA DISTAL MYOPATHY (AUTOSOMAL-RECESSIVE INCLUSION BODY MYOPATHY)/GNE MYOPATHY

Clinical Features

This autosomal recessive myopathy was initially reported in Japan,[395–398] but it occurs worldwide, and is allelic to autosomal recessive inclusion body *myopathy* (h-IBM type 1).[2,399–402] The preferred term nowadays is "GNE myopathy." Affected individuals usually develop weakness of the anterior compartment of the distal lower limb, leading to foot drop in the second or third decade of life. The posterior compartment of the legs and distal upper limb muscles are also affected early, but to a lesser degree. The proximal arm and leg muscles as well as the neck flexors may become weak over time. The quadriceps may become affected but usually remain relatively spared compared to other muscle groups, as are ocular and bulbar muscles. Sensation is normal. Muscle stretch reflexes can be normal or absent.

Laboratory Features

Serum CK is normal or only mildly elevated. Motor and sensory NCS are usually normal. EMG reveals positive sharp waves and early recruitment of small-amplitude, brief-duration MUAPs in weak muscles.

Histopathology

Muscle biopsies demonstrate rimmed vacuoles with muscle fibers as well as other nonspecific myopathic features, as described in the other forms of distal myopathy.[395–402] Because of the frequent rimmed vacuoles, the biopsy can be erroneously interpreted as sporadic inclusion body *myositis* (s-IBM). However, inflammation cell infiltrate and major histochemistry antigen 1 expression on muscle fibers are usually absent. EM can demonstrate 15–18-nm intranuclear and cytoplasmic tubulofilaments similar to that found in sporadic IBM.

Molecular Genetics and Pathogenesis

Nonaka myopathy and autosomal-recessive h-IBM are allelic disorders caused by mutations in the *GNE* gene on chromosome 9p1-q1 that encodes for UDP-*N*-acetylglucosamine 2-epimerase/*n*-acetylmannosamine kinase.[399,401,403] This may be involved in the post-translational glycosylation of proteins to form glycoproteins and in the production of sialic acid.

MIYOSHI DISTAL MYOPATHY

This recessively inherited myopathy is associated with early adult onset of calf atrophy and weakness and markedly elevated serum CKs. It is caused by mutations in the dysferlin gene and was discussed in greater detail in the section on LGMD 2B.

LAING DISTAL MYOPATHY

Clinical Features

Laing and colleagues initially described an Australian family with dominant inheritance (nine affected members over four generations) with weakness beginning in the anterior compartment of the distal lower limbs and neck flexors between the ages of 4 and 25 years.[404] Subsequently, this myopathy has been widely reported.[2,405–409] Over time, there is involvement of finger extensors and later, to a lesser extent, the shoulder and hip girdle muscles. Finger flexors and hand intrinsic muscles are spared. Scapular winging, scoliosis, pes cavus, ankle contractures, and/or lumbar hyperlordosis are seen in approximately 50% of patients. Hand tremor may occur.

Laboratory Features

Serum CK is normal or slightly elevated.[2,404,407,408] Motor and sensory NCS are normal. EMG reveals occasional fibrillation potentials and positive sharp waves and small-amplitude, short-duration, polyphasic MUAPs in distal more than proximal muscles.

Histopathology

Muscle biopsies demonstrate nonspecific myopathic features. Rimmed vacuoles are not seen. Large deposits of MyHC in the subsarcolemmal region of type 1 muscle fibers led some authorities to label this as a form of myosin storage myopathy.[19,410]

Molecular Genetics and Pathogenesis

Laing distal myopathy is caused by mutations in the slow/beta cardiac MyHC 1 gene, *MYH7*, located on chromosome 14q.[2,411–414] MyHC is the major myosin isoform expressed in type 1 muscle fibers. Of note, mutations have also been identified in the *MYH7* in hyaline body myopathy (discussed in Chapter 28). Mutations in *MYH7* are also a common cause of familial hypertrophic and dilated cardiomyopathy, although patients with the cardiomyopathy usually do not have much symptomatic skeletal muscle involvement and vice versa.[19] That said, we have followed patients with Laing myopathy, who also had a severe cardiomyopathy requiring transplantation, so cardiac evaluation in all patients is important.

WILLIAMS DISTAL MYOPATHY

Clinical Features

Williams distal myopathy is an autosomal dominant disorder that manifests as progressive, predominantly lower extremity weakness that can affect proximal or distal muscles either in the arms or legs with an onset in the teens to fifth decade of life.[2,415–418] Some patients develop a cardiomyopathy.

Laboratory Features

Serum CK is usually mildly elevated and EMG is myopathic.

Histopathology

Muscle biopsies may demonstrate features of MFM as will be discussed in a later section.

Molecular Genetics and Pathogenesis

William distal myopathy is caused by mutations in the *FLN-C* gene that encodes for filamin C, an actin-binding protein felt to be important in cytoskeletal formation.

► OTHER DISTAL MYOPATHIES

DISTAL MYOPATHY WITH NEBULIN MUTATIONS

Mutations in the nebulin gene (*NEB*), although usually associated with nemaline myopathy with a congenital onset, can cause a later onset distal myopathy with nemaline rods.[419,420] Such affected individuals develop slowly progressive weakness with foot drop along with finger extensor and neck flexor weakness later in childhood or in the teens. CK levels are normal or only slightly elevated. PFTs may reveal a reduced FVC.[419] Fatty degeneration in the anterior compartment of the lower legs may be apparent on skeletal muscle MRI.[419,420] The diagnosis is made by demonstration of nemaline bodies on muscle biopsy in patients with the characteristic phenotype and with confirmatory genetic testing.

DISTAL MYOPATHY WITH KELCH-LIKE HOMOLOGUE 9 (*KLHL9*) MUTATIONS

Mutations in *KLHL9* that encodes for KELCH-Like Homologue 9 is also associated with progressive foot drop followed by intrinsic hand weakness with onset in the first or second decade of life.[421] Inheritance is autosomal dominant. Weakness is slowly progressive such that affected individuals retained the ability to walk until the seventh decade. CK levels are normal or mildly elevated. Muscle biopsy reveals nonspecific dystrophic changes without rimmed vacuoles.

DISTAL MYOPATHY WITH VOCAL CORD PARALYSIS AND PHARYNGEAL WEAKNESS

Clinical Features

Late-onset, autosomal dominant vocal cord and pharyngeal distal myopathy (VCPDM) is a rare and controversial disorder, in regard to the localization of the lesion (i.e., motor neuron disease versus myopathy).[422–425] Weakness usually begins in the anterior tibial muscles in the fourth to sixth decade.

Weakness is asymmetric in some. Vocal cord and pharyngeal involvement develops after the limb weakness manifested. Ventillatory weakness can ensue.

The initial description of a large family in America was that of a vacuolar a myopathy.[422.423] Subsequently, some affected individuals developed progressive ventilatory failure resulting in death with 15 years of onset and examinations showed hyperreflexia of the lower limbs, indicative of upper motor neuron involvement as well as tongue fasciculations.[424] These clinical findings led to the reclassification of this disorder in this family by one group of authors as a form of slowly progressive familial amyotrophic lateral sclerosis (ALS21) rather than a myopathy.[424] However, a recent paper involving 6 other families with the same *MTR3* mutation reported a clearly progressive degenerative myopathy without any evidence of lower motor neuron defects by clinical examination, EMG, and histopathology.[425] This again calls into question the site of the localization, but we feel most cases are really a myopathy .

Laboratory Features

Serum CK levels are normal to moderately elevated. Motor and sensory NCS are usually normal but may reveal mild slowing of conduction velocities. EMG may reveal either myopathic or neurogenic features, but the description of these features was limited. Fibrillations and positive sharp waves have been described, but not fasciculation potentials.

Histopathology

Muscle biopsies demonstrated nonspecific myopathic features along with numerous rimmed vacuoles. Notably, fiber-type grouping and grouped angulated atrophic fibers have not been reported.

Molecular Genetics and Pathogenesis

This disorder is caused by mutations in *MTR3* that encodes for matrin-3.[423–425] Matrin-3 is a component of the nuclear matrix and appears to have roles in DNA replication, transcription, and RNA splicing. As mentioned, the localization of the site of pathology (motor neuron vs. muscle) is of debate. Perhaps, this may be similar to other disorders such as seen with mutations affecting similar genes such as *VCP*, *SQTM1*, *HNRNPA2B1*, and *HNRNPA1* that can all be associated with familial ALS or a h-IBM (also associated with rimmed vacuoles in muscle—see later section on h-IBMPFD).

▶ TREATMENT OF THE DISTAL MYOPATHIES

There is no specific medical treatment currently available for distal myopathies. Braces for lower limb weakness and other orthotic devices may be of benefit in improving gait and functional abilities.

▶ OTHER MUSCULAR DYSTROPHIES

MYOFIBRILLAR MYOPATHY

MFM is a clinically and genetically heterogeneous group of disorders, characterized by the pathologic finding of myofibrillar disruption on EM and excessive desmin accumulation in muscle fibers.[2,20,21,426–438] Because desmin is not the only protein that accumulates, the term "MFM" was suggested to be a more accurate description of the spectrum of the histologic abnormalities.[435] This myopathy has been reported as desmin storage myopathy, desmin myopathy, familial desminopathy, spheroid body myopathy, cytoplasmic body myopathy, Mallory body myopathy, familial cardiomyopathy with subsarcolemmal vermiform deposits, myopathy with intrasarcoplasmic accumulation of dense granulofilamentous material, and h-IBM with early respiratory failure.[426] In addition, some cases previously diagnosed with other forms of distal myopathy (Markesbery–Griggs distal myopathy) have MFM histopathology.[392] MFM has been classified by some in the past as congenital myopathies, but are probably best considered a form of muscular dystrophy.

Clinical Features

As mentioned, MFM is associated with a wide spectrum of clinical phenotypes.[2,426,429,431–438] Most affected individuals develop weakness between 25 and 45 years of age, although weakness may be noticeable in infancy or may present later in adulthood. Weakness can be predominantly proximal, distal, or generalized. In addition, some patients have a facioscapulohumeral or scapuloperoneal distribution of weakness. Facial and pharyngeal muscles can also be affected in some individuals. Rigidity of the spine can also be seen.

In addition to skeletal muscle, the heart can also be affected and cardiac arrhythmias and CHF may be the predominant features of the disease. In severe cardiomyopathies, pacemaker insertion or cardiac transplantation may be required. In addition, severe ventilatory muscle involvement can develop in MFM. Also, smooth muscle involvement may lead to intestinal pseudo-obstructions.

Laboratory Features

Serum CK is normal or usually only slightly increased in MFM.[2] EKGs may demonstrate conduction defects or arrhythmia, while echocardiograms may reveal a dilated or hypertrophic cardiomyopathy. NCS are usually normal, although low CMAP and SNAP amplitudes and slowing of conduction velocities can be seen. EMG reveals increased insertional and spontaneous activity with fibrillation potentials, positive sharp waves, pseudomyotonic potentials, complex repetitive discharges, and early recruitment of short-duration, small-amplitude, polyphasic MUAPs.[2]

Long-duration, large-amplitude MUAPs may also be seen, owing to the chronicity of the disorder.

Histopathology

Muscle biopsies reveal variability in fiber size, increased internalized nuclei, occasionally type 1 fiber predominance, and in some cases, scattered fibers with rimmed vacuoles.[2] In addition, Nakano et al. defined two major types of lesions on light and EM that characterize MFM: hyaline structures and nonhyaline lesions (Fig. 27-28).[434] The hyaline structures are cytoplasmic granular inclusions, which are typically eosinophilic on H&E and dark blue-green or occasionally red on modified Gomori trichrome stains. They do not stain for NADH. On EM, the hyaline lesions resemble cytoplasmic, spheroid, or Mallory bodies. The nonhyaline lesions appear as dark green areas of amorphous material on Gomori trichrome stains. On EM, these nonhyaline lesions correspond to foci of myofibrillar destruction and consist of disrupted myofilaments, Z-disc-derived bodies, dappled dense structures of Z-disc origin, and streaming of the Z-disc.[434,436] In addition, larger-size tubulofilaments (14–20 nm) typical of the inclusion body myopathies may accumulate.

Immunohistochemistry reveals that both the hyaline and the nonhyaline lesions contain desmin and numerous other proteins.[2,22,426–434,436,438] Abnormal accumulation of desmin is not specific for MFM and can be seen in a variety of neuromuscular conditions, including X-linked myotubular myopathy, congenital myotonic dystrophy, spinal muscular atrophy, nemaline rod myopathy, fetal myotubes, IBM, and in regenerating muscle fibers of any etiology. Abnormal accumulation of desmin has been demonstrated in cardiac muscles in MFM patients with cardiomyopathy. Immunohistochemistry also reveals that the nonhyaline lesions react strongly not only for desmin, but also for dystrophin, gelsolin, N terminus of β-amyloid precursor protein, and NCAM in addition to desmin. In addition, the nonhyaline lesions are depleted of actin, α-actinin, myosin, and, less consistently, titin and nebulin. In contrast, the hyaline structures are composed of compacted and degraded remnants of thick and thin filaments and react to actin, α-actinin, and myosin, in addition to dystrophin, gelsolin, filamin c, and the N terminus of β-amyloid precursor protein; they do not react to NCAM and react variably to desmin. Both types of lesions also react for αB-crystallin, α-1 antichymotrypsin, and ubiquitin and can be congophilic. The abnormal muscle fibers also abnormally express several cyclin-dependent kinases (CDC/CDK) in the cytoplasm, including CDC2, CDK2, CDK4, and CDK7.[426,438]

Nerve and intramuscular nerve biopsies have demonstrated enlarged axons with accumulation of intermediate-sized neurofilaments and formation of axonal spheroids in some patients.[439,440]

Molecular Genetics and Pathogenesis

The pathogenesis of MFM is likely related to disruption of the Z-disc.[2,20,21,426,435,436] Mutations have been identified in the genes that encode for desmin, αB-crystallin, myotilin, filamin c, BCL2-associated athanogene 3 (BAG3), FHL-1, ZASP (Z-band alternatively spliced PDX motif-containing protein), titin, selenoprotein N, DNAJB6, and transportin 3. Most of these proteins are Z-disc-related proteins. Most familial cases demonstrate autosomal-dominant inheritance, although autosomal-recessive (some desmin) and X-linked inheritance (FHL1) occur.

Mutations in the desmin gene, *DES*, located on chromosome 2q35 is associated with autosomal-dominant LGMD1E and recessive LGMD2R that have MFM histopathology as previously discussed.[2,129–138,428,432,436,441] Mutations in *DES* were demonstrated in the initial family reported with scapuloperoneal myopathy. Desmin is an intermediate filament protein of skeletal, cardiac, and some smooth muscle cells. This cytoskeletal protein links Z-bands with the sarcolemma and the nucleus. The intermediate filament network is important in the stability of the muscle fiber and during mitosis/regeneration of muscle cells. These abnormal desmin filaments form insoluble aggregates, which prevent the genesis of the normal filamentous network.[442]

Mutations in the αB-crystallin gene, *CRYAB*, on chromosome 11q21–23 have been demonstrated in some autosomal- dominant kinships.[435–437] Alpha B-crystallin possesses "molecular chaperone" activity and is felt to interact with desmin in the assembly of the intermediate filament network.

Missense mutations in the myotilin gene, *MYOT*, located on chromosome 5q22–31 cause late-onset MFM and are allelic to LGMD 1 A as previously discussed.[2,20,90–99] These patients had late onset of distal greater than proximal weakness, polyneuropathy, and cardiopathy. Myotilin is a component of the Z-disc where it interacts with α-actinin, actin, and filamin c and probably plays a fundamental role in myofibrillar assembly.

In addition, missense mutations in the *LDP3* gene located on chromosome 10q22.3–10q23.2 that encodes for ZASP are responsible for Markesbury–Griggs distal myopathy, which has MFM histopathology as previously discussed.[2,21,393] ZASP is expressed in skeletal and cardiac muscle and it binds to α-actinin, a component of the Z-disc that in turn cross-links thin filaments of adjacent sarcomeres.[21]

Mutations in *BAG3* located on chromosome 10q26.11 are associated with proximal and/or distal weakness, hypernasal speech, ventilatory weakness, and dilated cardiomyopathy with onset in the first or second decade.[394] BAG3 interacts with heat shock proteins and may have a role in cellular response to environmental stress.

Mutations in *FLN-C* located on chromosome 7q32 that encodes for filamin-C cause Williams distal myopathy,

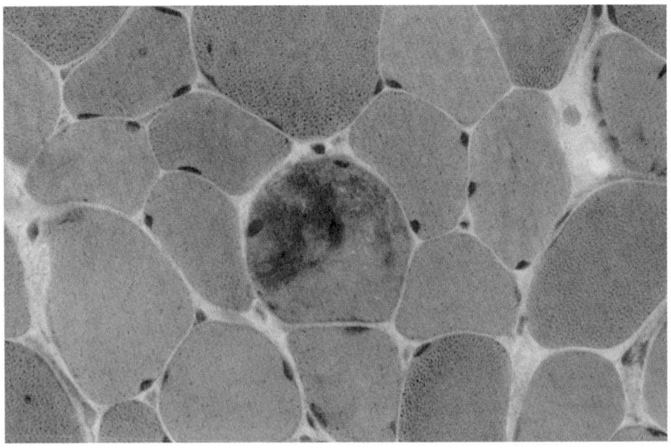

A

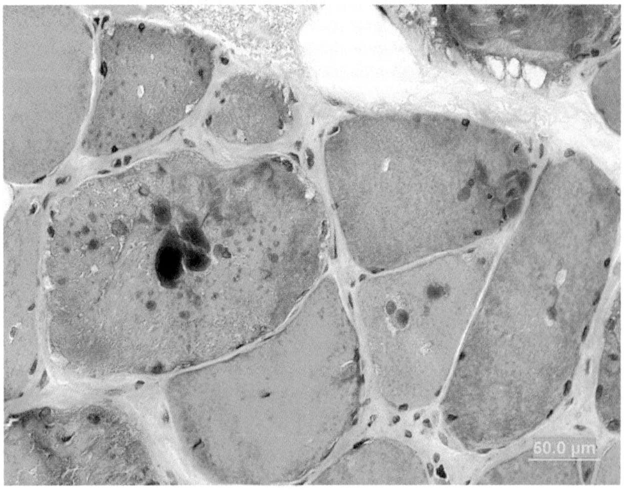

B

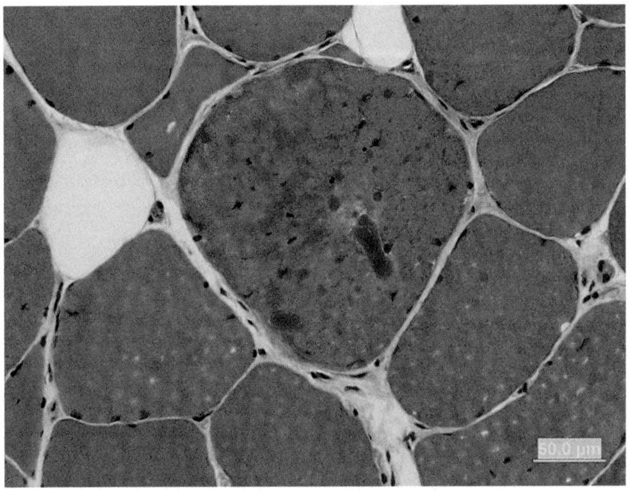

C

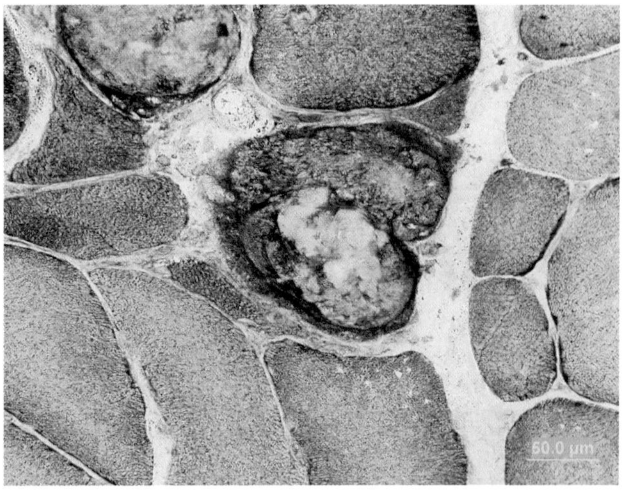

D

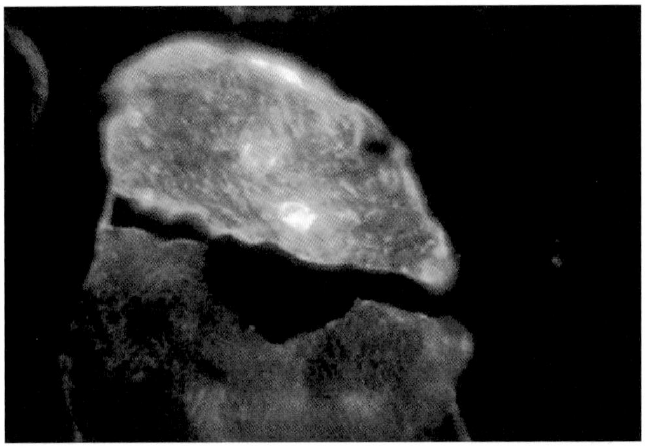

E

Figure 27-28. Myofibrillar myopathy. Nonhyaline lesions appear as amorphous accumulation of reddish-purple or dark green material **(A)**, while the hyaline lesions are denser and can have the appearance of cytoplasmic or spheroid bodies (**B**) on Trichrome stain. The hyaline lesions are eosinophilic on H&E but less well seen than on the trichrome stains **(C)**. The hyaline and nonhyaline lesions do not stain with NADH-TR (**D**). Immunostaining reveals that the lesions are immunoreactive to desmin (**E**).

as previously discussed.[2,22,415–418] Filamin-C binds actin and is involved in the formation of the Z-disc. In addition, filamin-c also binds γ- and δ-sarcoglycan at the sarcolemmal membrane and may also play a role in signaling pathways from the sarcolemma to the myofibril.[22]

Mutations in *FHL1* on Xq26.3 encoding for four and a half LIM protein some cases of scapuloperoneal dystrophy with reducing bodies and features of MFM on muscle biopsy.[2,329]

Mutations in the selenoprotein N gene (*SEPN1*) located on chromosome 1p36 were identified in autosomal-recessive

MFM associated with Mallory-body-like inclusions.[301] These patients have an early onset of axial muscle weakness, ventilatory weakness, and rigidity of the spine. Of note, mutations in *SEPN1* gene can cause MDC with rigid spine and multi/minicore myopathy, but can also have histopathology resembling MFM.

Finally, LGMD1D and LGMD1E caused by mutations in the genes encoding for DNAJB6 and transportin 3, respectively, can have MFM-like histopathology.[140]

Treatment

There is no proven medical therapy to improve skeletal muscle weakness. Antiarrhythmic and cardiotropic medications are sometimes necessary in patients with cardiopathy. Cardiac transplantation can be lifesaving in patients with severe cardiomyopathy.

HEREDITARY INCLUSION BODY MYOPATHIES

There are autosomal-dominant and autosomal-recessive forms of h-IBM.[2]

HEREDITARY INCLUSION BODY MYOPATHY 2 (h-IBM2) OR GNE MYOPATHY

Clinical Features

The most common form of autosomal recessive h-IBM2 is allelic Nonaka distal myopathy being caused by mutations in *GNE* that encodes for UDP-N-acetylglucosamine-2-epimerase/N-acetylmannosamine kinase.[2,395–402] As previously discussed, the preferred term now is "GNE myopathy." This myopathy was initially reported in Iranian Jews and other Middle Eastern Karaites and Arab Muslims of Palestinian and Bedouin origin as a form of hIBM, while Nonaka distal myopathy was the name given for similar patients reported in Japanese, Korean, and Chinese families. The age of onset and pattern of weakness in GNE myopathy are different from that of s-IBM. Most patients with s-IBM present over the age of 50 years with weakness of quadriceps and wrist and finger flexors. In contrast, most patients with GNE myopathy present in the late teens to early 40s with anterior tibial involvement leading to foot drop. There is insidious progression with gradual involvement of the iliopsoas, thigh adductors, and to a lesser extent the glutei muscles. Importantly, in differentiating from s-IBM, the quadriceps are usually normal or relatively spared.[399–402] However, rarely the quadriceps can be affected. The proximal arms and neck flexors can also become affected. There can be asymmetry of muscle weakness. Progression is variable, with some patients becoming wheelchair dependent within a few years of onset, while others are ambulatory several decades later.

There are a few reports of familial cases of s-IBM in which siblings, even twins, had the characteristic clinical phenotype and histological features of s-IBM.[402] These cases do not represent h-IBM. Rather, there may be a familial predisposition for development of s-IBM, similar to that described for other autoimmune disorders.

Laboratory Features

Serum CK levels are normal or only mildly elevated. Motor and sensory nerve conduction studies are usually normal. EMG demonstrates fibrillation potentials, positive sharp waves, and complex repetitive discharges. There is a mixture of small-amplitude, short-duration polyphasic MUAPs with large-amplitude, long-duration polyphasic MUAPs.

Histopathology

Muscle biopsies are similar to s-IBM, except for the lack of significant endomysial inflammation and invasion of non-necrotic muscle fibers.[2,399–402] Fiber size variability, split fibers, increased central nuclei, and fibers with rimmed vacuoles are evident. Amyloid and other "Alzheimer characteristic proteins" are seen in vacuolated muscle fibers, although they are much less frequent compared to s-IBM. As in s-IBM, EM demonstrates the abnormal accumulation of 15–18-nm tubulofilaments in the cytoplasm and nuclei of muscle fibers.

Molecular Genetics and Pathogenesis

Nonaka-type distal myopathy and autosomal-recessive h-IBM are allelic disorders caused by mutations in *GNE* on chromosome 9p1-q1 encoding UDP-N-acetylglucosamine-2-epimerase/N-acetylmannosamine kinase.[2,399–402] GNE is involved in the post-translational glycosylation of proteins to form glycoproteins. Disturbed glycosylation is therefore now recognized as a newly identified molecular genetic defect for muscular dystrophies. However, other mechanisms may be involved in the pathogenesis of this myopathy. GNE is an important enzyme in the sialic acid biosynthesis pathway.

Treatment

There is no medical treatment available for GNE myopathy. Patients with distal lower limb weakness may benefit from bracing.

HEREDITARY IBM TYPE 3

Clinical Features

This myopathy usually presents with congenital arthrogryposis and ophthalmoparesis with mild proximal weakness beginning in adulthood. Face and distal extremity weakness may occur. Some patients complain of muscle pain. As muscle biopsies may demonstrate rimmed vacuoles and tubulofilamentous inclusions, this disorder has also been called h-IBM type 3.[2,19,443,444]

Laboratory Features

Serum CK levels are usually.

Histopathology

Muscle biopsies reveal small and infrequent type II fibers, particularly type 2 A fibers, focal disorganization of the myofibrils, and rimmed vacuoles and inclusion consisting of 15- to 20-nm tubulofilaments.[2] Lobulated fibers and mini-cores have also been reported.

Molecular Genetics and Pathogenesis

Mutations have been identified in the *MYH2* gene located on chromosome 17p13.1, which encodes for MyHC IIa.[2,9,443,444] The MyHC IIa isoform of MyHCs is expressed in type 2 A muscle fibers.

H-IBM WITH CEREBRAL HYPOMYELINATION

This autosomal-recessive h-IBM is associated with an infantile onset of progressive proximal greater than distal weakness, legs worse than arms, and marked cerebral white matter abnormalities on CT and MRI.[445] Despite the apparent leukoencephalopathy on radiological imaging, intellectual function was normal in all the cases. Motor nerve conduction studies were mildly slow, suggesting dysmyelination of peripheral nerves as well.

H-IBM WITH PAGET DISEASE AND FRONTOTEMPORAL DEMENTIA

Clinical Features

h-IBM associated with Paget disease of the bone and frontotemporal dementia, or IBMPFD, is a rare autosomal-dominant disorder is usually caused by mutations in *VCP* that encodes for valosin-containing protein (VCP).[2,446–463] It is characterized by adult onset (range late first to ninth decade, with mean in the 40s) of limb-girdle, distal, or scapuloperoneal weakness. There also appears to be a mild asymmetry and variability in the patterns of muscle weakness. Frontotemporal dementia is seen in approximately 30–50% with onset approximately 10 years after weakness (average age 54 years). Paget disease of the bone (PDB) tends to occur earlier than in the more common sporadic forms of PDB and is seen with variable frequency. The complete triad of h-IBM, PDB, and frontotemporal dementia occurs in only about one-third of cases. In addition, mutations in the same gene cause a form of familial amyotrophic lateral sclerosis (fALS) with or without frontotemporal dementia.[464,465] A dilated cardiomyopathy may be seen in a quarter of patients.[459] Ultimately, the cause of death is through progressive muscle weakness and ventilatory failure. There is significant heterogeneity in clinical phenotype and severity both between and within families.

Laboratory Features

Serum CK levels are normal to slightly elevated. Serum alkaline phosphatase levels can be a screening test but may not be elevated in those without PDB. EMG shows myopathic changes with muscle membrane irritability.

Histopathology

Muscle biopsy reveal fibers with rimmed vacuoles and inclusions that immunostain with ubiquitin, TDP-43, and VCP.[2,455,456] Neurogenic features of type grouping and angulated fibers, which is notable *VCP* mutations can also be associated with motor neuron disease.[455,456] EM may show paired helical filaments in muscle and in PDB osteoclasts.

Molecular Genetics and Pathogenesis

h-IBMPFD is usually caused by mutations in the gene encoding VCP, a member of the AAA-ATPase superfamily.[2,446,447] VCP is associated with a variety of cellular activities, including cell-cycle control, membrane fusion, and the ubiquitin–proteasome degradation pathway. VCP normally localizes to nuclei and specifically near nucleoli. Mutations in VCP gene may disrupt in nuclear structure or normal translation of mRNA. In addition, mutations in *SQTM1*, *HNRPA2B1*, and *HNRNPA1*, have been noted to cause hIBM or fALS, while mutations in *SQTM1* can also cause PDB. Some have termed these disorders as "multisystem proteinopathies."[466,467].

▶SUMMARY

With so many different types of muscular dystrophies and the variability of clinical phenotypes associated with specific forms of dystrophy, even within individual families, the evaluation of patients presenting with weakness can be quite daunting. However, rather than ordering every genetic test possible or doing a muscle biopsy initially on every patient, an approach to ordering tests based on clinical phenotype (inheritance pattern, age of onset, pattern of weakness, and associated manifestations—early contractures and cardiac or ventilatory involvement) should be useful (Figs. 27-8, 27-10, 27-16, 27-19, 27-23, 27-27).[2,250] However, as next generation, whole genome, and whole exome sequencing become more widely available and less expensive, such large scale genetic testing will become a more accessible tool due to cost considerations. Nonetheless, accurate clinical assessment will remain a prerequisite in order to distinguish pathological mutations from the benign polymorphisms that this technology will uncover.

Unfortunately, there are limited beneficial medical treatments, other than corticosteroids for children with DMD. Still with supportive treatments (physical and occupational therapy, bracing, respiratory, and cardiac), quality of life can be improved in patients. More work needs to be done to further understand the pathogenesis of these disorders and discover targeted and better treatments.

REFERENCES

1. Wicklund MP. The muscular dystrophies. *Continuum (Minneap Minn)*. 2013;19(6 Muscle Disease):1535–1570.
2. Narayanaswami P, Weiss M, Selcen D, et al. Summary of evidence-based guideline: Diagnosis and treatment of limb-girdle and distal muscular dystrophies. *Neurology*. 2014;83 (16):1453–1463.
3. Hoffman EP, Brown RH Jr, Kunkel LM. Dystrophin: The protein product of the Duchenne muscular dystrophy locus. *Cell*. 1987;51(6):919–928.
4. Hoffman EP, Fischbeck KH, Brown RH, et al. Characterization of dystrophin in muscle-biopsy specimens from patients with Duchenne's or Becker's muscular dystrophy. *N Engl J Med*. 1988;318(21):1363–1368.
5. Koenig M, Hoffman EP, Bertelson CJ, Monaco AP, Feener C, Kunkel LM. Complete cloning of the Duchenne muscular dystrophy (DMD) cDNA and preliminary genomic organization of the DMD gene in normal and affected individuals. *Cell*. 1987;50(3):509–517.
6. Cohn RD, Campbell KP. Molecular basis of muscular dystrophies. *Muscle Nerve*. 2000;23(10):1456–1471.
7. Michele DE, Barresi R, Kanagawa M, et al. Post-translational disruption of dystroglycan–ligand interactions in congenital muscular dystrophies. *Nature*. 2002;418(6896):417–422.
8. Wewer UM, Engvall E. Merosin/laminin-2 and muscular dystrophy. *Neuromuscul Disord*. 1996;6(6):409–418.
9. Matsumura K, Yamada H, Saito F, Sunada Y, Shimizu T. Peripheral nerve involvement in merosin-deficient congenital muscular dystrophy and dy mouse. *Neuromuscul Disord*. 1997;7(1):7–12.
10. Vachon PH, Xu H, Liu L, et al. Integrins (alpha7beta1) in muscle function and survival. Disrupted expression in merosin-deficient congenital muscular dystrophy. *J Clin Invest*. 1997; 100(7):1870–1881.
11. Bansal D, Miyake K, Vogel SS, et al. Defective membrane repair in dysferlin-deficient muscular dystrophy. *Nature*. 2003; 423(6936):168–172.
12. Cenacchi G, Fanin M, De Giorgi LB, Angelini C. Ultrastructural changes in dysferlinopathy support defective membrane repair mechanism. *J Clin Pathol*. 2005;58(2):190–195.
13. Bashir R, Britton S, Strachan T, et al. A gene related to Caenorhabditis elegans spermatogenesis factor fer-1 is mutated in limb-girdle muscular dystrophy type 2B. *Nat Genet*. 1998;20 (1):37–42.
14. Matsuda C, Aoki M, Hayashi YK, Ho MF, Arahata K, Brown RH Jr. Dysferlin is a surface membrane-associated protein that is absent in Miyoshi myopathy. *Neurology*. 1999;53(5):1119–1122.
15. Carbone I, Bruno C, Sotgia F, et al. Mutation in the CAV3 gene causes partial caveolin-3 deficiency and hyperCKemia. *Neurology*. 2000;54(6):1373–1376.
16. Minetti C, Sotgia F, Bruno C, et al. Mutations in the caveolin-3 gene cause autosomal dominant limb-girdle muscular dystrophy. *Nat Genet*. 1998;18(4):365–368.
17. Sotgia F, Woodman SE, Bonuccelli G, et al. Phenotypic behavior of caveolin-3 R26Q, a mutant associated with hyperCKemia, distal myopathy, and rippling muscle disease. *Am J Physiol Cell Physiol*. 2003;285(5):C1150–C1160.
18. Woodman SE, Sotgia F, Galbiati F, Minetti C, Lisanti MP. Caveolinopathies: Mutations in caveolin-3 cause four distinct autosomal dominant muscle diseases. *Neurology*. 2004;62 (4):538–543.
19. Oldfors A, Tajsharghi H, Darin N, Lindberg C. Myopathies associated with myosin heavy chain mutations. *Acta Myol*. 2004;23(2):90–96.
20. Selcen D, Engel AG. Mutations in myotilin cause myofibrillar myopathy. *Neurology*. 2004;62(8):1363–1371.
21. Selcen D, Engel AG. Mutations in ZASP define a novel form of muscular dystrophy in humans. *Ann Neurol*. 2005;57(2):269–276.
22. Vorgerd M, van der Ven PF, Bruchertseifer V, et al. A mutation in the dimerization domain of filamin c causes a novel type of autosomal dominant myofibrillar myopathy. *Am J Hum Genet*. 2005;77(2):297–304.
23. Nagano A, Arahata K. Nuclear envelope proteins and associated diseases. *Curr Opin Neurol*. 2000;13(5):533–539.
24. Nagano A, Koga R, Ogawa M, et al. Emerin deficiency at the nuclear membrane in patients with Emery–Dreifuss muscular dystrophy. *Nat Genet*. 1996;12(3):254–259.
25. Ognibene A, Sabatelli P, Petrini S, et al. Nuclear changes in a case of X-linked Emery–Dreifuss muscular dystrophy. *Muscle Nerve*. 1999;22(7):864–869.
26. Sabatelli P, Lattanzi G, Ognibene A, et al. Nuclear alterations in autosomal-dominant Emery–Dreifuss muscular dystrophy. *Muscle Nerve*. 2001;24(6):826–829.
27. Bonne G, Mercuri E, Muchir A, et al. Clinical and molecular genetic spectrum of autosomal dominant Emery–Dreifuss muscular dystrophy due to mutations of the lamin A/C gene. *Ann Neurol*. 2000;48(2):170–180.
28. Felice KJ, Schwartz RC, Brown CA, Leicher CR, Grunnet ML. Autosomal dominant Emery–Dreifuss dystrophy due to mutations in rod domain of the lamin A/C gene. *Neurology*. 2000;55(2):275–280.
29. Frosk P, Weiler T, Nylen E, et al. Limb-girdle muscular dystrophy type 2 H associated with mutation in TRIM32, a putative E3-ubiquitin-ligase gene. *Am J Hum Genet*. 2002;70(3):663–672.
30. Brockington M, Blake DJ, Prandini P, et al. Mutations in the fukutin-related protein gene (FKRP) cause a form of congenital muscular dystrophy with secondary laminin alpha2 deficiency and abnormal glycosylation of alpha-dystroglycan. *Am J Hum Genet*. 2001;69(6):1198–1209.
31. Brockington M, Yuva Y, Prandini P, et al. Mutations in the fukutin-related protein gene (FKRP) identify limb girdle muscular dystrophy 2I as a milder allelic variant of congenital muscular dystrophy MDC1 C. *Hum Mol Genet*. 2001;10(25): 2851–2859.
32. Brown SC, Torelli S, Brockington M, et al. Abnormalities in alpha-dystroglycan expression in MDC1 C and LGMD2I muscular dystrophies. *Am J Pathol*. 2004;164(2):727–737.
33. Beltran-Valero de Bernabe D, Voit T, Longman C, et al. Mutations in the FKRP gene can cause muscle-eye-brain disease and Walker-Warburg syndrome. *J Med Genet*. 2004;41(5):e61.
34. Brockington M, Torelli S, Prandini P, et al. Localization and functional analysis of the LARGE family of glycosyltransferases: Significance for muscular dystrophy. *Hum Mol Genet*. 2005;14(5):657–665.
35. Longman C, Brockington M, Torelli S, et al. Mutations in the human LARGE gene cause MDC1D, a novel form of congenital muscular dystrophy with severe mental retardation and abnormal glycosylation of alpha-dystroglycan. *Hum Mol Genet*. 2003;12(21):2853–2861.
36. Bushby K, Finkel R, Birnkrant DJ, et al. Diagnosis and management of Duchenne muscular dystrophy, part 1: Diagnosis, and pharmacological and psychosocial management. *Lancet Neurol*. 2010;9(1):77–93.

37. Bushby K, Finkel R, Birnkrant DJ, et al. Diagnosis and management of Duchenne muscular dystrophy, part 2: Implementation of multidisciplinary care. *Lancet Neurol.* 2010;9(2):177–189.
38. Flanigan KM. Duchenne and Becker Muscular Dystrophies. *Neurol Clin.* 2014;32(3):671–688.
39. Emery AE. Population frequencies of inherited neuromuscular diseases-a world survey. *Neuromuscul Disord.* 1991;1(1):19–29.
40. Brooke MH, Fenichel GM, Griggs RC, et al. Duchenne muscular dystrophy: Patterns of clinical progression and effects of supportive therapy. *Neurology.* 1989;39(4):475–481.
41. Brooke MH, Griggs RC, Mendell JR, Fenichel GM, Shumate JB. The natural history of Duchenne muscular dystrophy: A caveat for therapeutic trials. *Trans Am Neurol Assoc.* 1981;106:195–199.
42. Farah MG, Evans EB, Vignos PJ Jr. Echocardiographic evaluation of left ventricular function in Duchenne's muscular dystrophy. *Am J Med.* 1980;69(2):248–254.
43. Perloff JK, Roberts WC, de Leon AC Jr, O'Doherty D. The distinctive electrocardiogram of Duchenne's progressive muscular dystrophy. An electrocardiographic-pathologic correlative study. *Am J Med.* 1967;42(2):179–188.
44. Sanyal SK, Johnson WW. Cardiac conduction abnormalities in children with Duchenne's progressive muscular dystrophy: Electrocardiographic features and morphologic correlates. *Circulation.* 1982;66(4):853–863.
45. Leibowitz D, Dubowitz V. Intellect and behaviour in Duchenne muscular dystrophy. *Dev Med Child Neurol.* 1981;23(5):577–590.
46. Arahata K, Engel AG. Monoclonal antibody analysis of mononuclear cells in myopathies. I: Quantitation of subsets according to diagnosis and sites of accumulation and demonstration and counts of muscle fibers invaded by T cells. *Ann Neurol.* 1984;16(2):193–208.
47. Bushby KM, Thambyayah M, Gardner-Medwin D. Prevalence and incidence of Becker muscular dystrophy. *Lancet.* 1991;337(8748):1022–1024.
48. Bushby KM, Gardner-Medwin D. The clinical, genetic and dystrophin characteristics of Becker muscular dystrophy. I. Natural history. *J Neurol.* 1993;240(2):98–104.
49. Sunohara N, Arahata K, Hoffman EP, et al. Quadriceps myopathy: Forme fruste of Becker muscular dystrophy. *Ann Neurol.* 1990;28(5):634–639.
50. Comi GP, Prelle A, Bresolin N, et al. Clinical variability in Becker muscular dystrophy. Genetic, biochemical and immunohistochemical correlates. *Brain.* 1994;117(Pt 1):1–14.
51. Gospe SM, Jr., Lazaro RP, Lava NS, Grootscholten PM, Scott MO, Fischbeck KH. Familial X-linked myalgia and cramps: A nonprogressive myopathy associated with a deletion in the dystrophin gene. *Neurology.* 1989;39(10):1277–1280.
52. Doriguzzi C, Palmucci L, Mongini T, Chiadò-Piat L, Restagno G, Ferrone M. Exercise intolerance and recurrent myoglobinuria as the only expression of Xp21 Becker type muscular dystrophy. *J Neurol.* 1993;240(5):269–271.
53. Muntoni F, Cau M, Ganau A, et al. Brief report: Deletion of the dystrophin muscle-promoter region associated with X-linked dilated cardiomyopathy. *N Engl J Med.* 1993;329(13):921–925.
54. Towbin JA, Hejtmancik JF, Brink P, et al. X-linked dilated cardiomyopathy. Molecular genetic evidence of linkage to the Duchenne muscular dystrophy (dystrophin) gene at the Xp21 locus. *Circulation.* 1993;87(6):1854–1865.
55. de Visser M, de Voogt WG, la Rivière GV. The heart in Becker muscular dystrophy, facioscapulohumeral dystrophy, and Bethlem myopathy. *Muscle Nerve.* 1992;15(5):591–596.
56. Kaido M, Arahata K, Hoffman EP, Nonaka I, Sugita H. Muscle histology in Becker muscular dystrophy. *Muscle Nerve.* 1991;14(11):1067–1073.
57. Hoffman EP, Kunkel LM, Angelini C, Clarke A, Johnson M, Harris JB. Improved diagnosis of Becker muscular dystrophy by dystrophin testing. *Neurology.* 1989;39(8):1011–1017.
58. Hoffman EP, Arahata K, Minetti C, Bonilla E, Rowland LP. Dystrophinopathy in isolated cases of myopathy in females. *Neurology.* 1992;42(5):967–975.
59. Arahata K, Ishihara T, Kamakura K, et al. Mosaic expression of dystrophin in symptomatic carriers of Duchenne's muscular dystrophy. *N Engl J Med.* 1989;320(3):138–142.
60. Clerk A, Rodillo E, Heckmatt JZ, Dubowitz V, Strong PN, Sewry CA. Characterisation of dystrophin in carriers of Duchenne muscular dystrophy. *J Neurol Sci.* 1991;102(2):197–205.
61. Minetti C, Chang HW, Medori R, et al. Dystrophin deficiency in young girls with sporadic myopathy and normal karyotype. *Neurology.* 1991;41(8):1288–1292.
62. Hyser CL, Doherty RA, Griggs RC, et al. Carrier assessment for mothers and sisters of isolated Duchenne dystrophy cases: The importance of serum enzyme determinations. *Neurology.* 1987;37(9):1476–1480.
63. Hyser CL, Griggs RC, Mendell JR, et al. Use of serum creatine kinase, pyruvate kinase, and genetic linkage for carrier detection in Duchenne and Becker dystrophy. *Neurology.* 1987;37(1):4–10.
64. Bakker E, Veenema H, Den Dunnen JT, et al. Germinal mosaicism increases the recurrence risk for 'new' Duchenne muscular dystrophy mutations. *J Med Genet.* 1989;26(9):553–559.
65. Prior TW, Bartolo C, Pearl DK, et al. Spectrum of small mutations in the dystrophin coding region. *Am J Hum Genet.* 1995;57(1):22–33.
66. Brooke MH, Fenichel GM, Griggs RC, et al. Clinical investigation of Duchenne muscular dystrophy. Interesting results in a trial of prednisone. *Arch Neurol.* 1987;44(8):812–817.
67. Fenichel GM, Florence JM, Pestronk A, et al. Long-term benefit from prednisone therapy in Duchenne muscular dystrophy. *Neurology.* 1991;41(12):1874–1877.
68. Griggs RC, Moxley RT 3rd, Mendell JR, et al. Prednisone in Duchenne dystrophy. A randomized, controlled trial defining the time course and dose response. Clinical Investigation of Duchenne Dystrophy Group. *Arch Neurol.* 1991;48(4):383–388.
69. Griggs RC, Moxley RT 3rd, Mendell JR, et al. Duchenne dystrophy: Randomized, controlled trial of prednisone (18 months) and azathioprine (12 months). *Neurology.* 1993;43(3 Pt 1):520–527.
70. Mendell JR, Moxley RT, Griggs RC, et al. Randomized, double-blind six-month trial of prednisone in Duchenne's muscular dystrophy. *N Engl J Med.* 1989;320(24):1592–1597.
71. Moxley RT 3rd, Ashwal S, Pandya S, et al. Practice parameter: Corticosteroid treatment of Duchenne dystrophy: Report of the Quality Standards Subcommittee of the American Academy of Neurology and the Practice Committee of the Child Neurology Society. *Neurology.* 2005;64(1):13–20.
72. Backman E, Henriksson KG. Low-dose prednisolone treatment in Duchenne and Becker muscular dystrophy. *Neuromuscul Disord.* 1995;5(3):233–241.
73. Connolly AM, Schierbecker J, Renna R, Florence J. High dose weekly oral prednisone improves strength in boys with Duchenne muscular dystrophy. *Neuromuscul Disord.* 2002;12(10):917–925.

74. Angelini C, Pegoraro E, Turella E, Intino MT, Pini A, Costa C. Deflazacort in Duchenne dystrophy: Study of long-term effect. *Muscle Nerve*. 1994;17(4):386–391.
75. Bonifati MD, Ruzza G, Bonometto P, et al. A multicenter, double-blind, randomized trial of deflazacort versus prednisone in Duchenne muscular dystrophy. *Muscle Nerve*. 2000;23(9):1344–1347.
76. Fenichel GM, Griggs RC, Kissel J, et al. A randomized efficacy and safety trial of oxandrolone in the treatment of Duchenne dystrophy. *Neurology*. 2001;56(8):1075–1079.
77. Tarnopolsky M, Martin J. Creatine monohydrate increases strength in patients with neuromuscular disease. *Neurology*. 1999;52(4):854–857.
78. Walter MC, Lochmuller H, Reilich P, et al. Creatine monohydrate in muscular dystrophies: A double-blind, placebo-controlled clinical study. *Neurology*. 2000;54(9):1848–1850.
79. Mendell JR, Kissel JT, Amato AA, et al. Myoblast transfer in the treatment of Duchenne's muscular dystrophy. *N Engl J Med*. 1995;333(13):832–838.
80. Fairclough RJ, Wood MJ, Davies KE. Therapy for Duchenne muscular dystrophy: Renewed optimism from genetic approaches. *Nat Rev Genet*. 2013;14:373–378.
81. Cirak S, Arechavala-Gomeza V, Guglieri M, et al. Exon skipping and dystrophin restoration in patients with Duchenne muscular dystrophy after systemic phosphorodiamidate morpholino oligomer treatment: An open-label, phase 2, dose-escalation study. *Lancet*. 2011;378(9791):595–605.
82. Mendell JR, Rodino-Klapac LR, Sahenk Z, et al. Eteplirsen for the treatment of Duchenne muscular dystrophy. *Ann Neurol*. 2013;74(5):637–647.
83. Goemans NM, Tulinius M, van den Akker JT, et al. Systemic administration of PRO051 in Duchenne's muscular dystrophy. *N Engl J Med*. 2011;364(16):1513–1522.
84. Bushby K, Finkel R, Wong B, et al. Ataluren treatment of patients with nonsense mutation dystrophinopathy. *Muscle Nerve*. 2014;50(4):477–487.
85. Darras BT, Francke U. Myopathy in complex glycerol kinase deficiency patients is due to 3 deletions of the dystrophin gene. *Am J Hum Genet*. 1988;43(2):126–130.
86. Guggenheim MA, McCabe ER, Roig M, et al. Glycerol kinase deficiency with neuromuscular, skeletal, and adrenal abnormalities. *Ann Neurol*. 1980;7(5):441–449.
87. Seltzer WK, Angelini C, Dhariwal G, Ringel SP, McCabe ER. Muscle glycerol kinase in Duchenne dystrophy and glycerol kinase deficiency. *Muscle Nerve*. 1989;12(4):307–313.
88. Gilchrist JM, Pericak-Vance M, Silverman L, Roses AD. Clinical and genetic investigation in autosomal dominant limb-girdle muscular dystrophy. *Neurology*. 1988;38(1):5–9.
89. Chutkow JG, Heffner RR Jr, Kramer AA, Edwards JA. Adult-onset autosomal dominant limb-girdle muscular dystrophy. *Ann Neurol*. 1986;20(2):240–248.
90. Hauser MA, Horrigan SK, Salmikangas P, et al. Myotilin is mutated in limb girdle muscular dystrophy 1A. *Hum Mol Genet*. 2000;9(14):2141–2147.
91. Olivé M, Goldfarb LG, Shatunov A, Fischer D, Ferrer I. Myotilinopathy: Refining the clinical and myopathological phenotype. *Brain*. 2005;128:2315–2326.
92. Pénisson-Besnier I, Talvinen K, Dumez C, et al. Myotilinopathy in a family with late onset myopathy. *Neuromuscul Disord*. 2006;16:427–431.
93. Schramm N, Born C, Weckbach S, Reilich P, Walter MC, Reiser MF. Involvement patterns in myotilinopathy and desminopathy detected by a novel neuromuscular whole-body MRI protocol. *Eur Radiol*. 2008;18:2922–2936.
94. Olivé M, Odgerel Z, Martínez A, et al. Clinical and myopathological evaluation of early- and late-onset subtypes of myofibrillar myopathy. *Neuromuscul Disord*. 2011;21:533–542.
95. Gilchrist JM, Pericak-Vance M, Silverman L, Roses AD. Clinical and genetic investigation in autosomal dominant limb-girdle muscular dystrophy. *Neurology*. 1988;38:5–9.
96. Marconi G, Pizzi A, Arimondi CG, Vannelli B. Limb girdle muscular dystrophy with autosomal dominant inheritance. *Acta Neurol Scand*. 1991;83(4):234–238.
97. Reilich P, Krause S, Schramm N, et al. A novel mutation in the myotilin gene (MYOT) causes a severe form of limb girdle muscular dystrophy 1 A (LGMD1 A). *J Neurol*. 2011;258(8):1437–1444.
98. McNeill A, Birchall D, Straub V, et al. Lower limb radiology of distal myopathy due to the S60 F myotilin mutation. *Eur Neurol*. 2009;62(3):161–166.
99. Schessl J, Bach E, Rost S, et al. Novel recessive myotilin mutation causes severe myofibrillar myopathy. *Neurogenetics*. 2014;15(3):151–156.
100. Fang W, Huang CC, Chu NS, Chen CJ, Lu CS, Wang CC. Childhood-onset autosomal-dominant limb-girdle muscular dystrophy with cardiac conduction block. *Muscle Nerve*. 1997;20(3):286–292.
101. van der Kooi AJ, Ledderhof TM, de Voogt WG, et al. A newly recognized autosomal dominant limb girdle muscular dystrophy with cardiac involvement. *Ann Neurol*. 1996;39(5):636–642.
102. Bonne G, Di Barletta MR, Varnous S, et al. Mutations in the gene encoding lamin A/C cause autosomal dominant Emery–Dreifuss muscular dystrophy. *Nat Genet*. 1999;21(3):285–288.
103. Bonne G, Mercuri E, Muchir A, et al. Clinical and molecular genetic spectrum of autosomal dominant Emery-Dreifuss muscular dystrophy due to mutations of the lamin A/C gene. *Ann Neurol*. 2000;48:170–180.
104. Jimenez-Escrig A, Gobernado I, Garcia-Villanueva M, Sanchez-Herranz A. Autosomal recessive Emery-Dreifuss muscular dystrophy caused by a novel mutation (R225Q) in the lamin A/C gene identified by exome sequencing. *Muscle Nerve*. 2012;45:605–610.
105. Rankin J, Auer-Grumbach M, Bagg W, et al. Extreme phenotypic diversity and nonpenetrance in families with the LMNA gene mutation R644 C. *Am J Med Genet A*. 2008;146A:1530–1542.
106. van der Kooi AJ, Bonne G, Eymard B, et al. Lamin A/C mutations with lipodystrophy, cardiac abnormalities, and muscular dystrophy. *Neurology*. 2002;59:620–623.
107. van der Kooi AJ, van Meegen M, Ledderhof TM, McNally EM, de Visser M, Bolhuis PA. Genetic localization of a newly recognized autosomal dominant limb-girdle muscular dystrophy with cardiac involvement (LGMD1B) to chromosome 1q11–21. *Am J Hum Genet*. 1997;60:891–895.
108. Vantyghem M, Pigny P, Maurage CA, et al. Patients with familial partial lipodystrophy of the Dunnigan type due to a LMNA R482 W mutation show muscular and cardiac abnormalities. *J Clin Endocrinol Metab*. 2004;89:5337–5346.
109. Carboni N, Mura M, Marrosu G, et al. Muscle imaging analogies in a cohort of patients with different clinical phenotypes caused by LMNA gene mutations. *Muscle Nerve*. 2010;41:458–463.
110. Deconinck N, Dion E, Ben Yaou R, et al. Differentiating Emery-Dreifuss muscular dystrophy and collagen VI-related myopathies using a specific CT scanner pattern. *Neuromuscul Disord*. 2010;20:517–523.

111. Mercuri E, Counsell S, Allsop J, et al. Selective muscle involvement on magnetic resonance imaging in autosomal dominant Emery-Dreifuss muscular dystrophy. *Neuropediatrics.* 2002;33:10–14.
112. Mercuri E, Clements E, Offiah A, et al. Muscle magnetic resonance imaging involvement in muscular dystrophies with rigidity of the spine. *Ann Neurol.* 2010;67:201–208.
113. Minetti C, Sotgia F, Bruno C, et al. Mutations in the caveolin-3 gene cause autosomal dominant limb-girdle muscular dystrophy. *Nat Genet.* 1998;18(4):365–368.
114. Aboumousa A, Hoogendijk J, Charlton R, et al. Caveolinopathy–new mutations and additional symptoms. *Neuromuscul Disord.* 2008;18(7):572–578.
115. González-Pérez P, Gallano P, González-Quereda L, et al. Phenotypic variability in a Spanish family with a Caveolin-3 mutation. *J Neurol Sci.* 2009;276:95–98.
116. Cagliani R, Bresolin N, Prelle A, et al. A CAV3 microdeletion differentially affects skeletal muscle and myocardium. *Neurology.* 2003;61:1513–1519.
117. Catteruccia, M, Sanna T, Santorelli FM, et al. Rippling muscle disease and cardiomyopathy associated with a mutation in the CAV3 gene. *Neuromuscul Disord.* 2009;19:779–783.
118. Dotti MT, Malandrini A, Gambelli S, Salvadori C, De Stefano N, Federico A. A new missense mutation in caveolin-3 gene causes rippling muscle disease. *J Neurol Sci.* 2006;243:61–64.
119. Fischer D, Schroers A, Blümcke I, et al. Consequences of a novel caveolin-3 mutation in a large German family. *Ann Neurol.* 2003;53:233–241.
120. Fulizio L, Nascimbeni AC, Fanin M, et al. Molecular and muscle pathology in a series of caveolinopathy patients. *Hum Mutat.* 2005;25:82–89.
121. Jacobi C, Ruscheweyh R, Vorgerd M, Weber MA, Storch-Hagenlocher B, Meinck HM. Rippling muscle disease: Variable phenotype in a family with five afflicted members. *Muscle Nerve.* 2010;41:128–132.
122. Ricker K, Moxley RT, Rohkamm R. Rippling muscle disease. *Arch Neurol.* 1989;46:405–408.
123. Sundblom J, Stålberg E, Osterdahl M, et al. Bedside diagnosis of rippling muscle disease in CAV3 p.A46 T mutation carriers. *Muscle Nerve.* 2010;41:751–757.
124. Vorgerd M, Bolz H, Patzold T, Kubisch C, Malin JP, Mortier W. Phenotypic variability in rippling muscle disease. *Neurology.* 1999;52:1453–1459.
125. Yabe I, Kawashima A, Kikuchi S, et al. Caveolin-3 gene mutation in Japanese with rippling muscle disease. *Acta Neurol Scand.* 2003;108:47–51.
126. Hackman P, Sandell S, Sarparanta J, et al. Four new Finnish families with LGMD1D; refinement of the clinical phenotype and the linked 7q36 locus. *Neuromuscul Disord.* 2011;21:338–344.
127. Sarparanta J, Jonson PH, Golzio C, et al. Mutations affecting the cytoplasmic functions of the co-chaperone DNAJB6 cause limb-girdle muscular dystrophy. *Nat Genet.* 2012;44:450–455, S1–S2.
128. Harms MB, Sommerville RB, Allred P, et al. Exome sequencing reveals DNAJB6 mutations in dominantly-inherited myopathy. *Ann Neurol.* 2012;71:407–416.
129. Goldfarb LG, Park KY, Cervenáková L, et al. Missense mutations in desmin associated with familial cardiac and skeletal myopathy. *Nat Genet.* 1998;19:402–403.
130. Bergman JE, Veenstra-Knol HE, van Essen AJ, et al. Two related Dutch families with a clinically variable presentation of cardioskeletal myopathy caused by a novel S13 F mutation in the desmin gene. *Eur J Med Genet.* 2007;50:355–366.
131. Dalakas MC, Dagvadorj A, Goudeau B, et al. Progressive skeletal myopathy, a phenotypic variant of desmin myopathy associated with desmin mutations. *Neuromuscul Disord.* 2003; 13:252–258.
132. Dalakas MC, Park KY, Semino-Mora C, Lee HS, Sivakumar K, Goldfarb LG. Desmin myopathy, a skeletal myopathy with cardiomyopathy caused by mutations in the desmin gene. *N Engl J Med.* 2000;342:770–780.
133. Walter MC, Reilich P, Huebner A, et al. Scapuloperoneal syndrome type Kaeser and a wide phenotypic spectrum of adult-onset, dominant myopathies are associated with the desmin mutation R350P. *Brain.* 2007;130:1485–1496.
134. Goudeau B, Rodrigues-Lima F, Fischer D, et al. Variable pathogenic potentials of mutations located in the desmin alpha-helical domain. *Hum Mutat.* 2006;27:906–913.
135. Bär H, Goudeau B, Wälde S, et al. Conspicuous involvement of desmin tail mutations in diverse cardiac and skeletal myopathies. *Hum Mutat.* 2007;28:374–376.
136. Dagvadorj A, Olivé M, Urtizberea JA, et al. A series of West European patients with severe cardiac and skeletal myopathy associated with a de novo R406 W mutation in desmin. *J Neurol.* 2004;251:143–149.
137. Olivé M, Armstrong J, Miralles F, et al. Phenotypic patterns of desminopathy associated with three novel mutations in the desmin gene. *Neuromuscul Disord.* 2007;17:443–450.
138. Greenberg SA, Salajegheh M, Judge DP, et al. Etiology of limb girdle muscular dystrophy 1D/1E determined by laser capture microdissection proteomics. *Ann Neurol.* 2012;71:141–145.
139. Palenzuela L, Andreu AL, Gàmez J, et al. A novel autosomal dominant limb-girdle muscular dystrophy (LGMD 1 F) maps to 7q32.1–32.2. *Neurology.* 2003;61(3):404–406.
140. Melià MJ, Kubota A, Ortolano S, et al. Limb-girdle muscular dystrophy 1 F is caused by a microdeletion in the transportin 3 gene. *Brain.* 2013;136:1508–1517.
141. Fardeau M, Eymard B, Mignard C, Tomé FM, Richard I, Beckmann JS. Chromosome 15-linked limb-girdle muscular dystrophy: Clinical phenotypes in Reunion Island and French metropolitan communities. *Neuromuscul Disord.* 1996; 6(6):447–453.
142. Fardeau M, Hillaire D, Mignard C, et al. Juvenile limb-girdle muscular dystrophy. Clinical, histopathological and genetic data from a small community living in the Reunion Island. *Brain.* 1996;119(Pt 1):295–308.
143. Kawai H, Akaike M, Kunishige M, et al. Clinical, pathological, and genetic features of limb-girdle muscular dystrophy type 2 A with new calpain 3 gene mutations in seven patients from three Japanese families. *Muscle Nerve.* 1998;21(11):1493–1501.
144. Penisson-Besnier I, Richard I, Dubas F, Beckmann JS, Fardeau M. Pseudometabolic expression and phenotypic variability of calpain deficiency in two siblings. *Muscle Nerve.* 1998;21(8):1078–1080.
145. Spencer MJ, Tidball JG, Anderson LV, et al. Absence of calpain 3 in a form of limb-girdle muscular dystrophy (LGMD2 A). *J Neurol Sci.* 1997;146(2):173–178.
146. Guglieri M, Magri F, D'Angelo MG, et al. Clinical, molecular, and protein correlations in a large sample of genetically diagnosed Italian limb girdle muscular dystrophy patients. *Hum Mutat.* 2008;29:258–266.
147. Norwood FL, Harling C, Chinnery PF, Eagle M, Bushby K, Straub V. Prevalence of genetic muscle disease in Northern

England: In-depth analysis of a muscle clinic population. *Brain.* 2009;132(Pt 11):3175–3186.
148. van der Kooi AJ, Frankhuizen WS, Barth PG, et al. Limb-girdle muscular dystrophy in the Netherlands: Gene defect identified in half the families. *Neurology.* 2007;68:2125–2128.
149. Krahn M, Lopez De Munain A, Streichenberger N, et al. CAPN3 mutations in patients with idiopathic eosinophilic myositis. *Ann Neurol.* 2006;59(6):905–911.
150. Amato AA. Adults with eosinophilic myositis and calpain-3 mutations. *Neurology.* 2008;70:730–731.
151. Jaka O, Azpitarte M, Paisán-Ruiz C, et al. Entire CAPN3 gene deletion in a patient with limb-girdle muscular dystrophy type 2 A. *Muscle Nerve.* 2014;50(3):448–453.
152. Degardin A, Morillon D, Lacour A, Cotten A, Vermersch P, Stojkovic T. Morphologic imaging in muscular dystrophies and inflammatory myopathies. *Skeletal Radiol.* 2010;39(12):1219–1227.
153. Mercuri E, Bushby K, Ricci E, et al. Muscle MRI findings in patients with limb girdle muscular dystrophy with calpain 3 deficiency (LGMD2 A) and early contractures. *Neuromuscul Disord.* 2005;15:164–171.
154. Beckmann JS, Richard I, Broux O, et al. Identification of muscle-specific calpain and beta-sarcoglycan genes in progressive autosomal recessive muscular dystrophies. *Neuromuscul Disord.* 1996;6(6):455–462.
155. Fanin M, Fulizio L, Nascimbeni AC, et al. Molecular diagnosis in LGMD2 A: Mutation analysis or protein testing? *Hum Mutat.* 2004;24(1):52–62.
156. Richard I, Broux O, Allamand V, et al. Mutations in the proteolytic enzyme calpain 3 cause limb-girdle muscular dystrophy type 2 A. *Cell.* 1995;81(1):27–40.
157. Richard I, Roudaut C, Saenz A, et al. Calpainopathy-a survey of mutations and polymorphisms. *Am J Hum Genet.* 1999; 64(6):1524–1540.
158. Luo SS, Xi JY, Zhu WH, et al. Genetic variability and clinical spectrum of Chinese patients with limb-girdle muscular dystrophy type 2 A. *Muscle Nerve.* 2012;46(5):723–729.
159. Fanin M, Pegoraro E, Matsuda-Asada C, Brown RH Jr, Angelini C. Calpain-3 and dysferlin protein screening in patients with limb-girdle dystrophy and myopathy. *Neurology.* 2001; 56(5):660–665.
160. Brown RH, Jr., Amato A. Calpainopathy and eosinophilic myositis. *Ann Neurol.* 2006;59(6):875–877.
161. Illa I, Serrano-Munuera C, Gallardo E, et al. Distal anterior compartment myopathy: A dysferlin mutation causing a new muscular dystrophy phenotype. *Ann Neurol.* 2001;49(1):130–134.
162. Illarioshkin SN, Ivanova-Smolenskaya IA, Tanaka H, et al. Clinical and molecular analysis of a large family with three distinct phenotypes of progressive muscular dystrophy. *Brain.* 1996;119(Pt 6):1895–1909.
163. Mahjneh I, Marconi G, Bushby K, Anderson LV, Tolvanen-Mahjneh H, Somer H. Dysferlinopathy (LGMD2B): A 23-year follow-up study of 10 patients homozygous for the same frameshifting dysferlin mutations. *Neuromuscul Disord.* 2001;11(1):20–26.
164. Mahjneh I, Passos-Bueno MR, Zatz M, et al. The phenotype of chromosome 2p-linked limb-girdle muscular dystrophy. *Neuromuscul Disord.* 1996;6(6):483–490.
165. Suzuki N, Aoki M, Takahashi T, et al. Novel dysferlin mutations and characteristic muscle atrophy in late-onset Miyoshi myopathy. *Muscle Nerve.* 2004;29(5):721–723.
166. Takahashi T, Aoki M, Tateyama M, et al. Dysferlin mutations in Japanese Miyoshi myopathy: Relationship to phenotype. *Neurology.* 2003;60(11):1799–1804.
167. Vilchez JJ, Gallano P, Gallardo E, et al. Identification of a novel founder mutation in the DYSF gene causing clinical variability in the Spanish population. *Arch Neurol.* 2005;62:1256–1259.
168. Ho M, Gallardo E, McKenna-Yasek D, De Luna N, Illa I, Brown RH Jr. A novel, blood-based diagnostic assay for limb girdle muscular dystrophy 2B and Miyoshi myopathy. *Ann Neurol.* 2002;51(1):129–133.
169. Paradas C, Llauger J, Diaz-Manera J, et al. Redefining dysferlinopathy phenotypes based on clinical findings and muscle imaging studies. *Neurology.* 2010;75:316–323.
170. Kesper K, Kornblum C, Reimann J, Lutterbey G, Schröder R, Wattjes MP. Pattern of skeletal muscle involvement in primary dysferlinopathies: A whole-body 3.0-T magnetic resonance imaging study. *Acta Neurol Scand.* 2009;120:111–118.
171. Brummer D, Walter MC, Palmbach M, et al. Long-term MRI and clinical follow-up of symptomatic and presymptomatic carriers of dysferlin gene mutations. *Acta Myol.* 2005;24:6–16.
172. Piccolo F, Moore SA, Ford GC, Campbell KP. Intracellular accumulation and reduced sarcolemmal expression of dysferlin in limb-girdle muscular dystrophies. *Ann Neurol.* 2000;48(6):902–912.
173. Gallardo E, Rojas-Garcia R, de Luna N, Pou A, Brown RH Jr, Illa I. Inflammation in dysferlin myopathy: Immunohistochemical characterization of 13 patients. *Neurology.* 2001;57(11):2136–2138.
174. Selcen D, Stilling G, Engel AG. The earliest pathologic alterations in dysferlinopathy. *Neurology.* 2001;56(11):1472–1481.
175. Spuler S, Carl M, Zabojszcza J, et al. Dysferlin-deficient muscular dystrophy features amyloidosis. *Ann Neurol.* 2008;63:323–328.
176. Liu J, Aoki M, Illa I, et al. Dysferlin, a novel skeletal muscle gene, is mutated in Miyoshi myopathy and limb girdle muscular dystrophy. *Nat Genet.* 1998;20(1):31–36.
177. Angelini C, Fanin M, Freda MP, Duggan DJ, Siciliano G, Hoffman EP. The clinical spectrum of sarcoglycanopathies. *Neurology.* 1999;52(1):176–179.
178. Duggan DJ, Gorospe JR, Fanin M, Hoffman EP, Angelini C. Mutations in the sarcoglycan genes in patients with myopathy. *N Engl J Med.* 1997;336(9):618–624.
179. Melacini P, Fanin M, Duggan DJ, et al. Heart involvement in muscular dystrophies due to sarcoglycan gene mutations. *Muscle Nerve.* 1999;22(4):473–479.
180. Angelini C, Fanin M, Menegazzo E, Freda MP, Duggan DJ, Hoffman EP. Homozygous alpha-sarcoglycan mutation in two siblings: One asymptomatic and one steroid-responsive mild limb-girdle muscular dystrophy patient. *Muscle Nerve.* 1998;21(6):769–775.
181. Bonnemann CG, Modi R, Noguchi S, et al. Beta-sarcoglycan (A3b) mutations cause autosomal recessive muscular dystrophy with loss of the sarcoglycan complex. *Nat Genet.* 1995; 11(3):266–273.
182. Campbell KP. Adhalin gene mutations and autosomal recessive limb-girdle muscular dystrophy. *Ann Neurol.* 1995;38(3): 353–354.
183. Duggan DJ, Fanin M, Pegoraro E, Angelini C, Hoffman EP. Alpha-Sarcoglycan (adhalin) deficiency: Complete deficiency patients are 5% of childhood-onset dystrophin-normal muscular dystrophy and most partial deficiency patients do not have gene mutations. *J Neurol Sci.* 1996;140(1-2):30–39.

184. Duggan DJ, Manchester D, Stears KP, Mathews DJ, Hart C, Hoffman EP. Mutations in the delta-sarcoglycan gene are a rare cause of autosomal recessive limb-girdle muscular dystrophy (LGMD2). *Neurogenetics*. 1997;1(1):49–58.
185. Ljunggren A, Duggan D, McNally E, et al. Primary adhalin deficiency as a cause of muscular dystrophy in patients with normal dystrophin. *Ann Neurol*. 1995;38(3):367–372.
186. McNally EM, Duggan D, Gorospe JR, et al. Mutations that disrupt the carboxyl-terminus of gamma-sarcoglycan cause muscular dystrophy. *Hum Mol Genet*. 1996;5(11):1841–1847.
187. Diniz G, Tosun Yildirim H, Akinci G, et al. Sarcolemmal alpha and gamma sarcoglycan protein deficiencies in Turkish siblings with a novel missense mutation in the alpha sarcoglycan gene. *Pediatr Neurol*. 2014;50:640–647.
188. Moreira ES, Vainzof M, Marie SK, Sertié AL, Zatz M, Passos-Bueno MR. The seventh form of autosomal recessive limb-girdle muscular dystrophy is mapped to 17q11–12. *Am J Hum Genet*. 1997;61(1):151–159.
189. Moreira ES, Wiltshire TJ, Faulkner G, et al. Limb-girdle muscular dystrophy type 2G is caused by mutations in the gene encoding the sarcomeric protein telethonin. *Nat Genet*. 2000;24(2):163–166.
190. Mues A, van der Ven PF, Young P, Fürst DO, Gautel M. Two immunoglobulin-like domains of the Z-disc portion of titin interact in a conformation-dependent way with telethonin. *FEBS Lett*. 1998;428(1-2):111–114.
191. Mayans O, van der Ven PF, Wilm M, et al. Structural basis for activation of the titin kinase domain during myofibrillogenesis. *Nature*. 1998;395(6705):863–869.
192. Weiler T, Greenberg CR, Zelinski T, et al. A gene for autosomal recessive limb-girdle muscular dystrophy in Manitoba Hutterites maps to chromosome region 9q31–q33: Evidence for another limb-girdle muscular dystrophy locus. *Am J Hum Genet*. 1998;63(1):140–147.
193. Schoser BG, Frosk P, Engel AG, Klutzny U, Lochmüller H, Wrogemann K. Commonality of TRIM32 mutation in causing sarcotubular myopathy and LGMD2 H. *Ann Neurol*. 2005;57(4):591–595.
194. Borg K, Stucka R, Locke M, et al. Intragenic deletion of TRIM32 in compound heterozygotes with sarcotubular myopathy/LGMD2 H. *Hum Mutat*. 2009;30(9):E831–E844.
195. Saccone V, Palmieri M, Passamano L, et al. Mutations that impair interaction properties of TRIM32 associated with limb-girdle muscular dystrophy 2 H. *Hum Mutat*. 2008;29:240–247.
196. Driss A, Amouri R, Ben Hamida C, et al. A new locus for autosomal recessive limb-girdle muscular dystrophy in a large consanguineous Tunisian family maps to chromosome 19q13.3. *Neuromuscul Disord*. 2000;10(4-5):240–246.
197. Mercuri E, Brockington M, Straub V, et al. Phenotypic spectrum associated with mutations in the fukutin-related protein gene. *Ann Neurol*. 2003;53(4):537–542.
198. Poppe M, Bourke J, Eagle M, et al. Cardiac and respiratory failure in limb-girdle muscular dystrophy 2I. *Ann Neurol*. 2004;56(5):738–741.
199. Poppe M, Cree L, Bourke J, et al. The phenotype of limb-girdle muscular dystrophy type 2I. *Neurology*. 2003;60(8):1246–1251.
200. Boito CA, Melacini P, Vianello A, et al. Clinical and molecular characterization of patients with limb-girdle muscular dystrophy type 2I. *Arch Neurol*. 2005;62:1894–1899.
201. Brockington M, Yuva Y, Prandini P, et al. Mutations in the fukutin-related protein gene (FKRP) identify limb girdle muscular dystrophy 2I as a milder allelic variant of congenital muscular dystrophy MDC1C. *Hum Mol Genet*. 2001;10(25):2851–2859.
202. Schwartz M, Hertz JM, Sveen ML, Vissing J. LGMD2I presenting with a characteristic Duchenne or Becker muscular dystrophy phenotype. *Neurology*. 2005;64(9):1635–1637.
203. Lindberg C, Sixt C, Oldfors A. Episodes of exercise-induced dark urine and myalgia in LGMD 2I. *Acta Neurol Scand*. 2012;125(4):285–287.
204. Mathews KD, Stephan CM, Laubenthal K, et al. Myoglobinuria and muscle pain are common in patients with limb-girdle muscular dystrophy 2I. *Neurology*. 2011;76(2):194–195.
205. Müller T, Krasnianski M, Witthaut R, Deschauer M, Zierz S. Dilated cardiomyopathy may be an early sign of the C826 A Fukutin-related protein mutation. *Neuromuscul Disord*. 2005;15(5):372–376.
206. Palmieri A, Manara R, Bello L, et al. Cognitive profile and MRI findings in limb-girdle muscular dystrophy 2I. *J Neurol*. 2011;258(7):1312–1320.
207. Matsumoto H, Noguchi S, Sugie K. Subcellular localization of fukutin and fukutin-related protein in muscle cells. *J Biochem (Tokyo)*. 2004;135(6):709–712.
208. Esapa CT, McIlhinney RA, Blake DJ. Fukutin-related protein mutations that cause congenital muscular dystrophy result in ER-retention of the mutant protein in cultured cells. *Hum Mol Genet*. 2005;14(2):295–305.
209. Udd B, Vihola A, Sarparanta J, Richard I, Hackman P. Titinopathies and extension of the M-line mutation phenotype beyond distal myopathy and LGMD2 J. *Neurology*. 2005;64(4):636–642.
210. Udd B. Limb-girdle type muscular dystrophy in a large family with distal myopathy: Homozygous manifestation of a dominant gene? *J Med Genet*. 1992;29(6):383–389.
211. Udd B, Rapola J, Nokelainen P, Arikawa E, Somer H. Nonvacuolar myopathy in a large family with both late adult onset distal myopathy and severe proximal muscular dystrophy. *J Neurol Sci*. 1992;113(2):214–221.
212. Udd B, Partanen J, Halonen P, et al. Tibial muscular dystrophy. Late adult-onset distal myopathy in 66 Finnish patients. *Arch Neurol*. 1993;50(6):604–608.
213. Udd B, Haravuori H, Kalimo H, et al. Tibial muscular dystrophy–from clinical description to linkage on chromosome 2q31. *Neuromuscul Disord*. 1998;8(5):327–332.
214. Van den Bergh PY, Bouquiaux O, Verellen C, et al. Tibial muscular dystrophy in a Belgian family. *Ann Neurol*. 2003;54(2):248–251.
215. Mahjneh I, Lamminen AE, Udd B, et al. Muscle magnetic resonance imaging shows distinct diagnostic patterns in Welander and tibial muscular dystrophy. *Acta Neurol Scand*. 2004;110(2):87–93.
216. Pénisson-Besnier I, Hackman P, Suominen T, et al. Myopathies caused by homozygous titin mutations: Limb-girdle muscular dystrophy 2 J and variations of phenotype. *J Neurol Neurosurg Psychiatry*. 2010;81(11):1200–1202.
217. Ohlsson M, Hedberg C, Brådvik B, et al. Hereditary myopathy with early respiratory failure associated with a mutation in A-band titin. *Brain*. 2012;135(Pt 6):1682–1694.
218. Pfeffer G, Elliott HR, Griffin H, et al. Titin mutation segregates with hereditary myopathy with early respiratory failure. *Brain*. 2012;135(Pt 6):1695–1713.
219. Carmignac V, Salih MA, Quijano-Roy S, et al. C-terminal titin deletions cause a novel early-onset myopathy with fatal cardiomyopathy. *Ann Neurol*. 2007;61(4):340–351.

220. Udd B, Kääriänen H, Somer H. Muscular dystrophy with separate clinical phenotypes in a large family. *Muscle Nerve.* 1991;14(11):1050–1058.
221. Godfrey C, Clement E, Mein R, et al. Refining genotype phenotype correlations in muscular dystrophies with defective glycosylation of dystroglycan. *Brain.* 2007;130(Pt 10):2725–2735.
222. Hicks D, Sarkozy A, Muelas N, et al. A founder mutation in Anoctamin 5 is a major cause of limb-girdle muscular dystrophy. *Brain.* 2011;134(Pt 1):171–182.
223. Penttilä S, Palmio J, Suominen T, et al. Eight new mutations and the expanding phenotype variability in muscular dystrophy caused by ANO5. *Neurology.* 2012;78(12):897–903.
224. Bolduc V, Marlow G, Boycott KM, et al. Recessive mutations in the putative calcium-activated chloride channel Anoctamin 5 cause proximal LGMD2 L and distal MMD3 muscular dystrophies. *Am J Hum Genet.* 2010;86(2):213–221.
225. Mahjneh I, Jaiswal J, Lamminen A, et al. A new distal myopathy with mutation in anoctamin 5. *Neuromuscul Disord.* 2010; 20(12):791–795.
226. Schessl J, Kress W, Schoser B. Novel ANO5 mutations causing hyper-CK-emia, limb girdle muscular weakness and Miyoshi type of muscular dystrophy. *Muscle Nerve.* 2012;45(5):740–742.
227. Sarkozy A, Hicks D, Hudson J, et al. ANO5 gene analysis in a large cohort of patients with anoctaminopathy: Confirmation of male prevalence and high occurrence of the common exon 5 gene mutation. *Hum Mutat.* 2013;34(8):1111–1118.
228. Jimenez-Mallebrera C, Torelli S, Feng L, et al. A comparative study of alpha-dystroglycan glycosylation in dystroglycanopathies suggests that the hypoglycosylation of alpha-dystroglycan does not consistently correlate with clinical severity. *Brain Pathol.* 2009;19(4):596–611.
229. Godfrey C, Escolar D, Brockington M, et al. Fukutin gene mutations in steroid-responsive limb girdle muscular dystrophy. *Ann Neurol.* 2006;60(5):603–610.
230. Biancheri R, Falace A, Tessa A, et al. POMT2 gene mutation in limb-girdle muscular dystrophy with inflammatory changes. *Biochem Biophys Res Commun.* 2007;363(4):1033–1037.
231. Clement EM, Godfrey C, Tan J, et al. Mild POMGnT1 mutations underlie a novel limb-girdle muscular dystrophy variant. *Arch Neurol.* 2008;65(1):137–141.
232. Hara Y, Balci-Hayta B, Yoshida-Moriguchi T, et al. A dystroglycan mutation associated with limb-girdle muscular dystrophy. *N Eng J Med.* 2011;364(10):939–946.
233. Banwell BL, Russel J, Fukudome T, Shen XM, Stilling G, Engel AG. Myopathy, myasthenic syndrome, and epidermolysis bullosa simplex due to plectin deficiency. *J Neuropathol Exp Neurol.* 1999;58(8):832–846.
234. Charlesworth A, Chiaverini C, Chevrant-Breton J, et al. Epidermolysis bullosa simplex with PLEC mutations: New phenotypes and new mutations. *Br J Dermatol.* 2013;168(4): 808–814.
235. Chavanas S, Pulkkinen L, Gache Y, et al. A homozygous nonsense mutation in the PLEC1 gene in patients with epidermolysis bullosa simplex with muscular dystrophy. *J Clin Invest.* 1996;98(10):2196–2200.
236. Forrest K, Mellerio JE, Robb S, et al. Congenital muscular dystrophy, myasthenic symptoms and epidermolysis bullosa simplex (EBS) associated with mutations in the PLEC1 gene encoding plectin. *Neuromuscul Disord.* 2010;20(11):709–711.
237. Gache Y, Chavanas S, Lacour JP, et al. Defective expression of plectin/HD1 in epidermolysis bullosa simplex with muscular dystrophy. *J Clin Invest.* 1996;97(10):2289–2298.
238. Pulkkinen L, Smith FJ, Shimizu H, et al. Homozygous deletion mutations in the plectin gene (PLEC1) in patients with epidermolysis bullosa simplex associated with late-onset muscular dystrophy. *Hum Mol Genet.* 1996;5(10):1539–1546.
239. Smith FJ, Eady RA, Leigh IM, et al. Plectin deficiency results in muscular dystrophy with epidermolysis bullosa. *Nat Genet.* 1996;13:450–457.
240. Yiu EM, Klausegger A, Waddell LB, et al. Epidermolysis bullosa with late-onset muscular dystrophy and plectin deficiency. *Muscle Nerve.* 2011;44:135–141.
241. Selcen D, Juel VC, Hobson-Webb LD, et al. Myasthenic syndrome caused by plectinopathy. *Neurology.* 2011;76(4):327–336.
242. Maselli RA, Arredondo J, Cagney O, et al. Congenital myasthenic syndrome associated with epidermolysis bullosa caused by homozygous mutations in PLEC1 and CHRNE. *Clin Genet.* 2011;80(5):444–451.
243. McMillan JR, Akiyama M, Rouan F, et al. Plectin defects in epidermolysis bullosa simplex with muscular dystrophy. *Muscle Nerve.* 2007;35(1):24–35.
244. Fine JD, Stenn J, Johnson L, Wright T, Bock HG, Horiguchi Y. Autosomal recessive epidermolysis bullosa simplex. Generalized phenotypic features suggestive of junctional or dystrophic epidermolysis bullosa, and association with neuromuscular diseases. *Arch Dermatol.* 1989;125:931–938.
245. Bolling MC, Pas HH, de Visser M, et al. PLEC1 mutations underlie adult-onset dilated cardiomyopathy in epidermolysis bullosa simplex with muscular dystrophy. *J Invest Dermatol.* 2010;130(4):1178–1181.
246. Gundesli H, Talim B, Korkusuz P, et al. Mutation in exon 1f of PLEC, leading to disruption of plectin isoform 1f, causes autosomal-recessive limb girdle muscular dystrophy. *Am J Hum Genet.* 2010;87(6):834–841.
247. Cetin N, Balci-Hayta B, Gundesli H, et al. A novel desmin mutation leading to autosomal recessive limb-girdle muscular dystrophy: Distinct histopathological outcomes compared with desminopathies. *J Med Genet.* 2013;50(7):437–443.
248. Henderson M, De Waele L, Hudson J, et al. Recessive desmin-null muscular dystrophy with central nuclei and mitochondrial abnormalities. *Acta Neuropathol.* 2013;125(6):917–919.
249. Bögershausen N, Shahrzad N, Chong JX, et al. Recessive TRAPPC11 mutations cause a disease spectrum of limb girdle muscular dystrophy and myopathy with movement disorder and intellectual disability. *Am J Hum Genet.* 2013;93(1):181–90.
250. Bönnemann CG, Wang CH, Quijano-Roy S, et al. Diagnostic approach to the congenital muscular dystrophies. *Neuromuscul Disord.* 2014;24(4):289–311.
251. Muntoni F, Voit T. The congenital muscular dystrophies in 2004: A century of exciting progress. *Neuromuscul Disord.* 2004;14(10):635–649.
252. Muntoni F, Voit T. 133rd ENMC International Workshop on Congenital Muscular Dystrophy (IXth International CMD Workshop) 21–23 January 2005, Naarden, the Netherlands. *Neuromuscul Disord.* 2005;15(11):794–801.
253. Philpot J, Cowan F, Pennock J, et al. Merosin-deficient congenital muscular dystrophy: The spectrum of brain involvement on magnetic resonance imaging. *Neuromuscul Disord.* 1999;9(2):81–85.
254. Prandini P, Berardinelli A, Fanin M, et al. LAMA2 loss-of-function mutation in a girl with a mild congenital muscular dystrophy. *Neurology.* 2004;63(6):1118–1121.

255. Sewry CA, Naom I, D'Alessandro M, et al. Variable clinical phenotype in merosin-deficient congenital muscular dystrophy associated with differential immunolabeling of two fragments of the laminin alpha 2 chain. *Neuromuscul Disord.* 1997;7(3):169–175.
256. Shorer Z, Philpot J, et al. Demyelinating peripheral neuropathy in merosin-deficient congenital muscular dystrophy. *J Child Neurol.* 1995;10(6):472–475.
257. Cohn RD, Herrmann R, Muntoni F, Sewry C, Dubowitz V, et al. Laminin alpha2 chain-deficient congenital muscular dystrophy: Variable epitope expression in severe and mild cases. *Neurology.* 1998;51(1):94–100.
258. Mora M, Moroni I, Uziel G, et al. Mild clinical phenotype in a 12-year-old boy with partial merosin deficiency and central and peripheral nervous system abnormalities. *Neuromuscul Disord.* 1996;6(5):377–381.
259. Morandi L, Di Blasi C, Farina L, et al. Clinical correlations in 16 patients with total or partial laminin alpha2 deficiency characterized using antibodies against 2 fragments of the protein. *Arch Neurol.* 1999;56(2):209–215.
260. Naom I, Sewry C, D'Alessandro M, et al. Prenatal diagnosis in merosin-deficient congenital muscular dystrophy. *Neuromuscul Disord.* 1997;7(3):176–179.
261. Pegoraro E, Marks H, Garcia CA, et al. Laminin alpha2 muscular dystrophy: Genotype/phenotype studies of 22 patients. *Neurology.* 1998;51(1):101–110.
262. Tan E, Topaloglu H, Sewry C, et al. Late onset muscular dystrophy with cerebral white matter changes due to partial merosin deficiency. *Neuromuscul Disord.* 1997;7(2):85–89.
263. Bushby K, Anderson LV, Pollitt C, Naom I, Muntoni F, Bindoff L. Abnormal merosin in adults. A new form of late onset muscular dystrophy not linked to chromosome 6 q2. *Brain.* 1998;121(Pt 4):581–588.
264. Mercuri E, Pennock J, Goodwin F, et al. Sequential study of central and peripheral nervous system involvement in an infant with merosin-deficient congenital muscular dystrophy. *Neuromuscul Disord.* 1996;6(6):425–429.
265. Sewry CA, D'Alessandro M, Wilson LA, et al. Expression of laminin chains in skin in merosin-deficient congenital muscular dystrophy. *Neuropediatrics.* 1997;28(4):217–222.
266. Guicheney P, Vignier N, Helbling-Leclerc A, et al. Genetics of laminin alpha 2 chain (or merosin) deficient congenital muscular dystrophy: From identification of mutations to prenatal diagnosis. *Neuromuscul Disord.* 1997;7(3):180–186.
267. Hayashi YK, Chou FL, Engvall E, et al. Mutations in the integrin alpha7 gene cause congenital myopathy. *Nat Genet.* 1998;19(1):94–97.
268. Yonekawa T, Nishino I. Ullrich congenital muscular dystrophy: Clinicopathological features, natural history and pathomechanism(s). *J Neurol Neurosurg Psychiatry.* 2015;86(3): 280–287.
269. Ishikawa H, Sugie K, Murayama K, et al. Ullrich disease due to deficiency of collagen VI in the sarcolemma. *Neurology.* 2004;62(4):620–623.
270. Baker NL, Morgelin M, Peat R, et al. Dominant collagen VI mutations are a common cause of Ullrich congenital muscular dystrophy. *Hum Mol Genet.* 2005;14(2):279–293.
271. Demir E, Ferreiro A, Sabatelli P, et al. Collagen VI status and clinical severity in Ullrich congenital muscular dystrophy: Phenotype analysis of 11 families linked to the COL6 loci. *Neuropediatrics.* 2004;35(2):103–112.
272. Meilleur KG, Zukosky K, Medne L, et al. Clinical, pathologic, and mutational spectrum of dystroglycanopathy caused by LARGE mutations. *J Neuropathol Exp Neurol.* 2014;73(5):425–441.
273. Manzani MC, Tambunan DE, Hill RS, et al. Exome sequencing and functional validation in zebrafish identify GTDC2 mutations as a cause of Walker-Warburg syndrome. *Am J Hum Genet.* 2012;91(3):541–547.
274. Buysse K, Riemersma M, Powell G, et al. Missense mutations in [beta]-1,3-N-acetylglucosaminyltransferase 1 (B3GNT1) cause Walker-Warburg syndrome. *Hum Mol Genet.* 2013;22(9): 1746–1754.
275. Stevens E, Carss KJ, Cirak S, et al. Mutations in B3GALNT2 cause congenital muscular dystrophy and hypoglycosylation of [alpha]-dystroglycan. *Am J Hum Genet.* 2013;92(3):354–365.
276. Hedberg C, Oldfors A, Darin N. B3GALNT2 is a gene associated with congenital muscular dystrophy with brain malformations. *Eur J Hum Genet.* 2014;22(5):707–710.
277. Vuillaumier-Barrot S, Bouchet-Séraphin C, Chelbi M, et al. Identification of mutations in TMEM5 and ISPD as a cause of severe cobblestone lissencephaly. *Am J Hum Genet.* 2012;91(6): 1135–1143.
278. Carss KJ, Stevens E, Foley AR, et al. Mutations in GDP-mannose pyrophosphorylase B cause congenital and limb-girdle muscular dystrophies associated with hypoglycosylation of [alpha]-dystroglycan. *Am J Hum Genet.* 2013;93(1):29–41.
279. Kim DS, Hayashi YK, et al. POMT1 mutation results in defective glycosylation and loss of laminin-binding activity in alpha-DG. *Neurology.* 2004;62(6):1009–1011.
280. Beltran-Valero de Bernabe D, Currier S, Steinbrecher A, et al. Mutations in the O-mannosyltransferase gene POMT1 give rise to the severe neuronal migration disorder Walker–Warburg syndrome. *Am J Hum Genet.* 2002;71(5):1033–1043.
281. Cormand B, Pihko H, Bayés M, et al. Clinical and genetic distinction between Walker–Warburg syndrome and muscle–eye–brain disease. *Neurology.* 2001;56(8):1059–1069.
282. Diesen C, Saarinen A, Pihko H, et al. POMGnT1 mutation and phenotypic spectrum in muscle–eye–brain disease. *J Med Genet.* 2004;41(10):e115.
283. Wewer UM, Durkin ME, Zhang X, et al. Laminin beta2 chain and adhalin deficiency in the skeletal muscle of Walker–Warburg syndrome (cerebro-ocular dysplasia-muscular dystrophy). *Neurology.* 1995;45(11):2099–2101.
284. Toda T, Kobayashi K, Kondo-Iida E, et al. The Fukuyama congenital muscular dystrophy story. *Neuromuscul Disord.* 2000;10(3):153–159.
285. Toda T, Yoshioka M, Nakahori Y, et al. Genetic identity of Fukuyama-type congenital muscular dystrophy and Walker–Warburg syndrome. *Ann Neurol.* 1995;37(1):99–101.
286. Kobayashi K, Nakahori Y, Miyake M, et al. An ancient retrotransposal insertion causes Fukuyama-type congenital muscular dystrophy. *Nature.* 1998;394(6691):388–392.
287. Yoshida A, Kobayashi K, Manya H, et al. Muscular dystrophy and neuronal migration disorder caused by mutations in a glycosyltransferase, POMGnT1. *Dev Cell.* 2001;1(5):717–724.
288. van Reeuwijk J, Janssen M, van den Elzen C, et al. POMT2 mutations cause alpha-dystroglycan hypoglycosylation and Walker Warburg syndrome. *J Med Genet.* 2005;42(12):907–912.
289. Balci B, Uyanik G, Dincer P, et al. An autosomal recessive limb girdle muscular dystrophy (LGMD2) with mild mental retardation is allelic to Walker–Warburg syndrome (WWS)

caused by a mutation in the POMT1 gene. *Neuromuscul Disord.* 2005;15(4):271–275.
290. Haltia M, Leivo I, Somer H, et al. Muscle–eye–brain disease: A neuropathological study. *Ann Neurol.* 1997;41(2):173–180.
291. Santavuori P, Somer H, Sainio K, et al. Muscle–eye–brain disease (MEB). *Brain Dev.* 1989;11(3):147–153.
292. Santavuori P, Valanne L, Autti T, Haltia M, Pihko H, Sainio K. Muscle–eye–brain disease: Clinical features, visual evoked potentials and brain imaging in 20 patients. *Eur J Paediatr Neurol.* 1998;2(1):41–47.
293. Louhichi N, Triki C, Quijano-Roy S, et al. New FKRP mutations causing congenital muscular dystrophy associated with mental retardation and central nervous system abnormalities. Identification of a founder mutation in Tunisian families. *Neurogenetics.* 2004;5(1):27–34.
294. Lotz BP, Stubgen JP. The rigid spine syndrome: A vacuolar variant. *Muscle Nerve.* 1993;16(5):530–536.
295. Mercuri E, Talim B, Moghadaszadeh B, et al. Clinical and imaging findings in six cases of congenital muscular dystrophy with rigid spine syndrome linked to chromosome 1p (RSMD1). *Neuromuscul Disord.* 2002;12(7–8):631–638.
296. Merlini L, Granata C, Ballestrazzi A, Marini ML. Rigid spine syndrome and rigid spine sign in myopathies. *J Child Neurol.* 1989;4(4):274–282.
297. Moghadaszadeh B, Topaloglu H, Merlini L, et al. Genetic heterogeneity of congenital muscular dystrophy with rigid spine syndrome. *Neuromuscul Disord.* 1999;9(6–7):376–382.
298. Reichmann H, Goebel HH, Schneider C, Toyka KV. Familial mixed congenital myopathy with rigid spine phenotype. *Muscle Nerve.* 1997;20(4):411–417.
299. Taylor J, Muntoni F, Robb S, Dubowitz V, Sewry C. Early onset autosomal dominant myopathy with rigidity of the spine: A possible role for laminin beta 1? *Neuromuscul Disord.* 1997;7(4):211–216.
300. Flanigan KM, Kerr L, Bromberg MB, et al. Congenital muscular dystrophy with rigid spine syndrome: A clinical, pathological, radiological, and genetic study. *Ann Neurol.* 2000;47(2): 152–161.
301. Ferreiro A, Ceuterick-de Groote C, Marks JJ, et al. Desmin-related myopathy with Mallory body-like inclusions is caused by mutations of the selenoprotein N gene. *Ann Neurol.* 2004;55 (5):676–686.
302. Tawil R, Van Der Maarel SM. Facioscapulohumeral muscular dystrophy. *Muscle Nerve.* 2006;34(1):1–15.
303. Personius KE, Pandya S, King WM, Tawil R, McDermott MP. Facioscapulohumeral dystrophy natural history study: Standardization of testing procedures and reliability of measurements. The FSH DY Group. *Phys Ther.* 1994;74(3):253–263.
304. Tawil R, McDermott MP, Mendell JR, Kissel J, Griggs RC. Facioscapulohumeral muscular dystrophy (FSHD): Design of natural history study and results of baseline testing. FSH-DY Group. *Neurology.* 1994;44(3 Pt 1):442–446.
305. Tawil R, McDermott MP, Pandya S, et al. A pilot trial of prednisone in facioscapulohumeral muscular dystrophy. FSHDY Group. *Neurology.* 1997;48(1):46–49.
306. van der Kooi AJ, Visser MC, Rosenberg N, et al. Extension of the clinical range of facioscapulohumeral dystrophy: Report of six cases. *J Neurol Neurosurg Psychiatry.* 2000;69(1):114–116.
307. Felice KJ, North WA, Moore SA, Mathews KD. FSH dystrophy 4q35 deletion in patients presenting with facial-sparing scapular myopathy. *Neurology.* 2000;54(10):1927–1931.
308. Wohlgemuth M, van der Kooi EL, van Kesteren RG, van der Maarel SM, Padberg GW. Ventilatory support in facioscapulohumeral muscular dystrophy. *Neurology.* 2004;63(1):176–178.
309. Laforet P, de Toma C, Eymard B, et al. Cardiac involvement in genetically confirmed facioscapulohumeral muscular dystrophy. *Neurology.* 1998;51(5):1454–1456.
310. Felice KJ, Jones JM, Conway SR. Facioscapulohumeral dystrophy presenting as infantile facial diplegia and late-onset limb-girdle myopathy in members of the same family. *Muscle Nerve.* 2005;32(3):368–372.
311. Munsat TL, Piper D, Cancilla P, Mednick J. Inflammatory myopathy with facioscapulohumeral distribution. *Neurology.* 1972;22(4):335–347.
312. Spuler S, Engel AG. Unexpected sarcolemmal complement membrane attack complex deposits on nonnecrotic muscle fibers in muscular dystrophies. *Neurology.* 1998;50(1):41–46.
313. Wijmenga C, Hewitt JE, Sandkuijl LA, et al. Chromosome 4q DNA rearrangements associated with facioscapulohumeral muscular dystrophy. *Nat Genet.* 1992;2(1):26–30.
314. Tawil R, Forrester J, Griggs RC, et al. Evidence for anticipation and association of deletion size with severity in facioscapulohumeral muscular dystrophy. The FSH-DY Group. *Ann Neurol.* 1996;39(6):744–748.
315. Lemmers RJ, Tawil R, Petek LM, et al. Digenic inheritance of an SMCHD1 mutation and an FSHD-permissive D4Z4 allele causes facioscapulohumeral muscular dystrophy type 2. *Nat Genet.* 2012;44(12), 1370–1374.
316. Sacconi S, Lemmers RJ, Balog J, et al. The FSHD2 gene SMCHD1 is a modifier of disease severity in families affected by FSHD1. *Am J Hum Genet.* 2013;93(4),744–751.
317. Kissel JT, McDermott MP, Natarajan R, et al. Pilot trial of albuterol in facioscapulohumeral muscular dystrophy. FSH-DY Group. *Neurology.* 1998;50(5):1402–1406.
318. Kissel JT, McDermott MP, Mendell JR, et al. Randomized, double-blind, placebo-controlled trial of albuterol in facioscapulohumeral dystrophy. *Neurology.* 2001;57(8):1434–1440.
319. Andrews CT, Taylor TC, Patterson VH. Scapulothoracic arthrodesis for patients with facioscapulohumeral muscular dystrophy. *Neuromuscul Disord.* 1998;8(8):580–584.
320. Letournel E, Fardeau M, Lytle JO, Serrault M, Gosselin RA. Scapulothoracic arthrodesis for patients who have fascioscapulohumeral muscular dystrophy. *J Bone Joint Surg Am.* 1990;72(1):78–84.
321. Chakrabarti A, Pearce JM. Scapuloperoneal syndrome with cardiomyopathy: Report of a family with autosomal dominant inheritance and unusual features. *J Neurol Neurosurg Psychiatry.* 1981;44(12):1146–1152.
322. Feigenbaum JA, Munsat TL. A neuromuscular syndrome of scapuloperoneal distribution. *Bull Los Angeles Neurol Soc.* 1970;35(2):47–57.
323. Kaeser HE. Scapuloperoneal muscular atrophy. *Brain.* 1965; 88(2):407–418.
324. Takahashi K, Nakamura H, Nakashima R. Scapuloperoneal dystrophy associated with neurogenic changes. *J Neurol Sci.* 1974;23(4):575–583.
325. Thomas PK, Schott GD, Morgan-Hughes JA. Adult onset scapuloperoneal myopathy. *J Neurol Neurosurg Psychiatry.* 1975;38(10):1008–1015.
326. Wilhelmsen KC, Blake DM, Lynch T, et al. Chromosome 12-linked autosomal dominant scapuloperoneal muscular dystrophy. *Ann Neurol.* 1996;39(4):507–520.

327. Tawil R, Myers GJ, Weiffenbach B, Griggs RC. Scapuloperoneal syndromes. Absence of linkage to the 4q35 FSHD locus. *Arch Neurol.* 1995;52(11):1069–1072.
328. Probst A, Ulrich J, Kaeser HE, Heitz P. Scapulo-peroneal muscular atrophy. Full autopsy report. Unusual findings in the anterior horn of the spinal cord. Lipid storage in muscle. *Eur Neurol.* 1977;16(1–6):181–196.
329. Quinzi CM, Vu TH, Min KC, et al. X-linked dominant scapuloperoneal myopathy is due to mutation in the gene encoding four-and-a-half-LIM protein 1. *Am J Hum Genet.* 2008;82:208–213.
330. Thomas PK, Calne DB, Elliott CF. X-linked scapuloperoneal syndrome. *J Neurol Neurosurg Psychiatry.* 1972;35(2):208–215.
331. Marques J, Duarte ST, Costa S, et al. Atypical phenotype in two patients with LAMA2 mutations. *Neuromuscul Disord.* 2014;24(5):419–424.
332. Emery AE, Dreifuss FE. Unusual type of benign x-linked muscular dystrophy. *J Neurol Neurosurg Psychiatry.* 1966;29(4):338–342.
333. Hopkins LC, Jackson JA, Elsas LJ. Emery–Dreifuss humeroperoneal muscular dystrophy: An x-linked myopathy with unusual contractures and bradycardia. *Ann Neurol.* 1981;10(3):230–237.
334. Kubo S, Tsukahara T, Takemitsu M, et al. Presence of emerinopathy in cases of rigid spine syndrome. *Neuromuscul Disord.* 1998;8(7):502–507.
335. Emery AE. Emery–Dreifuss muscular dystrophy—a 40 year retrospective. *Neuromuscul Disord.* 2000;10(4–5):228–232.
336. Schessl J, Columbus A, Hu Y, et al. Familial reducing body myopathy with cytoplasmic bodies and rigid spine revisited: Identification of a second LIM domain mutation in FHL1. *Neuropediatrics.* 2010;41(1):43–46.
337. Schoser B, Goebel HH, Janisch I, et al. Consequences of mutations within the C terminus of the FHL1 gene. *Neurology.* 2009;73(7):543–551.
338. Shalaby S, Hayashi YK, Nonaka I, Noguchi S, Nishino I. Novel FHL1 mutations in fatal and benign reducing body myopathy. *Neurology.* 2009;72(4):375–376.
339. Chen DH, Raskind WH, Parson WW, et al. A novel mutation in FHL1 in a family with X-linked scapuloperoneal myopathy: Phenotypic spectrum and structural study of FHL1 mutations. *J Neurol Sci.* 2010;296(1–2):22–29.
340. Selcen D, Bromberg MB, Chin SS, Engel AG. Reducing bodies and myofibrillar myopathy features in FHL1 muscular dystrophy. *Neurology.* 2011;77(22):1951–1959.
341. Shalaby S, Hayashi YK, Goto K, et al. Rigid spine syndrome caused by a novel mutation in four-and-a-half LIM domain 1 gene (FHL1). *Neuromuscul Disord.* 2008;18:959–961.
342. Bione S, Maestrini E, Rivella S, et al. Identification of a novel X-linked gene responsible for Emery–Dreifuss muscular dystrophy. *Nat Genet.* 1994;8(4):323–327.
343. van der Kooi AJ, van Meegen M, Ledderhof TM, McNally EM, de Visser M, Bolhuis PA. Genetic localization of a newly recognized autosomal dominant limb-girdle muscular dystrophy with cardiac involvement (LGMD1B) to chromosome 1q11–21. *Am J Hum Genet.* 1997;60(4):891–895.
344. Fatkin D, MacRae C, Sasaki T, et al. Missense mutations in the rod domain of the lamin A/C gene as causes of dilated cardiomyopathy and conduction-system disease. *N Engl J Med.* 1999;341(23):1715–1724.
345. Taylor J, Sewry CA, Dubowitz V, Muntoni F. Early onset, autosomal recessive muscular dystrophy with Emery–Dreifuss phenotype and normal emerin expression. *Neurology.* 1998;51(4):1116–1120.
346. Zhang Q, Bethmann C, Worth NF, et al. Nesprin-1 and -2 are involved in the pathogenesis of Emery Dreifuss muscular dystrophy and are critical for nuclear envelope integrity. *Hum Mol Genet.* 2007;16(23):2816–2833.
347. Liang WC, Mitsuhashi H, Keduka E, et al. TMEM43 mutations in Emery-Dreifuss muscular dystrophy-related myopathy. *Ann Neurol.* 2011;69(6):1005–1013.
348. Arts WF, Bethlem J, Volkers WS. Further investigations on benign myopathy with autosomal dominant inheritance. *J Neurol.* 1978;217(3):201–206.
349. Bertini E, Pepe G. Collagen type VI and related disorders: Bethlem myopathy and Ullrich scleroatonic muscular dystrophy. *Eur J Paediatr Neurol.* 2002;6(4):193–198.
350. Bethlem J, Wijngaarden GK. Benign myopathy, with autosomal dominant inheritance. A report on three pedigrees. *Brain.* 1976;99(1):91–100.
351. Haq RU, Speer MC, Chu ML, Tandan R. Respiratory muscle involvement in Bethlem myopathy. *Neurology.* 1999;52(1):174–176.
352. Jobsis GJ, Boers JM, Barth PG, de Visser M. Bethlem myopathy: A slowly progressive congenital muscular dystrophy with contractures. *Brain.* 1999;122(Pt 4):649–655.
353. Jobsis GJ, Keizers H, Vreijling JP, et al. Type VI collagen mutations in Bethlem myopathy, an autosomal dominant myopathy with contractures. *Nat Genet.* 1996;14(1):113–115.
354. Pepe G, Bertini E, Bonaldo P, et al. Bethlem myopathy (BETHLEM) and Ullrich scleroatonic muscular dystrophy: 100th ENMC international workshop, 23–24 November 2001, Naarden, the Netherlands. *Neuromuscul Disord.* 2002;12(10):984–993.
355. Pepe G, de Visser M, Bertini E, et al. Bethlem myopathy (BETHLEM) 86th ENMC international workshop, 10–11 November 2000, Naarden, the Netherlands. *Neuromuscul Disord.* 2002;12(3):296–305.
356. Mercuri E, Lampe A, Allsop J, et al., Muscle MRI in Ullrich congenital muscular dystrophy and Bethlem myopathy. *Neuromuscul Disord.* 2005;15(4), 303–310.
357. ten Dam L, van der Kooi AJ, van Wattingen M, de Haan RJ, de Visser M. Reliability and accuracy of skeletal muscle imaging in limb-girdle muscular dystrophies. *Neurology.* 2012;79(16), 2276–2277.
358. Pan TC, Zhang RZ, Pericak-Vance MA, et al. Missense mutation in a von Wille-brand factor type A domain of the alpha 3(VI) collagen gene (COL6A3) in a family with Bethlem myopathy. *Hum Mol Genet.* 1998;7(5):807–812.
359. Katz JS, Wolfe GI, Burns DK, et al. Isolated neck extensor myopathy: A common cause of dropped head syndrome. *Neurology.* 1996;46(4):917–921.
360. Rose MR, Levin KH, Griggs RC. The dropped head plus syndrome: Quantitation of response to corticosteroids. *Muscle Nerve.* 1999;22(1):115–118.
361. Serratrice G, Pouget J, Pellissier JF. Bent spine syndrome. *J Neurol Neurosurg Psychiatry.* 1996;60(1):51–54.
362. Suarez GA, Kelly JJ, Jr. The dropped head syndrome. *Neurology.* 1992;42(8):1625–1627.
363. Chahin N, Selcen D, Engel AG. Sporadic late onset nemaline myopathy. *Neurology.* 2005;65(8):1158–1164.

364. Biran I, Cohen O, Diment J, Peyser A, Bahnof R, Steiner I. Focal, steroid responsive myositis causing dropped head syndrome. *Muscle Nerve*. 1999;22(6):769–771.
365. Dominick J, Sheean G, Schleimer J, Wixom C. Response of the dropped head/bent spine syndrome to treatment with intravenous immunoglobulin. *Muscle Nerve*. 2006;33(6):824–826.
366. Duarte S, Oliveira J, Santos R, et al. Dominant and recessive RYR1 mutations in adults with core lesions and mild muscle symptoms. *Muscle Nerve*. 2011;44(1):102–108.
367. Løseth S, Voermans NC, Torbergsen T, et al. A novel late-onset axial myopathy associated with mutations in the skeletal muscle ryanodine receptor (RYR1) gene. *J Neurol*. 2013;260(6):1504–1510.
368. Brais B, Rouleau GA, Bouchard JP, Fardeau M, Tomé FM. Oculopharyngeal muscular dystrophy. *Semin Neurol*. 1999;19(1):59–66.
369. Hill ME, Creed GA, Bouchard JP, Fardeau M, Tomé FM. Oculopharyngeal muscular dystrophy: Phenotypic and genotypic studies in a UK population. *Brain*. 2001;124(Pt 3):522–526.
370. Blumen SC, Brais B, Korczyn AD, et al. Homozygotes for oculopharyngeal muscular dystrophy have a severe form of the disease. *Ann Neurol*. 1999;46(1):115–118.
371. Brais B, Bouchard JP, Xie YG, et al. Short GCG expansions in the PABP2 gene cause oculopharyngeal muscular dystrophy. *Nat Genet*. 1998;18(2):164–167.
372. Calado A, Tome FM, Brais B, et al. Nuclear inclusions in oculopharyngeal muscular dystrophy consist of poly(A) binding protein 2 aggregates which sequester poly(A) RNA. *Hum Mol Genet*. 2000;9(15):2321–2328.
373. Shanmugam V, Dion P, Rochefort D, Laganière J, Brais B, Rouleau GA. PABP2 polyalanine tract expansion causes intranuclear inclusions in oculopharyngeal muscular dystrophy. *Ann Neurol*. 2000;48(5):798–802.
374. Fukuhara N, Kumamoto T, Tsubaki T, Mayuzumi T, Nitta H. Oculopharyngeal muscular dystrophy and distal myopathy. Intrafamilial difference in the onset and distribution of muscular involvement. *Acta Neurol Scand*. 1982;65(5):458–467.
375. Goto I, Hayakawa T, Miyoshi T, Ino K, Kusunoki R. Case of oculo-pharyngo-distal myopathy with cardiopathy. *Rinsho Shinkeigaku*. 1973;13(9):529–536.
376. Amato AA, Jackson CE, Ridings LW, Barohn RJ. Childhood-onset oculopharyngodistal myopathy with chronic intestinal pseudo-obstruction. *Muscle Nerve*. 1995;18(8):842–847.
377. Vita G, Dattola R, Santoro M, Messina C. Familial oculopharyngeal muscular dystrophy with distal spread. *J Neurol*. 1983;230(1):57–64.
378. Dimachkie MM, Barohn RJ. Distal myopathies. *Neurol Clin*. 2014;32(3):817–842.
379. Barohn RJ, Amato AA, Griggs RC. Overview of distal myopathies: From the clinical to the molecular. *Neuromuscul Disord*. 1998;8(5):309–316.
380. Welander, L. Myopathia distalis tarda hereditaria; 249 examined cases in 72 pedigrees. *Acta Med Scand Suppl*. 1951;265:1–124.
381. Borg K, Ahlberg G, Borg J, Edström L. Welander's distal myopathy: Clinical, neurophysiological and muscle biopsy observations in young and middle aged adults with early symptoms. *J Neurol Neurosurg Psychiatry*. 1991;54(6):494–498.
382. Lindberg C, Borg K, Edström L, Hedström A, Oldfors A. Inclusion body myositis and We-lander distal myopathy: A clinical, neurophysiological and morphological comparison. *J Neurol Sci*. 1991;103(1):76–81.
383. Borg K, Solders G, Borg J, Edström L, Kristensson K. Neurogenic involvement in distal myopathy (Welander). Histochemical and morphological observations on muscle and nerve biopsies. *J Neurol Sci*. 1989;91(1–2):53–70.
384. Borg K, Tome FM, Edström L. Intranuclear and cytoplasmic filamentous inclusions in distal myopathy (Welander). *Acta Neuropathol (Berl)*. 1991;82(2):102–106.
385. Edstrom, L. Histochemical and histopathological changes in skeletal muscle in late-onset hereditary distal myopathy (Welander). *J Neurol Sci*. 1975;26(2):147–157.
386. Markesbery WR, Griggs RC, Herr B. Distal myopathy: Electron microscopic and histochemical studies. *Neurology*. 1977;27(8):727–735.
387. Hackman P, Sarparanta J, Lehtinen S, et al. Welander distal myopathy is caused by a mutation in the RNA-binding protein TIA1. *Ann Neurol*. 2013;73(4):500–9.
388. Klar J, Sobol M, Melberg A, et al. Welander distal myopathy caused by an ancient founder mutation in TIA1 associated with perturbed splicing. *Hum Mutat*. 2013;34(4):572–577.
389. Udd B, Bushby K, Nonaka I, Griggs R. 104th European Neuromuscular Centre (ENMC) International Workshop: Distal myopathies, 8–10th March 2002 in Naarden, the Netherlands. *Neuromuscul Disord*. 2002;12(9):897–904.
390. Udd B, Haravuori H, Kalimo H, et al. Tibial muscular dystrophy—from clinical description to linkage on chromosome 2q31. *Neuromuscul Disord*. 1998;8(5):327–332.
391. Hackman P, Vihola A, Haravuori H, et al. Tibial muscular dystrophy is a titinopathy caused by mutations in TTN, the gene encoding the giant skeletal-muscle protein titin. *Am J Hum Genet*. 2002;71(3):492–500.
392. Markesbery WR, Griggs RC, Leach RP, Lapham LW. Late onset hereditary distal myopathy. *Neurology*. 1974;24(2):127–134.
393. Griggs R, Vihola A, Hackman P, et al. Zaspopathy in a large classic late-onset distal myopathy family. *Brain*. 2007;130:1477–1484.
394. Lin X, Ruiz J, Bajraktari I, et al. Z-disc-associated, alternatively spliced, PDZ motif-containing protein (ZASP) mutations in the actin-binding domain cause disruption of skeletal muscle actin filaments in myofibrillar myopathy. *J Biol Chem*. 2014;289(19):13615–13626.
395. Mizusawa H, Kurisaki H, Takatsu M, et al. Rimmed vacuolar distal myopathy: A clinical, electrophysiological, histopathological and computed tomographic study of seven cases. *J Neurol*. 1987;234(3):129–136.
396. Nonaka I, Sunohara N, Ishiura S, Satoyoshi E. Familial distal myopathy with rimmed vacuole and lamellar (myeloid) body formation. *J Neurol Sci*. 1981;51(1):141–155.
397. Nonaka I, Sunohara N, Satoyoshi E, Terasawa K, Yonemoto K. Autosomal recessive distal muscular dystrophy: A comparative study with distal myopathy with rimmed vacuole formation. *Ann Neurol* 1985;17(1):51–59.
398. Sunohara N, Nonaka I, Kamei N, Satoyoshi E. Distal myopathy with rimmed vacuole formation. A follow-up study. *Brain*. 1989;112(Pt 1):65–83.
399. Argov Z, Eisenberg I, Grabov-Nardini G, et al. Hereditary inclusion body myopathy: The Middle Eastern genetic cluster. *Neurology*. 2003;60(9):1519–1523.
400. Argov Z, Yarom R. "Rimmed vacuole myopathy" sparing the quadriceps. A unique disorder in Iranian Jews. *J Neurol Sci*. 1984;64(1):33–43.
401. Eisenberg I, Grabov-Nardini G, Hochner H, et al. Mutations spectrum of GNE in hereditary inclusion body myopathy sparing the quadriceps. *Hum Mutat*. 2003;21(1):99.
402. Sivakumar K, Dalakas MC. The spectrum of familial inclusion body myopathies in 13 families and a description of a

quadriceps-sparing phenotype in non-Iranian Jews. *Neurology.* 1996;47(4):977–984.

403. Eisenberg I, Avidan N, Potikha T, et al. The UDP-N-acetylglucosamine 2-epimerase/N-acetylmannosamine kinase gene is mutated in recessive hereditary inclusion body myopathy. *Nat Genet.* 2001;29(1):83–87.
404. Laing NG, Laing BA, Meredith C, et al. Autosomal dominant distal myopathy: Linkage to chromosome 14. *Am J Hum Genet.* 1995;56(2):422–427.
405. Mastaglia FL, Phillips BA, Cala LA, et al. Early onset chromosome 14-linked distal myopathy (Laing). *Neuromuscul Disord.* 2002;12:350–357.
406. Meredith C, Herrmann R, Parry C, et al. Mutations in the slow skeletal muscle fiber myosin heavy chain gene (MYH7) cause laing early-onset distal myopathy (MPD1). *Am J Hum Genet.* 2004;75:703–708.
407. Muelas N, Hackman P, Lugue H, et al. MYH7 gene tail mutation causing myopathic profiles beyond Laing distal myopathy. *Neurology.* 2010;75:732–741.
408. Overeem S, Schelhaas HJ, Blijham PJ, et al. Symptomatic distal myopathy with cardiomyopathy due to a MYH7 mutation. *Neuromuscul Disord.* 2007;17:490–493.
409. Tasca G, Ricci E, Penttilä S, et al. New phenotype and pathology features in MYH7-related distal myopathy. *Neuromuscul Disord.* 2012;22:640–647.
410. Lamont PJ, Udd B, Mastaglia FL, et al. Laing early onset distal myopathy: Slow myosin defect with variable abnormalities on muscle biopsy. *J Neurol Neurosurg Psychiatry.* 2006;77(2):208–215.
411. Tajsharghi H, Thornell LE, Lindberg C, Lindvall B, Henriksson KG, Oldfors A. Myosin storage myopathy associated with a heterozygous missense mutation in MYH7. *Ann Neurol.* 2003;54(4):494–500.
412. Tajsharghi H, Oldfors A, Macleod DP, Swash M. Homozygous mutation in MYH7 in myosin storage myopathy and cardiomyopathy. *Neurology.* 2007;68:962.
413. Masuzugawa S, Kuzuhara S, Narita Y, Naito Y, Taniguchi A, Ibi T. Autosomal dominant hyaline body myopathy presenting as scapuloperoneal syndrome: Clinical features and muscle pathology. *Neurology.* 1997;48:253–257.
414. Bohlega S, Abu-Amero SN, Wakil SM, et al. Mutation of the slow myosin heavy chain rod domain underlies hyaline body myopathy. *Neurology.* 2004;62:518–521.
415. Williams DR, Reardon K, Roberts L, et al. A new dominant distal myopathy affecting posterior leg and anterior upper limb muscles. *Neurology.* 2005;64:1245–1254.
416. Duff RM, Tay V, Hackman P, et al. Mutations in the N-terminal actin-binding domain of filamin C cause a distal myopathy. *Am J Hum Genet.* 2011;88:729–740.
417. Guergueltcheva V, Peeters K, Baets J, et al. Distal myopathy with upper limb predominance caused by filamin C haploinsufficiency. *Neurology.* 2011;77:2105–2114.
418. Luan X, Hong D, Zhang W, Wang Z, Yuan Y. A novel heterozygous deletion-insertion mutation (2695–2712 del/GTTTGT ins) in exon 18 of the filamin C gene causes filaminopathy in a large Chinese family. *Neuromuscul Disord.* 2010;20:390–396.
419. Wallgren-Pettersson C, Lehtokari VL, Kalimo H, et al. Distal myopathy caused by homozygous missense mutations in the nebulin gene. *Brain.* 2007;130:1465–1476.
420. Lehtokari VL, Pelin K, Herczegfalvi A, et al. Nemaline myopathy caused by mutations in the nebulin gene may present as a distal myopathy. *Neuromuscul Disord.* 2011;21:556–562.
421. Cirak S, von Deimling F, Sachdev S, et al. Kelch-like homologue 9 mutation is associated with an early onset autosomal dominant distal myopathy. *Brain.* 2010;133:2123–2135.
422. Feit H, Silbergleit A, Schneider LB, et al. Vocal cord and pharyngeal weakness with autosomal dominant distal myopathy: Clinical description and gene localization to 5q31. *Am J Hum Genet.* 1998;63(6):1732–1742.
423. Senderek J, Garvey SM, Krieger M, et al. Autosomal-dominant distal myopathy associated with a recurrent missense mutation in the gene encoding the nuclear matrix protein, matrin 3. *Am J Hum Genet.* 2009;84:511–518.
424 Johnson JO, Pioro EP, Boehringer A, et al. Mutations in the Matrin 3 gene cause familial amyotrophic lateral sclerosis. *Nat Neurosci.* 2014;17(5):664–666.
425. Muller TJ, Kraya T, Stoltenburg-Didinger G, et al. Phenotype of the Matrin-3-distal myopathy in 16 German patients. *Ann Neurol.* 2014;76:669–680.
426. Amato AA, Kagan-Hallet K, Jackson CE, et al. The wide spectrum of myofibrillar myopathy suggests a multifactorial etiology and pathogenesis. *Neurology.* 1998;51(6):1646–1655.
424. Dalakas MC, Dagvadorj A, Goudeau B, et al. Progressive skeletal myopathy, a phenotypic variant of desmin myopathy associated with desmin mutations. *Neuromuscul Disord.* 2003;13(3):252–258.
428. Dalakas MC, Park KY, Semino-Mora C, Lee HS, Sivakumar K, Goldfarb LG. Desmin myopathy, a skeletal myopathy with cardiomyopathy caused by mutations in the desmin gene. *N Engl J Med.* 2000;342(11):770–780.
429. De Bleecker JL, Engel AG, Ertl BB. Myofibrillar myopathy with abnormal foci of desmin positivity. II. Immunocytochemical analysis reveals accumulation of multiple other proteins. *J Neuropathol Exp Neurol.* 1996;55(5):563–577.
430. Engel AG. Myofibrillar myopathy. *Ann Neurol.* 1999;46(5):681–683.
431. Goebel HH. Desmin-related neuromuscular disorders. *Muscle Nerve.* 1995;18(11):1306–1320.
432. Goldfarb LG, Park KY, Cervenáková L, et al. Missense mutations in desmin associated with familial cardiac and skeletal myopathy. *Nat Genet.* 1998;19(4):402–403.
433. Goldfarb LG, Vicart P, Goebel HH, Dalakas MC. Desmin myopathy. *Brain.* 2004;127(Pt 4):723–734.
434. Nakano S, Engel AG, Waclawik AJ, Emslie-Smith AM, Busis NA. Myofibrillar myopathy with abnormal foci of desmin positivity. I. Light and electron microscopy analysis of 10 cases. *J Neuropathol Exp Neurol.* 1996;55(5):549–562.
435. Selcen D, Engel AG. Myofibrillar myopathy caused by novel dominant negative alpha B-crystallin mutations. *Ann Neurol.* 2003;54(6):804–810.
436. Selcen D, Ohno K, Engel AG. Myofibrillar myopathy: Clinical, morphological and genetic studies in 63 patients. *Brain.* 2004;127(Pt 2):439–451.
437. Vicart P, Caron A, Guicheney P, et al. A missense mutation in the alphaBcrystallin chaperone gene causes a desmin-related myopathy. *Nat Genet.* 1998;20(1):92–95.
438. Nakano S, Engel AG, Akiguchi I, Kimura J. Myofibrillar myopathy. III. Abnormal expression of cyclin-dependent kinases and nuclear proteins. *J Neuropathol Exp Neurol.* 1997;56(8):850–856.
439. Bertini E, Biancalana V, Bolino A, et al. 118th ENMC International Workshop on Advances in Myotubular Myopathy, 26–28 September 2003, Naarden, the Netherlands (5th Workshop of the International Consortium on Myotubular Myopathy). *Neuromuscul Disord.* 2004;14(6):387–396.

440. Sabatelli M, Bertini E, Ricci E, et al. Peripheral neuropathy with giant axons and cardiomyopathy associated with desmin type intermediate filaments in skeletal muscle. *J Neurol Sci.* 1992;109(1):1–10.
441. Munoz-Marmol AM, Strasser G, Isamat M, et al. A dysfunctional desmin mutation in a patient with severe generalized myopathy. *Proc Natl Acad Sci U S A.* 1998;95(19):11312–11317.
442. Li M, Dalakas MC. Abnormal desmin protein in myofibrillar myopathies caused by desmin gene mutations. *Ann Neurol.* 2001;49(4):532–536.
443. Tajsharghi H, Darin N, Rekabdar E, et al. Mutations and sequence variation in the human myosin heavy chain IIa gene (MYH2). *Eur J Hum Genet.* 2005;13(5):617–622.
444. Martinsson T, Oldfors A, Darin N, et al. Autosomal dominant myopathy: Missense mutation (Glu-706 -> Lys) in the myosin heavy chain IIa gene. *Proc Natl Acad Sci U S A.* 2000;97: 14614–14619.
445. Cole AJ, Kuzniecky R, Karpati G, Carpenter S, Andermann E, Andermann F. Familial myopathy with changes resembling inclusion body myositis and periventricular leucoencephalopathy. A new syndrome. *Brain.* 1988;111(Pt 5):1025–1037.
446. Watts GD, Thorne M, Kovach MJ, Pestronk A, Kimonis VE. Clinical and genetic heterogeneity in chromosome 9p associated hereditary inclusion body myopathy: Exclusion of GNE and three other candidate genes. *Neuromuscul Disord.* 2003;13(7-8):559–567.
447. Watts GD, Wymer J, Kovach MJ, et al. Inclusion body myopathy associated with Paget disease of bone and frontotemporal dementia is caused by mutant valosin-containing protein. *Nat Genet.* 2004;36(4):377–381.
448. Watts GD, Thomasova D, Ramdeen SK, et al. Novel VCP mutations in inclusion body myopathy associated with Paget disease of bone and frontotemporal dementia. *Clin Genet.* 2007;72:420–426.
449. Watts GD. Inclusion body myopathy associated with Paget disease of bone and frontotemporal dementia is caused by mutant valosin-containing protein. *Nat Genet.* 2004;36:377–381.
450. Kimonis VE, Kovach MJ, Waggoner B, et al. Clinical and molecular studies in a unique family with autosomal dominant limb-girdle muscular dystrophy and Paget disease of bone. *Genet Med.* 2000;2:232–241.
451. Kimonis VE, Mehta SG, Fulchiero EC, et al. Clinical studies in familial VCP myopathy associated with Paget disease of bone and frontotemporal dementia. *Am J Med Genet A.* 2008;146A:745–757.
452. Kimonis VE, Watts GD. Autosomal dominant inclusion body myopathy, Paget disease of bone, and frontotemporal dementia. *Alzheimer Dis Assoc Disord.* 2005;19(Suppl 1):S44–S47.
453. Guyant-Maréchal L, Laquierrière A, Duyckaerts C, et al. Valosin-containing protein gene mutations: Clinical and neuropathologic features. *Neurology.* 2006;67:644–651.
454. Haubenberger D, Bittner RE, Rauch-Shorny S, et al. Inclusion body myopathy and Paget disease is linked to a novel mutation in the VCP gene. *Neurology.* 2005;65:1304–1305.
455. Miller TD, Jackson AP, Barresi R, et al. Inclusion body myopathy with Paget disease and frontotemporal dementia (IBMPFD): Clinical features including sphincter disturbance in a large pedigree. *J Neurol Neurosurg Psychiatry.* 2009;80:583–584.
456. Kim EJ, Park YE, Kim DS, et al. Inclusion body myopathy with Paget disease of bone and frontotemporal dementia linked to VCP p.Arg155Cys in a Korean family. *Arch Neurol.* 2011;68:787–796.
457. Kumar KR, Needham M, Mina K, et al. Two Australian families with inclusion-body myopathy, Paget's disease of bone and frontotemporal dementia: Novel clinical and genetic findings. *Neuromuscul Disord.* 2010;20:330–334.
458. Stojkovic T, Hammouda el H, Richard P, et al. Clinical outcome in 19 French and Spanish patients with valosin-containing protein myopathy associated with Paget's disease of bone and frontotemporal dementia. *Neuromuscul Disord.* 2009;19:316–323.
459. Viassolo V, Previtali SC, Schiatti E, et al. Inclusion body myopathy, Paget's disease of the bone and frontotemporal dementia: Recurrence of the VCP R155 H mutation in an Italian family and implications for genetic counselling. *Clin Genet.* 2008;74:54–60.
460. Waggoner B, Kovach MJ, Winkelman M, et al. Heterogeneity in familial dominant Paget disease of bone and muscular dystrophy. *Am J Med Genet.* 2002;108:187–191.
461. Shi Z, Hayashi YK, Mitsuhashi S, et al. Characterization of the Asian myopathy patients with VCP mutations. *Eur J Neurol.* 2012;19:501–509.
462. van der Zee J, Pirici D, Van Langenhove T, et al. Clinical heterogeneity in 3 unrelated families linked to VCP p.Arg159His. *Neurology.* 2009;73:626–632.
463. Palmio J, Sandell S, Suominen T, et al. Distinct distal myopathy phenotype caused by VCP gene mutation in a Finnish family. *Neuromuscul Disord.* 2011;21:551–555.
464. Johnson JO, Mandrioli J, Benatar M, et al. Exome sequencing reveals VCP mutations as a cause of familial ALS. *Neuron.* 2010;68(5):857–864.
465. González-Pérez P, Cirulli ET, Drory VE, et al. Novel mutation in VCP gene causes atypical amyotrophic lateral sclerosis. *Neurology.* 2012;79(22):2201–2208.
466. Kim HJ, Kim NC, Wang YD, et al. Mutations in prion-like domains in hnRNPA2B1 and hnRNPA1 cause multisystem proteinopathy and ALS. *Nature.* 2013;495:467–473.
467. Bucelli RC, Arhzaouy K, Pestronk A, et al. *SQSTM1* splice site mutation in distal myopathy with rimmed vacuoles. *Neurology.* 2015. (in-press)

CHAPTER 28

Congenital Myopathies

The term "congenital myopathy" was originally used to describe a group of myopathic disorders presenting preferentially, but not exclusively, at birth and being morphologically distinct from congenital muscular dystrophies (Table 28-1).[1–3] However, disorders that were once considered forms of muscular dystrophy are now known to be allelic to some types of congenital myopathy. For example, congenital muscular dystrophy with rigid spine syndrome, multi/minicore, and some cases of myofibrillar myopathy are caused by selenoprotein N1 mutations; sarcotubular myopathy and limb-girdle muscular dystrophy 2H (LGMD2H) are due to mutations in TRIM32; reducing body myopathy is now considered a type of LGMD. In addition, some disorders caused by mutations in sarcomeric proteins are classified as forms of LGMD (e.g., titinopathies, myotilinopathies, ZASPopathies), while others (e.g., actinomyosin, tropomyosin, α-actin, and troponin) are forms of congenital myopathy (nemaline myopathy). Thus, the nosology of what distinguishes a "congenital myopathy" from a "muscular dystrophy" on clinical and histopathologic grounds is not at all clear.

Usually, the congenital myopathies present in infancy as generalized hypotonia and weakness. Motor milestones are typically delayed. Affected infants are usually hypotonic and display delayed motor development. Some disorders with mutations in similar genes present later in childhood or even in adulthood. The congenital myopathies were initially considered as nonprogressive, although it is now clear that progressive weakness can occur.

Congenital myopathies can be inherited in an autosomal-dominant, autosomal-recessive, or X-linked pattern. Within families, there can be considerable variation with respect to disease presentation and degree of muscle involvement. The serum creatine kinase (CK) levels are either normal or usually mildly elevated. The classification of congenital myopathies has been based almost exclusively on clinical presentation and light/electron microscopic structural alterations of the muscle biopsy specimen (Table 28-1).

► CENTRAL CORE MYOPATHY

CLINICAL FEATURES

Central core myopathy usually manifests at birth or early childhood as generalized weakness and hypotonia.[1–7] The degree of muscle weakness can vary even within families.[3] Muscle weakness is stable or only slowly progressive. Motor milestones, such as the ability to sit and walk, are delayed. Some individuals who are affected never achieve independent ambulation, while others have only mild weakness. The proximal muscles, legs more than arms, are preferentially affected, leading to a wide-based hyperlordotic gait. Individuals who are affected may also demonstrate a Gowers sign when arising from the floor. There may be mild facial and neck flexor weakness. However, patients do not exhibit ptosis or extraocular muscle weakness—clinical features that can help distinguish central core myopathy clinically from centronuclear and nemaline myopathies. Muscle atrophy or hypertrophy are usually not seen in central core disease. Contractures are uncommon. Muscle stretch reflexes are normal or reduced. There are no apparent central nervous system abnormalities. Affected individuals may exhibit mild-to-moderate skeletal deformities including pes planus, pes cavus, kyphoscoliosis, and congenital hip dislocation. Mild ventilatory muscle weakness with reduced forced vital capacity and nocturnal hypoxemia is seen in some patients.[3]

LABORATORY FEATURES

The serum CK levels are normal or slightly elevated. Motor and sensory nerve conduction studies (NCS) are usually normal. Electromyography (EMG) may reveal fibrillation potentials and positive sharp waves and myopathic appearing motor unit action potentials (MUAPs) that recruit early in weak muscles.[8] Long-duration, polyphasic MUAPs and units with satellite potentials may also be appreciated. Skeletal muscle MRI reveals early involvement of the vasti, sartorius, and adductor magnus in the thigh with relative sparing of the rectus femoris, adductor longus, and hamstrings.[1]

HISTOPATHOLOGY

The characteristic histologic features are the structural alterations within the center of muscle fibers, so-called cores.[1–9] These cores appear only in type 1 muscle fibers and are particularly noticeable on nicotinamide adenine dinucleotide tetrazolium reductase (NADH-TR) stains, where the cores are devoid of stain (Fig. 28-1). The cores can occasionally be eccentric and multiple within a given muscle fiber. The distinction between central core and multi/minicore is that in central core myopathy the "cores" extend along the entire length of the muscle fibers on longitudinal section. However, in some cases, the distinction between central cores and multi/minicores is

▶ **TABLE 28-1. CONGENITAL MYOPATHIES**

Disease	Inheritance	Protein (Gene)	Clinical Features
Central core myopathy	AD (rare AR)	Ryanodine receptor (*RYR1*)	Onset: infancy or childhood, occasionally adulthood; proximal limbs and mild facial weakness; skeletal anomalies; risk for MH in those with RYR1 mutations
	AR	Muscle slow/β cardiac myosin heavy chain 7 gene (*MYH7*)	
	AD	α-Actin 1 (*ACTA1*)	
	AR	Titin (*TTN*)	
	AD	Coiled–coiled domain-containing 78 (*CCDC78*)	
Multi/minicore myopathy	AR	Selenoprotein N1/(*SEPN1*)	Onset: infancy or childhood; proximal and facial muscles; rare EOM weak; cardiomyopathy and respiratory weakness; skeletal anomalies; risk for MH in those with *RYR1* mutations
	AD/AR	Ryanodine receptor (*RYR1*)	
	AR	Titin (*TTN*)	
	AD	Muscle slow/β cardiac myosin heavy chain 7 gene (*MYH7*)	
	AR	Multiple EGF-like-domains 10 (*MEGF10*)	
Core–rod myopathy	AD/AR	α-Actin 1 (*ACTA1*)	Onset in infancy or childhood. Phenotypes can resemble those seen with nemaline myopathy
	AR	Nebulin (*NEB*)	
	AD	Kelch repeat and BTB/ (*KBTBD13*)	
Nemaline rod myopathy	AR	Nebulin (*NEB*)	*Infantile-onset form*: severe generalized hypotonia/weakness; respiratory weakness; skeletal anomalies; usually fatal in first year of life
	AD/AR	α-Actin (*ACTA1*)	
	AD/AR	α-Tropomyosin (*TMP3*)	
	AD/AR	β-Tropomyosin (*TPM2*)	*Mild early-onset form*: Most common subtype; onset in infancy or childhood; mild generalized hypotonia and weakness; facial muscles; rare ptosis, EOM weak; dysmorphic facies and skeletal anomalies
	AR	Slow troponin T (*TNNT1*)	
	AR	Cofilin-2 (*CFL2*)	
	AD	Kelch repeat and BTB Domain Containing 13 (*KBTBD13*)	*Adult-onset form*: onset in adult life; mild proximal and occasionally distal weakness; no facial or skeletal anomalies
	AR	Kelch-like family member 40 and 41 genes (*KLHL40* and *KLHL41*)	
Centronuclear/myotubular myopathy	X-linked	Myotubularin (*MTM1*)	Severe neonatal hypotonia and weakness; respiratory weakness; ptosis and EOM weak; poor prognosis in most
	AD	Dynamin-2 (DYN2)	
	AR	Ryanodine receptor (*RYR1*	
	AR	Amphiphysin 2 (*BIN2*)	Onset in late infancy or early childhood of generalized weakness and hypotonia; facial and EOM weakness, ptosis; facial anomalies
	AR	Titin (*TTN*)	Onset in late childhood or adulthood of mild proximal and/or distal weakness; ptosis is common; facial and EOM muscles variably involved; no skeletal or facial anomalies; mild sensory abnormalities
			Cases with *BIN2* mutations may have severe distal lower extremity weakness
Congenital fiber-type disproportion	AD	α-Tropomyosin (*TMP3*)	Onset in infancy to adulthood; generalized or proximal weakness; may have facial, respiratory or asymmetric weakness; skeletal anomalies
	AD	Ryanodine Receptor (*RYR1*)	
	AR	Rarely caused by mutations in *ACTA1, SEPN1, MYL2, TPM2, and MHC7*	
Reducing body myopathy	X-linked	Four and a half LIM (*FHL1*)	Onset in infancy or childhood; generalized nonprogressive weakness; occasional respiratory weakness; skeletal and facial anomalies
	AR	Desmin (*DES*)	
Fingerprint body myopathy	Unknown	Unknown	Infantile onset; slow or nonprogressive proximal weakness
Sarcotubular myopathy (allelic to LGMD 2 H)	AR	Tripartite motif-containing protein 32/(*TRIM 32*)	Onset: infancy; slow progressive proximal and/or distal weakness
Trilaminar myopathy	Unknown	Unknown	Infantile onset: generalized weakness; skeletal anomalies

▶ TABLE 28-1. **(CONTINUED)**

Disease	Inheritance	Protein (Gene)	Clinical Features
Hyaline body myopathy / familial myopathy with lysis of myofibrils / myosin storage myopathy	AD	Muscle slow/β cardiac myosin heavy chain 7 gene (*MYH7*)	Onset in infancy or adults; limb-girdle, scapuloperoneal, or distal weakness
H-IBM 3/myosin storage myopathy	AD	Myosin heavy chain type IIa (*MYH2*)	Congenital arthrogryposis; ophthalmoparesis; adult onset of mild proximal weakness and myalgias; rimmed vacuoles and inclusions on muscle biopsy (H-IBM type 3)
Cap myopathy	AD AD AD	β-Tropomyosin (*TPM2*) α-Tropomyosin *(TMP3)* α-Actin (*ACTA1)*	Onset in infancy; generalized weakness; skeletal anomalies
Zebra body myopathy	AR	α-Actin (*ACTA1)*	Onset in infancy or childhood; Generalized weakness—may be asymmetric and worse in arms
Tubular aggregate myopathy	AD AD AR AR	Stromal interaction molecule 1 (*STIM1*) Orai1 (*ORAI1)* UDP-N-acetylglucosamine-dolichyl-phosphate N-acetylglucosaminephosphotransferase 1 (*DPAGT1*) Glutamine-fructose-6-phosphate transaminase 1 (*GFPT1*)	Onset: childhood or early adulthood; limb-girdle weakness; immune deficiency; *ORAI1* mutations are also associated with miosis *GDPAGT1* and *GFPT1* mutations are associated with infantile onset of a myasthenic syndrome with fatigable weakness

AD, autosomal dominant; AR, autosomal recessive; EOM weakness, ophthalmoparesis; MH, malignant hyperthermia.

not clear, as there can be typical multi/minicores in patients with central core myopathy. Furthermore, repeat biopsies in patients initially diagnosed with minicores may subsequently reveal central cores.[10] In addition, muscle biopsies reveal variation in fiber size, increased internalized nuclei, and often a predominance of type 1 fibers that may be atrophic. Increased endomysial fibrosis and fat may be present,[9] but the other features help distinguish the disorder from muscular dystrophies.

On electron microscopy (EM), the cores may be "structured" or "unstructured" (Fig. 28-2). In structured cores,

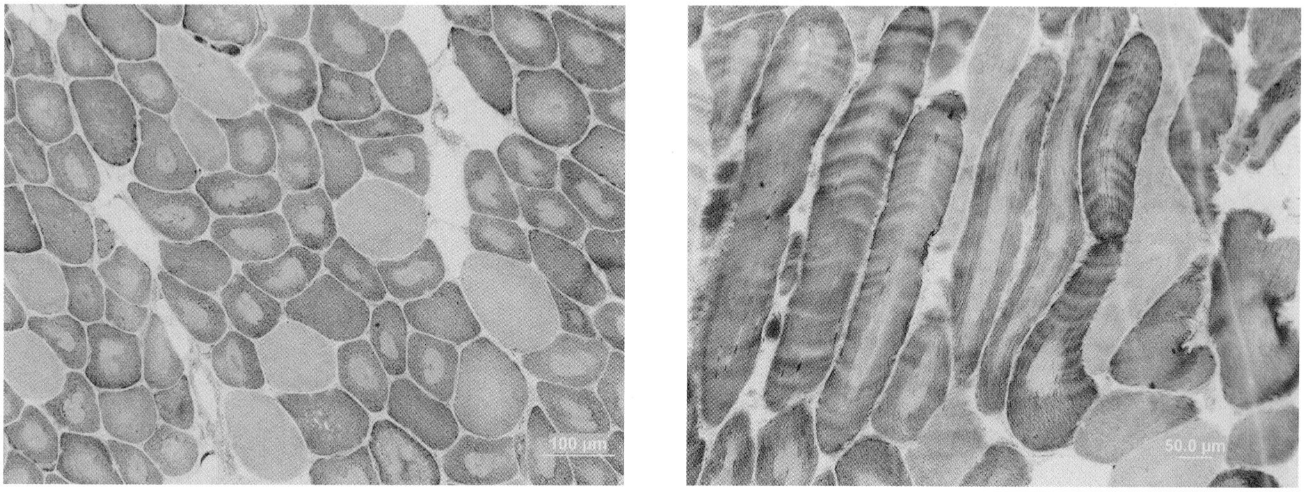

A B

Figure 28-1. Central core myopathy. Nicotinamide adenine dinucleotide tetrazolium reductase (NADH-TR) stain demonstrates areas devoid of oxidated enzyme activity in the center of the fibers or sometimes eccentric regions **(A)** that extend the length of the fiber longitudinally **(B)**.

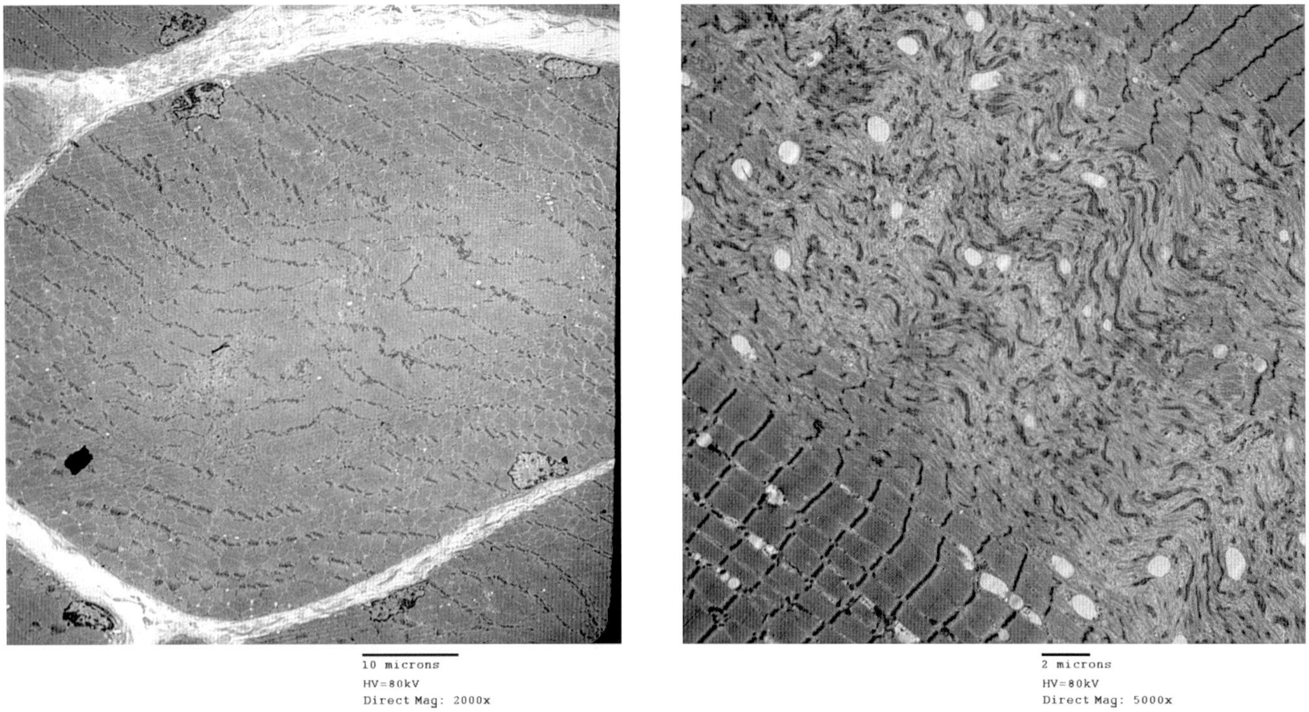

A B

Figure 28-2. Central core myopathy. Electron microscopy reveals areas with poorly aligned sarcomeres and reduced glycogen and mitochondrial in an "unstructured" core **(A)**. A core can be seen to extend over a large length of the fibers on a longitudinal section **(B)**.

there is streaming of the Z-band, but the sarcomeres are preserved. In unstructured cores, there is severe myofibrillar disruption and loss of the normal sarcomere organization. In both structured and unstructured cores, mitochondria and glycogen granules are reduced or absent. The cores appear to contain desmin, dystrophin, actin, α-actinin, gelsolin, nebulin, myotilin, β-amyloid precursor protein, NCAM, and various cyclin-dependent kinases based on immunocytochemistry; the cores are also variably congophilic.[11]

MOLECULAR GENETICS AND PATHOGENESIS

Central core myopathy is an autosomal-dominant disorder caused by mutations in the ryanodine receptor gene (*RYR1*) on chromosome 19q13.1 in the majority of cases.[1–3,12–15] Rarely, autosomal-recessive inheritance may occur with *RYR1* mutations.[16] Of note, mutations in the *RYR1* are responsible for one form of familial malignant hyperthermia; thus, patients with central core myopathy are at risk of malignant hyperthermia (Table 28-1).[17] Why these "cores" form in the center of the muscle fibers is unknown. The ryanodine receptor is a tetramer of RYR1 proteins, which bridges the gap between the sarcoplasmic reticulum and the T-tubules in skeletal muscle and forms a calcium-release channel. Thus, the ryanodine receptor likely plays an important role in excitation–contraction coupling. Most of the mutations associated with the classic phenotype are seen in the C-terminal domain that corresponds to the transmembrane domain of the protein.[1,2] In experimental studies of mutant myotubes, voltage-gated calcium release was reduced by approximately 90%, while caffeine-induced Ca^{2+} release was only marginally reduced in mutant myotubes, indicating the disruption of voltage-sensor activation of calcium release.[18,19]

Mutations in muscle slow/β cardiac myosin heavy chain 7 gene (*MYH7*) have been associated with eccentric cores and multi/minicores.[1,2,20] Mutations in the genes that encode actin 1 (*ACTA1*), titin (*TTN*), coiled–coiled domain-containing gene, *CCDC78*, have also been associated with core-like changes on muscle biopsy, while mutations in *NEB* that encodes nebulin and *KBTBD13* encoding Kelch repeat and BTB may cause cores and nemaline rods.[1–3,21,22]

TREATMENT

There is no specific medical treatment available for central core myopathy. Patients may benefit from physical therapy and orthotic devices. Patients with central core disease and their families should be informed of their risk of developing malignant hyperthermia with general anesthesia. Appropriate precautions and avoidance of certain anesthetic agents (e.g., halothane) and neuromuscular blocking agents (succinylcholine) need to be taken during surgical procedures.

▶ MULTI/MINICORE MYOPATHY

CLINICAL FEATURES

Although it is generally agreed that multi/minicore disease (MmD) constitutes a distinct entity, the morphologic lesions defining it are nonspecific, and the clinical expression of the disease is highly variable.[1–3,23–28] MmD usually presents in infancy or early childhood, but adult-onset cases have been reported as well. Affected infants are usually hypotonic and weak. Motor milestones are delayed, but ambulation is usually achieved. Most patients have generalized muscle weakness and atrophy predominantly affecting axial and proximal extremity muscles. Distal muscles are usually normal or only slightly involved. However, there may be a subgroup of MmD that manifests with predominantly distal hand weakness.[25,26] Facial muscle weakness, ptosis, and occasionally ophthalmoparesis can also be seen. It is unclear if these patients represent a distinct subgroup of MmD.

Muscle contractures and multiple skeletal deformities such as kyphoscoliosis, high-arched palate, and club feet are common findings. Weakness is usually stable or only slowly progressive.[26] Neck extensors and trunk muscles may be contracted, leading to rigidity of the spine. Cardiomyopathy and ventilatory muscle involvement can also develop.[27,28] Ventilatory involvement can be disproportionate to the degree of scoliosis.[2,26] Patients may require intermittent or continuous positive-pressure ventilation.

LABORATORY FEATURES

Serum CK is usually normal or only slightly elevated. Pulmonary function tests often reveal reduced forced vital capacities. Polysomnographic studies may disclose nocturnal oxygen desaturation and short apneic periods. NCS are normal. EMG usually reveals normal insertional and spontaneous activity, although early recruitment of short-duration, small-amplitude MUAPs may be appreciated.[8]

HISTOPATHOLOGY

Muscle biopsies reveal multiple small regions within muscle fibers of variable size (minicores) formed by disorganization of the myofibrils (Fig. 28-3).[25,26] These minicores are similar to central cores but are much smaller and do not extend the entire length of the muscle fiber as do central cores. In addition, minicores can occur in either type 1 or type 2 muscle fibers. Type 1 fiber predominance and atrophy as well as fiber size variation are also noted. There can be increased endomysial connective tissue as well. EM demonstrates myofibrillar disruption similar to that seen in central cores (Fig. 28-4).

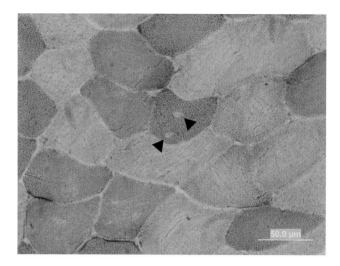

Figure 28-3. Multi/minicore myopathy. NADH stain demonstrates small areas devoid of oxidative enzyme activity (*arrowheads*).

MOLECULAR GENETICS AND PATHOGENESIS

This is a genetically heterogeneous group of disorders. The absence of clear dominant transmission in any well-established case and the presence of several consanguineous families strongly suggest that MmD is usually an

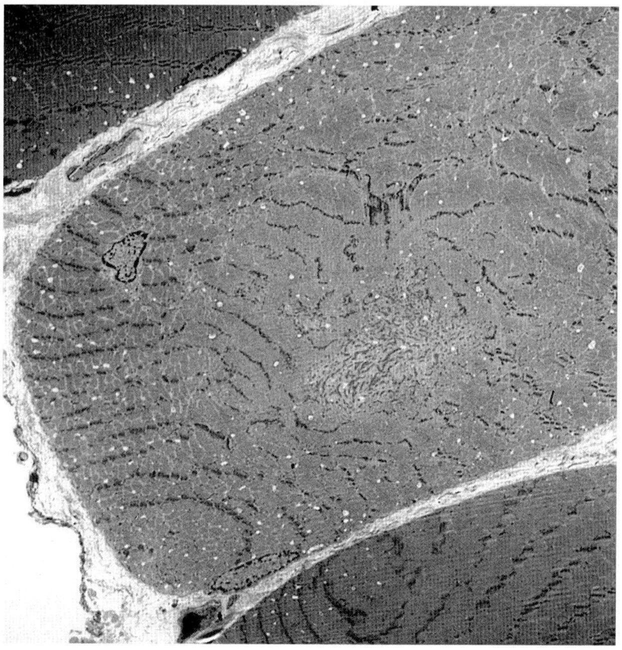

Figure 28-4. Multi/minicore myopathy. Electron microscopy reveals areas of myofibrillar disarray similar to central core myopathy but are much smaller.

autosomal-recessive entity or the result of spontaneous mutations.[1-3,26] Interestingly though, some patients with MmD (usually cases associated with external ophthalmoplegia and ptosis) have demonstrable mutations in the *RyR1* gene similar to central core myopathy.[1-3,10,29] Mutations in the selenoprotein N gene (*SEPN1*), which is located on chromosome 1p36, are the most common cause in individuals with classic MmD.[30] Of note, this is the same gene responsible for the congenital muscular dystrophy with rigid spine syndrome and some cases of myofibrillar myopathy.[30] The dystrophic changes and histologic features of myofibrillar myopathy apparent on some muscle biopsies and *SEPN1* mutations identified in some cases of MmD highlight the difficult nosologic boundaries between various types of congenital myopathies and muscular dystrophies. In addition, mutations in coifilin-2 gene, *CFL2*, encoded on chromosome 14q13 have been reported in two siblings that had nemaline rods and minicores on muscle biopsy. Mutations in myosin heavy chain 7 gene (*MYH7*)[31,32], titin (*TTN*)[33], and multiple EGF-like-domains 10 (*MEGF10*)[34] can be associated with minicores as well.

TREATMENT

No specific medical treatment is available. Patients may be at risk of malignant hyperthermia and should be counseled accordingly (see Central Core Myopathy).[35,36] Early-onset scoliosis is common and may require extensive arthrodesis. Patients may require intermittent or continuous positive-pressure ventilation.

▶ CORE–ROD MYOPATHY

CLINICAL FEATURES

Central core and nemaline rod myopathies are generally considered two genetically and histologically distinct disorders.[1-3,37-44] However, there are scattered reports in the literature of the simultaneous occurrence of both cores and rods in the same muscle biopsy. Onset of symptoms is variable (congenital or early adult life) as is severity. The weakness can be proximal, distal, or generalized. Some cases have ptosis and/or skeletal deformities (e.g., contractures, scoliosis).

LABORATORY FEATURES

The serum CK level can be normal or slightly elevated. NCS are usually normal. Early recruitment of small-amplitude, short-duration MUAPs are appreciated in weak muscles on EMG.

HISTOPATHOLOGY

Muscle biopsies, as implied by the name, can show both cores and rods along with type 1 fiber predominance (Figure 28-5).

MOLECULAR GENETICS AND PATHOGENESIS

Mutations in the ryanodine receptor gene (*RYR1*) account for most cases, however mutations in the genes that encode actin 1 (*ACTA1*), nebulin (*NEB*), and Kelch repeat and BTB (*KBTBD13*) have also been associated with muscle biopsies demonstrating both cores and nemaline rods.[1,2,37-44]

TREATMENT

No specific medical treatment is available. Those cases with RYR1 mutations should be counseled in regard to possible risk of malignant hyperthermia.

▶ OTHER PHENOTYPES ASSOCIATED WITH *RYR1* MUTATIONS

As previously discussed, the clinical phenotype associated with *RYR1* mutations is large and aside from central core and multi/minicore myopathies that usually occur early in life, also cause malignant hyperthermia. In addition, *RYR1* mutations have been identified as a cause of exertional myalgias and rhabdomyolysis in the absence of baseline weakness.[45] King–Denborough syndrome is a rare disorder characterized by a susceptibility to malignant hyperthermia, delayed motor development, short stature, cryptorchidism, skeletal abnormalities, and variable dysmorphic features that in some cases, but not all, have been associated with *RYR1* mutations.[46,47]

Furthermore, late-onset axial myopathy manifesting as bent spine syndrome (camptocormia) or neck extensor myopathy have been found to have *RYR1* mutations.[48-50] CKs are normal or slightly elevated. EMG may be normal in extremities and demonstrate fibrillation potentials and positive sharp waves only in axial/paraspinal muscles. In our experience, muscle biopsies of extremity muscles that are strong may be unrevealing while biopsy of upper trapezius or paraspinal muscles may demonstrate cores, multiminicores, or moth-eaten fibers.

▶ NEMALINE MYOPATHY

CLINICAL FEATURES

Nemaline myopathy is clinically and genetically heterogeneous. It can be inherited in an autosomal-dominant or autosomal-recessive fashion. There are three major clinical presentations of nemaline myopathy: (1) a severe infantile form, (2) a static or slowly progressive form, and (3) an adult-onset form.[51-64]

The severe infantile form is characterized by severe generalized weakness and hypotonia at birth. Muscle stretch and Moro reflexes are usually absent. Affected infants have a weak cry and suck. Because of ventilatory muscle

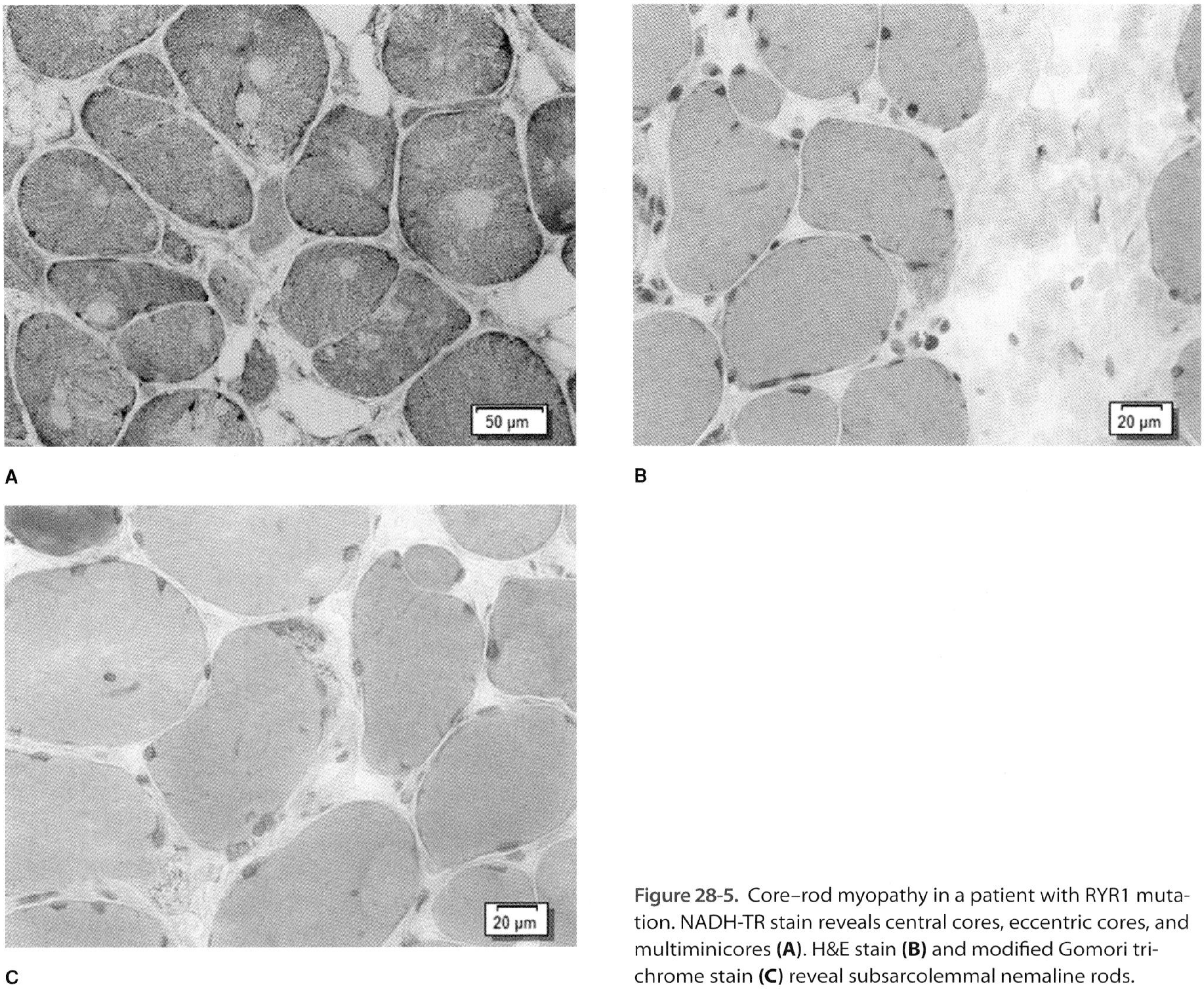

Figure 28-5. Core–rod myopathy in a patient with RYR1 mutation. NADH-TR stain reveals central cores, eccentric cores, and multiminicores **(A)**. H&E stain **(B)** and modified Gomori trichrome stain **(C)** reveal subsarcolemmal nemaline rods.

involvement, they often need to be mechanically ventilated. Most children with this severe infantile-onset form of nemaline myopathy die in the first year of life due to ventilatory complications. Arthrogryposis, neonatal ventilatory failure, and failure to achieve early motor milestones are associated with early mortality.[57] Most are inherited in an autosomal-recessive pattern, but autosomal-dominant inheritance also occurs.[1–3]

More commonly, nemaline myopathy manifests as mild, nonprogressive, or slowly progressive weakness beginning in infancy or early childhood. Both proximal and distal extremity muscles are affected and associated with generalized reduction in muscle bulk. Some patients have a facioscapuloperoneal distribution of weakness. Motor milestones are often delayed, and the children may exhibit a wide-based, waddling, hyperlordotic gait. Slight facial and masticatory muscle weakness may be appreciated, but ptosis and extraocular weakness are not typical. Many have a characteristic dysmorphic narrow facies with high-arched palate and micrognathia. In addition, multiple skeletal deformities such as pectus excavatum, kyphoscoliosis, temporal mandibular ankylosis, pes cavus, or club feet are common. Deep tendon reflexes are reduced or absent.

The adult-onset type of nemaline rod myopathy is associated with mild proximal and occasionally distally predominant muscle weakness presenting in adulthood. Some patients have minimal skeletal muscle weakness but manifest with a cardiomyopathy. The adult-onset form is not associated with dysmorphic facial features or skeletal deformities typical of the early-onset forms.

LABORATORY FEATURES

The serum CK level is normal or slightly elevated. NCS are usually normal. Early recruitment of small-amplitude, short-duration MUAPs are appreciated in weak muscles on EMG. In the severe infantile forms, EMG may demonstrate increased insertional and spontaneous activity in the form of

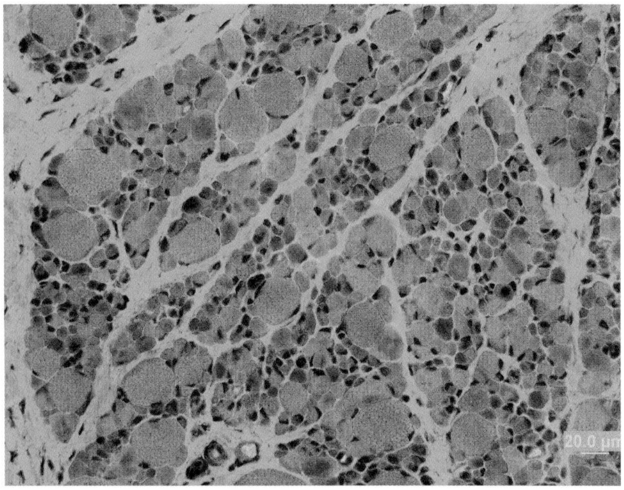

A

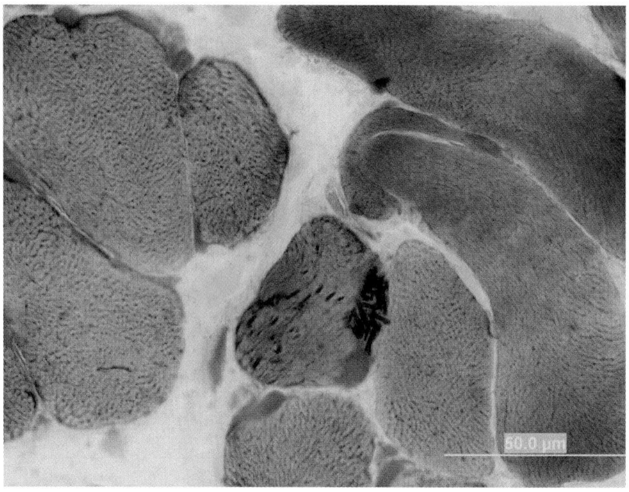

B

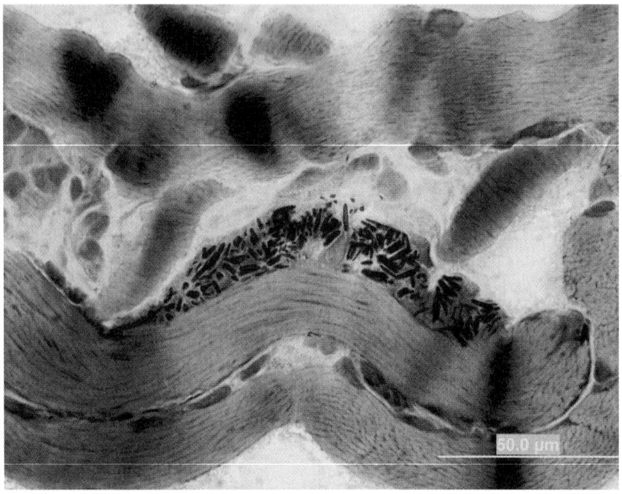

C

Figure 28-6. Nemaline myopathy. Infantile nemaline myopathy demonstrates many hypotrophic fibers **(A)**. In an adult-onset nemaline myopathy, high-power light microscopy reveals subsarcolemmal cluster of bluish-purple staining rods in cross section **(B)** and on longitudinal sections **(C)**. Modified Gomori trichrome stain.

fibrillation potentials and positive sharp waves. Such abnormal spontaneous activity is usually not appreciated in the more benign forms of the myopathy.

HISTOPATHOLOGY

Muscle biopsies often reveal type 1 fiber predominance and hypotrophy in the congenital forms but not in the adult-onset form of the disease. On routine histochemistry, the nemaline rods are best appreciated on modified Gomori trichrome stain, on which the rods appear as small, red or bluish purple staining bodies in the subsarcolemma and occasionally perinuclear regions (Fig. 28-6). On EM, the typical "rod bodies" measure 3–6 μm in length and 1–3 μm in diameter, giving the appearance of threads (nemaline: Greek for "thread like"). The nemaline rods have a density similar to the Z-disc (Fig. 28-7). Intranuclear rods may be observed, and early reports suggested that these represent a marker for this severe form of the disease (Fig. 28-8).[62–64] However, intranuclear rods are not demonstrated in all severe infantile cases and can also be found in milder adult-onset cases of nemaline myopathy.[56] Immunohistochemistry reveals that the rods and Z-disc are strongly immunoreactive for α-actinin.[65] Rods are not specific for congenital nemaline myopathy and have been reported following tenotomy, in HIV-associated myopathy, myofibrillar myopathy, inclusion body myositis, and hypothyroidism.

MOLECULAR GENETICS AND PATHOGENESIS

Nemaline rods arise secondary to a derangement of proteins necessary to maintain normal Z-disc structure. The myopathy is genetically heterogeneous, with mutations having been identified in the genes that encode nebulin (*NEB*), α-tropomyosin (*TPM3*), β-tropomyosin (*TPN2*), troponin T (*TNNT1*), α-actin (*ACTA1*), Cofilin-2/(*CFL2*), Kelch repeat and BTB 13 (*KBTBD13*), and Kelch-like family member 40 and 41 (*KLHL40* and *KLHL41*) (Table 28-1).[1–3,66–85]

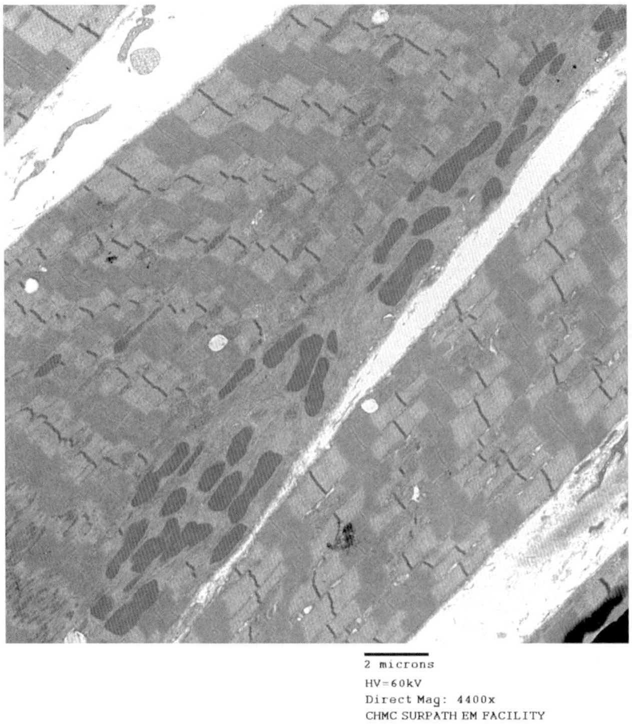

Figure 28-7. Nemaline myopathy. Electron microscopy reveals rods appearing as osmiophilic bodies, which have the same density as the Z discs.

Most of the autosomal-recessive cases (around 50%) are caused by mutations in the nebulin gene (*NEB*).[1–3,66–68] The clinical phenotype associated with nebulin mutations can be mild or severe. Mutations in the α-actin gene (*ACTA1*) can cause autosomal-recessive and autosomal-dominant nemaline myopathy.[1–3,53,69–72] *ACTA1* mutations are the second most common cause of nemaline myopathy (15–30%) but are responsible for about 50% of the severe lethal congenital-onset cases. The severity of the disease ranges from lack of spontaneous movements at birth requiring immediate mechanical ventilation to mild disease compatible with life to adulthood. There are rare reported cases with adult onset as well.[53] Mutations in the *ACTA1* gene are also responsible for previously reported cases of "congenital myopathy with excess of thin filaments."[1]

Mutations in the α-tropomyosin gene (*TPM3*) on chromosome 1q21–q23 can result in autosomal-dominant or autosomal-recessive nemaline myopathy.[73–75] The severity of cases with *TPM3* mutations vary from severe infantile to late childhood-onset, slowly progressive forms. A useful clue for *TPM3* mutations is when rods are only present in type 1 fibers as *TMP3* is not expressed in type 2 fibers. Mutations in the β-tropomyosin gene (*TPN2*) cause autosomal-dominant rod myopathy that may manifest with neck and distal lower extremity weakness (foot drop) and cardiomyopathy.[1,76] A severe, rare, infantile form of autosomal-recessive nemaline myopathy found in Amish communities is caused by mutations in the muscle troponin T (*TNNT1*) gene.[77] Mutations in the gene that encodes for the actin-binding protein, coiflin-2 (*CFL2*), have been identified nemaline myopathy and minicores.[78–80]

A recent study utilizing whole-exome sequencing found autosomal-recessive mutations in the Kelch-like family member 40 gene (*KLHL40*) in 28 apparently unrelated kindreds of various ethnicities with nemaline myopathy.[81] This accounted for 28% of the tested individuals in the Japanese cohort making *KLHL40* the most common cause of this severe form of nemaline myopathy in this population. Another study using whole-exome sequencing identified recessive small deletions and missense changes mutations in the Kelch-like family member 41 gene (*KLHL41*) in 5 unrelated individuals.[82] These studies along with cases of core–rod myopathy associated with mutations in Kelch repeat and BTB domain containing 13 (*KBTBD13*)[44] mutations suggest an importance of BTB-Kelch family members in maintenance of Z-disc and sarcomeric integrity.

As mentioned in the core–rod myopathy section, there are several other genes (*ACTA1, NEB, KBTBD13*) associated

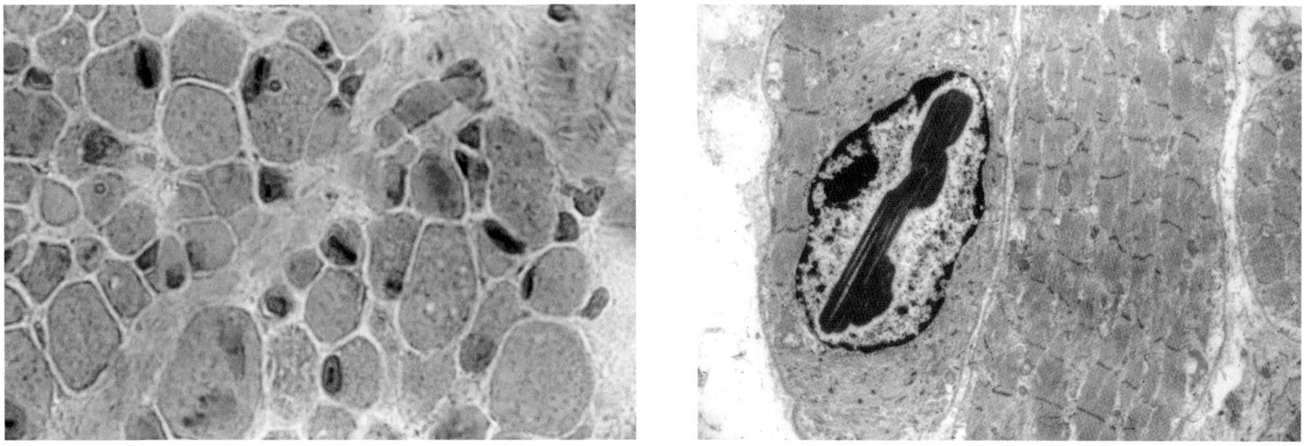

A B

Figure 28-8. Nemaline myopathy. Intranuclear rods are apparent on this modified Gomori trichrome stain **(A)** and on electron microscopy **(B)**.

with muscle biopsies showing both nemaline rods with cores. Further, both caps and nemaline rods were found in one patient caused by an autosomal-dominant mutation in the *TPM3* gene (discussed later in the Cap Myopathy section).[83]

TREATMENT

No specific medical treatment is available. Morbidity from respiratory tract infections and feeding difficulties frequently diminish with increasing age; therefore, aggressive early management is warranted in most cases of severe infantile nemaline myopathy. Individuals who are affected may benefit from physical therapy and bracing.

▶ LATE-ONSET NEMALINE MYOPATHY

CLINICAL FEATURES

This myopathy is likely distinct from the congenital, nemaline myopathy and is likely acquired as opposed to hereditary in nature. The myopathy usually presents after the age of 40 years and can begin as late as the ninth decade.[84–88] Some patients may present with isolated neck and paraspinal muscle weakness. Ventilatory muscle involvement may ensue and be cause of death, particularly in cases associated with a monoclonal gammopathy.

LABORATORY FEATURES

Serum CK is usually normal. Motor and sensory NCS are normal. EMG reveals increased insertional and spontaneous activity in the form of positive sharp waves, fibrillation potentials, and early recruitment of short-duration, small-amplitude MUAPs. About 50% of cases are associated with a monoclonal gammopathy of undetermined significance.[84–88]

HISTOPATHOLOGY

Routine light and electron microscopy demonstrates typical nemaline rods. The rods may be very short and therefore may be missed on routine light microscopy if thickness of the sections is greater than 3 μm.[84] However, the rods are almost always appreciated on EM.

MOLECULAR GENETICS AND PATHOGENESIS

This appears to be a sporadic disorder, and no genetic mutations have been reported. Thus, it may be an acquired myopathy as opposed to a hereditary disease. The relationship between the nemaline myopathy and the monoclonal gammopathy is not clear.

TREATMENT

The response to treatment with various immunotherapies in patients with late-onset nemaline myopathy with a monoclonal gammopathy is generally poor. However, some patients improved at least temporarily to intravenous immunoglobulin[86] or autologous stem cell transplantation.[87,88]

▶ CENTRONUCLEAR MYOPATHY

CLINICAL FEATURES

Spiro and colleagues first introduced the term "myotubular myopathy" to describe this myopathy, given its resemblance to myotubes on muscle biopsies.[89] However, this myopathy is not caused by an arrest of myotubes and the term "centronuclear myopathy" is more appropriate. At least three clinically different forms of the disease are recognized: (1) a slowly progressive, infantile–early childhood type; (2) a severe X-linked neonatal type; and (3) a late childhood- or adult-onset type.[1–3,89–93]

The slowly progressive, infantile–early childhood type is the most common presentation. These cases may be inherited in an autosomal-recessive or autosomal-dominant fashion. Children who are affected are usually the product of a normal pregnancy and delivery. Mild hypotonia and generalized weakness are apparent in infancy or early childhood and motor milestones are typically delayed. Ambulation is usually achieved, but the gait may be wide based and hyperlordotic. As with nemaline myopathy, generalized muscle atrophy, elongated narrow facies, and high-arched palate are often appreciated. Unlike other forms of congenital myopathy, ptosis and ophthalmoparesis are common in centronuclear myopathy. Muscle stretch reflexes are depressed or absent, but sensation is completely normal. Some children have mental retardation and seizures.

The X-linked recessive myotubular myopathy presents at birth with severe hypotonia and generalized weakness. Affected infants usually require ventilatory support and feeding tubes. Polyhydramnios is a frequent complication of the mother's pregnancy. Ptosis and ophthalmoparesis may not be apparent initially, but become more prominent after the newborn period. Arthrogryposis may be evident. X-linked myotubular myopathy is usually fatal in infancy; however, the prognosis is not invariably poor.[92,93] With aggressive medical intervention, the survival rate has increased.[93]

Interestingly, there have been a few well-described cases of manifesting females with proven X-linked (myotubularin deficiency) centronuclear myopathy.[94–96] Affected females can present with axial and proximal weakness, bilateral ptosis, and external ophthalmoplegia with onset in childhood or adult. The mechanism may be akin to skewed inactivation, as sometimes seen in manifesting female carriers of dystrophin mutations.

A more benign form of centronuclear myopathy can present in late childhood or adulthood. Muscle weakness

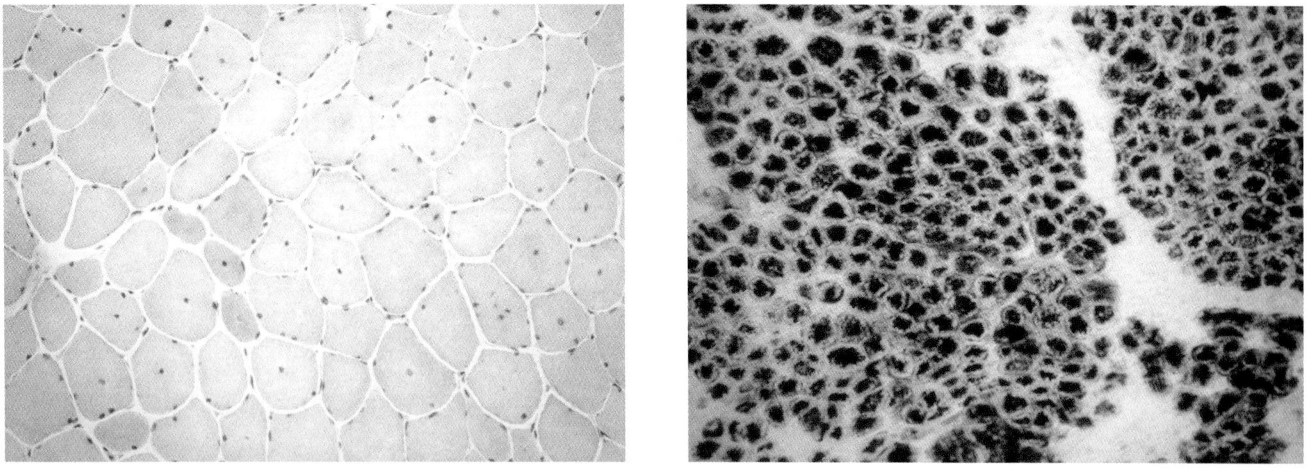

A B

Figure 28-9. Centronuclear myopathy. Increased number of internalized nuclei often in the center of the muscle fiber is appreciated **(A)**, hematoxylin and eosin (H&E). Late childhood- and adult-onset cases often have increased nuclei more randomly located throughout the fibers. Central areas appear dark on NADH-TR **(B)**.

is usually mild and only slowly progressive. The pattern of muscle weakness is quite variable, with some patients having predominantly proximal weakness, while distal muscles are more affected in others. Facial muscles may be weak, and some have ptosis and ophthalmoparesis. A facioscapulohumeral pattern of weakness has also been described.[97] Unlike infantile- and childhood-onset cases, dysmorphic facial features and skeletal anomalies are not associated with the adult-onset form of centronuclear myopathy. Some of these cases are felt to be autosomal-dominantly inherited.

LABORATORY FEATURES

Serum CK is normal or slightly elevated. Motor and sensory NCS are normal. However, EMG is usually very abnormal, particularly in the severe X-linked infantile-onset form, revealing increased insertional and spontaneous activity in the form of positive sharp waves, fibrillation potentials, complex repetitive discharges, and even myotonic discharges.[8] Early recruitment of short-duration, small-amplitude MUAPs are evident in weak muscles. Reduced amplitudes and mild slowing of motor and sensory NCS have been noted in some individuals with mutations in dynamin-2 gene (discussed in "Pathogenesis" section), which is not surprising, as this is also a cause of dominant intermediate Charcot–Marie–Tooth disease type B (DI-CMTB).

HISTOPATHOLOGY

Muscle biopsies reveal myonuclei in the center of muscle fibers, often forming chains when viewed longitudinally.[1–3,91] The type 1 fibers predominate and appear hypotrophic, while the type 2 fibers are normal in size. In cases associated with *BIN1* mutations, the nuclei often cluster in the center of the fiber rather than forming longitudinal chains. On transverse section, the number of muscle fibers with central nuclei range from 25% to 95% (Fig. 28-9A). The central nuclei appear in both fiber types. On ATPase stains, there is a small perinuclear halo devoid of ATPase activity. With oxidative enzyme stains, the center of muscle fibers appear dark (Fig. 28-9B). There can also be is a radial arrangement of the intermyofibrillar network, which resembles spokes on a wheel, in cases caused by dynamin-2 (*DYN2)* mutations (Fig. 28-10). Necklace fibers, in which there are rings/loops of oxidative enzyme staining internally within fibers, can be found in late-onset centronuclear myopathy and obligate

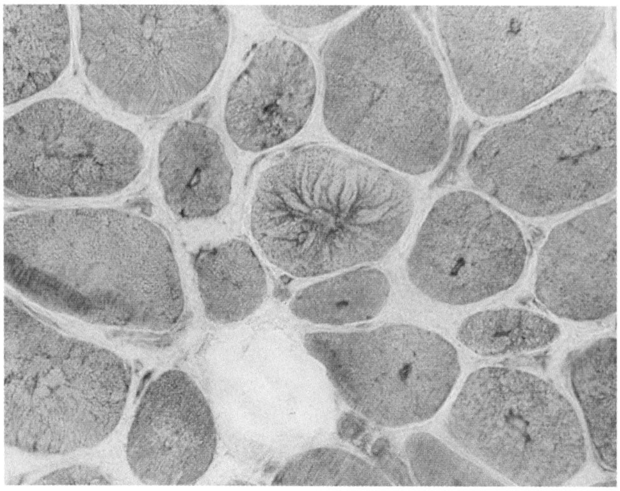

Figure 28-10. Radial spirals. Muscle biopsy in a patient with centronuclear myopathy caused by dynamin-2 (*DYN2)* mutations has radial spirals on NADH-TR. The radial arrangement of the intermyofibrillar network resembles spokes on a wheel.

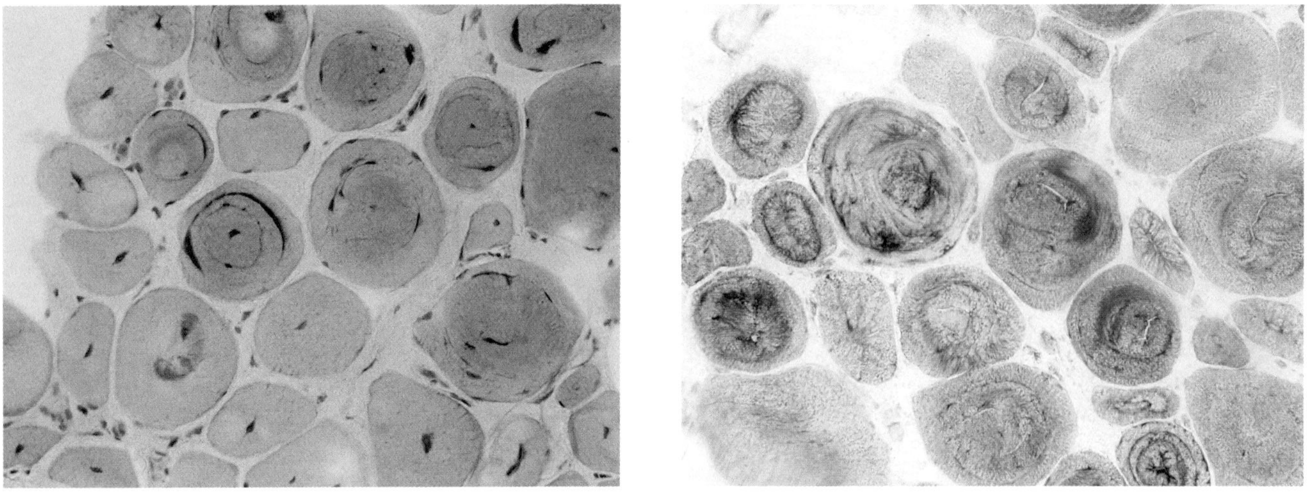

A B

Figure 28-11. Necklace fibers. Muscle biopsy of a patient with centronuclear myopathy caused by dynamin-2 *(DYN2)* mutations has necklace fibers that appear as internal rings/loops within fibers seen here on H&E **(A)** and NADH-TR **(B)** stains.

women carriers with myotubularin 1 (*MTM1*) mutations and in individuals with *DYN2* mutations (see below) (Fig. 28-11).[1-3,93] There can be increased endomysial connective tissue as can be seen in muscular dystrophies. On EM, there are reduced myofibrils and an excess of mitochondria and glycogen granules in the center of muscle fibers that are not occupied by nuclei.

MOLECULAR GENETICS AND PATHOGENESIS

As noted previously, there is genetic heterogeneity in centronuclear myopathy (Table 28-1). The severe X-linked neonatal form is caused by mutations in the myotubularin 1 gene (*MTM1*).[1-3,98,99] Myotubularin is a dual-specificity phosphatase, which plays a role in muscle cell growth and differentiation. Terminal muscle fiber differentiation is dependent on the hypophosphorylation of specific gene-regulating proteins.[100] Myotubularin is thought to dephosphorylate these regulating proteins, and mutations in the myotubularin gene lead to loss of function of this phosphatase activity, resulting in maturational disturbances of muscle.

Some autosomal-dominant cases of late-onset centronuclear myopathy characterized by prominent distal limb weakness and ptosis have been linked to mutations in the *DYN2* gene on chromosome 19p13.2, which encodes for dynamin-2.[90,101] Mutations in this gene have also been reported in cases of severe neonatal centronuclear myopathy. Of note, mutations in *DYN2* cause dominant intermediate Charcot–Marie–Tooth disease B (DI-CMTB),[102] thus explaining some of the overlapping features (distal weakness, mild sensory abnormalities) that might be seen. Dynamin-2 belongs to the family of large GTPases and is important in endocytosis, membrane trafficking, actin assembly, and centrosome cohesion.[90]

Rare cases of autosomal-recessive centronuclear myopathy have been reported associated with *RYR1*, amphiphysin 2 (*BIN2*), and titin (*TTN*) mutations.[1,2,103-106]

TREATMENT

Infants with the X-linked form of the disease often require mechanical ventilation and tube feedings to support life. With such aggressive medical intervention, the survival rate has increased.[92]

▶ CONGENITAL FIBER-TYPE DISPROPORTION

CLINICAL FEATURES

Congenital fiber-type disproportion usually manifests as generalized hypotonia and weakness along with a weak cry and suck in infancy.[1-3] Motor milestones are delayed, but muscle weakness is usually nonprogressive and functional status improves with age attained. However, there are cases with a progressive and sometimes fatal course secondary to ventilatory muscle insufficiency.[107] Some children who are affected display dysmorphic facial features with a high-arched palate, congenital hip dislocations, kyphoscoliosis, arthrogryposis, and a rigid spine. Muscle stretch reflexes are reduced. Approximately one-third of affected children have some type of central nervous system abnormalities; some of these cases may represent forms of congenital muscular dystrophy with impaired glycosylation of α-dystroglycan (see Chapter 27).

LABORATORY FEATURES

The serum CK is normal or mildly elevated. NCS are normal. EMG can be normal or can reveal increased insertional and spontaneous activity and early recruitment of myopathic MUAPs.[8]

HISTOPATHOLOGY

Muscle biopsies reveal disproportionate atrophy of type 1 compared to type 2 fibers.[107] While type 1 fibers are more numerous, they are typically less than 15% the diameter of type 2 fibers, which appear normal in size or slightly hypertrophic (Fig. 28-12). However, type 1 fiber predominance and hypotrophy are not specific for this myopathy, and these are also common in centronuclear, central core, nemaline, and fingerprint body myopathy and may also be found in congenital muscular dystrophies, spinal muscular atrophy, and central nervous system disease. With sequential muscle biopsies, nemaline rods or central nuclei may become apparent.[108] No consistent ultrastructural abnormalities have been noted.

MOLECULAR GENETICS AND PATHOGENESIS

Mutations in *TPM3* are the most common cause accounting for 25–50% of cases and are autosomal dominant in inheritance.[1-3] The second most common cause are mutations in *RYR1* that are inherited in an autosomal-recessive fashion and account for approximately 20% of cases.[1-3] Mutations in *ACTA1*, *SEPN1*, *MYL2*, and *TPM2* account for most of the remaining cases.[1-3,109-112]

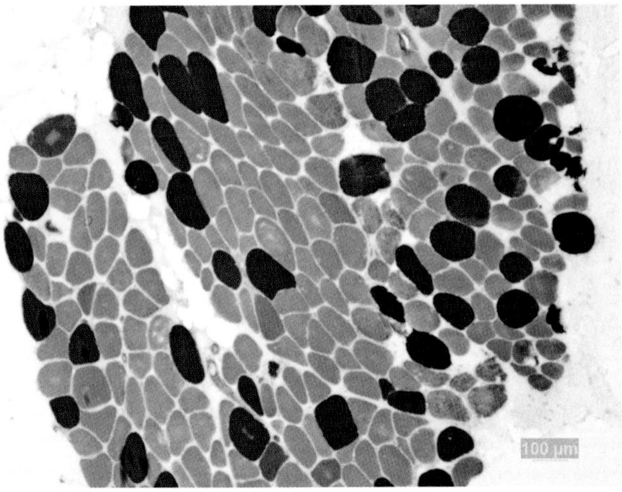

Figure 28-12. Congenital fiber-type disproportion. Type 1 fibers are more numerous but smaller in diameter than the type 2 fibers. However, type 1 fiber predominance and hypotrophy are not specific for this myopathy, and these are also common in other forms of congenital myopathy and congenital muscular dystrophy. ATPase 9.4.

TREATMENT

Supportive measures in regard to mechanical ventilation and tube feeding may be temporarily required in some patients. Physical therapy and orthotic devices may be beneficial.

► SARCOTUBULAR MYOPATHY

CLINICAL FEATURES

Sarcotubular myopathy was initially reported in two Hutterite brothers of a consanguineous marriage.[112] Subsequently, it has been demonstrated that this disorder is allelic to LGMD2H.[113] Patients can present with exertional myalgias or proximal muscle weakness in infancy or adult life. Scapular winging, calf hypertrophy, foot drop, and mild facial weakness may be appreciated. Muscle stretch reflexes are usually diminished.

LABORATORY FEATURES

Serum CK levels have ranged from normal to 20-fold elevated.[112,113] EMG may be normal or may reveal myopathic features.

HISTOPATHOLOGY

Muscle biopsy reveal increase in internal nuclei, muscle fiber splitting, and many fibers (mostly type 2) with small vacuoles.[112,113] These vacuoles, which abut T-tubules, appear to be membrane bound, and are empty or contain a small amount of amorphous debris on EM. The vacuoles immunostain for sarcoplasmic reticulum-associated ATPase.

MOLECULAR GENETICS AND PATHOGENESIS

Mutations in *TRIM32*, the gene encoding the tripartite motif-containing protein 32, have been demonstrated; thus, this disorder is allelic to LGMDH.[113] The TRIM 32 protein may be critical for the recognition of other protein(s) targeted to be ubiquitinated by this ligase enzyme.

TREATMENT

There is no specific medical treatment.

▶ FINGERPRINT BODY MYOPATHY

CLINICAL FEATURES

Fingerprint body myopathy is a rare disorder and typically presents as generalized hypotonia, weakness, and muscle atrophy in infancy or early childhood.[114–116] Muscle strength is stable or only slowly deteriorates over time. Muscle stretch reflexes are reduced or absent. Some individuals have a reduced intelligence and febrile seizures. In addition, kyphoscoliosis and pectus excavatum may be evident in some cases.

LABORATORY FEATURES

Serum CKs are normal or slightly elevated. NCS are normal. EMG may be normal or may demonstrate short-duration, low-amplitude MUAPs without abnormal insertional or spontaneous activity.

HISTOPATHOLOGY

Muscle biopsy reveals type 1 fiber predominance with type 1 fiber hypotrophy and type 2 fiber hypertrophy. On oxidative enzyme stains, there is reduced activity in the subsarcolemma and perinuclear regions in type 1 fibers. EM and phase-contrast microscopy demonstrate a complex lamellar pattern resembling fingerprints that are evident in these areas; these fingerprint bodies appear to be composed of cytoskeletal proteins.[114–116] Fingerprint bodies are nonspecific and have also been noted in myotonic dystrophy, various distal myopathies, nemaline myopathy, dermatomyositis, oculopharyngeal dystrophy, and muscle biopsies from patients with uremia and chronic pulmonary disease.

MOLECULAR GENETICS AND PATHOGENESIS

Most of the cases have been sporadic, although the disease was reported in a pair of male identical twins[114] and in two siblings.[116] The pathogenic mechanism for the formation of the fingerprint bodies is not known.

TREATMENT

There is no specific medical treatment.

▶ TRILAMINAR MYOPATHY

CLINICAL FEATURES

A single infant with rigidity of its trunk and limbs, decreased spontaneous movements, weak suck and swallowing, and numerous joint contractures has been reported with this disorder.[117] Sensation appeared normal and deep tendon reflexes were intact. By 10 months of age, the infant had some head control, but was still unable to sit. Subsequently, the patient was able to ambulate, albeit with difficulty.

LABORATORY FEATURES

Serum CK was markedly elevated at birth (approximately 40 times normal). EMG and NCS were normal.

HISTOPATHOLOGY

Muscle biopsy demonstrated variability in fiber size. The unique feature was that approximately 25% of fibers were hypertrophic and had three concentric zones that displayed a differential staining pattern.[117] The inner and outer zones stained intensely with Gomori trichrome and NADH stains, while the inverse pattern was seen on ATPase staining. On EM, the innermost zone demonstrated myofibrillar disarray and densely packed mitochondria, glycogen granules, and myofilaments. The intermediate zone revealed Z-band streaming. The outer zone was composed of disorganized myofibrils, mitochondria, lipid droplets, and vesicles.

MOLECULAR GENETICS AND PATHOGENESIS

The pathogenesis is unknown.

TREATMENT

No specific medical treatment is available.

▶ HYALINE BODY MYOPATHY/FAMILIAL MYOPATHY WITH LYSIS OF MYOFIBRILS/ MYOSIN STORAGE MYOPATHY

CLINICAL FEATURES

Hyaline body myopathy is a rare congenital myopathy, which can present in infancy to as late as the fifth decade of life with limb-girdle or scapuloperoneal pattern of weakness.[118–123] Muscle strength is stable or only slowly deteriorates and is nonprogressive. Rare patients have a cardiomyopathy.[123] Muscle stretch reflexes are preserved. Hyaline body myopathy has been reported as occurring sporadically as well as being inherited in an autosomal-dominant or autosomal-recessive fashion. There is variability in the severity of the course even within families.

LABORATORY FEATURES

Serum CK levels can be normal or mildly elevated, while EMG studies may be normal or may reveal an increased number of small-duration, low-amplitude, polyphasic MUAPs. Echocardiography may reveal a dilated cardiomyopathy with reduced ejection fraction.

HISTOPATHOLOGY

Muscle biopsies reveal subsarcolemmal "hyaline" bodies that stain pale green on modified Gomori trichrome and pale pink on H&E stains (Fig. 28-13).[118–123] The hyaline bodies occur in type 1 fibers, which are hypotrophic. The hyaline bodies do not stain with oxidative enzymes or periodic acid Schiff (PAS), but demonstrate intense ATPase activity. Angulated neurogenic fibers and fiber-type grouping may also be appreciated. Immunostaining demonstrates strong reactivity for slow myosin heavy chain (MyHC) in some but not all hyaline bodies.[120] The hyaline bodies are nonreactive for αB-crystallin, ubiquitin, tropomyosin, actins, desmin, and components of sarcolemma. On EM, the hyaline bodies appear to be composed of granulofilamentous debris often with fragments of sarcomeres and surrounded by a zone of sarcomeric disorganization.[120]

MOLECULAR GENETICS AND PATHOGENESIS

Missense mutations in the *MYH7* gene that encodes for slow/β-cardiac MyHC cause most cases of autosomal-dominant hyaline body myopathy.[119–123] Mutations in this gene also have been associated with a familial form of cardiomyopathy and Laing-type distal myopathy/dystrophy (see Chapter 27).

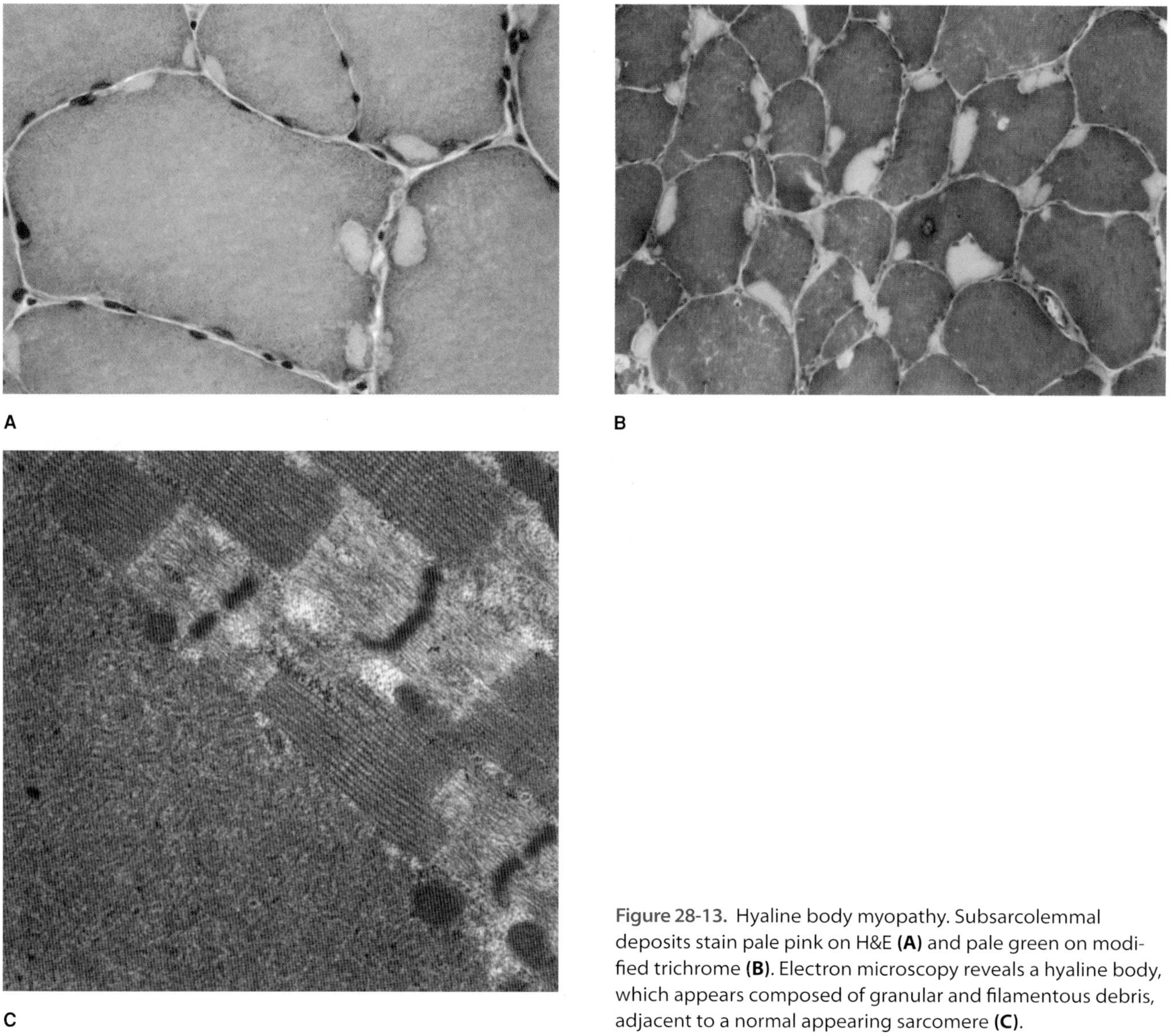

Figure 28-13. Hyaline body myopathy. Subsarcolemmal deposits stain pale pink on H&E **(A)** and pale green on modified trichrome **(B)**. Electron microscopy reveals a hyaline body, which appears composed of granular and filamentous debris, adjacent to a normal appearing sarcomere **(C)**.

Interestingly, despite extensive workup, cardiomyopathy has not been reported in patients with hyaline body myopathy harboring mutations in this gene.[119,123] *MYH7* encodes the major myosin isoform seen in type 1 muscle fibers and cardiac muscle. Within this region lies a candidate who exhibits homology to the MyHC. It appears that normal MyHC is essential for the assembly of thick filaments in skeletal muscle.

TREATMENT

There is no specific medical treatment available.

▶ OTHER MYOSIN STORAGE DISORDERS

Another autosomal-dominant myopathy characterized by mild weakness and myalgias with onset in childhood or early adult life has been linked to mutations in the *MYH2* gene, which encodes for MyHC IIa.[124,125] The MyHC IIa isoform of MyHCs is expressed in type 2 A muscle fibers. Other families present with congenital arthrogryposis, ophthalmoplegia, and mild proximal weakness beginning in adulthood. As muscle biopsies may demonstrate rimmed vacuoles and tubulofilamentous inclusions, this disorder has also been called hereditary inclusion body myopathy type 3 (see Chapter 27).[126,127]

▶ CAP MYOPATHY

CLINICAL FEATURES

The clinical features of this rare myopathy overlap with those seen in nemaline myopathy given the causal genes are similar. It is usually associated with neonatal onset of generalized muscle weakness and hypotonia associated with skeletal deformities and reduced muscle stretch reflexes.[1,2,128–136] Ventilatory muscles are also frequently affected.

LABORATORY FEATURES

Serum CK is normal. NCS are normal, while EMG demonstrates myopathic MUAPs.

HISTOPATHOLOGY

Muscle biopsies reveal many muscle fibers that contain a peripheral crescent that reacts strongly to NADH-TR, PAS, and phosphorylase, but not to SDH or myofibrillar ATPase. Immunohistochemistry reveals that these "caps" display increased fast-myosin activity, desmin, tropomyosin, and α-actinin.[129] On EM, there is widened Z-bands, disarray of the myofibrils, and lack of thick filaments.

MOLECULAR GENETICS AND PATHOGENESIS

This myopathy is most often caused by mutations in *TPM2*, but also has been reported with *TMP3* and *ACTA1* mutations each of which are more commonly associated with nemaline myopathy.[1,2,130–134] Both caps and nemaline rods were found in one patient caused by an autosomal-dominant mutation in the *TPM3* gene.[83]

TREATMENT

There is no specific medical treatment available.

▶ ZEBRA BODY MYOPATHY

CLINICAL FEATURES

Only a few of cases of zebra body myopathy have been reported.[137,138] One child presented with generalized weakness and atrophy from birth.[137] The second report involved a child with severe hypotonia, dysphagia, and asymmetric weakness of the upper limbs.[138] Muscle weakness was stable or only slowly progressive.

LABORATORY FEATURES

Serum CK is two to three times normal. EMG reveals myopathic units without abnormal spontaneous activity.

HISTOPATHOLOGY

Muscle biopsies demonstrate variability in muscle fiber size, increased internal nuclei, and occasional vacuoles. The Z-bodies appear on EM as osmiophilic 270-mm stria, with a periodicity such that these resemble stripes on a zebra.[137,138] The density of the stria is that of Z-discs and measuring up to 2 nm in length. Streaming of the Z-bands and nemaline rods may also be appreciated.

MOLECULAR GENETICS AND PATHOGENESIS

Zebra bodies are associated with mutations in *ACTA1*. However, they are not a specific abnormality and can be found in normal individuals at myotendinous junctions, in intrafusal fibers (muscle spindles), in extraocular muscles, and in cardiac muscles. These may also be found in other pathologic conditions (e.g., myofibrillar myopathy).

TREATMENT

There is no specific medical treatment available.

▶ TUBULAR AGGREGATE MYOPATHY

CLINICAL FEATURES

Tubular aggregates are a nonspecific histologic abnormality, which may be found in muscle biopsies of patients with hereditary periodic paralysis, hyperthyroidism, congenital myasthenia (slow channel syndrome), hypoxia, and some toxic myopathies. In addition, tubular aggregates are also found on muscle biopsy of patients with no symptoms or signs of a myopathy. However, there are at least three clinical syndromes in which the primary pathologic feature is tubular aggregates on muscle biopsy.[139–141] Individuals who are affected may have slow progressive limb-girdle weakness beginning in childhood or early adulthood. In addition, there is a form that resembles congenital myasthenia, which presents with slowly progressive muscle weakness from infancy.[140] These patients demonstrate fatigable weakness, which improves with anticholinesterase medications. Another clinical subgroup comprises patients with generalized myalgias, which are worse with exertion.[139] Muscle tone, bulk, and strength are normal as is the rest of the physical examination. In addition, there is a rare tubular aggregate myopathy associated with immunodeficiency—one such subtype also is associated with miosis.

LABORATORY FEATURES

Serum CK is normal or mildly increased. Routine motor and sensory NCS are normal. Patients with the myasthenic syndrome demonstrate a decremental response on repetitive stimulation, which improves with pyridostigmine. EMG can be normal or can demonstrate myopathic MUAPs and fibrillation potentials. Patients with the muscle-pain syndrome typically have completely normal electrodiagnostic findings.

HISTOPATHOLOGY

Tubular aggregates stain basophilic on H&E and are red on modified Gomori trichrome (Fig. 28-14A). These react intensely to NADH-TR (Fig. 28-14B), but not to SDH. Tubular aggregates are located in a subsarcolemmal position and are present only in type 2 muscle fibers in the syndromes associated with periodic paralysis and muscle pain but are evident in both fiber types in the limb-girdle syndrome. On EM, the aggregates are composed of bundles of tubules 60–80 nm in diameter, which course in various directions with respect to the long axis of the muscle fibers (Fig. 28-15).

MOLECULAR GENETICS AND PATHOGENESIS

Mutations in the gene that encodes for stromal interaction molecule 1, *STIM1*, cause a dominantly inherited tubular aggregate myopathy associated with immunodeficiency.[142,143] STIM1 regulates calcium in the endoplasmic reticulum. Mutations in the gene that encodes for Orai-1, *ORAI1*, are also associated with an autosomal-dominant tubular aggregate myopathy associated with immune deficiency along with miosis.[144] Some forms of congenital myasthenia, which can easily be mistaken for a congenital myopathy, if one does not appreciate fatigability or decrement on repetitive nerve stimulation, are associated with tubular aggregates.[145–147] These include mutations in the genes that encode for UDP-N-acetylglucosamine-dolichyl-phosphate, N-acetylglucosaminephosphotransferase 1 (*DPAGT1*)[145,146] and glutamine-fructose-6-phosphate transaminase 1 (*GFPT1*).[147]

TREATMENT

Patients with the congenital myasthenic syndrome may benefit from pyridostigmine. Individuals with the muscle pain syndrome may improve with dantrolene or tricyclic antidepressant medications.

▶ REDUCING BODY MYOPATHY

CLINICAL FEATURES

Reducing body myopathy is a rare disorder that has varied clinical presentations.[148–152] It can present in infancy with severe generalized weakness, hypotonia, and joint contractures. Ptosis may be apparent as well. There is an increased mortality due to associated ventilatory muscle weakness. Some affected individuals apparently develop muscle weakness later in childhood or in adulthood. The proximal or distal muscles may be preferentially affected, and involvement can be asymmetric, particularly in the arms. The course can vary from mild stable weakness to progressive deterioration of strength, leading to death. Some affected patients develop contractures of the major joints, scoliosis, and rigidity of the spine.

LABORATORY FEATURES

Serum CK levels are usually normal, although a few patients have demonstrated mild elevations. NCS are normal. EMG may demonstrate myopathic features.

HISTOPATHOLOGY

The characteristic feature on muscle biopsies are "reducing bodies," named such because of their unique ability to reduce nitroblue tetrazolium when mediated by menadione.[148–151] These reducing bodies stain purple with modified Gomori trichrome stain and pink on H&E stain and are devoid of oxidative enzyme staining. Immunohistochemistry reveals increased desmin at the periphery of some reducing bodies, but αB-crystallin, α-actinin, titin, and nebulin immunostains

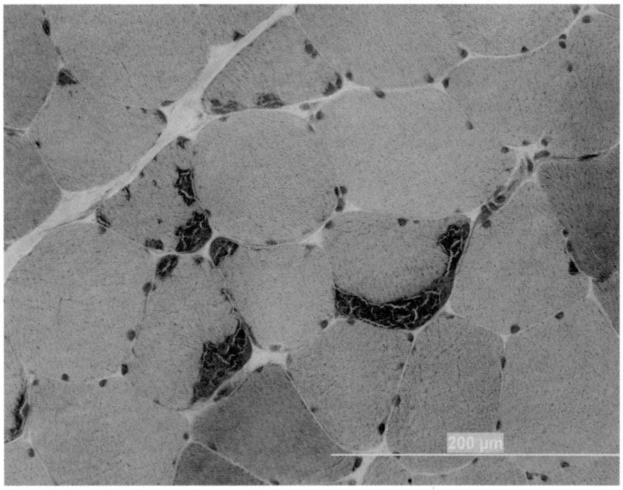

A

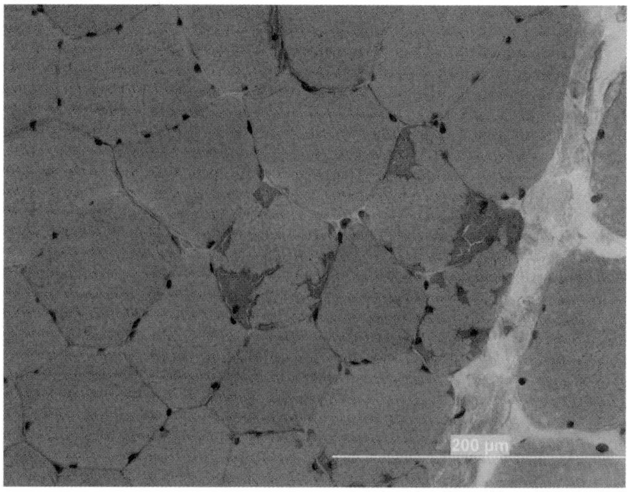

B

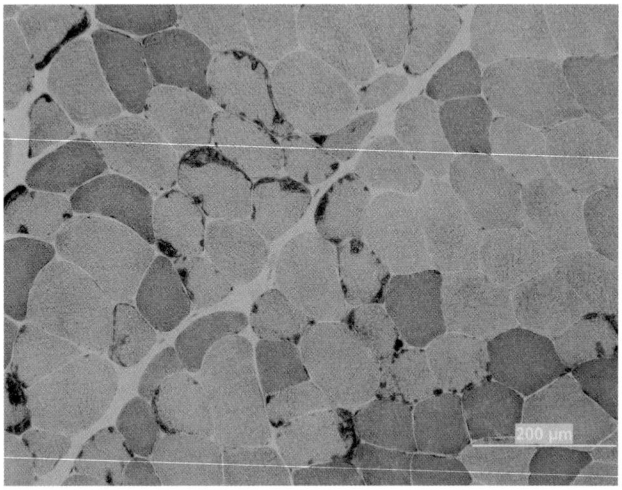

C

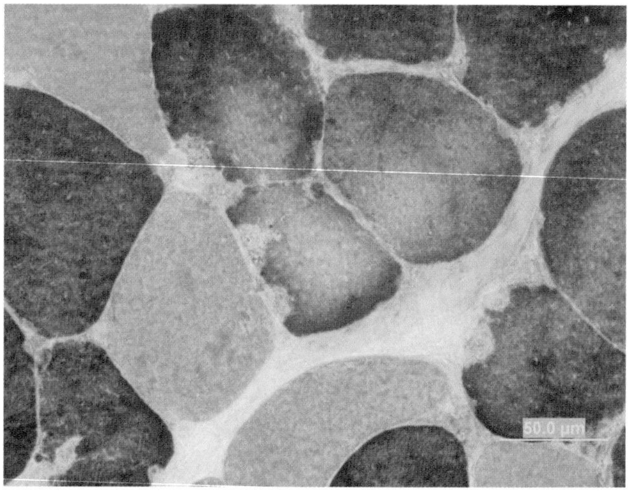

D

Figure 28-14. Tubular aggregates. Tubular aggregates appear as subsarcolemmal masses of reddish material on modified trichome **(A)** and are bluish on H&E **(B)**. The tubular aggregates occur only in type 2 fibers and appear densely staining on NADH-TR **(C)**, but do not stain with ATPase 9.4 **(D)**.

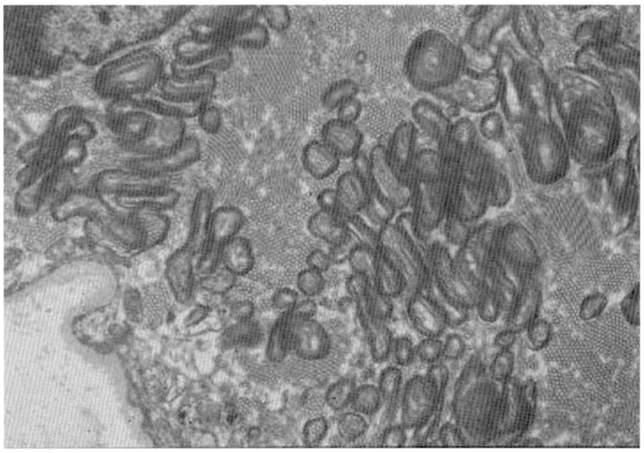

Figure 28-15. Tubular aggregates. On EM, tubular aggregates appear as subsarcolemmal aggregates of long, straight parallel tubules, which are somewhat haphazardly oriented in small bundles.

are normal. There is usually type 1 fiber predominance as seen in most other congenital myopathies, but the reducing bodies are evident in both fiber types. On EM, the reducing bodies appear to be composed of electron-dense granules and 12–17-nm tubulofilaments.

MOLECULAR GENETICS AND PATHOGENESIS

This rare disorder is usually caused by mutations in the four and a half LIM gene, (*FHL1*), located on chromosome Xq26.3 that encodes for four and a half LIM.[153–158] Rare cases of reducing body myopathy have also been reported with mutations in the desmin gene (*DES*).[159] In many ways the histopathology resembles in part what is in myofibrillar myopathy (discussed in Chapter 27).

TREATMENT

No specific treatment is available.

▶ MYOFIBRILLAR MYOPATHY

This is a genetically heterogeneous group of disorders, which are now considered to be forms of muscular dystrophy as opposed to congenital myopathies and are discussed in detail in Chapter 27.

▶ SUMMARY

As evident from this chapter, there is significant overlap in what have previously been termed congenital myopathies and congenital and limb-girdle dystrophies. Continued advances in molecular genetics have provided and will likely provide better insight into the classification of these myopathies. Unfortunately, there are no medications as yet available to successfully treat these disorders. However, physical and occupational therapy as outlined in Chapter 5 as well as supportive therapy for ventilatory or cardiac muscle involvement can be beneficial.

REFERENCES

1. North KN, Wang CH, Clarke N, et al. Approach to the diagnosis of congenital myopathies. *Neuromuscul Disord.* 2014;24(2): 97–116.
2. Romero NB, Clarke NF. Congenital myopathies. *Handb Clin Neurol.* 2013;113:1321–1336.
3. Iannaccone ST, Castro D. Congenital muscular dystrophies and congenital myopathies. *Continuum (Minneap Minn).* 2013; 19(6 Muscle Disease):1509–1534.
4. Isaacs H, Heffron JJ, Badenhorst M. Central core disease. A correlated genetic, histochemical, ultramicroscopic, and biochemical study. *J Neurol Neurosurg Psychiatry.* 1975;38(12):1177–1186.
5. Magee KR, Shy GM. A new congenital non-progressive myopathy. *Brain.* 1956;79(4):610–621.
6. Quinlivan RM, Muller CR, Davis M, et al. Central core disease: clinical, pathological, and genetic features. *Arch Dis Child.* 2003;88(12):1051–1055.
7. Bharucha-Goebel DX, Santi M, Medne L, et al. Severe congenital RYR1-associated myopathy: the expanding clinicopathologic and genetic spectrum. *Neurology.* 2013;80(17): 1584–1589.
8. Amato A, Dumitru D. *Hereditary Myopathies.* Philadelphia, PA: Hanley & Belfus; 2002.
9. Sewry CA, Muller C, Davis M, et al. The spectrum of pathology in central core disease. *Neuromuscul Disord.* 2002;12(10): 930–938.
10. Ferreiro A, Monnier N, Romero NB, et al. A recessive form of central core disease, transiently presenting as multi-minicore disease, is associated with a homozygous mutation in the ryanodine receptor type 1 gene. *Ann Neurol.* 2002;51(6):750–759.
11. De Bleecker JL, Ertl BB, Engel AG, et al. Patterns of abnormal protein expression in target formations and unstructured cores. *Neuromuscul Disord.* 1996;6(5):339–349.
12. Robinson R, Carpenter D, Shaw MA, Halsall J, Hopkins P. Mutations in RYR1 in malignant hyperthermia and central core disease. *Hum Mutat.* 2006;27:977–989.
13. Wu S, Ibarra MC, Malicdan MC, et al. Central core disease is due to RYR1 mutations in more than 90% of patients. *Brain.* 2006;129:1470–1480.
14. Monnier N, Marty I, Faure J, et al. Null mutations causing depletion of the type 1 ryanodine receptor (RYR1) are commonly associated with recessive structural congenital myopathies with cores. *Hum Mutat.* 2008;29:670–678.
15. Monnier N, Laquerriere A, Marret S, et al. First genomic rearrangement of the RYR1 gene associated with an atypical presentation of lethal neonatal hypotonia. *Neuromuscul Disord.* 2009;19:680–684.
16. Zhou H, Brockington M, Jungbluth H, et al. Epigenetic allele silencing unveils recessive RYR1 mutations in core myopathies. *Am J Hum Genet.* 2006;79:859–868.
17. Mathews KD, Moore SA. Multiminicore myopathy, central core disease, malignant hyperthermia susceptibility, and RYR1 mutations: one disease with many faces? *Arch Neurol.* 2004;61(1):27–29.
18. Avila G. Intracellular Ca^{2+} dynamics in malignant hyperthermia and central core disease: established concepts, new cellular mechanisms involved. *Cell Calcium.* 2005;37(2):121–127.
19. Avila G, O'Connell KM, Dirksen RT, et al. The pore region of the skeletal muscle ryanodine receptor is a primary locus for excitation-contraction uncoupling in central core disease. *J Gen Physiol.* 2003;121(4):277–286.
20. Romero NB, Xie T, Malfatti E, et al. Autosomal dominant eccentric core disease caused by a heterozygous mutation in the MYH7 gene. *J Neurol Neurosurg Psychiatry.* 2014;85(10):1149–1152.
21. Kaindl AM, Ruschendorf F, Krause S, et al. Missense mutations of ACTA1 cause dominant congenital myopathy with cores. *J Med Genet.* 2004;41:842–848.
22. Majczenko K, Davidson AE, Camelo-Piragua S, et al. Dominant mutation of CCDC78 in a unique congenital myopathy with prominent internal nuclei and atypical cores. *Am J Hum Genet.* 2012;91(2):365–371.
23. Engel AG, Gomez MR, Groover RV, et al. Multicore disease. A recently recognized congenital myopathy associated with multifocal degeneration of muscle fibers. *Mayo Clin Proc.* 1971;46(10):666–681.
24. Ferreiro A, Estournet B, Chateau D, et al. Multi-minicore disease–searching for boundaries: phenotype analysis of 38 cases. *Ann Neurol.* 2000;48(5):745–757.
25. Ferreiro A, Fardeau M. 80th ENMC international workshop on multi-minicore disease: 1st international MmD workshop. 12–13th May,. 2000, Soestduinen, The Netherlands. *Neuromuscul Disord.* 2002;12(1):60–68.
26. Jungbluth H, Beggs A, Bönnemann C, et al. 111th ENMC International Workshop on Multi-minicore Disease. 2nd International MmD Workshop, 9–11 November. 2002, Naarden, The Netherlands. *Neuromuscul Disord.* 2004;14(11):754–766.
27. Jungbluth H, Sewry C, Brown SC, et al. Minicore myopathy in children: a clinical and histopathological study of 19 cases. *Neuromuscul Disord.* 2000;10(4–5):264–273.
28. Zeman AZ, Dick DJ, Anderson JR, Watkin SW, Smith IE, Shneerson JM. Multicore myopathy presenting in adulthood with respiratory failure. *Muscle Nerve.* 1997;20(3):367–369.

29. Monnier N, Ferreiro A, Marty I, Labarre-Vila A, Mezin P, Lunardi J. A homozygous splicing mutation causing a depletion of skeletal muscle RYR1 is associated with multi-minicore disease congenital myopathy with ophthalmoplegia. *Hum Mol Genet.* 2003;12(10):1171–1178.
30. Ferreiro A, Quijano-Roy S, Pichereau C et al. Mutations of the selenoprotein N gene, which is implicated in rigid spine muscular dystrophy, cause the classical phenotype of multi-minicore disease: reassessing the nosology of early-onset myopathies. *Am J Hum Genet.* 2002;71(4):739–749.
31. Cullup T, Lamont PJ, Cirak S, et al. Mutations in MYH7 cause multi-minicore disease (MmD) with variable cardiac involvement. *Neuromuscul Disord.* 2012;22:1096–1104.
32. Clarke NF, Amburgey K, Teener J, et al. A novel mutation expands the genetic and clinical spectrum of MYH7-related myopathies. *Neuromuscul Disord.* 2013;23(5):432–436.
33. Carmignac V, Salih MA, Quijano-Roy S, et al. C-terminal titin deletions cause a novel early-onset myopathy with fatal cardiomyopathy. *Ann Neurol.* 2007;61:340–351.
34. Boyden SE, Mahoney LJ, Kawahara G, et al. Mutations in the satellite cell gene MEGF10 cause a recessive congenital myopathy with minicores. *Neurogenetics.* 2012;13(2):115–124.
35. Guis S, Figarella-Branger D, Monnier N, et al. Multiminicore disease in a family susceptible to malignant hyperthermia: histology, in vitro contracture tests, and genetic characterization. *Arch Neurol.* 2004;61(1):106–113.
36. Koch BM, Bertorini TE, Eng GD, Boehm R. Severe multicore disease associated with reaction to anesthesia. *Arch Neurol.* 1985;42(12):1204–1206.
37. Monnier N, Romero NB, Lerale J, et al. An autosomal dominant congenital myopathy with cores and rods is associated with a neomutation in the RYR1 gene encoding the skeletal muscle ryanodine receptor. *Hum Mol Genet.* 2000;9: 2599–2608.
38. Scacheri PC, Hoffman EP, Fratkin JD, et al. A novel ryanodine receptor gene mutation causing both cores and rods in congenital myopathy. *Neurology.* 2000;55:1689–1696.
39. Hernandez-Lain A, Husson I, Monnier N, et al. De novo RYR1 heterozygous mutation (I4898 T) causing lethal core-rod myopathy in twins. *EurJ Med Genet.* 2001;54:29–33.
40. Pallagi E, Molnár M, Molnár P, Diószeghy P. Central core and nemaline rods in the same patient. *Acta Neuropathol.* 1998;96:211–214.
41. Afifi AK, Smith JW, Zellweger H. Congenital nonprogressive myopathy: central core disease and nemaline myopathy in one family. *Neurology.* 1965;15:371–381.
42. Romero NB, Lehtokari V, Quijano-Roy S, et al. Core-rod myopathy caused by mutations in the nebulin gene. *Neurology.* 73:1159–1161.
43. Gommans IM, Davis M, Saar K, et al. A locus on chromosome 15q for a dominantly inherited nemaline myopathy with core-like lesions. *Brain.* 2003;126:1545–1551.
44. Sambuughin N, Yau KS, Olivé M, et al. Dominant mutations in KBTBD13, a member of the BTB/Kelch family, cause nemaline myopathy with cores. *Am J Hum Genet.* 2010;87:842–847.
45. Dlamini N, Voermans NC, Lillis S, et al. Mutations in RYR1 are a common cause of exertional myalgia and rhabdomyolysis. *Neuromuscul Disord.* 2013;23(7):540–548.
46. D'Arcy CE, Bjorksten A, Yiu EM, et al. King-Denborough syndrome caused by a novel mutation in the ryanodine receptor gene. *Neurology.* 2008;71(10):776–777.
47. Dowling JJ, Lillis S, Amburgey K, et al. King-Denborough syndrome with and without mutations in the skeletal muscle ryanodine receptor (RYR1) gene. *Neuromuscul Disord.* 2011; 21:420–427.
48. Duarte S. Oliveira J, Santos R, et al. Dominant and recessive RYR1 mutations in adults with core lesions and mild muscle symptoms. *Muscle Nerve.* 2011;44:102–108.
49. Løseth S, Voermans NC, Torbergsen T, et al. A novel late-onset axial myopathy associated with mutations in the skeletal muscle ryanodine receptor (RYR1) gene. *J Neurol.* 2013;260(6): 1504–1510.
50. Jungbluth H, Lillis S, Zhou H, et al. Late-onset axial myopathy with cores due to a novel heterozygous dominant mutation in the skeletal muscle ryanodine receptor (RYR1) gene. *Neuromuscul Disord.* 2009;19(5):344–347.
51. Shy GM, Engel WK, Somers JE, Wanko T. Nemaline myopathy. A new congenital myopathy. *Brain.* 1963;86:793–810.
52. Engel WK, Wanko T, Fenichel GM. Nemaline myopathy; a second case. *Arch Neurol.* 1964;11:22–39.
53. Agrawal PB, Strickland CD, Midgett C, et al. Heterogeneity of nemaline myopathy cases with skeletal muscle alpha-actin gene mutations. *Ann Neurol.* 2004;56(1):86–96.
54. Jungbluth H, Sewry CA, Brown SC, et al. Mild phenotype of nemaline myopathy with sleep hypoventilation due to a mutation in the skeletal muscle alpha-actin (ACTA1) gene. *Neuromuscul Disord.* 2001;11(1):35–40.
55. North KN, Laing NG, Wallgren-Pettersson C, et al. Nemaline myopathy: current concepts. The ENMC International Consortium and Nemaline Myopathy. *J Med Genet.* 1997;34 (9):705–713.
56. Ryan MM, Ilkovski B, Strickland CD, et al. Clinical course correlates poorly with muscle pathology in nemaline myopathy. *Neurology.* 2003;60(4):665–673.
57. Ryan MM, Schnell C, Strickland CD, et al. Nemaline myopathy: a clinical study of 143 cases. *Ann Neurol.* 2001;50(3):312–320.
58. Wallgren-Pettersson C. Congenital nemaline myopathy. A clinical follow-up of twelve patients. *J Neurol Sci.* 1989;89(1):1–14.
59. Wallgren-Pettersson C. Nemaline and myotubular myopathies. *Semin Pediatr Neurol.* 2002;9(2):132–144.
60. Wallgren-Pettersson C. Congenital myopathies. *Eur J Paediatr Neurol.* 2005;9(1):27–28.
61. Wallgren-Pettersson C, Laing NG. 138th ENMC Workshop: nemaline myopathy, 20–22 May. 2005, Naarden, The Netherlands. *Neuromuscul Disord.* 2006;16(1):54–60.
62. Barohn RJ, Jackson CE, Kagan-Hallet KS, et al. Neonatal nemaline myopathy with abundant intranuclear rods. *Neuromuscul Disord.* 1994;4(5–6):513–520.
63. Norton P, Ellison P, Sulaiman AR, Harb J. Nemaline myopathy in the neonate. *Neurology.* 1983;33(3):351–356.
64. Rifai Z, Kazee AM, Kamp C, Griggs RC. Intranuclear rods in severe congenital nemaline myopathy. *Neurology.* 1993;43 (11):2372–2377.
65. Wallgren-Pettersson C, Jasani B, Newman GR, et al. Alpha-actinin in nemaline bodies in congenital nemaline myopathy: immunological confirmation by light and electron microscopy. *Neuromuscul Disord.* 1995;5(2):93–104.
66. Gurgel-Giannetti J., Reed U, Bang ML, et al. Nebulin expression in patients with nemaline myopathy. *Neuromuscul Disord.* 2001;11(2):154–162.
67. Pelin K, Donner K, Holmberg M, Jungbluth H, Muntoni F, Wallgren-Pettersson C. Nebulin mutations in autosomal

recessive nemaline myopathy: an update. *Neuromuscul Disord.* 2002;12(7–8):680–686.
68. Pelin K, Hilpela P, Donner K, et al. Mutations in the nebulin gene associated with autosomal recessive nemaline myopathy. *Proc Natl Acad Sci U S A.* 1999;96(5):2305–2310.
69. Sparrow JC, Nowak KJ, Durling HJ, et al. Muscle disease caused by mutations in the skeletal muscle alpha-actin gene (ACTA1). *Neuromuscul Disord.* 2003;13(7–8):519–531.
70. Marston S, Mirza M, Abdulrazzak H, Sewry C. Functional characterisation of a mutant actin (Met132Val) from a patient with nemaline myopathy. *Neuromuscul Disord.* 2004;14(2): 167–174.
71. Nowak KJ, Wattanasirichaigoon D, Goebel HH, et al. Mutations in the skeletal muscle alpha-actin gene in patients with actin myopathy and nemaline myopathy. *Nat Genet.* 1999; 23(2):208–212.
72. Wallgren-Pettersson C, Pelin K, Nowak KJ, et al. Genotype phenotype correlations in nemaline myopathy caused by mutations in the genes for nebulin and skeletal muscle alpha-actin. *Neuromuscul Disord.* 2004;14(8–9):461–470.
73. Laing NG, Wilton SD, Akkari PA, et al. A mutation in the alpha tropomyosin gene TPM3 associated with autosomal dominant nemaline myopathy NEM1. *Nat Genet.* 1995;10(2):249.
74. Durling HJ, Reilich P, Müller-Höcker J, et al. De novo missense mutation in a constitutively expressed exon of the slow alpha-tropomyosin gene TPM3 associated with an atypical, sporadic case of nemaline myopathy. *Neuromuscul Disord.* 2002;12(10):947–951.
75. Wattanasirichaigoon D, Swoboda KJ, Takada F, et al. Mutations of the slow muscle alpha-tropomyosin gene, TPM3, are a rare cause of nemaline myopathy. *Neurology.* 2002;59(4):613–617.
76. Donner K, Ollikainen M, Ridanpää M, et al. Mutations in the beta-tropomyosin (TPM2) gene—a rare cause of nemaline myopathy. *Neuromuscul Disord.* 2002;12(2):151–158.
77. Jin JP, Brotto MA, Hossain MM, et al. Truncation by Glu180 nonsense mutation results in complete loss of slow skeletal muscle troponin T in a lethal nemaline myopathy. *J Biol Chem.* 2003;278(28):26159–26165.
78. Agrawal PB, Greenleaf RS, Tomczak KK, et al. Nemaline myopathy with minicores caused by mutation of the CFL2 gene encoding the skeletal muscle actin-binding protein, cofilin-2. *Am J Hum Genet.* 2007;80:162–167.
79. Ockeloen CW, Gilhuis HJ, Pfundt R, et al. Congenital myopathy caused by a novel missense mutation in the CFL2 gene. *Neuromuscul Disord.* 2012;22:632–639.
80. Ong RW, Alsaman A, Selcen D, et al. Novel cofilin-2 (CFL2) four base pair deletion causing nemaline myopathy. *J Neurol Neurosurg Psychiatry.* 2014;85(9):1058–1060.
81. Ravenscroft G, Miyatake S, Lehtokari VL, et al. Mutations in KLHL40 are a frequent cause of severe autosomal-recessive nemaline myopathy. *Am J Hum Genet.* 2013;93(1):6–18.
82. Gupta VA, Ravenscroft G, Shaheen R, et al. Identification of KLHL41 mutations implicates BTB-Kelch-mediated ubiquitination as an alternate pathway to myofibrillar disruption in nemaline myopathy. *Am J Hum Genet.* 2013;93(6):1108–1117.
83. Malfatti E, Schaeffer U, Chapon F, et al. Combined cap disease and nemaline myopathy in the same patient caused by an autosomal dominant mutation in the TPM3 gene. *Neuromuscul Disord.* 2013;23(12):992–997.
84. Chahin N, Selcen D, Engel AG. Sporadic late onset nemaline myopathy. *Neurology.* 2005;65(8):1158–1164.
85. Eymard B, Brouet JC, Collin H, Chevallay M, Bussel A, Fardeau M. Late-onset rod myopathy associated with monoclonal gammopathy. *Neuromuscul Disord.* 1993;3(5–6):557–560.
86. Milone M, Katz A, Amato AA, et al. Sporadic late onset nemaline myopathy responsive to IVIg and immunotherapy. *Muscle Nerve.* 2010;41:272–276.
87. Benveniste O, Laforet P, Dubourg O, et al. Stem cell transplantation in a patient with late-onset nemaline myopathy and gammopathy. *Neurology.* 2008;71:531–532.
88. Doppler K, Knop S, Einsele H, Sommer C, Wessig C. Sporadic late onset nemaline myopathy and immunoglobulin deposition disease. *Muscle Nerve.* 2013;48(6):983–988.
89. Spiro AJ, Shy GM, Gonatas NK. Myotubular myopathy. Persistence of fetal muscle in an adolescent boy. *Arch Neurol.* 1966;14(1):1–14.
90. Fischer D, Herasse M, Bitoun M, et al. Characterization of the muscle involvement in dynamin 2-related centronuclear myopathy. *Brain.* 2006;129(Pt 6):1463–1469.
91. Jeannet PY, Bassez G, Eymard B, et al. Clinical and histologic findings in autosomal centronuclear myopathy. *Neurology.* 2004;62(9):1484–1490.
92. McEntagart M, Parsons G, Buj-Bello A, et al. Genotype-phenotype correlations in X-linked myotubular myopathy. *Neuromuscul Disord.* 2002;12(10):939–946.
93. Wallgren-Pettersson C, Clarke A, Samson F, et al. The myotubular myopathies: differential diagnosis of the X linked recessive, autosomal dominant, and autosomal recessive forms and present state of DNA studies. *J Med Genet.* 1995;32(9):673–679.
94. Hammans SR, Robinson DO, Moutou C, et al. A clinical and genetic study of a manifesting heterozygote with X-linked myotubular myopathy. *Neuromuscul Disord.* 2000;10(2):133–137.
95. Jungbluth H, Sewry CA, Buj-Bello A, et al. Early and severe presentation of X-linked myotubular myopathy in a girl with skewed X-inactivation. *Neuromuscul Disord.* 2003;13(1):55–59.
96. Kristiansen M, Knudsen GP, Tanner SM, et al. X-inactivation patterns in carriers of X-linked myotubular myopathy. *Neuromuscul Disord.* 2003;13(6):468–471.
97. Felice KJ, Grunnet ML. Autosomal dominant centronuclear myopathy: report of a new family with clinical features simulating facioscapulohumeral syndrome. *Muscle Nerve.* 1997; 20(9):1194–1196.
98. Laporte J, Biancalana V, Tanner SM, et al. MTM1 mutations in X-linked myotubular myopathy. *Hum Mutat.* 2000;15(5): 393–409.
99. Laporte J, Guiraud-Chaumeil C, Vincent MC, et al. Mutations in the MTM1 gene implicated in X-linked myotubular myopathy. ENMC International Consortium on Myotubular Myopathy. European Neuro-Muscular Center. *Hum Mol Genet.* 1997;6(9):1505–1511.
100. Cui X, De Vivo I, Slany R, Miyamoto A, Firestein R, Cleary ML. Association of SET domain and myotubularin-related proteins modulates growth control. *Nat Genet.* 1998;18(4):331–337.
101. Bitoun M, Maugenre S, Jeannet PY, et al. Mutations in dynamin 2 cause dominant centronuclear myopathy. *Nat Genet.* 2005;37(11):1207–1209.
102. Zuchner S, Noureddine M, Kennerson M, et al. Mutations in the pleckstrin homology domain of dynamin 2 cause dominant intermediate Charcot–Marie–Tooth disease. *Nat Genet.* 2005;37(3):289–294.
103. Nicot AS, Toussaint A, Tosch V, et al. Mutations in amphiphysin 2 (BIN1) disrupt interaction with dynamin 2 and cause

autosomal recessive centronuclear myopathy. *Nat Genet*. 2007; 39:1134–1139.
104. Claeys KG, Maisonobe T, Böhm J, et al. Phenotype of a patient with recessive centronuclear myopathy and a novel BIN1 mutation. *Neurology*. 2010;74:519–521.
105. Böhm J, Yiş U, Ortaç R, et al. Case report of intrafamilial variability in autosomal recessive centronuclear myopathy associated to a novel BIN1 stop mutation. *Orphanet J Rare Dis*. 2010;5:35.
106. Ceyhan-Birsoy O, Agrawal PB, Hidalgo C, et al. Recessive truncating titin gene, TTN, mutations presenting as centronuclear myopathy. *Neurology*. 2013;81(14):1205–1214.
107. Cavanagh NP, Lake BD, McMeniman P, et al. Congenital fibre type disproportion myopathy. A histological diagnosis with an uncertain clinical outlook. *Arch Dis Child*. 1979;54(10):735–743.
108. Danon MJ, Giometti CS, Manaligod JR, Swisher C. Sequential muscle biopsy changes in a case of congenital myopathy. *Muscle Nerve*. 1997;20(5):561–569.
109. Laing NG, Clarke NF, Dye DE, et al. Actin mutations are one cause of congenital fibre type disproportion. *Ann Neurol*. 2004;56(5):689–694.
110. Brandis A, Aronica E, Goebel HH. TPM2 mutation. *Neuromuscul Disord*. 2008;18(12):1005.
111. Clarke NF, Kidson W, Quijano-Roy S, et al. SEPN1: associated with congenital fiber-type disproportion and insulin resistance. *Ann Neurol*. 2006;59:546–552.
112. Jerusalem F, Engel AG, Gomez MR. Sarcotubular myopathy. A newly recognized, benign, congenital, familial muscle disease. *Neurology*. 1973;23(9):897–906.
113. Schoser BG, Frosk P, Engel AG, Klutzny U, Lochmüller H, Wrogemann K. Commonality of TRIM32 mutation in causing sarcotubular myopathy and LGMD2 H. *Ann Neurol*. 2005;57(4):591–595.
114. Curless RG, Payne CM, Brinner FM. Fingerprint body myopathy: a report of twins. *Dev Med Child Neurol*. 1978;20(6):793–798.
115. Engel AG, Angelini C, Gomez MR. Fingerprint body myopathy, a newly recognized congenital muscle disease. *Mayo Clin Proc*. 1972;47(6):377–388.
116. Fardeau M, Tomé FM, Derambure S. Familial fingerprint body myopathy. *Arch Neurol*. 1976;33(10):724–725.
117. Ringel SP, Neville HE, Duster MC, Carroll JE, et al. A new congenital neuromuscular disease with trilaminar muscle fibers. *Neurology*. 1978;28(3):282–289.
118. Barohn RJ, Brumback RA, Mendell JR. Hyaline body myopathy. *Neuromuscul Disord*. 1994;4(3):257–262.
119. Bohlega S, Abu-Amero SN, Wakil SM, et al. Mutation of the slow myosin heavy chain rod domain underlies hyaline body myopathy. *Neurology*. 2004;62(9):1518–1521.
120. Bohlega S, Lach B, Meyer BF, et al. Autosomal dominant hyaline body myopathy: clinical variability and pathologic findings. *Neurology*. 2003;61(11):1519–1523.
121. Laing NG, Ceuterick-de Groote C, Dye DE, et al. Myosin storage myopathy: slow skeletal myosin (MYH7) mutation in two isolated cases. *Neurology*. 2005;64(3):527–529.
122. Masuzugawa S, Kuzuhara S, Narita Y, Naito Y, Taniguchi A, Ibi T. Autosomal dominant hyaline body myopathy presenting as scapuloperoneal syndrome: clinical features and muscle pathology. *Neurology*. 1997;48(1):253–257.
123. Tajsharghi H, Thornell LE, Lindberg C, Lindvall B, Henriksson KG, Oldfors A. Myosin storage myopathy associated with a heterozygous missense mutation in MYH7. *Ann Neurol*. 2003;54(4):494–500.
124. Oldfors A, Tajsharghi H, Darin N, Lindberg C. Myopathies associated with myosin heavy chain mutations. *Acta Myol*. 2004;23(2):90–96.
125. Tajsharghi H, Darin N, Rekabdar E, et al. Mutations and sequence variation in the human myosin heavy chain IIa gene (MYH2). *Eur J Hum Genet*. 2005;13(5):617–622.
126. Tajsharghi H, Thornell LE, Darin N, et al. Myosin heavy chain IIa gene mutation E706K is pathogenic and its expression increases with age. *Neurology*. 2002;58:780–786.
127. Martinsson T, Oldfors A, Darin N, et al. Autosomal dominant myopathy: missense mutation (Glu-706 → Lys) in the myosin heavy chain IIa gene. *Proc Natl Acad Sci U S A*. 2000;97(26): 14614–14619.
128. Fidzianska A, Badurska B, Ryniewicz B, Dembek I. "Cap disease": new congenital myopathy. *Neurology*. 1981;31(9):1113–1120.
129. Fidziańska A. Cap disease—a failure in the correct muscle fibre formation. *J Neurol Sci*. 2002;201(1–2):27–31.
130. Hung RM, Yoon G, Hawkins CE, Halliday W, Biggar D, Vajsar J. Cap myopathy caused by a mutation of the skeletal alpha-actin gene ACTA1. *Neuromuscul Disord*. 2010;20:238–240.
131. Lehtokari VL, Ceuterick-de Groote C, de Jonghe P, et al. Cap disease caused by heterozygous deletion of the beta-tropomyosin gene TPM2. *Neuromuscul Disord*. 2007;17:433–442.
132. Tajsharghi H, Ohlsson M, Lindberg C, Oldfors A. Congenital myopathy with nemaline rods and cap structures caused by a mutation in the beta-tropomyosin gene (TPM2). *Arch Neurol*. 2007;64:1334–1338.
133. Ohlsson M, Fidziańska A, Tajsharghi H, Oldfors A. TPM3 mutation in one of the original cases of cap disease. *Neurology*. 2009;72:1961–1963.
134. Waddell LB, Kreissl M, Kornberg A, et al. Evidence for a dominant negative disease mechanism in cap myopathy due to TPM3. *Neuromuscul Disord*. 2010;20:464–466.
135. Schreckenbach T, Schröder JM, Voit T, et al. Novel TPM3 mutation in a family with cap myopathy and review of the literature. *Neuromuscul Disord*. 2014;24:117–124.
136. Schaeffer U, Chapon F, Yang Y, et al. Combined cap disease and nemaline myopathy in the same patient caused by an autosomal dominant mutation in the TPM3 gene. *Neuromuscul Disord*. 2013;23(12):992–997.
137. Lake BD, Wilson J. Zebra body myopathy. Clinical, histochemical and ultrastructural studies. *J Neurol Sci*. 1975;24(4): 437–446.
138. Reyes MG, Goldbarg H, Fresco K, Bouffard A. Zebra body myopathy: a second case of ultrastructurally distinct congenital myopathy. *J Child Neurol*. 1987;2(4):307–310.
139. Martin JJ, Ceuterick C, Van Goethem G. On a dominantly inherited myopathy with tubular aggregates. *Neuromuscul Disord*. 1997;7(8):512–520.
140. Dobkin BH, Verity MA. Familial neuromuscular disease with type 1 fiber hypoplasia, tubular aggregates, cardiomyopathy, and myasthenic features. *Neurology*. 1978;28(11):1135–1140.
141. Morgan-Hughes JA, Mair WG, Lascelles PT. A disorder of skeletal muscle associated with tubular aggregates. *Brain*. 1970;93(4):873–880.
142. Böhm J, Chevessier F, Maues De Paula A, et al. Constitutive activation of the calcium sensor STIM1 causes tubular aggregate myopathy. *Am J Hum Genet*. 2013;92:271–278.
143. Hedberg C, Niceta M, Fattori F, et al. Childhood onset tubular aggregate myopathy associated with de novo STIM1 mutations. *J Neurol*. 2014;261(5):870–876.

144. Nesin V, Wiley G, Kousi M, et al. Activating mutations in STIM1 and ORAI1 cause overlapping syndromes of tubular myopathy and congenital miosis. *Proc Natl Acad Sci U S A*. 2014;111(11):4197–4202.
145. Selcen D, Shen XM, Brengman J, et al. DPAGT1 myasthenia and myopathy: genetic, phenotypic, and expression studies. *Neurology*. 2014;82(20):1822–1830.
146. Finlayson S, Palace J, Belaya K, et al. Clinical features of congenital myasthenic syndrome due to mutations in DPAGT1. *J Neurol Neurosurg Psychiatry*. 2013;84(10):1119–1125.
147. Selcen D, Shen XM, Milone M, et al. GFPT1-myasthenia: clinical, structural, and electrophysiologic heterogeneity. *Neurology*. 2013;81(4):370–378.
148. Brooke MH, Neville HE. Reducing body myopathy. *Neurology*. 1972;22(8):829–840.
149. Figarella-Branger D, Putzu GA, Bouvier-Labit C, Adult onset reducing body myopathy. *Neuromuscul Disord*. 1999;9(8): 580–586.
150. Nomizu S, Person DA, Saito C, Lockett LJ. A unique case of reducing body myopathy. *Muscle Nerve*. 1992;15(4):463–466.
151. Oh SJ, Meyers GJ, Wilson ER Jr, Alexander CB. A benign form of reducing body myopathy. *Muscle Nerve*. 1983;6(4): 278–282.
152. Bertini E, Salviati G, Apollo F, et al. Reducing body myopathy and desmin storage in skeletal muscle: morphological and biochemical findings. *Acta Neuropathol (Berl)*. 1994;87(1): 106–112.
153. Schessl J, Zou Y, McGrath MJ, et al. Proteomic identification of FHL1 as the protein mutated in human reducing body myopathy. *J Clin Invest*. 2008;118:904–912.
154. Schessl J, Taratuto AL, Sewry C, et al. Clinical, histological and genetic characterization of reducing body myopathy caused by mutations in FHL1. *Brain*. 2009;132:452–464.
155. Schessl J, Columbus A, Hu Y, et al. Familial reducing body myopathy with cytoplasmic bodies and rigid spine revisited: identification of a second LIM domain mutation in FHL1. *Neuropediatrics*. 2010;41:43–46.
156. Shalaby S, Hayashi YK, Nonaka I, Noguchi S, Nishino I. Novel FHL1 mutations in fatal and benign reducing body myopathy. *Neurology*. 2009;72:375–376.
157. Chen DH, Raskind WH, Parson WW, et al. A novel mutation in FHL1 in a family with X-linked scapuloperoneal myopathy: phenotypic spectrum and structural study of FHL1 mutations. *J Neurol Sci*. 2010;296:22–29.
158. Selcen D, Bromberg MB, Chin SS, Engel AG. Reducing bodies and myofibrillar myopathy features in FHL1 muscular dystrophy. *Neurology*. 2011;77:1951–1959.
159. Greenberg SA, Salajegheh M, Judge DP, et al. Etiology of limb girdle muscular dystrophy 1D/1E determined by laser capture microdissection proteomics. *Ann Neurol*. 2012;71:141–145.

CHAPTER 29

Metabolic Myopathies

The inherited metabolic myopathies are traditionally classified by their underlying biochemical abnormalities as disorders of (1) carbohydrate, (2) lipid, and (3) adenine nucleotide metabolism. A fourth possible category includes the mitochondrial encephalomyopathies. As mitochondrial disorders do not cause defects in a specific biochemical pathway, they are discussed in a separate chapter. The immediate source of energy for muscles comes from the hydrolysis of adenosine triphosphate (ATP). At rest, the major substrate for muscle in terms of ATP production comes from the metabolism of long-chain fatty acids. Therefore, any disorder impairing β-oxidation of long-chain fatty acids in the mitochondria can lead to a myopathy. During exercise, ATP is derived from the metabolism of carbohydrates, fatty acids, and ketones. Early in the course of exercise (e.g., up to 45 minutes), energy is derived mainly from free glucose or glucose made available via glycogenolysis. Subsequently, there is a shift toward the metabolism of fatty acids such that after a few hours 70% of energy is derived from lipid breakdown.

Metabolic myopathies can also be viewed as static or dynamic disorders. The static myopathies are defined by the presence of fixed or progressive weakness. On the other hand, the dynamic myopathies are associated with exercise intolerance (i.e., exertional myalgias, cramps, and myoglobinuria) as the dominant clinical features. Some metabolic defects are associated with both a dynamic and a static myopathy.

► DISORDERS OF CARBOHYDRATE METABOLISM

Carbohydrates are stored in liver and muscle as glycogen, a highly branched polymer of glucose. Normal synthesis and breakdown of glycogen is essential to maintain adequate glucose concentration in muscle that can be further metabolized and provide energy in the form of ATP. There are 16+ recognized glycogen storage diseases (GSDs), also called glycogenoses (Table 29-1). This is somewhat a misnomer because some of these glycogenoses do not result in the accumulation of glycogen in tissues.

The glycogenoses predominantly affect liver and muscle. Since there is differential metabolism of carbohydrates in these two tissues, the individual GSDs may produce strictly liver or muscle disease, or some combination of the two. Types I (glucose-6-phosphatase deficiency) and VI (liver phosphorylase deficiency) only cause liver disease and are not further discussed. Types II (lysosomal α-glucosidase deficiency), V (phosphorylase deficiency), VII [phosphofructokinase (PFK) deficiency], X [phosphoglycerate mutase (PGAM) deficiency], and XI (lactate dehydrogenase deficiency) produce almost exclusively muscle disease, while the remaining types produce a varying mixture of muscle disease with systemic disease.

The pathophysiological basis by which the varied enzymatic defects lead to muscle dysfunction remains largely unknown. The inability to metabolize a substrate reduces the ability of muscle cells to form ATP necessary for normal energy production. Further, the enzymatic defects may result in accumulation of metabolites, which may be toxic to muscle.

The exercise forearm test can be helpful diagnosing various disorders of glycolysis. The test can be adequately performed without blood pressure cuff insufflation. In fact, performing this test with the limb ischemic may be hazardous to the patient because it can induce profound muscle damage and myoglobinuria.[1] A butterfly needle is placed in the antecubital fossa and draw baseline lactate and ammonia levels are drawn. The forearm muscles are then exercised by having the patient rapidly and strenuously open and close the hand for 1 minute. Immediately after exercise and then 1, 2, 4, 6, and 10 minutes postexercise, blood samples are again taken and analyzed for lactate and ammonia. The normal response is for lactate and ammonia levels to raise three to four times the baseline levels. If neither the lactate nor the ammonia level increases, the test is inconclusive and implies that the muscles were not sufficiently exercised. A rise in lactate levels, but not ammonia, is diagnostic for myoadenylate deaminase (MAD) deficiency. In myophosphorylase, PFK, PGAM, phosphoglycerate kinase (PGK), phosphorylase b kinase (PBK), debranching enzyme, and lactate dehydrogenase deficiencies, the ammonia levels rise appropriately, but the lactic acid does not.

GLYCOGENOSIS TYPE 0 (GLYCOGEN SYNTHASE 1 DEFICIENCY)

Clinical Features

Only a few patients have been reported with this rare disorder.[2–4] Affected individuals presented with childhood onset of exercise intolerance and recurrent attacks of syncope of presumed cardiac origin. Prolonged QT syndrome and

▶ TABLE 29-1. **DISORDERS OF CARBOHYDRATE METABOLISM**

Disorder	Enzyme Defect	Inheritance	Clinical Features
Type 0	Glycogen synthase 1	Autosomal recessive	Childhood onset weakness, hypertrophic cardiomyopathy
Type I (von Gierke disease)	Glucose-6-phosphate	Autosomal recessive	No neuromuscular signs or symptoms
Type II (Pompe disease)	Acid maltase (α-1,4-glucosidase)	Autosomal recessive	Infancy: hypotonia, cardiomyopathy, respiratory failure, generalized weakness Childhood–adult: progressive weakness, respiratory failure
Type III (Cori–Forbes disease)	Debranching enzyme (amylo-1,6-glucosidase)	Autosomal recessive	Infancy: hypotonia, generalized weakness Childhood/adult: proximal or distal weakness, spasticity, dementia, incontinence
Type IV (Anderson disease)	Branching enzyme (amylo-1, 4–1,6-transglucosidase)	Autosomal recessive	Infancy: hypotonia, generalized weakness Childhood/adult: proximal or distal weakness
Type V (McArdle disease)	Myophosphorylase	Autosomal recessive	Infancy: rare weakness Childhood/adult: Exercise intolerance, rare weakness
Type VI	Liver phosphorylase	Autosomal recessive	No muscle involvement
Type VII (Tarui disease)	Phosphofructokinase	Autosomal recessive	Childhood: exercise intolerance, rare weakness
Type IXB	[a]Phosphorylase b kinase B subunit	Autosomal recessive	Infancy to adult: exercise intolerance, rare weakness
Type IXD	[a]Phosphorylase b kinase A subunit	X-linked	
Type X	Phosphoglycerate mutase	Autosomal recessive	Childhood–adult: exercise intolerance
Type XI	Lactate dehydrogenase	Autosomal recessive	Childhood–adult: exercise intolerance
Type XII	Aldolase A	Autosomal recessive	Infancy–childhood: exercise intolerance and weakness
Type XIII	β-Enolase	Autosomal recessive	Childhood–adult: exercise intolerance
Type XIV	Phosphoglucomutase	Autosomal recessive	Childhood: exercise intolerance and weakness
Type XV	Glycogenin 1	Autosomal recessive	Childhood onset of weakness
Other GSDs			
	Phosphoglycerate kinase 1	X-linked	Childhood: exercise intolerance, rare weakness, hemolytic anemia, mental retardation, seizures
	Triosephosphate isomerase	Autosomal recessive	Infancy: hypotonia, generalized weakness mental retardation

[a]Phosphorylase b kinase deficiency was previously termed GSD VIII. Both phosphorylase b kinase and phosphoglycerate kinase deficiencies have been termed GSD IX in the literature.

sudden cardiac death have occurred. However, loss of consciousness was gradual in one patient suggesting metabolic dysfunction within the central nervous system (CNS) as opposed to pure cardiac etiology.[4] Mild proximal weakness may be evident.

Laboratory Features

One report noted that exercise forearm test shows failure of lactate elevation and skeletal muscle magnetic resonance imaging (MRI) shows fatty degeneration of the gluteal and flexor muscles of the thigh.[4] Serum creatine kinase (CK) levels have not been reported.

Histopathology

Skeletal muscle and cardiac muscle as well as skin fibroblasts have depletion of glycogen. Phosphorylase activity may also be deficient in muscle fibers.[2–4]

Molecular Genetics and Pathogenesis

Synthesis of glycogen requires glycogen synthase 1 which catalyzes the addition of glucose monomers to the growing glycogen molecule through the formation of α-1,4-glycoside linkages. GSD 0 is caused by mutations in the *GYS1* gene that encodes glycogen synthase 1. Deficiency of this enzyme leads to the depletion of glycogen in skeletal and cardiac muscles.

Treatment

There are no specific medical therapies.

GLYCOGENOSIS TYPE II (POMPE DISEASE; ACID MALTASE DEFICIENCY; α-GLUCOSIDASE DEFICIENCY)

GSD II is an autosomal-recessive disorder caused by a deficiency of lysosomal acid α-glucosidase (Table 29-1, Fig. 29-1).

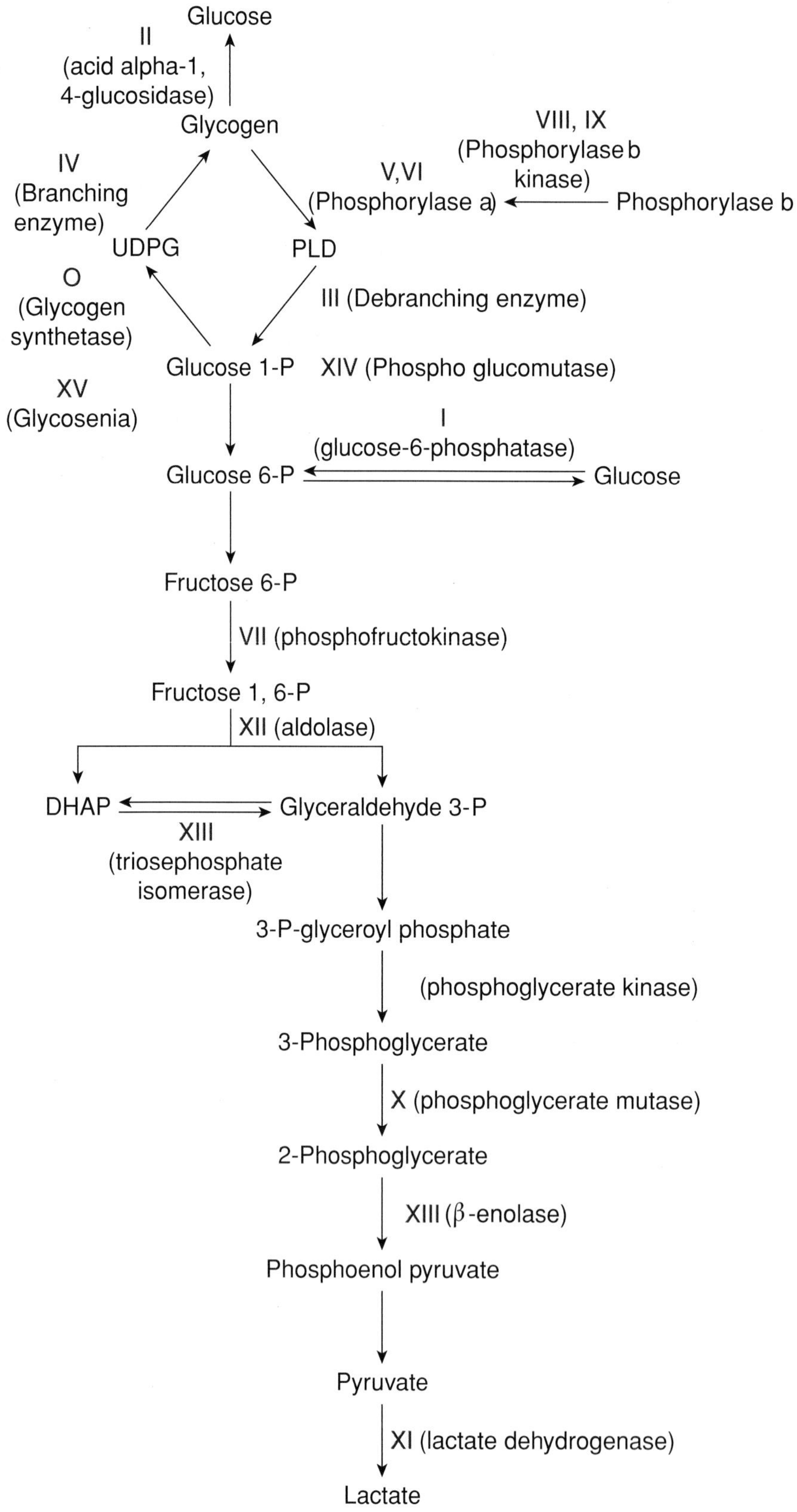

Figure 29-1. Glycolytic pathways. Glycogen metabolism disorders are caused by specific enzyme deficiencies involving each of the pathways illustrated with a Roman numeral. The enzymes corresponding to each numbered glycogen storage disorder are listed in Table 29-1. Diseases I and VI are not included, as these do not involve muscle. (Adapted with permission from Amato AA: sweet success—a treatment for McArdle's disease. *N Engl J Med*. 2003;349(26):2481–2482.)

GSD II, more commonly referred to as Pompe disease or acid maltase deficiency, may present in three major forms: a severe infantile form, a juvenile-onset type, and an adult-onset variant.[5–28] The incidence of infantile Pompe disease ranges from 1 in 31,000 to 1 in 138,000. The incidence of later onset forms has been purported to be as high as 1 in 53,000, but we think it is far less common in our experience.

Clinical Features

Infantile Pompe disease is characterized by generalized weakness and hypotonia, cardiomegaly, and mild-to-moderate hepatomegaly, with an onset in the first several months of life.[10,15–17] Infants often have an enlarged tongue (i.e., macroglossia). The weakness and cardiomyopathy are progressive. Feeding difficulties and ventilatory muscle weakness are common. The disease is invariably fatal by 2 years of age secondary to cardioventilatory failure.

The juvenile-onset acid maltase deficiency usually manifests in the first decade of life.[9,13,15,18,28] Motor milestones may be delayed. Weakness is slowly progressive and involves proximal greater than distal muscles in the legs and arms. Children often have hypertrophy of the calf muscles, a waddling gait, and significant lumbar lordosis and demonstrate a Gower maneuver to arise from the floor. Thus, affected children are not uncommonly misdiagnosed with Duchenne or some other form of limb-girdle muscular dystrophy. Rarely, acid maltase deficiency presents with rigidity of the spine.[21] Unlike the infantile-onset acid maltase deficiency, cardiomegaly, hepatomegaly, and macroglossia are uncommon. Nevertheless, it is relentlessly progressive, and ventilatory muscles are invariably affected leading to death in the second or third decade of life.

Adult-onset acid maltase deficiency usually manifests in the third or fourth decade (up to the eighth decade, mean 36.5 years).[7,9–11,15,21–24,28] Patients develop generalized proximal greater than distal muscle weakness resembling polymyositis or limb-girdle dystrophy. Some patients have a scapuloperoneal distribution of weakness.[3] Weakness is occasionally asymmetric and may involve the face or tongue.[23] Nearly half of the affected individuals complain of muscle pains, particularly in the thighs. Muscle stretch reflexes may be reduced. Hepatomegaly and cardiomegaly do not typically occur; however, electrocardiographic abnormalities and arrhythmias can be seen. As in the infantile and juvenile forms of the disease, there is a predilection for the involvement of ventilatory muscles. In this regard, 16–33% of patients present with symptoms related to ventilatory insufficiency (e.g., dyspnea, frequent nocturnal arousals, morning headaches, and excessive daytime sleepiness).[23,28]

Laboratory Features

Serum CK levels are moderately elevated in infantile-onset, but adults may have normal CK levels. α-Glucosidase activity may be assayed in muscle fibers, fibroblasts, leukocytes, lymphocytes, and urine. The reduction of activity generally correlates with the severity of the myopathy. Infantile-onset disease is associated with a severe deficiency of α-glucosidase activity, while the less severe adult-onset form has residual activity, up to 30% in muscle and 53% in lymphocytes.[24] Importantly, false-negative results on leukocyte assay can occur due to contamination with granulocytes or other sources of neutral glucosidase. A dried blood spot analysis of α-glucosidase activity is now the preferred initial screening test.[25–28] Of note, activity levels by dried blood spot do not correlate with severity of the myopathy. If the dried blood spot shows reduced enzyme activity, confirmatory testing may be performed by measuring α-glucosidase activity in cultured fibroblasts or muscle tissue or by genetic testing.

Computer tomography (CT) and MRI scans confirm the early and severe involvement of the adductor magnus and semimembranosus in the early stage of the disease and later fatty infiltration of the long head of the biceps femoris, semitendinosus, and the anterior thigh muscles. In advanced phases, selective sparing of sartorius, rectus, femoris, and gracilis muscles, and peripheral portions of the vastus lateralis are also evident.[29,30] Skeletal muscle MRI and CT also reveal early involvement of paravertebral and abdominal trunk muscular.[31]

Motor and sensory nerve conduction studies (NCS) are normal. Electromyography (EMG) reveals increased insertional and spontaneous activity in the form of fibrillation potentials, positive sharp waves, complex repetitive discharges, and even myotonic discharges. In mild forms of the disease, these irritative discharges may be evident only in the paraspinal muscles. Motor unit action potentials (MUAPs) are myopathic in appearance and recruit early.

Electrocardiograms (EKG) may demonstrate nonspecific abnormalities including left axis deviation, short PR interval, large QRS complexes, inverted T waves, ST depression, and persistent sinus tachycardia in both the severe and mild forms of GSD II.[23] Wolfe–Parkinson–White syndrome occurs in infantile and adult forms of the disease.[32,33] Echocardiograms may show hypertrophic cardiomyopathy. Pulmonary function tests show a restrictive defect with decreased forced vital capacity, reduced maximal inspiratory and expiratory pressures, and early fatigue of the diaphragm.[23,28]

Histopathology

Biopsies characteristically demonstrate glycogen-filled vacuoles within muscle fibers (Fig. 29-2).[15,24,28] These vacuoles are very prominent in the infantile form, but in the childhood and adult forms, these are apparent in only 25–75% of fibers in clinically affected muscles and may be absent in clinically unaffected muscle groups. Muscle biopsy may show only slight, nonspecific abnormalities in late-onset cases. When present, the vacuoles react strongly

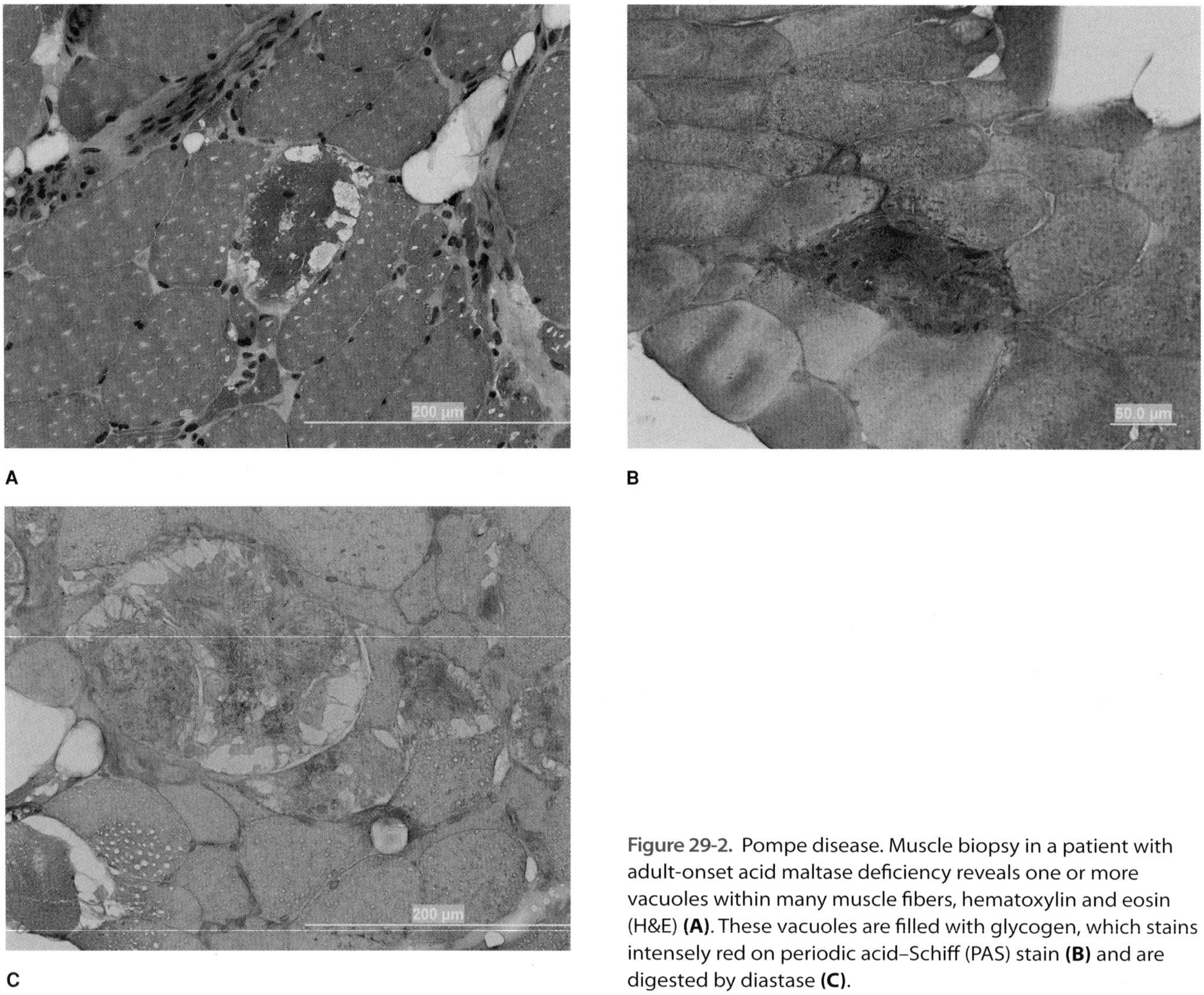

Figure 29-2. Pompe disease. Muscle biopsy in a patient with adult-onset acid maltase deficiency reveals one or more vacuoles within many muscle fibers, hematoxylin and eosin (H&E) **(A)**. These vacuoles are filled with glycogen, which stains intensely red on periodic acid–Schiff (PAS) stain **(B)** and are digested by diastase **(C)**.

to periodic acid–Schiff (PAS), are sensitive to diastase, and stain intensely with acid phosphatase, confirming that the vacuoles are secondary lysosomes filled with glycogen. Glycogen can also be found free in the cytoplasm on electron microscopy (EM). Muscle biopsies also reveal necrotic and regenerating muscle fibers, variation in fiber size and fiber splitting. In later stages, muscle fiber atrophy and increased endomysial connective tissue may be present. Occasionally, fiber-type grouping and group atrophy may be evident, owing to motor neuron degeneration. In this regard, glycogens accumulate in anterior horn cells and bulbar nuclei as well as Schwann cells accounting for the superimposed neurogenic findings in some patients.[34,35]

Molecular Genetics and Pathogenesis

Missense, nonsense, and frame-shift mutations have been identified in the α-glucosidase gene, *GAA*, located on chromosome 17q21–23 in infantile-, childhood-, and adult-onset cases.[36,37] Prenatal diagnosis is possible with amniocentesis or chorionic villus sampling.[36–38] Acid α-glucosidase is a lysosomal enzyme, which cleaves 1,4 and 1,6 linkages in glycogen, maltose, and isomaltose. Glycogen within lysosomes is degraded to glucose by α-glucosidase, and the deficiency of the enzyme results in glycogen accumulation. There appears to be an inverse correlation between residual acid α-glucosidase activity and the clinical severity. However, there are cases associated with an adult-onset Pompe disease that have very little residual enzyme activity, so the relationship between disease activity and clinical severity is not 100% accurate. Interestingly, there may be variability in phenotype and severity within families.[16,39]

How acid α-glucosidase leads to muscle fiber dysfunction is not completely understood. The accumulating glycogen that results from the deficiency may displace or replace important cellular organelles. Alternatively, the lysosomes filled with glycogen may rupture, thereby releasing proteases that degrade myofibrils and other important muscle proteins. Muscle catabolism is increased by 31% in Pompe disease compared to normal controls, and mean protein balance is reduced.[14] Furthermore, resting energy expenditure in Pompe disease is increased.[14] Patients do not exhibit exercise intolerance or myoglobinuria because metabolism of non-membrane-bound glycogen and glucose for energy metabolism is not impaired.

Treatment

In the past, there were no specific treatments for acid maltase deficiency other than supportive therapy for associated cardioventilatory complications. Low carbohydrate and ketogenic diets are ineffective. A small study reported that 4 out of 16 patients treated with high-protein diet demonstrated improvement in muscle and respiratory function.[14]

Enzyme replacement therapy (ERT) with intravenous recombinant α-glucosidase enzyme appears to be safe and beneficial in classic infantile Pompe disease though the results of clinical trials in late-onset acid maltase deficiency have demonstrated only a modest benefit in distance traveled in the 6-minute walk test and in forced vital capacity between the α-glucosidase and placebo-treated patients.[40–43] The recommended dose of α-glucosidase is 20 mg/kg every 2 weeks. As alluded above, not all patients, including infants with classic Pompe disease, respond to ERT. A poor prognostic factor among infants is cross-reactive immunologic material (CRIM) status; CRIM-negative is strongly correlated with a poor outcome.[44,45] Although most CRIM-negative infants initially respond to continuous use of ERT, a resurgence of the natural progression of weakness subsequently ensues. These CRIM-negative infants develop antibodies directed against the infused recombinant α-glucosidase. Presumably, those infants who do not produce even minute amount of α-glucosidase are at increased risk of mounting an antibody response against α-glucosidase, as it is seen to be a foreign protein by the immune system.

GLYCOGENOSIS TYPE III (DEBRANCHING ENZYME DEFICIENCY)

Clinical Features

GSD III, also known as Cori–Forbes disease, accounts for approximately 25% of GSD (Table 29-1, Fig. 29-1).[46–49] GSD III is caused by the deficiency of debranching enzyme. This enzyme has two separate catalytic functions: (1) oligo-1,4-1,4-glucanotransferase activity and (2) α-1,6 glucosidase activity. Both the transferase and the glucosidase activities are vital in breaking down glycogen into glucose, and a deficiency in either or both enzymatic functions lead to myopathy.

There are two principal and two less-common forms of GSD III. In GSD IIIa, debranching enzyme is deficient in both the liver and the muscle. In contrast, enzyme activity is abnormal only in the liver in GSD IIIb, and a myopathy does not occur in this form of the disease. In rare cases, selective loss of only one of the two debranching enzyme activities [glucosidase (type IIIc) or transferase (type IIId)] has also been demonstrated.[50]

Deficiency of the debranching enzyme in muscle leads to weakness in patients with GSD IIIa. Onset of muscle weakness may be appreciated in infancy or childhood, although it usually does not manifest until the third to fourth decade of life.[46–49,51–57] Severe atrophy and weakness of distal extremity muscles, particularly the peroneal and calf muscles, occur in about 50% of patients.[48] Tight heal cords are common, and patients may have the tendency to toe walk. This distal involvement can lead to an initial misdiagnosis of motor neuron disease or a peripheral neuropathy. Some patients do, in fact, have a superimposed mild sensorimotor polyneuropathy. Pseudohypertrophy, particularly of the more proximal muscle groups, may be seen.[54] Generalized muscle weakness can also occur. In addition, some patients develop progressive ventilatory muscle weakness with or without extremity weakness. Ventilatory failure can evolve fairly rapidly. Less commonly, some patients develop a cardiomyopathy with or without extremity weakness.[52,58–61] Finally, rare patients manifest with myalgias, cramps, exercise intolerance, or myoglobinuria.[48,53,55,56,62]

Laboratory Features

Deficiency of debranching enzyme can be demonstrated with biochemical assay of muscle, fibroblasts, or lymphocytes. Serum CK levels are elevated 2–20 times normal. Exercise forearm testing reveals normal increase in serum ammonia but not in lactate levels. EMG demonstrates abnormalities similar to that described with acid maltase deficiency. Pulmonary function tests show reduced forced vital capacity in patients with ventilatory muscle involvement. Echocardiogram reveals findings suggestive of hypertrophic obstructive cardiomyopathy in most patients with GSD IIIa, while conduction defects and arrhythmias are apparent on EKG.[46,58,61,62]

Histopathology

Muscle biopsies demonstrate a vacuolar myopathy with abnormal accumulation of glycogen in the subsarcolemmal and intermyofibrillar regions of muscle fibers.[51,53,54] These vacuoles stain intensely with PAS and are digested by diastase. In contrast to acid maltase deficiency, these vacuoles do not stain with acid phosphatase, suggesting that glycogen does not primarily accumulate in lysosomes. On EM, free pools of glycogen are apparent. Some glycogen appears in lysosomes, but not to the same extent as seen in acid maltase deficiency. Autopsy studies of the heart have revealed fibrosis, moderate to severe vacuolization of cardiac myocytes, mild-to-severe glycogen accumulation in the atrioventricular (AV), and glycogen accumulation in smooth muscle cells of intramyocardial arteries associated with smooth muscle hyperplasia and profoundly thickened vascular walls.[63] Abnormal glycogen accumulation can also be found in skin and peripheral nerves.[64–66]

Molecular Genetics and Pathogenesis

The mutations in the debranching enzyme gene, *AGL*, on chromosome 1p21 cause both GSD IIIa and GSD IIIb.[67–70] Prenatal diagnosis is possible.[71] The *AGL* gene is composed of 35 exons spanning 85 kb of genomic DNA. Alternative splicing and differential RNA transcription result in at least six distinct isoforms and underline the differential expression of the debranching enzyme.[72] Tissue-specific expression of different isoforms results from the presence of at least two promoter regions. Of note, mutations within exon 3 mutations appear to be specific for GSD IIIb.[70]

Deficiency of the enzyme leads to the accumulation of glycogen in muscle; the exact mechanism of muscle weakness is not known. Similar amounts of glycogen accumulation in muscle can be demonstrated in patients who do not manifest weakness. Accumulation of glycogen in peripheral nerves may account for some degree of weakness and atrophy, particularly of the distal muscles.

Treatment

Frequent low-carbohydrate meals and maintaining a high-protein intake may prevent fasting hypoglycemia. High-protein nocturnal intragastric feedings led to apparent improvement in exercise tolerance, muscle strength and mass, electromyographic findings, and growth in one patient,[57] but this observation has not been subsequently confirmed. Supportive therapy is required for patients with congestive heart failure. Liver transplantation has been done on patients with cirrhosis and hepatocellular carcinoma.[72] However, debranching enzyme activity has remained absent in leukocytes after transplantation and is not likely to normalize in muscle.

GLYCOGENOSIS TYPE IV (BRANCHING ENZYME DEFICIENCY)

Clinical Features

GSD IV is rare and caused by the deficiency of the enzyme that helps make the branched glycogen molecule (Table 29-1, Fig. 29-1).[73–90] There are several forms of branching enzyme deficiency. The classic and most common type of GSD IV, also known as Andersen disease, presents in infancy as progressive liver dysfunction with hepatomegaly, splenomegaly, and failure to thrive. Muscular weakness, atrophy, hypotonia, hyporeflexia, and contractures may occur but are overshadowed by the liver disease.[79,84] Most children succumb to severe liver failure by 5 years of age. There is also a benign hepatic form of GSD IV in which the liver disease does not progress.[70,88] Some patients with GSD IV manifests primarily with muscle weakness, atrophy, and cardiomyopathy in childhood or adult life.[70,74,82,83] Either proximal or distal muscle groups can be preferentially affected. In addition, a fatal infantile form is associated with congenital onset of severe weakness.[84–87] Finally, there is a variant of branching enzyme deficiency, known as polyglucosan body neuropathy, which usually presents in adults as progressive upper and lower motor neuron loss, sensory nerve involvement, cerebellar ataxia, neurogenic bladder, and dementia.[75,77,89,90] Occasionally, polyglucosan body neuropathy manifests in children.[78] There is a predilection for polyglucosan body neuropathy in the Ashkenazi population.

Laboratory Features

Depending on the subtype of GSD IV, deficiency of branching enzyme may be demonstrated in muscle, peripheral nerve, fibroblasts, or leukocytes.[74,75,80,89,90] In patients with primary neuromuscular involvement, the deficiency may be noted only in muscle.[74] Branching enzyme activity can be normal in the muscle in patients with adult polyglucosan body neuropathy.[75,77] The serum CK may be normal or slightly elevated. EMG reveals myopathic features and muscle membrane instability similar to that observed with GSDs II and III. In patients with polyglucosan body neuropathy, an axonal sensorimotor neuropathy is apparent, while the EMG abnormalities reflect a superimposed polyradiculopathy. EKG can demonstrate progressive conduction defects leading to complete AV block.[82] Echocardiogram may reveal a dilated cardiomyopathy.[82]

Histopathology

Routine light microscopy and EM reveals deposition of varying amounts of finely granular and filamentous polysaccharide (polyglucosan bodies) in the CNS, peripheral nerves (axons and Schwann cells), skin, liver, and cardiac and skeletal muscles.[74,77,78,81–83] These polyglucosan bodies are PAS-positive and diastase resistant, suggesting the accumulation of polysaccharides other than glycogen (Fig. 29-3). They are not specific for this disorder and can be seen occasionally in nerve biopsies from patients with other diseases. This polysaccharide resembles amylopectin in that it has longer than normal peripheral chains and few branch points.

Autopsy studies have demonstrated abnormal polysaccharide material in the liver, heart, skeletal muscle, and in neurons of the brain and the spinal cord. The abnormal polysaccharide material is more abundant in the motor neurons than in other nerve cells and affects all motor neurons of the brainstem and spinal cord.[91]

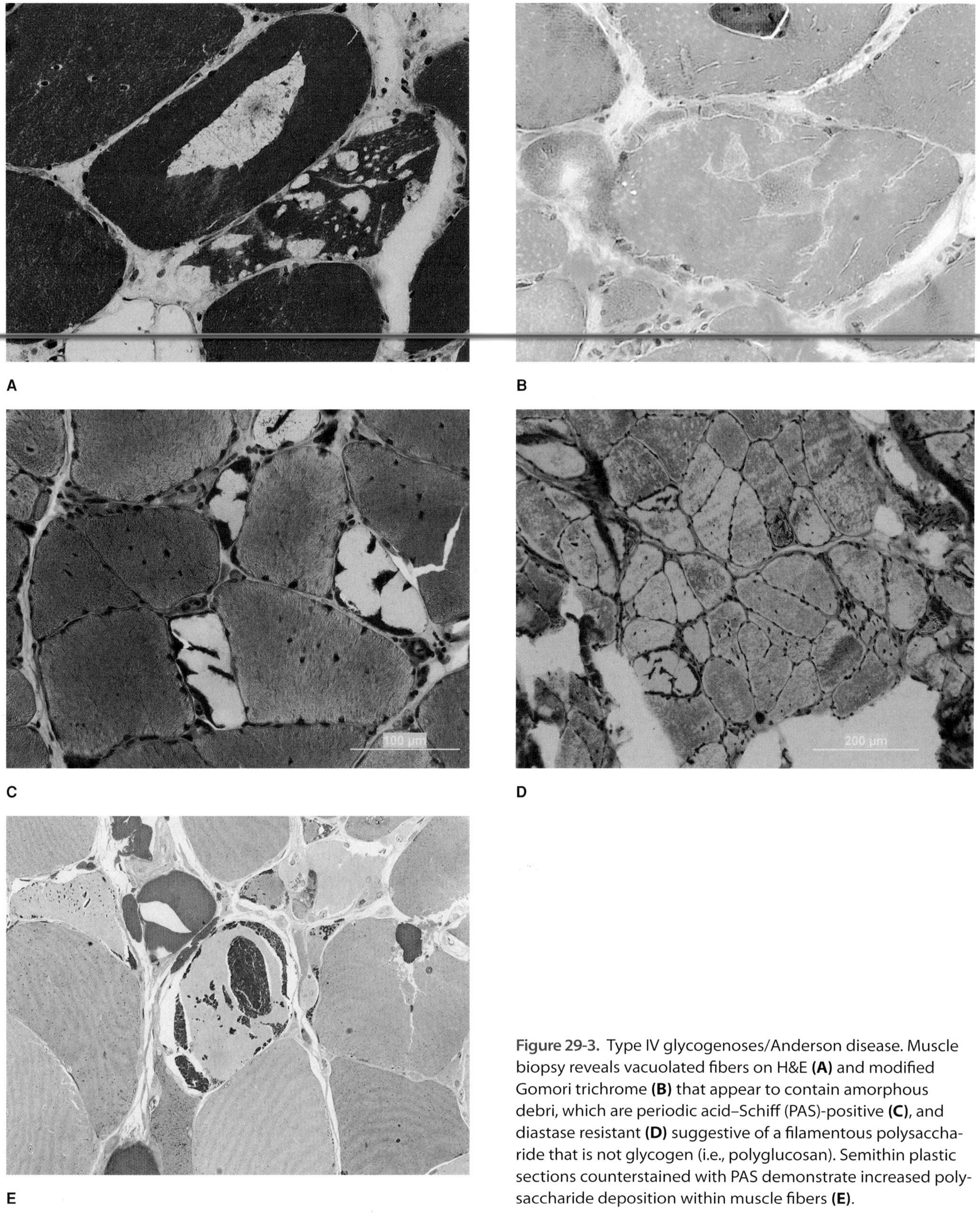

Figure 29-3. Type IV glycogenoses/Anderson disease. Muscle biopsy reveals vacuolated fibers on H&E **(A)** and modified Gomori trichrome **(B)** that appear to contain amorphous debri, which are periodic acid–Schiff (PAS)-positive **(C)**, and diastase resistant **(D)** suggestive of a filamentous polysaccharide that is not glycogen (i.e., polyglucosan). Semithin plastic sections counterstained with PAS demonstrate increased polysaccharide deposition within muscle fibers **(E)**.

Molecular Genetics and Pathogenesis

The disease is inherited in an autosomal-recessive manner. Deletions, nonsense, and missense mutations within the glycogen branching enzyme (*GBE1*) gene on chromosome 3p12 have been identified in the severe hepatic, benign hepatic, and the neuromuscular forms of GSD IV, including adult polyglucosan body disease.[73,76,89,90] There are phenotypic variability and differential expression of branching enzyme activity. The mechanism by which the abnormal accumulation of polysaccharide results in muscle damage is not known.

Treatment

Liver transplantation has been performed in some children with GSD IV with beneficial results.[92–94] Apparently, systemic microchimerism occurs after liver allotransplantation and can ameliorate pancellular enzyme deficiencies in this disease. Most of the patients became free of liver, neuromuscular, and cardiac dysfunction, with reduced polysaccharide accumulation in these tissues on long-term follow-up (mean 42 months). However, at least one child died from cardiomyopathy due to massive deposition of polysaccharide in the heart 2½ years after transplantation.[92] No other medical therapies have been demonstrated to be effective.

GLYCOGENOSIS TYPE V (MYOPHOSPHORYLASE DEFICIENCY)

Clinical Features

Glycogenosis type V (myophosphorylase deficiency), more commonly known as McArdle disease, is the most common neuromuscular disorder of carbohydrate metabolism. McArdle disease is an autosomal-recessive disorder that usually presents with exercise intolerance in childhood or young adults (Table 29-1, Fig. 29-1).[95–98] Patients complain of exertional muscle pain and cramps induced by brief, but very intense, activities (e.g., weight lifting and sprinting), but these can also occur following prolonged low-intensity exercises (e.g., swimming and jogging). If individuals who are affected ignore these symptoms and continue to exercise at a high level, the muscle pain and cramping can become quite intense and electrically silent contractures may develop. Some patients present with fatigue following exercise without associated cramps or muscle pain. Many patients note a second-wind phenomenon, in which after the onset of mild exertional myalgias or cramps (usually after 10 minutes of exercise), the muscle pain and sense of intolerance may dissipate. Subsequently, the individual may continue with the exercise at the previous or a slightly reduced level.[98] The second-wind phenomenon is the result of mobilization and use of blood-borne glucose.

Not everyone develops myoglobinuria and only about 50% of attacks of myoglobinuria are exertionally related. Myoglobinuria may not occur until the second or third decade, although it has developed in the 1st decade of life.[96,99] As many as 10% of attacks may be accompanied by acute renal failure, but this may be high as there probably are subclinical bouts of myoglobinuria that go unreported.[96]

Most patients have normal motor examinations between attacks of muscle cramping. However, fixed proximal weakness develops in as many as one-third of patients, perhaps as a result of recurrent bouts of rhabdomyolysis. Rare patients present with progressive proximal muscle atrophy and weakness in late-adult life rather than exercise intolerance.[100] Weakness may involve the arms more than the legs and can be asymmetric. Finally, a few cases have been reported with congenital weakness, some of which were rapidly progressive, leading to ventilatory failure within the first year of life.[101,102]

Laboratory Features

Serum CK levels are invariably elevated even while patients are asymptomatic. The exercise forearm test reveals a normal rise in serum ammonia but no significant rise in lactic acid.[103] EMG is usually normal in patients with McArdle disease.

Histopathology

Muscle biopsies demonstrate variability in fiber size, scattered necrotic and regenerating fibers, excessive accumulation of glycogen in the subsarcolemmal and intermyofibrillar areas, and absent myophosphorylase staining (see Fig. 3-6).[104,105] Biochemical assay for myophosphorylase reveals absent or significantly reduced activity.

Molecular Genetics and Pathogenesis

This disorder is inherited in an autosomal-recessive fashion and is caused by mutations in the *PYGM* gene that encodes myophosphorylase.[102,106,107] This enzyme initiates glycogen breakdown by phosphorylytically lysing α-1,4 glucosyl residues from the outer branches of glycogen, generating glucose-1-phosphate. Mutations result in little detectable protein or enzyme activity. Interestingly, the mutations associated with some of the rare cases of fatal infantile myopathy are the same as evident in the more common clinical presentation of McArdle disease.[102] A pseudodominant pattern of inheritance has been reported and felt to be secondary to heterozygotes who have low levels of residual myophosphorylase.[108] Another mechanism is the mating of a homozygote (or compound heterozygote) with a heterozygote.[108]

Although exercise intolerance and contractures had been postulated to be due to the inability to generate enough

ATP, studies have demonstrated that ATP is not depleted during exercise in McArdle disease, Tarui disease, or in the other disorders of glycogenolysis and glycolysis.[109] Exercise is associated with (1) an increase in adenosine diphosphate (ADP); (2) intracellular pH that does not acidify in response to exercise; (3) inorganic phosphate levels in muscle, which are 50% lower than normal muscle tissue; and (4) intracellular calcium concentrations at the onset of contracture, which is more than 10-fold greater than that found in normal control muscle ischemically exercised.[110] Perhaps the combination of increased intracellular ADP, reduced inorganic phosphate, and lack of acidification with impaired glycolysis increase sensitivity of the muscle fiber contractile apparatus to intracellular calcium. Further, the increased intracellular ADP may inhibit ADP dissociation from actin-myosin cross-bridges, thereby increasing the time spent in contraction.

In addition, patients with McArdle disease have reduced concentrations of the sodium–potassium ATPases pump, higher exercise-induced serum potassium concentrations, and a greater increase in heart rate during exercise.[111] Decreased sodium–potassium ATPases may lead to an exercise-induced increase in extracellular potassium because of impaired reuptake of potassium released during muscle contraction. Further, exercise intolerance leads to reduced physical activity, which may result in downregulation of the pump, and the increased ADP may decrease the transport rate of the remaining pumps. The increased concentration of extracellular potassium partially depolarizes the muscle membrane, thereby inactivating sodium channels and reducing membrane excitability.[111] Patients with McArdle disease also develop exaggerated tachycardia with exertion that can limit the exercise capacity of individuals who are affected.[111] It is not known why sodium–potassium pump concentrations in skeletal muscle in patients with McArdle disease are reduced. Reduced physical activity may downregulate the number of sodium–potassium ATPase pumps. Alternatively, myophosphorylase deficiency may reduce the pump concentration by disrupting the normal coupling of muscle glycogenolysis and pump activity.[111]

Treatment

A single-blind, placebo-controlled, crossover study of oral sucrose (75 g) in 12 patients with McArdle disease demonstrated marked improvement in exercise tolerance, supported by the subjects' reduced perceived exertion levels and their diminished maximum heart rates.[98] The limitation of oral sucrose loading is that the beneficial effect is short-lived. Repeated dosing may lead to weight gain, which in and of itself can reduce exercise tolerance. Furthermore, it can cause inhibition of fatty acid use, which also is an important fuel source with prolonged physical activity. Sucrose loading will also not be helpful in situations of unexpected exertional activity and prolonged physical activity or with static exercise (e.g., weight lifting).

A high-protein diet might help, but supplementing the diet with branched-chain amino acid supplementation can actually lower exercise capacity.[112] Creatine monohydrate has been studied but found to be of no significant benefit.[113] Surplus calories may lead to weight gain and subsequent decline in cardiovascular fitness. Some small studies have suggested that vitamin B6 supplementation (50 mg/day) can reduce exercise intolerance and enhance performance.[106] A recent Cochrane review of clinical trials reported that there was low quality evidence of improvement in some parameters with creatine, oral sucrose, ramipril, and a carbohydrate rich diet, although none indicated significant, clinical benefit.[97]

We instruct patients to avoid intense isometric exercises (e.g., weight lifting) and maximum aerobic exercises (e.g., sprinting). However, mild-to-moderate aerobic conditioning may be beneficial, as poor cardiovascular fitness results in a diminished delivery of blood-borne substrates necessary for muscle oxidative metabolism.[98,112] Patients should be instructed on how to moderate their physical activity in order to obtain a "second-wind" response. Any bout of moderate exercise should be preceded by 5–15 minutes of low-level warm-up activity to promote the transition to the second "wind."[112]

GLYCOGENOSIS TYPE VII (PFK DEFICIENCY)

Clinical Features

PFK deficiency or Tarui disease is an autosomal-recessive disease, caused by a deficiency in PFK in muscle and erythrocytes (Table 29-1, Fig. 29-1). PFK deficiency is much less common than McArdle disease. The clinical features are very similar to McArdle disease with respect to exercise intolerance, muscle pain, contractures, and relief of discomfort by rest. However, PFK deficiency is not associated with the warm-up phenomena, and there is a lower incidence of myoglobinuria.[114,115] In addition, some patients develop jaundice (due to mild hemolysis) and gouty arthritis due to PFK deficiency in erythrocytes.

The clinical phenotype can vary, and there are less common presentations. Some individuals who are affected manifest with hemolytic anemia without a myopathy. Others present later in adulthood with fixed weakness, which may predominantly affect the proximal or occasionally the scapuloperoneal muscles.[116,117] They may have had only mild exercise intolerance in their younger years but never have a history of cramps or myoglobinuria. In addition, PFK deficiency can present in infancy with severe generalized weakness and cardiomyopathy. Contractures, cortical blindness, and corneal opacifications are evident in some infants, but hemolytic anemia does not occur. Severely affected children may die from cardioventilatory failure in infancy or early childhood.

Laboratory Features

Serum CK is usually elevated, and mild anemia and increased reticulocyte count are often noted.[118] Exercise forearm testing reveals a normal increase in ammonia production but a blunted increase in lactic acid. EMG is usually normal.

Histopathology

Muscle biopsies demonstrate vacuoles and an abnormal accumulation of glycogen.[116] In addition, there is also an abnormal accumulation of polysaccharide, which stains intensely with PAS but is diastase resistant, especially in older patients. Muscle biopsies may reveal only nonspecific myopathic features without evidence of abnormal glycogen accumulation in the infantile form of disease. Definitive diagnosis of Tarui disease can be made by biochemical and histochemical analyses of muscle tissue, which reveal the deficiency of PFK activity and staining.

Molecular Genetics and Pathogenesis

PFK catalyzes the ATPase-dependent conversion of fructose 6-phosphate to fructose 1,6-diphosphate. Human PFK comprises three distinct isoenzyme subunits (M—muscle, L—liver, and P—platelet). Skeletal muscles contain only the M isoform, while erythrocytes contain a hybrid of M and L subunits. The gene responsible for the M isoform, PFK-M, was initially mapped to 1q32 but was subsequently reassigned to 12q13. The symptoms reflect inactivation of PFK in muscle and partial inactivation in red blood cells. Different molecular defects may explain the different clinical presentations; however, the biochemical and molecular basis for clinical heterogeneity remains unclear.

As in McArdle disease, there is ADP accumulation in exercised muscle, but whether or not there is also reduction in sodium–potassium pumps in Tarui disease is not known. The normal coupling of muscle glycogenolysis and sodium–potassium pump activity may be disrupted by increased ADP or reduction in pump concentration, as we described in the section on McArdle disease.

Treatment

Unlike in McArdle disease, glucose or fructose administration prior to activity does not help; rather it may be deleterious. Patients with PFK deficiency rely on free fatty acids as a fuel substrate during exercise. Therefore, they experience more exercise intolerance, if given a glucose infusion or they consume high-carbohydrate meals, because glucose reduces the blood levels of free fatty acids.[119] This is just the opposite of the second-wind phenomena and is sometime called the *out-of-wind phenomena*. An aerobic conditioning program similar to those given to patients with McArdle deficiency may improve exercise tolerance.

GLYCOGENOSIS TYPE VIII/IX (PHOSPHORYLASE B KINASE DEFICIENCY)

Muscle PBK or phosphorylase kinase (PHK) deficiency was formerly designated GSD VIII but now is more commonly referred to as GSD IX. PHK is a multimeric enzyme composed of four subunits. As will be discussed below, mutations involving PHKA1, encoding subunit α, cause the rare X-linked GSD IXa that is only associated with muscle involvement. Mutations in PHKB, encoding subunit β, cause the more common autosomal-recessive GSD IXb that involves both the liver and muscle. Mutations in other subunits are not associated with muscle involvement.

Clinical Features

PHK deficiency is associated with heterogeneous clinical manifestations.[120–123] It most commonly manifests as exercise intolerance with cramps and myoglobinuria (Table 29-1, Fig. 29-1). However, PHK deficiency can occasionally present in infancy or childhood with mild weakness and a delay in motor milestones. Rarely, a fatal cardiomyopathy can occur in infancy. Approximately 50% of patients develop proximal or distal weakness in adulthood.

Laboratory Features

Serum CK may be normal or mildly elevated. The exercise forearm test may be normal or abnormal. EMG is usually normal. Diagnosis is based on clinical findings, assay of PHK activity in erythrocytes, or liver or muscle tissues (depending upon presentation) and confirmatory findings on molecular genetic testing.

Histopathology

Muscle biopsy may be normal or may demonstrate variability in fiber size, scattered necrotic fibers, and slight subsarcolemmal accumulation of glycogen.[115] Biochemical analysis reveals decreased PHK activity.

Molecular Genetics and Pathogenesis

PHK catalyzes the conversion of inactive myophosphorylase to the active form and converts active glycogen synthetase to an inactive form. As mentioned above, PHK is a multimeric enzyme composed of four different subunits. Mutations in *PHKA1*, encoding subunit α, cause the less-common X-linked GSD IXa that is associated with muscle involvement only, while mutations in *PHKB*, encoding subunit β, cause autosomal-recessive GSD IXb that involves both liver and muscle.[124]

Treatment

There is no specific medical therapy. Patients should be instructed on a mild-to-moderate exercise program and to avoid vigorous activity.

GLYCOGENOSIS TYPE X (PHOSPHOGLYCERATE MUTASE DEFICIENCY)

Clinical Features

Phosphoglycerate mutatase (PGAM) deficiency presents in childhood or early adult life as exercise intolerance, cramps, and recurrent myoglobinuria (Table 29-1, Fig. 29-1).[125,126]

Laboratory Features

Serum CK is mildly elevated. The exercise forearm test is abnormal. EMG is normal.

Histopathology

Muscle biopsies reveal increased glycogen by PAS staining and on EM. Rarely, these are tubular aggregates in type 2B fibers. Biochemical assay demonstrates normal or only mildly elevated glycogen content and markedly diminished activity of PGAM (<10% of normal).

Molecular Genetics and Pathogenesis

Type X glycogenosis is an autosomal-recessive disorder caused by mutations in the PGAM-M gene encoded on chromosome 7p13–p12.3. PGAM catalyzes the interconversion of 2- and 3-phosphoglycerate. There are two subunits for PGAM: a muscle-specific subunit (PGAMM) and a non–muscle-specific or brain subunit (PGAMB). Mature muscle contains the homodimer MM form of PGAM, which has diminished enzymatic activity in type X glycogenosis.

Treatment

There is no definitive medical therapy. Dantrolene improved symptoms in one patient with severe cramps and tubular aggregates on muscle biopsy.[125] Nevertheless, dantrolene is not recommended as routine therapy. Patients should be instructed on avoiding strenuous activity and placed on a mild-to-moderate aerobic exercise program.

GLYCOGENOSIS TYPE XI (LACTATE DEHYDROGENASE DEFICIENCY)

Clinical Features

This rare autosomal-recessive disorder manifests as exercise intolerance, cramping, and recurrent myoglobinuria (Table 29-1, Fig. 29-1).[127] Muscle strength is normal. Patients may also develop a generalized, scaly, erythematous rash, particularly in the summer. Pregnancies may be complicated by uterine stiffness in early stages of delivery and often requires cesarean section. This complication has not been associated with other glycogenoses. Chronic renal failure can develop secondary to recurrent myoglobinuria.

Laboratory Features

Serum CK level is elevated. Serum LDH, which is usually markedly elevated during attacks of rhabdomyolysis, is normal in patients with LDH deficiency. A reduction in the LDH-M isoform (<5% of normal) in muscle and blood can be demonstrated on electrophoretic studies. On exercise forearm testing, lactate does not rise; however, there is a normal increase in pyruvate levels, because the enzymatic defect lies distal to the formation of pyruvate in the metabolic pathway. EMG is typically unremarkable.

Histopathology

Muscle biopsies can appear normal, but biochemical assay reveals reduced activity of LDH.

Molecular Genetics and Pathogenesis

There are five distinct LDH isoenzymes, each comprising tetramers composed of combinations of two different subunits, M and H. Thus far, only mutations involving the muscle M subunits encoded by the *LDH* gene, *LDHA*, on chromosome 11p15.4 have been associated with muscle disease.[127]

Treatment

There is no specific medical therapy. Obstetricians need to be made aware of potential complications of labor in affected pregnant females.

GLYCOGENOSIS TYPE XII (ALDOLASE A DEFICIENCY)

Clinical Features

This rare disorder has been reported in two young children who presented with rhabdomyolysis, exercise intolerance, and weakness, and episodes of hemolytic anemia- some following febrile illnesses (Table 29-1, Fig. 29-1).[128,129]

Laboratory Features

Serum CK was elevated in this singular case.

Histopathology

Muscle biopsy appeared normal on routine light microscopy, but EM revealed accumulation of lipid. Biochemical analysis revealed markedly reduced aldolase activity.

Molecular Genetics and Pathogenesis

Mutations in the aldolase gene located on chromosome 16q22–24 were reported.[128] Aldolase catalyzes the conversion of fructose 1,6-phosphate to dihydroxyacetone phosphate and glyceraldehyde 3-phosphate. The enzyme is expressed in red blood cells which probably accounts for the episodes of hemolytic anemia.

Treatment

There are no specific medical therapies.

GLYCOGENOSIS TYPE XIII (B-ENOLASE DEFICIENCY)

Clinical Features

This rare myopathy was reported in a 46-year-old man with exercise intolerance and myalgias (Table 29-1, Fig. 29-1).[130]

Laboratory Features

The serum CK levels were episodically elevated. No rise in lactic acid was noted on an exercise forearm test.

Histopathology

Muscle biopsy revealed abnormal accumulation of glycogen in the sarcoplasm. Selective β-enolase deficiency was demonstrated with immunohistochemistry and immunoblotting.

Molecular Genetics and Pathogenesis

Heterozygous mutations were identified within the β-enolase gene. β-Enolase catalyzes the step interconverting 2-phosphoglycerate and phosphoenolpyruvate.

Treatment

There are no specific medical therapies.

GLYCOGENOSIS TYPE XIV (PHOSPHOGLUCOMUTASE 1 DEFICIENCY)

Clinical Features

This rare myopathy is characterized by exercise-induced intolerance with episodes of rhabdomyolysis (Table 29-1, Fig. 29-1).[131,132] There is no second-wind phenomena.

Laboratory Features

CK at rest may be normal. Exercise forearm test reveals a normal elevation of lactate but also an exaggerated rise in ammonia.

Histopathology

Muscle biopsy revealed abnormal accumulation of glycogen in the sarcoplasm.

Molecular Genetics and Pathogenesis

Phosphoglucomutase 1 catalyzes the conversion of glucose-1-phosphate to glucose-6-phosphate. It is caused by mutations in *PGYM1*.

Treatment

There are no specific medical therapies.

GLYCOGENOSIS TYPE XV (GLYCOGENIN 1 DEFICIENCY)

Clinical Features

This rare myopathy was first reported in one patient who developed ventricular arrhythmia with exercise intolerance in early adulthood (Table 29-1, Fig. 29-1).[133] Examination in his 20s revealed mild proximal arm and neck flexion weakness along with dorsiflexion weakness. He had met early motor milestones but was unable to keep up with peers secondary to dyspnea on exertion.

A second recent report described seven unrelated adult patients with limb-girdle weakness with onset in childhood to mid 60s and no cardiomyopathy.[134]

Laboratory Features

Serum CKs can be normal or slightly elevated.[133,134] EMG may show increased insertional and spontaneous activity and early recruitment of small myopathic appearing motor units.[133,134] Echocardiography in one patient revealed a normal ejection fraction, while cardiac MRI demonstrated areas with late enhancement, and slightly increased left ventricular volume and mass.[133]

Histopathology

Skeletal and cardiac muscle biopsy revealed abnormal accumulation of glycogen in the sarcoplasm in the patient reported with a cardiomyopathy.[133] Type 1 fiber atrophy and predominance was appreciated on the skeletal muscle biopsy while the cardiocytes were hypertrophic; glycogen was depleted while glycogenin 1 was increased in muscle fibers. In contrast, in a recent series of seven patients with late-onset proximal weakness and no cardiomyopathy, the muscle biopsies were notable for abnormal accumulation of glycogen and polyglucosan bodies and depletion of glycogenin 1 in skeletal muscle biopsies.[134]

Molecular Genetics and Pathogenesis

Glycogenin 1 is encoded by *GYG1*. The enzyme catalyzes the formation of short glucose polymers of approximately 10 glucose residues, from uridine diphosphate glucose in an autoglucosylation reaction.[133,134] This enzymatic step is followed by elongation and branching of the polymer, catalyzed by glycogen synthase 1, which as discussed previously is abnormal in GSD type 0.

Treatment

There are no specific medical therapies.

▶ OTHER RELATED DISORDERS

TRIOSEPHOSPHATE ISOMERASE DEFICIENCY

Clinical Features

There is a report of an 8-year old with history of generalized hypotonia and weakness since infancy, mental retardation, and hemolytic anemia who was found to have triosephosphate isomerase deficiency (Table 29-1, Fig. 29-1).[135]

Laboratory Features

Serum CKs were normal but EMG was reportedly myopathic.

Histopathology

Muscle biopsy demonstrated increased glycogen on routine light microscopy and EM.

Molecular Genetics and Pathogenesis

Triosephosphate isomerase catalyzes the conversion of dihydroxyacetone phosphate into glyceraldehyde 3-phosphate.

Treatment

There are no specific medical therapies.

PHOSPHOGLYCERATE KINASE DEFICIENCY

Clinical Features

PGK deficiency is an X-linked disorder, which commonly presents in male children as hemolytic anemia and CNS disturbances (e.g., mental retardation and seizures) (Table 29-1, Fig. 29-1). In addition, some patients present with a myopathy.[136–139] Presentation with hemolytic anemia, CNS disturbances, and myopathy appears to occur in equal frequencies in patients with PGK deficiency.[140] The myopathy is characterized by exercise intolerance, cramps, and recurrent myoglobinuria. Slowly progressive proximal weakness has also been described.

Laboratory Features

Serum CK is two to three times normal. Most patients with the myopathy do not have hemolytic anemia, although it has been described.[139] Exercise forearm test fails to show a normal rise in lactate. EMG is usually normal.

Histopathology

Muscle biopsies are typically normal, but mild and diffuse PAS staining may be noted. Abnormal glycogen accumulation is usually apparent by EM. Enzymatic assays reveal reduced PGK enzyme activity.

Molecular Genetics and Pathogenesis

The disorder is caused by mutations in the PGK gene located on chromosome Xq13. PGK catalyzes the transfer of the acyl phosphate group of 1,3-diphosphoglycerate to ADP, with the formation of 3-phosphoglycerate and ATP in the terminal stage of the glycolysis.

Treatment

No specific medical therapy for the myopathy is available.

UBIQUITIN LIGASE (RBCK1) DEFICIENCY

Clinical Features

Ubiquitin ligase deficiency is a rare autosomal-recessive disorder reported in 10 patients whom presented in childhood to late teens with slowly progressive proximal leg weakness.[140] Patients with homozygous or compound heterozygous for truncating mutations have developed a rapidly progressive dilated cardiomyopathy with onset in adolescence that required cardiac transplantation. Hepatomegaly with abnormal accumulation of polyglucosan may also occur.

Laboratory Features

Serum CK was normal to sixfold elevated. Echocardiogram may demonstrate features of a dilated cardiomyopathy.

Histopathology

Skeletal and cardiac muscle biopsy fibers were typically devoid of normal glycogen, but contained abnormal accumulation of polyglucosan bodies that were PAS-positive that were resistant to diastase. The inclusions were also ubiquitinated and stained for ubiquitin-binding protein sequestosome-1 (p62).

Molecular Genetics and Pathogenesis

The disorder is caused by mutations in the *RBCK1* gene that encodes for ubiquitin ligase. *RBCK1* mutations are also known to be associated with recurrent infections and episodes of sepsis and possible autoimmune disorders. The enzyme appears to be involved in myogenesis. It also plays a role in regulating the nuclear factor κB (NFκB) pathways which may explain the recurrent infections and autoimmunity in some patients depending on the site of the mutation.

Treatment

No specific medical therapy for the myopathy is available, though medications treating congestive heart failure and cardiac transplantation have been used to treat the cardiomyopathy.

▶ OTHER VACUOLAR MYOPATHIES

We debated in which chapter to discuss Danon disease and X-linked myopathy with excessive autophagy (XMEA). Danon disease was initially reported as "lysosomal glycogen storage disease with normal acid maltase."[141] Some have termed this GSD IIb. XMEA shares similar histopathological features with Danon disease. As both are in the differential diagnosis of vacuolar myopathies with increased glycogen deposition, we decided to include discussion of these disorders in this chapter.

DANON DISEASE (X-LINKED VACUOLAR CARDIOMYOPATHY AND MYOPATHY)

Clinical Features

Danon initially described this rare disorder characterized by the triad of hypertrophic or dilated cardiomyopathy, myopathy, and mental retardation.[141–148] Males are more severely affected than females, but female carriers can also manifest with symptoms.[147,148] Individuals who are affected usually appear normal at birth but develop proximal muscle weakness and a cardiomyopathy in childhood or early adult life. Approximately 70% of males have some degree of mental retardation compared to less than 50% of women.[143,144] Either hypertrophic or dilated cardiomyopathy may occur that can be complicated by arrhythmia and sudden death.[144,147,148] In a recent review of 82 patients with Danon disease in the literature, the average ages of first symptom, cardiac transplantation, and death were 12.1, 17.9, and 19.0 years in males and 27.9, 33.7, and 34.6 years in females, respectively.[144]

Laboratory Features

Serum CK levels are moderately elevated. Echocardiograms often demonstrate a hypertrophic or dilated cardiomyopathy.[144,148] The most frequent EKG abnormality is Wolff–Parkinson–White syndrome, but AV block, bundle branch blocks, bradycardia, and atrial flutter/fibrillation may also be observed. Cardiac MRI may be useful in women harboring lysosome-associated membrane protein-2 (LAMP-2) mutations, as it may demonstrate early involvement and guide timely considerations of implantable cardioverter-defibrillator therapy.[148]

NCS are normal. Increased insertional and spontaneous activity in the form of fibrillation potentials, positive sharp waves, complex repetitive discharges, and myotonic discharges are evident on EMG.[141] There is early recruitment of small-amplitude, short-duration, polyphasic MUAPs.

Histopathology

Muscle biopsies demonstrate variability in fiber size with autophagic vacuoles.[141] Excess free glycogen between disorganized myofibrils and within membrane-bound sacs and vacuoles may be seen on EM. On EM, some of the vacuoles are bound by basal lamina. These histological features are similar to Pompe disease, although α-glucosidase activity is normal in Danon disease. The characteristic feature is the absence of LAMP-2 on immunostaining. Unlike X-linked myopathy with excessive autophagy (XMEA), which it can resemble, there is no deposition of membrane attack complex on muscle fibers.[149]

Molecular Genetics and Pathogenesis

Danon disease is caused by mutations in the gene that encodes for LAMP-2, which is located on the chromosome Xq24.[142] LAMP-2 is a major lysosomal membrane protein and mutations lead to defects in autophagy.

Treatment

There is no specific medical therapy at this time for the skeletal muscle weakness. Some patients require pacemakers, intracardiac defibrillators, or cardiac transplantation for the cardiomyopathy.[144,147,148]

X-LINKED MYOPATHY WITH EXCESSIVE AUTOPHAGY

Clinical Features

XMEA can present in infancy or early adult life with slowly progressive proximal weakness and atrophy.[149–153] Respiratory weakness can also ensue. Unlike Danon disease, which it can resemble, individuals with XMEA usually do not develop a cardiomyopathy or mental retardation. However, a case resembling XMEA was recently reported with cardiomyopathy.[152]

Laboratory Features

Serum CK levels may be normal or mildly elevated. Routine motor and sensory NCS are normal. EMG reveals increased insertional and spontaneous activity with fibrillation potentials, positive sharp waves, complex repetitive discharges, and myotonic discharges.[149–151] There is early recruitment of small-amplitude, short-duration, polyphasic MUAPs.

Histopathology

Muscle biopsies reveal muscle fiber size variation and many fibers with autophagic vacuoles (Fig. 29-4A and B).[149–153] Unlike Danon disease and acid maltase deficiency, these vacuoles are not PAS positive. Further, LAMP-2 is present in the vacuoles and within the cytoplasm in XMEA (Fig. 29-4C). Calcium and membrane attack complex (C5b-9) (Fig. 29-4D) deposit along the

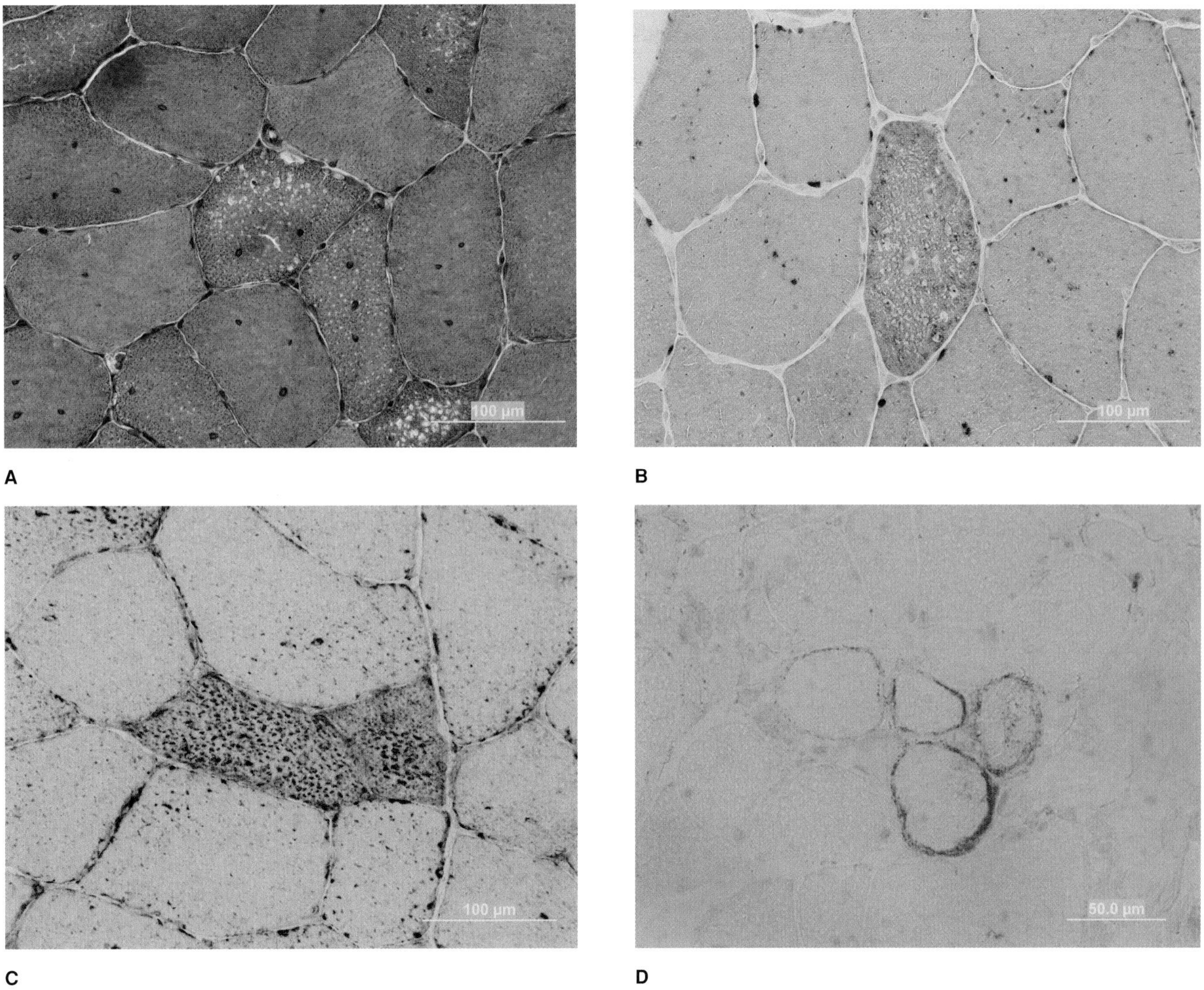

Figure 29-4. X-linked myopathy with excessive autophagia (XMEA). Muscle biopsies reveal fibers with autophagic vacuoles on modified Gomori trichrome **(A)**, which stain red with acid phosphatase stain **(B)**. Immunoperoxidase stain with antibodies directed against lysosome-associated membrane protein-2 (LAMP-2) demonstrates the presence of LAMP-2 in lysosomes **(C)**. Further, immunoperoxidase stain demonstrates membrane attack complex (C5b-9) deposition along the sarcolemma of abnormal muscle fibers **(D)**.

sarcolemma of abnormal muscle fibers.[149,153] On EM, some of the vacuoles are bound by basal lamina. These are often appreciated in the subsarcolemmal region where they appear to fuse with the cell membrane allowing expression of their contents into the extracellular space. Redundant folds of basal lamina surrounding muscle fibers are also characteristic.

Molecular Genetics and Pathogenesis

The XMEA is caused by mutations in the gene that encodes for VMA21 located on chromosome Xq28.[153] Vacuolar ATPases (V-ATPases) are composed of 14 subunits that act as a proton pumps which regulate the levels lysosomes. VMA21 is a chaperone protein that is essential to the assembly of V-ATPase. Defects in VMA21 lead to a rise in lysosomal pH which reduces degradation and blocks autophagy.

Treatment

There is no specific medical therapy for XMEA.

► DISORDERS OF PURINE NUCLEOTIDE METABOLISM

Disorders of purine metabolism more commonly cause hyperuricemic syndromes (gout and Lesch–Nyhan syndrome) or immunodeficiency disorders rather than a myopathy. A single disorder of nucleotide metabolism, MAD deficiency, has been linked to exercise intolerance and myoglobinuria in the past, but even this association has been questioned.

MYOADENYLATE DEAMINASE DEFICIENCY

Clinical Features

Patients with MAD deficiency may develop exertional muscle pain and fatigue[154–157] and perhaps myoglobinuria[155] in late adolescence to middle age. However, the relationship between MAD deficiency and the exercise intolerance and bouts of myoglobinuria is controversial. The neurological examination is normal. Many individuals with MAD deficiency are asymptomatic, and mild exertional muscle pain and fatigue are extremely common symptoms in the general population. MAD deficiency has been reported in 1–2% of muscle biopsies, making it the most common enzyme deficiency in muscle.[156] Additionally, muscle biopsies in patients with other types of neuromuscular disorders such as amyotrophic lateral sclerosis, spinal muscular atrophy, inflammatory myopathies, and various forms of muscular dystrophies have been found to have incidental deficiencies in MAD. Thus, although the frequency of MAD deficiency may be increased in muscle biopsies performed for evaluation of exertional myalgias,[154] a cause and effect relationship between the enzymatic deficiency and symptomatic muscle disease has yet to be established.

Laboratory Features

Serum CK is normal or only slightly elevated. The exercise forearm test is abnormal; serum lactate levels rise normally with exercise; however, ammonia levels remain relatively stable. EMG is normal.

Histopathology

The routine muscle biopsy is normal.[154] Specific biochemical assay or histological stain for MAD is essentially the only abnormality noted.

Molecular Genetics and Pathogenesis

MAD catalyzes the removal of an ammonia group from adenosine monophosphate (AMP) to form inosine monophosphate. AMP combines with ATP to form 2 ADP molecules (2 ADP $\leftrightarrow$ ATP + AMP). By catalyzing the conversion of AMP to inosine monophosphate, thereby reducing available AMP. MAD indirectly tilts the above equation in favor of the formation of ATP, maintaining energy supplies. Also, the production of ammonia by MAD buffers the lactic acid formed during exercise. Further, inosine monophosphate stimulates glycolysis by acting on PFK and aids in making fumarate, a substrate integral to the Kreb cycle. Thus, MAD deficiency potentially can have wide-reaching metabolic effects in multiple energy production cycles. Reduced phosphocreatine and ADP levels have been demonstrated in MAD deficiency patients compared to normal controls.[157] However, a study of sustained, isometric muscle contraction during ischemia in patients with MAD deficiency and normal controls found no difference in oxygen use, endurance time, resting, and postexercise lactate and phosphocreatine levels, suggesting a normal exercise capacity.[158]

Point mutations have been identified in primary MAD deficiency in the gene *AMPD1* (AMP deaminase 1), located on chromosome 1p13–21.[156,159] As noted above, MAD deficiency has been associated with a number of neuromuscular disorders. A study in the Dutch population revealed no significant differences in frequencies of the characteristic "mutation" in the MAD gene in patients with exercise intolerance, those with other neuromuscular disorders, and healthy volunteers.[156] It may be that the "mutations" that lead to MAD deficiency are no more than harmless polymorphisms.

Treatment

There is no specific medical treatment available.

► LIPID METABOLISM DISORDERS

The major source of fuel for muscles at rest and following prolonged or intense physical activity are free fatty acids, particularly long-chain fatty acids. β-Oxidation of free fatty acids occurs within the inner matrix of mitochondria and generates ATP. Fatty acids are divided into short-, medium-, long-, and very–long-chain fatty acids, depending on their size. Short- and medium-chain fatty acids are readily permeable to either the outer or the inner mitochondrial membranes. However, long-chain fatty acids must interact with various carrier proteins and be actively transported across the mitochondrial membranes (Fig. 29-5). First, the long-chain fatty acids combine with coenzyme A (CoA) in a reaction catalyzed by acyl-CoA-synthetase at the outer mitochondrial membrane, creating a long-chain acyl-CoA. Next, the long-chain acyl-CoA must link with carnitine in a reaction reversibly catalyzed by carnitine palmitoyltransferase 1 (CPT1), an enzyme located on the outer face of the outer mitochondrial membrane, in order to cross over the outer membrane. The long-chain acyl–carnitine complex within the intermembrane space is then transported across the inner mitochondrial membrane, in a reaction catalyzed by carnitine palmitoyltransferase 2 (CPT2) located on the inner surface of the inner membrane. This liberates carnitine from the long-chain acyl-CoA. The carnitine is then transported in the opposite direction, in a reaction catalyzed by carnitine/acylcarnitine translocase. The long-chain acyl-CoA, now within the mitochondrial matrix, can be metabolized by β-oxidation into ATP.

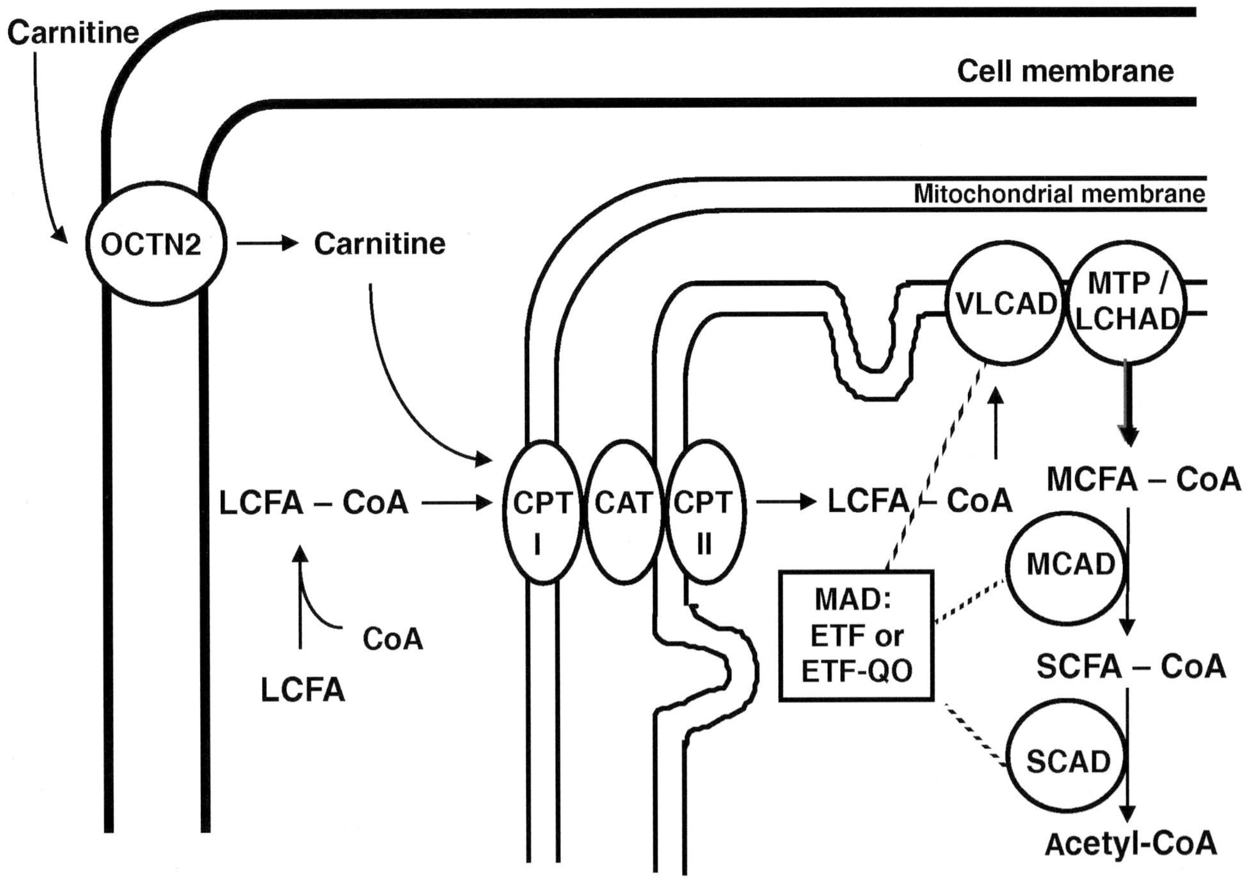

Figure 29-5. Simplified scheme of mitochondrial fatty acid oxidation. CAT, carnitine acylcarnitine translocase; CPT I, carnitine palmitoyl transferase I; CPT II, carnitine palmitoyl transferase II; LCFA, long-chain fatty acid; LCHAD, long-chain 3-hydroxyacyl-CoA dehydrogenase; MAD, multiple acyl-CoA dehydrogenase; MCAD, medium-chain acyl-CoA dehydrogenase; MCFA, medium-chain fatty acid; MTP, mitochondrial trifunctional protein; OCTN2, plasma membrane sodium-dependent carnitine transporter; SCAD, short-chain acyl-CoA dehydrogenase; SCFA, short-chain fatty acid; VLCAD, very–long-chain acyl-CoA dehydrogenase. (Reproduced with permission from Laforet P, Vianey-Sabab C. Disorders of muscle lipid metabolism: diagnostic and therapeutic changes. *Neuromuscul Disord*. 2010;20(11):693–700.)

β-Oxidation of the fatty acids within the mitochondria proceeds through repeated cycles consisting of four sequential enzymatic reactions (Fig. 29-6). First, flavin-dependent, length-specific acyl-CoA dehydrogenases [note that there are short-, medium-, long-, and very–long-chain acyl-CoA dehydrogenases (SCADs, MCADs, LCADs, and VLCADs)] convert the acyl-CoA substrates into enoyl-CoAs and reduce flavin adenine dinucleotide (FAD). Second, length-specific enoyl-CoA hydratase catalyzes the formation of 3-hydroxyacyl-CoA derivatives. Third, length-specific, NAD-dependent 3-hydroxyacyl-CoA dehydrogenases (HADs) catalyze the formation of 3-ketoacyl-CoA esters by a second dehydrogenation reaction. In the fourth and final step, length-dependent 3-ketothiolase catalyzes the conversion of the 3-ketoacyl-CoA ester to acetyl-CoA and fatty acyl-CoA, which are now two carbon atoms shorter than the acyl-CoA that entered

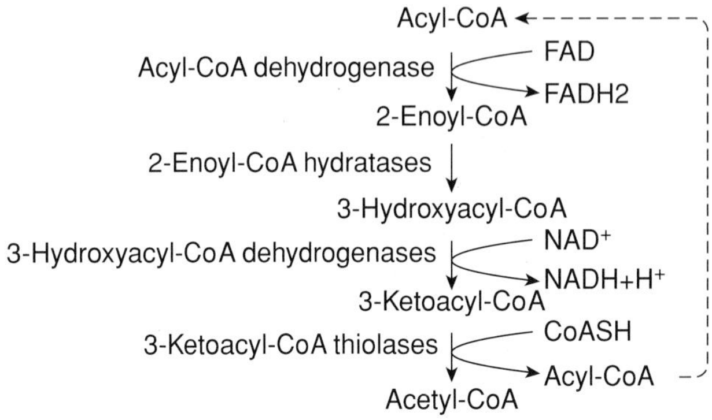

Figure 29-6. Β-oxidation of fatty acids pathway. There are four steps involved in the complete oxidation of fatty acids. The main defects in this pathway affecting muscle involve deficiencies of the acyl-CoA dehydrogenases. The details of each reaction are given in the text. (Reproduced with permission from Walsh RJ. Metabolic Myopathies. *Continuum*. 2006;12(3):76-120.)

the initial first step. This sequential cycle of four enzymatic reactions is then repeated.

Electrons transferred to $FADH_2$ and NADH are then transferred to the respiratory chain, which is composed of five multimeric protein complexes embedded in the inner mitochondrial membrane. FADH delivers its electrons to coenzyme Q via two flavoproteins: electron-transferring flavoprotein (ETF) and ETF-coenzyme Q oxidoreductase (ETF-QO). NADH delivers its electrons to complex I of the respiratory chain. The electrons are then transported down an energy gradient from one complex to another, generating a proton motive force, which is necessary to produce ATP.

Defects in the transport of long-chain fatty acids and lipid metabolism affect multiple organs, including muscle. Two major muscle manifestations are (1) progressive muscle weakness and hypotonia (e.g., as seen in carnitine transporter and carnitine/acylcarnitine defects) and (2) acute, recurrent rhabdomyolysis (e.g., as seen in deficiencies of CPT2, VLCAD, and trifunctional protein). Some defects result in both fixed weakness and recurrent bouts of rhabdomyolysis (e.g., VLCAD and trifunctional protein deficiencies).

Diagnostic workup depends on the clinical presentation.[160–163] In patients with fixed progressive weakness, other more common disorders as muscular dystrophy or congenital myopathy are typically suspected. The diagnosis of a lipid storage disease is often only suspected after a biopsy is performed and it shows a vacuolar myopathy with abnormal lipid accumulation (Fig. 29-7). The next step is to assess total and free carnitine levels and serum acylcarnitine. Typically the carnitine and acylcarnitine levels are markedly reduced in primary carnitine deficiency. In the acyl-CoA dehydrogenases deficiencies including multi–acyl-CoA dehydrogenase deficiency (MADD), specific patterns are seen on the acylcarnitine and urine organic acid profiles. If the carnitine levels, acylcarnitine profile, and the urine for organic acids are not remarkable, then one needs to consider a form of neutral lipid storage disease. In such cases, there is increase in triglycerides in the tissues

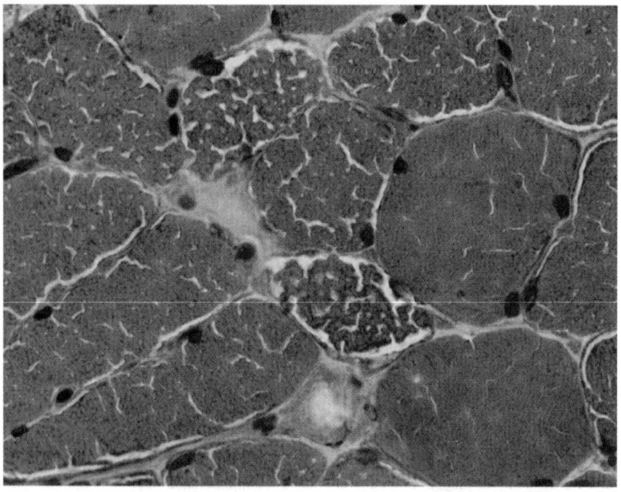

A

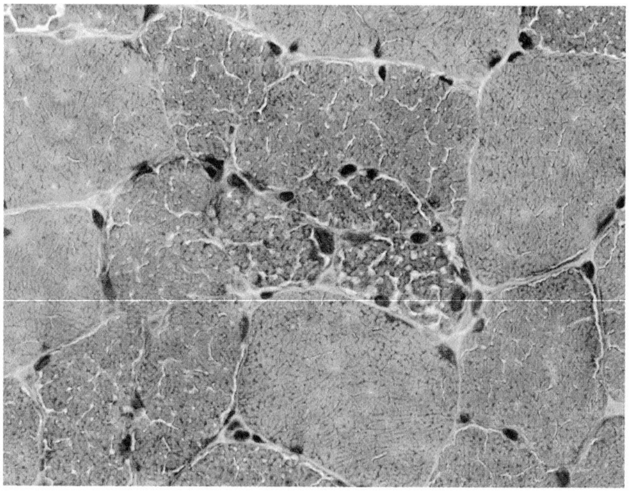

B

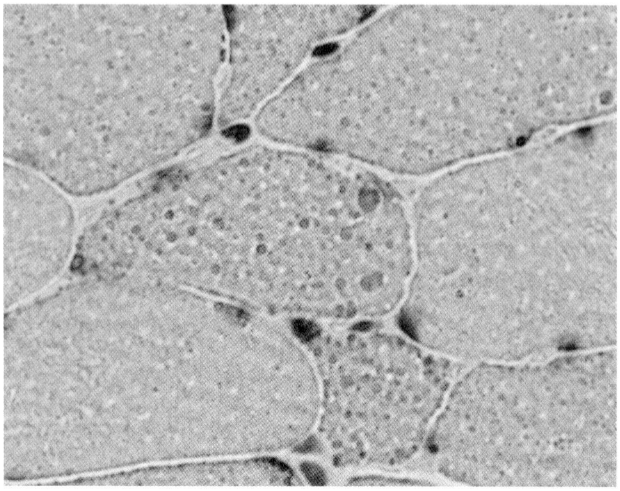

C

Figure 29-7. Multi-acyl-CoA dehydrogenase deficiency (MADD). Muscle biopsy demonstrates vacuoles within muscle fibers on H&E **(A)** and modified Gomori trichrome **(B)** that are filled by lipid deposition within fibers on oil red O stain **(C)**.

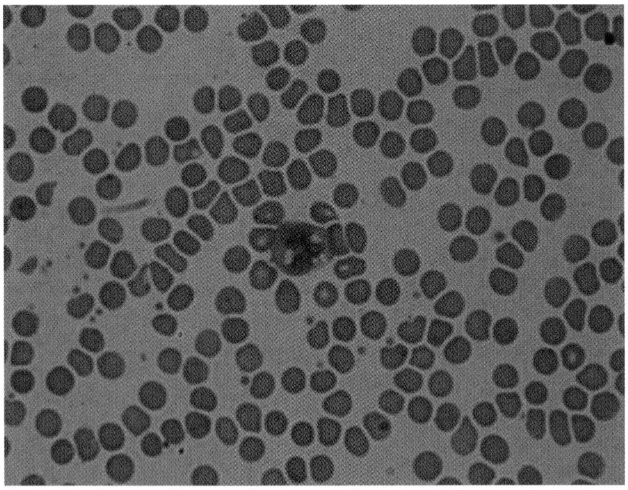

Figure 29-8. Jordan's anomaly. Blood smear demonstrates clear lipid droplets (triglyceride) within a polymorphonuclear cell in a case of neutral lipid storage disorder.

(not fatty acids). A blood smear may show the accumulation of triglyceride droplets, so-called Jordan's anomaly (Fig. 29-8).

Lipid storage disorders should also be suspected in cases of recurrent myoglobinuria following prolonged physical exertion—the time when fatty acid metabolism is needed for ATP production. Also, cases of myoglobinuria following a febrile illness or fasting should lead to consideration of a lipid storage disease. We usually start the workup with an exercise forearm test, which should be normal. Serum for acylcarnitine profile and urine for organic acid analysis are sent, and if abnormal may give a clue as to the exact enzyme defect and subsequent targeted genetic testing. The most common cause of recurrent myoglobinuria (when one is found) is CPT2 deficiency. Therefore, if the above tests are not revealing, the next step is to do genetic testing for the most common mutations associated with CPT2 deficiency. If this is normal then we usually proceed with a muscle biopsy or skin biopsy for fibroblasts and send specimens for analysis of various lipid enzymes. In children with recurrent episodes of myoglobinuria in the setting of febrile illness, who have normal serum acylcarnitine profile and urine organic acids, one needs to also consider lipin deficiency.

Please see the below discussion of specific lipid storage diseases for further details.

CARNITINE TRANSPORTER DEFICIENCY (PRIMARY CARNITINE DEFICIENCY)

Clinical Features

Primary systemic carnitine deficiency is a clinically heterogeneous disorder.[160–178] Some patients with primary carnitine deficiency develop symptoms and signs resembling Reye syndrome in early childhood with acute attacks of vomiting, altered mental status, hypoglycemia, and hepatomegaly.[161,163,170,172,173] These children may become weak, but the systemic manifestations tend to overshadow the myopathy. More commonly, individuals who are affected present with a hypertrophic or dilated cardiomyopathy and progressive proximal muscle weakness and atrophy in childhood or early adult life.[165,166,174–177] Rhabdomyolysis and respiratory weakness can occur.[179] Infantile onset has also been described. A few cases have worsened significantly during pregnancy or in the postpartum period.[178]

Secondary carnitine deficiency may result from a variety of disorders, including respiratory chain defects, organic aciduria, endocrinopathies, dystrophies, and renal and liver failure, malnutrition, and as a toxic effect of certain medications.[167,180] It is not known if the secondary deficiency of carnitine can in and of itself cause a myopathy.

Laboratory Features

Plasma and tissue (including muscle) carnitine levels are markedly diminished in primary carnitine deficiency, while the levels are only moderately reduced (25–50% normal) in secondary forms of carnitine deficiency.[160–163,167,174,181] Serum acylcarnitine levels are also reduced. Serum CK levels are normal in approximately 50% of patients with the myopathic form of the disease but can be elevated to as much as 15 times normal. In primary systemic carnitine deficiency, liver enzymes are also elevated. Fasting individuals with carnitine deficiency may develop hypoglycemia, acidosis, and elevated CK levels and liver function tests. However, ketones are not elevated in the urine during fasting.

EMG may reveal increased insertional activity with positive sharp waves, fibrillation potentials, and complex repetitive discharges. Early recruitment of short-duration, small-amplitude, and polyphasic MUAPs can be observed. An echocardiogram can demonstrate a dilated or hypertrophic cardiomyopathy.

Histopathology

Muscle biopsies reveal variability in muscle fiber size and abnormal accumulation of lipid in the subsarcolemma and intermyofibrillar regions (Fig. 29-9). Type 1 fibers are preferentially affected, as would be expected, given that oxidative metabolism primarily occurs in these fibers. EM also demonstrates increased lipid (Fig. 29-10). Muscle carnitine levels are dramatically decreased (<2–4% of normal) in patients with primary carnitine deficiency (this may serve to distinguish from patients with secondary deficiency).

Molecular Genetics and Pathogenesis

Primary carnitine deficiency is caused by mutations in the gene encoding for the sodium-dependent carnitine transporter protein, *OCTN2*, (also called *SLC22A5*) located on chromosome

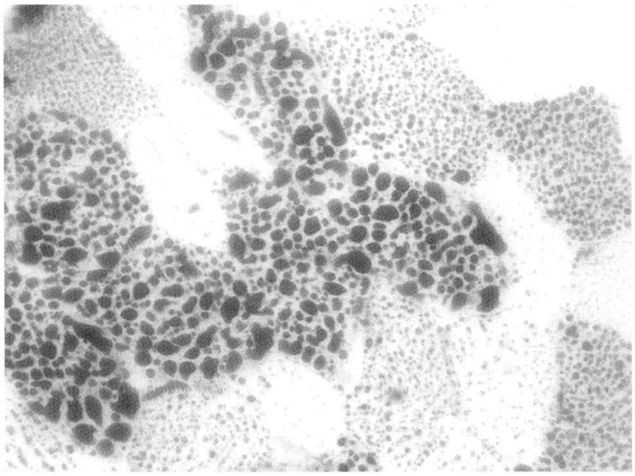

Figure 29-9. Carnitine deficiency. Muscle biopsy demonstrates increased lipid droplets within muscle fibers (*Oil red O*).

5q33.1.[182] Carnitine is supplied to tissues by diet and endogenous synthesis. Intracellular carnitine levels are maintained at 20–50 times the extra-cellular concentration by this active transport system (Fig. 29-5). The deficiency of carnitine impairs the transport of long-chain fatty acids into the inner mitochondrial matrix, thus severely affecting energy production from these fatty acids.

Treatment

Oral L-carnitine (100–200 mg/kg/day) benefits some, but not all patients, with carnitine deficiency.[160–162,168,174,179,183–185] There can be a dramatic clinical response to oral L-carnitine in patients with severe cardiomyopathy and muscle weakness.[174] However, only modest increases in muscle carnitine levels have been demonstrated, even in those who improved in muscle strength.[174] Perhaps, intracellular (muscle) concentration of carnitine only needs to be more than 2–4% of normal to allow for normal lipid metabolism.

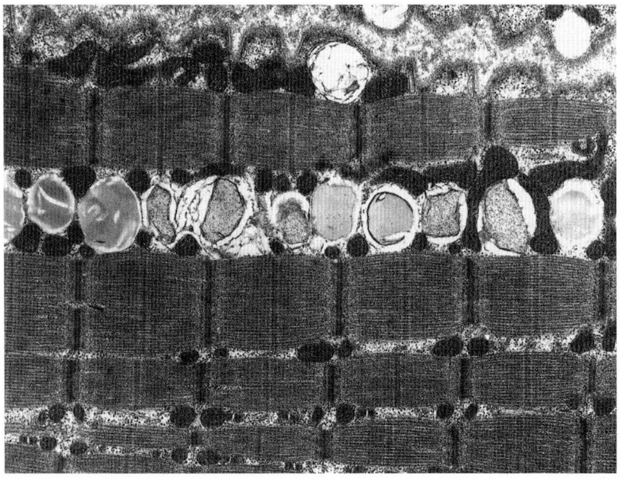

Figure 29-10. Electron microscopy reveals increased endomysial lipid droplets.

CPT2 DEFICIENCY

Clinical Features

CPT2 deficiency is inherited in an autosomal-recessive manner and typically presents in the second or third decade of life with muscular pain and myoglobinuria following intense or prolonged exertion.[160–162,186–189] Prolonged fasting and infection are other precipitating factors. The neuromuscular examination is usually normal between bouts of rhabdomyolysis. Rare cases of a CPT2 deficiency causing a fatal cardiomyopathy in infancy or early childhood have also been reported.

Laboratory Features

Serum CK levels are usually normal, except when the patient performs intense physical activities or fasts. Exercise forearm test is normal, which can also help distinguish CPT2 deficiency from the glycogen storage disorders which can also cause exercise-induced rhabdomyolysis. Muscle and serum carnitine levels are normal. EMG is usually unremarkable, although myopathic units may be seen. EKG is also normal.

Histopathology

There is usually no gross abnormality noted on light microscopic examination of muscle tissue. However, an increase in the lipid content of muscle may be apparent on EM.

Molecular Genetics and Pathogenesis

This disorder is caused by mutations in the *CPT2* gene located on chromosome 1p32.[188] The resultant deficiency of CPT2 impairs the transport of acylcarnitine across the inner mitochondrial membrane (Fig. 29-5). Thus, the generation of ATP from fatty acid metabolism is diminished. Interestingly, CPT1 deficiency does not usually cause a myopathy.

Treatment

A high-protein, low-fat diet with frequent meals should be advised. Avoidance of prolonged strenuous activity, cold temperatures, and fasting may prevent episodes of rhabdomyolysis. During febrile illness, patients should be instructed to increase their intake of complex carbohydrates and again avoid fasting.

VLCAD DEFICIENCY

Clinical Features

VLCAD deficiency is a clinically heterogeneous disorder with three major phenotypes.[190–199] The disorder most commonly manifests in childhood with an early onset of hypertrophic cardiomyopathy, recurrent episodes of hypoketotic hypoglycemia and dicarboxylic aciduria, and a high mortality rate (50–75%). There is a milder form characterized by episodes of hypoketotic hypoglycemia and dicarboxylic aciduria, minimal if any cardiac involvement, and low mortality. In addition, VLCAD deficiency can rarely present similar to CPT deficiency, with exercise-induced myoglobinuria beginning in early childhood to early adulthood.

Laboratory Features

Serum CK is elevated with myoglobinuria as expected. Between attacks, the CK may be normal. There can be a secondary deficiency of carnitine, in particular with muscle. There is an increase in plasma concentration of tetradecanoic acid ($C_{14:1}$) with normal levels of myristic acid ($C_{14:1}$), consistent with a defect in β-oxidation of long-chain fatty acids.[195,198] Reduced VLCAD activity can be demonstrated in cultured fibroblasts and lymphocytes.[198] EMG may reveal myopathic-appearing MUAPs.

Histopathology

Muscle biopsies may demonstrate abnormal accumulation of lipid.

Molecular Genetics and Pathogenesis

This myopathy is caused by mutations in the VLCAD gene, which is located on chromosome 17p11.2–p13.1.[190,191,197,198] Patients with this enzyme deficiency have impaired ability to metabolize very–long-chain fatty acids (Fig. 29-5). Some of the previously described cases of long-chain acyl-CoA deficiency probably in fact had very–long-chain CoA deficiency.[197]

Treatment

A low-fat/high-carbohydrate diet in which long-chain fatty acids are partially replaced by medium-chain triglycerides may be effective in preventing attacks of hypoketotic hypoglycemia, dicarboxylic aciduria, and myoglobinuria in some[194,199] but not all patients.[195] Individuals who are affected should be instructed to avoid fasting.

LCAD DEFICIENCY

Clinical Features

LCAD usually presents in infancy with failure to thrive, hepatomegaly, cardiomegaly, nonketotic hypoglycemia, and an encephalopathy resembling Reye syndrome.[200–202] Individuals who are affected may develop exercise intolerance with attacks of rhabdomyolysis and proximal weakness.

Laboratory Features

Serum CK is elevated during attacks of muscle pain and cramps. Total and free carnitine levels are reduced in the plasma, liver, and muscle, but long-chain acylcarnitine esters are increased. Diagnosis is suggested by demonstrating decreased LCAD activity in cultured fibroblasts.[200]

Histopathology

Muscle biopsies reportedly demonstrate abnormal accumulation of lipid.

Molecular Genetics and Pathogenesis

The *ACADL* gene localizes to 2q34–q35. However, as previously noted, some reported cases of LCAD deficiency were in fact patients with VLCAD deficiency.[197] LCAD acts on fatty acyl-CoA derivatives whose acyl residues contain more than 12 carbon atoms. Patients with LCAD deficiency have an impaired ability to metabolize long-chain fatty acids.

Treatment

Intravenous glucose has led to relief of the myalgias and lowering of the serum CK levels in some patients.[200] Carnitine can improve the cardiomyopathy but does not affect skeletal muscle strength.[200]

MCAD DEFICIENCY

Clinical Features

MCAD is the most common form of acyl-CoA deficiency, but unlike defects in long-chain fatty acid metabolism, this deficiency is only rarely associated with cardiac or skeletal muscle involvement.[203–207] However, rare episodes of rhabdomyolysis and acute encephalopathy have been reported in infancy and late in life.[203,206,208,209]

Laboratory Features

MCAD activity is diminished to <10% in muscle, fibroblasts, lymphocytes, and liver.[203,204,208] A secondary deficiency of carnitine may be evident in the plasma, liver, and muscle. Dicarboxylic, adipic, and sebacic acids are increased in the urine.

Histopathology

Muscle biopsy is notable only for excess lipid.

Molecular Genetics and Pathogenesis

The disorder is caused by mutations within the MCAD gene located on chromosome 1p31.[208] MCAD acts on fatty acyl-CoA derivatives whose acyl residues contain 4–14 carbon atoms.

Treatment

Carnitine may improve the hepatomegaly and urinary organic acid profile and prevent attacks of rhabdomyolysis and encephalopathy, although there is some concern that carnitine supplementation is ineffective and possibly dangerous.[207] Fasting should be avoided.

SCAD DEFICIENCY

Clinical Features

Patients with SCAD deficiency may manifest with a wide range of features, including dysmorphic facial features, feeding difficulties, failure to thrive, metabolic acidosis, ketotic hypoglycemia, lethargy, developmental delay, seizures, hypotonia, dystonia, and myopathy.[205,210–216] In regard to the myopathy, it presents as exercise intolerance, myalgias, or progressive proximal weakness, which may be present in infancy or may develop in early to mid adulthood. Facial weakness, ptosis, progressive external ophthalmoplegia, respiratory weakness, and cardiomyopathy have also been described.[211] Some infants present with failure to thrive and nonketotic hypoglycemia.

Laboratory Features

Serum CK and carnitine levels are usually normal. Serum acylcarnitine profile reveals increased butyrylcarnitine (C4) concentration.[213,214] There is increased urinary excretion of short-chain metabolites ethylmalonate and methylsuccinate.

Histopathology

The few reports of muscle biopsies have demonstrated excess lipid. Muscle carnitine levels may be secondarily reduced. SCAD deficiency can be demonstrated in muscle tissue. Multicore myopathy has also been reported in the setting of SCAD.[211]

Molecular Genetics and Pathogenesis

Genetic defects have been localized to the *ACADS* located at 12q22–qter, which encodes for SCAD.[216,217] The gene is 13 kb in length and consists of 10 exons. SCAD acts on fatty acyl-CoA derivatives whose acyl residues contain four to six carbon atoms.

Treatment

No specific medical therapy has been shown to be beneficial, including carnitine supplementation.

MITOCHONDRIAL TRIFUNCTIONAL PROTEIN DEFICIENCY/LONG-CHAIN HAD DEFICIENCY

Clinical Features

Mitochondrial trifunctional protein (MTP) is a complex of eight subunits, that includes long-chain HAD. MTP/long-chain HAD deficiency is clinically heterogeneous. It can present in infancy or early childhood with Reye-like syndrome, nausea, vomiting, seizures, hypoketotic hypoglycemia, respiratory failure, and cardiomyopathy.[218–225] Mortality is high (approximately 50%) due to the cardiomyopathy. Progressive weakness and recurrent episodes of myoglobinuria become more prevalent later in childhood. Some individuals who are affected develop a progressive sensorimotor polyneuropathy and pigmentary retinopathy.[223] Mothers of an affected fetus can develop distinctive complications of pregnancy: hemolysis, elevated liver enzymes, low platelets (HELLP) and acute fatty liver of pregnancy (AFLP).[221]

Laboratory Features

Serum CK and lactate levels may be elevated. Urinary organic acids reveal dicarboxylic aciduria and 3-hydroxydicarboxylic aciduria. Acylcarnitine profile demonstrates increased long chains. An assay of cultured fibroblasts can demonstrate the deficiency of long-chain HAD deficiency or genetic testing can be done to confirm the diagnosis.[137,206–211] NCS may reveal features suggestive of an axonal sensorimotor neuropathy, while myopathic MUAPS are apparent on EMG in weak muscles.

Histopathology

Muscle biopsies reveal an abnormal accumulation of lipids, although this increase is not as prominent as that observed in other disorders of β-oxidation. A nerve biopsy in one patient demonstrated marked loss of myelinated nerve fibers and axonal degeneration.

Molecular Genetics and Pathogenesis

The disorder is inherited in an autosomal-recessive pattern and the gene for HAD maps to 2p23. Long-chain HAD catalyzes the third step in β-oxidation: the conversion of 3-hydroxyacyl-CoA derivatives to 3-ketoacyl-CoA derivatives. Deficiency of the enzyme leads to impairment in metabolism of long-chain fatty acids (Fig. 29-5).

Treatment

Patients may benefit from a high-carbohydrate, low-fat protein diet with or without supplementation with medium-chain triglycerides, riboflavin, and L-carnitine supplementation.[218,225] Patients should avoid fasting.

MULTI-ACYL-CoA DEHYDROGENASE DEFICIENCY (MADD)

Clinical Features

MADD, also known as glutaric aciduria type II, usually manifests with progressive proximal weakness and atrophy associated with episodes of confusion, ataxia, tremor, nausea, vomiting, hypoketotic hypoglycemia, lethargy, and hepatomegaly in infancy or early childhood.[160–162,226–235] Some patients present with recurrent episodes of exercise-induced myoglobinuria later in childhood or adult life similar to CPT2 deficiency or with proximal or distal weakness.[229,230]

Laboratory Features

NCS demonstrate an axonal sensory neuropathy, while the EMG may reveal myopathic-appearing MUAPs. Serum acylcarnitine analysis usually reveals increased concentrations of all chain lengths, but mainly medium- and long-chain acylcarnitines. The plasma-free carnitine level is usually decreased, but can sometimes be normal. Urine organic acid demonstrates C5–C10 dicarboxylic aciduria and acylglycine derivatives. Reduced ETF-QO activity can be demonstrated in cultured fibroblasts.[228] Genetic testing is available to confirm a mutation.

Histopathology

Muscle biopsies reveal vacuoles with abnormal accumulation of lipid (Fig. 29-7).

Molecular Genetics and Pathogenesis

The disorder can result from deficiency of any of three subunits of the enzyme complex: the alpha or β subunits of ETF (ETFA or ETFB) and ETF dehydrogenase (ETF-QO). These genes map as follows: ETFA to 15q23–q25, ETFB to 19q13.3, and ETF-QO to 4q32–qter. ETF transfers electrons from reduced forms of acyl-CoA dehydrogenase to the respiratory chain via ETF-QO. ETF-QO transfers electrons from ETF to ubiquinone (Fig. 29-5). Defects in these enzymes result in the inability to oxidize the reduced forms of various dehydrogenases including VLCAD, LCAD, MCAD, and SCAD.

Treatment

Fasting should be avoided. Carnitine supplementation does not appear to help, although both low-fat diets[227,235] and riboflavin[228,231–234] have been reported to provide benefit.

NEUTRAL LIPID STORAGE DISEASE

Clinical Features

Neutral lipid storage disease is characterized by systemic accumulation of triglycerides (TG) in the cytoplasm and includes two distinct diseases: (1) neutral lipid storage disease with myopathy (NLSDM) (2) neutral lipid storage disease with ichthyosis (NLSDI) also called Chanarin–Dorfman syndrome (Fig. 29-11).[160–162,236–240] Patients with NLSDM may present with generalized weakness, distal myopathy, or cardiomyopathy. Patients with NLSDI present with similar weakness along with ichthyosis.

Laboratory Features

Serum CK is usually mildly elevated. EMG is myopathic and can show muscle membrane irritability. Plasma carnitine profile reveals normal or mildly reduced total and free carnitine. Plasma acylcarnitine profile and serum/urine organic acids are normal. Peripheral blood smear reveal lipid-containing vacuoles in leukocytes (Jordan's anomaly) (Fig. 29-8).

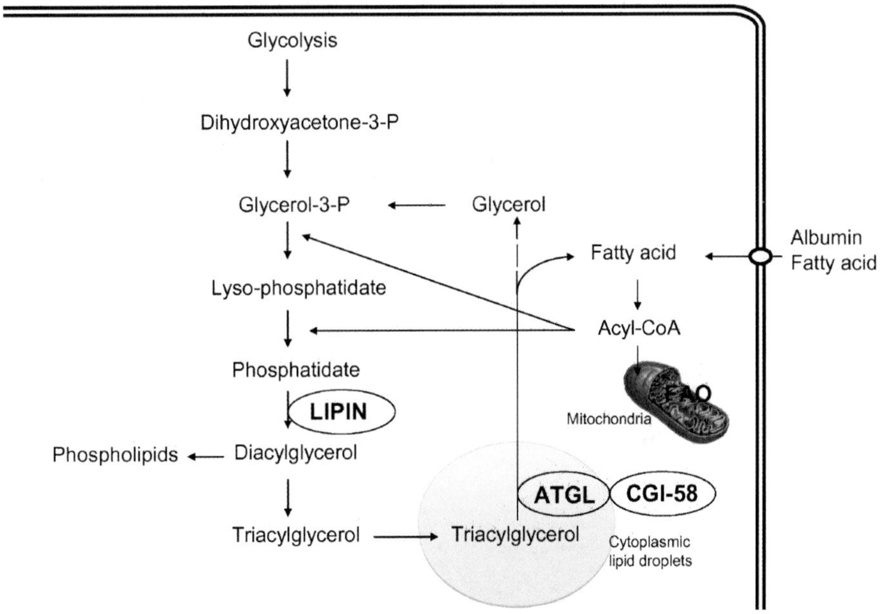

Figure 29-11. Simplified scheme of lipid metabolism. ATGL, adipose triglyceride lipase; CGI-58, activator of ATGL; FAO, fatty acid oxidation; LIPIN, phosphatidic acid phosphatase. (Reproduced with permission from Laforet P, Vianey-Sabab C. Disorders of muscle lipid metabolism: diagnostic and therapeutic changes. *Neuromuscul Disord.* 2010;20(11):693–700.)

Histopathology

Muscle biopsies reveal excess lipid.

Molecular Genetics and Pathogenesis

NLSDM is caused by mutations in a gene that encodes adipose triglyceride lipase (ATGL), which is also referred to as patatin-like phospholipase domain–containing protein 2 (PNPLA2).[238,239] This protein catalyzes the initial step in triglyceride hydrolysis. NLSDI is due to defects in the gene that encodes the co-activator of ATGL, comparative gene identification-58 (CGI-58), which is also known as abhydrolase domain–containing 5 (ABHD5).[240] Mutations in these genes lead to accumulation of triglycerides in muscle.

Treatment

There is no specific medical therapy.

PHOSPHATIDIC ACID PHOSPHATASE (LIPIN) DEFICIENCY

Clinical Features

Phosphatidic acid phosphatase (lipin) deficiency is another recently recognized disorder associated with triglyceride metabolism. It usually manifests in children with recurrent bouts of myoglobinuria in the setting of febrile illness but it has also been associated with exertional myalgias and has been reported in adults.[241–243] Clinical examination is otherwise unremarkable.

Laboratory Features

Serum CK is elevated. Total and free carnitine, plasma acylcarnitine profile, and urine organic acid levels are normal.

Histopathology

Muscle biopsies may reveal excess lipid or can be normal.

Molecular Genetics and Pathogenesis

Phosphatidic acid phosphatase (lipin) deficiency is caused by mutations in the *LPN1* gene. Phosphatidic acid phosphatase is important in triglyceride synthetase and catalyzes the conversion of phosphatidate to diacylglycerol (Fig. 29-11).

Treatment

There is no specific medical therapy.

▶SUMMARY

Evaluating patients with possible metabolic myopathies can be quite daunting. A basic understanding of carbohydrate and lipid metabolism and effects of exercise as provided in this chapter is necessary. We hope that clinicians will find our approach to these patients helpful.

REFERENCES

1. Meinck HM, Goebel HH, Rumpf KW, Kaiser H, Neumann P. The forearm ischaemic work test–hazardous to McArdle's patients? *J Neurol Neurosurg Psychiatry*. 1982;45:1144–1146.
2. Kollberg G, Tulinius M, Gilljam T, et al. Cardiomyopathy and exercise intolerance in muscle glycogen storage disease 0. *N Engl J Med*. 2007;357:1507–1514.
3. Cameron JM, Levandovskiy V, MacKay N, et al. Identification of a novel mutation in GYS1 (muscle-specific glycogen synthase) resulting in sudden cardiac death, that is diagnosable from skin fibroblasts. *Mol Genet Metab*. 2009;98:378–382.
4. Sukigara S, Liang WC, Komaki H, et al. Muscle glycogen storage disease 0 presenting recurrent syncope with weakness and myalgia. *Neuromuscul Disord*. 2012;22:162–165.
5. Barohn RJ, McVey AL, DiMauro S. Adult acid maltase deficiency. *Muscle Nerve*. 1993;16:672–676.
6. DiMauro S, Miranda AF, Sakoda S, et al. Metabolic myopathies. *Am J Med Genet*. 1986;25:635–651.
7. Engel AG. Acid maltase deficiency in adults: studies in four cases of a syndrome which may mimic muscular dystrophy or other myopathies. *Brain*. 1970;93:599–616.
8. Hogan GR, Gutmann L, Schmidt R, Gilbert E. Pompe's disease. *Neurology*. 1969;19:894–900.
9. Hudgson P, Gardner-Medwin D, Worsfold M, Pennington RJ, Walton JN. Adult myopathy from glycogen storage disease due to acid maltase deficiency. *Brain*. 1968;91:435–460.
10. Karpati G, Carpenter S, Engel AG, et al. The syndrome of systemic carnitine deficiency: clinical, morphologic, biochemical, and pathophysiologic features. *Neurology*. 1975;25:16–24.
11. Rosen EC, Engel AG. Acid maltase deficiency in adults presenting as respiratory failure. *Am J Med*. 1978;64:485–491.
12. Roth JC, Williams HE. The muscular variant of Pompe's disease. *J Pediatr*. 1967;71:567–573.
13. Smith J, Zellweger H, Afifi AK. Muscular form of glycogenosis, type II (Pompe). *Neurology*. 1967;17:537–549.
14. Bodamer OA, Leonard JV, Halliday D. Dietary treatment in late-onset acid maltase deficiency. *Eur J Pediatr*. 1997; 156(suppl 1):S39–S42.
15. Engel AG, Gomez MR, Seybold ME, Lambert EH. The spectrum and diagnosis of acid maltase deficiency. *Neurology*. 1975;23:95–106.
16. Loonen MC, Busch HF, Koster JF, et al. Family with different clinical forms of acid maltase deficiency (glycogenosis type II): biochemical and genetic studies. *Neurology*. 1981;31:1209–1216.
17. Pompe JC. Over idiopatsche hypertrophie van net hart. *Ned Tijdschr Geneeskd*. 1932;76:304–312.
18. Smith HL, Amick LD, Sidbury JB. Type II glycogenosis: report of a case with four-year survival and absence of acid maltase associated with abnormal glycogen. *Am J Dis Child*. 1966;111:475–481.
19. Swaiman KF, Kennedy WR, Sauls HS. Late infantile acid maltase deficiency. *Arch Neurol*. 1968;18:642–648.
20. Zellweger H, Brown BI, McCormick WF, Tu J. A mild form of muscular glycogenosis in two brothers with alpha-1,4-glucosidase deficiency. *Ann Pediatr (Paris)*. 1965;205:413.

21. Fadic R, Waclawik AJ, Brooks BR, Lotz BP. The rigid spine syndrome due to acid maltase deficiency. *Muscle Nerve.* 1997;20:364–366.
22. Engel AG, Dale AJD. Autophagic glycogenosis of late onset with mitochondrial abnormalities: light and electron microscopic observations. *Mayo Clin Proc.* 1968;43:233–238.
23. Felice KJ, Alesssi AG, Grunnet ML. Clinical variability in adult-onset acid maltase deficiency: report of affected sibs and review of the literature. *Medicine.* 1995;74:131–135.
24. Wokke JH, Ausems MG, van den Boogaard MJ, et al. Genotype–phenotype correlation in adult-onset acid maltase deficiency. *Ann Neurol.* 1995;38:450–454.
25. Umapathysivam K, Hopwood JJ, Meikle PJ. Determination of acid alpha-glucosidase activity in blood spots as a diagnostic test for Pompe disease. *Clin Chem.* 2001;47:1378–1383.
26. Kallwass H, Carr C, Gerrein J, et al. Rapid diagnosis of late-onset Pompe disease by fluorometric assay of alpha-glucosidase activities in dried blood spots. *Mol Genet Metab.* 2007;90: 449–452.
27. Vissing J, Lukacs Z, Straub V. Diagnosis of Pompe disease: muscle biopsy vs blood-based assays. *JAMA Neurol.* 2013;70:923–927.
28. American Association of Neuromuscular & Electrodiagnostic Medicine. Diagnostic criteria for late-onset (childhood and adult) Pompe disease. *Muscle Nerve.* 2009;40:149–160.
29. de Jager AE, van der Vliet TM, van der Ree TC, Oosterink BJ, Loonen MC. Muscle computer tomography in adult-onset acid maltase deficiency. *Muscle Nerve.* 1998;21:398–400.
30. Pichiecchio A, Uggetti C, Ravaglia S, et al. Muscle MRI in adult-onset acid maltase deficiency. *Neuromuscul Disord.* 2004; 14:51–55.
31. Alejaldre A, Díaz-Manera J, Ravaglia S, et al. Trunk muscle involvement in late-onset Pompe disease: study of thirty patients. *Neuromuscul Disord.* 2012;22(suppl 2):S148–S154.
32. Buckley BH, Hutchins GM. Pompe's disease presenting as hypertrophic myocardiopathy with Wolfe–Parkinson–White syndrome. *Am Heart J.* 1978;96:246–252.
33. Francesconi M, Auff E, Ursin C, Sluga E. WPW-syndrome kombiniert mit AV-block 2 bei einer adulten form einer glycogenose type II. *Wien Klin Wochenschr.* 1982;94:401.
34. Gambetti PL, DiMauro S, Baker L. Nervous system in Pompe's disease. *J Neuropathol Exp Neurol.* 1971;30:412–430.
35. Mancall EL, Aponte GE, Berry RG. Pompe's disease (diffuse glycogenosis) with neuronal storage. *J Neuropathol Exp Neurol.* 1965;24:85–96.
36. Raben N, Nichols RC, Boerkoel C, Plotz P. Genetic defects in patients with glycogenosis type II (acid maltase deficiency). *Muscle Nerve.* 1995;(suppl 3):S70–S74.
37. Reuser AJ, Kroos MA, Hermans MM, et al. Glycogenosis type II (acid maltase deficiency). *Muscle Nerve.* 1995;(suppl 3): S61–S69.
38. Kleijer WJ, van der Kraan M, Kroos MA, et al. Prenatal diagnosis of glycogen storage disease type II: enzyme assay or mutation analysis? *Pediatr Res.* 1995;38:103–106.
39. Kroos MA, Van der Kraan M, Van Diggelen OP, Klejer WJ, Reuser AJ. Two extremes of the clinical spectrum of glycogen storage disease type II in one family: a matter of genotype. *Hum Mutat.* 1997;9:17–22.
40. Kishnani PS, Corzo D, Nicolino M, et al. Recombinant human acid [alpha]-glucosidase: major clinical benefits in infantile-onset Pompe disease. *Neurology.* 2007;68:99–109.
41. van der Ploeg AT, Clemens P, Corzo D, et al. A randomized study of alglucosidase alfa in late-onset Pompe's disease. *N Engl J Med.* 2010;362:1396–1406.
42. Toscano A, Schoser B. Enzyme replacement therapy in late-onset Pompe disease: a systematic literature review. *J Neurol.* 2013;260:951–959.
43. Cupler EJ, Berger KI, Leshner RT, et al.; AANEM Consensus Committee on Late-onset Pompe Disease. Consensus treatment recommendations for late-onset Pompe disease. *Muscle Nerve.* 2012;45:319–333.
44. Kishnani PS, Goldenberg PC, DeArmey SL, et al. Cross-reactive immunologic material status affects treatment outcomes in Pompe disease infants. *Mol Genet Metab.* 2010;99:26–33
45. Banugaria SG, Prater SN, Ng YK, et al. The impact of antibodies on clinical outcomes in diseases treated with therapeutic protein: lessons learned from infantile Pompe disease. *Genet Med.* 2011;13:729–736.
46. Brunberg JA, McCormick WF, Schochet SS. Type III glycogenosis: an adult with diffuse weakness and muscle wasting. *Arch Neurol.* 1971;25:171–178.
47. Coleman RA, Winter HS, Wolf B, Gilchrist JM, Chen YT. Glycogen storage disease type III (glycogen debranching enzyme deficiency): correlation of biochemical defects with myopathy and cardiomyopathy. *Ann Intern Med.* 1992;116:896–900.
48. Cornelio G, Bresolin N, Singer PA, DiMauro S, Rowland LP. Clinical varieties of neuromuscular disease in debrancher deficiency. *Arch Neurol.* 1984;41:1027–1032.
49. Moses SW, Gadoth N, Bashan N, et al. Neuromuscular involvement in glycogen storage disease type III. *Acta Paediatr Scand.* 1986;75:289–296.
50. Ding JH, de Barsy T, Brown BI, Coleman RA, Chen YT. Immunoblot analyses of glycogen debranching enzyme in different subtypes of glycogen storage disease type III. *J Pediatr.* 1990;116(1):95–100.
51. DiMauro S, Hartwig GB, Hays A, et al. Debrancher deficiency: neuromuscular disorder in 5 adults. *Ann Neurol.* 1979;5:422–436.
52. Fukuda T, Sugie H, Ioto M, Tsurui S, Sugie Y, Igarashim Y. Nine cases of debrancher deficiency (glycogen storage disease type III) presenting with muscle weakness—study in clinicobiochemical analysis [Japanese]. *Rinsho Shika Clin Neurol.* 1996;36:540–543.
53. Hattori Y, Nohara C, Hirasawa E, Mori H, Imai H, Mizuno Y. A 21-year-old man with distal dominant progressive muscle atrophy (clinical conference) [Japanese]. *No To Shinei—Brain Nerve.* 1995;47(5):509–518.
54. Marbini A, Gemignani F, Saccardi F, Rimoldi M. Debrancher deficiency neuromuscular disorder with pseudohypertrophy in two brothers. *J Neurol.* 1989;236:418–420.
55. Murase T, Ikeda H, Muro T, Nakao K, Sugita H. Myopathy with type III glycogenosis. *J Neurol Sci.* 1973;20:287–295.
56. Ozand P, Tokatli M, Amiri S. Biochemical investigation of an unusual case of glycogenosis. *J Pediatr.* 1967;71:225–232.
57. Slonim AE, Weisberg C, Benke P, Evans OB, Burr IM. Reversal of debrancher deficiency myopathy by the use of high-protein nutrition. *Ann Neurol.* 1982;11:420–422.
58. Cuspidi C, Sampieri L, Pelizzoli S, et al. Obstructive hypertrophic cardiomyopathy in type III glycogen storage disease. *Acta Cardiol.* 1997;52:117–123.
59. Kiechl S, Kohlendorfer U, Thaler C, et al. Different clinical aspects of debrancher deficiency myopathy. *J Neurosurg Psychiatry.* 1999;67(3):364–368.

60. Miller CG, Alleyne GA, Brooks SE. Gross cardiac involvement in glycogen storage disease type III. *Br Heart J*. 1972;34:862–864.
61. Tada H, Kurita T, Ohe T, et al. Glycogen storage disease type III associated with ventricular tachycardia. *Am Heart J*. 1995;130:911–912.
62. Preisler N, Pradel A, Husu E, et al. Exercise intolerance in Glycogen Storage Disease Type III: weakness or energy deficiency? *Mol Genet Metab*. 2013;109:14–20.
63. Austin SL, Proia AD, Spencer-Manzon MJ, et al. Cardiac Pathology in Glycogen Storage Disease Type III. *JIMD Rep*. 2012;6:65–72.
64. Powell HC, Haas R, Hall CL, Wolff JA, Nyhan W, Brown BI. Peripheral nerve in type III glycogenosis: selective involvement of unmyelinated fiber Schwann cells. *Muscle Nerve*. 1985;8:667–671.
65. Sancho S, Navarro C, Fernandez JM, et al. Skin biopsy findings in glycogenosis III: clinical, biochemical, and electrophysiological correlations. *Ann Neurol*. 1990;27:480–486.
66. Ugawa Y, Inoue K, Takemura T, Iwamasa T. Accumulation of glycogen in sural nerve axons in adult-onset type III glycogenosis. *Ann Neurol*. 1986;19:294–296.
67. Okubo M, Hornishi A, Nakumura N, et al. A novel point mutation in an acceptor splice site of intron 32 (IVS32 A-12->G) but no exon 3 mutations in the glycogen debranching enzyme gene in a homozygous patient with glycogen storage disease type IIIb. *Hum Genet*. 1998;102(1):1–5.
68. Pavari R, Shen J, Hershkowitz E, Chen YT, Moses SW. Two new mutations in the 3 coding region of the glycogen debranching enzyme in a glycogen storage disease type IIIa Ashkenazi Jewish patient. *J Inherit Metab Dis*. 1998;21:141–148.
69. Shen J, Bao Y, Chen YT. A nonsense mutation due to a single base insertion in the 3′-coding region of glycogen debranching enzyme gene associated with a severe phenotype in a patient with glycogen storage disease type IIIa. *Hum Mutat*. 1997;9:37–40.
70. Shen J, Bao Y, Liu HM, Lee P, Leonard JV, Chen YT. Mutations in exon 3 of the glycogen debranching enzyme gene are associated with glycogen storage disease type III that is differentially expressed in liver and muscle. *J Clin Invest*. 1996;98:352–357.
71. Shen J, Liu HM, McConkie-Rosell A, Chen YT. Prenatal diagnosis and carrier detection for glycogen storage disease type III using polymorphic DNA markers. *Prenat Diagn*. 1998;18:61–64.
72. Haagsma EB, Smit GP, Niezen-Koning KE, et al. Type IIIb glycogen storage disease associated with end-stage cirrhosis and hepatocellular carcinoma. The liver transplant group. *Hepatology*. 1997;25:537–540.
73. Bao Y, Kishnani P, Wu JY, Chen YT. Hepatic and neuromuscular forms of glycogen storage disease IV caused by mutations in the same glycogen-branching enzyme gene. *J Clin Invest*. 1996;97:941–948.
74. Bornemann A, Besser R, Shin YS, Goebel HH. A mild adult myopathic variant of type IV glycogenosis. *Neuromuscul Disord*. 1996;6:95–99.
75. Bruno C, Servidei S, Shanske S, et al. Glycogen branching enzyme deficiency in adult polyglucosan body disease. *Ann Neurol*. 1993;33:88–93.
76. Bruno C, van Diggelen OP, Cassandrini D, et al. Clinical and genetic heterogeneity of branching enzyme deficiency (glycogenosis type IV). *Neurology*. 2004;63:1053–1058.
77. Cafferty MS, Lovelace RE, Hays AP, Servidei S, DiMauro S, Rowland LP. Polyglucosan body disease. *Muscle Nerve*. 1991;14:102–107.
78. Felice KJ, Grunnet ML, Rao KR, Wolfson LI. Childhood-onset spinocerebellar syndrome associated with massive polyglucosan body deposition. *Acta Neurol Scand*. 1997;95:60–64.
79. Fernandes J, Huijing F. Branching enzyme-deficiency glycogenosis: studies in therapy. *Arch Dis Child*. 1968;43:347–352.
80. Fishbein WN, Armbrustmacher VW, Griffin JL. Myoadenylate deaminase deficiency: a new disease of muscle. *Science*. 1978;200:545–548.
81. McMaster KR, Powers JM, Hennigar GR Jr, Wohltmann HJ, Farr GH Jr, et al. Nervous system involvement in type IV glycogenosis. *Arch Neurol*. 1979;103:105–111.
82. Nase S, Kunse KP, Sigmund M, Schoeder JM, Shin Y, Hanrath P. A new variant of type IV glycogenosis with primary cardiac manifestation and complete branching enzyme deficiency. In vivo detection by heart muscle biopsy. *Eur Heart J*. 1995;16:1695–1704.
83. Servidei S, Riepe RE, Langston C, et al. Severe cardiopathy in branching enzyme deficiency. *J Pediatr*. 1987;111:51–56.
84. Zellweger H, Mueller S, Ionasescu V, Schochet SS, McCormick WF. Glycogenosis IV: a new cause of infantile hypotonia. *J Pediatr*. 1972;80:842–844.
85. Taratuto AL, Akman HO, Saccoliti M, et al. Branching enzyme deficiency/glycogenosis storage disease type IV presenting as a severe congenital hypotonia: muscle biopsy and autopsy findings, biochemical and molecular genetic studies. *Neuromuscul Disord*. 2010;20:783–790.
86. Li SC, Hwu WL, Lin JL, et al. Association of the congenital neuromuscular form of glycogen storage disease type IV with a large deletion and recurrent frameshift mutation. *J Child Neurol*. 2012;27:204–208.
87. Escobar LF, Wagner S, Tucker M, Wareham J. Neonatal presentation of lethal neuromuscular glycogen storage disease type IV. *J Perinatol*. 2012;32:810–813.
88. McConkie-Rosell A, Wislon C, Picolli DA, et al. Clinical and laboratory findings in four patients with the non-progressive hepatic form of type IV glycogen storage disease. *J Inherit Metab Dis*. 1996;29:51–58.
89. Lossos A, Meiner Z, Barash V, et al. Adult polyglucosan body disease in Ashkenazi Jewish patients carrying the Tyr329 ser mutation in the glucogen-branching enzyme gene. *Ann Neurol*. 1998;44:867–872.
90. Ziemssen F, Sinderm E, Schroder JM, et al. Novel missense mutations in the glycogen-branching enzyme gene in adult polyglucosan body disease. *Ann Neurol*. 2000;47:536–540.
91. Tay SK, Akman HO, Wendy K, et al. Fatal infantile neuromuscular presentation of glycogen storage disease type IV. *Neuromuscul Disord*. 2004;14:253–260.
92. Rosenthal P, Podesta L, Grier R, et al. Failure of liver transplantation to diminish cardiac deposits of amylopectin and leukocyte inclusions in type IV glycogen storage disease. *Liver Transpl Surg*. 1995;1:373–376.
93. Selby R, Starzl TE, Yunis E, Brown BI, Kendall RS, Tzakis A. Liver transplantation for type IV glycogen storage disease. *N Engl J Med*. 1991;324:39–42.
94. Starzl TE, Demetris AJ, Trucco M, et al. Chimerism after liver transplantation for type IV glycogen storage disease and type 1 Gaucher's disease. *N Engl J Med*. 1993;328:745–749.
95. McArdle B. Myopathy due to a defect in muscle glycogen breakdown. *Clin Sci*. 1951;10:13–35.
96. Quinlivan R, Buckley J, James M, et al. McArdle disease: a clinical review. *J Neurol Neurosurg Psychiatry*. 2010;81:1182–1188.

97. Quinlivan R, Martinuzzi A, Schoser B. Pharmacological and nutritional treatment for McArdle disease (Glycogen Storage Disease type V). *Cochrane Database Syst Rev*. 2010;(12):CD003458.
98. Vissing J, Haller RG. The effect of oral sucrose on exercise tolerance in patients with McArdle's disease. *N Engl J Med*. 2003;349:2503–2509.
99. Kristjansson K, Tsujino S, DiMauro S. Myophosphorylase deficiency: an unusually severe form with myoglobinuria. *J Pediatr*. 1994;125:409–410.
100. Wolfe GI, Baker NS, Haller RG, Burns DK, Barohn RJ. McArdle's disease presenting with asymmetric, late-onset arm weakness. *Muscle Nerve*. 2000;23:641–645.
101. DiMauro S, Hartlage PL. Fatal infantile form of muscle phosphorylase deficiency. *Neurology*. 1978;28:1124–1129.
102. Tsujino S, Shanske S, DiMauro S. Molecular genetic heterogeneity of myophosphorylase deficiency (McArdle's disease). *N Engl J Med*. 1993;329:241–245.
103. Kazemi-Esfarjani P, Skomorowska E, Jensen TD, Haller RG, Vissing J. A nonischemic forearm exercise test for McArdle disease. *Ann Neurol*. 2002;52:153–159.
104. Brandt NJ, Buchthal F, Ebbesen F, Kamieniecka Z, Krarup C. Post-tetanic mechanical tension and evoked action potentials in McArdle's disease. *J Neurol Neurosurg Psychiatry*. 1977;40: 920–925.
105. Gruener R, McArdle B, Ryman BE, Weller RO. Contracture of phosphorylase deficient muscle. *J Neurol Neurosurg Psychiatry*. 1968;31:268–283.
106. Beynon RJ, Bartham C, Hopkins P, et al. McArdle's disease: molecular genetics and metabolic consequences of the phenotype. *Muscle Nerve*. 1995;(suppl 3):S18–S22.
107. Fernandez R, Navarro C, Andreu AL, et al. A novel missense mutation (W797R) in the myophosphorylase gene in Spanish patients with McArdle's disease. *Arch Neurol*. 2000;57:217–219.
108. Manfredi G, Silvestri G, Servidei S, et al. Manifesting heterozygotes in McArdle's disease: Clinical, morphological, and biochemical studies in a family. *J Neurol Sci*. 1992;115:91–94.
109. Ruff RL. Why do patients with McArdle's disease have decreased exercise capacity? *Neurology*. 1998;50:6–7.
110. Ruff RL. Elevated intracellular Ca2+ and myofibrillar Ca2+ sensitivity cause iodoacetate-induced muscle contractures. *J Appl Physiol*. 1996;81:1230–1239.
111. Haller RG, Clausen T, Vissing J. Reduced levels of skeletal muscle $Na^{+}K^{+}$-ATPase in McArdle disease. *Neurology*. 1998;50:37–40.
112. Haller RG. Treatment of McArdle disease. *Arch Neurol*. 2000;57:923–924.
113. Vorgerd M, Zange J, Kley R, et al. Effect of high-dose creatine therapy on symptoms of exercise intolerance in McArdle disease: double-blind, placebo-controlled crossover study. *Arch Neurol*. 2002;5997–6101.
114. Haller RG, Vissing J. No spontaneous second wind in muscle phosphofructokinase deficiency. *Neurology*. 2004;62(1):82–86.
115. Musumeci O, Bruno C, Mongini T, et al. Clinical features and new molecular findings in muscle phosphofructokinase deficiency (GSD type VII). *Neuromuscul Disord*. 2012;22:325–330.
116. Malfatti E, Birouk N, Romero NB, et al. Juvenile-onset permanent weakness in muscle phosphofructokinase deficiency. *J Neurol Sci*. 2012;316:173–177.
117. Hays AP, Hallett M, Delfs J, et al. Muscle phosphofructokinase deficiency: abnormal polysaccharide in a case of late-onset myopathy. *Neurology*. 1981;31:1077–1086.
118. DiMauro S, Spiegel R. Progress and problems in muscle glycogenoses. *Acta Myol*. 2011;30:96–102.
119. Haller RG, Lewis SF. Glucose-induced exertional fatigue in muscle phosphofructokinase deficiency. *N Engl J Med*. 1991; 324:364–369.
120. Abarbanel JM, Bashan N, Potashnik R, et al. Adult muscle phosphorylase "b" kinase deficiency. *Neurology*. 1986;36:560–562.
121. Clemens PR, Yamamoto M, Engel AG. Adult phosphorylase b kinase deficiency. *Ann Neurol*. 1990;28:529–538.
122. Van den Berg IE, Berger R. Phosphorylase b kinase deficiency in man: a review. *J Inherit Metab Dis*. 1990;13:442–451.
123. Wilkinson DA, Tonin P, Shanske S, Lombes A, Carlson GM, DiMauro S. Clinical and biochemical features of 10 adult patients with muscle phosphorylase kinase deficiency. *Neurology*. 1994;44:461–466.
124. Burwinkel B, Maichele AJ, Aagenaes O, et al. Autosomal glycogenosis of liver and muscle due to phosphorylase kinase deficiency is caused by mutations in the phosphorylase kinase beta subunit (PHKB). *Hum Mol Genet*. 1997;6:1109–1115.
125. Vissing J, Schmalbruch H, Haller RG, Clausen T. Muscle phosphoglycerate mutase deficiency with tubular aggregates: effect of dantrolene. *Ann Neurol*. 1999;46:274–277.
126. Naini A, Toscano A, Musumeci O, Vissing J, Akman HO, DiMauro S. Muscle phosphoglycerate mutase deficiency revisited. *Arch Neurol*. 2009;66(3):394–398.
127. Kanno T, Maekawa M. Lactate dehydrogenase M-subunit deficiencies: clinical features, metabolic background, and genetic heterogeneities. *Muscle Nerve*. 1995;(suppl 3):S54–S60.
128. Kreuder J, Borkhardt A, Repp R, et al. Inherited metabolic myopathy and hemolysis due to a mutation in aldolase A. *N Engl J Med*. 1996;334:1100–1104.
129. Yao DC, Tolan DR, Murray MF, et al. Hemolytic anemia and severe rhabdomyolysis caused by compound heterozygous mutations of the gene for erythrocyte/muscle isozyme of aldolase, ALDOA(Arg303X/Cys338Tyr). *Blood*. 2004;103:2401–2403.
130. Comi GP, Fortunato F, Lucchiari S, et al. Beta-enolase deficiency, a new metabolic myopathy of distal glycolysis. *Ann Neurol*. 2001;50:202–207.
131. Stojkovic T, Vissing J, Petit F, et al. Muscle glycogenosis due to phosphoglucomutase 1 deficiency. *N Engl J Med*. 2009;361: 425–427.
132. Preisler N, Laforêt P, Echaniz-Laguna A, et al. Fat and carbohydrate metabolism during exercise in phosphoglucomutase type 1 deficiency. *J Clin Endocrinol Metab*. 2013;98: E1235–E1240.
133. Moslemi AR, Lindberg C, Nilsson J, Tajsharghi H, Andersson B, Oldfors A. Glycogenin-1 deficiency and inactivated priming of glycogen synthesis.*N Engl J Med*. 2010;362:1203–1210.
134. Malfatt E, Nilsson J, Hedberg-Oldfors C, et al. A new muscle glycogen storage disease associated with glycogenin-1 deficiency. *Ann Neurology*. 2014;76:891–898.
135. Bardosi A, Eber SW, Hendrys M, Pelrun A. Myopathy with altered mitochondria due to a triosephosphate isomerase (TPI) deficiency. *Acta Neuropathol (Berl)*. 1990;79:387–394.
136. Fujii H, Kanno H, Hirono A, Shiomura T, Miwa S. A single amino acid substitution (157 Gly to Val) in a phosphoglycerate kinase variant (PGK Shizuoka) associated with chronic hemolysis and myoglobinuria. *Blood*. 1992;79:1582–1585.
137. Sugie H, Sugie Y, Nishida M, et al. Recurrent myoglobinuria in a child with mental retardation: phosphoglycerate kinase deficiency. *J Child Neurol*. 1989;4:95–99.

138. Tonin P, Shanske S, Miranda AF, et al. Phosphoglycerate kinase deficiency: biochemical and molecular genetic studies in a new myopathic variant (PGK Alberta). *Neurology.* 1993;43:387–391.
139. Tsujino S, Tonin P, Shanske S, et al. A splice junction mutation in a new myopathic variant of phosphoglycerate kinase deficiency (PGK North Carolina). *Ann Neurol.* 1994;35:349–353.
140. Nilsson J, Schoser B, Laforet P, et al. Polyglucosan body myopathy caused by defective ubiquitin ligase RBCK1. *Ann Neurol.* 2013;74(6):914–919.
141. Danon MJ, Oh SJ, DiMauro S, et al. Lysosomal glycogen storage disease with normal acid maltase. *Neurology.* 1981;31(1):51–57.
142. Nishino I, Fu J, Tanji K, et al. Primary LAMP-2 deficiency causes X-linked vacuolar cardiomyopathy and myopathy (Danon disease). *Nature.* 2000;406:906–910.
143. Sugie K, Yamatoto A, Murayama K, et al. Clinicopathological features of genetically confirmed Danon disease. *Neurology.* 2002;58:1773–1778.
144. Boucek D, Jirikowic J, Taylor M. Natural history of Danon disease. *Genet Med.* 2011;13:563–568.
145. Stevens-Lapsley JE, Kramer LR, Balter JE, Jirikowic J, Boucek D, Taylor M. Functional performance and muscle strength phenotypes in men and women with Danon disease. *Muscle Nerve.* 2010;42:908–914.
146. Kim H, Cho A, Lim BC, et al. A 13-year-old girl with proximal weakness and hypertrophic cardiomyopathy with Danon disease. *Muscle Nerve.* 2010;41:879–882.
147. Cheng Z, Fang Q. Danon disease: focusing on heart. *J Hum Genet.* 2012;57:407–410.
148. Miani D, Taylor M, Mestroni L, et al. Sudden death associated with Danon disease in women. *Am J Cardiol.* 2012;109:406–411.
149. Yamamoto A, Morisawa Y, Verloes A, et al. Infantile lysosomal glycogen storage disease with normal acid maltase is genetically distinct from Danon disease (X-linked vacuolar cardiomyopathy and myopathy). *Neurology.* 2001;57:903–905.
150. Kalimo H, Savonataus ML, Lang H, et al. X-linked myopathy with excessive autophagia: a new hereditary muscle disease. *Ann Neurol.* 1988;23:258–265.
151. Villanova M, Louboutin JP, Chateau D, et al. X-linked vacuolated myopathy: complement membrane attack complex on surface of injured muscle fibers. *Ann Neurol.* 1995;37:637–645.
152. Kaneda D, Sugie K, Yamatoto A, et al. A novel form of autophagic vacuolar myopathy with late-onset and multiorgan involvement. *Neurology.* 2003;61:128–131.
153. Ramachandran N, Munteanu I, Wang P, et al. VMA21 deficiency prevents vacuolar ATPase assembly and causes autophagic vacuolar myopathy. *Acta Neuropathol.* 2013;125(3):439–457.
154. Kelemen J, Rice DR, Bradley WG, Munsat TL, DiMauro S, Hogan EL. Familial myoadenylate deaminase deficiency and exertional myalgia. *Neurology.* 1982;32:857–863.
155. Tonin P, Lewis P, Servidei S, DiMauro S. Metabolic causes of myoglobinuria. *Ann Neurol.* 1990;27:181–185.
156. Verzijl HT, van Engelen BG, Luyten JA, et al. Genetic characteristics of myoadenylate deaminase deficiency. *Ann Neurol.* 1998;44:140–143.
157. Sabina RL, Swain JL, Olanow W, et al. Myoadenylate deaminase deficiency: functional and metabolic abnormalities associated with disruption of purine nucleotide cycle. *J Clin Invest.* 1984;73:720–730.
158. Vissing J, Lewis SF, Galbo H, Haller RG. Effect of deficient muscular glycogenolysis on extramuscular fuel production in exercise. *J Appl Physiol.* 1992;72:1773–1779.
159. Sabina RL, Fishbein WN, Pezeshkpour G, Clarke PR, Holmes EW. Molecular analysis of the myoadenylate deaminase deficiencies. *Neurology.* 1992;42:170–179.
160. Liang WC, Nishino I. Lipid storage myopathy. *Curr Neurol Neurosci Rep.* 2011;11:97–103.
161. Laforet P, Vianey-Sabab C. Disorders of muscle lipid metabolism: diagnostic and therapeutic changes. *Neuromuscular Dis.* 2010;20:693–700.
162. Ohkuma A, Noguchi S, Sugie H, et al. Clinical and genetic analysis of lipid storage myopathies. *Muscle Nerve.* 2009;39:333–342.
163. Di Donato S, Rimoldi M, Bertagnolio B, Uziel G, Wiesmann UN. A biochemical approach to lipid storage myopathies. *Biochem Exp Biol.* 1977;13(1):85–91.
164. Chapoy PF, Angelini C, Brown WJ, Stiff JE, Shug AL, Cederbaum SD. Systemic carnitine deficiency: a treatable inherited lipid storage disease presenting as Reye's syndrome. *N Engl J Med.* 1980;303:1389–1394.
165. Cornelio F, Di Donato S, Testa D, et al. Carnitine deficient myopathy and cardiomyopathy with fatal outcome. *Ital J Neurol Sci.* 1980;1(2):95–100.
166. Cornelio G, Di Donato S, Peluchetti D, et al. Fatal cases of lipid storage myopathy with carnitine deficiency. *J Neurol Neurosurg Psychiatry.* 1977;40:170–178.
167. Di Donato S. Primary and secondary carnitine deficiency in man. *Ital J Biochem.* 1984;33(4):285A–291A.
168. Di Donato S, Pelucchetti D, Rimoldi M, Mora M, Garavaglia B, Finocchiaro G. Systemic carnitine deficiency: clinical, biochemical, and morphological cure with L-carnitine. *Neurology.* 1984;34(2):157–162.
169. DiMauro S, Trevisan C, Hays A. Disorders of lipid metabolism in muscle. *Muscle Nerve.* 1980;3(5):369–388.
170. Engel AG, Banker BQ, Eiben RM. Carnitine deficiency: clinical, morphological, and biochemical observations in a fatal case. *J Neurol Neurosurg Psychiatry.* 1977;40:313–322.
171. Garavaglia B, Uziel G, Dworsak F, Carrar F, DiDonato S. Primary carnitine deficiency: heterozygote and intrafamilial phenotypic variation. *Neurology.* 1991;41:1691–1693.
172. Karpati G, Carpenter S, Eisen A, Aubé M, DiMauro S. The adult form of acid maltase (a-1,4-glucosidase) deficiency. *Ann Neurol.* 1977;1:276–280.
173. Morand P, Despert F, Carrier N, et al. Myopathie lipidique avec cardiomyopathie severe par deficit generalise en carnitine. *Arch Mal Coeur Vaiss.* 1979;5:536–544.
174. Stanley CA, DeLeeuw S, Coates PM, et al. Chronic cardiomyopathy and weakness or acute coma in children with a defect in carnitine uptake. *Ann Neurol.* 1991;30:709–716.
175. Bautista J, Rafel E, Martinez A, et al. Familial hypertrophic cardiomyopathy and muscle carnitine deficiency. *Muscle Nerve.* 1990;13:192–194.
176. Hart ZH, Chang CH, DiMauro S, Farooki Q, Ayyar R. Muscle carnitine deficiency and fatal cardiomyopathy. *Neurology.* 1978;28:147–151.
177. Markesbery WR, McQuillen MP, Procopis PG, Harrison AR, Engel AG. Muscle carnitine deficiency. *Arch Neurol.* 1974;31:320–324.
178. Angelini C, Govoni E, Bragaglia MM, Vergani L. Carnitine deficiency: acute postpartum crisis. *Ann Neurol.* 1978;4:558–562.
179. Prockop LD, Engel WK, Shug AL. Nearly fatal muscle carnitine deficiency with full recovery after replacement therapy. *Neurology.* 1983;33:1629–1631.

180. Engel AG, Rebouche CJ, Wilson DM, Glasgow AM, Romshe CA, Cruse RP. Primary systemic carnitine deficiency. II. Renal handling of carnitine. *Neurology*. 1981;31(7):819–825.
181. Treem WR, Stanley CA, Finegold DN, Hale DE, Coates PM. Primary carnitine deficiency due to a failure of carnitine transport in kidney, muscle, and fibroblasts. *N Engl J Med*. 1988;319(20):1331–1336.
182. Nezu JI, Tamai I, Oku A, et al. Primary systemic carnitine deficiency is caused by mutations in a gene encoding a sodium-dependent carnitine transporter. *Nat Genet*. 1999;21:91–94.
183. Angelini C, Lucke S, Cantarutti G. Carnitine deficiency of skeletal muscle: report of a treated case. *Neurology*. 1976;26:633–637.
184. Snyder TM, Little BW, Roman-Campos G, McQuillen JB. Successful treatment of familial idiopathic lipid storage myopathy with L-carnitine and modified lipid diet. *Neurology*. 1982;32:1106–1115.
185. Tripp ME, Katcher ML, Peters HA, et al. Systemic carnitine deficiency presenting as familial endocardial fibroelastosis: a treatable cardiomyopathy. *N Engl J Med*. 1981;305:385–390.
186. Angelini C, Trevisan C, Isaya G, Pegolo G, Vergani L. Clinical varieties of carnitine and carnitine palmitoyltransferase deficiency. *Clin Biochem*. 1987;20(1):1–7.
187. Demaugre F, Bonnefont JP, Mitchell G, et al. Hepatic and muscular presentations of carnitine palmitoyl transferase deficiency: two distinct entities. *Pediatr Res*. 1988;24(3):308–311.
188. Taroni F, Verderio E, Dworzak F, Willems PJ, Cavadini P, Di Donato S. Identification of a common mutation in the carnitine palmitoyltransferase II gene in familial recurrent myoglobinuria patients. *Nat Genet*. 1993;4:314–320.
189. Trevisan CP, Isaya G, Angelini C. Exercise-induced recurrent myoglobinuria: defective activity of inner carnitine palmitoyltransferase in muscle mitochondria of two patients. *Neurology*. 1987;37(7):1184–1188.
190. Andresen BS, Bross P, Vianey-Saban C, et al. Cloning and characterization of human very-long-chain acyl coenzyme. A dehydrogenase deficiency presenting with exercise-induced myoglobinuria. *Neurology*. 1996;44:467–473.
191. Aoyama T, Souri M, Ueno I, et al. Cloning of human very-long-chain acyl coenzyme A dehydrogenase and molecular characterization of its deficiency in two patients. *Am J Hum Genet*. 1995;57:273–283.
192. Brown-Harrison MC, Nada MA, Sprecher H, et al. Very long chain acyl-CoA dehydrogenase deficiency: successful treatment of acute cardiomyopathy. *Biochem Mol Med*. 1996;58(1):59–65.
193. Merinero B, Cerdra-Perez C, Garcia MJ, Vianey-Saban C, Duran M, Ugarte M. Mitochondrial very-long-chain acyl-CoA dehydrogenase deficiency with a mild course. *J Inherit Metab Dis*. 1996;19:173–176.
194. Minetti C, Garavaglia B, Bado M, et al. Very-long-chain acyl-coenzyme A dehydrogenase deficiency in a child with recurrent myoglobinuria. *Neuromuscul Disord*. 1998;8:3–6.
195. Smelt AH, Poorthuis BJ, Onkenhout W, et al. Very long chain acyl-coenzyme A dehydrogenase deficiency with adult onset. *Ann Neurol*. 1998;43(4):540–544.
196. Taroni F, Uziel G. Fatty-acid mitochondrial β-oxidation and hypoglycemia in children. *Curr Opin Neurol*. 1996;9:477–485.
197. Yamaguchi S, Indo Y, Coates PM, Hashimoto T, Tanaka K. Identification of a very-long-chain acyl-CoA dehydrogenase deficiency in three patients previously diagnosed with long-chain acyl-CoA dehydrogenase deficiency. *Pediatr Res*. 1993;34:111–113.
198. Laforêt P, Acquaviva-Bourdain C, Rigal O, et al. Diagnostic assessment and long-term follow-up of 13 patients with Very Long-Chain Acyl-Coenzyme A dehydrogenase (VLCAD) deficiency. *Neuromuscul Disord*. 2009;19:324–329.
199. Ogilvie I, Porfarzam M, Jackson S, Stockdale C, Bartlett K, Turnbull DM. Very long-chain acyl coenzyme A dehydrogenase deficiency presenting with exercise-induced myoglobinuria. *Neurology*. 1994;44(3 Pt 1):467–473.
200. Hale DE, Batshaw ML, Coates PM, et al. Long-chain acyl-CoA dehydrogenase deficiency in muscle of an adult with lipid myopathy. *Pediatr Res*. 1985;19:666–671.
201. Parini R, Garavaglia B, Saudubray JM, et al. Clinical diagnosis of long-chain acyl-coenzyme A-dehydrogenase deficiency: use of stress and fat-loading tests. *J Pediatr*. 1991;119(1 Pt 1):77–80.
202. Tein I, Vajsar J, MacMillan L, Sherwood WG. Long-chain L-3-hydroxyacyl-coenzyme A dehydrogenase deficiency neuropathy: response to cod liver oil. *Neurology*. 1999;52(3):640–643.
203. Zierz S, Engel AG, Romshe CA. Assay of acyl-CoA dehydrogenases in muscle and liver and identification of four new cases of medium-chain acyl-CoA dehydrogenase deficiency associated with systemic carnitine deficiency. *Adv Neurol*. 1988;48:231–237.
204. Coates PM, Hale DE, Stanley CA, Corkey BE, Cortner JA. Genetic deficiency of medium-chain acyl coenzyme A dehydrogenase: studies in cultured skin fibroblasts and peripheral mononuclear leukocytes. *Pediatr Res*. 1985;19(7):671–676.
205. Di Donato S, Gellera C. Short-chain and medium-chain acyl-CoA dehydrogenases are lowered in riboflavin-responsive lipid myopathies with multiple acyl-CoA dehydrogenase deficiency. *Prog Clin Biol Res*. 1990;321:325–332.
206. Ding JH, Roe CR, Iafolla AK, Chen YT. Medium-chain acyl-coenzyme A dehydrogenase deficiency and sudden infant death [letter]. *N Engl J Med*. 1991;325:61–62.
207. Treem WR, Stanley CA, Goodman SI. Medium-chain acyl-CoA dehydrogenase deficiency: metabolic effects and therapeutic efficacy of long-term carnitine supplementation. *J Inherit Metab Dis*. 1989;12:112–119.
208. Ruitenbeek W, Poels PJ, Turnbull DM, et al. Rhabdomyolysis and acute encephalopathy in late onset medium chain acyl-CoA dehydrogenase deficiency. *J Neurol Neurosurg Psychiatry*. 1995;58:209–214.
209. Zierz S, Engel AG, Romsche CA. Assay for acyl-CoA dehydrogenase in muscle and liver and identification of four cases of medium-chain acyl-CoA dehydrogenase deficiency associated with carnitine deficiency. In: Di Donato S, DiMauro S, Mamoli A, Rowland LP, eds. *Molecular Genetics of Neurological and Neuromuscular Diseases: Advances in Neurology*, Vol. 48. New York, NY: Raven Press; 1988:231–237.
210. Coates PM, Hale DE, Fiocchario G, Tanaka K, Winter SC. Genetic deficiency of short-chain acyl-coenzyme A dehydrogenase in cultured fibroblasts from a patient with muscle carnitine deficiency and severe muscle weakness. *J Clin Invest*. 1988;81:171–175.
211. Tein I, Haslam RH, Rhead WJ, Bennett MJ, Becker LE, Vockley J. Short-chain acyl-CoA dehydrogenase deficiency. A cause of ophthalmoplegia and multicore myopathy. *Neurology*. 1999;52:366–372.
212. Turnbull DM, Bartlett K, Stevens DL, et al. Short-chain acyl-CoA dehydrogenase deficiency associated with a lipid storage myopathy and secondary carnitine deficiency. *N Engl J Med*. 1984;311:1232–1236.

213. van Maldegem BT, Duran M, Wanders RJ, et al. Clinical, biochemical, and genetic heterogeneity in short-chain acyl-coenzyme A dehydrogenase deficiency. *JAMA*. 2006;296:943–952.
214. van Maldegem BT, Wanders JA, Wijburg FA. Clinical aspects of short-chain acyl-CoA dehydrogenase deficiency. *J Inherit Metab Dis*. 2010;33:507–511.
215. Baerlocher KE, Steinmann B, Aguzzi A, Krähenbühl S, Roe CR, Vianey-Saban C. Short-chain acyl-CoA dehydrogenase deficiency in a 16-year-old girl with severe muscle wasting and scoliosis. *J Inherit Metab Dis*. 1997;20(3):427–431.
216. Corydon MJ, Andresen BS, Bross P, et al. Structural organization of the human short-chain acyl-CoA dehydrogenase gene. *Mamm Genome*. 1997;8:922–926.
217. Naito E, Indo Y, Tanaka K. Short chain acyl-coenzyme A dehydrogenase (SCAD) deficiency: immunochemical demonstration of molecular heterogeneity due to variant SCAD with differing stability. *J Clin Invest*. 1989;84:1671–1674.
218. Jackson S, Baartlett K, Land J, et al. Long-chain 3-hydroxyacyl-CoA dehydrogenase deficiency. *Pediatr Res*. 1991;29:406–411.
219. Rocchiccioli F, Wanders RJ, Augburg P, et al. Deficiency of long-chain 3-hydroxyacyl-CoA dehydrogenase: a cause of lethal myopathy and cardiomyopathy in early childhood. *Pediatr Res*. 1990;28:657–662.
220. Thiel C, Baudach S, Schnackenberg U, Vreken P, Wanders RJ. Long-chain 3-hydroxyacyl-CoA dehydrogenase deficiency: neonatal manifestation at the first day of life presenting with tachypnoea. *J Inherit Metab Dis*. 1999;22:839–840.
221. Tyni T, Pihko H. Long-chain 3-hydroxyacyl-CoA dehydrogenase deficiency. *Acta Pediatr*. 1999;88:237–245.
222. Wanders RJ, IJlst L, van Gennip AH, et al. Long-chain 3-hydroxyacyl-CoA dehydrogenase deficiency: identification of a new inborn error of mitochondrial fatty acid beta-oxidation. *J Inherit Metab Dis*. 1990;13(3):311–314.
223. Bertini E, Dionisi-Vici C, Garavaglia B, et al. Peripheral sensory-motor neuropathy, pigmentary retinopathy, and fatal cardiomyopathy in long-chain 3-hydroxyacyl-CoA dehydrogenase deficiency. *Eur J Pediatr*. 1992;151(2):121–126.
224. Wanders RJ, Vreken P, den Boer ME, Wijburg FA, van Gennip AH, IJlst L. Disorders of mitochondrial fatty acyl-CoA beta-oxidation. *J Inherit Metab Dis*. 1999;22:442–487.
225. Korenke GC, Wanders RJ, Hanefeld F. Striking improvement of muscle strength under creatine therapy in a patient with long-chain 3-hydroxyacyl-CoA dehydrogenase deficiency. *J Inherit Metab Dis*. 2003;26(1):67–68.
226. Di Donato S, Frerman FE, Rimoldi M, Rinaldo P, Taroni F, Wiesmann UN. Systemic carnitine deficiency due to lack of electron transfer flavoprotein: ubiquinone oxidoreductase. *Neurology*. 1986;36(7):957–963.
227. Dusheiko G, Kew MC, Joffe BI, Lewin JR, Mantagos S, Tanaka K. Recurrent hypoglycemia associated with glutaric aciduria type II in an adult. *N Engl J Med*. 1979;301:1405–1409.
228. Gregersen N, Wintzensen H, Christensen SK, Christensen MF, Brandt NJ, Rasmussen K. C(6)-C(10)-dicarboxylic aciduria: investigations of a patient with riboflavin responsive multiple acyl-CoA dehydrogenation defects. *Pediatr Res*. 1982;16:861–868.
229. Izumi R, Suzuki N, Nagata M, et al. A case of late onset riboflavin-responsive multiple acyl-CoA dehydrogenase deficiency manifesting as recurrent rhabdomyolysis and acute renal failure. *Intern Med*. 2011;50:2663–2668.
230. Pollard LM, Williams NR, Espinoza L, et al. Diagnosis, treatment, and long-term outcomes of late-onset (type III) multiple acyl-CoA dehydrogenase deficiency. *J Child Neurol*. 2010;25:954–960.
231. Liang WC, Ohkuma A, Hayashi YK, et al. ETFDH mutations, CoQ10 levels, and respiratory chain activities in patients with riboflavin-responsive multiple acyl-CoA dehydrogenase deficiency. *Neuromuscul Disord*. 2009;19:212–216.
232. Olsen RK, Olpin SE, Andresen BS, et al. ETFDH mutations as a major cause of riboflavin-responsive multiple acyl-CoA dehydrogenation deficiency. *Brain* 2007;130:2045–2054.
233. Wen B, Dai T, Li W, et al. Riboflavin-responsive lipid-storage myopathy caused by ETFDH gene mutations. *J Neurol Neurosurg Psychiatry*. 2010;81:231–236.
234. Maillart E, Acquaviva-Bourdain C, Rigal O, et al. Multiple acyl-CoA dehydrogenase deficiency (MADD): a curable cause of genetic muscular lipidosis. *Rev Neurol*. 2010;166:289–294.
235. Mongini T, Doriguzzi C, Palmucci L, et al. Lipid storage myopathy in multiple acyl-CoA dehydrogenase deficiency: an adult case. *Eur Neurol*. 1992;32:170–176.
236. Dorfman ML, Hershko C, Eisenberg S, Sagher F. Ichthyosiform dermatosis with systemic lipidosis. *Arch Dermatol*. 1974;110:261–266.
237. Chanarin I, Patel A, Slavin G, Wills EJ, Andrews TM, Stewart G. Neutral-lipid storage disease: a new disorder of lipid metabolism. *Br Med J*. 1975;1:553–555.
238. Ohkuma A, Nonaka I, Malicdan MC, et al. Distal lipid storage myopathy due to PNPLA2 mutation. *Neuromuscul Disord*. 2008;18:671–674.
239. Fischer J, Lefevre C, Morava E, et al. The gene encoding adipose triglyceride lipase (PNPLA2) is mutated in neutral lipid storage disease with myopathy. *Nat Genet*. 2007;39:28–30.
240. Lefevre C, Jobard F, Caux F, et al. Mutations in CGI-58, the gene encoding a new protein of the esterase/lipase/thioesterase subfamily, in Chanarin-Dorfman syndrome. *Am J Hum Genet*. 2001;69:1002–1012.
241. Zeharia A, Shaag A, Houtkooper RH, et al. Mutations in LPIN1 cause recurrent acute myoglobinuria in childhood. *Am J Hum Genet*. 2008;83:489–494.
242. Michot C, Hubert L, Brivet M, et al. LPIN1 gene mutations: a major cause of severe rhabdomyolysis in early childhood. *Hum Mutat*. 2010;31:E1564–E73244.
243. Michot C, Hubert L, Romero NB, et al. Study of LPIN1, LPIN2 and LPIN3 in rhabdomyolysis and exercise-induced myalgia. *J Inherit Metab Dis*. 2012;35:1119–1128.

CHAPTER 30

Mitochondrial Disorders

Mitochondrial myopathies and neuropathies or neuromyopathies refer to a heterogeneous group of disorders caused by dysfunction of mitochondria.[1–10] Mitochondrial disorders can be classified according to the associated biochemical, genetic defects, or clinical phenotype (Tables 30-1 to 30-3). One difficulty in classifying patients by any particular scheme is the clinical-phenotypic heterogeneity associated with specific mitochondrial mutations and the genetic heterogeneity in well-defined clinical phenotypes that are seen with mitochondrial disorders.

The mitochondria are responsible for converting fuels (carbohydrates, lipids, and proteins) into energy for the cells. Fatty acids are metabolized into molecules of acetyl-CoA within the mitochondria. Amino acids are converted to pyruvate in the mitochondria. Carbohydrates are metabolized to pyruvate in the cytoplasm and then transported into the mitochondria. Pyruvate from either source is converted into acetyl-CoA. Acetyl-CoA, then enters into the Krebs cycle from which electrons are generated. Electrons derived from the Krebs cycle are shuttled to the respiratory chain and processed through complexes I–V to generate ATP molecules. Thus, mitochondrial disorders can be classified according to the metabolic defect present (1) transport, (2) substrate utilization, (3) Krebs cycle, (4) oxidation/phosphorylation coupling, and (5) respiratory chain (Table 30-1).

Some of the biochemical abnormalities seen in various mitochondrial disorders are nonspecific and the result of primary "upstream" defects in metabolic pathways. For example, cytochrome oxidase (COX) deficiency is seen in many types of mitochondrial myopathy and does not imply that the primary mutation lies in one of the genes encoding for subunits of COX. The rapid advances of molecular genetics may provide a better classification scheme. The mitochondrial disorders may be classified by their genetic defect (1) mitochondrial DNA (mtDNA), (2) nuclear DNA (nDNA) mutations directly or indirectly affecting the mitochondrial respiratory chain complex, or (3) nDNA mutations that are involved in mtDNA maintenance or mitochondrial dynamics (Table 30-2; Fig. 30-1).[1–6] Notably though, there is significant phenotypic variability even in patients with the same genetic mutation. Therefore, a combined classification scheme is currently favored because of phenotypical variability and problems inherent in current genotyping capabilities (Table 30-3). Prior to discussing specific disorders, we will review a few basic principles regarding the mitochondrial genome and different inheritance patterns of mitochondrial disorders.

▶ COMPOSITION OF MITOCHONDRIAL DNA AND PROTEINS

The mitochondrial genome comprises 16.5-kB circular double-stranded DNA that contains no noncoding regions (i.e., introns). In fact, contiguous mitochondrial genes overlap in some areas. There is a single promoter site, and transcription is polycistronic such that mitochondrial genes are transcribed as two large RNAs. These are subsequently cleaved into 13 respective messenger RNAs (mRNA), 2 ribosomal RNAs (rRNA), and 22 transfer RNAs (tRNA). Interestingly, the genetic code for translation of human mitochondrial genes differs from the standard code which governs the translation of human nuclear genes.

The 13 mRNAs are translated into 13 polypeptides that are subunits of the respiratory chain complexes. Also note that any mutation in a mitochondrial tRNA gene can impair the proper translation of the 13 mitochondrial mRNAs. Importantly, the 13 proteins encoded by the mitochondrial genome account for less than 5% of all mitochondrial proteins. Thus, the majority of mitochondrial proteins are encoded by the nuclear genome that are translated in the cytoplasm and subsequently are transported into the mitochondria. Furthermore, the nucleus appears to regulate replication of the mitochondrial genome.

The respiratory chain comprises five multienzyme complexes (complexes I–V) (Fig. 30-2). Complex I (NADH-CoQ reductase) contains 45 subunits, seven encoded by mtDNA; complex II [succinate dehydrogenase (SDH) CoQ reductase] comprises four subunits, each encoded by nuclear genes; complex III ($CoQH_2$-cytochrome c reductase) comprises 11 polypeptide units, one of which is encoded by mtDNA; complex IV (cytochrome c oxidase) has 13 subunits, three encoded by mtDNA; and complex V (ATPase synthetase) comprises 19 subunits, two encoded by mtDNA (Table 30-4).

▶ GENETICS OF MITOCHONDRIAL DISORDERS

A population-based study in Northern England found that 6.57 per 100,000 adults have a mitochondrial disease and 12.48 per 100,000 of children and adults are at risk for developing a mitochondrial disorder on the basis of identifiable mtDNA mutations.[11] Because this study included only disorders caused by mtDNA mutations and not nDNA mutations affecting mitochondria, the prevalence of mitochondrial

▶ TABLE 30-1. CLASSIFICATION OF THE MITOCHONDRIAL MYOPATHIES BY METABOLIC FUNCTION AFFECTED

Metabolic Function	Defects
Substrate transport	Carnitine palmitoyltransferase (CPT) Primary systemic/muscle carnitine deficiency Secondary carnitine deficiency Combined carnitine and CPT deficiency
Substrate utilization	Pyruvate decarboxylase deficiency Pyruvate dehydrogenase deficiency Pyruvate carboxylase deficiency Fatty acid β-oxidation defects
Kreb cycle	Fumarase α-Ketoglutarate dehydrogenase deficiency Dihydrolipoyl dehydrogenase
Oxidation/phosphorylation coupling	Luft's syndrome: Loose coupling with hypermetabolism
Respiratory chain	Complex I Complex II Complex III Complex IV Complex V Combinations of I–V

Reproduced with permission from Walsh RJ. Metabolic Myopathies. *Continuum*. 2006;12(3):76–120.

disorders is certainly higher. Remember that during fertilization, all the mitochondria are contributed by the mother. Hundreds of mitochondria are present in most cells in the body and every mitochondrion has several copies of mtDNA. Mutations involving mtDNA are more common and more likely to manifest clinically than mutations in nuclear genes because of the lack of introns and decreased DNA repair mechanisms in the mitochondrial genome. mtDNA mutations are randomly distributed in subsequent generations of somatic cells during mitosis and germ cells during meiosis. Therefore, some cells will have few or no mutant genomes (normal homoplasty), some will have a mixture of mutant and normal or wild-type mtDNA (heteroplasty), and some will have predominantly mutant genomes (mutant homoplasty). Phenotypic expression depends on the relative proportion of mutant and wild-type mitochondria within each cell within a given organ system. When the number of mitochondria bearing sufficient mutated mtDNA exceed a certain threshold, mitochondrial function becomes impaired and patients manifest clinical symptoms and signs of disease (threshold affect).

During mitosis and meiosis, the proportion of mutant mitochondria in daughter cells can shift, thus changing the genotype and possibly the phenotype (mitotic/meiotic segregation). In addition, mutant mitochondria may utilize the mitochondrial-encoded mRNAs and tRNAs from

▶ TABLE 30-2. CLASSIFICATION OF MITOCHONDRIAL DISORDERS BY GENETIC MUTATIONS

I. Mitochondrial DNA mutations
   A. Large scale deletions
      1. Kearns–Sayre syndrome
      2. PEO
   B. Mutations in mtDNA protein–coding genes
      1. ATP6 is associated with Leigh syndrome and NARP
      2. Cytochrome b is associated with exercise intolerance and recurrent myoglobinuria
      3. Cytochrome c oxidase is associated with fatal and benign infantile myopathies, Leigh syndrome, MELAS, recurrent rhabdomyolysis
   C. Mutations in mitochondrial tRNA and rRNA genes
      1. MERRF is usually associated with mutations in $tRNA^{Lys}$ gene. MERRF has also been associated with mutations in $tRNA^{Leu}$ and $tRNA^{Ser}$
      2. MELAS is usually associated with mutations in $tRNA^{Leu}$ gene. MELAS also occurs with mutations in $tRNA^{Val}$, $tRNA^{Cys}$, ND5 of complex 1, and in cytochrome b
II. Nuclear gene mutations
   A. Nuclear mutations associated with mtDNA maintenance and replication (multiple mtDNA deletions and mtDNA depletion)
      1. Thymidine phosphorylase gene (*TYMP*) is associated with autosomal recessive MNGIE
      2. Adenine nucleotide translocator 1 (*ANT1*) is associated with autosomal dominant PEO
      3. Twinkle (*C10orf2*) is associated with autosomal dominant PEO and SANDO
      4. Polymerase gamma (*POLG1* and *POLG2*) is associated with autosomal recessive and dominant PEO, SANDO, MIRAS
      5. Ribonucleotidase reductase (*RRM2B*) is associated with MNGIE and PEO
      6. Thymidine kinase 2 (*TK2*) is associated with severe myopathy
      7. DNA replication helicase/nuclease 2 (*DNA2*) is associated with PEO
      8. Deoxyguanosine kinase (*DGUOK*) is associated with PEO, recurrent rhabdomyolysis, and mtDNA depletion myopathy
      9. Paraplegin (*SGP7*) is usually associated with hereditary spastic paraglegia but can be associated with PEO and spasticity
   B. Nuclear mutations associated with abnormal mitochondrial fusion/fission
      1. Mitofusin 2 (*MFN2*) associated with CMT2A
      2. Ganglioside-induced differentiation associated-protein 1 (*GDAP1*) associated with CMT2K and CMT4A
      3. Optic atrophy 1 (*OPA1*) associated with optic atrophy 1 syndrome/CMT with optic atrophy
      4. Mitochondrial inner protein 17 (*MPV17*) associated with Navajo neurohepatopathy and PEO
   C. Nuclear DNA mutations directly affecting components of mitochondrial respiratory chain
      1. Leigh syndrome may be caused by mutations in SURF1 and several different subunits of Complexes I, II, IV of the respiratory chain encoded by nuclear genes
      2. NARP caused by mutations in *MTATP6*
      3. SDH mutations can be associated with exercise intolerance

▶ TABLE 30-3. **CLASSIFICATION OF MITOCHONDRIAL MYOPATHIES BY CLINICAL FEATURES AND GENOTYPE**

Disease	Mode of Inheritance	Mitochondrial DNA Mutation	Gene Location
Kearns–Sayre syndrome	Sporadic	Single large mtDNA mutation	Large area of mt genome
PEO	Sporadic	Single large mtDNA mutation	Large area of mt genome
PEO	Maternal	Point mutations of mtDNA	$tRNA^{Leu}$, $tRNA^{Ile}$, $tRNA^{Asn}$
PEOA	Autosomal dominant	Multiple mtDNA deletions	*POLG1*, C10*orf*2 (twinkle); less common: ANT1, *POLG2, TK2, OPA1, DGOUK, RRM2B*
PEOB	Autosomal recessive	Multiple mtDNA deletions	*POLG1*; less common: *TK2, DGOUK, RRM2B, MPV17, DNA2, SGP7*
ARCO	Autosomal recessive	Multiple mtDNA deletions	Unknown nuclear gene
MERRF	Maternal	Point mutations of mtDNA	$tRNA^{Lys}$, $tRNA^{Leu}$, $tRNA^{His}$, $tRNA^{Phe}$, $tRNA^{Ser}$, *MTND5*
MERRF	Autosomal recessive	Multiple mtDNA deletions	*POLG1*
MELAS	Maternal	Point mutations of mtDNA	$tRNA^{Leu}$, $tRNA^{Val}$, $tRNA^{Lys}$, $tRNA^{Phe}$, $tRNA^{Ser}$, *ND5, ND4, ND1, MTCYB*
MNGIE	Autosomal recessive	Multiple mtDNA deletions	*TYPM, POLG1, RRM2B*
MNGIE	Maternal	Point mutations of mtDNA	$tRNA^{Lys}$
Leigh syndrome	Maternal	Point mutations of mtDNA	MTND3, MTND5, MTND6, MTCO3, MTATP6, $tRNA^{Val}$, $tRNA^{Lys}$, $tRNA^{Trp}$, $tRNA^{Leu}$
Leigh syndrome	Autosomal recessive	None	*NDUFV1, NDUFS1, NDUFS3, NDUFS4, NDUFS7, NDUFS8, SDHA BCS1L, COX10, COX15, SCO2, SURF1, LRPPRC*
Leigh syndrome	X-linked	None	*PDHA1*
Leigh syndrome	Sporadic	Single large mtDNA mutation	Large area of mt genome
Recurrent myoglobinuria	Sporadic or autosomal recessive	Mutations and microdeletions of mtDNA	*MTCO1, 2, and 3, MTCYB, ND4*
Recurrent myoglobinuria	Maternal	Point mutations of mtDNA	$tRNA^{Phe}$
MLASA	Autosomal recessive	None	*PUS1*
SANDO	Autosomal recessive	Multiple mtDNA deletions	*POLG1, C10orf2*
SANDO	Autosomal dominant	Multiple mtDNA deletions	*C10orf2*
Navajo neurohepatopathy	Autosomal recessive	None	*MPV17*
Optic atrophy 1	Autosomal recessive	None	*OPA1*

PEO, progressive external ophthalmoplegia; ARCO, autosomal recessive cardiopathy and ophthalmoplegia; MELAS, mitochondrial encephalopathy, lactic acidosis, and strokes; MERRF, myoclonic epilepsy and ragged red fibers; MNGIE, myo-neuro-gastrointestinal encephalopathy; MLASA, mitochondrial myopathy and sideroblastic anemia; mtDNA, mitochondrial DNA; SANDO, sensory ataxic neuropathy, dysarthria/dysphagia, opthalmoplegia.

neighboring normal mitochondria in a process called complementation. Thus, there can be some degree of normal translation of mtDNA-encoded proteins even in mitochondria harboring large DNA deletions.

Different organs have differing susceptibility for mitochondrial abnormalities depending on their energy requirements. Because the central nervous system (CNS) is in constant demand for energy, small decreases in energy production can lead to severe abnormalities. In contrast, skeletal muscle has low energy demands at rest, but these demands drastically increase with exercise. This is the basis for exercise-intolerance in many patients with mitochondrial myopathies.

Primary mutations of mtDNA can only be inherited from the mother. Unlike X-linked disorders that are also passed on only from the mother, women and men are equally affected in inherited mitochondrial diseases, while men are generally more severely affected with an X-linked inheritance pattern. Further, based on the degree of mitochondrial segregation and heteroplasty, all the children of an affected mother may be affected to a variable degree, which is different from autosomal dominant and recessive inheritance patterns.

Mitochondrial disorders are not strictly inherited from an affected mother. Because over 95% of mitochondrial proteins are encoded from nuclear genes, mitochondrial disorders can be inherited in an autosomal dominant [e.g., some forms of progressive external ophthalmoplegia (PEO)], autosomal recessive [e.g., mitochondrial neurogastrointestinal encephalomyopathy (MNGIE) syndrome], and even X-linked (e.g., some forms of Leigh syndrome) fashion. In addition, the presence of mutations involving mtDNA does not imply a maternal/mitochondrial inheritance pattern. In this regard, Kearns–Sayre syndrome (KSS) is associated with large mtDNA deletions, but is sporadic in nature. In addition, as noted earlier there appears to be some nuclear control over the replication and/or maintenance mitochondrial

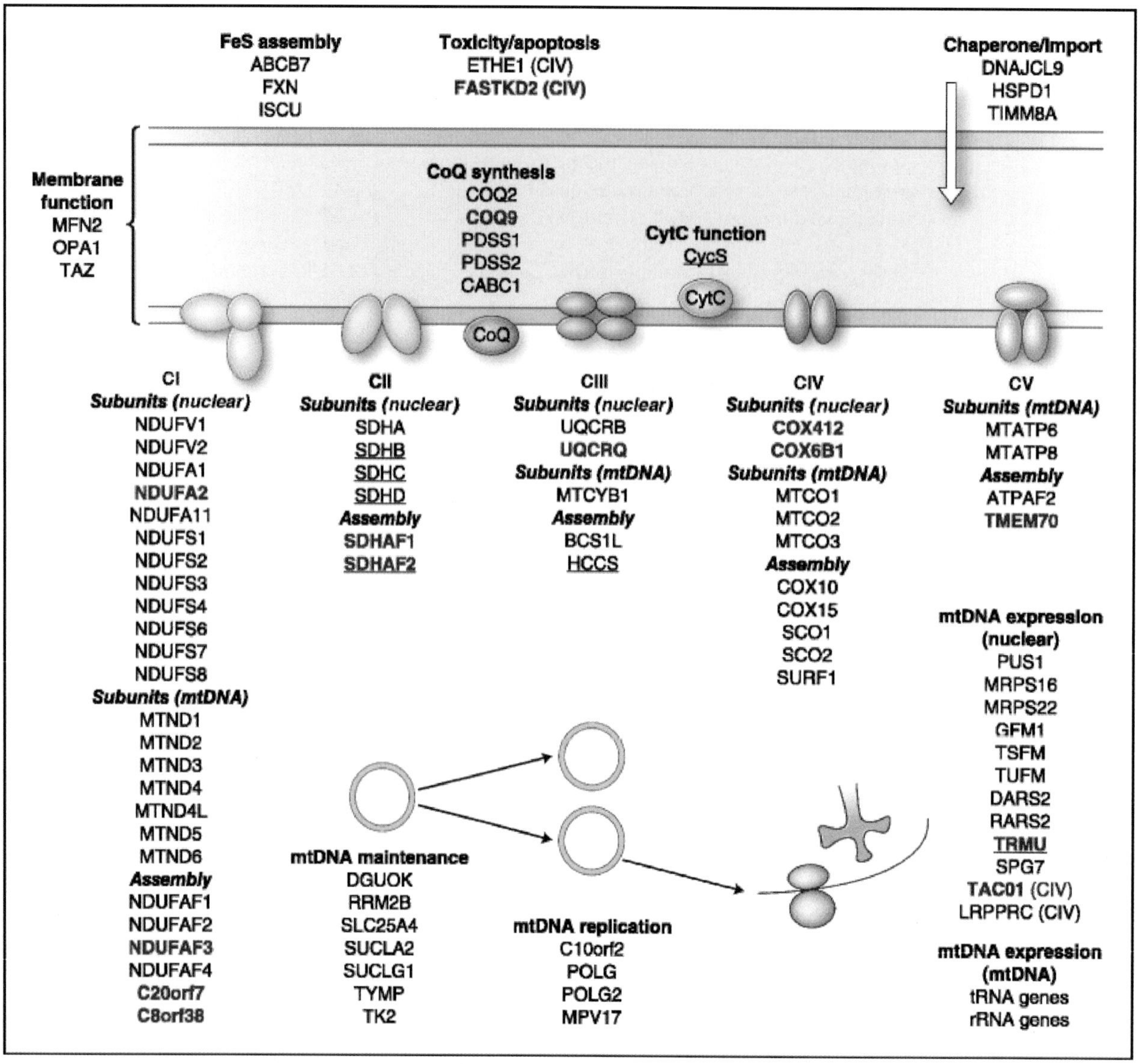

Figure 30-1. Genes associated with mitochondrial disease. Mutations have been identified in genes encoding CI, CII, CIII, CIV, and CV subunits and assembly factors; genes involved in mitochondrial DNA (mtDNA) maintenance (via nucleotide metabolism), mtDNA replication, and mtDNA expression; genes affecting the electron carriers coenzyme Q (CoQ) and cytochrome c (CytC); genes affecting FeS assembly; and genes involved in protein import, toxicity/apoptosis, and membrane function. Recently identified genes described in this review are highlighted in red. Genes affecting oxidative phosphorylation for which mutations are not reported to cause neuropathology are underlined. rRNA, ribosomal RNA; tRNA, transfer RNA. Currently, most cases of mitochondrial encephalopathy are untreatable, other than by relieving certain symptoms. Therefore, there is a great need to better understand the genetics of mitochondrial disease, which will enable prenatal diagnoses and will deliver the deeper understanding of mitochondrial function needed for the development of effective therapies. Recent advances in sequencing technology indicate that we may be on the cusp of a revolution in the way genetic diseases, such as mitochondrial encephalopathy, are diagnosed. (Reproduced with permission from Tucker EJ, Compton AG, Thorburn DR: recent advances in the genetics of mitochondrial encephalopathies. *Curr Neurol Neurosci Rep.* 2010;10(4):277–285.)

genome. Thus, mutations in some nuclear genes result in syndromes associated with depletion or multiple deletions of mtDNA. These disorders can demonstrate autosomal recessive or dominant inheritance patterns and are caused by defects in enzymes required for mtDNA replication and for maintaining the proper balance within mitochondria of deoxynucleoside triphosphates (dNTPs) that serve as the building blocks for mtDNA (Figs. 30-1 and 30-3). Replication of mtDNA requires the catalytic subunit of polymerase (encoded by the *POLG1* gene), the accessory subunit (encoded by *POLG2*), and the replicative helicases, twinkle (encoded by *PEO1*), and DNA replication helicase/nuclease 2 (encoded by *DNA2*). Mutations in these genes result in mtDNA depletion and/or multiple mtDNA deletions that

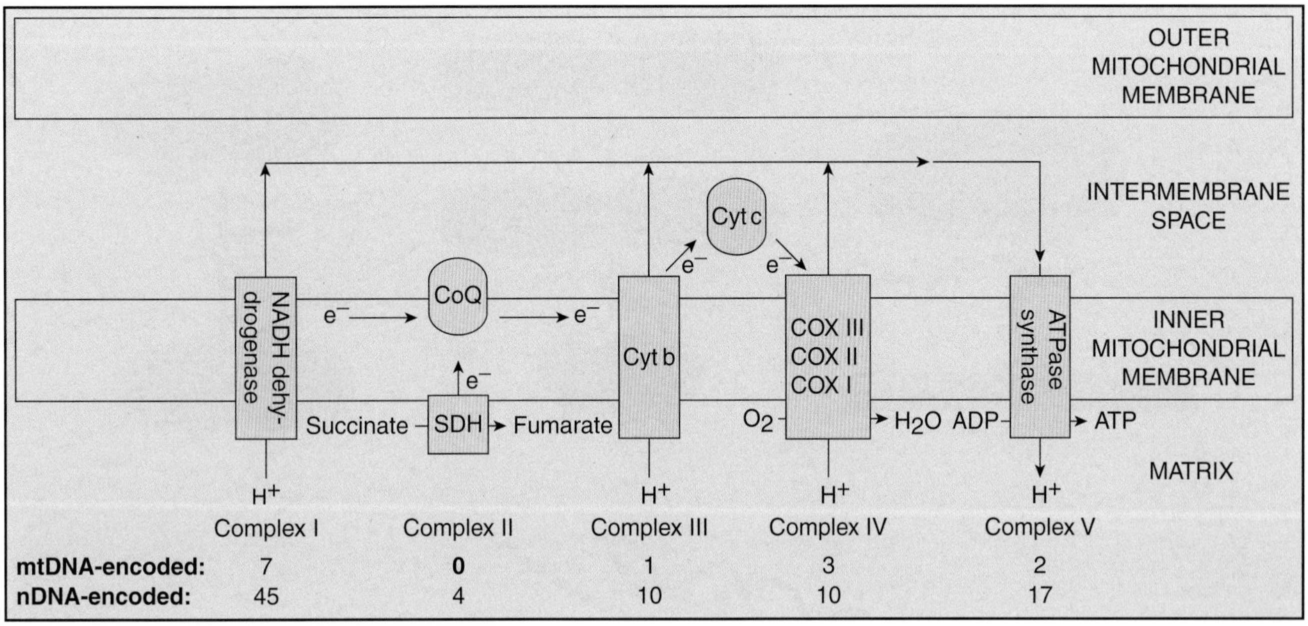

Figure 30-2. Schematic view of the respiratory chain. This diagram shows the number of subunits encoded by mitochondrial DNA (mtDNA) and nuclear DNA (nDNA) for each complex. All of the subunits for complex II are encoded by nDNA. Electrons (e−) flow down the respiratory chain and protons (H+) are pumped from the matrix to the intermembranous space through complexes I, III, and IV, then back into the matrix through complex V (ATPase synthase). Cytochrome c (Cyt c) and coenzyme Q (CoQ) are electron carriers. This process generates adenosine triphosphate (ATP). (Reproduced with permission from Walsh RJ. Metabolic Myopathies. *Continuum.* 2006;12(3):76–120.)

are found in various mitochondrial disorders [e.g., PEO, MNGIE, sensory ataxia neuropathy dysarthria/dysphagia ophthalmoplegia (SANDO)], which are discussed later.[1-6] A delicate balance of the 4 dNTPs (dATP, dGTP, dCTP, and dTTP) are also necessary for mtDNA replication. Several nuclear-encoded enzymes are key in preserving this balance (i.e., *TK2*, *DGUOK SUCLA2*, *SUCLG1*, *RRM2B*, *TYMP*, and *MPV17*). Mutations in these genes also lead to mtDNA depletion and cause various mitochondrial disorders (e.g., mitochondrial depletion myopathy, MNGIE, Navajo neurohepatopathy).[1-6] Furthermore, some nuclear genes are responsible for normal mitochondrial dynamics (Figs. 30-1 and 30-3). For example, fusion of mitochondria is dependent on nuclear-encoded profusion GTPases that are located in the mitochondrial membranes and mitofusin 1 and 2 (MFN1 and MFN2).[1-6]

► **TABLE 30-4. COMPOSITION AND GENETIC CONTROL OF THE MITOCHONDRIAL RESPIRATORY CHAIN**

	Respiratory Chain	
Complex	**Total Number Polypeptides**	**mtDNA Encoded**
I	45	7
II	4	0
III	11	1
IV	13	3
V	19	2

Modified with permission from Zeviani M, Bonilla E, DeVivo DC, DiMauro S. Mitochondrial Diseases. *Neurol Clin.* 1989;7:123–156.

There can be significant genetic heterogeneity even within well-defined clinical syndromes. For example, PEO can be associated with multiple mtDNA deletions, point mutations in various mitochondrial tRNA genes, or have no mtDNA mutations. In addition, specific mutations of mitochondrial-encoded genes can manifest with heterogeneous clinical phenotypes. For example, point mutations in the mitochondrial $tRNA^{Leu}$ can result in mitochondrial myopathy lactic acidosis and strokes (MELAS), PEO, encephalomyopathy, or a generalized myopathy with exercise intolerance. Variability in clinical phenotype can also be apparent within families with identical mtDNA mutations. The vast clinical and genetic heterogeneity of the various mitochondrial disorders can be explained by the different segregation patterns of mutant mitochondria, the degree of mutant heteroplasty, tissue-specific thresholds, and the severity of the biochemical impairment related to the specific mutations.

► LABORATORY FEATURES

Serum creatine kinase (CK), lactic acid, and pyruvate levels can be normal or elevated. In addition, lactic acid levels may also be elevated in cerebrospinal fluid (CSF). Some mitochondrial disorders (e.g., mtDNA depletion) can be associated with renal tubular defects characterized by glycosuria, proteinuria, and aminoaciduria.

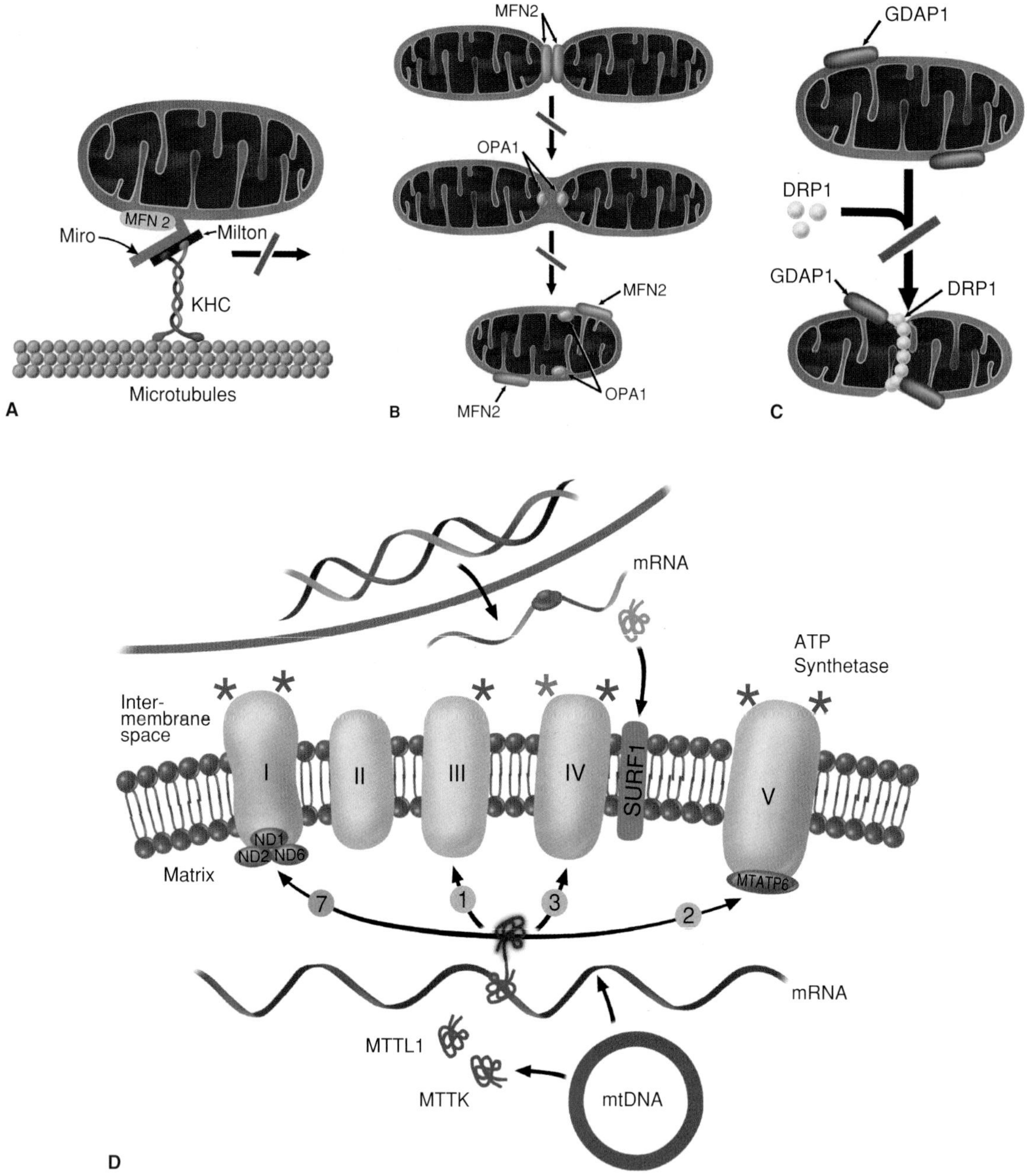

Figure 30-3. Overview of mechanisms underlying the main mitochondrial peripheral neuropathies. **(A)** MFN2 is located in the outer mitochondrial membrane and interacts with Miro and Milton proteins, which belong to the molecular complex that links mitochondria to kinesin (KHC) motors. **(B)** MFN2 participates in bringing the outer membranes of two mitochondria into close proximity. Thus, *MFN2* mutations can lead to defects in mitochondrial motility along the cytoskeletal microtubular tracks, and to dysfunction in fusion of the outer mitochondrial membranes of opposing mitochondria. Similarly, mutations in OPA1, which is located in the inner mitochondrial membrane, lead to dysfunction in the fusion process of the inner mitochondrial membrane. **(C)** Loss-of-function mutations in GDAP1, located in the outer mitochondrial membrane, can lead to dysfunction in the mitochondrial fission process, since GDAP1 might be a positive effector of assembly of the fission mediator DRP1. Dysfunction is shown by red oblique bars. **(D)** Dysfunctions in the respiratory chain can be due to the following: Direct mutations in mitochondrial protein-coding genes (red segment of circular mtDNA) *ND1*, *ND4*, and *ND6*, which encode for subunits of complex I (NADH dehydrogenase), and *MTATP6*, which encodes for a subunit of complex V (ATP-synthase); mutations in mitochondrial tRNA-coding genes (light blue segment) *MTTL1* and *MTTK*, which lead to dysfunction in transcription of mitochondrial protein-coding genes; or direct mutations in the nuclear gene *SURF1* (in green), which encodes an ancillary protein involved in complex IV (cytochrome c oxidase) assembly. Dysfunction in the corresponding respiratory chain complexes are shown by red, light blue, and green asterisks, respectively. Encircled numbers show the number of subunits encoded by mtDNA.

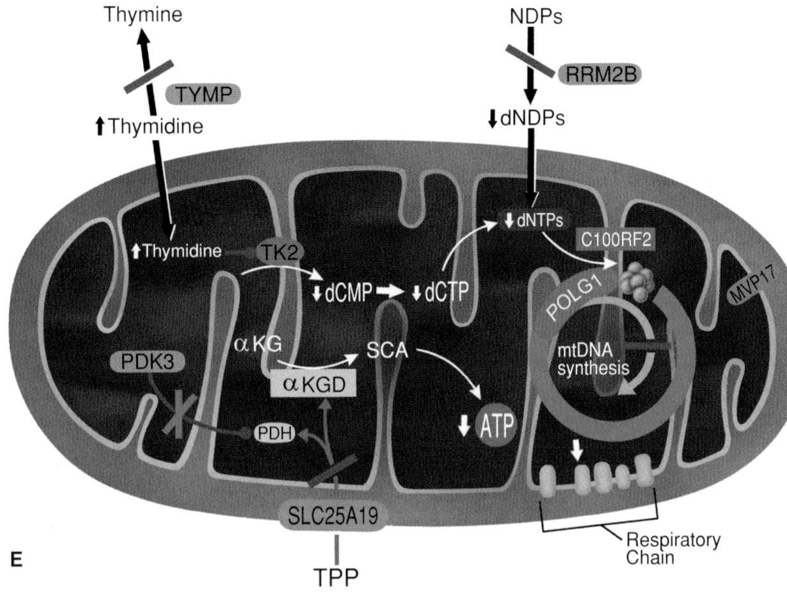

Figure 30-3. (*Continued*)**(E)** Dysfunctions of the respiratory chain can also occur as a result of changes in mtDNA synthesis (red oblique bar), which lead to mtDNA depletion or multiple mtDNA deletions. mtDNA synthesis might be disturbed by the following: Mutations in nuclear genes encoding components of the mitochondrial replisome—that is, polymerase gamma *POLG* and the helicase *C10orf2* genes; loss-of-function mutations (red oblique bar) in genes involved in the synthesis of nucleotides—that is, *RRM2B* and *TYMP*—which lead to nucleotide depletion (red lines show inhibition); or mutations in *MPV17*, a nuclear gene encoding an inner mitochondrial membrane protein of unknown function. Finally, mitochondrial peripheral neuropathies might result from changes in intermediary metabolism that eventually lead to decreased ATP synthesis. Mutations in *SLC25A19* inhibit the passage of TPP from the cytosol to the mitochondrial matrix, thus leading to lactate accumulation and an increase in αKG (an intermediate of the Krebs cycle), since TPP is an essential cofactor of PDH and αKGD (green lines show stimulation); similarly, a gain-of-function mutation (green tick mark) in *PDK3* might lock PDH in an inactive state, limiting glucose oxidation and favoring a switch toward anaerobic lactate production. mtDNA, mitochondrial DNA; NDPs, nucleoside diphosphates; dNDPs, deoxynucleoside diphosphates; dCTD, deoxycytidine; dCMP, deoxycytosine monophosphate; dCTP, deoxycytosine triphosphate; α-KG, α-ketoglutarate; α-KGD, α-ketoglutarate dehydrogenase; SCA, succinyl-CoA; TPP, thiamine pyrophosphate; PDH, pyruvate dehydrogenase.

Bicycle ergometry can sometimes be a useful test. Low levels of workload lead to an excessive rise in pulse rate and oxygen consumption. The degree of exercise intolerance correlates directly with the severity of impaired muscle oxidative phosphorylation as indicated by the peak capacity for muscle oxygen extraction and mitochondrial mutation load.[12,13] The diagnostic value of a constant workload protocol may be superior to an incremental cycle test, but the test is less sensitive for mitochondrial myopathies than simple testing of resting lactate and muscle morphology.[14]

A forearm exercise test can be performed where bicycle ergometry testing is not available.[15] The patient is instructed to open and close their hand (about once every 2 seconds at 40% of maximal voluntary contraction for 3 minutes). A butterfly needle can be placed in the antecubital fossa and venous oxygen and lactate levels can be measured at baseline and each minute during and immediately following exercise. Patients with mitochondrial myopathies and exercise intolerance often demonstrate excessive and prolonged lactate production and paradoxically increased venous oxygen saturation.[15] The range of elevated venous PO_2 during forearm exercise in mitochondrial myopathy patients (32–82 mm Hg) correlates closely with the severity of oxidative impairment as assessed during cycle exercise.[16] Thus, the measurement of venous PO_2 during aerobic forearm exercise provides an easily performed screening test that sensitively detects impaired oxygen use and accurately assesses the severity of oxidative impairment in patients with mitochondrial myopathy and exercise intolerance.

Nerve conduction studies (NCS) may be normal or abnormal. Some mitochondrial disorders are associated with a myopathy and/or a neuropathy. The neuropathy can be an axonal [i.e., neuropathy ataxia and retinitis pigmentosa (NARP)] or demyelinating in nature (e.g., MNGIE). Electromyography (EMG) is usually normal, although some myopathies are associated with increased insertional and spontaneous activity as well as early recruitment of small motor unit action potentials (MUAPs), while neurogenic disorders may be associated with decreased recruitment and large MUAPs. Conduction defects may be apparent on electrocardiograms (EKG).

Magnetic resonance imaging (MRI) and CT of the brain as well as electroencephalography (EEG) are typically abnormal in patients with a mitochondrial encephalomyopathy. MRI of skeletal muscle can reveal morphologic changes that resemble muscular dystrophies.[17] Magnetic resonance spectroscopy (MRS) with ^{31}P and ^{1}H compounds permits the analysis of ATP, creatine phosphate, inorganic phosphate, and pH in muscle and brain.[18,19] In mitochondrial disorders, there is a rapid fall in levels of creatine phosphate and an abnormal accumulation of inorganic phosphates in tissues with exercise. In addition, there is a delay in the recovery of phosphocreatine levels to normal after exercise. These techniques may also be potentially valuable in evaluating efficacy of various treatments.[20]

If a mitochondrial disorder is suspected from the clinical history and laboratory results, a muscle biopsy may be useful to confirm the diagnosis. Mutational analysis may be done on white blood cells. However, in certain syndromes, this is not as sensitive in finding mitochondrial mutations as in muscle tissue, particularly in those with large mtDNA deletions.

▶ HISTOPATHOLOGY

The histopathological abnormalities in nerve biopsies of the various mitochondrial disorders are nonspecific and generally not helpful. However, muscle biopsies are often useful in diagnosing a mitochondrial disorder, particularly if there is significant muscle involvement. The characteristic histological features are the presence of ragged red fibers on the modified-Gomori trichrome stain (Fig. 30-4). An increased number of lipid droplets are also often evident within these abnormal muscle fibers. Oxidative enzyme stains nicotinamide adenine dinucleotide dehydrogenase (NADH), SDH, and cytochrome c oxidase (COX) are also invaluable. The aggregated mitochondria intensely react to NADH and SDH stains forming ragged blue fibers (Fig. 30-4). Some patients with mitochondrial myopathies (in particular disorders not associated with mt-tRNA mutations) may have no ragged red fibers and normal NADH and SDH staining. COX stain (directed against one of the subunits encoded by mtDNA) appears to be the most sensitive stain and can demonstrate scattered muscle fibers with reduced or absent stain (Fig. 30-4). In addition, COX can highlight the subsarcolemmal accumulations of mitochondria. Reduced COX staining can be seen in both ragged red and otherwise normal-appearing muscle fibers. The variability of COX staining in combination with intense SDH staining is characteristic of disorders with mtDNA mutations. Remember, the SDH component of complex II is entirely encoded by nDNA, while 3 of 13 subunits of complex IV (COX) are encoded by mtDNA. Mutations of mtDNA often lead to a proliferation of mitochondria, perhaps in a compensatory response. Because SDH is encoded by nDNA, its transcription is generally increased in disorders caused by mtDNA mutations. The variability of COX staining reflects the heteroplasmic population of mutant and wild-type mitochondria. COX staining is not always abnormal in mitochondrial myopathies. Some patients with MELAS, point mutations in either ND genes or cytochrome b, or multiple mtDNA deletions (e.g., due to *POLG1* and other nDNA mutations) can have normal muscle histochemistry, including COX staining.[9]

Ultrastructural alterations in mitochondria are usually apparent on EM. These abnormalities include an increased number of normal-appearing mitochondria, enlarged mitochondria with abnormal cristae, and mitochondria with paracrystalline inclusions (Fig. 30-5). The paracrystalline inclusions are accumulations of dimeric mitochondrial creatine kinase (mtCK). This enzyme exists in both a dimeric and octamer form, but the increased radical generation in patients with mitochondrial disorders favors the production and crystallization of dimeric mtCK.[21]

▶ BIOCHEMICAL ANALYSIS OF MITOCHONDRIAL FUNCTION

Mitochondrial enzyme activities can be assayed in muscle biopsy specimens. This can be useful when the routine muscle histochemistry is unrevealing, but the diagnosis of a mitochondrial myopathy is still suspected because of the clinical phenotype. It can also be used to target genes for mutation screening. There is no standard method for performing mitochondrial metabolic analysis. Some centers prefer to assay only fresh muscle biopsy specimens (this is necessary for measurement of substrate oxidation). Rates of flux, substrate oxidation, and ATP production can be measured by polarography or using 14 C-labeled substrates. More commonly, measurement of enzyme activity of each of the individual respiratory complexes is performed on frozen muscle tissue.

▶ MOLECULAR GENETIC ANALYSIS

Mutation analysis of mtDNA and nuclear genes traditionally have been guided by the clinical phenotype, laboratory features, histochemistry, and biochemistry (Fig. 30-6).[1–10] In patients with classic clinical syndromes (e.g., MERRF, MELAS), one can proceed directly toward mutation screening for the most common mutations associated with these disorders. As will be discussed, however, there is wide genetic heterogeneity even within well-defined clinical phenotypes. If a mutation is not found in white blood cells, then a muscle biopsy and mitochondrial enzyme analysis can be performed. Then, screening for mutations can be done based on clinical phenotype aided by histochemical features and biochemical analysis. That said, recent advances in molecular genetics have allowed for less expensive and extensive screening of mtDNA and nDNA by next-generation sequencing and other techniques.

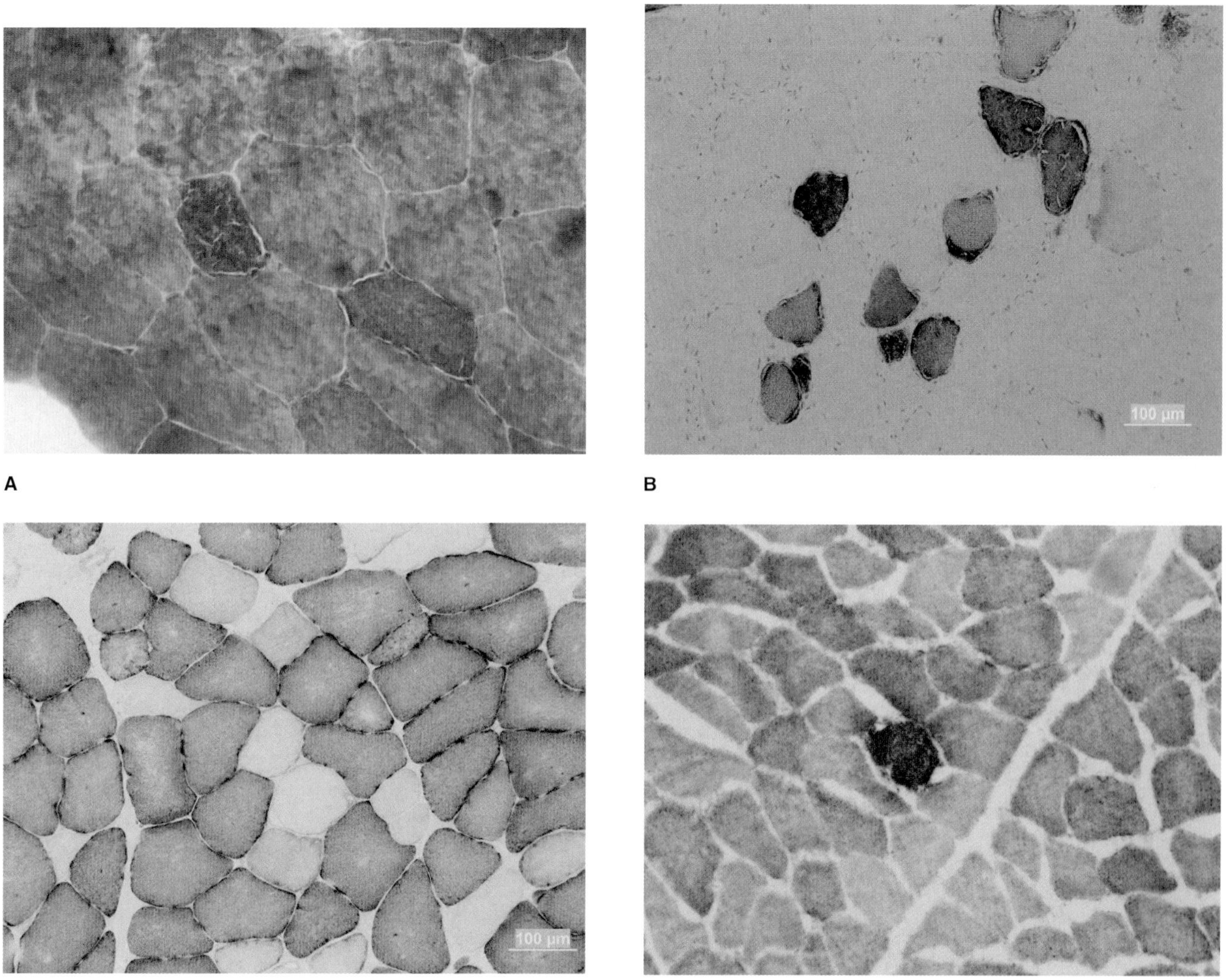

A B C D

Figure 30-4. Muscle biopsy demonstrates ragged red fibers resulting from the accumulation of abnormal mitochondrial below the sarcolemma of muscle fibers on modified Gomori-trichrome stain **(A)**. Mitochondrial myopathies associated with mtDNA mutations often spare SDH, which is entirely encoded by the nuclear genome. Therefore, muscle fibers with proliferating mitochondria stain intensely with SDH stain—so-called ragged blue fibers **(B)**. The most sensitive stain is for cytochrome c oxidase (COX). Scattered COX-negative fibers are often appreciated in mitochondrial myopathies **(C)**. Combining the COX and SDH stains is very helpful as well. The presence of COX negativity in an SDH-positive fiber (*blue staining*) is suggestive of an mtDNA mutation, though this may be secondary to mutations in nuclear genes regulating mtDNA **(D)**.

► SPECIFIC MITOCHONDRIAL DISORDERS

MYOCLONIC EPILEPSY AND RAGGED RED FIBERS

Clinical Features

Myoclonic epilepsy and ragged red fibers (MERRF) is characterized by myoclonus, generalized seizures (myoclonic and tonic–clonic), ataxia, dementia, sensorineural hearing loss, optic atrophy, and progressive muscular weakness developing in childhood or adult life.[1–3,22–31] The clinical spectrum is variable, which may be a reflection of the percentage of abnormal mitochondria that segregate into the respective tissues. Age of onset, spectrum and severity of involvement, and the course can vary, even within families. Muscle weakness and atrophy can be generalized, but there is a predilection for involvement of proximal arm and leg muscles. In addition, a generalized sensorimotor polyneuropathy and pes cavus deformities may be appreciated. The myoclonus is stimulus sensitive, but can be present at rest. The seizures may be photosensitive. Patients are often misdiagnosed as having juvenile myoclonic epilepsy,[32] until other signs or symptoms

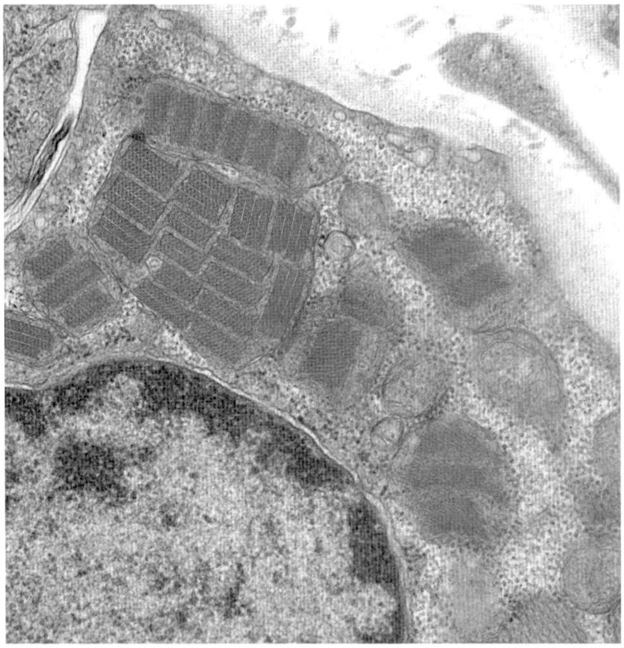

Figure 30-5. Electron microscopy. EM reveals increased numbers of mitochondria with abnormal paracrystalline inclusions.

(e.g., weakness, ataxia) manifest. Unlike KSS and PEO, individuals with MERRF do not usually ptosis, ophthalmoparesis, and pigmentary retinopathy. However, cardiomyopathy with conduction block or heart failure may also be seen in MERRF, particularly those cases presenting early.[28] MERRF can also be complicated by ventilatory muscle weakness and associated with life-threatening hypoventilation in the setting of surgery, sedation, or intercurrent infection.[28,33] Some patients also manifest with multiple symmetric lipomatosis.[34,35]

Laboratory Features

Serum CK can be normal or mildly elevated. Serum lactate can be normal or elevated as well. Generalized slowing of the background activity and bursts of spikes and slow waves may be apparent on EEG. MRI or CT scan of the brain often reveals cerebral and cerebellar atrophy. NCS may demonstrate reduced decreased amplitudes of sensory nerve action potentials consistent with a superimposed axonopathy in some patients.[23,36,37] EMG is usually normal, although early recruitment of small MUAPs might be evident in weak muscles.

Histopathology

Muscle histopathology is abnormal as noted previously. Many ragged red fibers and COX-negative fibers are evident as well as fibers with increased SDH staining. Neuronal loss and gliosis of the dentate nuclei, globus pallidus, red nuclei, substantia nigra, inferior olivary nuclei, optic nerves, and cerebellar cortex are apparent on autopsy.[24] In addition, demyelination and gliosis are evident in the corticospinal and spinothalamic tracts, and posterior columns.

Molecular Genetics and Pathogenesis

There is non-Mendelian maternal inheritance of MERRF. Approximately 80% of MERRF causes are caused by a point mutation at nucleotide position 8344 of the mitochondrial genome that results in an A to G transition in the $tRNA^{Lys}$ gene (*MTTK*).[30,38–40] Of note, there is clinical heterogeneity with this specific mutation as patients can present with PEO, Leigh syndrome, or multiple symmetric lipomatosis.[24,35] MERRF has also been described with mutations at other locations in the $tRNA^{Lys}$ gene (positions 8356 and 8366) and with mutations in the $tRNA^{Leu}$ (*MTTL1*) that is most commonly mutated in MELAS. Other tRNA mutations associated with MERRF include $tRNA^{His}$ (*MTTH*), $tRNA^{Phe}$ (*MTTF*), and $tRNA^{Ser}$ (*MTTS1*). In addition, an MERRF clinical phenotype can also be found in patients with multiple mtDNA deletions caused by mutations in the polymerase gamma 1 gene (*POLG1*) and in ND5 (*MTND5*). Mutations can be demonstrated by polymerase chain reaction of mtDNA in leukocytes or muscle specimens, but the frequency of abnormal mtDNA is greater in muscle.

As described previously, the mitochondrial tRNA gene mutations impair the translation of mitochondrial-DNA–encoded respiratory chain proteins. Assays of mitochondrial enzyme activity in biopsied muscle tissue reveals diminished activity of complex I and IV. At least 90% of the mitochondria must harbor mutations in order for clinical abnormalities to appear.[34]

Treatment

There is no specific therapy for MERRF other than treating the myoclonus (e.g., clonazepam) and the seizures with antiepileptic medications. A slight benefit was reported in a few patients with MERRF treated with creatine monohydrate (5–10 g/day).[41,42] Special care must be taken as patients with mitochondrial myopathies can develop marked alveolar hypoventilation in response to sedating medications and anesthetic agents.[43,44]

MITOCHONDRIAL MYOPATHY LACTIC ACIDOSIS AND STROKES

Clinical Features

MELAS is characterized by muscle weakness, high lactate levels in the serum or CSF, and stroke-like episodes.[1–3,44–48] Onset occurs in the first year of life in fewer than 10% with 60–80% developing symptoms and signs of the illness by the age of 15 years.[44,47] Rarely, MELAS can present as late as the eighth decade.[45] Most affected individuals have recurrent stroke-like episodes manifesting as migraine-type headaches

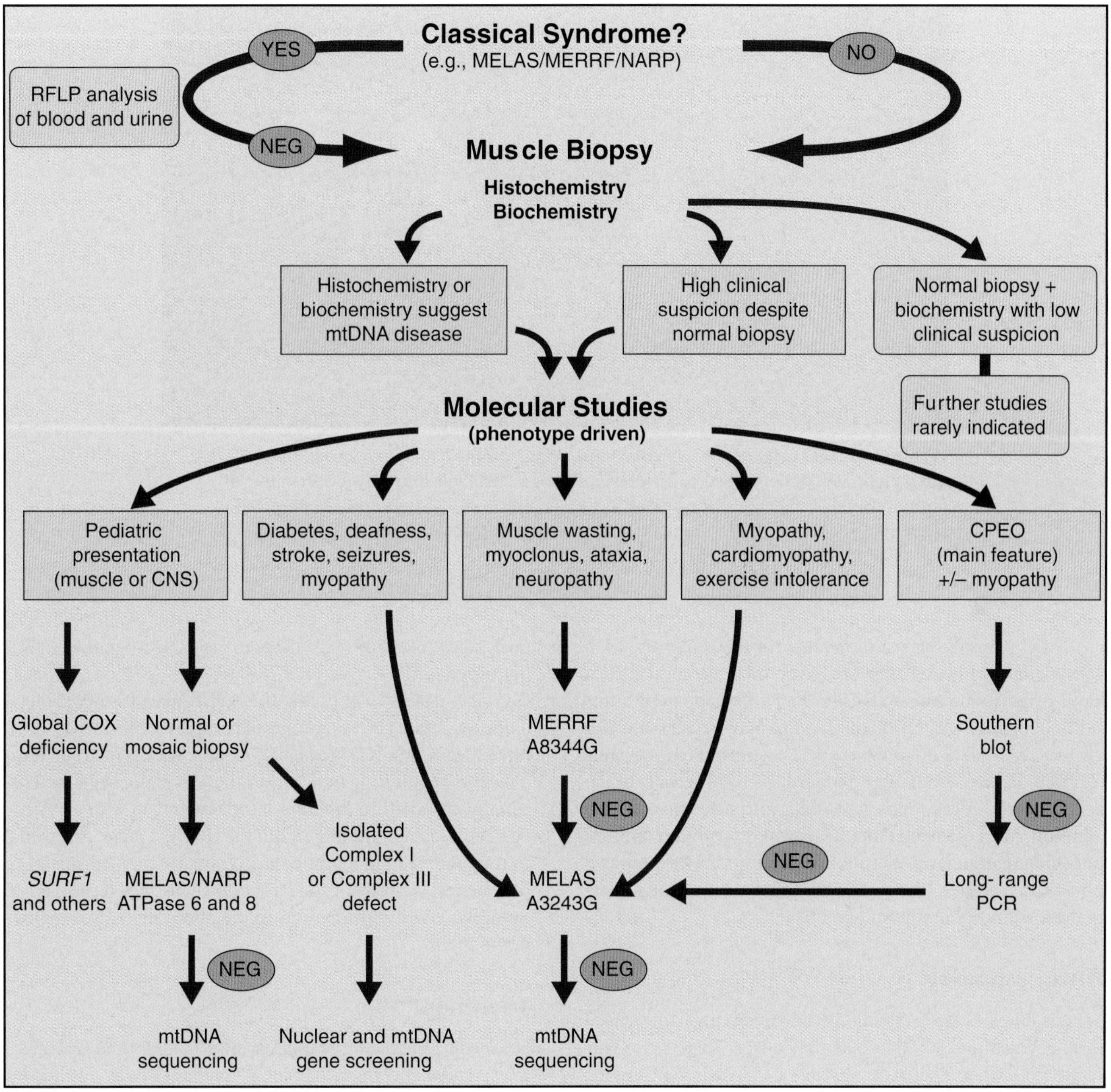

Figure 30-6. Flowchart illustrating routes of investigation in cases of suspected mitochondrial muscle disease. (Reproduced with permission from Taylor RW, Schaefer AM, Baron MJ,et al: the diagnosis of mitochondrial muscle disease. *Neuromuscul Disord.* 2004;14(4):237–245.)

with nausea and vomiting, hemiparesis, hemianopsia, or cortical blindness. These stroke-like attacks may be provoked by exercise or intercurrent infection. Progressive dementia may ensue. Most patients exhibit proximal muscle weakness and complain of easy fatigue and myalgias with exercise.

As with other mitochondrial disorders, many patients with MELAS are short-statured. Some affected individuals develop myoclonus, seizures, or ataxia and thus overlap clinically with MERRF. Ptosis, ophthalmoparesis, pigmentary retinopathy, and/or cardiomyopathy occur in less than 10% of patients. Rare individuals with the most common 3243 mutation in the *MTTL1* gene manifest with only diabetes mellitus and/or deafness.

Laboratory Features

Serum CK can be normal or elevated. Lactate levels are elevated in the serum and CSF in the majority of patients. EEG may demonstrate epileptiform activity. NCS are normal, but EMG may reveal early recruitment of myopathic-appearing MUAPs.

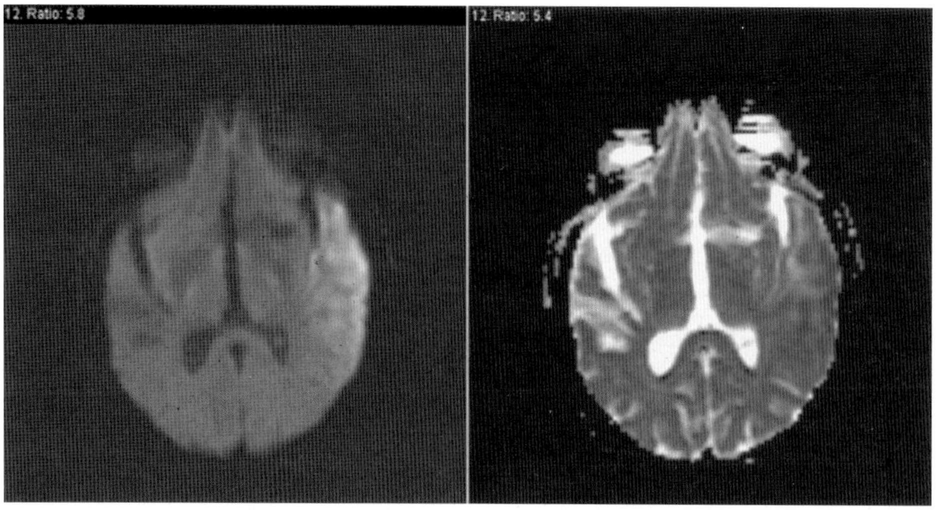

Figure 30-7. MRI in MELAS. The MRI brain imaging, during a stroke-like episode in a 61-year-old patient with genetically proven MELAS, shows a DWI high-intensity lesion in the left temporal lobe in the first image and absence of corresponding hypointensity on the corresponding ADC image. (Reproduced with permission from Walsh RJ. Metabolic Myopathies. *Continuum.* 2006;12(3):76–120.)

MRI scans of the brain reveal cortical atrophy and high T(2) signal and FLAIR abnormalities in the cerebral cortex, basal ganglia, and thalamus (Fig. 30-7). The apparent diffusion coefficient (ADC) of the lesions may be increased or decreased.[49] MRS of acute cortical lesions reveal severely elevated lactate levels and reduced concentrations of *N*-acetylaspartyl compounds, glutamate, and myo-inositol.[19] In addition, MRS of skeletal muscle may demonstrate a reduced phosphocreatine level, elevated concentrations of inorganic phosphate and free adenosine 5′-diphosphate, and an abnormally low phosphorylation potential.[19]

Histopathology

Muscle biopsies are indistinguishable from other mitochondrial myopathies as described previously. There are many ragged red fibers that have variable COX staining, ranging from increased reactivity to absent staining. This variability in COX staining is more prominent than that seen in MERRF. The COX-negative fibers intensely stain with SDH. Arterioles are also strongly SDH-reactive and an increased number of mitochondria are evident in the muscular walls of small blood vessels. Mitochondrial enzyme analysis of muscle tissue reveals reduced activities of complexes I, III, IV, and V.

Molecular Genetics and Pathogenesis

MELAS is inherited maternally in a non-Mendelian pattern. Over 70% of cases are caused by a mtDNA mutation, an A to G substitution, at nucleotide position 3243 in the gene (*MTTL1*) encoding for $tRNA^{Leu}$.[44] There is genetic heterogeneity of MELAS as mutations have also been identified at positions 3252, 3260, 3271, 3291 in the $tRNA^{Leu}$ gene as well as in the genes for $tRNA^{Val}$ (*MTTV*), $tRNA^{Lys}$ (*MTTK*), $tRNA^{Phe}$ (*MTTF*), $tRNA^{Ser}$ (*MTTS1*), the dehydrogenase-ubiquinone oxidoreductase (ND) subunits of complex I: ND1 (*MTND1*), ND4 (*MTND4*), ND5 (*MTND5*), and cytochrome b of complex III (*MTCYB*).[50] In addition there is phenotypic heterogeneity even within different family members who carry the common 3243 mutation within the $tRNA^{Leu}$ gene. Abnormal mitochondria in cerebral blood vessels or the neurons both may be responsible for the stroke-like episodes secondary to impaired energy production in metabolically active regions of the brain.

Treatment

No specific medical therapy is available other than treatment for seizures and myoclonus. Coenzyme Q does not appear to be of any significant benefit. A small study reported some improvement with dichloroacetate (DCA),[51] but a double-blind, placebo-controlled, randomized, 3-year crossover trial of DCA (25 mg/kg/day) in 30 patients demonstrated no efficacy with peripheral nerve toxicity.[52] Creatine monohydrate (5–10 g/day) modestly improved strength in a few patients with MELAS,[41,42,53] but again, blinded controlled studies are lacking.

KEARNS–SAYRE SYNDROME

Clinical Features

KSS is characterized by the clinical triad of PEO, pigmentary retinopathy, and cardiomyopathy with onset usually before the age of 20 years.[1-3,54-60] Other clinical features include short stature, proximal muscle weakness, sensorineural hearing loss, dementia, ataxia, depressed ventilatory drive, and multiple endocrinopathies (e.g., diabetes mellitus, hypothyroidism, hypoparathyroidism, delayed secondary sexual characteristics). Affected individuals are very sensitive to sedatives and anesthetic agents can provoke ventilatory failure.[61,62]

Laboratory Features

Serum CK level is typically normal; however, lactate and pyruvate levels may be elevated. CSF protein is usually increased. The EKG often reveals conduction defects. NCS are usually normal, although diminished amplitudes suggestive of an axonal sensory or sensorimotor polyneuropathy may be seen. EMG usually demonstrates normal insertional and spontaneous activity, but may reveal early recruitment of small polyphasic MUAPs in weak muscles.

Histopathology

Muscle biopsies demonstrate ragged red fibers; however, unlike MERRF and MELAS, there is little variability of COX staining with most of the ragged red fibers lacking COX reactivity.[44,63] The number of ragged red fibers and COX-negative fibers correlate with the percentage of mitochondria harboring large deletions. Autopsy may reveal spongy degeneration of the cerebral white matter.

Molecular Genetics and Pathogenesis

Single large mtDNA deletions (ranging from 1.3 to 8.8 kB) can be demonstrated in most patients with KSS.[56,58,60,63] As many as 43% of patients have a characteristic 4.9-kB deletion, suggesting there may be "hot spots" in the mitochondrial genome for these large deletions. One is more likely to find mtDNA mutations in muscle tissue than in peripheral white blood cells with the percentage of affected mitochondrial genomes in muscle biopsies ranging from 20% to 90%.[58] These large deletions most likely arise during oogenesis.[2] Mitochondrial disorders with single large deletions need to be differentiated from disorders with multiple deletions—see later). The large deletions usually involve several tRNA genes, thus impairing the adequate translation of mtDNA-encoded proteins. The single deletion mutations are usually sporadic in nature, although rare cases with familial occurrences have been reported.[28,56]

The clinical phenotype of individuals harboring single large mtDNA is again heterogeneous. Some patients develop migraines and stroke-like episodes with or without PEO, some have PEO with or without limb weakness, retinopathy, or deafness, others have an encephalopathy without PEO (including Leigh syndrome), while rare patients manifest only with diabetes mellitus, deafness, or Pearson syndrome.

Treatment

Some patients with KSS treated with creatine supplementation (0.08–0.35 g/kg body weight/day) have improved exercise capacity measured with bicycle ergometry.[53] Patients with cardiac conduction defects may require pacemaker insertion. Ptosis may be treated with eyelid surgery provided there is sufficient facial strength to allow full eye closure. Tarsorraphy should be undertaken judiciously, however, as there is risk for corneal injury due to exposure/trauma if the eyelids cannot completely close, and risk of ptosis recurrence. Patients and their physicians need to be made aware of the extreme sensitivity to CNS depressants and potential for decreased respiratory drive.[61,62]

PROGRESSIVE EXTERNAL OPHTHALMOPLEGIA

Clinical Features

Patients with PEO have ptosis and ophthalmoparesis (Fig. 30-8) with or without extremity weakness, but they lack pigmentary retinopathy, cardiac conduction defects, or other systemic manifestations (e.g., endocrinopathies).[1-3,56-58,63] Some cases that are sporadic in nature and associated with single large deletions of mtDNA probably represent a partial clinical expression of KSS. There are autosomal dominant and recessive forms as well as maternally (mitochondrial) inherited forms of PEO.

Laboratory Features

Serum CK, serum lactate, and CSF lactate can be normal or elevated. CSF protein may be increased. In contrast to classic KSS, the EKG does not demonstrate cardiac conduction defects. NCS are normal. EMG is also usually normal,

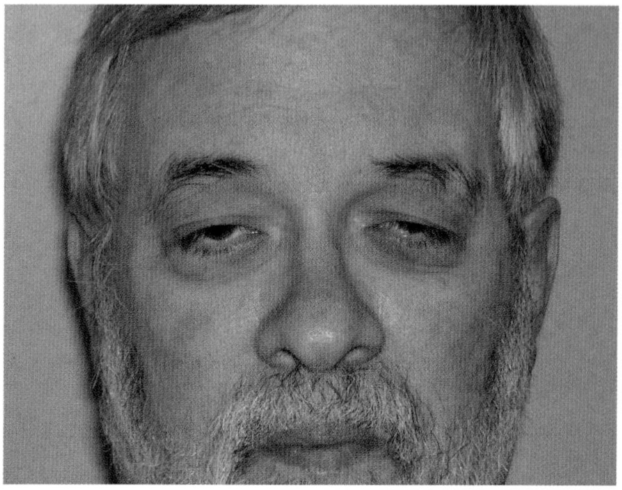

Figure 30-8. Progressive external ophthalmoplegia. A patient has ptosis and inability to move the eyes.

although myopathic MUAPs may be found in weak extremity muscles.

Histopathology

Muscle pathology is indistinguishable from KSS.

Molecular Genetics and Pathogenesis

Approximately 40–70% of patients with PEO have single large mtDNA deletions similar to KSS.[1–3,56–58,60,63] Such cases are generally sporadic in nature and PEO is not passed on to subsequent generations. Point mutations have been identified within various mitochondrial tRNAs (Leu, Ile, Asn, Trp) genes in several kinships with maternal inheritance of PEO.[64]

Autosomal dominant PEO is usually associated with multiple mtDNA deletions and is genetically heterogeneous (Table 30-2).[1–3,55,57,64–68] Several genes have been identified in autosomal dominant PEO (PEOA): PEOA1 due to mutations in the polymerase gamma 1 gene (*POLG1*); PEOA2 is caused by mutations in the *ANT1* gene that encodes for adenine nucleotide translocator (ANT); and PEOA3 caused by mutation in the twinkle gene (*C10orf2*). ANT is the most abundant mitochondrial protein and is responsible for transporting adenosine triphosphate across the inner mitochondrial membrane, while twinkle and POLG are involved in mtDNA replication. Less common, PEO has been associated with mutations in *POLG2, TK2, OPA1, DGOUK*, and *RRM2B*.

Autosomal recessive progressive external ophthalmoplegia (PEOB) is also most commonly caused by mutations in the *POLG1* gene. Mutations in this gene also have been implicated in Alper syndrome, which causes a clinical triad of psychomotor retardation, intractable epilepsy, and liver failure in infants and young children. Less common mutations have been identified in the *TK2, DGOUK, RRM2B, MPV17, DNA2*, and *SPG7* genes.[1–3,60,67,69]

Treatment

Surgery to correct ptosis may help. As with other mitochondrial disorders, individuals with PEO can develop hypoventilation in with infections and in response to sedatives or anesthetic agents.[61,62] Improvement in ventilatory muscle weakness has been reported with vitamin E treatment.[61,62]

AUTOSOMAL RECESSIVE CARDIOMYOPATHY AND OPHTHALMOPLEGIA (ARCO)

Clinical Features

Only a few patients have been reported with this rare syndrome characterized by childhood-onset PEO, facial and proximal limb weakness, and severe cardiomyopathy.[71,72] Affected individuals frequently complained of chest pain, dyspnea, and palpitations secondary to severe dilated cardiomyopathy and some require heart transplantation. The severe cardiomyopathy and autosomal recessive inheritance pattern help to distinguish this myopathy from autosomal dominant and maternally inherited PEO. The reported patients had no evidence of pigmentary retinopathy, hearing loss, ataxia, or peripheral neuropathy, although deep tendon reflexes were reduced.

Laboratory Features

Serum CK levels are mildly elevated. Serum lactate can be normal at rest but increases excessively during exercise. The EKG reveals cardiac conduction defects, while echocardiogram usually demonstrates dilated ventricles and a reduced ejection fraction. NCS are normal but EMG may reveal myopathic-appearing MUAPs.

Histopathology

Muscle biopsies reveal ragged red fibers which are strongly reactive to SDH but COX-negative.[71,72] However, there are also many COX-negative fibers which do not co-localize to ragged red and SDH-positive fibers. Biochemical assay have demonstrated decreased activity of respiratory chain enzymes containing mtDNA-encoded subunits, sparing the entirely nuclear-encoded SDH and citrate synthetase.

Molecular Genetics

Multiple mtDNA deletions may be found and the genetic defect is suspected to lie in nuclear genes involved in regulating the mitochondrial genome.

Treatment

Many patients will die from the severe cardiomyopathy within the first two decades of life, unless they receive cardiac transplantation.

MITOCHONDRIAL DNA DEPLETION MYOPATHY

Clinical Features

The mtDNA depletion syndromes (MDS) are a heterogeneous group of autosomal recessive disorders characterized by decreased mtDNA copy number in affected tissues (Table 30-2).[1–7,61,73–98] The MDS are associated with a severe myopathy that usually presents in infancy or early childhood, but milder cases manifesting in adult life have been reported. There is a predilection for proximal muscle involvement but ptosis and ophthalmoplegia are also common. Some also have a superimposed polyneuropathy. Muscle stretch reflexes are diminished or absent. In addition, some affected individuals can develop a cardiomyopathy, De Toni–Fanconi–Debré syndrome (a renal tubular defect), seizures, or liver failure. When the onset is in infancy, the muscle weakness is typically severe and progressive leading to feeding difficulties, respiratory failure, and death usually within the first year of life. Some forms of PEO (previously discussed) and MNGIE, mitochondria recessive ataxic syndrome (MIRAS), optic atrophy 1 (OA1), and Navajo neurohepatopathy (discussed in subsequent sections) are other mitochondrial disorders associated with MDS.

Laboratory Features

Serum CK can be normal or elevated as can serum lactate levels. The associated renal tubular defect results in glycosuria, proteinuria, and aminoaciduria. Cerebral atrophy and patchy areas of hypomyelination of subcortical white matter may be apparent on MRI scans.[80] Unlike most other mitochondrial myopathies, EMG may demonstrate numerous fibrillation potentials and positive sharp waves in those myopathies with mtDNA depletion. Motor units can have a mixed myopathic and neuropathic appearance. NCS can be normal or reveal features of an axonal or demyelinating sensorimotor neuropathy.

Histopathology

Muscle biopsies demonstrate many COX-negative fibers, although ragged red fibers may not be apparent.[74,80] EM shows enlarged mitochondria, some with concentric or whorled cristae, dense bodies, or paracrystalline inclusions. Biochemical assay of COX activity in skeletal muscle tissue of affected patients is greatly diminished or absent.

Molecular Genetics and Pathogenesis

MDS is associated with mutations in nuclear genes that control and maintain mtDNA.[1–7] At least half the cases are sporadic in nature but some are inherited in an autosomal recessive fashion. A depletion of mtDNA was first reported by Moraes et al. in 1991[81] and subsequently confirmed by others.[74,77–98] The quantity of mtDNA indirectly correlates with the clinical severity of the disorder. As much as a 99% reduction in mtDNA is present in the fatal infantile myopathy form of the disease, while the more benign myopathy has been demonstrated to have lesser depletions (36–88%) of mtDNA. Mitochondrial depletion myopathy is usually caused by mutations in the gene that encodes for thymidine kinase 2 (*TK2*),[77,86–97] but rare cases are caused by mutations in the deoxyguanosine kinase gene (*DGOUK*).[67,97,98]

Mitochondrial depletion can be seen by mutations in other genes that are associated with other clinical syndromes: thymidine phosphorylase (*TYMP*), *POLG1* and *2*, twinkle (*C10orf2*), mitochondrial inner membrane protein 17 (*MPV17*), ribonucleotidase reductase (*RRM2B*), optic atrophy 1 (*OPA1*), succinate-CoA ligase alpha subunit (*SUCLG1*), and succinate-CoA ligase ADP-forming, beta subunit (*SUCLA2*). Disorders associated with mutations in these genes are discussed in other sections.

Treatment

No specific medical therapy has been demonstrated to be effective.

MITOCHONDRIAL NEUROGASTROINTESTINAL ENCEPHALOMYOPATHY

Clinical Features

MNGIE, also referred to as POLIP syndrome, (*P*olyneuropathy, *O*phthalmoplegia, *L*eukoencephalopathy, and *I*ntestinal *P*seudo-obstruction) is an autosomal recessive mitochondrial disorder.[1–7,55,99–101] As the acronyms imply, the disorder is associated with a sensorimotor polyneuropathy, leukoencephalopathy on MRI of the brain, ragged red fibers on muscle biopsy, and chronic intestinal pseudo-obstruction. The disorder usually manifests before the age of 20 years (mean 13.9 years, range 2.5–32 years).[65] The course is progressive with severe disability or death by the third or fourth decade of life. The earliest symptoms are often caused by gastrointestinal dysmotility (i.e., dyspepsia, bloating, eructations, cramps, intolerance of large meals, and episodic nausea, vomiting, and diarrhea). Affected individuals gradually develop distal greater than proximal muscle weakness and atrophy, a stocking–glove distribution of sensory loss, and reduced muscle stretch reflexes throughout. Most patients have ptosis and extraocular muscle weakness. Despite the leukoencephalopathy apparent on MRI and on autopsies, most affected patients have little in the way of CNS symptoms or signs. However, rare patients have mental retardation. Other clinical features include pigmentary retinopathy, sensorineural hearing loss, facial weakness, hoarseness, or dysarthria.

Laboratory Features

Serum CK can be normal or mildly elevated. Lactate, pyruvate, and CSF protein levels are typically elevated. Thymidine phosphorylase activity is decreased in leukocytes and platelets, thymidine levels are increased in the plasma, and deoxyuridine is increased in serum and plasma in those cases caused by mutation in the *TYMP* gene that encodes for thymidine phosphorylase.[7]

Leukoencephalopathy of the cerebral and cerebellar white matter is apparent on MRI scans. Radiological studies also demonstrate dilatation and dysmotility of the esophagus, stomach, and small intestine. EKG has shown conduction defects in some patients, although they remained asymptomatic from a cardiac standpoint. Motor and sensory nerve conduction velocities may be slow to within the demyelinating range, while F-wave latencies are usually markedly prolonged.[65,101,102] Other cases are more suggestive of a primary axonopathy with reduced SNAP and CMAP amplitudes. EMG may reveal fibrillation potentials and positive sharp waves.[65] Recruitment of MUAPs can be decreased, suggestive of denervation in distal muscles. However, quantitative electromyography of proximal muscles may reveal small duration MUAPs suggesting a superimposed myopathic process. The generalized weakness coupled with the demyelinating polyneuropathy can lead to misdiagnosis as chronic inflammatory demyelinating polyneuropathy.[101]

Histopathology

Muscle biopsies may demonstrate ragged red fibers, ragged blue fibers with NADH and SDH staining, and COX-negative fibers.[65] Neurogenic atrophy may be apparent biopsies of distal muscles. Nerve biopsies have shown loss of myelinated nerve fibers, demyelination/remyelination, and rare onion-bulb formation, in addition to features of axonal degeneration. Abnormal mitochondria with paracrystalline inclusions occur in both muscle fibers and Schwann cells. Diminished COX and other respiratory complex activities can be demonstrated on enzymatic assays of muscle tissue.[65]

Autopsies have revealed widespread endoneurial fibrosis and demyelination in the peripheral nervous system and poorly defined white matter changes in the cerebral and cerebellar white matter.[101] Cranial nerves and spinal roots are less severely involved. Neurons of the brainstem and spinal cord appeared relatively intact. Interestingly, a loss of neurons and fibrotic changes of the autonomic ganglia and of the celiac and myenteric plexuses has been noted, which likely explains the associated gastrointestinal dysmotility.[101]

Molecular Genetics and Pathogenesis

Multiple mtDNA deletions similar to those found in some cases of autosomal dominant PEO have been demonstrated in some patients with autosomal recessive MNGIE.[1–7,64,100,103] Some cases of MNGIE are caused by mutations in the thymidine phosphorylase (*TYPM* or *ECGG1*) gene located on chromosome 22q13.32-qter.[100,103,104] Thymidine phosphorylase converts thymidine to 2-deoxy D-ribose 1-phosphate and may regulate thymidine availability for DNA synthesis. Interestingly, thymidine phosphorylase is not normally expressed in muscle tissue, so how it leads to multiple mtDNA deletions is unclear. It may lead to a reduction in the nucleotide pool within the mitochondria. Rare cases of MNGIE have been shown to be caused by mutations in *POLG1*, *RRM2B*, and the $tRNA^{Lys}$ (*MTTK*) gene.[7,105–107] Neuropathy is demyelinating in patients carrying *TYPM* or *RRM2B* mutations, whereas patients with *POLG1* mutations mainly have axonal electrodiagnostic (EDX) features.[7]

Treatment

No specific medical therapy is available. PEG tube or parenteral feedings for nutritional support are required in the majority of cases. Ankle foot orthotics may be beneficial in patients with foot drop.

SENSORY ATAXIA NEUROPATHY DYSARTHRIA/DYSPHAGIA OPHTHALMOPLEGIA

Clinical Features

SANDO (sensory ataxic neuropathy, dysarthria, ophthalmoplegia) is a disorder that may occur sporadically or in either a dominantly or recessively inherited fashion.[5–7,108–112] The onset of sensory ataxia is typically in early adulthood. Not all patients have each element of the SANDO syndrome. In addition to the phenotypic features described in the acronym, cerebellar ataxia, facial weakness, mild proximal weakness, exercise intolerance, Parkinsonism, myoclonus epilepsy, and hepatic failure have been described.[108,110]

Laboratory Features

NCS may reveal amplitude reduction and/or slowing of sensory SNAPs.[5–7,108–112]

Histopathology

Muscle biopsies may reveal ragged red and COX-negative muscle fibers. Sural nerve biopsy is not routinely performed but has revealed loss of large and small myelinated fibers and demonstrated onion-bulb formations.[5,6] Autopsy studies have shown axonal and dorsal column degeneration, suggesting involvement of dorsal root ganglia.[7]

Molecular Genetics and Pathogenesis

SANDO is usually autosomal recessively inherited and caused by mutations in *POLG1* that results in multiple mtDNA deletions and mtDNA depletion as mentioned previously.[109,111,112] SANDO can also result from mutations in *C10orf2*, which encodes twinkle helicase that also is involved in mtDNA replication.[113] Mutations in this gene can cause an autosomal dominant or recessive syndrome.

Treatment

No specific medical therapy is available.

MITOCHONDRIA RECESSIVE ATAXIC SYNDROME

MIRAS is very similar to SANDO and typically presents as a juvenile or adult onset ataxic neuropathy. Associated phenotypic features may include CPEO, dysarthria, seizures, nystagmus, cognitive impairment, involuntary movements, and psychiatric symptoms.[114–119] Like SANDO, it is usually caused by mutations in *POLG1*.

NEUROPATHY ATAXIA AND RETINITIS PIGMENTOSA

Clinical Features

NARP is associated with a childhood or adult onset axonal neuropathy, cerebellar ataxia, and retinitis pigmentosa. There may be proximal or distal weakness as well as pes cavus on examination.[5–7,120–123]

Laboratory Features

NCS reveal features suggestive of an axonal sensory neuropathy.

Histopathology

Muscle biopsy does not generally reveal ragged red or COX-negative fibers as the causal gene (see below) is involved only in the last step of ATP production. Nerve biopsy reveals loss of myelinated nerve fibers.[5,6]

Molecular Genetics and Pathogenesis

NARP is caused by mutations in mitochondrial-encoded ATPase 6 (*MTATP6*), which is also a cause of Leigh syndrome.

Treatment

No specific medical therapy is available.

NAVAJO NEUROHEPATOPATHY

Clinical Features

This manifests in infancy or early childhood with failure to thrive, diarrhea, vomiting, and signs of liver failure, including recurrent metabolic acidosis. In addition, infants have generalized hypotonia and weakness. Other neurological signs included microcephaly, seizures, ataxia, and dystonia. Those individuals who survive typically develop a severe sensorimotor polyneuropathy.[5–7,124–127] Loss of sensation leads to acromutilation and corneal ulcerations.

Laboratory Features

Serum transaminases and bilirubin are elevated while albumin is low. There may be evidence of a coagulopathy. Aminoaciduria is event on urine screen. MRI scans reveal increase signal in cortex and subcortical white matter as well as the dentate nuclei and cerebellar white matter.[5,6] NCS reveal slow of conduction velocities suggestive of a demyelinating sensorimotor polyneuropathy.[5–7,124,125]

Histopathology

Nerve biopsies have demonstrated loss of myelinated and unmyelinated nerve fibers.[124,127]

Molecular Genetics and Pathogenesis

This is caused by homozygous mutations (Arg50Trp) in the mitochondrial inner membrane protein gene (*MPV17*).[124,125]

Treatment

No specific medical therapy is available.

OPTIC ATROPHY 1 (OA1) SYNDROME

Clinical Features

OA1 usually manifests with progressive optic atrophy and is inherited in an autosomal dominant pattern.[7,128–132] It is allelic to what has also been called HMSN VI (CMT with optic atrophy). Approximately 20% of affective individuals develop neurological abnormalities, such as progressive external ophthalmoplegia, peripheral neuropathy, proximal myopathy, and hearing loss. The neuropathy is usually mild, and mostly sensory, but mild distal muscle atrophy and weakness along with pes cavus may be seen. Some patients have a sensory or cerebellar ataxia.

Laboratory Features

NCS are most suggestive of an axonal sensory greater than motor polyneuropathy.[129,132]

Histopathology

Muscle biopsy often shows multiple mtDNA deletions and sometimes depletion, ragged red fibers, and COX-negative fibers. Literature on nerve biopsy findings are lacking.

Molecular Genetics and Pathogenesis

This is caused my mutations in the *OPA1* gene, encoding a dynamin-related GTPase, which is important in mitochondrial fusion, fission, and cristae organization.[5,6,131,132]

Treatment

There is no specific medical treatment for OPA1.

LEIGH SYNDROME

Clinical Features

Leigh syndrome, or subacute necrotizing encephalomyopathy, usually presents in infancy or early childhood, but can rarely develop in adult life.[133,134] Affected individuals can manifest with recurrent vomiting, psychomotor retardation, hypotonia, generalized weakness and atrophy, ptosis, ophthalmoplegia, poor suck, respiratory failure, nystagmus, optic atrophy, hearing loss, involuntary movements, seizures, spasticity, ataxia, and peripheral neuropathy. The rate of progression varies, but the disorder is generally fatal.

Laboratory Features

Serum and CSF lactate levels are elevated as can be the lactate:pyruvate ratio. The syndrome is biochemically heterogeneous. Defects in activity of the pyruvate dehydrogenase (PDH), pyruvate decarboxylase (PDC), COX, and complex I have been described in some patients with Leigh syndrome. MRI demonstrates symmetric lesions in the thalamus, brainstem, cerebellum, and spinal cord reflecting the underlying pathology.

Histopathology

Muscle biopsy can demonstrate reduced or absent COX staining (mitochondrial and nuclear-encoded COX subunits) of muscle fibers, although ragged red fibers are usually not seen. Unlike fatal infantile myopathy, COX staining is also deficient in muscle spindles and in the smooth muscle of intramuscular blood vessels. Autopsy studies of the brain and spinal cord demonstrate symmetric cystic necrosis, spongioform changes, demyelination, and vascular proliferation in the thalamus, basal ganglia, brainstem, cerebellar white matter, dentate nuclei, and posterior columns.

Molecular Genetics and Pathogenesis

Leigh syndrome is genetically heterogeneous. Mutations have been identified in both nuclear- and mitochondrial-encoded genes. These genes are all involved in energy metabolism, including the generation of ATP, components of the PDH complex and mitochondrial respiratory chain complexes I, II, III, IV, and V, which are involved in oxidative phosphorylation.

Complex I comprises at least 45 subunits, of which seven are encoded by the mitochondrial genome (ND1–6, ND4 L) and the others are encoded by nuclear genes. Multiple complex I genes have been implicated in Leigh syndrome including mitochondrial-encoded *MTND3*, *MTND5*, and *MTND6*, and nuclear-encoded *NDUFV1*, *NDUFS1*, *NDUFS3*, *NDUFS4*, *NDUFS7*, and *NDUFS8* genes.[135,136]

From complex II, a mutation has been found in the nDNA gene flavoprotein subunit A (*SDHA*).[137] In complex III, a mutation has been found in the nDNA gene BCS1 L, which is involved in the assembly of complex III.

Complex IV mutated genes include mitochondrial-encoded cytochrome c oxidase subunit 3 (*MTCO3*) and nuclear-encoded cytochrome c oxidase assembly proteins 10 (*COX10*), and 15 (*COX15*). Two other nuclear-encoded genes with mutations are: (1) synthesis of cytochrome c oxidase 2 (*SCO2*), and (2) surfeit 1(*SURF1*). Surfeit1 is involved in the assembly of complex IV.[138] A mutation has also been found in a complex V gene, the mitochondrial-encoded ATPase 6 (*MTATP6*).[139] Of note, mutations in this gene are also responsible for the mitochondrial disorder termed NARP (neuropathy, ataxia, and retinitis pigmentosa) as previously discussed. When the proportion of mutated mtDNA is high (>90%), Leigh syndrome occurs; but NARP develops when the burden of mtDNA mutations is lower.

Mutations in multiple genes encoding mitochondrial tRNA proteins have also been identified in patients with maternally inherited Leigh syndrome: $TRNA^{Val}$ (*MTTV*), $tRNA^{Lys}$ (*MTTK*), $tRNA^{Trp}$ (*MTTW*), and $tRNA^{Leu}$ (*MTTL1*).[133,140] Single large deletions of mtDNA have also been demonstrated.[141]

Leigh syndrome may also be caused by mutations in components of the PDH complex. The gene *DLD* encodes for dihydrolipoamide dehydrogenase, which is a component not only of the PDH complex, but also of the alpha-ketoglutarate dehydrogenase complex, and the branched-chain alpha-keto acid dehydrogenase complex. Compound heterozygous mutations in *DLD* have been implicated in Leigh syndrome. X-linked Leigh syndrome is caused by mutation in the gene encoding the E1-alpha subunit of the PDH complex (*PDHA1*).[142–144]

The French-Canadian (or Saguenay-Lac Saint Jean) type of Leigh syndrome with COX deficiency (LSFC) is caused by mutation in the leucine-rich PPR motif-containing protein gene (*LRPPRC*). This gene encodes for an mRNA-binding protein involved in the processing and trafficking of mtDNA-encoded transcripts, but how this causes COX deficiency is not yet clear.

Treatment

There is no specific medical therapy available.

FOCAL MITOCHONDRIAL DEPLETION

Clinical Features

This disorder has been described in only a few patients.[145–146] A sister and brother presented in the second decade of life with exertional muscle pain and fatigue, myoglobinuria, and mild proximal weakness.[145] Their father of this pair was asymptomatic but had an elevated serum CK. Congenital weakness, hypotonia, delayed motor milestones, and mental retardation has also been reported.[146]

Laboratory Features

Serum CK levels are mild to moderately elevated and serum lactate levels are normal. A decreased selenium level has been described in one patient.[146] NCS are normal, but EMG may reveal myopathic MUAPs.

Histopathology

The most striking histologic feature, for which this disorder is named, is focal depletion of mitochondria in the center of the sarcoplasm in type 2 muscle fibers. At the periphery of muscle fibers, the mitochondria are enlarged. Scattered degenerating and regenerating fibers can be appreciated.

Molecular Genetics and Pathogenesis

This myopathy is presumably autosomal dominant. No molecular or quantitative defects of mtDNA have been reported in patients with this syndrome. Similar histological findings have been demonstrated in patients with myopathy felt to be related to selenium deficiency.[147]

Treatment

There is no specific medical therapy. A trial of selenium replacement should be considered in patients who are deficient in selenium.

MITOCHONDRIAL MYOPATHIES ASSOCIATED WITH EXERCISE INTOLERANCE/ RECURRENT MYOGLOBINURIA

Clinical Features

Some patients with mitochondrial myopathy manifest only with exercise-induced myalgias beginning in infancy or early adulthood.[1–3,148–159] They are typically short-statured and have generalized reduction in muscle bulk. Muscle strength may be normal or there can be mild proximal weakness. Recurrent episodes of myoglobinuria can also occur and be provoked by exercise and alcohol intake. However, provocative factors often are not present. We have seen patients with progressive deafness as well.

Laboratory Features

Serum lactate and pyruvate may be normal or slightly at rest but become significantly elevated with aerobic exercise. Serum CK can be normal or mildly elevated between episodes of myoglobinuria. EMG and NCS are typically normal.

Histopathology

Muscle biopsies may reveal scattered ragged red fibers, increased SDH and NADH stains (ragged blue fibers), as well as COX-negative fibers. However, COX stain can be normal, particularly in patients with mutations in *MTCO1, MTCO2, MTCO3, ND4,* and *MTCYB* (see below). Decreased COX activity has been found on enzyme analysis of muscle tissue in some,[148] but not all cases.[149] Abnormal mitochondria with paracrystalline inclusions can be detected on EM.

Molecular Genetics and Pathogenesis

This is a genetically heterogeneous group of disorders. Multiple mtDNA deletions were demonstrated in two brothers with presumed autosomal recessive inheritance.[138] In addition, point mutations in $tRNA^{Phe}$ have been found in kinships with and without recurrent myoglobinuria. Mutations within the gene encoding for subunits of cytochrome c oxidase (*MTCO1, MTCO2, MTCO3*) have been reported in sporadic cases.[2,142,150,151] Other cases of exercise intolerance and recurrent myoglobinuria have be ascribed to mutations in the mtDNA genes encoding for $tRNA^{Gly143}$ subunit 4 of NADH dehydrogenase (*ND4*),[154] and cytochrome b (*MTCYB*).[76,77,155,156] Mutations in *ND4*, may also produce Leber hereditary optic neuropathy[157] or Wolfram syndrome.[158] In addition, mutations in the gene encoding the iron-sulphur cluster assembly protein (*ISCU*) have been associated with exercise intolerance and myoglobinuria and muscle biopsies demonstrating succinate dehydrogenase deficiency and accumulation of iron in muscle fibers.[159]

Treatment

Attenuation of free-radical production and paracrystalline inclusions in muscle biopsies has been reported following a 5-week trial of creatine supplementation in a patient with a novel cytochrome b (*MTCYB*) mutation.[21] However, the patient did not feel any subjective improvement and there was no effect on his maximal oxygen consumption. There is no specific medical therapy other than treatment of myoglobinuria and avoidance of strenuous activity and alcohol.

Charcot–Marie Tooth Disease

There are at least three proteins involved in mitochondrial dynamics that cause forms of CMT: CMT2 A caused by mutations in the mitofusin 2 gene (*MFN2*). CMT2 K and CMT4 A are associated with mutations in ganglioside-induced differentiation associated-protein 1 (*GDAP1*), and OPA1 mutations are associated with CMT associated with optic atrophy as previously discussed (Fig. 30-3).[5–7] CMT caused by mutations involving MFN2 and GDAP1 are discussed in more detail in Chapter 11 (Charcot–Marie Tooth Disease and Related Disorders). MFN and GDAP1 are involved in the fusion and fission of mitochondria which are essential in controlling the shape, size, number, and transport of mitochondria within cells. Dynamin-like GTPases located in the outer membrane (e.g., MFN2) and inner membrane (e.g., OPA1) control mitochondrial fusion. MFN2 helps tether mitochondria during fusion, while OPA1 is important for fusion of the inner membrane and formation of cristae. GDAP1, located in the outer membrane, is important in mitochondrial fission.

► SUMMARY

There is a wide range of phenotypic and genotypic variability in patients with mitochondrial disorders. Due to high energy requirements, many of these disorders are associated with disorders of peripheral nerve and/or muscle. This phenotypic and genotypic heterogeneity makes definitive diagnosis (i.e., identifying specific genetic mutation) an often long and expensive process. Although there is a greater understanding regarding the molecular pathogenesis of the different forms of mitochondrial encephalomyopathies, these advances have not as yet led to easy diagnosis in many cases or effective medical treatments, other than supportive measures.

REFERENCES

1. DiMauro S, Schon EA, Carelli V, Hirano M. The clinical maze of mitochondrial neurology. *Nat Rev Neurol.* 2013;9(8):429–444.
2. Milone M, Wong LJ. Diagnosis of mitochondrial myopathies. *Mol Genet Metab.* 2013;110(1–2):35–41.
3. Pfeffer G, Chinnery PF. Diagnosis and treatment of mitochondrial myopathies. *Ann Med.* 2013;45(1):4–16.
4. Tucker EJ, Compton AG, Thorburn DR. Recent advances in the genetics of mitochondrial encephalopathies. *Curr Neurol Neurosci Rep.* 2010;10(4):277–285.
5. Finsterer J, Ahting U. Mitochondrial depletion syndromes in children and adults. *Can J Neurol Sci.* 2013;40:635–644.
6. Finsterer J. Inherited mitochondrial neuropathies. *J Neurol Sci.* 2011;304(1–2):9–16.
7. Pareyson D, Piscosquito G, Moroni I, Salsano E, Zeviani M. Peripheral neuropathy in mitochondrial disorders. *Lancet Neurol.* 2013;12(10):1011–1024.
8. Schmiedel J, Jackson S, Schafer J, Reichmann H. Mitochondrial cytopathies. *J Neurol.* 2003;250(3):267–277.
9. Taylor RW, Schaefer AM, Baron MJ, McFarland R, Turnbull DM. The diagnosis of mitochondrial muscle disease. *Neuromuscul Disord.* 2004;14:237–245.
10. Vu TH, Hirano M, DiMauro S. Mitochondrial diseases. *Neurol Clin.* 2002;20(3):809–839.
11. Chinnery PF, Johnson MA, Wardell TM, et al. The epidemiology of pathogenic mitochondrial DNA mutations. *Ann Neurol.* 2000;48:188–193.
12. Jeppesen TD, Schwartz M, Olsen DB, Vissing J. Oxidative capacity correlates with muscle mutation load in mitochondrial myopathy. *Ann Neurol.* 2003;54(1):86–92.
13. Taivassalo T, Jensen TD, Kennaway N, DiMauro S, Vissing J, Haller RG. The spectrum of exercise tolerance in mitochondrial myopathies: a study of 40 patients. *Brain.* 2003;126:413–423.
14. Jeppesen TD, Olsen D, Vissing J. Cycle ergometry is not a sensitive diagnostic test for mitochondrial myopathy. *J Neurol.* 2003;250(3):293–299.
15. Jensen TD, Kazemi-Esfarjani P, Skomorowska E, Vissing J. A forearm exercise screening test for mitochondrial myopathy. *Neurology.* 2002;58(10):1533–1538.
16. Taivassalo T, Abbott A, Wyrick P, Haller RG. Venous oxygen levels during aerobic forearm exercise: an index of impaired oxidative metabolism in mitochondrial myopathy. *Ann Neurol.* 2002;51(1):38–44.
17. Olsen DB, Langkilde AR, Orngreen MC, Rostrup E, Schwartz M, Vissing J. Muscle structural changes in mitochondrial myopathy relate to genotype. *J Neurol.* 2003;250(11):1328–1334.
18. Laforet P, Wary C, Duteil S, et al. [Exploration of exercise intolerance by 31P NMR spectroscopy of calf muscles coupled with MRI and ergometry]. *Rev Neurol.* 2003;159(1):56–67.
19. Moller HE, Wiedermann D, Kurlemann G, Hilbich T, Schuierer G. Application of NMR spectroscopy to monitoring MELAS treatment: a case report. *Muscle Nerve.* 2002;25(4):593–600.
20. Bendahan D, Mattei JP, Kozak-Ribbens G, Cozzone PJ. Non invasive investigation of muscle diseases using 31P magnetic resonance spectroscopy: potential in clinical applications. *Rev Neurol.* 2002;158(5 pt 1):527–540.
21. Tarnopolsky MA, Simon DK, Roy BD, et al. Attenuation of free radical production and paracrystalline inclusions by creatine supplementation in a patient with a novel cytochrome *b* mutation. *Muscle Nerve.* 2004;29:537–547.
22. Blumenthal DT, Shanske S, Schochet SS, et al. Myoclonus epilepsy with ragged red fibers and multiple mtDNA deletions. *Neurology.* 1998;50:524–525.
23. Fang W, Huang CC, Chu NS, et al. Myoclonic epilepsy with ragged-red fibers (MERRF) syndrome: report of a Chinese family with mitochondrial DNA point mutation in the $tRNA^{Lys}$ gene. *Muscle Nerve.* 1994;17:52–57.
24. Fukuhara N. Clinicopathological features of MERRF. *Muscle Nerve.* 1995;(suppl 3):S90–S94.
25. Fukuhara N. MERRF: a clinicopathological study. Relationships between myoclonus epilepsy and mitochondrial myopathies. *Rev Neurol.* 1991;147:476–479.
26. Fukuhara N, Tokiguchi S, Shirakawa K, Tsubaki T. Myoclonus epilepsy associated with ragged-red fibers (mitochondrial abnormalities): disease entity or a syndrome? *J Neurol Sci.* 1980;47:117–133.
27. Lombes A, Mendell JR, Nakase H, et al. Myoclonic epilepsy and ragged red fibers with cytochrome oxidase deficiency: neuropathology, biochemistry, and molecular genetics. *Ann Neurol.* 1989;26:20–33.
28. Ozawa M, Goto Y, Sakuta R, Tanno Y, Tsuji S, Nonaka I. The 8,344 mutation in mitochondrial DNA: a comparison between the proportion of mutant DNA and clinical pathologic findings. *Neuromuscul Disord.* 1995;5:483–488.
29. Rosing HS, Hopkins LC, Wallace DC, Epstein CM, Weidenheim K. Maternally inherited mitochondrial myopathy and myoclonic epilepsy. *Ann Neurol.* 1985;17:228–237.
30. Silvestri G, Ciafoni E, Santorelli FM, et al. Clinical features associated with the A→G transition at nucleotide 8344 of mtDNA ("MERRF mutation"). *Neurology.* 1993;43:1200–1206.
31. Tsairis P, Engel WK, Kark P. Familial myoclonic epilepsy syndrome associated with skeletal muscle mitochondrial abnormalities [abstract]. *Neurology.* 1973;23:408.
32. Greenberg DA, Durner M, Keddache M, et al. Reproducibility and complications in gene searches: linkage on chromosome 6, heterogeneity, association, and maternal inheritance in juvenile myoclonic epilepsy. *Am J Hum Genet.* 2000;66:508–516.
33. Bryne E, Dennet X, Trounce I. Burdon J. Mitochondrial myoneuropathy with respiratory failure and myoclonic epilepsy. *J Neurol Sci.* 1985;71:273–281.
34. Larsson NG, Tulinius MH, Holme E, Oldfors A. Pathologenetic aspects of the A8344G mutation of mitochondrial DNA associated with MERRF syndrome and multiple symmetric lipomas. *Muscle Nerve.* 1995;(suppl 3):S102–S106.
35. Muñoz-Málaga A, Bautista J, Salazar JA, et al. Lipomatosis, proximal myopathy, and the mitochondrial 8344 mutation. A lipid storage myopathy? *Muscle Nerve.* 2000;23:538–542.
36. Mizusawa H, Watanabe M, Kanazawa I, et al. Familial mitochondrial myopathy associated with peripheral neuropathy: partial deficiencies of complex I and complex IV. *J Neurol Sci.* 1988;86:171–184.
37. Pezeshkpour G, Krarup C, Buchthal F, DiMauro S, Bresolin N, McBurney J. Peripheral neuropathy in mitochondrial disease. *J Neurol Sci.* 1987;77:285–304.
38. Hammans SR, Sweeny MG, Brockington M, et al. The mitochondrial DNA transfer RNA^{Lys} $A \rightarrow G^{(8344)}$ mutation and

the syndrome of myoclonic epilepsy with ragged red fibres (MERRF). Relationship of the clinical phenotype to proportion of mutant mitochondrial DNA. *Brain.* 1993;116: 617–632.
39. Shoffner JM, Lott MT, Lezza AMS, Seibel P, Ballinger SW, Wallace DC. Myoclonic epilepsy and ragged-red fiber disease (MERRF) is associated with a mitochondrial DNA $tRNA^{Lys}$ mutation. *Cell.* 1990;61:931–937.
40. Yoneda M, Miyatake T, Attardi G. Heteroplasmic mitochondrial $tRNA^{Lys}$ mutation and its complementation in MERRF patient-derived mitochondrial transformants. *Muscle Nerve Suppl.* 1995;(suppl 3):S95–S101.
41. Tarnopolsky M, Martin J. Creatine monohydrate increases strength in patients with neuromuscular disease. *Neurology.* 1999;52:854–857.
42. Tarnopolsky MA, Roy BD, MacDonald JR. A randomized, controlled trial of creatine monohydrate in patients with mitochondrial cytopathies. *Muscle Nerve.* 1997;20:1502–1509.
43. Feit H, Kirkpatrick J, VanWoert MH, Pandian G. Myoclonus, ataxia, and hypoventilation: response to L-5-hydroxytrptophan. *Neurology.* 1983;33:109–112.
44. Ciafaloni E, Ricci E, Shanske S, et al. MELAS. Clinical features, biochemistry, and molecular genetics. *Ann Neurol.* 1992;31: 391–398.
45. Crimmins D, Morris JGL, Walker GL, et al. Mitochondrial encephalomyopathy: variable clinical expression within a single kindred. *J Neurol Neurosurg Psychiatry.* 1993;56:900–905.
46. Goto YI. Clinical features of MELAS and mitochondrial DNA mutations. *Muscle Nerve.* 1995;(suppl 3):A107–S112.
47. Goto Y, Horai S, Matsuoka T, et al. Mitochondrial myopathy, encephalopathy, lactic acidosis and stroke-like episodes (MELAS): correlative study of the clinical features and mitochondrial DNA mutation. *Neurology.* 1992;42:545–550.
48. Pavlakis SG, Phillips PC, DiMauro S, DeVivo DC, Rowland LP. Mitochondrial myopathy, encephalopathy, lactic acidosis, and stroke-like episode: a distinctive clinical syndrome. *Ann Neurol.* 1984;16:481–488.
49. Iizuka T, Sakai F, Kan S, Suzuki N. Slowly progressive spread of the stroke-like lesions in MELAS. *Neurology.* 2003;61(9): 1238–1244.
50. Servidei S. Mitochondrial encephalomyopathies: gene mutation. *Neuromuscul Disord.* 2000;10:10–15.
51. Saitoh S, Momoi MY, Yamagata T, Mori Y, Imai M. Effects of dochorpacetate in three patients with MELAS. *Neurology.* 1998;50:531–534.
52. Kaufmann P, Engelstad K, Wei Y, et al. Dichloroacetate causes toxic neuropathy in MELAS: a randomized, controlled clinical trial. *Neurology.* 2006;66(3):324–330.
53. Komura K, Hobbiebrunken E, Wilichowski EK, Hanefeld FA. Effectiveness of creatine monohydrate in mitochondrial encephalomyopathies. *Pediatr Neurol.* 2003;28(1):53–58.
54. Berenberg RA, Pellock JM, DiMauro S, et al. Lumping or splitting? "Ophthalmoplegia-plus" or Kearns-Sayre syndrome? *Ann Neurol.* 1977;1:37–54.
55. DiMauro S, Bonilla E, Lombes A, Shanske S, Minneti C, Moraes CT. Mitochondrial encephalomyopathies. *Neurol Clin.* 1990;8:483–506.
56. Holt IJ, Harding AE, Cooper JM, et al. Mitochondrial myopathies: clinical and biochemical features of 30 patients with major deletions of muscle mitochondrial DNA. *Ann Neurol.* 1989;26:699–708.
57. Laforêt P, Lombes A, Eymard B, et al. Chronic progressive external ophthalmoplegia with ragged-red fibers: clinical, morphological, and genetic investigations in 43 patients. *Neuromuscul Disord.* 1995;5:399–413.
58. Moraes CT, DiMauro S, Zeviani M, et al. Mitochondrial deletions in progressive external ophthalmoplegia and Kearns-Sayre syndrome. *N Engl J Med.* 1989;320:1293–1299.
59. Rowland LP. Progressive external ophthalmoplegia and ocular myopathies. In: Rowland LP, DiMauro S, eds. *Handbook of Clinical Neurology.* Vol 18(62). Amsterdam: Elsevier Science Publishers BV; 1992:287–329.
60. Zeviani M, Moraes CT, DiMauro S, et al. Deletions of mitochondrial DNA in Kearns-Sayre syndrome. *Neurology.* 1988;38:1339–1346.
61. Barohn RJ, Clanton T, Sahenk Z, Mendell JR. Recurrent respiratory insufficiency and depressed ventilatory drive complicating mitochondrial myopathies. *Neurology.* 1990;40:103–106.
62. Carroll JE, Zwillich C, Weil JV, Brooke MH. Depressed ventilatory response in oculocraniosomatic neuromuscular disease. *Neurology.* 1976;26:140–146.
63. Goto Y, Koga S, Horai S, Nonaka I. Chronic progressive external ophthalmoplegia: a correlative study of mitochondrial DNA deletions and their phenotypic expression in muscle biopsies. *J Neurol Sci.* 1990;100:63–69.
64. Servidei S, Zeviani M, Manfredi G, et al. Dominantly inherited mitochondrial myopathy with multiple deletions of mitochondrial DNA: clinical, morphologic, and biochemical studies. *Neurology.* 1991;41:1053–1059.
65. Hirano M, Silvestri G, Blake DM, et al. Mitochondrial neurogastrointestinal encephalomyopathy (MNGIE): clinical, biochemical, and genetic features of an autosomal recessive mitochondrial disorder. *Neurology.* 1994;44:721–727.
66. Kaukonen J, Juselius JK, Tiranti V, et al. Role of adenine nucleotide translocator 1 in mtDNA maintenance. *Science.* 2000;289:782–785.
67. Ronchi D, Garone C, Bordoni A. Next-generation sequencing reveals *DGUOK* mutations in adult patients with mitochondrial DNA multiple deletions. *Brain.* 2012:135:3404–3415.
68. Bakker HD, Scholte HR, Van den Bogert C, et al. Adenine nucleotide translocator deficiency in muscle: potential therapeutic value of vitamin E. *J Inherit Metab Dis.* 1993;16:548–552.
69. Ronchi D, Di Fonzo A, Lin W, et al. Mutations in DNA2 link progressive myopathy to mitochondrial DNA instability. *Am J Hum Genet.* 2013;92:293–300.
70. Pfeffer G, Gorman GS, Griffin H, et al. Mutations in the SPG7 gene cause chronic progressive external ophthalmoplegia through disordered mitochondrial DNA maintenance. *Brain.* 2014:137;1323–1336.
71. Bohlega S, Tanji K, Santorelli FM, Hirano M, al-Jishi A, DiMauro S. Multiple mitochondrial DNA deletions associated with autosomal recessive ophthalmoplegia and severe cardiomyopathy. *Neurology.* 1996;46:1329–1334.
72. Carrozzo R, Hirano M, Fromenty B, et al. Multiple mtDNA deletions in autosomal dominant and recessive diseases suggests distinct pathogeneses. *Neurology.* 1998;50:99–106.
73. Minchum PE, Dormer RL, Hughs IA, et al. Fatal infantile myopathy due to cytochrome c oxidase deficiency. *J Neurol Sci.* 1983;60:453–463.
74. Tritschler H-J, Andreetta F, Moraes CT, et al. Mitochondrial myopathy of childhood associated with depletion of mitochondrial DNA. *Neurology.* 1992;42:209–217.

75. Tritschler HJ, Bonilla E, Lombes A, et al. Differential diagnosis of fatal and benign cytochrome c oxidase deficient myopathies of infancy: an immunohistochemical approach. *Neurology.* 1991;41:300–305.
76. Zeviani M, Peterson P, Servidei S, et al. Benign reversible muscle cytochrome c oxidase deficiency: a second case. *Neurology.* 1987;37:64–67.
77. Mancuso M, Filosto M, Bonilla E, et al. Mitochondrial myopathy of childhood associated with mitochondrial DNA depletion and a homozygous mutation (T77M) in the TK2 gene. *Arch Neurol.* 2003;60(7):1007–1009.
78. Mancuso M, Filosto M, Stevens JC, et al. Mitochondrial myopathy and complex III deficiency in a patient with a new stop-codon mutation (G339X) in the cytochrome b gene. *J Neurol Sci.* 2003;209(1–2):61–63.
79. Campos Y, Martin MA, Garcia-Silva T, et al. Clinical heterogeneity associated with mitochondrial DNA depletion in muscle. *Neuromuscul Disord.* 1998;8:568–573.
80. Vu TH, Sciacco M, Tanji K, et al. Clinical manifestations of mitochondrial DNA depletion. *Neurology.* 1998;50:1783–1790.
81. Moraes CT, Shanske S, Tritschler HJ, et al. Mitochondrial DNA depletion with variable tissue specificity: a novel genetic abnormality in mitochondrial diseases. *Am J Hum Genet.* 1991;48:492–501.
82. Durham SE, Bonilla E, Samuels DC, DiMauro S, Chinnery PF. Mitochondrial DNA copy number threshold in mtDNA depletion myopathy. *Neurology.* 2005;65:453–455.
83. Figarella-Branger D, Pelssier JF, Scheiner C, Wernert F, Desnuelle C. Defects of the mitochondrial respiratory chain complexes in three pediatric cases with hypotonia and cardiac involvement. *J Neurol Sci.* 1992;108:105–113.
84. Mazziotta MR, Ricci E, Bertini E, et al. Fatal infantile liver failure associated with mitochondrial DNA depletion. *J Pediatr.* 1992;121:896–901.
85. Telerman-Toppet N, Biarent D, Bouton JM, et al. Fatal cytochrome c oxidase-deficient myopathy of infancy associated with mtDNA depletion: differential involvement of skeletal muscle and cultured fibroblasts. *J Inherit Metab Dis.* 1992;15:323–326.
86. Saada A, Ben-Shalom E, Zyslin R, Miller C, Mandel H, Elpeleg O. Mitochondrial deoxyribonucleoside triphosphate pools in thymidine kinase 2 deficiency. *Biochem Biophys Res Commun.* 2003;310(3):963–966.
87. Saada A, Shaag A, Elpeleg O. Mtdna depletion myopathy: elucidation of the tissue specificity in the mitochondrial thymidine kinase (TK2) deficiency. *Mol Genet Metab.* 2003;79(1):1–5.
88. Saada A, Shaag A, Mandel H, Nevo Y, Eriksson S, Elpeleg O. Mutation mitochondrial thymidine kinase in mitochondrial DNA depletion myopathy. *Nat Genet.* 2001;29:342–344.
89. Vila MR, Segovia-Silvestre T, Gamez J, et al. Reversion of mtDNA depletion in a patient with TK2 deficiency. *Neurology.* 2003;60(7):1203–1205.
90. Chanprasert S, Wang J, Weng SW, et al. Molecular and clinical characterization of the myopathic form of mitochondrial DNA depletion syndrome caused by mutations in the thymidine kinase (TK2) gene. *Mol Genet Metab.* 2013;110(1–2):153–161.
91. Paradas C, Gutiérrez Ríos P, Rivas E, Carbonell P, Hirano M, DiMauro S. TK2 mutation presenting as indolent myopathy. *Neurology.* 2013;80(5):504–506.
92. Béhin A, Jardel C, Claeys KG, et al. Adult cases of mitochondrial DNA depletion due to TK2 defect: an expanding spectrum. *Neurology.* 2012;78(9):644–648.
93. Lesko N, Naess K, Wibom R, et al. Two novel mutations in thymidine kinase-2 cause early onset fatal encephalomyopathy and severe mtDNA depletion. *Neuromuscul Disord.* 2010;20(3):198–203.
94. Collins J, Bove KE, Dimmock D, Morehart P, Wong LJ, Wong B. Progressive myofiber loss with extensive fibro-fatty replacement in a child with mitochondrial DNA depletion syndrome and novel thymidine kinase 2 gene mutations. *Neuromuscul Disord.* 2009;19(11):784–787.
95. Blakely E, He L, Gardner JL, et al. Novel mutations in the TK2 gene associated with fatal mitochondrial DNA depletion myopathy. *Neuromuscul Disord.* 2008;18(7):557–560.
96. Oskoui M, Davidzon G, Pascual J, et al. Clinical spectrum of mitochondrial DNA depletion due to mutations in the thymidine kinase 2 gene. *Arch Neurol.* 2006;63(8):1122–1126.
97. Wang L, Limongelli A, Vila MR, Carrara F, Zeviani M, Eriksson S. Molecular insight into mitochondrial DNA depletion syndrome in two patients with novel mutations in the deoxyguanosine kinase and thymidine kinase 2 genes. *Mol Genet Metab.* 2005;84(1):75–82.
98. Buchaklian AH, Helbling D, Ware SM, Dimmock DP. Recessive deoxyguanosine kinase deficiency causes juvenile onset mitochondrial myopathy. *Mol Genet Metab.* 2012;107(1–2):92–94.
99. Bardosi A, Creutzfeldt W, DiMauro S, et al. Myo-neuro-gastro-intestinal encephalopathy (MNGIE syndrome) due to partial deficiency of cytochrome C oxidase: a new mitochondrial multisystem disorder. *Acta Neuropathol (Berl).* 1987;74:248–258.
100. Nishino I, Spinazzola A, Papadimitriou A, et al. Mitochondral neurogastrointestinal encephalomyopathy: an autosomal recessive disorder due to thymidine phosphorylase mutations. *Ann Neurol.* 2000;47:729–800.
101. Simon LT, Horoupian DS, Dorfman LJ, et al. Polyneuropathy, ophthalmoplegia, leukoencephalopathy, and intestinal pseudo-obstruction: POLIP syndrome. *Ann Neurol.* 1990;28:349–360.
102. Bedlack RS, Vu T, Hammans S, et al. MNGIE neuropathy: five cases mimicking chronic inflammatory demyelinating polyneuropathy. *Muscle Nerve.* 2004;29(3):364–368.
103. Nishino I, Spinazzola A, Hirano M. Thymidine phosphorylase gene mutations in MNGIE: a human mitochondrial disorder. *Science.* 1999;283:689–692.
104. Hirano M, Garcia-de-Yebenes J, Jones AC, et al. Mitochondrial neurogastrointestinal encephalomyopathy syndrome maps to chromosome 22q13.32-qter. *Am J Hum Genet.* 1998;63:526–533.
105. Van Goethem G, Schwartz M, Lofgren A, Dermaut B, Van Broeckhoven C, Vissing J. Novel POLG mutations in progressive external ophthalmoplegia mimicking mitochondrial neurogastrointestinal encephalomyopathy. *Eur J Hum Genet.* 2003;11:547–549.
106. Tang S, Dimberg EL, Milone M, Wong LJ. Mitochondrial neurogastrointestinal encephalomyopathy (MNGIE)-like phenotype: an expanded clinical spectrum of POLG1 mutations. *J Neurol.* 2012;259:862–868.
107. Shaibani A, Shchelochkov OA, Zhang S, et al. Mitochondrial neurogastrointestinal encephalopathy due to mutations in RRM2B. *Arch Neurol.* 2009;66:1028–1032.
108. Fadic R, Russell JA, Russell JA. Sensory ataxic neuropathy as the presenting feature of a novel mitochondrial disease. *Neurology.* 1997;49:239–245.
109. Mancuso M, Filosto M, Bellan M, et al. POLG mutations causing ophthalmoplegia, sensorimotor polyneuropathy, ataxic and deafness. *Neurology.* 2004;62:316–318.

110. van Domburg PH, Gabreels-Festen AA, ter Laak H, et al. Mitochondrial cytopathy presenting as hereditary sensory neuropathy with progressive external ophthalmoplegia, ataxia and fatal myoclonic epileptic status. *Brain.* 1996;119:997–1010.
111. Milone M, Brunetti-Pierri N, Tang LY, et al. Sensory ataxic neuropathy with ophthalmoparesis caused by POLG mutations. *Neuromuscul Disord.* 2008;18;626–632.
112. Wong LJ, Naviaux RK, Brunetti-Pierri N, et al. Molecular and clinical genetics of mitochondrial diseases due to POLG mutations. *Hum Mutat.* 2008;29(9):E150–E172.
113. Martin-Negrier ML, Sole G, Jardel C, Vital C, Ferrer X, Vital A. TWINKLE gene mutation: report of a French family with an autosomal dominant progressive external ophthalmoplegia and literature review. *Eur J Neurol.* 2011;18:436–441.
114. Hakonen AH, Heiskanen S, Juvonen V, et al. Mitochondrial DNA polymerase W748 S mutation: a common cause of autosomal recessive ataxia with ancient European origin. *Am J Hum Genet.* 2005;77:430–441.
115. Wintgerthun S, Ferrari G, He L, et al. Autosomal recessive mitochondrial ataxic syndrome due to mitochondrial polymerase gamma mutations. *Neurology.* 2005;64:1204–1208.
116. Rantamaki MT, Soini HK, Finnila SM, Majamaa K, Udd B. Adult-onset ataxia and polyneuropathy caused by mitochondrial 8993 T>C mutation. *Ann Neurol.* 2005;58:337–340.
117. Van Goethem G, Luoma P, Rantamaki M, et al. POLG mutations in neurodegenerative disorders with ataxia but no muscle involvement. *Neurology.* 2004;63:1251–1257.
118. Luoma PT, Luo N, Loscher WN, et al. Functional defects due to spacer region mutations of human mitochondrial DNA polymerase in a family with an ataxia-myopathy syndrome. *Hum Mol Genet.* 2005;14:1907–1920.
119. Tzoulis C, Engelsen BA, Telstad W, et al. The spectrum of clinical disease caused by the A467 T and W748 S POLG mutations: a study of 26 cases. *Brain.* 2006;129:1685–1692.
120. Holt IJ, Harding AE, Petty RK, Morgan-Hughes JA. A new mitochondrial disease associated with mitochondrial DNA heteroplasmy. *Am J Hum Genet.* 1990;46:428–433.
121. Santorelli FM, Tanji K, Shanske S, DiMauro S. Heterogeneous clinical presentation of the mtDNA NARP/T8993G mutation. *Neurology.* 1997;49:270–273.
122. Childs AM, Hutchin T, Pysden K, et al. Variable phenotype including Leigh syndrome with a 9185TNC mutation in the MTATP6 gene. *Neuropediatrics.* 2007;38:313–316.
123. Gelfand JM, Duncan JL, Racine CA, et al. Heterogeneous patterns of tissue injury in NARP syndrome. *J Neurol.* 2011;258:440–448.
124. Karadimas CL, Vu TH, Holve SA, et al. Navajo neurohepatopathy is caused by a mutation in the MPV17 gene. *Am J Hum Genet.* 2006;79:544–548.
125. Spinazzola A, Viscomi C, Fernandez-Vizarra E, et al. MPV17 encodes an inner mitochondrial membrane protein and is mutated in infantile hepatic mitochondrial DNA depletion. *Nat Genet.* 2006;38:570–575.
126. Lawlor MW, Holve S, Stubbs EB Jr. Assessment of serum-mediated neurotoxicity in Navajo neuropathy. *Electromyogr Clin Neurophysiol.* 2000;40:211–214.
127. Appenzeller O, Kornfeld M, Snyder R. Acromutilating, paralyzing neuropathy with corneal ulceration in Navajo children. *Arch Neurol.* 1976;33:733–738.
128. Yu-Wai-Man P, Griffiths PG, Gorman GS, et al. Multi-system neurological disease is common in patients with OPA1 mutations. *Brain.* 2010;133:771–786.
129. Amati-Bonneau P, Valentino ML, Reynier P, et al. OPA1 mutations induce mitochondrial DNA instability and optic atrophy 'plus' phenotypes. *Brain.* 2008;131:338–351.
130. Hudson G, Amati-Bonneau P, Blakely EL, et al. Mutation of OPA1 causes dominant optic atrophy with external ophthalmoplegia, ataxia, deafness and multiple mitochondrial DNA deletions: a novel disorder of mtDNA maintenance. *Brain.* 2008;131:329–337.
131. Liguori M, La Russa A, Manna I, et al. A phenotypic variation of dominant optic atrophy and deafness (ADOAD) due to a novel OPA1 mutation. *J Neurol.* 2008;255:127–129.
132. Voo I, Allf BE, Udar N, Silva-Garcia R, Vance J, Small KW. Hereditary motor and sensory neuropathy type VI with optic atrophy. *Am J Ophthalmol.* 2003;136:670–677.
133. Chalmers RM, Lamont PJ, Nelson I, et al. A mitochondrial DNA $tRNA^{Val}$ point mutation associated with adult-onset Leigh syndrome. *Neurology.* 1997;49:589–592.
134. Lombes A, Nakase H, Tritschler HJ, et al. Biochemical and molecular analysis of cytochrome c oxidase deficiency in Leigh's syndrome. *Neurology.* 1991;41:491–498.
135. Loeffen J, Smeitink J, Triepels R, et al. The first nuclear-encoded complex 1 mutation in a patient with Leigh syndrome. *Am J Hum Genet.* 1998;63:1598–1604.
136. Triepels RH, Vanden Heuven L, Loeffen JL, et al. Leigh syndrome associated with a mutation in the NDUFS7 (PSST) nuclear encoded subunit of complex I. *Ann Neurol.* 1999;45:787–790.
137. Bougeron T, Roustin P, Chretien D, et al. Mutation of a nuclear succinate dehydrogenase gene results in mitochondrial respiratory chain deficiency. *Nat Genet.* 1995;11:144–149.
138. Ahu Z, Yao J, Johns T, et al. SURF1, encoding a factor involved in the biogenesis of cytochrome c oxidase, is mutated in Leigh syndrome. *Nat Genet.* 1998;20:337–343.
139. Shoffner JM, Fernhoff PM, Krawiecki NS, et al. Subacute necrotizing encephalopathy: oxidative phosphorylation defects and the ATPase 6 point mutation. *Neurology.* 1992;42:2168–2174.
140. Sweeney MG, Hammans SR, Duchen LW, et al. Mitochondrial DNA mutation underlying Leigh's syndrome: clinical, pathological, biochemical, and genetic studies of a patient presenting with progressive myoclonic epilepsy. *J Neurol Sci.* 1994;121:57–65.
141. Yamamoto M, Clemens PR, Engel AG. Mitochondrial DNA deletions in mitochondrial cytopathies: observations in 19 patients. *Neurology.* 1991;41:1822–1828.
142. DeVivo D. Complexities of the pyruvate dehydrogenase complex. *Neurology.* 1998;51:1247–1249.
143. Lissens W, Desguerre I, Benelli C, et al. Pyruvate dehydrogenase deficiency in a female due to a 4 base pair deletion in exon 10 of the E1 gene. *Hum Mol Genet.* 1995;4:307–308.
144. Matthews PM, Marchington DR, Squire M, Land J, Brown RM, Brown GK. Molecular genetic characterization of an X-linked form of Leigh's syndrome. *Ann Neurol.* 1993;33:652–655.
145. Genge A, Karpati G, Arnold D, Shoubridge EA, Carpenter S. Familial myopathy with conspicuous depletion of mitochondria in muscle fibers: a morphologically distinct disease. *Neuromuscul Disord.* 1995;5:139–144.
146. Nishino I, Kobayshi O, Goto Y-I, et al. A new distinct muscular dystrophy with mitochondrial structural abnormalities. *Muscle Nerve.* 1998;21:40–47.
147. Osaki Y, Nishino I, Murakami N, et al. Mitochondrial abnormalities in selenium-deficient myopathy. *Muscle Nerve.* 1998;21:637–639.

148. Saunier P, Chretien D, Wood C, et al. Cytochrome c oxidase deficiency presenting as recurrent neonatal myoglobinuria. *Neuromuscul Disord.* 1995;5:285–289.
149. Ohno K, Tanaka M, Sahashi K, et al. Mitochondrial DNA deletions in inherited recurrent myoglobinuria. *Ann Neurol.* 1991;29:364–369.
150. Chinnery PF, Johnson MA, Taylor RW, Durward WF, Turnbull DM. A novel mitochondrial tRNA isoleucine gene mutation causing chronic progressive external ophthalmoplegia. *Neurology.* 1997;49:1166–1168.
151. Moslemi AR, Lindberg C, Toft J, Holme E, Kollberg G, Oldfors A. A novel mutation in the mitochondrial tRNA(Phe) gene associated with mitochondrial myopathy. *Neuromuscul Disord.* 2004;14:46–50.
152. Keightley JA, Hoffbuhr KC, Burton MD, et al. A microdeletion in cytochrome c oxidase (COX) subunit III associated with COX deficiency and recurrent myoglobinuria. *Nat Genet.* 1996;12(4):410–416.
153. Nishigaki Y, Bonilla E, Shanske S, Gaskin DA, DiMauro S, Hirano M. Exercise-induced muscle "burning," fatigue, and hyper-CKemia: MtDNA T10010 C mutation in tRNA(Gly). *Neurology.* 2002;8(8):1282–1285.
154. Andreu AL, Tanji K, Bruno C, et al. Exercise intolerance due to a nonsense mutation in the mtDNA ND4 gene. *Ann Neurol.* 1999;45:820–823.
155. Andreu AL, Bruno C, Dunne TC, et al. A nonsense mutation (G15059 A) in the cytochrome *b* gene in a patient with exercise intolerance and myoglobinuria. *Ann Neurol.* 1999;45: 127–130.
156. Andreu AL, Bruno C, Shanske S, et al. Missense mutation in the mtDNA cytochrome *b* gene in a patient with myopathy. *Neurology.* 1998;51:1444–1447.
157. Wallace DC, Singh G, Lott MT, et al. Mitochondrial DNA mutation associated with Leber's hereditary optic neuropathy. *Science.* 1988;242:1427–1430.
158. Pilz D, Quarrell OW, Jones EW. Mitochondrial mutation commonly associated with Leber's hereditary optic neuropathy observed in a patient with Wolfram syndrome (DIDMOAD). *J Med Genet.* 1994;31:328–330.
159. Kollberg G, Melberg A, Holme E, Oldfors A. Transient restoration of succinate dehydrogenase activity after rhabdomyolysis in iron-sulphur cluster deficiency myopathy. *Neuromuscul Disord.* 2011;21:115–120.

CHAPTER 31

Myotonic Dystrophies

Myotonic dystrophy is the most common myotonic disorder (Table 31-1). There are at least two genetically distinct forms of myotonic dystrophy: Dystrophica myotonia type 1 (DM1) and dystrophica myotonia type 2 (DM2), the later of which is also known as proximal myotonic myopathy (PROMM).

► MYOTONIC DYSTROPHY (DM1)

CLINICAL FEATURES

DM1 in an autosomal dominant manner with a prevalence of 13.5 per 100,000.[1–4] DM1 can present at any age, including infancy. Limb weakness begins distally in the extremities and can progress slowly to affect proximal muscles. Wrist flexors are often weaker than wrist extensors. The neck flexors, including the sternocleidomastoids, are also affected early. Atrophy and weakness of temporalis and other facial muscles as well as the jaw muscles giving rise to the characteristic "hatchet face" appearance (Fig. 31-1). Ptosis is often evident. Some patients develop dysarthria and dysphagia due to pharyngeal and lingual muscles involvement.

Many patients do not complain or are not aware of their myotonia, although it is usually readily apparent on examination, particularly in the hands. Delayed relaxation of the fingers is seen following a forceful hand grip (action myotonia). The myotonia is lessened with repeated muscle contractions, a so-called warm-up phenomenon. Percussion of muscle groups, in particular of the thenar eminence or finger extensors also gives rise to delayed relaxation (percussion myotonia). Muscle reflexes are diminished, but sensory testing is normal.[5] Adult patients with DM1 may have a mild reduction in cognitive abilities, while severe mental retardation is associated with congenital myotonic dystrophy.[6,7]

Congenital myotonic dystrophy is much more severe than adult-onset DM1. Affected infants are invariably born to mothers with myotonic dystrophy.[8,9] It is important to examine mothers of floppy infants, as they may not even be aware that they have the disorder. Pregnancy may be complicated by polyhydramnios and diminished fetal movements. Infants with congenital myotonic dystrophy have severe generalized weakness and hypotonia and may also have arthrogryposis. Clinical myotonia is not apparent in the neonatal period and may not be noticeable until about 5 years of age. However, myotonic discharges can be appreciated on electromyography (EMG) before the appearance of clinical myotonia. Many infants require ventilatory assistance due to ventilatory insufficiency. The mortality rate in infancy is approximately 25%. Severe psychomotor abnormalities affect 75% of surviving children. Most will have some degree of mental retardation. Life expectancy is greatly reduced in DM1 patients, particularly those with early onset of the disease and significant proximal, in addition to distal, weakness.[10,11]

ASSOCIATED MANIFESTATIONS

DM1 is a systemic disorder affecting the gastrointestinal tract, the uterus, ventilatory muscles, cardiac muscle, the lens, and the endocrine system.[12] In addition to dysphagia, reduced gastrointestinal motility can lead to chronic pseudo-obstruction.[13,14] Alveolar hypoventilation can arise from involvement of the diaphragm and intercostal muscles. It is more severe in congenital myotonic dystrophy and may lead to ventilatory failure, but this certainly occurs in later onset cases as well.[9] It is unclear if decreased central drive contributes to hypoventilation.[15,16] Nonetheless, many patients develop symptoms suggestive of sleep apnea: frequent nocturnal arousals, excessive daytime hypersomnolence, and morning headaches. Pulmonary hypertension can develop and may lead to cor pulmonale.

Cardiac abnormalities are common with approximately 90% of patients having conduction defects on electrocardiograms (EKGs).[17] Sudden cardiac death secondary to arrhythmia is well documented. However, the severity of the cardiomyopathy does not necessarily correlate with the severity of skeletal muscle weakness. The size of the mutation (discussed in Pathogenesis section) and the severity of the skeletal muscle weakness do not correlate with the occurrence of cardiac conduction abnormalities or sudden death.[18] It seems that risk of sudden death increases with duration of disease and age, and that risk is higher in male patients.[18]

Neurobehavioral abnormalities are common in patients with DM1.[19,20] Neuropsychological testing demonstrates elements of obsessive–compulsive, passive–aggressive, dependent, and avoidant personality traits in many patients. Apathy and depression are also frequent. Cognitive impairment, particularly in memory and spatial orientation, may be demonstrated. The neuropsychological deficits appear to correlate with brain single photon emission computed tomography, which shows frontal and parieto-occipital hypoperfusion.[20]

Other systemic manifestations include posterior subscapular cataracts, frontal balding, testicular atrophy and impotence in men, and a high rate of fetal loss and complications of pregnancy in women. Hyperinsulinemia is common

▶ TABLE 31-1. **MYOTONIC DISORDERS**

Myotonic dystrophy type 1
Myotonic dystrophy type 2/proximal myotonic myopathy
Myotonia congenita
Paramyotonia congenita
Potassium-aggravated myotonia
Hyperkalemic periodic paralysis
Chondrodystrophic myotonia (Schwartz–Jampel syndrome)
Drug induced
Cholesterol-lowering agents (statin medications, fibrates)
Cyclosporine
Chloroquine

following glucose tolerance tests, however, the frequency of overt diabetes mellitus is not increased.[21]

Some epidemiological studies have reported an increased risk of cancer in patients with DM1. In a study of Swedish and Danish populations, the risk of malignancy was double that of the general population.[22] Specifically, they observed an increased risk of endometrial, ovarian, colon, and brain cancer. In a study from the Mayo Clinic, there was an increased risk of thyroid cancer and choroidal melanoma, as well as perhaps testicular and prostate cancer.[23] However, they found no increased risk of endometrial, ovarian, breast, colorectal, lung, renal, bladder, or brain cancers.

LABORATORY FEATURES

Serum creatine kinase (CK) may be normal or mildly increased. Motor and sensory nerve conduction studies (NCS) are usually normal. EMG demonstrates myotonic discharges (Fig. 31-2). It is important to sample multiple muscles as myotonic discharges are not necessarily appreciated in every muscle studied.[24] Facial and intrinsic hand muscles are the most commonly affected. In congenital myotonic dystrophy, electrical myotonia may be observed as early as 5 days to 3 weeks following birth and increases with age.[25,26] Fibrillation potentials, positive sharp waves, and myopathic motor unit action potentials (MUAPs) may also be seen but they can be obscured by the myotonic discharges.

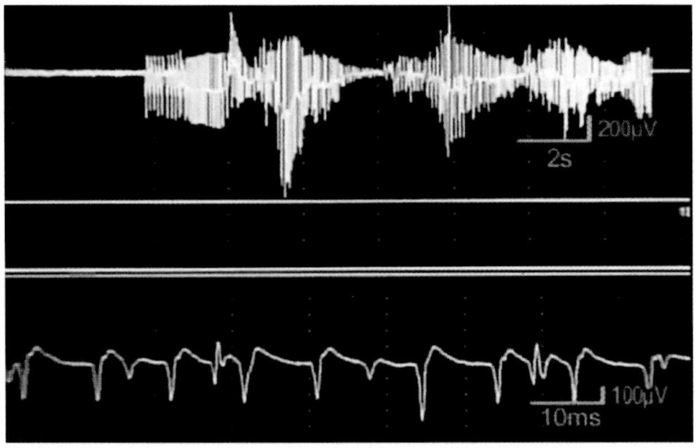

Figure 31-2. Myotonic dystrophy. Electromyography reveals myotonic discharges which wax and wane in frequency and amplitude.

HISTOPATHOLOGY

Muscle biopsies demonstrate an increased number of internalized nuclei in the muscle fibers (Fig. 31-3). Type 1 predominance and atrophy are very common. In addition, hypertrophic type 2 fibers, ring fibers, small angulated fibers, atrophic fibers with pyknotic nuclear clumps, and sarcoplasmic masses are also frequently observed. In contrast to other

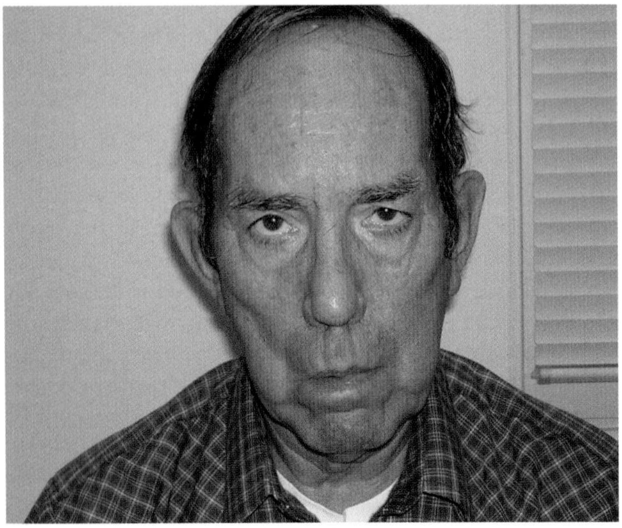

Figure 31-1. Myotonic dystrophy type 1. Note the typical myotonic facies of a DM 1 patient with frontal balding and temporal, jaw, and facial muscle atrophy, and weakness.

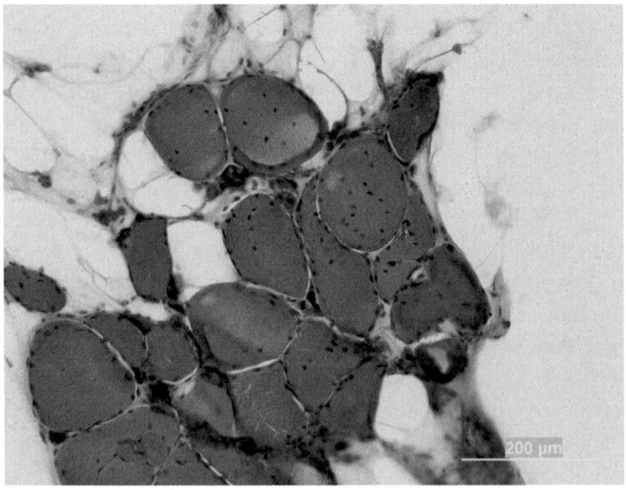

Figure 31-3. Myotonic dystrophy type 1. Muscle biopsies reveal adipose tissue and remaining muscle fibers with numerous internalized nuclei and atrophic fibers with pyknotic nuclear clumps.

muscular dystrophies, necrotic fibers and increased connective tissue are less conspicuous. Autopsy studies of the brain demonstrate neurofibrillary degeneration with abnormal tau expression.[27]

MOLECULAR GENETICS AND PATHOGENESIS

DM1 is caused by an expansion of unstable polymorphic cytosine–thymine–guanine (CTG) trinucleotide repeats in the 3′ untranslated region of the myotonin protein kinase gene, (*DMPK*), that is located on chromosome 19q13.2.[12,28–35] This CTG repeat is copied in the gene up to 27 times in normals, but 50 to more than 4,000 copies are found in DM1 patients. The severity of the myopathy directly correlates with the size of the CTG repeat, which is unstable. The mutation size usually expands from one generation to the next, which accounts for the anticipation phenomena (i.e., the earlier presentation and/or more severe disease in each generation). More marked expansion of the CTG repeat usually occurs in children of mothers with DM1, which explains the severe phenotype of congenital myotonic dystrophy.

It is not the abnormal expression of myotonin protein kinase itself that is responsible for the disorder. Rather, DM1 seems to be a consequence of nuclear retention of mutant mRNA containing expanded CTG repeats, rather than a specific lack or gain of function of the DMPK protein. Indeed, the myopathy and other systemic features appear to be due to a toxic gain of function of the mutant mRNA.[36]

The transcribed mRNA with expanded CTG (DM1) accumulates as abnormal focal collections in the nucleus that cannot be transported to the cytoplasm, where RNA translation into protein takes place.[37–40] Aggregates of mutated mRNA are directly toxic to cells by sequestering RNA-binding proteins (such as muscleblind proteins), which in turn, lead to abnormal splicing of pre-mRNA from various target genes (e.g., chloride ion channel, insulin receptor, tau protein, cardiac troponin, ryanodine receptor, and sarcoplasmic/endoplasmic reticulum Ca^{2+}-ATPase).[37–39,41–45] Therefore, there is abnormal translation of the RNAs into functional proteins, and this explains the multiple organ/systemic manifestations of DM1. Other studies have shown that mutant RNA binds and sequesters transcription factors with up to 90% depletion of selected transcription factors from active chromatin.[46] This leads to reduced expression of a variety of genes, including the chloride ion channel (CIC-1), which is also mutated in myotonia congenita and is the likely origin of the myotonic discharges that occur in both disorders.

TREATMENT

There are no medical therapies that clearly improve muscle strength. A small pilot study of dehydroepiandrosterone sulfate (DHEAS) in 11 patients with DM1 seemed to be beneficial in a few patients, but larger controlled trials are necessary before commenting on the possible efficacy.[47] Small trials of creatine monohydrate in DM1 failed to demonstrate efficacy.[48] A recent study of recombinant human insulin-like growth factor 1 (rhIGF-1) complexed with IGF-binding protein 3 (rhIGF-1/rhIGFBP-3) in patients with DM1 reported that drug was associated with increased lean body mass and improvement in metabolism, but not increased muscle strength or function.[49]

Patients are usually not so bothered by the myotonia to warrant treatment. Further, some drugs that may improve myotonia, such as quinine, procainamide, and tocainide, can also potentiate cardiac arrhythmias and should be avoided. A recent study demonstrated that mexiletine was helpful in reducing myotonia.[50] We initiate treatment with mexiletine 150 mg daily and gradually increase as tolerated and as necessary to control the symptoms, up to a maximum of 300 mg tid. We assess baseline EKG and with each increment of dosage. In addition, aerobic training is safe and may improve fitness effectively in patients with myotonic dystrophy.[51]

We obtain yearly EKGs to monitor for evidence of conduction defects/arrhythmias. If abnormalities are detected, we obtain a cardiology consultation, 24-hour Holter monitoring, and echocardiograms because some patients may require antiarrhythmic medication or pacemaker insertion. Pulmonary function tests are routinely performed. Patients with DM1 are at risk for pulmonary and cardiac complications from general anesthesia and neuromuscular blocking medications.[52–55] These agents should be used with extreme caution.

We obtain overnight polysomnography in patients with symptoms and signs of sleep apnea. Patients with significant hypoventilation or sleep apnea may benefit from noninvasive ventilatory assistance with BiPAP. Modafinil 200–400 mg per day is also effective in reducing the excessive daytime somnolence that is commonly associated with DM1.[56–58]

Some patients require excision of their cataracts. Occasionally for bothersome ptosis, we refer patients for blepharoplasty. However, it is important to discuss with patients the associated risk of inadvertent exposure keratitis. Physical and occupational therapy are important. Orthotic devices such as ankle braces are indicated in patients with foot drop to assist their gait.

Genetic counseling is of utmost importance. Patients need to know that the risk of passing the disease on to their children is 50% with each pregnancy. Further, the disease severity is generally worse from one generation to the next, particularly when the mother has DM1. Prenatal diagnosis is possible via amniocentesis or chorionic villus sampling.

► MYOTONIC DYSTROPHY TYPE 2 OR PROXIMAL MYOTONIC MYOPATHY

CLINICAL FEATURES

Myotonic dystrophy type 2 (DM2) is a multisystem, autosomal dominant disorder that resembles DM1 with myotonia, weakness, cataracts, testicular failure, glucose intolerance, hypogammaglobulinemia, and cardiac conduction defects.[2–4,12,21,40,59–69] In a study of 234 individuals with DM2, 90% had electrical myotonia, 82% weakness, 61% cataracts, 23% diabetes, and 19% cardiac involvement.[59] Most patients with DM2 become symptomatic between the ages of 20 and 60 years, although onset can occur in childhood. The initial symptoms are usually intermittent stiffness and pain of the thigh muscles in one or both legs. Myotonia may be evident in proximal and distal extremity muscles as well as facial muscles, however it is variable and not always present. Myotonia can initially manifest or worsen during pregnancy.[70,71] There is an associated "warm-up" phenomenon with decreased myotonia following repeated muscle contractions. The clinical myotonia does not exacerbate with cold temperature, although a few affected individuals have described worsening of symptoms with warm temperatures.[72]

Patients often describe pain that is episodic and disabling, with burning, tearing, or jabbing characteristics. This pain typically affects the thighs, shoulders, and upper arms and is not necessarily related to the myotonic stiffness of the muscles. They may complain of peculiar chest pains as well, leading to cardiac evaluations to rule out coronary artery disease.

Slowly progressive proximal and distal weakness develops in the majority of patients. The characteristic pattern of muscle weakness involves the neck flexors, elbow extensors, thumb and deep finger flexors, and hip flexors and extensors in the legs. In general, the proximal muscle is often affected earlier than one sees in DM1, thus the name "proximal myotonic myopathy." Some patients describe fluctuations of their weakness with episodes of increased weakness lasting hours or weeks.[64] During these periods of increased weakness, repeated activity can lead to transient improvement in strength. Significant loss of muscle bulk is not apparent early, however, approximately 9% of patients develop considerable atrophy of proximal muscles late in life.[59] Calf hypertrophy occurs in some patients, which can be asymmetric. Rarely, myoglobinuria can occur as a complication of DM2.

Symptoms and severity can vary within families. Studies have demonstrated an earlier onset of symptoms among offspring of affected individuals, suggesting that anticipation is also a feature of DM2.[59,64,67] However, in contrast to DM1, anticipation in DM2 is much milder and a congenital form has never been described.[59,67]

ASSOCIATED MANIFESTATIONS

Cataracts that are indistinguishable from those seen in DM1 are common in DM2.[12,59] These cataracts usually appear before the age of 50 years and have even developed in patients in their late childhood. Cardiac abnormalities may also develop.[12,59,73] Syncope, near-syncopal spells, or symptomatic tachycardia occur in 8%, cardiac conduction defects in 20%, and a potentially life-threatening cardiomyopathy occur in as many as 7% of individuals who are affected.[59] Unlike DM1, most series have not reported an increased incidence of alveolar hypoventilation in patients with DM2, however, some patients develop sleep apnea and excessive daytime somnolence.[72]

Also, in contrast to DM1, mental retardation is not a prominent feature. However, white matter abnormalities may be appreciated on magnetic resonance imaging (MRI) of the brain.[13] In addition, some affected individuals have stroke-like symptoms, seizures, parkinsonian features, and hypersomnia. Further, neuropsychological testing reveals lower scores on tests of frontal lobe function compared to normal along with avoidant personality traits; brain single photon emission and computed tomography can show frontal and parieto-occipital hypoperfusion similar to DM1.[20] Frontal balding has been reported in as many as 20–50% of men aged 21–34 years. Testicular atrophy with gonadal insufficiency can occur. Gastrointestinal hypomotility has not been described. Late-onset deafness was reported in one kinship with atypical DM2.

LABORATORY FEATURES

Serum CK levels are often mildly elevated. Low testosterone levels may be seen in as many as 29% of affected males and insulin insensitivity in 75% of patients.[59] A high GGT was demonstrated in 64%, low IgG in 65%, and low IgM in 11%.[59] Abnormalities are common in EKG as described earlier.

Motor and sensory NCS are normal. EMG reveals myotonic discharges even in patients without clinical myotonia, although these discharges can be difficult to detect in some patients. Despite the prominent proximal muscle involvement clinically, electrical myotonia is often more easily detected in distal muscles.

HISTOPATHOLOGY

Muscle biopsy reveals nonspecific myopathic features including a mild to moderate increase in internalized nuclei, variability of fiber size with atrophy of type 2 fibers, small angular fibers, and atrophic fibers with pyknotic nuclear clumps.[59,74,75] In contrast to that seen in DM1, selective type 1 fiber atrophy, sarcoplasmic masses, and ringed fibers are not usually appreciated on DM2 muscle biopsies. Autopsy studies demonstrate neurofibrillary degeneration with abnormal tau expression as in DM1.[27]

MOLECULAR GENETICS AND PATHOGENESIS

DM2 and PROMM are allelic disorders caused by CCTG repeat expansions in intron 1 of the zinc finger protein 9 gene, *(ZNF9)*, located on chromosome 3.[40,59] The transcribed mRNA with expanded CCTG repeats accumulates as abnormal focal collections in the nucleus similar to expanded CTG repeats seen in DM1.[37–40] As with DM1, the aggregates of mutated mRNA appear to exert their toxic effect on cells by sequestering RNA-binding proteins that leads to abnormal splicing of pre-mRNA from various target genes (e.g., chloride ion channel, insulin receptor, tau protein, cardiac troponin).[37–39,42,45] The subsequent abnormal translation of the RNAs into functional proteins explains the multiple organ/systemic manifestations of both DM1 and DM2.

TREATMENT

There is no specific treatment for DM2. A small randomized controlled trial of creatine monohydrate in DM2 was ineffective.[76] There is insufficient information regarding the efficacy of various antimyotonia agents, but mexiletine or carbamazepine, or phenytoin can be tried if the myotonia or muscle pain is bothersome to the patient.[72,77] Cataracts may need surgical excision. It seems prudent to carefully monitor patients during surgery and the postoperative period. One patient with PROMM developed increased muscle pain, myoglobinuria, and transient renal insufficiency after minor surgery.[64]

►SUMMARY

DM1 and DM2 are multi systemic disorders caused by expanded repeats in the noncoding regions of the *DMPK* and *ZNF9* genes, respectively. The novel pathogenic consequence of these mutations is not due to a loss of function created by loss of *DMPK* and *ZNF9* protein products, but rather a toxic effect on the cells by the accumulation of abnormal mRNA. The mutant mRNA sequesters necessary RNA-binding proteins and this results in abnormal splicing of pre-mRNA from various target genes (e.g., chloride ion channel, insulin receptor, tau protein, cardiac troponin), thus explaining the multisystemic manifestations of DM1 and DM2. There may be additional forms of myotonic dystrophy not localized to the DM1 and DM2 loci. Treatment of these disorders at this time is largely symptomatic.

REFERENCES

1. Emery AE. Population frequencies of inherited neuromuscular diseases–a world survey. *Neuromuscul Disord*. 1991;1:19–29.
2. Machuca-Tzili L, Brook D, Hilton-Jones D. Clinical and molecular aspects of the myotonic dystrophies: A review. *Muscle Nerve*. 2005;32(1):1–18.
3. Tramonte JJ, Burns TM. Myotonic dystrophy. *Arch Neurol*. 2005;62(8):1316–1319.
4. van Engelen BG, Eymard B, Wilcox D. 123rd ENMC International Workshop: Management and therapy in myotonic dystrophy, 6-8 February 2004, Naarden, The Netherlands. *Neuromuscul Disord*. 2005;15(5):389–394.
5. Messina C, Tonali P, Scoppetta C. The lack of deep reflexes in myotonic dystrophy: A neurophysiologic study. *J Neurol Sci*. 1976;30:303–311.
6. Bird TD, Follett C, Griep E. Cognitive and personality function in myotonic dystrophy. *J Neurol Neurosurg Psychiatry*. 1983;46:971–980.
7. Portwood MM, Wicks JJ, Lieberman JS, Duveneck MJ. Intellectual and cognitive function in adults with myotonic dystrophy. *Arch Phys Med Rehabil*. 1986;67:299–303.
8. Hageman AT, Gabreels FJ, Liem KD, Renkawek K, Boon JM. Congenital myotonic dystrophy; a report on thirteen cases and a review of the literature. *J Neurol Sci*. 1993;115:95–101.
9. Reardon W, Newcombe R, Fenton I, Sibert J, Hfarper PS. The natural history f congenital myotonic dystrophy: Mortality and long term clinical aspects. *Arch Dis Child*. 1993;68:177–181.
10. de Die-Smulders CE, Howeler CJ, Thijs C, et al. Age and causes of death in adult-onset myotonic dystrophy. *Brain*. 1998;121: 1557–1563.
11. Mathieu J, Allard P, Potvin L, Prevost C, Begin P. A 10 year study of mortality in a cohort of patients with myotonic dystrophy. *Neurology*. 1999;52:1658–1662.
12. Meola G. Genetic and clinical heterogeneity in myotonic dystrophies. *Muscle Nerve*. 2000;13:1789–1799.
13. Hund E, Jansen O, Koch MC, et al. Proximal myotonic myopathy with white matter abnormalities of the brain. *Neurology*. 1997;48:33–37.
14. Nowak TV, Anuras S, Brown BP, Ionasescu V, Green JB. Small intestine motility in myotonic dystrophy patients. *Gastroenterology*. 1984;86:808–813.
15. Begin R, Bureau MA, Lupien L, Lemiex B. Control and modulation of respiration in Steinert's myotonic dystrophy. *Am Rev Respir Dis*. 1980;121:281–289.
16. Hansotia P, Frens D. Hypersomnia associated with alveolar hypoventilation in myotonic dystrophy. *Neurology*. 1981;31: 1336–1337.
17. Motta J, Guilleminault C, Billingham M, Barry W, Mason J. Cardiac abnormalities in myotonic dystrophy. Electrophysiologic and histologic studies. *Am J Med*. 1979;67:467–473.
18. Sabovic M, Medica I, Logar N, Mandic E, Zidar J, Peterlin B. Relation of CTG expansion and clinical variables to electrocardiogram conduction abnormalities and sudden death in patients with myotonic dystrophy. *Neuromuscul Disord*. 2003;13(10):822–826.
19. Delaporte C. Personality patterns in patients with myotonic dystrophy. *Arch Neurol*. 1998;55:635–640.
20. Meola G, Sansone V, Perani D, et al. Executive dysfunction and avoidant personality trait in myotonic dystrophy type 1 (DM-1) and in proximal myotonic myopathy (PROMM/DM-2). *Neuromuscul Disord*. 2003;13(10):813–821.
21. Moxley RT 3rd, Griggs RC, Goldblatt D. VanGelder V, Herr BE, Thiel R. Decreased insulin sensitivity of forearm muscle in myotonic dystrophy. *J Clin Invest*. 1978;62:857–867.
22. Gadalla SM, Lund M, Pfeiffer RM, et al. Cancer risk among patients with myotonic muscular dystrophy. *JAMA*. 2011;306: 2480–2486.
23. Win AK, Perattur PG, Pulido JS, Pulido CM, Lindor NM. Increased cancer risks in myotonic dystrophy. *Mayo Clin Proc*. 2012;87(2):130–135.
24. Streib EW, Sun SF. Distribution of electrical myotonia in myotonic muscular dystrophy. *Ann Neurol*. 1983;14:80–82.
25. Dodge PR, Gamstrop I, Byers RK, Russell P. Myotonic dystrophy in infancy and childhood. *Pediatrics*. 1965;35:3–19.
26. Swift TR, Ignacio OJ, Dyken PR. Neonatal dystrophica myotonica. Electrophysiological studies. *Am J Dis Child*. 1975;129: 734–737.

27. Maurage CA, Udd B, Ruchoux MM, et al. Similar brain tau pathology in DM2/PROMM and DM1/Steinert disease. *Neurology*. 2005;65:1636–1638.
28. Brook JD, McCurrach ME, Harley HG, et al. Molecular basis of myotonic dystrophy: Expansion of a trinucleotide (CTG) repeat at the 3′ end of transcript encoding protein kinase family member. *Cell*. 1992;68:799–808.
29. Fischbeck KH. The mechanism of myotonic dystrophy. *Ann Neurol*. 1994;35:255–256.
30. Fu YH, Friedman DL, Richards S, et al. Decreased expression of myotonin-protein kinase messenger RNA and protein in adult form of myotonic dystrophy. *Science*. 1993;260:235–238.
31. Fu YH, Pizzuti A, Fenwick R Jr, et al. An unstable triplet repeat in a gene related to myotonic muscular dystrophy. *Science*. 1992;255:1256–1258.
32. Harper PS, Harley HG, Reardon W, Shaw DJ. Review article: Anticipation in myotonic dystrophy: New light on an old problem. *Am J Hum Genet*. 1992;51:10–16.
33. Mahadevan M, Tsilfidis C, Sabourin L, et al. Myotonic dystrophy mutation: An unstable CTG repeat in the 3′ untranslated region of the gene. *Science*. 1992;255:1253–1255.
34. Ptacek LJ, Johnson KJ, Griggs RC. Genetics and physiology of the myotonic disorders. *N Engl J Med*. 1993;328:482–489.
35. Shelbourne P, Davies J, Buxton J, et al. Direct diagnosis of myotonic dystrophy with a disease-specific DNA marker. *N Engl J Med*. 1993;328:471–475.
36. Tian B, White RJ, Xia T, et al. Expanded CUG repeat RNAs form hairpins that activate the double-stranded RNA-dependent protein kinase PKR. *RNA*. 2000;6:79–87.
37. Mankodi A, Takahashi MP, Jiang H, et al. Expanded CUG repeats trigger aberrant splicing of ClC-1 chloride channel pre-mRNA and hyperexcitability of skeletal muscle in myotonic dystrophy. *Mol Cell*. 2002;10:35–44.
38. Mankodi A, Teng-Umnauay P, Krym M, Hendierson D, Swanson M, Thornton CA. Ribonuclear inclusions in skeletal myotonic dystrophy types 1 and 2. *Ann Neurol*. 2003;54:760–768.
39. Mankodi A, Thornton CA. Myotonic syndromes. *Curr Opin Neurol*. 2002;15(5):545–552.
40. Udd B, Meola G, Krahe R, et al. Myotonic dystrophy type 2 (DM2) and related disorders report of the 180th ENMC workshop including guidelines on diagnostics and management 3–5 December 2010, Naarden, The Netherlands. *Neuromuscul Disord*. 2011;21:443–450.
41. Berg J, Jiang H, Thornton CA, Cannon SC. Truncated ClC-1 mRNA in myotonic dystrophy exerts a dominant-negative effect on the Cl current. *Neurology*. 2004;63(12):2371–2375.
42. Day JW, Ranum LP. RNA pathogenesis of the myotonic dystrophies. *Neuromuscul Disord*. 2005;15(1):5–16.
43. Kimura T, Nakamori M, Lueck JD, et al. Altered mRNA splicing of the skeletal muscle ryanodine receptor and sarcoplasmic/endoplasmic reticulum Ca^{2+}-ATPase in myotonic dystrophy type 1. *Hum Mol Genet*. 2005;14(15):2189–2200.
44. Pascual M, Vicente M, Monferrer L, Artero R. The Muscleblind family of proteins: An emerging class of regulators of developmentally programmed alternative splicing. *Differentiation*. 2006;74(2–3):65–80.
45. Kanadia RN, Johnstone KA, Mankodi A, et al. A muscleblind knockout model for myotonic dystrophy. *Science*. 2003;302:1978–1980.
46. Ebralidze A, Wang Y, Petkova V, Ebralidse K, Junghans RP. RNA leaching of transcription factors disrupts transcription in myotonic dystrophy. *Science*. 2004;303(5656):383–387.
47. Sugino M, Ohsawa N, Ito T, et al. A pilot study of dehydroepiandrosterone sulfate in myotonic dystrophy. *Neurology*. 1998;51(2):586–589.
48. Tarnopolsky M, Mahoney D, Thompson T, Naylor H, Doherty TJ. Creatine monohydrate supplementation does not increase muscle strength, lean body mass, or muscle phosphocreatine in patients with myotonic dystrophy type 1. *Muscle Nerve*. 2004;29(1):51–58.
49. Heatwole CR, Eichinger KJ, Friedman DI, et al. Open-label trial of recombinant human insulin-like growth factor 1/recombinant human insulin-like growth factor binding protein 3 in myotonic dystrophy type 1. *Arch Neurol*. 2011;68:37–44.
50. Logigian EL, Martens WB, Moxley RT 4th, et al. Mexiletine is an effective antimyotonia treatment in myotonic dystrophy type 1. *Neurology*. 2010;74:1441–1448.
51. Orngreen MC, Olsen DB, Vissing J. Aerobic training in patients with myotonic dystrophy type 1. *Ann Neurol*. 2005;57(5):754–757.
52. Aldridge LM. Anesthetic problems in myotonic dystrophy. A case report and review of the Aberdeen experience comprising 48 general anaesthetics in a further 16 patients. *Br J Anaesth*. 1985;57:1119–1130.
53. Brahams D. Postoperative monitoring in patients with muscular dystrophy. *Lancet*. 1989;2:1053–1054.
54. Harper PS. Postoperative complications in myotonic dystrophy. *Lancet*. 1989;2:1269.
55. Mathieu J, Allard P, Gobeil G, Girard M, De Braekeleer M, Begin P. Anesthetic and surgical complications in 219 cases of myotonic dystrophy. *Neurology*. 1997;49:1646–1650.
56. Damian MS, Gerlach A, Schmidt F, Lehman E, Reichmann H. Modafinil for excessive daytime sleepiness in myotonic dystrophy. *Neurology*. 2001;56:794–796.
57. MacDonald JR, Hill JD, Tarnopolsky MA. Modafinil reduces excessive somnolence and enhances mood in patients with myotonic dystrophy. *Neurology*. 2002;59(12):1876–1880.
58. Talbot K, Stradling J, Crosby J, Hilton-Jones D. Reduction in excess daytime sleepiness by modafinil in patients with myotonic dystrophy. *Neuromuscul Disord*. 2003;13(5):357–364.
59. Day JW, Ricker K, Jacobsen JF, et al. Myotonic dystrophy type 2: Molecular, diagnostic, and clinical spectrum. *Neurology*. 2003;60:657–664.
60. Meola G, Sansone V, Radice S, Skradski S, Ptacek L. A family with an unusual myotonic and myopathic phenotype and no CTG expansion (Proximal myotonic myopathic syndrome): A challenge for future molecular studies. *Neuromuscul Disord*. 1996;6:143–150.
61. Moxley RT 3rd. Proximal myotonic myopathy: Mini-review of a recently delineated clinical disorder. *Neuromuscul Disord*. 1996;6:87–93.
62. Ricker K, Grimm T, Koch MC, et al. Linkage of proximal myotonic myopathy to chromosome 3q. *Neurology*. 1999;52:170–171.
63. Ricker K, Koch MC, Lehmann-Horn F, et al. Proximal myotonic myopathy: A new dominant disorder with myotonia, muscle weakness, and cataracts. *Neurology*. 1994;44:1448–1452.
64. Ricker K, Koch MC, Lehmann-Horn F, et al. Proximal myotonic myopathy. Clinical features of a multisystemic disorder similar to myotonic dystrophy. *Arch Neurol*. 1995;52:25–31.
65. Ricker K, Moxley RT 3rd, Heine R, Lehmann-Horn F. Myotonia fluctuans. A third type of muscle sodium channel disease. *Arch Neurol*. 1994;44:500–1503.
66. Ricker K, Moxley RT 3rd, Heine R, Lehmann-Horne F. Myotonia fluctuans. A third type of muscle sodium channel disease. *Arch Neurol*. 1994;51:1095–1102.

67. Schneider C, Ziegler A, Ricker K, et al. Proximal myotonic myopathy. Evidence for anticipation in families with linkage to chromosome 3q. *Neurology*. 2000;55:383–388.
68. Thornton CA, Ashizawa T. Getting a grip on the myotonic dystrophies. *Neurology*. 1999;52:12–13.
69. Thornton CA, Griggs RC, Moxley RT 3rd. Myotonic dystrophy with no trinucleotide repeat expansion. *Ann Neurol*. 1994;35:269–272.
70. Newman B, Meola G, O'Donovan DG, Schapira AH, Kingston H. Proximal myotonic myopathy (PROMM) presenting as myotonia during pregnancy. *Neuromuscul Disord*. 1999;9:144–149.
71. Rudnik-Schoneborn S, Schneider-Gold C, Raabe U, Kress W, Zerres K, Schoser BG. Outcome and effect of pregnancy in myotonic dystrophy type 2. *Neurology*. 2006;66(4):579–580.
72. Sander HW, Tavoulareas G, Chokroverty S. Heat sensitive myotonia in proximal myotonic myopathy. *Neurology*. 1996;47:956–962.
73. Schoser BG, Ricker K, Schneider-Gold C, et al. Sudden cardiac death in myotonic dystrophy type 2. *Neurology*. 2004;63(12):2402–2404.
74. Schoser BG, Schneider-Gold C, Kress W, et al. Muscle pathology in 57 patients with myotonic dystrophy type 2. *Muscle Nerve*. 2004;29(2):275–281.
75. Vihola A, Bassez G, Meola G, et al. Histopathological differences of myotonic dystrophy type 1 (DM1) and PROMM/DM2. *Neurology*. 2003;60:1854–1857.
76. Schneider-Gold C, Beck M, Wessig C, et al. Creatine monohydrate in DM2/PROMM: A double-blind placebo-controlled clinical study. Proximal myotonic myopathy. *Neurology*. 2003;60(3):500–502.
77. Moxley RT 3rd. Myotonic disorders in childhood. Diagnosis and treatment. *J Child Neurol*. 1997;12:116–129.

CHAPTER 32

Nondystrophic Myotonias and Periodic Paralysis

In this chapter, we describe the pathophysiology, clinical presentation, laboratory findings, and treatment of the nondystrophic myotonias and periodic paralyses (Table 31-1).

There are several inherited myopathic disorders associated with clinical or electrical myotonia in which muscle is not dystrophic.[1–5] These disorders are caused by mutations in various ion channels, and are thus referred to here as muscle channelopathies. Mutations in the chloride channel cause myotonia congenita (MC). The sodium channelopathies include potassium-sensitive (hyperkalemic) periodic paralysis (HyperKPP), paramyotonia congenita (PMC), potassium-aggravated myotonias (PAM) (e.g., myotonia fluctuans, myotonia permanens, and acetazolamide-responsive myotonia), and familial hypokalemic periodic paralysis type 2 (HypoKPP2). HyperKPP and PMC are usually associated with episodes of transient generalized or focal weakness. Hypokalemic periodic paralysis type 1 (HypoKPP1) is not associated with myotonia clinically or electrically and is caused by mutations of muscle dihydropyridine (DHP) receptor (a type of calcium channel). Andersen–Tawil syndrome (ATS) is another rare form of hereditary periodic paralysis of which some forms are due to mutations in a potassium channel.

Electrophysiological studies, in particular the short- and long-exercise tests (SETs and LETs), also described in Chapter 2, can be useful in distinguishing subtypes of muscle channelopathy and thus deserve special comment (Tables 32-1 and 32-2).[1–9] The SET is performed by having the patient isometrically exercise a muscle (e.g., abductor digiti minimi) for 10 seconds, followed by measurement of compound muscle action potential (CMAP) amplitudes immediately after exercise and every 10 seconds thereafter up to 60 seconds. Fournier et al. modified the test by having the SET repeated twice more with a rest period of 60 seconds between trials. In addition, the SET should be done at room temperature and then with cooling of the muscle. In normal individuals, immediately after short exercise, there is a mild increase in the CMAP amplitudes compared to baseline (mean 4–5%, range −28% to +27%) with the amplitudes returning to baseline within 10 seconds.[8,9] If the SET is performed after cooling the limb (e.g., with an ice pack), the CMAP amplitudes decrease (−25% to −65%), but the durations of the CMAPs increase.

The LET is performed by having the patient isometrically exercise a muscle (e.g., abductor digiti minimi) for 5 minutes (with 3–4 seconds of rest every 30–45 seconds), while CMAP amplitudes are recorded every minute during the exercise period, immediately after cessation of exercise, then every minute for 5 minutes, and finally every 5 minutes for 40–45 minutes. In normal people, CMAP amplitudes only slightly decrease after the exercise period (range −16 to +5%), and the amplitudes then return to normal within the next 30–60 seconds and remain so during the next 40–50 minutes.[8,9]

Changes in CMAP amplitudes with the SET separates muscle channelopathies into five patterns (Table 32-2; Fig. 32-1).[8] The first three patterns help distinguish the nondystrophic myotonias, particularly when performed at room temperature and then in cold, while Patterns IV and V are useful in diagnosing periodic paralysis in combination with the LET.[6,8,9]

▶ CHLORIDE CHANNELOPATHIES

MYOTONIA CONGENITA

Clinical Features

The autosomal-dominant form of MC, or Thomsen disease, often presents in the first few years of life.[1–4,10–16] Affected infants may have difficulty opening their eyes after crying. Stiffness in the legs upon arising and taking the first few steps may lead to tripping and falling. As patients become older, their muscle stiffness may become more noticeable in the arms. Myotonia of muscles of mastication may result in difficulties in chewing and swallowing. As with most forms of myotonia, the stiffness in the muscles eases with repeated contractions, the so-called warm-up phenomena. Thus, although an affected individual may have initial stiffness in their legs when they begin to walk, within a short time ambulation becomes easier. After rest, the same stereotypical pattern of stiffness returns on initiation of physical activity. The myotonia can worsen with cold similar to that seen in PMC.[17] The severity of the myotonia can fluctuate and is variable even within affected family members. The stiffness may worsen during pregnancy. Of note, people with MC usually do not typically complain of muscle pain with their stiffness. In contrast to the myotonic dystrophies,

▶ TABLE 32-1. **NONDYSTROPHIC MYOTONIAS AND HEREDITARY PERIODIC PARALYSIS**

Disorder	Inheritance	Gene (Location)	Clinical or EMG Myotonia	Short Exercise Test	Long Exercise Test	Fournier Electro-physiologic Pattern
Myotonia congenita (MC)		*CLCN-1* (7q35)	Yes	±PEMPs; transient decrease in CMAP amplitudes after the first trial in AR-MC but less common with AD MC; reduction in amplitudes is less in the second and third trials. No change with cold in AR-MC, but reduction in amplitudes occurs after the first trial in AD-MC that improves with subsequent trials	Slight or no decrease in amplitudes immediately after exercise with no change over time	Pattern II
Thomsen disease	AD					
Becker disease	AR					
Hyperkalemic periodic paralysis (HyperKPP)	AD	*SCN4A* (17q13.1–13.3)	Maybe	No PEMPs; Increase in amplitudes after the first trial with further increase after the second and third trials	Transient increase in amplitudes immediately after exercise with subsequent gradual decrease in amplitudes over a prolonged period of time (as much as 40 minutes or more)	Pattern IV
Paramyotonia congenita (PMC)	AD	*SCN4A* (17q13.1–13.3)	Yes	PEMPs are common; amplitudes may increase or decrease with the initial trial but gradually decline after the second and third trials (most common with T1313M mutations—other forms of PMC usually have normal SET); reduction in amplitudes is more prominent in cold. PMC with Q270 m mutation may have normal SET at rest but has decrement with cooling	Decrease in amplitudes during and following exercise that may persist for hours	Pattern I
Potassium-aggravated myotonias Myotonia permanens Myotonia fluctuans Acetazolamide-responsive MC	AD	*SCN4A* (17q13.1–13.3)	Yes	No PEMPs; usually no change even with cooling	No change	Pattern III
Hypokalemic periodic paralysis type 1 (HypoKPP1)	AD	*CACNA1S* (1q31–32)	No	No PEMPs; usually no change even with cooling	Slight increase or no immediate change with exercise but gradually decline of amplitudes over time is seen in most	Pattern V
Hypokalemic periodic paralysis type 2 (HypoKPP2)	AD	*SCN4A* (17q13.1–13.3)	No	No PEMPs; usually no change even with cooling	A slight increase in amplitudes may be seen during and immediately after exercise followed by a delayed reduction in amplitudes after 10–20 minutes	Pattern V
Andersen–Tawil syndrome (ATS)	AD	*KCNJ2* (17q23.1–q24.2)	No	Unknown	A decrement in CMAP area and to a lesser extent the amplitude may be appreciated	
Schwartz–Jampel syndrome	AR	*HSPG2* (1p34.1–36.1)	Yes	Unknown	Unknown	

AD, autosomal-dominant; AR, autosomal recessive; PEMPs, postexercise myotonic potentials on the motor conduction studies.

▶ TABLE 32-2. ELECTRODIAGNOSTIC PATTERNS[7]

Patterns	SET	LET
I	Postexercise amplitude decrement that worsens with each trial	Postexercise amplitude decrement that does not return to baseline over 40 minutes
II	Postexercise amplitude decrement that improves with each trial	No postexercise amplitude change or small transient decrement
III	No postexercise amplitude change	No postexercise amplitude change
IV	Postexercise amplitude increment that increases with each trial	Transient postexercise amplitude increment followed by late continuous decrement over 40 minutes
V	No postexercise amplitude change	Late continuous postexercise amplitude decrement over 40 minutes

there are no systemic disorders (e.g., cataracts, endocrinopathies, cardiopathy, ventilatory muscle weakness) associated with MC or increased mortality. However, some individuals present later in life with stiffness and proximal weakness and resemble myotonic dystrophy type 2 (DM2) or proximal myotonic myopathy (PROMM).[4,17] There may be an increased risk of malignant hyperthermia (MH) with anesthetic agents.

On examination, affected individuals usually appear extremely muscular (e.g., Herculean). Muscle strength is usually normal, but some patients develop mild proximal weakness. Action myotonia can be elicited by having the

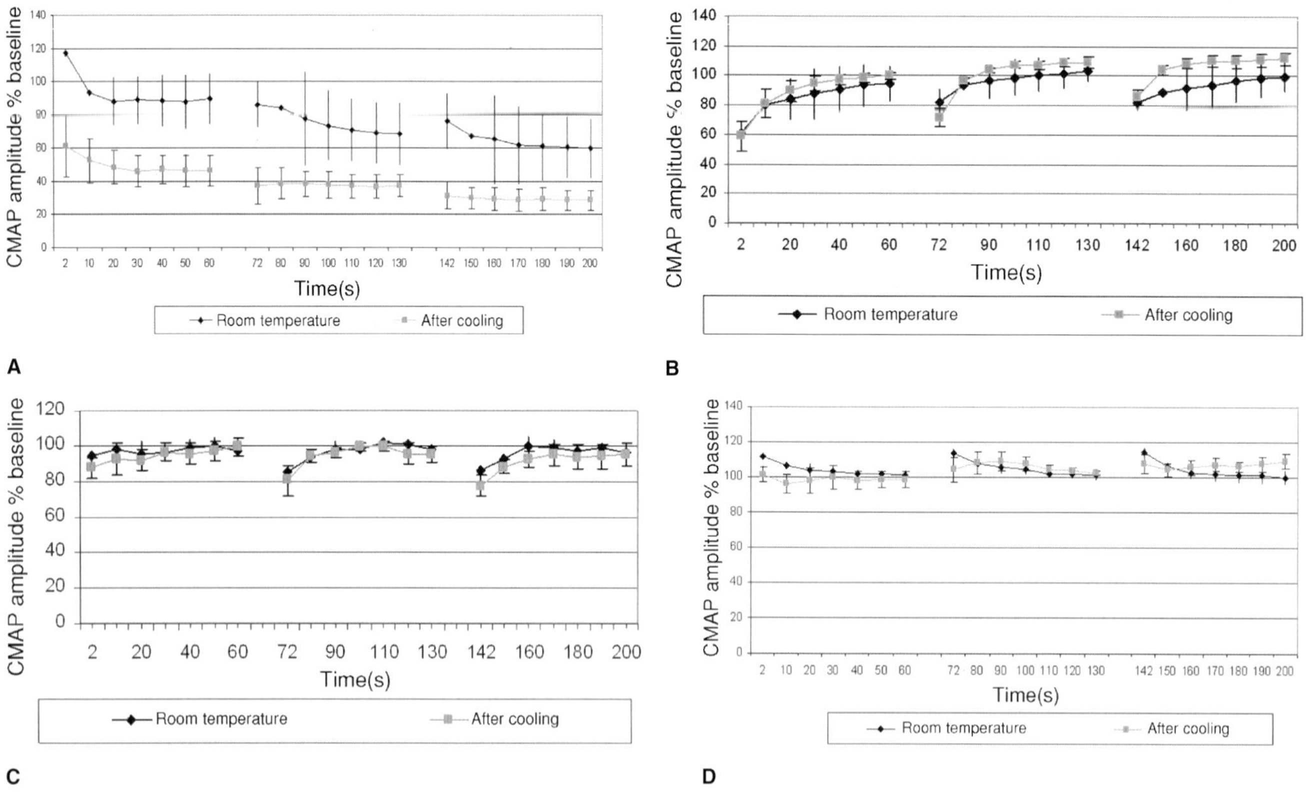

Figure 32-1. Short exercise test (SET) and Fournier Patterns in the nondystrophic myotonias. **(A)** Fournier Pattern I. Paramyotonia congenita associated with T1313M *SCN4A* mutation. The SET is associated with a decrease in CMAP amplitudes that worsens with repeated trials of short exercise at room temperature. SET with cooling shows even greater decrement of CMAP amplitude. PMC associated with **(B)** Fournier Pattern II. Autosomal recessive myotonia congenita. The SET is associated with a decrease in CMAP amplitudes immediately after exercise that returns to baseline after 20–40 seconds. The reduction in the CMAP amplitudes decreases with repeated trials of short exercise. **(C)** Autosomal-dominant myotonia congenita. SET at room temperature often shows no decrement, but with cooling there is reversion to Fournier Pattern II with decrement that improves with repeated activity. **(D)** Fournier Pattern III. SET at room temperature and after cooling is normal as seen in most cases of potassium-associated myotonia (PAM), PMC that are not associated with T1313M mutation, and in the myotonic dystrophies. (Reproduced with permission from Matthews E, Fialho D, Tan SV, et al: CINCH Investigators. The non-dystrophic myotonias: molecular pathogenesis, diagnosis and treatment. *Brain*. 2010;133(Pt 1):9–22.

patient make a strong grip and then try to relax their fingers, or by having patients forcefully close their eyes and then try to open them. One sees delayed relaxation, which improves with repeated activity due to the warm-up phenomena discussed above. In addition, myotonia can be demonstrated by percussing a muscle (e.g., the thenar eminence) with a reflex hammer (percussion myotonia).

Becker described the features of the autosomal recessive form of MC which bears his name. The clinical features of the autosomal recessive and dominant forms of MC are similar, but there are some differences.[1–4,10,11,14,15] The autosomal recessive or Becker type of MC usually presents between 4 and 12 years of age, somewhat later than that seen in the autosomal-dominant form, however, the severity of weakness is typically worse.[1,2,13] Transient muscle weakness, particularly in the distal arms, may occur following a severe bout of myotonia. On examination, muscle bulk is usually increased. Mild fixed weakness is apparent in proximal muscles of the arms and legs as well as in the neck. Systemic complications are not seen, though there is an increased risk of MH.

Laboratory Features

Skeletal muscle MRI is usually not that helpful as it may[18] or may not[19] demonstrate signal abnormalities, which if present are nonspecific. Serum creatine kinase (CK) is normal or only slightly elevated. Routine motor and sensory nerve conduction studies (NCS) are normal. On repetitive nerve stimulation, a decrement may be appreciated when a prolonged train of stimuli are delivered at 10 Hz or more. In such cases, the CMAP amplitudes may decrease to 65% of normal and even large degrees of decrement can occur with stimulation at higher rates.[6,20]

The SET is associated with a decrease in CMAP amplitude immediately after exercise that returns to baseline after 20–40 seconds, in 48–80% of individuals with MC, (Fig. 32-1B).[2,4,7,9] The reduction in the CMAP amplitude decreases with repeated trials of short exercise, corresponding to the clinical warm-up phenomena. Fournier et al.[7] called this Pattern II (Table 32-2). A greater than 40% decrement of SET is specific for MC.[4,9] More accurately though, it is the autosomal recessive cases that usually have the reduction in CMAP amplitudes, while the autosomal-dominant cases typically are not associated with significant change

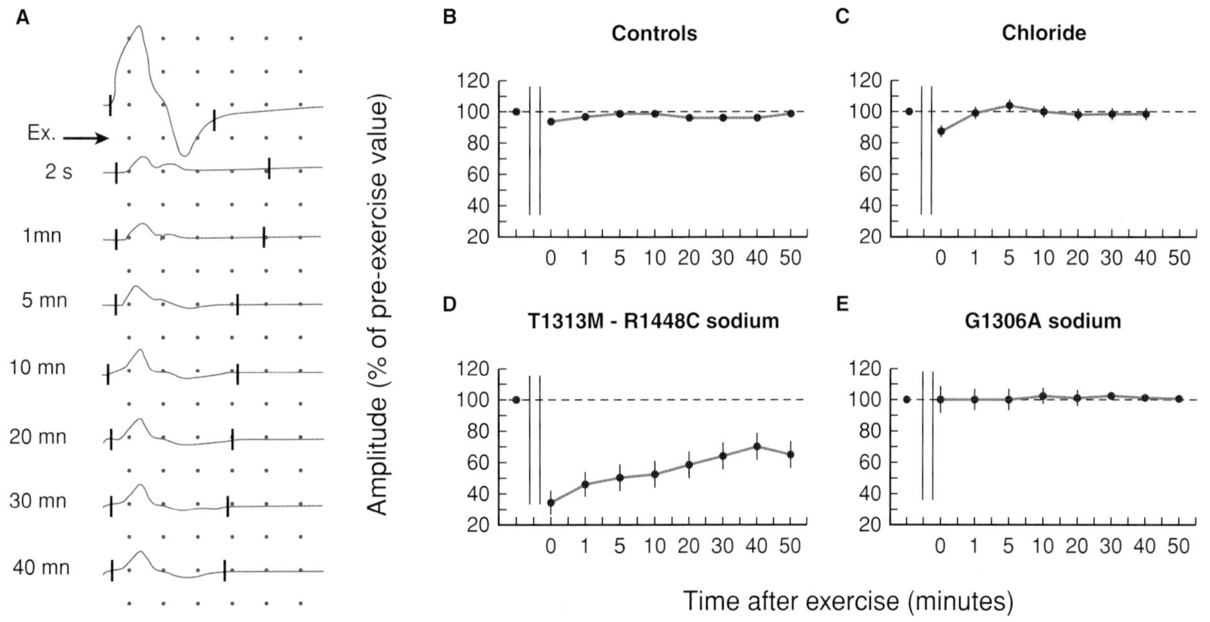

Figure 32-2. Long exercise test in myotonic syndromes. **(A)** Immediate and persistent decrease of compound muscle action potential (CMAP) amplitude (−85%) after long exercise in a paramyotonia congenita (PMC) patient with the T1313M sodium channel mutation. Pre-exercise (*top trace*) and postexercise recordings (*bottom trace*) at various times following the trial (Ex.) as indicated to the left of the tracings. Scale between two dots: 5 ms, 5 mV. Changes in CMAP amplitude of the abductor digiti minimi (ADM) muscle after long exercise (*double bars*) in 41 unaffected controls **(B)**, six myotonia congenita (MC) patients with chloride channel mutations **(C)**, 16 PMC patients with T1313M or R1448C sodium channel mutations **(D)**, and two patients with G1306A sodium channel mutations **(E)**. The amplitude of the CMAP, expressed as a percentage of its pre-exercise value, is plotted against the time elapsed after the exercise trial. (*symbols* and *vertical bars*) Means ± standard errors of the means. (Reproduced with permission from Fournier E., Arzel M, Sternberg D, et al. Electromyography guides toward subgroups of mutations in muscle channelopathies. *Ann Neurol.* 2004;56(5):650–661.)

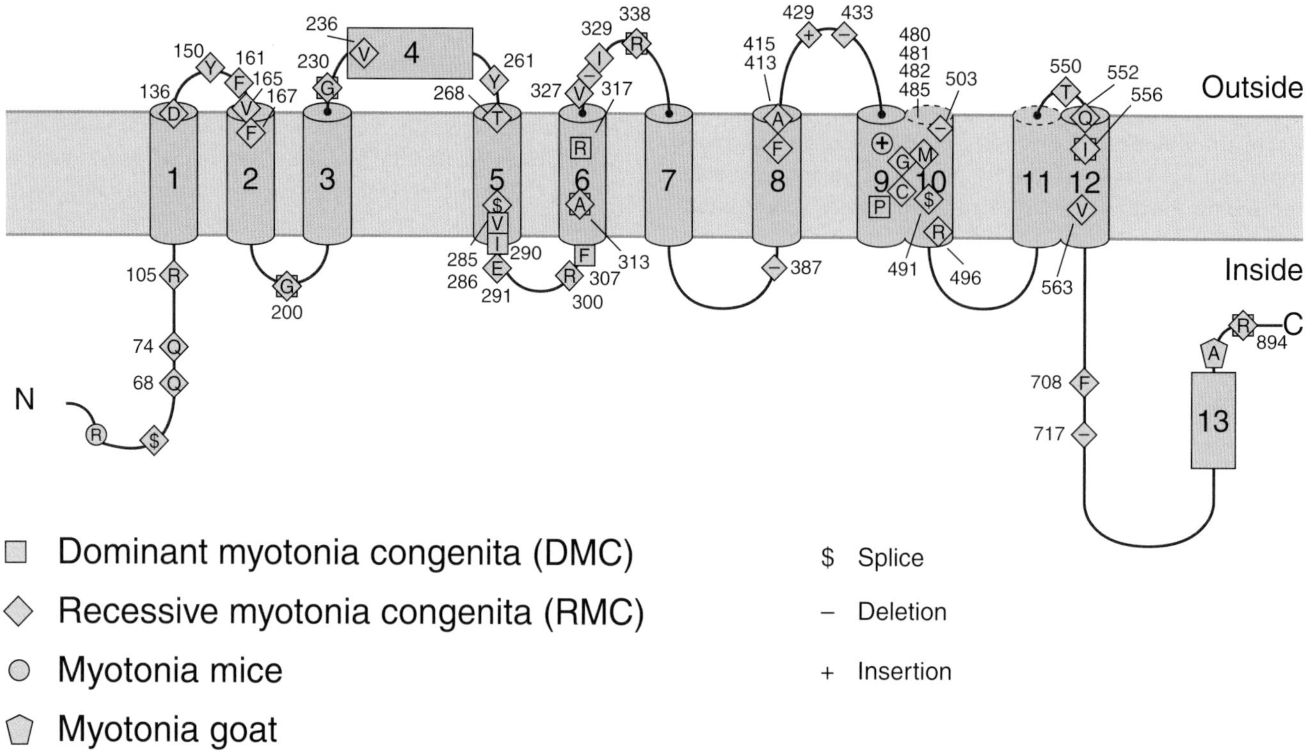

Figure 32-3. The chloride channel monomer, ClC 1, is functional as homodimeric channel complex. Different symbols used for known mutations leading to dominant Thomsen-type myotonia, recessive Becker-type myotonia, recessive myotonic mice, and dominant myotonic goat are explained on *bottom left*. Conventional one-letter abbreviations were used for replaced amino acids located at positions given by respective numbers of human protein. (Reproduced with permission from Lehmann-Horn F, Jurkat-Rott K. Voltage-gated ion channels and hereditary disease. *Physiol Rev.* 1999;79(4):1317–1372.)

in amplitude.[3,8,9] Performing the SET in a cooled limb in patients with autosomal-dominant MC may result in a drop in amplitude that improves with repeated short exercise (e.g., a conversion from normal to Pattern II with cold). In contrast, there is usually no significant difference in the results of the short exercise performed at room temperature, in comparison to cold in individuals with autosomal recessive MC (they remain with Pattern II).[4,8] Overall, Fournier Pattern II is seen in over 60% of autosomal recessive MC, but less than 30% of autosomal-dominant MC.[4,8] In addition, postexercise repetitive discharges or myotonic potentials (PEMPs) are seen in about one-third of MC patients after short exercise.[7] These PEMPs disappear within 10–30 seconds after exercise. The LET is usually normal, but 10–30% of patients with MC (usually AR-MC) have a and initial transient decrement greater than normal (Fig. 32-2).[7,9,21]

On needle electromyography (EMG), myotonic discharges are evident at rest and during volitional activity. Cooling a limb does not lead to exacerbation of the clinical or electrical myotonia or development of weakness, unlike that seen in PMC.[22] It may be difficult to appreciate motor unit action potential (MUAP) as the myotonic discharges obscure the voluntary MUAPs, but morphology and recruitment are usually normal. However, short duration, small amplitude MUAPs may occasionally be appreciated in weak muscles. Single fiber EMG reveals normal fiber density but slightly increased jitter.

Molecular Genetics and Pathogenesis

Both the autosomal-dominant form (Thomsen) and recessive form (Becker) of MC are caused by mutations in the muscle chloride channel gene (*CLCN1*) on chromosome 7q35 (Fig. 32-3).[1,5,23–25] Of note, there is a so-called painful variant of MC that resembles the Thomsen and Becker forms, except patients with this disorder more frequently complain of myalgias. This painful variant of MC is usually caused by mutations in the muscle sodium channel gene, *SCN4A*, (discussed later). Structurally, the chloride ion channel is a homotetramer with each subunit encoded by the *CLCN1* gene.[24] The function of the chloride ion channel is to maintain the high resting membrane conductance in muscle fibers.[26] Mutations of the *CLCN1* gene are associated with reduced chloride conductance. Because chloride ions are responsible for 70% of the skeletal muscle resting membrane potential, reduced chloride conductance leads to a decrease in the rate of muscle membrane repolarization. Thus, sodium channels are able to recover from inactivation faster. As a result of the muscle membrane being in a state of depolarization, recurrent firings of action potentials or myotonic discharges occur.[26]

Treatment

Many individuals with MC do not require medical treatment. However, when the myotonia is severe and impairs function, treatment with antiarrhythmic or antiepileptic medications (e.g., mexiletine, phenytoin, carbamazepine) that interfere with the muscle sodium channel can be beneficial. In this regard, a randomized, placebo-controlled trial demonstrated that mexiletine (200 mg three times daily) reduced muscle stiffness.[27] We have also found mexiletine diminishing the transient exacerbations of weakness that can accompany the myotonia. Prior to starting mexiletine, we obtain a baseline electrocardiogram (EKG) as the drug can prolong the QT interval. If the EKG reveals a significant abnormality, we obtain a cardiology consultation before beginning mexiletine. Light-headedness, diarrhea, and dyspepsia are dose-limiting side effects of mexiletine. Dantrolene, which blocks the release of calcium from the sarcoplasmic reticulum, may reduce myotonia as well, but is usually avoided because of side effects.

SODIUM CHANNELOPATHIES

The sodium channelopathies include HyperKPP, PMC, the PAMs (e.g., myotonia fluctuans, myotonia permanens, and acetazolamide responsive myotonia)[1–5,28–45] and familial HypoKPP2[1,32–34] They are myopathies that share some similar clinical and laboratory features but have differences (Table 32-1). These disorders are inherited in an autosomal-dominant fashion. They are all caused by missense mutations in the pore-forming subunit of the voltage-gated skeletal-muscle sodium channel $Na_V1.4$ (encoded by the *SCN4A* gene that is located on chromosome 17q23–25) (Fig. 32-4).[1,5,28,30–37] For the most part, each missense mutation in

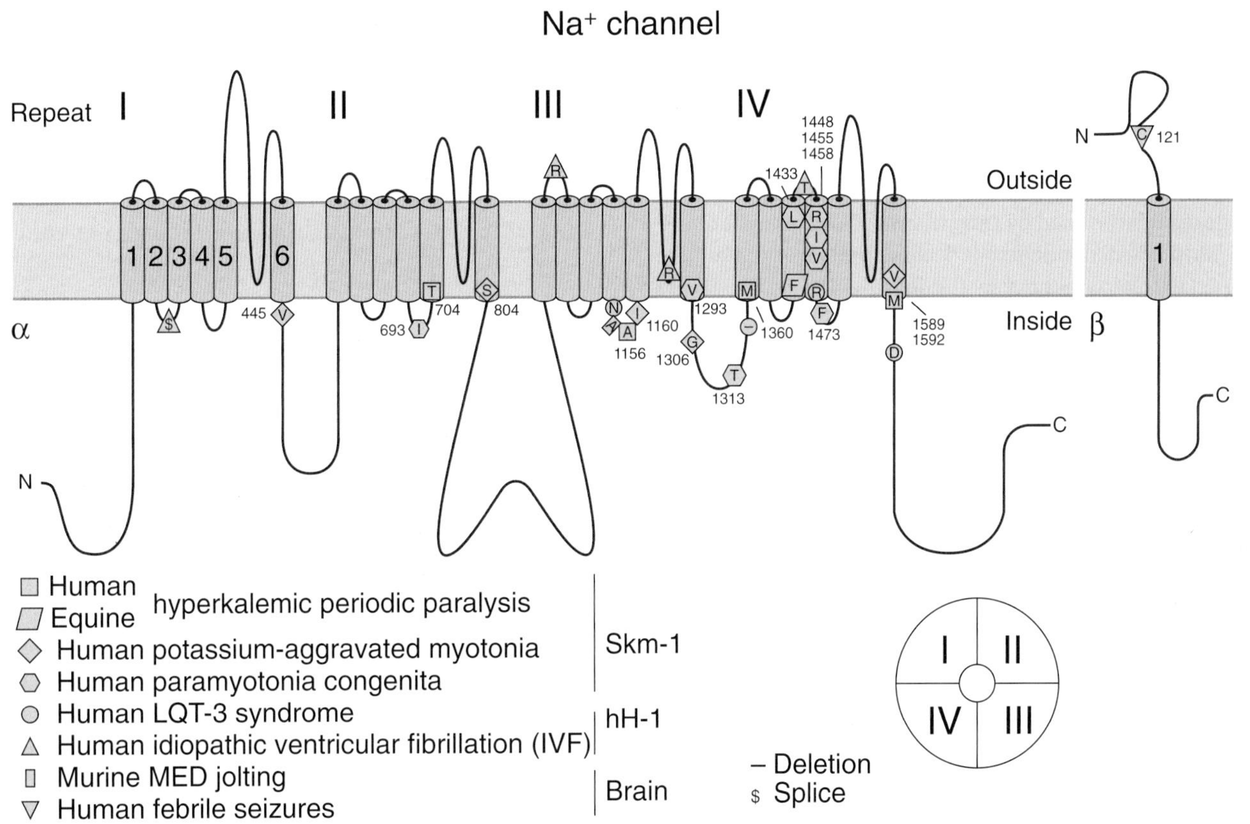

Figure 32-4. Subunits of voltage-gated sodium channel. α-subunit consists of four highly homologous domains (repeats I–IV) containing two transmembrane segments each (S1–S6). S5–S6 loops form ion-selective pores, and S4 segments contain positively charged residues conferring voltage dependence to the protein. Repeats are connected by intracellular loops; one of them, III–IV linker, contains supposed inactivation particle of channel. β1 and β2 are auxiliary subunits. When inserted in membrane, four repeats of protein fold to generate a central pore as schematically indicated on *bottom right*. Mutations have been described for α-subunits of various species and tissues: human and equine adult skeletal muscle (Skm-1), human heart (hH-1), and murine brain. So far, only one mutation has been reported for a sodium channel subunit, that is, one of human brain. Conventional one-letter abbreviations are used for replaced amino acids whose positions are given by respective numbers of human skeletal muscle channel. Different symbols used for point mutations indicate resulting diseases as explained at *bottom left*. (Reproduced with permission from Lehmann-Horn F, Jurkat-Rott K. Voltage-gated ion channels and hereditary disease. *Physiol Rev*. 1999;79(4):1317–1372.)

SCN4A is consistently associated with one of the four allelic sodium channel disorders, suggesting the presence of separate classes of functional defects. However, some variability exists and the distinction is often blurred between PMC and HyperKPP, even in affected members of the same family.

POTASSIUM-SENSITIVE OR HYPERKALEMIC PERIODIC PARALYSIS (ADYNAMIA EPISODICA HEREDITARIA)

Clinical Features

Potassium-sensitive periodic paralysis or hyperkalemic periodic paralysis (HyperKPP) is an autosomal-dominant disorder with a high degree of penetrance.[12,30,36–38,46,47–56] A recent large study in England revealed the prevalence to be 0.17 per 100,000.[5] HyperKPP manifests in three forms: (1) without myotonia, (2) with clinical or electrical myotonia, or (3) associated with paramyotonia. The course of the attacks of weakness is similar in each form, except that cooling triggers weakness in those with paramyotonia. Clinical myotonia is often mild, and can be elicited in the face (e.g., eyelids), tongue, forearm (e.g., finger extensors), and the thenar eminence with percussion or activity. The myotonia eases with repetitive activity, except in individuals with paramyotonia who exhibit paradoxical myotonia in which muscle stiffness is induced or worsened by exercise and cold temperature.

Most affected individuals become initially symptomatic with attacks of weakness in the first decade of life. These attacks usually develop in the morning, although can occur at any time, and are often precipitated by rest following exercise, intake of potassium rich food, fasting, and even by stress. The weakness can be mild or severe, with the latter more commonly occurring after strenuous physical activity. People may note paresthesia and achiness in the muscles prior to the development of weakness. The thigh and calf muscles are often affected and weakness may progress to other muscle groups. However, the weakness can also be focal. In contrast to HypoKPP, generalized flaccid paralysis is uncommon. Rarely, the bulbar and ventilatory muscles are affected. The sphincter muscles are unaffected during attacks.

The duration of weakness attacks is usually less than 2 hours, although mild weakness can persist for a few days. The frequency of attacks is highly variable, ranging from several times a day to less than once a year. In addition, there is great variation of attack severity and frequency within and between families. The frequency of paretic attacks often decreases with age. Sustained mild exercise after a period of strenuous activity may postpone or prevent weakness from developing in the exercising muscles, while resting muscle groups become weak. Following a bout of weakness, it is not uncommon for pain to be experienced in the affected muscles up to several days. During attacks, the reflexes are diminished or absent, while sensation remains normal. Between the attacks, sensation and muscle stretch reflexes are normal and lid lag or eyelid myotonia may be the only clinical signs present. Not infrequently, affected individuals develop fixed or slowly progressive weakness, independent of the episodic attacks, usually involving the more proximal muscles.

Laboratory Features

Skeletal muscle MRI scans may reveal nonspecific signal abnormalities in thigh and calf muscles.[18] Serum CK levels are usually mildly elevated. In between the attacks, serum potassium levels are within normal limits. Increase in serum potassium levels (usually to 5–6 mEq/L) are associated with attacks of weakness, though serum levels may remain within normal limits. Serum sodium levels can fall during episodes of weakness. During attacks, there is increased urinary excretion of potassium that can actually result in transient hypokalemia at the end of an attack. On EKG, the hyperkalemia can result in increased amplitudes of the precordial T waves.

Secondary causes of hyperkalemia can cause generalized weakness and must be excluded particularly in individuals with no family history (Table 32-3). Usually the serum potassium levels are greater than 7 mEq/L. Patients with secondary causes of hyperkalemic do not exhibit clinical or electrical myotonia. While provocative testing such as potassium challenge has been performed in the past when the diagnosis is unclear, there are obvious risks of such testing. The availability of commercial genetic testing and features on

TABLE 32-3. ETIOLOGIES OF SECONDARY HYPOKALEMIC AND HYPERKALEMIC PARALYSES

Hypokalemic paralysis
Thyrotoxic periodic paralysis
Renal tubular acidosis
Gitelman syndrome
Villous adenoma
Bartter syndrome
Hyperaldosteronism
Chronic or excessive use of diuretics, corticosteroids, licorice
Amphotericin B toxicity
Alcoholism
Toluene toxicity
Barium poisoning
Hyperkalemic paralysis
Addison disease
Hypoaldosteronism (hyporeninemic)
Isolated aldosterone deficiency
Excessive potassium supplementation
Potassium-sparing diuretics (e.g., spironolactone, triamterene)
Chronic renal failure
Rhabdomyolysis

Modified with permission from Amato AA, Dumitru D. Hereditary myopathies. In: Dumitru D, Amato AA, Swartz MJ, eds. *Electrodiagnostic Medicine*, 2nd ed. Philadelphia, PA: Hanley & Belfus, Inc.; 2002.

electrophysiological testing obviate the need for such provocative testing.

Routine motor and sensory NCS are normal between attacks of weakness.[53–56] However, during an attack of weakness, the CMAP amplitudes may be reduced in affected muscles. As previously mentioned, the SET and LET can be useful in distinguishing subtypes of channelopathies.[7–9] With the SET test, some patients with HyperKPP, depending on the exact mutation (e.g., T704M), have abnormal increased CMAP amplitudes that persist for a longer period of time than normal individuals.[7,9] Further, repetition of short exercise amplifies the increase in CMAP amplitudes. With the LET, during the exercise period and immediately afterwards, there is an initial increase in CMAP amplitudes from baseline that is followed by a progressive decline in the amplitudes over the next 40–50 minutes. Brief exercise (e.g., 10 seconds) during this paretic phase may induce an increment in the CMAP amplitudes (Fig. 32-5).[7] This constellation of findings on SET and LET is termed Fournier Pattern IV.

Needle EMG reveals variable findings. Myotonic discharges are found in 50–75% of affected individuals, though clinical myotonia is apparent in less than 20%.[7,57] In patients with myotonia, examination of the muscle between attacks of weakness reveals an increase in insertional activity, in the form of fibrillation potentials and positive sharp waves, in addition to myotonic discharges. These abnormal discharges reflect the hyperexcitability or instability of the muscle membrane and are not due to denervation. Reducing the limb temperature may exacerbate the runs of myotonic discharges. Analysis of MUAP parameters may reveal a slight increase in small amplitude, short duration, polyphasic potentials. In people with HyperKPP without myotonia, the insertional and spontaneous activity is normal between attacks of weakness. During an attack of weakness, the MUAPs decrease in duration and amplitude and may disappear altogether in plegic muscles.

Histopathology

Muscle biopsy in patients with HyperKPP frequently reveals nonrimmed vacuoles.[12,58,59]

Molecular Genetics and Pathogenesis

Potassium sensitive periodic paralysis is caused by mutations in the α-subunit of the voltage-dependent sodium channel gene (*SCN4A*) (Fig. 32-4).[5,13,38,41,60–62]

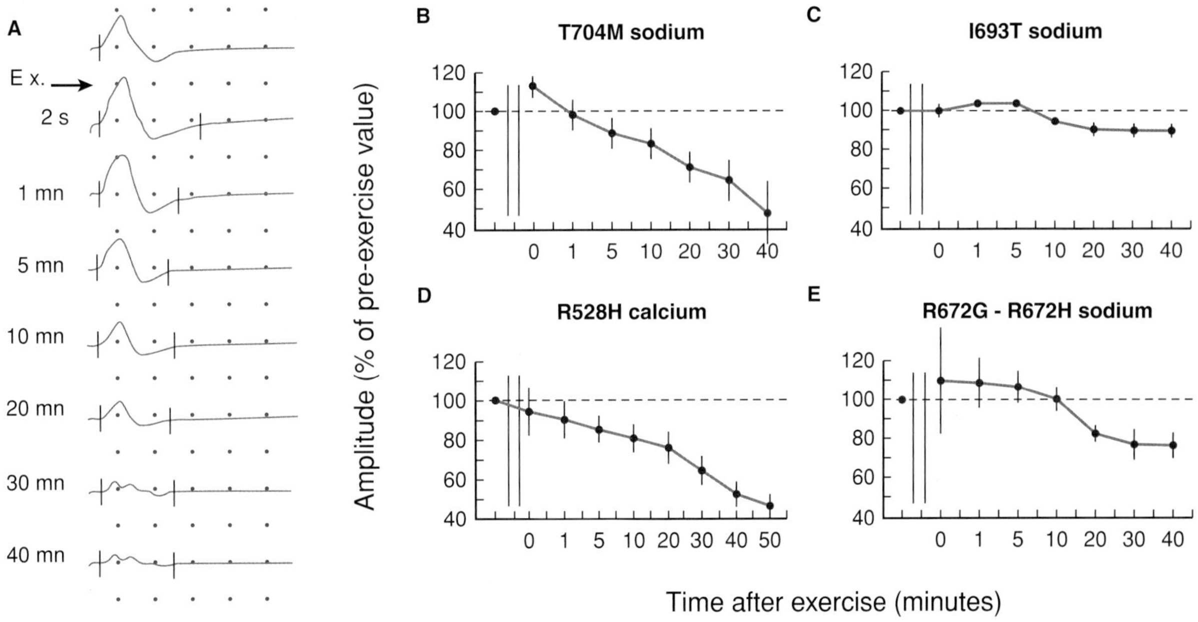

Figure 32-5. Long exercise test in periodic paralyses. **(A)** Early increase (+38%) and delayed decrease (−74%) of compound muscle action potential (CMAP) amplitude after long exercise in HyperKPP patient with the T704M sodium channel mutation. Pre-exercise (*top trace*) and postexercise recordings (*bottom trace*) at different times following the trial (Ex.) as indicated left of the traces. Scale between two dots: 5 ms, 5 mV. Changes in CMAP amplitude of the abductor digiti minimi (ADM) muscle after long exercise *(double bars)* in six HyperKPP patients with T704M sodium channel mutations **(B)**, six Myotonia-HyperKPP patients with the I693T mutation of the sodium channel **(C)**, 13 HypoKPP1 patients with the R528H calcium channel mutation **(D)**, and two HypoKPP2 patients with R672G or R672G sodium channel mutations **(E)**. The amplitude of the CMAP, expressed as a percentage of its pre-exercise value, is plotted against the time elapsed after the exercise trial *(symbols* and *vertical bars)*. Means ± standard errors of the means. (Reproduced with permission from Fournier E., Arzel M, Sternberg D, et al. Electromyography guides toward subgroups of mutations in muscle channelopathies. *Ann Neurol.* 2004;56(5):650–661.)

Treatment

Attack frequency may be reduced with a low-potassium, high-carbohydrate diet and avoidance of fasting, strenuous activity, and cold. Mild, short-lasting attacks of weakness usually do not require treatment. Sometimes a simple ingestion of simple carbohydrates (e.g., fruit juices, glucose-containing candies) decreases the serum potassium level by increasing insulin secretion and may improve strength. Beta-adrenergic agonists (e.g., metaproterenol, albuterol, salbutamol) also may increase strength but one needs to take care in regard to associated cardiac arrhythmias. Beta-adrenergic medications may have their effect through the sodium–potassium pump. Only in severe attacks of weakness is treatment with intravenous glucose, insulin, or calcium carbonate warranted. Prophylactic use of acetazolamide (125–1000 mg per day), chlorothiazide (250–1000 mg per day), or dichlorphenamide (50–150 mg per day) may be beneficial in reducing the frequency of attacks and perhaps the myotonia, though dichlorphenamide is no longer commercially available.[16,29,36] Mexiletine may be useful in managing myotonia when it is bothersome.

PARAMYOTONIA CONGENITA (EULENBURG DISEASE)

Clinical Features

PMC is an autosomal-dominant disorder with high penetrance that is allelic to potassium-sensitive periodic paralysis, which probably explains why many patients have clinical features of both disorders (paralysis periodica paramyotonia).[1–4,12,29,30,50,63–67] The name derives from the "para"-doxical reaction to exercise. In contrast to the warm-up phenomena observed in other myotonic syndromes, repeated exercise worsens the muscle stiffness in patients with PMC. Paramyotonia, particularly of the eyelids, is typically evident in most affected individuals. Myotonia is also exacerbated by exercise or cold exposure. A cold-induced attack of weakness can last for several hours even after return to a warm environment. Weakness can also be induced in some cases by potassium intake. Further attacks of weakness can be focal or generalized attacks of weakness.

Symptoms and signs of PMC usually manifest within the first decade of life. During a crying spell, infants may be noted to have difficulty opening their eyes secondary to the "exercise"-induced myotonia of the orbicularis oculi muscles. While percussion myotonia may be demonstrated, it is usually not prominent. Some people complain of mild muscle pain, but myalgias are usually not as prominent as that seen in patients with DM2/PROMM which PMC can resemble. In addition, fixed, progressive weakness muscle weakness of proximal or distal muscles can develop over time.

Laboratory Features

Serum CK levels are usually mildly to moderately elevated. Serum potassium levels may be normal or elevated in some patients during an attack of paralysis. Skeletal muscle MRI scans may reveal nonspecific signal abnormalities.[18]

Routine sensory and motor NCS are normal between attacks of weakness.[63] Prolonged repetitive stimulation at rates exceeding 5 Hz or repetitive stimulation following a minute or more of exercise can induce a decrement in the CMAP in some patients.[20,63] The SET may demonstrate several distinctive abnormalities (Tables 32-1 and 32-2).[4,7–9] Immediately after 10 seconds of exercise, repetitive after-discharges may be seen on recorded CMAPs evoked by a single supramaximal stimulus (PEMPs) (Fig. 32-6). Subsequent stimuli are associated with reduction of these PEMPs. Also, there is decrement in the amplitudes of the main CMAP waveforms compared to baseline with repeated stimuli following the short exercise in some patients. We repeat the SET with a 10-second break in between epochs to increase the yield of finding abnormalities. Upon repetition of the short exercise, even in those

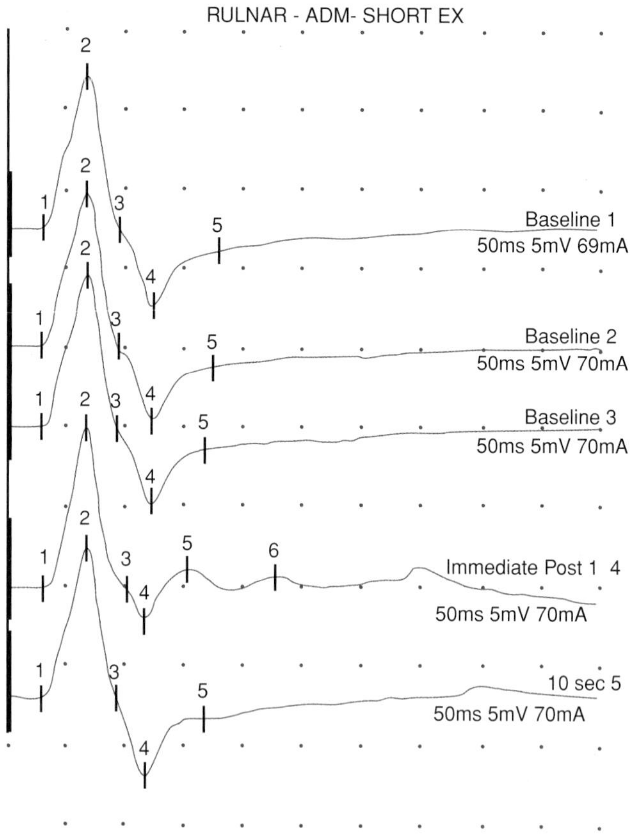

Figure 32-6. Postexercise myotonic potentials (PEMPs). PEMPs are seen following SET in a patient with paramyotonia congenita. The top three tracings are baseline compound muscle action potentials (CMAPs). Following short exercise of 10 seconds, the fourth trace from the top demonstrates PEMPs following the CMAP (labeled as 5 and 6 with tracer). The fifth CMAP 10 seconds no longer demonstrates any PEMPs.

patients who do not show any CMAP decline after the first trial, one may see marked reduction of CMAP amplitudes by the third trial (Fig. 32-1A). In some patients, there is also a gradual decrease in PEMPs. This so-called Fournier Pattern I is seen in approximately 90% of patients with PMC caused by a T1313M mutation in the *SCN4A* gene (Tables 32-1 and 32-2).[4,7,9] Fournier et al. reported patients with R1448C also had Pattern I, but other series reported no decrement on SET in individuals with this mutation.[4,7,9] This pattern is for the most part distinct from that seen in MC and DM2, which PMC may clinical resemble. Individuals with PMC mutations caused by Q270K mutations in the *SCN4A* gene may have SET that resemble those seen in MC (Fournier Pattern II).[8] To further increase the yield, the SET should be repeated after the extremity has been cooled.[4,8,9] Cooling may bring out further abnormalities (even more marked reduction in amplitudes that worsen with repetition of short exercises than seen when the SET is performed at room temperature). Upon cooling, the SET in patients with Q270M mutations may convert to Fournier Pattern I that is more typical of PMC. With the LET, the CMAP amplitudes are markedly reduced during and following the exercise compared to baseline.[4,7,9,22,63] The amplitudes remain reduced for prolonged periods, sometimes exceeding an hour.

EMG reveals normal MUAPs though they are often difficult to appreciate with the background of diffuse myotonic discharges.[4,7,65] In patients with PMC and periodic paralysis, local cooling of the muscle results in dense fibrillation potentials and the gradual reduction in MUAP activity. As the muscle becomes flaccid, the myotonic discharges abate and complete electrical silence is observed. In contrast, in patients with pure PMC without periodic paralysis, local cooling of the muscle results in increased myotonic discharges, but MUAP morphology and recruitment remain normal and the muscle strength remains normal. Single fiber EMG reveals a slight increase in jitter and fiber density.[66]

Histopathology

Muscle biopsy reveals nonspecific myopathic features and mild fiber size variation with a mixture of normal, atrophic and hypertrophic fibers.[67] Intracytoplasmic vacuoles may be appreciated, particularly in those individuals with superimposed periodic paralysis. Electron microscopy (EM) may show myofibrillar disarray and tubular aggregates.

Molecular Genetics and Pathogenesis

PMC with and without episodes of periodic paralysis are caused by mutations in *SCN4A* (Fig. 32-4).[1,5,39,41,68]

Treatment

A randomized, placebo-controlled trial of mexiletine (200 mg three times daily) was helpful in reducing muscle stiffness.[27] Cold-induced decrements of baseline CMAP amplitudes following exercise or repetitive stimulation may also improve with mexiletine.[69]

POTASSIUM-AGGRAVATED MYOTONIAS (MYOTONIA FLUCTUANS, MYOTONIA PERMANENS, AND ACETAZOLAMIDE-RESPONSIVE MYOTONIA)

PAM are also caused by mutations in the muscle sodium channel gene and are allelic to HyperKPP and PMC (Table 32-1).[1,4,7-9] Individuals with these disorders have myotonia without episodes of weakness. The electrophysiology of these disorders is more variable. Most of the time, SET is normal (Fig. 32-1D), but Fournier Patterns I and II may be seen. In those with normal SET at room temperature, cooling may result in reduced CMAP amplitudes that worsen with repeated short exercises similar to what is seen in PMC (conversion to Fournier Pattern I).[8] The LET in patients with PAM is usually normal. A randomized, placebo-controlled trial of mexiletine (200 mg three times daily) was helpful in reducing muscle stiffness in a study of nondystrophic myotonias that included PAM.[27]

MYOTONIA FLUCTUANS

Clinical Features

Myotonia fluctuans is characterized by (1) fluctuating myotonia of varying severity, (2) increased myotonia of delayed onset (several minutes) following exercise, (3) paramyotonia of eyelids, (4) warm-up phenomena of myotonia in the limbs, (5) no episodes of weakness nor weakness following potassium loading, exercise, or cold, and (6) increased myotonia with potassium but not with exposure to cold.[30,43,44,70] The fluctuating severity of the myotonia is unlike that seen in MC, PMC, and HyperKPP associated with myotonia. The severity of the myotonia can range from absolutely no stiffness to severe myotonia affecting the extraocular muscles, the muscles of mastication and swallowing, and the extremities. Myotonia fluctuans is also dissimilar from other myotonic disorders in that exercise induces myotonia, which is delayed in onset. The stiffness is not worse in the cold.

Laboratory Features

Serum CK levels are usually slightly elevated. The SET may be normal or shows mild reduction in amplitude that improves with repeated stimulation (i.e., Fournier Pattern II), similar to what is seen in MC without change in response to cooling.[7,8] The LET is normal.

Histopathology

Muscle biopsies may be normal or show increased internalized nuclei and fiber size variability.[44] Subsarcolemmal vacuoles may be appreciated on EM.[43]

Molecular Genetics and Pathogenesis

Myotonia fluctuans is caused by mutations in *SCN4A*.[13,43,44]

Treatment

Mexiletine[27] and avoidance of high-potassium foods may be helpful.

MYOTONIA PERMANENS

Clinical Features

Myotonia permanens is associated with constant muscle stiffness that is aggravated by potassium and following activity.[28,29,51,71] Affected people may develop dyspnea, acidosis, and hypoxia related to severe myotonia affecting ventilatory muscles. Neither episodic weakness nor exacerbation of myotonia with cold is seen.

Laboratory Features

Serum CK levels are normal or only mildly elevated.

Histopathology

Biopsy results have not been well described.

Molecular Genetics and Pathogenesis

Myotonia permanens is usually caused by G1306A mutations in *SCN4A*.[28,71]

Treatment

Mexiletine may be beneficial.[27]

ACETAZOLAMIDE-RESPONSIVE MYOTONIA

Clinical Features

Individuals with this disorder complain of painful muscle stiffness that begins in childhood but worsens with age into early adulthood.[13,32,72] The myotonia is most severe in the face and hands and is aggravated by potassium, fasting, and to a lesser extent by exercise. Muscle stiffness and pain may be eased by ingestion of high carbohydrate meals. Action and percussion myotonia are appreciated. Paradoxical myotonia may be found in the eyelids. Strength is normal.

Laboratory Features

Serum CK is usually mildly elevated. The SET may be normal or show mild reduction in amplitude that improves with repetitive activity (i.e., Fournier Pattern II) that is similar to what is seen in MC. There is no change with cooling.[7,8]

Histopathology

Muscle biopsies have been performed in only a few patients and have been normal or revealed generalized muscle fiber hypertrophy.

Molecular Genetics and Pathogenesis

Acetazolamide-responsive myotonia is also caused by mutations in *SCN4A*.[13,32,72]

Treatment

Acetazolamide may help diminish muscle stiffness and pain. We initiate treatment with acetazolamide 125 mg per day and titrated as tolerated to 250 mg three times daily. Mexiletine may also be helpful.

FAMILIAL HYPOKALEMIC PERIODIC PARALYSIS TYPE 2

Clinical Features

Most cases of familial HypoKPP are caused by mutations in the skeletal muscle voltage-gated calcium channel α-1 subunit (*CACNA1S*) gene (HypoKPP1).[5,12,35,36] However, several families have been identified with mutations in the *SCN4A* gene, so-called HypoKPP2.[5,12,33–36] HypoKPP2 is clinically similar to HypoKPP1. However, in a large retrospective series of molecularly defined HypoKPP1 and HypoKPP2 cases, the age of onset was earlier (average 10 years) and the duration of episodes longer (average 20 hours) in HypoKPP1 compared with HypoKPP2 (16 years of age and 1 hour of duration, respectively).[35] However, a study by a different group demonstrated a slightly older onset of symptoms in some cases of HypoKPP1 depending on the site of the mutation compared to HypoKPP2.[12] Greater than 70% of HypoKPP1 patients developed fixed proximal weakness compared with none of the HypoKPP2 patients.[35] Also, in regard to treatment, acetazolamide, which can be helpful in HypoKPP1, can occasionally exacerbate attacks of weakness in HypoKPP2.[35]

Laboratory Features

Serum potassium is reduced during the attacks. Serum CK may be normal or elevated. On the LET, a decrease of CMAP amplitudes are seen approximately 10–20 minutes after cessation of exercise (Table 32-1).[7] However, this decrement is less than what is typically observed in patients with a HyperKPP. EMG between attacks of muscle paralysis is usually normal and in particular, there are no myotonic discharges.[7,34,35]

Histopathology

While muscle biopsies in HypoKPP1 often demonstrate non-rimmed vacuoles within muscle fibers, biopsies in HypoKPP2 often reveal muscle fibers with tubular aggregates.[34,35]

Treatment

Some individuals with HypoKPP2 have a reduction of attacks with acetazolamide, but much fewer improve than in those with HypoKPP1[37] and some actually experience an exacerbation of weakness with acetazolamide rather than improvement.[35] Therefore, initiation of a trial of acetazolamide should be done cautiously in a patient with HypoKPP2 or HypoKPP in whom the genotype is unknown.

MOLECULAR GENETICS AND PATHOGENESIS/PATHOPHYSIOLOGY OF THE SODIUM CHANNELOPATHIES

The voltage-gated muscle sodium channel is a heterodimer composed of subunits that are encoded on chromosomes 17q23–25 and 19q13.1, respectively.[1,13,36] Point mutations in the subunit gene, *SCN4A*, are responsible for HyperKPP, PMC, and the various PAMs as previously discussed. No disorders are known to be caused by mutations in the β-subunit. The subunit has four homologous domains (I–IV) each containing six hydrophobic segments (S1–S6) that transverse the sarcolemmal membrane (Fig. 32-4).[1,13,26,30] An extracellular loop dips within the plasma membrane between S5 and S6 of each domain and participates in the formation of the pore. The S4 helix contains a repeating motif of positively charged amino acids at every third position suggesting that this region serves as the voltage sensor.[30] The S4 segment appears to be critical for inactivation of the open channel, while the S3 segment is important in the recovery of inactivated channels.[51] The interaction between the S3 and S4 segments is important for transition to and from inactivation states (Fig. 32-7).

Over 30 different point mutations in *SCN4A* have been reported and most are located in regions of the α-subunit critical for fast inactivation. Most of these missense mutations are associated with gain-of-function defects, which are either disrupted inactivation or enhanced activation. The notable exception is the mutations associated with HypoKPP2, which are all clustered in the voltage-sensor region of the second repeat (D2S4) and diminish activity by enhancing inactivation. The fast inactivation limits the number of sodium channels available for activation, which in turn leads to a refractory period, until there is repolarization of the muscle membrane.[1,8,28,51,60,73] The gain-of-function mutations associated with PMC and PAM typically slow the rate of inactivation three- to fivefold, resulting in a longer duration of the action potentials and increased availability of Na^+ channels (i.e., fraction not inactivated) at the end of each action potential that augment the membrane excitability and resulting myotonic discharges. In addition to slow inactivation, many PMC mutations also disrupt the final extent of inactivation. The steady inward Na current generated through the small fraction of mutant channels that have failed to inactivate, depolarizes the membrane to a new stable resting potential of approximately −50 mV. This results in inactivation of the wild-type and most of the mutant Na channels, resulting in a system that is refractory from generating an action potential, leading to a paralytic attack.[28,60,73] In these individuals, increased extracellular potassium results in further depolarization of the muscle membrane, thus leading to muscle fiber inexcitability.

In contrast, a process called "slow inactivation" limits the availability of sodium channels on a time scale of seconds to minutes, which can also affect muscle membrane excitability. Rare patients with *SCN4A* mutations manifesting as HyperKPP and myotonia have impaired slow inactivation, as opposed to defective fast inactivation.[74]

Patch clamp studies of intercostal muscles of patients with PMC demonstrate normal resting membrane potentials at 37°C, but cooling to 27°C leads to depolarization of the muscle membrane to approximately −40 mV.[60,73] As a result, spontaneous action potentials are generated secondary to the approximation of the resting membrane and threshold potentials that correlate with the cold-induced myotonia. Subsequently, the muscle membrane may remain in a depolarized state for a prolonged period of time such that it is no longer capable of generating further action potentials, and therefore, the muscles become weak.[28,60,73]

In HyperKPP, mutant sodium channels are associated with large persistent currents that further increase, when extracellular potassium levels are elevated.[28,60,73] Increased extracellular potassium leads to depolarization of the muscle membrane and increased late openings of the noninactivated sodium channels.[51] The continued sodium influx sustains the depolarization of the membrane, which in turn leads to inactivation of normal sodium channels and subsequent muscle fiber inexcitability.

In HypoKPP2, mutations in gating-charge–carrying argentine residues in an S4 segment induce a hyperpolarization-activated cationic leak through the voltage sensor of the skeletal muscle sodium channel.[75,76] A sustained proton leak may contribute to instability of ion conductance indirectly, by interfering with intracellular pH homeostasis.[76]

▶ CALCIUM CHANNELOPATHIES

PRIMARY HYPOKALEMIC PERIODIC PARALYSIS TYPE 1 (HYPOKPP1)

Clinical Features

HypoKPP1 is an autosomal-dominant disorder with reduced penetrance in women (a male to female ratio of 3 or 4 to 1) and an overall prevalence of 0.13 to 1/100,000.[5,13,36] Onset of episodic weakness usually occurs in the first two decades of life. Individuals with HypoKPP1 do not have clinical or electrophysiological myotonia or paramyotonia which may be useful in distinguishing from the HyperKPP and PMC.

Attacks of weakness may be precipitated by strenuous physical activity followed by rest or sleep, high carbohydrates

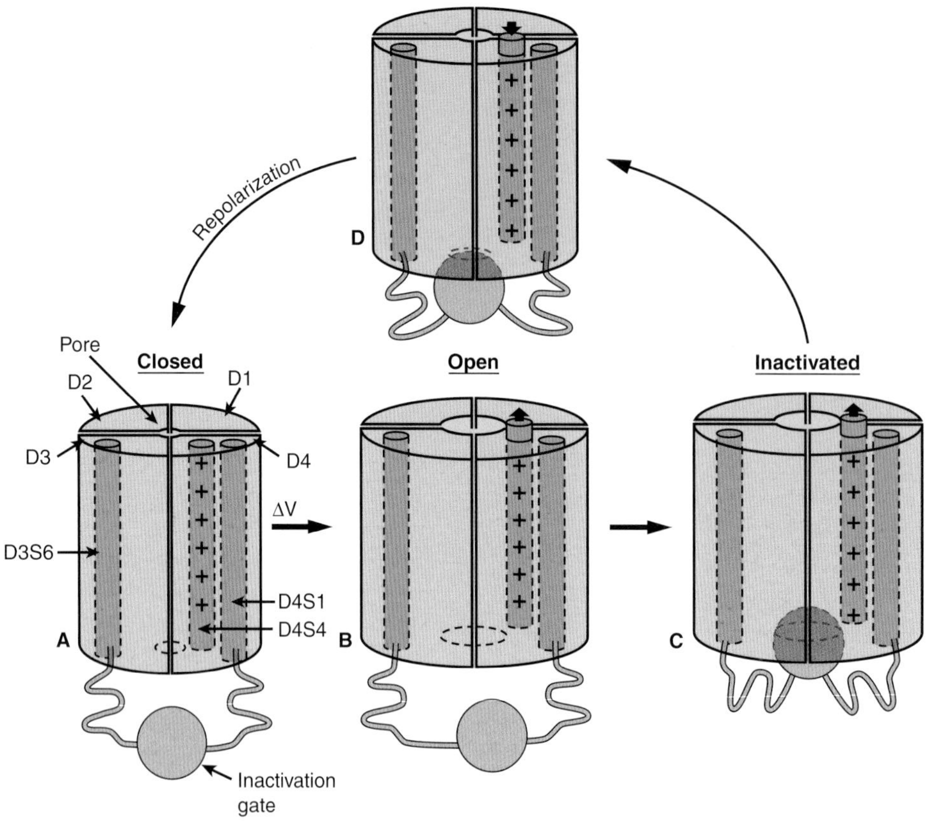

Figure 32-7. Cation channel model. voltage-gated sodium and calcium channels are believed to have similar structures and physiology. These cation channels have four domains (D1–D4) each containing six transmembrane segments. Cation channel model. This model shows the four domains (D1–D4, *blue*) of the cation channel arranged around the ion pore (*blue*) in the membrane. The S4 segments of cation channels contain a repeating motif of positively charged (+) amino acids (arginine or lysine) at every third position separated by two neutral amino acids. In the closed state **(A)**, the pore (*blue*) is closed and the inactivation gate (*brown*) is open. In response to depolarization, the S4 segments (*darker blue*) shown here move slightly under the influence of electrostatic forces. The S4 segment of domain 4 is the site of two of the recognized mutations in patients with paramyotonia congenita. Depolarization leads to a conformational shift that results in the pore (*blue*) opening **(B)**. Channel closing is thought to result from a "ball-valve" mechanism where the cytoplasmic loop (*brown*) between domains D3 and D4 falls into the ion pore, thus blocking it **(C)**. In this model, repolarization would then result in the protein assuming its closed conformation **(D)** and release of the inactivation gate. The channel is now in the closed state **(A)** and is ready to open in response to the next depolarization. (Reproduced with permission from Ptacek LJ. The familial periodic paralyses and nondystrophic myotonias. *Am J Med*. 1998;105(1):58–70.)

and sodium meals, alcohol consumption, emotional stress, concurrent viral illness, lack of sleep, and/or menstruation. Specific medications (e.g., beta agonists, corticosteroids, and insulin) are also triggers for attacks. Episodes of weakness can occur at any time of day, although most occur in the morning.

The severity of an attack can range from mild focal weakness of an isolated muscle group to severe generalized paralysis. Facial and ventilatory muscles as well as the sphincter muscles are typically spared or only minimally affected. Nevertheless, ventilatory muscle involvement and cardiac arrhythmia secondary to hypokalemia have occurred.[77] When weakness is profound, the muscle is electrically unexcitable. Reflexes are absent when muscles are severely affected. Severe muscle weakness usually last for several hours to more than a day, though many individuals note a residual weakness for several days following an attack. Typically, those muscles affected last are the first to recover.

The frequency of these attacks of weakness is also highly variable—they can occur several times a week to less than once a year. After the age of 30 years the frequency of the attacks often diminish and some individuals become free of attacks in their 40s or 50s. On the other hand, many patients develop permanent fixed or slowly progressive weakness over time.[12,36,78] Proximal muscles, especially in the legs, are more prone to developing fixed weakness.

Often an attack of periodic weakness is heralded by a sensation of heaviness or aching in the low back, thighs, and calves which spreads to involve other muscle groups, primarily those in the proximal upper limbs. Mild exercise during this prodrome may stave off the full-blown attack of weakness; however, this is not always successful.

Laboratory Features

Serum potassium levels are usually below 3.0 mEq/L during an attack of weakness though between attacks the serum potassium is normal. The EKG may demonstrate bradycardia, flattened T waves, prolonged PR and QT intervals, and notably U waves secondary to the hypokalemia. Serum CK levels are usually mildly elevated and increase during attacks of weakness. Provocative testing using intravenous glucose load, and sometimes insulin, was used in the past to lower the serum potassium to assist in diagnosis, but is not longer performed.

Sensory and motor NCS are normal between attacks of weakness.[78,79] However, surface recordings have revealed reduced muscle fiber conduction velocity between paralytic attacks.[80] During paralytic attacks, sensory studies remain normal, but the CMAP amplitudes are reduced secondary to muscle membrane inexcitability. Repetitive stimulation of mildly affected muscles demonstrates preservation of CMAP amplitudes to some degree, supporting the clinical impression that mild exercise can stave off an attack.

In contrast to individuals with HyperKPP, there are minimal changes in CMAP amplitudes immediately after the exercise phase of the SETs/LETs in those with HypoKPP (Table 32-1).[7,9] However, with the LET, there is usually a delayed decline in CMAP amplitudes ($-51 \pm 10\%$). The reduction in amplitudes is usually less in those with HypoKPP2 compared to HypoKPP1.[7]

EMG between attacks of muscle paralysis is usually normal.[79] However, EMG early in an attack of weakness reveals a slight increase in insertional and spontaneous potentials (e.g., fibrillation potentials and positive sharp waves), which are a reflection of the hyperirritable muscle membranes and not indicative of denervation. As the paralytic attack progresses, there is a decrease in the amplitude and duration of voluntary MUAPs as well as an overall decrease in the number of MUAPs contributing to the interference pattern. When the paralytic attack is maximal, there is marked reduction or complete absence of insertional activity, and there are minimal, if any, voluntary MUAPs. In patients who develop persistent muscle weakness, small amplitude, short duration, polyphasic MUAPs that recruit early may be appreciated in weak muscles along with rare fibrillation potentials and positive sharp waves.

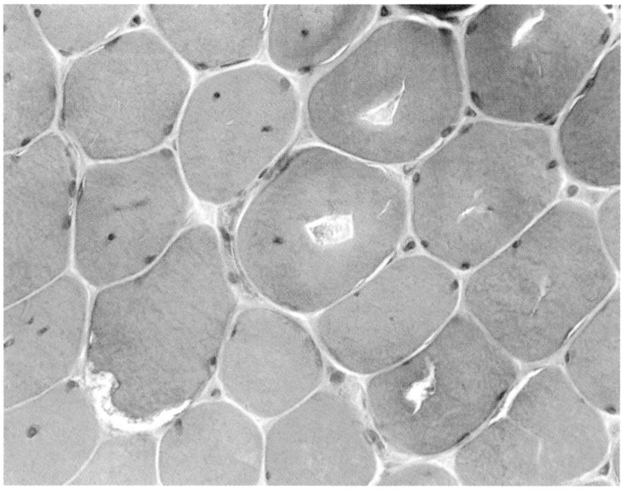

Figure 32-8. Muscle biopsy in a patient with HypoKPP reveals muscle fibers with vacuoles. Modified Gomori trichrome stain.

Between attacks, single fiber EMG shows normal jitter along with a slight increase in fiber density. The latter is likely the result of a mild myopathic process with muscle fiber splitting which can be appreciated on histopathology. During an attack, the reduction in muscle membrane excitability results in a dropout of single muscle fibers and a decrease in fiber density, compared to both normal and interattack values for the patients. This is accompanied by a slight increase in jitter with occasional blocking of potentials.[81]

Histopathology

Muscle biopsies may reveal intracellular vacuoles, tubular aggregates, and dilation of the sarcoplasmic reticulum (Fig. 32-8).[12,35,59] HypoKPP1 is more likely to be associated with vacuoles on biopsy, while tubular aggregates are more common in HypoKPP2.[12,35] Muscle fiber size variation, split fibers, hypertrophic, and some atrophic fibers can also be present. Rarely, necrotic and degenerating muscle fibers are noted.

Molecular Genetics and Pathogenesis

Approximately 70% of cases of familial HypoKPP1 are caused by mutations in the α-subunits of skeletal muscle l-type calcium channel gene, *CACNA1S*, located on chromosome 1q31–3245.[5,13,33,77] In 10% of affected individuals (HypoKPP2), the mutations are present in the α-subunits of skeletal muscle sodium channel gene, *SCN4A*, and no identifiable mutation is found in the remaining 20% of patients. For both HypoKPP1 and HypoKPP2, the mutations occur in highly conserved arginine residues in the voltage-sensing segments of the calcium channel.[13,33] In addition, rare cases of HypoKPP have been associated with mutations in another potassium channel gene, *KCNE3*.[82] Further, Gitelman syndrome, caused by mutations affecting the thiazide-sensitive sodium chloride co-transporter, may also cause hypokalemic paralysis.[83]

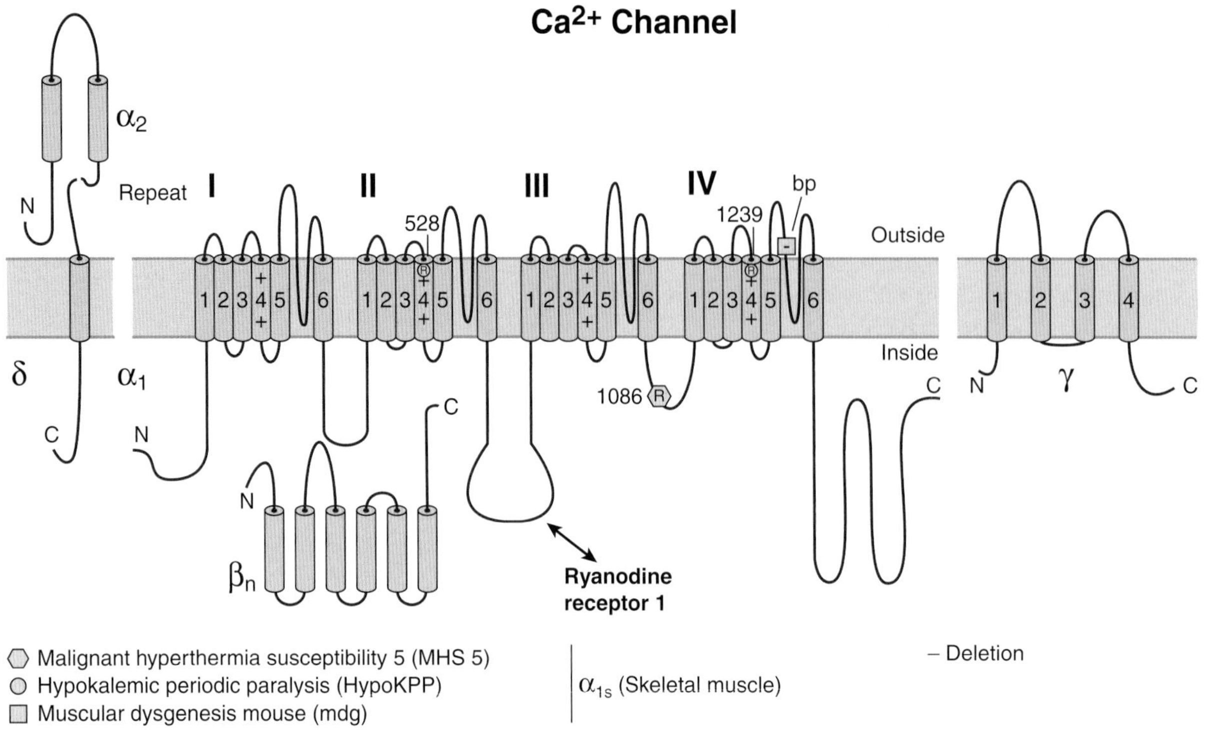

Figure 32-9. Subunits of voltage-gated calcium channel. α-subunit resembles that of sodium channel; however, function of various parts, for example, III–IV linker, may not be the same. α_2/δ, $\beta_1-\beta_4$, and γ are auxiliary subunits. Mutations shown here, α_{1S}-subunit of skeletal muscle L-type calcium channel (= dihydropyridine receptor), have been described for humans (HypoKPP, MHS 5) and mice (mdg). Conventional one-letter abbreviations are used for replaced amino acids whose positions are given by respective numbers of α_{1S}-subunit. Symbols used for point mutations indicate resulting diseases as explained at *bottom left*. (Reproduced with permission from Lehmann-Horn F, Jurkat-Rott K. Voltage-gated ion channels and hereditary disease. *Physiol Rev*. 1999;79:1317–1372.)

The voltage-gated calcium channel ($Ca_V1.1$), also known as the dihydropyridine receptor, is composed of five subunits (α1, α2, β, δ, and γ). The α1-subunit is composed of four domains, each containing six trans-membrane segments (S1–S6), and links to the ryanodine receptor (Fig. 32-9).[38] This receptor that functions not only as a calcium ion channel for the transverse tubules of skeletal muscle, but also as a voltage-sensor for excitation–contraction coupling (Fig. 32-10).[26] The other subunits of the calcium channel regulate the function of the α1-subunit.[38] The S4 segment of the α1-subunit confers the voltage-sensing properties to the channel, and is the site for most of the mutations identified in patients with HypoKPP1.

The mechanism for the induced attacks of weakness in HypoKPP1 is not completely understood.[13,77,84–87] Myofibers are depolarized and inexcitable during an attack. In vitro, muscle fibers from patients with HypoKPP1 exposed to low K solutions paradoxically depolarize. However, the source of the depolarizing current has remained elusive. The available data suggest a loss-of-function defect with reduced ionic current density. A study on fibers biopsied from a patient with an R528H calcium channel mutation detected a reduction in ATP-sensitive K current, more easily tying it to the depolarization seen with hypokalemia, and suggesting a secondary channelopathy resulting from altered calcium homeostasis. It has also been posited that reduced calcium influx through the T-tubule may be the cause of impaired excitation–contraction coupling.

The DHP receptor functions as a calcium channel as well as a voltage-sensor for excitation–contraction coupling. Electrophysiological recordings of myotubes expressing mutant calcium channels reveal diminished calcium current and a negative shift of the steady-state inactivation current.[77] Decreased calcium influx through the T-tubule may impair excitation–contraction coupling. Furthermore, the kinetics of the sodium channel also appear to be influenced by mutations involving *CACNA1S*. The sodium conductance is increased in the resting state leading depolarization of the resting membrane potential from about −80 mV to around −50 mV. In this partially depolarized state, the number of sodium channels available to activate is likely reduced, thus, creating an inexcitable membrane and clinical weakness.

Treatment

The primary mode of therapy is reducing exposure to known triggers (e.g., avoiding ingestion of high-carbohydrate

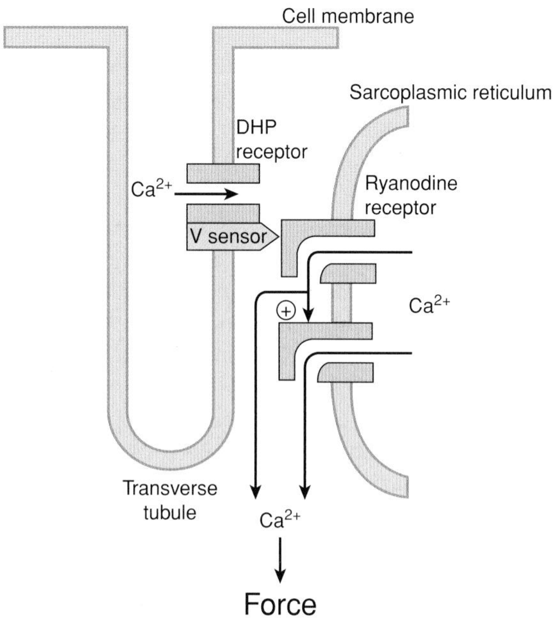

Figure 32-10. Triadic junction between a transverse tubule and sarcoplasmic reticulum: position of two calcium channels of skeletal muscle, L-type calcium channel, also called dihydropyridine (DHP) receptor, and calcium release channel, also called ryanodine receptor. Coupling between the two channels is not fully elucidated. Mutations in respective genes cause hypokalemic periodic paralysis, malignant hyperthermia, or central core disease. (Reproduced with permission from Lehmann-Horn F, Jurkat-Rott K. Voltage–gated ion channels and hereditary disease. *Physiol Rev*. 1999;79:1317–1372.)

meals, extremely strenuous exercise). Acetazolamide (125–1500 mg/day) and potassium salts (0.25–0.5 mEq/kg) are often prescribed prophylactically in order to prevent hypokalemia and reduce attacks of weakness. However, a large retrospective study found that only approximately 50% of genotyped patients with HyopKPP1 responded to acetazolamide and even fewer with HypoKPP2.[37] Importantly, acetazolamide may actually induce attacks of weakness in individuals with HypoKPP2 caused by *SCNA4* mutations.[12,36,37] Dichlorphenamide (50–150 mg/day) also may be effective in reducing attack frequency and severity, but unfortunately it is no longer available.[16] Triamterene (25–100 mg/day) or spironolactone (25–100 mg/day) may be used in an attempt to prevent attacks and perhaps to improve interattack weakness when acetazolamide is not effective. Acute attacks of weakness can be treated with oral potassium salts (0.25 mEq/kg body weight) every 30 minutes until strength improves.

In severe attacks and if the patient's condition precludes oral potassium, intravenous potassium (KCL bolus 0.05–0.1 mEq/kg body weight or 20–40 mEq/L of KCL in 5% mannitol) may be administered. Cardiac monitoring is essential throughout treatment. HypoKPP1 may be allelic with MH, so it is not surprising that MH without periodic paralysis has been described with mutation in *CACNA1S*. Hence, all HypoKPP patients undergoing surgery should be monitored for MH-like reactions (rigidity and marked elevation in CK). However, postoperative paralysis in this group of patients is more likely related to the stress of surgery.

SECONDARY HYPOKALEMIC PARALYSIS

Secondary HypoKPP needs to be excluded, particularly if there is no family history or in those with onset after the third decade of life (Table 32-3). Urinary or gastrointestinal dumping of potassium may precipitate attacks of weakness and cause a necrotizing myopathy. Muscle strength improves with correction of the hypokalemia.

THYROTOXIC PERIODIC PARALYSIS

Thyrotoxic periodic paralysis (TPP) resembles HypoKPP, except that there is typically no family history.[88] TPP is more common in Asian adults, but it occurs worldwide. Interestingly, although hyperthyroidism is more common in women, the majority of cases of TPP occur in men. Affected individuals can also develop progressive muscle weakness secondary to hyperthyroidism itself. The attacks of weakness dissipate with treatment and correction of the dysthyroid state but can recur with redevelopment of hyperthyroidism. Acetazolamide does not appear to have any significant benefit. However, β-blockers may be effective in reducing the frequency and severity of the paralytic attacks in thyrotoxic patients. Mutations in the *KCNJ18* gene that encodes an inwardly rectifying potassium (Kir) channel, Kir2.6, has been reported in about 33% of patients in the United States, France, and Brazil with TPP.[88,89] In addition, genome-wide screening of Asians with TPP found linkage to possible genetic mutation in *KCNJ2* which encodes for KIR2.1.[90–92]

▶ OTHER FORMS OF PERIODIC PARALYSIS

ANDERSEN–TAWIL SYNDROME (ANDERSEN SYNDROME OR KLEIN–LISAK–ANDERSEN SYNDROME)

Clinical Features

ATS is a rare ion channel disorder characterized by the clinical triad of periodic paralysis, ventricular arrhythmias associated with long QT, and skeletal developmental anomalies.[36,93–97] A diagnosis of ATS can be made when an individual exhibits two of these three cardinal features. Only about 60% of affected individuals manifest the complete triad, while approximately 80% express two of the three cardinal features. Inheritance is autosomal-dominant although de novo mutations are frequent, and phenotypic expression is extremely variable. A large, recent study found the prevalence in England to be approximately 0.08 per 100,000.[5]

The neuromuscular manifestations of ATS consist of episodic weakness that may arise spontaneously or be triggered by rest following exertion. The attacks of paralysis usually begin in the first or second decade of life and may be associated with elevated, normal or most commonly decreased serum potassium levels. The attacks vary in duration (hours to days), severity, and frequency ranging from a single lifetime event to daily bouts of weakness. Permanent proximal weakness often develops over time. Patients with ATS do not show evidence of myotonia or paramyotonia.

Cardiac manifestations include potentially life-threatening arrhythmias, including bidirectional ventricular tachycardia (VT), polymorphic VT, and torsades de pointes. The cardiac arrhythmias may be asymptomatic or manifest as palpitations, syncope, or even cardiac arrest necessitating defibrillator implantation. No specific triggers have been associated with the ventricular arrhythmias of ATS. One of the most common ECG findings is a long QT interval, which is recognized as an integral feature of ATS and may serve as a trigger for fatal ventricular arrhythmias. Thus, ATS must be considered in all individuals presenting with episodic weakness and/or a long QT syndrome.

Developmental anomalies associated with ATS include clinodactyly, hypertelorism, low set ears, mandibular hypoplasia, syndactyly, and scoliosis. Other features less commonly associated are short stature, a broad nose and forehead, cleft or high-arched palate, short digits, vaginal atresia, brachydactyly, cardiac valve abnormalities, and hypoplastic kidneys. Neurocognitive abnormalities may occur characterized by deficits in executive function and abstract reasoning.

Laboratory Features

Serum CK can be normal or only slightly elevated. Serum potassium levels may be normal, elevated or decreased during attacks of weakness. A prolonged QT interval is present in 80% of patients, while some have even more ominous ventricular tachyarrhythmias as previously discussed. Routine motor and sensory NCS are normal. The LET usually reveals a decrement in the CMAP area and to a lesser extent the amplitude.[9] EMG is usually normal as well between attacks of weakness. Myotonic discharges are not seen.

Histopathology

Tubular aggregates, similar to those observed in other forms of periodic paralysis, may be appreciated on muscle biopsies.

Molecular Genetics and Pathogenesis

Approximately two-thirds of ATS patients have missense mutations or small deletions in the *KCNJ2* gene (ATS1).[5,93,95,98,99] This gene encodes for the inwardly rectifying potassium channel (Kir2.1) and is predominantly expressed in heart, skeletal muscle, and brain. This mutation leads to impairment of muscle membrane and perhaps neuronal depolarization and repolarization, but its role in the associated skeletal developmental anomalies is not well understood. Kir2.1 channels help stabilize resting membrane potentials. The majority of *KCNJ2* mutations result in the failure of appropriate conduction, and many alter the binding of phosphatidylinositol 4, 5 bisphosphate, an important regulator of Kir2.1 channel function. It is postulated that reduced Kir2.1 channel function in skeletal muscle may result in sustained membrane depolarization, failure of action potential propagation, and flaccid paralysis. It may also prolong the most terminal phase of repolarization in the heart and lead to delayed after-depolarizations. Approximately 20% of patients with an ATS phenotype have no mutation of *KCJN2* (ATS2).

Treatment

It is important to be aware of and recognize the potential cardiac conduction abnormalities. Malignant arrhythmias may be treated with antiarrhythmic agents or pacemaker insertion. Small doses of acetazolamide may prevent paralytic attacks in some patients.

► OTHER SKELETAL MUSCLE CHANNELOPATHIES

OTHER POTASSIUM CHANNELOPATHIES

A few kindreds with periodic paralysis have been found to have mutations in another potassium channel gene, *KCNE3*.[82] Attacks of weakness have been associated with low serum potassium levels in some but not other cases.

OTHER CALCIUM CHANNELOPATHIES

Some cases of central core disease and MH are caused by mutations in the ryanodine receptor gene, *RYR1*, encoded on chromosome 19q13.1.[100] The ryanodine receptor is responsible for the release of calcium from the sarcoplasmic reticulum. Central core disease is discussed in Chapter 28 regarding Congenital Myopathies. MHS3 is caused by mutations in another calcium channel gene, *CACNA2D1*. Brody disease is caused by mutations in SERCA1 gene, *ATP2A1*, which encodes the fast-twitch skeletal muscle sarcoplasmic reticulum calcium ATPase, and is discussed in more detail in a later section.

MALIGNANT HYPERTHERMIA

Clinical Features

MH is a syndrome rather than a specific disorder that is characterized by severe muscle rigidity, myoglobinuria, fever, tachycardia, cyanosis, and cardiac arrhythmias precipitated by depolarizing muscle relaxants (e.g., succinylcholine) and fluorinated inhalational anesthetic agents (e.g., halothane).[101] The incidence of MH in patients exposed to general anesthesia varies from 0.5–0.0005%.[101] Importantly, at least 50% of patients who developed MH had previous anesthesia without any problem—so a negative history in this regard is not helpful. Signs of MH usually develop during surgery, but they can occur postoperatively. Rarely, attacks of MH have been induced following strenuous activity, ingestion of caffeine, or by stress.

Laboratory Features

Serum CK can be normal or mildly elevated between attacks. However, during an episode of MH, the serum CK levels become markedly elevated and myoglobinuria and renal insufficiency can ensue. In addition, metabolic and respiratory acidosis may develop with lactic acidosis, hypoxia, hypercarbia, and hyperkalemia. NCS and EMG are usually normal between episodes of MH unless the patient has a predisposing myopathic disorder, for example, PMC. Determining susceptibility to MH in the absence of genetic testing requires in vitro muscle contracture test. Unfortunately, this test is not readily available.[101]

Histopathology

Muscle biopsies demonstrate nonspecific myopathic features including fiber size variability, increased internal nuclei, moth-eaten fibers, and necrotic fibers after an attack of MH.

Pathogenesis and Molecular Genetics

MH susceptibility is genetically heterogeneous. MHS1 is caused by mutations in the *RYR1* gene located on chromosome 19q13.1.[100] These mutations may lead to an excessive release of calcium into the cytoplasm upon activation. Of note, mutations in this gene are also responsible for the congenital myopathy, central core disease. However, only a minority of patients with MH have mutations in the ryanodine receptor gene. MHS2 localizes to chromosome 17q11.2–q24 (possibly the gene for the subunit of the sodium channel). Thus, MHS2 may be allelic to HyperKPP, PMC, and PAM. MHS3 mutations in *CACNA2D1*, which also encodes a calcium channel subunit. MHS4 localizes to chromosome 3q13.1, but the gene has yet to be identified. MHS5 is allelic to HypoKPP1. Linkage to chromosome 5p has been demonstrated in still other families (MHS6). Besides these disorders, it is well known that patients with dystrophinopathies are susceptible to developing MH. Thus, it appears that MH may occur in various myopathic disorders affecting the structural proteins of the muscle membrane or ion channels.

Treatment

Anesthetic agents should be administered cautiously in people at risk for MH. If MH develops, the initial step is discontinuing the offending anesthetic agent while 100% oxygen is delivered.[101] Dantrolene 2–3 mg/kg every 5 minutes for a total of 10 mg/kg should be administered. The patient should be covered with cooling blankets and may even require lavage of the stomach, bladder, and lower gastrointestinal tract with iced saline solution. Acidosis and hyperkalemia are treated with sodium bicarbonate, hyperventilation, dextrose, insulin, and occasionally calcium chloride while the patient is monitored and treated for possible secondary cardiac arrhythmias. Urinary output must be maintained with hydration, furosemide, or mannitol.

BRODY DISEASE

Clinical Features

This rare disorder is characterized by impaired skeletal muscle relaxation following exercise.[102–104] Affected individuals complain of exercise-induced cramping and stiffness in the arms and legs. Recurrent myoglobinuria is an uncommon complication. Having the patient repeatedly open and close their fists or do several deep knee bends may induce delayed muscle relaxation that can be painful. Some patients also have impaired relaxation of the eyelids after forced eyelid closure. The muscle stiffness resembles paramyotonia as the stiffness worsens with activity. However, there is no percussion myotonia. Some people have mild proximal weakness on examination.

Laboratory Features

Serum CK levels are normal or only slightly elevated. Potassium levels are normal. Unlike the dynamic glycogen storage disorders, which it may mimic due to the exercise-induced cramps, an exercise forearm test reveals a normal rise in lactic acid and ammonia in Brody disease. NCS and EMG are normal.[102–104] Importantly, muscles exhibiting impaired relaxation are electrically silent, unlike what is observed in the myotonic disorders.

Histopathology

Muscle biopsies demonstrate type 2 muscle fiber atrophy and increased internalized nuclei. Decrease in calcium-ATPase in type 2 muscle fibers is appreciated with immunohistochemistry staining. On electron microscopy, swollen mitochondria with crystalline inclusions are rarely noted. As with MH, skeletal muscle fibers are extremely sensitive to caffeine.

Molecular Genetics and Pathogenesis

Brody disease is an autosomal recessive disorder caused by mutations in the *ATP2A1* gene located on chromosome 16p12.2–12.2.[102,104] This gene encodes for sarcoplasmic reticulum calcium-ATPase (SERCA1), a calcium channel present on the sarcoplasmic reticulum of type 2 muscle fibers. These mutations cause a decreased rate of ATP-dependent calcium transport across the channel. Normally, upon depolarization of the T tubules, calcium ions are released from the lateral cisterns of the sarcoplasmic reticulum into the sarcoplasm. Relaxation requires the calcium concentration in the sarcoplasm to return to baseline, which is accomplished by calcium-ATPase located in the sarcoplasmic reticulum membrane. This enzyme pumps calcium back into the sarcoplasmic reticulum, but the activity is reduced in Brody disease. This results in an increased intracellular calcium and impaired relaxation following phasic (fast-twitch) activity. Not all patients with Brody disease have been found to have mutations in the *ATP2A1* gene, thus, the disorder is genetically heterogeneous.[102]

Treatment

Dantrolene has been tried with variable success in a few patients as has verapamil. Dantrolene and verapamil were also demonstrated to improve muscle function in vitro in muscle biopsy specimens from patients with Brody disease.[103]

SCHWARTZ–JAMPEL SYNDROME (CHONDRODYSTROPHIC MYOTONIA)

Clinical Features

Schwartz–Jampel syndrome (SJS) is an autosomal recessive disorder associated with developmental skeletal abnormalities and myotonia.[104–114] Affected children often have dysmorphic facies with micrognathia, narrowed palpebral fissures, and low set ears. In addition, over time kyphoscoliosis, bowing of the diaphyses, irregular epiphyses, reduced stature, and pectus carinatum become apparent. Infants may have a decreased suck and a weak high-pitched cry. As seen in MC, facial muscles may distort during or following a crying spell due to myotonia. Muscles often appear hypertrophied and movement is slow due to stiffness related to the myotonia. Developmental motor milestones may be delayed.

Laboratory Features

Serum CK levels can be normal or mildly elevated. Routine motor and sensory NCS are usually normal. Needle EMG reveals complex repetitive,[114] myokymic,[112] pseudomyotonic (decrescendo runs of waning positive sharp waves), or myotonic discharges.[106–111,115]

Histopathology

Muscle biopsies reveal variation in fiber size with hypertrophic and atrophic fibers along with scattered degeneration and regenerating fibers.[114] Replacement of muscle fibers by fatty and connective tissue may be seen over tome.

Molecular Genetics and Pathogenesis

SJS results from mutations in the *HSPG2* gene located on chromosome 1p34–36.1, which encodes perlecan, the major heparan sulfate proteoglycan component of basement membranes.[116–119] Analyses of *HSPG2* messenger RNA (mRNA) and perlecan immunostaining on patients' cells revealed a hypomorphic effect of the studied mutations.[119] Truncating mutations result in instability of *HSPG2* mRNA through nonsense mRNA-mediated decay, whereas missense mutations involving cysteine residues lead to intracellular retention of perlecan.

How mutations in the *HSPG2* lead to myotonia is unclear but may indirectly affect the kinetics of the skeletal muscle sodium channel. Synchronous opening of sodium channels following a stimulus to the muscle membrane following repolarization of the membrane and delayed sodium channel activation have been demonstrated.[59]

Treatment

Procainamide or mexiletine may be beneficial in reducing the muscle stiffness associated with SJS.

▶ SUMMARY

Mutations affecting different muscle ion channels (sodium, calcium, chloride, and potassium) are associated with a variety of neuromuscular manifestations including clinical and electrical myotonia, periodic and sometimes progressive weakness, and occasionally skeletal deformities as seen in ATS. The overlapping features in these disorders can make them difficult to diagnose. The combination of a good clinical history (including family history), neuromuscular exam, and electrophysiological studies (EMG combined with SET performed at room temperature and with the extremity cooled) can be very helpful in guiding which genetic tests may be more useful in order to confirm the diagnosis for nondystrophic myotonias (Fig. 32-11). The LET can be helpful in diagnosing a hereditary periodic paralysis. Attacks of periodic paralysis may be reduced in some patients with acetazolamide, but this may make others worse (i.e., HypoKPP2). Mexiletine appears to be beneficial in alleviating bothersome myotonia in some patients.

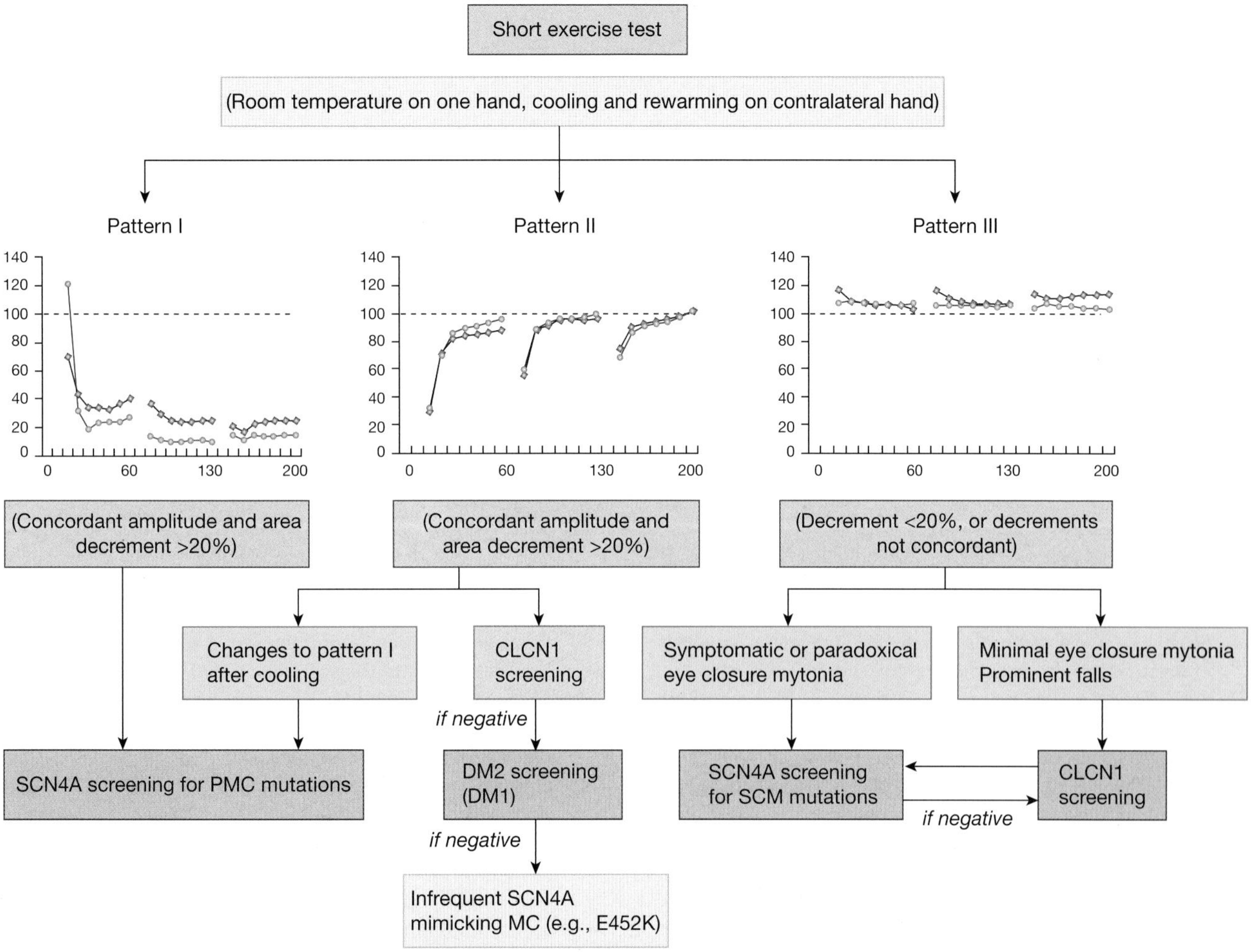

Figure 32-11. Suggested algorithm when using electrophysiological exercise tests for guiding genetic testing in patients with suspected nondystrophic myotonia. DM1, myotonic dystrophy type 1; DM2, myotonic dystrophy type 1 or proximal myotonic myopathy; MC, myotonia congenita; PMC, paramyotonia congenita; SCM, sodium channel myotonia. (Reproduced with permission from Tan SV, Matthews E, Barber M, et al: refined exercise testing can aid DNA-based diagnosis in muscle channelopathies. *Ann Neurol.* 2011;69(2):328–340.)

REFERENCES

1. Matthews E, Fialho D, Tan SV, et al; CINCH Investigators. The non-dystrophic myotonias: Molecular pathogenesis, diagnosis and treatment. *Brain.* 2010;133:9–22.
2. Trip J, Drost G, Ginjaar HB, et al. Redefining the clinical phenotypes of non-dystrophic myotonic syndromes. *J Neurol Neurosurg Psychiatry.* 2009;80:647–652.
3. Heatwole CR, Statland JM, Logigian EL. The diagnosis and treatment of myotonic disorders. *Muscle Nerve.* 2013;47:632–648.
4. Trivedi JR, Bundy B, Statland J, et al; CINCH Consortium. Non-dystrophic myotonia: Prospective study of objective and patient reported outcomes. *Brain.* 2013;136:2189–2200.
5. Horga A, Raja Rayan DL, Matthews E, et al. Prevalence study of genetically defined skeletal muscle channelopathies in England. *Neurology.* 2013;80:1472–1475.
6. Streib EW, Sun SF, Yarkowsky T. Transient paresis in myotonic syndromes: A simplified electrophysiologic approach. *Muscle Nerve.* 1982;5:719–723.
7. Fournier E, Arzel M, Sternberg D, et al. Electromyography guides toward subgroups of mutations in muscle channelopathies. *Ann Neurol.* 2004;56(5):650–661.
8. Fournier E, Viala K, Gervais H, et al. Cold extends electromyography distinction between ion channel mutations causing myotonia. *Ann Neurol.* 2006;60:356–365.
9. Tan SV, Matthews E, Barber M, et al. Refined exercise testing can aid DNA-based diagnosis in muscle channelopathies. *Ann Neurol.* 2011;69:328–340.
10. Colding-Jorgensen E. Phenotypic variability in myotonia congenita. *Muscle Nerve.* 2005;32:19–34.
11. Kuhn E, Fiehn W, Seiler D, Schroder JM. The autosomal recessive (Becker) form of myotonia congenita. *Muscle Nerve.* 1979; 2:109–117.
12. Miller TM, Dias da Silva MR, Miller HA, et al. Correlating phenotype and genotype in the periodic paralyses. *Neurology.* 2004;63(9):1647–1645.
13. Ptacek LJ. The familial periodic paralyses and nondystrophic myotonias. *Am J Med.* 1998;105:58–70.

14. Sanders DB. Myotonia congenita with painful muscle contractions. *Arch Neurol.* 1976;33:580–582.
15. Sun SF, Streib EW. Autosomal recessive generalized myotonia. *Muscle Nerve.* 1983;6:143–148.
16. Tawil R, McDermott MP, Brown R, Jr, et al. Randomized trial of dichlorphenamide in the periodic paralyses. *Ann Neurol.* 2000;47:46–53.
17. Schoser BG, Schroder JM, Grimm T, Sternberg D, Kress W. A large German kindred with cold-aggravated myotonia and a heterozygous A1481D mutation in the SCN4A gene. *Muscle Nerve.* 2007;35(5):59–606.
18. Morrow JM, Matthews E, Raja Rayan DL, et al. Muscle MRI reveals distinct abnormalities in genetically proven non-dystrophic myotonias. *Neuromuscul Disord.* 2013;23: 637–646.
19. Kornblum C, Lutterbey GG, Czermin B, et al. Whole-body high-field MRI shows no skeletal muscle degeneration in young patients with recessive myotonia congenita. *Acta Neurol Scand.* 2010;121:131–135.
20. Aminoff MJ, Layzer RB, Satya-Murti S, Faden AI. The declining electrical response of muscle to repetitive nerve stimulation in myotonia. *Neurology.* 1977;27:812–816.
21. Streib EW. AAEE minimonograph #27: Differential diagnosis of myotonic syndromes. *Muscle Nerve.* 1987;10:603–615.
22. Subramony SH, Malhotra CD, Mishras SK. Distinguishing paramyotonia congenita and myotonia congenita by electromyography. *Muscle Nerve.* 1983;6:374–379.
23. George AL Jr, Crackover MA, Abdalla JA, Hudson JA, Ebers GC. Molecular basis of Thomsen's disease (autosomal dominant myotonia congenital). *Nat Genet.* 1993;3:305–310.
24. Lorenz C, Meyer-Kleine C, Steinmeyer K, Koch MC, Jentsch TJ. Genomic organization of the human muscle chloride channel CIC-1 and analysis of novel mutations leading to Becker-type myotonia. *Hum Mol Genet.* 1994;3:941–946.
25. Wu FF, Ryan A, Devaney J, et al. Novel CLCN1 mutations with unique clinical and electrophysiological consequences. *Brain.* 2002;125(Pt 11):2392–2407.
26. Hoffman EP, Lehman-Horn F, Rudel R. Overexcited or inactive: Ion channels in muscle disease. *Cell.* 1995;80: 681–686.
27. Statland JM, Bundy BN, Wang Y, et al. Consortium for clinical investigation of neurologic channelopathies. Mexiletine for symptoms and signs of myotonia in nondystrophic myotonia: A randomized controlled trial. *JAMA.* 2012;308:1357–1365.
28. Cannon SC. From mutation to myotonia in sodium channel disorders. *Neuromuscul Disord.* 1997;7:241–249.
29. Moxley RT 3rd. Myotonic disorders in childhood. Diagnosis and treatment. *J Child Neurol.* 1997;12:116–129.
30. Ptacek LJ, Johnson KJ, Griggs RC. Genetics and physiology of the myotonic disorders. *N Engl J Med.* 1993;328:482–489.
31. Bulman DE, Scoggen KA, van Oene MD, et al. A novel sodium channel mutation in a family with hypokalemic periodic paralysis. *Neurology.* 1999;53:1932–1936.
32. Ptáĉek LJ, Tawil R, Griggs RC, et al. Sodium channel mutations in acetazolamide-responsive myotonia congenita, paramyotonia congenita, and hyperkalemic periodic paralysis. *Neurology.* 1994;44:150–1503.
33. Jurkat-Rott K, Mitrovic N, Hang C, et al. Voltage-sensor sodium channel mutations cause hypokalemic periodic paralysis type 2 by enhanced inactivation and reduced current. *Proc Natl Acad Sci USA.* 2000;97:9549–9554.
34. Ptácek LJ, Tawil R, Griggs RC, et al. Dihydropyridine receptor mutations cause hypokalemic periodic paralysis. *Cell.* 1994; 77:863–868.
35. Sternberg D, Maisonobe T, Jurkatt-Rott K, et al. Hypokalemic periodic paralysis type 2 caused by mutations at codon 672 in the muscle sodium channel gene SCNA4. *Brain.* 2001;124:1091–1099.
36. Venance SL, Cannon SC, Fialho D, et al; CINCH investigators. The primary periodic paralyses: Diagnosis, pathogenesis and treatment. *Brain.* 2006;129(Pt 1):8–17.
37. Matthews E, Portaro S, Ke Q, et al. Acetazolamide efficacy in hypokalemic periodic paralysis and the predictive role of genotype. *Neurology.* 2011;77:1960–1964.
38. Lehmann-Horn F, Jurkat-Rott K. Voltage-gated ion channels and hereditary diseases. *Physiol Rev.* 1999;79:1317–1372.
39. Ptacek LJ, George AL Jr, Barchi RL, et al. Mutations in an S4 segment of the adult skeletal muscle sodium channel cause paramyotonia congenita. *Neurology.* 1992;8:891–897.
40. Ptacek LJ, Tawil R, Griggs RC, Storvick D, Leppert M. Linkage of atypical myotonia congenital to a sodium channel locus. *Neurology.* 1992;42:431–433.
41. Ptacek LJ, Gouw L, Kwienciński H, et al. Sodium channel mutations in paramyotonia congenita and hyperkalemic periodic paralysis. *Ann Neurol.* 1993;33:300–307.
42. Ricker K, Camacho LM, Grafe P, Lehmann-Horn F, Rudel R. Adynamia episodica hereditaria: What causes the weakness? *Muscle Nerve.* 1989;12:883–891.
43. Ricker K, Lehmann-Horn F, Moxley RT. Myotonia fluctuans. *Arch Neurol.* 1990;47:268–272.
44. Ricker K, Moxley RT 3rd, Heine R, Lehmann-Horne F. Myotonia fluctuans. A third type of muscle sodium channel disease. *Arch Neurol.* 1994;51:1095–1102.
45. Rudel R, Ruppersberg JP, Spittelmeister W. Abnormalities of the fast sodium current in myotonic dystrophy, recessive generalized myotonia, and adynamia episodica. *Muscle Nerve.* 1989;12:281–287.
46. Bradley WG, Taylor R, Rice DR, Hausmanowa Petruzewicz I, Adelman LS, Jenkinson M. Progressive myopathy in hyperkalemic periodic paralysis. *Arch Neurol.* 1990;47:1013–1017.
47. Carson MJ, Pearson CM. Familial hyperkalemic periodic paralysis with myotonic features. *J Pediatr.* 1964;64:853–865.
48. Gamstorp I. Adynamia episodica hereditaria. *Acta Paediatr.* 1956;45(Suppl 108):1–126.
49. McArdle B. Adynamia episodica hereditaria and its treatment. *Brain.* 1960;85:121–148.
50. Rüdel R, Ricker K, Lehman-Horn F. Genotype-phenotype correlations in human skeletal muscle sodium channel diseases. *Arch Neurol.* 1993;50:1241–1248.
51. Rüdel R, Lehmann-Horn F. Workshop report. Paramyotonia, potassium-aggravated myotonias, and periodic paralyses. *Neuromuscul Disord.* 1997;7:127–132.
52. Subramony SH, Wee AS. Exercise and rest in hyperkalemic periodic paralysis. *Neurology.* 1986;36:173–177.
53. Bradley WG. Adynamia episodica hereditaria. *Brain.* 1969; 92:345–378.
54. Brooks JE. Hyperkalemic periodic paralysis. *Arch Neurol.* 1969;20:13–18.
55. Hoskins B, Vroom FQ, Jarrell MA. Hyperkalemic periodic paralysis. *Arch Neurol.* 1975;32:519–523.
56. Layzer RB, Lovelace RE, Rowland LP. Hyperkalemic periodic paralysis. *Arch Neurol.* 1967;16:445–472.

57. Amato AA, Dumitru D. Hereditary myopathies. In: Dumitru D, Amato AA, Swartz MJ, eds. *Electrodiagnostic Medicine*. 2nd ed. Philadelphia, PA: Hanley & Belfus, Inc.; 2002:1265–1370.
58. Meyers KR, Gilden DH, Rinaldi CF, Hansen JL. Periodic muscle weakness, normokalemia, and tubular aggregates. *Neurology*. 1972;22:269–279.
59. Tomé FMS, Borg K. Periodic paralysis and electrolyte disorders. In: Mastaglia FL, Walton JN, eds. *Skeletal Muscle Pathology*. Edinburgh: Churchill Livingstone; 1992:343–366.
60. Lehmann-Horn F, Kuther G, Ricker K, Grafe P, Ballany I, Rudel R. Adynamia episodica herediteria with myotonia: A noninactivating sodium current and the effect of extracellular pH. *Muscle Nerve*. 1987;10:363–374.
61. Lehmann-Horn F, Iaizzo PA, Hatt H, Franke C. Altered gating and conductance of Na+ channels in hyperkalemic periodic paralysis. *Pflugers Arch*. 1991;418:297–299.
62. Ptácek LJ, George AL Jr, Griggs RC, et al. Identification of a mutation in the gene causing hyperkalemic periodic paralysis. *Cell*. 1991;67:1021–1027.
63. Streib EW, Sun SF, Hanson M. Paramyotonia congenita: Clinical and electrophysiologic studies. *Electromyogr Clin Neurophysiol*. 1983;23:315–325.
64. Streib EW. Paramyotonia congenita. *Semin Neurol*. 1991;11: 249–257.
65. Lajoie WJ. Paramyotonia congenita, clinical features and electromyographic findings. *Arch Phys Med Rehabil*. 1961;42:507–512.
66. Lundberg PO, Stalberg E, Thiele B. Paralysis periodica paramyotonia: A clinical and neurophysiological study. *J Neurol Sci*. 1974;21:309–321.
67. Thrush DC, Morris CJ, Salmon MV. Paramyotonia congenita: A clinical, histochemical and pathologic study. *Brain*. 1972;95:537–552.
68. Jackson CE, Barohn RJ, Ptacek LJ. Paramyotonia congenita: Abnormal short exercise test, and improvement after mexiletine therapy. *Muscle Nerve*. 1994;17:763–768.
69. Streib EW. Paramyotonia congenita: Successful treatment with tocainide. Clinical and electrophysiologic findings in seven patients. *Muscle Nerve*. 1987;10:155–162.
70. Lennox G, Purves A, Marsden D. Myotonia fluctuans. *Arch Neurol*. 1992;49:1010–1011.
71. Colding-Jorgensen E, Duno M, Vissing J. Autosomal dominant monosymptomatic myotonia permanens. *Neurology*. 2006;67(1):153–155.
72. Trudell RG, Kaiser KK, Griggs RC. Acetazolamide responsive myotonia congenita. *Neurology*. 1987;37:488–491.
73. Lehmann-Horn F, Rudel R, Dengler R, Lorkovic H, Haass A, Ricker K. Membrane defects in paramyotonia congenita with and without a warm environment. *Muscle Nerve*. 1981;4: 396–406.
74. Haywood LJ, Sandoval GM, Cannon SC. Defective slow inactivation of sodium channels contributes to familial periodic paralysis. *Neurology*. 1999;52:1447–1453.
75. Sokolov S, Scheuer T, Catterall WA. Gating pore current in an inherited ion channelopathy. *Nature*. 2007;446(7131):76–78.
76. Struyk AF, Cannon SC. A Na+ Channel Mutation Linked to Hypokalemic Periodic Paralysis Exposes a Proton-selective Gating Pore. *J Gen Physiol*. 2007;130(1):11–20.
77. Lapie P, Lory P, Fontaine B. Hypokalemic periodic paralysis: An autosomal dominant muscle disorder caused by mutations in a voltage gated calcium channel. *Neuromusc Disord*. 1997;7:234–240.
78. Links TP, Zwarts MJ, Wilmink JT, Molenaar WM, Oosterhuis HJ. Permanent muscle weakness in familial hypokalemic periodic paralysis. *Brain*. 1990;113:1873–1889.
79. Gordon AM, Green JR, Lagunoff D. Studies on a patient with hypokalemic familial periodic paralysis. *Am J Med*. 1970;48: 185–195.
80. Links TP, Smit AJ, Molenaar WM, Zwarts MJ, Oosterhuis HJ. Familial hypokalemic periodic paralysis. Clinical, diagnostic, and therapeutic aspects. *J Neurol Sci*. 1994;122:33–43.
81. De Grandis D, Fiaschi A, Tomelleri G, Orrico D. Hypokalemic periodic paralysis: A single fiber study. *J Neurol Sci*. 1978; 37:107–112.
82. Abbot GW, Butler MH, Bendahhou S, Dalakas MC, Ptacek LJ, Goldstein SA. MiRP2 forms potassium channels in skeletal muscle with Kv3.4 and is associated with periodic paralysis. *Cell*. 2001:104:217–231.
83. Ng HY, Lin SH, Hsu CY, Tsai YZ, Chen HC, Lee CT. Hypokalemic paralysis due to Gitelman syndrome: A family study. *Neurology*. 2006;67(6):1080–1082.
84. Grafe P, Quasthoff S, Strupp M, Lehmann-Horn F. Enhancement of K +conductance improves in vitro the contraction force of skeletal muscle in hypokalemic periodic paralysis. *Muscle Nerve*. 1990;13:451–457.
85. Hoffmann WW, Smith RA. Hypokalemic periodic paralysis studies in vitro. *Brain*. 1970;93:445–474.
86. Rudel R, Lehmann-Horn F, Ricker K, Kuther G. Hypokalemic periodic paralysis: In vitro investigation of muscle fiber membrane parameters. *Muscle Nerve*. 1984;7:110–120.
87. Sipos I, Jurkat-Rott K, Harasztosi C, et al. Skeletal muscle DHP receptor mutations alter calcium currents in human hypokalemic periodic paralysis myotubes. *J Physiol*. 1995;483: 29–306.
88. Falhammar H, Thorén M, Calissendorff J. Thyrotoxic periodic paralysis: Clinical and molecular aspects. *Endocrine*. 2013; 43:274–284.
89. Ryan DP, da Silva MR, Soong TW, et al. Mutations in potassium channel Kir2.6 cause susceptibility to thyrotoxic hypokalemic periodic paralysis. *Cell*. 2010;140:88–98.
90. Jongjaroenprasert W, Phusantisampan T, Mahasirimongkol S, et al. A genome-wide association study identifies novel susceptibility genetic variation for thyrotoxic hypokalemic periodic paralysis. *J Hum Genet*. 2012;57:301–304.
91. Cheung CL, Lau KS, Ho AY, et al. Genome-wide association study identifies a susceptibility locus for thyrotoxic periodic paralysis at 17q24.3. *Nat Genet*. 2012;44:1026–1029.
92. Wang X, Chow CC, Yao X, et al. The predisposition to thyrotoxic periodic paralysis (TPP) is due to a genetic variant in the inward-rectifying potassium channel, KCNJ2. *Clin Endocrinol*. 2014;80(5):770–771.
93. Davies NP, Imbrici P, Fialho D, et al. Andersen–Tawil syndrome: New potassium channel mutations and possible phenotypic variation. *Neurology*. 2005;65(7):1083–1089.
94. Klein R, Ganelin R, Marks JF. Periodic paralysis with cardiac arrhythmia. *J Pediatr*. 1963;62:371–385.
95. Ma D, Tang XD, Rogers TB, Welling PA. An Andersen–Tawil syndrome mutation in Kir2.1 (V302M) alters the G-loop cytoplasmic K+ conduction pathway. *J Biol Chem*. 2007;282:5781–5789.
96. Salajegheh MK, Amato AA. Channelopathies: Paroxysmal paralysis. In: Squire LR, Albright TD, Bloom FE, eds. *New Encyclopedia of Neuroscience*. 2009;496–507.

97. Tawil R, Ptacek LJ, Pavlkis SG, et al. Andersen's syndrome: Potassium sensitive periodic paralysis, ventricular ectopy, and dysmorphic features. *Ann Neurol.* 1994;35:326–330.
98. Tan SV, Z'graggen WJ, Boërio D, et al. Membrane dysfunction in Andersen–Tawil syndrome assessed by velocity recovery cycles. *Muscle Nerve.* 2012;46:193–203.
99. Plaster NM, Tawil R, Trisani-Firouzi M, et al. Mutations in Kir2.1 cause the developmental and episodic electrical phenotypes of Andersen's syndrome. *Cell.* 2001;105:511–519.
100. Quane KA, Healy JM, Keating KE, et al. Mutations in the ryanodine receptor gene in central core disease and malignant hyperthermia. *Nat Genet.* 1993;5:51–55.
101. Bertorini TE. Myoglobinuria, malignant hyperthermia, neuroleptic malignant syndrome and serotonin syndrome. *Neurol Clin.* 1997;15:649–671.
102. Voermans NC, Laan AE, Oosterhof A, et al. Brody syndrome: A clinically heterogeneous entity distinct from Brody disease: A review of literature and a cross-sectional clinical study in 17 patients. *Neuromuscul Disord.* 2012;22:944–954.
103. Benders AA, Veerkamp JH, Oosterhof A. Ca^{2+} homeostasis in Brody's disease. A study in skeletal muscle and culture muscles cells and the effects of dantrolene and verapamil. *J Clin Invest.* 1996;94:741–748.
104. Odermatt A, Tashner PE, Khanna VK, et al. Mutations in the gene-encoding SERCA1, the fast-twitch skeletal muscle sarcoplasmic reticulum Ca^{2+} ATPase, are associated with Brody disease. *Nat Genet.* 1996;14:191–194.
105. Pavone L, Mollica F, Grasso A, Cao A, Gullotta F. Schwartz-Jampel syndrome in two daughters of first cousins. *J Neurol Neurosurg Psychiatry.* 1978;41:161–169.
106. Aberfeld DC, Namba T, Vye MV, Grob D. Chondrodystrophic myotonia: Report of two cases. *Arch Neurol.* 1970;22(5):455–462.
107. Brown SB, Carcia-Mullin R, Murai Y. The Schwartz-Jampel syndrome (myotonic chondrodystrophy) in the adult. *Neurology.* 1975;25:365–366.
108. Cadilhac J, Baldet P, Greze J, Duday H. EMG studies of two family cases of the Schwartz-Jampel syndrome (osteo-chondro-muscular dystrophy with myotonia). *Electromyogr Clin Neurophysiol.* 1975;15:5–12.
109. Cao A, Cianchetti C, Calisti L, de Virgiliis S, Ferreli A, Tangheroni W. Schwartz-Jampel syndrome. Clinical, electrophysiological and histopathological study of a severe variant. *J Neurol Sci.* 1978;35:175–187.
110. Fowler WM Jr, Layzer RB, Taylor RG, et al. The Schwartz-Jampel syndrome: Its clinical, physiological, and histological expression. *J Neurol Sci.* 1974;22:127–146.
111. Huttenlocher PR, Landwirth J, Hanson V, Gallagher BB, Bensch K. Osteo-chondro-muscular dystrophy: A disorder manifested by multiple skeletal deformities, myotonia, and dystrophic changes in muscle. *Pediatrics.* 1969;44: 945–958.
112. Pascuzzi RM, Gratianne R, Azzarelli B, Kincaid JC. Schwartz-Jampel syndrome with dominant inheritance. *Muscle Nerve.* 1990;13:1152–1163.
113. Pascuzzi RM. Schwartz–Jampel syndrome. *Semin Neurol.* 1991; 11:267–273.
114. Spanns F, Theunissen P, Reekers AD, Smit L, Veldman H. Schwartz–Jampel syndrome: I. Clinical, electromyographic and histologic studies. *Muscle Nerve.* 1990;13:516–527.
115. Taylor RG, Layzer RB, Davis HS, Fowler WM, Jr. Continuous muscle fiber activity in the Schwartz–Jampel syndrome. *Electroencephalogr Clin Neurophysiol.* 1972;33:497–509.
116. Arikawa-Hirasawa E, Le AH, Nishino I, et al. Structural and functional mutations of the perlecan gene cause Schwartz–Jampel syndrome, with myotonic myopathy and chondrodysplasia. *Am J Hum Genet.* 2002;70:1368–1375.
117. Nicole S, Davoine CS, Topaloglu H, et al. Perlecan, the major proteoglycan of basement membranes, is altered in patients with Schwartz–Jampel syndrome (chondrodystrophic myotonia). *Nat Genet.* 2000;26:480–483.
118. Stum M, Davoine CS, Fontaine B, Nicole S, Schwartz–Jampel syndrome and perlecan deficiency. *Acta Myol.* 2005;24:89–92.
119. Stum M, Davoine CS, Vicart S, et al. Spectrum of HSPG2 (Perlecan) mutations in patients with Schwartz–Jampel syndrome. *Hum Mutat.* 2006;27:1082–1091.

CHAPTER 33

Inflammatory Myopathies

There are four major categories of idiopathic inflammatory myopathy: dermatomyositis (DM), polymyositis (PM), immune-mediated necrotizing myopathy (IMNM), and inclusion body myositis (IBM), which are clinically, histologically, and pathogenically distinct (Tables 33-1 to 33-3).[1–12] These myositides may occur in isolation or in association with cancer, various connective tissue diseases (overlap syndromes), and autoantibodies. Other less common idiopathic myositides (i.e., granulomatous and myositis associated with infections) will also be discussed in this chapter. DM and IBM are rather homogeneous clinically and histologically. On the other hand, what has been called "PM" in the literature is likely a heterogeneous group of disorders. It is important to emphasize that not all myopathies with inflammation are classified as "inflammatory myopathies." In this regard, various muscular dystrophies (e.g., congenital, facioscapulohumeral, and dysferlinopathies) may be associated with profound inflammation and are not uncommonly misdiagnosed as PM.

There are a few reports of idiopathic inflammatory myopathy occurring in parents, children, and siblings of affected patients, suggesting a genetic predisposition to developing these disorders, possibly secondary to inherited human leukocyte antigens (HLA) haplotypes.[13–15] There are hereditary forms of inclusion body myopathy, but with rare exceptions, the muscle biopsies in these cases lack inflammation, and the clinical phenotype (i.e., age of onset and pattern of weakness) is different from sporadic IBM.

The annual incidence of the inflammatory myopathies as a whole has ranged between 0.1 and 1 per 100,000 person years,[3,5,16–21] with more recent studies suggesting the incidence may be greater than four cases per 100,000[22] with prevalence in the range of 14 to 32 per 100,000.[5,22–25] However, defining the actual incidence and prevalence of the individual myositides has been limited by the different diagnostic criteria employed in various epidemiological studies. Most published papers regarding epidemiology and treatment of DM and PM have used Bohan and Peter criteria (Table 33-4).[26–28] PM will be overdiagnosed with Bohan and Peter criteria. These criteria were fine in 1975, but these criteria do not require a muscle biopsy and the only feature that distinguishes PM from DM is the presence of a rash in DM. Further, the biopsy abnormalities as listed are nonspecific (except for perifascicular atrophy—a finding specific for DM, but not seen in PM) and do not help in distinguishing PM from DM or for that matter any myopathy with necrosis, including muscular dystrophies. Importantly, the Bohan and Peter histological criteria do not take into account the advances in histopathology and the distinct diagnoses of IBM and IMNM. This can have implications in regard to treatment strategies and prognosis as we will discuss.[29]

Criteria for diagnosis of the various inflammatory myopathies need to take into account the advances in understanding of the pathogeneses of these disorders. We emphasize that DM is not simply PM with a rash (or the converse: PM is not DM without a rash). Furthermore, IBM is not PM with inclusions (or the converse: IBM is not PM with inclusions). For this reason, revised criteria for the various idiopathic inflammatory myopathies have been devised to take into account the recent advancements in the field (Tables 33-2 and 33-3).[30–32] For definitive histopathological diagnosis of PM in the biopsy, some require endomysial infiltrates composed of CD8+ T cells and macrophages invading non-necrotic muscle fibers that express major histocompatibility-1 (MHC-1) antigen.[4,30–32] However, the sensitivity of this finding is low, and this biopsy feature is not diagnostic for PM, as it also is seen in IBM and rarely in dystrophies. Likewise, perivascular, perimysial, and endomysial inflammatory infiltrates are nonspecific findings and can be found in DM, PM, IBM, dystrophies, toxic, and metabolic myopathies. With the caveats noted above, we will begin our discussion of the individual inflammatory myopathies.

▶ DERMATOMYOSITIS

CLINICAL FEATURES

DM can present at any age, including infancy. Similar to most other autoimmune disorders, there is an increased incidence of DM in women compared to men.[11,16–19,33] Although the pathogenesis of childhood and adult DM is presumably similar, there are important differences in some of the clinical features and associated disorders. Weakness can develop rather acutely (over days or several weeks), or insidiously (over months).[17,34,35] Proximal leg and arm muscles as well as neck flexors are usually the earliest and most severely affected muscle groups. Thus, the earliest patient complaints are often difficulty lifting their arms over their heads, climbing steps, and arising from chairs. Distal muscles are also involved. Children are more likely to present with an insidious onset of muscle weakness and myalgias

▶ TABLE 33-1. **IDIOPATHIC INFLAMMATORY MYOPATHIES: CLINICAL AND LABORATORY FEATURES**

Disorder	Sex	Age of Onset	Rash	Pattern of Weakness	Serum CK	Muscle Biopsy	Cellular Infiltrate	Response to IS Therapy	Common Associated Conditions
DM	F > M	Childhood and adult	Yes	Proximal > distal	Normal or increased (up to 50× normal or higher)	Perimysial and perivascular inflammation; increase expression of IFN-1 regulated proteins on muscle fibers and capillaries; MAC, Ig, C deposition on capillaries	CD4+ dendritic cells; B cells; macrophages	Yes	Myocarditis, interstitial lung disease, malignancy, vasculitis, other connective tissue diseases (CTD)
PM	F > M	Adult	No	Proximal > distal	Increased (up to 50× normal or higher)	Endomysial inflammation	CD8+ T cells; macrophages; plasma cells	Yes	Myocarditis, interstitial lung disease, other connective tissue diseases
IBM	M > F	Elderly (>50 years)	No	Proximal = distal; predilection for: finger/wrist flexors, knee extensors	Normal or mildly increased (usually <10× normal)	Endomysial inflammation; rimmed vacuoles; amyloid deposits; EM: 15–18 nm tubulofilaments	CD8+ T cells; macrophages; plasma cells	None or minimal	Neuropathy autoimmune disorders - uncommon
NM	M = F	Adult and elderly	No	Proximal > distal	Elevated (>10 × normal or higher)	Necrotic muscle fibers; minimal inflammatory infiltrate; MHC1 and MAC expression on sarcolemma of non-necrotic muscle fibers	Mainly macrophages in necrotic fibers undergoing phagocytosis	Yes	Malignancy, CTD, possibly triggered by statin use

DM, dermatomyositis; PM, polymyositis; IBM, inclusion body myositis; NM, necrotizing myopathy; F, female; M, male; IS, immunosuppressive; Ig, immunoglobulin; MAC, membrane attack complex; C, complement; CK, creatine kinase; IFN-1, interferon-1.
Modified with permission from Amato AA, Barohn RJ. Idiopathic inflammatory myopathies. *Neurol Clin.* 1997;15(3):615–648.

▶ **TABLE 33-2. DIAGNOSTIC CRITERIA FOR POLYMYOSITIS, DERMATOMYOSITIS, IMMUNE-MEDIATED NECROTIZING MYOPATHY, AND NONSPECIFIC/UNSPECIFIED MYOSITIS**

I. *Polymyositis (PM)*
  1. Clinical features
    a. Inclusion criteria
      i. Onset usually over 18 year (post puberty)
      ii. Subacute or insidious onset
      iii. Pattern of weakness: symmetric proximal > distal weakness
    b. Exclusion criteria
      i. Clinical features of IBM (see Griggs et al.: asymmetric weakness, wrist/finger flexors same or worse than deltoids; knee extensors and/or ankle dorsiflexors same or worse than hip flexors)
      ii. Ocular weakness, isolated dysarthria, neck extensor > neck flexor weakness
    c. Exposure to myotoxic drugs, active endocrinopathy (hyperthyroid or hypothyroid and hyperparathyroid), amyloidosis, family history of muscular dystrophy or proximal motor neuropathies (e.g., SMA)
  2. Serum creatine kinase level must be elevated
  3. Other laboratory criteria (one of three): EMG criteria, skeletal muscle MRI, or presence of myositis-specific antibodies
    a. Electromyography:
      i. Inclusion criteria
        • Increased insertional and spontaneous activity in the form of fibrillation potentials, positive sharp waves, or complex repetitive discharges
        • Morphometric analysis reveals the presence of short-duration, small-amplitude, polyphasic MUAPs
      ii. Exclusion criteria
        • Prominent myotonic discharges that would suggest proximal myotonic dystrophy or other channelopathy
        • Morphometric analysis reveals predominantly long-duration, large-amplitude MUAPs
        • Decreased recruitment pattern of MUAPs
    b. Skeletal muscle MRI shows diffuse or patchy increased signal (edema) within muscle tissue on STIR images
    c. Myositis-specific antibodies are detected in the serum
  4. Muscle biopsy
    a. Definite PM requires endomysial inflammatory cell infiltrate (T cells) surrounding and invading non-necrotic muscle fibers
    b. Probable PM
      i. Endomysial CD8+ T cells surrounding and but no definite invasions of non-necrotic muscle fibers or
      ii. Ubiquitous MHC-1 expression
      iii. Also requires exclusion of "necrotizing myopathies" and dystrophies with immunopathology/electron microscopy and clinical history/examination
    c. Exclusion criteria
      i. Rimmed vacuoles, ragged red fibers, cytochrome oxidase-negative fibers that would suggest IBM
      ii. Perifascicular atrophy, deposition of MAC on small blood vessels, reduced capillary density, tubuloreticular inclusions in endothelial cells, or pipestem capillaries that would suggest dermatomyositis (DM) or another type of humorally mediated microangiopathy
      iii. Dystrophic features or MAC deposition on non-necrotic muscle fibers that would suggest a muscular dystrophy
  A. Definite PM
    1. All clinical criteria
    2. Elevated serum CK
    3. Muscle biopsy with features of histological features of definite PM
  B. Probable PM
    1. All clinical criteria
    2. Elevated serum CK
    3. Other laboratory criteria (one of three)
    4. Muscle biopsy with features of histological features of probable PM

II. *Dermatomyositis (DM)*
  1. Clinical features
    a. Inclusion criteria
      i. Onset in childhood (juvenile DM) or adulthood (adult DM)
      ii. Subacute or insidious onset
      iii. Pattern of weakness: symmetric proximal legs > arms, neck flexors > neck extensors
      iv. Rash suggestive of DM: heliotrope, Gottron's papules/sign, V-sign, shawl sign, holster sign
    b. Exclusion criteria
      i. Ocular weakness, isolated dysarthria, neck extensor > neck flexor weakness
      ii. Exclusion of other causes of weakness (see PM clinical exclusion criteria)

(continued)

▶ **TABLE 33-2. (CONTINUED)**

2. Muscle biopsy:
   a. Definite DM requires perifascicular atrophy
   b. Probable DM requires:
      Myxovirus resistance 1 protein (or other type 1–interferon-regulated proteins) deposition on small blood vessels or muscle fibers
      Or
      MAC deposition on small blood vessels
      Or
      Reduced capillary density
      Or
      Tubuloreticular inclusions in endothelial walls on EM
      Or
      MHC-1 expression of perifascicular fibers
      Or
      Perivascular, perimysial inflammatory cell infiltrate (this is a nonspecific abnormality in and of itself)

A. Definite DM
   1. All clinical criteria
   2. Muscle biopsy demonstrates perifascicular atrophy

B. Probable DM
   1. All clinical criteria
   2. Muscle biopsy fulfills probable DM histological criteria or elevated serum CK or other laboratory criteria (one of three: EMG, MRI, or MSA)

C. Amyopathic DM
   1. Rash typical of DM: heliotrope, Gottron's papules/sign, V-sign, shawl sign, and holster sign
   2. Skin biopsy demonstrates a reduced capillary density, deposition of MAC on small blood vessels along the dermal–epidermal junction, and variable keratinocyte decoration for MAC
   3. No subjective or objective muscle weakness
   4. Normal serum CK
   5. Normal EMG

D. Possible DM sine dermatitis
   1. Clinical criteria but classic DM rash is absent
   2. Muscle biopsy demonstrates:
      Perifascicular atrophy
      Or
      MxA deposition on small blood vessels or muscle fibers
      Or
      MAC deposition on small blood vessels
      Or
      Reduced capillary density
      Or
      Tubuloreticular inclusions in endothelial walls on EM
      Or
      MHC-1 expression of perifascicular fibers
   3. Elevated CK plus other laboratory criteria (one of three: EMG, MRI, or MSA)

III. *Nonspecific/unspecified myositis*
   1. Clinical features
      a. Inclusion criteria
         i. Onset in childhood or adulthood
         ii. Subacute or insidious onset
         iii. Pattern of weakness: symmetric proximal > distal weakness
      b. Exclusion criteria: Rash typical of DM; PM clinical exclusion criteria
   2. Muscle biopsy
      a. Perivascular, perimysial inflammatory cell infiltrate but there is no perifascicular atrophy, perifascicular MHC-1 expression, MAC deposition on small blood vessels, reduced capillary density, or tubuloreticular inclusions on EM
         Or
      b. Scattered endomysial CD8+ T cells infiltrate but that does not clearly surround or invade muscle fibers
         And
      c. Requires exclusion of "necrotizing myopathies," dystrophies, and "possible IBM" with immunopathology/electron microscopy and clinical history/examination
   3. Serum creatine kinase (CK) level is elevated
   4. Other laboratory criteria (one of three): EMG criteria, skeletal muscle MRI, or presence of myositis-specific antibodies

▶ TABLE 33-2. (CONTINUED)

IV. *Immune-mediated necrotizing myopathy*
1. Clinical features
   a. Inclusion criteria
      i. Onset usually over 18 year (post puberty)
      ii. Subacute or insidious onset
      iii. Pattern of weakness: symmetric proximal > distal weakness
   b. Exclusion criteria: Rash typical of DM; PM clinical exclusion criteria
2. Muscle biopsy
   a. The predominant abnormal histological feature of the muscle biopsy is the presence of many necrotic muscle fibers
   b. Inflammatory cells are sparse or only slightly perivascular; perimysial infiltrate is evident
   c. MAC deposition on small blood vessels may be seen
   d. Tubuloreticular inclusions in endothelial cells are uncommon or not evident
   e. Pipestem capillaries may be evident on EM
   f. No evidence of mononuclear inflammatory cells invading non-necrotic muscle fibers
   g. No perifascicular atrophy
3. Serum CK level must be elevated
4. Other laboratory criteria (one of three): EMG criteria, skeletal muscle MRI, or presence of myositis-specific antibodies

IBM, inclusion body myositis; MRI, magnetic resonance imaging; DM, dermatomyositis; MUAP, motor unit action potential; MHC-1, major histocompatibility-1; MAC, membrane attack complex; CK, creatine kinase; EM, electron microscopy; MSA, myositis-specific antibody; MxA, myxovirus resistance 1 protein.
Modified with permission from Hoogendijk JE, Amato AA, Lecky BR, et al. 119th ENMC international workshop: trial design in adult idiopathic inflammatory myopathies, with the exception of inclusion body myositis, 10–12 October 2003, Naarden, the Netherlands. *Neuromuscul Disord.* 2004;14(5):337–345.

that are often preceded by fatigue, low-grade fevers, and a rash. Dysphagia occurs in approximately 30% of patients with DM probably due to involvement of oropharyngeal and esophageal muscles.[3] Speech, chewing, and swallowing difficulties can arise secondary to involvement of the masseter muscle. We have even seen speech difficulties as a result of involvement of the pharyngeal, laryngeal, and the tongue muscles. Sensation is normal, and muscle stretch reflexes are preserved unless a severe degree of weakness has developed.

▶ TABLE 33-3. EUROPEAN NEUROMUSCULAR CENTER 2011 WORKSHOP CRITERIA FOR INCLUSION BODY MYOSITIS

Clinical & Laboratory Features	Classification	Pathological Features
Duration >12 months Age at onset >45 years Knee extension weakness ≥ hip flexion weakness And/Or Finger flexion weakness > shoulder abduction weakness CK no greater than 15× ULN	Clinicopathologically defined IBM	All of the following: Endomysial inflammatory infiltrate Rimmed vacuoles Protein accumulation[a] or 15–18 nm filaments
Duration >12 months Age at onset > 45 years Knee extension weakness ≥ hip flexion weakness And Finger flexion weakness > shoulder abduction weakness CK no greater than 15× ULN	Clinically defined IBM	One or more, but not all, of: Endomysial inflammatory infiltrate Upregulation of MHC class I Rimmed vacuoles Protein accumulation[a] or 15–18 nm filaments
Duration >12 months Age at onset >45 years Knee extension weakness ≥ hip flexion weakness Or Finger flexion weakness > shoulder abduction weakness CK no greater than 15× ULN	Probable IBM	One or more, but not all, of: Endomysial inflammatory infiltrate Upregulation of MHC class I Rimmed vacuoles Protein accumulation[a] or 15–18 nm filaments

[a]Demonstration of amyloid or other protein accumulation by established methods (e.g., for amyloid Congo red, crystal violet, thioflavin T/S, for other proteins p62, SMI-31, TDP-43).
Reproduced with permission from Rose MR, ENMC IBM Working Group. 188th ENMC International Workshop: Inclusion Body Myositis, 2–4 December 2011, Naarden, The Netherlands. *Neuromuscul Disord.* 2013;23(12):1044–1055.

TABLE 33-4. BOHAN AND PETER CRITERIA FOR PM AND DM

1. Symmetrical weakness of the limb-girdle muscles and anterior neck flexors, progressing over weeks to months, with or without dysphagia or ventilatory muscle involvement
2. Muscle biopsy evidence of necrosis of my fibers, phagocytosis, regeneration with basophilic, and large vesicular sarcolemmal nuclei, prominent nucleoli, atrophy in a perifascicular distribution, variation in fiber size, and an inflammatory exudate, often perivascular
3. Elevation in serum skeletal muscle enzymes, particularly the CK and often aldolase AST, ALT, and LDH
4. EMG triad of short, small polyphasic motor units; fibrillation potentials; positive sharp waves; insertional irritability; and complex repetitive discharges

Three of four of the above features are needed for the diagnosis of PM. The diagnosis of DM is made if the patient also has characteristic rash.
PM, polymyositis; DM, dermatomyositis; AST, aspartate aminotransferase; ALT, alanine aminotransferase.

DM is usually diagnosed earlier than other forms of myositis because of the characteristic rash, which typically accompanies or precedes the onset of muscle weakness.[1,3,34,36] However, the rash can develop years after the onset of weakness, which could lead to an erroneous diagnosis of PM. Some patients have the characteristic rash but never develop weakness (the so-called amyopathic DM or DM *sine* myositis).[36,37] Rare patients do not have an appreciable rash at the time they present with weakness. We have seen some patients with histopathological features characteristic of DM who have developed the rash months or years after onset of weakness or not at all (adermatopathic DM or DM *sine* dermatitis). These patients would be erroneously classified as PM using Bohan and Peter criteria.

The classical skin manifestations include a purplish discoloration of the eyelids (heliotrope rash) often associated with periorbital edema and a papular, erythematous rash over the knuckles (Gottron's papules) (Fig. 33-1). In addition, an erythematous, macular, sun-sensitive rash may appear on the face, neck and anterior chest (V-sign), shoulders and upper back (shawl sign), hips (holster sign), and extensor surfaces of elbows, knuckles, knees, and malleoli (Gottron's sign). The nail beds often have dilated capillary loops occasionally with thrombi or hemorrhage. The skin lesions can be subtle at times and difficult to appreciate in individuals who are darker skinned—another common reason for misdiagnosing patients with PM rather than DM.

Subcutaneous calcifications occur in 30–70% of children, but in our experience these are less common in adults (Fig. 33-2).[38,39] These lesions tend to develop over pressure points (buttocks, knees, and elbows) and can be complicated by ulceration of the overlying skin. Once the calcinosis appears, treatment is very difficult. Colchicine, probenecid, warfarin, and phosphate buffers have been tried with limited success. Surgery may be performed, but the lesions may recur or worsen.

ASSOCIATED MANIFESTATIONS

Cardiac

Conduction defects, arrhythmias, ventricular, and septal wall motion abnormalities, and reduced ejection fractions may be seen on electrocardiograms, echocardiography, and radionucleotide scintigraphy.[34,35,40–44] Nevertheless, most patients do not develop any cardiac symptoms. However, pericarditis, myocarditis, and congestive heart failure can occasionally develop secondary to involvement of cardiac muscle and may be lethal.[34,42]

Pulmonary

Interstitial lung disease (ILD) complicates approximately 10–20% of patients with DM.[34,45–48] Rarely, patients develop bronchiolitis obliterans with organizing pneumonia. ILD manifests clinically as dyspnea and nonproductive cough. It can begin abruptly or insidiously and even precede the development of the characteristic rash and muscle weakness. Chest radiographs reveal a diffuse reticulonodular pattern with a predilection for involvement at the lung bases. A diffuse alveolar pattern or ground-glass appearance is seen in the more fulminant cases.[45] A restrictive defect with reduced forced vital capacity and decreased diffusion capacity are evident on pulmonary function tests. Antibodies directed against t-histidyl transfer RNA synthetase, the so-called Jo-1 antibodies, are present in at least 50% of ILD cases associated with inflammatory myopathies.[49–51] A less common pulmonary complication is ventilatory muscle weakness, but it does occur. Furthermore, aspiration pneumonia can be a complication of oropharyngeal and esophageal weakness.

Gastrointestinal

Involvement of the skeletal and smooth muscles of the gastrointestinal tract can lead to dysphagia, aspiration, and delayed gastric emptying. Vasculopathy affecting the gastrointestinal tract is a serious complication that appears to be much more common in juvenile DM compared to adult DM. The vasculopathy can result in mucosal ulceration, perforation, and life-threatening hemorrhage.

Joints

Arthralgias of large and small joints with or without arthritis are common. Joint and muscle pain often eases when the limbs are flexed, and this can lead to the formation of

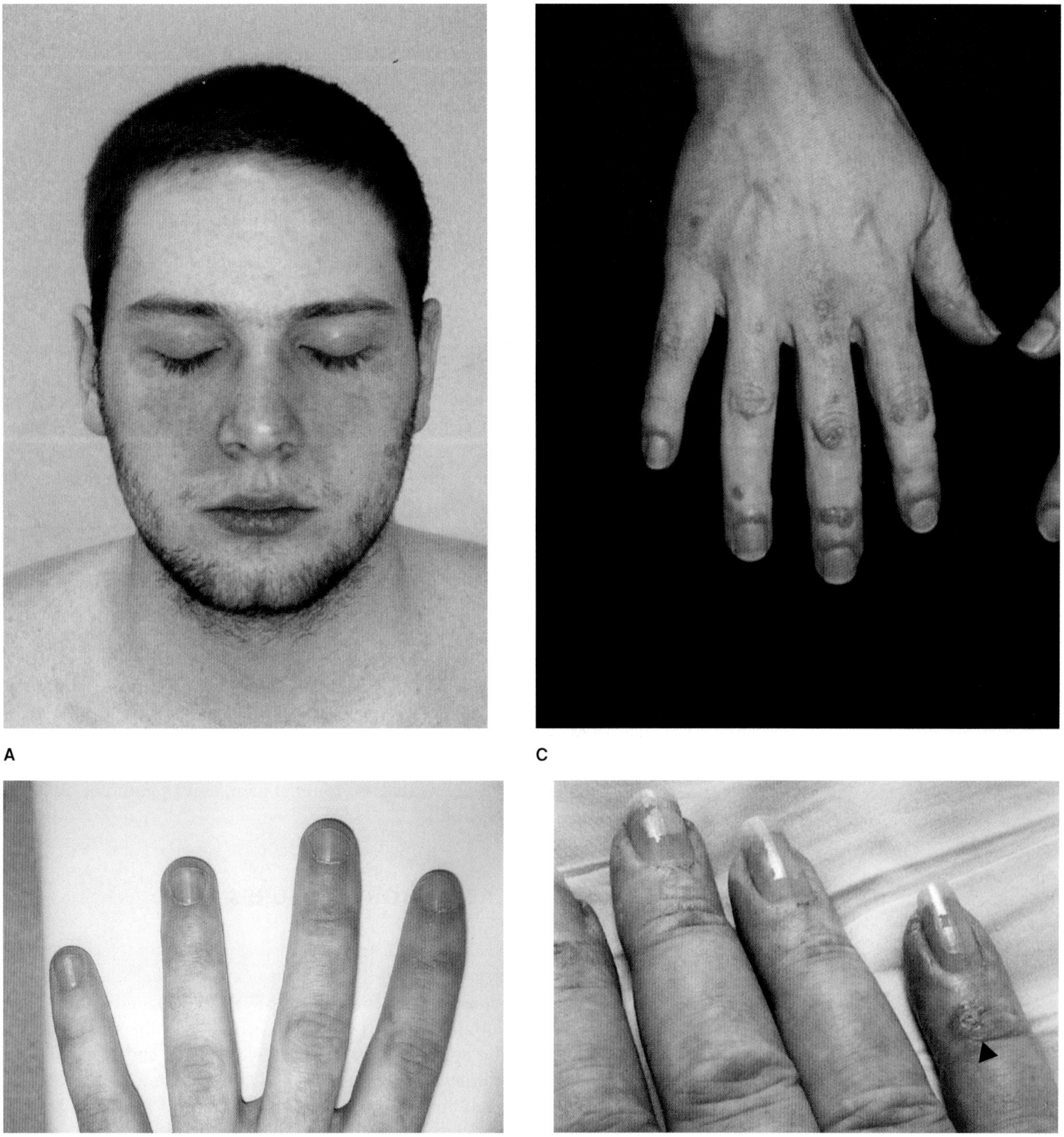

A C B D

Figure 33-1. Dermatomyositis. Moderate erythematous rash is appreciated along the hairline of the scalp, the malar region of the face, and the eyelids—later the heliotrope rash **(A)**. Macular erythematous rash is seen over the extensor surface of the knuckles (Gottron's sign) **(B)**. Gottron's papules are the papular lesions seen here on the knuckles **(C)**. Dilated capillary loops are evident in the nail bed changes as well as a small ulceration involving the distal aspect of the little finger **(D)**.

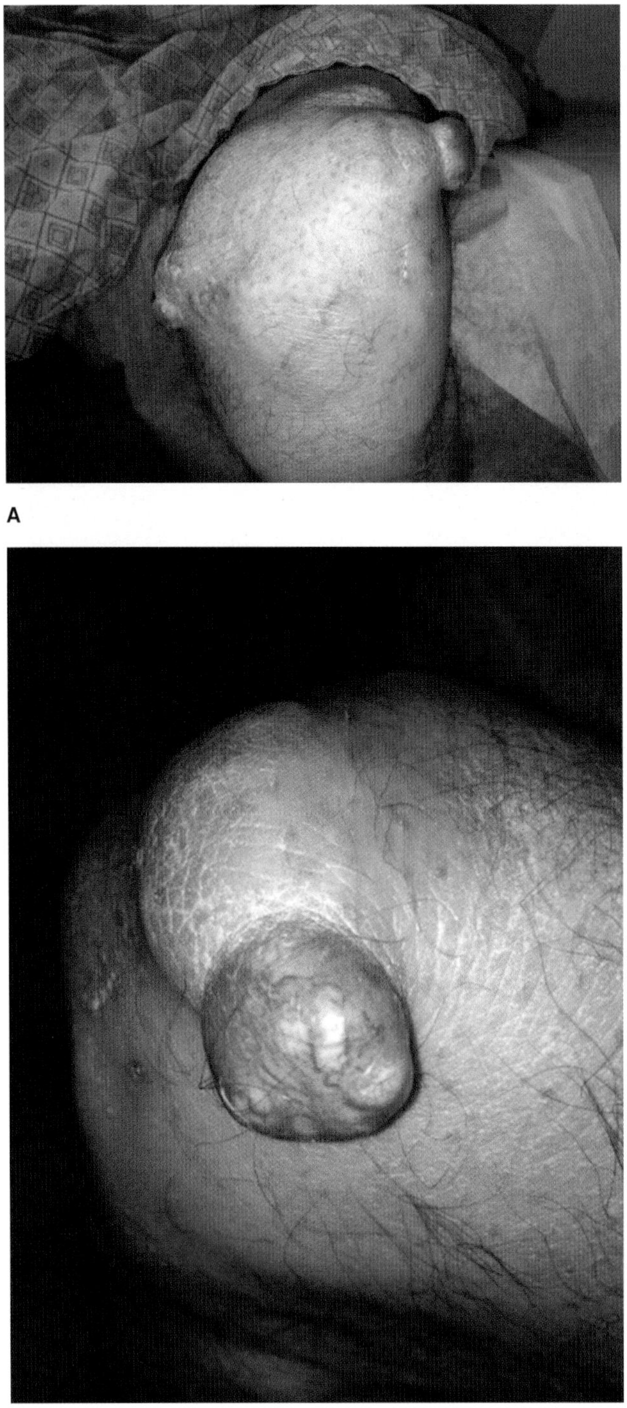

A

B

Figure 33-2. Calcinosis. This adult patient, who had under treated juvenile dermatomyositis as a child, has severe calcinosis on the medial and lateral aspects of the left knee **(A)**; lateral lesion is seen at higher magnification **(B)**.

flexion contractures across the major joints. This emphasizes the importance of early physical therapy and range of motion exercises to prevent contractures from developing. Flexion contractures at the ankles leading to toe walking are a common early finding in childhood DM.

Vasculopathy

A vasculopathy affects the skin, muscle, and gastrointestinal system. Rarely, massive muscle infarction can lead to myoglobinuria and acute renal tubular necrosis.

Malignancy

There is an increased incidence of cancer ranging from 6–45% in DM.[27,28,34,35,52,53] The association with cancer has not been demonstrated in juvenile DM and the increased risk is predominantly seen in adults over the age of 40 years. Although women are more likely to develop DM than men, the risk of malignancy is equal in both sexes. Most malignancies are identified within 2 years of the presentation of the myositis. The clinical severity of rash or muscle weakness does not appear to correlate with the presence or absence of a neoplasm. Treatment of the underlying malignancy sometimes results in improvement of muscle strength.

We perform a comprehensive history and annual physical examination with breast and pelvic examinations for women and testicular and prostate examinations for men to search for an underlying malignancy. In addition, we obtain a complete blood count (CBC), routine blood chemistries, urinalysis, and stool specimens for occult blood. Computerized tomographic (CT) scans of the chest, abdomen, and pelvis and mammography are also ordered. Colonoscopy should be done on all patients over the age of 50 years or in those who have attributable gastrointestinal symptoms (e.g., abdominal pain, constipation, or blood in the stool).

LABORATORY FEATURES

Necrosis of muscle fibers usually leads to increased serum creatine kinase (CK), aldolase, myoglobin, lactate dehydrogenase, aspartate aminotransferase (AST), and alanine aminotransferase (ALT) levels. Serum CK is the most sensitive and specific marker for muscle damage and is elevated in at least 90% of patients with DM.[27,34,35] However, serum CK levels do not correlate with the severity of weakness. The CK level can be normal even in individuals who are markedly weak, particularly in childhood DM, in patients with slow, insidious disease, and in those with little residual muscle mass. In approximately 10% of cases with a normal CK, the aldolase level is elevated.[54–56] Erythrocyte sedimentation rate (ESR) is usually normal or only mildly elevated and is not a reliable indicator of disease severity.

Antinuclear antibodies (ANAs) are detected in 24–60% of patients with DM.[34,50,51] These antibodies are much more common in patients with overlap syndromes (to be discussed later). Some patients have the so-called "myositis-associated antibodies" or "myositis-specific antibodies" (MSAs) (Table 33-5).[5,34,50,51,57–74] Autoantibodies

▶ TABLE 33-5. **AUTOANTIBODIES ASSOCIATED WITH INFLAMMATORY MYOPATHIES**

Antisynthetase Autoantibodies	Autoantigen	Clinical Features
Anti–Jo-1	Histidyl t-RNA synthetase	PM, DM + ILD, Raynaud, arthritis, mechanic hands
Anti–PL-7	Threonyl t-RNA synthetase	PM, DM + ILD. Raynaud, arthritis, mechanic hands
Anti–PL-12	Alanyl t-RNA synthetase	ILD > PM, DM
Anti-EJ	Glycyl t-RNA synthetase	PM > DM + ILD. Raynaud, arthritis, mechanic hands
Anti-OJ	Isoleucylt-RNA synthetase	ILD + PM/DM, Raynaud, arthritis, mechanic hands
Anti-KS	Asparaginyl t-RNA synthetase	ILD > PM, DM, Raynaud, arthritis, mechanic hands
Anti-Zo	Phenylalanyl t-RNA synthetase	ILD + PM, DM, Raynaud, arthritis, mechanic hands
Anti-Ha	Tyrosyl t-RNA synthetase	ILD + PM, DM, Raynaud, arthritis, mechanic hands
Dermatomyositis Autoantibodies		
Anti-Mi-2	Chromatin remodeling enzyme	Severe skin disease, treatment responsive
Anti-MDA5	Melanoma differentiation-associated gene 5	ILD, palmar lesions, rash > myopathy
Anti-TIF1 γ	Transcriptional intermediary factor 1 γ	Cancer-associated dermatomyositis
Anti–NXP-2	Nuclear matrix protein	Severe muscle weakness
Anti-SAE	Small ubiquitin-like modifier-activating enzyme	Rapidly progressive, ILD, rash > myopathy
IMNM Autoantibodies		
Anti-SRP	Signal recognition particle	Severe, treatment-resistant, myopathy, cardiac involvement
Anti-HMGCR	HMGCR	Severe myopathy that continues despite stopping statin
Inclusion body myositis Autoantibody		
Anti-cN1A/anti-Mup44	Cytosolic 5′-nucleotidase	Inclusion body myositis

PM, polymyositis; DM, dermatomyositis; ILD, interstitial lung disease; HMGCR, HMG-CoA reductase; cN1 A, cytosolic 5′-nucleotidase.
Reproduced with permission from Ciafaloni E, Chinnery P, Griggs R: *Evaluation and Treatment of Myopathies*. 2nd ed. Oxford, UK: Oxford University Press; 2014.

to various aminoacyl tRNA synthetases (ARSs) constitute the majority of the MSA of which Jo-1 antibodies (directed against histidyl t-RNA synthetase) are the most common. Jo-1 are demonstrated in as many as 20% of patients with inflammatory myopathy and are strongly associated with ILD.[5,49–51] Some patients have ILD but no myositis, so one can argue that these antibodies are not necessarily specific for myositis. The other antisynthetases are much less common and are each found in <23% of patients with inflammatory myopathy. It has been suggested that the presence of Jo-1 antibodies is associated with only a moderate response to treatment and a poor long-term prognosis.[59–61] However, there has not been a prospective study of treatment outcomes comparing patients with myositis associated ILD with Jo-1 antibodies with patients without these antibodies. Nevertheless there is a constellation of features that constitute the so-called "antisynthetase syndrome" including ILD, myositis, Raynaud's syndrome, arthritis, and mechanic hands which can be useful in diagnosis.

Mi-2 antibodies are found in 15–20% of patients with DM. Mi-2 is a 240-kD nuclear protein of unknown function. The Mi-2 antibodies are typically associated with an acute onset, a florid rash, a good response to therapy, and a favorable prognosis.[5,50,51,59–61] However, again it is not known if patients with DM patients with Mi-2 antibodies respond differently than DM without the antibody.

Antibodies directed against melanoma differentiation-association protein 5 (anti-MDA5), also known as anti-CADM-140 antibodies, are found in 10–20%of DM patients and up to 65% of patients with clinically amyopathic DM and are associated with rapidly progressive ILD, particularly in Asians.[62–67] Anti-MDA-5 antibody levels closely correlate with the severity of skin ulcerations, ILD, and disease prognosis.

Autoantibodies targeting transcriptional intermediary factor 1-γ (TIF1-γ), also known p155 antibodies, are found in adult cancer-associated DM with an 89% specificity and 70% sensitivity.[73] Antibodies directed against nuclear matrix protein NXP-2 (also known as MORC3) have been found in as many as 17% of patients with DM and are also associated with cancer.[73]

Magnetic resonance imaging (MRI) can provide information on the pattern of muscle involvement by looking at the cross-sectional area of axial and limb muscles.[74–79] MRI may demonstrate signal abnormalities in affected muscles secondary to inflammation and edema or replacement by fibrotic tissue. However, the changes on MRI are not usually specific for myositis. Some have advocated MRI as a method to guide which muscle to biopsy.[78] However, we have found that MRI usually adds little to a good clinical examination and EMG in defining the pattern of muscle involvement and determining the muscle for biopsy.

ELECTROPHYSIOLOGICAL FEATURES

The characteristic electromyography (EMG) abnormalities observed in patients with myositis include (1) increased insertional and spontaneous activity with fibrillation potentials, positive sharp waves, and occasionally pseudomyotonic discharges (e.g., decrescendo waves of positive waves that do not wax or wane in frequency and amplitude) or complex repetitive discharges; (2) small-duration, low-amplitude, polyphasic motor unit action potentials (MUAPs); and (3) MUAPs that recruit early but at normal frequencies.[80] Recruitment may be decreased (fast firing MUAPs) in advanced disease, if there is marked loss of muscle fibers. Decreased insertional activity may be seen in chronic disease secondary to fibrosis. In addition, large-duration, polyphasic MUAPs may also be evident later in longstanding disease due to muscle fiber splitting and regeneration rather than a superimposed neurogenic process.

The degree of abnormal spontaneous EMG activity reflects the ongoing disease activity. EMG can be used to assist determining which muscle to biopsy in patients with only mild weakness. In addition, EMG may also be useful in the assessment of previously responsive patients with myositis who become weaker by differentiating an increase in disease activity from weakness secondary to type 2 muscle fiber atrophy from disuse or chronic steroid administration. Abnormal insertional and spontaneous activity is expected in active myositis, while isolated type 2 muscle fiber atrophy is not associated with such abnormal activity on EMG. Along these lines, it is our opinion that a multifocal or diffuse pattern of abnormal insertional and spontaneous activity without obvious changes in MUAP morphology or recruitment is much more likely to represent an acute myopathy, like DM, than a neurogenic disorder.

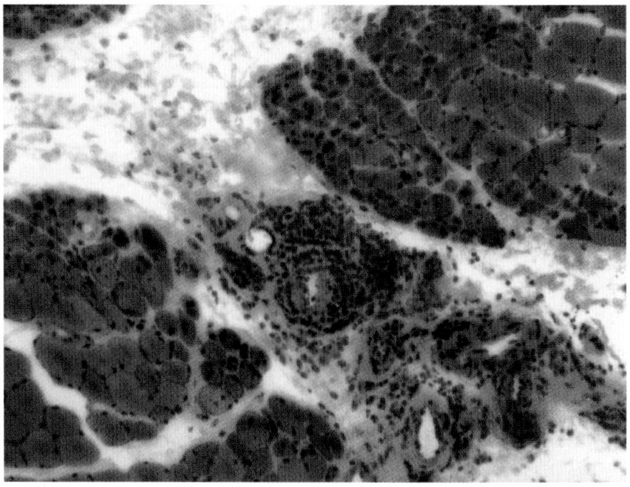

A

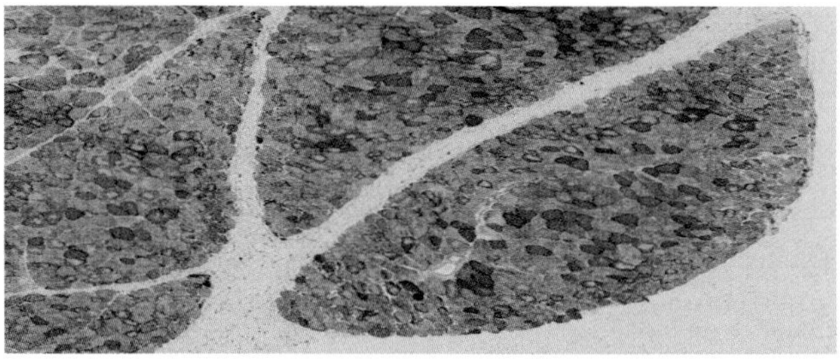

B

Figure 33-3. Dermatomyositis. Muscle biopsy demonstrates classic perifascicular atrophy of muscle fibers and perivascular inflammation within the perimysium **(A)**, hematoxylin and eosin (H&E). Combined cytochrome oxidase/succinic dehydrogenase (COX/SDH) stain demonstrates COX-negative/SDH-positive staining of perifascicular muscle fibers **(B)**.

HISTOPATHOLOGY

The pathological process is multifocal, and the frequency and severity of histological abnormalities can vary within the muscle biopsy specimens. The pathognomonic histological feature is perifascicular atrophy (Fig. 33-3A), although this is a late finding and in our experience is found in <50% of adult-onset cases (it is somewhat more frequent in juvenile-onset DM). The perifascicular area contains small regenerating and degenerating fibers. Oxidative enzyme stains highlight the microvacuolation within these fibers. Combined COX/SDH stain may demonstrate COX-negative/SDH-positive staining perifascicular muscle fibers (Fig. 33-3B). Scattered necrotic fibers and much less frequently, wedge-shaped microinfarcts may be evident. Even though DM is an inflammatory myopathy, inflammatory cell infiltrates are not evident with routine histochemistry in some patients. The inflammatory infiltrate is composed primarily of macrophages, B cells, and CD4+ cells in the perivascular and perimysial regions around blood vessels (perivascular).[32,81] These CD4+ cells are mainly plasmacytoid dendritic cells (PDCs) and not T-helper cells as they are often CD3 negative.[82] Importantly, in contrast to PM and IBM (discussed later), invasion of non-necrotic fibers is not prominent. Immunohistochemistry (IHC) staining demonstrate that muscle fibers express MHC-1 antigen, STAT1, and various interferon-α/β inducible proteins, including myxovirus resistance 1 (MxA) and ISG15 on the sarcolemma, particularly in the perifascicular regions (Fig. 33-4), and can be seen even before the development of perifascicular atrophy.[82,83] However, there is no overexpression of interferon-gamma inducible proteins on muscle fibers.

DM is associated with a reduction in the capillary density (number of capillaries per area of muscle) and compensatory dilation of the remaining small vessels.[84] One of the earliest demonstrable histological abnormalities in DM is deposition of the C5b-9 complement membrane attack complex (MAC) around small blood vessels (Fig. 33-5).[84–86] Deposition of MAC precedes inflammatory

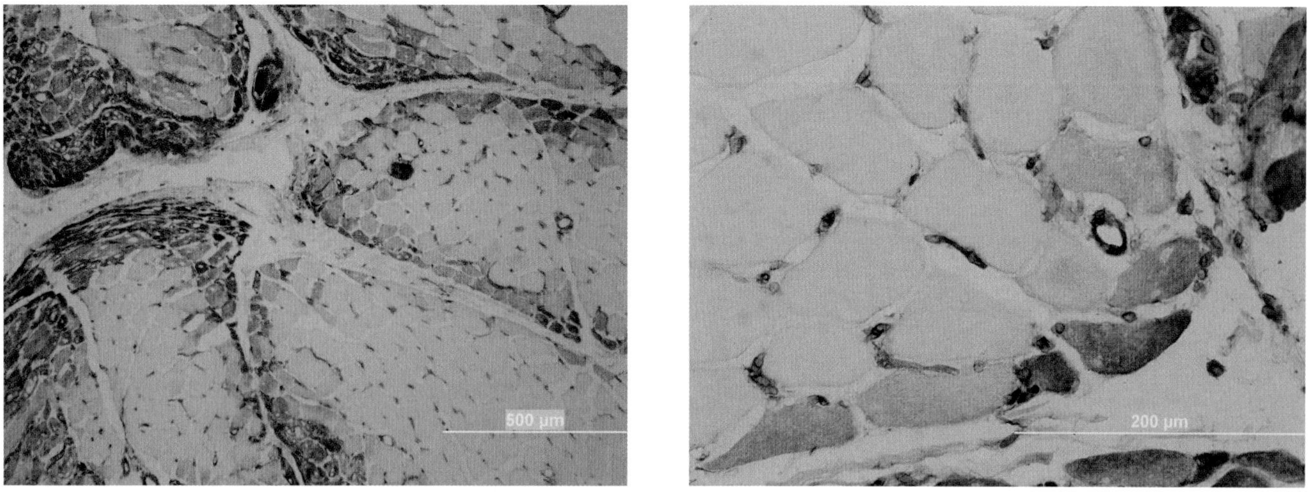

A B

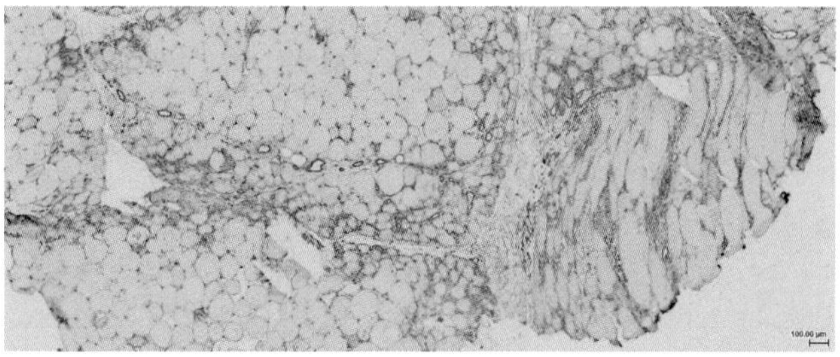

C

Figure 33-4. Dermatomyositis. Immunoperoxidase stain reveals the expression of the interferon-α/β-inducible myxovirus resistance 1 (MxA) protein on perifascicular muscle fibers **(A)** as well as small arterioles and capillaries **(B)**. There is also increased expression of major histocompatibility antigen 1 (MHC1) on the perifascicular muscle fibers **(C)**. Note that MHC1 is not normally expressed on muscle fibers, but is normally expressed on blood vessels.

cell infiltration and other structural abnormalities (e.g., perifascicular atrophy) in the muscle on light microscopy and is relatively specific for DM.[84] Other complement components (C3 and C9) and immunoglobulins (IgM and less often IgG) are also deposited on or around the walls of intramuscular blood vessels.[87] These observations have led to the hypothesis that DM is caused by deposition of immunoglobulins on capillaries, subsequent activation of complement, and MAC-induced necrosis of the vessels, which then lead to ischemic damage of muscle. However, as discussed in section "Pathogenesis", this hypothesis is purely speculative. In addition to expression of MxA on muscle fibers, MxA also is expressed on capillaries in DM (Fig. 33-4).

Electron microscopy (EM) reveals small intramuscular blood vessels (arterioles and capillaries) with endothelial hyperplasia, microvacuoles, and tubuloreticular cytoplasmic inclusions.[12,88]

PATHOGENESIS

Immunological studies and other histological features on muscle biopsies have suggested that DM may be at least in part a humorally/complement mediated microangiopathy, although this is far from proven.[89] Although the presence of MAC is well established, its frequency is not, and this is important with regard to the possibility of varied mechanisms of disease and distinct subtypes of DM. Its presence on blood vessels could be due to either immune complex deposition, or complement activation by either the classical antibody-mediated or alternative pathways. Even classical pathway activation, which is antibody dependent, can still be relatively antigen nonspecific; some IgM antibodies

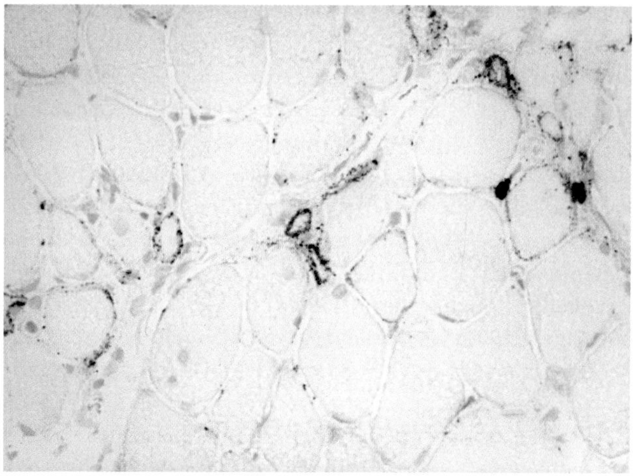

Figure 33-5. Dermatomyositis. Immunoperoxidase stain demonstrates deposition of membrane attack complex (MAC) around small blood vessels and capillaries.

are highly polyclonal, binding with low avidity to many self-antigens. The specificity of MAC presence is also in question, as it is present in abnormal vascular tissue (e.g., atherosclerotic coronary arteries). It may be that the microvasculature is damaged by some other mechanism (e.g., interferon- or other cytokine-related toxicity), and the deposition of immunoglobulins and complement on the damaged vascular tissue might be a secondary phenomenon. That some individuals have developed DM with hereditary complement deficiencies argues against primary destruction of capillaries by complement and MAC.[90,91]

The microangiopathy has been postulated to cause ischemic damage and occasionally infarction of muscle fibers. It has been suggested that the perifascicular atrophy is the result of hypoperfusion to the watershed region of muscle fascicles. However, it has never been demonstrated that the perifascicular region is indeed the watershed area in muscle fibers and that perifascicular fibers are more prone to ischemic damage.[92] Perifascicular atrophy and endomysial capillary MAC deposition were found, in one study, to be inversely correlated,[85] and another study found no correlation between perifascicular atrophy and capillary depletion.[84] Furthermore, perifascicular atrophy has not been reported in vasculitis, a condition with known muscle ischemia and infarction, nor has perifascicular atrophy been found in experimental models of skeletal muscle ischemia.[92] In another model of ischemic myopathy, resulting from microarterial embolization with particles 20–80 m in diameter, the pathological changes were located centrally within fascicles and the perifascicular regions were instead preferentially spared.[93], Finally, perifascicular atrophy is not evident in ischemic muscle in animal models when muscle is rendered ischemic from vasculitis or other small vessel injury.

Gene microarray studies of biopsied muscle tissue demonstrate an increased expression of genes induced by type 1 interferons.[82,94,95] Although this is not specific, it is compatible with the hypothesis of a viral infection triggering the autoimmune attack as interferons have a well-defined role in antiviral innate immunity. However, there are other possibilities. Type 1 interferons (i.e., interferon-α and interferon-β) are synthesized by PDCs in response to a serum factor(s) containing immune complexes of antibody, double-stranded DNA, or RNA viruses. Abundant PDCs are evident in the muscle biopsies of patients with DM.[82] PDCs are CD4+ and comprise a large component of the inflammatory cell infiltrate in DM. These CD4+ cells were originally thought to be CD4+ T-helper cells, but it was subsequently demonstrated that most are CD3-. Therefore, these CD4+ cells are predominantly PDCs and not lymphocytes. Increased expression of interferon-α/β inducible protein MxA is evident on blood vessels and muscle fibers (with a predilection for the perifascicular fibers). Interestingly, one postulated function of MxA is to form tubuloreticular inclusions around RNA viruses. These inclusions have the same morphology as the tubuloreticular inclusions seen on EM in blood vessels in DM. Using immunoelectron microscopy, MxA was demonstrated within inclusions in vessels in DM muscle biopsies.[82] Interestingly, increased expression of type 1 interferon regulated genes are also evident in the peripheral blood and on skin biopsies of patients with active DM, similar to what has been described in systemic lupus erythematosus (SLE). Further, expression levels in the blood appear to correlate with disease activity. We suspect that dysregulated interferon-α/β production plays a major role in the pathogenesis of DM and could be directly toxic to the small blood vessels and muscle fibers themselves.

PROGNOSIS

In the absence of malignancy, prognosis is generally favorable in patients with DM. Poor prognostic features are increased age, associated ILD, cardiac disease, and late or previous inadequate treatment with 5-year survival rates ranging from 70% to 93%.[35,59,96,97]

▶ POLYMYOSITIS

PM, as reported in the literature, is likely to be a heterogeneous group of disorders rather than a distinct entity. A major source of debate among clinicians who primarily take care of patients with PM (e.g., neurologists and rheumatologists) is the criteria for diagnosing PM. The most commonly employed criteria were developed by Bohan and Peter in 1975 (Table 33-4),[26,27] but these do not take into account advancements in our understanding of the immunopathogenesis of the various inflammatory myopathies or even the existence of IBM and IMNM. Revised criteria for the various idiopathic inflammatory myopathies have been proposed (Tables 33-2 and 33-3). For definitive histopathological diagnosis of PM, these criteria require CD8+ T cells invading *non-necrotic* muscle fibers that express MHC-1 antigen.[9,30,31] Even so, this biopsy feature is not diagnostic for PM, as it also is seen in IBM and rarely in dystrophies. Further, mononuclear cell invasion of non-necrotic muscle fibers is uncommon in suspected cases of PM, and some argue that it is not necessary for the diagnosis of PM.[58,98] More frequently on biopsy we appreciate perivascular/perimysial inflammatory cell infiltrates or endomysial inflammatory cells, but no actual invasion on non-necrotic muscle fibers.[11,31] Whether or not these cases represent "PM," with the absence of CD8+ T cells invading non-necrotic muscle fibers or a distinct type of inflammatory myopathy, is unclear. Such perivascular, perimysial inflammation is common, particularly in patients with overlap myositis, but can be seen in DM and IBM and, occasionally, in dystrophies.

For the various reasons listed above, it is impossible to extract from the literature the true incidence and prognosis of PM or its subtypes and the associated laboratory abnormalities, medical conditions (e.g., connective tissue disorder [CTD], ILD, myocarditis, and cancer). We need prospective studies using contemporary clinical, laboratory, and histopathological criteria for PM to address these issues. Nevertheless, we will summarize the available literature regarding "PM."

CLINICAL FEATURES

PM generally presents in patients over the age of 20 years. Unlike DM, idiopathic PM in absence of an underlying connective tissue disease is rare in childhood in our experience. As in DM and other autoimmune disorders, PM is more prevalent in women.[16–28,34,35] The diagnosis of PM is often delayed compared to DM. As with DM, patients present with symmetric proximal arm and leg weakness that typically develops over several weeks or months. Distal muscles may also become involved but are not as weak as the more proximal muscles. Muscle pain and tenderness are frequently noted but these are not the primary symptoms—weakness is the primary complaint. Approximately one-third of patients complain of swallowing difficulties. Mild facial weakness occasionally may be demonstrated on examination. Sensation is normal and muscle stretch reflexes are usually preserved.

ASSOCIATED MANIFESTATIONS

The cardiac and pulmonary complications of PM are reportedly similar to that described in the DM section. Myositis with secondary congestive heart failure or conduction abnormalities occur in up to one-third of patients, but again histopathological confirmation of definite PM using more up-to-date criteria is lacking in most of these studies.[34,35,40–44] Anti-signal recognition particle (SRP) antibodies have been associated with myocarditis and were felt to be specific for PM, although the histopathology is more often that of a necrotizing myopathy.[99,100] In studies of SRP-myositis in which detailed immunohistochemistries were performed, the biopsies were not suggestive of PM (i.e., inflammatory infiltrate was scant), but rather revealed features suggestive of a microvasculopathy.[82,101] ILD has been reported to occur in at least 10% of patient with PM, with at least half having Jo-1 antibodies.[34,45–48,50,51,61] Muscle biopsies from patients with Jo-1 antibodies demonstrated perimysial abnormalities (fragmentation and increase staining with alkaline phosphatase of the perimysial connective tissue, atrophy and degeneration of perifascicular muscle fibers, and perivascular/perimysial inflammation without endomysial inflammatory cells invading non-necrotic muscle fibers.[10,101] This suggests to us that anti-SRP and anti–Jo-1 myositis cases are probably distinct from idiopathic PM.

Polyarthritis has been reported in as many as 45% of patients with PM at the time of diagnosis.[35] The risk of malignancy with PM seems to be lower than that seen in DM, but is slightly higher than expected in the general population.[28,35,52,53]

LABORATORY FEATURES

Serum CK level is elevated fivefold or more in most PM cases.[27,28,34,35] Unlike DM and IBM (to be discussed later) in which the CK can be normal, the serum CK should be elevated in active PM. Serum CK can be useful in monitoring response to therapy, but only in conjunction with the physical examination, as the CK level does not necessarily correlate with the degree of weakness. ESR is normal in most patients and does not correlate with disease activity or severity.

Positive ANAs are reportedly present in 16–40% of patients with PM.[27,34,35,50] However, again the exact relationship of ANAs and CTD in patients with histologically defined PM is unclear. The relationships of various MSAs to PM were previously addressed (Table 33-5).

MRI may demonstrate T2 signal abnormalities in affected muscles secondary to inflammation and edema or T1 abnormalities as a result of replacement by fibrotic tissue (Fig. 33-6).[74–78]

ELECTROPHYSIOLOGICAL FEATURES

EMG is usually abnormal in PM with increased insertional and spontaneous activity, small polyphasic MUAPs, and early recruitment.[80] These abnormal features do not distinguish PM from other inflammatory myopathies or myopathies with muscle membrane instability.

HISTOPATHOLOGY

The histological features of PM are distinct from DM. The predominant histological features in PM are variability in fiber size, scattered necrotic and regenerating fibers, and inflammatory cell infiltrates. However, as mentioned previously, the specific characteristics of this inflammatory cell infiltrate have been the subject of recent debate. Small studies of PM reported that muscle biopsies demonstrate CD8+ T cells and macrophages invading non-necrotic muscle fibers expressing MHC-1 antigen (Fig. 33-7).[31,32,81,102] Subsequently, some have argued that this histopathological feature is required for the diagnosis of definite PM.[4,30,31] However, other authorities argue that invasion of non-necrotic muscle fibers is not necessary and perivascular, perimysial, or endomysial inflammation without actual invasion of non-necrotic muscle fibers can suffice for the diagnosis of PM in the proper clinical context.[58,98] In our opinion, demonstrating invasion of non-necrotic endomysial muscle fibers by T cells is very helpful in making a diagnosis of PM on *histopathological* grounds, as the sole findings of perivascular, perimysial, and even endomysial inflammatory cell infiltrates can be seen in DM, some dystrophies, and rhabdomyolysis from metabolic and toxic myopathies. Importantly, invasion of non-necrotic muscle fibers is not diagnostic for PM and is actually more commonly seen in IBM as will be discussed later. That said, invasion of non-necrotic muscle fibers is not mandatory to make a clinical diagnosis of PM in the appropriate situation.

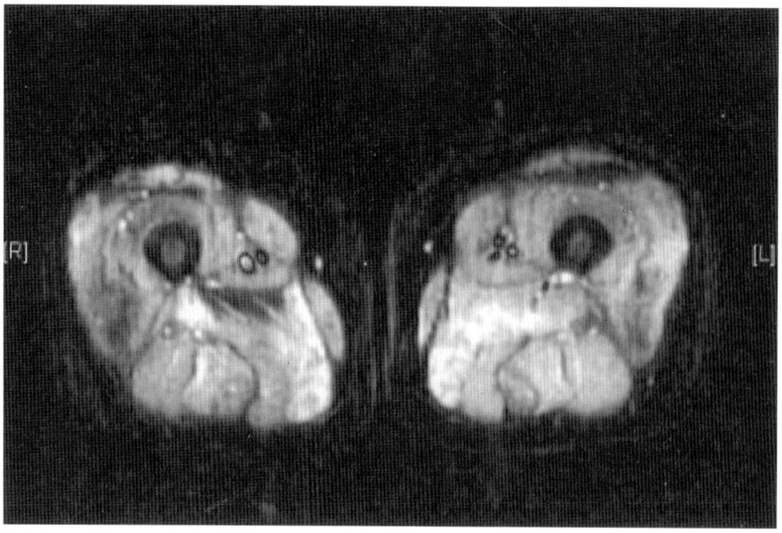

Figure 33-6. Polymyositis. Skeletal muscle MRI (STIR image) reveals patchy areas of increased signal consistent with edema/inflammation in the semitendinosus and semimembranosus in the posterior thigh and to a lesser extent in the quadriceps muscles on both legs.

The endomysial inflammatory cells consist primarily of activated CD8+ (cytotoxic), *alpha, and beta* T cells and macrophages.[32,81,102] Rare cases of PM with CD4- and CD8- *gamma/delta* T-cell infiltrates have been reported.[103–105] The T-cell receptors of endomysial T cells have an oligoclonal pattern of gene rearrangements and a restricted motif in the CD3R region, suggesting that the immune response is antigen specific.[106,107] Further, there are many myeloid dendritic cells in the endomysium that appear to surround non-necrotic muscle fibers and may serve to present antigens to cytotoxic T cells. Although B cells are rare, plasma cells are common in the endomysium and likely account for the increased expression of immunoglobulin genes on microarray experiments.[108] There is also evidence of oligoclonal pattern of gene rearrangements in plasma cells in PM muscle biopsies. Unlike DM, MAC, complement, or immunoglobulins are not deposited on the microvasculature in PM.

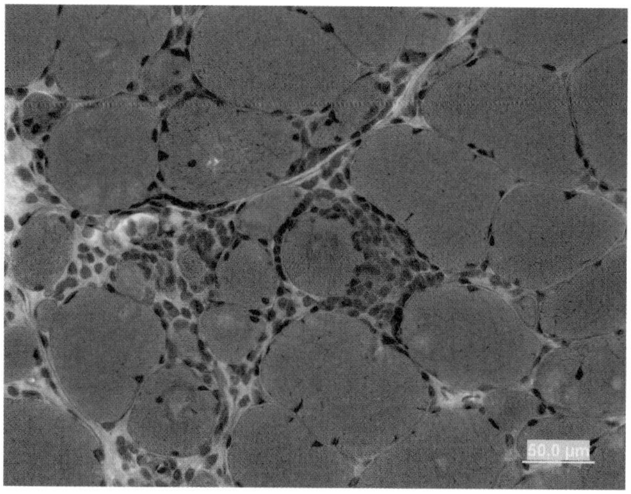

A

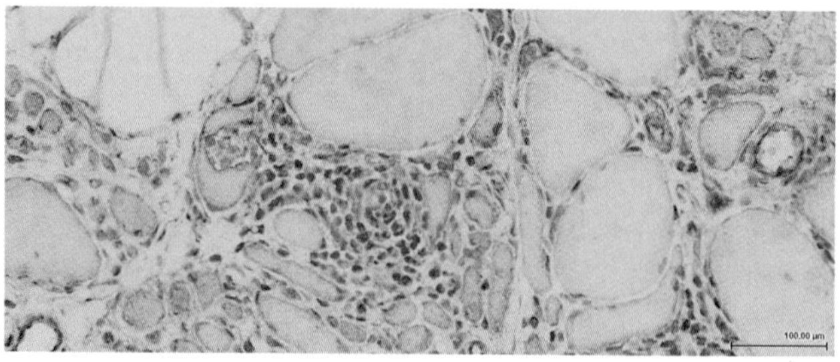

B

Figure 33-7. Polymyositis. Muscle biopsy demonstrates endomysial mononuclear inflammatory cell infiltrate surrounding and invading non-necrotic muscle fibers, H&E **(A)**. Immunoperoxidase stain demonstrates perivascular and endomysial inflammatory cells surrounding and appearing to invade non-necrotic muscle fibers expressing major histocompatibility antigen type 1(MHC1) on the sarcolemma **(B)**.

PATHOGENESIS

PM is believed to be the result of an HLA-restricted, antigen-specific, cell-mediated immune response directed against muscle fibers. The trigger of this autoimmune attack is not known, but viral infections have been speculated. However, there is no conclusive evidence supporting this hypothesis.[109] MHC-1 molecules on the surface of cells usually express endogenous self-peptides rather than viral particles. Neither viral proteins nor DNA have been identified in muscle fibers. Thus, the autoimmune response may be directed against endogenous self-antigens rather than processed viral antigens. Nonetheless, a viral infection could indirectly trigger an immune response secondary to antigenic mimicry with muscle proteins, altering the expression of proteins on the surface of muscle fibers such that these become antigenic, or by the loss of physiological self-tolerance. Myositis may complicate human immunodeficiency virus (HIV) and human T-lymphocyte virus-1 (HTLV-1) infections.[110] In these cases, the myositis appears to be the result of such indirect triggering of the immune response against muscle fibers.

The cytotoxic T cells appear to destroy muscle fibers via the perforin pathway. These autoinvasive T cells contain perforin granules oriented next to the sarcolemma of muscle fibers.[111] Upon release of these granules by exocytosis, pore formations are induced on the sarcolemma, leading to osmolysis of muscle fibers.

DIFFERENTIAL DIAGNOSIS

A diagnosis of PM relies on a thorough search to exclude other causes of weakness (Table 33-6).[29,112] A detailed clinical examination of an appreciation of the pattern of weakness can help differentiate IBM and muscular dystrophies with inflammation from PM. Serum CK should be elevated in PM, while it is normal in patients with "fibromyalgia" and polymyalgia rheumatica and can be normal in IBM. Skeletal muscle MRI is often interpreted as showing "myositis." However, these increased signal abnormalities are not specific and can be seen in dystrophies, rhabdomyolysis from toxic medications (e.g., statins) metabolic myopathy, and muscle infarcts from various causes (e.g., vasculitis and diabetic vasculopathy). The specific pattern of muscle involvement and extensive fatty replacement in the absence of edematous changes on MRI scans would be helpful, suggesting a dystrophy as opposed to PM. EMG can be useful, as the presence of diffuse myotonic discharges should lead to the consideration of proximal myotonic myopathy or late-onset acid maltase deficiency—conditions that we have seen misdiagnosed as PM.

Importantly, the diagnosis of PM requires a muscle biopsy. It is important to look for histopathological features that would suggest IBM (e.g., rimmed vacuoles, inclusions, ragged red fibers, etc.). However, the absence of these findings does not exclude the diagnosis of IBM. Muscle biopsy is essential to look for features that might suggest a dystrophy, metabolic myopathy such as acid maltase deficiency, or necrotizing myopathy.

▶ **TABLE 33-6. DISORDERS THAT CAN RESEMBLE POLYMYOSITIS**

Inclusion body myositis
Dermatomyositis *sine* dermatitis
Necrotizing myopathy
Inflammatory myopathy associated with infections (e.g., HIV, HTLV-1, and hepatitis B and C)
Muscular dystrophies (e.g., facioscapulohumeral, congenital, dysferlinopathies, and other limb-girdle dystrophies) and late-onset congenital myopathies
Proximal myotonic myopathy (myotonic dystrophy type 2)
Amyloid myopathy (light chain or familial)
Metabolic and mitochondrial myopathies
Endocrine myopathies (e.g., hypothyroidism, hyperparathyroidism, and diabetic muscle infarction)
Drug-induced myopathies (e.g., cholesterol lowering agents, cyclosporine, chloroquine, amiodarone, colchicine, and D-penicillamine)
Juvenile or adult-onset spinal muscular atrophy (including Kennedy's disease)
Polymyalgia rheumatica

HIV, human immunodeficiency virus; HTLV-1, human T-lymphocyte virus-1.
Data from Amato AA, Griggs RC. Unicorns, dragons, polymyositis, and other mythological beasts. *Neurology.* 2003;61(3):288–289.

PROGNOSIS

Most patients with PM improve with immunosuppressive therapies but usually require life-long treatment.[34,59,96] Some retrospective studies suggest that PM does not respond to immunosuppressive agents as well as DM. However, interpretation of the results of these retrospective series is difficult, as the diagnosis of PM was usually made based on the Bohan and Peter criteria rather than on more up-to-date criteria based on strict clinical and histological criteria.

▶ OVERLAP SYNDROMES

The term "overlap syndrome" is applied when DM or PM is associated with other well-defined CTDs such as scleroderma, mixed connective tissue disease (MCTD), Sjögren's syndrome, SLE, or rheumatoid arthritis.[1,3,4,11] In our experience[82,83,94] and others,[11,31] the muscle biopsies in patients with overlap syndrome resemble DM, a necrotizing myopathy, or are associated with nonspecific (e.g., perivascular and perimysial) inflammatory cell infiltrates as opposed to PM (at least if defined by CD8+ cells invading nonnecrotic muscle fibers). These features correspond to what some have termed myopathy with perimysial pathology.[10] The prognoses in these patients are related in part to the underlying CTD. Retrospective series of patients that suggest that myositis associated with overlap syndromes is more responsive to immunosuppressive treatment than isolated DM and PM, but again prospective studies are lacking.[10,34,49,59,96]

SCLERODERMA

Weakness is common in scleroderma. Most patients have normal serum CKs and EMG, while muscle biopsies demonstrate only mild variability in fiber size with atrophy of type 2 muscle fibers and perimysial fibrosis. However,

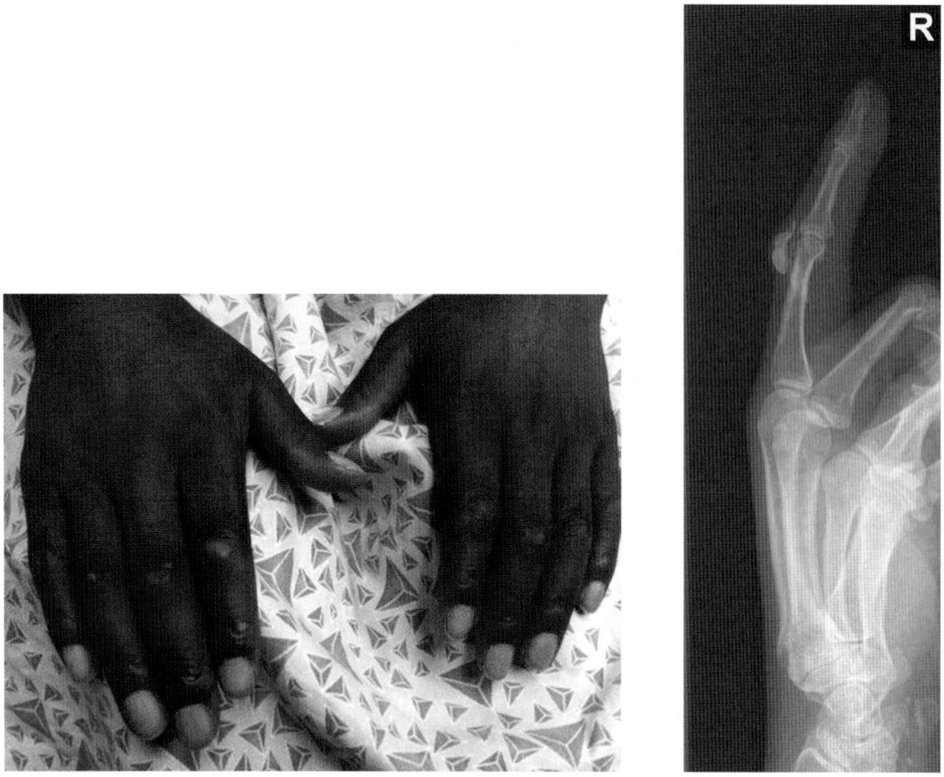

A B

Figure 33-8. Scleroderma associated myositis. Sclerodactyly is appreciated along with discoloration of the skin on some of the knuckles **(A)**. An x-ray reviews calcinosis involving a finger **(B)**.

5–17% of patients with scleroderma have myositis which can occur in either of its two major forms—progressive systemic sclerosis or CREST (Calcinosis, Raynaud's phenomena, Esophageal dysmotility, Sclerodactyly, Telangiectasia) syndrome (Fig. 33-8).[35,113–116] Patients with scleroderma myositis may have mildly increased serum CK levels and irritable and myopathic EMGs. Detailed descriptions of the immunohistopathology on muscle biopsies are lacking, and therefore it is difficult to ascertain if these have features of DM or PM.

Most patients with CREST syndrome have anticentromere antibodies, while anti-Scl-70 antibodies are common in patients with progressive systemic sclerosis. Some patients with scleroderma myositis have anti-PMScl (also called anti-PM-1) antibodies.[51,117]

SJÖGREN'S SYNDROME

Sjögren's syndrome is characterized by dryness of the eyes and mouth (sicca syndrome) and other mucosal membranes. Muscle pain and weakness are common in Sjögren's syndrome, but true myositis is rare. Muscle weakness is usually due to disuse atrophy secondary to arthritis and pain. Nonetheless, myositis can occur with Sjögren's syndrome.[35,118–120] About 90% of patients have ANAs directed against ribonucleoproteins, specifically SS-A (Ro) and less commonly SS-B (La) antibodies.

SYSTEMIC LUPUS ERYTHEMATOSUS

SLE is an autoimmune disorder affecting multiple organ systems. As with other CTDs, weakness is not unusual in SLE but is most often the result of disuse atrophy. Nevertheless, myositis can occur with SLE.[35,82,121,122]

Most patients with SLE have positive ANA titers that are directed against native DNA (highly specific for SLE) and ribonuclear proteins (RNPs). The anti-RNP antibodies are present in less than half of patients with SLE and include anti-SS-A and anti-SS-B (also present in Sjögren's syndrome), anti-U1 RNP (also present in MCTD), and anti-Sm (specific for SLE).

Of note, gene expression studies in peripheral blood of patients with SLE demonstrated an upregulation of type 1 interferon-inducible genes, similar to what is seen in gene expression studies of muscle biopsies in DM.[82] In this regard, MxA is highly expressed in both SLE blood and DM muscle. Both disorders are also associated with tubular reticular inclusions in endothelial cells on EM. Thus, DM and SLE likely share a similar pathogenic basis with abnormalities involving the innate immune system.

RHEUMATOID ARTHRITIS

The most common etiology of weakness in RA is type 2 muscle fiber atrophy from chronic steroids or disuse secondary to arthritis, but myositis can infrequently occur.[35]

MIXED CONNECTIVE TISSUE DISEASE

Patients with MCTD have clinical features of scleroderma, SLE, rheumatoid arthritis, and myositis.[123] In terms of the myositis, DM is reported more commonly than PM.[35,82,113,123] This is certainly our experience. Necrotizing myopathy can also complicate MCTD. High titers of anti-U1 RNP antibodies are common in MCTD but are nonspecific, as these can also be detected in SLE.

▶ INCLUSION BODY MYOSITIS

CLINICAL FEATURES

IBM is characterized clinically by the insidious onset of slowly progressive proximal and distal weakness, which generally develops after the age of 40 years (and usually after 50 years) (Tables 33-1 and 33-3).[1–3,9,124–132] IBM appears to be the most common myopathy (apart from sarcopenia of aging) in patients over the age of 50 years. The slow progressive nature of the myopathy probably accounts in part for the delay in diagnosis that averages 6–7 years after the onset of symptoms. Men are much more commonly affected than women, in contrast to the female predominance seen in DM and PM.

The clinical hallmark of IBM is early weakness and atrophy of the quadriceps, flexor forearm muscles (i.e., wrist and finger flexors) (Fig. 33-9), and ankle dorsiflexors.[1–3,9,126–128] This pattern of weakness is present in as many as two-thirds of patients with IBM, but not all.[132] With manual muscle testing,

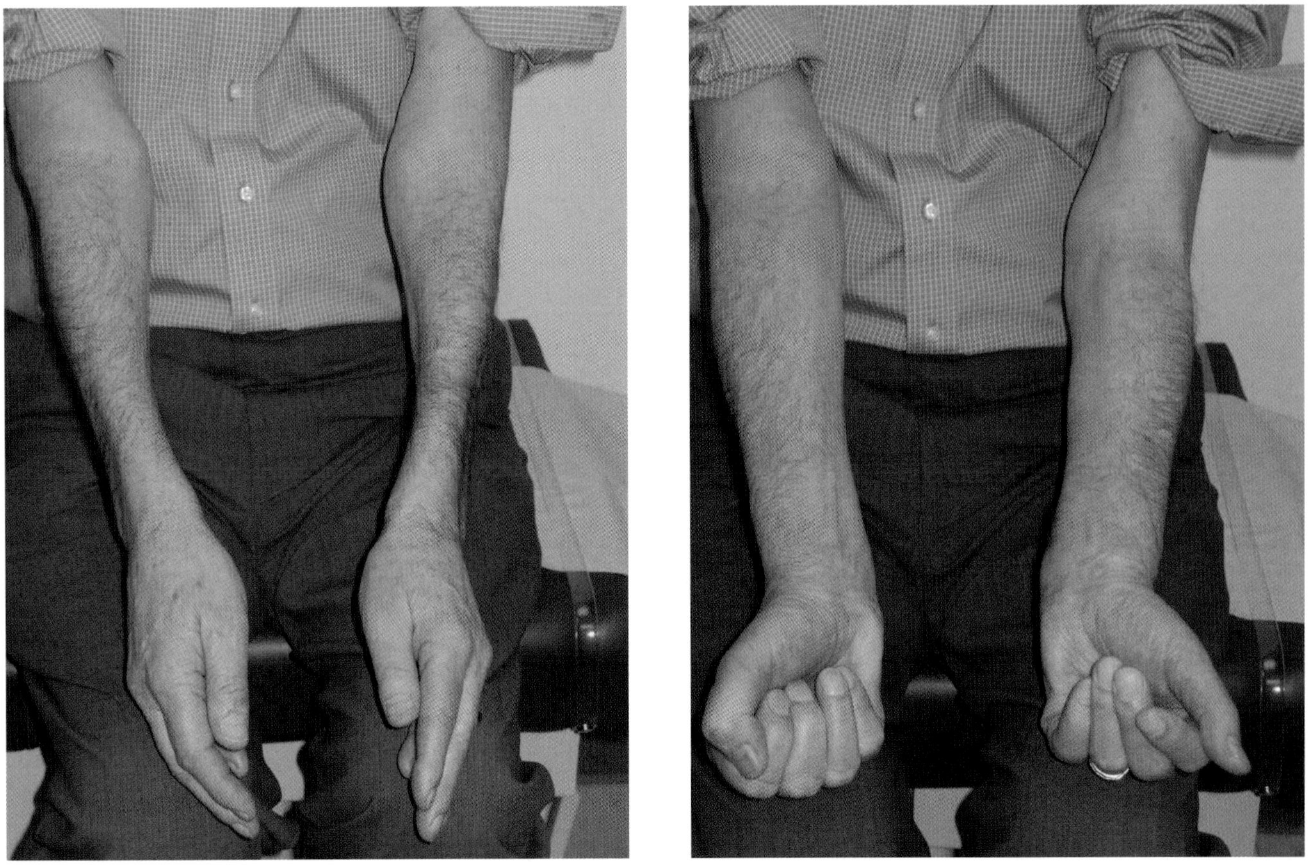

A B

Figure 33-9. Inclusion body myositis. The clinical hallmark of IBM is early, and often asymmetric, atrophy flexor forearm muscles **(A)**. This patient was asked to make a grip (flex the fingers) and one can see the asymmetrical weakness flexing the fingers of the left hand, particularly the deep finger flexors and flexor pollicis longus **(B)**. (Reproduced with permission from Amato AA, Barohn RJ. Inclusion body myositis: old and new concepts. *J Neurol Neurosurg Psychiatry*. 2009;80(11):1186–1193.)

the MRC grades of the finger and wrist flexors (in particular the deep finger flexors such as the flexor pollicis longus) are usually lower than those of the shoulder abductors, and the muscle scores of the knee extensors and ankle dorsiflexors may be the same or lower than those of the hip flexors in patients with IBM.[2,129–132] In contrast, the proximal muscles (shoulder abductors and hip flexors) are usually weaker than distal muscle groups by manual muscle testing grades in DM and PM. In addition, muscle involvement in IBM is often asymmetric, in contrast to the symmetrical involvement in DM and PM. The asymmetric involvement of muscle, not uncommonly, leads to the misdiagnosis of amyotrophic lateral sclerosis (ALS). However, the muscle groups affected early are different in IBM compared to ALS. Again in IBM, there is an atrophy of the flexor forearm compartment, but the hand intrinsics (thenar and hypothenar eminence) are spared, in contrast to ALS in which atrophy in the upper limbs usually is first seen in the hand intrinsics. The presence of slowly progressive, asymmetric, quadriceps and wrist/finger flexor weakness, and atrophy in a patient over 50 years of age strongly suggests the diagnosis of IBM even in the absence of histological confirmation.[2,129–132] Although slowly progressive, IBM is very debilitating. Longitudinal studies have reported that 37% of patients used a wheelchair after 14 years,[128] while others have reported 47% of IBM patients being completely confined to a wheelchair after only 12 years.[127]

Swallowing difficulties develop in up to 60% of patients due to esophageal and pharyngeal muscle involvement. This can lead to weight loss or aspiration. In severe cases, cricopharyngeal myotomy may be beneficial.[126,133,134] We have followed a number of patients in whom dysphagia was the presenting feature of the disease. Only after following patients for several years did they develop weakness in the extremities that are more characteristic of IBM. Mild facial weakness is evident in one-third of cases.[2,126] Rare patients may have severe facial diplegia.[135] In keeping with other inflammatory myopathies, neck flexor weakness is the rule, but some patients manifest with atypical features such as with head drop or bent spine syndrome/camptocormia owing to severe paraspinal muscle involvement.[136,137] Most patients have no sensory symptoms, but as many as 30% have evidence of a generalized sensory peripheral neuropathy on clinical examination and electrophysiological testing.[2] Muscle stretch reflexes are normal or slightly decreased. In particular, the patellar reflexes are lost early.

ASSOCIATED MANIFESTATIONS

Unlike DM and PM, IBM is not associated with myocarditis, lung disease, or an increased risk of malignancy. However, as many as 15% of patients with IBM have underlying autoimmune disorders such as Sjögren's syndrome, SLE, scleroderma, sarcoidosis, variable immunoglobulin deficiency, or thrombocytopenia.[1,3,138]

LABORATORY FEATURES

Serum CK is normal or only mildly elevated (usually less than 10-fold above normal).[2,9,126] Positive ANAs and a monoclonal gammopathy of unclear significance are found in approximately 20% of patients with IBM. Antibodies directed against cytosolic 5′ nucleotidase 1 A (cN1A) have been detected in as many as two-thirds of IBM patients, whereas this antibody is very uncommon in other neuromuscular disorders.[139,140] Therefore, cN1A antibody testing may well be useful as a screening test to complement the clinical examination and muscle biopsy, particularly when not all the characteristic features of IBM are present clinically or on muscle biopsy. There is a significant incidence of the HLA DR3 phenotype (*0301/0302) in IBM.[141] Skeletal muscle MRI scans demonstrate atrophy and signal abnormalities in affected muscle groups (Fig. 33-10).[75,142] Video-swallow studies in individuals with dysphagia often demonstrate prominence of the cricopharyngeal muscle (Fig. 33-11).

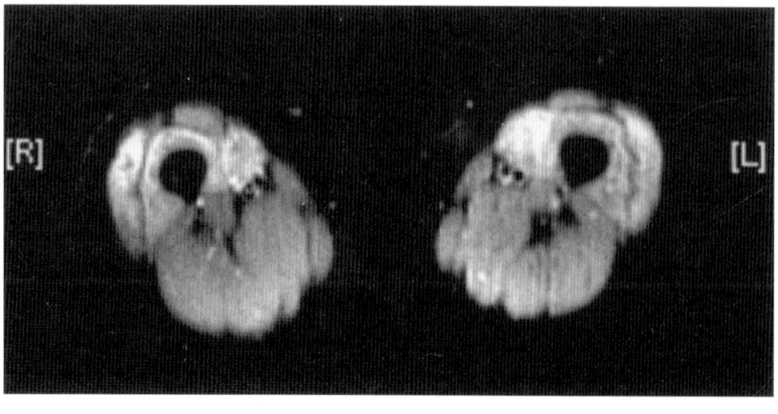

Figure 33-10. Inclusion body myositis. Skeletal muscle MRI (STIR images) reveals patchy areas of increased signal in the vastus lateralis and vastus medialis with relative sparing of the rectus femoris in both thighs.

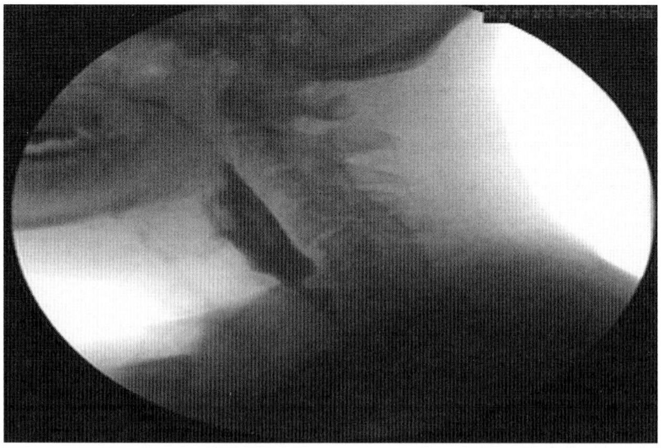

Figure 33-11. Video-swallow studies in an IBM patient with dysphagia demonstrates prominence of the cricopharyngeal muscle that narrows the esophagus.

ELECTROPHYSIOLOGICAL STUDIES

Nerve conduction studies reveal evidence of a mild axonal sensory neuropathy in up to 30% of patients.[2] EMG demonstrates increased spontaneous and insertional activity, small polyphasic MUAPs, and early recruitment.[80,126] In addition, large polyphasic MUAPs can also be demonstrated in one-third of patients, which has led to the misinterpretation of a neurogenic process and misdiagnosis in some patients as having ALS.[126,143,144] However, large polyphasic MUAPs can also be seen in myopathies and probably reflects the chronicity of the disease process rather than a neurogenic etiology.

HISTOPATHOLOGY

Muscle biopsy characteristically reveals endomysial inflammation, small groups of atrophic fibers, eosinophilic cytoplasmic inclusions, and muscle fibers with one or more rimmed vacuoles lined with granular material (Fig. 33-12).[2,9,126,145–151] Amyloid deposition in vacuolated muscle fibers and to a lesser extent within nuclei can be demonstrated on Congo-red staining using polarized light or fluorescence techniques (Fig. 33-13).[145,146] The number of vacuolated and amyloid-positive fibers may increase with time in individual patients.[147] An increased number of ragged red fibers and COX-negative fibers are also evident in patients with IBM compared to patients with DM and PM and age-matched controls (Fig. 33-12).[148] The myonuclei also appear strikingly abnormal. Some are enlarged, contain eosinophilic inclusions, or are located within the vacuoles and appear to be exploding into the vacuoles themselves.

IHC may reveal inclusions react to antibodies directed against p62 (Fig. 33-13), B amyloid, C- and N-terminal epitopes of B-amyloid precursor protein, neurofilament heavy chain, prion protein, apolipoprotein E, 1-antichymotrypsin, and ubiquitin within muscle fibers.[9,131,153] In addition,

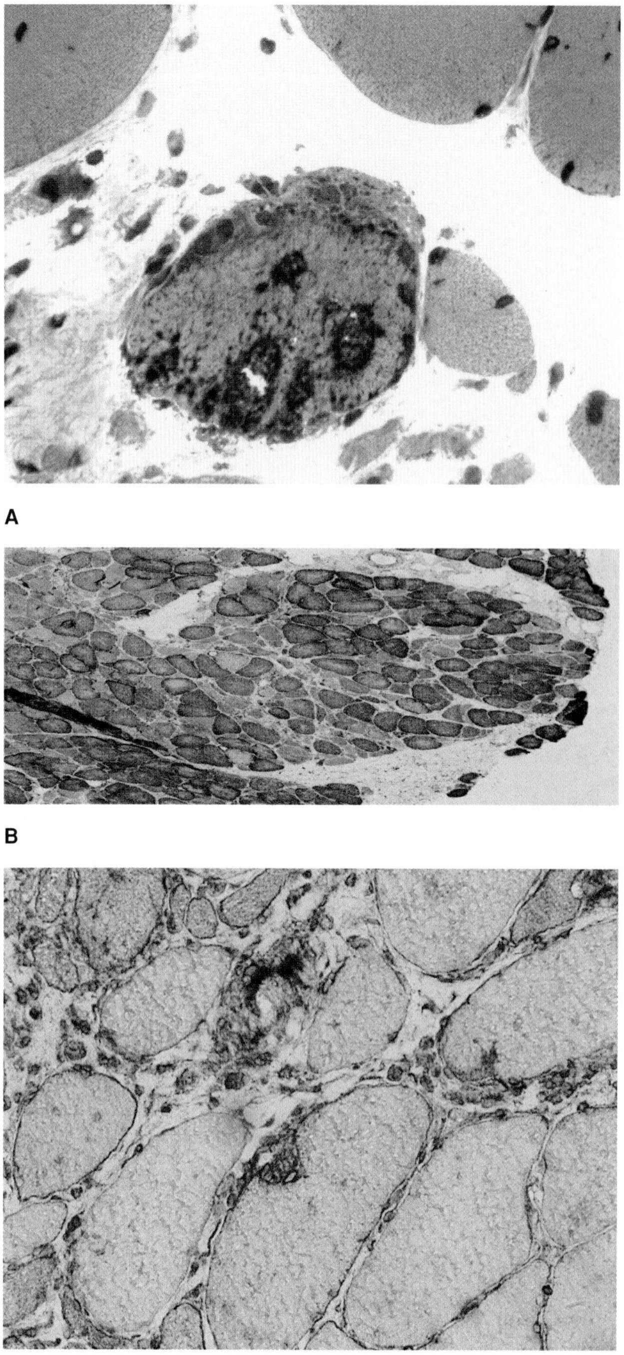

Figure 33-12. Inclusion body myositis. Muscle biopsy reveals muscle fiber with rimmed vacuoles, H&E **(A)**. There is also an increased number of cytochrome oxidase negative fibers as seen here on a combined cytochrome oxidase/succinic dehydrogenase stain in which the COX-negative fibers stain more blue **(B)** Endomysial inflammatory cells appear to surround and invade non-necrotic muscle fibers that express major histocompatibility antigen type 1 or MHC1 on the sarcolemma **(C)**.

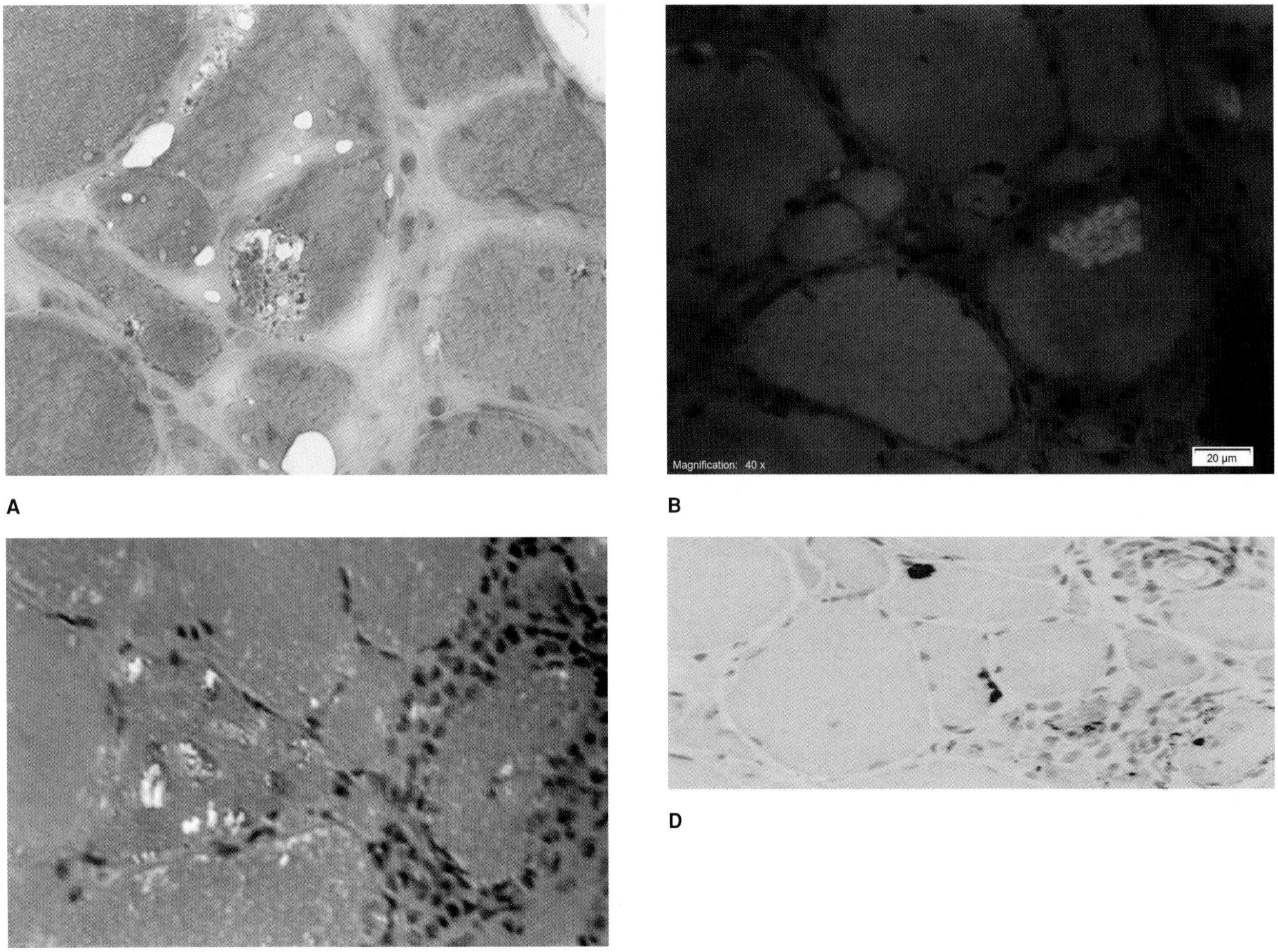

Figure 33-13. Inclusion body myositis. The vacuolated muscle fibers may contain intracytoplasmic **(A)** eosinophilic inclusions (H&E stain), that can appear intensely red on Congo-red stain under rhodamine immunofluorescence (Texas-red filter) **(B)**, and as small apple-green birefringent deposits with Congo-red stain under polarized light **(C)** as well as p62 **(D)**.

IHC demonstrates that rimmed vacuoles are lined with the nuclear membrane proteins lamin A/C and emerin, as well as other nuclear proteins (histone H1, histone 2AX, DNA-PK, Hu70, and Hu80).[6,154] An accumulation of mislocalized nucleic acid binding proteins (including TDP-43, a predominantly nuclear heterogeneous nuclear ribonucleoprotein [hnRNP] that undergoes nucleocytoplasmic shuttling and associates with translation machinery in the cytoplasm) has also identified in IBM nuclear sarcoplasm.[155–157] A recent study showed that both LC3 and p62 were sensitive markers of IBM.[158] In contrast, TDP-43 immunopositivity was highly specific for IBM, but the sensitivity of this test was lower, with definitive staining present in just 67% of IBM cases.[158]

On EM, 15–21-nm cytoplasmic and intranuclear tubulofilaments are found in vacuolated muscle fibers, although a minimum of three vacuolated fibers often need to be scrutinized to confirm their presence (Fig. 33-14).[126] Vacuolated fibers also contain cytoplasmic clusters of 6–10-nm amyloid-like fibrils. Because of sampling error, repeat muscle biopsies may be required to demonstrate the rimmed vacuoles and abnormal tubulofilament or amyloid accumulation, in order to histologically confirm the diagnosis of "definite" IBM.[2] This sampling error may account for many cases of IBM being misdiagnosed as PM.

As with PM, in IBM there is endomysial inflammatory cell infiltrate composed of macrophages and CD8+ cytotoxic/suppressor T lymphocytes, which surround and invade non-necrotic fibers.[9,81] In addition, there are many myeloid dendritic cells in the endomysium that appear to surround non-necrotic muscle fibers and may serve to present antigens to cytotoxic T cells. MHC class 1 antigens are expressed on necrotic and non-necrotic muscle fibers (Fig. 33-12C).[102] The T-cell receptor repertoire of the inflammatory cells has an oligoclonal pattern of gene rearrangement, although there is heterogeneity in the CDR3 domain.[107,149] These findings suggest that the T-cell response is not directed against a muscle-specific

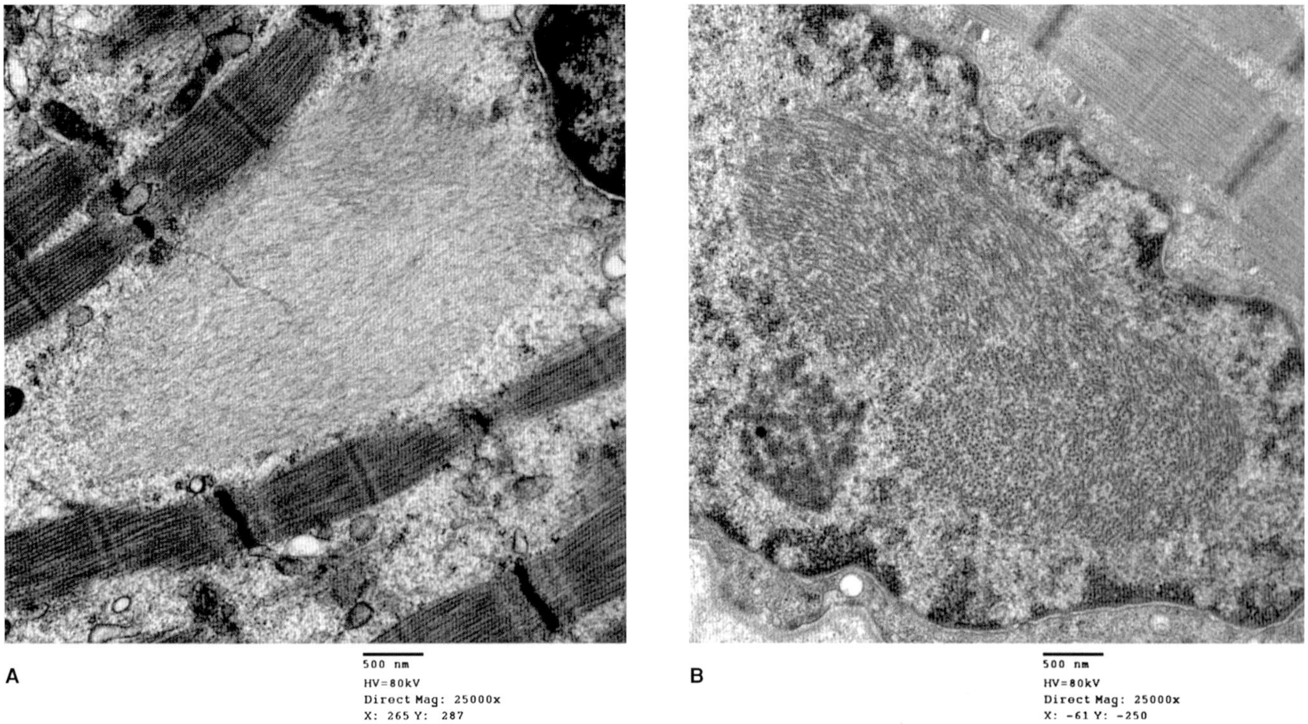

Figure 33-14. Inclusion body myositis. Electron microscopy demonstrates 15–21-nm tubulofilamentous inclusions in the cytoplasm **(A)** and nucleus **(B)**. (Courtesy of Dr. Steven A. Greenberg.)

antigen, although a superantigen could trigger the response. However, Dalakas and colleagues have found persistent clonal restriction of T-cell receptors in infiltrating lymphocytes on repeated muscle biopsies in some individual patients, suggesting that there is a continuous antigen-driven attack against the muscle fibers.[150] Plasma cells are also quite prominent in the endomysium.[108] Autoantibodies directed against desmin has been demonstrated in some muscle biopsies.[151]

PATHOGENESIS

The pathogenesis of IBM is unknown. It is unclear if IBM is a primary inflammatory myopathy like DM and PM, or a primary degenerative myopathy with a secondary inflammatory response (such as seen in a variety of muscular dystrophies). The clonally restricted inflammatory cell infiltrate is suggestive of an autoimmune disorder mediated by cytotoxic T cells. The frequency of muscle fibers invaded by inflammatory cells is usually greater than necrotic or amyloidogenic fibers, suggesting that the inflammatory response plays a more important role than the accumulation of vacuoles or amyloidogenic filaments in the pathogenesis of IBM.[152] The autoinvasive T cells in IBM release perforin granules; pores form on the muscle membrane, resulting in osmolysis. RNA expression studies demonstrate an increase in immunoglobulin-related genes.[94] This may be explained by the prominent plasma cell infiltration in the endomysium. However, the pathogenic role, if any, of these plasma cells and immunoglobulins is unclear. No abnormal deposition of immunoglobulins or complement has been demonstrated on muscle fibers or the vasculature in IBM (as opposed to DM).

However, the lack of significant clinical response with various immunosuppressive agents argues against IBM being a primary autoimmune disorder. We treated eight patients with IBM for 6–24 months with immunosuppressive medications.[147] None of the patients improved in strength or function despite lower serum CK levels and reduced inflammation on the post-treatment muscle biopsies. Interestingly, the amounts of vacuolated muscle fibers and fibers with amyloid deposition were increased in the follow-up biopsies. We suggested that inflammation may play a secondary role in the pathogenesis of IBM.

IBM could be a degenerative disorder of muscle. Although "Alzheimer-characteristic proteins" accumulate in vacuolated muscle fibers by IHC,[9,153] similar degrees of increased mRNA of these proteins are also seen in muscle biopsies of patients with PM and DM.[94] Thus, the increased expression of these proteins in IBM is not likely secondary to increased transcription of mRNA but involves a more distal mechanism. Perhaps, one or more of these proteins become modified post translation, causing misfiling and impaired elimination by the proteasomes.[153]

Ragged red fibers and mitochondrial DNA mutations are more frequent in patients with IBM than in the other inflammatory myopathies and in age-matched controls but are thought to be secondary abnormalities.[9,148,159] Vacuolated muscle fibers express increased nitro tyrosine and both the inducible and the nuclear forms of nitric oxide syntheses, suggesting that nitric oxide–induced oxidative stress (NOS) may play a role in muscle fiber destruction in IBM.[160] Of note, B-crystalline, a member of the heat-shock protein family, is also overexpressed in both normal and abnormal muscle fibers, indicating that the pathological stress is acting upstream from the development of rimmed vacuoles and the accumulation of Alzheimer-like proteins, NOS expression, and mitochondrial mutations.[161]

As mentioned, the myonuclei are very abnormal in IBM. Filamentous inclusions are evident within some myonuclei, rimmed vacuoles immunostain with antibodies directed against various nuclear membrane proteins as well as nucleic acid–binding proteins (including TDP-43 and hnRNP), and furthermore nucleic acid–binding proteins seem to be extruded out of the nuclei and accumulate as deposits in the sarcoplasm. These features suggest that abnormalities in RNA processing play a role in the pathology of this disease, as has been suggested in some of the hereditary neurodegenerative disorders of the central nervous system (e.g., some forms of familial ALS and frontotemporal dementia) and in some forms of hereditary inclusion body myopathy (see Chapter 27).

A viral etiology has been speculated to be involved in the pathogenesis of IBM but has never been proven. Chronic persistent mumps was previously hypothesized based on immunostaining of inclusions by antimumps antibodies[162] but was subsequently rejected after in situ hybridization and polymerase chain reaction (PCR) studies failed to confirm mumps infection.[163,164] Interestingly, patients with retroviral infections (HIV and HTLV-1) and postpolio syndrome can have histological abnormalities on muscle biopsy similar to IBM.[165,166]

DIFFERENTIAL DIAGNOSIS

Most of the patients that we have seen with IBM were previously diagnosed as having PM or ALS. It is important to remember that because of sampling error, histopathological confirmation of IBM is not always possible. The presence of slowly progressive, asymmetric quadriceps and wrist/finger flexor weakness and atrophy in a patient over 50 years of age strongly suggests the diagnosis of IBM even in the absence of histological confirmation (Table 33-3). That said, there are occasional patients with IBM that manifest initially with only hip girdle weakness such that they mimic PM.

As alluded above, the asymmetric muscle atrophy and distal weakness unfortunately may lead to the misdiagnosis of ALS. However, the muscle groups affected early are different in IBM compared to ALS. Again in IBM, there is atrophy of the flexor forearm compartment but the hand intrinsics (thenar and hypothenar eminence) are spared, in contrast to ALS in which atrophy in the arms usually is first seen in the hand intrinsics.

Rimmed vacuoles, amyloid/TDP-43/SMI-31/p62 deposition, and tubulofilamentous inclusions are not usually seen in other forms of inflammatory myopathy, but can be observed in patients with various forms of hereditary inclusion body *myopathy* (h-IBM discussed in Chapter 27). The age of onset is usually in early adult life and the pattern of weakness differs (preferential involvement of the tibialis anterior muscles) in patients with autosomal-recessive h-IBM. Autosomal-dominant h-IBM is less common, and the clinical phenotype is more variable but usually predominantly affects the shoulder and hip girdle. One form of autosomal-dominant h-IBMs caused by mutations in the valosin-containing protein gene is associated with Paget disease and frontotemporal dementia.[167] Rimmed vacuoles are also commonly seen in other types of muscular dystrophy, including limb-girdle muscular dystrophy type 1 A (LGMD 1 A) (myotilinopathies), LGMD2G (telethoninopathy), LGMD 2 J (titinopathy), oculopharyngeal dystrophy, Welander distal myopathy, and the myofibrillar myopathies. However, there is a lack of inflammatory cells invading non-necrotic muscle fibers in these myopathies and in the h-IBMs.

PROGNOSIS

Life expectancy is not significantly altered in IBM. The myopathy is slowly progressive, and unfortunately it is not responsive to immunosuppressive or immunomodulating therapies. As mentioned above many patients require a scooter or wheelchair within 10–15 years of onset of symptoms.[126–128]

▶ IMMUNE-MEDIATED NECROTIZING MYOPATHY

CLINICAL FEATURES

Despite the paucity of inflammatory cells, IMNM is best categorized as an inflammatory myopathy due to its suspected autoimmune nature.[4,5,11,31,100,168–179] Nearly 20% of inflammatory myopathy patients in a recent series had necrotizing myopathy.[31] Patients present with proximal weakness, which may begin acutely or more insidiously. Some patients complain of myalgias. Patients may have an underlying connective tissue disease (usually scleroderma or MCTD), cancer (paraneoplastic necrotizing myopathy), or the cause may be idiopathic. The most common associated malignancies are gastrointestinal tract adenocarcinomas and small and nonsmall cell carcinomas of the lung. Muscular dystrophies and toxic myopathies (e.g., statin myopathies) need to be excluded. That said, we have seen a large number of necrotizing myopathies that developed in the setting of a patient taking a statin medication but continued to progress for 6 or more months after discontinuation of the statin. These patients only improved once they were treated with immunosuppressive therapy and often relapsed when these medications were tapered. Thus, we feel that statin medications may rarely induce an autoimmune necrotizing myopathy, besides the more typical toxic myopathy that may also be necrotizing in appearance. Patients with necrotizing myopathies generally improve with immunosuppressive and immunomodulating therapies but, in our experience, they are more difficult to treat than patients with DM or PM.

LABORATORY FEATURES

Serum CK is usually markedly elevated. Positive ANAs suggestive of an underlying CTD may be found. Patients with IMNM may have anti-SRP antibodies, which are associated with severe weakness, dilated cardiomyopathy, and poor responsiveness to standard immunosuppression.[5,11,100,168–179] Recent studies have demonstrated that patients with statin-associated IMNM, particularly if over 50 years of age, often have autoantibodies directed, interestingly enough, against 3-hydroxy-3-methylglutaryl coenzyme A (HMG-CoA) reductase.[173–179] The levels may correlate with serum CK and strength of patients.[179] Importantly, these antibodies are not typically found in patients who take statins but have no symptoms or in those who have myopathic symptoms/signs that reverse upon discontinuation of statins.[178]

EMG demonstrates increased insertional and spontaneous activity, myopathic MUAPs, and early recruitment similar to the other described inflammatory myopathies.

HISTOPATHOLOGY

The most prominent features on muscle biopsy are scattered necrotic muscle fibers (Fig. 33-15A).[4,5,11,100,168–177] By Bohan and Peter criteria, patients with necrotizing myopathy could be diagnosed as PM. Nevertheless, the pathogenic basis appears to be quite distinct from PM and, in other reported cases, more closely resembles a microangiopathy. The so-called pipestem capillaries may be evident on routine histochemistry and EM.[169] Deposition of MAC on small blood vessels and depletion of capillaries can be seen, although not as prominent as that noted in DM. There is usually expression of MAC and MHC1 on the sarcolemma of non-necrotic fibers (Fig. 33-15B and C). There is no perifascicular atrophy, perivascular inflammation is sparse, and tubuloreticular inclusions in endothelium are not commonly seen on EM.

PATHOGENESIS

The pathogenesis of this necrotizing myopathy is unknown; however, the deposition of MAC on small arterioles and capillaries with thickened endothelial walls and on the sarcolemma suggests that in some cases complement-mediated damage may be playing a role.

TREATMENT

In our experience, the IMNM are more difficult to treat than DM and PM. We typically always start treatment with corticosteroids plus a second-line immunosuppressive agent (e.g., methotrexate). Furthermore, it is not uncommon that we need to add IVIG or rituximab.

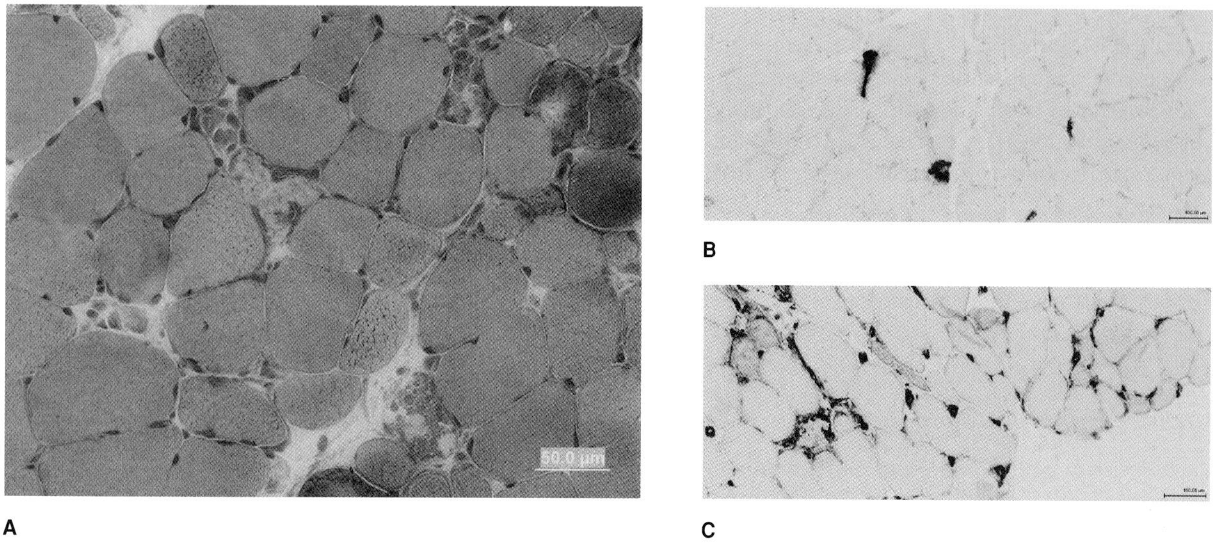

Figure 33-15. Necrotizing myositis. Muscle biopsy reveals scattered necrotic fibers, some in the process of undergoing phagocytosis **(A)**. Unlike polymyositis, there is scant, if any, inflammatory cell infiltrate, except in fibers undergoing phagocytosis. Immunohistochemistry may reveal deposition of membrane attack complex (MAC) on small vessels **(B)** and of major histocompatibility antigen 1 (MHC1) on the sarcolemma of non-necrotic muscle fibers **(C)**. MAC deposits may also be appreciated on the sarcolemma of non-necrotic fibers and diffusely in necrotic fibers. Note that blood vessels normally stain for MHC1.

▶ OTHER IDIOPATHIC INFLAMMATORY MYOPATHIES

EOSINOPHILIC MYOPATHY

Clinical Features

Eosinophilic myopathy may occur as part of the hypereosinophilic syndrome (HES) and has been subclassified into focal eosinophilic myositis, eosinophilic PM, and eosinophilic perimyositis.[180–185] The diagnostic criteria for a HES are (1) persistent eosinophilia of 1,500 eosinophils/mm^3 for at least 6 months, (2) no evidence of parasitic or other recognized causes of eosinophilia, and (3) signs and symptoms of organ system involvement related to infiltration of eosinophils. Patients with focal eosinophilic myositis and eosinophilic PM present with focal or generalized muscle weakness with or without myalgias and skin changes, while those with perimyositis typically have myalgias without significant weakness. Patients may have other systemic manifestations of HES, including encephalopathy, peripheral neuropathy, myocarditis/pericarditis (manifesting as CHF or arrhythmia), pulmonary (i.e., fibrosis, pleuritis, and asthma), renal and gastrointestinal involvement, and skin changes (i.e., petechial rash, splinter hemorrhages of the nail beds, livedo reticularis, and Raynaud's phenomena). The constellation of clinical and laboratory features suggest that eosinophilic PM, HES, and the Churg–Strauss syndrome may fall into the spectrum of the same or similar disease process.

Laboratory Features

Serum CK is usually elevated in focal eosinophilic myositis and eosinophilic PM, but is often normal in eosinophilic perimyositis. Hypereosinophilia is generally present. Hypergammaglobulinemia, anemia, and rheumatoid factor may also be seen. ESR is elevated in <50%. Serum ANA is usually negative. EKG may demonstrate cardiac arrhythmia, and chest x-rays may reveal pulmonary infiltrates. Increased insertional and spontaneous activity (i.e., fibrillation potentials and PSWs) with early recruitment of small polyphasic MUAPs are observed on EMG. In addition, there may be evidence of superimposed multiple mononeuropathies, which may also be evident on EMG/NCS.

Histopathology

Muscle biopsies in patients with focal eosinophilic myositis and eosinophilic PM reveal an endomysial inflammatory cell infiltrate, often but not invariably, including eosinophils. Inflammatory cells may appear to surround and invade muscle fibers (Fig. 33-16). Nodular granulomas may also be seen. In patients with eosinophilic perimyositis, muscle biopsies reveal an inflammatory cell infiltrate (eosinophils are not a constant feature) restricted to the fascia and superficial perimysium.

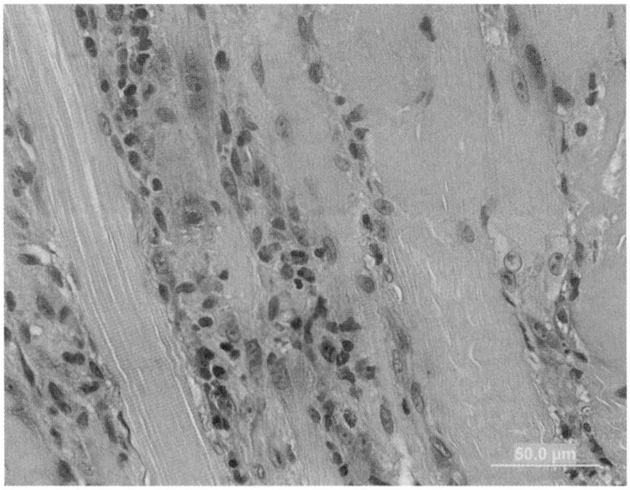

Figure 33-16. Eosinophilic myositis. Muscle biopsy demonstrates necrotic fibers and endomysial inflammatory cell infiltrate that includes many eosinophils. Paraffin-embedded tissue with H&E stain.

Pathogenesis

The etiology of HES and the eosinophilic myopathies is unknown. Eosinophilia may be the result of a perverse effect on T-cell clones.[186,187] T lymphocytes secrete interleukin-5 and interleukin-3, cytokines that are required for the growth and differentiation of eosinophils.[183] Eosinophils, in turn, damage muscle fibers by their release of the eosinophilic major basic protein, which causes lysis of the membranes of target cells.[183]

Of note, a couple of recent series have reported children and adults incorrectly diagnosed as having eosinophilic myositis who had mutations in the calpain-3 gene.[188] Thus, these patients actually had LGMD 2 A.

Differential Diagnosis

The differential diagnosis of myopathies associated with eosinophilia includes parasitic infection, vasculitides (e.g., Churg–Straus syndrome), nonhematological and hematological malignancies (T-cell lymphomas and aplastic anemia), toxic oil and L-tryptophan-induced eosinophilic-myalgia syndrome, idiopathic eosinophilic fasciitis (Shulman syndrome), HES, and eosinophilic myopathy as well as LGMD 2 A. Peripheral blood eosinophil count is elevated in each condition.

Prognosis and Treatment

A poor prognosis for long-term survival with fewer than 20% of patients surviving 3 years was suggested in early reports, but these series of patients may have been biased by the inclusion of autopsied cases. Response to corticosteroids is variable, but some patients do respond. Most patients require the addition of second-line cytotoxic agents (see section "Treatment"). Bone marrow transplantation may be required for refractory cases. Certainly, in childhood cases and refractory adult cases, patients should be screened for mutations in the calpain-3 gene to make sure that they do not have this form of muscular dystrophy.

DIFFUSE FASCIITIS WITH EOSINOPHILIA

Clinical Features

Diffuse fasciitis with eosinophilia or Shulman's syndrome is characterized by diffuse fasciitis and peripheral eosinophilia.[189,190] Men are affected more commonly than women in a 2:1 ratio. Most patients are between 30 and 60 years of age; however, children can be affected. Patients complain of myalgias, muscle tenderness, arthralgias, and low-grade fever. On examination, proximal muscles may be weak, although the motor examination is often limited due to decreased effort because of the pain. Joint contractures may develop in the hands, elbows, and knees and, less commonly, at the shoulders and hips secondary to immobilization due to severe pain. Dermatological assessment reveals thickening of the skin with edema and dimpling (the so-called "peau d'orange") in the extremities and occasionally in the trunk. Unlike HES with eosinophilic PM, the heart, lungs, kidneys, and other visceral organs are usually not involved. However, there do appear to be a disproportionate number of hematological complications including aplastic anemia, idiopathic thrombocytopenia, leukemia, lymphoma, and other lymphoproliferative disorders.

Laboratory Features

Over two-thirds have peripheral eosinophilia >7%, while hypergammaglobulinemia and elevated ESR are evident in at least one-third of patients.[189,190] ANAs are detected in about 25% of patients. Serum CK is usually normal. EMG may demonstrate myopathic MUAPs and muscle membrane instability in the superficial subfascial layers. Skeletal muscle MRI reveals increased signal in the fascia overlying the muscle fibers (Fig. 33-17).

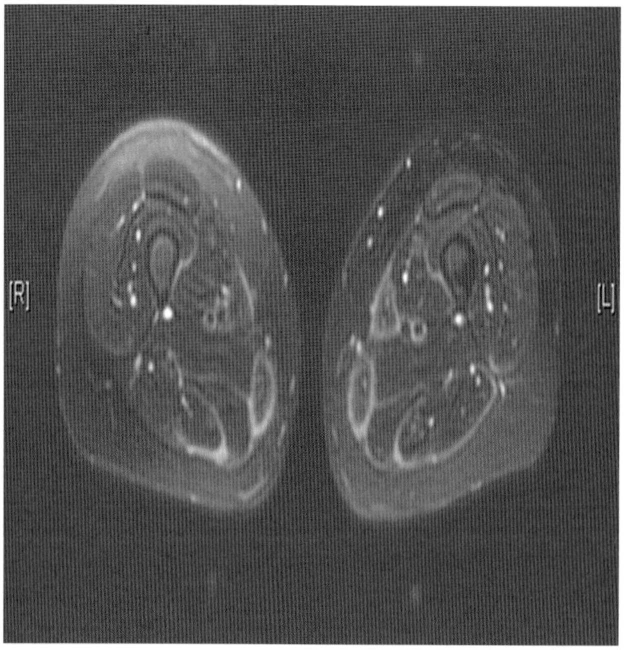

Figure 33-17. Skeletal muscle MRI (T-2 with fat saturation) of the thigh in a patient with fasciitis demonstrates increased signal in fascia surrounding individual large muscle groups, particularly in the posterior compartment.

Histopathology

A full-thickness biopsy extending from the skin to muscle reveals that the fascia is thickened and contains many lymphocytes, macrophages, plasma cells, and eosinophils (Fig. 33-18).[189,190] Immunoglobulin and C3 deposition in the

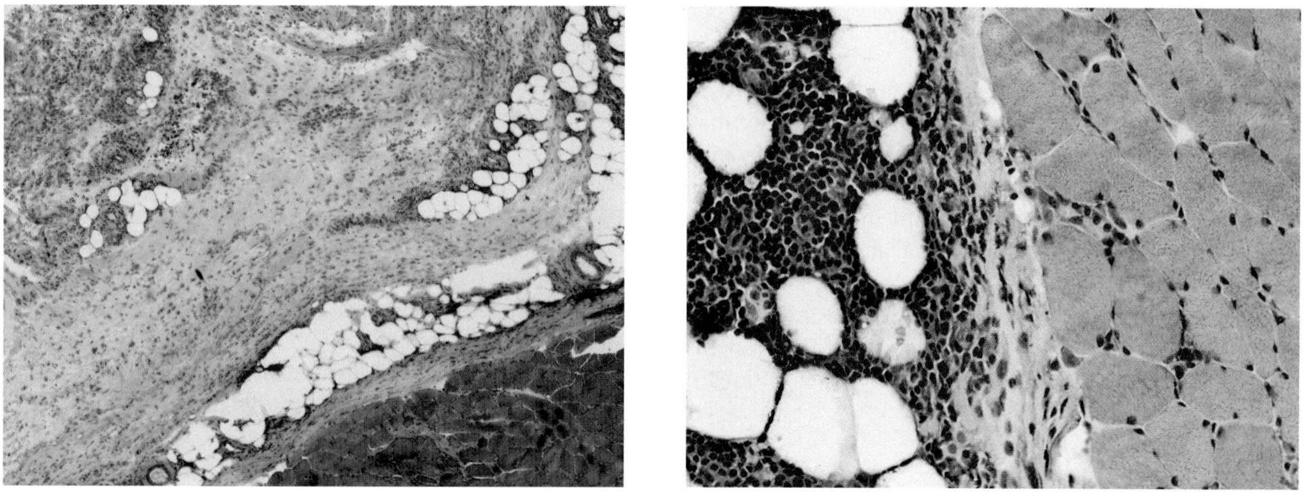

A B

Figure 33-18. Muscle and fascia biopsy reveals inflammatory cell infiltrate including eosinophils in the fascia with sparing of the underlying muscle at low power (**A**, modified Gomori trichrome) and at higher power (**B**, H&E).

fascia have also been reported in some patients. The inflammatory infiltrate may invade the adjacent subcutaneous tissues, perimysium, and endomysium. In addition, scattered necrotic fibers and perifascicular atrophy may be seen.

Pathogenesis

The etiology of diffuse fasciitis with eosinophilia is not known but likely has an autoimmune basis. The clinical and histological features overlap with the eosinophilic myalgia syndrome[191] and toxic oil syndromes,[192] which are caused by the ingestion of tryptophan and denatured rapeseed, respectively. This suggests the possibility of a toxin-induced fasciitis; however, the majority of patients with eosinophilic fasciitis report no known toxic exposures.

Prognosis and Treatment

Corticosteroid treatment usually leads to a rapid improvement. Spontaneous remission may have also been reported. Relapses occur in a minority of patients. The prognosis is not as favorable in cases with hematological complications.

GRANULOMATOUS AND GIANT CELL MYOSITIS

Clinical Features

Granulomatous or giant cell myositis most commonly occurs in patients who also have myasthenia gravis and/or thymoma.[193,194] The myositis may develop before or after the diagnosis of myasthenia gravis or thymoma, and the thymoma can be benign or malignant. In addition to proximal weakness, patients with concomitant myasthenia gravis also often have diplopia, ptosis, and bulbar dysfunction. Importantly, there is also an association with a severe and sometimes deadly granulomatous myocarditis.

Laboratory Features

Serum CK is usually elevated. Myasthenic patients may also have acetylcholine receptor and striated muscle antibodies. EMG demonstrates myopathic MUAPs and muscle membrane instability. In patients with myasthenia gravis, repetitive nerve stimulation may reveal an abnormal decrement. Chest CT should be ordered to look for a thymoma. Echocardiogram can reveal reduced ejection fraction and ventricular wall motion abnormalities, and EKG may demonstrate conduction block or arrhythmia in patients with myocarditis.

Histopathology

Skeletal and often cardiac muscle biopsies reveal granulomatous inflammation and multinucleated giant cells (Fig. 33-19).

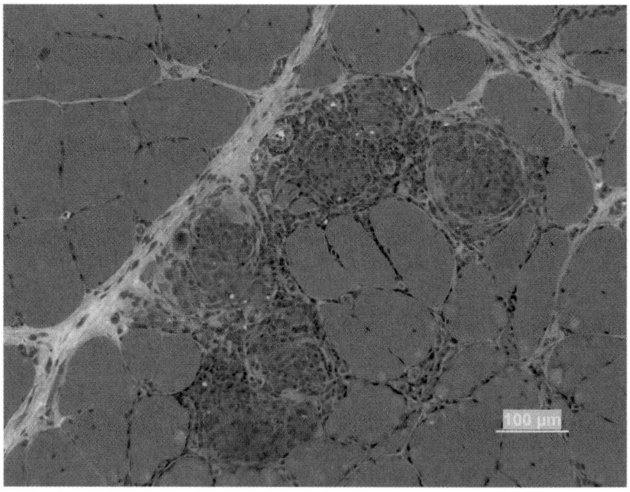

Figure 33-19. Granulomatous myositis. Muscle biopsy reveals granuloma formation in the endomysium, H&E.

Pathogenesis

The etiology of this disorder is unknown, but the granulomatous inflammation and giant cell formation suggest a disorder of cell-mediated immunity. However, the frequent occurrence of myasthenia gravis supports the fact that aberrant humorally mediated immunity may play a role as well.

Prognosis and Treatment

Some patients improve with corticosteroids; however, the response does not seem to be as favorable as is evident in the more common idiopathic PM. This poorer response may be attributed to the frequent myocardial involvement and the superimposed myasthenia gravis and thymoma. Patients generally need aggressive immunosuppressive therapy with high-dose corticosteroids and a second-line agent.

SARCOID MYOPATHY

Clinical Features

Incidental granulomas can be seen in muscle biopsies of patients with sarcoidosis even when they lack symptoms or signs of a myopathy.[195–197] The granulomas may even be palpated within the muscle. Weakness can be mainly proximal or distal. Some patients develop focal myalgias, tenderness, and atrophy. Other patients with sarcoid myopathy also have clinical and histological features of DM or IBM. Signs and symptoms of a superimposed neuropathy due to sarcoidosis can also be seen.

Sarcoidosis is more prevalent in blacks than in whites and in women more than in men, and, although uncommon, it can occur in children. The majority of patients present with pulmonary symptoms and lymphadenopathy. Erythema nodosum and arthralgias are also early features.

Laboratory Features

Serum CK is usually normal or only mildly elevated.[195–197] Serum angiotensin-converting enzyme levels can be normal or elevated. Patients are frequently anergic to antigen skin testing. Chest films may demonstrate hilar lymphadenopathy and parenchymal involvement of the lungs. EMG can be normal or show myopathic features. Mixed myopathic and neurogenic MUAPs may be found in patients with a chronic myopathy or with a superimposed neuropathy.

Histopathology

Muscle biopsy reveals noncaseating granulomas consisting of clusters of epithelioid cells, lymphocytes, and giant cells usually around blood vessels in the perimysium and also in the endomysium.[195–197]

Pathogenesis

The exact pathogenic mechanism of sarcoidosis is unknown but likely involves abnormal cell-mediated immunity, given the presence of granulomas and the T-cell anergy in vitro and in vivo.

Prognosis and Treatment

Treatment of sarcoidosis is usually focused on other systemic manifestations, as the myositis is typically asymptomatic. Corticosteroids are usually effective in treating the myositis, although methotrexate, cyclosporine, or TNF-alpha blockade is occasionally required. In refractory patients, one should consider IBM and perform a repeat biopsy, as we have seen several cases of patients with both sarcoidosis and histologically confirmed IBM. In such cases, the granulomas may have been incidental with the weakness actually due to IBM.

BEHCET'S DISEASE

Clinical Features

Behcet's disease is a multisystemic disorder characterized by recurrent mucocutaneous and ocular lesions (e.g., oral and genital ulcers, hypopyon, and iritis), erythema nodosum, thrombophlebitis, colitis, meningoencephalitis, and peripheral neuropathy. Onset can occur in childhood or late adult life. In addition, patients may develop focal or generalized myalgias with or without weakness due to myositis.[198–202] The lower extremities, particularly the calves, are primarily affected. Myocarditis may occur.

Laboratory Features

Serum CK levels are normal or mildly elevated. Usually there is leukocytosis, elevated ESR, and increased C-reactive protein levels. Approximately 50% of patients are HLA-B5 positive.[147]

Histopathology

Muscle biopsy may reveal macrophages along with CD4+ and CD8+ lymphocytes and neutrophils surrounding and invading non-necrotic muscles and widespread expression of MHC-1 antigen on muscle fibers similar to PM.[202] In addition, deposits of complement factor C3 and immunoglobulins have been demonstrated in blood vessel walls as seen in DM.[202]

Pathogenesis

The immunohistological findings reveal a cell-mediated attack directed against muscle fibers, but the enhanced neutrophil migration and immune complex deposition on blood vessels support a leukocytoclastic vasculitis or vasculopathy in the pathogenesis of the disease.

Prognosis and Treatment

The myositis is responsive to immunosuppressive therapy.

FOCAL MYOSITIS

Clinical Features

Focal myositis is a rare disorder, which usually manifests as a solitary, painful, and rapidly expanding skeletal muscle mass.[203–207] It can develop at any age. The most common site of involvement is the leg, but focal myositis can also occur in the upper extremities, abdomen, head, and neck. Focal myositis may be mistaken for a malignant soft tissue tumor (i.e., sarcoma). Rarely, focal myositis generalizes to more typical PM.[205] The disorder needs to be distinguished from focal muscle infarction (most commonly seen in diabetes), sarcoidosis, Behcet's syndrome, vasculitis, soft tissue tumors, and focal infections such as pyomyositis (bacterial infection of muscle seen in immunosuppressed patients). The lesions may resolve spontaneously or with corticosteroid treatment.

Laboratory Features

Serum CK and ESR are usually normal. MRI and CT imaging demonstrate edema within the affected muscle groups (Fig. 33-20).[203,206,207]

Histopathology

Muscle biopsies reveal CD4+ and CD8+ T lymphocytes and macrophages in the endomysium along with necrosis and phagocytosis of muscle fibers.[203] In addition, fiber size variability, split fibers, increased centronuclei, and endomysial fibrosis are seen. One report noted that MHC class 1 antigens were not expressed on muscle fibers, in contrast to PM in which these antigens are typically abnormally expressed on the fibers.[203]

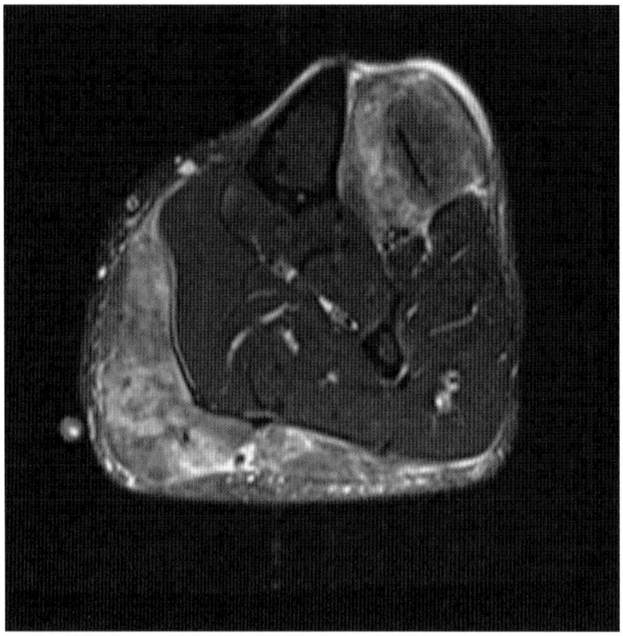

Figure 33-20. Focal myositis. Skeletal muscle MRI (STIR) reveals increased signal in the tibialis anterior and medial gastrocnemius muscles in a patient with focal myositis.

Pathogenesis

The etiology is unknown. Immunological studies suggest that the disorder is distinct from PM and not the result of a cell-mediated attack directed against a muscle-specific antigen.

▶ MYOSITIS ASSOCIATED WITH INFECTIONS

VIRAL INFECTIONS

Human Immunodeficiency Virus

Clinical Features

Patients with HIV infection may develop an inflammatory myopathy (Table 33-7).[110,208] This complication is more common in adults compared to children with HIV infection. Inflammatory myopathy usually develops in patients with AIDS, but can occur in the early stages of HIV infection. The clinical presentation is similar to idiopathic PM with subacute or chronic, progressive, symmetrical proximal weakness, and myalgias. Occasionally, patients with HIV have muscle biopsies that resemble IBM. Patients may have concurrent HIV-related neuropathy and may complain also of sensory loss and painful paresthesia. Rhabdomyolysis has also been reported as a rare complication of HIV infection usually but not always in association with antiretroviral therapies and/or statin medications.[209–212] HIV-related myositis needs to be distinguished from zidovudine (AZT) myotoxicity, HIV-wasting syndrome, and other neuromuscular diseases that can complicate HIV infection (e.g., HIV-related myositis is usually associated with higher CK and more abnormal insertional and spontaneous activity on EMG).[110,212–216]

▶ TABLE 33-7. INFLAMMATORY MYOPATHY ASSOCIATED WITH INFECTIONS

Viral
Human immunodeficiency virus (HIV)
Human T-leukemia virus 1 (HTLV-1)
Influenza types A, B, and C (rare)
Hepatitis B and C
Less common: adenovirus, coxsackie virus, echovirus, parainfluenza virus, Epstein–Barr virus, arbovirus, respiratory syncytial virus, and cytomegalovirus herpes simplex
Bacterial
Staphylococcus aureus
Streptococci
Escherichia coli
Yersinia
Legionella
Leptospirosis
Lyme disease
Fungal
Candida
Cryptococcus
Sporotrichosis
Actinomycosis
Histoplasmosis
Parasites
Protozoans
Toxoplasmosis
Sarcocystis
Trypanosomiasis
Cestodes (tapeworms)
Cysticercosis
Hydatidosis
Coenurosis
Sparganosis
Nematodes (unsegmented roundworms)
Trichinosis
Visceral/cutaneous larva migrans
Dracunculiasis

Laboratory Features

Serum CK is elevated in most patients. EMG demonstrates muscle membrane instability (i.e., fibrillation potentials, PSWs, and complex repetitive discharges) and early recruitment of small myopathic-appearing MUAPs.

Histopathology

Muscle biopsies reveal perimysial and endomysial inflammation consisting mainly of CD8+ cytotoxic T cells and macrophages, which surround and invade non-necrotic muscle fibers.[208] Perivascular inflammation is common, but actual necrotizing vasculitis is not seen. Occasional ragged red fibers, nemaline rods, and cytoplasmic bodies are found.[216] Rare patients may have rimmed vacuoles typical of IBM.[165]

Pathogenesis

HIV has been detected by PCR in muscle biopsy specimens; however, the virus is evident by ultrastructural studies only in inflammatory cells.[217] The myositis is not a direct effect of infection of muscle by HIV. Rather, the HIV infection triggers a T-cell-mediated and MHC-1-restricted immune response against unknown antigen(s) on muscle fibers.

Prognosis and Treatment

There are no large uncontrolled studies assessing the efficacy of various treatment options in HIV-related myositis. A trial of antiretroviral medications may be of benefit, if these are not already prescribed. In our experience, IVIG has not been all that effective in improving strength. Corticosteroids are the most effective treatment, but need to be used with caution, given the risk of further immunosuppression in the patient who is already immunocompromised.

Human T-Cell Leukemia Virus Type 1

Clinical Features

HTLV-1 infection can cause adult T-cell leukemia and tropical spastic paraparesis (TSP).[218–220] In addition, a myositis may occur in patients who are infected with or without leukemia or TSP. Patients develop progressive proximal muscle weakness and myalgias similar to HIV-related myositis. In a patient with TSP, concurrent myositis should be suspected, if the patient has concurrent proximal upper extremity and neck weakness in addition to leg weakness and spasticity.

Laboratory Features

Serum CK is usually elevated. EMG demonstrates typical myopathic features. In addition, an upper motor neuron pattern of recruitment can be seen in patients who also have TSP (i.e., inadequate activation of MUAPS resulting in a reduced interference pattern without rapidly firing MUAPS).

Histopathology

Muscle biopsy is similar to that observed in idiopathic PM and HIV myositis.[218–220] In addition, rimmed vacuoles similar to IBM can be seen.[165]

Pathogenesis

As with HIV-related myositis, HTLV-1 can be demonstrated within some inflammatory cells, but not in the muscle fibers themselves. A T-cell-mediated and MHC-1-restricted cytotoxic process similar to HIV is suspected.

Prognosis and Treatment

Although there are only a small number of patients reported who were treated with immunosuppressive agents, the myositis may improve with corticosteroid treatment. In contrast, the myelopathy is relatively refractory to immunosuppression.

Influenza Viruses

Clinical Features

Influenza A, B, and rarely C are associated with upper respiratory infection. As most of us who have experienced the common cold or flu know, myalgias are common when fever and other constitutional symptoms of influenza infection appear. The myalgias are usually an indirect effect of influenza infection, probably related to the systemic release of cytokines. Nevertheless, active myositis can develop, and the associated clinical syndromes appear different in children and adults.[221–225]

In children, the myositis manifests as severe pain, swelling, and tenderness of the calves when the upper respiratory infection symptoms begin to reside.[221,222,225] Because of the severe muscle pain, affected children may prefer to walk on the toes or crawl and limit their movements. Importantly, prolonged inactivity can lead to muscle contractures. The severe pain limits adequate assessment of muscle strength. Most cases are self-limited, with symptoms lasting less than a week. Myoglobinuria can complicate associated influenza infection, particularly if there is an underlying metabolic defect such as carnitine palmitoyltransferase deficiency.[226]

Influenza virus myositis tends to be more severe in adults.[223,224] Generalized or proximal weakness develops in half the adult patients with myositis. Myoglobinuria is more common in adults and can be complicated by renal failure. Patients complain of generalized muscle pain, but this a less prominent symptom than seen in children.

Laboratory Features

CK is usually elevated in patients with acute myositis, while it is typically normal in uncomplicated influenza infection. EMG may show the typical features of an active necrotizing myopathy.

Histopathology

In children, biopsies have revealed scattered necrotic and regenerating muscle fibers with interstitial mononuclear and polymorphonuclear inflammatory cells.[221] EM has not demonstrated any viral-like particles in the muscle biopsies. Viral cultures are only rarely positive.[227]

In adults, the muscle biopsies have demonstrated scattered necrotic and regenerating fibers; however, mononuclear inflammatory cell infiltration is scant. Rare muscle fibers containing viral particles within membrane-bound vacuoles near the sarcolemma have been seen on EM.[228] In addition, intranuclear inclusions consisting of 7–9-nm parallel filaments were present in fibers that did not contain viral particles.[228]

Pathogenesis

It is not known why only rare patients with influenza infection develop myositis. It is possible that the muscle destruction is a direct effect of the viral infection or alternatively an indirect effect secondary to altering the immune system.

Prognosis and Treatment

The disorder is usually self-limiting, although rare patients have been reported with recurrences associated with infection of different influenza types.[225] Treatment is supportive with bed rest and hydration to avoid renal failure from myoglobinuria. Acetaminophen and nonsteroidal anti-inflammatory drugs (NSAIDs) (avoid aspirin in children) can be used to treat myalgias and fever.

Other Viral-Related Myositis

Acute viral myositis can also occur in infections with coxsackie virus, parainfluenza, mumps, measles, adenovirus, herpes simplex, cytomegalovirus, hepatitis B and C, Epstein–Barr virus, respiratory syncytial virus, echovirus, and possibly arboviruses. Diagnosis requires acute and convalescent titers (3 or 4 weeks after infection) titers being measured in the serum. The blood, stool, urine, and throat can be cultured in an attempt to isolate the virus. As in influenza, the myositis associated with these other viruses is usually self-limited and requires only supportive therapy and treatment of myoglobinuria to prevent renal failure.

BACTERIAL INFECTIONS

Clinical Features

The term "pyomyositis" is used to describe focal or multifocal abscesses associated with bacterial infection of the muscle. Pyomyositis is more common in the tropics but has been increasing in frequency in developed countries secondary to HIV infection[229,230] and intravenous drug abuse.[231] Patients present with focal muscle pain, tenderness, and fever. The most common sites of the abscesses are the quadriceps, glutei, and deltoids.[232] If not treated early, the patients can become septic.

Laboratory Features

Serum CK may be normal or elevated. Neutrophilic pleocytosis and elevated ESRs are the rule. Initially, blood cultures may show no growth or organisms until the patient becomes septic.[233] Ultrasound, CT, and MRI of skeletal muscle can be useful in localizing pyogenic abscesses for fine-needle aspiration and diagnosis.[233,234]

Histopathology

Muscle biopsy reveals necrotic tissue containing neutrophils, macrophages, lymphocytes, and occasionally eosinophils.[229,231,232,234] Bacterial infection may be difficult to visualize on light microscopy, but the organisms can be cultured from the drained abscesses.

Pathogenesis

Staphylococcus aureus, streptococci, *Escherichia coli*, *Yersinia*, and *Legionella* are the most common organisms responsible for pyomyositis.[232–234] Pyomyositis usually arises as an extension of the infection from adjacent tissues or via hematological spread of the organisms. Infection of the muscle does not usually develop in the absence of primary infection elsewhere.

Prognosis and Treatment

Early in the course of the illness, microabscesses may respond to appropriate antibiotics. More severe infections require incision and drainage of the abscesses in addition to antibiotics. Despite aggressive treatment, mortality rates range from 1–10% in cases complicated by sepsis.[232]

MYOSITIS ASSOCIATED WITH LYME DISEASE

Clinical Features

Lyme disease is often associated with the central nervous system and peripheral nerve manifestations. Rarely, myositis can complicate Lyme disease.[235–240] Clinical features can resemble DM.[236] Rhabdomyolysis can complicate severe myositis.[237] Patients with myositis usually present with focal or generalized weakness and myalgias and may have concomitant manifestations such as rash, arthritis, myocarditis, or more typical neurologic syndromes (e.g., cranial neuropathy, radiculopathy) associated with Lyme disease.

Laboratory Features

Serum CK levels are normal or only slightly increased in the majority of patients; very high levels are rare.[237] Lyme antibody testing may be positive.

Electrophysiological Features

EMG demonstrates myopathic findings often with concomitant polyradiculoneuropathy.[237,240]

Histopathology

Muscle biopsies of suspected Lyme-associated myositis have demonstrated focal nodular infiltrates, perimysial inflammation, and necrotic muscle fibers. Diffuse mononuclear infiltration and invasion of non-necrotic muscle fibers are usually not seen. Interstitial lymphohistiocytic infiltrates with plasma cells are found predominantly in the vicinity of small endomysial vessels. Immunohistology shows infiltrates that mainly consist of CD4+ T lymphocytes and macrophages and fewer CD8+ T and B cells. Occasionally, the organisms can be seen with silver stains. We have seen a case with perifascicular atrophy characteristic of DM.

Pathogenesis

The histopathological features are suggestive of a vasculopathy.

Prognosis and Treatment

Corticosteroids can help with the myalgias, but the infection needs to be treated with appropriate antibiotics to ultimately improve muscle strength and function.

FUNGAL MYOSITIS

Fungal infection of the muscles is uncommon unless the patient is immunosuppressed. *Candida* is the most common fungal organism and almost always occurs in the setting of diffuse candidiasis.[241,242] Patients manifest with diffuse myalgias, tenderness, weakness, fever, and a papular erythematous rash. However, the myositis is often overshadowed by other systemic involvement. Muscle biopsy demonstrates infiltration of the muscle by hyphal and yeast forms of the organism, inflammation, and hemorrhagic necrosis. Myositis has also been reported complicating actinomycosis, histoplasmosis, sporotrichosis, and cryptococcal infection.[243,244]

PARASITIC INFECTIONS

Trichinosis

Clinical Features

Trichinosis is caused by the nematode *Trichinella spiralis* and is the most common parasitic disease of skeletal muscle. Two to twelve days following ingestion of inadequately cooked meat (usually pork), larvae disseminate through the blood stream and invade muscle tissue. The most frequent muscles involved in order of frequency are the diaphragm, extraocular, tongue, laryngeal, jaw, intercostal, trunk, and limbs.[245,246] Patients complain of generalized muscle pain and weakness, fever, abdominal pain, and diarrhea. In addition, periorbital edema, ptosis, subconjunctival hemorrhage, and an erythematous urticarial or petechial rash are often evident. Myalgias and weakness peak in the third week of the infection but can last for several months. Occasionally, the parasite invades the heart muscle leading to myocarditis and the central nervous system causing meningoencephalitis.

Laboratory Features

Most patients have eosinophilic leukocytosis and elevated serum CK. Serum antibodies against *T. spiralis* can be demonstrated 3–4 weeks after infection.[246]

Histopathology

Muscle biopsies reveal prominent infiltration of the muscle by eosinophils and polymorphonuclear leukocytes in the early stage of infection.[245,246] In chronic stages of infection, mononuclear inflammatory cells become more prevalent. Larvae, cysts, focal calcification of the cysts, fibrosis, and granulomas may be observed (Fig. 33-21).

Pathogenesis

Following ingestion of meat infected with encysted larvae, gastric juices liberate the larvae that infect the gut. Maturation of the parasite occurs in the gut. Subsequently, second-generation larvae disseminate into the bloodstream and lymphatics to invade muscle and provoke the inflammatory response.

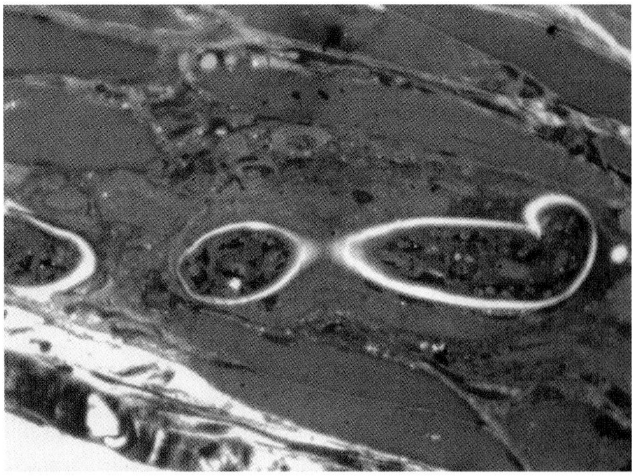

Figure 33-21. Trichinosis. Muscle biopsy demonstrates the parasite cut multiple times. Toluidine blue.

Prognosis and Treatment

The treatment of choice for the larvae and adult nematode is thiabendazole, but efficacy has not been established against the encysted larvae. Mebendazole may be effective against both circulating and encysted larvae. A 2-week course of prednisone is recommended because a Herxheimer-like reaction may develop as the larvae degenerate. Most patients respond quickly to treatment.

Cysticercosis

Clinical Features

Cysticercosis is caused by the tape worm—*Taenia solium*. Infection of skeletal muscles is manifested by myalgias; tenderness; pseudohypertrophy of infected muscles, especially the tongue and calves, and mild weakness.[247,248] Involvement of the central nervous system may cause focal neurologic deficits, encephalopathy, and seizures.

Laboratory Features

Serum CK and peripheral eosinophil counts are usually increased.

Histopathology

Muscle biopsies reveal eosinophils, plasma cells, macrophages, lymphocytes, and occasionally giant cells along with larvae surrounded by fibrotic changes.[247,248] The encysted larvae eventually calcify.

Pathogenesis

Infection results from ingestion of undercooked meat, mainly pork, which contains the larva form of *T. solium*. The tape worms mature in the small intestine and release ova. Ingestion of food or water contaminated by these ova results in hematogenous spread and infection of the muscle.

Prognosis and Treatment

Praziquantel reduces the size and number of cysts in the central nervous system, but efficacy in myositis has not been established. Niclosamide and paromomycin are the drugs of choice for removing the adult tapeworm. Concomitant administration of corticosteroids is helpful in decreasing the inflammatory reaction directed against degenerating parasites.

Toxoplasmosis

Clinical Features

Toxoplasmosis is caused by the protozoa *Toxoplasma gondii* and manifests as fever, lymphadenopathy, meningoencephalitis, hepatosplenomegaly, uveitis, pneumonia, myocarditis, and/or rash. It is more common in patients who are immunosuppressed. Myositis is uncommon but can occur in isolation or associated with systemic symptoms and presents as fever, myalgias, and weakness.[249–251]

Laboratory Features

Serum CK is usually elevated. The diagnosis of toxoplasmosis can be confirmed with serologic studies (i.e., Sabin–Feldman dye, complement fixation, indirect hemagglutination, and indirect fluorescent antibody). EMG reveals typical features of an inflammatory myopathy.

Histopathology

Muscle biopsies reveal lymphocytes, macrophages, and occasionally giant cells in the endomysium and perimysium. Cysts containing the bradyzoite stage of *T. gondii* are more commonly identified in muscle than the free tachyzoite form.

Pathogenesis

The most common mode of infection is by ingestion of food contaminated by oocysts or ingestion of cysts containing bradyzoites in undercooked food. The organism usually matures to the tachyzoite form and invades the bloodstream and lymphatics and disseminates to other tissues. Systemic disease is most common in patients who are immunosuppressed.

Prognosis and Treatment

The combination of pyrimethamine and sulfadiazine or trisulfapyrimidines are treatments of choice. Combination therapy is effective against the trophozoites but not against encysted protozoa.

▶ TREATMENT OF INFLAMMATORY MYOPATHIES

There are many published retrospective studies and small case reports regarding the use of various immunosuppressive and immunomodulating therapies in different types of inflammatory myopathy (Table 33-8; also see Chapter 5). Unfortunately, most of these older studies are difficult to interpret because they group adult and childhood DM together with PM, IBM, and necrotizing myopathy. Many of these reports were retrospective and unblinded and lacked placebo controls. Further, in several reports, patients with subjective improvement or lower serum CK levels were defined as positive responses rather than the more important objective improvement in muscle strength and function. There have been only a few published prospective, double-blinded, placebo-controlled trials in the treatment of PM,[252,253] DM,[253–255] and IBM.[256–261] Nevertheless, there has been a trend in recent years to perform more rigorous studies. Despite the paucity of prospective, double-blinded, placebo-controlled trials, it is clear to experienced clinicians that various modes of immunotherapy are helpful in DM and PM in improving muscle strength and function. In contrast, IBM is generally refractory to immunosuppressive therapy.

CORTICOSTEROIDS

Prednisone is our first-line treatment of choice for DM, PM, and IMNM.[1,5,7,29] In patients with severe weakness, we often initiate treatment with a short course of intravenous methylprednisolone (1 g daily for 3 days) prior to starting oral agents. High-dose prednisone appears to reduce morbidity and improve muscle strength and function.[35,59,96,97] Retrospective series report that 58–100% of patients with DM at least partially improve, while 30–66% respond completely with prednisone.[2,59] Over 80% of patients with PM at least partially improve, but only 10–33% completely respond to prednisone.[2,59] Noticeable clinical improvement begins within 3–6 months of starting prednisone in most patients with DM or PM.[2,35] IMNM is more refractory, often requires more than just prednisone alone, and usually takes longer to see a beneficial effect. When no response is noted after an adequate trial of high-dose prednisone, other alternative diagnoses (e.g., IBM or an inflammatory muscular dystrophy) and repeat muscle biopsy should be considered.

Most authorities have found minimal, if any, clinically significant improvement in strength of function with prednisone or other second-line agents in patients with IBM.[2,3,126–128,147,262] However, a few retrospective, unblinded studies reported mild or transient improvement with prednisone.[59,263] A partial response to prednisone was noted in 40–58% of patients with IBM, although none had complete return of strength. Careful review of these retrospective, unblinded studies shows that the investigators considered *subjective* improvement or lower serum CK levels with treatment a "positive" response. No demonstration of objective improvement in muscle strength was evident. One recent large retrospective series reported that IBM patients treated with immunotherapy actually fared worse than those who were not treated.[128]

In patients with DM, PM, presumed autoimmune necrotizing myopathy, and other idiopathic inflammatory myositides other than IBM (i.e., sarcoidosis), we initiate treatment with single-dose prednisone (0.75–1.5 mg/kg up

▶ TABLE 33-8. **IMMUNOSUPPRESSIVE THERAPY FOR NEUROMUSCULAR DISORDERS**

Therapy	Route	Dose	Side Effects	Monitor
Prednisone	Oral	0.75–1.5 mg kg per day to start	Hypertension, fluid and weight gain, hyperglycemia, hypokalemia, cataracts, gastric irritation, osteoporosis, infection, aseptic femoral necrosis	Weight, blood pressure, serum glucose/potassium, cataract formation
Methylprednisolone	Intravenous	1 g in 100 mL/normal saline over 1–2 hours, daily or every other day for 3–6 doses	Arrhythmia, flushing, dysgeusia, anxiety, insomnia, fluid and weight gain, hyperglycemia, hypokalemia, infection	Heart rate, blood pressure, serum glucose/ potassium
Azathioprine	Oral	2–3 mg/kg per day; single a.m. dose	Flu-like illness, hepatotoxicity, pancreatitis, leukopenia, macrocytosis, neoplasia, infection, teratogenicity	Blood count, liver enzymes
Methotrexate	Oral	7.5–20 mg weekly, single or divided doses; one day a week dosing	Hepatotoxicity, pulmonary fibrosis, infection, neoplasia, infertility, leukopenia, alopecia, gastric irritation, stomatitis, teratogenicity	Liver enzymes, blood count
	Subcutaneously	20–50 mg weekly; one day a week dosing	Same as oral.	Same as p.o.
Cyclophosphamide	Oral intravenous	1.5–2 mg/kg per day; single a.m. dose 0.5–1.0 g/m^2 per month × 6–12 months	Bone marrow suppression, infertility, hemorrhagic cystitis, alopecia, infections, neoplasia, teratogenicity	Blood count, urinalysis
Cyclosporine	Oral	4–6 mg/kg per day, split into two daily doses	Nephrotoxicity, hypertension, infection, hepatotoxicity, hirsutism, tremor, gum hyperplasia, teratogenicity,	Blood pressure, creatinine/BUN, liver enzymes, cyclosporine levels,
Tacrolimus	Oral	0.1–0.2 mg/kg per day in two divided doses	Nephrotoxicity, hypertension, infection, hepatotoxicity, hirsutism, tremor, gum hyperplasia, teratogenicity,	Blood pressure, creatinine/BUN, liver enzymes, tacrolimus levels
Mycophenolate mofetil	Oral	Adults (1 g BID to 1.5 g BID) Children (600 mg/m^2/dose BID (no more than 1 g per day in patients with renal failure)	Bone marrow suppression, hypertension, tremor, diarrhea, nausea, vomiting, headache, sinusitis, confusion, amblyopia, cough, teratogenicity, infection, neoplasia	Blood count
Intravenous Immunoglobulin	Intravenous	2 g/kg over 2–5 days; then 1 gm/kg every 4–8 weeks as needed	Hypotension, arrhythmia, diaphoresis, flushing, nephrotoxicity, headache, aseptic meningitis, anaphylaxis, stroke	Heart rate, blood pressure, creatinine/BUN
Rituximab	Intravenous	A course is typically 750 mg/m^2 (up to 1 g) and repeated in 2 weeks or 375 mg/m^2 weekly Courses are then repeated usually every 6–18 months	Infusion reactions (as per IVIG), infection, progressive multifocal leukoencephalopathy	Some check B-cell count prior to subsequent courses (but this may not be warranted)

to 100 mg) every morning (the most common dose used in adults is 60 mg daily).[1,3,5,6,29,264–266] Some studies have suggested that treating patients with alternate steroids or intermittent pulses of intravenous corticosteroids may be equally efficacious and associated with fewer side effects than daily steroids.[266,267] So, one can treat patients with daily prednisone for about 2 weeks and then switch to alternate day prednisone (e.g., 100 mg every other day). Some patients do not tolerate alternate day dosing or it is challenging in the setting of diabetes in trying to control blood sugar with this regimen, so daily dosing is necessary. We typically follow patients initially at every 2–4 weeks. We maintain the high-dose prednisone until patients are back to normal strength or until improvement in strength has reached a plateau (usually 4–6 months). Subsequently, we slowly taper the prednisone by 5–10 mg every 2–4 weeks. Once the dose is reduced to 10 mg every day or 20 mg every other day, we usually taper prednisone by 2.5–5 mg every 2–4 weeks.

Although most patients improve, the response may not be complete and most will require at least a small dose of prednisone or a second-line agent to have a sustained remission. In those patients who do not respond at all to high-dose prednisone, the clinician needs to consider alternative disorders (e.g., IBM or an inflammatory muscular dystrophy).

We monitor the serum CK levels; however, adjustments of prednisone and other immunosuppressive agents should be based on the objective clinical examination and not the CK levels or the patients' subjective response. Serum CKs can be elevated in patients with no objective weakness or can be normal or only mildly elevated in patients with active disease. An increasing serum CK can herald a relapse, but without objective clinical deterioration, we usually do not increase the dose of the immunosuppressive agent. However, we may hold the dose or the slow the taper. A maintenance dose of prednisone may be required to sustain the clinical response. We try to get patients to 10 mg daily (20 mg every other day) or less of prednisone.

Relapse of the myositis needs to be distinguished from steroid myopathy. This quandary may occur in patients who initially improved but then start developing progressive muscle weakness following long-term corticosteroid treatment because it can cause type 2 muscle fiber atrophy. Features that would suggest a "steroid myopathy" as opposed to relapse of myositis would be a normal serum CK, other clinical features of steroid excess such as ecchymoses and "moon facies," and absence of muscle membrane irritability on EMG. In contrast, patients who become weaker during prednisone taper, have increasing serum CK levels, and abnormal spontaneous activity on EMG are more likely experiencing a flare of the myositis.

CONCURRENT MANAGEMENT

We obtain a chest x-ray and, in at-risk individuals, a PPD skin test prior to initiating immunosuppressive medications. Patients with prior history of tuberculosis or a positive PPD may need to be treated prophylactically with isoniazid. If patients have ILD and are to be placed on prednisone plus another immunosuppressive agent, we also start an antibiotic (e.g., Bactrim) for pneumocystis prophylaxis.

We measure bone density with dual-energy x-ray absorptiometry at baseline and yearly while patients are receiving corticosteroids. A bone density score of less than 2.5 standard deviations below normal is considered positive for osteoporosis. Calcium supplementation (1 g per day) and vitamin D (400–800 IU per day) are started for prophylaxis against steroid-induced osteoporosis. Postmenopausal women are also started on a bisphosphonate for prevention and treatment of osteoporosis. We prescribe alendronate 35 mg per week (or another bisphosphonate) as prophylaxis against steroid-induced osteoporosis or 70 mg per week in those with osteoporosis. Because the long-term side effects of bisphosphonates are not known, particularly in men and young premenopausal women, we prophylactically treat (alendronate 35 mg per week) these individuals, only if the dual-energy x-ray absorptiometry scan demonstrates a density between 1 and 2.5 standard deviations below normal at baseline or if significant bone loss occurs on follow-up scans. If bone densities are in the osteoporosis range, we treat with alendronate 70 mg per week. Alendronate can cause severe esophagitis, and absorption is impaired if taken with meals. Therefore, patients must be instructed to remain upright and not to eat for at least 30 minutes following the dose of alendronate in the morning.

Antihistamine-H_2 blockers are not routinely started, unless the patient develops gastrointestinal discomfort or has a history of peptic ulcer disease. We instruct patients to start a low-sodium, low-carbohydrate, high-protein diet to prevent excessive weight gain. Physical therapy and an aerobic exercise program are helpful in fending off side effects of prednisone (e.g., weight gain) and preventing contractures and calcinosis that may result from immobility. Blood pressure is measured at each visit as accelerated hypertension and renal failure may occur, particularly in patients with scleroderma or MCTD.[113] In addition, periodic eye examinations for cataracts and glaucoma should be performed. We periodically check fasting blood glucose and serum potassium levels, while they are on high doses of prednisone. Potassium supplementation may be required, if the patient becomes hypokalemic.

SECOND-LINE THERAPIES

These agents are used primarily in patients poorly responsive to prednisone or who relapse during prednisone taper as well as for their potential steroid-sparing effect (Table 33-8). There is equipoise regarding when to start second-line agents (e.g., methotrexate, azathioprine, mycophenolate, or immunoglobulin). The clinician must review with the patient the increased risks of immunosuppression versus possible benefits (e.g., faster improvement, steroid-sparing effect and/or avoidance of the morbidities associated with long-term steroid use). We usually start a second-line agent along with corticosteroids in patients with severe weakness or other organ system involvement (e.g., myocarditis, ILD), those with increased risk of steroid complications (e.g., diabetics, patients with osteoporosis, or postmenopausal women), and patients, who we know from experience have difficulty to treat myositis (e.g., IMNM). A second-line agent should also be strongly considered in patients who fail to significantly improve after 2–4 months of treatment or if there is an exacerbation during treatment with prednisone. In patients who relapse during the taper, we double the dose of prednisone (no more than 100 mg per day). Once a patient has regained their strength, we resume the prednisone taper at a slower rate. We instruct patients taking immunosuppressant medications to use sunscreen and be vigilant because of the increased risk of cancer, in particular of the skin.

INTRAVENOUS IMMUNOGLOBULIN

IVIG has become increasingly popular in the treatment of refractory myositis. Small, uncontrolled studies have reported beneficial response in DM and PM.[261,269–270] A prospective, double-blind, placebo-controlled study of IVIG in 15 patients with DM demonstrated significant clinical improvement with IVIG.[255] In support of the clinical observations, repeat biopsies in five of the responsive patients revealed an increase in muscle fiber diameter, increase in the number and decrease in the diameter of capillaries, resolution of complement on capillaries, and a reduction in the expression of intercellular adhesion molecule 1 (ICAM-1) and MHC-1 antigens.

Mild improvement in muscle strength was reported in three of four patients with IBM treated with IVIG.[271] However, we were unable to document any significant clinical improvement in nine patients with IBM treated with IVIG.[263] Subsequently several prospective, double-blind, placebo-controlled studies of IVIG in IBM have revealed no significant improvement.[257,258]

We initiate IVIG (2 g/kg) slowly over 2–5 days and repeat infusions at monthly intervals for at least 3 months. Subsequently, we try to decrease or spread out the dose: 2 g/kg every 2 months or 1 g/kg per month. Treatment needs to be individualized. Our own anecdotal experience suggests that IVIG is effective for DM and necrotizing myopathies but is less effective for PM and not at all for IBM. We generally give IVIG in combination with prednisone. There is little evidence that it is effective as a monotherapy. Patients should also have renal function checked beforehand, especially those with diabetes mellitus, because of a risk of IVIG-induced renal failure. Flu-like symptoms—headaches, myalgias, fever, chills, nausea, and vomiting—are common and occur in as many as half the patients. Rash, aseptic meningitis, and stroke can also occur.

METHOTREXATE

There are no prospective, blinded, controlled studies of methotrexate in DM or PM. However, retrospective studies report that as many as 71–88% of patients with DM and PM, including those refractory to prednisone, improve at least partially with the addition of methotrexate.[59,272–276] Methotrexate appears to reduce morbidity in refractory childhood DM,[219] but its side-effect profile has limited its use in children. Methotrexate was not shown to be beneficial in a randomized, placebo-controlled trial in IBM patients.[256]

Methotrexate is administered only 1 day a week. We usually begin methotrexate orally at 5.0 mg per week. The dose is gradually increased by 2.5 mg each week up to 20 mg per week given in three divided doses 12 hours apart. The dose should be reduced and used cautiously in patients with renal insufficiency. If there is no improvement after 1 month of 20 mg per week of oral methotrexate, we switch to weekly parenteral (usually subcutaneous) methotrexate and increase the dose by 5 mg every week up to 60 mg per week. The major side effects of methotrexate are alopecia, stomatitis, ILD, teratogenicity, oncogenicity, risk of infection, and pulmonary fibrosis, along with bone marrow, renal, and liver toxicity. Doses over 50 mg per week require leucovorin rescue, although we rarely use such high doses. However, all patients are concomitantly treated with folate.

Because methotrexate can cause pulmonary fibrosis, we do not recommend its use in patients with myositis who already have the associated ILD and try to avoid its use in patients with Jo-1 antibodies. We obtain baseline and periodic pulmonary function tests including forced vital capacity and diffusion capacity and repeat these periodically on patients treated with methotrexate. We monitor CBC and liver function tests (LFTs)—AST, ALT, bilirubin, and gamma-glutamyl transpeptidase (GGT) every 2 weeks until the patient is on a stable dose of methotrexate, then every 1–3 months. It is important to check the GGT, as it is the most reliable indicator of hepatic dysfunction, because the AST and ALT can be elevated from muscle involvement.

AZATHIOPRINE

Retrospective studies indicate that azathioprine is an effective therapy in DM and PM.[35,59] In one study, the addition of azathioprine was associated with improvement in 64% of patients with DM and PM, although a complete response occurred in only 11%.[59] Not surprisingly, patients who previously responded to prednisone were more likely than patients who are prednisone-refractory to improve with the addition of azathioprine. A prospective, double-blind study comparing azathioprine (2 mg/kg) in combination with prednisone to placebo plus prednisone found no significant difference in objective improvement at 3 months.[252] However, in the open-label follow-up period, patients on the combination of azathioprine and prednisone did better than those on prednisone alone and required lower doses of prednisone.[277] Azathioprine appears to be effective in some cases of childhood DM but is generally avoided, given its oncogenic potential with long-term use.

Prior to beginning azathioprine, patients can be screened for thiopurine methyltransferase (TPMT) deficiency. Patients who are heterozygous for a mutation in TPMT may be able to tolerate azathioprine at lower dosages, but those who are homozygous for TPMT mutations should not receive the drug as they cannot metabolize it and may have severe bone marrow toxicity. In those patients without TPMT mutations, we initiate azathioprine at a dose of 50 mg per day in adults and increase the dose by 50 mg every 2 weeks up to 2–3 mg/kg per day. Approximately 12% of patients develop a systemic reaction characterized by fever, abdominal pain, nausea, vomiting, and anorexia that requires discontinuation of the drug.[270] This systemic reaction generally occurs within the first few weeks of therapy and resolves within a few days of discontinuing the medication. Recurrence of the systemic reaction usually follows restarting azathioprine. Other major side effects of azathioprine are bone marrow suppression, hepatic toxicity, pancreatitis, teratogenicity, oncogenicity, and increased risk of infection. Allopurinol should be avoided, because combination with azathioprine increases the risk of bone marrow and liver toxicity. A major drawback of azathioprine is that it may take 6–18 months to be effective.

CBCs and LFTs need to be followed closely. If the white blood count (WBC) falls below 4,000/mm^3, we decrease the dose. Azathioprine is held if the WBC declines to 2,500/mm^3 or the absolute neutrophil count falls to 1,000/mm^3. Leukopenia can develop as early as 1 week or as late as 2 years after initiating azathioprine. The leukopenia usually reverses within 1 month, and it is possible to then rechallenge the patient with azathioprine without recurrence of the severe leukopenia.[270] In addition, we discontinue azathioprine if the LFTs increase more than twice the baseline values. Liver toxicity generally develops within the first several months of treatment and can take several months to resolve. Patients can occasionally be successfully rechallenged with azathioprine after LFTs return to baseline without recurrence of hepatic dysfunction.[270]

MYCOPHENOLATE MOFETIL

Mycophenolate mofetil inhibits the proliferation of T and B lymphocytes by blocking purine synthesis in only lymphocytes. Mycophenolate has been used in patients who require transplant to prevent rejection and has recently been tried in a few patients with myositis with reported benefit. The starting dose is 1.0 g twice daily and can be increased to 3 g daily in divided doses if necessary. Mycophenolate is renally excreted; therefore, the dose should be decreased (no more than 1 g per day total dose) in patients with renal insufficiency. A benefit of mycophenolate compared to other immunosuppressive agents is the lack of renal or liver toxicity. Mycophenolate appears to be beneficial in some patients; however, we have seen a number of severe infections as a complication.[278–281] The most frequent side effect is diarrhea. Less common side effects include abdominal discomfort, nausea, peripheral edema, fever, and leukopenia.

RITUXIMAB

Rituximab is a monoclonal antibody directed against CD20+ B cells, which it depletes for 6 months or more. A number of small series have suggested that rituximab may be effective in DM, PM, and necrotizing myopathies.[282–285] A large prospective, double-blind, NIH trial found no benefit but there were significant flaws in the study design.[253] A subset of patients do likely respond,[286] and it has been our experience that rituximab can be beneficial in patients with refractory DM, PM, and IMNM. We use it in patients who are refractory to prednisone and at least one of the other second-line agents discussed above. The typical dosage is 750 mg/m^2 (up to 1 g) IV and then repeat the infusion in two weeks. Alternatively, patients can be treated with a 4-week course (375 mg/m^2 weekly × 4 weeks). A course of rituximab as above is usually repeated every 6–18 months depending on how well they are doing. There is a very small risk of progressive multifocal leukoencephalopathy, which is discussed with patients before prescribing.

CYCLOPHOSPHAMIDE

Some reports note improvement in individual patients with oral and intravenous cyclophosphamide.[35,287–291] However, other reports have found increased morbidity with intravenous cyclophosphamide without significant benefit.[292,293] Cyclophosphamide has been advocated for use in myositis associated with ILD or vasculitis, but clinical studies are lacking. Given the controversy regarding the efficacy and the toxicity profile of cyclophosphamide, we reserve it for patients who are refractory to prednisone, methotrexate, azathioprine, mycophenolate, IVIG, and rituximab. When used, we usually pulse patients with cyclophosphamide at 0.5–1 g intravenously/m^2 per month for 6–12 months. Cyclophosphamide can be given orally at a dose of 1.0–2.0 mg/kg per day, but there may be a greater risk of hemorrhagic cystitis. The major side effects are gastrointestinal upset, bone marrow toxicity, alopecia, hemorrhagic cystitis, teratogenicity, sterilization, and increased risk of infection and secondary malignancy. Hydration with intravenous fluids prior to intravenous treatment, maintaining a high fluid intake (oral or intravenous therapy), and treatment with mesna are important precautions to help avoid hemorrhagic cystitis. Urinalysis and CBCs are monitored closely (every 1–2 weeks at the onset of therapy and then at least monthly). The dose of cyclophosphamide should be decreased if the WBC decreases below 4,000/mm^3. Cyclophosphamide is held if the WBC declines below 3,000/mm^3, the absolute neutrophil count falls below 1,000/mm^3, or there is evidence of hematuria. It can be restarted at a lower dose once the leukopenia has resolved, but we do not restart the medication in patients with hematuria.

CHLORAMBUCIL

Chlorambucil is uncommonly used because of the significant side effects, which include bone marrow suppression, increased risk of cancer, infection, hepatotoxicity, Stevens–Johnson syndrome, and gastrointestinal disturbance. However, there are a few reports of chlorambucil being used to treat PM and DM.[272,294,295] CBCs and LFTs need to be monitored closely in patients treated with chlorambucil.

CYCLOSPORINE AND TACROLIMUS

Cyclosporine (2.5–10 mg/kg per day) may be effective in some patients with DM and PM, including childhood DM.[122,296–303]

Improvement in strength may be seen within 2–6 weeks, and it may also serve as a steroid-sparing agent. However, the cost and potential side effects have limited its use in most patients with myositis. Tacrolimus has also been reported to help patients with refractory myositis.[304] Side effects of cyclosporine and tacrolimus are renal toxicity, hypertension, electrolyte imbalance, gastrointestinal upset, hypertrichosis, gingival hyperplasia, oncogenicity, tremor, and risk of infection.

We start cyclosporine at a dose of 3.0–4.0 mg/kg per day in two divided doses and gradually increase to 6.0 mg/kg per day as necessary. The cyclosporine dose should initially be titrated to maintain trough serum cyclosporine levels of 50–200 ng/mL. Blood pressure, electrolytes and renal function, and trough cyclosporine levels need to be monitored closely.

Tacrolimus is started at a dose of 0.1 mg/kg and increased up to 0.2 mg/kg (in two divided doses daily). Dosing is titrated to maintain a trough level of 5–15 mg/mL. Blood pressure, electrolytes, and renal function need to be monitored closely and doses adjusted should renal insufficiency develop. With both of these agents, patients should be given a list of drugs to avoid that may increase the risk of renal toxicity.

INFLIXIMAB AND ETANERCEPT

These agents block TNF-alpha and are effective treatments in rheumatoid arthritis and other autoimmune disorders. A few small reports suggest that these medications may be effective in PM and DM.[254,305–311] However, others small reports have found no benefit, and some individuals worsening.[312–315] Therefore, we save TNF-alpha blockers as a last resort in refractory patients.

PLASMAPHERESIS AND LEUKOPHERESIS

Uncontrolled series have reported improvement in DM, PM, and IBM with plasmapheresis or leukapheresis.[316–318] However, a controlled trial of 36 patients with DM and PM comparing plasmapheresis with leukapheresis and with sham apheresis demonstrated no improvement with either plasmapheresis or leukapheresis over the sham apheresis.[319]

TOTAL BODY IRRADIATION

There are a few case reports of refractory cases of DM and PM improving following total body irradiation.[320–322] Others have not found total body irradiation to be effective in PM.[323] Total body irradiation is ineffective in IBM and may actually aggravate the disease.[324]

THYMECTOMY

Thymectomy has been performed on a small number of patients with PM and DM with improvement.[325]

▶ SUMMARY

DM, PM, NM, and IBM are clinically, histologically, and pathogenically distinct categories of idiopathic inflammatory myopathy. Features of DM, PM, and IMNM can overlap with those of other autoimmune connective tissue diseases. Other types of inflammatory myopathy are much less common but are clinically and histologically distinguishable. DM is an immune-mediated microangiopathy, perhaps due to over expression of type 1 interferons that may be directly toxic to muscle fibers as well. PM is a T-cell-mediated disorder directed against muscle fibers. The pathogenesis of IMNM and IBM are unknown. DM, PM, NM are responsive to immunosuppressive therapy, in contrast to IBM, which is generally refractory to therapy. Prospective, double-blind, placebo-controlled trials are necessary to determine prognostic features for treatment responsiveness and the best treatment options for the different disorders.

REFERENCES

1. Amato AA, Barohn RJ. Idiopathic inflammatory myopathies. *Neurol Clin.* 1997;15(3):615–648.
2. Amato AA, Gronseth GS, Jackson CE, et al. Inclusion body myositis: clinical and pathological boundaries. *Ann Neurol.* 1996;40:581–586.
3. Dalakas MC. Polymyositis, dermatomyositis and inclusion-body myositis. *N Engl J Med.* 1991;325(21):1487–1498.
4. Hoogendijk JE, Amato AA, Lecky BR, et al. 119th ENMC international workshop: trial design in adult idiopathic inflammatory myopathies, with the exception of inclusion body myositis, 10–12 October 2003, Naarden, the Netherlands. *Neuromuscul Disord.* 2004;14(5):337–345.
5. Mammen A, Amato AA. Inflammatory myopathies. In: Griggs RC, Tawil R, eds. *Evaluation and Treatment of Myopathies.* 2nd ed. Philadelphia, PA: F.A. Davis Company; 2014.
6. Amato AA, Greenberg SA. Inflammatory myopathies. *Continuum (Minneap Minn).* 2013;19(6 Muscle Disease):1615–1633.
7. Amato AA, Barohn RJ. Evaluation and treatment of inflammatory myopathies. *J Neurol Neurosurg Psychiatry.* 2009;80(10):1060–1068.
8. Amato AA, Barohn RJ. Inclusion body myositis: old and new concepts. *J Neurol Neurosurg Psychiatry.* 2009;80(11):1186–1193.
9. Griggs RC, Askanas V, DiMauro S, et al. Inclusion body myositis and myopathies. *Ann Neurol.* 1995;38(5):705–713.
10. Pestronk A. Acquired immune and inflammatory myopathies: pathologic classification. *Curr Opin Rheumatol.* 2011;23(6):595–604.
11. Fernandez C, Bardin N, De Paula AM, et al. Correlation of clinicoserologic and pathologic classifications of inflammatory myopathies: study of 178 cases and guidelines for diagnosis. *Medicine.* 2013;92(1):15–24.
12. Banker BQ. Dermatomyostis of childhood, ultrastructural alterations of muscle and intramuscular blood vessels. *J Neuropathol Exp Neurol.* 1975;34(1):46–75.
13. Harati Y, Niakan E, Bergman EW. Childhood dermatomyositis in monozygotic twins. *Neurology.* 1986;36(5):721–723.
14. Lewkonia RM, Buxton PH. Myositis in father and daughter. *J Neurol Neurosurg Psychiatry.* 1973;36(5):820–825.

15. Amato AA, Shebert RT. Inclusion body myositis in twins. *Neurology*. 1998;51:598–600.
16. Medsger TA Jr, Dawson WN Jr, Masi AT. The epidemiology of polymyositis. *Am J Med*. 1970;48(6):715–723.
17. Vargas-Leguas H, Selva-O'Callaghan A, Campins-Marti M, et al. Polymyositis-dermatomyositis: incidence in Spain (1997–2004). *Med Clin (Barc)*. 2007;129(19):721–724.
18. Flachenecker P. Epidemiology of neuroimmunological diseases. *J Neurol*. 2006;253(suppl 5):V2–V8.
19. Gaubitz M. Epidemiology of connective tissue disorders. *Rheumatology (Oxford)*. 2006;45(suppl 3):iii3–iii4.
20. Prieto S, Grau JM. The geoepidemiology of autoimmune muscle disease. *Autoimmun Rev*. 2010;9(5):A330–A334.
21. Hengstman GJ, van Venrooij WJ, Vencovsky J, Moutsopoulos HM, van Engelen BG. The relative prevalence of dermatomyositis and polymyositis in Europe exhibits a latitudinal gradient. *Ann Rheum Dis*. 2000;59(2):141–142.
22. Smoyer Tomic KE, Amato AA, Fernandes AW. Incidence and prevalence of idiopathic inflammatory myopathies among commercially insured, Medicare supplemental insured, and Medicaid enrolled populations: an administrative claims analysis. *BMC Musculoskelet Disord*. 2012;13(1):103.
23. Bernatsky S, Joseph L, Pineau CA, et al. Estimating the prevalence of polymyositis and dermatomyositis from administrative data: age, sex and regional differences. *Ann Rheum Dis*. 2009;68(7):1192–1196.
24. Ohta A, Nagai M, Nishina M, Tomimitsu H, Kohsaka H. Prevalence and incidence of polymyositis and dermatomyositis in Japan. *Mod Rheumatol*. 2014;24(3):477–480.
25. Furst DE, Amato AA, Iorga ŞR, Gajria K, Fernandes AW. Epidemiology of adult idiopathic inflammatory myopathies in a U.S. managed care plan. *Muscle Nerve*. 2012;45:676–683.
26. Bohan A, Peter JB. Polymyositis and dermatomyositis (first of two parts). *N Engl J Med*. 1975;292(7):344–347.
27. Bohan A, Peter JB. Polymyositis and dermatomyositis (second of two parts). *N Engl J Med*. 1975;292(8):403–407.
28. Bohan A, Peter JB, Bowman RL, Pearson CM. Computer-assisted analysis of 153 patients with polymyositis and dermatomyositis. *Medicine (Baltimore)*. 1977;56(4):255–286.
29. Briemberg HR, Amato AA. Dermatomyositis and Polymyositis. *Curr Treat Options Neurol*. 2003;5(5):349–356.
30. Dalakas MC, Hohlfeld R. Polymyositis and dermatomyositis. *Lancet*. 2003;362(9388):971–982.
31. van der Meulen MF, Bronner IM, Hoogendijk JE, et al. Polymyositis: an over diagnosed entity. *Neurology*. 2003;61(3):316–321.
32. Arahata K, Engel AG. Monoclonal antibody analysis of mononuclear cells in myopathies. I: quantitation of subsets according to diagnosis and sites of accumulation and demonstration and counts of muscle fibers invaded by T cells. *Ann Neurol*. 1984;16(2):193–208.
33. Bruguier A, Texier P, Clement MC, Dulac O, Ponsot G, Arthuis M. Pediatric dermatomyositis. Apropos of 28 cases. *Arch Fr Pediatr*. 1984;41(1):9–14.
34. Hochberg MC, Feldman D, Stevens MB. Adult onset polymyositis/dermatomyositis: an analysis of clinical and laboratory features and survival in 76 patients with a review of the literature. *Semin Arthritis Rheum*. 1986;15(3):168–178.
35. Tymms KE, Webb J. Dermatopolymyositis and other connective tissue diseases: a review of 105 cases. *J Rheumatol*. 1985;12(6):1140–1148.
36. Sontheimer RD. Cutaneous features of classic dermatomyositis and amyopathic dermatomyositis. *Curr Opin Rheumatol*. 1999;11(6):475–482.
37. Euwer RL, Sontheimer RD. Amyopathic dermatomyositis: a review. *J Invest Dermatol*. 1993;100(1):124S–127S.
38. Cohen MG, Nash P, Webb J. Calcification is rare in adult-onset dermatopolymyositis. *Clin Rheumatol*. 1986;5(4):512–516.
39. Pachman LM. Juvenile dermatomyositis: immunogenetics, pathophysiology, and disease expression. *Rheum Dis Clin North Am*. 2002;28(3):579–602, vii.
40. Askari AD. Inflammatory disorders of muscle. Cardiac abnormalities. *Clin Rheum Dis*. 1984;10(1):131–149.
41. Denbow CE, Lie JT, Tancredi RG, Bunch TW. Cardiac involvement in polymyositis: a clinicopathologic study of 20 autopsied patients. *Arthritis Rheum*. 1979;22(10):1088–1092.
42. Gottdiener JS, Sherber HS, Hawley RJ, Engel WK. Cardiac manifestations in polymyositis. *Am J Cardiol*. 1978;41(7):1141–1149.
43. Haupt HM, Hutchins GM. The heart and cardiac conduction system in polymyositis-dermatomyositis: a clinicopathologic study of 16 autopsied patients. *Am J Cardiol*. 1982;50(5):998–1006.
44. Strongwater SL, Annesley T, Schnitzer TJ. Myocardial involvement in polymyositis. *J Rheumatol*. 1983;10(3):459–463.
45. Dickey BF, Myers AR. Pulmonary disease in polymyositis/dermatomyositis. *Semin Arthritis Rheum*. 1984;14(1):60–76.
46. Frazier AR, Miller RD. Interstitial pneumonitis in association with polymyositis and dermatomyositis. *Chest*. 1974;65(4):403–407.
47. Park S, Nyhan WL. Fatal pulmonary involvement in dermatomyositis. *Am J Dis Child*. 1975;129(6):723–726.
48. Schwarz MI, Matthay RA, Sahn SA, Stanford RE, Marmorstein BL, Scheinhorn DJ. Interstitial lung disease in polymyositis and dermatomyositis: analysis of six cases and review of the literature. *Medicine (Baltimore)*. 1976;55(1):89–104.
49. Hochberg MC, Feldman D, Stevens MB, Arnett FC, Reichlin M. Antibody to Jo-1 in polymyositis/dermatomyositis: association with interstitial pulmonary disease. *J Rheumatol*. 1984;11(5):663–665.
50. Love LA, Leff RL, Fraser DD, et al. A new approach to the classification of idiopathic inflammatory myopathy: myositis specific autoantibodies define useful homogeneous patient groups. *Medicine (Baltimore)*. 1991;70(6):360–374.
51. Targoff IN, Miller FW, Medsger TA Jr, Oddis CV. Classification criteria for the idiopathic inflammatory myopathies. *Curr Opin Rheumatol*. 1997;9(6):527–535.
52. Callen JP. Relationship of cancer to inflammatory muscle diseases. Dermatomyositis, polymyositis, and inclusion body myositis. *Rheum Dis Clin North Am*. 1994;20(4):943–953.
53. Sigurgeirsson B, Lindelof B, Edhag O, Allander E. Risk of cancer in patients with dermatomyositis or polymyositis. A population-based study. *N Engl J Med*. 1992;326(6):363–367.
54. Carter JD, Kanik KS, Vasey FB, Valeriano-Marcet J. Dermatomyositis with normal creatine kinase and elevated aldolase levels. *J Rheumatol*. 2001;28(10):2366–2367.
55. Nozaki K, Pestronk A. High aldolase with normal creatine kinase in serum predicts a myopathy with perimysial pathology. *J Neurol Neurosurg Psychiatry*. 2009;80(8):904–908.
56. Casciola-Rosen L, Hall JC, Mammen AL, Christopher-Stine L, Rosen A. Isolated elevation of aldolase in the serum of myositis patients: a potential biomarker of damaged early regenerating muscle cells. *Clin Exp Rheumatol*. 2012;30(4):548–553.
57. Hengstman GJ, Brouwer R, Egberts WT, et al. Clinical and serological characteristics of 125 Dutch myositis patients. Myositis

specific autoantibodies aid in the differential diagnosis of the idiopathic inflammatory myopathies. *J Neurol.* 2002;249(1):69–75.
58. Hengstman GJ, van Engelen BG. Polymyositis, invasion of non-necrotic muscle fibres, and the art of repetition. *BMJ.* 2004;329(7480):1464–1467.
59. Joffe MM, Love LA, Leff RL, et al. Drug therapy of the idiopathic inflammatory myopathies: predictors of response to prednisone, azathioprine, and methotrexate and a comparison of their efficacy. *Am J Med.* 1993;94(4):379–387.
60. Miller FW. Myositis-specific autoantibodies. Touchstones for understanding the inflammatory myopathies. *JAMA.* 1993;270(15):1846–1849.
61. Plotz PH, Rider LG, Targoff IN, Raben N, O'Hanlon TP, Miller FW. NIH conference. Myositis: immunologic contributions to understanding cause, pathogenesis, and therapy. *Ann Intern Med.* 1995;122(9):715–724.
62. Sato S, Hirakata M, Kuwana M, et al. Autoantibodies to a 140-kd polypeptide, CADM-140, in Japanese patients with clinically amyopathic dermatomyositis. *Arthritis Rheum.* 2005; 52(5):1571–1576.
63. Sato S, Hoshino K, Satoh T, et al. RNA helicase encoded by melanoma differentiation-associated gene 5 is a major autoantigen in patients with clinically amyopathic dermatomyositis: association with rapidly progressive interstitial lung disease. *Arthritis Rheum.* 2009;60(7):2193–2200.
64. Nakashima R, Imura Y, Kobayashi S, et al. The RIG-I-like receptor IFIH1/MDA5 is a dermatomyositis-specific autoantigen identified by the anti-CADM-140 antibody. *Rheumatology (Oxford).* 2010;49(3):433–440.
65. Fiorentino D, Chung L, Zwerner J, Rosen A, Casciola-Rosen L. The mucocutaneous and systemic phenotype of dermatomyositis patients with antibodies to MDA5 (CADM-140): a retrospective study. *J Am Acad Dermatol.* 2011;65(1):25–34.
66. Chaisson NF, Paik J, Orbai AM, et al. A novel dermato-pulmonary syndrome associated with MDA-5 antibodies: report of 2 cases and review of the literature. *Medicine (Baltimore).* 2012;91(4):220–228.
67. Cao H, Pan M, Kang Y, et al. Clinical manifestations of dermatomyositis and clinically amyopathic dermatomyositis patients with positive expression of anti-melanoma differentiation-associated gene 5 antibody. *Arthritis Care Res (Hoboken).* 2012;64(10):1602–1610.
68. Targoff IN, Mamyrova G, Trieu EP, et al. A novel autoantibody to a 155-kd protein is associated with dermatomyositis. *Arthritis Rheum.* 2006;54(11):3682–3689.
69. Kaji K, Fujimoto M, Hasegawa M, et al. Identification of a novel autoantibody reactive with 155 and 140 kDa nuclear proteins in patients with dermatomyositis: an association with malignancy. *Rheumatology (Oxford).* 2007;46(1):25–28.
70. Trallero-Araguas E, Rodrigo-Pendas JA, Selva-O'Callaghan A, et al. Usefulness of anti-p155 autoantibody for diagnosing cancer-associated dermatomyositis: a systematic review and meta-analysis. *Arthritis Rheum.* 2012;64(2):523–532.
71. Ghirardello A, Bassi N, Palma L, et al. Autoantibodies in polymyositis and dermatomyositis. *Curr Rheumatol Rep.* 2013;15(6):335.
72. Casciola-Rosen L, Mammen AL. Myositis autoantibodies. *Curr Opin Rheumatol.* 2012;24(6):602–608.
73. Fiorentino DF, Chung LS, Christopher-Stine L, et al. Most patients with cancer-associated dermatomyositis have antibodies to nuclear matrix protein NXP-2 or transcription intermediary factor 1γ. *Arthritis Rheum.* 2013;65(11):2954–2962.
74. Fraser DD, Frank JA, Dalakas M, Miller FW, Hicks JE, Plotz P. Magnetic resonance imaging in the idiopathic inflammatory myopathies. *J Rheumatol.* 1991;18(11):1693–1700.
75. Fraser DD, Frank JA, Dalakas MC. Inflammatory myopathies: MR imaging and spectroscopy. *Radiology.* 1991;179(2):341–342; discussion 343–344.
76. Hernandez RJ, Sullivan DB, Chenevert TL, Keim DR. MR imaging in children with dermatomyositis: musculoskeletal findings and correlation with clinical and laboratory findings. *AJR Am J Roentgenol.* 1993;161(2):359–366.
77. Mastaglia FL, Laing NG. Investigation of muscle disease. *J Neurol Neurosurg Psychiatry.* 1996;60(3):256–274.
78. Pitt AM, Fleckenstein JL, Greenlee RG Jr, Burns DK, Bryan WW, Haller R. MRI-guided biopsy in inflammatory myopathy: initial results. *Magn Reson Imaging.* 1993;11(8):1093–1099.
79. Del Grande F, Carrino JA, Del Grande M, Mammen AL, Christopher Stine L. Magnetic resonance imaging of inflammatory myopathies. *Top Magn Reson Imaging.* 2011;22(2):39–43.
80. Amato A, Dumitru D. *Acquired Myopathies.* Philadelphia, PA: Hanley & Belfus; 2002.
81. Engel AG, Arahata K. Monoclonal antibody analysis of mononuclear cells in myopathies. II: phenotypes of autoinvasive cells in polymyositis and inclusion body myositis. *Ann Neurol.* 1984;16(2):209–215.
82. Greenberg SA, Pinkus JL, Pinkus GS, et al. Interferon-alpha/beta-mediated innate immune mechanisms in dermatomyositis. *Ann Neurol.* 2005;57(5):664–678.
83. Salajegheh M, Kong SW, Pinkus JL, et al. Interferon-stimulated gene 15 (ISG15) conjugates proteins in dermatomyositis muscle with perifascicular atrophy. *Ann Neurol.* 2010;67:53–63.
84. Emslie-Smith AM, Engel AG. Microvascular changes in early and advanced dermatomyositis: a quantitative study. *Ann Neurol.* 1990;27(4):343–356.
85. Kissel JT, Halterman RK, Rammohan KW, Mendell JR. The relationship of complement-mediated microvasculopathy to the histologic features and clinical duration of disease in dermatomyositis. *Arch Neurol.* 1991;48(1):26–30.
86. Kissel JT, Mendell JR, Rammohan KW. Microvascular deposition of complement membrane attack complex in dermatomyositis. *N Engl J Med.* 1986;314(6):329–334.
87. Whitaker JN, Engel WK. Vascular deposits of immunoglobulin and complement in idiopathic inflammatory myopathy. *N Engl J Med.* 1972;286(7):333–338.
88. De Visser M, Emslie-Smith AM, Engel AG. Early ultrastructural alterations in adult dermatomyositis. Capillary abnormalities precede other structural changes in muscle. *J Neurol Sci.* 1989;94(1–3):181–192.
89. Greenberg SA, Amato AA. Uncertainties in the pathogenesis of adult dermatomyositis. *Curr Opin Neurol.* 2004;17(3):359–364.
90. Ichikawa E, Furuta J, Kawachi Y, Imakado S, Otsuka F. Hereditary complement (C9) deficiency associated with dermatomyositis. *Br J Dermatol.* 2001;144(5):1080–1083.
91. Leddy JP, Griggs RC, Klemperer MR, Frank MM. Hereditary complement (C2) deficiency with dermatomyositis. *Am J Med.* 1975;58(1):83–91.
92. Karpati G, Carpenter S, Melmed C, Eisen AA. Experimental ischemic myopathy. *J Neurol Sci.* 1974;23(1):129–161.
93. Hathaway PW, Engel WK, Zellweger H. Experimental myopathy after microarterial embolization; comparison with childhood x-linked pseudohypertrophic muscular dystrophy. *Arch Neurol.* 1970;22(4):365–378.

94. Greenberg SA, Sanoudou D, Haslett JN, et al. Molecular profiles of inflammatory myopathies. *Neurology*. 2002;59(8):1170–1182.
95. Tezak Z, Hoffman EP, Lutz JL, et al. Gene expression profiling in DQA1*0501+ children with untreated dermatomyositis: a novel model of pathogenesis. *J Immunol*. 2002;168(8):4154–4163.
96. Hochberg MC, Lopez-Acuna D, Gittelsohn AM. Mortality from polymyositis and dermatomyositis in the United States, 1968–1978. *Arthritis Rheum*. 1983;26(12):1465–1471.
97. Murabayashi K, Saito E, Okada S, Ogawa T, Kinoshita M. Prognosis of life in polymyositis/dermatomyositis. *Ryumachi*. 1991;31(4):391–397.
98. Hengstman GJ, van Engelen BG. Polymyositis: an over-diagnosed entity. *Neurology*. 2004;63(2):402–403; author reply 403.
99. Hengstman GJ, van Engelen BG, van Venrooij WJ. Myositis specific autoantibodies: changing insights in pathophysiology and clinical associations. *Curr Opin Rheumatol*. 2004;16(6):692–699.
100. Miller T, Al-Lozi MT, Lopate G, Pestronk A. Myopathy with antibodies to the signal recognition particle: clinical and pathological features. *J Neurol Neurosurg Psychiatry*. 2002;73(4):420–428.
101. Mozaffar T, Pestronk A. Myopathy with anti-Jo-1 antibodies: pathology in perimysium and neighbouring muscle fibres. *J Neurol Neurosurg Psychiatry*. 2000;68(4):472–478.
102. Emslie-Smith AM, Arahata K, Engel AG. Major histocompatibility complex class I antigen expression, immunolocalization of interferon subtypes, and T cell-mediated cytotoxicity in myopathies. *Hum Pathol*. 1989;20(3):224–231.
103. Mor F. Polymyositis mediated by lymphocytes expressing the gamma/delta receptor. *N Engl J Med*. 1991;325(8):587–588.
104. Hohlfeld R, Engel AG, Ii K, Harper MC. Polymyositis mediated by T lymphocytes that express the gamma/delta receptor. *N Engl J Med*. 1991;324(13):877–881.
105. O'Hanlon TP, Messersmith WA, Dalakas MC, Plotz PH, Miller FW. Gamma delta T cell receptor gene expression by muscle-infiltrating lymphocytes in the idiopathic inflammatory myopathies. *Clin Exp Immunol*. 1995;100(3):519–528.
106. Hofbauer M, Wiesener S, Babbe H, et al. Clonal tracking of autoaggressive T cells in polymyositis by combining laser microdissection, single-cell PCR, and CDR3-spectratype analysis. *Proc Natl Acad Sci USA*. 2003;100(7):4090–4095.
107. Mantegazza R, Andreetta F, Bernasconi P, et al. Analysis of T cell receptor repertoire of muscle-infiltrating T lymphocytes in polymyositis. Restricted V alpha/beta rearrangements may indicate antigen-driven selection. *J Clin Invest*. 1993;91(6):2880–2886.
108. Greenberg SA, Bradshaw EM, Pinkus JL, et al. Plasma cells in muscle in inclusion body myositis and polymyositis. *Neurology*. 2005;65(11):1782–1787.
109. Leff RL, Love LA, Miller FW, et al. Viruses in idiopathic inflamma-tory myopathies: absence of candidate viral genomes in muscle. *Lancet*. 1992;339(8803):1192–1195.
110. Dalakas MC, Pezeshkpour GH, Gravell M, Sever JL. Polymyositis associated with AIDS retrovirus. *JAMA*. 1986; 256(17):2381–2383.
111. Goebels N, Michaelis D, Engelhardt M, et al. Differential expression of perforin in muscle-infiltrating T cells in polymyositis and dermatomyositis. *J Clin Invest*. 1996;97(12):2905–2910.
112. Amato AA, Griggs RC. Unicorns, dragons, polymyositis, and other mythological beasts. *Neurology*. 2003;61(3):288–289.
113. Greenberg SA, Amato AA. Inflammatory myopathy associated with mixed connective tissue disease and scleroderma renal crisis. *Muscle Nerve*. 2001;24(11):1562–1566.
114. Follansbee WP, Zerbe TR, Medsger TA Jr. Cardiac and skeletal muscle disease in systemic sclerosis (scleroderma): a high risk association. *Am Heart J*. 1993;125(1):194–203.
115. Marguerie C, Bunn CC, Copier J, et al. The clinical and immunogenetic features of patients with autoantibodies to the nucleolar antigen PM-Scl. *Medicine (Baltimore)*. 1992;71(6): 327–336.
116. Ringel RA, Brick JE, Brick JF, Gutmann L, Riggs JE. Muscle involvement in the scleroderma syndromes. *Arch Intern Med*. 1990;150(12):2550–2552.
117. Brouwer R, Vree Egberts WT, Hengstman GJ, et al. Autoantibodies directed to novel components of the PM/Scl complex, the human exosome. *Arthritis Res*. 2002;4(2):134–138.
118. Denko CW, Old JW. Myopathy in the Sicca syndrome (Sjogren's syndrome). *Am J Clin Pathol*. 1969;51(5):631–637.
119. Ponge T, Mussini JM, Ponge A, et al. Primary Gougerot–Sjogren syndrome with necrotizing polymyositis: favorable effect of hydroxychloroquine. *Rev Neurol (Paris)*. 1987;143(2):147–148.
120. Ringel SP, Forstot JZ, Tan EM, Wehling C, Griggs RC, Butcher D. Sjogren's syndrome and polymyositis or dermatomyositis. *Arch Neurol*. 1982;39(3):157–163.
121. Foote RA, Kimbrough SM, Stevens JC. Lupus myositis. *Muscle Nerve*. 1982;5(1):65–68.
122. Goei The HS, Jacobs P, Houben H. Cyclosporine in the treatment of intractable polymyositis. *Arthritis Rheum*. 1985;28 (12):1436–1437.
123. Sharp GC, Irvin WS, Tan EM, Gould RG, Holman HR. Mixed connective tissue disease—an apparently distinct rheumatic disease syndrome associated with a specific antibody to an extractable nuclear antigen (ENA). *Am J Med*. 1972;52(2):148–159.
124. Chou S. Myxovirus-like structures in a case of human chronic polymyositis. *Science*. 1967;158:1453–1455.
125. Yunis EJ, Samaha FJ. Inclusion body myositis. *Lab Invest*. 1971;25(3):240–248.
126. Lotz BP, Engel AG, Nishino H, Stevens JC, Litchy WJ. Inclusion body myositis. Observations in 40 patients. *Brain*. 1989;112(pt 3): 727–747.
127. Cox FM, Titulaer MJ, Sont JK, Wintzen AR, Verschuuren JJ, Badrising UA. A 12-year follow-up in sporadic inclusion body myositis: an end stage with major disabilities. *Brain*. 2011;134(pt 11):3167–3175.
128. Benveniste O, Guiguet M, Freebody J, et al. Long-term observational study of sporadic inclusion body myositis. *Brain*. 2011;134(pt 11):3176–3184.
129. Brady S, Squier W, Hilton-Jones D. Clinical assessment determines the diagnosis of inclusion body myositis independently of pathological features. *J Neurol Neurosurg Psychiatry*. 2013;84(11):1240–1246.
130. Chahin N, Engel AG. Correlation of muscle biopsy, clinical course, and outcome in PM and sporadic IBM. *Neurology*. 2008;70(6):418–424.
131. Rose MR, ENMC IBM Working Group. 188th ENMC international workshop: inclusion body myositis, 2–4 december 2011, Naarden, The Netherlands. *Neuromuscul Disord*. 2013; 23:1044–1055.
132. Lloyd TE, Mammen AL, Amato AA, Weiss MD, Needham M, Greenberg SA. Evaluation and construction of diagnostic criteria for inclusion body myositis. *Neurology*. 2014;83(5):426–433.
133. Darrow DH, Hoffman HT, Barnes GJ, Wiley CA. Management of dysphagia in inclusion body myositis. *Arch Otolaryngol Head Neck Surg*. 1992;118(3):313–317.

134. Verma A, Bradley WG, Adesina AM, Sofferman R, Pendlebury WW. Inclusion body myositis with cricopharyngeus muscle involvement and severe dysphagia. *Muscle Nerve*. 1991;14(5):470–473.
135. Ghosh PS, Laughlin RS, Engel AG. Inclusion-body myositis presenting with facial diplegia. *Muscle Nerve*. 2014;49(2): 287–289.
136. Ma H, McEvoy KM, Milone M. Sporadic inclusion body myositis presenting with severe camptocormia. *J Clin Neurosci* 2013;20(11):1628–1629.
137. Goodman BP, Liewluck T, Crum BA, Spinner RJ. Camptocormia due to inclusion body myositis. *J Clin Neuromuscul Dis*. 2012;14(2):78–81.
138. Danon MJ, Perurena OH, Ronan S, Manaligod JR. Inclusion body myositis associated with systemic sarcoidosis. *Can J Neurol Sci*. 1986;13(4):334–336.
139. Pluk H, van Hoeve BJ, van Dooren SH, et al. Autoantibodies to cytosolic 5′-nucleotidase 1 A in inclusion body myositis. *Ann Neurol*. 2013;73(3):397–407.
140. Larman HB, Salajegheh M, Nazareno R, et al. Cytosolic 5′-nucleotidase 1 A autoimmunity in sporadic inclusion body myositis. *Ann Neurol*. 2013;73(3):408–418.
141. Garlepp MJ, Laing B, Zilko PJ, et al. HLA associations with inclusion body myositis. *Clin Exp Immunol*. 1994;98(1):40–45.
142. Sekul EA, Chow C, Dalakas MC. Magnetic resonance imaging of the forearm as a diagnostic aid in patients with sporadic inclusion body myositis. *Neurology*. 1997;48(4):863–866.
143. Eisen A, Berry K, Gibson G. Inclusion body myositis (IBM): myopathy or neuropathy? *Neurology*. 1983;33(9):1109–1114.
144. Joy JL, Oh SJ, Baysal AI. Electrophysiological spectrum of inclusion body myositis. *Muscle Nerve*. 1990;13(10):949–951.
145. Askanas V, Engel WK, Alvarez RB. Enhanced detection of Congo-red-positive amyloid deposits in muscle fibers of inclusion body myositis and brain of Alzheimer's disease using fluorescence technique. *Neurology*. 1993;43(6):1265–1267.
146. Mendell JR, Sahenk Z, Gales T, Paul L. Amyloid filaments in inclusion body myositis. Novel findings provide insight into nature of filaments. *Arch Neurol*. 1991;48(12):1229–1234.
147. Barohn RJ, Amato AA, Sahenk Z, Kissel JT, Mendell JR. Inclusion body myositis: explanation for poor response to immunosuppressive therapy. *Neurology*. 1995;45(7):1302–1304.
148. Rifai Z, Welle S, Kamp C, Thornton CA. Ragged red fibers in normal aging and inflammatory myopathy. *Ann Neurol*. 1995;37(1):24–29.
149. O'Hanlon TP, Dalakas MC, Plotz PH, Miller FW. The alpha beta T-cell receptor repertoire in inclusion body myositis: diverse patterns of gene expression by muscle-infiltrating lymphocytes. *J Autoimmun*. 1994;7(3):321–333.
150. Amemiya K, Granger RP, Dalakas MC. Clonal restriction of T-cell receptor expression by infiltrating lymphocytes in inclusion body myositis persists over time. Studies in repeated muscle biopsies. *Brain*. 2000;123(pt 10):2030–2039.
151. Ray A, Amato AA, Bradshaw EM, et al. Autoantibodies produced at the site of tissue damage provide evidence of humoral autoimmunity in inclusion body myositis. *PLoS One*. 2012;7(10):e46709.
152. Pruitt JN 2nd, Showalter CJ, Engel AG. Sporadic inclusion body myositis: counts of different types of abnormal fibers. *Ann Neurol*. 1996;39(1):139–143.
153. Askanas V, Engel WK. Proposed pathogenetic cascade of inclusion-body myositis: importance of amyloid-beta, misfolded proteins, predisposing genes, and aging. *Curr Opin Rheumatol*. 2003;15(6):737–744.
154. Greenberg SA, Pinkus JL, Amato AA. Nuclear membrane proteins are present within rimmed vacuoles in inclusion-body myositis. *Muscle Nerve*. 2006;34:406–416.
155. Salajegheh M, Pinkus JL, Taylor JP, et al. Sarcoplasmic redistribution of nuclear TDP-43 in inclusion body myositis. *Muscle Nerve*. 2009;40(1):19–31.
156. Olive M, Janue A, Moreno D, Gamez J, Torrejon-Escribano B, Ferrer I. TAR DNA-binding protein 43 accumulation in protein aggregate myopathies. *J Neuropathol Exp Neurol*. 2009;68(3):262–273.
157. Kusters B, van Hoeve BJ, Schelhaas HJ, Ter Laak H, van Engelen BG, Lammens M. TDP-43 accumulation is common in myopathies with rimmed vacuoles. *Acta Neuropathol*. 2009;117(2):209–211.
158. Hiniker A, Daniels BH, Lee HS, Margeta M. Comparative utility of LC3, p62 and TDP-43 immunohistochemistry in differentiation of inclusion body myositis from polymyositis and related inflammatory myopathies. *Acta Neuropathol Commun*. 2013;1(1):29.
159. Oldfors A, Larsson NG, Lindberg C, Holme E. Mitochondrial DNA deletions in inclusion body myositis. *Brain*. 1993;116 (pt 2):325–336.
160. Yang CC, Alvarez RB, Engel WK, Askanas V. Increase of nitric oxide synthases and nitrotyrosine in inclusion-body myositis. *Neuroreport*. 1996;8(1):153–158.
161. Banwell BL, Engel AG. AlphaB-crystallin immunolocalization yields new insights into inclusion body myositis. *Neurology*. 2000;54(5):1033–1041.
162. Chou SM. Inclusion body myositis: a chronic persistent mumps myositis? *Hum Pathol*. 1986;17(8):765–777.
163. Kallajoki M, Hyypia T, Halonen P, Orvell C, Rima BK, Kalimo H. Inclusion body myositis and paramyxoviruses. *Hum Pathol*. 1991;22(1):29–32.
164. Nishino H, Engel AG, Rima BK. Inclusion body myositis: the mumps virus hypothesis. *Ann Neurol*. 1989;25(3):260–264.
165. Cupler EJ, Leon-Monzon M, Miller J, Semino-Mora C, Anderson TL, Dalakas MC. Inclusion body myositis in HIV-1 and HTLV-1 infected patients. *Brain*. 1996;119(pt 6):1887–1893.
166. Semino-Mora C, Dalakas MC. Rimmed vacuoles with beta-amyloid and ubiquitinated filamentous deposits in the muscles of patients with long-standing denervation (postpoliomyelitis muscular atrophy): similarities with inclusion body myositis. *Hum Pathol*. 1998;29(10):1128–1133.
167. Watts GD, Wymer J, Kovach MJ, et al. Inclusion body myopathy associated with Paget disease of bone and frontotemporal dementia is caused by mutant valosin-containing protein. *Nat Genet*. 2004;36(4):377–381.
168. Bronner IM, Hoogendijk JE, Wintzen AR, et al. Necrotising myopathy, an unusual presentation of a steroid-responsive myopathy. *J Neurol*. 2003;250(4):480–485.
169. Emslie-Smith AM, Engel AG. Necrotizing myopathy with pipestem capillaries, microvascular deposition of the complement membrane attack complex (MAC), and minimal cellular infiltration. *Neurology*. 1991;41(6):936–939.
170. Levin MI, Mozaffar T, Al-Lozi MT, Pestronk A. Paraneoplastic necrotizing myopathy: clinical and pathological features. *Neurology*. 1998;50(3):764–767.
171. Vosskamper M, Korf B, Franke F, Schachenmayr W. Paraneoplastic necrotizing myopathy: a rare disorder to be differentiated from polymyositis. *J Neurol*. 1989;236(8):489–490.

172. Hengstman GJ, ter Laak HJ, Vree Egberts WT, et al. Anti-signal recognition particle autoantibodies: marker of a necrotising myopathy. *Ann Rheum Dis.* 2006;65(12):1635–1638.
173. Needham M, Fabian V, Knezevic W, Panegyres P, Zilko P, Mastaglia FL. Progressive myopathy with up-regulation of MHC-I associated with statin therapy. *Neuromuscul Disord.* 2007;17(2):194–200.
174. Grable-Esposito P, Katzberg HD, Greenberg SA, Srinivasan J, Katz J, Amato AA. Immune-mediated necrotizing myopathy associated with statins. *Muscle Nerve.* 2010;41(2):185–190.
175. Mammen AL, Amato AA. Statin myopathy: a review of recent progress. *Curr Opin Rheumatol.* 2010;22(6):644–650.
176. Christopher-Stine L, Casciola-Rosen LA, Hong G, Chung T, Corse AM, Mammen AL. A novel autoantibody recognizing 200-kd and 100-kd proteins is associated with an immune-mediated necrotizing myopathy. *Arthritis Rheum.* 2010;62:2757–2766.
177. Mammen AL, Chung T, Christopher-Stine L,et al. Autoantibodies against 3-hydroxy-3-methylglutaryl-coenzyme A reductase in patients with statin-associated autoimmune myopathy. *Arthritis Rheum.* 2011;63(3):713–721.
178. Mammen AL, Pak K, Williams EK, et al. Rarity of anti-3-hydroxy-3-methylglutaryl-coenzyme A reductase antibodies in statin users, including those with self-limited musculoskeletal side effects. *Arthritis Care Res (Hoboken).* 2012;64(2):269–272.
179. Werner J, Christopher-Stine L, Ghazarian SR, et al. Antibody levels correlate with creatine kinase levels and strength in anti-HMG-CoA reductase-associated autoimmune myopathy. *Arthritis Rheum.* 2012;64(12):4087–4093.
180. Kobayashi Y, Fujimoto T, Shiiki H, Kitaoka K, Murata K, Dohi K. Focal eosinophilic myositis. *Clin Rheumatol.* 2001; 20(5):369–371.
181. Layzer RB, Shearn MA, Satya-Murti S. Eosinophilic polymyositis. *Ann Neurol.* 1977;1(1):65–71.
182. Moore PM, Harley JB, Fauci AS. Neurologic dysfunction in the idiopathic hypereosinophilic syndrome. *Ann Intern Med.* 1985;102(1):109–114.
183. Murata K, Sugie K, Takamure M, Fujimoto T, Ueno S. Eosinophilic major basic protein and interleukin-5 in eosinophilic myositis. *Eur J Neurol.* 2003;10(1):35–38.
184. Serratrice G, Pellissier JF, Cros D, Gastaut JL, Brindisi G. Relapsing eosinophilic perimyositis. *J Rheumatol.* 1980;7(2):199–205.
185. Serratrice G, Pellissier JF, Roux H, Quilichini P. Fasciitis, perimyositis, myositis, polymyositis, and eosinophilia. *Muscle Nerve.* 1990;13(5):385–395.
186. Dunand M, Lobrinus JA, Spertini O, Kuntzer T. Eosinophilic perimyositis as the presenting feature of a monoclonal T-cell expansion. *Muscle Nerve.* 2005;31(5):646–651.
187. Simon HU, Plotz SG, Simon D, Dummer R, Blaser K. Clinical and immunological features of patients with interleukin-5-producing T cell clones and eosinophilia. *Int Arch Allergy Immunol.* 2001;124(1-3):242–245.
188. Amato AA. Adults with eosinophilic myositis and calpain-3 mutations. *Neurology.* 2008;70(9):730–731.
189. Lakhanpal S, Ginsburg WW, Michet CJ, Doyle JA, Moore SB. Eosinophilic fasciitis: clinical spectrum and therapeutic response in 52 cases. *Semin Arthritis Rheum.* 1988;17(4):221–231.
190. Shulman LE. Diffuse fasciitis with eosinophilia: a new syndrome? *Trans Assoc Am Physicians.* 1975;88:70–86.
191. Hertzman PA, Blevins WL, Mayer J, Greenfield B, Ting M, Gleich GJ. Association of the eosinophilia-myalgia syndrome with the ingestion of tryptophan. *N Engl J Med.* 1990;322(13):869–873.
192. Kilbourne EM, Rigau-Perez JG, Heath CW Jr, et al. Clinical epidemiology of toxic-oil syndrome. Manifestations of a new illness. *N Engl J Med.* 1983;309(23):1408–1414.
193. Namba T, Brunner NG, Grob D. Idiopathic giant cell polymyositis. Report of a case and review of the syndrome. *Arch Neurol.* 1974;31(1):27–30.
194. Pascuzzi RM, Roos KL, Phillips LH 2nd. Granulomatous inflammatory myopathy associated with myasthenia gravis. A case report and review of the literature. *Arch Neurol.* 1986;43(6):621–623.
195. Mozaffar T, Lopate G, Pestronk A. Clinical correlates of granulomas in muscle. *J Neurol.* 1998;245(8):519–524.
196. Silverstein A, Siltzbach LE. Muscle involvement in sarcoidosis. Asymptomatic, myositis, and myopathy. *Arch Neurol.* 1969; 21(3):235–241.
197. Stjernberg N, Cajander S, Truedsson H, Uddenfeldt P. Muscle involvement in sarcoidosis. *Acta Med Scand.* 1981;209(3): 213–216.
198. Afifi AK, Frayha RA, Bahuth NB, Tekian A. The myopathology of Behcet's disease—a histochemical, light-, and electron-microscopic study. *J Neurol Sci.* 1980;48(3):333–342.
199. Di Giacomo V, Carmenini G, Meloni F, Valesini G. Myositis in Behcet's disease. *Arthritis Rheum.* 1982;25(8):1025.
200. Finucane P, Doyle CT, Ferriss JB, Molloy M, Murnaghan D. Behcet's syndrome with myositis and glomerulonephritis. *Br J Rheumatol.* 1985;24(4):372–375.
201. Lingenfelser T, Duerk H, Stevens A, Grossmann T, Knorr M, Saal JG. Generalized myositis in Behcet disease: treatment with cyclosporine. *Ann Intern Med.* 1992;116(8):651–653.
202. Worthmann F, Bruns J, Türker T, Gosztonyi G. Muscular involvement in Behcet's disease: case report and review of the literature. *Neuromuscul Disord.* 1996;6(4):247–253.
203. Caldwell CJ, Swash M, Van der Walt JD, Geddes JF. Focal myositis: a clinico-pathological study. *Neuromuscul Disord.* 1995;5(4):317–321.
204. Colding-Jorgensen E, Laursen H, Lauritzen M. Focal myositis of the thigh: report of two cases. *Acta Neurol Scand.* 1993;88(4):289–292.
205. Heffner RR Jr, Barron SA. Polymyositis beginning as a focal process. *Arch Neurol.* 1981;38(7):439–442.
206. Moreno-Lugris C, Gonzalez-Gay MA, Sanchez-Andrade A, et al. Magnetic resonance imaging: a useful technique in the diagnosis and follow up of focal myositis. *Ann Rheum Dis.* 1996;55(11):856.
207. Moskovic E, Fisher C, Westbury G, Parsons C. Focal myositis, a benign inflammatory pseudotumour: CT appearances. *Br J Radiol.* 1991;64(762):489–493.
208. Illa I, Nath A, Dalakas M. Immunocytochemical and virological characteristics of HIV-associated inflammatory myopathies: similarities with seronegative polymyositis. *Ann Neurol.* 1991;29(5):474–481.
209. Callens S, De Roo A, Colebunders R. Fanconi-like syndrome and rhabdomyolysis in a person with HIV infection on highly active antiretroviral treatment including tenofovir. *J Infect.* 2003;47(3):262–263.
210. Mahe A, Bruet A, Chabin E, Fendler JP. Acute rhabdomyolysis coincident with primary HIV-1 infection. *Lancet.* 1989; 2(8677):1454–1455.
211. McDonagh CA, Holman RP. Primary human immunodeficiency virus type 1 infection in a patient with acute rhabdomyolysis. *South Med J.* 2003;96(10):1027–1030.

212. Rastegar D, Claiborne C, Fleisher A, Matsumoto A. A patient with primary human immunodeficiency virus infection who presented with acute rhabdomyolysis. *Clin Infect Dis*. 2001;32(3):502–504.
213. Arnaudo E, Dalakas M, Shanske S, Moraes CT, DiMauro S, Schon EA. Depletion of muscle mitochondrial DNA in AIDS patients with zidovudine-induced myopathy. *Lancet*. 1991;337(8740):508–510.
214. Cupler EJ, Danon MJ, Jay C, Hench K, Ropka M, Dalakas MC. Early features of zidovudine-associated myopathy: histopathological findings and clinical correlations. *Acta Neuropathol (Berl)*. 1995;90(1):1–6.
215. Dalakas M. HIV or zidovudine myopathy? *Neurology*. 1994; 44(2):360–361; author reply 362–364.
216. Dalakas MC, Pezeshkpour GH, Flaherty M. Progressive nemaline (rod) myopathy associated with HIV infection. *N Engl J Med*. 1987;317(25):1602–1603.
217. Pezeshkpour G, Illa I, Dalakas MC. Ultrastructural characteristics and DNA immunocytochemistry in human immunodeficiency virus and zidovudine-associated myopathies. *Hum Pathol*. 1991;22(12):1281–1288.
218. Caldwell CJ, Barrett WY, Breuer J, Farmer SF, Swash M. HTLV-1 polymyositis. *Neuromuscul Disord*. 1996;6(3):151–154.
219. Evans BK, Gore I, Harrell LE, Arnold T, Oh SJ. HTLV-I-associated myelopathy and polymyositis in a US native. *Neurology*. 1989;39(12):1572–1575.
220. Morgan OS, Rodgers-Johnson P, Mora C, Char G. HTLV-1 and polymyositis in Jamaica. *Lancet*. 1989;2(8673):1184–1187.
221. Mejlszenkier JD, Safran AP, Healy JJ, Embree L, Ouellette EM. The myositis of influenza. *Arch Neurol*. 1973;29(6):441–443.
222. Middleton PJ, Alexander RM, Szymanski MT. Severe myositis during recovery from influenza. *Lancet*. 1970;2(7672):533–535.
223. Minow RA, Gorbach S, Johnson BL Jr, Dornfeld L. Myoglobinuria associated with influenza A infection. *Ann Intern Med*. 1974;80(3):359–361.
224. Morgensen JL. Myoglobinuria and renal failure associated with influenza. *Ann Intern Med*. 1974;80(3):362–363.
225. Ruff RL, Secrist D. Viral studies in benign acute childhood myositis. *Arch Neurol*. 1982;39(5):261–263.
226. Christenson JC, San Joaquin VH. Influenza-associated rhabdomyolysis in a child. *Pediatr Infect Dis J*. 1990;9(1):60–61.
227. Farrell MK, Partin JC, Bove KE. Epidemic influenza myopathy in Cincinnati in 1977. *J Pediatr*. 1980;96(3 pt 2):545–551.
228. Gamboa ET, Eastwood AB, Hays AP, Maxwell J, Penn AS. Isolation of influenza virus from muscle in myoglobinuric polymyositis. *Neurology*. 1979;29(10):1323–1335.
229. Antony SJ, Kernodle DS. Nontropical pyomyositis in patients with AIDS. *J Natl Med Assoc*. 1996;88(9):565–569.
230. Rodgers WB, Yodlowski ML, Mintzer CM. Pyomyositis in patients who have the human immunodeficiency virus. Case report and review of the literature. *J Bone Joint Surg Am*. 1993;75(4):588–592.
231. Hsueh PR, Hsiue TR, Hsieh WC. Pyomyositis in intravenous drug abusers: report of a unique case and review of the literature. *Clin Infect Dis*. 1996;22(5):858–860.
232. Chiedozi LC. Pyomyositis. Review of 205 cases in 112 patients. *Am J Surg*. 1979;137(2):255–259.
233. Akman I, Ostrov B, Varma BK, Keenan G. Pyomyositis: report of three patients and review of the literature. *Clin Pediatr (Phila)*. 1996;35(8):397–401.
234. O'Neill DS, Baquis G, Moral L. Infectious myositis. A tropical disease steals out of its zone. *Postgrad Med*. 1996;100(2): 193–194, 199–200.
235. Atlas E, Novak SN, Duray PH, Steere AC. Lyme myositis: muscle invasion by Borrelia burgdorferi. *Ann Intern Med*. 1988;109(3):245–246.
236. Horowitz HW, Sanghera K, Goldberg N, et al. Dermatomyositis associated with Lyme disease: case report and review of Lyme myositis. *Clin Infect Dis*. 1994;18(2):166–171.
237. Jeandel C, Perret C, Blain H, Jouanny P, Penin F, Laurain MC. Rhabdomyolysis with acute renal failure due to Borrelia burgdorferi. *J Intern Med*. 1994;235(2):191–192.
238. Muller-Felber W, Reimers CD, de Koning J, Fischer P, Pilz A, Pongratz DE. Myositis in Lyme borreliosis: an immunohistochemical study of seven patients. *J Neurol Sci*. 1993;118(2):207–212.
239. Reimers CD, de Koning J, Neubert U, et al. Borrelia burgdorferi myositis: report of eight patients. *J Neurol*. 1993;240(5):278–283.
240. Schmutzhard E, Willeit J, Gerstenbrand F. Meningopolyneuritis Bannwarth with focal nodular myositis. A new aspect in Lyme borreliosis. *Klin Wochenschr*. 1986;64(22):1204–1208.
241. Arena FP, Perlin M, Brahman H, Weiser B, Armstrong D. Fever, rash, and myalgias of disseminated candidiasis during antifungal therapy. *Arch Intern Med*. 1981;141(9):1233.
242. Jarowski CI, Fialk MA, Murray HW, et al. Fever, rash, and muscle tenderness. A distinctive clinical presentation of disseminated candidiasis. *Arch Intern Med*. 1978;138(4):544–546.
243. Halverson PB, Lahiri S, Wojno WC, Sulaiman AR. Sporotrichal arthritis presenting as granulomatous myositis. *Arthritis Rheum*. 1985;28(12):1425–1429.
244. Wrzolek MA, Sher JH, Kozlowski PB, Rao C. Skeletal muscle pathology in AIDS: an autopsy study. *Muscle Nerve*. 1990; 13(6):508–515.
245. Davis MJ, Cilo M, Plaitakis A, Yahr MD. Trichinosis: severe myopathic involvement with recovery. *Neurology*. 1976; 26(1):37–40.
246. Gross B, Ochoa J. Trichinosis: clinical report and histochemistry of muscle. *Muscle Nerve*. 1979;2(5):394–398.
247. Jacob JC, Mathew NT. Pseudohypertrophic myopathy in cysticercosis. *Neurology*. 1968;18(8):767–771.
248. Sawhney BB, Chopra JS, Banerji AK, Wahi PL. Pseudohypertrophic myopathy in cysticerosis. *Neurology*. 1976;26(3):270–272.
249. Gherardi R, Baudrimont M, Lionnet F, et al. Skeletal muscle toxoplasmosis in patients with acquired immunodeficiency syndrome: a clinical and pathological study. *Ann Neurol*. 1992;32(4):535–542.
250. Pollock JL. Toxoplasmosis appearing to be dermatomyositis. *Arch Dermatol*. 1979;115(6):736–737.
251. Rowland LP, Greer M. Toxoplasmic polymyositis. *Neurology*. 1961;11:367–370.
252. Bunch TW, Worthington JW, Combs JJ, Ilstrup DM, Engel AG. Azathioprine with prednisone for polymyositis. A controlled, clinical trial. *Ann Intern Med*. 1980;92(3):365–369.
253. Oddis CV, Reed AM, Aggarwal R, et al. Rituximab in the treatment of refractory adult and juvenile dermatomyositis and adult polymyositis: a randomized, placebo-phase trial. *Arthritis Rheum*. 2013;65:314–324.
254. Muscle Study Group. A randomized, pilot trial of etanercept in dermatomyositis. *Ann Neurol*. 2011;70(3):427–436.
255. Dalakas MC, Illa I, Dambrosia JM, et al. A controlled trial of high-dose intravenous immune globulin infusions as treatment for dermatomyositis. *N Engl J Med*. 1993;329(27):1993–2000.
256. Badrising UA, Maat-Schieman ML, Ferrari MD, et al. Comparison of weakness progression in inclusion body myositis during treatment with methotrexate or placebo. *Ann Neurol*. 2002;51(3):369–372.

257. Dalakas MC, Koffman B, Fujii M, et al. A controlled study of intravenous immunoglobulin combined with prednisone in the treatment of IBM. *Neurology*. 2001;56(3):323–327.
258. Dalakas MC, Sonies B, Dambrosia J, Sekul E, Cupler E, Sivakumar K. Treatment of inclusion-body myositis with IVIG: a double-blind, placebo-controlled study. *Neurology*. 1997;48(3):712–716.
259. Muscle Study Group. A randomized trial of ßINF1 a (Avonex) in patients with inclusion body myositis (IBM). *Neurology*. 2001;57:1566–1570.
260. Muscle Study Group. Randomized pilot trial of high dose ßINF1 a in patients with inclusion body myositis. *Neurology*. 2004;63:718–720.
261. Gordon PA, Winer JB, Hoogendijk JE, Choy EH. Immunosuppressant and immunomodulatory treatment for dermatomyositis and polymyositis. *Cochrane Database Syst Rev*. 2012;8:CD003643.
262. Amato AA, Barohn RJ, Jackson CE, Pappert EJ, Sahenk Z, Kissel JT. Inclusion body myositis: treatment with intravenous immunoglobulin. *Neurology*. 1994;44(8):1516–1518.
263. Leff RL, Miller FW, Hicks J, Fraser DD, Plotz PH. The treatment of inclusion body myositis: a retrospective review and a randomized, prospective trial of immunosuppressive therapy. *Medicine (Baltimore)*. 1993;72(4):225–235.
264. Oddis CV. Idiopathic inflammatory myopathies: a treatment update. *Curr Rheumatol Rep*. 2003;5(6):431–436.
265. Uchino M, Araki S, Yoshida O, Uekawa K, Nagata J. High single-dose alternate-day corticosteroid regimens in treatment of polymyositis. *J Neurol*. 1985;232(3):175–178.
266. Uchino M, Yamashita S, Uchino K, et al. Long-term outcome of polymyositis treated with high single-dose alternate-day prednisolone therapy. *Eur Neurol*. 2012;68(2):117–21.
267. van de Vlekkert J, Hoogendijk JE, de Haan RJ, et al. Oral dexamethasone pulse therapy versus daily prednisolone in subacute onset myositis, a randomised clinical trial. *Neuromuscul Disord*. 2010;20(6):382–389.
268. Wang DX, Shu XM, Tian XL, et al. Intravenous immunoglobulin therapy in adult patients with polymyositis/dermatomyositis: a systematic literature review. *Clin Rheumatol*. 2012;31(5):801–806.
269. Patwa HS, Chaudhry V, Katzberg H, Rae-Grant AD, So YT. Evidence-based guideline: intravenous immunoglobulin in the treatment of neuromuscular disorders: report of the Therapeutics and Technology Assessment Subcommittee of the American Academy of Neurology. *Neurology*. 2012;78(13):1009–1015.
270. Kissel JT, Levy RJ, Mendell JR, Griggs RC. Azathioprine toxicity in neuro-muscular disease. *Neurology*. 1986;36(1):35–39.
271. Soueidan SA, Dalakas MC. Treatment of inclusion-body myositis with high-dose intravenous immunoglobulin. *Neurology*. 1993;43(5):876–879.
272. Cagnoli M, Marchesoni A, Tosi S. Combined steroid, methotrexate and chlorambucil therapy for steroid-resistant dermatomyositis. *Clin Exp Rheumatol*. 1991;9(6):658–659.
273. Giannini M, Callen JP. Treatment of dermatomyositis with methotrexate and prednisone. *Arch Dermatol*. 1979;115(10):1251–1252.
274. Metzger AL, Bohan A, Goldberg LS, Bluestone R, Pearson CM. Polymyositis and dermatomyositis: combined methotrexate and corticosteroid therapy. *Ann Intern Med*. 1974;81(2):182–189.
275. Sokoloff MC, Goldberg LS, Pearson CM. Treatment of corticosteroid-resistant polymyositis with methotrexate. *Lancet*. 1971;1(7688):14–16.
276. Miller LC, Sisson BA, Tucker LB, DeNardo BA, Schaller JG. Methotrexate treatment of recalcitrant childhood dermatomyositis. *Arthritis Rheum*. 1992;35(10):1143–1149.
277. Bunch TW. Prednisone and azathioprine for polymyositis: long-term followup. *Arthritis Rheum*. 1981;24(1):45–48.
278. Rowin J, Amato AA, Deisher N, Cursio J, Meriggioli MN. Mycophenolate mofetil in dermatomyositis: is it safe? *Neurology*. 2006;66(8):1245–1247.
279. Schneider C, Gold R, Schafers M, Toyka K. Mycophenolate mofetil in the therapy of polymyositis associated with a polyautoimmune syndrome. *Muscle Nerve*. 2002;25(2):286–288.
280. Majithia V, Harisdangkul V. Mycophenolate mofetil (Cellcept): an alternative therapy for autoimmune inflammatory myopathy. *Rheumatology*. 2005;44(3):386–389.
281. Tausche AK, Meurer M. Mycophenolate mofetil for dermatomyositis. *Dermatology*. 2001;202:341–343.
282. Levine TD. Rituximab in the treatment of dermatomyositis: an open-label pilot study. *Arthritis Rheum*. 2005;52(2):601–607.
283. Mok CC, Ho LY, To CH. Rituximab for refractory polymyositis: an open-label prospective study. *J Rheumatol* 2007;34(9):1864–1868.
284. Valiyil R, Casciola-Rosen L, Hong G, Mammen A, Christopher-Stine L. Rituximab therapy for myopathy associated with anti-signal recognition particle antibodies: a case series. *Arthritis Care Res (Hoboken)*. 2010;62(9):1328–1334.
285. Mahler EA, Blom M, Voermans NC, van Engelen BG, van Riel PL, Vonk MC. Rituximab treatment in patients with refractory inflammatory myopathies. *Rheumatology*. 2011;50(12):2206–2213.
286. Aggarwal R, Bandos A, Reed AM, et al. Predictors of clinical improvement in rituximab-treated refractory adult and juvenile dermatomyositis and adult polymyositis. *Arthritis Rheum*. 2013;66(3):740–749. doi: 10.1002/art.38270.
287. Bombardieri S, Hughes GR, Neri R, Del Bravo P, Del Bono L. Cyclophosphamide in severe polymyositis. *Lancet*. 1989;1(8647):1138–1139.
288. Haga HJ, D'Cruz D, Asherson R, Hughes GR. Short term effects of intravenous pulses of cyclophosphamide in the treatment of connective tissue disease crisis. *Ann Rheum Dis*. 1992;51(7):885–888.
289. Kono DH, Klashman DJ, Gilbert RC. Successful IV pulse cyclophosphamide in refractory PM in 3 patients with SLE. *J Rheumatol*. 1990;17(7):982–983.
290. Leroy JP, Drosos AA, Yiannopoulos DI, Youinou P, Moutsopoulos HM. Intravenous pulse cyclophosphamide therapy in myositis and Sjogren's syndrome. *Arthritis Rheum*. 1990;33(10):1579–1581.
291. Niakan E, Pitner SE, Whitaker JN, Bertorini TE. Immunosuppressive agents in corticosteroid-refractory childhood dermatomyositis. *Neurology*. 1980;30(3):286–291.
292. Cronin ME, Miller FW, Hicks JE, Dalakas M, Plotz PH. The failure of intravenous cyclophosphamide therapy in refractory idiopathic inflammatory myopathy. *J Rheumatol*. 1989;16(9):1225–1228.
293. Fries JF, Sharp GC, McDevitt HO, Holman HR. Cyclophosphamide therapy in systemic lupus erythematosus and polymyositis. *Arthritis Rheum*. 1973;16(2):154–162.

294. Sinoway PA, Callen JP. Chlorambucil. An effective corticosteroid-sparing agent for patients with recalcitrant dermatomyositis. *Arthritis Rheum*. 1993;36(3):319–324.
295. Wallace DJ, Metzger AL, White KK. Combination immunosuppressive treatment of steroid-resistant dermatomyositis/polymyositis. *Arthritis Rheum*. 1985;28(5):590–592.
296. Borleffs JC. Cyclosporine as monotherapy for polymyositis? *Transplant Proc*. 1988;20(3 suppl 4):333–334.
297. Correia O, Polonia J, Nunes JP, Resende C, Delgado L. Severe acute form of adult dermatomyositis treated with cyclosporine. *Int J Dermatol*. 1992;31(7):517–519.
298. Girardin E, Dayer JM, Paunier L. Cyclosporine for juvenile dermatomyositis. *J Pediatr*. 1988;112(1):165–166.
299. Heckmatt J, Hasson N, Saunders C, et al. Cyclosporin in juvenile dermatomyositis. *Lancet*. 1989;1(8646):1063–1066.
300. Jones DW, Snaith ML, Isenberg DA. Cyclosporine treatment for intractable polymyositis. *Arthritis Rheum*. 1987;30(8): 959–960.
301. Lueck CJ, Trend P, Swash M. Cyclosporin in the management of polymyositis and dermatomyositis. *J Neurol Neurosurg Psychiatry*. 1991;54(11):1007–1008.
302. Mehregan DR, Su WP. Cyclosporine treatment for dermatomyositis/polymyositis. *Cutis*. 1993;51(1):59–61.
303. Pistoia V, Buoncompagni A, Scribanis R, et al. Cyclosporin A in the treatment of juvenile chronic arthritis and childhood polymyositis-dermatomyositis. Results of a preliminary study. *Clin Exp Rheumatol*. 1993;11(2):203–208.
304. Oddis CV, Sciurba FC, Elmagd KA, Starzl TE. Tacrolimus in refractory polymyositis with interstitial lung disease. *Lancet*. 1999;353(9166):1762–1763.
305. Hengstman GJ, van den Hoogen FH, Barrera P, et al. Successful treatment of dermatomyositis and polymyositis with anti-tumor-necrosis-factor-alpha: preliminary observations. *Eur Neurol*. 2003;50(1):10–15.
306. Hengstman GJ, van den Hoogen FH, van Engelen BG. Treatment of dermatomyositis and polymyositis with anti-tumor necrosis factor-alpha: long-term follow-up. *Eur Neurol*. 2004;52(1):61–63.
307. Efthimiou P, Schwartzman S, Kagen LJ. Possible role for tumour necrosis factor inhibitors in the treatment of resistant dermatomyositis and polymyositis: a retrospective study of eight patients. *Ann Rheum Dis*. 2006;65(9):1233–1236.
308. Riley P, McCann LJ, Maillard SM, Woo P, Murray KJ, Pilkington CA. Effectiveness of infliximab in the treatment of refractory juvenile dermatomyositis with calcinosis. *Rheumatology (Oxford)*. 2008;47(6):877–880.
309. Korkmaz C, Temiz G, Cetinbas F, Büyükkidan B. Successful treatment of alveolar hypoventilation due to dermatomyositis with anti-tumour necrosis factor-alpha. *Rheumatology (Oxford)*. 2004;43(7):937–938.
310. Labioche I, Liozon E, Weschler B, Loustaud-Ratti V, Soria P, Vidal E. Refractory polymyositis responding to infliximab: extended follow-up. *Rheumatology (Oxford)*. 2004;43(4):531–532.
311. Sprott H, Glatzel M, Michel BA. Treatment of myositis with etanercept (Enbrel), a recombinant human soluble fusion protein of TNF-alpha type II receptor and IgG1. *Rheumatology (Oxford)*. 2004;43(4):524–526.
312. Dastmalchi M, Grundtman C, Alexanderson H, et al. A high incidence of disease flares in an open pilot study of infliximab in patients with refractory inflammatory myopathies. *Ann Rheum Dis*. 2008;67(12):1670–1677.
313. Hengstman GJ, De Bleecker JL, Feist E, et al. Open-label trial of anti-TNF-alpha in dermato- and polymyositis treated concomitantly with methotrexate. *Eur Neurol*. 2008;59:159–163.
314. Klein R, Rosenbach M, Kim EJ, Kim B, Werth VP, Dunham J. Tumor necrosis factor inhibitor-associated dermatomyositis. *Arch Dermatol*. 2010;146:780–784.
315. Iannone F, Scioscia C, Falappone PC, Covelli M, Lapadula G. Use of etanercept in the treatment of dermatomyositis: a case series. *J Rheumatol*. 2006;33(9):1802–1804.
316. Brewer EJ Jr, Giannini EH, Rossen RD, Patten B, Barkley E. Plasma exchange therapy of a childhood onset dermatomyositis patient. *Arthritis Rheum*. 1980;23(4):509–513.
317. Dau PC. Plasmapheresis in idiopathic inflammatory myopathy. Experience with 35 patients. *Arch Neurol*. 1981;38(9):544–552.
318. Herson S, Cherin P, Coutellier A. The association of plasma exchange synchronized with intravenous gamma globulin therapy in severe intractable polymyositis. *J Rheumatol*. 1992;19(5):828–829.
319. Miller FW, Leitman SF, Cronin ME, et al. Controlled trial of plasma exchange and leukopheresis in polymyositis and dermatomyositis. *N Engl J Med*. 1992;326(21):1380–1384.
320. Hubbard WN, Walport MJ, Halnan KE, Beaney RP, Hughes GR. Remission from polymyositis after total body irradiation. *Br Med J (Clin Res Ed)*. 1982;284(6333):1915–1916.
321. Kelly JJ, Madoc-Jones H, Adelman LS, Andres PL, Munsat TL. Response to total body irradiation in dermatomyositis. *Muscle Nerve*. 1988;11(2):120–123.
322. Morgan SH, Bernstein RM, Coppen J, Halnan KE, Hughes GR. Total body irradiation and the course of polymyositis. *Arthritis Rheum*. 1985;28(7):831–835.
323. Cherin P, Herson S, Coutellier A, Bletry O, Piette JC. Failure of total body irradiation in polymyositis: report of three cases. *Br J Rheumatol*. 1992;31(4):282–283.
324. Kelly JJ Jr, Madoc-Jones H, Adelman LS, Andres PL, Munsat TL. Total body irradiation not effective in inclusion body myositis. *Neurology*. 1986;36(9):1264–1266.
325. Cumming WJ. Thymectomy in refractory dermatomyositis. *Muscle Nerve*. 1989;12(5):424.

CHAPTER 34

Myopathies Associated with Systemic Disease

Myopathies can occur in the setting of a variety of systemic diseases. Previous chapters have discussed inflammatory myopathies that can occur in the setting of connective tissue diseases (e.g., systemic lupus erythematosus, mixed connective tissue disease, Sjögren syndrome, and rheumatoid arthritis) and systemic infections (e.g., HIV). Myopathies occurring as complications of medications (toxic myopathies) are also dealt with elsewhere in the book. In this chapter, we will focus on myopathies related to endocrine disturbances, electrolyte imbalance, nutritional deficiency, and amyloidosis. We also discuss some other less well-defined syndromes such as fibromyalgia.

► ENDOCRINE MYOPATHIES

Myopathies can complicate various endocrinopathies.[1,2] In this section, we review myopathies associated with thyroid, parathyroid, adrenal, pituitary, and pancreatic disorders.

THYROID DISORDERS

Both hyperthyroidism and hypothyroidism can be associated with myopathy. In addition, polyneuropathy and neuromuscular junction disorders can occur with dysthyroid states and these need to be differentiated from one another.

THYROTOXIC MYOPATHY

Clinical Features

The mean age of onset of thyrotoxicosis is in the fifth decade. The severity of the myopathy does not necessarily relate to the severity of the thyrotoxicosis. Muscle symptoms usually appear several months after the onset of other clinical symptoms associated with mild hyperthyroidism.[3] Interestingly, thyrotoxicosis is more common in females; however, thyrotoxic myopathy occurs more commonly in men. Anywhere from 61% to 82% of patients with thyrotoxicosis have some degree of detectable weakness on examination, but only about 5% of patients with thyrotoxicosis present with muscle weakness as their chief complaint.[1,3–5]

Thyrotoxic myopathy is characterized by proximal muscle weakness and atrophy.[2–4,6,7] Some individuals have severe shoulder-girdle atrophy and scapular winging.[2] Distal extremity weakness can be the predominant feature in approximately 20% of patients.[4] Myalgias and fatigue are common. Some patients develop dysphagia, dysphonia, and respiratory distress due to involvement of bulbar, esophageal–pharyngeal muscles, and ventilatory muscles.[8,9] Weakness of extraocular muscles and proptosis occur in the setting of Graves' disease but the sphincters are spared in hyperthyroidism. Rarely, rhabdomyolysis with myoglobinuria can develop in severe thyrotoxicosis.[10]

Muscle stretch tendon reflexes are often brisk. In addition, fasciculations and myokymia are occasionally seen which probably reflects thyrotoxicosis-induced irritability of anterior horn cells or peripheral nerves.[11–13] Peripheral neuropathy in hyperthyroidism is quite rare, but a demyelinating polyneuropathy has been reported.[11]

Other manifestations of hyperthyroidism include nervousness, anxiety, psychosis, tremor, increased perspiration, heat intolerance, palpitations, insomnia, diarrhea, increased appetite, and weight loss. Common signs include goiter, tachycardia, atrial fibrillation, widened pulse pressure, as well as warm, thin, and moist skin.

Myasthenia gravis can develop in association with Graves' disease. It can be a challenge distinguishing which neuromuscular symptoms are related to Graves' disease or to myasthenia gravis. Muscle weakness associated with hyperthyroidism does not fluctuate or significantly improve with anticholinesterase medications.

Thyrotoxicosis is also associated with an unusual form of hypokalemic periodic paralysis. Thyrotoxic periodic paralysis (TPP) may occur sporadically, although a dominantly inherited mutation in a potassium channel has been recently identified in some patients. TPP has been commonly reported in Asians, but it is not restricted to this population.[2,5] TPP is also more common in males. The attacks of weakness are similar in onset, frequency, duration, and pattern to familial hypokalemic periodic paralysis (Chapter 32). The one distinguishing feature is that familial hypokalemic periodic paralysis typically has its onset within the first three decades of life, while the onset of TPP usually develops later in adult life. Serum potassium levels tend to be low during the attacks of weakness, but levels can be normal. Muscle strength returns with treatment and normalization of thyroid function. β-adrenergic blocking agents also improve the myopathy.

Laboratory Features

Serum creatine kinase (CK) levels are usually normal in hyperthyroidism and can even be on the low side. Thyroid stimulating hormone (TSH) level is low in primary hyperthyroidism, while the thyroxine (T4) level and, occasionally, only the triiodothyronine (T3) level are elevated. In TTP serum potassium levels also are usually decreased. Routine motor and sensory nerve conduction studies (NCS) are normal.[12,16] Electromyography (EMG) is usually normal, although fasciculation potentials and MUAP multiplets may be evident due to motor nerve hyperactivity.

Histopathology

Routine muscle biopsies are usually unremarkable, however, mild fatty infiltration, muscle fiber atrophy (types 1 and 2), variability in muscle fiber size, scattered isolated necrotic fibers, decreased glycogen, and increased internal nuclei can be noted.[12,14–16] Nonspecific ultrastructural findings on electron microscopy (EM) may be seen including Z-band streaming, focal swelling of the T tubules, elongated mitochondria, decreased mitochondria, and subsarcolemmal glycogen deposition.[17]

In patients with TPP, muscle biopsies can reveal changes similar to that seen in familial hypokalemic periodic paralysis: Vacuoles may be appreciated, on routine light microscopy, while subsarcolemmal blebs filled with glycogen and dilated terminal cisternae of the sarcoplasmic reticulum might be apparent on EM.

Pathogenesis

The thyroid gland produces T4 that is converted to the more active T3 hormone in the periphery. These thyroid hormones are largely bound to plasma proteins. Free thyroid hormones bind to cytoplasmic receptors on target cells and are internalized into the nucleus, where they regulate the transcription of specific genes. Type 1 muscle fibers have a greater density of these thyroid receptors than do type 2 fibers.[18]

The pathogenic basis of thyrotoxic myopathy is unknown but is thought to be due to enhanced muscle catabolism. There is an increase in the basal metabolic rate with enhanced mitochondrial consumption of oxygen, pyruvate, and malate.[18] Glucose uptake and glycolysis are stimulated in muscle independent of insulin.[19] This can lead to an insulin-resistant state with fasting hyperglycemia and glucose intolerance and subsequent depletion of glycogen and reduced ATP production. Insulin resistance also may interfere with insulin's anabolic effect on amino acid and protein metabolism.[20] There is an inadequate level of protein synthesis to meet the demands of accelerated breakdown, which in turn, may be driven by increased lysosomal protease activity.[21,22]

A mutation in the *KCNJ18* gene that encodes an inwardly rectifying potassium channel, Kir2.6 has been discovered in a cohort of TPP patients.[23] Mutations were present in up to 33% of the unrelated TPP patients from the United States, Brazil, and France, but in only one of 83 patients from Hong Kong and 0 of 31 Thai patients. Thus, TPP is genetically heterogeneous. The demonstrated mutations appear to lead to muscle membrane inexcitability. In addition, thyroid hormones increase potassium efflux from muscle, which can lead to an increase in the number and activity of sodium-potassium ATPase pumps.[24] This, in turn, results in partial depolarization of the muscle membrane, rendering it less excitable. Depolarization-induced sodium-channel inactivation[6] and impaired propagation of the action potential across altered T tubules further renders the muscle membrane less excitable.[25]

Treatment

Muscle strength improves gradually over several months with treatment of the hyperthyroidism.[2] Propranolol can prevent and lessen the attacks of TPP. Unlike the familial form of hypokalemic periodic paralysis, acetazolamide is ineffective in preventing attacks of weakness associated with thyrotoxicosis.

Extraocular muscle weakness associated with Graves' disease can persist for months or years after treatment. Artificial tears and ophthalmic ointments may be beneficial in preventing drying of the cornea and exposure keratitis that can result from severe lid retraction. Immunosuppression with corticosteroids and cyclosporine can be helpful in some patients but may be associated with significant side effects.[26]

HYPOTHYROID MYOPATHY

Clinical Features

Approximately one-third of individuals with hypothyroidism develop proximal arm and leg weakness along with myalgias, cramps, and generalized fatigue.[2,7,27] Rare patients develop muscle hypertrophy; rhabdomyolysis may occur. Further, ventilatory muscles may be affected in severe cases.[28]

Delayed relaxation of the muscle stretch reflexes may be demonstrated, particularly at the ankle. This finding is best appreciated by having the patient kneel on a chair or bench while striking the Achilles tendon. Myoedema refers to painless and electrically silent mounding of muscle tissue when firmly percussed and is observed in approximately one-third of affected individuals.[29] Myasthenia gravis can also occur in association with hypothyroidism.[30]

Laboratory Features

The serum CK levels are elevated as much as 10–100 times of normal. A TSH level should be checked in any patient with idiopathic CK-emia. In primary hypothyroidism, serum

T4 and T3 levels are low, while TSH levels are elevated. The motor and sensory NCS are usually normal, unless they have a concomitant polyneuropathy. Needle EMG is also usually normal, although short-duration, low-amplitude polyphasic motor unit action potentials (MUAPs) may be appreciated in severely affected muscles.[31–35]

Histopathology

Muscle biopsy abnormalities are nonspecific and may include variability in muscle fiber size with atrophy of type 2 and occasionally type 1 fibers, hypertrophic muscle fibers, rare necrotic fibers, increased internalized nuclei, ring fibers, glycogen accumulation, vacuoles, and increased connective tissue.[15,36,37] Mitochondrial swellings and inclusions, myofibrillar disarray with central core-like changes, autophagic vacuoles, glycogen accumulation, excess lipid, dilated sarcoplasmic reticulum, and T-tubule proliferation may be appreciated on EM.[36]

Pathogenesis

Hypothyroidism leads to reduced anaerobic and mitochondrial aerobic metabolism of carbohydrates and fatty acids decreasing ATP production. [38,39] Hypothyroidism also impairs adrenergic function and produces a concomitant insulin-resistant state. Protein synthesis and catabolism are reduced.

Treatment

The myopathy improves with treatment of the hypothyroidism. However, some degree of weakness can persist even 1 year after return to a euthyroid state.

PARATHYROID DISORDERS

Myopathies are common in disorders of calcium and phosphate homeostasis. The regulation of calcium and phosphate levels requires a complex interaction of intestinal, renal, hepatic, endocrine, skin, and skeletal functions.[2] Vitamin D regulates calcium absorption in the intestines. There are several forms of vitamin D: (1) vitamin D3 or cholecalciferol, which is derived from the skin; (2) vitamin D2 or ergocalciferol, which is dietary and absorbed through the intestines; and (3) 25-hydroxy-vitamin D, which is made in the liver and converted to the more potent metabolite 1,25-dihydroxy-vitamin D in the kidneys. Parathyroid hormone (PTH) assists in the regulation of serum calcium levels by promoting bone resorption, increasing renal calcium absorption and phosphate excretion, and enhancing 1,25-vitamin D conversion. Diet, intestinal absorption, and renal excretion contribute to serum phosphate levels. Increased PTH leads to increased levels of 1,25-dihydroxy-vitamin D, hypercalcemia, and hypophosphatemia. Persistently elevated PTH results in resorption of minerals within bone and replacement by fibrous tissue, a condition termed "osteitis fibrosa" or "osteitis fibrosa cystica" in severe forms.[2]

HYPERPARATHYROIDISM AND OSTEOMALACIA

Clinical Features

Muscle weakness is very common in osteomalacia, caused by vitamin D deficiency and secondary hyperparathyroidism in adults, occurring in as many as 72% of patients.[40] Weakness develops however in only 2–10% of patients with isolated hyperparathyroidism.[40,41] The earlier diagnosis and treatment of hyperparathyroidism and osteomalacia have led to fewer and less severe neuromuscular complications than appreciated in the past.[40–45]

The myopathy associated with primary hyperparathyroidism or osteomalacia is characterized by symmetric proximal weakness and atrophy, which are worse in the lower extremities. Concomitant bone pain is common due to associated microfractures. Involvement of the neck extensor muscles can lead to the so-called "dropped head syndrome." There are rare reports of hoarseness, dysphagia, ventilatory involvement, and spasticity,[41,46–49] although the majority of these cases were likely patients with amyotrophic lateral sclerosis and coincidental hyperparathyroidism.[49]

Muscle stretch reflexes are often brisk, but plantar responses are flexor. As many as 50% of patients complain of cramps and paresthesia. In addition, in 29–57% of patients there is stocking-glove loss of pain or vibratory sensation and decreased muscle stretch reflexes suggestive of an associated peripheral neuropathy.[41] Finally, hypercalcemia can be associated with neurobehavioral abnormalities (memory loss, poor concentration, personality changes, inappropriate behavior including catatonia, anxiety, and hallucinations).

Secondary hyperparathyroidism and muscle weakness can develop in patients with chronic renal failure.[50] Multifocal muscle infarcts and myoglobinuria due to calcification of the arteries (calciphylaxis) can develop in this setting.[51–53] Calciphylaxis can also occur in patients with renal failure without overt hyperparathyroidism.[54]

Laboratory Features

Serum CK levels are usually normal in primary and secondary hyperparathyroidism and osteomalacia. CK may be slightly elevated in patients with muscle infarcts due to calciphylaxis.[53] In primary hyperparathyroidism, serum calcium levels are usually elevated and serum phosphate levels are low, while urinary excretion of calcium is low and excretion of phosphate is high. In patients with concurrent hypoalbuminemia, serum calcium levels may be normal, so it is imperative to measure the ionized calcium levels which are typically elevated. Increased urinary excretion of cyclic adenosine monophosphate in the presence of hypercalcemia is also seen in hyperparathyroidism. Serum PTH levels and 1,25-dihydroxy-vitamin D levels are elevated in primary hyperparathyroidism. In contrast, 1,25-dihydroxy-vitamin D levels are low in secondary hyperparathyroidism due to renal failure. Noninvasive imaging techniques, such as ultrasound, thallium/technetium scintigraphy, computed tomography, and magnetic resonance imaging (MRI), may be useful in localizing abnormal parathyroid glands.[55]

Serum calcium level is low or normal, serum phosphate is variably low, and 25 OH vitamin D levels are also usually low in patients with osteomalacia. 1,25 OH vitamin D levels may be normal, however, as the body attempts to convert remaining vitamin D to this more potent form. Serum PTH levels are elevated in an attempt to normalize serum calcium levels that are reduced in response to vitamin D deficiency. Urinary excretion of calcium is low in an attempt to preserve serum calcium levels (except in cases secondary to renal tubular acidosis), while excretion of phosphate is high in response to secondary hyperthyroidism. In addition, serum alkaline phosphatase levels are elevated in 80–90% of cases of osteomalacia, again due to the body's attempt to normalize serum calcium by increasing bone resorption.[56] Skeletal survey reveals decreased bone density along with loss of trabeculae, blurring of trabecular margins, variably thinned cortices and microfractures that are most evident in the pelvis and proximal femur.[42] EMG and NCS are normal unless the patients have a neuropathy related to their renal failure.

Histopathology

Muscle biopsies usually demonstrate nonspecific myopathic features with atrophy predominantly of type 2 fibers, but occasionally also of type 1 fibers. Muscle biopsies may reveal multifocal infarcts and calcium deposition primarily within vessel walls in patients with calciphylaxis.[53]

Pathogenesis

Primary hyperparathyroidism can be caused by parathyroid adenomas or hyperplasia as well as pituitary adenomas. Secondary hyperparathyroidism usually occurs in the setting of chronic renal failure which results in the reduction of 1,25-dihydroxy-vitamin D conversion or in malabsorption of vitamin D in disorders such as celiac disease. Vitamin D deficiency leads to diminished intestinal absorption of calcium and decreased renal phosphate clearance, which promotes secondary hyperparathyroidism and osteomalacia. In addition to acquired forms, there are hereditary forms of primary hyperparathyroidism[57] and of vitamin D deficiency and osteomalacia.[42]

The mechanism(s) of weakness in hyperparathyroidism and osteomalacia are not known. PTH stimulates proteolysis in muscle[58] and impairs energy production, transfer, and utilization.[2,59] In addition, PTH may reduce the sensitivity of contractile myofibrillar proteins to calcium and activate a cytoplasmic protease, thus impairing the bioenergetics of muscle.[1] Calcium and phosphate levels do not correlate well with the severity of muscle weakness.[40,41,60] Vitamin D also has a direct effect on muscle by increasing muscle adenosine triphosphatase concentration, accelerating amino acid incorporation into muscle proteins,[2,61] and enhancing the uptake of calcium by the sarcoplasmic reticulum and mitochondria.[62,63]

Treatment

Hyperparathyroidism is diagnosed earlier than in the past because of routine screening of serum calcium levels. Thus, affected individuals are frequently asymptomatic or only mildly affected when they are diagnosed. Medical therapies and surgery are very effective for improvement of muscle weakness when detected within a few months.[2,41,55,64]

The treatment of choice of symptomatic patients with primary hyperparathyroidism is parathyroidectomy.[55] If a patient has a parathyroid adenoma, the affected gland is removed, while additional glands may be biopsied. Individuals with hyperplasia of all four glands generally have subtotal (three and a half glands) parathyroidectomies. Those who are asymptomatic or have significant perioperative risk may be managed medically.[64] Secondary hyperparathyroidism improves with vitamin D and calcium replacement or renal transplantation, if it is due to end-stage renal failure.[65] Occasionally, subtotal parathyroidectomy may need to be performed in patients with secondary hyperparathyroidism. Likewise, the myopathy associated with osteomalacia responds well to vitamin D and calcium replacement and to treatment of the underlying responsible condition.[40,42–44,56,66,67]

HYPERPARATHYROIDISM AND MOTOR NEURON DISEASE

Some authors have suggested that hyperparathyroidism can cause a neuromuscular syndrome that mimics amyotrophic lateral sclerosis and that patients may improve following resection of parathyroid adenomas.[41,47] However, we suspect most of these patients who improved with parathyroidectomy did not have a motor neuron disorder, but rather, hyperparathyroid-related myopathy.[49] In our experience, hyperparathyroidism in patients, who meet clinical and electrophysiologic criteria for amyotrophic lateral sclerosis, is rare and coincidental. These patients do not improve with parathyroidectomy.[49]

HYPOPARATHYROIDISM

Clinical Features

Hypoparathyroidism does not typically cause a myopathy, although a few patients do develop mild proximal weakness.[68–70] In addition, painless myoglobinuria without objective weakness or tetany has been reported.[71] On the other hand, paresthesia and tetany can develop in hypoparathyroidism secondary to hypocalcemia. The examiner may be able to demonstrate Chvostek sign (ipsilateral facial contraction upon tapping the facial nerve at the external auditory meatus) and Trousseau sign (thumb adduction, metacarpophalangeal joint flexion, and interphalangeal joint extension) in these hypocalcemic patients.

Laboratory Features

Serum CK may be normal or mildly elevated in patients.[72,73] Hypoparathyroidism is associated with low serum PTH and calcium levels and high serum phosphate levels. Motor and sensory NCS are normal. Needle EMG may reveal normal insertional activity. Fasciculation potentials result from motor nerve hyperexcitability induced by the hypocalcemia.[74–76] Multiplets (clusters of MUAPs activated with voluntary effort with interdischarge intervals between 2 and 20 ms) are another manifestation of nerve hyperexcitability and is the most characteristic electrodiagnostic abnormality seen in hypoparathyroidism or tetany. Otherwise, MUAP morphology and recruitment are normal.

Histopathology

Muscle biopsies may be normal or demonstrate mild variability in fiber size and increased internalized nuclei that reflect previous muscle damage caused by episodes of tetany.[2,15] Decreased glycogen phosphorylase activity of muscle biopsy specimens has also been described.[1]

Pathogenesis

Hypoparathyroidism is seen in a number of conditions including osteomalacia, complications of surgery, hypomagnesemia or hypermagnesemia, irradiation, drugs, sepsis, infiltrative diseases of the parathyroid, and autoimmune, hereditary, or developmental disorders of the parathyroid glands.[77] Decreased PTH leads to reduced synthesis of 1,25-dihydroxyvitamin D, hypocalcemia, and hyperphosphatemia.

The pathogenic mechanism of muscle weakness associated with hypoparathyroidism is poorly understood. Decreased serum calcium concentration causes a shift in the resting membrane potential closer to threshold.[71,78–80] Therefore, less current is required to elicit an action potential, which can lead to tetany. Elevated serum CK and mild histologic abnormalities on muscle biopsy are generally considered secondary to muscle damage from tetany.

Treatment

Muscle weakness improves following correction of the hypocalcemia and hyperphosphatemia with vitamin D and calcium administration.[70]

ADRENAL DISORDERS

The adrenal gland comprises three major regions: (1) zona fasciculata, (2) zona glomerulosa, and (3) zona reticularis.[2] The zona fasciculata produces and secretes glucocorticoids, which when produced in excess by an adrenal tumor can cause a myopathy. Mineralocorticoids such as aldosterone are generated by the zona glomerulosa and when produced in excess can cause hypokalemia which in turn leads to muscle weakness. The zona reticularis generates androgens but excess or deficiency of these hormones does not result in a muscle weakness. In contrast, these so-called anabolic steroids may increase muscle strength and mass. In the following section, we discuss myopathies associated with glucocorticoid excess or deficiency.

STEROID MYOPATHY

Steroid myopathy is the most common endocrine-related myopathy. An excess of glucocorticoids may arise directly from adrenal tumors, indirectly from pituitary tumors or from iatrogenic sources (corticosteroid medications).

Clinical Features

Approximately 50–80% of patients with Cushing disease develop some degree of proximal weakness prior to treatment.[2,81] Distal extremity, oculobulbar, and facial muscles are spared. Patients classically have an increase in truncal adipose tissue, a rounded facial appearance, and thin, frequently ecchymotic and hyperpigmented skin (i.e., the so-called Cushingoid appearance).

The incidence of iatrogenic steroid myopathy is not at all clear. Women appear to be more at risk for developing a steroid myopathy than men, approximately 2:1 but the reasons are unclear. An increased risk of the myopathy is seen with prednisone doses of 30 mg/day or more (or equivalent doses of other corticosteroids).[2] Fluorinated corticosteroids have a greater propensity for producing muscle weakness than the nonfluorinated compounds (e.g., risk for myopathy: Triamcinolone > betamethasone > dexamethasone).[82] Alternate day therapy may reduce the risk of corticosteroid-induced weakness but this has never been proven in a clinical study. Weakness can develop within several weeks of starting high doses of corticosteroids but more typically develops after chronic administration. In addition, an acute onset of severe generalized weakness can occur in patients receiving high dosages of intravenous corticosteroids (e.g., 1 g of methylprednisolone/day for multiple consecutive days) with or without concomitant administration of neuromuscular blocking agents (see section on acute quadriplegic myopathy/critical illness myopathy in Chapter 35).

Laboratory Features

Serum CK is normal. Serum potassium can be low and sodium may be elevated. Motor and sensory NCS and EMG are normal.

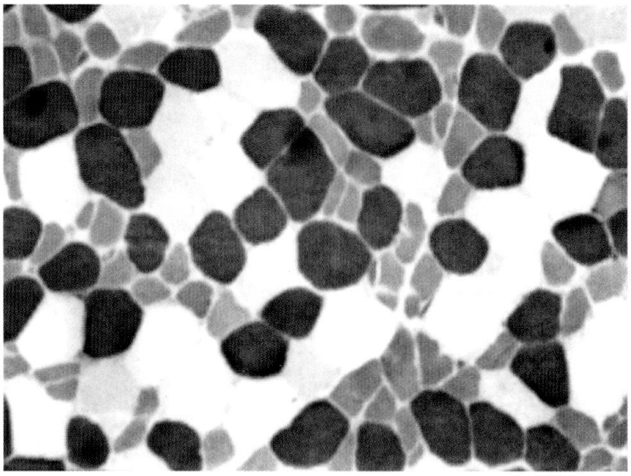

Figure 34-1. Steroid myopathy. Atrophy of type 2B fibers, which are intermediate staining, are appreciated on ATPase 4.5.

Histopathology

Muscle biopsy characteristically reveals preferential atrophy of type 2B fibers (Fig. 34-1).[15,83] Milder degrees of atrophy and increased lipid deposition of type 1 muscle may be seen as well.

Pathogenesis

Corticosteroids bind to receptors on target cells and are subsequently internalized into the nuclei, where they regulate the transcription of specific genes. It is not known how corticosteroids lead to muscle dysfunction. Corticosteroids may result in diminished protein synthesis, increased protein degradation, altered carbohydrate metabolism, impaired mitochondrial function, or decreased sarcolemmal membrane excitability (i.e., in the setting of acute quadriplegic myopathy).[1,2] In addition, hypokalemia associated with excess corticosteroid can also cause muscle weakness.

Treatment

In cases of adrenal tumors, treatment is surgical when possible. In patients with iatrogenic steroid myopathy, treatment requires reduction in the corticosteroid dose, switching to an alternate day regimen, and encouraging exercise to prevent concomitant disuse atrophy.[2] Experimental studies suggest that insulin-like growth factor-1 may have a prophylactic effect on preventing steroid myopathy.[84] Increasing the dietary protein content of the diet is a suggested treatment of unproven benefit.

A common dilemma that physicians face is renewed or exacerbated weakness in a patient receiving corticosteroids for treatment of an immune-mediated neuromuscular disorder (e.g., inflammatory myopathy, inflammatory neuropathies, or myasthenia gravis).[85,86] Following an initial improvement in their strength with corticosteroid treatment, some patients later experience a subsequent decline in muscle function. The question then arises: Is this a relapse/exacerbation of the disease or a steroid myopathy? Several clinical and laboratory features may be helpful in these situations. Patients with steroid myopathy usually have other manifestations of steroid excess, such as a Cushingoid appearance. If the weakness developed while the patient was tapering the corticosteroids, a relapse of the underlying disease process should be considered. In contrast, if weakness occurred while the patient was on a chronic high doses of steroids, a steroid myopathy is then perhaps more likely. In the case of an inflammatory myopathy, an increasing serum CK would point to an exacerbation of the myositis.[87] An EMG can be useful in that it is usually normal in steroid myopathy, while abnormal insertion and spontaneous activity along with early recruitment of myopathic MUAPs would be expected in exacerbation of inflammatory myopathy. Abnormally increased signal on STIR images of skeletal muscle MRI scans would also favor active myositis. Likewise, in myasthenia gravis flare, one might expect to find fluctuation of clinical deficits on examination (ptosis and ophthalmoplegia are not seen in steroid myopathy) and an increase in decrement with repetitive stimulation tests, or increased jitter and blocking on single fiber EMG. Steroid myopathy typically affects the proximal muscles of the lower extremities first in a symmetric fashion, which can also help to distinguish it from aggravation of steroid responsive diseases. However, sometimes it is impossible to state with certainty whether the new weakness is related to a relapse of the underlying disease or secondary to the corticosteroid treatment. In such cases, the best approach is to taper the corticosteroid medication and closely observe the patient. If improvement in strength follows, one can assume the patient had a steroid myopathy. If the patient deteriorates, the worsening weakness is more likely related to the underlying autoimmune neuromuscular disorder, and they may require increased doses of corticosteroids or other forms of immunotherapy.

ADRENAL INSUFFICIENCY

Adrenal insufficiency can result from adrenal or pituitary dysfunction and may be associated with subjective weakness (asthenia) and fatigue.[2] Objective weakness is usually the result of electrolyte disturbances (e.g., hyperkalemia) or concurrent endocrinopathies.[2] Serum CK levels, EMG, and muscle biopsies are usually normal. Symptoms improve with proper replacement of adrenal hormones.

► PITUITARY DISORDERS

ACROMEGALY

Clinical Features

Patients with acromegaly may develop slowly progressive proximal arm and leg weakness without muscle atrophy.[2,88] If anything, muscle hypertrophy is appreciated. Acromegaly can cause bony overgrowth leading to nerve root or spinal cord compression. In addition, there is a predisposition for developing multiple entrapment neuropathies such as carpal and cubital tunnel syndromes. Degenerative joint changes can produce pain that limits activity which may result in disuse muscle atrophy as well.

Laboratory Features

Serum CK levels can be normal or mildly elevated. Motor and sensory NCS can be normal or demonstrate features of a mononeuropathy (i.e., carpal tunnel syndrome).[89–91] Short-duration and low-amplitude MUAPs may be detected on EMG of proximal muscles of the arms and legs owing to the myopathy.[88] In addition, the EMG can reveal neurogenic features of involved muscle groups, if a patient has a mononeuropathy or radiculopathy related to their acromegaly.

HISTOPATHOLOGY

Muscle biopsies reveal variation in muscle fiber size with hypertrophy and atrophy of all fiber types.[92,93] Hypertrophy of satellite cells is often appreciated. In addition, rare necrotic fibers may be seen. Myofibrillar loss and abnormal glycogen accumulation may be found on EM.

Pathogenesis

The development and severity of muscle weakness correlate with the duration of acromegaly rather than the levels of serum growth hormone.[88,94] Growth hormone increases protein synthesis within muscle fibers and may lead to muscle fiber hypertrophy.[95,96] However, the pathogenic basis for the muscle weakness that develops despite increased muscle bulk is not known. Studies have demonstrated that the respiratory quotient of resting forearms muscles of patients with acromegaly is lower than normal (0.68 vs. 0.76).[97] Administration of growth hormone increases fatty acid oxidation and decreases glucose utilization.[98] It appears that growth hormone causes muscle to preferentially metabolize lipid as opposed to carbohydrates and this could alter dynamic muscle activity and fatigue. In addition, growth hormone may reduce myofibrillar ATPase activity.[99] In addition, muscle membranes are slightly depolarized compared to normal resting activity which would make them less excitable.[1]

Treatment

Surgical resection of the pituitary adenoma with subsequent reduction of the growth hormone levels leads to improved muscle strength.[88]

PANHYPOPITUITARISM

Pituitary failure in adults commonly leads to muscle weakness and fatigue, probably due to secondary deficiencies of thyroid and glucocorticoid hormones.[100] The myopathy improves with replacement of these hormones. Prepubertal panhypopituitarism is associated with dwarfism and lack of sexual and muscular development. Deficiency of growth hormone may contribute to muscle weakness in this condition, as administration of only thyroid and adrenal hormones does not result in improved strength unless growth hormone is also replaced.[101] However, it is less clear if growth hormone deficiency can contribute to muscle weakness in adults with panhypopituitarism.

DIABETES MELLITUS

Neuromuscular complications of diabetes are usually referable to peripheral neuropathies (see Chapter 21). The only myopathic disorder clearly associated with diabetes is muscle infarction.

DIABETIC MUSCLE INFARCTION

Clinical Features

Diabetic muscle infarction usually occurs in the setting of poorly controlled diabetes. Most patients have other evidence of end-organ damage (retinopathy, nephropathy, neuropathy).[102–109] Patients most commonly present with acute pain and swelling in one thigh. Occasionally, the calf is affected and rarely an upper extremity. A tender mass may be palpated in the quadriceps (most often the vastus lateralis), biceps femoris, or thigh adductors, and occasionally in the gastrocnemius muscle. The focal swelling and MRI changes often lead to a misdiagnosis of a sarcoma or focal myositis. Muscle biopsy should be avoided, if possible, because of the risk of subsequent hemorrhage into the tissue.[54]

Laboratory Features

Serum CK levels may be normal or elevated. Hemoglobin A1C level and erythrocyte sedimentation rate (ESR) are elevated in the majority of patients. MRI or CT of the leg demonstrates signal abnormalities in areas of infarcted muscle. EMG demonstrates fibrillation potentials and positive sharp waves as well as small, polyphasic MUAPs with early recruitment in the involved muscles.[103]

Histopathology

Muscle biopsies demonstrate large areas of necrosis, edema, hemorrhage, and inflammatory infiltrate consistent with muscle infarction (Fig. 34-2). This infarcted area is later replaced by connective and adipose tissue. Thickening of the basement membranes, hyperplasia of the media, and lumens occluded by fibrin, calcium, and lipid of small- and medium-sized blood vessels may be appreciated.[54]

Pathogenesis

Ischemic damage and secondary hemorrhagic infarction result from long-standing, diabetic vasculopathy.

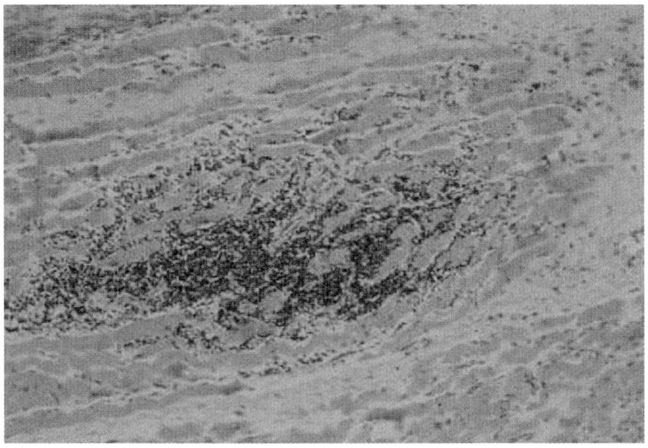

Figure 34-2. Diabetic muscle infarct. Quadriceps muscle biopsy reveals widespread necrosis and endomysial inflammatory cell infiltrate. Paraffin section, stained with hematoxylin and eosin.

Treatment

The muscle pain and swelling resolve after several weeks, although symptoms may recur in the contralateral leg. Treatment consists of immobilization and pain control. Sometimes we give a short course of prednisone to help with the pain by reducing edema and release of cytokines. However, one must closely monitor the serum glucose levels in such cases.

▶ MYOPATHIES ASSOCIATED WITH ELECTROLYTE IMBALANCE

DISORDERS OF POTASSIUM (HYPOKALEMIA)

Clinical Features

Hypokalemia is the most common electrolyte abnormality that causes muscle weakness.[110] Clinical, laboratory, and electrophysiological features are similar to familial hypokalemic periodic paralysis (see Chapter 32). Patients must be evaluated for other etiologies of hypokalemia (Table 34-1) before assuming a diagnosis of familial hypokalemic periodic paralysis. Patients usually present with acute to subacute symmetric proximal or generalized weakness, although asymmetric muscle weakness can be seen. The presentation can be mistaken for Guillain–Barré syndrome. Weakness is often accompanied by complaints of myalgias and cramps. A severe complication of hypokalemia is rhabdomyolysis with myoglobinuria and secondary renal failure.

Laboratory Features

Usually the potassium levels are less than 2.5 mEq/L before any muscle breakdown and weakness occur. Serum CK levels are usually elevated in patients with hypokalemic myopathy. NCS are normal. EMG of weak muscles may demonstrate fibrillation potentials and positive sharp waves as well as early recruitment of small-duration, low-amplitude MUAPs. The EKG may demonstrate bradycardia, flattened T waves, prolonged PR and QT intervals, and notable U waves.

▶ TABLE 34-1. **ETIOLOGIES OF SECONDARY HYPOKALEMIC AND HYPERKALEMIC PARALYSES**

Hypokalemic Paralysis
Thyrotoxic periodic paralysis
Renal tubular acidosis
Villous adenoma
Bartter syndrome
Hyperaldosteronism
Chronic or excessive use of diuretics, corticosteroids, licorice
Amphotericin B toxicity
Alcoholism
Toluene toxicity
Barium poisoning
Hyperkalemic Paralysis
Addison disease
Hypoaldosteronism (hyporeninemic)
Isolated aldosterone deficiency
Excessive potassium supplementation
Potassium-sparing diuretics (e.g., spironolactone, triamterene)
Chronic renal failure
Rhabdomyolysis

Histopathology

Biopsies of very weak muscles may demonstrate vacuoles and scattered necrotic fibers.

Pathogenesis

The mechanism of muscle fiber destruction and weakness is not fully known. Reduced extracellular potassium concentration may render the muscle membrane less excitable. Hypokalemia may also diminish blood flow and suppress the synthesis and storage of glycogen in muscles.

Treatment

Muscle strength returns with correction of the hypokalemia. The patients need a medical workup to elucidate the underlying cause of the hypokalemia.

HYPERKALEMIA

Clinical Features

Hyperkalemia can also cause generalized muscle weakness. In addition, there is evidence of increased neuronal or muscle membrane excitability as manifested by the presence of

Chvostek sign or myotonic lid lag. There are a number of causes of hyperkalemia that must be excluded before concluding a patient has familial hyperkalemic periodic paralysis (Table 34-1).

Laboratory Features

Most patients with severe generalized weakness have serum potassium levels greater than 7 mEq/L. Renal insufficiency and acidosis may accompany the hyperkalemia but serum CK levels are usually normal. EKG may demonstrate tall, peaked T waves.

Routine NCS are normal. EMG may demonstrate early recruitment of small "myopathic" MUAPs, but fibrillation potentials and positive sharp waves are atypical. Unlike, familial potassium-sensitive periodic paralysis, myotonic discharges are never seen in the acquired forms of hyperkalemic myopathy.

Histopathology

Muscle biopsies are typically normal.

Pathogenesis

Hyperkalemia causes a prolonged depolarization of the muscle membrane that in turn inactivates the sodium channel, inactivation reduces the excitability of the muscle membrane.

Treatment

Muscle strength returns with correction of hyperkalemia. The underlying cause of the hyperkalemia must be elucidated and treated.

DISORDERS OF CALCIUM

The muscle symptoms of hypercalcemia and hypocalcemia were discussed in the section regarding parathyroid myopathies. Hypercalcemia in the absence of parathormone excess usually manifests with primarily central nervous system rather than neuromuscular symptoms.

DISORDERS OF PHOSPHATE

Hypophosphatemia

Hypophosphatemia can occur in diabetic ketoacidosis, acute alcohol intoxication, hyperalimentation with phosphate-poor preparations, severe diarrhea, and in patients taking phosphate-binding antacids. Serum phosphate levels less than 0.4 mM/L may lead to generalized muscle weakness potentially severe enough to produce ventilatory failure, rhabdomyolysis, and myoglobinuria.[111] Some patients develop paresthesia and diminished muscle stretch reflexes. Severe hypophosphatemia is another potential Guillain–Barré syndrome mimic. In the authors, experience of a single case, the electrophysiologic signature was that of a sensorimotor axonopathy with muscle biopsy demonstrating type 2 fiber atrophy. Symptoms resolve with correction of the serum phosphate levels.

DISORDERS OF MAGNESIUM

Hypermagnesemia most often occurs secondary to over usage of magnesium-containing laxatives, particularly if the patient has renal insufficiency.[112] It can also develop during treatment of eclampsia with magnesium sulfate. Severe generalized and ventilatory muscle weakness may ensue but resolves with correction of the serum magnesium levels.

Muscle and nerve hyperexcitability, as characterized by Chvostek and Trousseau signs as well as tetany, may be seen in hypomagnesemia. However, hypocalcemia and other electrolyte disturbances typically accompany hypomagnesemia, and therefore, it is difficult to attribute the neuromuscular abnormality solely to the low serum magnesium levels.

▶ MYOPATHIES ASSOCIATED WITH MALIGNANCY

Patients with malignancies frequently develop generalized weakness, although most do not represent a true paraneoplastic syndrome. Muscle weakness in patients with cancer are much more likely related to impaired nutrition, increased catabolic state induced by the tumor, disuse atrophy, and perhaps toxic effects of chemotherapeutic agents. There are a few well-defined paraneoplastic syndromes, including sensory neuronopathies or sensorimotor neuropathies (e.g., anti-Hu syndrome as discussed in Chapter 19) and Lambert–Eaton syndrome (see Chapter 26), resulting in generalized weakness. Inflammatory and necrotizing myopathies can occur in the setting of cancer (as discussed in more detail in Chapter 33). Rarely, patients with malignancy can have spread of the tumor into a region of muscle.[113,114] Any muscle group can be invaded by resulting in pain, swelling, and weakness in the local region. EMG of the affected muscles may reveal membrane instability and MUAPs with short duration and low amplitudes. Muscle biopsy can demonstrate evidence of tumor emboli.

▶ OTHER MYOPATHIES SECONDARY TO SYSTEMIC DISEASE

AMYLOID MYOPATHY

Clinical Features

Amyloid myopathy usually occurs in the setting of primary amyloidosis (light-chain amyloidosis, AL).[115–122] and is less frequent with familial amyloidosis.[123,124] Amyloid myopathy does not typically occur in secondary amyloidosis (AA), however we have seen it in rare cases of senile amyloidosis.

With primary and familial amyloidosis, cardiac muscles, peripheral nerves, skin, kidneys, and other organs can also be affected in addition to skeletal muscle. In fact, most patients present with non–muscle-related symptoms. Approximately 20% of patients have a coexistent generalized peripheral neuropathy; mononeuropathies such as carpal tunnel syndrome and ulnar neuropathy also occur.[112] Amyloid myopathy usually manifests with an insidious onset of progressive proximal weakness, although distal muscles can also be affected.[120,122] The distal muscle weakness may be in part related to a superimposed amyloid neuropathy. Hypertrophy of involved muscle groups can be appreciated; the tongue is often involved with notable macroglossia. However, other patients develop atrophic muscles; again this could be related to the associated neuropathy. Rare patients have been reported presenting with neck extensor weakness (dropped head syndrome).[125] Ventilatory failure can occur due to involvement of the diaphragm muscle and phrenic nerves. Muscle induration, stiffness, and pain are also variably present.

Laboratory Features

Serum CK is usually elevated two- to fivefold but has been as high as 70-fold in a patient with familial amyloidosis due to gelsolin mutation FA.[120] AL is associated with monoclonal light chain immunoglobulins (λ greater than κ) in the serum or urine. Renal insufficiency and proteinuria result from amyloid deposition in the kidneys.

NCS are abnormal in patients with coexistent peripheral neuropathy. They often reveal reduced motor and sensory amplitudes and mild slowing of conduction velocities.[117,119–121] Superimposed carpal tunnel syndrome is a common finding. EMG reveals muscle membrane irritability with frequent fibrillation potentials and positive sharp waves, particularly in the paraspinal and proximal extremity muscles.[115,117–122,126] Complex repetitive discharges and myotonic discharges may also be appreciated. Early recruitment of short-duration, low-amplitude, polyphasic MUAPs is present in weak proximal muscles. In addition, patients with superimposed amyloid neuropathy often have decreased recruitment of long-duration, large-amplitude potential MUAPs in distal muscles.

MRI scans may reveal hypointense reticulum in the subcutaneous fat with or without increased T2 and STIR signal in affected extremities.[127–130] Furthermore, MRI may show decreased T1 signaling in the bone marrow, suggesting hematologic malignancies.[127]

Histopathology

Muscle biopsies demonstrate variability in fiber size with an admixture of hypertrophic and atrophic fibers.[120] Scattered necrotic and regenerating fibers and increased internalized nuclei may be seen. Group atrophy related to denervation may be appreciated. Amyloid deposition is best visualized using rhodamine optics on Congo-red stained section (Fig. 34-3).[120] After employing this technique in the routine evaluation of all muscle specimens, the Mayo Clinic demonstrated a 10-fold increase in the diagnosis of amyloid myopathy, suggesting it is probably an underdiagnosed entity.[120]

The amyloid deposits are best appreciated surrounding small arterioles and venules. In addition, muscle fibers are also partially or completely encased by amyloid deposits. In primary amyloidosis, immunohistochemical studies reveal that the amyloid deposits are composed of λ or κ light chains.[120] Immunohistochemistry employing antibodies directed against gelsolin and transthyretin are useful in excluding or diagnosing familial amyloidosis. Mass spectroscopy can also be utilized to identify the subtype of the amyloid deposits. Membrane attack complex may colocalize with amyloid deposition. ApoE was deposited in all patients regardless of the type

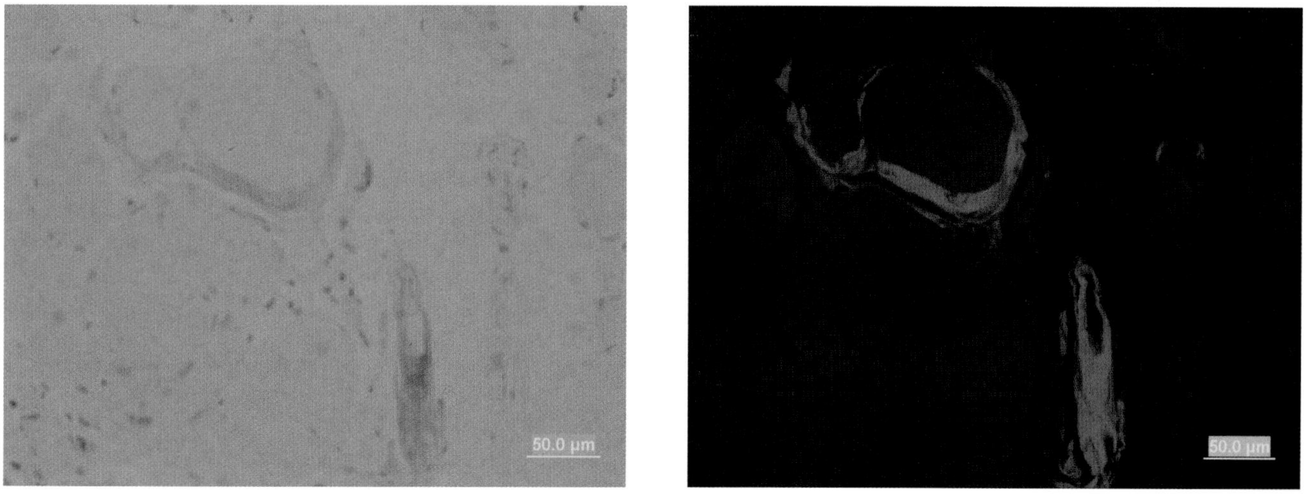

A B

Figure 34-3. Amyloid myopathy. Amyloid deposition is appreciated surrounding blood vessels and occasionally encasing individual muscle fibers on Congo red staining. The deposits are pink on routine light microscopy **(A)** and bright red using rhodamine optics **(B)**.

to systemic amyloidosis in one large series of patients.[120] EM confirms the deposition of short, nonbranching 10-nm amyloid filaments around small blood vessel and muscle fibers.

Pathogenesis

The exact mechanism by which amyloid deposition causes muscle fiber damage is not known. Ischemic damage may arise due to deposition of amyloid in blood vessel walls. Encasement of muscle fibers by the amyloid may interfere with the transport of oxygen, nutrients, and wastes into and out of muscle fibers. There may also be mechanical interference of muscle contraction secondary to amyloid infiltration. Alternatively, the amyloid may interfere with electrical conduction along the sarcolemma.

Treatment

Although autologous stem bone marrow transplant has been attempted, there is no proven effective medical therapy for the myopathy secondary to systemic amyloidosis.

CRITICAL ILLNESS MYOPATHY/ACUTE QUADRIPLEGIC MYOPATHY

This entity is usually associated with high dose steroids with or without nondepolarizing neuromuscular agents and is discussed in detail in Chapter 35 regarding Toxic Myopathies.

▶ ILL-DEFINED DISORDERS

POLYMYALGIA RHEUMATICA

Clinical Features

Polymyalgia rheumatica usually occurs in patients over the age of 50 years (peak incidence of 70–79 years).[7,131,132] The prevalence is approximately of 1 case for every 133 people older than 50 years.[133] There is a female predilection for the development of polymyalgia rheumatica. Patients usually complain of an insidious or acute onset of diffuse nonarticular pain and stiffness, particularly in the morning, beginning about the neck and shoulder region. Other body regions may be affected. A low-grade fever, anorexia, and malaise may accompany the myalgias. Affected individuals may complain of feeling weak or fatigued but on manual muscle testing their strength should be normal. Approximately 16% of patients develop temporal arteritis which can be complicated by acute vision loss.[131] Temporal artery biopsy should be performed on all such patients with headaches or visual disturbances to look for evidence in giant-cell arteritis.

Laboratory Features

The ESR is usually abnormal and elevated; typically over of 40 mm/h. Serum CK should be normal. Likewise, EMG and NCS should be normal.

Histopathology

The muscle biopsies should be normal, but mild nonspecific findings (e.g., type 2 fiber atrophy, fiber size variation, and moth-eaten fibers) have been reported.[132] Also note there is no evidence of significant inflammation in the muscle or overlying fascia.

Pathogenesis

The exact pathogenic basis for polymyalgia rheumatica is unclear. The elevated ESR and excellent response to corticosteroids suggest an immunologic mechanism. Some cases are clearly associated with arteritis/vasculitis but it is not usually related to a true myositis or fasciitis.

Treatment

The administration of corticosteroids, usually at low dose, results in considerable symptom relief within a few days.

FIBROMYALGIA

Fibromyalgia and myofascial pain syndrome, and the fatigue that often accompany them, are commonly diagnosed disorders that are controversial in regard to their nature because of the lack of objective evidence of organic disease.[134,135] Fibromyalgia is often dominated by subjective complaints of generalized muscle pain in addition to other somatic complains including headaches, fatigue, and abdominal cramps. In this regard, it shares many features with the somatoform disorders and the dubious "chronic fatigue syndrome."[136,137]

There is no "gold standard" for diagnosing fibromyalgia. Fibromyalgia may be diagnosed if a sufficient although arbitrary number of "tender points" at specific locations on the body are found.[138] Unfortunately, the study by which these criteria were based was scientifically flawed.[134,135] The investigators predetermined that tender points were necessary for the diagnosis and they each received training in how to identify such tender points. Patients diagnosed with fibromyalgia based on the presence of tender points were then evaluated by other investigators to confirm their presence. That these tender points were reproducible (good intraobserver reliability), served as a validation of the diagnosis for the investigators. Skeptics criticized the study for confirming the established bias of the investigators.[134,135,139] Detecting tender points is dependent on the patient's subjective input and is in no way a truly objective marker. The neurological examination including muscle strength testing and laboratory evaluation is otherwise normal in fibromyalgia. Likewise, serum CK, NCS, and electromyography (even of in the areas of tender points) are normal. Finally, there is no difference in the frequency of abnormal histologic findings compared to control populations.

Myofacial pain syndrome (MPS) is similar to fibromyalgia, but the pain is described as being more focal as opposed to generalized.[134,135] Rather than tender points, advocates of the disorder suggest patients have "trigger points." These trigger points have been associated with "taut bands," "nodules," and "local twitch responses." However, blinded, controlled studies have demonstrated a low sensitivity and specificity of this so-called diagnostic marker of MPS.[140] One study described abnormal "spontaneous EMG" activity in the area of the trigger points.[141] However, review of the published figures suggest this was just normal end plate spike activity. The majority of electromyographers, including ourselves, have not been able to verify the presence of any abnormalities in MPS.[134,135] As with fibromyalgia, the clinical examination, serum CK, EMG, and NCS, and muscle biopsies are normal.

Regardless of the organicity of the pain related to fibromyalgia or MPS, the patients' symptoms are often quite distressing and disabling to them. We often recommend treatment with tricyclic antidepressant medications, pregabalin, or gabapentin, as we do with other chronic pain syndromes, in addition to maintenance of as normal a lifestyle as possible. Patients may also benefit from physical therapy program to increase their endurance and tolerance.

▶ SUMMARY

Many systemic disorders can be associated with a myopathy. The myopathy may be a direct effect of the systemic process or may be toxic related to drugs used to treat the underlying condition. The regenerative capability of muscle allows for improvement in strength with effective treatment of the underlying cause in many cases. This underlines the importance of a detailed evaluation in patients referred for possible myopathy.

REFERENCES

1. Kaminski HJ, Ruff RL. Endocrine myopathies (hyper- and hypofunction of adrenal, thyroid, pituitary, and parathyroid glands and iatrogenic corticosteroid myopathy). In: Engel AG, Franzini-Armstrong C, eds. *Myology*, 2nd ed. New York, NY: McGraw-Hill; 1994:1726–1753.
2. Kissel JT, Mendell JR. The endocrine myopathies. In Rowland LP, DiMauro S, eds. *Handbook of Clinical Neurology*, Vol 18(62). Amsterdam: Elsevier Science Publishers BV; 1992:527–551.
3. Ramsay I. *Thyroid Disease and Muscle Dysfunction*. Chicago, IL: William Heinemann Medical Books; 1974.
4. Puvanendran K, Cheah JS, Naganathan N, Wong PK. Thyrotoxic myopathy: a clinical and quantitative analytic electromyographic study. *J Neurol Sci*. 1979;42:441–451.
5. Sataysohi E, Murakami K, Kowa H, Kinishita M, Nishiyama Y. Periodic paralysis in hyperthyroidism. *Neurology*. 1963;13:746–752.
6. Ruff RL, Weissmann J. Endocrine myopathies. *Neurol Clin*. 1988;6:575–592.
7. Ludin HP, Spiess H, Koenig MP. Neuromuscular dysfunction associated with thyrotoxicosis. *Eur Neurol*. 1969;2:269–278.
8. McElvaney GN, Wilcox PG, Fairborn MS, et al. Respiratory muscle weakness and dyspnea in thyrotoxic patients. *Am Rev Respir Dis*. 1990;141(5 pt 1):1221–1227.
9. Mier A, Brophy C, Wass JA, Besser GM, Green M. Reversible muscle weakness in hyperthyroidism. *Am Rev Respir Dis*. 1989;139:529–533.
10. Bennet WR, Huston DP. Rhabdomyolysis in thyroid storm. *Am J Med*. 1984;77:733–735.
11. Feibel JH, Campa JF. Thyrotoxic neuropathy (Basedow's paraplegia). *J Neurol Neurosurg Psychiatry*. 1976;39:491–497.
12. Havard CW, Campbell ED, Ross HB, Spence AW. Electromyographic and histologic findings in the muscles of patients with thyrotoxicosis. *Q J Med*. 1963;32:145–163.
13. McCommas AJ, Sica RE, McNabb AR, Goldberg WM, Upton AR. Evidence for reversible motoneurone dysfunction in thyrotoxicosis. *J Neurol Neurosurg Psychiatry*. 1974;37:548–558.
14. Engel AG. Neuromuscular manifestations of Grave's disease. *Mayo Clin Proc*. 1972;47:919–925.
15. Hudgson P, Kendall-Taylor P. Endocrine myopathies. In: Mastaglia FL, Walton JN, eds. *Skeletal Muscle Pathology*. Edinburgh: Churchill Livingstone; 1992:493–509.
16. Waldstein SS, Bronsky D, Shrifter HB, Oester YT.et al. The electromyogram in myxedema. *AMA Arch Intern Med*. 1958;101:97–102.
17. Engel AG. Electron microscopic observations in thyrotoxic and corticosteroid-induced myopathies. *Mayo Clin Proc*. 1966;41:785–796.
18. Janssen JW, Delange-Berkout IW, Van Hardeveld C, Kassenaar AA. The disappearance of l-thyroxine and triiodothyronine from plasma, red and white skeletal muscle after administration of one subcutaneous dose of l-thyroxin to hyperthyroid and euthyroid rats. *Acta Endocrinol (Copenh)*. 1981;97:226–230.
19. Celsing F, Blomstrand E, Melichna J, et al. Effect of hyperthyroidism in fibre-type composition, fibre area, glycogen content, and enzyme activity in human muscle protein activity in human skeletal muscle. *Clin Physiol*. 1986;6:171–181.
20. Dubaniewicz A, Kaciuba-Uscilko H, Nazar K, Budohoski L. Sensitivity of the soleus to insulin in resting and exercising with experimental hypo- and hyperthyroidism. *Biochem J*. 1989;263:243–247.
21. Brown JG, Millward DJ. The influence of thyroid status on skeletal muscle protein metabolism. *Biochem Soc Trans*. 1980;8:366–367.
22. Morrison WL, Gibson JN, Jung RT, Rennie MJ. Skeletal muscle and whole body protein turnover in thyroid disease. *Eur J Clin Invest*. 1988;18:62–68.
23. Ryan DP, da Silva MR, Soong TW, et al. Mutations in potassium channel Kir2.6 cause susceptibility to thyrotoxic hypokalemic periodic paralysis. *Cell*. 2010;140:88–98.
24. Everts ME, Dørup I, Flyvberg A, Marshall SM, Jørgensen KD. Na(+)-K(+) pump in rat muscle: Effects of hypophysectomy, growth hormone, and thyroid hormone. *Am J Physiol*. 1990;259(2 pt 1):E278–E283.
25. Dulhunty AF, Gage PW, Lamb GD. Differential effects of thyroid hormone on T-tubules and terminal cisternae in rat muscles: an electrophysiological and morphometric analysis. *J Muscle Res Cell Motil*. 1986;7:225–236.
26. Prummel MF, Mourits MP, Berout A, et al. Prednisone and cyclosporine in the treatment of severe Graves' disease. *N Engl J Med*. 1989;321:1353–1359.

27. Salick AI, Colachis SC Jr, Pearson CM. Myxedema myopathy: Clinical, electrodiagnostic, and pathologic findings in advanced case. *Arch Phys Med Rehabil.* 1968;49:230–237.
28. Martinez FJ, Bermudez-Gomez M, Celli BR. Hypothyroidism. A reversible cause of diaphragmatic dysfunction. *Chest.* 1989;96:1059–1063.
29. Salick AI, Pearson CM. Electrical silence of myoedema. *Neurology.* 1967;17(9):899–901.
30. Takamori M, Gutman L, Crosby TW, Martin JD. Myasthenic syndromes in hypothyroidism. Electrophysiological study of neuromuscular transmission and muscle contraction in two patients. *Arch Neurol.* 1972;26:326–335.
31. Afifi AK, Najjar SS, Mire-Salam J, Bergman RA. The myopathology of the Kocher-Debre'-Se'me'laigne syndrome: Electromyography, light- and electron-microscopic study. *J Neurol Sci.* 1974;22:445–470.
32. Astrom KE, Kugelberg E, Muller R. Hypothyroid myopathy. *Arch Neurol.* 1961;5:472–482.
33. Emser W, Schimrigk K. Myxedema myopathy: A case report. *Eur Neurol.* 1977;16:286–291.
34. Klein I, Parker M, Shebert R, Ayyar DR, Levey GS. Hypothyroidism presenting as muscle stiffness and pseudohypertrophy: Hoffman's syndrome. *Am J Med.* 1981;70:891–894.
35. Norris FH Jr, Panner BJ. Hypothyroid myopathy. *Arch Neurol.* 1966;14:574–589.
36. Evans RM, Watanabe I, Singer PA. Central changes in hypothyroid myopathy: A case report. *Muscle Nerve.* 1990;13:952–956.
37. Laycock MA, Pascuzzi RM. The neuromuscular effects of hypothyroidism. *Semin Neurol.* 1991;11:288–294.
38. Ho KL. Basophilic bodies of skeletal muscle in hypothyroidism: enzyme histochemical and ultrastructural studies. *Hum Pathol.* 1989;20:1119–1124.
39. Schwartz HL, Oppenheimer JH. Physiologic and biochemical actions of thyroid hormone. *Pharmacol Ther B.* 1978;3:349–376.
40. Smith R, Stern G. Muscular weakness in osteomalacia and hyperparathyroidism. *J Neurol Sci.* 1969;8:511–520.
41. Patten BM, Bilezikian JP, Mallette LE, Prince A, Engel WK, Aurbach GD. Neuromuscular disease in primary hyperparathyroidism. *Ann Intern Med.* 1974;80:182–193.
42. Goldring SR, Krane SM, Avioli LV. Disorders of calcification: Osteomalacia and rickets. In: De Groot, ed. *Endocrinology.* 3rd ed. Philadelphia, PA: WB Saunders; 1994:1204–1227.
43. Mallette LE, Patten BM, Engel WK. Neuromuscular disease in secondary hyperparathyroidism. *Ann Intern Med.* 1975;82:474–483.
44. Smith R, Stern G. Myopathy, osteomalacia and hyperparathyroidism. *Brain.* 1967;90:593–602.
45. Vicale CT. The diagnostic features of a muscular syndrome resulting from hyperparathyroidism, osteomalacia, owing to renal tubular acidosis, and perhaps to related disorders of calcium metabolism. *Trans Am Neurol Assoc.* 1949;74:143–147.
46. Berenbaum F, Rajzbaum G, Bonnchon P, Amor B. Une hyperparathyroide revelee une chute de la tete. *Rev Rhum Mal Osteoartic.* 1993;60:467–469.
47. Gelinas DF, Miller RG, McVey AL. Reversible neuromuscular dysfunction associated with hyperparathyroidism [abstract]. *Neurology.* 1994;44(Suppl 2):A348.
48. Gentric A, Pennec YL. Fatal primary hyperparathyroidism with myopathy involving respiratory muscles. *J Am Geriatr Soc.* 1994;42:1306.
49. Jackson CE, Amato AA, Bryan WW, Wolfe GI, Sakhee K, Barohn RJ. Primary hyperparathyroidism and ALS. Is there a relation? *Neurology.* 1998;50:1795–1799.
50. Floyd M, Ayyar DR, Barwick DD, Hudson P, Weightman D. Myopathy in chronic renal failure. *Q J Med.* 1974;53:509–524.
51. Richardson JA, Herron G, Reitz R, Layzer R. Ischemic ulcerations of the skin and necrosis of muscle in azotemic hyperparathyroidism. *Ann Intern Med.* 1969;71:129–138.
52. Randall DP, Fisher MA, Thomas C. Rhabdomyolysis as the presenting manifestation of calciphylaxis. *Muscle Nerve.* 2000;23:289–293.
53. De Luca GC, Eggers SD. A rare complication of azotemic hyperparathyroidism: Ischemic calcific myopathy. *Neurology.* 2010;75:1942.
54. Banker BQ, Chester CS. Infarction of thigh muscle in the diabetic patient. *Neurology.* 1973;23:667–677.
55. Norton JA, Sugg SL. Surgical management of hyperparathyroidism. In: De Groot, ed. *Endocrinology.* 3rd ed. Philadelphia, PA: WB Saunders; 1994:1106–1122.
56. Russell JA. Osteomalacic myopathy. *Muscle Nerve.* 1994;17(6):578–580.
57. Habener J, Arnold A, Potts JT. Hyperparathyroidism. In: De Groot, ed. *Endocrinology.* 3rd edn. Philadelphia, PA: WB Saunders; 1994:1044–1060.
58. Garber AJ. Effects of parathyroid hormone on skeletal muscle protein and amino acid metabolism in the rat. *J Clin Invest.* 1983;71:1806–1821.
59. Baczynski R, Massry SG, Magott M, El-Belbessi S, Kohan R, Brautbar N. Effect of parathyroid hormone on energy metabolism of skeletal muscle. *Kidney Int.* 1985;28:722–727.
60. Frame B, Heinze EG Jr, Block MA, Manson GA. Myopathy in primary hyperparathyroidism. Observations in three patients. *Ann Intern Med.* 1968;68:1022–1027.
61. Birge SG, Haddad JG. 25-hydroxycholecalciferol stimulation of muscle metabolism. *J Clin Invest.* 1975;56:1100–1107.
62. Curry OB, Basten JF, Francis MJ, Smith R. Calcium up-take by the sarcoplasmic reticulum of muscle from vitamin D deficiency in rabbits. *Nature.* 1974;249:83–84.
63. Pointon JJ, Francis MJO, Smith R. Effect of vitamin D deficiency on sarcoplasmic reticulum and troponin C concentration of rabbit skeletal muscle. *Clin Sci (Lond).* 1979;57:257–263.
64. Nussbaum SR, Neer RM, Potts JT Jr. Medical management of hyperparathyroidism and hypercalcemia. In: De Groot, ed. *Endocrinology.* 3rd ed. Philadelphia, PA: WB Saunders; 1994:1094–1105.
65. Probhala A, Garg R, Dandona P. Severe myopathy associated with vitamin D deficiency in western New York. *Arch Intern Med.* 2000;160(8):1119–1203.
66. Irani PF. Electromyography in nutritional osteomalacic myopathy. *J Neurol Neurosurg Psychiatry.* 1976;39:686–693.
67. Schott GD, Wills MR. Myopathy in hypophosphataemic osteomalacia presenting in adult life. *J Neurol Neurosurg Psychiatry.* 1975;38:297–304.
68. Kruse K, Scheunemann W, Baier W, Schaub J. Hypocalcemic myopathy in idiopathic hypoparathyroidism. *Eur J Pediatr.* 1982;138:280–282.
69. Snowdon JA, Macfie AC, Pearce JB. Hypocalcemic myopathy and parathyroid psychosis. *J Neurol Neurosurg Psychiatry.* 1976;38:48–52.

70. Yamaguchi H, Okamoto K, Shooji M, Morimatsu M, Hirai S. Muscle histology of hypocalcemic myopathy in hypoparathyroidism . *J Neurol Neurosurg Psychiatry*. 1987;50:817–818.
71. Akmal M. Rhabdomyolysis in a patient with hypocalcemia due to hypoparathyroidism. *Am J Nephrol*. 1993;13:61–63.
72. Hower J, Struck H, Tackman W, Stolecke H. CPK activity in hypoparathyroidism. *N Engl J Med*. 1972;287:1098.
73. Shane E, McClane KA, Olarte MR, Bilezikian JP. Hypoparathyroidism and elevated serum enzymes. *Neurology*. 1980; 30:192–195.
74. Kugelberg E. Neurologic mechanism for certain phenomena in tetany. *Arch Neurol Psychiatry*. 1946;56:507–521.
75. Kugelberg E. Activation of human nerves by ischemia; Trousseau's phenomenon in tetany. *Arch Neurol Psychiatry*. 1948;60:140–164.
76. Kugelberg E. Activation of human nerves by hyperventilation and hypocalcemia. *Arch Neurol Psychiatry*. 1948;60:153–164.
77. Fitzpatrick LA, Arnold A. Hypoparathyroidism. In: De Groot, ed. *Endocrinology*. 3rd ed. Philadelphia, PA: WB Saunders; 1994:1123–1135.
78. Brink F. The role of calcium ion in neural processes. *Pharmacol Rev*. 1954;6:243–298.
79. Frankenhaeuser B. The effect of calcium on the myelinated nerve fiber. *J Physiol*. 1957;137:245–260.
80. Frankenhaeuser B, Hodgkin AL. The action of calcium on the electric properties of squid axons. *J Physiol*. 1957;137:218–244.
81. Muller R, Kugelberg E. Myopathy in Cushing's syndrome. *J Neurol Neurosurg Psychiatry*. 1959;22:314–319.
82. Faludi G, Gotlieb J, Meyers J. Factors influencing the development of steroid-induced myopathy. *Ann N Y Acad Sci*. 1966;138:62–72.
83. Pleasure DE, Walsh GO, Engel WK. Atrophy of skeletal muscle in patients with Cushing's syndrome. *Arch Neurol*. 1970;22: 118–125.
84. Kanda F, Takatani K, Okuda S, Matsushi T, Chihara K. Preventive effects of insulin-like growth factor-1 on steroid-induced muscle atrophy. *Muscle Nerve*. 1999;22:213–217.
85. Afifi AK, Bergman RA, Harvey JC. Steroid myopathy. *Johns Hopkins Med J*. 1968;123:158–173.
86. MacLean K, Schurr PH. Reversible amyotrophy complicating treatment with fludrocortisone. *Lancet*. 1959;1:701–702.
87. Askari A, Vignos PJ Jr, Moskowitz RW. Steroid myopathy in connective tissue disease. *Am J Med*. 1976;61:485–492.
88. Pickett JB, Layzer RB, Levin SR, Scheider V, Campbell MJ, Sumner AJ. Neuromuscular complications of acromegaly. *Neurology*. 1975;25:638–645.
89. Low PA, McLeod JG, Turtle JR, Donnelly P, Wright RG. Peripheral neuropathy in acromegaly. *Brain*. 1974;97:139–152.
90. Lundberg PO, Osterman PO, Stalberg E. Neuromuscular signs and symptoms in acromegaly. In: Walton JN, Canal N, Scarlato G, eds. Muscle Diseases: Proceedings of an International Congress Milan, 19–21, May, 1969. Amsterdam: Excerpta Medica; 1970:531–534.
91. Stewart BM. The hypertrophic neuropathy of acromegaly. *Arch Neurol*. 1966;14:107–110.
92. Mastaglia FL, Barwick DD, Hall R. Myopathy in acromegaly. *Lancet*. 1970;2:907–909.
93. Stern LZ, Payne CM, Hannapel LK. Acromegaly: Histochemical and electron microscopic changes in deltoid and intercostal muscle. *Neurology*. 1974;24:589–593.
94. Naglesparen M, Trickey R, Davies MJ, Jenkins JS. Muscle changes in acromegaly. *Br Med J*. 1976;2:914–915.
95. Bigland B, Jehring B. Muscle performance in rats, normal and treated with growth hormone. *J Physiol*. 1952;116:129–136.
96. Prysor-Jones RA, Jenkins JS. Effect of excessive secretion of growth hormone ion tissues of the rat, with particular reference to the heart and skeletal muscle. *J Endocrinol*. 1980;85:75–82.
97. Rabinowitz D, Zierler KL. Differentiation of active from inactive acromegaly by studies of forearm metabolism and response to intra-arterial insulin. *Bull Johns Hopkins Hosp*. 1963;113:211–224.
98. Winckler B, Steele R, Altszuller N, De Bodo RC. Effect of growth hormone on free fatty acid metabolism. *Am J Physiol*. 1964;206:174–178.
99. Florini JR, Ewton DZ. Skeletal muscle fiber types and myosin ATPase activity do not change with age or growth hormone administration. *J Gerontol*. 1989;44:B110–B117.
100. Brasel JA, Wright JC, Wilkins L, Blizzard RM. An evaluation of seventy-five patients with hypopituitarism. *Am J Med*. 1965;38:484–498.
101. Raben MS. Growth hormone: 2. Clinical use of growth hormone. *N Engl J Med*. 1962;266:82–86.
102. Anglada M, Vidaller A, Bolao F, Ferrer I, Olive M. Diabetic muscular infarction. *Muscle Nerve*. 2000;23:825–826.
103. Barohn RJ, Kissel JT. Painful thigh mass in a young woman: diabetic thigh infarction. *Muscle Nerve*. 1992;15:850–855.
104. Bjornskowve EK, Carry MR, Katz FH, Lefkowitz J, Ringel SP. Diabetic muscle infarction: a new perspective on pathogenesis and management. *Neuromuscul Disord*. 1995;5(1):39–45.
105. Bodner RA, Younger DS, Rosoklija G. Diabetic muscle infarction. *Muscle Nerve*. 1994;17:949–950.
106. Chester CS, Banker BQ. Focal infarctions of muscle in diabetics. *Diabetic Care*. 1986;9:623–630.
107. Umpierrez GE, Stiles RG, Kleinbart J, Krendel DA, Watts NB. Diabetic muscle infarction. *Am J Med*. 1996;101:245–250.
108. Huang BK, Monu JU, Doumanian J. Diabetic myopathy: MRI patterns and current trends. *AJR Am J Roentgenol*. 2010;195: 198–204.
109. Joshi R, Reen B, Sheehan H. Upper extremity diabetic muscle infarction in three patients with end-stage renal disease: a case series and review. *J Clin Rheumatol*. 2009;15:81–84.
110. Comi G, Testa D, Cornelio F, Comola M, Canal M. Potassium depletion myopathy: a clinical and morphological study of six cases. *Muscle Nerve*. 1985;8:17–21.
111. Knochel JP. The clinical status of hypophosphatemia: an update. *N Engl J Med*. 1985;313:447–449.
112. Mordes JP, Wacker WE. Excess magnesium. *Pharmacol Rev*. 1977;29:273–300.
113. Doshi R, Fowler T. Proximal myopathy due to discrete carcinomatous metastases in muscle. *J Neurol Neurosurg Psychiatry*. 1983;46:358–360.
114. Heffner RR Jr. Myopathy of embolic origin in patients with carcinoma. *Neurology*. 1971;21:840–846.
115. Jennekens FG, Wokke JH. Proximal weakness of the extremities as a main feature of amyloid myopathy. *J Neurol Neurosurg Psychiatry*. 1987;50:1353–1358.
116. Nardkarni N, Freimer M. Mendell JR. Amyloidosis causing a progressive myopathy. *Muscle Nerve*. 1995;18:1016–1018.
117. Ringel SP, Claman HN. Amyloid-associated muscle pseudohypertrophy. *Arch Neurol*. 1982;39:413–417.
118. Roke ME, Brown WF, Boughner D, Ang LC, Rice GP. Myopathy in primary systemic amyloidosis. *Can J Neurol Sci*. 1988;15:314–316.

119. Rubin DI, Hermann RC. Electrophysiologic findings in amyloid myopathy. *Muscle Nerve*. 1999;22:355–359.
120. Spuler S, Emslie-Smith A, Engel AG. Amyloid myopathy: an underdiagnosed entity. *Ann Neurol*. 1998;43:719–728.
121. Whitaker JN, Hashimoto K, Quinones M. Skeletal muscle pseudohypertrophy in primary amyloidosis. *Neurology*. 1977; 27:47–54.
122. Smetstad C, Monstad P, Lindboe CF, Mygalns A. Amyloid myopathy present with distal atrophic weakness. *Muscle Nerve*. 2004;29:605–609.
123. Bruni J, Bilbao JM, Prtzker PH. Myopathy associated with amyloid angiopathy. *Can J Neurol Sci*. 1977;4:77–80.
124. Yamada M, Tsukagoshi H, Hatakeyama S. Skeletal muscle amyloid deposition in AL- (primary or myeloma-associated), AA- (secondary), and prealbumin-type amyloidosis. *J Neurol Sci*. 1988;85:223–232.
125. Chuquilin M, Al-Lozi M. Primary amyloidosis presenting as "dropped head syndrome". *Muscle Nerve*. 2011;43:905–909.
126. Chapin JE, Kornfeld M, Harris A. Amyloid myopathy: characteristic features of a still underdiagnosed disease. *Muscle Nerve*. 2005;31(2):266–272.
127. Hull KM, Griffith L, Kuncl RW, Wigley FM. A deceptive case of amyloid myopathy. Clinical and magnetic resonance imaging features. *Arthritis Rheum*. 2001;8:1954–1958.
128. Mandl LA, Folkerth RD, Pick MA, Weinblatt ME, Gravallese EM. Amyloid myopathy masquerading as polymyositis. *J Rheumatol*. 2000;27:949–952.
129. Metzler JP, Fleckenstein JL, White CL 3rd, Haller RG, Frenkel EP, Greenlee RG Jr. MRI evaluation of amyloid myopathy. *Skeletal Radiol*. 1992;21:463–465.
130. Tuomaala H, Kärppä M, Tuominen H, Remes AM. Amyloid myopathy: A diagnostic challenge. *Neurol Int*. 2009;1:e7.
131. Chuang TY, Hunder GG, Ilstrup DM, Kurland LT. Polymyalgia rheumatica. A 10-year epidemiologic and clinical study. *Ann Intern Med*. 1982;97:672–680.
132. Coomes EN. The rate of recovery of reversible myopathies and the effects of anabolic agents in steroid myopathy. *Neurology*. 1965;18:523–530.
133. Salvarani C, Cantini F, Boiardi L, Hunder GG. Polymyalgia rheumatica and giant-cell arteritis. *N Engl J Med*. 2002;347(4): 261–271.
134. Bohr T. Problems with myofascial pain syndrome and fibromyalgia syndrome. *Neurology*. 1996;46:593–597.
135. Bohr TW. Fibromyalgia syndrome and myofascial pain syndrome: Do they exist? *Neurol Clin*. 1995;13:365–384.
136. Goldenberg DL. Fibromyalgia, chronic fatigue syndrome, and myofascial pain syndrome. *Curr Opin Rheumatol*. 1993;5: 199–208.
137. Komaroff AL, Goldenberg D. The chronic fatigue syndrome: Definition, current studies, and lessons for fibromyalgia research. *J Rheumatol*. 1989;16:23–27.
138. Wolfe F, Smythe HA, Yunus MB, et al. The American College of Rheumatology. 1990 Criteria for the Classification of Fibromyalgia. Report of the Multicenter Criteria Committee. *Arthritis Rheum*. 1990;33(2):160–172.
139. Cohen ML, Quinter JL. Fibromyalgia syndrome, a problem of tautology. *Lancet*. 1993;342:906–909.
140. Wolfe F, Simons DG, Fricton J, et al. The fibromyalgia and myofascial pain syndromes: A preliminary study of tender points and trigger points in persons with fibromyalgia, myofascial pain syndrome and no disease. *J Rheumatol*. 1992;19(6):944–951.
141. Hubbard D, Berkoff G. Myofascial trigger points show spontaneous needle EMG activity. *Spine (Phila Pa 1976)*. 1993; 18:1803–1807.

CHAPTER 35

Toxic Myopathies

Many drugs can cause a myopathy.[1–10] The pathophysiological mechanisms are diverse and, in many instances, unclear. Medications can have either a direct or an indirect adverse effect on muscle. The direct effect can be focal, as might occur secondary to a drug being injected into tissue, or more commonly generalized. Indirect toxic effects may result from the agent creating an electrolyte imbalance or inducing an immunological reaction. Muscle fibers may undergo necrosis as a result of the drug directly disrupting the sarcolemma, nuclear or mitochondria function, or that of other organelles. In this chapter, we classify the toxic myopathies according to their presumed pathogenic mechanisms (Table 35-1).

► NECROTIZING MYOPATHIES

A number of drugs can cause a generalized necrotizing myopathy. Affected individuals may complain of myalgias or weakness, or they might just have asymptomatic elevations of their serum creatine kinase (CK) levels. Severe necrotizing myopathy may be complicated by myoglobinuria and renal failure. The degree of serum CK elevation is proportionate to the amount of muscle damaged.

CHOLESTEROL-LOWERING DRUGS

Cholesterol-lowering medications including 3-hydroxy-3-methylglutaryl-coenzyme A (3-HMG-CoA) reductase inhibitors,[11–19] fibric acid derivatives,[16,20–30] niacin,[31,32] and ezetimibe[33–36] may cause a toxic myopathy. Most patients just have mild elevations in serum CK without any symptoms. Others have myalgias and less frequently weakness. Myoglobinuria is a rare event but can be complicated by death. With discontinuation of the offending agent, the myalgias, weakness, and elevated serum CK levels tend to completely resolve, but it may take several days to months. However, rarely these agents may trigger an immune-mediated inflammatory myopathy, usually necrotizing, that requires treatment with immunosuppressive medications.

HMG-CoA REDUCTASE INHIBITORS

Clinical Features

Statin agents inhibit 3-HMG-CoA reductase, the rate controlling enzyme in cholesterol synthesis (Fig. 35-1). Adverse side effects including asymptomatic hyper-CK-emia, myalgias, proximal weakness, and, less commonly, myoglobinuria occur with all of the major HMG-CoA reductase inhibitors: lovastatin,[13,16,18,19,32,37,38] simvastatin,[12,14,15,38,39] provastatin,[17,38] atorvastatin,[11,38,40] fluvastatin,[38] and cerivastatin.[38,41,42] The nomenclature regarding statin-induced toxic myopathies in the published literature is unfortunately quite unsatisfactory, listing "myalgias," "myositis," and "myopathy" as three independent types of muscle disorders caused by statin use, when these three subtypes may just reflect the spectrum of severity of the myopathy.[43–45]

Reviews discussing statin myopathies cite a 2–7% incidence of myalgias, 0.1–1.0% incidence of weakness or elevated CK, and myoglobinuria developing in <0.5% of patients.[1,43,46–49] The National Heart Lung and Blood Institute advisory panel estimated the incidence of severe myopathy to be approximately 0.08% for lovastatin, simvastatin, and pravastatin.[44] The risk of toxic myopathy increases with the concomitant use of fibric acids,[18,19,27,31,32,40] niacin,[31,32] cyclosporine,[18,19] ezetimibe,[33–36] triazole antibiotics,[50] rapamycin,[51] and sirolimus[48] as well as in the presence of renal insufficiency or hepatobiliary dysfunction. In this regard, 5% of patients taking both lovastatin and gemfibrozil developed a severe myopathy,[27] while a severe myopathy complicated as many as 30% of patients receiving both lovastatin and cyclosporine.[13,18,19]

Most patients with a statin myopathy improve within a few weeks of stopping the agent. One dilemma we face is if patients who exhibited symptoms or signs of statin-intolerance might be rechallenged once the muscle symptoms have resolved. In one study of 51 patients, who previously experienced myalgias or elevated transaminase levels on a variety of different statins, 37 (72.5%) were able to tolerate every other day rosuvastatin.[52]

Although the term "myositis" has been used to denote cases associated with markedly elevated serum CK levels, histopathological confirmation is lacking in most cases. "Myositis" denotes an autoimmune attack on muscle. True cases of myositis, particularly dermatomyositis, have been described in association with statin use.[17,53–60] More recently, an immune-mediated necrotizing myopathy has been reported to occur in the setting of statin use (discussed in greater detail in Chapter 33).[49,61–64] In these cases weakness continues to progress despite discontinuation of the statin, and only improves if the patients are treated with immunosuppressive agents. Furthermore, disease activity often flares, if the immunosuppressive medications are discontinued.

▶ TABLE 35-1. **TOXIC MYOPATHIES**

Pathogenic Classification	Drug	Clinical Features	Laboratory Features	Histopathology
Necrotizing myopathy	Cholesterol-lowering agents Cyclosporine Labetalol Propofol Alcohol	Acute or insidious onset Proximal weakness Myalgias	Elevated serum CK EMG: fibs, PSWs, myotonia (statins, cyclosporine), myopathic MUAPs	Many necrotic muscle fibers No evidence of endomysial inflammatory cell infiltrate invading non-necrotic muscle fibers
Amphiphilic	Chloroquine Hydroxychloro-quine Amiodarone	Acute or insidious onset Proximal and distal weakness Myalgias Sensorimotor neuropathy Hypothyroid (amiodarone)	Elevated serum CK EMG: fibs, PSWs, myotonia (choroquine), myopathic MUAPs NCS: axonal sensorimotor neuropathy	Autophagic vacuoles and inclusions are apparent in some muscle fibers and in Schwann cells
Antimicrotubular	Colchicine Vincristine	Acute or insidious onset Proximal and distal weakness Myalgias Sensorimotor neuropathy	Normal or elevated CK EMG: fibs, PSWs, myotonia (colchicine), myopathic MUAPs NCS: axonal sensorimotor neuropathy	Autophagic vacuoles and inclusions are evident in some muscle fibers Nerve biopsies demonstrate axonal degeneration
Mitochondrial myopathy	Zidovudine Other HIV-related antiretrovirals?	Acute or insidious onset Proximal weakness Myalgias Rhabdomyolysis Painful sensory neuropathy	Normal or elevated CK EMG: normal or myopathic NCS: axonal sensory neuropathy/ neuronopathy	Muscle biopsies reveal ragged red fibers, COX-negative fibers May also see inflammatory cell infiltrates, cytoplasmic bodies, nemaline rods
Inflammatory myopathy	L-tryptophan D-penicillamine Cimetidine L-Dopa Phenytoin Lamotrigine Alpha-interferon Tumor necrosis alpha blockers Hydroxyurea Imatinib	Acute or insidious onset Proximal weakness Myalgias	Elevated serum CK EMG: fibs, PSWs, myopathic MUAPs	Perivascular, perimysial, or endomysial inflammatory cell infiltrates
Hypokalemic myopathy	Diuretics Laxatives Amphotericin Toluene abuse Licorice Corticosteroids Alcohol abuse	Acute proximal or generalized weakness Myalgias	Serum CK may be elevated Low serum potassium	May see scattered necrotic fibers and vacuoles
Critical illness myopathy	Corticosteroids Nondepolarizing neuromuscular blocking agents	Acute generalized weakness including respiratory muscles	Serum CK can be normal or elevated NCS: low amplitude CMAPs with relatively normal SNAPs EMG: fibs, PSWs, myopathic MUAPs or no voluntary MUAPs	Atrophy of muscle fibers, scattered necrotic fibers; absence of myosin thick filaments
Unknown	Omeprazole	Acute or insidious onset Proximal weakness Myalgias Sensorimotor neuropathy	Normal or slightly elevated serum CK EMG: myopathic MUAPs NCS: axonal sensorimotor neuropathy	Type II muscle fiber atrophy may be seen
	Isotretinoin	Acute or insidious onset Proximal weakness Myalgias	Normal or elevated CK	Atrophy of fibers
	Finasteride	Proximal weakness and atrophy	Serum CK is normal EMG: myopathic MUAPs	Variability in fiber size, type II fiber atrophy, increased internalized nuclei
	Emetine	Acute or insidious onset Proximal weakness Myalgias	Serum CKs mild to moderately elevated	Myofibrillar myopathy

Modified with permission from Amato AA, Dumitru D. Acquired myopathies. In: Dumitru D, Amato AA, Zwarts MJ, eds. *Electrodiagnostic Medicine*. 2nd ed. Philadelphia, PA: Hanley & Belfus, Inc.; 2002:1371–1432.

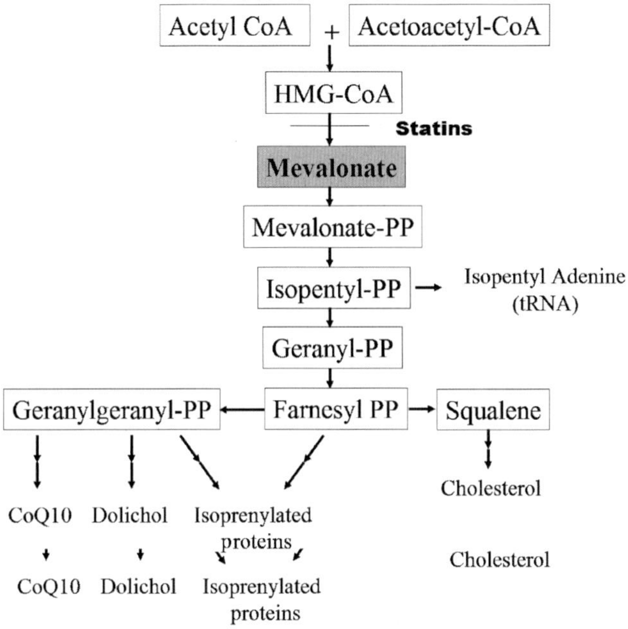

Figure 35-1. Hydroxy-3methyl-glutaryl-coenzyme A pathway. (Reproduced with permission from Greenberg SA, Amato AA. Statin myopathies. *Continuum*. 2006;12(3):169–184.)

Laboratory Features

Asymptomatic elevation of serum CK is common in patients taking statin medications. Marked elevations of CK occur in patients with severe weakness and myoglobinuria. Routine motor and sensory nerve conduction studies (NCS) are normal. Fibrillation potentials, positive sharp waves, and myotonic discharges with early recruitment of small-duration motor unit action potentials (MUAPs) are apparent in weak muscles.[65] Electromyography (EMG) in patients with asymptomatic serum CK elevations is often normal.

Interestingly, autoantibodies directed against HMG-CoA reductase have been reported in cases of statin-associated immune-mediated necrotizing myopathies.[61,62] These antibodies are not usually seen in patients who just take statin medications or those that have the more typical statin myotoxicity that resolves upon discontinuation of the offending medication.

Histopathology

Muscle biopsies reveal muscle fiber necrosis with phagocytosis and small regenerating fibers in patients with elevated serum CKs and weakness or myalgias (Fig. 35-2). Lipid-filled vacuoles within myofibers and cytochrome oxidase–negative myofibers may be appreciated, but these are not consistent findings.[66] Patients with statin-induced necrotizing myopathy often have increased expression of major histocompatibility antigen 1 (MHC1) and membrane attack complex deposition on the sarcolemma of non-necrotic muscle fibers.[61–64]

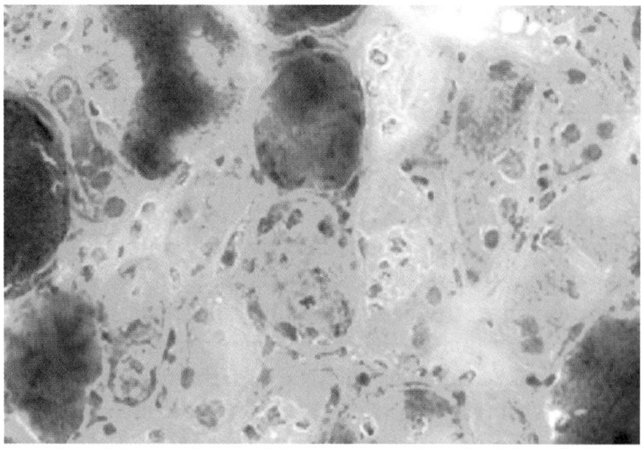

Figure 35-2. Statin myopathy. Muscle biopsy demonstrates scattered necrotic muscle fibers. Modified Gomori trichrome.

Pathogenesis

The pathogenesis of the myopathy secondary to HMG-CoA reductase inhibitors is unclear, as several pathways may potentially be interrupted downstream (Fig. 35-1).[1,49,67] Mevalonate is the immediate product of HMG-CoA reductase metabolism. Subsequently, mevalonate is metabolized to farnesol, which is converted to either squalene or geranylgeraniol. Squalene is the first metabolite committed to the synthesis of cholesterol. In contrast, geranylgeraniol is important in the biosynthesis of coenzyme Q_{10} [a mitochondrial enzyme important in the production of adenosine triphosphate (ATP)], dolichol (important in glycoprotein synthesis), and isopentylamine (a component of tRNA), and in the activation of regulatory proteins (G-proteins). It is possible that statins could diminish cholesterol within muscle membranes, thereby predisposing the muscle fibers to rhabdomyolysis. However, the depletion of metabolites of geranylgeraniol, and not the inhibition of cholesterol synthesis, may be the primary cause of myotoxicity. In this regard, HMG-CoA reductase inhibitors decrease the levels of coenzyme Q, which could impair energy production.

A couple genome-wide association study conducted in patients with suspected statin-induced toxic myopathy revealed a strong association of myopathy with a single nucleotide polymorphism (SNP), rs4363657, located within the *SLCO1B1* gene on chromosome 12.[68] This gene encodes a protein that regulates the hepatic uptake of statins. Of note, more than 60% statin myopathy patients carried this SNP. No SNPs in any other region were clearly associated with myopathy, including those genes associated with metabolic myopathies.

There are several reports of patients treated with statins who developed dermatomyositis[55–57,59,60] or polymyositis.[17,53,54,58] The most common myositis that we and others have seen in patients on a statin medication is a necrotizing myopathy.[61–64] Unlike polymyositis, muscle biopsies in these cases many necrotic fibers without much in the way of endomysial inflammation, except around and within the necrotic fibers. In many instances, the myositis does not improve following discontinuation of the statin medication (after 6 months or more) and only improves after treatment with an immunosuppressant medication. In addition, the myopathy may worsen after discontinuation of the immunosuppressant agent and improve once again upon reinstituting immunotherapy. In addition, as noted previously, autoantibodies directed against the HMG-CoA reductase have been reported in these cases of statin-associated necrotizing myopathies.[61,62] These features suggest that these rare cases of necrotizing myopathy do not represent a "toxic" myopathy per se, but a distinct immune-mediated process.

FIBRIC ACID DERIVATIVES

Clinical Features

Clofibrate and gemfibrozil are branched-chain fatty acid esters, which are used to treat hyperlipidemia. These fibric acid derivatives can cause a myopathy that typically presents within 2 or 3 months after starting the drug.[16,20–30,40] However, the toxic myopathy may develop up to 2 years following initiation of treatment. Affected individuals complain of generalized weakness, myalgias, and cramps. Myoglobinuria is also a rare complication. Patients with renal insufficiency, those taking both clofibrate and gemfibrozil, and especially also those receiving an HMG-CoA inhibitor, are particularly at increased risk of developing myotoxicity.

Laboratory Features

Elevated serum CK levels are usually noted. Motor and sensory NCS are normal.[22,24,28] Needle EMG may demonstrate fibrillation potentials, positive sharp waves, complex repetitive discharges, myotonic discharges, and short-duration, small-amplitude polyphasic MUAPs in affected muscle groups.[20,21,25,29,69]

Histopathology

Muscle biopsies demonstrate scattered necrotic muscle fibers. In animal models, clofibrate is also known to result in noninflammatory necrosis of muscle tissue with fiber size variation and groups of small atrophic muscle fibers.[70]

Pathogenesis

The pathogenic mechanism of the myopathy associated with fibric acid derivatives is not known. These medications might somehow destabilize the lipophilic muscle membrane leading to muscle fiber degeneration.[27]

NIACIN

Rarely, niacin use is complicated by myalgias and cramps.[31] Serum CK levels can be elevated as much as 10-fold. The symptoms improve and CK levels normalize after discontinuation of niacin. Electrodiagnostic studies and muscle biopsies have not been reported in detail. In most cases, rhabdomyolysis occurred in patients who were also taking a statin agent.[31] Of note, niacin can inhibit HMG-CoA reductase; therefore, the pathogenic mechanism of the myopathy is likely similar to that of the statins.

EZETIMIBE

Ezetimibe selectively inhibits the absorption of intestinal cholesterol. There are a few reports of ezetimibe-induced myopathy.[33,36,71] Similar to other cholesterol-lowering agents, patients may develop hyper-CK-emia with or without myalgias or weakness. Most cases occur in patients who are already on a statin agent, but some occur with Ezetimibe monotherapy. The toxic myopathy usually resolves within a few weeks after the medication is discontinued. However, we have also seen rare cases of what appear to be an immune-mediated necrotizing myopathy as discussed in the statin section in which the myopathy improved only after the affected patients were treated with immunosuppressive agents.

USE OF CHOLESTEROL-LOWERING AGENTS IN PATIENTS WITH KNOWN MYOPATHIES

A common question posed to neuromuscular specialists is if patients with known myopathies (e.g., muscular dystrophy, metabolic myopathies, polymyositis) can be treated with cholesterol-lowering agents to control their hypercholesterolemia. There is very little evidence that there is increased risk of statin-induced myotoxicity in patients with an underlying myopathy (aside from those that have the rare statin-induced immune-mediated necrotizing myopathy). Furthermore, there is no strong evidence that statin medications (or other lipid-lowering agents) can exacerbate any underlying myopathy. Given the well-known benefits of statins in patients at risk for cardiovascular disease and lack of any strong evidence of increased risk of these medications in patients with underlying myopathy, we again see no contraindication to their use in most patients. We do tend to follow them closer and periodically check their CK levels.

CYCLOSPORINE AND TACROLIMUS

Clinical Features

The immunophilins (i.e., cyclosporine and tacrolimus) are commonly used as immunosuppressive agents, especially in patients requiring transplantation.[72] Rarely, generalized myalgias and proximal muscle weakness develop within months after starting these medications.[72–77] Myoglobinuria can also occur, particularly in patients receiving cyclosporine or tacrolimus concurrent with cholesterol-lowering agents or colchicine.[18,19,78–81] Tacrolimus has also been associated with hypertrophic cardiomyopathy and congestive heart failure.[82] Myalgias, muscle strength, and cardiac function improve with reduction or discontinuation of the offending cyclophilin.

Laboratory Features

Serum CK is usually elevated. NCS are normal. EMG often reveals increased muscle membrane instability with fibrillation potentials, positive sharp waves, and myotonic potentials.[74] Early recruitment of small-amplitude, short-duration MUAPs may be demonstrated in weak muscle groups.

Histopathology

Muscle biopsies demonstrate necrosis, vacuoles, and type 2 muscle fiber atrophy.

Pathogenesis

The pathogenic basis of immunophilin-induced myopathy and cardiomyopathy is not known. Perhaps, the agents destabilize the lipophilic muscle membrane leading to muscle fiber degeneration, similar to the cholesterol-lowering agents. In this regard, cyclosporine itself has a cholesterol-lowering effect. This may explain the increased risk of myopathy in patients receiving cyclosporine and the more classic lipid-lowering agents (e.g., fibric acid derivatives and statins).

LABETALOL

Clinical Features

There are a few reports of necrotizing myopathy associated with the use of the antihypertensive agent, labetalol.[83,84] Patients can develop acute or insidious onset of proximal weakness or myalgias, which resolve following discontinuation of the medication.

Laboratory Features

Serum CK can be markedly elevated. EMG may demonstrate increased insertional and spontaneous activity with fibrillation potentials and positive sharp waves. Short-duration, small-amplitude, polyphasic MUAPs, which recruit early, are evident.

Histopathology

Routine light microscopy can be normal[83] or can reveal necrotic and regenerating fibers.[84] Electron microscopy (EM) revealed subsarcolemmal vacuoles in one case.[83]

Pathogenesis

The pathogenic etiology for the muscle necrosis seen is not known.

PROPOFOL

Clinical Features

Propofol is an anesthetic agent that is frequently used for sedating patients who are mechanically ventilated and sometimes for the treatment of status epilepticus. Myoglobinuria, metabolic acidosis, hypoxia, and myocardial arrest are rare adverse events associated with the use of propofol.[85–87] Propofol does not appear to be associated with malignant hyperthermia. Acute quadriplegic myopathy (AQM) in the intensive care unit (ICU) has also developed in patients treated with propofol in combination with high-dose intravenous corticosteroids.[88] The myopathy in these individuals could be explained by the high-dose corticosteroids rather than the use of propofol. It remains to be determined if propofol is an independent risk factor for the development of AQM.

Laboratory Features

Serum CK levels are markedly elevated. Electrophysiologic studies have not been performed or were not reported in the cases associated with rhabdomyolysis in children. The adult patients with AQM have low-amplitude compound muscle action potentials (CMAPs), profuse fibrillation potentials, positive sharp waves, and early recruitment of short-duration, small-amplitude polyphasic MUAPs.[88]

Histopathology

Muscle biopsies reveal necrosis of skeletal and cardiac muscle.[85–87] Patients with AQM, may have prominent necrosis and loss of thick filaments.[88]

Pathogenesis

The mechanism for muscle destruction is unknown.

Treatment

Propofol should be discontinued and supportive therapy instituted for myoglobinuria, metabolic acidosis, hyperkalemia, and renal failure.

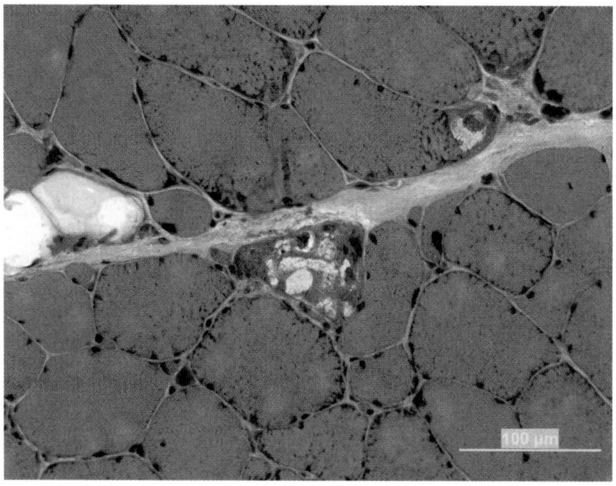

A

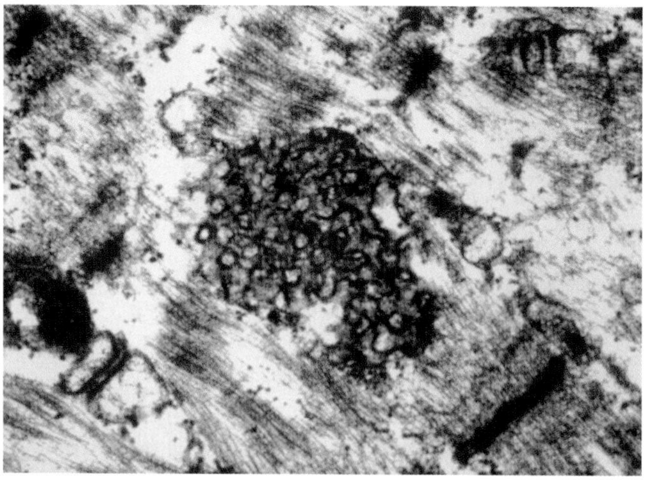

B

Figure 35-3. Chloroquine myopathy. Chloroquine can cause a vacuolar myopathy **(A)**, hematoxylin and eosin (H&E). Electron microscopy reveals a bundle of dilated tubules **(B)**. (Reproduced with permission from Wasay M, Wolfe GI, Herrold JM, Burns DK, Barohn RJ. Chloroquine myopathy and neuropathy with elevated CSF protein. *Neurology.* 1998;51(4):1226–1227.)

AMPHIPHILIC DRUG MYOPATHY (DRUG-INDUCED AUTOPHAGIC LYSOSOMAL MYOPATHY)

Amphiphilic drugs contain separate hydrophobic and hydrophilic regions, which allow the drugs to interact with the anionic phospholipids of cell membranes and organelles. In addition to a myopathy, these agents can also cause a toxic neuropathy that is even more severe than the direct toxicity on muscle.

CHLOROQUINE

Clinical Features

Chloroquine, a quinoline derivative, is used to treat malaria, sarcoidosis, systemic lupus erythematosus (SLE), and other connective tissue diseases.[7,8,89–92] Some patients develop slowly progressive, painless, proximal weakness and atrophy, which affect the legs more than the arms. A cardiomyopathy can also occur. Sensation is often reduced as are muscle stretch reflexes, particularly at the ankles, secondary to a concomitant neuropathy. This "neuromyopathy" usually does not occur unless patients take 500 mg a day for a year or more but has been reported with doses as low as 200 mg/day. The neuromyopathy improves after chloroquine discontinuation.

Laboratory Features

Serum CK levels are usually elevated. Motor and sensory NCS reveal mild-to-moderate reduction in the amplitudes with slightly slow velocities in patients with a superimposed neuropathy.[90,92] Individuals with only the myopathy usually have normal motor and sensory studies.[89] Increased insertional activity in the form of positive sharp waves, fibrillation potentials, and myotonic discharges are seen primarily, but not exclusively, in the proximal limb muscles.[89,90,92] Early recruitment of small-amplitude, short duration polyphasic MUAPs are appreciated in weak proximal muscles. Neurogenic appearing units and reduced recruitment may be seen in distal muscles that are more affected by the toxic neuropathy.

Histopathology

Autophagic vacuoles are evident in as many as 50% of skeletal and cardiac muscle fibers (Fig. 35-3).[7,8,89,91,92] Type 1 fibers appear to be preferentially affected. The vacuoles stain positive for acid phosphatase, suggesting lysosomal origin. On EM, the vacuoles are noted to contain concentric lamellar myeloid debris and curvilinear structures. Autophagic vacuoles are also evident in nerve biopsies.

Pathogenesis

Chloroquine is believed to interact with lipid membranes, forming drug–lipid complexes that are resistant to digestion by lysosomal enzymes. This results in the formation of the autophagic vacuoles filled with myeloid debris.

HYDROXYCHLOROQUINE

Hydroxychloroquine is structurally similar to chloroquine and can cause a neuromyopathy.[90] The myopathy is usually not as severe as seen in chloroquine. Vacuoles are less appreciated on routine light microscopy, but EM still usually demonstrates the abnormal accumulation of myeloid and curvilinear bodies.

AMIODARONE

Clinical Features

Amiodarone is an antiarrhythmic medication that can also cause a neuromyopathy.[93–97] The neuromyopathy is characterized by severe proximal and distal weakness along with distal sensory loss and reduced muscle stretch reflexes. The legs are more affected than the arms. Some patients develop tremor or ataxia. Amiodarone can also cause hypothyroidism, which may also contribute to proximal weakness. Patients with renal insufficiency are predisposed to developing the toxic neuromyopathy. Muscle strength gradually improves following discontinuation of amiodarone.

Laboratory Features

Serum CK levels are elevated. Motor and sensory NCS reveal reduced amplitudes and slow conduction velocities, particularly in the lower extremities.[96,97] EMG demonstrates fibrillation potentials and positive sharp waves in proximal and distal muscles. In proximal muscles, MUAPs are typically polyphasic, short in duration, small in amplitude, and recruit early. Distal muscles are more likely to have large-amplitude, long-duration polyphasic MUAPs with decreased recruitment.

Histopathology

Muscle biopsies demonstrate scattered fibers with autophagic vacuoles. In addition, neurogenic atrophy can also be appreciated, particularly in distal muscles. EM reveals myofibrillar disorganization and autophagic vacuoles filled with myeloid debris. Myeloid inclusions are also apparent on nerve biopsies. These lipid membrane inclusions may be evident in muscle and nerve biopsies as long as 2 years following discontinuation of amiodarone.

Pathogenesis

The pathogenesis is presumably similar to other amphiphilic medications (e.g., chloroquine).

▶ ANTIMICROTUBULAR MYOPATHIES

COLCHICINE

Clinical Features

Colchicine is commonly prescribed for individuals with gout. Colchicine can also cause a generalized toxic neuromyopathy. It is weakly amphiphilic, but its toxic effect is believed to arise secondary to its binding with tubulin and prevention of tubulin's polymerization into microtubular structures.[5,8,9] The neuromyopathy usually develops after chronic administration, but it can also develop secondary to acute intoxication.[5,98–100] Chronic renal failure and age over 50 years are risk factors for the development of neuromyopathy. Patients usually manifest with progressive proximal muscle weakness over several months. Clinical myotonia has been described.[101] A superimposed toxic neuropathy leads to distal sensory loss as well as diminished reflexes. The neuromyopathy weakness typically resolves within 4–6 months after discontinuing the colchicine.

Laboratory Features

Serum CK level is elevated up to 50-fold in symptomatic patients. Serum CK may also be mildly elevated in asymptomatic patients taking colchicine. NCS reveal reduced amplitudes, slightly prolonged latencies, and mildly slow conduction velocities of motor and sensory nerves in the arms and legs.[98–100,102] Needle EMG demonstrates positive sharp waves, fibrillation potentials, and complex repetitive discharges, which are detected with ease in all muscle regions. Myotonic discharges may also be seen.[101] The myopathic MUAP abnormalities can be masked in the distal limb muscles secondary to the superimposed peripheral neuropathy.

Histopathology

Muscle biopsy demonstrates acid phosphatase–positive autophagic vacuoles containing membranous debris (Fig. 35-4). In addition, nerve biopsies can reveal evidence suggestive of a mild axonal neuropathy.

Pathogenesis

The abnormal assembly of microtubules most likely disrupts intracellular movement or localization of lysosomes, leading to the accumulation of autophagic vacuoles.[99]

VINCRISTINE

Clinical Features

Vincristine is a chemotherapeutic agent, which disrupts gene transcription and also promotes the polymerization of tubulin into microtubules.[8] The dose limiting side effect of vincristine is a toxic axonal sensorimotor polyneuropathy that is associated with distal muscle weakness and sensory loss. Proximal muscle weakness and myalgias are less common.[103]

Laboratory Features

Serum CK levels have not been reported in patients suspected of having a superimposed myopathy. NCS demonstrate markedly reduced amplitudes of SNAPs and CMAPs, while the distal latencies are slightly prolonged, and conduction velocities are mildly slow.[103] Needle EMG demonstrates positive sharp waves, fibrillation potentials, and neurogenic appearing MUAPs in the distally located muscles of the upper and lower extremities.

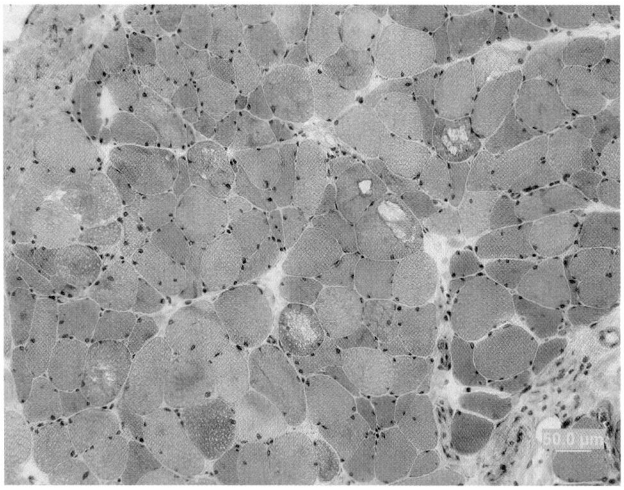

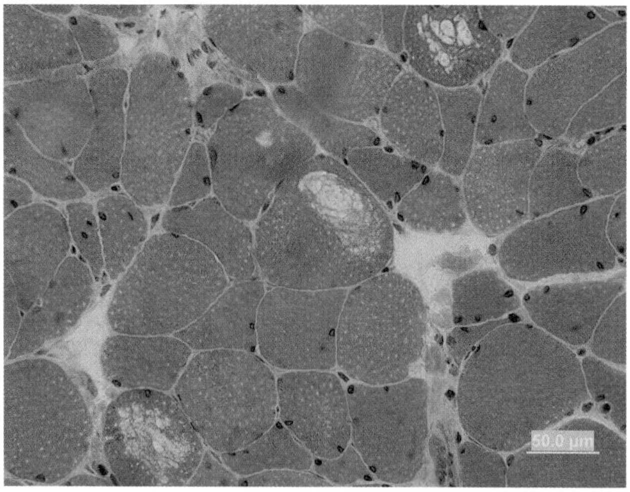

A B

Figure 35-4. Colchicine myopathy. Colchicine can cause a vacuolar myopathy as evident on modified Gomori trichrome stain **(A)** and hematoxylin and eosin stain **(B)**.

Histopathology

Biopsies of distal muscles demonstrate evidence of neurogenic atrophy and, occasionally, the accumulation of lipofuscin granules. Proximal muscle biopsies reveal scattered necrotic fibers.[103] On EM, there is prominent myofibrillar disarray and subsarcolemmal accumulation of osmiophilic material. In addition, some myonuclei contain membrane-bound inclusions. Autophagic vacuoles with spheromembranous debris have been noted in research animals[104,105] but have not been appreciated in humans.[103]

Pathogenesis

The pathogenic basis of the neuromyopathy is presumably similar to that of colchicine.

▶ DRUG-INDUCED MITOCHONDRIAL MYOPATHY

ZIDOVUDINE (AZIDOTHYMIDINE)

Clinical Features

Patients with azidothymidine (AZT) myopathy usually present with an insidious onset of progressive proximal muscle weakness and myalgias.[106–116] However, these clinical features do not help in distinguishing AZT myopathy from other HIV-related myopathies. Other myopathies related to HIV infection are heterogeneous and include inflammatory myopathy, microvasculitis, noninflammatory necrotizing myopathy, and type 2 muscle fiber atrophy secondary to disuse or wasting due to their chronic debilitated state.[107,110–112,114–124] Furthermore, weakness in an HIV-infected patient can also be secondary to peripheral neuropathy (e.g., chronic inflammatory demyelinating polyneuropathy) or myasthenia gravis. Clinically, AZT myopathy and the other myopathic disorders associated with HIV infection are indistinguishable, compounding the diagnostic difficulty. Regardless of etiology of the myopathy, patients manifest with progressive proximal muscle weakness and myalgias. In addition, muscle weakness may be multifactorial.

Laboratory Features

Serum CK levels are normal or only mildly elevated in AZT myopathy. However, similar elevations are evident in other forms of HIV-related myopathy. An elevated serum CK (e.g., greater than five times the upper limited of normal) is more suggestive of an HIV-associated myositis. Motor and sensory NCS are normal, unless there is a concomitant peripheral neuropathy. Needle EMG may demonstrate positive sharp waves and fibrillation potentials and early recruitment of short-duration, small-amplitude polyphasic MUAPs.[114,119,122,125] In addition, small polyphasic MUAPs with early recruitment but no abnormal spontaneous activity was reported in patients with AIDS, along with ultrastructural mitochondrial abnormalities but no inflammation or nemaline rods on biopsy.[112]

Histopathology

Muscle biopsies are remarkable for the presence of ragged red fibers, suggesting mitochondrial abnormalities in AZT myopathy (Fig. 35-5). The number of ragged red fibers correlates with the cumulative dose of AZT.[110,111] In addition, necrotic fibers, cytoplasmic bodies, nemaline rods, and fibers with microvacuolation may be seen in addition to ragged red fibers.[107,110,111] In contrast to HIV-associated inflammatory myopathy, significant endomysial inflammation with or

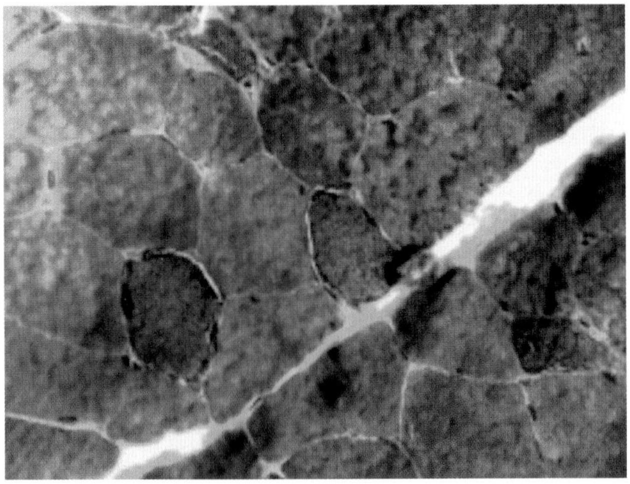

Figure 35-5. Azidothymidine myopathy. Ragged red fibers suggestive of abnormal mitochondria are evident on modified Gomori trichrome stain.

without invasion of non-necrotic fibers should not be present in cases of pure AZT myopathy. EM reveals abnormalities of the mitochondria and myofilaments.

Pathogenesis

AZT acts as a false substitute for the viral reverse transcriptase, thereby inhibiting its enzymatic activity and replication of the HIV virus. However, AZT also inhibits the activity of mitochondrial DNA polymerase, which probably accounts for the mitochondrial abnormalities. When treated with AZT, patients with HIV have a decrease in quantity of mitochondrial DNA and decline in respiratory chain enzymatic activity, compared to untreated infected patients.[121,126] The histological and molecular abnormalities on repeated muscle biopsies resolve coinciding with clinical improvement following discontinuation of AZT.[127] Although, AZT is responsible for at least some of the mitochondrial abnormalities evident on muscle biopsy, the contribution of these mitochondrial abnormalities to the muscle weakness remains controversial.

Treatment

In the past, anywhere from 18% to 100% of patients with "AZT" myopathy improved following discontinuation of the medication.[107,110,112,114,116,119,120,128] AZT is not used as much anymore as other antiviral agents are typical used nowadays in the treatment of HIV (see below).

OTHER ANTIVIRAL AGENTS

The risk of mitochondrial myopathy with other nucleoside reverse transcriptase inhibitors (e.g., lamivudine), zalcitabine, didanosine is probably less than that of AZT.[129,130] However, these agents are clearly associated with mitochondrial toxicity, and patients may develop associated hyperlactemia and hepatic steatosis on these medications. The AIDS Clinical Trial group randomized 2,467 patients to receive one of four single or combination regimens with AZT, didanosine, zalcitabine, and their respective placebo.[123] Approximately 10% of patients had myalgias prior to treatment and 7% developed myalgia during treatment. There was no significant difference between treatment arms and the rate of myalgia or muscle weakness in any group. Five patients (0.5%) had elevated serum CK (>4× normal) prior to treatment, and 52 (5%) developed increased CK during treatment. Serum CK levels were significantly higher in the AZT-zalcitabine group, but this did not correlate with symptoms of myopathy. Unfortunately, there was no comment on muscle biopsies, and thus it is unclear if the myopathies were secondary to mitochondrial toxicity or myositis.

The main treatment of HIV infection currently is with highly active antiretroviral therapy (HAART) consisting of a combination of nucleoside reverse transcriptase inhibitors and protease inhibitors. Rare cases of rhabdomyolysis and myoglobinuria occur in patients taking other HAART medications including tenofovir[131] and ritonavir.[132] A review of 563 patients between 1995 and 1998 demonstrated a prevalence of "HIV-associated myopathy" in 1.5% of patients treated with HAART.[91] It was not clearly stated how the myopathy was defined (e.g., clinical symptoms or signs, elevated serum CK, EMG, or biopsy). Further, it is unclear if the myopathy was felt to be due to mitochondrial toxicity, myositis, or wasting syndrome.

▶ DRUG-INDUCED INFLAMMATORY MYOPATHIES

CHOLESTEROL-LOWERING AGENTS

As discussed in the Necrotizing Myopathies section, dermatomyositis, polymyositis, and in particular, an immune-mediated necrotizing myopathy rarely occur in patients taking statin medications and occasionally the other cholesterol lowering agents.[61–64] These inflammatory myopathies do not improve with the discontinuation of the cholesterol-lowering agent. Rather, patients need to be treated with immunotherapy.

L-TRYPTOPHAN/EOSINOPHILIA–MYALGIA SYNDROME

Clinical Features

Eosinophilia–myalgia syndrome was described in the late 1980s and early 1990s and was found to be caused by a contaminant used in the production of L-tryptophan.[133–139] The clinical, laboratory, electrophysiological, and histopathological features were similar to that seen in diffuse fasciitis with eosinophilia (Shulman syndrome).[140] Patients developed a subacute onset of generalized muscle pain and tenderness with variable degrees of weakness. Onset could have been within a few weeks or after several years of starting tryptophan. Numbness, paresthesias, arthralgias, lymphadenopathy, dyspnea, abdominal pain, mucocutaneous ulcers, and an erythematous rash were also common. Some patients developed a severe generalized sensorimotor polyneuropathy mimicking Guillain–Barré syndrome[138,141] or multiple mononeuropathies suggestive of a vasculitis.[142]

Laboratory Features

Serum CK level are normal or elevated. Autoantibodies are absent and ESR is usually normal. The absolute eosinophil count was elevated ($>1 \times 10^9$ cells/L). Decreased amplitudes of compound muscle and sensory nerve action potentials (SNAPs) with normal or mildly reduced conduction velocities are evident in patients with a polyneuropathy.[138,143] A few patients with severe Guillain–Barré syndrome had electrophysiologic studies showing multifocal conduction block and slowing of conduction velocities.[141] Needle EMG revealed muscle membrane instability in the form of fibrillation potentials, positive sharp waves, and complex repetitive discharges.[136,138,141] Small and large polyphasic MUAPs with early recruitment are seen as a result of the chronic myopathy.[136,138] Large polyphasic MUAPs with decreased recruitment are seen in patients with severe neuropathy.[138] The electrophysiological abnormalities improve with discontinuation of tryptophan.

Histopathology

Muscle biopsies demonstrated diffuse or perivascular inflammatory infiltrate in the fascia, perimysium, and, to a lesser extent, in the endomysium.[138] The majority of inflammatory cells are CD8+ T cells and macrophages, while eosinophils and B cells comprised <3% of the infiltrating cells. Unlike DM, there is no deposition of membrane attack complex on small blood vessels. Nerve biopsies show predominately perivascular inflammatory infiltrates, mainly mononuclear, with occasional eosinophils in the epineurium, endoneurium, and/or perineurium with axonal degeneration.[136,138,141,143,144]

Pathogenesis

The disorder was caused by a contaminant(s) in the manufacture of tryptophan. Two trace adulterants have been identified as the possible toxins: 3-phenylaminoalanine and 1,1′-ethylidenebis tryptophan.[145] The mechanism by which this contaminant resulted in the disorder is unknown, but the eosinophilia and eosinophilic infiltrate in tissues suggest some form of allergic reaction.

Treatment

Discontinuation of L-tryptophan and treatment with high-dose corticosteroids were usually effective in the prior epidemic. Some patients experienced relapses upon withdrawal of steroids.

TOXIC OIL SYNDROME

The toxic oil syndrome occurred as a single epidemic in Spain and has not recurred since 1981. It was quite similar to the eosinophilia–myalgia syndrome associated with tryptophan.[146] The disorder was linked to the ingestion of illegally marked, denatured rapeseed oil as a cooking substitute for olive oil. Interestingly, the toxic contaminant in the rapeseed oil, 3-phenylamino-1, 2-propanediol, is chemically similar to 3-phenylaminoalanine, the presumed adulterant in tryptophan causing the eosinophilia–myalgia syndrome.[145]

D-PENICILLAMINE

D-Penicillamine is rarely used nowadays to treat Wilson disease, rheumatoid arthritis (RA), and other connective tissue disorders. Approximately 0.2–1.4% of patients treated with D-penicillamine developed an inflammatory myopathy reminiscent of polymyositis or dermatomyositis.[147–150] It has also been associated with myasthenia. Discontinuation of the drug results in resolution of the symptoms. The medication may be restarted at a lower dosage without recurrence of the inflammatory myopathy.

CIMETIDINE

Rare cases of inflammatory myopathy have been reported with cimetidine, a histamine H_2 receptor antagonist.[151] One patient developed generalized weakness and myalgias associated with CK elevations up to 40,000 U/L and interstitial nephritis. The muscle biopsy revealed perivascular inflammation, predominantly consisting of CD8+ lymphocytes. No deposition of immunoglobulin or complement on small blood vessels was noted, nor did the patients have a cutaneous rash to suggest dermatomyositis. However, cases of cutaneous vasculitis have been described with cimetidine use.[152]

PROCAINAMIDE

Proximal muscle weakness and myalgias rarely occur with procainamide usage.[41,153] Serum CK levels are elevated, and EMG has been reported as being consistent with a "patchy" myopathy. Muscle biopsies demonstrate perivascular inflammation and rare necrotic muscle fibers. The pathogenesis may be related to lupus-like vasculitis, which can occur in patients treated with procainamide. The myopathy resolves following withdrawal of procainamide.

L-DOPA

A single case of proximal muscle weakness and myalgias has been reported in a patient with Parkinson disease treated with L-Dopa.[154] The patient developed the muscle symptoms after treatment with L-Dopa for over 4 years. The serum CK was elevated 10-fold. Gastrocnemius and quadriceps muscle biopsies revealed perivascular inflammation and rare necrotic fibers. The authors suggested that the patient developed a hypersensitivity vasculitis to the L-Dopa; however, it is more likely that the myositis occurred incidentally.

PHENYTOIN

Myalgias and weakness may develop in patients treated with phenytoin due to hypersensitivity reactions.[155] Serum CK levels can be elevated, and muscle biopsies show scattered necrotic and regenerating muscle fibers. EMG can reveal increased spontaneous activity with fibrillation potentials and positive sharp waves. Small-amplitude, short-duration, polyphasic MUAPs, which recruit early may be observed. The myopathy improves with discontinuation of the phenytoin and a short course of corticosteroids.

LAMOTRIGINE

We have seen a case of severe myoglobinuria and renal failure associated with a generalized rash, anemia, leukopenia, and thrombocytopenia shortly after the patient was started on lamotrigine. The clinical and laboratory features resembled thrombocytic thrombocytopenic purpura. The patient improved with plasmapheresis and discontinuation of lamotrigine.

ALPHA-INTERFERON

Alpha-interferon is used in the treatment of viral hepatitis and certain malignancies [e.g., chronic myelogenous leukemia (CML) and melanoma]. A rare side effect of alpha-interferon is the occurrence of autoimmune disorders including myasthenia gravis and myositis.[156–158] Further, as discussed in Chapter 33, the overproduction of type 1 interferons, such as alpha-interferon, have been implicated in the pathogenesis of dermatomyositis.

TUMOR NECROSIS FACTOR-ALPHA BLOCKERS

Tumor necrosis factor alpha (TNF-α) blockers are used to treat RA, ankylosing spondylitis, and psoriatic arthritis. Side effects of TNF-α blockers include induction of other autoimmune disorders such as SLE and autoimmune neuropathies. Some patients with myositis patients treated with various TNF-α blockers improve, while others worsen.[159] In addition, there are reports of patients with previous history of myositis, who develop an inflammatory myopathy while being treated with a TNF-α blocker.[160,161]

IMATINIB MESYLATE (GLEEVEC)

Imatinib mesylate is a tyrosine kinase inhibitor used to treat patients with CML. Imatinib inhibits the tyrosine kinase activity of the BCR-ABL oncoprotein in CML. Imatinib is well tolerated, but myalgias occur in 21–52% of patients. We reported a patient with CML who developed polymyositis while taking imatinib.[162] CML28 antibodies were detected in the patient's serum. CML28 is identical to hRrp46p, a component of the human exosome, a multiprotein complex involved in processing of RNA. Antibodies directed against hRrp46p and other components of the human exosome (e.g., PM-Scl 100 and PMScl 75) have been noted in patients with polymyositis (see Chapter 33). The patient's strength and serum CK normalized with discontinuation of the imatinib and a course of corticosteroids.

Tyrosine kinases are involved in signal transduction, cell growth, and differentiation. The mechanism by which imatinib therapy could cause myositis is unclear. The previous use of an immunomodulatory agent (i.e., alpha-interferon) followed by imatinib leads to rapid apoptosis of leukemic cells. The subsequent release of a large bolus of leukemia antigens may have cross-reactivity with muscle antigens and generate an autoimmune response.

► MYOPATHIES SECONDARY TO IMPAIRED PROTEIN SYNTHESIS OR INCREASED CATABOLISM

STEROID MYOPATHY

Clinical Features

Steroid myopathy manifests as proximal muscle weakness and atrophy affecting the legs more than the arms.[163–170] The distal extremities, oculobulbar, and facial muscles are normal as are sensation and muscle stretch reflexes. Most patients exhibit a Cushingoid appearance with facial edema and increased truncal adipose tissue. Prednisone at doses of 30 mg/day or more (or equivalent doses of other corticosteroids) is associated with an increased risk of myopathy.[167] Any synthetic glucocorticoid can cause the myopathy, but those that are fluorinated (triamcinolone > betamethasone > dexamethasone) are more likely to result in muscle weakness than the nonflourinated compounds.[171] Women appear to be more at risk than men (approximately 2:1) of developing a steroid myopathy. Alternate-day dosing may reduce the risk of corticosteroid-induced weakness.

Muscle weakness can develop within several weeks following the administration of corticosteroids; however, it more commonly occurs as a complication of chronic administration of oral high–dose corticosteroids. Acute onset of severe generalized weakness can occur in patients receiving high dosages of intravenous corticosteroids with or without concomitant administration of neuromuscular blocking agents or sepsis (see section regarding Acute Quadriplegic Myopathy).

Laboratory Features

Serum CK is normal. Serum potassium can be low as a result of glucocorticoid excess and can cause some degree of weakness. Motor and sensory nerve conductions are normal in steroid myopathy.[172] Repetitive stimulation studies should not demonstrate a significant decrement or increment. Needle EMG is normal as well.

The paucity of abnormalities is understandable, as corticosteroids preferentially affect type 2 muscle fibers. The first recruited motor units are comprised of type 1 muscle fibers. Because these are not affected as severely as type 2 fibers, there is little in the way of electrophysiological abnormality to observe.

Histopathology

Muscle biopsies reveal atrophy of type 2 fibers, especially the fast-twitch, glycolytic-type 2B fibers (Fig. 35-6).[166,167,173,174] There may also be a lesser degree of atrophy of type 1 muscle fibers. Lipid droplets are commonly noted in type 1 fibers, and rare mitochondrial abnormalities have been seen on EM.

Pathogenesis

Corticosteroids bind to receptors on target cells and are subsequently internalized into the nuclei, where these regulate the transcription of specific genes. How corticosteroids cause a myopathy is not known, but could be the result of decreased protein synthesis, increased protein degradation, alterations in carbohydrate metabolism, mitochondrial alterations, or reduced sarcolemmal excitability.[166,167]

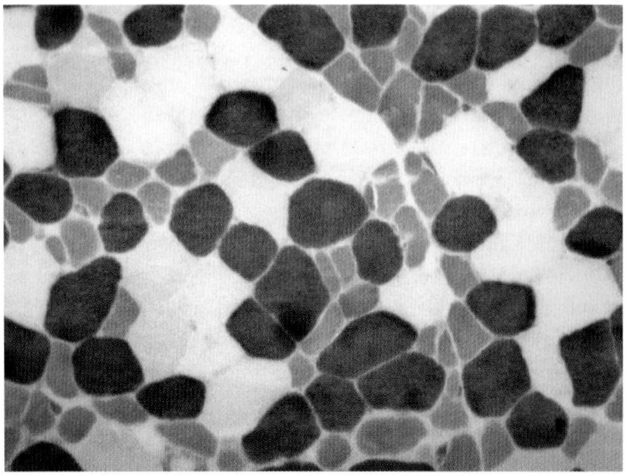

Figure 35-6. Steroid myopathy. Selective atrophy of the intermediately staining type 2B fibers is evident. ATPase pH 4.5.

Treatment

Reduction in the dose, tapering to an alternate-day regimen, or switching to a nonflourinated steroid along with a low carbohydrate diet and exercise to prevent concomitant disuse atrophy are major modes of therapy.[167,171,175]

Of particular concern is to distinguish steroid myopathy from an exacerbation of underlying immune-mediated neuromuscular disorder (e.g., inflammatory myopathy, myasthenia gravis, and chronic inflammatory demyelinating polyneuropathy) in a patient being treated with corticosteroids.[169,175–177] If the weakness occurs while the patient is tapering the corticosteroid, relapse of the underlying disease process would be most likely. In contrast, if weakness developed while the patient was on chronic high doses of steroids, a steroid myopathy should be considered. In the case of an inflammatory myopathy, an increasing serum CK and an EMG with prominent increase in insertional and spontaneous activity would point to an exacerbation of the myositis.[175] In some cases, it is impossible to state with certainty whether the new weakness is related to a relapse of the underlying disease or secondary to the corticosteroid treatment. In such cases, we taper the corticosteroid medication and closely observe the patient. If muscle strength improves presumably, the patient had a steroid myopathy. If patient's strength declines then more likely the weakness is caused by an exacerbation of the underlying autoimmune disease and requires increased doses of corticosteroids or other immunosuppressive medication.

FINASTERIDE

Clinical Features

Finasteride is used to treat benign prostatic hypertrophy. It is a 4-azasteroid that inhibits 5α-reductase, and thus blocks dihydrotestosterone production and androgen action in the prostate and skin. One patient developed severe proximal greater than distal weakness and atrophy while being treated with finasteride (5 mg qd).[178] Sensation and muscle stretch reflexes were normal.

Laboratory Features

Serum CK levels were normal.

Electrophysiological Findings

NCS were normal, while the EMG demonstrated showed small polyphasic MUAPs.

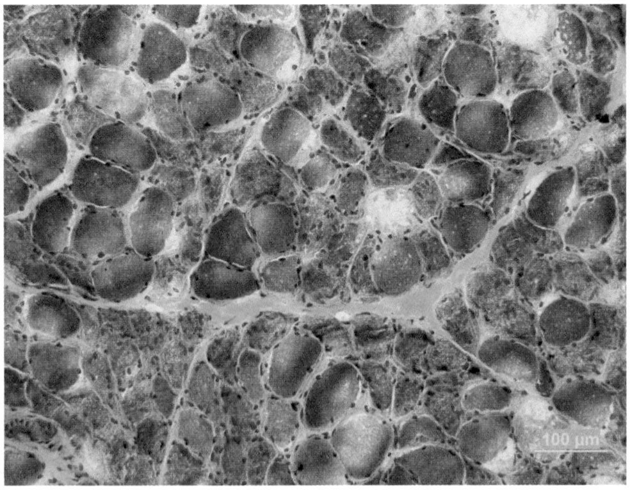

A

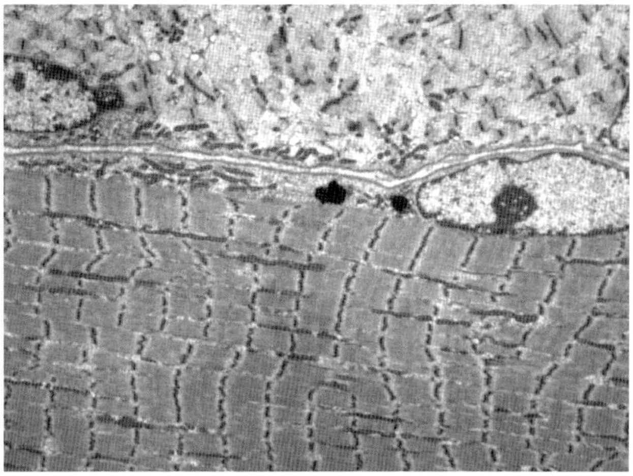

B

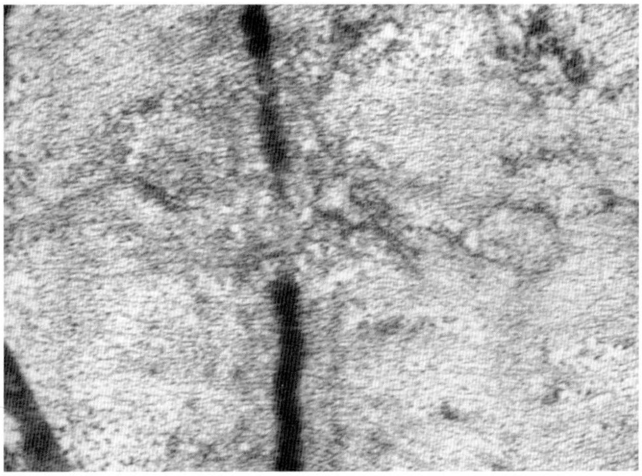

C

Figure 35-8. Critical illness/acute quadriplegic myopathy. Muscle biopsy demonstrates marked degeneration and atrophy of muscle fibers on modified Gomori trichrome **(A)**. Electron microscopy demonstrates a muscle fiber with a preserved sarcomeres adjacent to a degenerating muscle fiber **(B)**. Higher power view on EM reveals the preserved Z-disc and thin filaments but the loss of the myosin thick filaments **(C)**.

Scattered necrotic muscle fibers may be seen.[194,197,200,205,207] Focal or diffuse loss of reactivity for myosin ATPase activity in type 1 fibers more than type 2 fibers, corresponding to the loss of thick filaments (myosin) apparent on EM, is typically observed (Fig. 32-6).[187,189,190,192–194,200,205] Other structural proteins (actin, titin, and nebulin) are relatively spared.[200]

Pathogenesis

The variable laboratory, histological, and electrophysiological features suggest that the pathogenesis is multifactorial. Some biopsies demonstrate widespread necrosis, which certainly can account for the muscle weakness observed in patients. The mechanism of muscle fiber necrosis is not known, and, importantly, not all patients have this feature on biopsy. Myosin is selectively lost in some but not all patients. Calcium-activated proteases (calpains) may be responsible for proteolysis of myosin.[200] Perhaps, glucocorticoids, nondepolarizing neuromuscular agents, or the milieu of critical illness induces the expression of calpains. In addition, the enhanced expression of cytokines during sepsis may, in turn, lead to a catabolic state in muscle with breakdown of proteins, glycogen, and lipid.

The reduced muscle membrane excitability may be the result of a combination of several factors: (1) partial depolarization of the resting membrane potential, (2) reduced muscle membrane resistance, and (3) decreased sodium currents.[198,199,209,211] Denervation and neuromuscular blockade normally decrease the resting membrane muscle potential, increase membrane resistance secondary to decreased chloride conductance, and increase the number of sodium channels on the muscle membrane. In denervated rats treated with corticosteroids, the resting membrane potential does not significantly decrease but muscle membrane resistance decreases (rather than increase) as a result of increased chloride conductance. The reduced membrane resistance decreases the depolarization caused by the opening of sodium channels. In addition, there is diminished sodium current secondary to a reduction in the number of sodium channels, decreased sodium channel conductance, or impaired voltage-dependent gating.

Treatment

Supportive care and treating underlying systemic abnormalities (e.g., antibiotics in sepsis and dialysis in renal failure) are the only modes of therapy. Corticosteroids or nondepolarizing neuromuscular blockers should be discontinued if possible. Patients require extensive physical and occupational therapy to prevent contractures and help regain muscle strength and functional abilities.

OMEPRAZOLE

Clinical Features

Omeprazole inhibits the H^+/K^+ ATPase enzyme system (the proton pump) at the secretory surface of the gastric parietal cell and is used for the treatment of gastric and duodenal ulcers and reflux. Rare cases of neuromyopathy have been reported with the use of omeprazole.[212,213] Patients develop proximal weakness and myalgias along with paresthesias and a stocking distribution of sensory loss, predominantly in the legs. Muscle reflexes are diminished or absent.

Laboratory Features

Serum CK levels are normal or mildly elevated. NCS may be normal or reveal an axonal sensorimotor polyneuropathy.[212] EMG can be normal or show small polyphasic MUAPs.[213]

Histopathology

Muscle biopsies in the two reported patients revealed only type 2 muscle fiber atrophy.[212,213] Superficial peroneal nerve biopsy in one patient demonstrated axonal degeneration.[212]

Pathogenesis

The pathogenic mechanism for the neuromyopathy is unknown.

Treatment

Muscle strength and sensation improve and serum CK levels normalize following discontinuation of omeprazole. Symptoms may recur if omeprazole is restarted.

ISOTRETINOIN CLINICAL FEATURES

Isotretinoin (Accutane) is used for treatment of severe acne. Exercise-induced myalgias and proximal weakness can occur.[214–216]

Laboratory Features

Serum CK levels can be normal or elevated 100-fold.[214,215] Decreased serum carnitine levels may be seen. EMG can demonstrate small polyphasic MUAPs.

Histopathology

Muscle biopsy in a single reported patient demonstrated only atrophy of muscle fibers.

Pathogenesis

The basis for the myopathy is not clear. The diminished carnitine levels and response to L-carnitine in some patients suggest that perturbation of lipid metabolism may be contributory.

Treatment

The myalgias, weakness, and CK elevations improve with discontinuation of isotretinoin.

DRUG-INDUCED HYPOKALEMIC MYOPATHY

Hypokalemia can be a complication of a variety of medications (e.g., diuretics, laxatives, mineralocorticoids, amphotericin, and lithium). Further, excessive eating of licorice may have an aldosterone-like effect and cause hypokalemia. Hypokalemic myopathy has also been associated with alcohol abuse and inhalation of toluene. The clinical, laboratory, histopathological, and electrophysiologic features of hypokalemic myopathy are similar, regardless of the etiology of the hypokalemia. Affected individuals develop acute or subacute generalized weakness that can resemble Guillain–Barré syndrome. Weakness usually does not occur unless the serum potassium levels are less than 2 mEq/L. The serum CK levels are elevated. EMGs can be normal or demonstrate mild irritability in the form of fibrillation potentials and positive sharp waves in severely weakened muscles. Muscle biopsies are not typically performed as the diagnosis is apparent with the appropriate laboratory testing. However, muscle biopsies may demonstrate scattered necrotic and regenerating muscle fibers as well as vacuoles that arise from T-tubules. The weakness improves with correction of the hypokalemia.

▶ MYOPATHIES ASSOCIATED WITH ANESTHETIC AGENTS AND CENTRALLY ACTING MEDICATIONS

MALIGNANT HYPERTHERMIA

Clinical Features

Malignant hyperthermia is a genetically heterogeneous group of disorders characterized by severe muscle rigidity, myoglobinuria, fever, tachycardia, cyanosis, and cardiac arrhythmias precipitated by depolarizing muscle relaxants (e.g., succinylcholine) and inhalational anesthetic agents (e.g., halothane).[217] The incidence of malignant hyperthermia ranges from 0.5% to 0.0005%.[217] At least 50% of patients have had previous anesthesia without any problems.[4] The signs of malignant hyperthermia usually appear during surgery but can develop in the postoperative period. Rarely, attacks of malignant hyperthermia have been triggered by exercise, ingestion of caffeine, and stress.[218]

Laboratory Features

Serum CK can be normal or mildly elevated between attacks in patients susceptible to malignant hyperthermia. During attacks of malignant hyperthermia, serum CK levels are markedly elevated and myoglobinuria can develop. Hyperkalemia is also usually present. Metabolic and respiratory acidosis is evident with lactic acidosis, hypoxia, and hypercarbia. NCS and EMG are usually normal in the interictal periods. However, EMG performed shortly after an attack of malignant hyperthermia may demonstrate increased spontaneous activity and, perhaps, small polyphasic MUAPs that recruit early.

The in vitro muscle contracture test can be performed to assess the susceptibility of malignant hyperthermia in individuals who may be at risk (i.e., family members with history of malignant hyperthermia).[217] However, the test is not routinely available and false-positive and false-negative tests occur. Varying concentrations of halothane and caffeine are applied to strips of muscle that are stimulated at 0.1–0.2 Hz for 1–5 seconds, while tension is measured by a stain gauge. In patients susceptible to malignant hyperthermia, much lower concentrations of caffeine and halothane produce muscle contractions than are required to produce a similar in normal muscle tissue.

Histopathology

Muscle biopsies demonstrate nonspecific myopathic features including fiber size variability, increased internal nuclei, moth-eaten fibers, and necrotic fibers after an attack of malignant hyperthermia.

Pathogenesis and Molecular Genetics

At least some cases of malignant hyperthermia probably arise secondary to excessive calcium release by the sarcoplasmic reticulum calcium channels. Increased intracytoplasmic calcium leads to excessive muscle contraction, increased use of oxygen and ATP, and overproduction of heat. Why various anesthetic agents and depolarizing muscle relaxants trigger this exaggerated release of calcium from the sarcoplasmic reticulum in predisposed individuals is not known.

Malignant hyperthermia susceptibility is genetically very heterogeneous, as families have been linked to different chromosomes and genes. The first mutations were discovered in the ryanodine receptor gene located on chromosome 19q13.1 (MHS1).[142,219,220] The ryanodine receptor bridges the gap between the sarcoplasmic reticulum and the T tubule. Mutations in the ryanodine receptor may result in a functional alteration of the associated calcium channel such that there is an excessive release of calcium into the cytoplasm upon activation. Of note, mutations in this gene also cause the congenital myopathy, central core disease. Mutations in the ryanodine receptor gene account for only a minority of patients with malignant hyperthermia; other genetic loci have been identified. MHS2 localizes to chromosome 17q11.2–q24 (possibly the gene for the subunit of the sodium channel).[221] Thus, MHS2 may be allelic to potassium-sensitive periodic paralysis, paramyotonia congenita, and related disorders. MHS3 links to chromosome 7q21–q22 (possibly to a gene *CACNA2D1*, encoding a subunit of the calcium channel).[222] MHS4 localizes to chromosome 3q13.1, but the gene has yet to be identified.[223] Mutations in the dihydropteridine receptor gene on chromosome 1q31 (allelic to hypokalemic periodic paralysis type 1) cause MHS5.[224] Linkage to chromosome 5p has been demonstrated in still other families (MHS6).[225] In addition, patients with muscular dystrophies, myotonic dystrophies, mitochondrial myopathies, and other channelopathies are susceptible to developing malignant hyperthermia.[226] Thus, it appears that malignant hyperthermia may occur in various myopathic disorders, affecting the structural proteins of the muscle membrane or ion channels.

Treatment

Individuals at risk of malignant hyperthermia should not be given known triggering anesthetic agents if possible. Malignant hyperthermia is a medical emergency, requiring several therapeutic steps.[217] The anesthetic agent must be discontinued, while 100% oxygen is delivered. Dantrolene 2–3 mg/kg every 5 minutes for a total of 10 mg/kg should be administered. The stomach, bladder, and lower gastrointestinal tract are lavaged with iced saline solution, and cooling blankets are applied. Acidosis and hyperkalemia are treated with sodium bicarbonate, hyperventilation, dextrose, insulin, and occasionally calcium chloride. Urinary output must be maintained with hydration, furosemide, or mannitol. The patient must be monitored and treated for cardiac arrhythmias.

► MYOPATHIES SECONDARY TO DRUGS OF ABUSE

ALCOHOLIC MYOPATHY

Chronic alcohol abuse is more often attributed to causing neuropathy than myopathy.[9] However, several forms of a toxic myopathy due to alcohol have been described: (1) acute necrotizing myopathy, (2) acute hypokalemic myopathy, (3) chronic alcoholic myopathy, (4) asymptomatic alcoholic myopathy, and (5) alcoholic cardiomyopathy.[227–231]

An acute necrotizing myopathy manifests as acute muscle pain, tenderness to palpation, cramping, swelling, and weakness following or during a recent particularly intense binge. The severity of the myopathy is highly variable. Severe cases can be associated with myoglobinuria and acute renal failure. The muscle cramps resolve over the course of several days, while the remainder of symptoms may last several weeks. Serum CK levels are markedly elevated during these attacks. Muscle biopsies reveal widespread muscle fiber necrosis and occasionally fibers with tubular aggregates. Disorganization of the sarcomeres and degeneration of mitochondria may be appreciated on EM. Patents require appropriate supportive medical care and nutritional supplementation as many are malnourished.

Alcohol abuse can lead to acute hypokalemia, which can cause generalized weakness. Muscle weakness evolves over the time period of 1 or 2 days. Serum potassium is very low, <2 mEq/L, and the CK levels are elevated. Muscle biopsy performed in the acute time frame may reveal vacuoles with the muscle fibers. The myopathy resolves with correction of the serum potassium.

Some alcoholics develop the insidious onset of primarily proximal limb-girdle weakness, especially of the lower limbs, which has been attributed to a chronic alcoholic myopathy. Muscle biopsy may reveal scattered muscle fiber atrophy, necrosis, and regeneration. Whether the muscle weakness is caused by a toxic influence of alcohol on muscle, a toxic peripheral neuropathy, or malnutrition is unclear.

An asymptomatic alcoholic myopathy has been suggested in some patients on the basis of an elevated serum CK levels found coincidentally. There is no complaint of weakness, and the physical examination does not reveal striking evidence of a myopathic disorder. Histological findings are not available for this class of patients, and the true nature of this presumed form of alcoholic myopathy is questionable. The elevated serum CK may be related to subclinical necrotizing myopathy, hypokalemia, or muscle trauma.

Laboratory Features

Serum CK levels may be normal or slightly elevated and potassium levels may be reduced or normal. Reduced amplitudes of the sensory and, occasionally, motor nerve conductions studies may be seen, if patients have a concomitant alcoholic neuropathy. Needle EMG may reveal positive sharp waves, fibrillation potentials, and early recruitment of short-duration, low-amplitude MUAPs firing at high rates with minimal force production in weak muscles in patients with a necrotizing alcoholic myopathy.[227–231]

Pathogenesis

The pathogenic basis for the various forms of alcoholic myopathies is not known. The metabolism of alcohol may lead to the accumulation of toxic metabolites (e.g., acetaldehyde) or free radicals that may be toxic to lipid membranes.

▶ MYOPATHIES SECONDARY TO ILLICIT DRUGS

Illicit drugs including opioids (e.g., heroin, meperidine, cocaine, pentazocine, piritramide, amphetamines, etc.) may be myotoxic.[232–235] Muscle injury can be related to direct muscle trauma (e.g., needle injury), rhabdomyolysis secondary to pressure and ischemic necrosis related to prolonged loss of consciousness, ischemia due to vasoconstriction, rhabdomyolysis caused by generalized status epilepticus, or the direct toxic effects of the drugs (or adulterants) on muscle tissue. Serum CK levels should be markedly elevated, and muscle biopsies reveal widespread necrosis in such cases.

Inhalation of volatile agents (e.g., toluene) can also cause generalized muscle weakness and, occasionally, myoglobinuria. Toluene causes distal renal tubular acidosis with associated severe hypokalemia, hypophosphatemia, and mild hypocalcemia. Muscle strength returns after correction of the electrolyte abnormalities and abstinence from further exposure.

▶ SUMMARY

Various drugs can cause muscle damage and from a variety of different mechanisms. It is imperative to take a good medical history including current and previous medication history (as well as history of illicit drug use and alcohol abuse), as stopping the offending agent usually leads to improvement of the myopathy. However, continued use can be associated with significant morbidity and even death (e.g., from myoglobinuria). The most common toxic myopathy is associated with statin use in keeping with how frequently these medications are prescribed. That said, most individuals treated with statin medications and other medications known to cause toxic myopathy have no complications.

REFERENCES

1. Amato AA, Dumitru D. Acquired myopathies. In: Dumitru D, Amato AA, Zwarts MJ, eds. *Electrodiagnostic Medicine.* 2nd ed. Philadelphia, PA: Hanley & Belfus; 2002:1371–1432.
2. Argov Z, Mastaglia FL. Drug-induced neuromuscular disorders in man. In: Walton JN, ed. *Disorders of Voluntary Muscle.* 5th ed. Edinburgh: Churchill-Livingstone; 1988:981–1014.
3. Baker PC. Drug-induced and toxic myopathies. *Semin Neurol.* 1983;3:265–273.
4. Griggs RC, Mendell JR, Miller RG. Myopathies of systemic disease. In: *Evaluation and Treatment of Myopathies.* Philadelphia, PA: FA Davis; 1995:355–385.
5. Kuncl RW, Wiggins WW. Toxic myopathies. *Neurol Clin.* 1988;6:593–619.
6. Lane RJM, Mastaglia FL. Drug-induced myopathies in man. *Lancet.* 1978;2:562–565.
7. Mastaglia FL. Adverse effects of drugs on muscle. *Drugs.* 1982;24:304–321.
8. Mastaglia FL. Toxic myopathies. In: Rowland LP, DiMauro S, eds. *Handbook of Clinical Neurology.* Vol 18, No. 62: Myopathies. Amsterdam: Elsevier Science Publishers BV; 1992:595–622.
9. Victor M, Sieb JP. Myopathies due to drugs, toxins, and nutritional deficiency. In: Engel AG, Franzini-Armstrong C, eds. *Myology.* 2nd ed. New York, NY: McGraw-Hill; 1994:1697–1725.

10. Mastaglia FL. Iatrogenic myopathies. *Curr Opin Neurol.* 2010;23:445–449.
11. Bakker-Arema RG, Best J, Fayyad R, et al. A brief review paper on the efficacy and safety of atorvastatin in early clinical trials. *Atherosclerosis.* 1997;131:17–23.
12. Berland Y, Coponat H, Durand C, Baz M, Laugier R, Musso JL. Rhabdomyolysis and simvastatin use. *Nephron.* 1991;57:365–366.
13. Corpier C, Jones P, Suki W, et al. Rhabdomyolysis and renal injury with lovastatin use. *JAMA.* 1988;260:239–241.
14. Davidson MH, Stein EA, Dujoven CA, et al. The efficacy and six week tolerability of simvastatin 80 and 160 mg/day. *Am J Cardiol.* 1997;79:38–42.
15. Deslypere J, Vermuelen A. Rhabdomyolysis and simvastatin. *Ann Intern Med.* 1991;114:342.
16. Marais GE, Larson KK. Rhabdomyolysis and acute renal failure induced by combination lovastatin and gemfibrozil therapy. *Ann Intern Med.* 1990;112:228–230.
17. Schalke BB, Schmidt B, Toyka K, Hartung HP. Pravastatin-associated inflammatory myopathy. *N Engl J Med.* 1992;327: 649–650.
18. Tobert J. Efficacy and long-term adverse effect pattern of lovastatin. *Am J Cardiol.* 1988;62:28J–33J.
19. East C, Alivizatos PA, Grundy SM, Jones PH, Farmer JA. Rhabdomyolysis in patients receiving lovastatin after cardiac transplantation. *N Engl J Med.* 1988;318:48.
20. Abourizk N, Khalil BA, Bahuth N, Afifi AK. Clofibrate induced muscular syndrome. *J Neurol Sci.* 1979;42:1–9.
21. Denizot M, Fabre J, Pometa D, Wildi E. Clofibrate, nephrotic syndrome, and histological changes in muscle. *Lancet.* 1973;1:1326.
22. Gabriel R, Pearce JM. Clofibrate induced myopathy and neuropathy. *Lancet.* 1976;2:906.
23. Kwiecinski H. Myotonia induced with clofibrate in rats. *J Neurol.* 1978;219:107–116.
24. Langer T, Levy RI. Acute muscular syndrome associated with administration of clofibrate. *N Engl J Med.* 1968;279:856–858.
25. London F, Gross KF, Ringel SP. Cholesterol-lowering agent myopathy (CLAM). *Neurology.* 1991;41:1159–1160.
26. Magarian GJ, Lucas LM. Gemfibrozil-induced myopathy. *Arch Intern Med.* 1991;151:1873–1874.
27. Pierce LR, Wysowski DK, Gross TP. Myopathy and rhabdomyolysis associated with lovastatin-gemfibrozil combination therapy. *JAMA.* 1990;264:71–75.
28. Pierides AM, Alvarez-Ude F, Kerr DN. Clofibrate induced muscle damage in patients with chronic renal failure. *Lancet.* 1975;2:1279–1282.
29. Rush P, Baron M, Kapusta M. Clofibrate myopathy: a case report and a review of the literature. *Semin Arthritis Rheum.* 1986;15:226–229.
30. Shepherd J. Fibrates and statins in the treatment of hyperlipidemia: an appraisal of their efficacy and safety. *Eur Heart J.* 1995;16:5–13.
31. Litin SC, Andersone CF. Nicotinic acid-associated myopathy: a report of three cases. *Am J Med.* 1989;86:481–483.
32. Reaven P, Witzum J. Lovastatin, nicotinic acid and rhabdomyolysis [letter]. *Ann Intern Med.* 1988;109:597–598.
33. Fux R, Morike K, Gundel UF, Hartmann R, Gleiter CH. Ezetimibe and statin-associated myopathy. *Ann Intern Med.* 2004;140(8):671–672.
34. Havranek JM, Wolfsen AR, Warnke GA, Phillips PS. Monotherapy with ezetimibe causing myopathy. *Am J Med.* 2006;119 (3):285–286.
35. Simard C, Poirier P. Ezetimibe-associated myopathy in monotherapy and in combination with a 3-hydroxy-3-methylglutaryl coenzyme A reductase inhibitor. *Can J Cardiol.* 2006;22(2):141–144.
36. Perez-Calvo J, Civeira-Murillo F, Cabello A. Worsening myopathy associated with ezetimibe in a patient with McArdle disease. *QJM.* 2005;98(6):461–462.
37. Dujovne CA, Chremos AN, Pool JL, et al. Expanded Clinical Evaluation of Lovastatin (EXCEL) study results. IV. Additional perspectives on the tolerability of lovastatin. *Am J Med.* 1991;91(suppl 1B):25–30.
38. Jones P, Kafonek S, Laurora I, Hunningshake D. Comparative dose efficacy study of atorvastatin versus simvastatin, provastatin, lovastatin, and fluvastatin in patients with hypercholesterolemia (the CURVES Study). *Am J Cardiol.* 1998;81:582–587.
39. Galper JB. Increase incidence of myositis in patients treated with high dose simvastatin. *Am J Cardiol.* 1998;81:259.
40. Duell PB, Connor WE, Illingsworth DR. Rhabdomyolysis after taking atorvastatin with gemfibrozil. *Am J Cardiol.* 1998;81:368–369.
41. Furberg CD, Pitt B. Commentary: withdrawal of cervistatin from the world market. *Curr Control Trials Cardiovasc Med.* 2001;2:205–207.
42. von Keutz E, Schluter G. Preclinical safety evaluation of cerivastation, a novel HMG-CoA reductase inhibitor. *Am J Cardiol.* 1998;82(4B):11J–17J.
43. Hamilton-Craig I. Statin-associated myopathy. *Med J Aust.* 2001;175:486–489.
44. Pasternak RC, Smith SC, Bairey-Merz CN, Grundy S, Cleeman J, Lenfant C. ACC/AHA/NHLBI clinical advisory on the use and safety of statins. *J Am Coll Cardiol.* 2002;40: 556–572.
45. Ucar M, Mjorndal T, Dahlqvist R. HMG-CoA reductase inhibitors and myotoxicity. *Drug Saf.* 2000;22:441–457.
46. Hodel C. Myopathy and rhabdomyolysis with lipid-lowering drugs. *Toxicol Lett.* 2002;128:159–168.
47. Thompson PD, Clarkson P, Karas RH. Statin-associated myopathy. *JAMA.* 2003;289:1681–1690.
48. dos Santos AG, Guardia AC, Pereira TS, et al. Rhabdomyolysis as a clinical manifestation of association with ciprofibrate, sirolimus, cyclosporine, and pegylated interferon-α in liver-transplanted patients: A case report and literature review. *Transplant Proc.* 2014;46:1887–1888.
49. Mammen AL, Amato AA. Statin myopathy: a review of recent progress. *Curr Opin Rheumatol.* 2010;22:644–650.
50. Shanmugam VK, Matsumoto C, Pien E, et al. Voriconazole associated myositis. *J Clin Rheumatol.* 2009;15:350–353.
51. Basic-Jukic N, Kes P, Bubic-Filipi L, Vranjican Z. Rhabdomyolysis and acute kidney injury secondary to concomitant use of fluvastatin and rapamycin in a renal transplant recipient. *Nephrol Dial Transplant.* 2010;25:2036.
52. Backes JM, Venero CV, Gibson CA, et al. Effectiveness and tolerability of every-other-day rosuvastatin dosing in patients with prior statin intolerance. *Ann Pharmacother.* 2008;42: 341–346.
53. Fauchais AL, Iba Ba J, Maurage P, et al. Polymyositis induced or associated with lipid-lowering drugs: five cases. *Rev Med Interne.* 2004;25(4):294–298.
54. Giordano N, Senesi M, Mattii G, Battisti E, Villanova M, Gennari C. Polymyositis associated with simvastatin. *Lancet.* 1997;349(9065):1600–1601.

55. Hill C, Zeitz C, Kirkham B. Dermatomyositis with lung involvement in a patient treated with simvastatin. *Aust N Z J Med.* 1995;25(6):745–746.
56. Khattak FH, Morris IM, Branford WA. Simvastatin-associated dermatomyositis. *Br J Rheumatol.* 1994;33(2):199.
57. Noel B, Cerottini JP, Panizzon RG. Atorvastatin-induced dermatomyositis. *Am J Med.* 2001;110(8):670–671.
58. Riesco-Eizaguirre G, Arpa-Gutierrez FJ, Gutierrez M, Toribio E. Severe polymyositis with simvastatin use. *Rev Neurol.* 2003;37(10):934–936.
59. Rodriguez-Garcia JL, Serrano Commino M. Lovastatin-associated dermatomyositis. *Postgrad Med J.* 1996;72(853): 694.
60. Vasconcelos OM, Campbell WW. Dermatomyositis-like syndrome and HMG-CoA reductase inhibitor (statin) in-take. *Muscle Nerve.* 2004;30(6):803–807.
61. Christopher-Stine L, Casciola Rosen L, Hong G, Chung T, Corse AM, Mammen AL. A novel autoantibody recognizing 200 and 100 kDa proteins is associated with an immune mediated necrotizing myopathy. *Arthritis Rheum.* 2010;62: 2757–2766.
62. Mammen AL, Chung T, Christopher-Stine L, et al. Autoantibodies against 3-hydroxy-3-methylglutaryl-coenzyme A reductase in patients with statin-associated autoimmune myopathy. *Arthritis Rheum.* 2011;63:713–721.
63. Needham M, Fabian V, Knezevic W, Panegyres P, Zilko P, Mastaglia FL. Progressive myopathy with up-regulation of MHC-I associated with statin therapy. *Neuromuscul Disord.* 2007;17(2):194–200.
64. Grable-Esposito P, Katzberg HD, Greenberg SA, Srinivasan J, Katz J, Amato AA. Immune-mediated necrotizing myopathy associated with statins. *Muscle Nerve.* 2010;41:185–190.
65. Meriggioli MN, Barboi A, Rowin J, Cochran EJ. HMGCoA reductase inhibitor myopathy: clinical, electrophysiologic, and pathologic data in five patients. *J Clin Neuromuscul Dis.* 2001;2:129–134.
66. Phillips PS, Haas RH, Bannykh S, et al. Statin-associated myopathy with normal creatine kinase levels. *Ann Intern Med.* 2002;137:581–585.
67. Greenberg SA, Amato AA. Statin myopathies. In: Amato AA, ed. *Continuum: Muscle Diseases.* Vol 12. 2006, pp. 169–184.
68. SEARCH Collaborative Group; Link E, Parish S, Armitage J, et al. SLCO1B1 variants and statin-induced myopathy: a genomewide study. *N Engl J Med.* 2008;359:789–799.
69. Kra SJ. Muscle syndrome with clofibrate usage. *Conn Med.* 1974;38:348–349.
70. Afifi AK, Hajj SS, Tekian A, et al. Clofibrate-induced myotoxicity in rats. *Eur Neurol.* 1984;23:182–197.
71. Slim H, Thompson PD. Ezetimibe-related myopathy: a systematic review. *J Clin Lipidol.* 2008;2:328–234.
72. Amato AA, Barohn RJ. Neurological complications of transplantations. In: Harati Y, Rolack LA, eds. *Practical Neuroimmunology.* Boston, MA: Butterworth-Heineman; 1997:341–375.
73. Arellano F, Krup P. Muscular disorders associated with cyclosporine [letter]. *Lancet.* 1991;337:915.
74. Costigan DA. Acquired myotonia, weakness and vacuolar myopathy secondary to cyclosporine [abstract]. *Muscle Nerve.* 1989;12:761.
75. Goy JJ, Stauffer JC, Deruaz JP, et al. Myopathy as a possible side effect cyclosporine. *Lancet.* 1989;1:1446–1449.
76. Grezard O, Lebranchu Y, Birmele B, Sharobeem R, Nivet H, Bagros P. Cyclosporine-induced muscular toxicity. *Lancet.* 1990;1:177.
77. Noppen D, Verlkeriers B, Dierckx R, Bruyland M, Vanhaelst L. Cyclosporine and myopathy. *Ann Intern Med.* 1987;107: 945–946.
78. Hibi S, Hisawa A, Tamai M, et al. Severe rhabdomyolysis with tacrolimus [letter]. *Lancet.* 1995;346:702.
79. Norman D, Illingworth DR, Munson J, Hosenpud J. Myolysis and acute renal failure in heart transplant recipient receiving lovastatin. *N Engl J Med.* 1988;318:46–47.
80. Rieger EH, Halasz NA, Wahlstrom HE. Colchicine neuromyopathy after renal transplantation. *Transplantation.* 1990; 49:1196–1198.
81. Volin L, Jarventie G, Ruut U. Fatal rhabdomyolysis as a complication of bone marrow transplantation. *Bone Marrow Transplant.* 1990;6:59–60.
82. Atkinson P, Joubert G, Barron A, et al. Hypertrophic cardiomyopathy with tacrolimus in paediatric transplant patient. *Lancet.* 1995;345:894–896.
83. Teicher A, Rosenthal T, Kissen E, Sarova I. Labetalol-induced toxic myopathy. *Br Med J.* 1981;282:1824–1825.
84. Willis JK, Tilton AH, Harkin JC, Boineau FG. Reversible myopathy due to labatolol. *Pediatr Neurol.* 1990;6:275–276.
85. Hanna JP, Ramundo ML. Rhabdomyolysis and hypoxia associated with prolonged propofol infusion in children. *Neurology.* 1988;50:301–303.
86. Parke TJ, Steven JE, Rice AS, et al. Metabolic acidosis and myocardial failure after propofol infusion in children: five case reports. *Br Med J.* 1992;305:613–616.
87. Strickland RA, Murray MJ. Fatal metabolic acidosis in pediatric patient receiving and infusion of propofol in the intensive care unit: is there a relationship? *Crit Care Med.* 1995;23:405–409.
88. Hanson P, Dive A, Brucher JM, Bisteau M, Dangoisse M, Deltombe T. Acute corticosteroid myopathy in intensive care patients. *Muscle Nerve.* 1997;20:1371–1380.
89. Eadie MJ, Ferrier TM. Chloroquine myopathy. *J Neurol Neurosurg Psychiatry.* 1966;29:331–337.
90. Estes ML, Ewing-Wilson D, Chou SM, et al. Chloroquine neuromyotoxicity. Clinical and pathological perspective. *Am J Med.* 1987;82:447–455.
91. Maschke M, Kastrup O, Esser S, Ross B, Hengge U, Hufnagel A. Incidence and prevalence of neurological disorders associated with HIV since the introduction of highly active antiretroviral therapy (HAART). *J Neurol Sci.* 2000;69: 376–380.
92. Mastaglia FL, Papadimitriou JM, Dawkins RL, Beveridge B. Vacuolar myopathy associated with chloroquine, lupus erythematosus and thymoma. *J Neurol Sci.* 1977;34:315–328.
93. Alderson K, Griffin JW, Cornblath DR, Levine JH, Kuncl RW, Griffin LSC. Neuromuscular complications of amiodarone therapy. *Neurology.* 1987;37(suppl):355.
94. Costa-Jussa FR, Jacobs JM. The pathology of amiodarone neurotoxicity. I. Experimental changes with reference to changes in other tissues. *Brain.* 1985;108:735–752.
95. Jacobs JM, Costa-Jussa FR. The pathology of amiodarone neurotoxicity. II. Peripheral neuropathy in man. *Brain.* 1985;108:753–769.
96. Meier C, Kauer B, Muller U, Ludin HP. Neuromyopathy during amiodarone treatment: a case report. *J Neurol.* 1979;220: 231–239.

97. Roth R, Itabashi H, Louie J, Anderson T, Narahara KA. Amiodarone toxicity: myopathy and neuropathy. *Am Heart J.* 1990;119:1223–1225.
98. Kuncl RW, Duncan G, Watson D, Alderson K, Rogawski MA, Peper M. Colchicine myopathy and neuropathy. *N Engl J Med.* 1987;316:1562–1568.
99. Kuncl RW, Cornblath DR, Avila O, Duncan G. Electrodiagnosis of human colchicine myoneuropathy. *Muscle Nerve.* 1989;12:360–364.
100. Riggs JE, Schochet SS, Gutmann L, Crosby TW, DiBartolomeo AG. Chronic colchicine neuropathy and myopathy. *Arch Neurol.* 1986;43:521–523.
101. Rutkove SB, De Girolami U, Preston DC, et al. Myotonia in colchicine myoneuropathy. *Muscle Nerve.* 1996;19:870–875.
102. Kontos HA. Myopathy associated with chronic colchicine toxicity. *N Engl J Med.* 1962;266:38–39.
103. Bradley WG, Lassman LP, Pearce GW, Walton JN. The neuromyopathy of Vincristine in man: clinical, electrophysiological and pathological studies. *J Neurol Sci.* 1970;10:107–131.
104. Anderson P, Song S, Slotwiner P. The fine structure of spheromembranous degeneration of skeletal muscle induced by vincristine. *J Neuropathol Exp Neurol.* 1967;26:15–24.
105. Slotwiner P, Song S, Andersone P. Spheromembranous degeneration of muscle induced by vincristine. *Arch Neurol.* 1966; 15:172–176.
106. Dalakas M. HIV or zidovudine myopathy? [letter]. *Neurology.* 1994;44:360–361.
107. Dalakas MC, Illa I, Pezeshkpour GH, Laukaitis JP, Cohen B, Griffin JL. Mitochondrial myopathy caused by long-term zidovudine therapy. *N Engl J Med.* 1990;322:1098–1105.
108. Gherardi R, Chariot P. HIV or zidovudine myopathy [letter]? *Neurology.* 1994;44:361–362.
109. Grau JM, Casademont J. HIV or zidovudine myopathy? [letter]. *Neurology.* 1994;44:361.
110. Grau JM, Masanes F, Pedreo E, Casdemont J, FernandezSola J, Urbano-Marquez A. Human immunodeficiency virus type 1 infection and myopathy: clinical relevance of zidovidine therapy. *Ann Neurol.* 1993;34:206–211.
111. Mhiri C, Baudrimont M, Bonne G, et al. Zidovudine myopathy: a distinctive disorder associated with mitochondrial dysfunction. *Ann Neurol.* 1991;29:606–614.
112. Peters BS, Winer J, Landon DN, Stoffer A, Pinching AJ. Mitochondrial myopathy associated with chronic zidovudine therapy in AIDS. *Q J Med.* 1993;86:5–15.
113. Richman DD, Fischl MA, Grieco HM, et al. The toxicity of azidothymidine (AZT) in the treatment of patients with AIDS and AIDS-related complex. *N Engl J Med.* 1987;317: 192–197.
114. Simpson DM, Bender AN. Human immunodeficiency virus-associated myopathy: analysis of 11 patients. *Ann Neurol.* 1988;24:79–84.
115. Simpson DM, Bender AN, Farraye J, Mendelson SG, Wolfe DE. Human immunodeficiency virus wasting syndrome represents a treatable myopathy. *Neurology.* 1990;40: 535–538.
116. Simpson DM, Slasor P, Dafni U, Berger J, Fischl MA, Hall C. Analysis of myopathy in a placebo-controlled zidovudine trial. *Muscle Nerve.* 1997;20:382–385.
117. Bailey RO, Turok DI, Jaufmann BP, Singh JK. Myositis and acquired immunodeficiency syndrome. *Hum Pathol.* 1987;18: 749–751.
118. Bessen LJ, Green JB, Louie E, Seitzman P, Weinberg H. Severe polymyositis-like syndrome associated with zidovudine therapy of AIDS and ARC. *N Engl J Med.* 1988;318:708.
119. Chalmers AC, Greco CM, Miller RG. Prognosis in AZT myopathy. *Neurology.* 1991;41:1181–1184.
120. Manji H, Harrison MJ, Round JM, et al. Muscle disease, HIV and zidovudine: the spectrum of muscle disease in HIV-infected individuals treated with zidovudine. *J Neurol.* 1993;240:479–488.
121. Reyes MG, Casanova J, Varricchio F, Sequeira W, Fresco K. Zidovudine myopathy. *Neurology.* 1992;42:1252.
122. Simpson DM, Citak KA, Godfrey E, Godbold J, Wolfe D. Myopathies associated with human immunodeficiency virus and zidovudine: can their effects be distinguished? *Neurology.* 1993;43:971–976.
123. Simpson DA, Katzenstein DA, Hughes MD, et al. Neuromuscular function in HIV infection: analysis of a placebo-controlled combination antiviral trial. AIDS Clinical Group 175/801 Study Team. *AIDS.* 1998;12:2425–2432.
124. Till M, McDonnel KB. Myopathy with human immunodeficiency virus type 1 (HIV) infection. HIV-1 or zidovudine? *Ann Intern Med.* 1990;113:492–494.
125. Panegyres PK, Papadimitriou JM, Hollingsworth PN, Armstrong JA, Kakulas BA. Vesicular changes in the myopathies of AIDS. Ultrastructural observations and their relationship to zidovudine treatment. *J Neurol Neurosurg Psychiatry.* 1990;53:649–655.
126. Arnaudo E, Dalakas M, Shanske S, Moraes CT, DiMauro S, Schon EN. Depletion of mitochondrial DNA in AIDS patients with zidovudine-induced myopathy. *Lancet.* 1991;1:508–510.
127. Masanes F, Barrientos A, Cebrian M, et al. Clinical, histological, and molecular reversibility of zidovudine myopathy. *J Neurol Sci.* 1998;159:225–228.
128. Jay CA, Hench K, Ropka M. Improvement of AZT myopathy after change to dideoxyinosine (ddI) or dideoxycytosine (ddC) [abstract]. *Neurology.* 1993;43(suppl 2):A373–A374.
129. Benbrik E, Chariot P, Boanvaud S, et al. Cellular and mitochondrial toxicity of zidovudine (AZT), didanosione (ddI), and zacitabine (ddC) on cultured human muscle cells. *J Neurol Sci.* 1997;149:19–25.
130. Pedrol E, Masanes F, Fernandez-Sola J, et al. Lack of myotoxicity with didanosine (dI). Clinical and experimental studies. *J Neurol Sci.* 1996;138:42–48.
131. Callens S, De Roo A. Fanconi-like syndrome and rhabdomyolysis in a person with HIV infection on highly active antiretroviral treatment occluding tenofovir [letter]. *J Infect Dis.* 2003;47:262–263.
132. Mah Ming JB, Gill MJ. Drug-induced rhabdomyolysis after concomitant use of clarithermycine, atorvastatin, lopinivir/ritanovir in a patient with HIV. *AIDS Patient Care STDS.* 2003;17:207–210.
133. Belongia EA, Hedberg CW, Gleich GJ, et al. An investigation of the case of the eosinophilia myalgia syndrome associated with tryptophan use. *N Engl J Med.* 1990;323:357–365.
134. Donofrio PD, Stanton C, Miller VS, et al. Demyelinating polyneuropathy in eosinophilia-myalgia syndrome. *Muscle Nerve.* 1992;15:796–805.
135. Hertzman PA, Blevins WL, Mayer J, Greenfield B, Ting M, Gleich GJ. Association of the eosinophilia-myalgia syndrome with the ingestion of tryptophan. *N Engl J Med.* 1990;322: 869–873.

136. Sagman DL, Melamed JC. L-Tryptophan induced eosinophilia-myalgia syndrome and myopathy. *Neurology*. 1990;40: 1629–1630.
137. Sakimoto K. The cause of the eosinophilia-myalgia syndrome associated with tryptophan use. *N Engl J Med*. 1990;323:992.
138. Smith BE, Dyck PJ. Peripheral neuropathy in the eosinophilic-myalgia syndrome associated with Ltryptophan ingestion. *Neurology*. 1990;40:1035–1040.
139. Tanhehco JL, Wiechers DO, Golbus J, Neely SE. Eosinophilia-myalgia syndrome: myopathic electrodiagnostic characteristics. *Muscle Nerve*. 1992;15:561–567.
140. Shulman LE. Diffuse fasciitis with eosinophilia: a new syndrome? *Trans Assoc Am Physicians*. 1975;88:70–86.
141. Heiman-Patterseon TD, Bird SJ, Parry GJ, et al. Peripheral neuropathy associated with eosinophilia-myalgia syndrome. *Ann Neurol*. 1990;28:522–528.
142. Quane KA, Keating KE, Manning BM, et al. Detection of a common mutation in the ryanodine receptor gene in malignant hyperthermia: implication for diagnosis and heterogenetic studies. *Hum Mol Genet*. 1994;3:471–476.
143. Selwa JF, Feldman EL, Blaivas M. Mononeuropathy multiplex in tryptophan-associated eosinophilic-myalgia syndrome. *Neurology*. 1990;40:1632–1633.
144. Turi GK, Solitaire GB, James N, Dicker R. Eosinophiliamyalgia syndrome (L-tryptophan-associated neuromyopathy). *Neurology*. 1990;40:1793–1796.
145. Mayeno AN, Belongia EA, Lin F, Lundy SK, Gleich GJ. 3-(Phenylamino) alanine—a novel aniline-derived aminoacid associated with the eosinophilic-myalgia syndrome: a link to the toxic oil syndrome. *Mayo Clin Proc*. 1992;67:1134.
146. Kilbourne EM, Rigau-Perez JG, Heath CW, et al. Clinical epidemiology of toxic-oil syndrome. *N Engl J Med*. 1983;309: 1408–1414.
147. Dawkins RL, Zilko PJ, Carrano J, Garlepp MJ, McDonald BL. Immunobiology of D-penicillamine. *J Rheumatol*. 1981; 8(suppl):56–61.
148. Hall JT, Fallahi S, Koopman WJ. Penicillamine-induced myositis: observations and unique features in two patients and review of the literature. *Am J Med*. 1984;77:719.
149. Takahashi K, Ogita T, Okudaira H, Yoshinoya S, Yoshizawa H, Miyamoto T. D-penicillamine induced polymyositis in patients with rheumatoid arthritis. *Arthritis Rheum*. 1986;29: 560–564.
150. Taneja V, Mehra N, Singh YN, Kumar A, Malaviya A, Singh RR. HLA-D region genes and susceptibility to D-penicillamine-induced polymyositis. *Arthritis Rheum*. 1990;33:1445–1447.
151. Watson AJ, Dalbow MH, Stachura I, et al. Immunologic studies in cimetidine-induced nephropathy and polymyositis. *N Engl J Med*. 1983;308:142–145.
152. Mitchell CG, Magnussen AR, Weiler JM. Cimetidine-induced cutaneous vasculitis. *Am J Med*. 1983;75:875.
153. Lewis CA, Boheimer N, Rose P, Jackson G. Myopathy after short term administration of procainamide. *Br Med J*. 1986;292: 593–597.
154. Wolf S, Goldberg LS, Verity MA. Neuromyopathy and periarteriolitis in a patient receiving levodopa. *Arch Intern Med*. 1976;136:1055–1057.
155. Harney J, Glasberg MR. Myopathy and hypersensitivity to phenytoin. *Neurology*. 1983;33:790–791.
156. Cirigliano G, Della RA, Tavoni A, Tavoni A, Vicava P, Bombardieri S. Polymyositis occurring during alpha-interferon treatment for malignant melanoma: a case report and review of the literature. *Rheumatol Int*. 1999;19:65–67.
157. Dietrich L, Bridges AJ, Albertini MR. DM after interferon alpha treatment. *Med Oncol*. 2000;17:64–69.
158. Hengstman GJ, Vogels OJ, ter Laak HJ, de Witte T, van Engelen BG. Myositis during ling-term interferon-alpha treatment. *Neurology*. 2000;54:2186.
159. The Muscle Study Group. A randomized, pilot trial of etanercept in dermatomyositis. *Ann Neurol*. 2011;70(3):427–436.
160. Klein R, Rosenbach M, Kim EJ, Kim B, Werth VP, Dunham J. Tumor necrosis factor inhibitor-associated dermatomyositis. *Arch Dermatol*. 2010;146:780–784.
161. Ishikawa Y, Yukawa N, Ohmura K, et al. Etanercept-induced anti-Jo-1-antibody-positive polymyositis in a patient with rheumatoid arthritis: a case report and review of the literature. *Clin Rheumatol*. 2010;29:563–566.
162. Srinivasan J, Wu C, Amato AA. Inflammatory myopathy associated with imitinab therapy. *J Clin Neuromuscul Dis*. 2004; 5:119–121.
163. Coomes EN. The rate of recovery of reversible myopathies and the effects of anabolic agents in steroid myopathy. *Neurology*. 1965;18:523–530.
164. Engel AG. Metabolic and endocrine myopathies. In: Walton JN, ed. *Disorders of Voluntary Muscle*. 5th ed. Edinburgh: Churchill-Livingstone; 1988:811–868.
165. Golding DN, Murray SM, Pearce GW, Thompson M. Corticosteroid myopathy. *Ann Phys Med*. 1962;6:171–177.
166. Kaminski HJ, Ruff RL. Endocrine myopathies (hyper- and hypofunction of adrenal, thyroid, pituitary, and parathyroid glands and iatrogenic corticosteroid myopathy). In: Engel AG, Franzini-Armstrong C, eds. *Myology*. 2nd ed. New York, NY: McGraw-Hill; 1994:1726–1753.
167. Kissel JT, Mendell JR. The endocrine myopathies. In: Rowland LP, DiMauro S, eds. *Handbook of Clinical Neurology*. Vol 18. No. 62: Myopathies. Amsterdam: Elsevier Science Publishers BV; 1992:527–551.
168. Muller R, Kugelberg E. Myopathy in Cushing's syndrome. *J Neurol Neurosurg Psychiatry*. 1959;22:314–319.
169. Williams RS. Triamcinolone myopathy. *Lancet*. 1959;516: 698–700.
170. Yates DAH. Steroid myopathy. In: Walton JN, Canal N, Scarlato G, eds. *Muscle Diseases: Proceedings of an International Congress Milan*. 19–21 May, 1969. Amsterdam: Excerpta Medica; 1970:482–488.
171. Faludi G, Gotlieb J, Meyers J. Factors influencing the development of steroid-induced myopathy. *Ann NY Acad Sci*. 1967; 138:61–72.
172. Buchthal F. Electrophysiological abnormalities in metabolic myopathies and neuropathies. *Acta Neurol Scand*. 1970;46(suppl 43):129–176.
173. Hudgson P, Kendall-Taylor P. Endocrine myopathies. In: Mastaglia FL, Walton JN, eds. *Skeletal Muscle Pathology*. Edinburgh: Churchill Livingstone; 1992:493–509.
174. Pleasure DE, Walsh GO, Engel WK. Atrophy of skeletal muscle in patients with Cushing's syndrome. *Arch Neurol*. 1970;22:118–125.
175. Amato AA, Barohn RJ. Idiopathic Inflammatory myopathies. *Neurol Clin*. 1997;15:615–648.
176. Afifi AK, Bergman RA, Harvey JC. Steroid myopathy. *Johns Hopkins Med J*. 1968;123:158–174.

177. MacLean D, Schurr PH. Reversible amyotrophy complicating treatment with fluodrocortisone. *Lancet*. 1959;516:701–702.
178. Haan J, Hollander JM, van Duinin SG, Sacena PR, Wintzen AR. Reversible severe myopathy during treatment with finasteride. *Muscle Nerve*. 1997;20:502–504.
179. Bennett HS, Spiro AJ, Pollack MA, Zucker P. Ipecac-induced myopathy simulating dermatomyositis. *Neurology*. 1982;32:91–94.
180. Mateer JE, Farrell BJ, Chou SS, Gutmann L. Reversible ipecac myopathy. *Arch Neurol*. 1985;42:188–190.
181. Palmer EP, Guay AT. Reversible myopathy secondary to abuse of ipecac in patients with major eating disorders. *N Engl J Med*. 1985;313:1457–1459.
182. Amato AA, Jackson CE, Lampin S, Kaggan-Hallet K. Myofibrillar myopathy: no evidence of apoptosis by TUNEL. *Neurology*. 1999;52(4):861–863.
183. Amato AA, Kagan-Hallet K, Jackson CE, et al. The wide spectrum of myofibrillar myopathy suggests a multifactorial etiology and pathogenesis. *Neurology*. 1998;51(6):1646–1655.
184. Bolton CF, Gilbert JJ, Hahn AF, Sibbald WJ. Polyneuropathy in critically ill patients. *J Neurol Neurosurg Psychiatry*. 1984;47:1223–1231.
185. Zochodne DW, Bolton CF, Wells GF, et al. Critical illness polyneuropathy. A complication of sepsis and multiorgan failure. *Brain*. 1987;110:819–842.
186. Barohn RJ, Jackson CE, Rogers SJ, Ridings LW, McVey AL. Prolonged paralysis due to nondepolarizing neuromuscular blocking agents and corticosteroids. *Muscle Nerve*. 1994;17:647–654.
187. Gooch JL. AAEM case report #29: prolonged paralysis after neuromuscular blockade. *Muscle Nerve*. 1995;18:937–942.
188. Al-Lozi MT, Pestronk A, Yee WC, Flaris N, Cooper J. Rapidly evolving myopathy with myosin-deficient fibers. *Ann Neurol*. 1994;35:273–279.
189. Danon MJ, Carpenter S. Myopathy with thick filament (myosin) loss following prolonged paralysis with vecuronium during steroid treatment. *Muscle Nerve*. 1991;14:1131–1139.
190. Deconinck N, Van Parijs V, Beckers-Bleukx G, Van den Bergh P. Critical illness myopathy unrelated to corticosteroids or neuromuscular blocking agents. *Neuromuscul Disord*. 1998;8:186–192.
191. Gutmann L, Blumenthal D, Schochet SS. Acute type II myofiber atrophy in critical illness. *Neurology*. 1996;46:819–821.
192. Hirano M, Ott BR, Rapps EC, et al. Acute quadriplegic myopathy: a complication of treatment with steroids, nondepolarizing blocking agents, or both. *Neurology*. 1992;42:2082–2087.
193. Lacomis D, Giuliani MJ, Van Cott A, Kramer DJ. Acute myopathy of the intensive care: clinical, electromyographic, and pathological aspects. *Ann Neurol*. 1996;40:645–654.
194. Lacomis D, Petrella JT, Giuliani MJ. Causes of neuromuscular weakness in the intensive care unit: a study of ninety-two patients. *Muscle Nerve*. 1998;21:610–617.
195. Lacomis D, Smith TW, Chad DA. Acute myopathy and neuropathy in status asthmaticus: Case report and literature review. *Muscle Nerve*. 1993;16:84–90.
196. McFarlane IA, Rosenthal FD. Severe myopathy after status asthmaticus. *Lancet*. 1977;2:615.
197. Ramsay DA, Zochodne DW, Robertson DM, Nag S, Ludwin SK. A syndrome of acute severe muscle necrosis in intensive care unit patients. *J Neuropathol Exp Neurol*. 1993;52:387–398.
198. Rich MM, Bird SJ, Raps EC, McClaskey LF, Teener JW. Direct muscle stimulation in acute quadriplegic myopathy. *Muscle Nerve*. 1997;20:665–673.
199. Rich MM, Teener JW, Raps EC, Schotland DL, Bird SJ. Muscle is electrically inexcitable in acute quadriplegic myopathy. *Neurology*. 1996;46:731–736.
200. Showalter CJ, Engel AG. Acute quadriplegic myopathy: analysis of myosin isoforms and evidence for calpain-mediated proteolysis. *Muscle Nerve*. 1997;20:316–322.
201. Sitwell LD, Weishenker BG, Monipetit V, Reid D. Complete ophthalmoplegia as a complication of acute corticosteroid- and pancuronium-associated myopathy. *Neurology*. 1991;41:921–922.
202. Op de Coul AA, Lambregts PC, Koeman J, van Puyenbroek MJ, Ter Laak HJ, Gabreels-Festen AA. Neuromuscular complications in patients given Pavulon (pancuronium bromide) during artificial ventilation. *Clin Neurol Neurosurg*. 1985;87:17–22.
203. Witt NJ, Zochodne DW, Bolton CF, et al. Peripheral nerve function in sepsis and multiorgan failure. *Chest*. 1991;99:176–184.
204. Latronico N, Fenzi F, Recupero D, et al. Critical illness myopathy and neuropathy. *Lancet*. 1996;347:1579–1582.
205. Campellone JV, Lacomis D, Kramer DJ, Van Cott AC, Giuliani MJ. Acute myopathy after liver transplantation. *Neurology*. 1998;50:46–53.
206. Road J, Mackie G, Jiang TX, Stewart H, Eisen A. Reversible paralysis with status asthmaticus, steroids, and pancuronium: clinical electrophysiological correlates. *Muscle Nerve*. 1997;20:1587–1590.
207. Zochodne DW, Ramsey DA, Saly V, Shelley S, Moffatt S. Acute necrotizing myopathy of the intensive care: electrophysiological studies. *Muscle Nerve*. 1994;17:285–292.
208. Douglass JA, Tuxen DV, Horne M, et al. Myopathy in severe asthma. *Am Rev Respir Dis*. 1992;146:517–519.
209. Rich MM, Pinter MJ, Kraner SD, Barchi RL. Loss of electrical excitability in an animal model of acute quadriplegic myopathy. *Ann Neurol*. 1998;43:171–179.
210. Allen DC, Arunachalam R, Mills KR. Critical illness myopathy: further evidence from muscle-fiber excitability studies of an acquired channelopathy. *Muscle Nerve*. 2008;37:14–22.
211. Ruff RL. Why do ICU patients become paralyzed? *Ann Neurol*. 1998;43:154–155.
212. Faucheux JM, Tourneize P, Viguier A, Arne-Bes MC, Larrue M, Geraud G. Neuromyopathy secondary to omeprazole treatment. *Muscle Nerve*. 1998;21:261–262.
213. Garrot FJ, Lacambrac D, Del Sert T, García Díaz B, Obeso G, Solís J. Subacute myopathy during omeprazole therapy [letter]. *Lancet*. 1994;340:672.
214. Sarifakioglu E, Onur O, Kart H, Yilmaz AE. Acute myopathy and acne fulminans triggered by isotretinoin therapy. *Eur J Dermatol*. 2011;21(5):794–795.
215. Chroni E, Monastirli A, Tsambaos D. Neuromuscular adverse effects associated with systemic retinoid dermatotherapy: monitoring and treatment algorithm for clinicians. *Drug Saf*. 2010;33:25–34.
216. Kaymak Y. Creatine phosphokinase values during isotretinoin treatment for acne. *Int J Dermatol*. 2008;47:398–340.
217. Bertorini TE. Myoglobinuria, malignant hyperthermia, neuroleptic malignant syndrome and serotonin syndrome. *Neurol Clin*. 1997;15:649–671.

218. Nelson TE, Flewellen EH. Current concepts: the malignant hyperthermia syndrome. *N Engl J Med.* 1983;309:416–418.
219. MacLennan DH, Phillips MS. Malignant hyperthermia. *Science.* 1992;256:789–794.
220. McCarthy TV, Healy JM, Heffron JJ, et al. Localization of the malignant hyperthermia susceptibility locus to human chromosome 19q12–13.2. *Nature.* 1990;343:562–564.
221. Moslehi R, Lanlois S, Yam I, Fiedman J. Linkage of malignant hyperthermia and hyperkalemic periodic paralysis to the adult skeletal muscle sodium channel (SCNa4) gene in a large pedigree. *Am J Hum Genet.* 1998;76:21–27.
222. Iles DE, Lehman-Horn F, Scherer SW, et al. Localization of the gene encoding the d2/d-subunits of the L-type voltage dependent calcium channel to chromosome 7q and analysis of the segregation of flanking markers in malignant hyperthermia susceptible families. *Hum Mol Genet.* 1994;3:969–975.
223. Subrak R, Procaccio V, Klasusnitzer M, et al. Mapping of a further malignant hyperthermia susceptibility locus to chromosome 3q13.1. *Am J Hum Genet.* 1995;56:684–691.
224. Monnier N, Procaccio V, Stieglitz P, Lunardi J. Malignant hyperthermia susceptibility is associated with a mutation of the a1-subunit of the human dihydropyridine-sensitive L-type voltage -dependent calcium-channel receptor in skeletal muscle. *Am J Hum Genet.* 1997;60:1316–1325.
225. Robinson RL, Monnier N, Jung M, et al. A genome wide search for susceptibility loci in three European malignant hyperthermia pedigrees. *Hum Mol Genet.* 1997;6:953–961.
226. Sethna NF, Rockoff MA, Worthen HM, Rosnow JM. Anesthesia-related complications of children with Duchenne muscular dystrophy. *Anesthesiology.* 1988;68:462–465.
227. Ekbom K, Hed R, Kirstein L, Astrom KE. Muscular affections in chronic alcoholism. *Arch Neurol.* 1964;10:449–458.
228. Mayer RF, Garcia-Mullin R, Eckholdt JW. Acute alcoholic myopathy. *Neurology.* 1968;18:275.
229. Oh SJ. Chronic alcoholic myopathy: an entity difficult to diagnose. *South Med J.* 1972;65:449–452.
230. Perkoff GT, Dioso MM, Bleisch V, Klinkerfuss G. A spectrum of myopathy associated with alcoholism. I. Clinical and laboratory features. *Ann Intern Med.* 1967;67:481–492.
231. Rubenstein AE, Wainapel SF. Acute hypokalemic myopathy in alcoholism: a clinical entity. *Arch Neurol.* 1977;34:553–555.
232. Cogen FC, Rigg G, Simmons JL, Domino EF. Phencyclidine-associated acute rhabdomyolysis. *Ann Intern Med.* 1978;88:210–212.
233. Richter RW, Challenor YB, Pearson J, Kagen LJ, Hamilton LL, Ramsey WH. Acute myoglobinuria associated with heroin addiction. *J Am Med Assoc.* 1971;216:1172–1176.
234. Richter RW, Pearson J, Bruun B, Challenor YB, Brust JC, Baden MM. Neurological complications of heroin addiction. *Bull N Y Acad Med.* 1973;49:1–21.
235. Van den Bergh PY, Guettat L, Vande Berg BC, Martine JJ. Focal myopathy associated with chronic intramuscular injection of piritramide. *Muscle Nerve.* 1997;20(12):1598–1600.

CHAPTER 36

Neuromuscular Mimics

Sabrina Paganoni and Erik Ensrud

We define "neuromuscular mimic" as any musculoskeletal condition that presents with pain and apparent weakness, and can mimic a neuromuscular etiology such as radiculopathy or entrapment neuropathy. "Limb pain" is a common reason for referral to the clinic and EMG laboratory and the identification of the underlying pain generator is often challenging. For example, in two series of patients referred for electrodiagnostic testing for suspected cervical or lumbosacral radiculopathy, the prevalence of musculoskeletal disorders was 42% and 32%, respectively.[1,2] Thus, musculoskeletal disorders are common in patients suspected of having a radiculopathy. They can mimic radiculopathy or coexist with it in many individuals.[1,2] Importantly, neuromuscular mimics can often be diagnosed quickly at the bedside and are eminently treatable. Their prompt recognition may avoid unnecessary and expensive diagnostic procedures and result in more efficient clinical practice. It is common for physicians from many specialties to be unfamiliar with recognizing these conditions.[3]

In this chapter, we will describe the most common mimics of radiculopathy and neuropathy in the upper and lower limbs (Table 36-1). We will not perform an exhaustive review of these pathologies. Rather, this chapter will serve as an entry point for physicians with minimal musculoskeletal training with the goal of providing them with time-efficient and resource-efficient tools to screen for these common conditions in their busy daily practice.

A few key "pearls" are worth remembering when performing a musculoskeletal examination. First, it is important to check the bilateral limbs for side-to-side comparison, starting from the noninvolved side first, whenever possible. If the test maneuver elicits pain, one needs to ask the patient whether the elicited pain is the same that he/she has been experiencing. This is important in order to avoid overcalling pathology as musculoskeletal examination maneuvers can trigger some discomfort even in healthy individuals, particularly if palpation and provocative tests are performed too vigorously. Finally, when assessing whether the maneuver reproduces the patient's chief complaint, it is very helpful to look for the "wince sign," with the patient blinking and grimacing as the pain is reproduced.

▶ TOP MIMICS IN THE UPPER LIMBS

SUPRASPINATUS TENDINOPATHY

Supraspinatus tendinopathy is a common cause of shoulder pain and can mimic C5/6/7 radiculopathy.

Symptoms

The rotator cuff consists of four muscles that are responsible for securing the arm into the glenohumeral (shoulder) joint. These muscles are the supraspinatus, infraspinatus, teres minor, and subscapularis. The tendon most commonly injured within the rotator cuff is the supraspinatus.[4] Risk factors include older age, repetitive overhead activity, whether work- or sport-related, anatomic variants, instability of the glenohumeral joint, and periscapular muscle weakness and imbalance.[5–7] The latter are common in people with underlying neurologic diseases.

Patients complain of shoulder pain that is aggravated by arm movement, especially overhead. Painful daily activities may include putting on a shirt or brushing hair. The pain may be localized to the deltoid area, but may also radiate upward toward the neck or distally down the arm, thus mimicking cervical radiculopathy, most often in a C5–C7 distribution. Often, patients have difficulty sleeping on the side of the affected shoulder due to pain.

Diagnosis

Shoulder examination includes inspection, range of motion (ROM), strength testing, palpation, and special tests.[8] With long-standing rotator cuff tendinopathy, inspection may reveal atrophy of the supra- and infraspinatus muscles. ROM above 90 degrees of abduction, either actively or passively, is often painful. Active ROM may be limited by pain, but passive ROM is preserved. There may be tenderness to palpation over the affected muscles or focal subacromial tenderness at the posterolateral border of the acromion. Pain may also be elicited by one of the many special tests that are available to examine the shoulder.[8,9] A simple and sensitive screening test for supraspinatus tendinopathy is the Hawkins test (Fig. 36-1). Reduced passive ROM and weakness with resisted abduction and/or external rotation suggest the presence of adhesive capsulitis and rotator cuff tear, respectively. Musculoskeletal ultrasound and magnetic resonance imaging (MRI) can be considered if further investigation and confirmation of the etiology are desired.[10]

Treatment

Conservative treatment for supraspinatus tendinopathy includes rest, activity modification, ice, nonsteroidal anti-inflammatory drugs (NSAIDs), and physical therapy. Physical therapy is directed to preserving ROM while restoring proper

▶ TABLE 36-1. NEUROMUSCULAR MIMICS

Upper Limb Mimics
Supraspinatus tendinopathy
Biceps tendinopathy
Lateral epicondylitis
De Quervain syndrome
Carpometacarpal (CMC) joint osteoarthritis
Lower Limb Mimics
Hip joint osteoarthritis
Greater trochanteric bursitis
Pes anserine bursitis
Plantar fasciitis

muscle activation and strength balance among the muscles of the rotator cuff.[11,12] A subacromial steroid injection may reduce pain and enable earlier participation in ROM exercises and rehabilitation.[13] Referral to orthopedics, physiatry, or rheumatology for further diagnostic and therapeutic management is warranted if there is no response to several weeks of conservative management or if additional pathology is suspected.

BICEPS TENDINOPATHY

Biceps tendinopathy is a common cause of anterior shoulder pain and can mimic C5/C6 cervical radiculopathy.

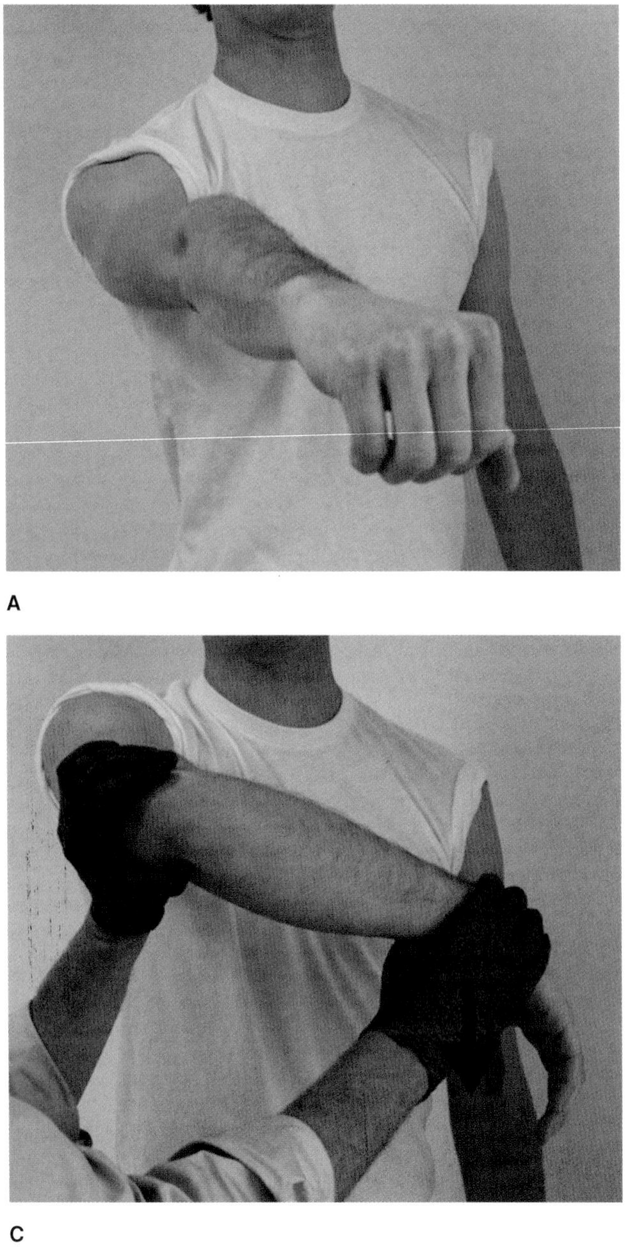

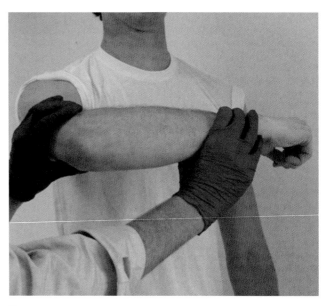

Figure 36-1. Hawkins test. Correct positioning is important to perform the test. The patient forward flexes the arm to 90 degrees **(A)** and the examiner flexes the elbow to 90 degrees **(B)**. The examiner then forcibly internally rotates the shoulder **(C)**. The maneuver drives the greater tuberosity of the humerus farther under the coracoacromial ligament. Pain with this maneuver is considered positive for impingement of the supraspinatus tendon under the acromion.

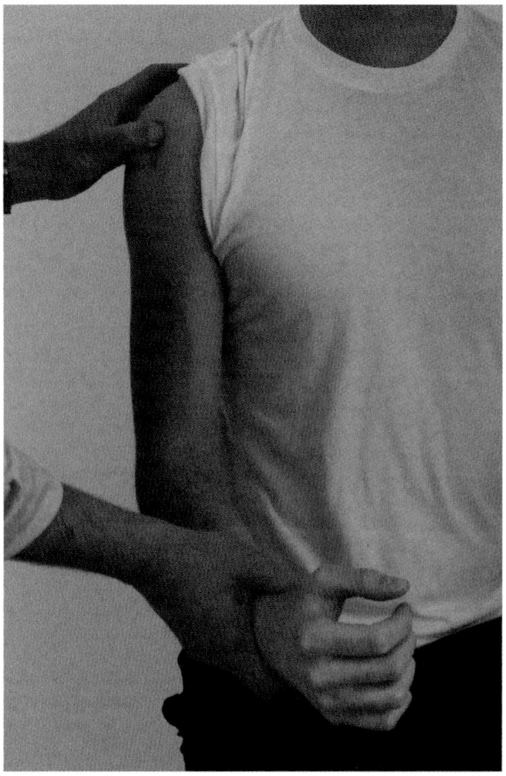

Figure 36-2. **Yergason test.** The long head of the biceps tendon is palpated for tenderness in the bicipital groove, between the greater and lesser tuberosities of the humeral head. Localization of the bicipital groove is aided by internally and externally rotating the shoulder with the elbow flexed at 90 degrees while feeling for the tuberosities.

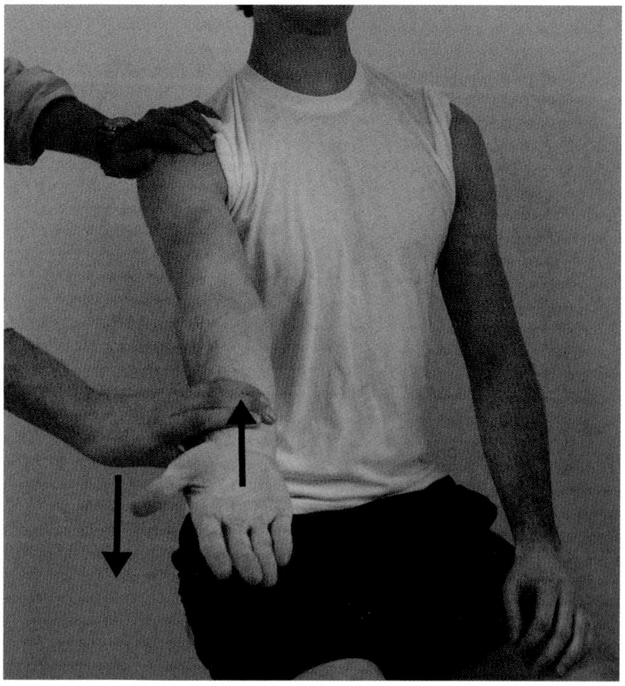

Figure 36-3. **Speed test.** The patient is asked to flex the shoulder against resistance from the examiner while the elbow is extended and the forearm is supinated. The test is positive for biceps tendon pathology when pain is localized to the bicipital groove.

Symptoms

The tendon of the long head of the biceps, with its synovial lining, lies within the bicipital groove which is located in the anterior upper humerus and is bordered laterally by the greater tuberosity and medially by the lesser tuberosity. The bicipital groove is easily palpable in the anterior upper arm when the arm is externally rotated (Fig. 36-2). Tendinopathy occurs where the tendon passes through the bicipital groove and over the head of the humerus just like a rope through a pulley. The underlying pathology may involve inflammation of the tendon and tendon sheath (tendonitis, tenosynovitis) and/or chronic overuse injury and degeneration (tendinosis).[14]

Affected individuals complain of a deep, throbbing ache in the anterior shoulder. Tenderness is usually localized to the bicipital groove, but may radiate to the deltoid region or downward to the anterolateral arm making it difficult to distinguish from upper cervical radicular pain. The pain often worsens at night, especially if sleeping on the affected side, and may increase with lifting, pulling, or repetitive overhead reaching. The risk of developing biceps tendinopathy increases with age and is higher in people who routinely perform activities that require repetitive overhead movements. Importantly, biceps tendinopathy often coexists with other pathologies of the shoulder, including rotator cuff tendinopathy and tears, as well as intra-articular injuries such as a labral tear.[15,16]

Diagnosis

Clinical diagnosis includes assessing for Yergason test, which is tenderness identified by palpation of the long head of the biceps tendon in the bicipital groove while internally and externally rotating the humerus (Fig. 36-2).[17] Another helpful test is the Speed test.[18] For the Speed test, the patient is asked to flex the arm (lift upward) against resistance from the examiner with the elbow extended and the forearm fully supinated (Fig. 36-3). The test is considered positive when pain is localized to the bicipital groove, implying biceps tendonitis and/or tenosynovitis. Of note, the Speed test may be positive with other shoulder degenerative pathologies. Ultrasound[19] and/or MRI[20] are not needed for the diagnosis of biceps tendinopathy, but may be considered in patients who are suspected of having additional concurrent shoulder pathologies or are refractory to treatment.

Treatment

Conservative treatment is appropriate for most patients with biceps tendinopathy.[21,22] Treatment includes rest and activity modification to allow the tendon to heal. Oral or

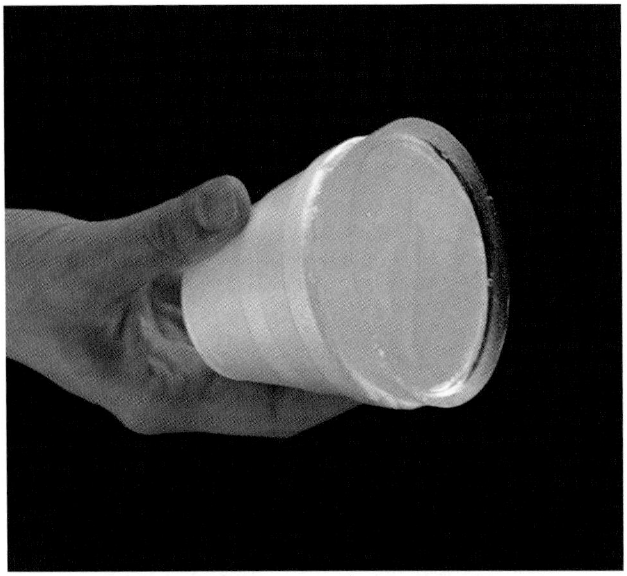

Figure 36-4. **Frozen paper cup for ice therapy.** A paper cup is filled with water and placed in a freezer. When the water is frozen, the top of the cup can be peeled away to expose the ice. Ice massage is then performed by placing the cup over the injury in a circular pattern allowing the ice to melt away.

topical NSAIDs and modalities, such as ice therapy, help reduce pain and inflammation. The superficial location of the biceps tendon as it runs through the bicipital groove makes it particularly amenable to ice massage. Patients can be instructed to ice the tender area by directly applying ice to the skin using gentle stroking motions ("ice massage"). The paper cup method is a comfortable, convenient, and inexpensive method of performing ice massage. Water is frozen in a paper cup and ice is exposed by tearing the top rim of paper (Fig. 36-4). Ice is then applied to the affected area multiple times a day until the area is numb, which usually occurs within 5 minutes.

If symptoms do not improve with use of rest, activity modification, NSAIDs, and ice therapy, referral to a musculoskeletal medicine expert (from physiatry, sports medicine or orthopedic surgery) may be considered. Physical therapy is used to improve muscle strength and tendon stability. An ultrasound-guided injection of steroid in the biceps tendon sheath is an option for both diagnostic and therapeutic purposes.[23,24] Ultrasound guidance is needed to avoid injecting the tendon with resulting risk of rupture. Surgical intervention is used only in selected patients and includes tenotomy and tenodesis.[20,25]

LATERAL EPICONDYLITIS

Lateral epicondylitis (colloquially known as "tennis elbow") is a common tendinopathy that presents as lateral elbow pain. Pain may radiate distally along the forearm, mimicking C6 cervical radiculopathy or ulnar neuropathy.

Symptoms

The lateral epicondyle of the humerus is located lateral to the olecranon process and is the origin of the wrist and finger extensors. Overuse and poor mechanics can lead to an overload of the extensor tendons.[26,27] The underlying pathology is not inflammatory, but rather degenerative and consists of tendon microtearing.[28] Pathology most often involves the extensor carpi radialis brevis, approximately 1–2 cm distal to the attachment to the lateral epicondyle, but can affect the other extensors as well.

In most cases, the pain begins shortly after a period of overuse and slowly worsens over weeks and months. There is usually no specific injury associated with the start of symptoms. The point of maximal pain and tenderness is typically located just distal to the lateral epicondyle over the extensor tendon mass, however pain can extend into the distal forearm mimicking C6 radiculopathy. Pain is exacerbated by arm use, especially repetitive wrist extension and pronation/supination activities. There may be perceived weakness in grip strength. Lateral epicondylitis is most often associated with tennis and other racquet sports. Poor technique including improper backhand, string tension, and grip size are contributing factors.[29] However, any activity that places excessive repetitive stress on the lateral forearm musculature can cause this condition.[30,31]

Diagnosis

Clinical diagnosis includes assessing for tenderness by palpation over the lateral epicondyle and 1–2 cm distal to it over the common extensor tendon which usually represents the point of maximal tenderness in lateral epicondylitis. The provocative maneuver or "tennis elbow test" consists of resisted radial wrist extension with the forearm in pronation (Fig. 36-5). The examiner stabilizes the elbow with a thumb over the lateral epicondyle. The test is positive if pain is elicited when the patient makes a fist and extends the wrist against resistance by the examiner. The pain is usually worse with the elbow in extension than with the elbow in flexion. Imaging is generally not needed to diagnose this condition, but a plain x-ray of the elbow may be considered to rule out intra-articular pathology and/or loose body fragments. In addition, an x-ray may reveal calcification over the lateral epicondyle. Ultrasound and MRI may be considered if there is no response to conservative treatment.

Treatment

Despite the prevalence of lateral epicondylitis and the availability of different treatment options, only few high-quality clinical trials are available to support evidence-based management algorithms for this condition. Activity modification is an important first step in management and includes correcting training or technique errors such as grip size of the tennis racket when appropriate. Initial conservative management also includes pain control by using a short course of topical or oral NSAIDs[32] and ice massage (as described above). Wrist

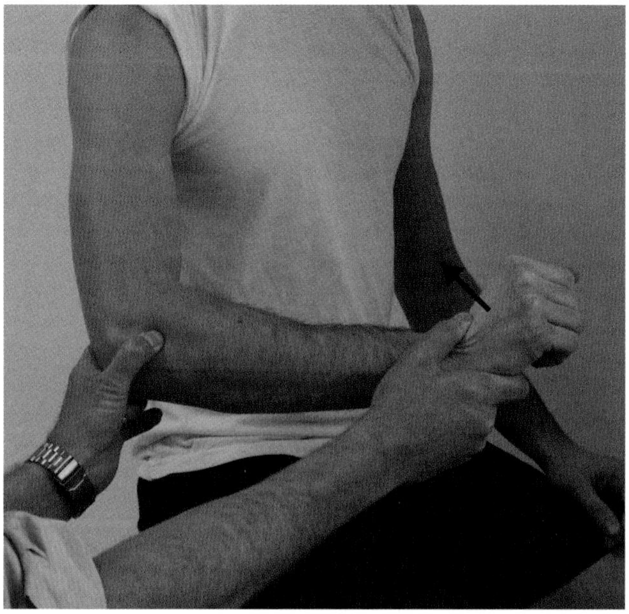

Figure 36-5. **Tennis elbow test.** The examiner stabilizes the elbow while palpating along the lateral epicondyle. With the elbow pronated and a closed fist, the patient extends the wrist against the examiner's resistance. The point of maximal tenderness is generally located one fingerbreadth distal to the lateral epicondyle over the extensor tendon mass. The pain is usually worse with the elbow in extension than with the elbow in flexion.

extensor stretching (Fig. 36-6)[33] and bracing[34] are often helpful. Bracing consists of using a counterforce elbow strap. Elbow or "tennis straps" are placed on the forearm a few centimeters distal to the elbow joint, are easy to use and inexpensive. Counterforce bracing may reduce tendon and muscle strain at the origin of the forearm extensor muscles, thus relieving pain during activities. Physical therapy has been found to be effective in lateral epicondylitis.[35,36] Therapy includes progressive isometric and eccentric strengthening and incorporates stretching and modalities as needed. Eccentric exercise occurs when muscles contract while lengthening. Application of

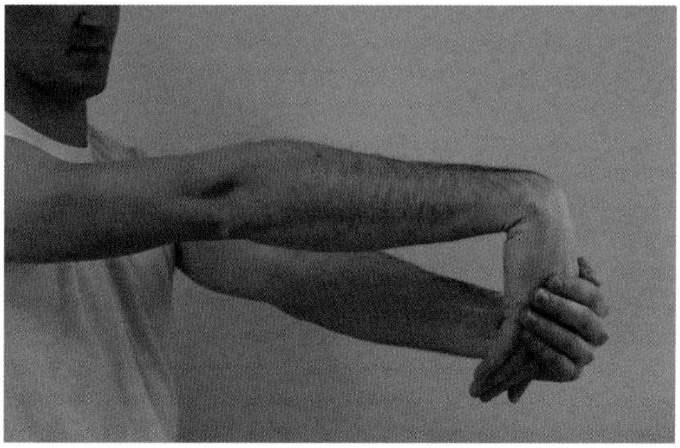

Figure 36-6. Wrist extensor stretch.

this technique for lateral epicondylitis involves contracting the wrist extensors against the resistance of an exercise band.[37,38] Steroid injections have also been used to treat "tennis elbow."[39] Their use, however, is controversial.[40] Trials have found that corticosteroid injections improve short-term outcomes in lateral epicondylitis, but do not prevent recurrence and may actually lead to worse long-term outcomes.[36,41,42]

DE QUERVAIN SYNDROME

De Quervain syndrome is a common cause of wrist pain and can mimic carpal tunnel syndrome, C6 cervical radiculopathy, and superficial radial sensory neuropathy.

Symptoms

De Quervain syndrome is the most common tenosynovitis of the wrist. It results from inflammation of the fluid-filled sheath (synovium) that surrounds the tendons of the abductor pollicis longus (APL) and extensor pollicis brevis (EPB) in the first dorsal compartment of the wrist. These tendons run over the dorsal aspect of the radial styloid process.

The exact causes of De Quervain syndrome are unclear, but they probably include shear and repetitive microtrauma. Postures where the thumb is held in abduction and extension are considered predisposing factors[43,44] although evidence regarding a possible relation with certain occupations is controversial. A systematic review of potential risk factors did not find evidence of an association with specific occupation-related activities.[45] Women are affected more than men[46] and the syndrome commonly occurs during and after pregnancy, due to hormonal changes and possibly lifting the newborn repetitively in a cradled position thus putting stress on the wrist and thumb. Because of the latter postulated risk factor, De Quervain syndrome is also known as "mother's wrist."

Patients with this condition present with insidious onset of pain over the dorsal radial aspect of the wrist which may be accompanied by swelling. The pain may radiate distally into the thumb or proximally along the radial aspect of the forearm. Symptoms are exacerbated by grasping or ulnar deviation of the wrist.

Diagnosis

De Quervain syndrome can be easily diagnosed on physical examination. Patients usually have tenderness to palpation over the dorsal radial wrist. Finkelstein test is pathognomonic for the condition (Fig. 36-7). To perform the test, the patient is first asked to wrap the fingers around the thumb. To avoid having tight finger flexor tendons splint and immobilize the wrist, it is helpful to ask the patient to wrap the fingers around the thumb lightly, as if the thumb were an egg. The examiner then ulnarly deviates the wrist. A positive test occurs when the patient experiences sharp and intense pain over the radial styloid process, exactly where the tendon

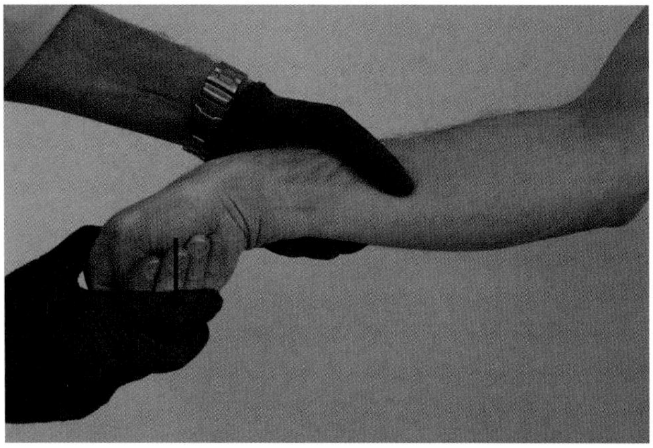

Figure 36-7. **Finkelstein test.** The patient is asked to make a fist over the thumb. The examiner ulnarly deviates the wrist. A positive test is indicated by exquisite pain in the region of the radial styloid.

sheath takes its course. De Quervain tenosynovitis is a clinical diagnosis and imaging is not needed.

Treatment

Conservative treatment includes rest, ice, anti-inflammatory medications (oral or topical), steroid injections, and a thumb spica splint. The splint is worn during the day, but the patient should remove it several times a day to perform gentle ROM exercises to prevent the complications of prolonged immobilization. Iontophoresis can help with inflammation and pain control. Steroid injections are very effective in providing pain relief and have a favorable side effect profile.[47] They work best when used in conjunction with a thumb spica splint.[48] Ultrasound guidance for steroid injection is recommended to more precisely localize the site of injection.[49] Surgery is rarely indicated and carries a small risk of injury to the superficial radial nerve.[50]

CARPOMETACARPAL JOINT OSTEOARTHRITIS

Carpometacarpal (CMC) joint osteoarthritis (OA) (colloquially known as "thumb arthritis") is a common cause of hand pain and can mimic carpal tunnel syndrome.

Symptoms

The CMC joint of the thumb connects the trapezium to the first metacarpal bone and plays an important role in the normal functioning of the thumb (Fig. 36-8). Degenerative changes in this joint result in "thumb arthritis" which can cause severe hand pain, swelling, decreased ROM, and reduced grip strength.[51] Pain and swelling occur at the base of the thumb. The discomfort is exacerbated by activities that involve using the thumb to apply force or grasping an object. Thumb arthritis can make it difficult to perform simple household tasks, such as opening jars, pulling a zipper, and turning doorknobs.[52] Patients may complain of reduced grip strength.[52]

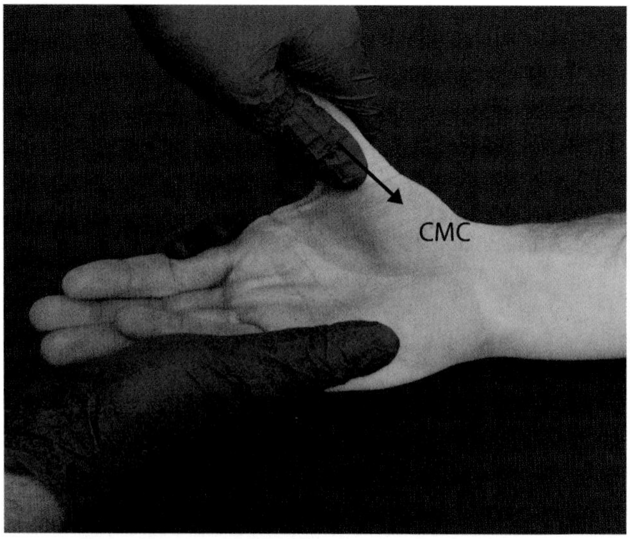

Figure 36-8. **Thumb osteoarthritis.** The location of the first CMC joint at the base of the thumb is demonstrated in the figure. The grind test is performed by gripping the metacarpal bone of the thumb, loading it with axial forces to push it against the carpal bone (trapezium), and rotating it in circular motion.

The condition is more common in postmenopausal women.[53] Risk factors include genetic predisposition,[54] history of prior trauma to the joint, occupations involving repetitive thumb use,[55] history of rheumatoid arthritis or articular hypermobility,[56] and the presence of OA in other joints.[57,58]

Diagnosis

Thumb OA can be easily diagnosed by using the grind test (Fig. 36-8).[59] The examiner holds the wrist in one hand and grasps the first metacarpal bone in the other hand. Axial pressure toward the wrist is applied while rotating the metacarpal bone in a wide circular arc, resulting in compression of the CMC joint. The test is considered positive if the patient reports pain at the base of the thumb. In a positive test, the examiner will also note a grinding or catch sensation while rotating the metacarpal bone in the circular arc. In addition, the CMC joint may appear enlarged from osteoarthritic hypertrophy. Radiographic evaluation has higher sensitivity than the grind test, but the presence of radiographic OA only has a modest association with clinical symptoms such as hand pain and disability.[60]

Treatment

Treatment for thumb arthritis includes both nonsurgical and surgical options. Activity modification can be tried first to reduce the activities that most exacerbate pain. As an example, one can use pens with a bigger grip, change door knobs to latches, and use jar openers. Splints can be effective in early stages and can be used at night and/or during the day depending on the patient's job and needs. Different splints are available to support the thumb, place the joint in a resting position, and decrease pain.[61–63] No one splint is superior to the other. Customized braces may provide a better fit and have been associated with improved outcomes, but are more expensive.[62] Oral acetaminophen and NSAIDs can be used to manage pain. If a combination of splinting and oral medications is not effective, an intra-articular steroid injection can reduce inflammation and provide pain relief for a few months.[64,65] In severe cases, surgical treatment may be needed and includes different procedures that are tailored to the extent of arthritic involvement.[66] Surgery may include metacarpal osteotomy, trapeziectomy, arthrodesis (joint fusion), and arthroplasty[67] (joint replacement). Recovery after surgery includes 6 weeks of bracing and about 3 months of hand therapy to work on ROM and flexibility of the thumb.[68] Most patients regain their strength and return to normal activities at the 6-month time point.

▶ TOP MIMICS IN THE LOWER LIMBS

HIP JOINT OSTEOARTHRITIS

Hip OA is a common[69] cause of hip, groin, and thigh pain and can mimic L2/3/4 radiculopathy.

Symptoms

The characteristic symptoms of hip OA include anterior hip and groin pain that is exacerbated by weight bearing/physical activity and improves with rest. These characteristics help differentiate hip OA from greater trochanteric bursitis which presents with lateral hip pain aggravated by direct pressure. The pain of hip OA can radiate down the thigh and may also involve the groin area, knee region, and buttock area. Patients may complain of difficulty walking and leg "stiffness." The pain can either be stabbing and sharp or it can be a dull ache. While the causes of hip OA are not completely known, risk factors include increasing age, genetic predisposition, prior hip injury or developmental deformities, heavy manual labor, participation in weight-bearing sports, and being overweight.[70–73]

Diagnosis

The key clinical finding suggestive of hip OA on examination is the ability to reproduce the patient's pain when ranging the femur into full internal rotation (Fig. 36-9).[74] Furthermore, with hip OA, internal rotation is generally limited more than external rotation. The reason underlying these findings is that sharp forceful internal rotation of the femur compresses the joint space, approximating the bony acetabulum and femoral

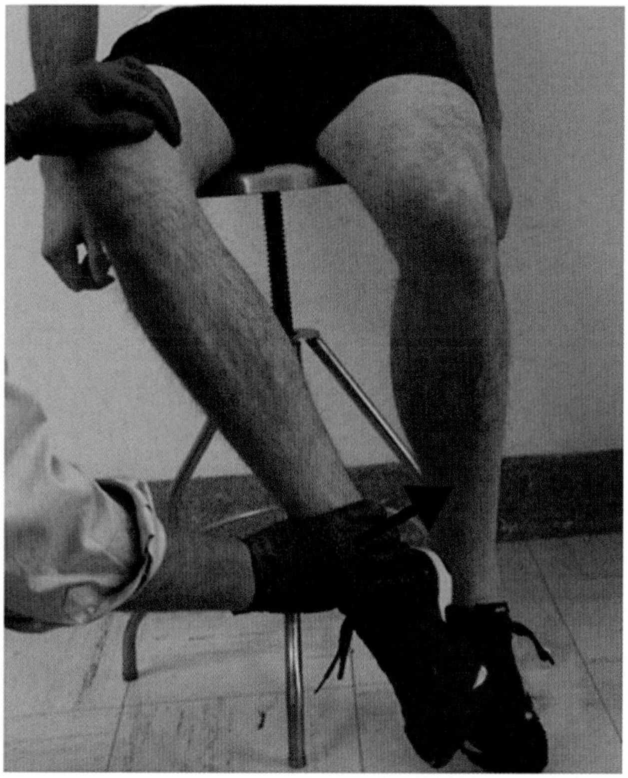

A

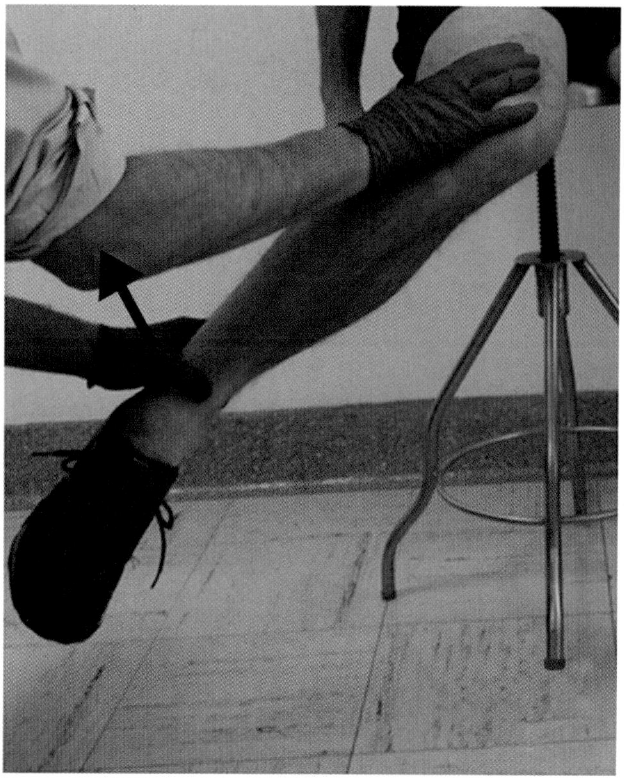

B

Figure 36-9. **Hip internal and external rotation.** Hip external rotation **(A)** is not typically associated with pain in hip osteoarthritis, whereas hip internal rotation **(B)** does reproduce the patient's pain. Hip range of motion can be tested in a sitting position, as demonstrated here, or with the patient lying down on the examination table.

head, which is uncomfortable when the articular cartilage is degenerated. External rotation is generally better tolerated. Patients may also develop an antalgic gait because they tend to spend a shorter time weight bearing on the affected side due to pain. Diagnosis can be confirmed by weight-bearing anteroposterior (AP) pelvis x-ray to assess the articular width of the hip joints. Joint space narrowing, sclerosis of the joint space margins, and periarticular osteophyte formation are consistent with OA.[75] An ultrasound-guided intra-articular anesthetic and/or steroid injection can be a valuable diagnostic tool when there are questions about the location of the pain generator.[76,77]

Treatment

Treatment of hip OA starts with education about joint protection, weight loss (if appropriate), use of modalities for pain reduction, physical therapy[78,79] to preserve strength and ROM, and use of mobility aids as needed.[80,81] A cane held on the nonaffected side helps to off load the affected hip resulting in improved pain and gait mechanics. Pharmacologic treatment includes acetaminophen, NSAIDs, and ultrasound-guided intra-articular steroid injections.[82] Surgical intervention (either hip resurfacing or replacement) followed by rehabilitation may ultimately be needed to ensure optimal pain control and function in advanced cases.[81]

GREATER TROCHANTERIC BURSITIS

Greater trochanteric bursitis causes lateral hip/thigh pain and can mimic L3/L4/L5 radiculopathy.[83]

Symptoms

Greater trochanteric bursitis presents as tenderness to palpation over the greater trochanter, in the lateral hip and thigh.[84,85] Some prefer the term "greater trochanteric pain syndrome," which may be more accurate because the etiology of this condition is not fully understood. The pain generator may be related to an inflammation of the trochanteric bursa located on the outer side of the femur. However, contributing pain generators may include the gluteus medius and gluteus minimus muscles, their attachments into the greater trochanter of the femur and the femoral shaft, and overlying tissue such as the iliotibial (IT) band.[86–89] All of these structures are associated with the greater trochanter and may be affected by abnormal lower limb biomechanics and disturbances in gait, which are common occurrences in people with underlying neurologic diseases.[83,90–92] Gait abnormalities affect the biomechanics around the greater trochanter and lead to altered pressure on the bursae and friction in the tendons and other soft tissue structures, which ultimately result in local pain and tenderness.[90]

Patients typically complain of lateral hip pain that may radiate into the buttock and outer thigh into the knee. Patients may rub their thigh when describing the pain. The pain is characteristically exacerbated by direct pressure to the point that patients may describe intolerance to sleeping on the affected side. Pain can also be aggravated by walking, especially climbing stairs and can be disabling with a negative impact on quality of life.[93]

Diagnosis

The diagnosis is based on history and clinical findings of exquisite pain on direct palpation of the region of the greater trochanter.[94] Palpation can be performed in the lateral decubitus position with the affected side placed upward. The trochanteric process is the most prominent portion of the femur. Side-to-side comparison can be easily accomplished by palpating the outer thighs and hips with the patient in a seated position facing the examiner (Fig. 36-10). The examiner palpates along the lateral femurs from distal to proximal until reaching the greater trochanters (Fig. 36-10). Note that palpation of the lateral thigh can elicit some discomfort in people with tight IT bands. However, when trochanteric bursitis is present, direct

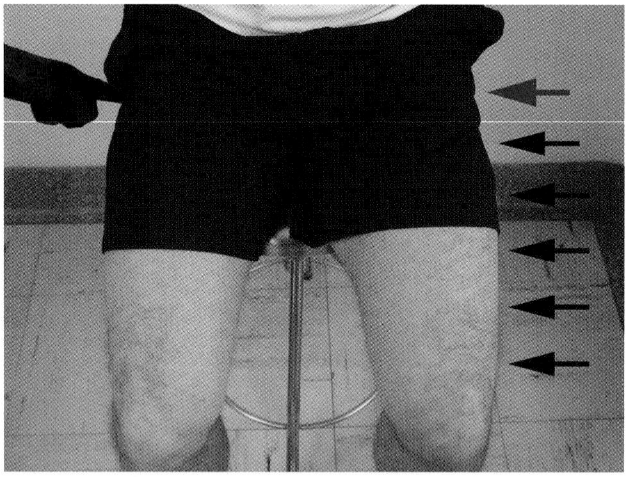

Figure 36-10. **Greater trochanter palpation.** To localize the greater trochanter, the examiner palpates the lateral thigh starting distally (*arrows*) and moving proximally until the greater trochanter of the femur is identified (as indicated by the examiner in the picture). Palpating the greater trochanter will elicit pain in patients with greater trochanteric bursitis. Performing the maneuver in sitting, as demonstrated here, allows a quick side-to-side comparison. Note that palpation of the lateral thigh can elicit some discomfort in people with tight iliotibial bands. However, when greater trochanteric bursitis is present, there will be additional, sharp pain localized to the greater trochanter. The maneuver can also be performed with the patient lying down on the examination table and the affected leg placed upward. Lying down on the side of the affected leg produces exquisite pain in patients with greater trochanteric bursitis.

palpation will elicit prominent sharp pain that reproduces the patient's pain.

Pain relief with local anesthetic and/or steroid injection corroborates the diagnosis and provides excellent pain relief.[95,96] Plain radiographs of the hip can be performed to exclude structural abnormalities, while ultrasound and MRI can be considered in refractory cases.[87]

Treatment

NSAIDs and ice therapy help relieve pain and reduce the inflammation. Ice therapy to the lateral hip every 4–6 hours can be accomplished by ice massage with a paper cup (Fig. 36-4) or by using flexible frozen gels or a bag of frozen peas against the hip to cover a larger area. Typical, uncomplicated greater trochanteric pain syndrome responds very well to local injections of an anesthetic and/or steroid.[91,95,96] The pain may actually worsen for 1 or 2 days immediately following the procedure before improving. Injection aftercare is critical to the success of the injection. The patient should rest, avoid direct pressure and repetitive bending, and use NSAIDs and ice as needed for pain relief. In order to help prevent recurrence, predisposing factors should be addressed as much as possible. Physical therapy can be helpful to stretch the back and IT band and strengthening the hip muscles can relieve tension in the hip and reduce friction. Daily stretches should be incorporated into an individualized home exercise program (HEP) for best results. Stretches are most effective and best tolerated after the steroid injection of the bursae has been performed.

PES ANSERINE BURSITIS

Bursitis is a common cause of lower extremity pain. Pes anserine bursitis presents as medial knee and leg pain and can mimic L4 lumbar radiculopathy.

Symptoms

The pes anserinus ("goose's foot") is the insertion of the conjoined tendons of three muscles (semitendinosus, sartorius, and gracilis) onto the anteromedial surface of the proximal tibia. It lies superficial to the superficial fibers of the medial collateral ligament (MCL) of the knee. Inflammation of the anserine bursa that lies just under the tendons near their insertion is termed pes anserine bursitis.[97]

Pes anserine bursitis should be suspected when pain occurs in the medial knee region over the upper tibia.[98] Pain is exacerbated by repetitive knee flexion such as when ascending stairs and climbing. Sports that involve side-to-side cutting activity (e.g., tennis and soccer) as well as underlying knee medial compartment OA and obesity may predispose to bursitis. Muscle imbalances involving the hip adductors, hip flexors, and hamstrings may cause an abnormal pull at the insertion point of the three tendons resulting in pes anserine bursitis.[99,100]

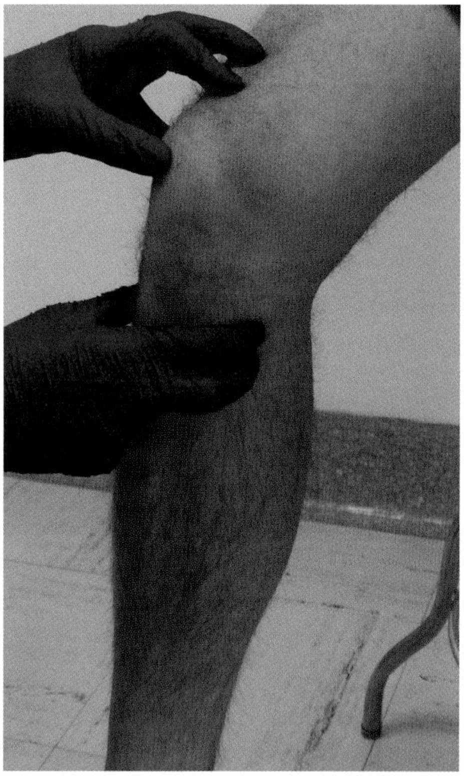

Figure 36-11. **Pes anserine bursa.** The figure depicts the location of the anserine bursa in the medial leg.

Diagnosis

The diagnosis of pes anserine bursitis is made clinically by direct palpation of the bursa, which elicits localized tenderness (Fig. 36-11). The entire tibial plateau needs to be palpated to differentiate between the localized tenderness of anserine bursitis and medial joint line tenderness from an intra-articular injury. In addition, there may be more extensive tenderness along the medial femoral epicondyle to the medial tibia which is present with MCL injury. Imaging is usually not indicated unless there is suspicion for stress fracture or intra-articular pathology such as meniscal injury or knee OA.

Treatment

In the acute phase, treatment includes rest, ice massage (as described above), and a short course of topical or oral NSAIDs to reduce the pain and swelling in the bursa. Activity modification to "rest" the bursa include avoiding direct pressure (which can be accomplished at night by using a pillow between the knees) as well as activities such as squatting, repetitive knee bending, and crossing the legs.[101] A corticosteroid injection into the bursa can be used both as a diagnostic and therapeutic tool and often provides quick relief.[102] A rehabilitation program is needed to treat any underlying cause of anterior to posterior and medial to lateral muscle imbalance. Therapy focuses on maximizing flexibility, strength, and endurance of the muscles whose tendons form the pes anserinus as well as addressing any muscle imbalances of the entire kinetic chain. Core control should be maximized to allow for proper hamstring and hip adductor and flexion function. Running shoes and inserts need to be appropriate for each individual biomechanics characteristics. Surgery (bursectomy) is rarely needed.

PLANTAR FASCIITIS

Plantar fasciitis is a common cause of plantar foot pain. It can occur on both sides and mimic the pain associated with distal sensory polyneuropathy. It can also present unilaterally mimicking S1 radiculopathy.

Symptoms

The plantar fascia is a band of thick connective tissue that originates on the calcaneus (or heel bone) and fans out on the sole of the foot to connect it to the base of the toes and support the arch of the foot. It is also related to the Achilles tendon, with connecting fibers between the two from the distal aspect of the Achilles tendon to the origin of the plantar fascia at the calcaneal tubercle.[103] Poor foot biomechanics can cause increased tension on the fascia and pain. This can occur in patients with pes planus, pes cavus, increased subtalar pronation, limited ankle dorsiflexion, decreased intrinsic foot muscle strength, and tight heel cords, all conditions that place stress on the plantar fascia.[104,105] Therefore plantar fasciitis can coexist with many underlying neuromuscular conditions that are associated with foot deformity and weakness. Obesity, pregnancy, and prolonged standing are additional risk factors.[104,106]

Patients typically describe the worst pain as occurring with weight bearing after getting out of bed in the morning or after a period of inactivity. Pain can be gnawing, stabbing, or burning. History of pain when taking the first steps in the morning helps differentiate this condition from the pain experienced by patients with sensory polyneuropathy whose foot pain is characteristically worse at night when off their feet. In some patients, the pain may radiate to the dorsolateral foot due to the patient offloading the pressure on the heel and walking on the outside of the foot creating an overuse condition to the lateral foot and ankle.

Diagnosis

The history and clinical examination are the mainstay of diagnosis. On physical examination there is tenderness to palpation on the medial plantar aspect of the heel bone (Fig. 36-12). This area corresponds to the site of the plantar fascia insertion on the calcaneus. Palpation of the medial slip of the plantar fascia may also reveal tightness and discomfort (Fig. 36-13), but the area of maximal tenderness

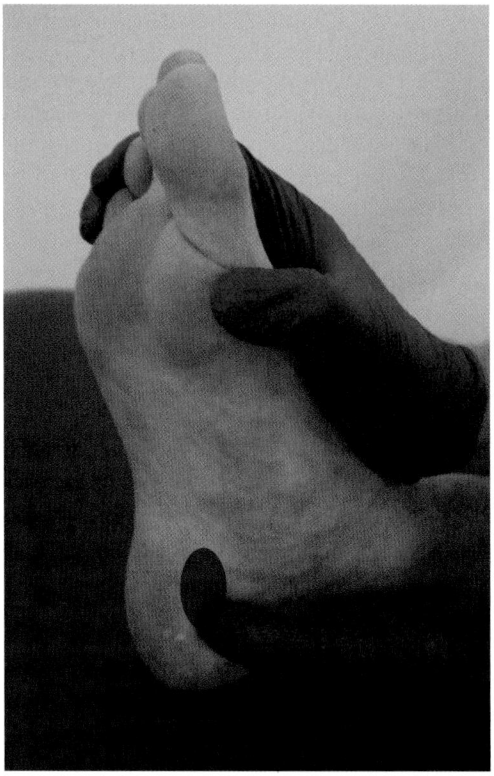

Figure 36-12. **Medial calcaneus palpation.** This maneuver reveals the area of maximal tenderness in plantar fasciitis at the site of the plantar fascia insertion on the heel bone (*shaded area*).

corresponds to the medial tubercle of the calcaneus (Fig. 36-12). Discomfort in the proximal plantar fascia can also be elicited by passive ankle and toe dorsiflexion. Diagnostic imaging is rarely needed for the initial diagnosis. Ultrasound and MRI are reserved for cases that do not respond to treatment or to exclude other heel pathology.[107,108] Plain x-rays of the foot can reveal a calcaneal heel spur in many individuals.[108] The heel spur, however, is not pathognomonic of plantar fasciitis and is not the cause of pain in this condition. Rather, the heel spur is thought to represent a byproduct of the chronic pulling of the fascia off the calcaneus and exists in many patients without symptoms of plantar fasciitis.

Treatment

Plantar fasciitis is a self-limiting condition that usually improves within 1 year regardless of treatment. Conservative treatment usually starts with patient-directed therapies. If these are not effective within a few weeks to a few months, management is advanced to include physician-prescribed interventions.

Initial patient-directed modalities include rest, activity modification, ice massage, oral analgesics (acetaminophen or NSAIDs), and stretching.[109,110] Ice massage is performed

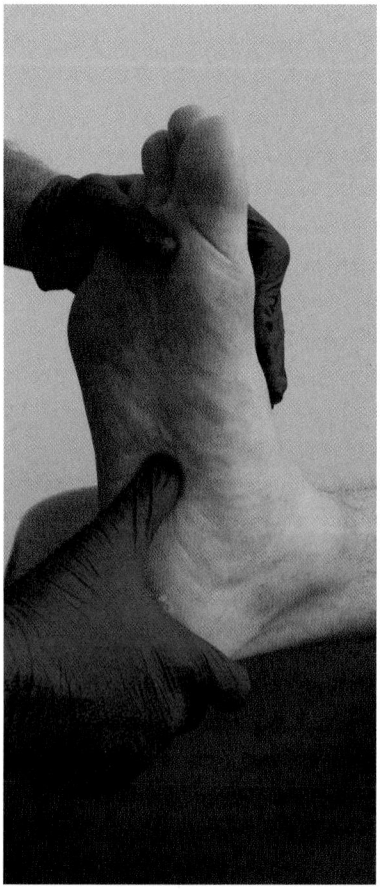

Figure 36-13. **Plantar fascia palpation.** Palpating the plantar fascia in the arch of the foot can elicit pain in people with plantar fasciitis.

by having the patient roll the arch of the foot over a frozen soda can or plastic bottle until numb. Treatment can be repeated multiple times a day. Stretching is performed both in bed before getting up in the morning and several times during the day. Before getting up, the patient is asked to stretch the Achilles tendon by dorsiflexing the foot and holding on to it for at least 30 seconds. This exercise is repeated 10 times and can be modified by including a large towel if limited flexibility prevents the patient from reaching the foot. While seated, the patient is also asked to stretch the plantar fascia by dorsiflexing the toes, holding the metatarsophalangeals and stretching the fascia in the arch region. During the day, the patient may stretch by leaning against a wall and performing wall leans, alternating between knee bent and knee extended while the heel is on the ground. Again each stretch is held for a minimum of 30 seconds and repeated several times. Intrinsic foot and calf strengthening exercises can help as well.

If pain persists, physician-prescribed treatments should be considered. These include shoe inserts, night splinting, physical therapy, and corticosteroid injections. Shoe inserts are commonly recommended for people with plantar fasciitis to aid in limiting overpronation of the foot and to unload the tensile forces on the plantar fascia. These include heel cups, prefabricated longitudinal arch supports, and custom-made full-length shoe insoles.[111–113] Night splints can be used to prevent foot plantar flexion during sleep by keeping the foot and ankle in a neutral 90-degree position. Night splints have been shown to improve plantar fasciitis pain,[113] but poor compliance because of sleep disturbance and foot discomfort has limited their long-term use. Multiple physical therapy modalities may be used, often in combination. Deep myofascial massage and iontophoresis can be performed by a physical therapist. In iontophoresis, electrical pulses are used to cause absorption of topical medications into the soft tissues beneath the skin. A small study found iontophoresis of acetic acid or dexamethasone to be helpful in plantar fasciitis.[114] Corticosteroid injections have been found to be effective in the treatment of plantar fasciitis and may be part of the initial approach in patients who desire an expedited return to normal activity.[115,116] Possible risks associated with corticosteroid injection include fat pad atrophy and plantar fascia rupture. In recent years, platelet-rich plasma injections have been proposed as an alternative treatment for plantar fasciitis and are currently being tested in clinical trials to determine their efficacy.[117,118] Patients with recalcitrant plantar fasciitis can consider extracorporeal shock wave therapy (ESWT) or, as a last resort, plantar fasciotomy. ESWT is thought to promote neovascularization and induce tissue repair. The technique is commonly used as it is noninvasive and has a good side effect profile although clinical trials have resulted in conflicting evidence.[119–122]

▶ SUMMARY

Musculoskeletal disorders are a common cause of limb pain and are likely to be encountered in daily practice, whether in the neuromuscular clinic or in the EMG laboratory. Musculoskeletal problems can "mimic" radiculopathy or entrapment neuropathy, thus posing a diagnostic challenge. In addition, musculoskeletal pain can complicate chronic neuromuscular diseases such as motor neuron disease and muscular dystrophy. Importantly, many common musculoskeletal problems can be diagnosed quickly at the bedside and are eminently treatable. Therefore, their prompt recognition has the potential to improve clinical flow and patient outcomes.

▶ ACKNOWLEDGMENTS

We would like to thank Farah Hameed, MD (Columbia University Medical Center, Department of Rehabilitation and Regenerative Medicine) for helpful comments and suggestions, and Andrew Sandefer (EMG Laboratory, VA Boston Healthcare) for technical assistance during the drafting of this chapter.

REFERENCES

1. Cannon DE, Dillingham TR, Miao H, Andary MT, Pezzin LE. Musculoskeletal disorders in referrals for suspected cervical radiculopathy. *Arch Phys Med Rehabil.* 2007;88:1256–1259.
2. Cannon DE, Dillingham TR, Miao H, Andary MT, Pezzin LE. Musculoskeletal disorders in referrals for suspected lumbosacral radiculopathy. *Am J Phys Med Rehabil.* 2007;86:957–961.
3. Stockard AR1, Allen TW. Competence levels in musculoskeletal medicine: comparison of osteopathic and allopathic medical graduates. *J Am Osteopath Assoc.* 2006;106(6):350–355.
4. Fu FH, Harner CD, Klein AH. Shoulder impingement syndrome. A critical review. *Clin Orthop Relat Res.* 1991;269:162–173.
5. Yi Y, Shim JS, Kim K, et al. Prevalence of the rotator cuff tear increases with weakness in hemiplegic shoulder. *Ann Rehabil Med.* 2013;37:471–478.
6. Gumina S, Carbone S, Campagna V, Candela V, Sacchetti FM, Giannicola G. The impact of aging on rotator cuff tear size. *Musculoskelet Surg.* 2013;97(suppl 1):69–72.
7. Bodin J, Ha C, Petit Le Manac'h A, et al. Risk factors for incidence of rotator cuff syndrome in a large working population. *Scand J Work Environ Health.* 2012;38:436–446.
8. Jain NB, Wilcox RB 3rd, Katz JN, Higgins LD. Clinical examination of the rotator cuff. *PM R.* 2013;5:45–56.
9. Hegedus EJ, Goode AP, Cook CE, et al. Which physical examination tests provide clinicians with the most value when examining the shoulder? Update of a systematic review with meta-analysis of individual tests. *Br J Sports Med.* 2012;46:964–978.
10. Teefey SA, Rubin DA, Middleton WD, Hildebolt CF, Leibold RA, Yamaguchi K. Detection and quantification of rotator cuff tears. Comparison of ultrasonographic, magnetic resonance imaging, and arthroscopic findings in seventy-one consecutive cases. *J Bone Joint Surg Am.* 2004;86-A:708–716.
11. Green S, Buchbinder R, Hetrick S. Physiotherapy interventions for shoulder pain. *Cochrane Database Syst Rev.* 2003;(2):CD004258.
12. Gebremariam L, Hay EM, van der Sande R, Rinkel WD, Koes BW, Huisstede BM. Subacromial impingement syndrome–effectiveness of physiotherapy and manual therapy. *Br J Sports Med.* 2014;48(16):1202–1208.
13. Dogu B, Yucel SD, Sag SY, Bankaoglu M, Kuran B. Blind or ultrasound-guided corticosteroid injections and short-term response in subacromial impingement syndrome: A randomized, double-blind, prospective study. *Am J Phys Med Rehabil.* 2012;91:658–665.
14. Mazzocca AD, McCarthy MB, Ledgard FA, et al. Histomorphologic changes of the long head of the biceps tendon in common shoulder pathologies. *Arthroscopy.* 2013;29:972–981.
15. Beall DP, Williamson EE, Ly JQ, et al. Association of biceps tendon tears with rotator cuff abnormalities: Degree of correlation with tears of the anterior and superior portions of the rotator cuff. *AJR Am J Roentgenol.* 2003;180:633–639.
16. Murthi AM, Vosburgh CL, Neviaser TJ. The incidence of pathologic changes of the long head of the biceps tendon. *J Shoulder Elbow Surg.* 2000;9:382–385.
17. Gazzillo GP, Finnoff JT, Hall MM, Sayeed YA, Smith J. Accuracy of palpating the long head of the biceps tendon: An ultrasonographic study. *PM R.* 2011;3:1035–1040.
18. Bennett WF. Specificity of the Speed's test: Arthroscopic technique for evaluating the biceps tendon at the level of the bicipital groove. *Arthroscopy.* 1998;14:789–796.
19. Chen HS, Lin SH, Hsu YH, Chen SC, Kang JH. A comparison of physical examinations with musculoskeletal ultrasound in the diagnosis of biceps long head tendinitis. *Ultrasound Med Biol.* 2011;37:1392–1398.
20. Schaeffeler C, Waldt S, Holzapfel K, et al. Lesions of the biceps pulley: Diagnostic accuracy of MR arthrography of the shoulder and evaluation of previously described and new diagnostic signs. *Radiology.* 2012;264:504–513.
21. Longo UG, Loppini M, Marineo G, Khan WS, Maffulli N, Denaro V. Tendinopathy of the tendon of the long head of the biceps. *Sports Med Arthrosc.* 2011;19:321–332.
22. Snyder GM, Mair SD, Lattermann C. Tendinopathy of the long head of the biceps. *Med Sport Sci.* 2012;57:76–89.
23. Zhang J, Ebraheim N, Lause GE. Ultrasound-guided injection for the biceps brachii tendinitis: Results and experience. *Ultrasound Med Biol.* 2011;37:729–733.
24. Hashiuchi T, Sakurai G, Morimoto M, Komei T, Takakura Y, Tanaka Y. Accuracy of the biceps tendon sheath injection: Ultrasound-guided or unguided injection? A randomized controlled trial. *J Shoulder Elbow Surg.* 2011;20:1069–1073.
25. Galasso O, Gasparini G, De Benedetto M, Familiari F, Castricini R. Tenotomy versus tenodesis in the treatment of the long head of biceps brachii tendon lesions. *BMC Musculoskelet Disord.* 2012;13:205.
26. Chourasia AO, Buhr KA, Rabago DP, et al. Relationships between biomechanics, tendon pathology, and function in individuals with lateral epicondylosis. *J Orthop Sports Phys Ther.* 2013;43:368–378.
27. Lucado AM, Kolber MJ, Cheng MS, Echternach JL Sr. Upper extremity strength characteristics in female recreational tennis players with and without lateral epicondylalgia. *J Orthop Sports Phys Ther.* 2012;42:1025–1031.
28. Regan W, Wold LE, Coonrad R, Morrey BF. Microscopic histopathology of chronic refractory lateral epicondylitis. *Am J Sports Med.* 1992;20:746–749.
29. Abrams GD, Renstrom PA, Safran MR. Epidemiology of musculoskeletal injury in the tennis player. *Br J Sports Med.* 2012;46:492–498.
30. Titchener AG, Fakis A, Tambe AA, Smith C, Hubbard RB, Clark DI. Risk factors in lateral epicondylitis (tennis elbow): A case-control study. *J Hand Surg Eur.* 2013;38:159–164.
31. Shiri R, Viikari-Juntura E, Varonen H, Heliovaara M. Prevalence and determinants of lateral and medial epicondylitis: A population study. *Am J Epidemiol.* 2006;164:1065–1074.
32. Pattanittum P, Turner T, Green S, Buchbinder R. Non-steroidal anti-inflammatory drugs (NSAIDs) for treating lateral elbow pain in adults. *Cochrane Database Syst Rev.* 2013;5:CD003686.
33. Sölveborn SA. Radial epicondylalgia ('tennis elbow'): Treatment with stretching or forearm band. A prospective study with long-term follow-up including range-of-motion measurements. *Scand J Med Sci Sports.* 1997;7:229–237.
34. Sadeghi-Demneh E, Jafarian F. The immediate effects of orthoses on pain in people with lateral epicondylalgia. *Pain Res Treat.* 2013;2013:353597.
35. Nilsson P, Baigi A, Swärd L, Möller M, Månsson J. Lateral epicondylalgia: A structured programme better than corticosteroids and NSAID. *Scand J Occup Ther.* 2012;19(5):404–410.
36. Olaussen M, Holmedal O, Lindbaek M, Brage S, Solvang H. Treating lateral epicondylitis with corticosteroid injections or

non-electrotherapeutical physiotherapy: A systematic review. *BMJ Open*. 2013;3:e003564.
37. Svernlov B, Adolfsson L. Non-operative treatment regime including eccentric training for lateral humeral epicondylalgia. *Scand J Med Sci Sports*. 2001;11:328–334.
38. Martinez-Silvestrini JA, Newcomer KL, Gay RE, Schaefer MP, Kortebein P, Arendt KW. Chronic lateral epicondylitis: Comparative effectiveness of a home exercise program including stretching alone versus stretching supplemented with eccentric or concentric strengthening. *J Hand Ther*. 2005;18(4):411–419, quiz 420.
39. Titchener AG, Booker SJ, Bhamber NS, Tambe AA, Clark DI. Corticosteroid and platelet-rich plasma injection therapy in tennis elbow (lateral epicondylalgia): A survey of current UK specialist practice and a call for clinical guidelines. *Br J Sports Med*. 2013.
40. Krogh TP, Bartels EM, Ellingsen T, et al. Comparative effectiveness of injection therapies in lateral epicondylitis: A systematic review and network meta-analysis of randomized controlled trials. *Am J Sports Med*. 2013;41:1435–1446.
41. Coombes BK, Bisset L, Brooks P, Khan A, Vicenzino B. Effect of corticosteroid injection, physiotherapy, or both on clinical outcomes in patients with unilateral lateral epicondylalgia: A randomized controlled trial. *JAMA*. 2013;309:461–469.
42. Krogh TP, Fredberg U, Stengaard-Pedersen K, Christensen R, Jensen P, Ellingsen T. Treatment of lateral epicondylitis with platelet-rich plasma, glucocorticoid, or saline: A randomized, double-blind, placebo-controlled trial. *Am J Sports Med*. 2013; 41:625–635.
43. Armstrong TJ, Fine LJ, Goldstein SA, Lifshitz YR, Silverstein BA. Ergonomics considerations in hand and wrist tendinitis. *J Hand Surg Am*. 1987;12:830–837.
44. Luopajarvi T, Kuorinka I, Virolainen M, Holmberg M. Prevalence of tenosynovitis and other injuries of the upper extremities in repetitive work. *Scand J Work Environ Health*. 1979; 5(suppl 3):48–55.
45. Stahl S, Vida D, Meisner C, et al. Systematic review and meta-analysis on the work-related cause of de Quervain tenosynovitis: A critical appraisal of its recognition as an occupational disease. *Plast Reconstr Surg*. 2013;132(6):1479–1491.
46. Hartwell SW Jr, Larsen RD, Posch JL. Tenosynovitis in Women in Industry. *Cleve Clin Q*. 1964;31:115–118.
47. Ashraf MO, Devadoss VG. Systematic review and meta-analysis on steroid injection therapy for de Quervain's tenosynovitis in adults. *Eur J Orthop Surg Traumatol*. 2014;24(2):149–157.
48. Mardani-Kivi M, Karimi Mobarakeh M, Bahrami F, Hashemi-Motlagh K, Saheb-Ekhtiari K, Akhoondzadeh N. Corticosteroid injection with or without thumb spica cast for de quervain tenosynovitis. *J Hand Surg Am*. 2014;39:37–41.
49. McDermott JD, Ilyas AM, Nazarian LN, Leinberry CF. Ultrasound-guided injections for de Quervain's tenosynovitis. *Clin Orthop Relat Res*. 2012;470:1925–1931.
50. Kang HJ, Koh IH, Jang JW, Choi YR. Endoscopic versus open release in patients with de Quervain's tenosynovitis: A randomised trial. *Bone Joint J*. 2013;95-B:947–951.
51. Gehrmann SV, Tang J, Li ZM, Goitz RJ, Windolf J, Kaufmann RA. Motion deficit of the thumb in CMC joint arthritis. *J Hand Surg Am*. 2010;35:1449–1453.
52. Zhang Y, Niu J, Kelly-Hayes M, Chaisson CE, Aliabadi P, Felson DT. Prevalence of symptomatic hand osteoarthritis and its impact on functional status among the elderly: The Framingham Study. *Am J Epidemiol*. 2002;156:1021–1027.
53. Wilder FV, Barrett JP, Farina EJ. Joint-specific prevalence of osteoarthritis of the hand. *Osteoarthritis Cartilage*. 2006;14:953–957.
54. Jonsson H, Manolescu I, Stefansson SE, et al. The inheritance of hand osteoarthritis in Iceland. *Arthritis Rheum*. 2003;48:391–395.
55. Fontana L, Neel S, Claise JM, Ughetto S, Catilina P. Osteoarthritis of the thumb carpometacarpal joint in women and occupational risk factors: A case-control study. *J Hand Surg Am*. 2007;32:459–465.
56. Jonsson H, Valtysdottir ST, Kjartansson O, Brekkan A. Hypermobility associated with osteoarthritis of the thumb base: A clinical and radiological subset of hand osteoarthritis. *Ann Rheum Dis*. 1996;55:540–543.
57. Kessler S, Stove J, Puhl W, Sturmer T. First carpometacarpal and interphalangeal osteoarthritis of the hand in patients with advanced hip or knee OA. Are there differences in the aetiology? *Clin Rheumatol*. 2003;22:409–413.
58. Chaisson CE, Zhang Y, McAlindon TE, et al. Radiographic hand osteoarthritis: Incidence, patterns, and influence of pre-existing disease in a population based sample. *J Rheumatol*. 1997;24:1337–1343.
59. Merritt MM, Roddey TS, Costello C, Olson S. Diagnostic value of clinical grind test for carpometacarpal osteoarthritis of the thumb. *J Hand Ther*. 2010;23:261–267; quiz 268.
60. Dahaghin S, Bierma-Zeinstra SM, Ginai AZ, Pols HA, Hazes JM, Koes BW. Prevalence and pattern of radiographic hand osteoarthritis and association with pain and disability (the Rotterdam study). *Ann Rheum Dis*. 2005;64:682–687.
61. Sillem H, Backman CL, Miller WC, Li LC. Comparison of two carpometacarpal stabilizing splints for individuals with thumb osteoarthritis. *J Hand Ther*. 2011;24(3):216–225; quiz 126; discussion 227–230.
62. Bani MA, Arazpour M, Kashani RV, Mousavi ME, Hutchins SW. Comparison of custom-made and prefabricated neoprene splinting in patients with the first carpometacarpal joint osteoarthritis. *Disabil Rehabil Assist Technol*. 2013;8:232–237.
63. Egan MY, Brousseau L. Splinting for osteoarthritis of the carpometacarpal joint: A review of the evidence. *Am J Occup Ther*. 2007;61:70–78.
64. Maarse W, Watts AC, Bain GI. Medium-term outcome following intra-articular corticosteroid injection in first CMC joint arthritis using fluoroscopy. *Hand Surg*. 2009;14:99–104.
65. Joshi R. Intraarticular corticosteroid injection for first carpometacarpal osteoarthritis. *J Rheumatol*. 2005;32:1305–1306.
66. Hentz VR. Surgical treatment of trapeziometacarpal joint arthritis: A historical perspective. *Clin Orthop Relat Res*. 2014;472(4):1184–1189.
67. Badia A, Sambandam SN. Total joint arthroplasty in the treatment of advanced stages of thumb carpometacarpal joint osteoarthritis. *J Hand Surg Am*. 2006;31:1605–1614.
68. Ataker Y, Gudemez E, Ece SC, Canbulat N, Gulgonen A. Rehabilitation protocol after suspension arthroplasty of thumb carpometacarpal joint osteoarthritis. *J Hand Ther*. 2012; 25(4):374–382; quiz 383.
69. Nho SJ, Kymes SM, Callaghan JJ, Felson DT. The burden of hip osteoarthritis in the United States: Epidemiologic and economic considerations. *J Am Acad Orthop Surg*. 2013;21 (suppl 1):S1–S6.
70. Evangelou E, Kerkhof HJ, Styrkarsdottir U, et al. A meta-analysis of genome-wide association studies identifies novel

variants associated with osteoarthritis of the hip. *Ann Rheum Dis*. 2014;73(12):2130–2136.
71. Richmond SA, Fukuchi RK, Ezzat A, Schneider K, Schneider G, Emery CA. Are joint injury, sport activity, physical activity, obesity, or occupational activities predictors for osteoarthritis? A systematic review. *J Orthop Sports Phys Ther*. 2013;43: 515–B19.
72. Prieto-Alhambra D, Judge A, Javaid MK, Cooper C, Diez-Perez A, Arden NK. Incidence and risk factors for clinically diagnosed knee, hip and hand osteoarthritis: Influences of age, gender and osteoarthritis affecting other joints. *Ann Rheum Dis*. 2014;73(9):1659–1664.
73. Franklin J, Ingvarsson T, Englund M, Lohmander S. Association between occupation and knee and hip replacement due to osteoarthritis: A case-control study. *Arthritis Res Ther*. 2010;12:R102.
74. Chong T, Don DW, Kao MC, Wong D, Mitra R. The value of physical examination in the diagnosis of hip osteoarthritis. *J Back Musculoskelet Rehabil*. 2013;26:397–400.
75. Xu L, Hayashi D, Guermazi A, et al. The diagnostic performance of radiography for detection of osteoarthritis-associated features compared with MRI in hip joints with chronic pain. *Skeletal Radiol*. 2013;42:1421–1428.
76. Yoong P, Guirguis R, Darrah R, Wijeratna M, Porteous MJ. Evaluation of ultrasound-guided diagnostic local anaesthetic hip joint injection for osteoarthritis. *Skeletal Radiol*. 2012;41:981–985.
77. Deshmukh AJ, Thakur RR, Goyal A, Klein DA, Ranawat AS, Rodriguez JA. Accuracy of diagnostic injection in differentiating source of atypical hip pain. *J Arthroplasty*. 2010;25:129–133.
78. Svege I, Nordsletten L, Fernandes L, Risberg MA. Exercise therapy may postpone total hip replacement surgery in patients with hip osteoarthritis: A long-term follow-up of a randomised trial. *Ann Rheum Dis*. 2015;74(1):164–169.
79. Jensen C, Roos EM, Kjaersgaard-Andersen P, Overgaard S. The effect of education and supervised exercise vs. education alone on the time to total hip replacement in patients with severe hip osteoarthritis. A randomized clinical trial protocol. *BMC Musculoskelet Disord*. 2013;14:21.
80. Zhang W, Moskowitz RW, Nuki G, et al. OARSI recommendations for the management of hip and knee osteoarthritis, Part II: OARSI evidence-based, expert consensus guidelines. *Osteoarthritis Cartilage*. 2008;16:137–162.
81. Hochberg MC, Altman RD, April KT, et al. American College of Rheumatology. 2012 recommendations for the use of nonpharmacologic and pharmacologic therapies in osteoarthritis of the hand, hip, and knee. *Arthritis Care Res (Hoboken)*. 2012;64:465–474.
82. Lambert RG, Hutchings EJ, Grace MG, Jhangri GS, Conner-Spady B, Maksymowych WP. Steroid injection for osteoarthritis of the hip: A randomized, double-blind, placebo-controlled trial. *Arthritis Rheum*. 2007;56:2278–2287.
83. Swezey RL. Pseudo-radiculopathy in subacute trochanteric bursitis of the subgluteus maximus bursa. *Arch Phys Med Rehabil*. 1976;57:387–390.
84. Schapira D, Nahir M, Scharf Y. Trochanteric bursitis: A common clinical problem. *Arch Phys Med Rehabil*. 1986;67:815–817.
85. Shbeeb MI, Matteson EL. Trochanteric bursitis (greater trochanter pain syndrome). *Mayo Clin Proc*. 1996;71:565–569.
86. Bird PA, Oakley SP, Shnier R, Kirkham BW. Prospective evaluation of magnetic resonance imaging and physical examination findings in patients with greater trochanteric pain syndrome. *Arthritis Rheum*. 2001;44:2138–2145.
87. Blankenbaker DG, Ullrick SR, Davis KW, De Smet AA, Haaland B, Fine JP. Correlation of MRI findings with clinical findings of trochanteric pain syndrome. *Skeletal Radiol*. 2008;37: 903–909.
88. Fearon AM, Scarvell JM, Cook JL, Smith PN. Does ultrasound correlate with surgical or histologic findings in greater trochanteric pain syndrome? A pilot study. *Clin Orthop Relat Res*. 2010;468:1838–1844.
89. Long SS, Surrey DE, Nazarian LN. Sonography of greater trochanteric pain syndrome and the rarity of primary bursitis. *AJR Am J Roentgenol*. 2013;201:1083–1086.
90. Segal NA, Felson DT, Torner JC, et al; Multicenter Osteoarthritis Study Group. Greater trochanteric pain syndrome: Epidemiology and associated factors. *Arch Phys Med Rehabil*. 2007;88:988–992.
91. Sayegh F, Potoupnis M, Kapetanos G. Greater trochanter bursitis pain syndrome in females with chronic low back pain and sciatica. *Acta Orthop Belg*. 2004;70:423–428.
92. Sloan RL. Greater trochanteric pain syndrome, another cause of hip or thigh pain in multiple sclerosis. *Pract Neurol*. 2009;9:163–165.
93. Fearon AM, Cook JL, Scarvell JM, Neeman T, Cormick W, Smith PN. Greater trochanteric pain syndrome negatively affects work, physical activity and quality of life: A case control study. *J Arthroplasty*. 2014;29(2):383–386.
94. Karpinski MR, Piggott H. Greater trochanteric pain syndrome. A report of 15 cases. *J Bone Joint Surg Br*. 1985;67:762–763.
95. McEvoy JR, Lee KS, Blankenbaker DG, del Rio AM, Keene JS. Ultrasound-guided corticosteroid injections for treatment of greater trochanteric pain syndrome: Greater trochanter bursa versus subgluteus medius bursa. *AJR Am J Roentgenol*. 2013; 201:W313–W317.
96. Brinks A, van Rijn RM, Willemsen SP, et al. Corticosteroid injections for greater trochanteric pain syndrome: A randomized controlled trial in primary care. *Ann Fam Med*. 2011;9:226–234.
97. Forbes JR, Helms CA, Janzen DL. Acute pes anserine bursitis: MR imaging. *Radiology*. 1995;194:525–527.
98. Rennie WJ, Saifuddin A. Pes anserine bursitis: Incidence in symptomatic knees and clinical presentation. *Skeletal Radiol*. 2005;34:395–398.
99. Alvarez-Nemegyei J. Risk factors for pes anserinus tendinitis/bursitis syndrome: A case control study. *J Clin Rheumatol*. 2007;13:63–65.
100. Devan MR, Pescatello LS, Faghri P, Anderson J. A prospective study of overuse knee injuries among female athletes with muscle imbalances and structural abnormalities. *J Athl Train*. 2004;39:263–267.
101. Butcher JD, Salzman KL, Lillegard WA. Lower extremity bursitis. *Am Fam Physician*. 1996;53:2317–2324.
102. Cardone DA, Tallia AF. Diagnostic and therapeutic injection of the hip and knee. *Am Fam Physician*. 2003;67:2147–2152.
103. Stecco C, Corradin M, Macchi V, et al. Plantar fascia anatomy and its relationship with Achilles tendon and paratenon. *J Anat*. 2013;223:665–676.
104. Riddle DL, Pulisic M, Pidcoe P, Johnson RE. Risk factors for Plantar fasciitis: A matched case-control study. *J Bone Joint Surg Am*. 2003;85-A:872–877.
105. Bolivar YA, Munuera PV, Padillo JP. Relationship between tightness of the posterior muscles of the lower limb and plantar fasciitis. *Foot Ankle Int*. 2013;34:42–48.

106. Werner RA, Gell N, Hartigan A, Wiggerman N, Keyserling WM. Risk factors for plantar fasciitis among assembly plant workers. *PM R*. 2010;2:110–116; quiz 1 p following 167.
107. Karabay N, Toros T, Hurel C. Ultrasonographic evaluation in plantar fasciitis. *J Foot Ankle Surg*. 2007;46:442–446.
108. McMillan AM, Landorf KB, Barrett JT, Menz HB, Bird AR. Diagnostic imaging for chronic plantar heel pain: A systematic review and meta-analysis. *J Foot Ankle Res*. 2009;2:32.
109. Donley BG, Moore T, Sferra J, Gozdanovic J, Smith R. The efficacy of oral nonsteroidal anti-inflammatory medication (NSAID) in the treatment of plantar fasciitis: A randomized, prospective, placebo-controlled study. *Foot Ankle Int*. 2007;28:20–23.
110. Digiovanni BF, Nawoczenski DA, Malay DP, et al. Plantar fascia-specific stretching exercise improves outcomes in patients with chronic plantar fasciitis. A prospective clinical trial with two-year follow-up. *J Bone Joint Surg Am*. 2006;88:1775–1781.
111. Lee SY, McKeon P, Hertel J. Does the use of orthoses improve self-reported pain and function measures in patients with plantar fasciitis? A meta-analysis. *Phys Ther Sport*. 2009;10:12–18.
112. Hawke F, Burns J, Radford JA, du Toit V. Custom-made foot orthoses for the treatment of foot pain. *Cochrane Database Syst Rev*. 2008;3:CD006801.
113. Roos E, Engstrom M, Soderberg B. Foot orthoses for the treatment of plantar fasciitis. *Foot Ankle Int*. 2006;27:606–611.
114. Osborne HR, Allison GT. Treatment of plantar fasciitis by LowDye taping and iontophoresis: Short term results of a double blinded, randomised, placebo controlled clinical trial of dexamethasone and acetic acid. *Br J Sports Med*. 2006;40:545–549; discussion 549.
115. McMillan AM, Landorf KB, Gilheany MF, Bird AR, Morrow AD, Menz HB. Ultrasound guided corticosteroid injection for plantar fasciitis: Randomised controlled trial. *BMJ*. 2012;344:e3260.
116. Schulhofer SD. Short-term benefits of ultrasound-guided corticosteroid injection in plantar fasciitis. *Clin J Sport Med*. 2013;23:83–84.
117. Kim E, Lee JH. Autologous platelet-rich plasma versus dextrose prolotherapy for the treatment of chronic recalcitrant plantar fasciitis. *PM R*. 2014;6(2):152–158.
118. Peerbooms JC, van Laar W, Faber F, Schuller HM, van der Hoeven H, Gosens T. Use of platelet rich plasma to treat plantar fasciitis: Design of a multi centre randomized controlled trial. *BMC Musculoskelet Disord*. 2010;11:69.
119. Buchbinder R, Ptasznik R, Gordon J, Buchanan J, Prabaharan V, Forbes A. Ultrasound-guided extracorporeal shock wave therapy for plantar fasciitis: A randomized controlled trial. *JAMA*. 2002;288:1364–1372.
120. Kudo P, Dainty K, Clarfield M, Coughlin L, Lavoie P, Lebrun C. Randomized, placebo-controlled, double-blind clinical trial evaluating the treatment of plantar fasciitis with an extracoporeal shockwave therapy (ESWT) device: A North American confirmatory study. *J Orthop Res*. 2006;24:115–123.
121. Dizon JN, Gonzalez-Suarez C, Zamora MT, Gambito ED. Effectiveness of extracorporeal shock wave therapy in chronic plantar fasciitis: A meta-analysis. *Am J Phys Med Rehabil*. 2013;92:606–620.
122. Speed C. A systematic review of shockwave therapies in soft tissue conditions: Focusing on the evidence. *Br J Sports Med*. 2014;48(21):1538–1542.

INDEX

Note: Page number followed by f and t indicates figure and table respectively.

B

C

D

E

F

G

I

M

N

O

P

T